NANDA-I Diagnoses

NURSING DIAGNOSIS HANDBOOK

An Evidence-Based Guide to Planning Care

Betty J. Ackley, MSN, EdS, RN
Gail B. Ladwig, MSN, RN
Mary Beth Flynn Makic, PhD, RN, CCNS, FAAN, FNAP
Marina Reyna Martinez-Kratz, MS, RN, CNE
Melody Zanotti, BA, RN, LSW

Twelfth Edition

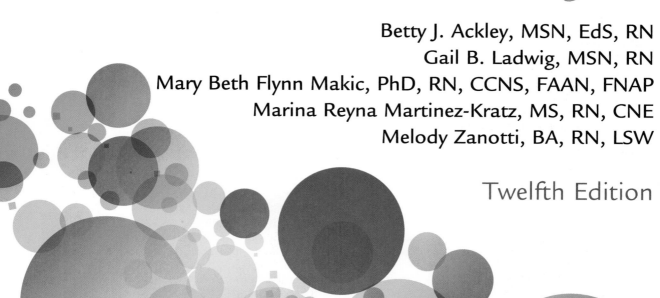

ELSEVIER

NURSING DIAGNOSIS HANDBOOK, TWELFTH EDITION

ISBN: 978-0-323-55112-0

Previous editions copyrighted 2017, 2014, 2011, 2008, 2006, 2004, 2002, 1999, 1997, 1995, and 1993.

International Standard Book Number: 978-0-323-55112-0

Senior Content Strategist: Sandra Clark
Senior Content Development Specialist: Jennifer Wade
Publishing Services Manager: Julie Eddy
Book Production Specialist: Clay S. Broeker
Design Direction: Amy Buxton

Printed in Canada

Last digit is the print number: 9 8 7 6 5 4 3 2 1

ELSEVIER

3251 Riverport Lane
St. Louis, Missouri 63043

 Working together
to grow libraries in
developing countries

www.elsevier.com • www.bookaid.org

To Jerry Ladwig, my wonderful husband who, after 54 years, is still supportive and helpful; he has been my "right-hand man" in every revision of this book. Also, to my very special children, their spouses, and all of my grandchildren ... Jerry, Kathy, Alexandra, Elizabeth, and Benjamin Ladwig; Christine, John, Sean, Ciara, and Bridget McMahon; Jennifer, Jim, Abby, Katelyn, Blake, and Connor Martin; Amy, Scott, Ford, and Vaughn Bertram ... the greatest family anyone could ever hope for. A special thank you to my grandson Sean for his work on checking and incorporating the correct/new NANDA language for the diagnoses that I worked on.
Gail B. Ladwig

Thank you to my husband, Zlatko, and children, Alexander and Erik, whose unconditional love and support are ever present in my life. To my parents and sisters for always encouraging me to follow my passion. To Gail, for her incredible leadership and mentorship throughout the rigorous process of revising this essential text. And finally, to Betty, for her unwavering commitment to the profession of nursing through her roles as an expert teacher and prolific author. You are missed but your spirit continues to inform nursing practice excellence.
Mary Beth Flynn Makic

To my best friend and the love of my life, Kent Martinez-Kratz. To my children, Maxwell, Jesse, and Sierra, whose love, inspiration, and wit make my life complete. To my first fans, my parents and siblings. To Gail, for being the absolute best nursing professor, mentor, and comadre. And finally, to Betty's memory, for inspiring excellence in nursing education and practice.
Marina Reyna Martinez-Kratz

Thank you to my husband Marty for his infinite patience and encouragement in all my endeavors. Thank you to my amazing children, their spouses, and my grandchildren ... Rachael, Frank, Corey, Zak, Dominic, and Dylan ... for their unconditional love and inspiration. Thank you to my friend and mentor Gail Ladwig for offering me the opportunity to contribute to this incredible textbook. Your gifts of friendship, knowledge, and positivity will stay with me forever. Your lifelong dedication and commitment to the field of nursing are truly inspiring.
Melody Zanotti

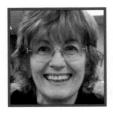

Betty Ackley was co-author of *Nursing Diagnosis: Guide to Planning Care*, which has been a successful text for 20 years, and co-author for four editions of *Mosby's Guide to Nursing Diagnosis*. She was also a lead co-author/editor of *Evidence-Based Nursing Care Guidelines: Medical-Surgical Interventions*. This text is designed to help nurses easily find and use evidence to provide excellence in nursing care. The text was published in 2008 and was named AJN book of the year.

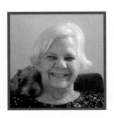

Gail B. Ladwig has a long career in teaching and practicing nursing. Gail is co-author of *Nursing Diagnosis: Guide to Planning Care*, which has been a very successful text for more than 25 years, and she has been co-author for all editions of *Mosby's Guide to Nursing Diagnosis*, now in its fifth edition. She is also a co-author/editor of *Evidence-Based Nursing Care Guidelines: Medical-Surgical Interventions*. This text was published in 2008 and was named AJN book of the year. Gail has been an active member and supporter of NANDA-I for many, many years. Gail is the mother of 4 children and grandmother of 12 and loves to spend time with her grandchildren. She has been married to her husband Jerry for 54 years and is passionate about her family and the profession of nursing.

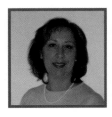

Mary Beth Flynn Makic is a Professor at the University of Colorado, College of Nursing, Aurora, Colorado, where she teaches in the undergraduate, graduate, and doctoral programs. She is the director of the Clinical Nurse Specialist graduate program at the College of Nursing. She has worked predominately in critical care for 30 years. Mary Beth is best known for her publications and presentations, regionally and nationally, as an expert on evidence-based practice in nursing. Her practice expertise and research focus on the care of the trauma, general surgical, and burn-injured patient populations; acute wound healing; pressure ulcer prevention; and hospital-acquired conditions (HACs). She is passionate about nurses' understanding and translating current best evidence into practice to optimize patient and family outcomes. She is

co-author of *Trauma Nursing: from Resuscitation through Rehabilitation* and a section editor of *American Association of Critical Care Nurses Procedure Manual for Critical Care*. She is actively involved in several professional nursing and inter-professional organizations.

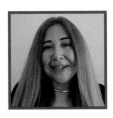

Marina Reyna Martinez-Kratz is a professor of nursing at Jackson College, Jackson, Michigan. She is a registered nurse with 30 years of experience and is a Certified Nurse Educator. She received her nursing degrees from Jackson Community College and the University of Michigan. Her expertise in nursing practice has focused on psychiatric nursing, professional issues, and nutrition. In 1998, Marina joined the faculty at Jackson Community College and currently teaches nursing courses in Behavioral Health, Leadership, and Nutrition. In addition, Marina serves on the Nursing Assessment and Professional Development Committees and is a Mandated Reporter Trainer. She has served as a behavioral health consultant for several health care facilities, contributes to and reviews many academic publications, and has presented at the state and national level. Marina belongs to many professional organizations and serves as Board Secretary for the Jackson Council for the Prevention of Child Abuse and Child Neglect and the NLN Ambassador for Jackson College. Marina's passion is helping students learn to think like nurses! Marina is the proud mother of 3 children and has been married to her partner and best friend Kent for 28 years.

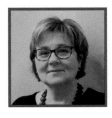

Melody Zanotti has enjoyed a diverse career in health care and education for over 30 years. She worked as a staff nurse in MICU, SICU and stepdown units for many years. She was instrumental in establishing a nurse triage and resource call center for a major health care system in Ohio. She worked as a school nurse before pursuing a degree in Social Work. Melody received a BA in Social Work and worked as a school social worker for over 10 years. While working as an LSW, she co-developed a truancy prevention program, partnering the school district with local municipalities. Melody currently volunteers her time for many causes. She has done medical missionary work in Africa and is working on a health education program empowering young women in Uganda.

Contributors

Betty J. Ackley, MSN, EdS, RN[†]
President and Owner
The Betty Ackley LLC
Consultant in Nursing Process, Evidence-Based Nursing,
    and Pilates
Jackson, Michigan

**Michelle Acorn, DNP, NP PHC/Adult, BA, BScN/
PHCNP, MN/ACNP, GNC(C), CGP**
Nurse Practitioner
University of Toronto
Toronto, Canada

Keith Anderson, PhD, MSW
Associate Professor
School of Social Work
University of Montana
Missoula, Montana

Amanda Andrews, BSc (Hons), MA
Senior Teaching Fellow
Pre Qualifying Department
Birmingham City University
Birmingham, United Kingdom

Kathaleen C. Bloom, PhD, CNM
Professor and Associate Director
School of Nursing
University of North Florida
Jacksonville, Florida

**Kathleen Patricia Buckheit, MPH, BSN, RN, CEN,
COHN-S/CM, CCM, FAAOHN**
Director of Education
American Association of Occupational Health Nurses, Inc.
    (AAOHN)
Chicago, Illinois

Elyse Bueno, MS, ACCNS-AG, CCRN
Nurse Manager
Surgical Trauma Intensive Care Unit
University of Colorado Hospital
Aurora, Colorado

Elizabeth Burkhart, PhD, RN, ANEF
Associate Professor
Marcella Niehoff School of Nursing
Loyola University
Chicago, Illinois

**Melodie Cannon, DNP, MSc/FNP, BHScN, RN(EC),
NP-PHC, CEN, GNC(C)**
Nurse Practitioner
Internal Medicine/Emergency Department/GI
Scarborough Rouge Hospital, Centenary Site
Toronto, Canada
Adjunct Lecturer
Lawrence S. Bloomberg Faculty of Nursing
University of Toronto
Toronto, Canada

Stacey M. Carroll, PhD, APRN-BC
Assistant Professor
Nursing
Anna Maria College
Paxton, Massachusetts

Krystal Chamberlain, BSN, RN, CCRN
Clinical Nurse Educator
Neurosurgical ICU
University of Colorado Hospital
Aurora, Colorado

Nadia Charania, PhD, RN
Clinical Assistant Professor
School of Nursing
University of Michigan
Ann Arbor, Michigan

Nichol Chesser, RN, CNM, DNP
Assistant Professor
OB/GYN
University of Colorado
Aurora, Colorado

Jo Ann Coar, BSN, RN-BC, CWOCN, COS-C
Wound Healing Center
Education Department
Chilton Medical Center
Pompton Plains, New Jersey

[†]Deceased.

Maureen F. Cooney, DNP, FNP-BC
Pain Management Nurse Practitioner
Westchester Medical Center
Valhalla, New York
Adjunct Associate Professor
Pace University
College of Health Professions
Lienhard School of Nursing
New York, New York

Tara Cuccinelli, RN, MS, AGCNS-BC
Clinical Nurse Specialist
Emergency Department
UCHealth Memorial
Colorado Springs, Colorado

Ruth M. Curchoe, RN, BSN, MSN, CIC
Independent Consultant
Infection Prevention
Rochester, New York

Mary Rose Day, DN, MA, PGDip PHN, BSc, Dip Management (RCSI), RPHN, RM, RGN
School of Nursing and Midwifery
University College
Cork, Ireland

Mary Alice DeWys, RN, BS, CIMI
Infant Development and Feeding Specialist (Retired)
Pediatric and Neonatal Nursing
Spectrum Health
Infant Developmental and Feeding Specialist
Hassle Free Feeding Program Division of Harmony Through Touch
Infant Developmental and Feeding Specialist
Pediatric Nursing
Grand Valley State University (Research Team for Premature, Young Infant Developmental Assessment Tool)
Grand Rapids, Michigan

Susan M. Dirkes, RN, MS, CCRN
Staff Nurse
Nursing Department
University of Michigan
Ann Arbor, Florida
Clinical Educator
Nursing Department
NxStage Medical, Lawrence
Sarasota, Massachusetts

Julianne E. Doubet, BSN, RN, EMT-B
Paramedic Instructor (Retired)
Emergency Department
Bethesda North Hospital
Mason, Ohio

Lorraine Duggan, MSN, ACNP-BC
Nurse Practitioner
HouseCalls
Optum Health/United Healthcare Group
Delaware, Maryland

Dawn Fairlie, PhD, NP
Assistant Professor
School of Health Sciences, Department of Nursing
College of Staten Island, City University of New York
Staten Island, New York

Arlene T. Farren, PhD, RN, AOCN, CTN-A, CNE
Associate Professor
Nursing
College of Staten Island
Staten Island, New York
Associate Professor
Nursing
City University of New York Graduate Center
New York, New York

Judith Ann Floyd, PhD, RN, FNAP, FAAN
Professor
College of Nursing
Wayne State University
Detroit, Michigan

Katherine Foss, MSN, RN
Instructor
Clinical Education Center
University of Colorado, College of Nursing
Supervisor, Clinical Entry Programs
Professional Development
University of Colorado Hospital
Aurora, Colorado

Shari D. Froelich, DNP, MSN, MSBA, ANP-BC, ACHPN, PMHNP-BC
Nurse Practitioner
Alcona Health Center
Alpena, Michigan

Tracy P. George, DNP, APRN-BC, CNE
Assistant Professor
Nursing
Francis Marion University
Florence, South Carolina

Susanne W. Gibbons, PhD, C-ANP/GNP
Clinical Nurse Practitioner
Adult and Geriatric
Centennial Medical Group
Elkridge, Maryland

Barbara A. Given, PhD, RN, FAAN
University Distinguished Professor
College of Nursing
Michigan State University
East Lansing, Michigan

Pauline McKinney Green, PhD, RN, CNE
Professor Emerita
Nursing
Howard University College of Nursing and Allied Health
    Sciences
Washington, District of Columbia

Sherry A. Greenberg, PhD, RN, GNP-BC
Senior Training Specialist
Hartford Institute for Geriatric Nursing and Nurses
    Improving Care for Healthsystem Elders
New York University Rory Meyers College of Nursing
New York, New York

Marloes Harkema, BA
Academie voor Verpleegkunde
Hanzehoge School
Groningen, Netherlands

Dianne F. Hayward, RN, MSN, WHNP
Adjunct Faculty
Nursing
Oakland Community College
Waterford, Michigan

Dina M. Hewett, PhD, RN, NEA-BC, CCRN-A
Director and Professor of Nursing
Mary Inez Grindle School of Nursing
Brenau University
Gainesville, Georgia

Patricia Hindin, PhD, CNM
Associate Professor
Advanced Nursing Practice
Rutgers University School of Nursing
Newark, New Jersey

Jacqueline A. Hogan, RD, CSO, LD
Senior Dietitian
Clinical Nutrition
University of Texas MD Anderson
Houston, Texas

Paula D. Hopper, MSN, RN, CNE
Professor of Nursing Emeritus
Jackson College
Lecturer
Eastern Michigan University
Jackson, Michigan

Wendie A. Howland, MN, RN-BC, CRRN, CCM, CNLCP, LNCC
Principal
Legal Nurse Consulting and Life Care Planning
Howland Health Consulting
Cape Cod, Massachusetts

Teri Hulett, RN, BSN, CIC, FAPIC
Infection Prevention Consultant and Educator
Infection Prevention Strategies, LLC
Thornton, Colorado

Olga F. Jarrín, PhD, RN
Assistant Professor
School of Nursing
Rutgers University
Newark, New Jersey
Assistant Professor
Institute for Health, Health Care Policy, and Aging Research
Rutgers University
New Brunswick, New Jersey
Adjunct Assistant Professor
School of Nursing
University of Pennsylvania
Philadelphia, Pennsylvania

Rebecca Johnson, PhD, RN, FAAN, FNAP
Millsap Professor of Gerontological Nursing and Public
    Policy
Sinclair School of Nursing
Professor
College of Veterinary Medicine
University of Missouri
Columbia, Missouri

Catherine Kleiner, PhD, MSN, BSN
Director of Research, Innovation, and Professional Practice
Children's Hospital of Colorado
Aurora, Colorado

Gail B. Ladwig, MSN, RN
Professor Emeritus
Jackson Community College
Jackson, Michigan
Consultant in Guided Imagery, Healing Touch, and Nursing
    Diagnosis
Hilton Head, South Carolina

Rosemary Koehl Lee, DNP, ARNP, ACNP-BC, CCNS, CCRN
Clinical Nurse Specialist
Critical Care
Homestead Hospital
Homestead, Florida
Adjunct Faculty
College of Nursing
Nova Southeastern University
Palm Beach Gardens, Florida

Ellen MacKinnon, MS, RN, CNRN, AGCNS-BC
Clinical Nurse Specialist
Pulmonary Department
National Jewish Health
Denver, Colorado

Mary Beth Flynn Makic, PhD, RN, CCNS, FAAN, FNAP
Professor
College of Nursing
University of Colorado
Aurora, Colorado

Marina Reyna Martinez-Kratz, MS, RN, CNE
Professor
Department of Nursing
Jackson College
Jackson, Michigan

Lauren McAlister, MSN, FNP, DNP Candidate
School of Nursing
University of North Florida
Jacksonville, Florida

Marsha McKenzie, MA Ed, BSN, RN
Coordinator of Pathways and Curriculum Development
Academic Affairs
Big Sandy Community and Technical College
Prestonsburg, Kentucky

Kimberly S. Meyer, PhD, ACNP-BC, CNRN
Neurotrauma/Cerebrovascular Nurse Practitioner
Neurosurgery
AGACNP Track Coordinator
School of Nursing
University of Louisville
Louisville, Kentucky

Annie Muller, DNP, APRN-BC
Associate Professor
School of Health Sciences
Francis Marion University
Florence, South Carolina

Morgan Nestingen, MSN, AGCNS, ONS
Regional Oncology Navigation Manager
Nursing Administration
Centura Health, St. Anthony Hospital
Lakewood, Colorado

Katherina A. Nikzad-Terhune, PhD, MSW
Assistant Professor
Department of Counseling, Social Work, and Leadership
Northern Kentucky University
Highland Heights, Kentucky

Darcy O'Banion, RN, MS, APN, ACCNS-AG
Senior Instructor
Department of Neurology
University of Colorado School of Medicine
Aurora, Colorado

Mary E. Oesterle, MA, CCC-SLP
Speech Language Pathologist
Rehabilitation
Chelsea Hospital, St. Joseph Mercy Health System
Chelsea, Michigan

Wolter Paans, PhD
Professor of Nursing Diagnostics
School of Nursing
Hanze University
Groningen, Netherlands

Margaret Elizabeth Padnos, RN, AB, BSN, MA
Registered Nurse (Retired)
Former NICU Transition Team
Spectrum Health
Grand Rapids, Michigan

Kathleen L. Patusky, MA, PhD, RN, CNS
Associate Professor
School of Nursing
Rutgers University
Newark, New Jersey

Kim Paxton, DNP, APRN, ANP-BC, LHIT-C
Adult Geriatric Primary Care Nurse Practitioner Specialty Director
College of Nursing
University of Colorado
Aurora, Colorado

Ann Will Poteet, MS, RN, CNS, AGNP-C
Nurse Practitioner
Cardiology—Adult Congenital Heart Disease
University of Colorado, School of Medicine
Aurora, Colorado

Kerri J. Reid, RN, MS, CNS, CCRN-K
Senior Instructor of Clinical Teaching
Clinical Education Center and Simulation
College of Nursing
University of Colorado
Aurora, Colorado

Lori M. Rhudy, PhD, RN, CNRN, ACNS-BC
Clinical Associate Professor
School of Nursing
University of Minnesota
Minneapolis, Minnesota
Nurse Scientist
Nursing Research Division
Mayo Clinic
Rochester, Minnesota

Shelley Sadler, BSN, MSN, APRN, WHNP-BC
Instructor of Nursing
Department of Nursing
Morehead State University
Morehead, Kentucky

Debra Siela, PhD, RN, CCNS, ACNS-BC, CCRN-K, CNE, RRT
Associate Professor
School of Nursing
Ball State University
Muncie, Indiana

Kimberly Silvey, MSN, RN, RAC-CT
Minimum Data Set Coordinator
Clinical Reimbursement
Signature Healthcare
Lexington, Kentucky

Tammy Spencer, DNP, RN, CNE, AGCNS-BC, CCNS
Assistant Professor
College of Nursing
University of Colorado
Aurora, Colorado

Bernie St. Aubyn, BSc (Hons), MSc
Senior Lecturer
Pre Qualifying Department
Birmingham City University
Birmingham, United Kingdom

Elaine E. Steinke, PhD, APRN, CNS-BC, FAHA, FAAN
Professor Emeritus
School of Nursing
Wichita State University
Wichita, Kansas

Denise Sullivan, MSN, ANP-BC
Associate Director of Nursing and Nurse Practitioner
Anesthesiology/Pain Medicine Service
NYC Health + Hospitals/Jacobi
Bronx, New York

Cynthia DeLeon Thelen, MSN, BSN, RN
Adjunct Professor
School of Human Services
Spring Arbor University
Spring Arbor, Michigan
State Administrative Manager
Licensing and Regulatory Affairs, Bureau of Community
    and Health Systems
State of Michigan
Lansing, Michigan

**Rosemary Timmerman, DNP, APRN, CCNS,
    CCRN-CSC-CMC**
Clinical Nurse Specialist
Intensive Care Unit
Providence Alaska Medical Center
Anchorage, Alaska

Janelle M. Tipton, MSN, RN, AOCN
Manager and Oncology Clinical Nurse Specialist
Cancer Center
Volunteer Faculty
College of Nursing and College of Medicine
University of Toledo
Toledo, Ohio

Stephanie Turrise, PhD, MSN, BSN
Assistant Professor
School of Nursing
University of North Carolina Wilmington
Wilmington, North Carolina

Carolien van der Velde
Academie voor Verpleegkunde
Hanzehogeschool, Roden
Drenthe, Netherlands

Anna van der Woude, BSN
Hanzehogeschool, Groningen
Groningen, Netherlands

Barbara Baele Vincensi, PhD, RN, FNP
Associate Professor
Nursing
Hope College
Holland, Michigan

Kerstin West-Wilson, BS, MS, BSN, RN, IBCLC
Neonatal Intensive Care
Children's Hospital at Saint Francis
Tulsa, Oklahoma

Barbara J. Wheeler, RN, BN, MN, IBCLC, RN
Clinical Nurse Specialist
Woman and Child Program
St. Boniface Hospital
Professional Affiliate
Manitoba Centre for Nursing and Health Research
Instructor II
College of Nursing
University of Manitoba
Winnipeg, Canada

Suzanne White, MSN, RN, PHCNS, BC
Associate Professor
Nursing
Morehead State University
Morehead, Kentucky

Linda S. Williams, MSN, BSN
Professor Emeritus
Nursing
Jackson College
Jackson, Michigan

**Ruth A. Wittmann-Price, PhD, RN, CNS, CHSE, CNE,
    ANEF, FAAN**
Dean and Professor of Nursing
School of Health Sciences
Francis Marion University
Florence, South Carolina

Melody Zanotti, BA, RN, LSW
Retired
Cleveland, Ohio

Milou Zemering, BN
Academie voor Verpleegkunde
Hanzehogeschool, Groningen
Groningen, Netherlands

Reviewers

Diane Benefiel, EdD, MSN, RN
Nursing Faculty
Nursing Education
Fresno City College
Adjunct Nursing Faculty
Nursing Education
Fresno Pacific University
Fresno, California

Anna M. Bruch, RN, MSN
Nursing Professor
Health Professions
Illinois Valley Community College
Oglesby, Illinois

Kim Clevenger, EdD, MSN, RN, BC
Associate Professor of Nursing
Morehead State University
Morehead, Kentucky

Wanda Hayes, RN, DNP
Nursing Program Director
Judson College
Marion, Alabama

Julia E. Robinson, DNP, MSN, APRN, FNP-C, GCNS-BC, PHN
Associate Professor, Assistant Department Chairperson, and Assistant Program Director
Nursing Education
Palomar Community College
San Marcos, California

Nursing Diagnosis Handbook: An Evidence-Based Guide to Planning Care is a convenient reference to help the practicing nurse or nursing student make a nursing diagnosis and write a care plan with ease and confidence. This handbook helps nurses correlate nursing diagnoses with known information about clients on the basis of assessment findings; established medical, surgical, or psychiatric diagnoses; and the current treatment plan.

Making a nursing diagnosis and planning care are complex processes that involve diagnostic reasoning and critical thinking skills. Nursing students and practicing nurses cannot possibly memorize the extensive list of defining characteristics, related factors, and risk factors for the 244 diagnoses approved by NANDA-International (NANDA-I). There are also two additional diagnoses that the authors think are significant: Hearing Loss and Vision Loss. These diagnoses are contained in Appendix E. This book correlates suggested nursing diagnoses with what nurses know about clients and offers a care plan for each nursing diagnosis.

Section I, Nursing Process, Clinical Reasoning, Nursing Diagnosis, and Evidence-Based Nursing, is divided into two parts. Part A includes an overview of the nursing process. This section provides information on how to make a nursing diagnosis and directions on how to plan nursing care. It also includes information on using clinical reasoning skills and eliciting the "client's story." Part B includes advanced nursing concepts: concept mapping, QSEN (quality and safety education for nurses), evidence-based nursing care, quality nursing care, patient-centered care, safety, informatics in nursing, and team/collaborative work with an interprofessional team.

In **Section II, Guide to Nursing Diagnoses,** the nurse can look up symptoms and problems and their suggested nursing diagnoses for more than 1450 client symptoms; medical, surgical, and psychiatric diagnoses; diagnostic procedures; surgical interventions; and clinical states.

In **Section III, Guide to Planning Care,** the nurse can find care plans for all nursing diagnoses suggested in Section II. We have included the suggested nursing outcomes from the Nursing Outcomes Classification (NOC) and interventions from the Nursing Interventions Classification (NIC) by the Iowa Intervention Project. We believe this work is a significant addition to the nursing process to further define nursing practice with standardized language.

Scientific rationales based on research are included for most of the interventions. This is done to make the evidence base of nursing practice apparent to the nursing student and practicing nurse.

New special features of the twelfth edition of *Nursing Diagnosis Handbook: An Evidence-Based Guide to Planning Care* include the following:
- Labeling of classic older research studies that are still relevant as Classic Evidence-Based (CEB)
- Seventy-two revised nursing diagnoses approved by NANDA-I
- Addition of the terms At-Risk Populations and Associated Conditions to the diagnostic indicators as approved by NANDA-I
- NANDA-I approved change for the definition of the Health Promotion Diagnoses
- Seventeen new nursing diagnoses recently approved by NANDA-I, along with retiring eight nursing diagnoses: Risk for disproportionate growth, Noncompliance, Readiness for enhanced fluid balance, Readiness for enhanced urinary elimination, Risk for impaired cardiovascular function, Risk for ineffective gastrointestinal perfusion, Risk for ineffective renal perfusion, and Risk for imbalanced body temperature
- Eleven revisions of nursing diagnoses made by NANDA-I in existing nursing diagnoses
  - **Old diagnosis:** Deficient diversional activity
    Revised diagnosis: Decreased diversional activity engagement
  - **Old diagnosis:** Insufficient breast milk
    Revised diagnosis: Insufficient breast milk production
  - **Old diagnosis:** Neonatal jaundice
    Revised diagnosis: Neonatal hyperbilirubinemia
  - **Old diagnosis:** Risk for neonatal jaundice
    Revised diagnosis: Risk for hyperbilirubinemia
  - **Old diagnosis:** Impaired oral mucous membrane
    Revised diagnosis: Impaired oral mucous membrane integrity
  - **Old diagnosis:** Risk for impaired oral mucous membrane
    Revised diagnosis: Risk for impaired oral mucous membrane integrity
  - **Old diagnosis:** Risk for sudden infant death syndrome
    Revised diagnosis: Risk for sudden infant death
  - **Old diagnosis:** Risk for trauma
    Revised diagnosis: Risk for physical trauma
  - **Old diagnosis:** Risk for allergy response
    Revised diagnosis: Risk for allergic reaction
  - **Old diagnosis:** Latex allergy response
    Revised diagnosis: Latex allergic reaction

- **Old diagnosis**: Risk for latex allergy response
  Revised diagnosis: Risk for latex allergic reaction
- Further addition of pediatric and critical care interventions to appropriate care plans
- An associated Evolve Online Course Management System that includes a care plan constructor, critical thinking case studies, Nursing Interventions Classification (NIC) and Nursing Outcomes Classification (NOC) labels, PowerPoint slides, review questions for the NCLEX-RN® exam, and appendixes for Nursing Diagnoses Arranged by Maslow's Hierarchy of Needs, Nursing Diagnoses Arranged by Gordon's Functional Health Patterns, Motivational Interviewing for Nurses, Wellness-Oriented Diagnostic Categories, and Nursing Care Plans for Hearing Loss and Vision Loss

The following features of *Nursing Diagnosis Handbook: A Guide to Planning Care* are also available:

- Suggested nursing diagnoses for more than 1450 clinical entities, including signs and symptoms, medical diagnoses, surgeries, maternal-child disorders, mental health disorders, and geriatric disorders
- Labeling of nursing research as EBN (Evidence-Based Nursing) and clinical research as EB (Evidence-Based) to identify the source of evidence-based rationales
- An Evolve Online Courseware System with a Care Plan Constructor that helps the student or nurse write a nursing care plan
- Rationales for nursing interventions that are (for the most part) based on nursing research
- Nursing references identified for each care plan
- A complete list of NOC Outcomes on the Evolve website
- A complete list of NIC Interventions on the Evolve website
- Nursing care plans that contain many holistic interventions
- Care plans written by leading national nursing experts from throughout the United States, along with international contributors, who together represent all of the major nursing specialties and have extensive experience with nursing diagnoses, the nursing process, and evidence-based practice. Several contributors are the original submitters/authors of the nursing diagnoses established by NANDA-I.
- A format that facilitates analyzing signs and symptoms by the process already known by nurses, which involves using defining characteristics of nursing diagnoses to make a diagnosis
- Use of NANDA-I terminology and approved diagnoses
- An alphabetical format for Sections II and III, which allows rapid access to information
- Nursing care plans for all nursing diagnoses listed in Section II
- Specific geriatric interventions in appropriate plans of care
- Specific client/family teaching interventions in each plan of care
- Information on culturally competent nursing care included where appropriate
- Inclusion of commonly used abbreviations (e.g., AIDS, MI, HF) and cross-references to complete terms in Section II

We acknowledge the work of NANDA-I, which is used extensively throughout this text. The original NANDA-I work can be found in *NANDA-I Nursing Diagnoses: Definitions & Classification 2018-2020*, eleventh edition.

We and the consultants and contributors trust that nurses will find this twelfth edition of *Nursing Diagnosis Handbook: An Evidence-Based Guide to Planning Care* a valuable tool that simplifies the process of identifying appropriate nursing diagnoses for clients and planning for their care, thus allowing nurses more time to provide evidence-based care that speeds each client's recovery.

Gail B. Ladwig
Mary Beth Flynn Makic
Marina Reyna Martinez-Kratz
Melody Zanotti

Acknowledgments

We would like to thank the following people at Elsevier: Sandy E. Clark, Senior Content Strategist, who supported us with this twelfth edition of the text with intelligence and kindness; Jennifer Wade, Senior Content Development Specialist, who was a continual source of support; and a special thank you to Clay Broeker for the project management of this edition.

With gratitude, we acknowledge nurses and student nurses, who are always an inspiration for us to provide fresh and accurate material. We are honored that they continue to value this text and to use it in their studies and practice.

We would like to thank all of the dedicated contributors who are experts in their fields of nursing. We appreciate all of their hard work.

Care has been taken to confirm the accuracy of information presented in this book. However, the authors, editors, and publisher cannot accept any responsibility for consequences resulting from errors or omissions of the information in this book and make no warranty, express or implied, with respect to its contents. The reader should use practices suggested in this book in accordance with agency policies and professional standards. Every effort has been made to ensure the accuracy of the information presented in this text.

We hope you find this text useful in your nursing practice.

Gail B. Ladwig
Mary Beth Flynn Makic
Marina Reyna Martinez-Kratz
Melody Zanotti

How to Use *Nursing Diagnosis Handbook: An Evidence-Based Guide to Planning Care*

STEP 1: ASSESS

Following the guidelines in Section I, begin to formulate your nursing diagnosis by gathering and documenting the objective and subjective information about the client.

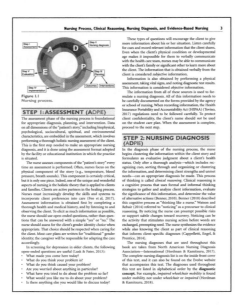

STEP 2: DIAGNOSE

Turn to Section II, Guide to Nursing Diagnoses, and locate the client's symptoms, clinical state, medical or psychiatric diagnoses, and anticipated or prescribed diagnostic studies or surgical interventions (listed in alphabetical order). Note suggestions for appropriate nursing diagnoses.

Then use Section III, Guide to Planning Care, to evaluate each suggested nursing diagnosis and "related to" (r/t) etiology statement. Section III is a listing of care plans according to NANDA-I, arranged alphabetically by diagnostic concept, for each nursing diagnosis referred to in Section II. Determine the appropriateness of each nursing diagnosis by comparing the Defining Characteristics and/or Risk Factors to the client data collected.

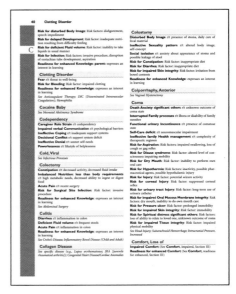

STEP 3: DETERMINE OUTCOMES

Use Section III, Guide to Planning Care, to find appropriate outcomes for the client. Use either the NOC Outcomes with the associated rating scales or Client Outcomes as desired.

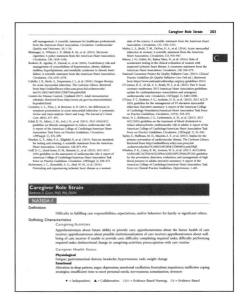

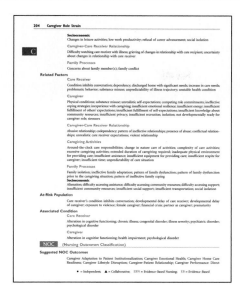

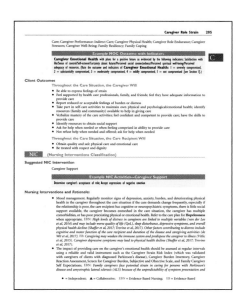

PLAN INTERVENTIONS

Use Section III, Guide to Planning Care, to find appropriate interventions for the client. Use the Nursing Interventions as found in that section.

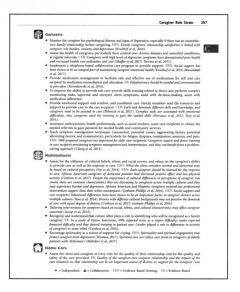

GIVE NURSING CARE

Administer nursing care following the plan of care based on the interventions.

EVALUATE NURSING CARE

Evaluate nursing care administered using either the NOC Outcomes or Client Outcomes. If the outcomes were not met and the nursing interventions were not effective, reassess the client and determine if the appropriate nursing diagnoses were made.

DOCUMENT

Document all of the previous steps using the format provided in the clinical setting.

Contents

NURSING
DIAGNOSIS
HANDBOOK

An Evidence-Based Guide to Planning Care

Nursing Process, Clinical Reasoning, Nursing Diagnosis, and Evidence-Based Nursing

Gail B. Ladwig, MSN, RN,

Mary Beth Flynn Makic, PhD, RN, CCNS, FAAN, FNAP, and

Marina Martinez-Kratz, MS, RN, CNE

Section I is divided into two parts. Part A includes an overview of the nursing process. This section provides information on how to make a nursing diagnosis and directions on how to plan nursing care. It also includes information on using clinical reasoning skills and eliciting the "patient's story." Part B includes advanced nursing concepts.

Part A: The Nursing Process: Using Clinical Reasoning Skills to Determine Nursing Diagnosis and Plan Care

1. **A**ssessing: performing a nursing assessment
2. **D**iagnosing: making nursing diagnoses
3. **P**lanning: formulating and writing outcome statements and determining appropriate nursing interventions based on appropriate best evidence (research)
4. **I**mplementing care
5. **E**valuating the outcomes and the nursing care that has been implemented. Make necessary revisions in care interventions as needed

Part B: Advanced Nursing Concepts

- Concept mapping
- Quality and Safety Education for Nurses (QSEN)
- Evidence-based nursing care
- Quality nursing care
- Patient-centered care
- Safety
- Informatics in nursing
- Team/collaborative work with interprofessional team

The Nursing Process: Using Clinical Reasoning Skills to Determine Nursing Diagnoses and Plan Care

The primary goals of nursing are to (1) determine client/family responses to human problems, level of wellness, and need for assistance; (2) provide physical care, emotional care, teaching, guidance, and counseling; and (3) implement interventions aimed at prevention and assisting the client to meet his or her own needs and health-related goals. The nurse must always focus on assisting clients and families to their highest level of functioning and self-care. The care that is provided should be structured in a way that allows clients the ability to influence their health care and accomplish their self-efficacy goals. The nursing process, which is a problem-solving approach to the identification and treatment of client problems, provides a framework for assisting clients and families to their optimal level of functioning. The nursing process involves five dynamic and fluid phases: **assessment, diagnosis, planning, implementation,** and **evaluation.** Within each of these phases, the client and family story is embedded and is used as a foundation for knowledge, judgment, and actions brought to the client care experience. A description of the "patient's story" and each aspect of the nursing process follow.

THE "PATIENT'S STORY"

The "patient's story" is a term used to describe objective and subjective information about the client that describes who the client is as a person in addition to their usual medical history. Specific aspects of the story include physiological, psychological, and family characteristics; available resources; environmental and social context; knowledge; and motivation. Care is influenced, and often driven, by what the client states—verbally or through their physiological state. The "patient's story" is fluid and must be shared and understood throughout the client's health care experience.

There are multiple sources for obtaining the patient's story. The primary source for eliciting this story is through communicating directly with the client and the client's family. It is important to understand how the illness (or wellness) state has affected the client physiologically, psychologically, and spiritually. The client's perception of his or her health state is important to understand and may have an impact on subsequent interventions. At times, clients will be unable to tell their story verbally, but there is still much they can communicate through their physical state. The client's family (as the client defines them) is a valuable source of information and can provide a rich perspective on the client. Other valuable sources of the "patient's story" include the client's health record. Every time a piece of information is added to the health record, it becomes a part of the "patient's story." All nursing care is driven by the client's story. The nurse must have a clear understanding of the story to effectively complete the nursing process. Understanding the full story also provides an avenue for identifying mutual goals with the client and family aimed at improving client outcomes and goals.

Note: The "patient's story" is terminology that is used to describe a holistic assessment of information about the client, including the client's and the family's input as much as possible. In this text, we use the term "patient's story" in quotes whenever we refer to the specific process. In all other places, we use the term *client* in place of the word *patient*; we think labeling the person as a client is more respectful and empowering for the person. *Client* is also the term that is used in the National Council Licensure Examination (NCLEX-RN) test plan (National Council of State Boards of Nursing, 2016).

Understanding the "patient's story" is critically important, in that psychological, socioeconomic, and spiritual characteristics play a significant role in the client's ability and desire to access health care. Also knowing and understanding the "patient's story" is an integral first step in giving client-centered care. In today's health care world, the focus is on the client, which leads to increased satisfaction with care. Improving the client's health care experience is tied to reimbursement through value-based purchasing of care to reward providers for the quality of care they provide (Centers for Medicare and Medicaid Services, 2018).

THE NURSING PROCESS

The nursing process is an organizing framework for professional nursing practice, which is a critical thinking process for the nurse to use to give the best care possible to the client. It is very similar to the steps used in scientific reasoning and problem solving. This section is designed to help the nursing student learn how to use this thinking process, or the nursing process. Key components of the process include the steps listed subsequently. An easy, convenient way to remember the steps of the nursing process is to use an acronym, **ADPIE** (Figure I.1):

1. **A**ssess: perform a nursing assessment.
2. **D**iagnose: make nursing diagnoses.
3. **P**lan: formulate and write outcome/goal statements and determine appropriate nursing interventions based on the client's reality and evidence (research).
4. **I**mplement care.
5. **E**valuate the outcomes and the nursing care that has been implemented. Make necessary revisions in care interventions as needed.

The next section is an overview and practical application of the steps of the nursing process. The steps are listed in the usual order in which they are performed.

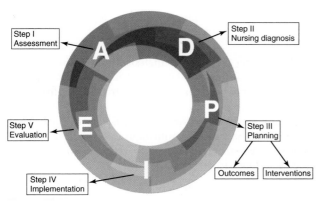

Figure 1.1
Nursing process.

STEP 1: ASSESSMENT (ADPIE)

The assessment phase of the nursing process is foundational for appropriate diagnosis, planning, and intervention. Data on all dimensions of the "patient's story," including biophysical, psychological, sociocultural, spiritual, and environmental characteristics, are embedded in the assessment, which involves performing a thorough holistic nursing assessment of the client. This is the first step needed to make an appropriate nursing diagnosis, and it is done using the assessment format adopted by the facility or educational institution in which the practice is situated.

The nurse assesses components of the "patient's story" every time an assessment is performed. Often, nurses focus on the physical component of the story (e.g., temperature, blood pressure, breath sounds). This component is certainly critical, but it is only one piece. Indeed, one of the unique and wonderful aspects of nursing is the holistic theory that is applied to clients and families. Clients are active partners in the healing process. Nurses must increasingly develop the skills and systems to incorporate client preferences into care (Feo et al, 2017). Assessment information is obtained first by completing a thorough health and medical history, and by listening to and observing the client. To elicit as much information as possible, the nurse should use open-ended questions, rather than questions that can be answered with a simple "yes" or "no." The nurse should assess for the client's gender identity choice when appropriate. That choice should be respected when caring for the client. Most care plans are written for "traditional " gender identity; the caregiver will be responsible for adapting the care accordingly.

In screening for depression in older clients, the following open-ended questions are useful (Lusk & Fater, 2013):
• What made you come here today?
• What do you think your problem is?
• What do you think caused your problem?
• Are you worried about anything in particular?
• What have you tried to do about the problem so far?
• What would you like me to do about your problem?
• Is there anything else you would like to discuss today?

These types of questions will encourage the client to give more information about his or her situation. Listen carefully for cues and record relevant information that the client shares. Even when the client's physical condition or developmental age makes it impossible for them to verbally communicate with the health care team, nurses may be able to communicate with the client's family or significant other to learn more about the client. The information that is obtained verbally from the client is considered *subjective* information.

Information is also obtained by performing a physical assessment, taking vital signs, and noting diagnostic test results. This information is considered *objective* information.

The information from all of these sources is used to formulate a nursing diagnosis. All of this information needs to be carefully documented on the forms provided by the agency or school of nursing. When recording information, the Health Insurance Portability and Accountability Act (HIPAA) (Tovino, 2017) regulations need to be followed carefully. To protect client confidentiality, the client's name should *not* be used on the student care plan. When the assessment is complete, proceed to the next step.

STEP 2: NURSING DIAGNOSIS (ADPIE)

In the diagnosis phase of the nursing process, the nurse begins clustering the information within the client story and formulates an evaluative judgment about a client's health status. Only after a thorough analysis—which includes recognizing cues, sorting through and organizing or clustering the information, and determining client strengths and unmet needs—can an appropriate diagnosis be made. This process of thinking is called *clinical reasoning*. Clinical reasoning is a cognitive process that uses formal and informal thinking strategies to gather and analyze client information, evaluate the significance of this information, and determine the value of alternative actions (Benner, 2010). Benner (2010) described this cognitive process as "thinking like a nurse." Watson and Rebair (2014) referred to "noticing" as a precursor to clinical reasoning. By noticing the nurse can preempt possible risks or support subtle changes toward recovery. Noticing can be the activity that stimulates nursing action before words are exchanged, preempting need. The nurse synthesizes the evidence while also knowing the client as part of clinical reasoning that informs client-specific diagnoses (Cappelletti, Engel, & Prentice, 2014).

The nursing diagnoses that are used throughout this book are taken from North American Nursing Diagnosis Association—International (Herdman & Kamitsuru, 2017). The complete nursing diagnosis list is on the inside front cover of this text, and it can also be found on the Evolve website that accompanies this text. The diagnoses used throughout this text are listed in alphabetical order by the **diagnostic concept.** For example, *impaired wheelchair mobility* is found under *mobility,* not under *wheelchair* or *impaired* (Herdman & Kamitsuru, 2018).

The holistic assessment of the client helps determine the type of diagnosis that follows. For example, if during the assessment a client is noted to have unsteady gait and balance disturbance and states, "I'm concerned I will fall while walking down my stairs," but has not fallen previously, then the client would be identified as having a "risk" nursing diagnosis.

Once the diagnosis is determined, the next step is to determine related factors and defining characteristics. The process for formulating a nursing diagnosis with related factors and defining characteristics is found in the next section. A client may have many nursing and medical diagnoses, and determining the priority with which each should be addressed requires clinical reasoning and application of knowledge.

Formulating a Nursing Diagnosis With Related Factors and Defining Characteristics

A working nursing diagnosis may have two or three parts. The two-part system consists of the nursing diagnosis and the "related to" (r/t) statement: "Related factors are etiologies, circumstances, facts, or influences that have some type of relationship with the nursing diagnosis (e.g., cause, contributed factor)." (Herdman & Kamitsuru, 2018).

The two-part system is often used when the defining characteristics, or signs and symptoms identified in the assessment, may be obvious to those caring for the client.

The three-part system consists of the nursing diagnosis, the r/t statement, and the defining characteristics, which are "observable cues/inferences that cluster as manifestations of an actual or wellness nursing diagnosis" (Herdman & Kamitsuru, 2018).

Some nurses refer to the three-part diagnostic statement as the **PES system**:

P (problem)—The nursing diagnosis label: a concise term or phrase that represents a pattern of related cues. The nursing diagnosis is taken from the official NANDA-I list.
E (etiology)—"Related to" (r/t) phrase or etiology: related cause or contributor to the problem.
S (symptoms)—Defining characteristics phrase: symptoms that the nurse identified in the assessment.

Here we use the example of a beginning nursing student who is attempting to understand the nursing process and how to make a nursing diagnosis:

Problem: Use the nursing diagnosis label deficient **Knowledge** from the NANDA-I list. Remember to check the definition: "Absence or deficiency of cognitive information related to a specific topic" (Herdman & Kamitsuru, 2018).
Etiology: r/t unfamiliarity with information about the nursing process and nursing diagnosis. At this point the beginning nurse would not be familiar with available resources regarding the nursing process.
Symptoms: Defining characteristics, as evidenced by (aeb) verbalization of lack of understanding: "I don't understand this, and I really don't know how to make a nursing diagnosis."

When using the **PES** system, look at the **S** first, and then formulate the three-part statement. (You would have gotten the **S**, symptoms, which are defining characteristics, from your assessment.)

Therefore, the three-part nursing diagnosis is: deficient **Knowledge** r/t unfamiliarity with information about the nursing process and nursing diagnosis aeb verbalization of lack of understanding.

Types of Nursing Diagnoses

There are three different types of nursing diagnoses.

Problem-Focused Diagnosis. "A clinical judgment concerning an undesirable human response to a health condition/life process that exists in an individual, family, group or community" (Herdman & Kamitsuru, 2018, p 35).

"Related factors are an integral part of all problem-focused diagnoses. Related factors are etiologies, circumstances, facts or influences that have some type of relationship with the nursing diagnosis (e.g., cause, contributed factor)" (Herdman & Kamitsuru, 2018, p 39).

Example of a Problem-Focused Nursing Diagnosis. **Overweight** related to excessive intake in relation to metabolic needs, concentrating food intake at the end of the day aeb weight 20% over ideal for height and frame. Note: This is a three-part nursing diagnosis.

Risk Nursing Diagnosis. Risk nursing diagnosis is a "clinical judgment concerning the susceptibility of an individual, family, group, or community for developing an undesirable human response to health conditions/life processes" (Herdman & Kamitsuru, 2018, p 35). "Risk factors are influences that increase the vulnerability of an individual, family, group, or community to an unhealthy event" (Herdman & Kamitsuru, 2018, p 39). Defining characteristics and related factors are observable cues and circumstances or influences that have some type of relationship with the nursing diagnosis that may contribute to a health problem. Identification of related factors allows nursing interventions to be implemented to address the underlying cause of a nursing diagnosis (Herdman & Kamitsuru, 2018, p 39).

Example of a Risk Nursing Diagnosis. Risk for **Overweight:** Risk factor: concentrating food at the end of the day. Note: This is a two-part nursing diagnosis.

Health Promotion Nursing Diagnosis. A clinical judgment concerning motivation and desire to increase well-being and to actualize health potential. These responses are expressed by a readiness to enhance specific health behaviors, and can be used in any health state. Health promotion responses may exist in an individual, family, group, or community (Herdman & Kamitsuru, 2018, p 35). Health promotion is different from prevention in that health promotion focuses on being as healthy as possible, as opposed to preventing a disease or problem. The difference between health promotion and disease prevention is that the reason for the health behavior should always be a positive one. *With a health promotion diagnosis, the outcomes and interventions should be focused on enhancing health.*

   Example of a Health Promotion Nursing Diagnosis. Readiness for enhanced **Nutrition** aeb willingness to change eating pattern and eat healthier foods. Note: This is a two-part nursing diagnosis.

Application and Examples of Making a Nursing Diagnosis

When the assessment is complete, identify common patterns/symptoms of response *to actual or potential health problems from the assessment* and select an appropriate nursing diagnosis label using clinical reasoning skills. Use the steps with Case Study 1. (The same steps can be followed using an actual client assessment in the clinical setting or in a student assessment.)
A. Highlight or underline the relevant symptoms (defining characteristics). As you review your assessment information, ask: Is this normal? Is this an ideal situation? Is this a problem for the client? You may go back and validate information with the client.
B. Make a list of the symptoms (underlined or highlighted information).
C. Cluster similar symptoms.
D. Analyze/interpret the symptoms. (What do these symptoms mean or represent when they are together?)
E. Select a nursing diagnosis label from the NANDA-I list that fits the appropriate defining characteristics and nursing diagnosis definition.

Case Study I—Older Client with Breathing Problems

A. Underline the Symptoms (Defining Characteristics)

A 73-year-old man has been admitted to the unit with a diagnosis of chronic obstructive pulmonary disease (COPD). He states that he has "difficulty breathing when walking short distances." He also states that his "heart feels like it is racing" (heart rate is 110 beats per minute) at the same time. He states that he is "tired all the time," and while talking to you about his story, he is continually wringing his hands and looking out the window.

B. List the Symptoms (Subjective and Objective)

"Difficulty breathing when walking short distances"; "heart feels like it is racing"; heart rate is 110 beats per minute; "tired all the time"; continually wringing his hands and looking out the window.

C. Cluster Similar Symptoms

"Difficulty breathing when walking short distances"
"Heart feels like it is racing"; heart rate = 110 beats per minute
"Tired all the time"
Continually wringing his hands
Looking out the window

D. Analyze
Interpret the Subjective Symptoms (What the Client Has Stated)
- "Difficulty breathing when walking short distances" = exertional discomfort: a defining characteristic of **Activity** intolerance
- "Heart feels like it is racing" = abnormal heart rate response to activity: a defining characteristic of **Activity** intolerance
- "Tired all the time" = verbal report of weakness: a defining characteristic of **Activity** intolerance

Interpret the Objective Symptoms (Observable Information)
- Continually wringing his hands = extraneous movement, hand/arm movements: a defining characteristic of **Anxiety**
- Looking out the window = poor eye contact, glancing about: a defining characteristic of **Anxiety**
- Heart rate = 110 beats per minute

E. Select the Nursing Diagnosis Label

In Section II, look up *dyspnea (difficulty breathing)* or *dysrhythmia (abnormal heart rate or rhythm)*, which are chosen because they are high priority, and you will find the nursing diagnosis **Activity** intolerance listed with these symptoms. Is this diagnosis appropriate for this client?

   To validate that the diagnosis **Activity** intolerance is appropriate for the client, turn to Section III and read the NANDA-I definition of the nursing diagnosis **Activity** intolerance: "Insufficient physiological or psychological energy to endure or complete required or desired daily activities" (Herdman & Kamitsuru, 2018, p 228). When reading the definition, ask, "Does this definition describe the symptoms demonstrated by the client?" "Is any more assessment information needed?" "Should I take his blood pressure or take an apical pulse rate?" If the appropriate nursing diagnosis has been selected, the definition should describe the condition that has been observed.

   The client may also have defining characteristics for this particular diagnosis. Are the client's symptoms that you identified in the list of defining characteristics (e.g., verbal report of fatigue, abnormal heart rate response to activity, exertional dyspnea)?

   Another way to use this text and to help validate the diagnosis is to look up the client's medical diagnosis in Section II. This client has a medical diagnosis of COPD. Is **Activity** intolerance listed with this medical diagnosis? Consider whether the nursing diagnosis makes sense given the client's medical diagnosis (in this case, COPD). There may be times when a nursing diagnosis is not directly linked to a medical diagnosis (e.g., ineffective **Coping**) but is nevertheless appropriate given nursing's holistic approach to the client/family.

   The process of identifying significant symptoms, clustering or grouping them into logical patterns, and then choosing an appropriate nursing diagnosis involves diagnostic reasoning (critical thinking) skills that must be learned in the process of becoming a nurse. This text serves as a tool to help the learner in this process.

"Related to" Phrase or Etiology

The second part of the nursing diagnosis is the "related to" (r/t) phrase. Related factors are those that appear to show some type of patterned relationship with the nursing diagnosis. Such factors may be described as antecedent to, associated with, related to, contributing to, or abetting. Pathophysiological and psychosocial changes, such as developmental age and cultural and environmental situations, may be causative or contributing factors.

Often, a nursing diagnosis is complementary to a medical diagnosis and vice versa. Ideally the etiology (r/t statement), or cause, of the nursing diagnosis is something that can be treated independently by a nurse. When this is the case, the diagnosis is identified as an independent nursing diagnosis.

If medical intervention is also necessary, it might be identified as a collaborative nursing diagnosis. A carefully written, individualized r/t statement enables the nurse to plan nursing interventions and refer for diagnostic procedures, medical treatments, pharmaceutical interventions, and other interventions that will assist the client/family in accomplishing goals and return to a state of optimum health. Diagnoses and treatments provided by the multidisciplinary team all contribute to the client/family outcome. The coordinated effort of the team can only improve outcomes for the client/family and decrease duplication of effort and frustration among the health care team and the client/family.

The etiology is *not* the medical diagnosis. It may be the underlying issue contributing to the nursing diagnosis, but a medical diagnosis is *not* something the nurse can treat independently, without health care provider orders. In the case of the man with COPD, think about what happens when someone has COPD. How does this affect the client? What is happening to him because of this diagnosis?

For each suggested nursing diagnosis, the nurse should refer to the statements listed under the heading Related Factors (r/t) in Section III. These r/t factors may or may not be appropriate for the individual client. If they are not appropriate, the nurse should develop and write an r/t statement that is appropriate for the client. For the client from Case Study 1, a two-part statement could be made here:

Problem = Activity intolerance
Etiology = r/t imbalance between oxygen supply and demand

It was already determined that the client had **Activity** intolerance. With the respiratory symptoms identified from the assessment, imbalance between oxygen supply and demand is appropriate.

Defining Characteristics Phrase

The defining characteristics phrase is the third part of the three-part diagnostic system, and it consists of the signs and symptoms that have been gathered during the assessment phase.

The phrase "as evidenced by" (aeb) may be used to connect the etiology (r/t) with the defining characteristics. The use of identifying defining characteristics is similar to the process that the health care provider uses when making a medical diagnosis. For example, the health care provider who observes the following signs and symptoms—diminished inspiratory and expiratory capacity of the lungs, complaints of dyspnea on exertion, difficulty in inhaling and exhaling deeply, and sometimes chronic cough—may make the medical diagnosis of COPD. This same process is used to identify the nursing diagnosis of **Activity** intolerance.

Put It All Together: Writing the Three-Part Nursing Diagnosis Statement

Problem—Choose the label (nursing diagnosis) using the guidelines explained previously. A list of nursing diagnosis labels can be found in Section II and on the inside front cover.

Etiology—Write an r/t phrase (etiology). These can be found in Section II.

Symptoms—Write the defining characteristics (signs and symptoms), or the "as evidenced by" (aeb) list. A list of the signs and symptoms associated with each nursing diagnosis can be found in Section III.

Case Study 1—73-Year-Old Male Client with Chronic Obstructive Pulmonary Disease (Continued)

Using the information from the earlier case study/example, the nursing diagnostic statement would be as follows:

Problem—**Activity** intolerance.
Etiology—r/t imbalance between oxygen supply and demand.
Symptoms—Verbal reports of fatigue, exertional dyspnea ("difficulty breathing when walking"), and abnormal heart rate response to activity ("racing heart"), heart rate 110 beats per minute.

Therefore, the nursing diagnostic statement for the client with COPD is **Activity** intolerance r/t imbalance between oxygen supply and demand aeb verbal reports of fatigue, exertional dyspnea, and abnormal heart rate in response to activity.

Consider a second case study:

Case Study 2—Woman with Insomnia

As before, the nurse always begins with an assessment. To make the nursing diagnosis, the nurse follows the steps below.

A. Underline the Symptoms

A 45-year-old woman comes to the clinic and asks for medication to help her sleep. She states that she is worrying too much and adds, "It takes me about an hour to get to sleep, and it is very hard to fall asleep. I feel like I can't do anything because I am so tired. My job has become very stressful because of a new boss and too much work."

B. List the Symptoms (Subjective and Objective)

Asks for medication to help her sleep; states she is worrying about too much; "It takes me about an hour to get to sleep"; "it is very hard to fall asleep"; "I feel like I can't do anything because I am so tired"; "My job has become very stressful because of a new boss and too much work."

C. Cluster Similar Symptoms

Asks for medication to help her sleep
"It takes me about an hour to get to sleep."
"It is very hard to fall asleep."
"I feel like I can't do anything because I am so tired."
"I am worrying too much."
"My job is stressful."
"Too much work."

D. Analyze/Interpret the Symptoms
Subjective Symptoms

- Asks for medication to help her sleep; "It takes me about an hour to get to sleep"; "it is very hard to fall asleep"; "I feel like I can't do anything because I am so tired." (All defining characteristics = verbal complaints of difficulty with sleeping.)
- States she is worrying too much (anxiety): "My job is stressful."

Objective Symptoms

- None

E. Select a Nursing Diagnosis with Related Factors and Defining Characteristics

Look up "sleep" in Section II. Listed under the heading "**Sleep pattern, disturbed**" in Section II is the following information:

Insomnia (nursing diagnosis) r/t anxiety and stress

This client states she is worrying too much, which may indicate anxiety; she also recently has increased job stress.

Look up **Insomnia** in Section III. Check the definition: "A disruption in amount and quality of sleep that impairs functioning" (Herdman & Kamitsuru, 2017, p 213). Does this describe the client in the case study? What are the related factors? What are the symptoms? Write the diagnostic statement:

Problem—**Insomnia**
Etiology—r/t anxiety, stress
Symptoms—Difficulty falling asleep, "I am so tired, I can't do anything."

The nursing diagnostic statement is written in this format:
Insomnia r/t anxiety and stress aeb difficulty falling asleep.

Note: There are more than 30 case studies available for both student and faculty use on the Evolve website that accompanies this text.

After the diagnostic statement is written, proceed to the next step: planning.

STEP 3: PLANNING (ADPIE)

The planning phase of the nursing process includes the identification of priorities and determination of appropriate client-specific outcomes and interventions. The nurse in collaboration with the client and family (as applicable) and the rest of the health care team must determine the urgency of the identified problems and prioritize client needs. *Mutual goal setting,* along with *symptom pattern recognition* and *triggers,* helps prioritize interventions and determine which interventions are going to provide the greatest impact. *Symptom pattern recognition* and/or *triggers* is a process of identifying symptoms that clients have related to their illness, understanding which symptom patterns require intervention, and identifying the associated time frame to intervene effectively. For example, a client with heart failure is noted to gain 5 pounds overnight. Coupling this symptom with other symptoms of edema and shortness of breath while walking can be referred to as "symptom pattern recognition"—in this case, that the client is retaining fluid. The nurse, and often the client/family, recognize these symptoms as an immediate *cause* and that more action/intervention is needed to avoid a potential adverse outcome.

Nursing diagnoses should be prioritized based on urgent needs, diagnoses with high level of congruence with defining characteristics, related factors, or risk factors (Herdman & Kamitsuru, 2018, p 41). Use of ABC (airway, breathing, and circulation) and safety is a method to rank threats to the client's immediate survival or safety. The highest priority can also be determined by using Maslow's hierarchy of needs. In this hierarchy, priority is given to immediate problems that may be life-threatening (thus ABC). For example, ineffective **Airway** clearance, aeb the symptoms of increased secretions and increased use of inhaler related to asthma, creates an immediate cause compared to the nursing diagnosis of **Anxiety,** a love and belonging or security need, which makes it a lesser priority than ineffective **Airway** clearance. Refer to Appendix A on Evolve for assistance in prioritizing nursing diagnoses.

The planning phase should be done, whenever possible, with the client/family and the multidisciplinary team to maximize efforts and understanding, and increase compliance with the proposed plan and outcomes. For a successful plan of care, measurable goals and outcomes, including nursing interventions, must be identified.

SMART Outcomes

When writing outcome statements, it can be helpful to use the acronym SMART, which means the outcome must be:

Specific
Measurable
Attainable
Realistic
Timed

The SMART acronym is used in business, education, and health care settings. This method assists the nurse in identifying patient outcomes more effectively.

Once priorities are established, outcomes for the client can be easily identified. Client-specific outcomes are determined based on the mutually set goals. Outcomes refer to the measurable degree of the client's response. The client's response/outcome may be intentional and favorable, such as leaving the hospital 2 days after surgery without any complications. The client's outcome can be negative and unintentional, such as demonstrating a surgical site infection. Generally, outcomes are described in relation to the client's response to interventions; for example, the client's cough becomes more productive after the client begins using the controlled coughing technique.

Based on the "patient's story," the nursing assessment, the mutual goals and outcomes identified by the caregiving team and the client/family, and the clinical reasoning that the nurse uses to prioritize his or her work, the nurse then decides what interventions to use. Based on the nurse's clinical judgment and knowledge, nursing interventions are defined as *all treatments that a nurse performs to enhance client outcomes.*

The selection of appropriate, effective interventions can be individualized to meet the mutual goals established by the client/family. It is then the nurses' education, experiences, and skills that allow them to select and carry out interventions to meet that mutual goal.

Outcomes

After the appropriate priority setting of the nursing diagnoses and interventions is determined, outcomes are developed or examined and decided on. This text includes standardized Nursing Outcomes Classification (NOC) outcomes written by a large team of University of Iowa College of Nursing faculty and students in conjunction with clinicians from a variety of settings (Moorhead et al, 2018). "Nursing-sensitive outcome (NOC) is an individual, family or community state, behavior or perception that is measured along a continuum in response to nursing interventions. The outcomes are stated as concepts that reflect a client, caregiver, family, or community state, perception of behavior rather than as expected goals" (Moorhead et al, 2018).

It is very important for the nurse to *involve* the client and/or family in determining appropriate outcomes. The use of outcomes information creates a continuous feedback loop that is essential to improve nursing quality, ensure patient safety, and secure the best possible client outcomes (Sim et al, 2018). The minimum requirements for rating an outcome are when the outcome is selected (i.e., the baseline measure) and when care is completed (i.e., the discharge summary). This may be sufficient in short-stay, acute-care settings. Depending on how rapidly the client's condition is expected to change, some settings may evaluate once a day or once a shift. Community agencies may evaluate every visit or every other visit, for example. Because measurement times are not standardized, they can be individualized for the client and the setting (Moorhead et al, 2018).

Development of appropriate outcomes can be done one of two ways: using the NOC list or developing an appropriate outcome statement, both of which are included in Section III. There are suggested outcome statements for each nursing diagnosis in this text that can be used as written or modified as necessary to meet the needs of the client.

The Evolve website includes a list of additional NOC outcomes. The use of NOC outcomes can be helpful to the nurse because they contain a five-point, Likert-type rating scale that can be used to evaluate progress toward achieving the outcome. In this text, the rating scale is listed, along with some of the more common indicators; for example, see the rating scale for the outcome **Sleep** (Table I.1).

Because the NOC outcomes are specific, they enhance the nursing process by helping the nurse measure and record the outcomes before and after interventions have been performed. The nurse can choose to have clients rate their own progress using the Likert-type rating scale. This involvement can help increase client motivation to progress *toward* outcomes.

After client outcomes are selected or written, and *discussed* with a client, the nurse plans nursing care with the client and establishes a means that will help the client achieve the selected outcomes. The usual means are nursing interventions.

Interventions

Interventions are like road maps directing the best ways to provide nursing care. The more clearly a nurse writes an intervention, the easier it will be to complete the journey and arrive at the destination of desired client outcomes.

Section III includes suggested interventions for each nursing diagnosis. The interventions are identified as independent (autonomous actions that are initiated by the nurse in response to a nursing diagnosis) or collaborative (actions that the nurse performs in collaboration with other health care professionals, and that may require a health care provider's order and may be in response to both medical and nursing diagnoses). The nurse may choose the interventions appropriate for the client and individualize them accordingly, or determine additional interventions.

This text also contains several suggested Nursing Interventions Classification (NIC) interventions for each nursing diagnosis to help the reader see how NIC is used along with NOC and nursing diagnoses. The NIC interventions are a comprehensive, standardized classification of treatments that nurses perform. The classification includes both physiological and psychosocial interventions, and covers all nursing specialties. A list of NIC interventions is included on the Evolve website. For more information about NIC interventions, refer to the NIC text (Butcher & Bulechek, 2018).

Putting It All Together—Recording the Care Plan

The nurse must document the actual care plan, including prioritized nursing diagnostic statements, outcomes, and interventions. This may be done electronically or in writing. To ensure continuity of care, the plan must be documented

TABLE 1.1

Example NOC Outcome

Sleep—0004

Domain—Functional Health (I)   Care Recipient:

Class—Energy Maintenance (A)   Data Source:

Scale(s)—Severely Compromised to Not Compromised (a) and Severe to None (n)
Definition: Natural periodic suspension of consciousness during which the body is restored.
Outcome Target Rating: Maintain at_____   Increase to _____

Sleep Overall Rating	Severely Compromised 1	Substantially Compromised 2	Moderately Compromised 3	Mildly Compromised 4	Not Compromised 5	
INDICATORS:						
000401 Hours of sleep	1	2	3	4	5	NA
000402 Observed hours of sleep	1	2	3	4	5	
000403 Sleep pattern	1	2	3	4	5	NA
000404 Sleep quality	1	2	3	4	5	NA
000405 Sleep efficiency	1	2	3	4	5	NA
000407 Sleep routine	1	2	3	4	5	NA
000418 Sleeps through the night consistently	1	2	3	4	5	NA
000408 Feelings of rejuvenation after sleep	1	2	3	4	5	NA
000410 Wakeful at appropriate times	1	2	3	4	5	NA
000419 Comfortable bed	1	2	3	4	5	NA
000420 Comfortable temperature in room	1	2	3	4	5	NA
000411 Electroencephalogram findings	1	2	3	4	5	NA
000412 Electromyogram findings	1	2	3	4	5	NA
000413 Electrooculogram findings	1	2	3	4	5	NA

	Severe	Substantial	Moderate	Mild	None	
000421 Difficulty getting to sleep	1	2	3	4	5	NA
000406 Interrupted sleep	1	2	3	4	5	NA
000409 Inappropriate napping	1	2	3	4	5	NA
000416 Sleep apnea	1	2	3	4	5	NA
000417 Dependence on sleep aids	1	2	3	4	5	NA
000422 Nightmares	1	2	3	4	5	NA
000423 Nocturia	1	2	3	4	5	NA
000424 Snoring	1	2	3	4	5	NA
000425 Pain	1	2	3	4	5	NA

Adapted from Moorhead, S., Johnson, M., Maas, M. L., et al. (Eds.). (2018). *Nursing outcomes classification (NOC)* (6th ed.). St Louis: Elsevier.

and shared with all health care personnel caring for the client. This text provides rationales, most of which are research based, to validate that the interventions are appropriate and workable.

The Evolve website includes an electronic care plan constructor that can be easily accessed, updated, and individualized. Many agencies are using electronic records, and this is an ideal resource. See the inside front cover of this text for information regarding access to the Evolve website, or go to http://evolve.elsevier.com/Ackley/NDH.

STEP 4: IMPLEMENTATION (ADPIE)

The implementation phase includes the "carrying out" of the specific, individualized, jointly agreed on interventions in the plan of care. Often, the interventions implemented are focused on *symptom management*, which is alleviating symptoms. Typically, nursing care does not involve "curing" the medical condition causing the symptom; rather, nursing care focuses on caring for the client/family so they can function at their highest level.

The implementation phase of the nursing process is the point at which you actually give nursing care. You perform the interventions that have been individualized to the client. All the hard work you put into the previous steps (ADP) can now be actualized to assist the client. As the interventions are performed, make sure that they are appropriate for the client. Consider that the client who was having difficulty breathing was also older. He may need extra time to carry out any activity. Check the rationale or research that is provided to determine why the intervention is being used. The evidence should support the individualized actions that you are implementing.

Client outcomes are achieved by the performance of the nursing interventions in collaboration with other disciplines and the client/family. During this phase, the nurse continues to assess the client to determine whether the interventions are effective and the desired outcomes are met.

STEP 5: EVALUATION (ADPIE)

The final phase of the nursing process is evaluation. Evaluation occurs not only at the end of the nursing process, but throughout the process. Evaluation of an intervention is, in essence, another nursing assessment; hence, the dynamic feature of the nursing process. The nurse reassesses the client, taking into consideration where the client was before the intervention (i.e., baseline) and where the client is after the intervention.

Nurses are also in a great place (at the bedside) to evaluate how clients respond to other, multidisciplinary interventions, and their assessment of the client's response is valuable to determine whether the client's plan of care needs to be altered or not. For example, the client may receive 2 mg of morphine intravenously for pain (a pharmaceutical intervention to treat pain), and the nurse is the member of the health care team who can best assess how the client responded to that medication. Did the client receive relief from pain? Did the client develop any side effects? The nurse's documented evaluation of the client's response will be very helpful to the entire health care team.

The client/family can often tell the nurse how the intervention helped or did not help. This reassessment requires the nurse to revisit the mutual outcomes/goals set earlier and ask, "Are we moving toward that goal, or does the goal seem unreachable after the intervention?" If the outcomes were not met, the nurse begins again with assessment and determines the reason they were not met. Consider the **SMART** acronym and Case Study 1. Were the outcomes **S**pecific? Were the outcomes **M**easurable? Did the client's heart rate decrease? Did the client indicate that it was easier to breathe when walking from his bed to the bathroom? Were the outcomes **A**ttainable and **R**ealistic? Did he still report "being tired"? Did you allow adequate **T**ime for a positive outcome? Also ask yourself whether you identified the correct nursing diagnosis. Should the interventions be changed? At this point, the nurse can look up any new symptoms or conditions that have been identified and adjust the care plan as needed. Decisions about implementing additional interventions may be necessary; if so, they should be made in collaboration with the client/family if possible.

In some instances, the client/family/nurse triad will establish new, achievable goals and continue to cycle through the nursing process until the mutual goals are achieved.

Another important part of the evaluation phase is documentation. The nurse should use the facility's tool for documentation and record the nursing activity that was performed as well as the results of the nursing interventions. Many facilities use problem-oriented charting, in which the nurse evaluates the care and client outcomes as part of charting. Documentation is also necessary for legal reasons, because in a legal dispute, *if it wasn't charted/recorded, it wasn't done.*

Many health care providers use critical pathways or care maps to plan nursing care. The use of nursing diagnoses should be an integral part of any critical pathway/care map to ensure that nursing care needs are being assessed and appropriate nursing interventions are planned and implemented.

Advanced Nursing Process Concepts

Conceptual Mapping and the Nursing Process

Conceptual mapping is an active learning strategy that promotes critical thinking and clinical judgment, and helps increase clinical competency (George et al, 2014; Jamison & Lis, 2014; Kaddoura, Van-Dyke, & Yang, 2016). Nurses identify complex client problems that require critical thinking to identify priority interventions based on current best evidence to impact client outcomes. (Kaddoura, Van-Dyke, & Yang, 2016). Concept mapping facilitates critical thinking and encourages deeper understanding of the complexity of concepts that influence nursing practice interventions (Lee et al, 2013). The process involves developing a diagram or pictorial representation of newly generated ideas. A concept map begins with a central theme or concept, and then related information is diagrammed radiating from the center theme. A concept map can be used to diagram the critical thinking strategy involved in applying the nursing process in practice.

Start with a blank sheet of paper; the client should be at the center of the paper. The next step involves linking to the person, via lines, the symptoms (defining characteristics) from the assessment to help determine the appropriate nursing diagnosis.

Figure I.2 is an example of how a concept map can be used to begin the nursing diagnostic process.

After the symptoms are visualized, similar ones can be put together to formulate a nursing diagnosis using another concept map (Figure I.3).

The central theme in this concept map is the nursing diagnosis: **Activity** intolerance, with the defining characteristics/client symptoms as concepts that lead to and support the nursing diagnosis. The conceptual map can then be used as a method for determining outcomes and interventions as desired. The nursing process is a thinking process. Using conceptual mapping is a method to help the nurse or nursing student think more effectively about the client.

Quality and Safety Education for Nurses

The QSEN (2018) project represents the nursing profession's response to the five health care competencies articulated by the Institute of Medicine (now called the National Academy of Medicine) (2003). These competencies were adopted by nursing leaders to guide nursing education to better meet the evolving needs of clients and the health care system. (Cronenwett et al, 2007). The QSEN project defined the six competencies for nursing: patient-centered care, teamwork and collaboration, evidence-based practice (EBP), quality improvement, safety, and informatics (Cronenwett et al, 2007). The objective of the QSEN project is to provide nurses with the knowledge, skills,

and attitudes critical for improving the quality and safety of health care systems. Initially, QSEN was developed to enhance nursing education, but it has since been incorporated into practice settings (Lyle-Edrosolo & Waxman, 2016). Additionally, the core elements of QSEN map to key practice initiatives identified by The Joint Commission (TJC) and The American Nurses Credentialing Center Magnet (Magnet) recognition program (The Joint Commission, 2018). A crosswalk of the similarities of the QSEN competencies to TJC and Magnet demonstrates the alignment of the QSEN competencies to guide nursing practice excellence to improve the quality and safety of health care (Lyle-Edrosolo & Waxman, 2016; QSEN, 2018). The following are the competencies that were identified.

Patient-Centered Care

Patient-centered care is the ability to "recognize the patient or designee as the source of control and full partner in providing compassionate and coordinated care based on respect for patient's preferences, values, and needs" (QSEN, 2018). Patient-centered care begins with the nurse learning as much as possible about the client, including their "client's story" as explained in Part A of this text. The nursing process, using

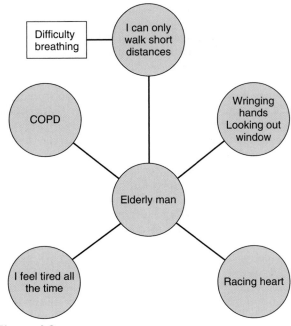

Figure I.2
Example of a concept map.

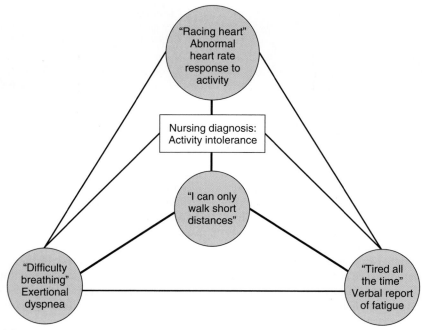

Figure 1.3
Formulating a nursing diagnosis using a concept map.

nursing diagnosis, is intrinsically all about patient-centered care when the nurse engages the client/family as a full partner in the entire process: assessment, nursing diagnosis selection, outcomes, interventions, and evaluation. This competency is about providing care in partnership with the client and family. The client, family, nurse, health care provider, and other health care workers form a team to collaborate with the client and family in every way possible to achieve health.

Client education needs to be centered on the needs of the client, addressing behavior-changing techniques to accomplish the defined goals. At present, too often new health information is given to clients in the form of a lecture, handout, admonishment, or direction where the client is powerless. Conversations need to occur between the client and nurse to understand behavioral changes that can be implemented to achieve goals. Motivational interviewing is a technique based on reinforcement of the client's present thoughts and motivations on behavior change, and based on respect for the client as an individual (Miller & Rollnick, 2013). This technique has been used for almost 30 years and has an extensive research base showing effectiveness by engaging in conversations to empower clients to identify strategies and tools to achieve health care goals. To learn more about motivational interviewing, refer to Appendix C on Evolve.

Addressing the unique cultural needs of clients is another example of patient-centered care. Nurses who are culturally competent base care planning on cultural awareness and assessments, which enables them to identify client values, beliefs, and preferences. Cultural awareness can ensure safe and quality outcomes for all clients by assisting clients to become "safety allies" who can alert professionals to their preferences and deviations from their usual routines (Sherwood & Zomorodi, 2014). This text provides the addition of multicultural interventions that reflect the client's cultural preferences, values, and needs.

Patient-centered care can help nurses change attitudes toward clients, especially when caring for older clients (Pope, 2012). Caring for the retired school teacher who raised four children can be different from just caring for the client woman in Room 234 who has her call light on frequently and is incontinent of urine at too-frequent intervals. Including the client and family in the bedside report and care decisions is key to patient satisfaction and enhances overall quality of care (Flagg, 2015).

Teamwork and Collaboration

Teamwork and collaboration are defined as the ability to "function effectively within nursing and interprofessional teams, fostering open communication, mutual respect, and shared decision-making to achieve quality client care" (QSEN, 2018). Interprofessional collaboration has the potential to shift the attitudes and perceptions of health care providers so there is an increased awareness of each other's roles, values, and disciplinary knowledge (Wilson et al, 2014). The need for collaboration by health care professionals is a reality of contemporary health care practice and is identified within each nursing diagnosis in this text. Many nursing interventions are referrals to other health care personnel to best meet the client's needs; thus collaborative interventions are designated with a triangular symbol ▲.

Evidence-Based Practice

QSEN defines EBP as the integration of best current evidence with clinical expertise and client/family preferences and values for delivery of optimal health care (QSEN, 2018). It is well established that EBP results in higher quality care for clients than care that is based on traditional nursing knowledge (Makic et al, 2014; Buccheri et al, 2017). It is imperative that each nurse and nursing student develops clinical inquiry skills, which means the nurse continually questions whether care is being given in the best way possible based on a review of the quality and strength of the evidence (Buccheri et al, 2017). Basing nursing practice on evidence, inclusive of research and other forms of evidence, is a concept that is incorporated throughout this text. EBP is a systematic process that uses current evidence in making decisions about the care of clients, including evaluation of quality and applicability of existing research, client preferences, clinical expertise, and available health care resources (Melnyk & Fineout-Overholt, 2015). To determine the best way of giving care, the use of EBP is needed. To make this happen, nurses need ready access to the evidence.

This text includes evidence-based rationales whenever possible. An effort is made to provide research-based rationales. The evidence ranges along a continuum from a case study about a single client to a systematic review performed by experts to quality improvement reports that provide information to guide nursing care. Every attempt has been made to supply the most current evidence for the nursing interventions. In Section III, the abbreviation **EBN** is used when interventions have a scientific rationale supported by nursing research. The abbreviation **EB** is used when interventions have a scientific rationale supported by research that has been obtained from disciplines other than nursing. **CEB** is used as a heading for classic research that has not been replicated or is older. It may be either nursing research or research from other disciplines. Many times the **CEB**-labeled research will be the seminal studies that were conducted addressing client concern or nursing care intervention.

When using **EBP,** it is vitally important that the client's concerns and individual situations be taken into consideration. The nurse must always use critical thinking when applying evidence-based guidelines to any particular nursing situation. Each client is unique in his or her needs and capabilities. To improve outcomes, clinicians and clients should collaborate to formulate a treatment plan that incorporates both evidence-based data and client preferences within the context of each client's specific clinical situation (Mackey and Bassendowski, 2017). This text integrates current best evidence and the nursing process, and it assists the nurse in increasing the use of evidence-based interventions in the clinical setting.

Quality Improvement

Quality improvement has been used for many years, with processes in place to ensure that the client receives appropriate care. The QSEN quality improvement competency is defined as the ability of the nurse to use data to monitor the outcomes of care processes and use improvement methods to design and test changes to continuously improve the quality and safety of health care systems (QSEN, 2018). QSEN resources supporting quality improvement initiatives are available at their website http://qsen.org/competencies/quality-improvement-resources-2/. As with EBP, quality improvement initiatives need to critically examine research and other forms of strong evidence in supporting process changes. Research is the basis on which best practice should be supported (Odom-Forren, 2013) Research in addition to other forms of evidence, such as quality improvement studies, provide a growing body of evidence to guide practice.

It is essential for nurses to participate in the work of quality and performance improvement to attain and sustain excellence in nursing care. As nurses are educated about performance and quality measures, they are more likely to value these activities and make quality improvement part of their nursing practice (Nelson, 2014). Although there is potential overlap of work in quality departments and EBP/research departments, the hope is that quality departments collaborate closely with EBP/research departments to improve the practice of nursing. Best evidence should be used to guide nursing practice interventions, and quality improvement critically evaluates and enhances the process of care to ensure effective delivery of high quality, evidence-based care to clients.

Safety

Safety is defined as minimizing risk of harm to clients and providers through both system effectiveness and individual performance (QSEN, 2018). Client safety is a priority when health care is delivered. Nurses are required to adhere to established standards of care as a guideline for providing safe client care. Internal organizational policies and procedures established by health care institutions should be based on the most relevant and current evidence to guide safe practice standards. External standards of care are established by regulatory agencies (e.g., TJC), professional organizations (e.g., the American Nurses Association), and health care organizations. QSEN competencies align well with external agencies guiding safe practice expectations (Lyle-Edrosolo & Waxman, 2016).

Client safety was identified as a priority of care by TJC through the launch of National Patient Safety Goals in 2002. TJC continually reviews and establishes standards for improving client safety that include the need for increased handwashing, better client identification before receiving medications or treatments, and protection of suicidal clients from self-harm. Many of the safety standards have been incorporated into the care plans in this text.

Informatics

QSEN defines informatics as the nurse's ability to use information and technology to communicate, manage knowledge, mitigate error, and support decision-making (QSEN, 2018). The use of information technology is a critical part of the nurse's professional role, and every nurse must be computer literate (Technology Informatics Guiding Education Reform

[TIGER], 2018). Key technology and computer proficiencies for nursing practice should include basic computer system and desktop skills; the ability to search for client information; communication using email; ability to search electronic health care databases; and use of technology for client education, client documentation, and client monitoring (Hubner et al, 2017; TIGER, 2018).

In addition to computer literacy, nurses must also acquire informatic knowledge that addresses client privacy and the security of health care information as it applies to the use of technology (Hubner et al, 2017; TIGER, 2018). Because nurses document on the electronic medical record and use smartphones for access to information on medications, diagnoses, and treatments, there are constant threats to client confidentiality, which needs to be maintained through secure access systems. Nurses also use clinical decision support systems in many facilities that contain order sets tailored for conditions or types of clients. These systems include information vital to nurses and also may provide alerts about potentially dangerous situations when giving client care.

Nurses need access to technology to effectively bring evidence to the client bedside because evidence is constantly evolving. Use of informatics is integral in the use of EBP. As evidence changes, practice should also change. Moving best evidence consistently into practice requires behavior changes by the clinician and system to effectively implement best evidence into practice. Similarly, habits in practice that result in unnecessary care need to be deimplemented. (van Bodegrom-Vos, Dvidoff, & Marang-van de Mheen, 2017). The Choosing Wisely campaign primarily focused on deimplementing unnecessary medical tests or treatments that were found to not provide benefit to patients (Levinson et al, 2015). Similarly, there are interventions that nurses should question because these interventions may not be beneficial for clients. The American Academy of Nursing maintains a list of nursing interventions that should be questioned as to client benefit. Continually reviewing the evidence to implement best practice while deimplementing interventions that are no longer supported by evidence or may no longer be truly necessary requires the nurses to remain actively engaged in EBP as a practice norm (American Academy of Nursing, 2015).

EBP, safety initiatives, informatics, patient-centered care, teamwork, and quality work together in a synergistic manner lead to excellence in nursing care. Quality care needs to be more than safe; the care should result in the best outcome possible for the client. For this to happen, the client should receive care that is based on evidence of the effectiveness of the nursing care interventions.

The nursing process is continually evolving. This text is all about *thinking* for the nurse to help the client in any way possible. Our goal is to present state-of-the art information to help the nurse and nursing student provide the best care possible.

REFERENCES

American Academy of Nursing. (2015). *Choosing wisely: Twenty things nurses and patients should question*. Retrieved from http://www.aannet.org/initiatives/choosing-wisely. (Accessed 17 March 2018).

Benner, P. (2010). *Educating nurses: A call for radical transformation*. San Francisco: Jossey-Bass.

Buccheri, R. K., & Sharifi, C. (2017). Critical appraisal of tools and reporting guidelines for evidence-based practice. *World Views on Evidence-Based Nursing*, 14(6), 463–472.

Butcher, H., Bulechek, G., et al. (2018). *Nursing interventions classification (NIC) e-book* (7th ed.). St Louis: Mosby/Elsevier.

Cappelletti, A., Engel, J. E., & Prentice, D. (2014). Systematic review of clinical judgment and reasoning in nursing. *The Journal of Nursing Education*, 53(8), 453–458.

Centers for Medicare and Medicaid Services. (2018). *Hospital value-based purchasing*. Retrieved from https://www.cms.gov/Medicare/Quality-Initiatives-Patient-Assessment-Instruments/HospitalQualityInits/Hospital-Value-Based-Purchasing-.html. (Accessed 20 March 2018).

Cronenwett, L., Sherwood, G., Barnsteiner, J., et al. (2007). Quality and safety education for nurses. *Nursing Outlook*, 55, 121–131.

Feo, R., et al. (2017). Using holistic interpretive synthesis to create practice-relevant guidance for person-centred fundamental care delivered by nurses. *Nursing Inquiry*, 24(2), 1–11. doi:10.1111/nin.12152.

Flagg, A. J. (2015). The role of patient centered care in nursing. *The Nursing Clinics of North America*, 50(1), 75–86

George, A., Geethakrishnan, R., & D'Souza, P. (2014). Concept mapping. *Holistic Nursing Practice*, 28(1), 43–47.

Herdman, T. H., & Kamitsuru, S. (Eds.). (2018). *NANDA international nursing diagnoses: Definitions & classification (2018–2020)*. New York: Thieme.

Hubner, U., Shaw, T., Thye, J., et al. (2017). *Towards an international framework for recommendations of core competencies in nursing and interprofessional informatics: The TIGER competency synthesis project*. Retrieved from http://www.himss.org/library/towards-international-framework-recommendations-core-competencies-nursing-and-interprofessional. (Accessed 17 March 2018).

Institute of Medicine (IOM). (2003). *Health professions education: a bridge to quality*. Washington, DC: National Academies Press. Retrieved from https://www.ncbi.nlm.nih.gov/books/NBK221528/pdf/Bookshelf_NBK221528.pdf. (Accessed 10 March 2018).

Jamison, T., & Lis, G. A. (2014). Engaging the learning by bridging the gap between theory and clinical competence. *The Nursing Clinics of North America*, 49(1), 69–80.

The Joint Commission. (2018). *2018 National patient safety goals*. Retrieved from https://www.jointcommission.org/standards_information/npsgs.aspx. (Accessed 17 March 2018).

Kaddoura, M., Van-Dyke, O., & Yang, Q. (2016). Impact of a concept map teaching approach on nursing students' critical thinking skills. *Nursing and Health Sciences*, 18(3), 350–354.

Lee, W., Chiang, C. H., Liao, I. C., et al. (2013). The longitudinal effect of concept map teaching on critical thinking of nursing students. *Nurse Education Today*, 33(10), 1219–1223.

Levinson, W., Kallewaard, M., Bhatia, S. R., et al. (2015). Choosing wisely: A growing international campaign. *BMJ Quality and Safety*, 24(12), 167–174.

Lusk, J. M., & Fater, K. (2013). A concept analysis of patient-centered care. *Nursing Forum, 48*(2), 89–98.

Lyle-Edrosolo, G., & Waxman, K. T. (2016). Aligning healthcare safety and quality competencies: Quality and safety education for nurses, the Joint Commissions, and American Nurses Credentialing Center, Magnet Standards Crosswalk. *Nurse Leader, 7*(2), 70–75.

Mackey, A., Bassendowski, S. (2017). The history of evidence-based practice in nursing education and practice. *Journal of Professional Nursing, 33*(1), 51–55.

Makic, M. B., Rauen, C., Watson, R., et al. (2014). Examining the evidence to guide practice: Challenging practice habits. *Critical Care Nurse, 34*(2), 28–45.

Melnyk, B., & Fineout-Overholt, E. (2015). *Evidence-based practice in nursing & healthcare: A guide to best practice* (3rd ed.). Philadelphia: Wolters Kluwer Health.

Miller, W. R., & Rollnick, S. (2013). *Motivational interviewing: Helping people change* (3rd ed.). New York: Guilford Press.

Moorhead, S., Johnson, M., Maas, M. L., et al. (Ed.), (2018). *Nursing outcomes classification (NOC): Measurement of health outcomes* (6th ed.). St Louis: Elsevier.

National Council of State Boards of Nursing. (2016). *NCLEX-RN examination, detailed test plan.* Retrieved from https://www.ncsbn.org/2016_RN_DetTestPlan_Educator.pdf. (Accessed 18 March 2018).

Nelson, A. M. (2014). Best practice in nursing: A concept analysis. *International Journal of Nursing Studies, 51*(11), 1507–1516.

Odom-Forren, J. (2013). Research: The foundation for evidence. *Journal of Perianesthesia Nursing, 28*(6), 331–332.

Pope, T. (2012). How person-centered care can improve nurses' attitudes to hospitalized older patients. *Nursing Older People, 24*(1), 32–36.

Population health implications of the Affordable Care Act: Workshop summary. (2014). Washington, DC: The National Academies Press.

Quality and Safety Education for Nurses (QSEN). (2018). Retrieved from qsen.org/competencies/pre-licensure-ksas/. (Accessed 16 March 2018).

Sherwood, G., & Zomorodi, M. (2014). A new mindset for quality and safety: The QSEN competencies redefine nurses' roles in practice. *Nephrology Nursing Journal: Journal of the American Nephrology Nurses' Association, 41*(1), 15–22, 72.

Sim, J. et al. (2018). Measuring the outcomes of nursing practice: A Delphi study. *Journal of Clinical Nursing, 27*(1–2), e368–e378. doi:10.1111/jocn.13971.

Technology Informatics Guiding Education Reform (TIGER). (2018). *The TIGER initiative: Informatics competencies for every practicing nurse: Recommendations from the TIGER Collaborative.* Retrieved from http://www.himss.org/professionaldevelopment/tiger -initiative. (Accessed 17 March 2018).

Tovino, S. A. (2017). Teaching the HIPAA privacy rule. *Saint Louis University Law Journal, 61*(3), 469–494.

Van Bodegrom-Vos, L., Davidoff, F., & Marang-van de Mheen, P. (2017). Implementation and de-implementation: Two sides of the same coin? *BMJ Quality & Safety, 26*(8), 495–501.

Watson, F., & Rebair, A. (2014). The art of noticing: Essential to nursing practice. *The British Journal of Nursing, 23*(10), 514–517.

Wilson, L., Callender, B., Hall, T. L., et al. (2014). Identifying global health competencies to prepare 21st century global health professionals: Report from the global health competency subcommittee of the consortium of universities for global health. *The Journal of Law, Medicine & Ethics: A Journal of the American Society of Law, Medicine & Ethics, 42*, 26–31.

Guide to
Nursing Diagnosis

Betty J. Ackley, MSN, EdS, RN, Gail B. Ladwig, MSN, RN,

Mary Beth Flynn Makic, PhD, RN, CCNS, FAAN, FNAP,

Marina Martinez-Kratz, MS, RN, CNE, and Melody Zanotti, BA, RN, LSW

Section II is an alphabetical listing of client symptoms, client problems, medical diagnoses, psychosocial diagnoses, and clinical states. Each of these will have a list of possible nursing diagnoses. You may use this section to find suggestions for nursing diagnoses for your client.

- Assess the client using the format provided by the clinical setting.

- Locate the client's symptoms, problems, clinical state, diagnoses, surgeries, and diagnostic testing in the alphabetical listing contained in this section.

- Note suggestions given for appropriate nursing diagnoses.

- Evaluate the suggested nursing diagnoses to determine whether they are appropriate for the client and have information that was found in the assessment.

- Use Section III (which contains an alphabetized list of all NANDA-I approved nursing diagnoses) to validate this information and check the definition, related factors, and defining characteristics. Determine whether the nursing diagnosis you have selected is appropriate for the client.

A

Abdominal Distention

Constipation r/t decreased activity, decreased fluid intake, decreased fiber intake, pathological process

Dysfunctional Gastrointestinal motility r/t decreased perfusion of intestines, medication effect

Nausea r/t irritation of gastrointestinal tract

Imbalanced Nutrition: less than body requirements r/t nausea, vomiting

Acute Pain r/t retention of air, gastrointestinal secretions

Delayed Surgical recovery r/t retention of gas, secretions

Abdominal Hysterectomy

See Hysterectomy

Abdominal Pain

Dysfunctional Gastrointestinal motility r/t decreased perfusion, medication effect

Acute Pain r/t injury, pathological process

Abdominal Surgery

Constipation r/t decreased activity, decreased fluid intake, anesthesia, opioids

Dysfunctional Gastrointestinal motility r/t medication or anesthesia effect, trauma from surgery

Imbalanced Nutrition: less than body requirements r/t high metabolic needs, decreased ability to ingest or digest food

Acute Pain r/t surgical procedure

Ineffective peripheral Tissue Perfusion r/t immobility, abdominal surgery

Risk for delayed Surgical recovery: Risk factor: extensive surgical procedure

Risk for Surgical Site Infection: Risk factor: invasive procedure

Risk for Venous Thromboembolism: Risk factor: immobility, surgery

Readiness for enhanced Knowledge: expresses an interest in learning

See Surgery, Perioperative Care; Surgery, Postoperative Care; Surgery, Preoperative Care

Abdominal Trauma

Disturbed Body Image r/t scarring, change in body function, need for temporary colostomy

Ineffective Breathing pattern r/t abdominal distention, pain

Deficient Fluid volume r/t hemorrhage, active fluid volume loss

Dysfunctional Gastrointestinal motility r/t decreased perfusion

Acute Pain r/t abdominal trauma

Risk for Bleeding: Risk factor: trauma and possible contusion/rupture of abdominal organs

Risk for Infection: Risk factor: possible perforation of abdominal structures

Ablation, Radiofrequency Catheter

Fear r/t invasive procedure

Risk for decreased Cardiac tissue perfusion: Risk factor: catheterization of heart

Abortion, Induced

Compromised family Coping r/t unresolved feelings about decision

Acute Pain r/t surgical intervention

Chronic low Self-Esteem r/t feelings of guilt

Chronic Sorrow r/t loss of potential child

Risk for Bleeding: Risk factor: trauma from abortion

Risk for delayed Development: Risk factors: unplanned or unwanted pregnancy

Risk for Infection: Risk factors: open uterine blood vessels, dilated cervix

Risk for Post-Trauma syndrome: Risk factor: psychological trauma of abortion

Risk for Spiritual distress: Risk factor: perceived moral implications of decision

Readiness for enhanced Health literacy: expresses desire to enhance personal health care decisions

Readiness for enhanced Knowledge: expresses an interest in learning

Abortion, Spontaneous

Disturbed Body Image r/t perceived inability to carry pregnancy, produce child

Disabled family Coping r/t unresolved feelings about loss

Ineffective Coping r/t personal vulnerability

Interrupted Family processes r/t unmet expectations for pregnancy and childbirth

Fear r/t implications for future pregnancies

Grieving r/t loss of fetus

Acute Pain r/t uterine contractions, surgical intervention

Situational low Self-Esteem r/t feelings about loss of fetus

Chronic Sorrow r/t loss of potential child

Risk for Bleeding: Risk factor: trauma from abortion

Risk for Infection: Risk factors: septic or incomplete abortion of products of conception, open uterine blood vessels, dilated cervix

Risk for Post-Trauma syndrome: Risk factor: psychological trauma of abortion

Risk for Spiritual distress: Risk factor: loss of fetus

Readiness for enhanced Knowledge: expresses an interest in learning

Abruptio Placentae <36 Weeks

Anxiety r/t unknown outcome, change in birth plans

Death Anxiety r/t unknown outcome, hemorrhage, or pain

Interrupted Family processes r/t unmet expectations for pregnancy and childbirth

Fear r/t threat to well-being of self and fetus

Impaired Gas exchange: placental r/t decreased uteroplacental area

Acute Pain r/t irritable uterus, hypertonic uterus

Impaired Tissue integrity: maternal r/t possible uterine rupture

Risk for Bleeding: Risk factor: separation of placenta from uterus causing bleeding

Risk for Infection: Risk factor: partial separation of placenta

Risk for disturbed Maternal–Fetal dyad: Risk factors: trauma of process, lack of energy of mother

Risk for Shock: Risk factor: separation of placenta from uterus

Readiness for enhanced Knowledge: expresses an interest in learning

Abscess Formation

Ineffective Protection r/t inadequate nutrition, abnormal blood profile, drug therapy, depressed immune function

Impaired Tissue integrity r/t altered circulation, nutritional deficit or excess

Readiness for enhanced Knowledge: expresses an interest in learning

Abuse, Child

See Child Abuse

Abuse, Spouse, Parent, or Significant Other

Anxiety r/t threat to self-concept, situational crisis of abuse

Caregiver Role Strain r/t chronic illness, self-care deficits, lack of respite care, extent of caregiving required

Impaired verbal Communication r/t psychological barriers of fear

Compromised family Coping r/t abusive patterns

Defensive Coping r/t low self-esteem

Dysfunctional Family processes r/t inadequate coping skills

Insomnia r/t psychological stress

Post-Trauma syndrome r/t history of abuse

Powerlessness r/t lifestyle of helplessness

Chronic low Self-Esteem r/t negative family interactions

Risk for impaired emancipated Decision-Making: Risk factor: inability to verbalize needs and wants

Risk for Female Genital Mutilation: Risk factor: lack of family knowledge about impact of practice on physical health

Risk for self-directed Violence: Risk factor: history of abuse

Accessory Muscle Use (to Breathe)

Ineffective Breathing pattern (See **Breathing** pattern, ineffective, Section III)

See Asthma; Bronchitis; COPD (Chronic Obstructive Pulmonary Disease); Respiratory Infections, Acute Childhood (Croup, Epiglottis, Pertussis, Pneumonia, Respiratory Syncytial Virus)

Accident Prone

Frail Elderly syndrome r/t history of falls

Acute Confusion r/t altered level of consciousness

Ineffective Coping r/t personal vulnerability, situational crises

Ineffective Impulse control (See **Impulse** control, ineffective, Section III)

Risk for Injury: Risk factor: history of accidents

Achalasia

Ineffective Coping r/t chronic disease

Acute Pain r/t stasis of food in esophagus

Impaired Swallowing r/t neuromuscular impairment

Risk for Aspiration: Risk factor: nocturnal regurgitation

Acid-Base Imbalances

Risk for Electrolyte imbalance: Risk factors: renal dysfunction, diarrhea, treatment-related side effects (e.g., medications, drains)

Acidosis, Metabolic

Acute Confusion r/t acid-base imbalance, associated electrolyte imbalance

Impaired Memory r/t effect of metabolic acidosis on brain function

Imbalanced Nutrition: less than body requirements r/t inability to ingest, absorb nutrients

Risk for Electrolyte imbalance: Risk factor: effect of metabolic acidosis on renal function

Risk for Injury: Risk factors: disorientation, weakness, stupor

Risk for decreased Cardiac tissue perfusion: Risk factor: dysrhythmias from hyperkalemia

Risk for Shock: Risk factors: abnormal metabolic state, presence of acid state impairing function, decreased tissue perfusion

Acidosis, Respiratory

Activity intolerance r/t imbalance between oxygen supply and demand

Impaired Gas exchange r/t ventilation-perfusion imbalance

Impaired Memory r/t hypoxia

Risk for decreased Cardiac tissue perfusion: Risk factor: dysrhythmias associated with respiratory acidosis

Acne

Disturbed Body Image r/t biophysical changes associated with skin disorder

Ineffective Health management r/t insufficient knowledge of therapeutic regimen

Impaired Skin integrity r/t hormonal changes (adolescence, menstrual cycle)

Acromegaly

Activity intolerance (See **Activity** intolerance, Section III)

Ineffective Airway clearance r/t airway obstruction by enlarged tongue

Disturbed Body Image r/t changes in body function and appearance

Impaired physical Mobility r/t joint pain

Risk for decreased Cardiac tissue perfusion: Risk factor: increased atherosclerosis from abnormal health status

Risk for unstable blood Glucose level: Risk factor: abnormal physical health status

Sexual dysfunction r/t changes in hormonal secretions

Risk for Overweight: Risk factor: energy expenditure less than energy intake

A

Activity Intolerance, Potential to Develop

Activity intolerance (See **Activity** intolerance, Section III)

Acute Abdominal Pain

Deficient Fluid volume r/t air and fluids trapped in bowel, inability to drink

Acute Pain r/t pathological process

Risk for dysfunctional Gastrointestinal motility: Risk factor: ineffective gastrointestinal tissue perfusion

See Abdominal Pain

Acute Alcohol Intoxication

Ineffective Breathing pattern r/t depression of the respiratory center from excessive alcohol intake

Acute Confusion r/t central nervous system depression

Dysfunctional Family processes r/t abuse of alcohol

Risk for Aspiration: Risk factor: depressed reflexes with acute vomiting

Risk for Infection: Risk factor: impaired immune system from malnutrition associated with chronic excessive alcohol intake

Risk for Injury: Risk factor: chemical (alcohol)

Acute Back Pain

Anxiety r/t situational crisis, back injury

Constipation r/t decreased activity, effect of pain medication

Ineffective Coping r/t situational crisis, back injury

Impaired physical Mobility r/t pain

Acute Pain r/t back injury

Readiness for enhanced Knowledge: expresses an interest in learning

Acute Confusion

See Confusion, Acute

Acute Coronary Syndrome

Decreased Cardiac output r/t cardiac disorder

Risk for decreased Cardiac tissue perfusion (See **Cardiac** tissue perfusion, risk for decreased, Section III)

See Angina; Myocardial Infarction (MI)

Acute Lymphocytic Leukemia (ALL)

See Cancer; Chemotherapy; Child with Chronic Condition; Leukemia

Acute Renal Failure

See Renal Failure

Acute Respiratory Distress Syndrome

See ARDS (Acute Respiratory Distress Syndrome)

Acute Substance Withdrawal Syndrome

Anxiety r/t unknown outcome of withdrawal sequence, physiological effects

Imbalanced Energy Field r/t hyperactivity of energy flow

Impaired Comfort r/t restlessness and agitation

Acute Confusion r/t effects of substance withdrawal

Ineffective Coping r/t situational crisis, withdrawal

Labile Emotional Control r/t lack of control over the progression of withdrawal process

Fear r/t threat to well-being of self

Insomnia r/t physical and psychological effects of substance withdrawal

Imbalanced Nutrition: less than body requirements r/t nausea, anxiety

Powerlessness r/t loss of ability to control withdrawal process

Risk for acute Confusion: Risk factor: possible alteration in level of consciousness

Risk for Injury: Risk factor: alteration in sensory perceptual functioning

Risk for Suicide: Risk factor: psychic pain

Risk for other-directed Violence: Risk factors: poor impulse control, hallucinations

Risk for self-directed Violence: Risk factors: poor impulse control, hallucinations

Adams–Stokes Syndrome

See Dysrhythmia

Addiction

See Alcoholism; Substance Abuse

Addison's Disease

Activity intolerance r/t weakness, fatigue

Disturbed Body Image r/t increased skin pigmentation

Deficient Fluid volume r/t failure of regulatory mechanisms

Imbalanced Nutrition: less than body requirements r/t chronic illness

Risk for Injury: Risk factor: weakness

Readiness for enhanced Knowledge: expresses an interest in learning

Adenoidectomy

Acute Pain r/t surgical incision

Ineffective Airway clearance r/t hesitation or reluctance to cough as a result of pain, fear

Nausea r/t anesthesia effects, drainage from surgery

Acute Pain r/t surgical incision

Risk for Aspiration: Risk factors: postoperative drainage, impaired swallowing

Risk for Bleeding: Risk factor: surgical incision

Risk for deficient Fluid volume: Risk factors: decreased intake as a result of painful swallowing, effects of anesthesia

Risk for Dry Mouth: Risk factor: mouth breathing due to nasal congestion

Risk for imbalanced Nutrition: less than body requirements: Risk factor: reluctance to swallow

Readiness for enhanced Knowledge: expresses an interest in learning

Adhesions, Lysis of

See Abdominal Surgery

Adjustment Disorder

Anxiety r/t inability to cope with psychosocial stressor

Labile Emotional Control r/t emotional disturbance

Risk-prone Health behavior r/t assault to self-esteem

Disturbed personal Identity r/t psychosocial stressor (specific to individual)

Situational low Self-Esteem r/t change in role function

Impaired Social interaction r/t absence of significant others or peers

Adjustment Impairment

Risk-prone Health behavior (See **Health** behavior, risk-prone, Section III)

Adolescent, Pregnant

Anxiety r/t situational and maturational crisis, pregnancy

Disturbed Body Image r/t pregnancy superimposed on developing body

Decisional Conflict: keeping child versus giving up child versus abortion r/t lack of experience with decision-making, interference with decision-making, multiple or divergent sources of information, lack of support system

Disabled family Coping r/t highly ambivalent family relationships, chronically unresolved feelings of guilt, anger, despair

Ineffective Coping r/t situational and maturational crisis, personal vulnerability

Ineffective Denial r/t fear of consequences of pregnancy becoming known

Ineffective adolescent Eating dynamics r/t lack of knowledge of nutritional needs during pregnancy

Interrupted Family processes r/t unmet expectations for adolescent, situational crisis

Fear r/t labor and delivery

Deficient Knowledge r/t pregnancy, infant growth and development, parenting

Imbalanced Nutrition: less than body requirements r/t lack of knowledge of nutritional needs during pregnancy and as growing adolescent

Ineffective Role performance r/t pregnancy

Situational low Self-Esteem r/t feelings of shame and guilt about becoming or being pregnant

Impaired Social interaction r/t self-concept disturbance

Social isolation r/t absence of supportive significant others

Risk for impaired Attachment: Risk factor: anxiety associated with the parent role

Risk for delayed Development: Risk factor: unplanned or unwanted pregnancy

Risk for urge urinary Incontinence: Risk factor: pressure on bladder by growing uterus

Risk for disturbed Maternal–Fetal dyad: Risk factors: immaturity, substance use

Risk for impaired Parenting: Risk factors: adolescent parent, unplanned or unwanted pregnancy, single parent

Readiness for enhanced Childbearing process: reports appropriate prenatal lifestyle

Readiness for enhanced Health literacy: expresses desire to enhance social support for health

Readiness for enhanced Knowledge: expresses an interest in learning

Adoption, Giving Child Up for

Decisional Conflict r/t unclear personal values or beliefs, perceived threat to value system, support system deficit

Ineffective Coping r/t stress of loss of child

Interrupted Family processes r/t conflict within family regarding relinquishment of child

Grieving r/t loss of child, loss of role of parent

Insomnia r/t depression or trauma of relinquishment of child

Social isolation r/t making choice that goes against values of significant others

Chronic Sorrow r/t loss of relationship with child

Risk for Spiritual distress: Risk factor: perceived moral implications of decision

Readiness for enhanced Spiritual well-being: harmony with self-regarding final decision

Adrenocortical Insufficiency

Deficient Fluid volume r/t insufficient ability to reabsorb water

Ineffective Protection r/t inability to tolerate stress

Delayed Surgical recovery r/t inability to respond to stress

Risk for Shock: Risk factors: deficient fluid volume, decreased cortisol to initiate stress response to insult to body

See Addison's Disease; Shock, Hypovolemic

Advance Directives

Death Anxiety r/t planning for end-of-life health decisions

Decisional Conflict r/t unclear personal values or beliefs, perceived threat to value system, support system deficit

Grieving r/t possible loss of self, significant other

Readiness for enhanced Spiritual well-being: harmonious interconnectedness with self, others, higher power, God

Affective Disorders

See Depression (Major Depressive Disorder); Dysthymic Disorder; Manic Disorder, Bipolar I; SAD (Seasonal Affective Disorder)

Age-Related Macular Degeneration

See Macular Degeneration

Aggressive Behavior

Fear r/t real or imagined threat to own well-being

Risk for other-directed Violence (See **Violence**, other-directed, risk for, Section III)

Aging

Death Anxiety r/t fear of unknown, loss of self, impact on significant others

Impaired Dentition r/t ineffective oral hygiene

Risk for Frail Elderly syndrome: Risk factors: >70 years, activity intolerance, impaired vision

Grieving r/t multiple losses, impending death

A

Ineffective Health maintenance r/t powerlessness

Hearing Loss r/t exposure to loud noises, aging

Functional urinary Incontinence r/t impaired vision, impaired cognition, neuromuscular limitations, altered environmental factors

Impaired Resilience r/t aging, multiple losses

Sleep deprivation r/t aging-related sleep-stage shifts

Risk for Caregiver Role Strain: Risk factor: inability to handle increasing needs of significant other

Risk for Impaired emancipated Decision-Making: Risk factor: inability to process information regarding health care decisions

Risk for Injury: Risk factors: vision loss, hearing loss, decreased balance, decreased sensation in feet

Risk for Loneliness: Risk factors: inadequate support system, role transition, health alterations, depression, fatigue

Risk for Ineffective Thermoregulation: Risk factor: aging

Readiness for enhanced community Coping: providing social support and other resources identified as needed for elderly client

Readiness for enhanced family Coping: ability to gratify needs, address adaptive tasks

Readiness for enhanced Health management: knowledge about medication, nutrition, exercise, coping strategies

Readiness for enhanced Knowledge: specify need to improve health

Readiness for enhanced Nutrition: need to improve health

Readiness for enhanced Relationship: demonstrates understanding of partner's insufficient function

Readiness for enhanced Sleep: need to improve sleep

Readiness for enhanced Spiritual well-being: one's experience of life's meaning, harmony with self, others, higher power, God, environment

Agitation

Acute Confusion r/t side effects of medication, hypoxia, decreased cerebral perfusion, alcohol abuse or withdrawal, substance abuse or withdrawal, sensory deprivation or overload

Sleep deprivation r/t sustained inadequate sleep hygiene, sundown syndrome

Agoraphobia

Anxiety r/t real or perceived threat to physical integrity

Ineffective Coping r/t inadequate support systems

Fear r/t leaving home, going out in public places

Impaired Social interaction r/t disturbance in self-concept

Social isolation r/t altered thought process

Agranulocytosis

Delayed Surgical recovery r/t abnormal blood profile

Risk for Infection: Risk factor: abnormal blood profile

Readiness for enhanced Knowledge: expresses an interest in learning

AIDS (Acquired Immunodeficiency Syndrome)

Death Anxiety r/t fear of premature death

Disturbed Body Image r/t chronic contagious illness, cachexia

Caregiver Role Strain r/t unpredictable illness course, presence of situation stressors

Diarrhea r/t inflammatory bowel changes

Interrupted Family processes r/t distress about diagnosis of human immunodeficiency virus (HIV) infection

Fatigue r/t disease process, stress, decreased nutritional intake

Fear r/t powerlessness, threat to well-being

Grieving: family/parental r/t potential or impending death of loved one

Grieving: individual r/t loss of physical and psychosocial well-being

Hopelessness r/t deteriorating physical condition

Imbalanced Nutrition: less than body requirements r/t decreased ability to eat and absorb nutrients as a result of anorexia, nausea, diarrhea; oral candidiasis

Chronic Pain r/t tissue inflammation and destruction

Impaired Resilience r/t chronic illness

Situational low Self-Esteem r/t crisis of chronic contagious illness

Ineffective Sexuality pattern r/t possible transmission of disease

Social isolation r/t self-concept disturbance, therapeutic isolation

Chronic Sorrow r/t chronic illness

Spiritual distress r/t challenged beliefs or moral system

Risk for deficient Fluid volume: Risk factors: diarrhea, vomiting, fever, bleeding

Risk for Infection: Risk factor: inadequate immune system

Risk for Loneliness: Risk factor: social isolation

Risk for impaired Oral Mucous Membrane integrity: Risk factor: immunological deficit

Risk for impaired Skin integrity: Risk factors: immunological deficit, diarrhea

Risk for Spiritual distress: Risk factor: physical illness

Readiness for enhanced Health literacy: expresses desire to enhance understanding of health information to make health care choices

Readiness for enhanced Knowledge: expresses an interest in learning

See AIDS, Child; Cancer; Pneumonia

AIDS, Child

Impaired Parenting r/t congenital acquisition of infection secondary to intravenous (IV) drug use, multiple sexual partners, history of contaminated blood transfusion

See AIDS (Acquired Immunodeficiency Syndrome); Child with Chronic Condition; Hospitalized Child; Terminally Ill Child, Adolescent; Terminally Ill Child, Infant/Toddler; Terminally Ill Child, Preschool Child; Terminally Ill Child, School-Age Child/Preadolescent; Terminally Ill Child/Death of Child, Parent

AIDS Dementia

Chronic Confusion r/t viral invasion of nervous system

See Dementia

Airway Obstruction/Secretions

Ineffective Airway clearance (See **Airway** clearance, ineffective, Section III)

Alcohol Withdrawal

Anxiety r/t situational crisis, withdrawal

Acute Confusion r/t effects of alcohol withdrawal

Ineffective Coping r/t personal vulnerability

Dysfunctional Family processes r/t abuse of alcohol

Insomnia r/t effect of alcohol withdrawal, anxiety

Imbalanced Nutrition: less than body requirements r/t poor dietary habits

Chronic low Self-Esteem r/t repeated unmet expectations

Acute Substance Withdrawal syndrome: Risk factor: developed dependence to alcohol

Risk for deficient Fluid volume: Risk factors: excessive diaphoresis, agitation, decreased fluid intake

Risk for other-directed Violence: Risk factor: substance withdrawal

Risk for self-directed Violence: Risk factor: substance withdrawal

Readiness for enhanced Knowledge: expresses an interest in learning

Alcoholism

Anxiety r/t loss of control

Risk-prone Health behavior r/t lack of motivation to change behaviors, addiction

Acute Confusion r/t alcohol abuse

Chronic Confusion r/t neurological effects of chronic alcohol intake

Defensive Coping r/t denial of reality of addiction

Disabled family Coping r/t codependency issues due to alcoholism

Ineffective Coping r/t use of alcohol to cope with life events

Labile Emotional Control r/t substance abuse

Ineffective Denial r/t refusal to acknowledge addiction

Dysfunctional Family processes r/t alcohol abuse

Impaired Home maintenance r/t memory deficits, fatigue

Insomnia r/t irritability, nightmares, tremors

Impaired Memory r/t alcohol abuse

Self-Neglect r/t effects of alcohol abuse

Imbalanced Nutrition: less than body requirements r/t anorexia, inappropriate diet with increased carbohydrates

Powerlessness r/t alcohol addiction

Ineffective Protection r/t malnutrition, sleep deprivation

Chronic low Self-Esteem r/t failure at life events

Social isolation r/t unacceptable social behavior, values

Acute Substance Withdrawal syndrome: Risk factor: developed dependence to alcohol

Risk for Injury: Risk factor: alteration in sensory or perceptual function

Risk for Loneliness: Risk factor: unacceptable social behavior

Risk for Acute Substance Withdrawal syndrome: Risk factor: developed dependence to alcohol

Risk for other-directed Violence: Risk factors: reactions to substances used, impulsive behavior, disorientation, impaired judgment

Risk for self-directed Violence: Risk factors: reactions to substances used, impulsive behavior, disorientation, impaired judgment

Alcoholism, Dysfunctional Family Processes

Dysfunctional Family processes (See **Family** processes, dysfunctional, Section III)

Alkalosis

See Metabolic Alkalosis

ALL (Acute Lymphocytic Leukemia)

See Cancer; Chemotherapy; Child with Chronic Condition; Leukemia

Allergies

Latex Allergic reaction r/t hypersensitivity to natural rubber latex

Risk for Allergic reaction: Risk factors: chemical factors, dander, environmental substances, foods, insect stings, medications

Risk for Latex Allergic reaction: Risk factor: repeated exposure to products containing latex

Readiness for enhanced Knowledge: expresses an interest in learning

Alopecia

Disturbed Body Image r/t loss of hair, change in appearance

Readiness for enhanced Knowledge: expresses an interest in learning

ALS (Amyotrophic Lateral Sclerosis)

See Amyotrophic Lateral Sclerosis (ALS)

Altered Mental Status

See Confusion, Acute; Confusion, Chronic; Memory Deficit

Alzheimer's Disease

Caregiver role strain r/t duration and extent of caregiving required

Chronic Confusion r/t loss of cognitive function

Compromised family Coping r/t interrupted family processes

Frail Elderly syndrome r/t alteration in cognitive functioning

Impaired Home maintenance r/t impaired cognitive function, inadequate support systems

Hopelessness r/t deteriorating condition

Insomnia r/t neurological impairment, daytime naps

Impaired Memory r/t neurological disturbance

Impaired physical Mobility r/t severe neurological dysfunction

Self-Neglect r/t loss of cognitive function

Powerlessness r/t deteriorating condition

Self-Care deficit: specify r/t loss of cognitive function, psychological impairment

Social isolation r/t fear of disclosure of memory loss

Wandering r/t cognitive impairment, frustration, physiological state

Risk for chronic functional Constipation: Risk factor: impaired cognitive functioning

Risk for Injury: Risk factor: confusion

A

Risk for Loneliness: Risk factor: potential social isolation

Risk for Relocation stress syndrome: Risk factors: impaired psychosocial health, decreased health status

Risk for other-directed Violence: Risk factors: frustration, fear, anger, loss of cognitive function

Readiness for enhanced Knowledge: Caregiver: expresses an interest in learning

See Dementia

AMD (Age-Related Macular Degeneration)

See Macular Degeneration

Amenorrhea

Imbalanced Nutrition: less than body requirements r/t inadequate food intake

See Sexuality, Adolescent

AMI (Acute Myocardial Infarction)

See MI (Myocardial Infarction)

Amnesia

Acute Confusion r/t alcohol abuse, delirium, dementia, drug abuse

Dysfunctional Family processes r/t alcohol abuse, inadequate coping skills

Impaired Memory r/t excessive environmental disturbance, neurological disturbance

Post-Trauma syndrome r/t history of abuse, catastrophic illness, disaster, accident

Amniocentesis

Anxiety r/t threat to self and fetus, unknown future

Decisional Conflict r/t choice of treatment pending results of test

Risk for Infection: Risk factor: invasive procedure

Amnionitis

See Chorioamnionitis

Amniotic Membrane Rupture

See Premature Rupture of Membranes

Amputation

Disturbed Body Image r/t negative effects of amputation, response from others

Grieving r/t loss of body part, future lifestyle changes

Impaired physical Mobility r/t musculoskeletal impairment, limited movement

Acute Pain r/t surgery, phantom limb sensation

Chronic Pain r/t surgery, phantom limb sensation

Ineffective peripheral Tissue Perfusion r/t impaired arterial circulation

Impaired Skin integrity r/t poor healing, prosthesis rubbing

Risk for Bleeding: Risk factor: vulnerable surgical site

Risk for Impaired Tissue integrity: Risk factor: mechanical factors impacting site

Readiness for enhanced Knowledge: expresses an interest in learning

Amyotrophic Lateral Sclerosis (ALS)

Death Anxiety r/t impending progressive loss of function leading to death

Ineffective Breathing pattern r/t compromised muscles of respiration

Impaired verbal Communication r/t weakness of muscles of speech, deficient knowledge of ways to compensate and alternative communication devices

Decisional Conflict: ventilator therapy r/t unclear personal values or beliefs, lack of relevant information

Impaired Resilience r/t perceived vulnerability

Chronic Sorrow r/t chronic illness

Impaired Swallowing r/t weakness of muscles involved in swallowing

Impaired spontaneous Ventilation r/t weakness of muscles of respiration

Risk for Aspiration: Risk factor: impaired swallowing

Risk for Spiritual distress: Risk factor: chronic debilitating condition

See Neurological Disorders

Anal Fistula

See Hemorrhoidectomy

Anaphylactic Shock

Deficient Fluid volume r/t compromised regulatory mechanism

Ineffective Airway clearance r/t laryngeal edema, bronchospasm

Latex Allergic reaction r/t abnormal immune mechanism response

Impaired spontaneous Ventilation r/t acute airway obstruction from anaphylaxis process

Anaphylaxis Prevention

Risk for Allergic reaction (See **Allergic reaction**, risk for, Section III)

Anasarca

Excess Fluid volume r/t excessive fluid intake, cardiac/renal dysfunction, loss of plasma proteins

Risk for decreased Cardiac Output: Risk factor: imbalanced fluid volume

Risk for impaired Skin integrity: Risk factor: impaired circulation to skin from edema

Anemia

Anxiety r/t cause of disease

Impaired Comfort r/t feelings of always being cold from decreased hemoglobin and decreased metabolism

Fatigue r/t decreased oxygen supply to the body, increased cardiac workload

Impaired Memory r/t change in cognition from decreased oxygen supply to the body

Delayed Surgical recovery r/t decreased oxygen supply to body, increased cardiac workload

Risk for Bleeding (See **Bleeding,** risk for, Section III)

Risk for Injury: Risk factor: alteration in peripheral sensory perception

Readiness for enhanced Knowledge: expresses an interest in learning

Anemia, in Pregnancy

Anxiety r/t concerns about health of self and fetus

Fatigue r/t decreased oxygen supply to the body, increased cardiac workload

Risk for delayed Development: Risk factor: reduction in the oxygen-carrying capacity of blood

Risk for Infection: Risk factor: reduction in oxygen-carrying capacity of blood

Risk for disturbed Maternal–Fetal dyad: Risk factor: compromised oxygen transport

Readiness for enhanced Knowledge: expresses an interest in learning

Anemia, Sickle Cell

See Anemia; Sickle Cell Anemia/Crisis

Anencephaly

See Neural Tube Defects (Meningocele, myelomeningocele, Spina Bifida, Anencephaly)

Aneurysm, Abdominal Aortic Repair Surgery

Risk for deficient Fluid volume: Risk factor: hemorrhage r/t potential abnormal blood loss

Risk for Surgical Site Infection: Risk factor: invasive procedure

See Abdominal Surgery

Aneurysm, Cerebral

See Craniectomy/Craniotomy; Subarachnoid Hemorrhage

Anger

Anxiety r/t situational crisis

Defensive Coping r/t inability to acknowledge responsibility for actions and results of actions

Labile Emotional Control r/t stressors

Fear r/t environmental stressor, hospitalization

Grieving r/t significant loss

Risk-prone Health behavior r/t assault to self-esteem, disability requiring change in lifestyle, inadequate support system

Powerlessness r/t health care environment

Risk for compromised Human Dignity: Risk factors: inadequate participation in decision-making, perceived dehumanizing treatment, perceived humiliation, exposure of the body, cultural incongruity

Risk for Post-Trauma syndrome: Risk factor: inadequate social support

Risk for other-directed Violence: Risk factors: history of violence, rage reaction

Risk for self-directed Violence: Risk factors: history of violence, history of abuse, rage reaction

Angina

Activity intolerance r/t acute pain, dysrhythmias

Anxiety r/t situational crisis

Decreased Cardiac output r/t myocardial ischemia, medication effect, dysrhythmia

Ineffective Coping r/t personal vulnerability to situational crisis of new diagnosis, deteriorating health

Ineffective Denial r/t deficient knowledge of need to seek help with symptoms

Grieving r/t pain, loss of health

Acute Pain r/t myocardial ischemia

Ineffective Sexuality pattern r/t disease process, medications, loss of libido

Readiness for enhanced Knowledge: expresses an interest in learning

See MI (Myocardial Infarction)

Angiocardiography (Cardiac Catheterization)

See Cardiac Catheterization

Angioplasty, Coronary

Fear r/t possible outcome of interventional procedure

Ineffective peripheral Tissue Perfusion r/t vasospasm, hematoma formation

Risk for Bleeding: Risk factors: possible damage to coronary artery, hematoma formation

Risk for decreased Cardiac tissue perfusion: Risk factors: ventricular ischemia, dysrhythmias

Readiness for enhanced Knowledge: expresses an interest in learning

Anomaly, Fetal/Newborn (Parent Dealing with)

Anxiety r/t threat to role functioning, situational crisis

Decisional Conflict: interventions for fetus or newborn r/t lack of relevant information, spiritual distress, threat to value system

Disabled family Coping r/t chronically unresolved feelings about loss of perfect baby

Ineffective Coping r/t personal vulnerability in situational crisis

Interrupted Family processes r/t unmet expectations for perfect baby, lack of adequate support systems

Fear r/t real or imagined threat to baby, implications for future pregnancies, powerlessness

Grieving r/t loss of ideal child

Hopelessness r/t long-term stress, deteriorating physical condition of child, lost spiritual belief

Deficient Knowledge r/t limited exposure to situation

Impaired Parenting r/t interruption of bonding process

Powerlessness r/t complication threatening fetus or newborn

Parental Role conflict r/t separation from newborn, intimidation with invasive or restrictive modalities, specialized care center policies

Situational low Self-Esteem r/t perceived inability to produce a perfect child

Social isolation r/t alterations in child's physical appearance, altered state of wellness

Chronic Sorrow r/t loss of ideal child, inadequate bereavement support

Spiritual distress r/t test of spiritual beliefs

Risk for impaired Attachment: Risk factor: ill infant unable to effectively initiate parental contact as result of altered behavioral organization

Risk for disorganized Infant behavior: Risk factor: congenital disorder

Risk for impaired Parenting: Risk factors: interruption of bonding process; unrealistic expectations for self, infant, or partner; perceived threat to own emotional survival; severe stress; lack of knowledge

Risk for Spiritual distress: Risk factor: lack of normal child to raise and carry on family name

Anorectal Abscess

Disturbed Body Image r/t odor and drainage from rectal area

Acute Pain r/t inflammation of perirectal area

Risk for Constipation: Risk factor: fear of painful elimination

Readiness for enhanced Knowledge: expresses an interest in learning

Anorexia

Deficient Fluid volume r/t inability to drink

Imbalanced Nutrition: less than body requirements r/t loss of appetite, nausea, vomiting, laxative abuse

Delayed Surgical recovery r/t inadequate nutritional intake

Risk for delayed Surgical recovery: Risk factor: inadequate nutritional intake

Anorexia Nervosa

Activity intolerance r/t fatigue, weakness

Disturbed Body Image r/t misconception of actual body appearance

Constipation r/t lack of adequate food, fiber, and fluid intake

Defensive Coping r/t psychological impairment, eating disorder

Disabled family Coping r/t highly ambivalent family relationships

Ineffective Denial r/t fear of consequences of therapy, possible weight gain

Diarrhea r/t laxative abuse

Interrupted Family processes r/t situational crisis

Ineffective adolescent Eating dynamics r/t food refusal

Ineffective family Health management r/t family conflict, excessive demands on family associated with complexity of condition and treatment

Imbalanced Nutrition: less than body requirements r/t inadequate food intake, excessive exercise

Chronic low Self-Esteem r/t repeated unmet expectations

Ineffective Sexuality pattern r/t loss of libido from malnutrition

Risk for Infection: Risk factor: malnutrition resulting in depressed immune system

Risk for Spiritual distress: Risk factor: low self-esteem

See Maturational Issues, Adolescent

Anosmia (Smell, Loss of Ability to)

Imbalanced Nutrition: less than body requirements r/t loss of appetite associated with loss of smell

Antepartum Period

See Pregnancy, Normal; Prenatal Care, Normal

Anterior Repair, Anterior Colporrhaphy

Urinary Retention r/t edema of urinary structures

Risk for urge urinary Incontinence: Risk factor: trauma to bladder

Readiness for enhanced Knowledge: expresses an interest in learning

See Vaginal Hysterectomy

Anticoagulant Therapy

Risk for Bleeding: Risk factor: altered clotting function from anticoagulant

Risk for deficient Fluid volume: hemorrhage: Risk factor: altered clotting mechanism

Readiness for enhanced Knowledge: expresses an interest in learning

Antisocial Personality Disorder

Defensive Coping r/t excessive use of projection

Ineffective Coping r/t frequently violating the norms and rules of society

Labile Emotional Control r/t psychiatric disorder

Hopelessness r/t abandonment

Impaired Social interaction r/t sociocultural conflict, chemical dependence, inability to form relationships

Spiritual distress r/t separation from religious or cultural ties

Ineffective Health management r/t excessive demands on family

Risk for Loneliness: Risk factor: inability to interact appropriately with others

Risk for impaired Parenting: Risk factors: inability to function as parent or guardian, emotional instability

Risk for Self-Mutilation: Risk factors: self-hatred, depersonalization

Risk for other-directed Violence: Risk factor: history of violence, altered thought patterns

Anuria

See Renal Failurec

Anxiety

See **Anxiety**, Section III

Anxiety Disorder

Ineffective Activity planning r/t unrealistic perception of events

Anxiety r/t unmet security and safety needs

Death Anxiety r/t fears of unknown, powerlessness

Decisional Conflict r/t low self-esteem, fear of making a mistake

Defensive Coping r/t overwhelming feelings of dread

Disabled family Coping r/t ritualistic behavior, actions

Imbalanced Energy Field r/t feelings of restlessness and apprehension

Impaired Mood Regulation r/t functional impairment, impaired social functioning, alteration in sleep pattern

Ineffective Coping r/t inability to express feelings appropriately

Ineffective Denial r/t overwhelming feelings of hopelessness, fear, threat to self

Insomnia r/t psychological impairment, emotional instability

Labile Emotional Control r/t emotional instability

Powerlessness r/t lifestyle of helplessness

Self-Care deficit r/t ritualistic behavior, activities

Sleep deprivation r/t prolonged psychological discomfort

Risk for Spiritual distress: Risk factor: psychological distress

Readiness for enhanced Knowledge: expresses an interest in learning

Aortic Valvular Stenosis

See Congenital Heart Disease/Cardiac Anomalies

Aphasia

Anxiety r/t situational crisis of aphasia

Impaired verbal Communication r/t decrease in circulation to brain

Ineffective Coping r/t loss of speech

Ineffective Health maintenance r/t deficient knowledge regarding information on aphasia and alternative communication techniques

Aplastic Anemia

Activity intolerance r/t imbalance between oxygen supply and demand

Fear r/t ability to live with serious disease

Risk for Bleeding: Risk factor: inadequate clotting factors

Risk for Infection: Risk factor: inadequate immune function

Readiness for enhanced Knowledge: expresses an interest in learning

Apnea in Infancy

See Premature Infant (Child); Premature Infant (Parent); SIDS (Sudden Infant Death)

Apneustic Respirations

Ineffective Breathing pattern r/t perception or cognitive impairment, neurological impairment

Appendectomy

Deficient Fluid volume r/t fluid restriction, hypermetabolic state, nausea, vomiting

Acute Pain r/t surgical incision

Delayed Surgical recovery r/t rupture of appendix

Risk for Infection: Risk factors: perforation or rupture of appendix, peritonitis

Risk for Surgical Site Infection: Risk factor: surgical incision

Readiness for enhanced Knowledge: expresses an interest in learning

See Hospitalized Child; Surgery, Postoperative Care

Appendicitis

Deficient Fluid volume r/t anorexia, nausea, vomiting

Acute Pain r/t inflammation

Risk for Infection: Risk factor: possible perforation of appendix

Readiness for enhanced Knowledge: expresses an interest in learning

Apprehension

Anxiety r/t threat to self-concept, threat to health status, situational crisis

Death Anxiety r/t apprehension over loss of self, consequences to significant others

ARDS (Acute Respiratory Distress Syndrome)

Ineffective Airway clearance r/t excessive tracheobronchial secretions

Death Anxiety r/t seriousness of physical disease

Impaired Gas exchange r/t damage to alveolar capillary membrane, change in lung compliance

Impaired spontaneous Ventilation r/t damage to alveolar capillary membrane

See Ventilated Client, Mechanically

Arrhythmia

See Dysrhythmia

Arterial Insufficiency

Ineffective peripheral Tissue Perfusion r/t interruption of arterial flow

Delayed Surgical recovery r/t ineffective tissue perfusion

Arthritis

Activity intolerance r/t chronic pain, fatigue, weakness

Disturbed Body Image r/t ineffective coping with joint abnormalities

Impaired physical Mobility r/t joint impairment

Chronic Pain r/t progression of joint deterioration

Self-Care deficit: specify r/t pain with movement, damage to joints

Readiness for enhanced Knowledge: expresses an interest in learning

See JRA (Juvenile Rheumatoid Arthritis)

Arthrocentesis

Acute Pain r/t invasive procedure

Arthroplasty (Total Hip Replacement)

See Total Joint Replacement (Total Hip/Total Knee/Shoulder); Surgery, Perioperative Care; Surgery, Postoperative Care; Surgery, Preoperative Care

Arthroscopy

Impaired physical Mobility r/t surgical trauma of knee

Readiness for enhanced Knowledge: expresses an interest in learning

Ascites

Ineffective Breathing pattern r/t increased abdominal girth

Imbalanced Nutrition: less than body requirements r/t loss of appetite

A

Chronic Pain r/t altered body function

Readiness for enhanced Knowledge: expresses an interest in learning

See Ascites; Cancer; Cirrhosis

Asperger's Syndrome

Ineffective Relationship r/t poor communication skills, lack of empathy

See Autism

Asphyxia, Birth

Ineffective Breathing pattern r/t depression of breathing reflex secondary to anoxia

Ineffective Coping r/t uncertainty of child outcome

Fear (parental) r/t concern over safety of infant

Impaired Gas exchange r/t poor placental perfusion, lack of initiation of breathing by newborn

Grieving r/t loss of perfect child, concern of loss of future abilities

Impaired spontaneous Ventilation r/t brain injury

Risk for impaired Attachment: Risk factors: ill infant who is unable to initiate parental contact, hospitalization in critical care environment

Risk for delayed Development: Risk factor: lack of oxygen to brain

Risk for disorganized Infant behavior: Risk factor: lack of oxygen to brain

Risk for Injury: Risk factor: lack of oxygen to brain

Risk for ineffective Cerebral tissue perfusion: Risk factor: poor placental perfusion or cord compression resulting in lack of oxygen to brain

Aspiration, Danger of

Risk for Aspiration (See **Aspiration,** risk for, Section III)

Assault Victim

Post-Trauma syndrome r/t assault

Rape-Trauma syndrome r/t rape

Impaired Resilience r/t frightening experience, post-trauma stress response

Risk for Post-Trauma syndrome: Risk factors: perception of event, inadequate social support, unsupportive environment, diminished ego strength, duration of event

Risk for Spiritual distress: Risk factors: physical, psychological stress

Assaultive Client

Risk for Injury: Risk factors: confused thought process, impaired judgment

Risk for other-directed Violence: Risk factors: paranoid ideation, anger

Asthma

Activity intolerance r/t fatigue, energy shift to meet muscle needs for breathing to overcome airway obstruction

Ineffective Airway clearance r/t tracheobronchial narrowing, excessive secretions

Anxiety r/t inability to breathe effectively, fear of suffocation

Disturbed Body Image r/t decreased participation in physical activities

Ineffective Breathing pattern r/t anxiety

Ineffective Coping r/t personal vulnerability to situational crisis

Ineffective Health management (See **Health** management, ineffective, in Section III)

Impaired Home maintenance r/t deficient knowledge regarding control of environmental triggers

Sleep deprivation r/t ineffective breathing pattern, cough

Readiness for enhanced Health management (See **Health** management, readiness for enhanced, in Section III)

Readiness for enhanced Knowledge: expresses an interest in learning

See Child with Chronic Condition; Hospitalized Child

Ataxia

Anxiety r/t change in health status

Disturbed Body Image r/t staggering gait

Impaired physical Mobility r/t neuromuscular impairment

Risk for Falls: Risk factors: gait alteration, instability

Atelectasis

Ineffective Breathing pattern r/t loss of functional lung tissue, depression of respiratory function or hypoventilation because of pain

Impaired Gas exchange r/t decreased alveolar-capillary surface

Anxiety r/t alteration in respiratory pattern

See Atelectasis

Atherosclerosis

See MI (Myocardial Infarction); CVA (Cerebrovascular Accident); Peripheral Vascular Disease (PVD)

Athlete's Foot

Impaired Skin integrity r/t effects of fungal agent

Readiness for enhanced Knowledge: expresses an interest in learning

See Pruritus

ATN (Acute Tubular Necrosis)

See Renal Failure

Atrial Fibrillation

See Dysrhythmia

Atrial Septal Defect

See Congenital Heart Disease/Cardiac Anomalies

Attention Deficit Disorder

Risk-prone Health behavior r/t intense emotional state

Disabled family Coping r/t significant person with chronically unexpressed feelings of guilt, anxiety, hostility, and despair

Ineffective Impulse control r/t (See **Impulse** control, ineffective, Section III)

Chronic low Self-Esteem r/t difficulty in participating in expected activities, poor school performance

Social isolation r/t unacceptable social behavior

Risk for delayed Development: Risk factor: behavior disorders

Risk for Falls: Risk factor: rapid non-thinking behavior

Risk for Loneliness: Risk factor: social isolation

Risk for impaired Parenting: Risk factor: lack of knowledge of factors contributing to child's behavior

Risk for Spiritual distress: Risk factor: poor relationships

Autism

Impaired verbal Communication r/t speech and language delays

Compromised family Coping r/t parental guilt over etiology of disease, inability to accept or adapt to child's condition, inability to help child and other family members seek treatment

Disturbed personal Identity r/t inability to distinguish between self and environment, inability to identify own body as separate from those of other people, inability to integrate concept of self

Self-Neglect r/t impaired socialization

Impaired Social interaction r/t communication barriers, inability to relate to others, failure to develop peer relationships

Risk for delayed Development: Risk factor: autism

Risk for Loneliness: Risk factor: difficulty developing relationships with other people

Risk for Self-Mutilation: Risk factor: autistic state

Risk for other-directed Violence: Risk factors: frequent destructive rages toward others secondary to extreme response to changes in routine, fear of harmless things

Risk for self-directed Violence: Risk factors: frequent destructive rages toward self, secondary to extreme response to changes in routine, fear of harmless things

See Child with Chronic Condition

Autonomic Dysreflexia

Autonomic Dysreflexia r/t bladder distention, bowel distention, noxious stimuli

Risk for Autonomic Dysreflexia: Risk factors: bladder distention, bowel distention, noxious stimuli

Autonomic Hyperreflexia

See Autonomic Dysreflexia

B

Baby Care

Readiness for enhanced Childbearing process: demonstrates appropriate feeding and baby care techniques, along with attachment to infant and providing a safe environment

Anxiety r/t situational crisis, back injury

Ineffective Coping r/t situational crisis, back injury

Impaired physical Mobility r/t pain

Acute Pain r/t back injury

Chronic Pain r/t back injury

Risk for Constipation: Risk factors: decreased activity, side effect of pain medication

Risk for Disuse syndrome: Risk factor: severe pain

Readiness for enhanced Knowledge: expresses an interest in learning

Bacteremia

Risk for Infection: Risk factor: compromised immune system

Risk for Shock: Risk factor: development of systemic inflammatory response from presence of bacteria in bloodstream

Balanced Energy Field

Imbalanced Energy Field (See **Energy Field**, imbalanced, Section III)

Barrel Chest

See Aging (if appropriate); COPD (Chronic Obstructive Pulmonary Disease)

Bathing/Hygiene Problems

Impaired Mobility r/t chronic physically limiting condition

Self-Neglect (See **Self-Neglect**, Section III)

Bathing Self-Care deficit (See **Self-Care** deficit, bathing, Section III)

Battered Child Syndrome

Dysfunctional Family processes r/t inadequate coping skills

Sleep deprivation r/t prolonged psychological discomfort

Chronic Sorrow r/t situational crises

Risk for Post-Trauma syndrome: Risk factors: physical abuse, incest, rape, molestation

Risk for Self-Mutilation: Risk factors: feelings of rejection, dysfunctional family

Risk for Suicide: Risk factor: childhood abuse

See Child Abuse

Battered Person

See Abuse, Spouse, Parent, or Significant Other

Bedbugs, Infestation

Impaired Home maintenance r/t deficient knowledge regarding prevention of bedbug infestation

Impaired Skin integrity r/t bites of bedbugs

See Pruritus

Bed Mobility, Impaired

Impaired bed Mobility (See **Mobility**, bed, impaired, Section III)

Bed Rest, Prolonged

Decreased Diversional activity engagement r/t prolonged bed rest

Impaired bed Mobility r/t neuromuscular impairment

Social isolation r/t prolonged bed rest

Risk for chronic functional Constipation: Risk factor: insufficient physical activity

Risk for Disuse syndrome: Risk factor: prolonged immobility

Risk for Frail Elderly syndrome: Risk factor: prolonged immobility

Risk for Loneliness: Risk factor: prolonged bed rest

Risk for Overweight: Risk factor: energy expenditure below energy intake

Risk for Pressure ulcer: Risk factor: prolonged immobility

Risk for Venous Thromboembolism: Risk factor: prolonged immobility

Bedsores

See Pressure Ulcer

Bedwetting

Ineffective Health maintenance r/t unachieved developmental level, neuromuscular immaturity, diseases of the urinary system

Bell's Palsy

Disturbed Body Image r/t loss of motor control on one side of face

Imbalanced Nutrition: less than body requirements r/t difficulty with chewing

Acute Pain r/t inflammation of facial nerve

Risk for Injury (eye): Risk factors: decreased tears, decreased blinking of eye

Readiness for enhanced Knowledge: expresses an interest in learning

Benign Prostatic Hypertrophy

See BPH (Benign Prostatic Hypertrophy); Prostatic Hypertrophy

Bereavement

Grieving r/t loss of significant person

Insomnia r/t grief

Risk for complicated Grieving: Risk factor: emotional instability, lack of social support

Risk for Spiritual distress: Risk factor: death of a loved one

Biliary Atresia

Anxiety r/t surgical intervention, possible liver transplantation

Impaired Comfort r/t inflammation of skin, itching

Imbalanced Nutrition: less than body requirements r/t decreased absorption of fat and fat-soluble vitamins, poor feeding

Risk for Bleeding: Risk factors: vitamin K deficiency, altered clotting mechanisms

Risk for ineffective Breathing pattern: Risk factors: enlarged liver, development of ascites

Risk for impaired Skin integrity: Risk factor: pruritus

See Child with Chronic Condition; Cirrhosis; Hospitalized Child

Biliary Calculus

See Cholelithiasis

Biliary Obstruction

See Jaundice

Bilirubin Elevation in Neonate

See Hyperbilirubinemia, Neonatal

Biopsy

Fear r/t outcome of biopsy

Readiness for enhanced Knowledge: expresses an interest in learning

Bioterrorism

Contamination r/t exposure to bioterrorism

Risk for Infection: Risk factor: exposure to harmful biological agent

Risk for Post-Trauma syndrome: Risk factor: perception of event of bioterrorism

Bipolar Disorder I (Most Recent Episode, Depressed or Manic)

Ineffective Activity planning r/t unrealistic perception of events

Fatigue r/t psychological demands

Risk-prone Health behavior: Risk factor: low state of optimism

Ineffective Health maintenance r/t lack of ability to make good judgments regarding ways to obtain help

Self-Care deficit: specify r/t depression, cognitive impairment

Chronic low Self-Esteem r/t repeated unmet expectations

Social isolation r/t ineffective coping

Risk for complicated Grieving: Risk factor: lack of previous resolution of former grieving response

Risk for Loneliness: Risk factors: stress, conflict

Risk for Spiritual distress: Risk factor: mental illness

Risk for Suicide: Risk factors: psychiatric disorder, poor support system

See Depression (Major Depressive Disorder); Manic Disorder, Bipolar I

Birth Asphyxia

See Asphyxia, Birth

Birth Control

See Contraceptive Method

Bladder Cancer

Urinary Retention r/t clots obstructing urethra

See Cancer; TURP (Transurethral Resection of the Prostate)

Bladder Distention

Urinary Retention r/t high urethral pressure caused by weak detrusor, inhibition of reflex arc, blockage, strong sphincter

Bladder Training

Disturbed Body Image r/t difficulty maintaining control of urinary elimination

Functional urinary Incontinence r/t altered environment; sensory, cognitive, mobility deficit

Stress urinary Incontinence r/t degenerative change in pelvic muscles and structural supports

Urge urinary Incontinence r/t decreased bladder capacity, increased urine concentration, overdistension of bladder

Readiness for enhanced Knowledge: expresses an interest in learning

Bladder Training, Child

See Toilet Training

Bleeding Tendency

Risk for Bleeding (See **Bleeding**, risk for, Section III)

Risk for delayed Surgical recovery: Risk factor: bleeding tendency

Blepharoplasty

Disturbed Body Image r/t effects of surgery

Readiness for enhanced Knowledge: expresses an interest in learning

Blindness

Interrupted Family processes r/t shift in health status of family member (change in visual acuity)

Impaired Home maintenance r/t decreased vision

Ineffective Role performance r/t alteration in health status (change in visual acuity)

Self-Care deficit: **specify** r/t inability to see to be able to perform activities of daily living

Risk for delayed Development: Risk factor: vision impairment

Risk for Injury: Risk factor: sensory dysfunction

Readiness for enhanced Knowledge: expresses an interest in learning

Blood Disorder

Ineffective Protection r/t abnormal blood profile

Risk for Bleeding: Risk factor: abnormal blood profile

See ITP (Idiopathic Thrombocytopenic Purpura); Hemophilia; Lacerations; Shock, Hypovolemic

Blood Glucose Control

Risk for unstable blood Glucose level (See **Glucose** level, blood, unstable, risk for, Section III)

Blood Pressure Alteration

See Hypotension; HTN (Hypertension)
See **Unstable Blood Pressure**, Risk for, Section III

Blood Transfusion

Anxiety r/t possibility of harm from transfusion
See Anemia

Body Dysmorphic Disorder

Anxiety r/t perceived defect of body

Disturbed Body Image r/t over involvement in physical appearance

Chronic low Self-Esteem r/t lack of self-valuing because of perceived body defects

Social isolation r/t distancing self from others because of perceived self-body defects

Risk for Suicide: Risk factor: perceived defects of body affecting self-valuing and hopes

Body Image Change

Disturbed Body Image (See **Body Image**, disturbed, Section III)

Body Temperature, Altered

Ineffective Thermoregulation (See **Thermoregulation**, ineffective, Section III)

Bone Marrow Biopsy

Fear r/t unknown outcome of results of biopsy

Acute Pain r/t bone marrow aspiration

Readiness for enhanced Knowledge: expresses an interest in learning

See Disease necessitating bone marrow biopsy (e.g., Leukemia)

Borderline Personality Disorder

Ineffective Activity planning r/t unrealistic perception of events

Anxiety r/t perceived threat to self-concept

Defensive Coping r/t difficulty with relationships, inability to accept blame for own behavior

Ineffective Coping r/t use of maladjusted defense mechanisms (e.g., projection, denial)

Powerlessness r/t lifestyle of helplessness

Social isolation r/t immature interests

Ineffective family Health management r/t manipulative behavior of client

Risk for Caregiver Role Strain: Risk factors: inability of care receiver to accept criticism, care receiver taking advantage of others to meet own needs or having unreasonable expectations

Risk for Self-Mutilation: Risk factors: ineffective coping, feelings of self-hatred

Risk for Spiritual distress: Risk factor: poor relationships associated with abnormal behaviors

Risk for self-directed Violence: Risk factors: feelings of need to punish self, manipulative behavior

Boredom

Decreased Diversional activity engagement r/t environmental lack of diversional activity

Impaired Mood regulation r/t emotional instability

Social isolation r/t altered state of wellness

Botulism

Deficient Fluid volume r/t profuse diarrhea

Readiness for enhanced Knowledge: expresses an interest in learning

Bowel Incontinence

Bowel Incontinence r/t decreased awareness of need to defecate, loss of sphincter control, fecal impaction

Readiness for enhanced Knowledge: expresses an interest in learning

Bowel Obstruction

Constipation r/t decreased motility, intestinal obstruction

Deficient Fluid volume r/t inadequate fluid volume intake, fluid loss in bowel

B

Imbalanced Nutrition: less than body requirements r/t nausea, vomiting

Acute Pain r/t pressure from distended abdomen

Bowel Resection

See Abdominal Surgery

Bowel Sounds, Absent or Diminished

Constipation r/t decreased or absent peristalsis

Deficient Fluid volume r/t inability to ingest fluids, loss of fluids in bowel

Delayed Surgical recovery r/t inability to obtain adequate nutritional status

Risk for dysfunctional Gastrointestinal motility (See **Gastrointestinal** motility, dysfunctional, risk for, Section III)

Bowel Sounds, Hyperactive

Diarrhea r/t increased gastrointestinal motility

Bowel Training

Bowel Incontinence r/t loss of control of rectal sphincter

Readiness for enhanced Knowledge: expresses an interest in learning

Bowel Training, Child

See Toilet Training

BPH (Benign Prostatic Hypertrophy)

Ineffective Health maintenance r/t deficient knowledge regarding self-care with prostatic hypertrophy

Insomnia r/t nocturia

Urinary Retention r/t obstruction of urethra

Risk for urge urinary Incontinence: Risk factors: detrusor muscle instability with impaired contractility, involuntary sphincter relaxation

Risk for Infection: Risk factors: urinary residual after voiding, bacterial invasion of bladder

Readiness for enhanced Knowledge: expresses an interest in learning

See Prostatic Hypertrophy

Bradycardia

Decreased Cardiac output r/t slow heart rate supplying inadequate amount of blood for body function

Risk for ineffective Cerebral tissue perfusion: Risk factors: decreased cardiac output secondary to bradycardia, vagal response

Readiness for enhanced Knowledge: expresses an interest in learning

Bradypnea

Ineffective Breathing pattern r/t neuromuscular impairment, pain, musculoskeletal impairment, perception or cognitive impairment, anxiety, fatigue or decreased energy, effects of drugs

See Sleep apnea (See **Airway** clearance, ineffective, Section III)

Brain Injury

See Intracranial Pressure, Increased

Risk for ineffective Thermoregulation: Risk factor: post traumatic inflammation or infection

Brain Surgery

See Craniectomy/Craniotomy

Brain Tumor

Acute Confusion r/t pressure from tumor

Fear r/t threat to well-being

Grieving r/t potential loss of physiosocial-psychosocial well-being

Decreased Intracranial adaptive capacity r/t presence of brain tumor

Acute Pain r/t pressure from tumor

Vision Loss r/t tumor growth compressing optic nerve and/or brain tissue

Risk for Injury: Risk factors: sensory-perceptual alterations, weakness

Risk for ineffective Thermoregulation: Risk factor: changes in metabolic activity of the brain

See Cancer; Chemotherapy; Child with Chronic Condition; Craniectomy/Craniotomy; Hospitalized Child; Radiation Therapy; Terminally Ill Child, Adolescent; Terminally Ill Child, Infant/Toddler; Terminally Ill Child, Preschool Child; Terminally Ill Child, School-Age Child/Preadolescent; Terminally Ill Child/Death of Child, Parent

Braxton Hicks Contractions

Activity intolerance r/t increased contractions with increased gestation

Anxiety r/t uncertainty about beginning labor

Fatigue r/t lack of sleep

Stress urinary Incontinence r/t increased pressure on bladder with contractions

Insomnia r/t contractions when lying down

Ineffective Sexuality pattern r/t fear of contractions associated with loss of infant

Breast Biopsy

Fear r/t potential for diagnosis of cancer

Risk for Spiritual distress: Risk factor: fear of diagnosis of cancer

Readiness for enhanced Knowledge: expresses an interest in learning

Breast Cancer

Death Anxiety r/t diagnosis of cancer

Ineffective Coping r/t treatment, prognosis

Fear r/t diagnosis of cancer

Sexual dysfunction r/t loss of body part, partner's reaction to loss

Chronic Sorrow r/t diagnosis of cancer, loss of body integrity

Risk for Spiritual distress: Risk factor: fear of diagnosis of cancer

Readiness for enhanced Health literacy: expresses desire to enhance understanding of health information to make health care choices

Readiness for enhanced Knowledge: expresses an interest in learning

See Cancer; Chemotherapy; Mastectomy; Radiation Therapy

Breast Examination, Self

See SBE (Self-Breast Examination)

Breast Lumps

Fear r/t potential for diagnosis of cancer

Readiness for enhanced Knowledge: expresses an interest in learning

Breast Pumping

Risk for Infection: Risk factors: possible contaminated breast pump, incomplete emptying of breast

Risk for impaired Skin integrity: Risk factor: high suction

Readiness for enhanced Knowledge: expresses an interest in learning

Breastfeeding, Effective

Readiness for enhanced Breastfeeding (See **Breastfeeding**, readiness for enhanced, Section III)

Breastfeeding, Ineffective

Ineffective Breastfeeding (See **Breastfeeding**, ineffective, Section III)

See Infant Feeding Pattern, Ineffective; Painful Breasts, Engorgement; Painful Breasts, Sore Nipples

Breastfeeding, Interrupted

Interrupted Breastfeeding (See **Breastfeeding**, interrupted, Section III)

Breast Milk Production, Insufficient

Insufficient Breast Milk Production (See **Breast Milk Production**, insufficient, Section III)

Breath Sounds, Decreased or Absent

See Atelectasis; Pneumothorax

Breathing Pattern Alteration

Ineffective Breathing pattern r/t neuromuscular impairment, pain, musculoskeletal impairment, perception or cognitive impairment, anxiety, decreased energy or fatigue

Breech Birth

Fear: **maternal** r/t danger to infant, self

Impaired Gas exchange: **fetal** r/t compressed umbilical cord

Risk for Aspiration: **fetal**: Risk factor: birth of body before head

Risk for delayed Development: Risk factor: compressed umbilical cord

Risk for impaired Tissue integrity: **fetal**: Risk factor: difficult birth

Risk for impaired Tissue integrity: **maternal**: Risk factor: difficult birth

Bronchitis

Ineffective Airway clearance r/t excessive thickened mucus secretion

Readiness for enhanced Health management: wishes to stop smoking

Readiness for enhanced Knowledge: expresses an interest in learning

Bronchopulmonary Dysplasia

Activity intolerance r/t imbalance between oxygen supply and demand

Excess Fluid volume r/t sodium and water retention

Imbalanced Nutrition: less than body requirements r/t poor feeding, increased caloric needs as a result of increased work of breathing

See Child with Chronic Condition; Hospitalized Child; Respiratory Conditions of the Neonate

Bronchoscopy

Risk for Aspiration: Risk factor: temporary loss of gag reflex

Risk for Injury: Risk factors: complication of pneumothorax, laryngeal edema, hemorrhage (if biopsy done)

Bruits, Carotid

Risk for ineffective Cerebral tissue perfusion: Risk factors: interruption of carotid blood flow to brain

Bryant's Traction

See Traction and Casts

Buck's Traction

See Traction and Casts

Buerger's Disease

See Peripheral Vascular Disease (PVD)

Bulimia

Disturbed Body Image r/t misperception about actual appearance, body weight

Compromised family Coping r/t chronically unresolved feelings of guilt, anger, hostility

Defensive Coping r/t eating disorder

Diarrhea r/t laxative abuse

Fear r/t food ingestion, weight gain

Imbalanced Nutrition: less than body requirements r/t induced vomiting, excessive exercise, laxative abuse

Ineffective adolescent Eating dynamics r/t overeating, leading to purge

Powerlessness r/t urge to purge self after eating

Chronic low Self-Esteem r/t lack of positive feedback

See Maturational Issues, Adolescent

Bullying

Anxiety r/t specific or nonspecific threat to self

Impaired Social interaction r/t dysfunctional interactions with others

Fear r/t perceived threat to self

Risk for compromised Human Dignity: Risk factors: dehumanizing treatment, humiliation

Risk for other-directed Violence: Risk factors: social isolation, unresolved interpersonal conflicts

Risk for Powerlessness: Risk factor: ineffective coping strategies

C

Risk for impaired Resilience: Risk factor: insufficient familial and social support

Risk for self-directed violence: Risk factors: unresolved interpersonal conflicts, social isolation

Risk for chronic low Self-Esteem: Risk factors: ineffective coping strategies, absence of sense of belonging, inadequate respect from others

Bunion

Readiness for enhanced Knowledge: expresses an interest in learning

Bunionectomy

Impaired physical Mobility r/t sore foot

Impaired Walking r/t pain associated with surgery

Risk for Surgical Site Infection: Risk factors: surgical incision

Readiness for enhanced Knowledge: expresses an interest in learning

Burn Risk

Risk for Thermal injury (See **Thermal** injury, risk for, Section III)

Burns

Anxiety r/t burn injury, treatments

Disturbed Body Image r/t altered physical appearance

Decreased Diversional activity engagement r/t long-term hospitalization

Fear r/t pain from treatments, possible permanent disfigurement

Deficient Fluid volume r/t loss of protective skin

Grieving r/t loss of bodily function, loss of future hopes and plans

Hypothermia r/t impaired skin integrity

Impaired physical Mobility r/t pain, musculoskeletal impairment, contracture formation

Imbalanced Nutrition: less than body requirements r/t increased metabolic needs, anorexia, protein and fluid loss

Acute Pain r/t burn injury, treatments

Chronic Pain r/t burn injury, treatments

Ineffective peripheral Tissue Perfusion r/t circumferential burns, impaired arterial/venous circulation

Post-Trauma syndrome r/t life-threatening event

Impaired Skin integrity r/t injury of skin

Delayed Surgical recovery r/t ineffective tissue perfusion

Risk for ineffective Airway clearance: Risk factors: potential tracheobronchial obstruction, edema

Risk for deficient Fluid volume: Risk factors: loss from skin surface, fluid shift

Risk for Infection: Risk factors: loss of intact skin, trauma, invasive sites

Risk for Peripheral Neurovascular dysfunction: Risk factor: eschar formation with circumferential burn

Risk for Post-Trauma syndrome: Risk factors: perception, duration of event that caused burns

Risk for ineffective Thermoregulation: Risk factor: disruption of skin integrity

Readiness for enhanced Knowledge: expresses an interest in learning

See Hospitalized Child; Safety, Childhood

Bursitis

Impaired physical Mobility r/t inflammation in joint

Acute Pain r/t inflammation in joint

Bypass Graft

See Coronary Artery Bypass Grafting (CABG)

C

CABG (Coronary Artery Bypass Grafting)

See Coronary Artery Bypass Grafting (CABG)

Cachexia

Frail Elderly syndrome r/t fatigue, feeding self-care deficit

Imbalanced Nutrition: less than body requirements r/t inability to ingest food because of physiological factors

Risk for Infection: Risk factor: inadequate nutrition

Calcium Alteration

See Hypercalcemia; Hypocalcemia

Cancer

Activity intolerance r/t side effects of treatment, weakness from cancer

Death Anxiety r/t unresolved issues regarding dying

Disturbed Body Image r/t side effects of treatment, cachexia

Decisional Conflict r/t selection of treatment choices, continuation or discontinuation of treatment, "do not resuscitate" decision

Constipation r/t side effects of medication, altered nutrition, decreased activity

Compromised family Coping r/t prolonged disease or disability progression that exhausts supportive ability of significant others

Ineffective Coping r/t personal vulnerability in situational crisis, terminal illness

Ineffective Denial r/t complicated grieving process

Fear r/t serious threat to well-being

Grieving r/t potential loss of significant others, high risk for infertility

Ineffective Health maintenance r/t deficient knowledge regarding prescribed treatment

Hopelessness r/t loss of control, terminal illness

Insomnia r/t anxiety, pain

Impaired physical Mobility r/t weakness, neuromusculoskeletal impairment, pain

Imbalanced Nutrition: less than body requirements r/t loss of appetite, difficulty swallowing, side effects of chemotherapy, obstruction by tumor

Impaired Oral Mucous Membrane integrity r/t chemotherapy, effects of radiation, oral pH changes, decreased oral secretions

Chronic Pain r/t metastatic cancer

Powerlessness r/t treatment, progression of disease

Ineffective Protection r/t cancer suppressing immune system

Ineffective Role performance r/t change in physical capacity, inability to resume prior role

Self-Care deficit: specify r/t pain, intolerance to activity, decreased strength

Impaired Skin integrity r/t immunological deficit, immobility

Social isolation r/t hospitalization, lifestyle changes

Chronic Sorrow r/t chronic illness of cancer

Spiritual distress r/t test of spiritual beliefs

Risk for Bleeding: Risk factor: bone marrow depression from chemotherapy

Risk for Disuse syndrome: Risk factors: immobility, fatigue

Risk for impaired Home maintenance: Risk factor: lack of familiarity with community resources

Risk for Infection: Risk factor: inadequate immune system

Risk for compromised Resilience: Risk factors: multiple stressors, pain, chronic illness

Risk for Spiritual distress: Risk factor: physical illness of cancer

Readiness for enhanced Knowledge: expresses an interest in learning

Readiness for enhanced Spiritual well-being: desire for harmony with self, others, higher power, God, when faced with serious illness

See Chemotherapy; Child with Chronic Condition; Hospitalized Child; Leukemia; Radiation Therapy; Terminally Ill Child, Adolescent; Terminally Ill Child, Infant/Toddler; Terminally Ill Child, Preschool Child; Terminally Ill Child, School-Age Child/Preadolescent; Terminally Ill Child/Death of Child, Parent

Candidiasis, Oral

Readiness for enhanced Knowledge: expresses an interest in learning

Impaired Oral Mucous Membrane integrity r/t overgrowth of infectious agent, depressed immune function

Acute Pain r/t oral condition

Capillary Refill Time, Prolonged

Impaired Gas exchange r/t ventilation perfusion imbalance

Ineffective peripheral Tissue Perfusion r/t interruption of arterial flow

See Shock, Hypovolemic

Carbon Monoxide Poisoning

See Smoke Inhalation

Cardiac Arrest

Post-Trauma syndrome r/t experiencing serious life event

See Dysrhythmia; MI (Myocardial Infarction)

Cardiac Catheterization

Fear r/t invasive procedure, uncertainty of outcome of procedure

Risk for Injury: hematoma: Risk factor: invasive procedure

Risk for decreased Cardiac tissue perfusion: Risk factors: ventricular ischemia, dysrhythmia

Risk for Peripheral Neurovascular dysfunction: Risk factor: vascular obstruction

Risk for Impaired Tissue integrity: Risk factor: invasive procedure

Readiness for enhanced Knowledge: expresses an interest in learning postprocedure care, treatment, and prevention of coronary artery disease

Cardiac Disorders in Pregnancy

Activity intolerance r/t cardiac pathophysiology, increased demand for cardiac output because of pregnancy, weakness, fatigue

Death Anxiety r/t potential danger of condition

Compromised family Coping r/t prolonged hospitalization or maternal incapacitation that exhausts supportive capacity of significant others

Ineffective Coping r/t personal vulnerability

Interrupted Family processes r/t hospitalization, maternal incapacitation, changes in roles

Fatigue r/t physiological, psychological, and emotional demands

Fear r/t potential maternal effects, potential poor fetal or maternal outcome

Powerlessness r/t illness-related regimen

Ineffective Role performance r/t changes in lifestyle, expectations from disease process with superimposed pregnancy

Situational low Self-Esteem r/t situational crisis, pregnancy

Social isolation r/t limitations of activity, bed rest or hospitalization, separation from family and friends

Risk for decreased Cardiac tissue perfusion: Risk factor: strain on compromised heart from work of pregnancy, delivery

Risk for delayed Development: Risk factor: poor maternal oxygenation

Risk for deficient Fluid volume: Risk factor: sudden changes in circulation after delivery of placenta

Risk for excess Fluid volume: Risk factors: compromised regulatory mechanism with increased afterload, preload, circulating blood volume

Risk for impaired Gas exchange: Risk factor: pulmonary edema

Risk for disturbed Maternal–Fetal dyad: Risk factor: compromised oxygen transport

Risk for compromised Resilience: Risk factors: multiple stressors, fear

Risk for Spiritual distress: Risk factor: fear of diagnosis for self and infant

Readiness for enhanced Knowledge: expresses an interest in learning

Cardiac Dysrhythmia

See Dysrhythmia

Cardiac Output, Decreased

Decreased Cardiac output r/t cardiac dysfunction

Decreased Cardiac output (See **Cardiac** output, decreased, Section III)

Oliguria r/t cardiac dysfunction

Risk for decreased Cardiac output (See **Cardiac** output, risk for decreased, Section III)

Cardiac Tamponade

Decreased Cardiac output r/t fluid in pericardial sac

See Pericarditis

Cardiogenic Shock

See Shock, Cardiogenic

Caregiver Role Strain

Caregiver Role Strain (See **Caregiver Role Strain**, Section III)

Risk for compromised Resilience: Risk factor: stress of prolonged caregiving

Carious Teeth

See Cavities in Teeth

Carotid Endarterectomy

Fear r/t surgery in vital area

Risk for ineffective Airway clearance: Risk factor: hematoma compressing trachea

Risk for Bleeding: Risk factor: possible hematoma formation, trauma to region

Risk for ineffective Cerebral tissue perfusion: Risk factors: hemorrhage, clot formation

Readiness for enhanced Knowledge: expresses an interest in learning

Carpal Tunnel Syndrome

Impaired physical Mobility r/t neuromuscular impairment

Chronic Pain r/t unrelieved pressure on median nerve

Self-Care deficit: bathing, dressing, feeding r/t pain

Carpopedal Spasm

See Hypocalcemia

Casts

Decreased Diversional activity engagement r/t physical limitations from cast

Impaired physical Mobility r/t limb immobilization

Self-Care deficit: bathing, dressing, feeding r/t presence of cast(s) on upper extremities

Self-Care deficit: toileting r/t presence of cast(s) on lower extremities

Impaired Walking r/t cast(s) on lower extremities, fracture of bones

Risk for Peripheral Neurovascular dysfunction: Risk factors: mechanical compression from cast, trauma from fracture

Risk for impaired Skin integrity: Risk factor: unrelieved pressure on skin from cast

Readiness for enhanced Knowledge: expresses an interest in learning

See Traction and Casts

Cataract Extraction

Anxiety r/t threat of permanent vision loss, surgical procedure

Vision Loss r/t edema from surgery (*see Appendix E on Evolve*)

Risk for Injury: Risk factors: increased intraocular pressure, accommodation to new visual field

Readiness for enhanced Knowledge: expresses an interest in learning

Catatonic Schizophrenia

Impaired verbal Communication r/t cognitive impairment

Impaired Memory r/t cognitive impairment

Impaired physical Mobility r/t cognitive impairment, maintenance of rigid posture, inappropriate or bizarre postures

Imbalanced Nutrition: less than body requirements r/t decrease in outside stimulation, loss of perception of hunger, resistance to instructions to eat

Social isolation r/t inability to communicate, immobility

See Schizophrenia

Catheterization, Urinary

Risk for Infection: Risk factor: invasive procedure

Readiness for enhanced Knowledge: expresses an interest in learning

Cavities in Teeth

Impaired Dentition r/t ineffective oral hygiene, barriers to self-care, economic barriers to professional care, nutritional deficits, dietary habits

Celiac Disease

Diarrhea r/t malabsorption of food, immune effects of gluten on gastrointestinal system

Imbalanced Nutrition: less than body requirements r/t malabsorption caused by immune effects of gluten

Readiness for enhanced Knowledge: expresses an interest in learning

Cellulitis

Acute Pain r/t inflammatory changes in tissues from infection

Impaired Tissue integrity r/t inflammatory process damaging skin and underlying tissue

Ineffective peripheral Tissue Perfusion r/t edema of extremities

Risk for Vascular Trauma: Risk factor: infusion of antibiotics

Readiness for enhanced Knowledge: expresses an interest in learning

Cellulitis, Periorbital

Acute Pain r/t edema and inflammation of skin/tissues

Impaired Skin integrity r/t inflammation or infection of skin, tissues

Vision Loss r/t decreased visual field secondary to edema of eyelids (*see Appendix E on Evolve*)

Readiness for enhanced Knowledge: expresses an interest in learning

See Hospitalized Child

Central Line Insertion

Risk for Infection: Risk factor: invasive procedure

Risk for Vascular Trauma (See **Vascular Trauma**, risk for, Section III)

Readiness for enhanced Knowledge: expresses an interest in learning

Cerebral Aneurysm

See Craniectomy/Craniotomy; Intracranial Pressure, Increased; Subarachnoid Hemorrhage

Cerebral Palsy

Impaired verbal Communication r/t impaired ability to articulate or speak words because of facial muscle involvement

Decreased Diversional activity engagement r/t physical impairments, limitations on ability to participate in recreational activities

Impaired physical Mobility r/t spasticity, neuromuscular impairment or weakness

Imbalanced Nutrition: less than body requirements r/t spasticity, feeding or swallowing difficulties

Self-Care deficit: specify r/t neuromuscular impairments, sensory deficits

Impaired Social interaction r/t impaired communication skills, limited physical activity, perceived differences from peers

Chronic Sorrow r/t presence of chronic disability

Risk for Falls: Risk factor: impaired physical mobility

Risk for Injury: Risk factors: muscle weakness, inability to control spasticity

Risk for impaired Parenting: Risk factor: caring for child with overwhelming needs resulting from chronic change in health status

Risk for Spiritual distress: Risk factor: psychological stress associated with chronic illness

See Child with Chronic Condition

Cerebral Perfusion

Risk for ineffective Cerebral tissue perfusion (See **Cerebral** tissue perfusion, ineffective, risk for, Section III)

Cerebrovascular Accident (CVA)

See CVA (Cerebrovascular Accident)

Cervicitis

Ineffective Health maintenance r/t deficient knowledge regarding care and prevention of condition

Ineffective Sexuality pattern r/t abstinence during acute stage

Risk for Infection: Risk factors: spread of infection, recurrence of infection

Cesarean Delivery

Disturbed Body Image r/t surgery, unmet expectations for childbirth

Interrupted Family processes r/t unmet expectations for childbirth

Fear r/t perceived threat to own well-being, outcome of birth

Impaired physical Mobility r/t pain

Acute Pain r/t surgical incision

Ineffective Role performance r/t unmet expectations for childbirth

Situational low Self-Esteem r/t inability to deliver child vaginally

Risk for Bleeding: Risk factor: surgery

Risk for imbalanced Fluid volume: Risk factors: loss of blood, fluid shifts

Risk for Surgical Site Infection: Risk factor: surgical incision

Risk for Urinary Retention: Risk factor: regional anesthesia

Readiness for enhanced Childbearing process: a pattern of preparing for, maintaining, and strengthening care of newborn

Readiness for enhanced Knowledge: expresses an interest in learning

Chemical Dependence

See Alcoholism; Substance Abuse

Chemotherapy

Death Anxiety r/t chemotherapy not accomplishing desired results

Disturbed Body Image r/t loss of weight, loss of hair

Fatigue r/t disease process, anemia, drug effects

Nausea r/t effects of chemotherapy

Imbalanced Nutrition: less than body requirements r/t side effects of chemotherapy

Impaired Oral Mucous Membrane integrity r/t effects of chemotherapy

Ineffective Protection r/t suppressed immune system, decreased platelets

Risk for Bleeding: Risk factors: tumor eroding blood vessel, stress effects on gastrointestinal system

Risk for Infection: Risk factor: immunosuppression

Risk for Vascular Trauma: Risk factor: infusion of irritating medications

Readiness for enhanced Knowledge: expresses an interest in learning

See Cancer

Chest Pain

Fear r/t potential threat of death

Acute Pain r/t myocardial injury, ischemia

Risk for decreased Cardiac tissue perfusion: Risk factor: ventricular ischemia

See Angina; MI (Myocardial Infarction)

Chest Tubes

Ineffective Breathing pattern r/t asymmetrical lung expansion secondary to pain

Impaired Gas exchange r/t decreased functional lung tissue

Acute Pain r/t presence of chest tubes, injury

Risk for Injury: Risk factor: presence of invasive chest tube

Cheyne-Stokes Respiration

Ineffective Breathing pattern r/t critical illness

Chickenpox

See Communicable Diseases, Childhood

Child Abuse

Interrupted Family processes r/t inadequate coping skills

Fear r/t threat of punishment for perceived wrongdoing

C

Insomnia r/t hypervigilance, fear

Imbalanced Nutrition: less than body requirements r/t inadequate caretaking

Acute Pain r/t physical injuries

Impaired Parenting r/t psychological impairment, physical or emotional abuse of parent, substance abuse, unrealistic expectations of child

Ineffective child Eating dynamics r/t hostile parental relationship

Post-Trauma syndrome r/t physical abuse, incest, rape, molestation

Chronic low Self-Esteem r/t lack of positive feedback, excessive negative feedback

Impaired Skin integrity r/t altered nutritional state, physical abuse

Social isolation: family imposed r/t fear of disclosure of family dysfunction and abuse

Risk for delayed Development: Risk factors: shaken baby syndrome, abuse

Risk for Poisoning: Risk factors: inadequate safeguards, lack of proper safety precautions, accessibility of illicit substances because of impaired home maintenance

Risk for Suffocation: Risk factors: unattended child, unsafe environment

Risk for Physical Trauma: Risk factors: inadequate precautions, cognitive or emotional difficulties

Childbearing Problems

Ineffective Childbearing process (See **Childbearing** process, ineffective, Section III)

Risk for ineffective Childbearing process: (See **Childbearing** process, risk for ineffective, Section III)

Child Neglect

See Child Abuse; Failure to Thrive

Child with Chronic Condition

Activity intolerance r/t fatigue associated with chronic illness

Compromised family Coping r/t prolonged overconcern for child; distortion of reality regarding child's health problem, including extreme denial about its existence or severity

Disabled family Coping r/t prolonged disease or disability progression that exhausts supportive capacity of significant others

Ineffective Coping: child r/t situational or maturational crises

Decisional Conflict r/t treatment options, conflicting values

Decreased Diversional activity engagement r/t immobility, monotonous environment, frequent or lengthy treatments, reluctance to participate, self-imposed social isolation

Interrupted Family processes r/t intermittent situational crisis of illness, disease, hospitalization

Ineffective Health maintenance r/t exhausting family resources (finances, physical energy, support systems)

Impaired Home maintenance r/t overtaxed family members (e.g., exhausted, anxious)

Hopelessness: child r/t prolonged activity restriction, long-term stress, lack of involvement in or passively allowing care as a result of parental overprotection

Insomnia: child or parent r/t time-intensive treatments, exacerbation of condition, 24-hour care needs

Deficient Knowledge r/t knowledge or skill acquisition regarding health practices, acceptance of limitations, promotion of maximal potential of child, self-actualization of rest of family

Imbalanced Nutrition: less than body requirements r/t anorexia, fatigue from physical exertion

Risk for Overweight r/t effects of steroid medications on appetite

Chronic Pain r/t physical, biological, chemical, or psychological factors

Powerlessness: child r/t health care environment, illness-related regimen, lifestyle of learned helplessness

Parental Role conflict r/t separation from child as a result of chronic illness, home care of child with special needs, interruptions of family life resulting from home care regimen

Chronic low Self-Esteem r/t actual or perceived differences; peer acceptance; decreased ability to participate in physical, school, and social activities

Ineffective Sexuality pattern: parental r/t disrupted relationship with sexual partner

Impaired Social interaction r/t developmental lag or delay, perceived differences

Social isolation: family r/t actual or perceived social stigmatization, complex care requirements

Chronic Sorrow r/t developmental stages and missed opportunities or milestones that bring comparisons with social or personal norms, unending caregiving as reminder of loss

Risk for delayed Development: Risk factor: chronic illness

Risk for Infection: Risk factor: debilitating physical condition

Risk for impaired Parenting: Risk factors: impaired or disrupted bonding, caring for child with perceived overwhelming care needs

Readiness for enhanced family Coping: impact of crisis on family values, priorities, goals, or relationships; changes in family choices to optimize wellness

Childbirth

Readiness for enhanced Childbearing process (See **Childbearing** process, readiness for enhanced, Section III)

See Labor, Normal; Postpartum, Normal Care

Childhood Obesity

Obesity r/t disordered eating behaviors

Risk for Activity intolerance: Risk factors: sedentary lifestyle, exertional discomfort

Risk for unstable blood Glucose Level: Risk factor: excessive weight gain

Risk for Metabolic Imbalance syndrome: Risk factors: obesity, sedentary lifestyle

Readiness for enhanced Knowledge: expresses desire to make healthier nutrition choices

Chills

Hyperthermia r/t infectious process

Chlamydia Infection

See STD (Sexually Transmitted Disease)

Chloasma

Disturbed Body Image r/t change in skin color

Choking or Coughing with Eating

Impaired Swallowing r/t neuromuscular impairment

Risk for Aspiration: Risk factors: depressed cough and gag reflexes

Cholecystectomy

Imbalanced Nutrition: less than body requirements r/t high metabolic needs, decreased ability to digest fatty foods

Acute Pain r/t trauma from surgery

Risk for deficient Fluid volume: Risk factors: restricted intake, nausea, vomiting

Risk for Surgical Site Infection: Risk factor: invasive procedure

Readiness for enhanced Knowledge: expresses an interest in learning

See Abdominal Surgery

Cholelithiasis

Nausea r/t obstruction of bile

Imbalanced Nutrition: less than body requirements r/t anorexia, nausea, vomiting

Acute Pain r/t obstruction of bile flow, inflammation in gallbladder

Readiness for enhanced Knowledge: expresses an interest in learning

Chorioamnionitis

Anxiety r/t threat to self and infant

Grieving r/t guilt about potential loss of ideal pregnancy and birth

Hyperthermia r/t infectious process

Situational low Self-Esteem r/t guilt about threat to infant's health

Risk for Infection: Risk factors: infection transmission from mother to fetus; infection in fetal environment

Chronic Confusion

See Confusion, Chronic

Chronic Functional Constipation

(See **Constipation**, chronic functional, section III)

(See **Constipation**, chronic functional, risk for, section III)

Chronic Lymphocytic Leukemia

See Cancer; Chemotherapy; Leukemia

Chronic Obstructive Pulmonary Disease (COPD)

See COPD (Chronic Obstructive Pulmonary Disease)

Chronic Pain

See Pain Management, Chronic

Chronic Renal Failure (Chronic Renal Disease)

See Renal Failure

Chvostek's Sign

See Hypocalcemia

Circumcision

Acute Pain r/t surgical intervention

Risk for Bleeding: Risk factor: surgical trauma

Risk for Infection: Risk factor: surgical wound

Readiness for enhanced Knowledge: parent: expresses an interest in learning

Cirrhosis

Chronic Confusion r/t chronic organic disorder with increased ammonia levels, substance abuse

Defensive Coping r/t inability to accept responsibility to stop substance abuse

Fatigue r/t malnutrition

Ineffective Health maintenance r/t deficient knowledge regarding correlation between lifestyle habits and disease process

Nausea r/t irritation to gastrointestinal system

Imbalanced Nutrition: less than body requirements r/t loss of appetite, nausea, vomiting

Chronic Pain r/t liver enlargement

Chronic low Self-Esteem r/t chronic illness

Chronic Sorrow r/t presence of chronic illness

Risk for Bleeding: Risk factors: impaired blood coagulation, bleeding from portal hypertension

Risk for Injury: Risk factors: substance intoxication, potential delirium tremens

Risk for impaired Oral Mucous Membrane integrity: Risk factors: altered nutrition, inadequate oral care

Risk for impaired Skin integrity: Risk factors: altered nutritional state, altered metabolic state

Cleft Lip/Cleft Palate

Ineffective Airway clearance r/t common feeding and breathing passage, postoperative laryngeal, incisional edema

Ineffective Breastfeeding r/t infant anomaly

Impaired verbal Communication r/t inadequate palate function, possible hearing loss from infected eustachian tubes

Fear: parental r/t special care needs, surgery

Grieving r/t loss of perfect child

Ineffective infant Feeding dynamic r/t fear resulting in inadequate feeding

Ineffective infant Feeding pattern r/t cleft lip, cleft palate

Impaired physical Mobility r/t imposed restricted activity, use of elbow restraints

Impaired Oral Mucous Membrane integrity r/t surgical correction

Acute Pain r/t surgical correction, elbow restraints

Impaired Skin integrity r/t incomplete joining of lip, palate ridges

Chronic Sorrow r/t birth of child with congenital defect

Risk for Aspiration: Risk factor: common feeding and breathing passage

C

Risk for disturbed Body Image: Risk factors: disfigurement, speech impediment

Risk for delayed Development: Risk factor: inadequate nutrition resulting from difficulty feeding

Risk for deficient Fluid volume: Risk factor: inability to take liquids in usual manner

Risk for Infection: Risk factors: invasive procedure, disruption of eustachian tube development, aspiration

Readiness for enhanced Knowledge: parent: expresses an interest in learning

Clotting Disorder

Fear r/t threat to well-being

Risk for Bleeding: Risk factor: impaired clotting

Readiness for enhanced Knowledge: expresses an interest in learning

See Anticoagulant Therapy; DIC (Disseminated Intravascular Coagulation); Hemophilia

Cocaine Baby

See Neonatal Abstinence Syndrome

Codependency

Caregiver Role Strain r/t codependency

Impaired verbal Communication r/t psychological barriers

Ineffective Coping r/t inadequate support systems

Decisional Conflict r/t support system deficit

Ineffective Denial r/t unmet self-needs

Powerlessness r/t lifestyle of helplessness

Cold, Viral

See Infectious Processes

Colectomy

Constipation r/t decreased activity, decreased fluid intake

Imbalanced Nutrition: less than body requirements r/t high metabolic needs, decreased ability to ingest or digest food

Acute Pain r/t recent surgery

Risk for Surgical Site Infection: Risk factor: invasive procedure

Readiness for enhanced Knowledge: expresses an interest in learning

See Abdominal Surgery

Colitis

Diarrhea r/t inflammation in colon

Deficient Fluid volume r/t frequent stools

Acute Pain r/t inflammation in colon

Readiness for enhanced Knowledge: expresses an interest in learning

See Crohn's Disease; Inflammatory Bowel Disease (Child and Adult)

Collagen Disease

See specific disease (e.g., Lupus erythematosus; JRA [juvenile rheumatoid arthritis]); Congenital Heart Disease/Cardiac Anomalies

Colostomy

Disturbed Body Image r/t presence of stoma, daily care of fecal material

Ineffective Sexuality pattern r/t altered body image, self-concept

Social isolation r/t anxiety about appearance of stoma and possible leakage of stool

Risk for Constipation: Risk factor: inappropriate diet

Risk for Diarrhea: Risk factor: inappropriate diet

Risk for impaired Skin integrity: Risk factor: irritation from bowel contents

Readiness for enhanced Knowledge: expresses an interest in learning

Colporrhaphy, Anterior

See Vaginal Hysterectomy

Coma

Death Anxiety: significant others r/t unknown outcome of coma state

Interrupted Family processes r/t illness or disability of family member

Functional urinary Incontinence r/t presence of comatose state

Self-Care deficit: r/t neuromuscular impairment

Ineffective family Health management r/t complexity of therapeutic regimen

Risk for Aspiration: Risk factors: impaired swallowing, loss of cough or gag reflex

Risk for Disuse syndrome: Risk factor: altered level of consciousness impairing mobility

Risk for Dry Mouth: Risk factor: inability to perform own oral care

Risk for Hypothermia: Risk factors: inactivity, possible pharmaceutical agents, possible hypothalamic injury

Risk for Injury: Risk factor: potential seizure activity

Risk for corneal Injury: Risk factor: suppressed corneal reflex

Risk for urinary tract Injury: Risk factor: long-term use of urinary catheter

Risk for impaired Oral Mucous Membrane integrity: Risk factors: dry mouth, inability to do own mouth care

Risk for Pressure ulcer: Risk factor: prolonged immobility

Risk for impaired Skin integrity: Risk factor: immobility

Risk for Spiritual distress: significant others: Risk factors: loss of ability to relate to loved one, unknown outcome of coma

Risk for impaired Tissue integrity: Risk factor: impaired physical mobility

See Head Injury; Subarachnoid Hemorrhage; Intracranial Pressure, Increased

Comfort, Loss of

Impaired Comfort (See **Comfort**, impaired, Section III)

Readiness for enhanced Comfort (See **Comfort**, readiness for enhanced, Section III)

Communicable Diseases, Childhood (e.g., Measles, Mumps, Rubella, Chickenpox, Scabies, Lice, Impetigo)

Impaired Comfort r/t pruritus, inflammation or infection of skin, subdermal organisms

Decreased Diversional activity engagement r/t imposed isolation from peers, disruption in usual play activities, fatigue, activity intolerance

Ineffective Health maintenance r/t nonadherence to appropriate immunization schedules, lack of prevention of transmission of infection

Acute Pain r/t impaired skin integrity, edema

Risk for Infection: transmission to others: Risk factor: contagious organisms

See Meningitis/Encephalitis; Respiratory Infections, Acute Childhood

Communication

Readiness for enhanced Communication (See **Communication**, readiness for enhanced, Section III)

Communication Problems

Impaired verbal Communication (See **Communication**, verbal, impaired, Section III)

Community Coping

Ineffective community Coping (See **Coping**, community, ineffective, Section III)

Readiness for enhanced community Coping: community sense of power to manage stressors, social supports available, resources available for problem solving

Community Health Problems

Deficient community Health (See **Health**, deficient, community, Section III)

Companion Animal

Anxiety r/t environmental and personal stressors

Impaired Comfort r/t insufficient environmental control

Compartment Syndrome

Fear r/t possible loss of limb, damage to limb

Acute Pain r/t pressure in compromised body part

Ineffective peripheral Tissue Perfusion r/t increased pressure within compartment

Compulsion

See OCD (Obsessive-Compulsive Disorder)

Conduction Disorders (Cardiac)

See Dysrhythmia

Confusion, Acute

Acute Confusion r/t older than 70 years of age with hospitalization, alcohol abuse, delirium, dementia, substance abuse

Frail Elderly syndrome r/t impaired memory

Risk for acute Confusion: Risk factor: alteration in level of consciousness

Confusion, Chronic

Chronic Confusion r/t dementia, Korsakoff's psychosis, multi-infarct dementia, cerebrovascular accident, head injury

Frail Elderly syndrome r/t impaired memory

Impaired Memory r/t fluid and electrolyte imbalance, neurological disturbances, excessive environmental disturbances, anemia, acute or chronic hypoxia, decreased cardiac output

Impaired Mood regulation r/t emotional instability

See Alzheimer's Disease; Dementia

Congenital Heart Disease/Cardiac Anomalies

Activity intolerance r/t fatigue, generalized weakness, lack of adequate oxygenation

Ineffective Breathing pattern r/t pulmonary vascular disease

Decreased Cardiac output r/t cardiac dysfunction

Excess Fluid volume r/t cardiac dysfunction, side effects of medication

Impaired Gas exchange r/t cardiac dysfunction, pulmonary congestion

Imbalanced Nutrition: less than body requirements r/t fatigue, generalized weakness, inability of infant to suck and feed, increased caloric requirements

Risk for delayed Development: Risk factor: inadequate oxygen and nutrients to tissues

Risk for deficient Fluid volume: Risk factor: side effects of diuretics

Risk for disorganized Infant behavior: Risk factor: invasive procedures

Risk for Poisoning: Risk factor: potential toxicity of cardiac medications

Risk for ineffective Thermoregulation: Risk factor: neonatal age

See Child with Chronic Condition; Hospitalized Child

Congestive Heart Failure (CHF)

See Heart Failure

Conjunctivitis

Acute Pain r/t inflammatory process

Vision Loss r/t change in visual acuity resulting from inflammation

Consciousness, Altered Level of

Acute Confusion r/t alcohol abuse, delirium, dementia, drug abuse, head injury

Chronic Confusion r/t multi-infarct dementia, Korsakoff's psychosis, head injury, cerebrovascular accident, neurological deficit

Functional urinary Incontinence r/t neurological dysfunction

Decreased Intracranial adaptive capacity r/t brain injury

Impaired Memory r/t neurological disturbances

Self-Care deficit: specify r/t neuromuscular impairment

Risk for Aspiration: Risk factors: impaired swallowing, loss of cough or gag reflex

Risk for Disuse syndrome: Risk factor: impaired mobility resulting from altered level of consciousness

C

C

Risk for Dry Mouth: Risk factor: inability to perform own oral care

Risk for Falls: Risk factor: diminished mental status

Risk for impaired Oral Mucous Membrane integrity: Risk factors: dry mouth, interrupted oral care

Risk for ineffective Cerebral tissue perfusion: Risk factors: increased intracranial pressure, altered cerebral perfusion

Risk for impaired Skin integrity: Risk factor: immobility

See Coma; Head Injury; Subarachnoid Hemorrhage; Intracranial Pressure, Increased

Constipation

Constipation (See **Constipation**, Section III)

Constipation, Chronic Functional

Constipation (See **Constipation**, chronic functional, Section III)

Constipation, Perceived

Perceived Constipation (See perceived **Constipation**, Section III)

Constipation, Risk for

Risk for Constipation (See **Constipation**, risk for, Section III)

Risk for chronic functional Constipation (See **Constipation**, chronic functional, risk for, Section III)

Contamination

Contamination (See **Contamination**, Section III)

Risk for Contamination (See **Contamination**, risk for, Section III)

Continent Ileostomy (Kock Pouch)

Ineffective Coping r/t stress of disease, exacerbations caused by stress

Imbalanced Nutrition: less than body requirements r/t malabsorption from disease process

Risk for Injury: Risk factors: failure of valve, stomal cyanosis, intestinal obstruction

Readiness for enhanced Knowledge: expresses an interest in learning

See Abdominal Surgery; Crohn's Disease

Contraceptive Method

Decisional Conflict: method of contraception r/t unclear personal values or beliefs, lack of experience or interference with decision-making, lack of relevant information, support system deficit

Ineffective Sexuality pattern r/t fear of pregnancy

Readiness for enhanced Health management: requesting information about available and appropriate birth control methods

Convulsions

Anxiety r/t concern over controlling convulsions

Impaired Memory r/t neurological disturbance

Risk for Aspiration: Risk factor: impaired swallowing

Risk for delayed Development: Risk factor: seizures

Risk for Injury: Risk factor: seizure activity

Readiness for enhanced Knowledge: expresses an interest in learning

See Seizure Disorders, Adult; Seizure Disorders, Childhood

COPD (Chronic Obstructive Pulmonary Disease)

Activity intolerance r/t imbalance between oxygen supply and demand

Ineffective Airway clearance r/t bronchoconstriction, increased mucus, ineffective cough, infection

Anxiety r/t breathlessness, change in health status

Death Anxiety r/t seriousness of medical condition, difficulty being able to "catch breath," feeling of suffocation

Interrupted Family processes r/t role changes

Impaired Gas exchange r/t ventilation-perfusion inequality

Ineffective Health management (See **Health** management, ineffective, Section III)

Imbalanced Nutrition: less than body requirements r/t decreased intake because of dyspnea, unpleasant taste in mouth left by medications, increased need for calories from work of breathing

Powerlessness r/t progressive nature of disease

Self-Care deficit: r/t fatigue from the increased work of breathing

Chronic low Self-Esteem r/t chronic illness

Sleep deprivation r/t breathing difficulties when lying down

Impaired Social interaction r/t social isolation because of oxygen use, activity intolerance

Chronic Sorrow r/t presence of chronic illness

Risk for Infection: Risk factor: stasis of respiratory secretions

Readiness for enhanced Health management (See **Health** management, readiness for enhanced, Section III)

Coping

Readiness for enhanced Coping (See **Coping**, readiness for enhanced, Section III)

Risk for Complicated Immigration Transition: Risk factors: insufficient knowledge about the process to access resources in the host country, insufficient social support in the host country, overt discrimination

Coping Problems

Compromised family Coping (see **Coping**, compromised family, Section III)

Defensive Coping (See **Coping**, defensive, Section III)

Disabled family Coping (See **Coping**, disabled family, Section III)

Ineffective Coping (See **Coping**, ineffective, Section III)

Ineffective community Coping (see **Coping**, ineffective community, Section III)

Corneal Injury

Risk for corneal Injury (See corneal **Injury**, risk for, Section III)

Corneal Reflex, Absent

Risk for Injury: Risk factors: accidental corneal abrasion, drying of cornea

Corneal Transplant

Risk for Surgical Site Infection: Risk factors: invasive procedure, surgery

Readiness for enhanced Health management: describes need to rest and avoid strenuous activities during healing phase

Coronary Artery Bypass Grafting (CABG)

Decreased Cardiac output r/t dysrhythmia, depressed cardiac function, change in preload, contractility or afterload

Fear r/t outcome of surgical procedure

Deficient Fluid volume r/t intraoperative blood loss, use of diuretics in surgery

Acute Pain r/t traumatic surgery

Risk for Perioperative Positioning injury: Risk factors: hypothermia, extended supine position

Risk for Surgical Site Infection: Risk factor: surgical incision

Risk for Impaired Tissue integrity: Risk factor: surgical procedure

Readiness for enhanced Knowledge: expresses an interest in learning

Costovertebral Angle Tenderness

See Kidney Stone; Pyelonephritis

Cough, Ineffective

Ineffective Airway clearance r/t decreased energy, fatigue, normal aging changes

See Bronchitis; COPD (Chronic Obstructive Pulmonary Disease); Pulmonary Edema

Crackles in Lungs, Coarse

Ineffective Airway clearance r/t excessive secretions in airways, ineffective cough

See Heart Failure; Pneumonia; Pulmonary Edema

Crackles in Lungs, Fine

Ineffective Breathing pattern r/t fatigue, surgery, decreased energy

See Bronchitis or Pneumonia (if from pulmonary infection); Congestive Heart Failure (CHF) (if cardiac in origin); Infection, potential for

Craniectomy/Craniotomy

Frail Elderly syndrome r/t alteration in cognition

Fear r/t threat to well-being

Decreased Intracranial adaptive capacity r/t brain injury, intracranial hypertension

Impaired Memory r/t neurological surgery

Acute Pain r/t recent brain surgery, increased intracranial pressure

Risk for ineffective Cerebral tissue perfusion: Risk factors: cerebral edema, increased intracranial pressure

Risk for Injury: Risk factor: potential confusion

See Coma (if relevant)

Crepitation, Subcutaneous

See Pneumothorax

Crisis

Anxiety r/t threat to or change in environment, health status, interaction patterns, situation, self-concept, or role functioning; threat of death of self or significant other

Death Anxiety r/t feelings of hopelessness associated with crisis

Compromised family Coping r/t situational or developmental crisis

Ineffective Coping r/t situational or maturational crisis

Fear r/t crisis situation

Grieving r/t potential significant loss

Impaired individual Resilience r/t onset of crisis

Situational low Self-Esteem r/t perception of inability to handle crisis

Stress overload (See **Stress** overload, Section III)

Risk for Spiritual distress: Risk factors: physical or psychological stress, natural disasters, situational losses, maturational losses

Crohn's Disease

Anxiety r/t change in health status

Ineffective Coping r/t repeated episodes of diarrhea

Diarrhea r/t inflammatory process

Ineffective Health maintenance r/t deficient knowledge regarding management of disease

Imbalanced Nutrition: less than body requirements r/t diarrhea, altered ability to digest and absorb food

Acute Pain r/t increased peristalsis

Powerlessness r/t chronic disease

Risk for deficient Fluid volume: Risk factor: abnormal fluid loss with diarrhea

Croup

See Respiratory Infections, Acute Childhood (Croup, Epiglottitis, Pertussis, Pneumonia, Respiratory)

Cryosurgery for Retinal Detachment

See Retinal Detachment

Cushing's Syndrome

Activity intolerance r/t fatigue, weakness

Disturbed Body Image r/t change in appearance from disease process

Excess Fluid volume r/t failure of regulatory mechanisms

Sexual dysfunction r/t loss of libido

Impaired Skin integrity r/t thin vulnerable skin from effects of increased cortisol

Risk for Infection: Risk factor: suppression of immune system caused by increased cortisol levels

Risk for Injury: Risk factors: decreased muscle strength, brittle bones

Readiness for enhanced Knowledge: expresses an interest in learning

Cuts (Wounds)

See Lacerations

CVA (Cerebrovascular Accident)

Anxiety r/t situational crisis, change in physical or emotional condition

Disturbed Body Image r/t chronic illness, paralysis

Caregiver Role Strain r/t cognitive problems of care receiver, need for significant home care

Impaired verbal Communication r/t pressure damage, decreased circulation to brain in speech center informational sources

Chronic Confusion r/t neurological changes

Constipation r/t decreased activity

Ineffective Coping r/t disability

Interrupted Family processes r/t illness, disability of family member

Frail Elderly syndrome r/t alteration in cognitive functioning

Grieving r/t loss of health

Impaired Home maintenance r/t neurological disease affecting ability to perform activities of daily living

Functional urinary Incontinence r/t neurological dysfunction

Reflex urinary Incontinence r/t loss of feeling to void

Impaired Memory r/t neurological disturbances

Impaired physical Mobility r/t loss of balance and coordination

Unilateral Neglect r/t disturbed perception from neurological damage

Self-Care deficit: specify r/t decreased strength and endurance, paralysis

Impaired Social interaction r/t limited physical mobility, limited ability to communicate

Impaired Swallowing r/t neuromuscular dysfunction

Impaired Transfer Ability r/t limited physical mobility

Vision Loss r/t pressure damage to visual centers in the brain (*see Appendix E on Evolve*)

Impaired Walking r/t loss of balance and coordination

Risk for Aspiration: Risk factors: impaired swallowing, loss of gag reflex

Risk for chronic functional Constipation: Risk factor: immobility

Risk for Disuse syndrome: Risk factor: paralysis

Risk for Falls: Risk factor: paralysis, decreased balance

Risk for Injury: Risk factors: vision loss, decreased tissue perfusion with loss of sensation

Risk for ineffective Cerebral tissue perfusion: Risk factor: clot, emboli, or hemorrhage from cerebral vessel

Risk for impaired Skin integrity: Risk factor: immobility

Readiness for enhanced Knowledge: expresses an interest in learning

Cyanosis, Central with Cyanosis of Oral Mucous Membranes

Impaired Gas exchange r/t alveolar-capillary membrane changes

Cyanosis, Peripheral with Cyanosis of Nail Beds

Ineffective peripheral Tissue Perfusion r/t interruption of arterial flow, severe vasoconstriction, cold temperatures

Cystic Fibrosis

Activity intolerance r/t imbalance between oxygen supply and demand

Ineffective Airway clearance r/t increased production of thick mucus

Anxiety r/t dyspnea, oxygen deprivation

Disturbed Body Image r/t changes in physical appearance, treatment of chronic lung disease (clubbing, barrel chest, home oxygen therapy)

Impaired Gas exchange r/t ventilation-perfusion imbalance

Impaired Home maintenance r/t extensive daily treatment, medications necessary for health

Imbalanced Nutrition: less than body requirements r/t anorexia; decreased absorption of nutrients, fat; increased work of breathing

Chronic Sorrow r/t presence of chronic disease

Risk for Caregiver Role Strain: Risk factors: illness severity of care receiver, unpredictable course of illness

Risk for deficient Fluid volume: Risk factors: decreased fluid intake, increased work of breathing

Risk for Infection: Risk factors: thick, tenacious mucus; harboring of bacterial organisms; immunocompromised state

Risk for Spiritual distress: Risk factor: presence of chronic disease

See Child with Chronic Condition; Hospitalized Child; Terminally Ill Child, Adolescent; Terminally Ill Child, Infant/Toddler; Terminally Ill Child, Preschool Child; Terminally Ill Child, School-Age Child/Preadolescent; Terminally Ill Child/Death of Child, Parent

Cystitis

Acute Pain: dysuria r/t inflammatory process in bladder and urethra

Impaired Urinary elimination: frequency r/t urinary tract infection

Urge urinary Incontinence: Risk factor: infection in bladder

Readiness for enhanced Knowledge: expresses an interest in learning

Cystocele

Stress urinary Incontinence r/t prolapsed bladder

Readiness for enhanced Knowledge: expresses an interest in learning

Cystoscopy

Urinary Retention r/t edema in urethra obstructing flow of urine

Risk for Infection: Risk factor: invasive procedure

Readiness for enhanced Knowledge: expresses an interest in learning

D

Deafness

Impaired verbal Communication r/t impaired hearing

Hearing Loss r/t alteration in sensory reception, transmission, integration

Risk for delayed Development: Risk factor: impaired hearing

Risk for Injury: Risk factor: alteration in sensory perception

Death

Risk for Sudden Infant Death (See **Sudden Infant Death**, risk for, Section III)

Death, Oncoming

Death Anxiety r/t unresolved issues surrounding dying

Compromised family Coping r/t client's inability to provide support to family

Ineffective Coping r/t personal vulnerability

Fear r/t threat of death

Grieving r/t loss of significant other

Powerlessness r/t effects of illness, oncoming death

Social isolation r/t altered state of wellness

Spiritual distress r/t intense suffering

Readiness for enhanced Spiritual well-being: desire of client and family to be in harmony with each other and higher power, God

See Terminally Ill Child, Adolescent; Terminally Ill Child, Infant/ Toddler; Terminally Ill Child, Preschool Child; Terminally Ill Child, School-Age Child/Preadolescent; Terminally Ill Child/Death of Child, Parent

Decisions, Difficulty Making

Decisional Conflict r/t support system deficit, perceived threat to value system, multiple or divergent sources of information, lack of relevant information, unclear personal values or beliefs

Risk for impaired Emancipated Decision-Making: Risk factor: insufficient self-confidence in decision-making

Readiness for enhanced Decision-Making (See **Decision-Making**, readiness for enhanced, Section III)

Decubitus Ulcer

See Pressure Ulcer

Deep Vein Thrombosis (DVT)

See DVT (Deep Vein Thrombosis); Venous Thromboembolism

Defensive Behavior

Defensive Coping r/t nonacceptance of blame, denial of problems or weakness

Ineffective Denial r/t inability to face situation realistically

Dehiscence, Abdominal

Fear r/t threat of death, severe dysfunction

Acute Pain r/t stretching of abdominal wall

Impaired Skin integrity r/t altered circulation, malnutrition, opening in incision

Delayed Surgical recovery r/t altered circulation, malnutrition, opening in incision

Impaired Tissue integrity r/t exposure of abdominal contents to external environment

Risk for deficient Fluid volume: Risk factor: altered circulation associated with opening of wound and exposure of abdominal contents

Risk for Surgical Site Infection: Risk factors: loss of skin integrity, open surgical wound

Dehydration

Deficient Fluid volume r/t active fluid volume loss

Impaired Oral Mucous Membrane integrity r/t decreased salivation, fluid deficit

Risk for chronic functional Constipation: Risk factor: decreased fluid volume

Risk for Dry Mouth: Risk factor: decreased fluid volume

Risk for ineffective Thermoregulation: Risk factor: decreased fluid volume

Risk for unstable Blood Pressure: Risk factor: hypotension caused by insufficient fluid volume

See Burns; Heat Stroke; Vomiting; Diarrhea

Delirium

Acute Confusion r/t effects of medication, response to hospitalization, alcohol abuse, substance abuse, sensory deprivation or overload, infection, polypharmacy

Impaired Memory r/t delirium

Sleep deprivation r/t sustained inadequate sleep hygiene

Risk for Injury: Risk factor: altered level of consciousness

Delirium Tremens (DT)

See Alcohol Withdrawal

Delivery

See Labor, Normal

Delusions

Impaired verbal Communication r/t psychological impairment, delusional thinking

Acute Confusion r/t alcohol abuse, delirium, dementia, substance abuse

Ineffective Coping r/t distortion and insecurity of life events

Fear r/t content of intrusive thoughts

Risk for other-directed Violence: Risk factor: delusional thinking

Risk for self-directed Violence: Risk factor: delusional thinking

Dementia

Chronic Confusion r/t neurological dysfunction

Interrupted Family processes r/t disability of family member

Frail Elderly syndrome r/t alteration in cognitive functioning

Impaired Home maintenance r/t inadequate support system, neurological dysfunction

D

Imbalanced Nutrition: less than body requirements r/t neurological impairment

Functional urinary Incontinence r/t neurological dysfunction

Insomnia r/t neurological impairment, naps during the day

Impaired physical Mobility r/t alteration in cognitive function

Self-Neglect r/t cognitive impairment

Self-Care deficit: specify r/t psychological or neuromuscular impairment

Chronic Sorrow: Significant other r/t chronic long-standing disability, loss of mental function

Impaired Swallowing r/t neuromuscular changes associated with long-standing dementia

Risk for Caregiver Role Strain: Risk factors: number of caregiving tasks, duration of caregiving required

Risk for Chronic Functional Constipation: Risk factor: decreased fluid intake

Risk for Falls: Risk factor: diminished mental status

Risk for Frail Elderly syndrome: Risk factors: cognitive impairment

Risk for Injury: Risk factors: confusion, decreased muscle coordination

Risk for impaired Skin integrity: Risk factors: altered nutritional status, immobility

Denial of Health Status

Ineffective Denial r/t lack of perception about the health status effects of illness

Ineffective Health management r/t denial of seriousness of health situation

Dental Caries

Impaired Dentition r/t ineffective oral hygiene, barriers to self-care, economic barriers to professional care, nutritional deficits, dietary habits

Ineffective Health maintenance r/t lack of knowledge regarding prevention of dental disease

Depression (Major Depressive Disorder)

Death Anxiety r/t feelings of lack of self-worth

Constipation r/t inactivity, decreased fluid intake

Fatigue r/t psychological demands

Ineffective Health maintenance r/t lack of ability to make good judgments regarding ways to obtain help

Hopelessness r/t feeling of abandonment, long-term stress

Impaired Mood Regulation r/t emotional instability

Insomnia r/t inactivity

Self-Neglect r/t depression, cognitive impairment

Powerlessness r/t pattern of helplessness

Chronic low Self-Esteem r/t repeated unmet expectations

Sexual dysfunction r/t loss of sexual desire

Social isolation r/t ineffective coping

Chronic Sorrow r/t unresolved grief

Risk for complicated Grieving: Risk factor: lack of previous resolution of former grieving response

Risk for Suicide: Risk factor: grieving, hopelessness

Dermatitis

Anxiety r/t situational crisis imposed by illness

Impaired Comfort r/t itching

Impaired Skin integrity r/t side effect of medication, allergic reaction

Readiness for enhanced Knowledge: expresses an interest in learning

See Itching

Despondency

Hopelessness r/t long-term stress

See Depression (Major Depressive Disorder)

Destructive Behavior Toward Others

Risk-prone Health behavior r/t intense emotional state

Ineffective Coping r/t situational crises, maturational crises, disturbance in pattern of appraisal of threat

Risk for other-directed Violence (See **Violence**, other-directed, risk for, Section III)

Developmental Concerns

Risk for delayed Development (See **Development**, delayed, risk for, Section III)

See Growth and Development Lag

Diabetes in Pregnancy

See Gestational Diabetes (Diabetes in Pregnancy)

Diabetes Insipidus

Deficient Fluid volume r/t inability to conserve fluid

Ineffective Health maintenance r/t deficient knowledge regarding care of disease, importance of medications

Diabetes Mellitus

Ineffective Health maintenance r/t complexity of therapeutic regimen

Ineffective Health management (See **Health** management, ineffective, Section III)

Imbalanced Nutrition: less than body requirements r/t inability to use glucose (type 1 [insulin-dependent] diabetes)

Risk for Overweight: Risk factor: excessive intake of nutrients (type 2 diabetes)

Ineffective peripheral Tissue perfusion r/t impaired arterial circulation

Powerlessness r/t perceived lack of personal control

Sexual dysfunction r/t neuropathy associated with disease

Vision Loss r/t ineffective tissue perfusion of retina

Risk for unstable blood Glucose level (See **Glucose** level, blood, unstable, risk for, Section III)

Risk for Infection: Risk factors: hyperglycemia, impaired healing, circulatory changes

Risk for Injury: Risk factors: hypoglycemia or hyperglycemia from failure to consume adequate calories, failure to take insulin

Risk for dysfunctional Gastrointestinal motility: Risk factor: complication of diabetes

Risk for Metabolic Imbalance syndrome: Risk factor: complication of diabetes

Risk for impaired Skin integrity: Risk factor: loss of pain perception in extremities

Risk for delayed Surgical recovery: Risk factor: impaired healing due to circulatory changes

Readiness for enhanced Health literacy: expresses desire to enhance understanding of health information to make health care choices

Readiness for enhanced Health management (See **Health** management, readiness for enhanced, Section III)

Readiness for enhanced Knowledge: expresses an interest in learning

See Hyperglycemia; Hypoglycemia

Diabetes Mellitus, Juvenile (Insulin-Dependent Diabetes Mellitus Type 1)

Risk-prone Health behavior r/t inadequate comprehension, inadequate social support, low self-efficacy, impaired adjustment attributable to adolescent maturational crises

Disturbed Body Image r/t imposed deviations from bio-physical and psychosocial norm, perceived differences from peers

Impaired Comfort r/t insulin injections, peripheral blood glucose testing

Ineffective Health maintenance r/t (See **Health** maintenance, ineffective, Section III)

Imbalanced Nutrition: less than body requirements r/t inability of body to adequately metabolize and use glucose and nutrients, increased caloric needs of child to promote growth and physical activity participation with peers

Risk for Metabolic Imbalance syndrome: Risk factor: complication of diabetes

Readiness for enhanced Knowledge: expresses an interest in learning

See Diabetes Mellitus; Child with Chronic Condition; Hospitalized Child

Diabetic Coma

Acute Confusion r/t hyperglycemia, presence of excessive metabolic acids

Deficient Fluid volume r/t hyperglycemia resulting in polyuria

Ineffective Health management r/t lack of understanding of preventive measures, adequate blood glucose control

Risk for unstable blood Glucose level (See **Glucose** level, blood, unstable, risk for, Section III)

Risk for Infection: Risk factors: hyperglycemia, changes in vascular system

See Diabetes Mellitus

Diabetic Ketoacidosis

See Ketoacidosis, Diabetic

Diabetic Neuropathy

See Neuropathy, Peripheral

Diabetic Retinopathy

Grieving r/t loss of vision

Ineffective Health maintenance r/t deficient knowledge regarding preserving vision with treatment if possible, use of low-vision aids

See Vision Impairment; Blindness

Dialysis

See Hemodialysis; Peritoneal Dialysis

Diaphragmatic Hernia

See Hiatal Hernia

Diarrhea

Diarrhea r/t infection, change in diet, gastrointestinal disorders, stress, medication effect, impaction

Deficient Fluid volume r/t excessive loss of fluids in liquid stools

Risk for Electrolyte imbalance: Risk factor: effect of loss of electrolytes from frequent stools

DIC (Disseminated Intravascular Coagulation)

Fear r/t threat to well-being

Deficient Fluid volume: hemorrhage r/t depletion of clotting factors

Risk for Bleeding: Risk factors: microclotting within vascular system, depleted clotting factors

Digitalis Toxicity

Decreased Cardiac output r/t drug toxicity affecting cardiac rhythm, rate

Ineffective Health management r/t deficient knowledge regarding action, appropriate method of administration of digitalis

Dignity, Loss of

Risk for compromised Human Dignity (See **Human Dignity**, compromised, risk for, Section III)

Dilation and Curettage (D&C)

Acute Pain r/t uterine contractions

Risk for Bleeding: Risk factor: surgical procedure

Risk for Surgical Site Infection: Risk factor: surgical procedure

Risk for ineffective Sexuality pattern: Risk factors: painful coitus, fear associated with surgery on genital area

Readiness for enhanced Knowledge: expresses an interest in learning

Dirty Body (for Prolonged Period)

Self-Neglect r/t mental illness, substance abuse, cognitive impairment

Discharge Planning

Impaired Home Maintenance r/t family member's disease or injury interfering with home maintenance

D

Deficient Knowledge r/t lack of exposure to information for home care

Relocation stress syndrome: Risk factors: insufficient predeparture counseling, insufficient support system, unpredictability of experience

Readiness for enhanced Health literacy: expresses desire to enhance understanding of health information to make health care choices

Readiness for enhanced Knowledge: expresses an interest in learning

Discomforts of Pregnancy

Disturbed Body Image r/t pregnancy-induced body changes

Impaired Comfort r/t enlarged abdomen, swollen feet

Fatigue r/t hormonal, metabolic, body changes

Stress urinary Incontinence r/t enlarged uterus, fetal movement

Insomnia r/t psychological stress, fetal movement, muscular cramping, urinary frequency, shortness of breath

Nausea r/t hormone effect

Acute Pain: headache r/t hormonal changes of pregnancy

Acute Pain: leg cramps r/t nerve compression, calcium/phosphorus/potassium imbalance

Risk for Constipation: Risk factors: decreased intestinal motility, inadequate fiber in diet

Risk for Injury: Risk factors: faintness and/or syncope caused by vasomotor lability or postural hypotension, venous stasis in lower extremities

Dislocation of Joint

Acute Pain r/t dislocation of a joint

Self-Care deficit: r/t inability to use a joint

Risk for Injury: Risk factor: unstable joint

Dissecting Aneurysm

Fear r/t threat to well-being

See Abdominal Surgery; Aneurysm, Abdominal Aortic Repair

Disseminated Intravascular Coagulation (DIC)

See DIC (Disseminated Intravascular Coagulation)

Dissociative Identity Disorder (Not Otherwise Specified)

Anxiety r/t psychosocial stress

Ineffective Coping r/t personal vulnerability in crisis of accurate self-perception

Disturbed personal Identity r/t inability to distinguish self-caused by multiple personality disorder, depersonalization, disturbance in memory

Impaired Memory r/t altered state of consciousness

See Multiple Personality Disorder (Dissociative Identity Disorder)

Distress

Anxiety r/t situational crises, maturational crises

Death Anxiety r/t denial of one's own mortality or impending death

Disuse Syndrome, Potential to Develop

Risk for Disuse syndrome: Risk factors: paralysis, mechanical immobilization, prescribed immobilization, severe pain, altered level of consciousness

Diversional Activity Engagement, Lack of

Decreased Diversional activity engagement r/t environmental lack of diversional activity as in frequent hospitalizations, lengthy treatments

Diverticulitis

Constipation r/t dietary deficiency of fiber and roughage

Diarrhea r/t increased intestinal motility caused by inflammation

Deficient Knowledge r/t diet needed to control disease, medication regimen

Imbalanced Nutrition: less than body requirements r/t loss of appetite

Acute Pain r/t inflammation of bowel

Risk for deficient Fluid Volume: Risk factor: diarrhea

Dizziness

Decreased Cardiac output r/t alteration in heart rate and rhythm, altered stroke volume

Deficient Knowledge r/t actions to take to prevent or modify dizziness and prevent falls

Impaired physical Mobility r/t dizziness

Risk for Falls: Risk factor: difficulty maintaining balance

Risk for ineffective Cerebral tissue perfusion: Risk factor: interruption of cerebral arterial blood flow

Domestic Violence

Impaired verbal Communication r/t psychological barriers of fear

Compromised family Coping r/t abusive patterns

Defensive Coping r/t low self-esteem

Dysfunctional Family processes r/t inadequate coping skills

Fear r/t threat to self-concept, situational crisis of abuse

Insomnia r/t psychological stress

Post-Trauma syndrome r/t history of abuse

Powerlessness r/t lifestyle of helplessness

Situational low Self-Esteem r/t negative family interactions

Risk for compromised Resilience: Risk factor: effects of abuse

Risk for other-directed Violence: Risk factor: history of abuse

Down Syndrome

See Child with Chronic Condition; Intellectual Disability

Dress Self (Inability to)

Dressing Self-Care deficit r/t intolerance to activity, decreased strength and endurance, pain, discomfort, perceptual or cognitive impairment, neuromuscular impairment, musculoskeletal impairment, depression, severe anxiety

Dribbling of Urine

Overflow urinary Incontinence r/t degenerative changes in pelvic muscles and urinary structures

Stress urinary Incontinence r/t degenerative changes in pelvic muscles and urinary structures

Drooling

Impaired Swallowing r/t neuromuscular impairment, mechanical obstruction

Risk for Aspiration: Risk factor: impaired swallowing

Dropout from School

Impaired individual Resilience (See **Resilience**, individual, impaired, Section III)

Anxiety r/t conflict about life goals

Ineffective Coping r/t inadequate resources

Drug Abuse

See Substance Abuse

Drug Withdrawal

See Acute Substance Withdrawal Syndrome

Dry Eye

Risk for dry Eye: Risk factors: (See dry **Eye**, risk for, Section III)

Risk for Corneal Injury: Risk factor: suppressed corneal reflex

Readiness for enhanced Knowledge: expresses an interest in learning

See Conjunctivitis; Keratoconjunctivitis Sicca (Dry Eye Syndrome)

Dry Mouth

Risk for Dry Mouth: Risk factors: (See **Dry Mouth**, risk for, Section III)

Risk for impaired Oral Mucous Membrane integrity: Risk factor: reduced quality or quantity of saliva caused by decreased fluid volume

DT (Delirium Tremens)

See Alcohol Withdrawal

DVT (Deep Vein Thrombosis)

Constipation r/t inactivity, bed rest

Impaired physical Mobility r/t pain in extremity

Acute Pain r/t vascular inflammation, edema

Ineffective peripheral Tissue perfusion r/t deficient knowledge of aggravating factors

Delayed Surgical recovery r/t impaired physical mobility

Readiness for enhanced Knowledge: expresses an interest in learning

Risk for ineffective Thermoregulation: Risk factor: inactivity

See Anticoagulant Therapy; Venous Thromboembolism, risk for (See Section III)

Dying Client

See Terminally Ill Adult; Terminally Ill Adolescent; Terminally Ill Child, Infant/Toddler; Terminally Ill Child, Preschool Child; Terminally Ill Child, School-Age Child/Preadolescent; Terminally Ill Child/Death of Child, Parent

Dysfunctional Eating Pattern

Imbalanced Nutrition: less than body requirements r/t psychological factors

Risk for Overweight: Risk factor: psychological factors

See Anorexia Nervosa; Bulimia; Maturational Issues, Adolescent; Obesity

Dysfunctional Family Unit

See Family Problems

Dysfunctional Ventilatory Weaning

Dysfunctional Ventilatory weaning response r/t physical, psychological, situational factors

Dysmenorrhea

Nausea r/t prostaglandin effect

Acute Pain r/t cramping from hormonal effects

Readiness for enhanced Knowledge: expresses an interest in learning

Dyspareunia

Sexual Dysfunction r/t lack of lubrication during intercourse, alteration in reproductive organ function

Dyspepsia

Anxiety r/t pressures of personal role

Acute Pain r/t gastrointestinal disease, consumption of irritating foods

Readiness for enhanced Knowledge: expresses an interest in learning

Dysphagia

Impaired Swallowing r/t neuromuscular impairment

Risk for Aspiration: Risk factor: loss of gag or cough reflex

Dysphasia

Impaired verbal Communication r/t decrease in circulation to brain

Impaired Social interaction r/t difficulty in communicating

Dyspnea

Activity intolerance r/t imbalance between oxygen supply and demand

Ineffective Breathing pattern r/t compromised cardiac or pulmonary function, decreased lung expansion, neurological impairment affecting respiratory center, extreme anxiety

Fear r/t threat to state of well-being, potential death

Impaired Gas exchange r/t alveolar-capillary damage

Insomnia r/t difficulty breathing, positioning required for effective breathing

Sleep deprivation r/t ineffective breathing pattern

Dysrhythmia

Activity intolerance r/t decreased cardiac output

Decreased Cardiac output r/t alteration in heart rate, rhythm

Fear r/t threat of death, change in health status

Risk for ineffective Cerebral tissue perfusion: Risk factor: decreased blood supply to the brain from dysrhythmia

Risk for unstable Blood Pressure r/t cardiac arrhythmia and electrolyte imbalance

Readiness for enhanced Knowledge: expresses an interest in learning

Dysthymic Disorder

Ineffective Coping r/t impaired social interaction

Ineffective Health maintenance r/t inability to make good judgments regarding ways to obtain help

Insomnia r/t anxious thoughts

Chronic low Self-Esteem r/t repeated unmet expectations

Ineffective Sexuality pattern r/t loss of sexual desire

Social Isolation r/t ineffective coping

See Depression (Major Depressive Disorder)

Dystocia

Anxiety r/t difficult labor, deficient knowledge regarding normal labor pattern

Ineffective Coping r/t situational crisis

Fatigue r/t prolonged labor

Grieving r/t loss of ideal labor experience

Acute Pain r/t difficult labor, medical interventions

Powerlessness r/t perceived inability to control outcome of labor

Risk for Bleeding: Risk factor: hemorrhage secondary to uterine atony

Risk for ineffective Cerebral tissue perfusion (fetal): Risk factor: difficult labor and birth

Risk for delayed Development: infant: Risk factor: difficult labor and birth

Risk for Infection: Risk factor: prolonged rupture of membranes

Risk for impaired Tissue integrity (maternal and fetal): Risk factor: difficult labor

Dysuria

Impaired Urinary elimination r/t infection/inflammation of the urinary tract

Risk for urge urinary Incontinence: Risk factor: detrusor hyperreflexia from infection in the urinary tract

Acute Pain r/t infection/inflammation of the urinary tract

E

Ear Surgery

Acute Pain r/t edema in ears from surgery

Hearing Loss r/t invasive surgery of ears, dressings

Risk for delayed Development: Risk factor: hearing impairment

Risk for Falls: Risk factor: dizziness from excessive stimuli to vestibular apparatus

Readiness for enhanced Knowledge: expresses an interest in learning

See Hospitalized Child

Earache

Acute Pain r/t trauma, edema, infection

Hearing Loss r/t altered sensory reception, transmission

Eating Dynamics, Adolescent

Imbalanced Nutrition: less than body requirements r/t negative perception of one's body

Ineffective Adolescent Eating Dynamics r/t altered family dynamics, eating disorder, excessive stress

Risk for Overweight: Risk factor: Media influence resulting in unhealthy choices, insufficient interest in physical activity

Readiness for enhanced Health literacy: expresses desire to learn to make healthy food choices

Eating Dynamics, Child

Imbalanced Nutrition: less than body requirements r/t excessive of parental control over quantity and choices of foods

Ineffective Child Eating Dynamics r/t bribing child to eat, forcing child to eat

Risk for delayed Development: Risk factor: inadequate nutrition to meet metabolic needs for normal development

Risk for Overweight: Risk factors: unhealthy choices, frequent snacking, low physical activity

Eating Dynamics, Infant

See Feeding Dynamics, Infant

Eclampsia

Interrupted Family processes r/t unmet expectations for pregnancy and childbirth

Fear r/t threat of well-being to self and fetus

Risk for Aspiration: Risk factor: seizure activity

Risk for ineffective Cerebral tissue perfusion: fetal: Risk factor: uteroplacental insufficiency

Risk for delayed Development: Risk factor: uteroplacental insufficiency

Risk for excess Fluid volume: Risk factor: decreased urine output as a result of renal dysfunction

Risk for unstable Blood Pressure: Risk factor: hypertension caused by excess fluid volume

ECMO (Extracorporeal Membrane Oxygenator)

Death Anxiety r/t emergency condition, hemorrhage

Decreased Cardiac output r/t altered contractility of the heart

Impaired Gas exchange (See **Gas** exchange, impaired, Section III)

See Respiratory Conditions of the Neonate

ECT (Electroconvulsive Therapy)

Decisional Conflict r/t lack of relevant information

Fear r/t real or imagined threat to well-being

Impaired Memory r/t effects of treatment

See Depression (Major Depressive Disorder)

Ectopic Pregnancy

Death Anxiety r/t emergency condition, hemorrhage

Disturbed Body Image r/t negative feelings about body and reproductive functioning

Fear r/t threat to self, surgery, implications for future pregnancy

Acute Pain r/t stretching or rupture of implantation site

Ineffective Role performance r/t loss of pregnancy

Situational low Self-Esteem r/t loss of pregnancy, inability to carry pregnancy to term

Chronic Sorrow r/t loss of pregnancy, potential loss of fertility

Risk for Bleeding: Risk factor: possible rupture of implantation site, surgical trauma

Risk for ineffective Coping: Risk factor: loss of pregnancy

Risk for interrupted Family processes: Risk factor: situational crisis

Risk for Infection: Risk factors: traumatized tissue, surgical procedure

Risk for Spiritual distress: Risk factor: grief process

Eczema

Disturbed Body Image r/t change in appearance from inflamed skin

Impaired Comfort: pruritus r/t inflammation of skin

Impaired Skin integrity r/t side effect of medication, allergic reaction

Readiness for enhanced Knowledge: expresses an interest in learning

ED (Erectile Dysfunction)

See Erectile Dysfunction (ED); Impotence

Edema

Excess Fluid volume r/t excessive fluid intake, cardiac dysfunction, renal dysfunction, loss of plasma proteins

Ineffective Health maintenance r/t deficient knowledge regarding treatment of edema

Risk for impaired Skin integrity: Risk factors: impaired circulation, fragility of skin

See Heart Failure; Renal Failure

Elder Abuse

See Abuse, Spouse, Parent, or Significant Other

Elderly

See Aging; Frail Elderly Syndrome

Electroconvulsive Therapy

See ECT (Electroconvulsive Therapy)

Electrolyte Imbalance

Risk for Electrolyte imbalance (See **Electrolyte imbalance**, risk for, Section III)

Risk for unstable Blood Pressure: Risk factor: fluid volume changes

Emaciated Person

Frail Elderly syndrome r/t living alone, malnutrition, alteration in cognitive functioning

Imbalanced Nutrition: less than body requirements r/t inability to ingest food, digest food, absorb nutrients because of biological, psychological, economic factors

Emancipated Decision-Making, Impaired

Risk for impaired emancipated Decision-Making: Risk factor: inability or unwillingness to verbalize needs and wants

Readiness for enhanced emancipated Decision-Making: expresses desire to enhance decision-making process

Embolectomy

Fear r/t threat of great bodily harm from embolus

Ineffective peripheral Tissue Perfusion r/t presence of embolus

Risk for Bleeding: Risk factors: postoperative complication, surgical area

See Surgery, Postoperative Care

Emboli

See Pulmonary Embolism (PE)

Embolism in Leg or Arm

Ineffective peripheral Tissue Perfusion r/t arterial/venous obstruction from clot

See DVT (Deep Vein Thrombosis)

Emesis

Nausea (See **Nausea**, Section III)

See Vomiting

Emotional Problems

See Coping Problems

Empathy

Readiness for enhanced community Coping: social supports, being available for problem solving

Readiness for enhanced family Coping: basic needs met, desire to move to higher level of health

Readiness for enhanced Spiritual Well-Being: desire to establish interconnectedness through spirituality

Emphysema

See COPD (Chronic Obstructive Pulmonary Disease)

Emptiness

Social isolation r/t inability to engage in satisfying personal relationships

Chronic Sorrow r/t unresolved grief

Spiritual distress r/t separation from religious or cultural ties

Encephalitis

See Meningitis/Encephalitis

Endocardial Cushion Defect

See Congenital Heart Disease/Cardiac Anomalies

Endocarditis

Activity intolerance r/t reduced cardiac reserve, prescribed bed rest

E

E

Decreased Cardiac output r/t inflammation of lining of heart and change in structure of valve leaflets, increased myocardial workload

Risk for imbalanced Nutrition: less than body requirements: Risk factors: fever, hypermetabolic state associated with fever

Risk for ineffective Cerebral tissue perfusion: Risk factor: possible presence of emboli in cerebral circulation

Risk for ineffective peripheral Tissue perfusion: Risk factor: possible presence of emboli in peripheral circulation

Readiness for enhanced Knowledge: expresses an interest in learning

Endometriosis

Grieving r/t possible infertility

Nausea r/t prostaglandin effect

Acute Pain r/t onset of menses with distention of endometrial tissue

Sexual dysfunction r/t painful intercourse

Readiness for enhanced Knowledge: expresses an interest in learning

Endometritis

Anxiety r/t, fear of unknown

Ineffective Thermoregulation r/t infectious process

Acute Pain r/t infectious process in reproductive tract

Readiness for enhanced Knowledge: expresses an interest in learning

Enuresis

Ineffective Health maintenance r/t unachieved developmental task, neuromuscular immaturity, diseases of urinary system

See Toilet Training

Environmental Interpretation Problems

See Chronic Confusion

Epididymitis

Anxiety r/t situational crisis, pain, threat to future fertility

Acute Pain r/t inflammation in scrotal sac

Ineffective Sexuality pattern r/t edema of epididymis and testes

Readiness for enhanced Knowledge: expresses an interest in learning

Epiglottitis

See Respiratory Infections, Acute Childhood (Croup, Epiglottitis, Pertussis, Pneumonia, Respiratory Syncytial Virus)

Epilepsy

Anxiety r/t threat to role functioning

Ineffective Health management r/t deficient knowledge regarding seizure control

Impaired Memory r/t seizure activity

Risk for Aspiration: Risk factors: impaired swallowing, excessive secretions

Risk for delayed Development: Risk factor: seizure disorder

Risk for Injury: Risk factor: environmental factors during seizure

Readiness for enhanced Knowledge: expresses an interest in learning

See Seizure Disorders, Adult; Seizure Disorders, Childhood (Epilepsy, Febrile Seizures, Infantile Spasms)

Episiotomy

Anxiety r/t fear of pain

Disturbed Body Image r/t fear of resuming sexual relations

Impaired physical Mobility r/t pain, swelling, tissue trauma

Acute Pain r/t tissue trauma

Sexual dysfunction r/t altered body structure, tissue trauma

Impaired Skin integrity r/t perineal incision

Risk for Infection: Risk factor: tissue trauma

Epistaxis

Fear r/t large amount of blood loss

Risk for deficient Fluid volume: Risk factor: excessive blood loss

Epstein-Barr Virus

See Mononucleosis

Erectile Dysfunction (ED)

Situational low Self-Esteem r/t physiological crisis, inability to practice usual sexual activity

Sexual dysfunction r/t altered body function

Readiness for enhanced Knowledge: information regarding treatment for erectile dysfunction

See Impotence

Escherichia coli Infection

Fear r/t serious illness, unknown outcome

Deficient Knowledge r/t how to prevent disease; care of self with serious illness

See Gastroenteritis; Gastroenteritis, Child; Hospitalized Child

Esophageal Varices

Fear r/t threat of death from hematemesis

Risk for Bleeding: Risk factors: portal hypertension, distended variceal vessels that can easily rupture

See Cirrhosis

Esophagitis

Acute Pain r/t inflammation of esophagus

Readiness for enhanced Knowledge: expresses an interest in learning

Evisceration

See Dehiscence, Abdominal

Exhaustion

Impaired individual Resilience (See **Resilience**, individual, impaired, Section III)

Disturbed Sleep pattern (See **Sleep** pattern, disturbed, Section III)

Exposure to Hot or Cold Environment

Hyperthermia r/t exposure to hot environment, abnormal reaction to anesthetics

Hypothermia r/t exposure to cold environment

Risk for ineffective Thermoregulation: Risk factors: extremes of environmental temperature, inappropriate clothing for environmental temperature

External Fixation

Disturbed Body Image r/t trauma, change to affected part

Risk for Infection: Risk factor: presence of pins inserted into bone

See Fracture

Extracorporeal Membrane Oxygenator (ECMO)

See ECMO (Extracorporeal Membrane Oxygenator)

Eye Discomfort

Risk for dry Eye (See **Eye,** dry, risk for, Section III)

Risk for corneal Injury: Risk factors: exposure of the eyeball, blinking less than five times per minute

Eye Surgery

Anxiety r/t possible loss of vision

Self-Care deficit: specify r/t impaired vision

Vision Loss r/t surgical procedure, eye pathology

Risk for Injury: Risk factor: impaired vision

Readiness for enhanced Knowledge: expresses an interest in learning

See Hospitalized Child

F

Failure to Thrive, Child

Disorganized Infant behavior (See **Infant** behavior, disorganized, Section III)

Ineffective Child Eating dynamics r/t lack of knowledge or resources regarding nutritional needs of child

Ineffective Infant Feeding dynamics r/t lack of knowledge regarding nutritional needs of infant

Insomnia r/t inconsistency of caretaker; lack of quiet, consistent environment

Imbalanced Nutrition: less than body requirements r/t inadequate type or amounts of food for infant or child, inappropriate feeding techniques

Impaired Parenting r/t lack of parenting skills, inadequate role modeling

Chronic low Self-Esteem: parental r/t feelings of inadequacy, support system deficiencies, inadequate role model

Social isolation r/t limited support systems, self-imposed situation

Risk for impaired Attachment: Risk factor: inability of parents to meet infant's needs

Risk for delayed Development (See **Development**, delayed, risk for, Section III)

Readiness for enhanced Knowledge: parent expresses willingness to learn how to meet **infant/child nutritional needs**

Falls, Risk for

Risk for Falls (See **Falls,** risk for, Section III)

Family Problems

Compromised family Coping (See **Coping,** family, compromised, Section III)

Disabled family Coping (See **Coping,** family, disabled, Section III)

Interrupted Family processes r/t situation transition and/or crises, developmental transition and/or crises

Ineffective family Health management (See family **Health** management, ineffective, Section III)

Readiness for enhanced family Coping: needs sufficiently gratified, adaptive tasks effectively addressed to enable goals of self-actualization to surface

Family Process

Dysfunctional Family processes (See **Family** processes, dysfunctional, Section III)

Interrupted Family processes (See **Family** processes, interrupted, Section III)

Readiness for enhanced Family processes (See **Family** processes, readiness for enhanced, Section III)

Readiness for enhanced Relationship (See **Relationship,** readiness for enhanced, Section III)

Fatigue

Fatigue (See **Fatigue,** Section III)

Fear

Death Anxiety r/t fear of death

Fear r/t identifiable physical or psychological threat to person

Febrile Seizures

See Seizure Disorders, Childhood (Epilepsy, Febrile Seizures, Infantile Spasms)

Fecal Impaction

See Impaction of Stool

(See **Constipation,** Section III)

(See **Constipation,** chronic functional, Section III)

Fecal Incontinence

Bowel Incontinence r/t neurological impairment, gastrointestinal disorders, anorectal trauma, weakened perineal muscles

Feeding Dynamics, Infant

Ineffective Infant Eating Dynamics r/t inappropriate transition to sold foods

Risk for Caregiver Role Strain: Risk factor: fatigue leading to ineffective or insufficient feeding

Risk for impaired Attachment: Risk factor: inability physically or psychologically to meet nutritional needs of newborn

Risk for impaired Parenting: Risk factors: stress, sleep deprivation, insufficient knowledge, and/or social isolation

Readiness for enhanced Health literacy: expresses a desire to enhance knowledge of appropriate feeding dynamics for each developmental stage (See **Ineffective Feeding Dynamics,** Infant, Section III)

F

Feeding Problems, Newborn

Ineffective Breastfeeding (See **Breastfeeding**, ineffective, Section III)

Ineffective Infant Feeding Dynamics r/t attachment issues, lack of knowledge of appropriate methods of feeding infant for each stage of development

Insufficient Breast Milk Production (See **Breast Milk Production**, insufficient, Section III)

Disorganized Infant behavior r/t prematurity, immature neurological system

Ineffective Infant Feeding dynamics r/t parental lack of knowledge of appropriate feeding methods for each stage of development

Ineffective infant Feeding pattern r/t prematurity, neurological impairment or delay, oral hypersensitivity, prolonged nothing-by-mouth status

Impaired Swallowing r/t prematurity

Neonatal Abstinence syndrome: At-risk population: in utero substance exposure secondary to maternal substance use

Risk for delayed Development: Risk factor: inadequate nutrition

Risk for deficient Fluid volume: Risk factor: inability to take in adequate amount of fluids

Female Genital Mutilation

Acute Pain r/t traumatic surgical procedure

Anxiety r/t situational crisis

Disturbed Body Image r/t scarring, changes in body function

Fear r/t threat to well-being

Powerlessness r/t absence of control of decision-making

Impaired Skin Integrity r/t traumatic surgical procedure

Impaired Tissue Integrity r/t wound, potential for infection

Risk for compromised Human Dignity: Risk factor: dehumanizing treatment

Risk for Infection: Risk factor: invasive procedure

Risk for Post-Trauma Syndrome: Risk factor: experiencing traumatic surgery

Risk for chronic low Self-Esteem: Risk factor: cultural incongruence (See **Female Genital Mutilation**, Risk for, Section III)

Femoral Popliteal Bypass

Anxiety r/t threat to or change in health status

Acute Pain r/t surgical trauma, edema in surgical area

Ineffective peripheral Tissue Perfusion r/t impaired arterial circulation

Risk for Bleeding: Risk factor: surgery on arteries

Risk for Surgical Site Infection: Risk factor: invasive procedure

Fetal Alcohol Syndrome

See Neonatal Abstinence Syndrome

Fetal Distress/Nonreassuring Fetal Heart Rate Pattern

Fear r/t threat to fetus

Ineffective peripheral Tissue Perfusion: fetal r/t interruption of umbilical cord blood flow

Fever

Ineffective Thermoregulation r/t infectious process

Fibrocystic Breast Disease

See Breast Lumps

Filthy Home Environment

Impaired Home maintenance (See **Home** maintenance, impaired, Section III)

Self-Neglect r/t mental illness, substance abuse, cognitive impairment

Financial Crisis in the Home Environment

Impaired Home maintenance r/t insufficient finances

Fistulectomy

See Hemorrhoidectomy

Flail Chest

Ineffective Breathing pattern r/t chest trauma

Fear r/t difficulty breathing

Impaired Gas exchange r/t loss of effective lung function

Impaired spontaneous Ventilation r/t paradoxical respirations

Flashbacks

Post-Trauma syndrome r/t catastrophic event

Flat Affect

Hopelessness r/t prolonged activity restriction creating isolation, failing or deteriorating physiological condition, long-term stress, abandonment, lost belief in transcendent values or higher power or God

Risk for Loneliness: Risk factors: social isolation, lack of interest in surroundings

See Depression (Major Depressive Disorder); Dysthymic Disorder

Fluid Volume Deficit

Deficient Fluid volume r/t active fluid loss, vomiting, diarrhea, failure of regulatory mechanisms

Risk for Shock: Risk factors: hypovolemia, sepsis, systemic inflammatory response syndrome (SIRS)

Risk for unstable Blood Pressure: Risk factor: hypotension, excessive loss or insufficient intake of fluid

Fluid Volume Excess

Excess Fluid volume r/t compromised regulatory mechanism, excess sodium intake

Risk for unstable Blood Pressure: Risk factor: hypertension, excessive intake or retention of fluid

Fluid Volume Imbalance, Risk for

Risk for imbalanced Fluid volume: Risk factor: major invasive surgeries

Food Allergies

Diarrhea r/t immune effects of offending food on gastrointestinal system

Risk for Allergic reaction: Risk factor: specific foods

Readiness for enhanced Knowledge: expresses an interest in learning

See Anaphylactic Shock

Foodborne Illness

Diarrhea r/t infectious material in gastrointestinal tract

Deficient Fluid volume r/t active fluid loss from vomiting and diarrhea

Deficient Knowledge r/t care of self with serious illness, prevention of further incidences of foodborne illness

Nausea r/t contamination irritating stomach

Risk for dysfunctional Gastrointestinal motility: Risk factor: contaminated food

See Gastroenteritis; Gastroenteritis, Child; Hospitalized Child; Escherichia coli Infection

Food Intolerance

Risk for dysfunctional Gastrointestinal motility: Risk factor: food intolerance

Foreign Body Aspiration

Ineffective Airway clearance r/t obstruction of airway

Ineffective Health maintenance r/t parental deficient knowledge regarding high-risk items

Risk for Suffocation: Risk factor: inhalation of small objects

See Safety, Childhood

Formula Feeding of Infant

Grieving: maternal r/t loss of desired breastfeeding experience

Ineffective Infant Feeding Dynamics r/t lack of knowledge of appropriate methods of feeding infant for each stage of development

Risk for Constipation: infant: Risk factor: iron-fortified formula

Risk for Infection: infant: Risk factors: lack of passive maternal immunity, supine feeding position, contamination of formula

Readiness for enhanced Knowledge: expresses an interest in learning

Fracture

Decreased Diversional activity engagement r/t immobility

Impaired physical Mobility r/t limb immobilization

Acute Pain r/t muscle spasm, edema, trauma

Post-Trauma syndrome r/t catastrophic event

Impaired Walking r/t limb immobility

Risk for ineffective peripheral Tissue Perfusion: Risk factors: immobility, presence of cast

Risk for Peripheral Neurovascular dysfunction: Risk factors: mechanical compression, treatment of fracture

Risk for impaired Skin integrity: Risk factors: immobility, presence of cast

Risk for Venous Thromboembolism: Risk factors: trauma, immobility

Readiness for enhanced Knowledge: expresses an interest in learning

Fractured Hip

See Hip Fracture

Frail Elderly Syndrome

Activity intolerance r/t sensory changes

Risk for Frail Elderly syndrome (see **Frail Elderly** syndrome, risk for, Section III)

Risk for Injury: Risk factors: impaired vision, impaired gait

Risk for Powerlessness: Risk factor: inability to maintain independence

Frequency of Urination

Stress urinary Incontinence r/t degenerative change in pelvic muscles and structural support

Urge urinary Incontinence r/t decreased bladder capacity, irritation of bladder stretch receptors causing spasm, alcohol, caffeine, increased fluids, increased urine concentration, overdistended bladder

Impaired Urinary elimination r/t urinary tract infection

Urinary retention r/t high urethral pressure caused by weak detrusor, inhibition of reflex arc, strong sphincter, blockage

Friendship

Readiness for enhanced Relationship: expresses desire to enhance communication between partners

Frostbite

Acute Pain r/t decreased circulation from prolonged exposure to cold

Ineffective peripheral Tissue Perfusion r/t damage to extremities from prolonged exposure to cold

Impaired Tissue integrity r/t freezing of skin and tissues

Risk for ineffective Thermoregulation: Risk factor: prolonged exposure to cold

See Hypothermia

Frothy Sputum

See CHF (Congestive Heart Failure); Pulmonary Edema; Seizure Disorders, Adult; Seizure Disorders, Childhood (Epilepsy, Febrile Seizures, Infantile Spasms)

Fusion, Lumbar

Anxiety r/t fear of surgical procedure, possible recurring problems

Impaired physical Mobility r/t limitations from surgical procedure, presence of brace

Acute Pain r/t discomfort at bone donor site, surgical operation

Risk for Injury: Risk factor: improper body mechanics

Risk for Perioperative Positioning injury: Risk factor: immobilization during surgery

Readiness for enhanced Knowledge: expresses an interest in learning

G

Gag Reflex, Depressed or Absent

Impaired Swallowing r/t neuromuscular impairment

Risk for Aspiration: Risk factors: depressed cough or gag reflex

Gallop Rhythm

Decreased Cardiac output r/t decreased contractility of heart

Gallstones

See Cholelithiasis

G

G

Gang Member

Impaired individual Resilience (See **Resilience**, individual, impaired, Section III)

Gangrene

Fear r/t possible loss of extremity

Ineffective peripheral Tissue perfusion r/t obstruction of arterial flow

See Diabetes Mellitus; Peripheral Vascular Disease

Gas Exchange, Impaired

Impaired Gas exchange r/t ventilation-perfusion imbalance

Gastric Ulcer

See GI Bleed (Gastrointestinal Bleeding); Ulcer, Peptic (Duodenal or Gastric)

Gastritis

Imbalanced Nutrition: less than body requirements r/t vomiting, inadequate intestinal absorption of nutrients, restricted dietary regimen

Acute Pain r/t inflammation of gastric mucosa

Risk for deficient Fluid volume: Risk factors: excessive loss from gastrointestinal tract from vomiting, decreased intake

Gastroenteritis

Diarrhea r/t infectious process involving intestinal tract

Deficient Fluid volume r/t excessive loss from gastrointestinal tract from diarrhea, vomiting

Nausea r/t irritation to gastrointestinal system

Imbalanced Nutrition: less than body requirements r/t vomiting, inadequate intestinal absorption of nutrients, restricted dietary intake

Acute Pain r/t increased peristalsis causing cramping

Risk for Electrolyte imbalance: Risk factor: loss of gastrointestinal fluids high in electrolytes

Readiness for enhanced Knowledge: expresses an interest in learning

See Gastroenteritis, Child

Gastroenteritis, Child

Impaired Skin integrity: diaper rash r/t acidic excretions on perineal tissues

Readiness for enhanced Knowledge: expresses an interest in learning

Acute Pain r/t increased peristalsis causing cramping

See Gastroenteritis; Hospitalized Child

Gastroesophageal Reflux (GERD)

Ineffective Airway clearance r/t reflux of gastric contents into esophagus and tracheal or bronchial tree

Ineffective Health maintenance r/t deficient knowledge regarding anti-reflux regimen (e.g., positioning, change in diet)

Acute Pain r/t irritation of esophagus from gastric acids

Risk for Aspiration: Risk factor: entry of gastric contents in tracheal or bronchial tree

Gastroesophageal Reflux, Child

Ineffective Airway clearance r/t reflux of gastric contents into esophagus and tracheal or bronchial tree

Anxiety: parental r/t possible need for surgical intervention

Deficient Fluid volume r/t persistent vomiting

Imbalanced Nutrition: less than body requirements r/t poor feeding, vomiting

Risk for Aspiration: Risk factor: entry of gastric contents in tracheal or bronchial tree

Risk for impaired Parenting: Risk factors: disruption in bonding as a result of irritable or inconsolable infant; lack of sleep for parents

Readiness for enhanced Knowledge: expresses an interest in learning

See Child with Chronic Condition; Hospitalized Child

Gastrointestinal Bleeding (GI Bleed)

See GI Bleed (Gastrointestinal Bleeding)

Gastrointestinal Hemorrhage

See GI Bleed (Gastrointestinal Bleeding)

Gastrointestinal Surgery

Risk for Injury: Risk factor: inadvertent insertion of nasogastric tube through gastric incision line

See Abdominal Surgery

Gastroschisis/Omphalocele

Ineffective Airway clearance r/t complications of anesthetic effects

Impaired Gas exchange r/t effects of anesthesia, subsequent atelectasis

Grieving r/t threatened loss of infant, loss of perfect birth or infant because of serious medical condition

Risk for deficient Fluid volume: Risk factors: inability to feed because of condition, subsequent electrolyte imbalance

Risk for Infection: Risk factor: disrupted skin integrity with exposure of abdominal contents

Risk for Injury: Risk factors: disrupted skin integrity, ineffective protection

Gastrostomy

Risk for impaired Skin integrity: Risk factor: presence of gastric contents on skin

See Tube Feeding

Gender Dysphoria

Anxiety r/t conflict between physical (assigned) gender and gender they identify with

Decisional Conflict r/t uncertainty about choices regarding gender reassignment

Disturbed Body Image r/t alteration in self-perception, inability to identify with own body

Ineffective Denial r/t insufficient emotional support

Fear r/t victimization

Disturbed Personal Identity r/t gender confusion

Ineffective Sexuality Pattern r/t conflict surrounding gender identity

Risk for Compromised Human Dignity: Risk factor: cultural incongruence, humiliation

Readiness for enhanced Decision-Making: expresses desire to enhance understanding of choices for decision-making

Genital Herpes

See Herpes Simplex II

Genital Warts

See STD (Sexually Transmitted Disease)

GERD

See Gastroesophageal Reflux (GERD)

Gestational Diabetes (Diabetes in Pregnancy)

Anxiety r/t threat to self and/or fetus

Impaired Nutrition: less than body requirements r/t decreased insulin production and glucose uptake in cells

Risk for Overweight: fetal: r/t excessive glucose uptake

Impaired Nutrition: more than body requirements: fetal r/t excessive glucose uptake

Risk for delayed Development: fetal: Risk factor: endocrine disorder of mother

Risk for unstable blood Glucose: Risk factor: excessive intake of carbohydrates

Risk for disturbed Maternal–Fetal dyad: Risk factor: impaired glucose metabolism

Risk for impaired Tissue integrity: fetal: Risk factors: large infant, congenital defects, birth injury

Risk for impaired Tissue integrity: maternal: Risk factor: delivery of large infant

Readiness for enhanced Knowledge: expresses an interest in learning

See Diabetes Mellitus

GI Bleed (Gastrointestinal Bleeding)

Fatigue r/t loss of circulating blood volume, decreased ability to transport oxygen

Fear r/t threat to well-being, potential death

Deficient Fluid volume r/t gastrointestinal bleeding, hemorrhage

Imbalanced Nutrition: less than body requirements r/t nausea, vomiting

Acute Pain r/t irritated mucosa from acid secretion

Risk for ineffective Coping: Risk factors: personal vulnerability in crisis, bleeding, hospitalization

Readiness for enhanced Knowledge: expresses an interest in learning

Gingivitis

Impaired Oral Mucous Membrane integrity r/t ineffective oral hygiene

Glaucoma

Deficient Knowledge r/t treatment and self-care for disease

See Vision Impairment

Glomerulonephritis

Excess Fluid volume r/t renal impairment

Imbalanced Nutrition: less than body requirements r/t anorexia, restrictive diet

Acute Pain r/t edema of kidney

Readiness for enhanced Knowledge: expresses an interest in learning

Gluten Allergy

See Celiac Disease

Gonorrhea

Acute Pain r/t inflammation of reproductive organs

Risk for Infection: Risk factor: spread of organism throughout reproductive organs

Readiness for enhanced Knowledge: expresses an interest in learning

See STD (Sexually Transmitted Disease)

Gout

Impaired physical Mobility r/t musculoskeletal impairment

Chronic Pain r/t inflammation of affected joint

Readiness for enhanced Knowledge: expresses an interest in learning

Grandiosity

Defensive Coping r/t inaccurate perception of self and abilities

Grand Mal Seizure

See Seizure Disorders, Adult; Seizure Disorders, Childhood (Epilepsy, Febrile Seizures, Infantile Spasms)

Grandparents Raising Grandchildren

Anxiety r/t change in role status

Decisional Conflict r/t support system deficit

Parental Role conflict r/t change in parental role

Compromised family Coping r/t family role changes

Interrupted Family processes r/t family roles shift

Ineffective Role performance r/t role transition, aging

Ineffective family Health management r/t excessive demands on individual or family

Risk for impaired Parenting: Risk factor: role strain

Risk for Powerlessness: Risk factors: role strain, situational crisis, aging

Risk for Spiritual distress: Risk factor: life change

Readiness for enhanced Parenting: physical and emotional needs of children are met

Graves' Disease

See Hyperthyroidism

Grieving

Grieving r/t anticipated or actual significant loss, change in life status, style, or function

Imbalanced Energy Field r/t blockage of the energy flow

G

Grieving, Complicated

Complicated Grieving r/t expected or sudden death of a significant other with whom there was a volatile relationship, emotional instability, lack of social support

Risk for complicated Grieving: Risk factors: death of a significant other with whom there was a volatile relationship, emotional instability, lack of social support

Groom Self (Inability to)

Bathing Self-Care deficit (See **Self-Care** deficit, bathing, Section III)

Dressing Self-Care deficit (See **Self-Care** deficit, dressing, Section III)

Growth and Development Lag

See Failure to Thrive, Child

Guillain-Barré Syndrome

Impaired Spontaneous Ventilation r/t weak respiratory muscles

Risk for Aspiration: Risk factors: ineffective cough; depressed gag reflex

See Neurologic Disorders

Guilt

Grieving r/t potential loss of significant person, animal, prized material possession, change in life role

Impaired individual Resilience (See **Resilience**, individual, impaired, Section III)

Situational low Self-Esteem r/t unmet expectations of self

Risk for complicated Grieving: Risk factors: actual loss of significant person, animal, prized material possession, change in life role

Risk for Post-Trauma syndrome: Risk factor: exaggerated sense of responsibility for traumatic event

Readiness for enhanced Spiritual well-being: desire to be in harmony with self, others, higher power or God

H

Hair Loss

Disturbed Body Image r/t psychological reaction to loss of hair

Imbalanced Nutrition: less than body requirements r/t inability to ingest food because of biological, psychological, economic factors

Halitosis

Impaired Dentition r/t ineffective oral hygiene

Impaired Oral Mucous Membrane integrity r/t ineffective oral hygiene

Hallucinations

Anxiety r/t threat to self-concept

Acute Confusion r/t alcohol abuse, delirium, dementia, mental illness, substance abuse

Ineffective Coping r/t distortion and insecurity of life events

Risk for Self-Mutilation: Risk factor: command hallucinations

Risk for other-directed Violence: Risk factors: catatonic excitement, manic excitement, rage or panic reactions, response to violent internal stimuli

Risk for self-directed Violence: Risk factors: catatonic excitement, manic excitement, rage or panic reactions, response to violent internal stimuli

Headache

Acute Pain r/t lack of knowledge of pain control techniques or methods to prevent headaches

Ineffective Health management r/t lack of knowledge, identification, elimination of aggravating factors

Head Injury

Ineffective Breathing pattern r/t pressure damage to breathing center in brainstem

Acute Confusion r/t increased intracranial pressure

Decreased Intracranial adaptive capacity r/t increased intracranial pressure

Risk for ineffective Cerebral tissue perfusion: Risk factors: effects of increased intracranial pressure, trauma to brain

See Neurologic Disorders

Health Behavior, Risk-Prone

Risk-prone Health behavior: Risk factors (See **Health** behavior, risk-prone, Section III)

Risk for Metabolic Imbalance syndrome r/t obesity

Health Maintenance Problems

Ineffective Health maintenance (See **Health** maintenance, ineffective, Section III)

Ineffective Health management (See **Health** management, ineffective, Section III)

Health-Seeking Person

Readiness for enhanced Health literacy (See **Health** literacy, readiness for enhanced, Section III)

Readiness for enhanced Health management (See **Health** management, readiness for enhanced, Section III)

Hearing Impairment

Impaired verbal Communication r/t inability to hear own voice

Hearing Loss *(see Appendix E on Evolve)*

Social isolation r/t difficulty with communication

Heart Attack

See MI (Myocardial Infarction)

Heartburn

Nausea r/t gastrointestinal irritation

Acute Pain: heartburn r/t inflammation of stomach and esophagus

Risk for imbalanced Nutrition: less than body requirements: Risk factor: pain after eating

Readiness for enhanced Knowledge: expresses an interest in learning

See Gastroesophageal Reflux (GERD)

Heart Failure

Activity intolerance r/t weakness, fatigue, shortness of breath

Decreased Cardiac output r/t impaired cardiac function, increased preload, decreased contractility, increased afterload

Constipation r/t activity intolerance

Fatigue r/t disease process with decreased cardiac output

Fear r/t threat to one's own well-being

Excess Fluid volume r/t impaired excretion of sodium and water

Impaired Gas exchange r/t excessive fluid in interstitial space of lungs

Powerlessness r/t illness-related regimen

Risk for Shock (cardiogenic): Risk factors: decreased contractility of heart, increased afterload

Readiness for enhanced Health management (See **Health** management, readiness for enhanced, Section III)

See Child with Chronic Condition; Congenital Heart Disease/Cardiac Anomalies; Hospitalized Child

Heart Surgery

See Coronary Artery Bypass Grafting (CABG)

Heat Stroke

Deficient Fluid volume r/t profuse diaphoresis from high environmental temperature

Hyperthermia r/t vigorous activity, high environmental temperature, inappropriate clothing

Hematemesis

See GI Bleed (Gastrointestinal Bleeding)

Hematuria

See Kidney Stone; UTI (Urinary Tract Infection)

Hemianopia

Anxiety r/t change in vision

Unilateral Neglect r/t effects of disturbed perceptual abilities

Risk for Injury: Risk factor: disturbed sensory perception

Hemiplegia

Anxiety r/t change in health status

Disturbed Body Image r/t functional loss of one side of body

Impaired physical Mobility r/t loss of neurological control of involved extremities

Self-Care deficit: specify: r/t neuromuscular impairment

Impaired Sitting r/t partial paralysis

Impaired Standing r/t partial paralysis

Impaired Transfer ability r/t partial paralysis

Unilateral Neglect r/t effects of disturbed perceptual abilities

Impaired Walking r/t loss of neurological control of involved extremities

Risk for Falls: Risk factor: impaired mobility

Risk for impaired Skin integrity: Risk factors: alteration in sensation, immobility; pressure over bony prominence

See CVA (Cerebrovascular Accident)

Hemodialysis

Ineffective Coping r/t situational crisis

Interrupted Family processes r/t changes in role responsibilities as a result of therapy regimen

Excess Fluid volume r/t renal disease with minimal urine output

Powerlessness r/t treatment regimen

Risk for Caregiver Role Strain: Risk factor: complexity of care receiver treatment

Risk for Electrolyte imbalance: Risk factor: effect of metabolic state on renal function

Risk for deficient Fluid volume: Risk factor: excessive removal of fluid during dialysis

Risk for Infection: Risk factors: exposure to blood products, risk for developing hepatitis B or C, impaired immune system

Risk for Injury: Risk factors: clotting of blood access, abnormal surface for blood flow

Risk for impaired Tissue integrity: Risk factor: mechanical factor associated with fistula formation

Readiness for enhanced Knowledge: expresses an interest in learning

See Renal Failure; Renal Failure, Child with Chronic Condition

Hemodynamic Monitoring

Risk for Infection: Risk factor: invasive procedure

Risk for Injury: Risk factors: inadvertent wedging of catheter, dislodgment of catheter, disconnection of catheter

Risk for impaired Tissue integrity: Risk factor: invasive procedure

See Shock, Cardiogenic; Shock, Hypovolemic; Shock, Septic

Hemolytic Uremic Syndrome

Fatigue r/t decreased red blood cells

Fear r/t serious condition with unknown outcome

Deficient Fluid volume r/t vomiting, diarrhea

Nausea r/t effects of uremia

Risk for Injury: Risk factors: decreased platelet count, seizure activity

Risk for impaired Skin integrity: Risk factor: diarrhea

See Hospitalized Child; Renal Failure, Acute/Chronic, Child

Hemophilia

Fear r/t high risk for AIDS infection from contaminated blood products

Impaired physical Mobility r/t pain from acute bleeds, imposed activity restrictions, joint pain

Acute Pain r/t bleeding into body tissues

Risk for Bleeding: Risk factors: deficient clotting factors, child's developmental level, age-appropriate play, inappropriate use of toys or sports equipment

Readiness for enhanced Knowledge: expresses an interest in learning

H

See Child with Chronic Condition; Hospitalized Child; Maturational Issues, Adolescent

Hemoptysis

Fear r/t serious threat to well-being

Risk for ineffective Airway clearance: Risk factor: obstruction of airway with blood and mucus

Risk for deficient Fluid volume: Risk factor: excessive loss of blood

Hemorrhage

Fear r/t threat to well-being

Deficient Fluid volume r/t massive blood loss

See Hypovolemic Shock

Hemorrhoidectomy

Anxiety r/t embarrassment, need for privacy

Constipation r/t fear of pain with defecation

Acute Pain r/t surgical procedure

Urinary retention r/t pain, anesthetic effect

Risk for Bleeding: Risk factors: inadequate clotting, trauma from surgery

Readiness for enhanced Knowledge: expresses an interest in learning

Hemorrhoids

Impaired Comfort r/t itching in rectal area

Constipation r/t painful defecation, poor bowel habits

Impaired Sitting r/t pain and pressure

Readiness for enhanced Knowledge: expresses an interest in learning

Hemothorax

Deficient Fluid volume r/t blood in pleural space

See Pneumothorax

Hepatitis

Activity intolerance r/t weakness or fatigue caused by infection

Decreased Diversional activity engagement r/t isolation

Fatigue r/t infectious process, altered body chemistry

Imbalanced Nutrition: less than body requirements r/t anorexia, impaired use of proteins and carbohydrates

Acute Pain r/t edema of liver, bile irritating skin

Social isolation r/t treatment-imposed isolation

Risk for deficient Fluid volume: Risk factor: excessive loss of fluids from vomiting and diarrhea

Readiness for enhanced Knowledge: expresses an interest in learning

Hernia

See Hiatal Hernia; Inguinal Hernia Repair

Herniated Disk

See Low Back Pain

Herniorrhaphy

See Inguinal Hernia Repair

Herpes in Pregnancy

Fear r/t threat to fetus, impending surgery

Situational low Self-Esteem r/t threat to fetus as a result of disease process

Risk for Infection: infant: Risk factors: transplacental transfer during primary herpes, exposure to active herpes during birth process

See Herpes Simplex II

Herpes Simplex I

Impaired Oral Mucous Membrane integrity r/t inflammatory changes in mouth

Herpes Simplex II

Ineffective Health maintenance r/t deficient knowledge regarding treatment, prevention, spread of disease

Acute Pain r/t active herpes lesion

Situational low Self-Esteem r/t expressions of shame or guilt

Sexual dysfunction r/t disease process

Impaired Tissue integrity r/t active herpes lesion

Impaired Urinary elimination r/t pain with urination

Herpes Zoster

See Shingles

HHNS (Hyperosmolar Hyperglycemic Nonketotic Syndrome)

See Hyperosmolar Hyperglycemic Nonketotic Syndrome (HHNS)

Hiatal Hernia

Ineffective Health maintenance r/t deficient knowledge regarding care of disease

Nausea r/t effects of gastric contents in esophagus

Imbalanced Nutrition: less than body requirements r/t pain after eating

Acute Pain r/t gastroesophageal reflux

Hip Fracture

Acute Confusion r/t sensory overload, sensory deprivation, medication side effects, advanced age, pain

Constipation r/t immobility, opioids, anesthesia

Fear r/t outcome of treatment, future mobility, present helplessness

Impaired physical Mobility r/t surgical incision, temporary absence of weight bearing, pain when walking

Acute Pain r/t injury, surgical procedure, movement

Powerlessness r/t health care environment

Self-Care deficit: specify r/t musculoskeletal impairment

Impaired Transfer ability r/t immobilization of hip

Impaired Walking r/t temporary absence of weight bearing

Risk for Bleeding: Risk factors: postoperative complication, surgical blood loss

Risk for Surgical Site Infection: Risk factor: invasive procedure

Risk for Injury: Risk factors: activities such as greater than 90-degree flexion of hips that can result in dislodged prosthesis, unsteadiness when ambulating

Risk for Perioperative Positioning injury: Risk factors: immobilization, muscle weakness, emaciation

Risk for Peripheral Neurovascular dysfunction: Risk factors: trauma, vascular obstruction, fracture

Risk for impaired Skin integrity: Risk factor: immobility

Risk for Venous Thromboembolism: Risk factors: immobility, trauma

Hip Replacement

See Total Joint Replacement (Total Hip/Total Knee/Shoulder)

Hirschsprung's Disease

Constipation: bowel obstruction r/t inhibited peristalsis as a result of congenital absence of parasympathetic ganglion cells in distal colon

Grieving r/t loss of perfect child, birth of child with congenital defect even though child expected to be normal within 2 years

Imbalanced Nutrition: less than body requirements r/t anorexia, pain from distended colon

Acute Pain r/t distended colon, incisional postoperative pain

Impaired Skin integrity r/t stoma, potential skin care problems associated with stoma

Readiness for enhanced Knowledge: expresses an interest in learning

See Hospitalized Child

Hirsutism

Disturbed Body Image r/t excessive hair

Hitting Behavior

Acute Confusion r/t dementia, alcohol abuse, drug abuse, delirium

Risk for other-directed Violence (See **Violence,** other-directed, risk for, Section III)

HIV (Human Immunodeficiency Virus)

Fear r/t possible death

Ineffective Protection r/t depressed immune system

Readiness for enhanced Health literacy: expresses desire to enhance understanding of health information to make health care choices

See AIDS (Acquired Immunodeficiency Syndrome)

Hodgkin's Disease

See Anemia; Cancer; Chemotherapy

Homelessness

Impaired Home maintenance r/t impaired cognitive or emotional functioning, inadequate support system, insufficient finances

Home Maintenance Problems

Impaired Home maintenance (See **Home** maintenance, impaired, Section III)

Self-Neglect r/t mental illness, substance abuse, cognitive impairment

Powerlessness r/t interpersonal interactions

Risk for Physical Trauma: Risk factor: being in high-crime neighborhood

Hope

Readiness for enhanced Hope (See **Hope,** readiness for enhanced, Section III)

Hopelessness

Hopelessness (See **Hopelessness,** Section III)

Hospitalized Child

Activity intolerance r/t fatigue associated with acute illness

Anxiety: separation (child) r/t familiar surroundings and separation from family and friends

Compromised family Coping r/t possible prolonged hospitalization that exhausts supportive capacity of significant people

Ineffective Coping: parent r/t possible guilt regarding hospitalization of child, parental inadequacies

Decreased Diversional activity engagement r/t immobility, monotonous environment, frequent or lengthy treatments, reluctance to participate, therapeutic isolation, separation from peers

Interrupted Family processes r/t situational crisis of illness, disease, hospitalization

Fear r/t deficient knowledge or maturational level with fear of unknown, mutilation, painful procedures, surgery

Hopelessness: child r/t prolonged activity restriction, uncertain prognosis

Insomnia: child or parent r/t 24-hour care needs of hospitalization

Acute Pain r/t treatments, diagnostic or therapeutic procedures, disease process

Powerlessness: child r/t health care environment, illness-related regimen

Risk for impaired Attachment: Risk factor: separation

Risk for delayed Development: regression: Risk factors: disruption of normal routine, unfamiliar environment or caregivers, developmental vulnerability of young children

Risk for Injury: Risk factors: unfamiliar environment, developmental age, lack of parental knowledge regarding safety (e.g., side rails, IV site/pole)

Risk for imbalanced Nutrition: less than body requirements: Risk factors: anorexia, absence of familiar foods, cultural preferences

Readiness for enhanced family Coping: impact of crisis on family values, priorities, goals, relationships in family

See Child with Chronic Condition

Hostile Behavior

Risk for other-directed Violence: Risk factor: antisocial personality disorder

HTN (Hypertension)

Ineffective Health management (See **Health** management, ineffective, Section III)

Readiness for enhanced Health management (See **Health** management, readiness for enhanced, Section III)

Risk for Overweight: Risk factor: lack of knowledge of relationship between diet and disease process

Human Energy Field

Energy Field, Imbalanced (See **Imbalanced Energy Field,** Section III)

Humiliating Experience

Risk for compromised Human Dignity (See **Human Dignity,** compromised, risk for, Section III)

Huntington's Disease

Decisional Conflict r/t whether to have children

See Neurologic Disorders

Hydrocele

Acute Pain r/t severely enlarged hydrocele

Ineffective Sexuality pattern r/t recent surgery on area of scrotum

Hydrocephalus

Decisional Conflict r/t unclear or conflicting values regarding selection of treatment modality

Interrupted Family processes r/t situational crisis

Imbalanced Nutrition: less than body requirements r/t inadequate intake as a result of anorexia, nausea, vomiting, feeding difficulties

Risk for delayed Development: Risk factor: sequelae of increased intracranial pressure

Risk for Infection: Risk factor: sequelae of invasive procedure (shunt placement)

Risk for ineffective Cerebral tissue perfusion: Risk factors: interrupted flow, hypervolemia of cerebral ventricles

Risk for Falls: Risk factors: acute illness, alteration in cognitive functioning

See Normal Pressure Hydrocephalus (NPH); Child with Chronic Condition; Hospitalized Child; Premature Infant (Child); Premature Infant (Parent)

Hygiene, Inability to Provide Own

Frail Elderly syndrome r/t living alone

Self-Neglect (See **Self-Neglect,** Section III)

Bathing Self-Care deficit (See **Self-Care** deficit, bathing, Section III)

Hyperactive Syndrome

Decisional Conflict r/t multiple or divergent sources of information regarding education, nutrition, medication regimens; willingness to change own food habits; limited resources

Parental Role conflict: when siblings present r/t increased attention toward hyperactive child

Compromised family Coping r/t unsuccessful strategies to control excessive activity, behaviors, frustration, anger

Ineffective Impulse control r/t disorder of development, environment that might cause frustration or irritation

Ineffective Role performance: parent r/t stressors associated with dealing with hyperactive child, perceived or projected blame for causes of child's behavior, unmet needs for support or care, lack of energy to provide for those needs

Chronic low Self-Esteem r/t inability to achieve socially acceptable behaviors; frustration; frequent reprimands, punishment, or scolding for uncontrolled activity and behaviors; mood fluctuations and restlessness; inability to succeed academically; lack of peer support

Impaired Social interaction r/t impulsive and overactive behaviors, concomitant emotional difficulties, distractibility and excitability

Risk for delayed Development: Risk factor: behavior disorders

Risk for impaired Parenting: Risk factor: disruptive or uncontrollable behaviors of child

Risk for other-directed Violence: parent or child: Risk factors: frustration with disruptive behavior, anger, unsuccessful relationships

Hyperbilirubinemia, Neonatal

Anxiety: parent r/t threat to infant, unknown future

Parental Role conflict r/t interruption of family life because of care regimen

Neonatal Hyperbilirubinemia r/t abnormal breakdown of red blood cells following birth

Imbalanced Nutrition: less than body requirements (infant) r/t disinterest in feeding because of jaundice-related lethargy

Risk for Injury: infant: Risk factors: kernicterus, phototherapy lights

Risk for ineffective Thermoregulation: Risk factor: phototherapy

Readiness for enhanced Health management (parents): expresses desire to manage treatment: assessment of jaundice when infant is discharged from the hospital, when to call the physician, and possible preventive measures such as frequent breastfeeding (See Neonatal **Hyperbilirubinemia,** Risk for, Section III)

Hypercalcemia

Decreased Cardiac output r/t bradydysrhythmia

Impaired physical Mobility r/t decreased muscle tone

Imbalanced Nutrition: less than body requirements r/t gastrointestinal manifestations of hypercalcemia (nausea, anorexia, ileus)

Risk for Disuse syndrome: Risk factor: comatose state impairing mobility

Hypercapnia

Fear r/t difficulty breathing

Impaired Gas exchange r/t ventilation-perfusion imbalance, retention of carbon dioxide

See ARDS (Adult Respiratory Distress Syndrome); COPD (Chronic Obstructive Pulmonary Disorder); Sleep Apnea

Hyperemesis Gravidarum

Anxiety r/t threat to self and infant, hospitalization

Deficient Fluid volume r/t excessive vomiting

Impaired Home maintenance r/t chronic nausea, inability to function

Nausea r/t hormonal changes of pregnancy

Imbalanced Nutrition: less than body requirements r/t excessive vomiting

Powerlessness r/t health care regimen

Social isolation r/t hospitalization

Risk for Electrolyte imbalance: Risk factor: vomiting

Hyperglycemia

Ineffective Health management r/t complexity of therapeutic regimen, decisional conflicts, economic difficulties, unsupportive family, insufficient cues to action, deficient knowledge, mistrust, lack of acknowledgment of seriousness of condition

Risk for unstable blood Glucose level (See **Glucose** level, blood, unstable, risk for, Section III)

See Diabetes Mellitus

Hyperkalemia

Risk for Activity intolerance: Risk factor: muscle weakness

Risk for decreased Cardiac tissue perfusion: Risk factor: abnormal electrolyte level affecting heart rate and rhythm

Risk for excess Fluid volume: Risk factor: untreated renal failure

Hypernatremia

Risk for deficient Fluid volume: Risk factors: abnormal water loss, inadequate water intake

Hyperosmolar Hyperglycemic Nonketotic Syndrome (HHNS)

Acute Confusion r/t dehydration, electrolyte imbalance

Deficient Fluid volume r/t polyuria, hyperglycemia, inadequate fluid intake

Risk for Electrolyte imbalance: Risk factor: effect of metabolic state on kidney function

Risk for Injury: seizures: Risk factors: hyperosmolar state, electrolyte imbalance

See Diabetes Mellitus; Diabetes Mellitus, Juvenile (Insulin-Dependent Diabetes Mellitus Type 1)

Hyperphosphatemia

Deficient Knowledge r/t dietary changes needed to control phosphate levels

See Renal Failure

Hypersensitivity to Slight Criticism

Defensive Coping r/t situational crisis, psychological impairment, substance abuse

Hypertension (HTN)

See HTN (Hypertension)

Risk for decreased Cardiac output: Risk factors: decreased contractility and altered conductivity associated with myocardial damage

Risk for unstable Blood Pressure: (See **Unstable Blood Pressure,** Risk for, Section III)

Hyperthermia

Hyperthermia (See **Hyperthermia,** Section III)

Hyperthyroidism

Anxiety r/t increased stimulation, loss of control

Diarrhea r/t increased gastric motility

Insomnia r/t anxiety, excessive sympathetic discharge

Imbalanced Nutrition: less than body requirements r/t increased metabolic rate, increased gastrointestinal activity

Risk for Injury: eye damage: Risk factor: protruding eyes without sufficient lubrication

Risk for unstable Blood Pressure r/t hyperthyroidism

Readiness for enhanced Knowledge: expresses an interest in learning

Hyperventilation

Ineffective Breathing pattern r/t anxiety, acid-base imbalance

See Anxiety Disorder; Dyspnea; Heart Failure

Hypocalcemia

Activity intolerance r/t neuromuscular irritability

Ineffective Breathing pattern r/t laryngospasm

Imbalanced Nutrition: less than body requirements r/t effects of vitamin D deficiency, renal failure, malabsorption, laxative use

Hypoglycemia

Acute Confusion r/t insufficient blood glucose to brain

Ineffective Health management r/t deficient knowledge regarding disease process, self-care

Imbalanced Nutrition: less than body requirements r/t imbalance of glucose and insulin level

Risk for unstable blood Glucose level (See **Glucose** level, blood, unstable, risk for, Section III)

See Diabetes Mellitus; Diabetes Mellitus, Juvenile (IDDM Type 1)

Hypokalemia

Activity intolerance r/t muscle weakness

Risk for decreased Cardiac tissue perfusion: Risk factor: possible dysrhythmia from electrolyte imbalance

Hypomagnesemia

Imbalanced Nutrition: less than body requirements r/t deficient knowledge of nutrition, alcoholism

See Alcoholism

Hypomania

Insomnia r/t psychological stimulus

See Manic Disorder, Bipolar I

Hyponatremia

Acute Confusion r/t electrolyte imbalance

Excess Fluid volume r/t excessive intake of hypotonic fluids

Risk for Injury: Risk factors: seizures, new onset of confusion

Hypoplastic Left Lung

See Congenital Heart Disease/Cardiac Anomalies

Hypotension

Decreased Cardiac output r/t decreased preload, decreased contractility

Risk for deficient Fluid volume: Risk factor: excessive fluid loss

Risk for ineffective Cerebral tissue perfusion: Risk factors: hypovolemia, decreased contractility, decreased afterload

Risk for Shock (See **Shock,** risk for, Section III)

Risk for unstable Blood Pressure (See **Unstable Blood Pressure,** Risk for, Section III)

See Dehydration; Heart Failure; MI (Myocardial Infarction)

Hypothermia

Hypothermia (See **Hypothermia,** Section III)

Risk for Hypothermia (see **Hypothermia,** risk for, Section III)

Hypothyroidism

Activity intolerance r/t muscular stiffness, shortness of breath on exertion

Constipation r/t decreased gastric motility

Impaired Gas exchange r/t respiratory depression

Impaired Skin integrity r/t edema, dry or scaly skin

Risk for Overweight: Risk factor: decreased metabolic process

Hypovolemic Shock

See Shock, Hypovolemic

Hypoxia

Acute Confusion r/t decreased oxygen supply to brain

Fear r/t breathlessness

Impaired Gas exchange r/t altered oxygen supply, inability to transport oxygen

Risk for Shock (See **Shock,** risk for, Section III)

Hysterectomy

Constipation r/t opioids, anesthesia, bowel manipulation during surgery

Ineffective Coping r/t situational crisis of surgery

Grieving r/t change in body image, loss of reproductive status

Acute Pain r/t surgical injury

Sexual dysfunction r/t disturbance in self-concept

Urinary retention r/t edema in area, anesthesia, opioids, pain

Risk for Bleeding: Risk factor: surgical procedure

Risk for Constipation: Risk factors: opioids, anesthesia, bowel manipulation during surgery

Risk for ineffective peripheral Tissue perfusion: Risk factor: deficient knowledge of aggravating factors

Risk for Surgical Site Infection: Risk factor: invasive procedure

Readiness for enhanced Knowledge: Expresses an interest in learning

See Surgery, Perioperative Care; Surgery, Preoperative Care; Surgery, Postoperative Care

I

IBS (Irritable Bowel Syndrome)

Constipation r/t low-residue diet, stress

Diarrhea r/t increased motility of intestines associated with disease process, stress

Ineffective Health management r/t deficient knowledge, powerlessness

Chronic Pain r/t spasms, increased motility of bowel

Risk for Electrolyte imbalance: Risk factor: diarrhea

Readiness for enhanced Health management: expresses desire to manage illness and prevent onset of symptoms

ICD (Implantable Cardioverter/Defibrillator)

Anxiety r/t possible dysrhythmia, threat of death

Decreased Cardiac output r/t possible dysrhythmia

Readiness for enhanced Knowledge: expresses an interest in learning

IDDM (Insulin-Dependent Diabetes)

See Diabetes Mellitus

Identity Disturbance/Problems

Disturbed personal Identity r/t situational crisis, psychological impairment, chronic illness, pain

Risk for disturbed personal Identity (See **Identity,** personal, risk for disturbed in Section III)

Idiopathic Thrombocytopenic Purpura (ITP)

See ITP (Idiopathic Thrombocytopenic Purpura)

Ileal Conduit

Disturbed Body Image r/t presence of stoma

Ineffective Health management r/t new skills required to care for appliance and self

Ineffective Sexuality pattern r/t altered body function and structure

Social isolation r/t alteration in physical appearance, fear of accidental spill of urine

Risk for Latex Allergic reaction: Risk factor: repeated exposures to latex associated with treatment and management of disease

Risk for impaired Skin integrity: Risk factor: difficulty obtaining tight seal of appliance

Readiness for enhanced Knowledge: expresses an interest in learning

Ileostomy

Disturbed Body Image r/t presence of stoma

Diarrhea r/t dietary changes, alteration in intestinal motility

Deficient Knowledge r/t limited practice of stoma care, dietary modifications

Ineffective Sexuality pattern r/t altered body function and structure

Social isolation r/t alteration in physical appearance, fear of accidental spill of ostomy contents

Risk for impaired Skin integrity: Risk factors: difficulty obtaining tight seal of appliance, caustic drainage

Readiness for enhanced Knowledge: expresses an interest in learning

Ileus

Deficient Fluid volume r/t loss of fluids from vomiting, fluids trapped in bowel

Dysfunctional Gastrointestinal motility r/t effects of surgery, decreased perfusion of intestines, medication effect, immobility

Nausea r/t gastrointestinal irritation

Acute Pain r/t pressure, abdominal distention

Readiness for enhanced Knowledge: expresses an interest in learning

Immigration Transition, Risk for Complicated

Anxiety r/t changes in safety and security needs

Fear r/t unfamiliar environment, separation from support system, possible language barrier

Impaired Social interaction r/t possible communication or sociocultural barriers

Risk for Loneliness: Risk factor: separation from support system

Risk for Powerlessness: Risk factor: insufficient social support

Risk for Relocation stress syndrome: Risk factors: insufficient support system, social isolation, and potential communication barriers

Risk for Impaired Resilience: Risk factor: decreased ability to adapt to adverse or changing situations

Readiness for enhanced Coping: expresses desire to enhance social support

Readiness for enhanced Knowledge: expresses a desire to become familiar with resources within their environment

Immobility

Ineffective Breathing pattern r/t inability to deep breathe in supine position

Acute Confusion: elderly r/t sensory deprivation from immobility

Constipation r/t immobility

Risk for Frail Elderly syndrome: Risk factors: low physical activity, bed rest

Impaired physical Mobility r/t medically imposed bed rest

Ineffective peripheral Tissue Perfusion r/t interruption of venous flow

Powerlessness r/t forced immobility from health care environment

Impaired Walking r/t limited physical mobility, deconditioning of body

Risk for Disuse syndrome: Risk factor: immobilization

Risk for impaired Skin integrity: Risk factors: pressure over bony prominences, shearing forces when moved; pressure from devices

Risk for Impaired Tissue Integrity: Risk factors: mechanical factors from pressure over bony prominences, shearing forces when moved; pressure from devices

Risk for Overweight: Risk factor: energy expenditure less than energy intake

Risk for Venous Thromboembolism: Risk factor: lack of physical activity

Readiness for enhanced Knowledge: expresses an interest in learning

Immunization

See **Readiness for enhanced Health literacy**, Section III
See **Readiness for enhanced Health management**, Section III

Immunosuppression

Risk for Infection: Risk factors: immunosuppression; exposure to disease outbreak

Impaired Social interaction r/t therapeutic isolation

Impaction of Stool

Constipation r/t decreased fluid intake, less than adequate amounts of fiber and bulk-forming foods in diet, medication effect, or immobility

Impaired Sitting

Impaired physical Mobility r/t musculoskeletal, cognitive, or neuromuscular disorder

Impaired Standing

Activity intolerance r/t insufficient physiological or psychological energy

Powerlessness r/t loss of function

Imperforate Anus

Anxiety r/t ability to care for newborn

Deficient Knowledge r/t home care for newborn

Impaired Skin integrity r/t pruritus

Impetigo

Impaired Skin integrity r/t infectious disease

Readiness for enhanced Knowledge: expresses an interest in learning

See *Communicable Diseases, Childhood (e.g., Measles, Mumps, Rubella, Chickenpox, Scabies, Lice)*

Implantable Cardioverter/Defibrillator (ICD)

See *ICD (Implantable Cardioverter/Defibrillator)*

Impotence

Situational low Self-Esteem r/t physiological crisis, inability to practice usual sexual activity

Sexual dysfunction r/t altered body function

Readiness for enhanced Knowledge: treatment information for erectile dysfunction

See *Erectile Dysfunction (ED)*

Impulsiveness

Ineffective Impulse control r/t (See **Impulse** control, ineffective in Section III)

Inactivity

Activity intolerance r/t imbalance between oxygen supply and demand, sedentary lifestyle, weakness, immobility

I

Hopelessness r/t deteriorating physiological condition, long-term stress, social isolation

Impaired physical Mobility r/t intolerance to activity, decreased strength and endurance, depression, severe anxiety, musculoskeletal impairment, perceptual or cognitive impairment, neuromuscular impairment, pain, discomfort

Risk for Constipation: Risk factor: insufficient physical activity

Incompetent Cervix

See Premature Dilation of the Cervix (Incompetent Cervix)

Incontinence of Stool

Disturbed Body Image r/t inability to control elimination of stool

Bowel Incontinence r/t decreased awareness of need to defecate, loss of sphincter control

Toileting Self-Care deficit r/t cognitive impairment, neuromuscular impairment, perceptual impairment, weakness

Situational low Self-Esteem r/t inability to control elimination of stool

Risk for impaired Skin integrity: Risk factor: presence of stool

Incontinence of Urine

Functional urinary Incontinence r/t altered environment; sensory, cognitive, or mobility deficits

Overflow urinary Incontinence r/t relaxation of pelvic muscles and changes in urinary structures

Reflex urinary Incontinence r/t neurological impairment

Stress urinary Incontinence (See **Incontinence**, urinary, stress, Section III)

Urge urinary Incontinence (See **Incontinence**, urinary, urge, Section III)

Toileting Self-Care deficit r/t cognitive impairment

Situational low Self-Esteem r/t inability to control passage of urine

Risk for impaired Skin integrity: Risk factor: presence of urine on perineal skin

Indigestion

Nausea r/t gastrointestinal irritation

Imbalanced Nutrition: less than body requirements r/t discomfort when eating

Induction of Labor

Anxiety r/t medical interventions, powerlessness

Decisional Conflict r/t perceived threat to idealized birth

Ineffective Coping r/t situational crisis of medical intervention in birthing process

Acute Pain r/t contractions

Situational low Self-Esteem r/t inability to carry out normal labor

Risk for Injury: maternal and fetal: Risk factors: hypertonic uterus, potential prematurity of newborn

Readiness for enhanced Family processes: family support during induction of labor

Infant Apnea

See Premature Infant (Child); Respiratory Conditions of the Neonate; Sudden Infant Death Syndrome (SIDS)

Infant Behavior

Disorganized Infant behavior r/t pain, oral/motor problems, feeding intolerance, environmental overstimulation, lack of containment or boundaries, prematurity, invasive or painful procedures

Risk for disorganized Infant behavior: Risk factors: pain, oral/motor problems, environmental overstimulation, lack of containment or boundaries

Readiness for enhanced organized Infant behavior: stable physiologic measures, use of some self-regulatory measures

Infant Care

Readiness for enhanced Childbearing process: a pattern of preparing for, maintaining, and strengthening care of newborn infant

Infant Feeding Pattern, Ineffective

Ineffective infant Feeding pattern r/t prematurity, neurological impairment or delay, oral hypersensitivity, prolonged nothing-by-mouth order

Infant of Diabetic Mother

Decreased Cardiac output r/t cardiomegaly

Deficient Fluid volume r/t increased urinary excretion and osmotic diuresis

Imbalanced Nutrition: less than body requirements r/t hypotonia, lethargy, poor sucking, postnatal metabolic changes from hyperglycemia to hypoglycemia and hyperinsulinism

Risk for delayed Development: Risk factor: prolonged and severe postnatal hypoglycemia

Risk for impaired Gas exchange: Risk factors: increased incidence of cardiomegaly, prematurity

Risk for unstable blood Glucose level: Risk factor: metabolic change from hyperglycemia to hypoglycemia and hyperinsulinism

Risk for disturbed Maternal–Fetal dyad: Risk factor: impaired glucose metabolism

See Premature Infant (Child); Respiratory Conditions of the Neonate

Infant of Substance-Abusing Mother

See Neonatal Abstinence Syndrome

Infantile Polyarteritis

See Kawasaki Disease

Infection, Potential for

Risk for Infection (See **Infection**, risk for, Section III)

Infectious Processes

Impaired Comfort r/t distressing symptoms

Diarrhea r/t gastrointestinal inflammation

Ineffective Health maintenance r/t knowledge deficit regarding transmission, symptoms, and treatment

Ineffective Health Management r/t lack of knowledge regarding preventative immunizations

Ineffective Protection r/t inadequate nutrition, abnormal blood profiles, drug therapies, treatments

Impaired Social interaction r/t therapeutic isolation

Risk for Electrolyte Imbalance: Risk factors: vomiting, diarrhea

Risk for deficient Fluid Volume: Risk factors: vomiting, diarrhea, inadequate fluid intake

Risk for Infection: Risk factor: increased environmental exposure when in close proximity to infected persons

Risk for Surgical Site Infection r/t immunosuppression

Risk for ineffective Thermoregulation: Risk factor: infectious process

Readiness for enhanced Knowledge: expresses desire for information regarding prevention and treatment

Infertility

Ineffective Health management r/t deficient knowledge about infertility

Powerlessness r/t infertility

Chronic Sorrow r/t inability to conceive a child

Spiritual distress r/t inability to conceive a child

Inflammatory Bowel Disease (Child and Adult)

Ineffective Coping r/t repeated episodes of diarrhea

Diarrhea r/t effects of inflammatory changes of the bowel

Deficient Fluid volume r/t frequent and loose stools

Imbalanced Nutrition: less than body requirements r/t anorexia, decreased absorption of nutrients from gastrointestinal tract

Acute Pain r/t abdominal cramping and anal irritation

Impaired Skin integrity r/t frequent stools, development of anal fissures

Social isolation r/t diarrhea

See Child with Chronic Condition; Crohn's Disease; Hospitalized Child; Maturational Issues, Adolescent

Influenza

See Infectious Processes

Inguinal Hernia Repair

Impaired physical Mobility r/t pain at surgical site and fear of causing hernia to rupture

Acute Pain r/t surgical procedure

Urinary retention r/t possible edema at surgical site

Risk for Surgical Site Infection: Risk factor: surgical procedure

Injury

Risk for Falls: Risk factors: orthostatic hypotension, impaired physical mobility, diminished mental status

Risk for Injury: Risk factor: environmental conditions interacting with client's adaptive and defensive resources

Risk for corneal Injury: Risk factors: blinking less than five times per minute, mechanical ventilation, pharmaceutical agent, prolonged hospitalization

Risk for Thermal injury: Risk factors: cognitive impairment, inadequate supervision, developmental level

Risk for urinary tract Injury: Risk factor: inflammation and/ or infection from long-term use of urinary catheter

Insomnia

(See **Insomnia**, Section III)

Insulin Shock

See Hypoglycemia

Intellectual Disability

Impaired verbal Communication r/t developmental delay

Interrupted Family processes r/t crisis of diagnosis and situational transition

Grieving r/t loss of perfect child, birth of child with congenital defect or subsequent head injury

Deficient community Health r/t lack of programs to address developmental deficiencies

Impaired Home maintenance r/t insufficient support systems

Self-Neglect r/t learning disability

Self-Care deficit: bathing, dressing, feeding, toileting r/t perceptual or cognitive impairment

Self-Mutilation r/t inability to express tension verbally

Social isolation r/t delay in accomplishing developmental tasks

Spiritual distress r/t chronic condition of child with special needs

Stress overload r/t intense, repeated stressor (chronic condition)

Impaired Swallowing r/t neuromuscular impairment

Risk for ineffective Activity planning r/t inability to process information

Risk for delayed Development: Risk factor: cognitive or perceptual impairment

Risk for impaired Religiosity: Risk factor: social isolation

Risk for Self-Mutilation: Risk factors: separation anxiety, depersonalization

Readiness for enhanced family Coping: adaptation and acceptance of child's condition and needs

See Child with Chronic Condition; Safety, Childhood

Intermittent Claudication

Deficient Knowledge r/t lack of knowledge of cause and treatment of peripheral vascular diseases

Acute Pain r/t decreased circulation to extremities with activity

Ineffective peripheral Tissue Perfusion r/t interruption of arterial flow

Risk for Injury: Risk factor: tissue hypoxia

Readiness for enhanced Knowledge: prevention of pain and impaired circulation

See Peripheral Vascular Disease (PVD)

Internal Cardioverter/Defibrillator (ICD)

See ICD (Implantable Cardioverter/Defibrillator)

Internal Fixation

Impaired Walking r/t repair of fracture

Risk for Infection: Risk factors: traumatized tissue, broken skin

See Fracture

I

I

Interstitial Cystitis

Acute Pain r/t inflammatory process

Impaired Urinary elimination r/t inflammation of bladder

Risk for Infection: Risk factor: suppressed inflammatory response

Readiness for enhanced Knowledge: expresses an interest in learning

Intervertebral Disk Excision

See Laminectomy

Intestinal Obstruction

See Ileus; Bowel Obstruction

Intestinal Perforation

See Peritonitis

Intoxication

Anxiety r/t loss of control of actions

Acute Confusion r/t alcohol abuse

Ineffective Coping r/t use of mind-altering substances as a means of coping

Impaired Memory r/t effects of alcohol on mind

Risk for Aspiration: Risk factors: diminished mental status, vomiting

Risk for Falls: Risk factor: diminished mental status

Risk for other-directed Violence: Risk factor: inability to control thoughts and actions

Intraaortic Balloon Counterpulsation

Anxiety r/t device providing cardiovascular assistance

Decreased Cardiac output r/t heart dysfunction needing counterpulsation

Compromised family Coping r/t seriousness of significant other's medical condition

Impaired physical Mobility r/t restriction of movement because of mechanical device

Risk for Peripheral Neurovascular dysfunction: Risk factors: vascular obstruction of balloon catheter, thrombus formation, emboli, edema

Risk for Infection: Risk factor: invasive procedure

Risk for impaired Tissue integrity: Risk factor: invasive procedure

Intracranial Pressure, Increased

Ineffective Breathing pattern r/t pressure damage to breathing center in brainstem

Acute Confusion r/t increased intracranial pressure

Decreased Intracranial adaptive capacity r/t sustained increase in intracranial pressure

Impaired Memory r/t neurological disturbance

Vision Loss r/t pressure damage to sensory centers in brain

Risk for ineffective Cerebral tissue perfusion: Risk factors: body position, cerebral vessel circulation deficits

See Head Injury; Subarachnoid Hemorrhage

Intrauterine Growth Retardation

Anxiety: maternal r/t threat to fetus

Ineffective Coping: maternal r/t situational crisis, threat to fetus

Impaired Gas exchange r/t insufficient placental perfusion

Imbalanced Nutrition: less than body requirements r/t insufficient placenta

Situational low Self-Esteem: maternal r/t guilt about threat to fetus

Spiritual distress r/t unknown outcome of fetus

Risk for Powerlessness: Risk factor: unknown outcome of fetus

Intravenous Therapy

Risk for Vascular Trauma: Risk factor: infusion of irritating chemicals

Intubation, Endotracheal or Nasogastric

Disturbed Body Image r/t altered appearance with mechanical devices

Impaired verbal Communication r/t endotracheal tube

Imbalanced Nutrition: less than body requirements r/t inability to ingest food because of the presence of tubes

Impaired Oral Mucous Membrane r/t presence of tubes

Acute Pain r/t presence of tube

Iodine Reaction with Diagnostic Testing

Risk for adverse reaction to iodinated Contrast Media (See Reaction to iodinated **Contrast Media**, risk for adverse, Section III)

Irregular Pulse

See Dysrhythmia

Irritable Bowel Syndrome (IBS)

See IBS (Irritable Bowel Syndrome)

Isolation

Impaired individual Resilience (See **Resilience**, individual, impaired, Section III)

Social isolation (See **Social** isolation, Section III)

Itching

See Pruritus

ITP (Idiopathic Thrombocytopenic Purpura)

Decreased Diversional activity engagement r/t activity restrictions, safety precautions

Ineffective Protection r/t decreased platelet count

Risk for Bleeding: Risk factors: decreased platelet count, developmental level, age-appropriate play

See Hospitalized Child

J

Jaundice

Imbalanced Nutrition: less than body requirements r/t decreased appetite with liver disorder

Risk for Bleeding: Risk factor: impaired liver function

Risk for impaired Liver function: Risk factors: possible viral infection, medication effect

Risk for impaired Skin integrity: Risk factors: pruritus, itching

See Cirrhosis; Hepatitis

Jaundice, Neonatal

See Hyperbilirubinemia, Neonatal

Jaw Pain and Heart Attacks

See Angina; Chest Pain; MI (Myocardial Infarction)

Jaw Surgery

Deficient Knowledge r/t emergency care for wired jaws (e.g., cutting bands and wires), oral care

Imbalanced Nutrition: less than body requirements r/t jaws wired closed, difficulty eating

Acute Pain r/t surgical procedure

Impaired Swallowing r/t edema from surgery

Risk for Aspiration: Risk factor: wired jaws

Jittery

Anxiety r/t unconscious conflict about essential values and goals, threat to or change in health status

Death Anxiety r/t unresolved issues relating to end of life

Risk for Post-Trauma syndrome: Risk factors: occupation, survivor's role in event, inadequate social support

Jock Itch

Ineffective Health management r/t prevention and treatment of disorder

Impaired Skin integrity r/t moisture and irritating or tight-fitting clothing

See Pruritus

Joint Dislocation

See Dislocation of Joint

Joint Pain

See Arthritis; Bursitis; JRA (Juvenile Rheumatoid Arthritis); Osteoarthritis; Rheumatoid Arthritis (RA)

Joint Replacement

Risk for Peripheral Neurovascular dysfunction: Risk factor: orthopedic surgery

Risk for impaired Tissue integrity: Risk factor: invasive procedure

See Total Joint Replacement (Total Hip/Total Knee/Shoulder)

JRA (Juvenile Rheumatoid Arthritis)

Impaired Comfort r/t altered health status

Fatigue r/t chronic inflammatory disease

Impaired physical Mobility r/t pain, restricted joint movement

Acute Pain r/t swollen or inflamed joints, restricted movement, physical therapy

Self-Care deficit: feeding, bathing, dressing, toileting r/t restricted joint movement, pain

Risk for compromised Human Dignity: Risk factors: perceived intrusion by clinicians, invasion of privacy

Risk for Injury: Risk factors: impaired physical mobility, splints, adaptive devices, increased bleeding potential from antiinflammatory medications

Risk for compromised Resilience: Risk factor: chronic condition

Risk for situational low Self-Esteem: Risk factor: disturbed body image

Risk for impaired Skin integrity: Risk factors: splints, adaptive devices

See Child with Chronic Condition; Hospitalized Child

K

Kaposi's Sarcoma

Risk for complicated Grieving: Risk factor: loss of social support

Risk for impaired Religiosity: Risk factors: illness/hospitalization, ineffective coping

Risk for impaired Resilience: Risk factor: serious illness

See AIDS (Acquired Immunodeficiency Syndrome)

Kawasaki Disease

Anxiety: parental r/t progression of disease, complications of arthritis, and cardiac involvement

Impaired Comfort r/t altered health status

Hyperthermia r/t inflammatory disease process

Imbalanced Nutrition: less than body requirements r/t impaired oral mucous membrane integrity

Impaired Oral Mucous Membrane integrity r/t inflamed mouth and pharynx; swollen lips that become dry, cracked, fissured

Acute Pain r/t enlarged lymph nodes; erythematous skin rash that progresses to desquamation, peeling, denuding of skin

Impaired Skin integrity r/t inflammatory skin changes

Risk for imbalanced Fluid volume: Risk factor: hypovolemia

Risk for decreased Cardiac tissue perfusion: Risk factor: cardiac involvement

Risk for Dry Mouth: Risk factor: decreased fluid intake

See Hospitalized Child

Keloids

Disturbed Body Image r/t presence of scar tissue at site of a healed skin injury

Readiness for enhanced Health management: desire to have information to manage condition

K

Keratoconjunctivitis Sicca (Dry Eye Syndrome)

Risk for dry Eye: Risk factors: aging, staring at a computer screen for long intervals

Risk for Infection: Risk factor: dry eyes that are more vulnerable to infection

Risk for corneal Injury: Risk factors: dry eye, exposure of the eyeball

See Conjunctivitis

Keratoplasty

See Corneal Transplant

Ketoacidosis, Alcoholic

See Alcohol Withdrawal; Alcoholism

Ketoacidosis, Diabetic

Deficient Fluid volume r/t excess excretion of urine, nausea, vomiting, increased respiration

Impaired Memory r/t fluid and electrolyte imbalance

Imbalanced Nutrition: less than body requirements r/t body's inability to use nutrients

Risk for unstable blood Glucose level: Risk factor: deficient knowledge of diabetes management (e.g., action plan)

Risk for Powerlessness: Risk factor: illness-related regimen

Risk for impaired Resilience: Risk factor: complications of disease

See Diabetes Mellitus

Keyhole Heart Surgery

See MIDCAB (Minimally Invasive Direct Coronary Artery Bypass)

Kidney Disease Screening

Readiness for enhanced Health management: seeks information for screening

Kidney Failure

See Renal Failure

Kidney Failure Acute/Chronic, Child

See Renal Failure, Acute/Chronic, Child

Kidney Failure, Nonoliguric

See Renal Failure, Nonoliguric

Kidney Stone

Acute Pain r/t obstruction from kidney calculi

Impaired Urinary elimination: urgency and frequency r/t anatomical obstruction, irritation caused by stone

Risk for Infection: Risk factor: obstruction of urinary tract with stasis of urine

Readiness for enhanced Knowledge: expresses an interest in learning about prevention of stones

Kidney Transplant

Ineffective Protection r/t immunosuppressive therapy

Readiness for enhanced Decision-Making: expresses desire to enhance understanding of choices

Readiness for enhanced Family processes: adapting to life without dialysis

Readiness for enhanced Health management: desire to manage the treatment and prevention of complications after transplantation

Readiness for enhanced Spiritual well-being: heightened coping, living without dialysis

See Renal Failure, Kidney Transplantation, Donor; Kidney Transplantation, Recipient; Nephrectomy; Surgery, Perioperative Care; Surgery, Postoperative Care; Surgery, Preoperative Care

Kidney Transplantation, Donor

Impaired emancipated Decision-Making r/t harvesting of kidney from traumatized donor

Moral Distress r/t conflict among decision makers, end-of-life decisions, time constraints for decision-making

Spiritual distress r/t grieving from loss of significant person

Risk for Surgical Site Infection: Risk factor: surgical procedure

Readiness for enhanced Communication: expressing thoughts and feelings about situation

Readiness for enhanced family Coping: decision to allow organ donation

Readiness for enhanced emancipated Decision-Making: expresses desire to enhance understanding and meaning of choices

Readiness for enhanced Resilience: decision to donate organs

Readiness for enhanced Spirituality: inner peace resulting from allowance of organ donation

See Nephrectomy

Kidney Transplantation, Recipient

Anxiety r/t possible rejection, procedure

Ineffective Health maintenance r/t long-term home treatment after transplantation, diet, signs of rejection, use of medications

Deficient Knowledge r/t specific nutritional needs, possible paralytic ileus, fluid or sodium restrictions

Impaired Urinary elimination r/t possible impaired renal function

Risk for Bleeding: Risk factor: surgical procedure

Risk for Infection: Risk factor: use of immunosuppressive therapy to control rejection

Risk for Surgical Site Infection: Risk factor: surgical procedure

Risk for Shock: Risk factor: possible hypovolemia

Risk for Spiritual distress: Risk factor: obtaining transplanted kidney from someone's traumatic loss

Readiness for enhanced Spiritual well-being: acceptance of situation

Kidney Tumor

See Wilms' Tumor

Kissing Disease

See Mononucleosis

Knee Replacement

See Total Joint Replacement (Total Hip/Total Knee/Shoulder)

Knowledge

Readiness for enhanced Knowledge (See **Knowledge,** readiness for enhanced, Section III)

Knowledge, Deficient

Ineffective Health maintenance r/t lack of or significant alteration in communication skills (written, verbal, and/or gestural)

Deficient Knowledge (See **Knowledge,** deficient, Section III)

Readiness for enhanced Knowledge (See **Knowledge,** readiness for enhanced, Section III)

Kock Pouch

See Continent Ileostomy (Kock Pouch)

Korsakoff's Syndrome

Acute Confusion r/t alcohol abuse

Dysfunctional Family processes r/t alcoholism as possible cause of syndrome

Impaired Memory r/t neurological changes associated with excessive alcohol intake

Self-Neglect r/t cognitive impairment from chronic alcohol abuse

Risk for Falls: Risk factor: cognitive impairment from chronic alcohol abuse

Risk for Injury: Risk factors: sensory dysfunction, lack of coordination when ambulating from chronic alcohol abuse

Risk for impaired Liver function: Risk factor: substance abuse (alcohol)

Risk for imbalanced Nutrition: less than body requirements: Risk factor: lack of adequate balanced intake from chronic alcohol abuse

L

Labor, Induction of

See Induction of Labor

Labor, Normal

Anxiety r/t fear of the unknown, situational crisis

Impaired Comfort r/t labor

Fatigue r/t childbirth

Deficient Knowledge r/t lack of preparation for labor

Labor Pain r/t uterine contractions, stretching of cervix and birth canal

Impaired Tissue integrity r/t passage of infant through birth canal, episiotomy

Risk for ineffective Childbearing process (See **Childbearing** process, Section III)

Risk for Falls: Risk factors: excessive loss or shift in intravascular fluid volume, orthostatic hypotension

Risk for deficient Fluid volume: Risk factor: excessive loss of blood

Risk for Infection: Risk factors: multiple vaginal examinations, tissue trauma, prolonged rupture of membranes

Risk for Injury: fetal: Risk factor: hypoxia

Risk for Post-Trauma syndrome: Risk factors: trauma or violence associated with labor pains, medical or surgical interventions, history of sexual abuse

Readiness for enhanced Childbearing process: responds appropriately, is proactive, bonds with infant, uses support systems

Readiness for enhanced family Coping: significant other provides support during labor

Readiness for enhanced Health management: prenatal care and childbirth education birth process

Readiness for enhanced Power: expresses readiness to enhance participation in choices regarding treatment during labor

Labor Pain

Labor Pain r/t uterine contractions, stretching of cervix and birth canal

Labyrinthitis

Ineffective Health management r/t delay in seeking treatment for respiratory and ear infections

Risk for Injury r/t dizziness

Readiness for enhanced Health management: management of episodes

See Ménière's Disease

Lacerations

Readiness for enhanced Health management: appropriate care of injury

Risk for Infection: Risk factor: broken skin

Risk for Physical Trauma: Risk factor: children playing with dangerous objects

Lactation

See Breastfeeding, Ineffective; Breastfeeding, Interrupted

Lactic Acidosis

Decreased Cardiac output r/t altered heart rate/rhythm, preload, and contractility

Risk for Electrolyte imbalance: Risk factor: impaired regulatory mechanism

Risk for decreased Cardiac tissue perfusion: Risk factor: hypoxia

See Ketoacidosis, Diabetic

Lactose Intolerance

Readiness for enhanced Knowledge: interest in identifying lactose intolerance, treatment, and substitutes for milk products

See Abdominal Distention; Diarrhea

Laminectomy

Anxiety r/t change in health status, surgical procedure

Impaired Comfort r/t surgical procedure

Deficient Knowledge r/t appropriate postoperative and postdischarge activities

Impaired physical Mobility r/t neuromuscular impairment

Acute Pain r/t localized inflammation and edema

Urinary retention r/t competing sensory impulses, effects of opioids or anesthesia

Risk for Bleeding: Risk factor: surgery

Risk for Surgical Site Infection: Risk factor: invasive procedure, surgery

Risk for Perioperative Positioning injury: Risk factor: prone position

See Surgery, Perioperative Care; Surgery, Postoperative Care; Surgery, Preoperative Care

Language Impairment

See Speech Disorders

Laparoscopic Laser Cholecystectomy

See Cholecystectomy; Laser Surgery

Laparoscopy

Urge urinary Incontinence r/t pressure on the bladder from gas

Acute Pain: shoulder r/t gas irritating the diaphragm

Laparotomy

See Abdominal Surgery

Large Bowel Resection

See Abdominal Surgery

Laryngectomy

Ineffective Airway clearance r/t surgical removal of glottis, decreased humidification

Death Anxiety r/t unknown results of surgery

Disturbed Body Image r/t change in body structure and function

Impaired Comfort r/t surgery

Impaired verbal Communication r/t removal of larynx

Interrupted Family processes r/t surgery, serious condition of family member, difficulty communicating

Grieving r/t loss of voice, fear of death

Ineffective Health management r/t deficient knowledge regarding self-care with laryngectomy

Imbalanced Nutrition: less than body requirements r/t absence of oral feeding, difficulty swallowing, increased need for fluids

Impaired Oral Mucous Membrane r/t absence of oral feeding

Chronic Sorrow r/t change in body image

Impaired Swallowing r/t edema, laryngectomy tube

Risk for Electrolyte imbalance: Risk factor: fluid imbalance

Risk for complicated Grieving: Risk factors: loss, major life event

Risk for compromised Human Dignity: Risk factor: inability to communicate

Risk for Surgical Site Infection: Risk factors: invasive procedure, surgery

Risk for Powerlessness: Risk factors: chronic illness, change in communication

Risk for impaired Resilience: Risk factor: change in health status

Risk for situational low Self-Esteem: Risk factor: disturbed body image

Laser Surgery

Impaired Comfort r/t surgery

Constipation r/t laser intervention in vulval and perianal areas

Deficient Knowledge r/t preoperative and postoperative care associated with laser procedure

Acute Pain r/t heat from laser

Risk for Bleeding: Risk factor: surgery

Risk for Infection: Risk factor: delayed heating reaction of tissue exposed to laser

Risk for Injury: Risk factor: accidental exposure to laser beam

LASIK Eye Surgery (Laser-Assisted in Situ Keratomileusis)

Impaired Comfort r/t surgery

Decisional Conflict r/t decision to have surgery

Risk for Infection: Risk factor: invasive procedure/surgery

Readiness for enhanced Health management: surgical procedure preoperative and postoperative teaching and expectations

Latex Allergic Reaction

Latex Allergic reaction (See **Latex Allergic** reaction, Section III)

Risk for Latex Allergic reaction (See **Latex Allergic** reaction, risk for, Section III)

Readiness for enhanced Knowledge: prevention and treatment of exposure to latex products

Laxative Abuse

Perceived Constipation r/t health belief, faulty appraisal, impaired thought processes

Lead Poisoning

Contamination r/t flaking, peeling paint in presence of young children

Impaired Home maintenance r/t presence of lead paint

Risk for delayed Development: Risk factor: lead poisoning

Left Heart Catheterization

See Cardiac Catheterization

Legionnaires' Disease

Contamination r/t contaminated water in air-conditioning systems

See Pneumonia

Lens Implant

See Cataract Extraction; Vision Impairment

Lethargy/Listlessness

Frail Elderly syndrome r/t alteration in cognitive function

Fatigue r/t decreased metabolic energy production

Insomnia r/t internal or external stressors

Risk for ineffective Cerebral tissue perfusion: Risk factor: carbon dioxide retention and/or lack of oxygen supply to brain

Leukemia

Ineffective Protection r/t abnormal blood profile

Fatigue r/t abnormal blood profile and/or side effects of chemotherapy treatment

Risk for imbalanced Fluid volume: Risk factors: nausea, vomiting, bleeding, side effects of treatment

Risk for Infection: Risk factor: ineffective immune system

Risk for impaired Resilience: Risk factor: serious illness

See Cancer; Chemotherapy

Leukopenia

Ineffective Protection r/t leukopenia

Risk for Infection: Risk factor: low white blood cell count

Level of Consciousness, Decreased

See Confusion, Acute; Confusion, Chronic

Lice

Impaired Comfort r/t inflammation, pruritus

Readiness for enhanced Health management: preventing and treating infestation

Impaired Home maintenance r/t close unsanitary, overcrowded conditions

Self-Neglect r/t lifestyle

See Communicable Diseases, Childhood (e.g., Measles, Mumps, Rubella, Chickenpox, Scabies, Lice)

Lifestyle, Sedentary

Sedentary lifestyle (See **Sedentary** lifestyle, Section III)

Risk for ineffective peripheral Tissue Perfusion: Risk factor: lack of movement

Lightheadedness

See Dizziness; Vertigo

Limb Reattachment Procedures

Anxiety r/t unknown outcome of reattachment procedure, use and appearance of limb

Disturbed Body Image r/t unpredictability of function and appearance of reattached body part

Grieving r/t unknown outcome of reattachment procedure

Spiritual distress r/t anxiety about condition

Stress overload r/t multiple coexisting stressors, physical demands

Risk for Bleeding: Risk factor: severed vessels

Risk for Perioperative Positioning injury: Risk factor: immobilization

Risk for Peripheral Neurovascular dysfunction: Risk factors: trauma, orthopedic and neurovascular surgery, compression of nerves and blood vessels

Risk for Powerlessness: Risk factor: unknown outcome of procedure

Risk for impaired Religiosity: Risk factors: suffering, hospitalization

See Surgery, Postoperative Care

Liposuction

Disturbed Body Image r/t dissatisfaction with unwanted fat deposits in body

Risk for impaired Resilience: Risk factor: body image disturbance

Readiness for enhanced Decision-Making: expresses desire to make decision regarding liposuction

Readiness for enhanced Self-Concept: satisfaction with new body image

See Surgery, Perioperative Care; Surgery, Postoperative Care; Surgery, Preoperative Care

Lithotripsy

Readiness for enhanced Health management: expresses desire for information related to procedure and aftercare and prevention of stones

See Kidney Stone

Liver Biopsy

Anxiety r/t procedure and results

Risk for deficient Fluid volume: Risk factor: hemorrhage from biopsy site

Risk for Infection: Risk factor: invasive procedure

Risk for Powerlessness: Risk factor: inability to control outcome of procedure

Liver Cancer

Risk for Bleeding: Risk factor: liver dysfunction

Risk for Falls: Risk factor: confusion associated with liver dysfunction

Risk for impaired Liver function: Risk factor: disease process

Risk for impaired Resilience: Risk factor: serious illness

See Cancer; Chemotherapy; Radiation Therapy

Liver Disease

See Cirrhosis; Hepatitis

Liver Function

Risk for impaired Liver function (See **Liver** function, impaired, risk for, Section III)

Liver Transplant

Impaired Comfort r/t surgical pain

Decisional Conflict r/t acceptance of donor liver

Ineffective Protection r/t immunosuppressive therapy

Risk for impaired Liver function: Risk factors: possible rejection, infection

Readiness for enhanced Family processes: change in physical needs of family member

Readiness for enhanced Health management: desire to manage the treatment and prevention of complications after transplantation

L

Readiness for enhanced Spiritual well-being: heightened coping

See Surgery, Perioperative Care; Surgery, Postoperative Care; Surgery, Preoperative Care

Living Will

Moral Distress r/t end-of-life decisions

Readiness for enhanced Decision-Making: expresses desire to enhance understanding of choices for decision-making

Readiness for enhanced Relationship: shares information with others

Readiness for enhanced Religiosity: request to meet with religious leaders or facilitators

Readiness for enhanced Resilience: uses effective communication

Readiness for enhanced Spiritual well-being: acceptance of and preparation for end of life

See Advance Directives

Lobectomy

See Thoracotomy

Loneliness

Spiritual distress r/t loneliness, social alienation

Risk for Loneliness (See **Loneliness,** risk for, Section III)

Risk for impaired Religiosity: Risk factor: lack of social interaction

Readiness for enhanced Hope: expresses desire to enhance interconnectedness with others

Readiness for enhanced Relationship: expresses satisfaction with complementary relationship between partners

Loose Stools (Bowel Movements)

Diarrhea r/t increased gastric motility

Risk for dysfunctional Gastrointestinal motility (See **Gastrointestinal** motility, dysfunctional, risk for, Section III)

See Diarrhea

Loss of Bladder Control

See Incontinence of Urine

Loss of Bowel Control

See Incontinence of Stool

Lou Gehrig's Disease

See Amyotrophic Lateral Sclerosis (ALS)

Low Back Pain

Impaired Comfort r/t back pain

Ineffective Health maintenance r/t deficient knowledge regarding self-care with back pain

Impaired physical Mobility r/t back pain

Chronic Pain r/t degenerative processes, musculotendinous strain, injury, inflammation, congenital deformities

Urinary Retention r/t possible spinal cord compression

Risk for Powerlessness: Risk factor: living with chronic pain

Readiness for enhanced Health management: expresses desire for information to manage pain

Low Blood Glucose

See Hypoglycemia

Low Blood Pressure

See Hypotension

Lower GI Bleeding

See GI Bleed (Gastrointestinal Bleeding)

Lumbar Puncture

Anxiety r/t invasive procedure and unknown results

Deficient Knowledge r/t information about procedure

Acute Pain r/t possible loss of cerebrospinal fluid

Risk for ineffective Cerebral tissue perfusion: Risk factor: treatment-related side effects

Risk for Infection: Risk factor: invasive procedure

Lumpectomy

Decisional Conflict r/t treatment choices

Readiness for enhanced Knowledge: preoperative and postoperative care

Readiness for enhanced Spiritual well-being: hope of benign diagnosis

See Cancer

Lung Cancer

See Cancer; Chemotherapy; Radiation Therapy; Thoracotomy

Lung Surgery

See Thoracotomy

Lupus Erythematosus

Disturbed Body Image r/t change in skin, rash, lesions, ulcers, mottled erythema

Fatigue r/t increased metabolic requirements

Ineffective Health maintenance r/t deficient knowledge regarding medication, diet, activity

Acute Pain r/t inflammatory process

Powerlessness r/t unpredictability of course of disease

Impaired Religiosity r/t ineffective coping with disease

Chronic Sorrow r/t presence of chronic illness

Spiritual distress r/t chronicity of disease, unknown etiology

Risk for decreased Cardiac tissue perfusion: Risk factor: altered circulation

Risk for impaired Resilience: Risk factor: chronic disease

Risk for impaired Skin integrity: Risk factors: chronic inflammation, edema, altered circulation

Lyme Disease

Impaired Comfort r/t inflammation

Fatigue r/t increased energy requirements

Deficient Knowledge r/t lack of information concerning disease, prevention, treatment

L

Acute Pain r/t inflammation of joints, urticaria, rash

Risk for decreased Cardiac output: Risk factor: dysrhythmia

Risk for Powerlessness: Risk factor: possible chronic condition

Lymphedema

Disturbed Body Image r/t change in appearance of body part with edema

Excess Fluid volume r/t compromised regulatory system; inflammation, obstruction, or removal of lymph glands

Deficient Knowledge r/t management of condition

Risk for Infection: Risk factors: abnormal lymphatic system allowing stasis of fluids with decreased resistance to infection

Risk for situational low Self-Esteem: Risk factor: disturbed body image

Lymphoma

See Cancer

M

Macular Degeneration

Ineffective Coping r/t visual loss

Compromised family Coping r/t deteriorating vision of family member

Risk-prone Health behavior r/t deteriorating vision while trying to maintain usual lifestyle

Hopelessness r/t deteriorating vision

Sedentary lifestyle r/t visual loss

Self-Neglect r/t change in vision

Social isolation r/t inability to drive because of visual changes

Risk for Falls: Risk factor: visual difficulties

Risk for Injury: Risk factor: inability to distinguish traffic lights and safety signs

Risk for Powerlessness: Risk factor: deteriorating vision

Risk for impaired Religiosity: Risk factor: possible lack of transportation to church

Risk for impaired Resilience: Risk factor: changing vision

Readiness for enhanced Health management: appropriate choices of daily activities for meeting the goals of a treatment program

Magnetic Resonance Imaging (MRI)

See MRI (Magnetic Resonance Imaging)

Major Depressive Disorder

See Depression (Major Depressive Disorder)

Malabsorption Syndrome

Diarrhea r/t lactose intolerance, gluten sensitivity, resection of small bowel

Dysfunctional Gastrointestinal motility r/t disease state

Deficient Knowledge r/t lack of information about diet and nutrition

Imbalanced Nutrition: less than body requirements r/t inability of body to absorb nutrients because of physiological factors

Risk for Electrolyte imbalance: Risk factors: hypovolemia, hyponatremia, hypokalemia

Risk for imbalanced Fluid volume: Risk factors: diarrhea, hypovolemia

See Abdominal Distention

Maladaptive Behavior

See Crisis; Post-Trauma Syndrome; Suicide Attempt

Malaise

See Fatigue

Malaria

Contamination r/t geographic area

Risk for Contamination: Risk factors: increased environmental exposure (not wearing protective clothing, not using insecticide or repellant on skin, clothing, and in room in areas in which infected mosquitoes are present); inadequate defense mechanisms (inappropriate use of prophylactic regimen)

Risk for impaired Liver function: Risk factor: complications of disease

Readiness for enhanced community Coping: uses resources available for problem-solving

Readiness for enhanced Health management: expresses desire to enhance immunization status/vaccination status

Readiness for enhanced Resilience: immunization status

See Anemia

Male Infertility

See Erectile Dysfunction (ED); Infertility

Malignancy

See Cancer

Malignant Hypertension (Arteriolar Nephrosclerosis)

Decreased Cardiac output r/t altered afterload, altered contractility

Fatigue r/t disease state, increased blood pressure

Excess Fluid volume r/t decreased kidney function

Risk for ineffective Cerebral tissue perfusion: Risk factor: elevated blood pressure damaging cerebral vessels

Risk for acute Confusion: Risk factors: increased blood urea nitrogen or creatinine levels

Risk for imbalanced Fluid volume: Risk factors: hypertension, altered kidney function

Risk for unstable Blood Pressure: Risk factor: damaged vessels due to disease process

Readiness for enhanced Health management: expresses desire to manage the illness, high blood pressure

Malignant Hyperthermia

Hyperthermia r/t anesthesia reaction associated with inherited condition

Readiness for enhanced Health management: knowledge of risk factors

Malnutrition

Insufficient Breast Milk Production r/t (See **Breast Milk,** insufficient production, Section III)

Frail Elderly syndrome r/t undetected malnutrition

Deficient Knowledge r/t misinformation about normal nutrition, social isolation, lack of food preparation facilities

Imbalanced Nutrition: less than body requirements r/t inability to ingest food, digest food, or absorb nutrients because of biological, psychological, or economic factors; institutionalization (i.e., lack of menu choices)

Ineffective Protection r/t inadequate nutrition

Ineffective Health management r/t inadequate nutrition

Self-Neglect r/t inadequate nutrition

Risk for Powerlessness: Risk factor: possible inability to provide adequate nutrition

Mammography

Readiness for enhanced Health management: follows guidelines for screening

Readiness for enhanced Resilience: responsibility for self-care

Manic Disorder, Bipolar I

Anxiety r/t change in role function

Ineffective Coping r/t situational crisis

Ineffective Denial r/t fear of inability to control behavior

Interrupted Family processes r/t family member's illness

Risk-prone Health behavior r/t low self-efficacy

Ineffective Health management r/t unpredictability of client, excessive demands on family, chronic illness, social support deficit

Impaired Home maintenance r/t altered psychological state, inability to concentrate

Disturbed personal Identity r/t manic state

Insomnia r/t constant anxious thoughts

Imbalanced Nutrition: less than body requirements r/t lack of time and motivation to eat, constant movement

Impaired individual Resilience r/t psychological disorder

Ineffective Role performance r/t impaired social interactions

Self-Neglect r/t manic state

Sleep deprivation r/t hyperagitated state

Risk for ineffective Activity planning r/t inability to process information

Risk for Caregiver Role Strain: Risk factor: unpredictability of condition

Risk for imbalanced Fluid volume: Risk factor: hypovolemia

Risk for Powerlessness: Risk factor: inability to control changes in mood

Risk for Spiritual distress: Risk factor: depression

Risk for Suicide: Risk factor: bipolar disorder

Risk for self-directed Violence: Risk factors: hallucinations, delusions

Risk for other-directed Violence: Risk factor: pathologic intoxication

Readiness for enhanced Hope: expresses desire to enhance problem-solving goals

Manipulative Behavior

Defensive Coping r/t superior attitude toward others

Ineffective Coping r/t inappropriate use of defense mechanisms

Self-Mutilation r/t use of manipulation to obtain nurturing relationship with others

Self-Neglect r/t maintaining control

Impaired Social interaction r/t self-concept disturbance

Risk for Loneliness: Risk factor: inability to interact appropriately with others

Risk for situational low Self-Esteem: Risk factor: history of learned helplessness

Risk for Self-Mutilation: Risk factor: inability to cope with increased psychological or physiological tension in healthy manner

Marfan Syndrome

Decreased Cardiac output r/t dilation of the aortic root, dissection or rupture of the aorta

Risk for decreased Cardiac tissue perfusion: Risk factor: heart-related complications from Marfan syndrome

Readiness for enhanced Health management: describes reduction of risk factors

See Mitral Valve Prolapse; Scoliosis

Mastectomy

Disturbed Body Image r/t loss of sexually significant body part

Impaired Comfort r/t altered body image; difficult diagnosis

Death Anxiety r/t threat of mortality associated with breast cancer

Fatigue r/t increased metabolic requirements

Fear r/t change in body image, prognosis

Deficient Knowledge r/t self-care activities

Nausea r/t chemotherapy

Acute Pain r/t surgical procedure

Sexual dysfunction r/t change in body image, fear of loss of femininity

Chronic Sorrow r/t disturbed body image, unknown long-term health status

Spiritual distress r/t change in body image

Risk for Surgical Site Infection: Risk factors: surgical procedure, broken skin

Risk for impaired physical Mobility: Risk factors: nerve or muscle damage, pain

Risk for Post-Trauma syndrome: Risk factors: loss of body part, surgical wounds

Risk for Powerlessness: Risk factor: fear of unknown outcome of procedure

Risk for impaired Resilience: Risk factor: altered body image

See Cancer; Modified Radical Mastectomy; Surgery, Perioperative Care; Surgery, Postoperative Care; Surgery, Preoperative Care

M

Mastitis

Anxiety r/t threat to self, concern over safety of milk for infant

Ineffective Breastfeeding r/t breast pain, conflicting advice from health care providers

Deficient Knowledge r/t antibiotic regimen, comfort measures

Acute Pain r/t infectious disease process, swelling of breast tissue

Ineffective Role performance r/t change in capacity to function in expected role

Maternal Infection

Ineffective Protection r/t invasive procedures, traumatized tissue

See Postpartum, Normal Care

Maturational Issues, Adolescent

Ineffective Coping r/t maturational crises

Risk-prone Health behavior r/t inadequate comprehension, negative attitude toward health care

Interrupted Family processes r/t developmental crises of adolescence resulting from challenge of parental authority and values, situational crises from change in parental marital status

Deficient Knowledge: potential for enhanced health maintenance r/t information misinterpretation, lack of education regarding age-related factors

Impaired Social interaction r/t ineffective, unsuccessful, or dysfunctional interaction with peers

Social isolation r/t perceived alteration in physical appearance, social values not accepted by dominant peer group

Risk for Ineffective Activity planning: Risk factor: unrealistic perception of personal competencies

Risk for disturbed personal Identity: Risk factor: maturational issues

Risk for Injury: Risk factor: thrill-seeking behaviors

Risk for chronic low Self-Esteem: Risk factor: lack of sense of belonging in peer group

Risk for situational low Self-Esteem: Risk factor: developmental changes

Readiness for enhanced Communication: expressing willingness to communicate with parental figures

Readiness for enhanced Relationship: expresses desire to enhance communication with parental figures

See Sexuality, Adolescent; Substance Abuse (if relevant)

Maze III Procedure

See Dysrhythmia; Open Heart Surgery

MD (Muscular Dystrophy)

See Muscular Dystrophy (MD)

Measles (Rubeola)

See Communicable Diseases, Childhood (e.g., Measles, Mumps, Rubella, Chickenpox, Scabies, Lice)

Meconium Aspiration

See Respiratory Conditions of the Neonate

Meconium Delayed

Risk for neonatal hyperbilirubinemia: Risk factor: delayed meconium

Medical Marijuana

Imbalanced Nutrition: less than body requirements r/t eating disorder, appetite loss, effects of chemotherapy

Chronic Pain Syndrome r/t persistence of pain as a result of physical injury or condition

Nausea r/t effects of chemotherapy

Melanoma

Disturbed Body Image r/t altered pigmentation, surgical incision

Fear r/t threat to well-being

Ineffective Health maintenance r/t deficient knowledge regarding self-care and treatment of melanoma

Acute Pain r/t surgical incision

Chronic Sorrow r/t disturbed body image, unknown long-term health status

Readiness for enhanced Health management: describes reduction of risk factors; protection from sunlight's ultraviolet rays

See Cancer

Melena

Fear r/t presence of blood in feces

Risk for imbalanced Fluid volume: Risk factor: hemorrhage

See GI Bleed (Gastrointestinal Bleeding)

Memory Deficit

Impaired Memory (See **Memory,** impaired, Section III)

Ménière's Disease

Risk for Injury: Risk factor: symptoms of disease

Readiness for enhanced Health management: expresses desire to manage illness

See Dizziness; Nausea; Vertigo

Meningitis/Encephalitis

Ineffective Airway clearance r/t seizure activity

Impaired Comfort r/t altered health status

Excess Fluid volume r/t increased intracranial pressure, syndrome of inappropriate secretion of antidiuretic hormone

Decreased Intracranial adaptive capacity r/t sustained increase in intracranial pressure

Impaired Mobility r/t neuromuscular or central nervous system insult

Acute Pain r/t biological injury

Risk for Aspiration: Risk factor: seizure activity

Risk for acute Confusion: Risk factor: infection of brain

Risk for Falls: Risk factors: neuromuscular dysfunction and confusion

Risk for Injury: Risk factor: seizure activity

Risk for impaired Resilience: Risk factor: illness

M

Risk for Shock: Risk factor: infectious process
Risk for ineffective Cerebral tissue perfusion: Risk factors: cerebral tissue edema and inflammation of meninges, increased intracranial pressure; infection
Risk for ineffective Thermoregulation: Risk factor: infectious process
See Hospitalized Child

Meningocele

See Neural Tube Defects

Menopause

Impaired Comfort r/t symptoms associated with menopause
Insomnia r/t hormonal shifts
Impaired Memory r/t change in hormonal levels
Sexual dysfunction r/t menopausal changes
Ineffective Sexuality pattern r/t altered body structure, lack of lubrication, lack of knowledge of artificial lubrication
Ineffective Thermoregulation r/t changes in hormonal levels
Risk for urge urinary Incontinence: Risk factor: changes in hormonal levels affecting bladder function
Risk for Overweight: Risk factor: change in metabolic rate caused by fluctuating hormone levels
Risk for Powerlessness: Risk factor: changes associated with menopause
Risk for impaired Resilience: Risk factor: menopause
Risk for situational low Self-Esteem: Risk factors: developmental changes, menopause
Readiness for enhanced Health management: verbalized desire to manage menopause
Readiness for enhanced Self-Care: expresses satisfaction with body image
Readiness for enhanced Spiritual well-being: desire for harmony of mind, body, and spirit

Menorrhagia

Fear r/t loss of large amounts of blood
Risk for deficient Fluid volume: Risk factor: excessive loss of menstrual blood

Mental Illness

Defensive Coping r/t psychological impairment, substance abuse
Ineffective Coping r/t situational crisis, coping with mental illness
Compromised family Coping r/t lack of available support from client
Disabled family Coping r/t chronically unexpressed feelings of guilt, anxiety, hostility, or despair
Ineffective Denial r/t refusal to acknowledge abuse problem, fear of the social stigma of disease
Risk-prone Health behavior r/t low self-efficacy
Disturbed personal Identity r/t psychoses
Ineffective Relationship r/t effects of mental illness in partner relationship
Chronic Sorrow r/t presence of mental illness
Stress overload r/t multiple coexisting stressors

Ineffective family Health management r/t chronicity of condition, unpredictability of client, unknown prognosis
Risk for Loneliness: Risk factor: social isolation
Risk for Powerlessness: Risk factor: lifestyle of helplessness
Risk for impaired Resilience: Risk factor: chronic illness
Risk for chronic low Self-Esteem: Risk factor: presence of mental illness/repeated negative reinforcement

Metabolic Acidosis

See Ketoacidosis, Alcoholic; Ketoacidosis, Diabetic

Metabolic Alkalosis

Deficient Fluid volume r/t fluid volume loss, vomiting, gastric suctioning, failure of regulatory mechanisms

Metabolic Imbalance Syndrome

Ineffective Health Maintenance r/t deficient knowledge regarding basic health practice
Obesity r/t energy expenditure below energy intake
Risk for unstable blood Glucose level: Risk factor: variations in serum glucose levels

Metastasis

See Cancer

Methicillin-Resistant *Staphylococcus aureus* (MRSA)

See MRSA (Methicillin-Resistant Staphylococcus aureus)

MI (Myocardial Infarction)

Activity intolerance r/t imbalance between oxygen supply and demand
Anxiety r/t threat of death, possible change in role status
Death Anxiety r/t seriousness of medical condition
Constipation r/t decreased peristalsis from decreased physical activity, medication effect, change in diet
Ineffective family Coping r/t spouse or significant other's fear of partner loss
Ineffective Denial r/t fear, deficient knowledge about heart disease
Interrupted Family processes r/t crisis, role change
Fear r/t threat to well-being
Ineffective Health maintenance r/t deficient knowledge regarding self-care and treatment
Acute Pain r/t myocardial tissue damage from inadequate blood supply
Situational low Self-Esteem r/t crisis of MI
Ineffective Sexuality pattern r/t fear of chest pain, possibility of heart damage
Risk for Powerlessness: Risk factor: acute illness
Risk for Shock: Risk factors: hypotension, myocardial dysfunction, hypoxia
Risk for Spiritual distress: Risk factor: physical illness
Risk for decreased Cardiac output: Risk factors: alteration in heart rate, rhythm, and contractility
Risk for decreased Cardiac tissue perfusion: Risk factors: coronary artery spasm, hypertension, hypotension, hypoxia

Readiness for enhanced Knowledge: expresses an interest in learning about condition
See Angioplasty, Coronary; Coronary Artery Bypass Grafting (CABG)

MIDCAB (Minimally Invasive Direct Coronary Artery Bypass)

Risk for Bleeding: Risk factor: surgery

Readiness for enhanced Health management: preoperative and postoperative care associated with surgery

Risk for Surgical Site Infection: Risk factor: surgical procedure
See Angioplasty, Coronary; Coronary Artery Bypass Grafting (CABG)

Midlife Crisis

Ineffective Coping r/t inability to deal with changes associated with aging

Powerlessness r/t lack of control over life situation

Spiritual distress r/t questioning beliefs or value system

Risk for disturbed personal Identity: Risk factor: alteration in social roles

Risk for chronic low Self-Esteem: Risk factor: ineffective coping with loss

Readiness for enhanced Relationship: meets goals for lifestyle change

Readiness for enhanced Spiritual well-being: desire to find purpose and meaning to life

Migraine Headache

Ineffective Health maintenance r/t deficient knowledge regarding prevention and treatment of headaches

Readiness for enhanced Health management: expresses desire to manage illness

Acute Pain: headache r/t vasodilation of cerebral and extra-cerebral vessels

Risk for impaired Resilience: Risk factors: chronic illness, disabling pain

Military Families, Personnel

Anxiety r/t apprehension and helplessness caused by uncertainty of family members' situation

Interrupted Family Processes r/t possible change in family roles, decrease in available emotional support

Relocation stress syndrome r/t unpredictability of experience, powerlessness, significant environmental change

Milk Intolerance
See Lactose Intolerance

Minimally Invasive Direct Coronary Bypass (MIDCAB)
See MIDCAB (Minimally Invasive Direct Coronary Artery Bypass)

Miscarriage
See Pregnancy Loss

Mitral Stenosis

Activity intolerance r/t imbalance between oxygen supply and demand

Anxiety r/t possible worsening of symptoms, activity intolerance, fatigue

Decreased Cardiac output r/t incompetent heart valves, abnormal forward or backward blood flow, flow into a dilated chamber, flow through an abnormal passage between chambers

Fatigue r/t reduced cardiac output

Ineffective Health maintenance r/t deficient knowledge regarding self-care with disorder

Risk for decreased Cardiac tissue perfusion: Risk factor: incompetent heart valve

Risk for Infection: Risk factors: invasive procedure, risk for endocarditis

Mitral Valve Prolapse

Anxiety r/t symptoms of condition: palpitations, chest pain

Fatigue r/t abnormal catecholamine regulation, decreased intravascular volume

Fear r/t lack of knowledge about mitral valve prolapse, feelings of having heart attack

Ineffective Health maintenance r/t deficient knowledge regarding methods to relieve pain and treat dysrhythmia and shortness of breath, need for prophylactic antibiotics before invasive procedures

Acute Pain r/t mitral valve regurgitation

Risk for ineffective Cerebral tissue perfusion: Risk factor: postural hypotension

Risk for Infection: Risk factor: invasive procedures

Risk for Powerlessness: Risk factor: unpredictability of onset of symptoms

Readiness for enhanced Knowledge: expresses interest in learning about condition

Mobility, Impaired Bed

Impaired bed Mobility (See **Mobility,** bed, impaired, Section III)

Mobility, Impaired Physical

Impaired physical Mobility (See **Mobility,** physical, impaired, Section III)

Risk for Falls: Risk factor: impaired physical mobility

Mobility, Impaired Wheelchair

Impaired wheelchair Mobility (See **Mobility,** wheelchair, impaired, Section III)

Modified Radical Mastectomy

Readiness for enhanced Communication: willingness to enhance communication
See Mastectomy

Mononucleosis

Activity intolerance r/t generalized weakness

Impaired Comfort r/t sore throat, muscle aches

Fatigue r/t disease state, stress

Ineffective Health maintenance r/t deficient knowledge concerning transmission and treatment of disease

Acute Pain r/t enlargement of lymph nodes, oropharyngeal edema

Impaired Swallowing r/t enlargement of lymph nodes, oropharyngeal edema

Risk for Injury: Risk factor: possible rupture of spleen

Risk for Loneliness: Risk factor: social isolation

Mood Disorders

Caregiver Role Strain r/t overwhelming needs of care receiver, unpredictability of mood alterations

Labile Emotional Control r/t (See Labile **Emotional Control**, Section III)

Risk-prone Health behavior r/t hopelessness, altered locus of control

Impaired Mood regulation r/t (See **Mood** regulation, impaired, Section III)

Self-Neglect r/t inability to care for self

Social isolation r/t alterations in mental status

Risk for situational low Self-Esteem: Risk factor: unpredictable changes in mood

Readiness for enhanced Communication: expresses feelings

See specific disorder: Depression (Major Depressive Disorder); Dysthymic Disorder; Hypomania; Manic Disorder, Bipolar I

Moon Face

Disturbed Body Image r/t change in appearance from disease and medication(s)

Risk for situational low Self-Esteem: Risk factor: change in body image

See Cushing's Syndrome

Moral/Ethical Dilemmas

Impaired emancipated Decision-Making r/t questioning personal values and belief, which alter decision

Moral Distress r/t conflicting information guiding moral or ethical decision-making

Risk for Powerlessness: Risk factor: lack of knowledge to make a decision

Risk for Spiritual distress: Risk factor: moral or ethical crisis

Readiness for enhanced emancipated Decision-Making: expresses desire to enhance congruency of decisions with personal values and goals

Readiness for enhanced Religiosity: requests assistance in expanding religious options

Readiness for enhanced Resilience: vulnerable state

Readiness for enhanced Spiritual well-being: request for interaction with others regarding difficult decisions

Morning Sickness

See Hyperemesis Gravidarum; Pregnancy, Normal

Motion Sickness

See Labyrinthitis

Mottling of Peripheral Skin

Ineffective peripheral Tissue Perfusion r/t interruption of arterial flow, decreased circulating blood volume

Risk for Shock: Risk factor: inadequate circulation to perfuse body

Mourning

See Grieving

Mouth Lesions

See Mucous Membrane Integrity, Impaired Oral

MRI (Magnetic Resonance Imaging)

Anxiety r/t fear of being in closed spaces

Readiness for enhanced Health management: describes reduction of risk factors associated with exam

Deficient Knowledge r/t unfamiliarity with information resources; exam information

Readiness for enhanced Knowledge: expresses interest in learning about exam

MRSA (Methicillin-Resistant *Staphylococcus aureus*)

Impaired Skin integrity r/t infection

Delayed Surgical recovery r/t infection

Ineffective Thermoregulation r/t severe infection stimulating immune system

Impaired Tissue integrity r/t wound, infection

Risk for Loneliness: Risk factor: physical isolation

Risk for impaired Resilience: Risk factor: illness

Risk for Shock: Risk factor: sepsis

MS (Multiple Sclerosis)

See Multiple Sclerosis

Mucocutaneous Lymph Node Syndrome

See Kawasaki Disease

Mucous Membrane Integrity, Impaired Oral

Impaired Oral Mucous Membrane integrity (See **Oral Mucous Membrane** integrity, impaired, Section III)

Multi-Infarct Dementia

See Dementia

Multiple Gestations

Anxiety r/t uncertain outcome of pregnancy

Death Anxiety r/t maternal complications associated with multiple gestations

Insufficient Breast Milk Production r/t multiple births

Ineffective Childbearing process r/t unavailable support system

Fatigue r/t physiological demands of a multifetal pregnancy and/or care of more than one infant

Impaired Home maintenance r/t fatigue

Stress urinary Incontinence r/t increased pelvic pressure

Insomnia r/t impairment of normal sleep pattern; parental responsibilities

Deficient Knowledge r/t caring for more than one infant

Neonatal Hyperbilirubinemia r/t feeding pattern not well established

Deficient Knowledge r/t caring for more than one infant

M

Imbalanced Nutrition: less than body requirements r/t physiological demands of a multifetal pregnancy

Stress overload r/t multiple coexisting stressors, family demands

Impaired Walking r/t increased uterine size

Risk for ineffective Breastfeeding: Risk factors: lack of support, physical demands of feeding more than one infant

Risk for delayed Development: fetus: Risk factor: multiple gestations

Risk for neonatal hyperbilirubinemia: Risk factors: abnormal weight loss, prematurity, feeding pattern not well-established

Readiness for enhanced Childbearing process: demonstrates appropriate care for infants and mother

Readiness for enhanced Family processes: family adapting to change with more than one infant

Multiple Personality Disorder (Dissociative Identity Disorder)

Anxiety r/t loss of control of behavior and feelings

Disturbed Body Image r/t psychosocial changes

Defensive Coping r/t unresolved past traumatic events, severe anxiety

Ineffective Coping r/t history of abuse

Hopelessness r/t long-term stress

Disturbed personal Identity r/t severe child abuse

Chronic low Self-Esteem r/t rejection, failure

Risk for Self-Mutilation: Risk factor: need to act out to relieve stress

Readiness for enhanced Communication: willingness to discuss problems associated with condition

See Dissociative Identity Disorder (Not Otherwise Specified)

Multiple Sclerosis (MS)

Ineffective Activity planning r/t unrealistic perception of personal competence

Ineffective Airway clearance r/t decreased energy or fatigue

Impaired physical Mobility r/t neuromuscular impairment

Self-Neglect r/t functional impairment

Powerlessness r/t progressive nature of disease

Self-Care deficit: specify r/t neuromuscular impairment

Sexual dysfunction r/t biopsychosocial alteration of sexuality

Chronic Sorrow r/t loss of physical ability

Spiritual distress r/t perceived hopelessness of diagnosis

Urinary Retention r/t inhibition of the reflex arc

Risk for Disuse syndrome: Risk factor: physical immobility

Risk for Injury: Risk factors: altered mobility, sensory dysfunction

Risk for imbalanced Nutrition: less than body requirements: Risk factors: impaired swallowing, depression

Risk for Powerlessness: Risk factor: chronic illness

Risk for impaired Religiosity: Risk factor: illness

Risk for Thermal Injury: Risk factor: neuromuscular impairment

Readiness for enhanced Health management: expresses a desire to manage condition

Readiness for enhanced Self-Care: expresses desire to enhance knowledge of strategies and responsibility for self-care

Readiness for enhanced Spiritual well-being: struggling with chronic debilitating condition

See Neurologic Disorders

Mumps

See Communicable Diseases, Childhood (e.g., Measles, Mumps, Rubella, Chickenpox, Scabies, Lice)

Murmurs

Decreased Cardiac output r/t altered preload/afterload

Risk for decreased Cardiac tissue perfusion: Risk factor: incompetent valve

Risk for Fatigue: Risk factor: decreased cardiac output

Muscular Atrophy/Weakness

Risk for Disuse syndrome: Risk factor: impaired physical mobility

Risk for Falls: Risk factor: impaired physical mobility

Muscular Dystrophy (MD)

Activity intolerance r/t fatigue, muscle weakness

Ineffective Activity planning r/t unrealistic perception of personal competence

Ineffective Airway clearance r/t muscle weakness and decreased ability to cough

Constipation r/t immobility

Fatigue r/t increased energy requirements to perform activities of daily living

Impaired physical Mobility r/t muscle weakness and development of contractures

Imbalanced Nutrition: less than body requirements r/t impaired swallowing or chewing

Self-Care deficit: feeding, bathing, dressing, toileting r/t muscle weakness and fatigue

Self-Neglect r/t functional impairment

Impaired Transfer ability r/t muscle weakness

Impaired Swallowing r/t neuromuscular impairment

Impaired Walking r/t muscle weakness

Risk for Aspiration: Risk factor: impaired swallowing

Risk for decreased Cardiac tissue perfusion: Risk factor: hypoxia associated with cardiomyopathy

Risk for Disuse syndrome: Risk factor: complications of immobility

Risk for Falls: Risk factor: muscle weakness

Risk for Infection: Risk factor: pooling of pulmonary secretions as a result of immobility and muscle weakness

Risk for Injury: Risk factors: muscle weakness and unsteady gait

Risk for Overweight: Risk factor: inactivity

Risk for Powerlessness: Risk factor: chronic condition

Risk for impaired Religiosity: Risk factor: illness

Risk for impaired Resilience: Risk factor: chronic illness

Risk for situational low Self-Esteem: Risk factor: presence of chronic condition

M

Readiness for enhanced Self-Concept: acceptance of strength and abilities

Risk for impaired Skin integrity: Risk factors: immobility, braces, or adaptive devices

See Child with Chronic Condition; Hospitalized Child

MVC (Motor Vehicle Crash)

See Fracture; Head Injury; Injury; Pneumothorax

Myasthenia Gravis

Ineffective Airway clearance r/t decreased ability to cough and swallow

Interrupted Family processes r/t crisis of dealing with diagnosis

Fatigue r/t paresthesia, aching muscles, weakness of muscles

Impaired physical Mobility r/t defective transmission of nerve impulses at the neuromuscular junction

Imbalanced Nutrition: less than body requirements r/t difficulty eating and swallowing

Impaired Swallowing r/t neuromuscular impairment

Risk for Caregiver Role Strain: Risk factors: severity of illness of client, overwhelming needs of client

Risk for impaired Religiosity: Risk factor: illness

Risk for impaired Resilience: Risk factor: new diagnosis of chronic, serious illness

Readiness for enhanced Spiritual well-being: heightened coping with serious illness

See Neurologic Disorders

Mycoplasma Pneumonia

See Pneumonia

Myelocele

See Neural Tube Defects

Myelomeningocele

See Neural Tube Defects

Myocardial Infarction (MI)

See MI (Myocardial Infarction)

Myocarditis

Activity intolerance r/t reduced cardiac reserve and prescribed bed rest

Decreased Cardiac output r/t altered preload/afterload

Deficient Knowledge r/t treatment of disease

Risk for decreased Cardiac tissue perfusion: Risk factors: hypoxia, hypovolemia, cardiac tamponade

Readiness for enhanced Knowledge: treatment of disease

See Heart Failure, if appropriate

Myringotomy

Fear r/t hospitalization, surgical procedure

Ineffective Health maintenance r/t deficient knowledge regarding care after surgery

Acute Pain r/t surgical procedure

Risk for Surgical Site Infection: Risk factor: invasive procedure

See Ear Surgery

Myxedema

See Hypothyroidism

N

Narcissistic Personality Disorder

Defensive Coping r/t grandiose sense of self

Impaired emancipated Decision-Making r/t lack of realistic problem-solving skills

Interrupted Family processes r/t taking advantage of others to achieve own goals

Risk-prone Health behavior r/t low self-efficacy

Disturbed personal Identity r/t psychological impairment

Ineffective Relationship r/t lack of mutual support/respect between partners

Impaired individual Resilience r/t psychological disorders

Impaired Social interaction r/t self-concept disturbance

Risk for Loneliness: Risk factors: emotional deprivation, social isolation

Narcolepsy

Anxiety r/t fear of lack of control over falling asleep

Disturbed Sleep pattern r/t uncontrollable desire to sleep

Risk for Physical Trauma: Risk factor: falling asleep during potentially dangerous activity

Readiness for enhanced Sleep: expresses willingness to enhance sleep

Narcotic Use

See Opioid Use (preferred terminology)

Nasogastric Suction

Impaired Oral Mucous Membrane integrity r/t presence of nasogastric tube

Risk for Electrolyte imbalance: Risk factor: loss of gastrointestinal fluids that contain electrolytes

Risk for imbalanced Fluid volume: Risk factor: loss of gastrointestinal fluids without adequate replacement

Risk for dysfunctional Gastrointestinal motility: Risk factor: decreased intestinal motility

Nausea

Nausea (See **Nausea,** Section III)

Near-Drowning

Ineffective Airway clearance r/t aspiration of fluid

Aspiration r/t aspiration of fluid into lungs

Fear: parental r/t possible death of child, possible permanent and debilitating sequelae

Impaired Gas exchange r/t laryngospasm, holding breath, aspiration, inflammation

Grieving r/t potential death of child, unknown sequelae, guilt about accident

Ineffective Health maintenance r/t parental deficient knowledge regarding safety measures appropriate for age

Hypothermia r/t central nervous system injury, prolonged submersion in cold water

Risk for delayed Development: Risk factors: hypoxemia, cerebral anoxia

Risk for complicated Grieving: Risk factors: potential death of child, unknown sequelae, guilt about accident

Risk for Infection: Risk factors: aspiration, invasive monitoring

Risk for ineffective Cerebral tissue perfusion: Risk factor: hypoxia

Readiness for enhanced Spiritual well-being: struggle with survival of life-threatening situation

See Child with Chronic Condition; Hospitalized Child; Safety, Childhood; Terminally Ill Child/Death of Child, Parent

Nearsightedness

Readiness for enhanced Health management: need for correction of myopia

Nearsightedness; Corneal Surgery

See LASIK Eye Surgery (Laser-Assisted in Situ Keratomileusis)

Neck Vein Distention

Decreased Cardiac output r/t decreased contractility of heart resulting in increased preload

Excess Fluid volume r/t excess fluid intake, compromised regulatory mechanisms

See Congestive Heart Failure (CHF); Heart Failure

Necrosis, Kidney Tubular; Necrosis, Acute Tubular

See Renal Failure

Necrotizing Enterocolitis

Ineffective Breathing pattern r/t abdominal distention, hypoxia

Diarrhea r/t infection

Deficient Fluid volume r/t vomiting, gastrointestinal bleeding

Neonatal Hyperbilirubinemia r/t feeding pattern not well established

Imbalanced Nutrition: less than body requirements r/t decreased ability to absorb nutrients, decreased perfusion to gastrointestinal tract

Risk for dysfunctional Gastrointestinal motility: Risk factor: infection

Risk for Infection: Risk factors: bacterial invasion of gastrointestinal tract, invasive procedures

See Hospitalized Child; Premature Infant (Child)

Negative Feelings About Self

Chronic low Self-Esteem r/t long-standing negative self-evaluation

Self-Neglect r/t negative feelings

Readiness for enhanced Self-Concept: expresses willingness to enhance self-concept

Neglect, Unilateral

Unilateral Neglect (See **Unilateral Neglect,** Section III)

Neglectful Care of Family Member

Caregiver Role Strain r/t overwhelming care demands of family member, lack of social or financial support

Disabled family Coping r/t highly ambivalent family relationships, lack of respite care

Interrupted Family processes r/t situational transition or crisis

Deficient Knowledge r/t care needs

Impaired individual Resilience r/t vulnerability from neglect

Risk for compromised Human Dignity: Risk factor: inadequate participation in decision-making

Neonatal Abstinence Syndrome

Ineffective Airway clearance r/t pooling of secretions from lack of adequate cough reflex, effects of viral or bacterial lower airway infection as a result of altered protective state

Interrupted Breastfeeding r/t use of drugs or alcohol by mother

Ineffective Childbearing process r/t inconsistent prenatal health visits, suboptimal maternal nutrition, substance abuse

Impaired Comfort r/t irritability and inability to relax

Diarrhea r/t effects of withdrawal, increased peristalsis from hyperirritability

Disorganized infant Behavior r/t exposure and/or withdrawal from toxic substances (alcohol or drugs), lack of attachment

Ineffective infant Feeding pattern r/t uncoordinated or ineffective sucking reflex

Imbalanced Nutrition: less than body requirements r/t feeding problems; uncoordinated or ineffective suck and swallow; effects of diarrhea, vomiting, or colic associated with maternal substance abuse

Impaired Parenting r/t impaired or absent attachment behaviors, inadequate support systems

Ineffective infant Feeding Pattern r/t neurological delay

Disturbed Sleep Pattern r/t hyperirritability or hypersensitivity to environmental stimuli

Risk for impaired Attachment: Risk factor: (parent) substance misuse, inability to meet infant's needs

Risk for delayed Development: Risk factor: effects of prenatal substance abuse

Risk for Infection: Risk factor: stress effects of withdrawal

Risk for Disturbed Maternal–Fetal Dyad: Risk factor: substance abuse

Risk for Sudden Infant Death: Risk factor: prenatal illicit drug exposure

Risk for ineffective Thermoregulation: Risk factor: immature nervous system

See Anomaly, Fetal/Newborn (Parent Dealing with); Cerebral Palsy; Child with Chronic Condition; Failure to Thrive; Hospitalized Child; Hyperactive Syndrome; Premature Infant/Child; Sudden Infant Death, Risk for

N

Neonatal Hyperbilirubinemia

Neonatal Hyperbilirubinemia (See neonatal **Hyperbilirubinemia,** Section III)

Neonate

Readiness for enhanced Childbearing process: appropriate care of newborn

See Newborn, Normal; Newborn, Postmature; Newborn, Small for Gestational Age (SGA)

Neoplasm

Fear r/t possible malignancy

See Cancer

Nephrectomy

Anxiety r/t surgical recovery, prognosis

Ineffective Breathing pattern r/t location of surgical incision

Constipation r/t lack of return of peristalsis

Acute Pain r/t incisional discomfort

Spiritual distress r/t chronic illness

Risk for Bleeding: Risk factor: surgery

Risk for imbalanced Fluid volume: Risk factors: vascular losses, decreased intake

Risk for Surgical Site Infection: Risk factor: surgical procedure

Nephrostomy, Percutaneous

Acute Pain r/t invasive procedure

Impaired Urinary elimination r/t nephrostomy tube

Risk for Infection: Risk factor: invasive procedure

Nephrotic Syndrome

Activity intolerance r/t generalized edema

Disturbed Body Image r/t edematous appearance and side effects of steroid therapy

Excess Fluid volume r/t edema resulting from oncotic fluid shift caused by serum protein loss and kidney retention of salt and water

Imbalanced Nutrition: less than body requirements r/t anorexia, protein loss

Imbalanced Nutrition: more than body requirements r/t increased appetite attributable to steroid therapy

Social isolation r/t edematous appearance

Risk for Infection: Risk factor: altered immune mechanisms caused by disease and effects of steroids

Risk for impaired Skin integrity: Risk factor: edema

See Child with Chronic Condition; Hospitalized Child

Neural Tube Defects (Meningocele, Myelomeningocele, Spina Bifida, Anencephaly)

Chronic functional Constipation r/t immobility or less than adequate mobility

Grieving r/t loss of perfect child, birth of child with congenital defect

Reflex urinary Incontinence r/t neurogenic impairment

Total urinary Incontinence r/t neurogenic impairment

Urge urinary Incontinence r/t neurogenic impairment

Impaired Mobility r/t neuromuscular impairment

Chronic low Self-Esteem r/t perceived differences, decreased ability to participate in physical and social activities at school

Impaired Skin integrity r/t incontinence

Risk for delayed Development: Risk factor: inadequate nutrition

Risk for Latex Allergic reaction: Risk factor: multiple exposures to latex products

Risk for imbalanced Nutrition: more than body requirements: Risk factors: diminished, limited, or impaired physical activity

Risk for Powerlessness: Risk factor: debilitating disease

Risk for impaired Skin integrity: lower extremities: Risk factor: decreased sensory perception

Readiness for enhanced family Coping: effective adaptive response by family members

Readiness for enhanced Family processes: family supports each other

See Child with Chronic Condition; Premature Infant (Child)

Neuralgia

See Trigeminal Neuralgia

Neuritis (Peripheral Neuropathy)

Activity intolerance r/t pain with movement

Ineffective Health maintenance r/t deficient knowledge regarding self-care with neuritis

Acute Pain r/t stimulation of affected nerve endings, inflammation of sensory nerves

See Neuropathy, Peripheral

Neurogenic Bladder

Reflex urinary Incontinence r/t neurological impairment

Urinary Retention r/t interruption in the lateral spinal tracts

Risk for Latex Allergic reaction: Risk factor: repeated exposures to latex associated with possible repeated catheterizations

Neurologic Disorders

Ineffective Airway clearance r/t perceptual or cognitive impairment, decreased energy, fatigue

Acute Confusion r/t dementia, alcohol abuse, drug abuse, delirium

Ineffective Coping r/t disability requiring change in lifestyle

Interrupted Family processes r/t situational crisis, illness, or disability of family member

Grieving r/t loss of usual body functioning

Impaired Home maintenance r/t client's or family member's disease

Risk for corneal Injury: Risk factor: lack of spontaneous blink reflex

Impaired Memory r/t neurological disturbance

Impaired physical Mobility r/t neuromuscular impairment

Imbalanced Nutrition: less than body requirements r/t impaired swallowing, depression, difficulty feeding self

Powerlessness r/t progressive nature of disease

Self-Care deficit: specify r/t neuromuscular dysfunction

Sexual dysfunction r/t biopsychosocial alteration of sexuality

Social isolation r/t altered state of wellness

Impaired Swallowing r/t neuromuscular dysfunction

Risk for Disuse syndrome: Risk factors: physical immobility, neuromuscular dysfunction

Risk for Injury: Risk factors: altered mobility, sensory dysfunction, cognitive impairment

Risk for ineffective Cerebral tissue perfusion: Risk factor: cerebral disease/injury

Risk for impaired Religiosity: Risk factor: life transition

Risk for impaired Skin integrity: Risk factors: altered sensation, altered mental status, paralysis

See specific condition: Alcohol Withdrawal; Amyotrophic Lateral Sclerosis (ALS); CVA (Cerebrovascular Accident); Delirium; Dementia; Guillain-Barré Syndrome; Head Injury; Huntington's Disease; Spinal Cord Injury; Myasthenia Gravis; Muscular Dystrophy (MD); Parkinson's Disease

Neuropathy, Peripheral

Chronic Pain r/t damage to nerves in the peripheral nervous system as a result of medication side effects, vitamin deficiency, or diabetes

Ineffective Thermoregulation r/t decreased ability to regulate body temperature

Risk for Injury: Risk factors: lack of muscle control, decreased sensation

Risk for impaired Skin integrity: Risk factor: poor perfusion

Risk for Thermal Injury: Risk factor: nerve damage

See Peripheral Vascular Disease (PVD)

Neurosurgery

See Craniectomy/Craniotomy

Newborn, Normal

Breastfeeding r/t normal oral structure and gestational age greater than 34 weeks

Ineffective Thermoregulation r/t immaturity of neuroendocrine system

Risk for Sudden Infant Death: Risk factors: lack of knowledge regarding infant sleeping in prone or side-lying position, prenatal or postnatal infant smoke exposure, infant overheating or overwrapping, loose articles in the sleep environment

Risk for Infection: Risk factors: open umbilical stump, immature immune system

Risk for Injury: Risk factors: immaturity, need for caretaking

Readiness for enhanced Childbearing process: appropriate care of newborn

Readiness for enhanced organized Infant behavior: demonstrates adaptive response to pain

Readiness for enhanced Parenting: providing emotional and physical needs of infant

Newborn, Postmature

Hypothermia r/t depleted stores of subcutaneous fat

Impaired Skin integrity r/t cracked and peeling skin as a result of decreased vernix

Risk for ineffective Airway clearance: Risk factor: meconium aspiration

Risk for unstable blood Glucose level: Risk factor: depleted glycogen stores

Newborn, Small for Gestational Age (SGA)

Neonatal Hyperbilirubinemia r/t neonate age and difficulty feeding

Imbalanced Nutrition: less than body requirements r/t history of placental insufficiency

Ineffective Thermoregulation r/t decreased brown fat, subcutaneous fat

Risk for delayed Development: Risk factor: history of placental insufficiency

Risk for Injury: Risk factors: hypoglycemia, perinatal asphyxia, meconium aspiration

Risk for Sudden Infant Death: Risk factor: low birth weight

Nicotine Addiction

Risk-prone Health behavior r/t smoking

Ineffective Health maintenance r/t lack of ability to make a judgment about smoking cessation

Risk for impaired Skin integrity: Risk factor: poor tissue perfusion associated with nicotine

Powerlessness r/t perceived lack of control over ability to give up nicotine

Readiness for enhanced emancipated Decision-Making: expresses desire to enhance understanding and meaning of choices

Readiness for enhanced Health literacy: expresses desire to enhance understanding of health information to make health care choices

Readiness for enhanced Health management: expresses desire to learn measures to stop smoking

NIDDM (Non–Insulin-Dependent Diabetes Mellitus)

Readiness for enhanced Health management: expresses desire for information on exercise and diet to manage diabetes
See Diabetes Mellitus

Nightmares

Post-Trauma syndrome r/t disaster, war, epidemic, rape, assault, torture, catastrophic illness, or accident

Nipple Soreness

Impaired Comfort r/t physical condition
See Painful Breasts, Sore Nipples; Sore Nipples, Breastfeeding

Nocturia

Urge urinary Incontinence r/t decreased bladder capacity, irritation of bladder stretch receptors causing spasm, alcohol, caffeine, increased fluids, increased urine concentration, overdistention of bladder

N

Impaired Urinary elimination r/t sensory motor impairment, urinary tract infection

Risk for Powerlessness: Risk factor: inability to control nighttime voiding

Nocturnal Myoclonus

See Restless Leg Syndrome; Stress

Nocturnal Paroxysmal Dyspnea

See PND (Paroxysmal Nocturnal Dyspnea)

Non–Insulin-Dependent Diabetes Mellitus (NIDDM)

See Diabetes Mellitus

Normal Pressure Hydrocephalus (NPH)

Impaired verbal Communication r/t obstruction of flow of cerebrospinal fluid affecting speech

Acute Confusion r/t increased intracranial pressure caused by obstruction to flow of cerebrospinal fluid

Impaired Memory r/t neurological disturbance

Risk for ineffective Cerebral tissue perfusion: Risk factor: fluid pressing on the brain

Risk for Falls: Risk factor: unsteady gait as a result of obstruction of cerebrospinal fluid

NSTEMI (non–ST-elevation myocardial infarction)

See MI (Myocardial Infarction)

Nursing

See Breastfeeding, Effective; Breastfeeding, Ineffective; Breastfeeding, Interrupted

Nutrition

Readiness for enhanced Nutrition (See **Nutrition,** readiness for enhanced, Section III)

Nutrition, Imbalanced

Imbalanced Nutrition: less than body requirements (See **Nutrition:** less than body requirements, imbalanced, Section III)

Obesity (See **Obesity,** Section III)

Overweight (See **Overweight,** Section III)

Risk for Dry Mouth r/t depression

Risk for Overweight (See **Overweight,** risk for, Section III)

O

Obesity

Disturbed Body Image r/t eating disorder, excess weight

Risk-prone Health behavior: r/t negative attitude toward health care

Obesity (See **Obesity,** Section III)

Chronic low Self-Esteem r/t ineffective coping, overeating

Risk for Metabolic Imbalance syndrome: Risk factor: obesity

Risk for ineffective peripheral Tissue Perfusion: Risk factor: sedentary lifestyle

Readiness for enhanced Nutrition: expresses willingness to enhance nutrition

OBS (Organic Brain Syndrome)

See Organic Mental Disorders; Dementia

Obsessive-Compulsive Disorder (OCD)

See OCD (Obsessive-Compulsive Disorder)

Obstruction, Bowel

See Bowel Obstruction

Obstructive Sleep Apnea

Insomnia r/t blocked airway

Obesity r/t excessive intake related to metabolic need

See PND (Paroxysmal Nocturnal Dyspnea)

OCD (Obsessive-Compulsive Disorder)

Ineffective Activity planning r/t unrealistic perception of events

Anxiety r/t threat to self-concept, unmet needs

Impaired emancipated Decision-Making r/t inability to make a decision for fear of reprisal

Disabled family Coping r/t family process being disrupted by client's ritualistic activities

Ineffective Coping r/t expression of feelings in an unacceptable way, ritualistic behavior

Risk-prone Health behavior r/t inadequate comprehension associated with repetitive thoughts

Powerlessness r/t unrelenting repetitive thoughts to perform irrational activities

Impaired individual Resilience r/t psychological disorder

Risk for situational low Self-Esteem: Risk factor: inability to control repetitive thoughts and actions

Occupational Injury

Fatigue r/t lack of sleep

Deficient Knowledge r/t inadequate training, improper use of equipment

Stress Overload r/t feelings of pressure

Risk for Occupational Injury (See **Risk for Occupational Injury,** Section III)

ODD (Oppositional Defiant Disorder)

Anxiety r/t feelings of anger and hostility toward authority figures

Ineffective Coping r/t lack of self-control or perceived lack of self-control

Disabled Family coping r/t feelings of anger, hostility; defiant behavior toward authority figures

Risk-prone Health behavior r/t multiple stressors associated with condition

Ineffective Impulse control r/t anger/compunction to engage in disruptive behaviors

Chronic or situational low Self-Esteem r/t poor self-control and disruptive behaviors

Impaired Social interaction r/t being touchy or easily annoyed, blaming others for own mistakes, constant trouble in school

Social isolation r/t unaccepted social behavior

Ineffective family Health management r/t difficulty in limit setting and managing oppositional behaviors

Risk for ineffective Activity planning: Risk factors: unrealistic perception of events, hedonism, insufficient social support

Risk for impaired Parenting: Risk factors: children's difficult behaviors and inability to set limits

Risk for Powerlessness: Risk factor: inability to deal with difficult behaviors

Risk for Spiritual distress: Risk factors: anxiety and stress in dealing with difficult behaviors

Risk for other-directed Violence: Risk factors: history of violence, threats of violence against others, history of antisocial behavior, history of indirect violence

Older Adult

See Aging

Oliguria

Deficient Fluid volume r/t active fluid loss, failure of regulatory mechanism, inadequate intake

See Cardiac Output, Decreased; Renal Failure; Shock, Hypovolemic

Omphalocele

See Gastroschisis/Omphalocele

Oophorectomy

Risk for ineffective Sexuality pattern: Risk factor: altered body function

See Surgery, Perioperative Care; Surgery, Postoperative Care; Surgery, Preoperative Care

OPCAB (Off-Pump Coronary Artery Bypass)

See Angioplasty, Coronary; Coronary Artery Bypass Grafting (CABG)

Open Heart Surgery

Risk for decreased Cardiac tissue perfusion: Risk factor: cardiac surgery

See Coronary Artery Bypass Grafting (CABG); Dysrhythmia

Open Reduction of Fracture with Internal Fixation (Femur)

Anxiety r/t outcome of corrective procedure

Impaired physical Mobility r/t postoperative position, abduction of leg, avoidance of acute flexion

Powerlessness r/t loss of control, unanticipated change in lifestyle

Risk for Surgical Site Infection: Risk factor: surgical procedure

Risk for Perioperative Positioning injury: Risk factor: immobilization

Risk for peripheral neurovascular dysfunction: Risk factors: mechanical compression, orthopedic surgery, immobilization

Risk for venous thromboembolism: Risk factor: impaired mobility

See Surgery, Postoperative Care

Opioid Addiction

See Substance Abuse

Opioid Use

Acute Pain r/t physical injury or surgical procedure

Chronic Pain syndrome r/t prolonged use of opioids

Risk for Constipation: Risk factor: effects of opioids on peristalsis

See Substance Abuse; Substance Withdrawal; Pain Management, Acute; Pain Management, Chronic

Opportunistic Infection

Delayed Surgical recovery r/t abnormal blood profiles, impaired healing

Risk for Infection: Risk factor: abnormal blood profiles

See AIDS (Acquired Immunodeficiency Syndrome); HIV (Human Immunodeficiency Virus)

Oppositional Defiant Disorder (ODD)

See ODD (Oppositional Defiant Disorder)

Oral Mucous Membrane Integrity, Impaired

Impaired Oral Mucous Membrane integrity (See **Oral Mucous Membrane** integrity, impaired, Section III)

Oral Thrush

See Candidiasis, Oral

Orchitis

Readiness for enhanced Health management: follows recommendations for mumps vaccination

See Epididymitis

Organic Mental Disorders

Chronic Confusion r/t progressive impairment in cognitive functioning

Frail Elderly syndrome r/t alteration in cognitive function

Impaired Social interaction r/t disturbed thought processes

Risk for disturbed personal Identity: Risk factor: delusions/fluctuating perceptions of stimuli

See Dementia

Orthopedic Traction

Ineffective Role performance r/t limited physical mobility

Impaired Social interaction r/t limited physical mobility

Impaired Transfer ability r/t limited physical mobility

Risk for impaired Religiosity: Risk factor: immobility

See Traction and Casts

Orthopnea

Ineffective Breathing pattern r/t inability to breathe with head of bed flat

Decreased Cardiac output r/t inability of heart to meet demands of body

O

Orthostatic Hypotension

See Dizziness

Osteoarthritis

Acute Pain r/t movement

Impaired Walking r/t inflammation and damage to joints

See Arthritis

Osteomyelitis

Decreased Diversional activity engagement r/t prolonged immobilization, hospitalization

Fear: parental r/t concern regarding possible growth plate damage caused by infection, concern that infection may become chronic

Ineffective Health maintenance r/t continued immobility at home, possible extensive casts, continued antibiotics

Impaired physical Mobility r/t imposed immobility as a result of infected area

Acute Pain r/t inflammation in affected extremity

Ineffective Thermoregulation r/t infectious process

Risk for Constipation: Risk factor: immobility

Risk for Infection: Risk factor: inadequate primary and secondary defenses

Risk for impaired Skin integrity: Risk factor: irritation from splint or cast

See Hospitalized Child

Osteoporosis

Deficient Knowledge r/t diet, exercise, need to abstain from alcohol and nicotine

Impaired physical Mobility r/t pain, skeletal changes

Imbalanced Nutrition: less than body requirements r/t inadequate intake of calcium and vitamin D

Acute Pain r/t fracture, muscle spasms

Risk for Injury: fracture: Risk factors: lack of activity, risk of falling resulting from environmental hazards, neuromuscular disorders, diminished senses, cardiovascular responses to drugs

Risk for Powerlessness: Risk factor: debilitating disease

Readiness for enhanced Health management: expresses desire to manage the treatment of illness and prevent complications

Ostomy

See Child with Chronic Condition; Colostomy; Ileal Conduit; Ileostomy

Otitis Media

Acute Pain r/t inflammation, infectious process

Risk for delayed Development: speech and language: Risk factor: frequent otitis media

Risk for Infection: Risk factors: eustachian tube obstruction, traumatic eardrum perforation, infectious process

Readiness for enhanced Knowledge: information on treatment and prevention of disease

Ovarian Carcinoma

Death Anxiety r/t unknown outcome, possible poor prognosis

Fear r/t unknown outcome, possible poor prognosis

Ineffective Health Maintenance r/t deficient knowledge regarding self-care, treatment of condition

Readiness for enhanced Family Processes: family functioning meets needs of client

Readiness for enhanced Resilience: participates in support groups

See Chemotherapy; Hysterectomy; Radiation Therapy

P

Pacemaker

Anxiety r/t change in health status, presence of pacemaker

Death Anxiety r/t worry over possible malfunction of pacemaker

Deficient Knowledge r/t self-care program, when to seek medical attention

Acute Pain r/t surgical procedure

Risk for Bleeding: Risk factor: surgery

Risk for decreased Cardiac tissue perfusion: Risk factor: pacemaker malfunction

Risk for Infection: Risk factors: invasive procedure, presence of foreign body (catheter and generator)

Risk for Powerlessness: Risk factor: presence of electronic device to stimulate heart

Readiness for enhanced Health management: appropriate health care management of pacemaker

Paget's Disease

Disturbed Body Image r/t possible enlarged head, bowed tibias, kyphosis

Deficient Knowledge r/t appropriate diet high in protein and calcium, mild exercise

Chronic Sorrow r/t chronic condition with altered body image

Risk for Physical Trauma: fracture: Risk factor: excessive bone destruction

Pain Management, Acute

Acute Pain r/t injury or surgical procedure

Imbalanced Energy Field r/t unpleasant sensory and emotional feelings

Pain Management, Chronic

Chronic Pain (See **Pain,** chronic, Section III)

Chronic Pain Syndrome r/t persistent pain affecting daily living

Risk for Constipation: Risk factor: effects of meds on peristalsis

Readiness for enhanced Knowledge: expresses a desire to learn alternative methods of non-pharmaceutical pain control

See Substance Abuse

Painful Breasts, Engorgement

Acute Pain r/t distention of breast tissue

Ineffective Role performance r/t change in physical capacity to assume role of breastfeeding mother

Impaired Tissue integrity r/t excessive fluid in breast tissues

Risk for ineffective Breastfeeding: Risk factors: pain, infant's inability to latch on to engorged breast

Risk for Infection: Risk factor: milk stasis

Painful Breasts, Sore Nipples

Insufficient Breast Milk Production r/t long breastfeeding time/pain response

Ineffective Breastfeeding r/t pain

Acute Pain r/t cracked nipples

Ineffective Role performance r/t change in physical capacity to assume role of breastfeeding mother

Impaired Skin integrity r/t mechanical factors involved in suckling, breastfeeding management

Risk for Infection: Risk factor: break in skin

Pallor of Extremities

Ineffective peripheral Tissue Perfusion r/t interruption of vascular flow

See Shock; Peripheral Vascular disease (PVD)

Palpitations (Heart Palpitations)

See Dysrhythmia

Pancreatic Cancer

Death Anxiety r/t possible poor prognosis of disease process

Ineffective family Coping r/t poor prognosis

Fear r/t poor prognosis of the disease

Grieving r/t shortened life span

Deficient Knowledge r/t disease-induced diabetes, home management

Spiritual distress r/t poor prognosis

Risk for impaired Liver function: Risk factor: complications from underlying disease

See Cancer; Chemotherapy; Radiation Therapy; Surgery, Perioperative Care; Surgery, Postoperative Care; Surgery, Preoperative Care

Pancreatitis

Ineffective Breathing pattern r/t splinting from severe pain, disease process and inflammation

Ineffective Denial r/t ineffective coping, alcohol use

Diarrhea r/t decrease in pancreatic secretions resulting in steatorrhea

Deficient Fluid volume r/t vomiting, decreased fluid intake, fever, diaphoresis, fluid shifts

Ineffective Health maintenance r/t deficient knowledge concerning diet, alcohol use, medication

Nausea r/t irritation of gastrointestinal system

Imbalanced Nutrition: less than body requirements r/t inadequate dietary intake, increased nutritional needs as a result of acute illness, increased metabolic needs caused by increased body temperature, disease process

Acute Pain r/t irritation and edema of the inflamed pancreas

Chronic Sorrow r/t chronic illness

Readiness for enhanced Comfort: expresses desire to enhance comfort

Panic Disorder (Panic Attacks)

Ineffective Activity planning r/t unrealistic perception of events

Anxiety r/t situational crisis

Ineffective Coping r/t personal vulnerability

Risk-prone Health behavior r/t low self-efficacy

Disturbed personal Identity r/t situational crisis

Post-Trauma syndrome r/t previous catastrophic event

Social isolation r/t fear of lack of control

Risk for Loneliness: Risk factor: inability to socially interact because of fear of losing control

Risk for Post-Trauma syndrome: Risk factors: perception of the event, diminished ego strength

Risk for Powerlessness: Risk factor: ineffective coping skills

Readiness for enhanced Coping: seeks problem-oriented and emotion-oriented strategies to manage condition

See Anxiety; Anxiety Disorder

Paralysis

Disturbed Body Image r/t biophysical changes, loss of movement, immobility

Impaired Comfort r/t prolonged immobility

Constipation r/t effects of spinal cord disruption, inadequate fiber in diet

Ineffective Health maintenance r/t deficient knowledge regarding self-care with paralysis

Impaired Home maintenance r/t physical disability

Reflex urinary Incontinence r/t neurological impairment

Impaired physical Mobility r/t neuromuscular impairment

Impaired wheelchair Mobility r/t neuromuscular impairment

Self-Neglect r/t functional impairment

Powerlessness r/t illness-related regimen

Self-Care deficit: specify r/t neuromuscular impairment

Sexual dysfunction r/t loss of sensation, biopsychosocial alteration

Chronic Sorrow r/t loss of physical mobility

Impaired Transfer ability r/t paralysis

Risk for Autonomic Dysreflexia: Risk factor: cause of paralysis

Risk for Disuse syndrome: Risk factor: paralysis

Risk for Falls: Risk factor: paralysis

Risk for Injury: Risk factors: altered mobility, sensory dysfunction

Risk for Latex Allergic reaction: Risk factor: possible repeated urinary catheterizations

Risk for Post-Trauma syndrome: Risk factor: event causing paralysis

Risk for impaired Religiosity: Risk factors: immobility, possible lack of transportation

Risk for impaired Resilience: Risk factor: chronic disability

Risk for situational low Self-Esteem: Risk factor: change in body image and function

Risk for impaired Skin integrity: Risk factors: altered circulation, altered sensation, immobility

Risk for Venous Thromboembolism: Risk factor: prolonged immobility

P

Readiness for enhanced Self-Care: expresses desire to enhance knowledge and responsibility for strategies for self-care
See Child with Chronic Condition; Hemiplegia; Hospitalized Child; Neural Tube Defects (Meningocele, Myelomeningocele, Spina Bifida, Anencephaly); Spinal Cord Injury

Paralytic Ileus

Constipation r/t decreased gastrointestinal motility

Deficient Fluid volume r/t loss of fluids from vomiting, retention of fluid in bowel

Dysfunctional Gastrointestinal motility r/t recent abdominal surgery, electrolyte imbalance

Nausea r/t gastrointestinal irritation

Acute Pain r/t pressure, abdominal distention, presence of nasogastric tube
See Bowel Obstruction

Paranoid Personality Disorder

Ineffective Activity planning r/t unrealistic perception of events

Anxiety r/t uncontrollable intrusive, suspicious thoughts

Risk-prone Health behavior r/t intense emotional state

Disturbed personal Identity r/t difficulty with reality testing

Impaired individual Resilience r/t psychological disorder

Chronic low Self-Esteem r/t inability to trust others

Social isolation r/t inappropriate social skills

Risk for Loneliness: Risk factor: social isolation

Risk for other-directed Violence: Risk factor: being suspicious of others and their actions

Paraplegia

See Spinal Cord Injury

Parathyroidectomy

Anxiety r/t surgery

Risk for ineffective Airway clearance: Risk factors: edema or hematoma formation, airway obstruction

Risk for Bleeding: Risk factor: surgery

Risk for impaired verbal Communication: Risk factors: possible laryngeal damage, edema

Risk for Infection: Risk factor: surgical procedure
See Hypocalcemia

Parent Attachment

Risk for impaired Attachment (See **Attachment,** impaired, risk for, Section III)

Readiness for enhanced Childbearing process: demonstrates appropriate care of newborn
See Parental Role Conflict

Parental Role Conflict

Parental Role conflict (See **Role** conflict, parental, Section III)

Ineffective Relationship r/t unrealistic expectations

Chronic Sorrow r/t difficult parent–child relationship

Risk for Spiritual distress: Risk factor: altered relationships

Readiness for enhanced Parenting: willingness to enhance parenting

Parenting

Readiness for enhanced Parenting (See **Parenting,** readiness for enhanced, Section III)

Parenting, Impaired

Impaired Parenting (See **Parenting,** impaired, Section III)

Chronic Sorrow r/t difficult parent–child relationship

Risk for Spiritual distress: Risk factor: altered relationships

Parenting, Risk for Impaired

Risk for impaired Parenting (See **Parenting,** impaired, risk for, Section III)
See Parenting, Impaired

Paresthesia

Risk for Injury: Risk factors: inability to feel temperature changes, pain

Risk for impaired Skin integrity: Risk factor: impaired sensation

Risk for Thermal injury: Risk factor: neuromuscular impairment

Parkinson's Disease

Impaired verbal Communication r/t decreased speech volume, slowness of speech, impaired facial muscles

Constipation r/t weakness of muscles, lack of exercise, inadequate fluid intake, decreased autonomic nervous system activity

Frail Elderly syndrome r/t chronic illness

Imbalanced Nutrition: less than body requirements r/t tremor, slowness in eating, difficulty in chewing and swallowing

Chronic Sorrow r/t loss of physical capacity

Risk for Injury: Risk factors: tremors, slow reactions, altered gait
See Neurologic Disorders

Paroxysmal Nocturnal Dyspnea (PND)

See PND (Paroxysmal Nocturnal Dyspnea)

Patent Ductus Arteriosus (PDA)

See Congenital Heart Disease/Cardiac Anomalies

Patient-Controlled Analgesia (PCA)

See PCA (Patient-Controlled Analgesia)

Patient Education

Deficient Knowledge r/t lack of exposure to information misinterpretation, unfamiliarity with information resources to manage illness

Readiness for enhanced emancipated Decision-Making: expresses desire to enhance understanding of choices for decision-making

Readiness for enhanced Knowledge (specify): interest in learning

Readiness for enhanced Health management: expresses desire for information to manage the illness

PCA (Patient-Controlled Analgesia)

Deficient Knowledge r/t self-care of pain control

Nausea r/t side effects of medication

P

Risk for Injury: Risk factors: possible complications associated with PCA

Risk for Vascular Trauma: Risk factors: insertion site and length of insertion time

Readiness for enhanced Knowledge: appropriate management of PCA

Pectus Excavatum

See Marfan Syndrome

Pediculosis

See Lice

PEG (Percutaneous Endoscopic Gastrostomy)

See Tube Feeding

Pelvic Inflammatory Disease (PID)

See PID (Pelvic Inflammatory Disease)

Penile Prosthesis

Ineffective Sexuality pattern r/t use of penile prosthesis

Risk for Surgical Site Infection: Risk factor: invasive surgical procedure

Risk for situational low Self-Esteem: Risk factor: ineffective sexuality pattern

Readiness for enhanced Health management: seeks information regarding care and use of prosthesis

See Erectile Dysfunction (ED); Impotence

Peptic Ulcer

See Ulcer, Peptic (Duodenal or Gastric)

Percutaneous Transluminal Coronary Angioplasty (PTCA)

See Angioplasty, Coronary

Pericardial Friction Rub

Decreased **Cardiac** output

Acute Pain r/t inflammation, effusion

Risk for decreased Cardiac tissue perfusion: Risk factors: inflammation in pericardial sac, fluid accumulation compressing heart

Pericarditis

Activity intolerance r/t reduced cardiac reserve, prescribed bed rest

Decreased Cardiac output r/t impaired cardiac function from inflammation of pericardial sac

Risk for decreased Cardiac tissue perfusion: Risk factor: inflammation in pericardial sac

Deficient Knowledge r/t unfamiliarity with information sources

Risk for imbalanced Nutrition: less than body requirements: Risk factors: fever, hypermetabolic state associated with fever

Acute Pain r/t biological injury, inflammation

Periodontal Disease

Risk for impaired Oral Mucous Membrane integrity (See **Oral Mucous Membrane** integrity, impaired, risk for, Section III)

Perioperative Hypothermia

Risk for Perioperative Hypothermia (See **Perioperative Hypothermia**, risk for, Section III)

Perioperative Positioning

Risk for Perioperative Positioning injury (See **Perioperative Positioning** injury, risk for, Section III)

Peripheral Neuropathy

See Neuropathy, Peripheral

Peripheral Neurovascular Dysfunction

Risk for Peripheral Neurovascular dysfunction (See **Peripheral Neurovascular** dysfunction, risk for, Section III)

See Neuropathy, Peripheral; Peripheral Vascular disease (PVD)

Peripheral Vascular Disease (PVD)

Ineffective Health maintenance r/t deficient knowledge regarding self-care and treatment of disease

Chronic Pain: intermittent claudication r/t ischemia

Ineffective peripheral Tissue Perfusion r/t disease process

Risk for Falls: Risk factor: altered mobility

Risk for Injury: Risk factors: tissue hypoxia, altered mobility, altered sensation

Risk for Peripheral Neurovascular dysfunction: Risk factor: possible vascular obstruction

Risk for impaired Tissue integrity: Risk factor: altered circulation or sensation

Readiness for enhanced Health management: self-care and treatment of disease

See Neuropathy, Peripheral; Peripheral Neurovascular Dysfunction

Peritoneal Dialysis

Ineffective Breathing pattern r/t pressure from dialysate

Impaired Comfort r/t instillation of dialysate, temperature of dialysate

Impaired Home maintenance r/t complex home treatment of client

Deficient Knowledge r/t treatment procedure, self-care with peritoneal dialysis

Chronic Sorrow r/t chronic disability

Risk for ineffective Coping: Risk factor: disability requiring change in lifestyle

Risk for unstable blood Glucose level: Risk factors: increased concentrations of glucose in dialysate, ineffective medication management

Risk for imbalanced Fluid volume: Risk factor: medical procedure

Risk for Infection: peritoneal: Risk factors: invasive procedure, presence of catheter, dialysate

Risk for Powerlessness: Risk factors: chronic condition and care involved

P

See Child with Chronic Condition; Hemodialysis; Hospitalized Child; Renal Failure; Renal Failure, Acute/Chronic, Child

Peritonitis

Ineffective Breathing pattern r/t pain, increased abdominal pressure

Constipation r/t decreased oral intake, decrease of peristalsis

Deficient Fluid volume r/t retention of fluid in bowel with loss of circulating blood volume

Nausea r/t gastrointestinal irritation

Imbalanced Nutrition: less than body requirements r/t nausea, vomiting

Acute Pain r/t inflammation and infection of gastrointestinal system

Risk for dysfunctional Gastrointestinal motility: Risk factor: gastrointestinal disease

Pernicious Anemia

Diarrhea r/t malabsorption of nutrients

Fatigue r/t imbalanced nutrition: less than body requirements

Impaired Memory r/t lack of adequate red blood cells

Nausea r/t altered oral mucous membrane; sore tongue, bleeding gums

Imbalanced Nutrition: less than body requirements r/t lack of appetite associated with nausea and altered oral mucous membrane

Impaired Oral Mucous Membrane integrity r/t vitamin deficiency; inability to absorb vitamin B_{12} associated with lack of intrinsic factor

Risk for Falls: Risk factors: dizziness, lightheadedness

Risk for Peripheral Neurovascular dysfunction: Risk factor: anemia

Persistent Fetal Circulation

See Congenital Heart Disease/Cardiac Anomalies

Personal Identity Problems

Disturbed personal Identity (See **Identity,** personal, disturbed, Section III)

Risk for disturbed personal Identity (See disturbed personal **Identity,** risk for, Section III)

Personality Disorder

Ineffective Activity planning r/t unrealistic perception of events

Impaired individual Resilience r/t psychological disorder

See specific disorder: Antisocial Personality Disorder; Borderline Personality Disorder; OCD (Obsessive-Compulsive Disorder); Paranoid Personality Disorder

Pertussis (Whooping Cough)

Risk for impaired emancipated Decision-Making: Risk factor: indecision regarding administration of usual childhood vaccinations

See Respiratory Infections, Acute Childhood

Pesticide Contamination

Contamination r/t use of environmental contaminants; pesticides

Risk for Allergic reaction: Risk factor: repeated exposure to pesticides

Petechiae

See Anticoagulant Therapy; Clotting Disorder; DIC (Disseminated Intravascular Coagulation); Hemophilia

Petit Mal Seizure

Readiness for enhanced Health management: wears medical alert bracelet; limits hazardous activities such as driving, swimming, working at heights, operating equipment

See Epilepsy

Pharyngitis

See Sore Throat

Phenylketonuria (PKU)

See PKU (Phenylketonuria)

Pheochromocytoma

Anxiety r/t symptoms from increased catecholamines—headache, palpitations, sweating, nervousness, nausea, vomiting, syncope

Ineffective Health maintenance r/t deficient knowledge regarding treatment and self-care

Insomnia r/t high levels of catecholamines

Nausea r/t increased catecholamines

Risk for decreased Cardiac tissue perfusion: Risk factor: hypertension

See Surgery, Perioperative Care; Surgery, Postoperative Care; Surgery, Preoperative Care

Phlebitis

See Thrombophlebitis

Phobia (Specific)

Fear r/t presence or anticipation of specific object or situation

Powerlessness r/t anxiety about encountering unknown or known entity

Impaired individual Resilience r/t psychological disorder

Readiness for enhanced Power: expresses readiness to enhance identification of choices that can be made for change

See Anxiety; Anxiety Disorder; Panic Disorder (Panic Attacks)

Photosensitivity

Ineffective Health maintenance r/t deficient knowledge regarding medications inducing photosensitivity

Risk for dry Eye: Risk factors: pharmaceutical agents, sunlight exposure

Risk for impaired Skin integrity: Risk factor: exposure to sun

Physical Abuse

See Abuse, Child; Abuse, Spouse, Parent, or Significant Other

Pica

Anxiety r/t stress

Imbalanced Nutrition: less than body requirements r/t eating nonnutritive substances

Impaired Parenting r/t lack of supervision, food deprivation

Risk for Constipation: Risk factor: presence of undigestible materials in gastrointestinal tract

Risk for dysfunctional Gastrointestinal motility: Risk factor: abnormal eating behavior

Risk for Infection: Risk factor: ingestion of infectious agents via contaminated substances

Risk for Poisoning: Risk factor: ingestion of substances containing lead

See Anemia

PID (Pelvic Inflammatory Disease)

Ineffective Health maintenance r/t deficient knowledge regarding self-care, treatment of disease

Acute Pain r/t biological injury; inflammation, edema, congestion of pelvic tissues

Ineffective Sexuality pattern r/t medically imposed abstinence from sexual activities until acute infection subsides, change in reproductive potential

Risk for Infection: Risk factors: insufficient knowledge to avoid exposure to pathogens; proper hygiene, nutrition, other health habits

See Maturational Issues, Adolescent; STD (Sexually Transmitted Disease)

PIH (Pregnancy-Induced Hypertension/Preeclampsia)

Anxiety r/t fear of the unknown, threat to self and infant, change in role functioning

Death Anxiety r/t threat of preeclampsia

Decreased Diversional activity engagement r/t bed rest

Interrupted Family processes r/t situational crisis

Impaired Home maintenance r/t bed rest

Deficient Knowledge r/t lack of experience with situation

Impaired physical Mobility r/t medically prescribed limitations

Impaired Parenting r/t prescribed bed rest

Powerlessness r/t complication threatening pregnancy, medically prescribed limitations

Ineffective Role performance r/t change in physical capacity to assume role of pregnant woman or resume other roles

Situational low Self-Esteem r/t loss of idealized pregnancy

Impaired Social interaction r/t imposed bed rest

Risk for imbalanced Fluid volume: Risk factors: hypertension, altered kidney function

Risk for Injury: fetal: Risk factors: decreased uteroplacental perfusion, seizures

Risk for Injury: maternal: Risk factors: vasospasm, high blood pressure

Risk for unstable Blood Pressure: Risk factor: hypertension, imbalanced fluid volume

Readiness for enhanced Knowledge: exhibits desire for information on managing condition

Piloerection

Hypothermia r/t exposure to cold environment

Pink Eye

See Conjunctivitis

Pinworms

Impaired Comfort r/t itching

Impaired Home maintenance r/t inadequate cleaning of bed linen and toilet seats

Insomnia r/t discomfort

Readiness for enhanced Health management: proper handwashing; short, clean fingernails; avoiding hand, mouth, nose contact with unwashed hands; appropriate cleaning of bed linen and toilet seats

Pituitary Tumor, Benign

See Cushing's Disease

PKU (Phenylketonuria)

Risk for delayed Development: Risk factors: not following strict dietary program; eating foods extremely low in phenylalanine; avoiding eggs, milk, any foods containing aspartame (e.g., NutraSweet)

Readiness for enhanced Health management: testing for PKU and following prescribed dietary regimen

Placenta Abruptio

Death Anxiety r/t threat of mortality associated with bleeding

Fear r/t threat to self and fetus

Ineffective Health maintenance r/t deficient knowledge regarding treatment and control of hypertension associated with placenta abruptio

Acute Pain: abdominal/back r/t premature separation of placenta before delivery

Risk for Bleeding: Risk factor: placenta abruptio

Risk for deficient Fluid volume: Risk factor: maternal blood loss

Risk for Powerlessness: Risk factors: complications of pregnancy and unknown outcome

Risk for Shock: Risk factor: hypovolemia

Risk for Spiritual distress: Risk factor: fear from unknown outcome of pregnancy

Placenta Previa

Death Anxiety r/t threat of mortality associated with bleeding

Disturbed Body Image r/t negative feelings about body and reproductive ability, feelings of helplessness

Ineffective Coping r/t threat to self and fetus

Decreased Diversional activity engagement r/t long-term hospitalization

Interrupted Family processes r/t maternal bed rest, hospitalization

Fear r/t threat to self and fetus, unknown future

Impaired Home maintenance r/t maternal bed rest, hospitalization

Impaired physical Mobility r/t medical protocol, maternal bed rest

Ineffective Role performance r/t maternal bed rest, hospitalization

Situational low Self-Esteem r/t situational crisis

Spiritual distress r/t inability to participate in usual religious rituals, situational crisis

Risk for Bleeding: Risk factor: placenta previa

Risk for Constipation: Risk factors: bed rest, pregnancy

Risk for deficient Fluid volume: Risk factor: maternal blood loss

Risk for imbalanced Fluid volume: Risk factor: maternal blood loss

Risk for Injury: fetal and maternal: Risk factors: threat to uteroplacental perfusion, hemorrhage

Risk for disturbed Maternal–Fetal dyad: Risk factor: complication of pregnancy

Risk for impaired Parenting: Risk factors: maternal bed rest, hospitalization

Risk for ineffective peripheral Tissue Perfusion: placental: Risk factors: dilation of cervix, loss of placental implantation site

Risk for Powerlessness: Risk factors: complications of pregnancy, unknown outcome

Risk for Shock: Risk factor: hypovolemia

Plantar Fasciitis

Impaired Comfort r/t inflamed structures of feet

Impaired physical Mobility r/t discomfort

Acute Pain r/t inflammation

Chronic Pain r/t inflammation

Pleural Effusion

Ineffective Breathing pattern r/t pain

Excess Fluid volume r/t compromised regulatory mechanisms; heart, liver, or kidney failure

Acute Pain r/t inflammation, fluid accumulation

Pleural Friction Rub

Ineffective Breathing pattern r/t pain

Acute Pain r/t inflammation, fluid accumulation

Pleural Tap

See Pleural Effusion

Pleurisy

Ineffective Breathing pattern r/t pain

Impaired Gas exchange r/t ventilation perfusion imbalance

Acute Pain r/t pressure on pleural nerve endings associated with fluid accumulation or inflammation

Impaired Walking r/t activity intolerance, inability to "catch breath"

Risk for ineffective Airway clearance: Risk factors: increased secretions, ineffective cough because of pain

Risk for Infection: Risk factor: exposure to pathogens

PMS (Premenstrual Syndrome)

Fatigue r/t hormonal changes

Excess Fluid volume r/t alterations of hormonal levels inducing fluid retention

Deficient Knowledge r/t methods to deal with and prevent syndrome

Acute Pain r/t hormonal stimulation of gastrointestinal structures

Risk for Powerlessness: Risk factors: lack of knowledge and ability to deal with symptoms

Risk for impaired Resilience: Risk factor: PMS symptoms

Readiness for enhanced Communication: willingness to express thoughts and feelings about PMS

Readiness for enhanced Health management: desire for information to manage and prevent symptoms

PND (Paroxysmal Nocturnal Dyspnea)

Anxiety r/t inability to breathe during sleep

Ineffective Breathing pattern r/t increase in carbon dioxide levels, decrease in oxygen levels

Insomnia r/t suffocating feeling from fluid in lungs on awakening from sleep

Sleep deprivation r/t inability to breathe during sleep

Risk for decreased Cardiac tissue perfusion: Risk factor: hypoxia

Risk for Powerlessness: Risk factor: inability to control nocturnal dyspnea

Readiness for enhanced Sleep: expresses willingness to learn measures to enhance sleep

Pneumonectomy

See Thoracotomy

Pneumonia

Activity intolerance r/t imbalance between oxygen supply and demand

Ineffective Airway clearance r/t inflammation and presence of secretions

Impaired Gas exchange r/t decreased functional lung tissue

Ineffective Health management r/t deficient knowledge regarding self-care and treatment of disease

Imbalanced Nutrition: less than body requirements r/t loss of appetite

Impaired Oral Mucous Membrane integrity r/t dry mouth from mouth breathing, decreased fluid intake

Ineffective Thermoregulation r/t infectious process

Risk for acute Confusion: Risk factors: underlying illness, hypoxia

Risk for deficient Fluid volume: Risk factor: inadequate intake of fluids

Risk for Vascular Trauma: Risk factor: irritation from intravenous antibiotics

See Respiratory Infections, Acute Childhood

Pneumothorax

Fear r/t threat to own well-being, difficulty breathing

Impaired Gas exchange r/t ventilation-perfusion imbalance, decreased functional lung tissue

Acute Pain r/t recent injury, coughing, deep breathing

Risk for Injury: Risk factor: possible complications associated with closed chest drainage system

See Chest Tubes

Poisoning, Risk for

Risk for Poisoning (See **Poisoning,** risk for, Section III)

Poliomyelitis

See Paralysis

Polydipsia

See Diabetes Mellitus

Polyphagia

Readiness for enhanced Nutrition: knowledge of appropriate diet for diabetes

See Diabetes Mellitus

Polyuria

See Diabetes Mellitus

Postoperative Care

See Surgery, Postoperative Care

Postpartum Depression

Anxiety r/t new responsibilities of parenting

Disturbed Body Image r/t normal postpartum recovery

Ineffective Childbearing process r/t depression/lack of support system

Ineffective Coping r/t hormonal changes

Fatigue r/t childbirth, postpartum state, crying child

Risk-prone Health behavior r/t lack of support systems

Impaired Home maintenance r/t fatigue, care of newborn

Hopelessness r/t stress, exhaustion

Deficient Knowledge r/t lifestyle changes

Impaired Parenting r/t hormone-induced depression

Ineffective Role performance r/t new responsibilities of parenting

Sexual dysfunction r/t fear of another pregnancy, postpartum pain, lochia flow

Sleep deprivation r/t environmental stimulation of newborn

Impaired Social interaction r/t change in role functioning

Risk for disturbed personal Identity: Risk factor: role change/depression/inability to cope

Risk for situational low Self-Esteem: Risk factor: decreased power over feelings of sadness

Risk for Spiritual distress: Risk factors: altered relationships, social isolation

Readiness for enhanced Hope: expresses desire to enhance hope and interconnectedness with others

See Depression (Major Depressive Disorder)

Postpartum Hemorrhage

Activity intolerance r/t anemia from loss of blood

Death Anxiety r/t threat of mortality associated with bleeding

Disturbed Body Image r/t loss of ideal childbirth

Insufficient Breast Milk Production r/t fluid volume depletion

Interrupted Breastfeeding r/t separation from infant for medical treatment

Decreased Cardiac output r/t hypovolemia

Fear r/t threat to self, unknown future

Deficient Fluid volume r/t uterine atony, loss of blood

Impaired Home maintenance r/t lack of stamina

Deficient Knowledge r/t lack of exposure to situation

Acute Pain r/t nursing and medical interventions to control bleeding

Ineffective peripheral Tissue Perfusion r/t hypovolemia

Risk for Bleeding: Risk factor: postpartum complications

Risk for impaired Childbearing: Risk factor: postpartum complication

Risk for imbalanced Fluid volume: Risk factor: maternal blood loss

Risk for Infection: Risk factors: loss of blood, depressed immunity

Risk for impaired Parenting: Risk factor: weakened maternal condition

Risk for Powerlessness: Risk factor: acute illness

Risk for Shock: Risk factor: hypovolemia

Postpartum, Normal Care

Anxiety r/t change in role functioning, parenting

Effective Breastfeeding r/t basic breastfeeding knowledge, support of partner and health care provider

Fatigue r/t childbirth, new responsibilities of parenting, body changes

Acute Pain r/t episiotomy, lacerations, bruising, breast engorgement, headache, sore nipples, epidural or intravenous site, hemorrhoids

Sexual dysfunction r/t recent childbirth

Impaired Tissue integrity r/t episiotomy, lacerations

Sleep deprivation r/t care of infant

Impaired Urinary elimination r/t effects of anesthesia, tissue trauma

Risk for Constipation: Risk factors: hormonal effects on smooth muscles, fear of straining with defecation, effects of anesthesia

Risk for Infection: Risk factors: tissue trauma, blood loss

Readiness for enhanced family Coping: adaptation to new family member

Readiness for enhanced Hope: desire to increase hope

Readiness for enhanced Parenting: expresses willingness to enhance parenting skills

Post-Trauma Syndrome

Post-Trauma syndrome (See **Post-Trauma** syndrome, Section III)

Post-Trauma Syndrome, Risk for

Risk for Post-Trauma syndrome (See **Post-Trauma** syndrome, risk for, Section III)

P

Post-Traumatic Stress Disorder (PTSD)

See PTSD (Post-Traumatic Stress Disorder)

Potassium, Increase/Decrease

See Hyperkalemia; Hypokalemia

Power/Powerlessness

Powerlessness (See **Powerlessness,** Section III)

Risk for Powerlessness (See **Powerlessness,** risk for, Section III)

Readiness for enhanced Power (See **Power,** readiness for enhanced, Section III)

Preeclampsia

See PIH (Pregnancy-Induced Hypertension/Preeclampsia)

Pregnancy, Cardiac Disorders

See Cardiac Disorders in Pregnancy

Pregnancy-Induced Hypertension/ Preeclampsia (PIH)

See PIH (Pregnancy-Induced Hypertension/Preeclampsia)

Pregnancy Loss

Anxiety r/t threat to role functioning, health status, situational crisis

Compromised family Coping r/t lack of support by significant other because of personal suffering

Ineffective Coping r/t situational crisis

Grieving r/t loss of pregnancy, fetus, or child

Acute Pain r/t surgical intervention

Ineffective Role performance r/t inability to assume parenting role

Ineffective Sexuality pattern r/t self-esteem disturbance resulting from pregnancy loss and anxiety about future pregnancies

Chronic Sorrow r/t loss of a fetus or child

Spiritual distress r/t intense suffering from loss of child

Risk for deficient Fluid volume: Risk factor: blood loss

Risk for complicated Grieving: Risk factor: loss of pregnancy

Risk for Infection: Risk factor: retained products of conception

Risk for Powerlessness: Risk factor: situational crisis

Risk for ineffective Relationship: Risk factor: poor communication skills in dealing with the loss

Risk for Spiritual distress: Risk factor: intense suffering

Readiness for enhanced Communication: willingness to express feelings and thoughts about loss

Readiness for enhanced Hope: expresses desire to enhance hope

Readiness for enhanced Spiritual well-being: desire for acceptance of loss

Pregnancy, Normal

Anxiety r/t unknown future, threat to self secondary to pain of labor

Disturbed Body Image r/t altered body function and appearance

Interrupted Family processes r/t developmental transition of pregnancy

Fatigue r/t increased energy demands

Fear r/t labor and delivery

Deficient Knowledge r/t primiparity

Nausea r/t hormonal changes of pregnancy

Imbalanced Nutrition: less than body requirements r/t growing fetus, nausea

Imbalanced Nutrition: more than body requirements r/t deficient knowledge regarding nutritional needs of pregnancy

Sleep deprivation r/t uncomfortable pregnancy state

Impaired Urinary elimination r/t frequency caused by increased pelvic pressure and hormonal stimulation

Risk for Constipation: Risk factor: pregnancy

Risk for Sexual dysfunction: Risk factors: altered body function, self-concept, body image with pregnancy

Readiness for enhanced Childbearing process: appropriate prenatal care

Readiness for enhanced family Coping: satisfying partner relationship, attention to gratification of needs, effective adaptation to developmental tasks of pregnancy

Readiness for enhanced Family processes: family adapts to change

Readiness for enhanced Health management: seeks information for prenatal self-care

Readiness for enhanced Nutrition: desire for knowledge of appropriate nutrition during pregnancy

Readiness for enhanced Parenting: expresses willingness to enhance parenting skills

Readiness for enhanced Relationship: meeting developmental goals associated with pregnancy

Readiness for enhanced Spiritual well-being: new role as parent

See Discomforts of Pregnancy

Premature Dilation of the Cervix (Incompetent Cervix)

Ineffective Activity planning r/t unrealistic perception of events

Ineffective Coping r/t bed rest, threat to fetus

Decreased Diversional activity engagement r/t bed rest

Fear r/t potential loss of infant

Grieving r/t potential loss of infant

Deficient Knowledge r/t treatment regimen, prognosis for pregnancy

Impaired physical Mobility r/t imposed bed rest to prevent preterm birth

Powerlessness r/t inability to control outcome of pregnancy

Ineffective Role performance r/t inability to continue usual patterns of responsibility

Situational low Self-Esteem r/t inability to complete normal pregnancy

Sexual dysfunction r/t fear of harm to fetus

Impaired Social interaction r/t bed rest

Risk for Infection: Risk factor: invasive procedures to prevent preterm birth

Risk for Injury: fetal: Risk factors: preterm birth, use of anesthetics

Risk for Injury: maternal: Risk factor: surgical procedures to prevent preterm birth (e.g., cerclage)

Risk for impaired Resilience: Risk factor: complication of pregnancy

Risk for Spiritual distress: Risk factors: physical/psychological stress

Premature Infant (Child)

Insufficient Breast Milk Production r/t ineffective sucking, latching on of the infant

Impaired Gas exchange r/t effects of cardiopulmonary insufficiency

Disorganized Infant behavior r/t prematurity

Insomnia r/t noisy and noxious intensive care environment

Neonatal Hyperbilirubinemia r/t infant experiences difficulty making transition to extrauterine life

Imbalanced Nutrition: less than body requirements r/t delayed or understimulated rooting reflex, easy fatigue during feeding, diminished endurance

Impaired Swallowing r/t decreased or absent gag reflex, fatigue

Ineffective Thermoregulation r/t large body surface/weight ratio, immaturity of thermal regulation, state of prematurity

Risk for delayed Development: Risk factor: prematurity

Risk for Infection: Risk factors: inadequate, immature, or undeveloped acquired immune response

Risk for Injury: Risk factor: prolonged mechanical ventilation, retinopathy of prematurity (ROP) secondary to 100% oxygen environment

Risk for Neonatal Hyperbilirubinemia: Risk factor: late preterm birth

Readiness for enhanced organized Infant behavior: use of some self-regulatory measures

Premature Infant (Parent)

Ineffective Breastfeeding r/t disrupted establishment of effective pattern secondary to prematurity or insufficient opportunities

Decisional Conflict r/t support system deficit, multiple sources of information

Compromised family Coping r/t disrupted family roles and disorganization, prolonged condition exhausting supportive capacity of significant persons

Ineffective infant Feeding dynamics r/t insufficient knowledge of nutritional needs

Grieving r/t loss of perfect child possibly leading to complicated grieving

Complicated Grieving (prolonged) r/t unresolved conflicts

Parental Role conflict r/t expressed concerns, expressed inability to care for child's physical, emotional, or developmental needs

Chronic Sorrow r/t threat of loss of a child, prolonged hospitalization

Spiritual distress r/t challenged belief or value systems regarding moral or ethical implications of treatment plans

Risk for impaired Attachment: Risk factors: separation, physical barriers, lack of privacy

Risk for disturbed Maternal–Fetal dyad: Risk factor: complication of pregnancy

Risk for Powerlessness: Risk factor: inability to control situation

Risk for impaired Resilience: Risk factor: premature infant

Risk for Spiritual distress: Risk factor: challenged belief or value systems regarding moral or ethical implications of treatment plans

Readiness for enhanced Family process: adaptation to change associated with premature infant

See Child with Chronic Condition; Hospitalized Child

Premature Rupture of Membranes

Anxiety r/t threat to infant's health status

Disturbed Body Image r/t inability to carry pregnancy to term

Ineffective Coping r/t situational crisis

Grieving r/t potential loss of infant

Situational low Self-Esteem r/t inability to carry pregnancy to term

Risk for ineffective Childbearing process: Risk factor: complication of pregnancy

Risk for Infection: Risk factor: rupture of membranes

Risk for Injury: fetal: Risk factor: risk of premature birth

Premenstrual Tension Syndrome (PMS)

See PMS (Premenstrual Tension Syndrome)

Prenatal Care, Normal

Readiness for enhanced Childbearing process: appropriate prenatal lifestyle

Readiness for enhanced Knowledge: appropriate prenatal care

Readiness for enhanced Spiritual well-being: new role as parent

See Pregnancy, Normal

Prenatal Testing

Anxiety r/t unknown outcome, delayed test results

Acute Pain r/t invasive procedures

Risk for Infection: Risk factor: invasive procedures during amniocentesis or chorionic villus sampling

Risk for Injury: Risk factor: invasive procedures

Preoperative Teaching

See Surgery, Preoperative Care

Pressure Ulcer

Impaired bed Mobility r/t intolerance to activity, pain, cognitive impairment, depression, severe anxiety, severity of illness

Imbalanced Nutrition: less than body requirements r/t limited access to food, inability to absorb nutrients because of biological factors, anorexia

Acute Pain r/t tissue destruction, exposure of nerves

Impaired Skin integrity: stage I or II pressure ulcer r/t physical immobility, mechanical factors, altered circulation, skin irritants, excessive moisture

P

Impaired Tissue integrity: stage III or IV pressure ulcer r/t altered circulation, impaired physical mobility, excessive moisture

Risk for Infection: Risk factors: physical immobility, mechanical factors (shearing forces, pressure, restraint, altered circulation, skin irritants, excessive moisture, open wound)

Risk for Pressure ulcer (See **Pressure** ulcer, risk for, Section III)

Preterm Labor

Anxiety r/t threat to fetus, change in role functioning, change in environment and interaction patterns, use of tocolytic drugs

Ineffective Coping r/t situational crisis, preterm labor

Decreased Diversional activity engagement r/t long-term hospitalization

Grieving r/t loss of idealized pregnancy, potential loss of fetus

Impaired Home maintenance r/t medical restrictions

Impaired physical Mobility r/t medically imposed restrictions

Ineffective Role performance r/t inability to carry out normal roles secondary to bed rest or hospitalization, change in expected course of pregnancy

Situational low Self-Esteem r/t threatened ability to carry pregnancy to term

Sexual dysfunction r/t actual or perceived limitation imposed by preterm labor and/or prescribed treatment, separation from partner because of hospitalization

Sleep deprivation r/t change in usual pattern secondary to contractions, hospitalization, treatment regimen

Impaired Social interaction r/t prolonged bed rest or hospitalization

Risk for Injury: fetal: Risk factors: premature birth, immature body systems

Risk for Injury: maternal: Risk factor: use of tocolytic drugs

Risk for Powerlessness: Risk factor: lack of control over preterm labor

Risk for Vascular Trauma: Risk factor: intravenous medication

Readiness for enhanced Childbearing process: appropriate prenatal lifestyle

Readiness for enhanced Comfort: expresses desire to enhance relaxation

Readiness for enhanced Communication: willingness to discuss thoughts and feelings about situation

Problem-Solving Dysfunction

Defensive Coping r/t situational crisis

Impaired Emancipated Decision-Making r/t problem-solving dysfunction

Risk for chronic low Self-Esteem: Risk factor: repeated failures

Readiness for enhanced Communication: willing to share ideas with others

Readiness for enhanced Relationship: shares information and ideas between partners

Readiness for enhanced Resilience: identifies available resources

Readiness for enhanced Spiritual well-being: desires to draw on inner strength and find meaning and purpose to life

Projection

Anxiety r/t threat to self-concept

Defensive Coping r/t inability to acknowledge that own behavior may be a problem, blaming others

Chronic low Self-Esteem r/t failure

Impaired Social interaction r/t self-concept disturbance, confrontational communication style

Risk for Loneliness: Risk factor: blaming others for problems

See Paranoid Personality Disorder

Prolapsed Umbilical Cord

Fear r/t threat to fetus, impending surgery

Ineffective peripheral Tissue Perfusion: fetal r/t interruption in umbilical blood flow

Risk for ineffective Cerebral tissue perfusion: fetal: Risk factor: cord compression

Risk for Injury: Risk factor: (maternal) emergency surgery

See TURP (Transurethral Resection of the Prostate)

Prostatic Hypertrophy

Ineffective Health maintenance r/t deficient knowledge regarding self-care and prevention of complications

Sleep deprivation r/t nocturia

Urinary Retention r/t obstruction

Risk for Infection: Risk factors: urinary residual after voiding, bacterial invasion of bladder

See BPH (Benign Prostatic Hypertrophy)

Prostatitis

Impaired Comfort r/t inflammation

Ineffective Health maintenance r/t deficient knowledge regarding treatment

Urge urinary Incontinence r/t irritation of bladder

Ineffective Protection r/t depressed immune system

Pruritus

Impaired Comfort r/t inflammation of skin causing itching

Deficient Knowledge r/t methods to treat and prevent itching

Risk for impaired Skin integrity: Risk factors: scratching, dry skin

Psoriasis

Disturbed Body Image r/t lesions on body

Impaired Comfort r/t irritated skin

Ineffective Health maintenance r/t deficient knowledge regarding treatment modalities

Powerlessness r/t lack of control over condition with frequent exacerbations and remissions

Impaired Skin integrity r/t lesions on body

Psychosis

Ineffective Activity planning r/t compromised ability to process information

Ineffective Health maintenance r/t cognitive impairment, ineffective individual and family coping

Self-Neglect r/t mental disorder

Impaired individual Resilience r/t psychological disorder

Situational low Self-Esteem r/t excessive use of defense mechanisms (e.g., projection, denial, rationalization)

Risk for disturbed personal Identity: Risk factor: psychosis

Impaired Mood regulation r/t psychosis

Risk for Post-Trauma syndrome: Risk factor: diminished ego strength

See Schizophrenia

PTCA (Percutaneous Transluminal Coronary Angioplasty)

See Angioplasty, Coronary

PTSD (Posttraumatic Stress Disorder)

Anxiety r/t exposure to internal or external cues that symbolize or resemble an aspect of the traumatic event

Chronic Sorrow r/t chronic disability (e.g., physical, mental)

Death Anxiety r/t psychological stress associated with traumatic event

Ineffective Breathing pattern r/t hyperventilation associated with anxiety

Ineffective Coping r/t extreme anxiety

Ineffective Impulse control r/t thinking of initial trauma experience

Insomnia r/t recurring nightmares

Post-Trauma syndrome r/t exposure to a traumatic event

Sleep deprivation r/t nightmares interrupting sleep associated with traumatic event

Spiritual distress r/t feelings of detachment or estrangement from others

Risk for impaired Resilience: Risk factor: chronicity of existing crisis

Risk for Powerlessness: Risk factors: flashbacks, reliving event

Risk for ineffective Relationship: Risk factor: stressful life events

Risk for self- or other-directed Violence: Risk factors: fear of self or others

Readiness for enhanced Comfort: expresses desire to enhance relaxation

Readiness for enhanced Communication: willingness to express feelings and thoughts

Readiness for enhanced Spiritual well-being: desire for harmony after stressful event

Pulmonary Edema

Anxiety r/t fear of suffocation

Ineffective Airway clearance r/t presence of tracheobronchial secretions

Decreased Cardiac output r/t increased preload, infective forward perfusion

Impaired Gas exchange r/t extravasation of extravascular fluid in lung tissues and alveoli

Ineffective Health maintenance r/t deficient knowledge regarding treatment regimen

Sleep deprivation r/t inability to breathe

Risk for acute Confusion: Risk factor: hypoxia

See Heart Failure

Pulmonary Embolism (PE)

Anxiety r/t fear of suffocation

Decreased Cardiac output r/t right ventricular failure secondary to obstructed pulmonary artery

Fear r/t severe pain, possible death

Impaired Gas exchange r/t altered blood flow to alveoli secondary to embolus

Deficient Knowledge r/t activities to prevent embolism, self-care after diagnosis of embolism

Acute Pain r/t biological injury, lack of oxygen to cells

Ineffective peripheral Tissue Perfusion r/t deep vein thrombus formation

See Anticoagulant Therapy

Pulmonary Stenosis

See Congenital Heart Disease/Cardiac Anomalies

Pulse Deficit

Risk for Decreased Cardiac output r/t dysrhythmia

See Dysrhythmia

Pulse Oximetry

Readiness for enhanced Knowledge: information about treatment regimen

See Hypoxia

Pulse Pressure, Increased

See Intracranial Pressure, Increased

Pulse Pressure, Narrowed

See Shock, Hypovolemic

Pulses, Absent or Diminished Peripheral

Ineffective peripheral Tissue Perfusion r/t interruption of arterial flow

Risk for Peripheral Neurovascular dysfunction: Risk factors: fractures, mechanical compression, orthopedic surgery trauma, immobilization, burns, vascular obstruction

Purpura

See Clotting Disorder

Pyelonephritis

Ineffective Health maintenance r/t deficient knowledge regarding self-care, treatment of disease, prevention of further urinary tract infections

Acute Pain r/t inflammation and irritation of urinary tract

Disturbed Sleep pattern r/t urinary frequency

Impaired Urinary elimination r/t irritation of urinary tract

Pyloric Stenosis

Imbalanced Nutrition: less than body requirements r/t vomiting secondary to pyloric sphincter obstruction

Acute Pain r/t abdominal fullness

P

Risk for decreased Fluid volume: Risk factors: vomiting, dehydration

See Hospitalized Child

Pyloromyotomy (Pyloric Stenosis Repair)

See Surgery Preoperative Care, Perioperative Care, Postoperative Care

R

RA (Rheumatoid Arthritis)

See Rheumatoid Arthritis (RA)

Rabies

Ineffective Health maintenance r/t deficient knowledge regarding care of wound, isolation, and observation of infected animal

Acute Pain r/t multiple immunization injections

Risk for ineffective Cerebral tissue perfusion: Risk factor: rabies virus

Radial Nerve Dysfunction

Acute Pain r/t trauma to hand or arm

See Neuropathy, Peripheral

Radiation Therapy

Activity intolerance r/t fatigue from possible anemia

Disturbed Body Image r/t change in appearance, hair loss

Diarrhea r/t irradiation effects

Fatigue r/t malnutrition from lack of appetite, nausea, and vomiting; side effect of radiation

Deficient Knowledge r/t what to expect with radiation therapy, how to do self-care

Nausea r/t side effects of radiation

Imbalanced Nutrition: less than body requirements r/t anorexia, nausea, vomiting, irradiation of areas of pharynx and esophagus

Impaired Oral Mucous Membrane integrity r/t irradiation effects

Ineffective Protection r/t suppression of bone marrow

Risk for Dry Mouth: Risk factor: possible side effect of radiation treatments

Risk for impaired Oral Mucous Membrane integrity: Risk factor: radiation treatments

Risk for Powerlessness: Risk factors: medical treatment and possible side effects

Risk for impaired Resilience: Risk factor: radiation treatment

Risk for impaired Skin integrity: Risk factor: irradiation effects

Risk for Spiritual distress: Risk factors: radiation treatment, prognosis

Radical Neck Dissection

See Laryngectomy

Rage

Risk-prone Health behavior r/t multiple stressors

Labile Emotional Control r/t psychiatric disorders and mood disorders

Impaired individual Resilience r/t poor impulse control

Stress overload r/t multiple coexisting stressors

Risk for Self-Mutilation: Risk factor: command hallucinations

Risk for Suicide: Risk factor: desire to kill self

Risk for other-directed Violence: Risk factors: panic state, manic excitement, organic brain syndrome

Rape-Trauma Syndrome

Rape-Trauma syndrome (See **Rape-Trauma** syndrome, Section III)

Chronic Sorrow r/t forced loss of virginity

Risk for ineffective Childbearing process r/t to trauma and violence

Risk for Post-Trauma syndrome: Risk factor: trauma or violence associated with rape

Risk for Powerlessness: Risk factor: inability to control thoughts about incident

Risk for ineffective Relationship: Risk factor: trauma and violence

Risk for chronic low Self-Esteem: Risk factors: perceived lack of respect from others, feeling violated

Risk for Spiritual distress: Risk factor: forced loss of virginity

Rash

Impaired Comfort r/t pruritus

Impaired Skin integrity r/t mechanical trauma

Risk for Infection: Risk factors: traumatized tissue, broken skin

Risk for Latex Allergic reaction: Risk factor: allergy to products associated with latex

Rationalization

Defensive Coping r/t situational crisis, inability to accept blame for consequences of own behavior

Ineffective Denial r/t fear of consequences, actual or perceived loss

Impaired individual Resilience r/t psychological disturbance

Risk for Post-Trauma syndrome: Risk factor: survivor's role in event

Readiness for enhanced Communication: expresses desire to share thoughts and feelings

Readiness for enhanced Spiritual well-being: possibility of seeking harmony with self, others, higher power, God

Rats, Rodents in Home

Impaired Home maintenance r/t lack of knowledge, insufficient finances

Risk for Allergic reaction: Risk factor: repeated exposure to environmental contamination

See Filthy Home Environment

Raynaud's Disease

Deficient Knowledge r/t lack of information about disease process, possible complications, self-care needs regarding disease process and medication

Ineffective peripheral Tissue Perfusion r/t transient reduction of blood flow

Acute Pain r/t transient reduction in blood flow

RDS (Respiratory Distress Syndrome)

See Respiratory Conditions of the Neonate

Rectal Fullness

Chronic functional Constipation r/t decreased activity level, decreased fluid intake, inadequate fiber in diet, decreased peristalsis, side effects of antidepressant or antipsychotic therapy

Risk for chronic functional Constipation: Risk factor: habitual denial of or ignoring urge to defecate

Rectal Lump

See Hemorrhoids

Rectal Pain/Bleeding

Chronic functional Constipation r/t pain on defecation

Deficient Knowledge r/t possible causes of rectal bleeding, pain, treatment modalities

Acute Pain r/t pressure of defecation

Risk for Bleeding: Risk factor: rectal disease

Rectal Surgery

See Hemorrhoidectomy

Rectocele Repair

Chronic functional Constipation r/t painful defecation

Ineffective Health maintenance r/t deficient knowledge of postoperative care of surgical site, dietary measures, exercise to prevent constipation

Acute Pain r/t surgical procedure

Urinary retention r/t edema from surgery

Risk for Bleeding: Risk factor: surgery

Risk for Surgical Site Infection: Risk factors: surgical procedure, possible contamination of area with feces

Reflex Incontinence

Reflex urinary Incontinence (See **Incontinence,** urinary, reflex, Section III)

Regression

Anxiety r/t threat to or change in health status

Defensive Coping r/t denial of obvious problems, weaknesses

Self-Neglect r/t functional impairment

Powerlessness r/t health care environment

Impaired individual Resilience r/t psychological disturbance

Ineffective Role performance r/t powerlessness over health status

See Hospitalized Child; Separation Anxiety

Regretful

Anxiety r/t situational or maturational crises

Death Anxiety r/t feelings of not having accomplished goals in life

Risk for Spiritual distress: Risk factor: inability to forgive

Rehabilitation

Ineffective Coping r/t loss of normal function

Impaired physical Mobility r/t injury, surgery, psychosocial condition warranting rehabilitation

Self-Care deficit: specify r/t impaired physical mobility

Risk for Falls: Risk factor: physical deconditioning

Readiness for enhanced Comfort: expresses desire to enhance feeling of comfort

Readiness for enhanced Self-Concept: accepts strengths and limitations

Readiness for enhanced Health Management: expresses desire to manage rehabilitation

Relationship

Ineffective Relationship (See ineffective **Relationship,** Section III)

Readiness for enhanced Relationship (See Risk for enhanced **Relationship,** Section III)

Relaxation Techniques

Anxiety r/t situational crisis

Readiness for enhanced Comfort: expresses desire to enhance relaxation

Readiness for enhanced Health management: desire to manage illness

Readiness for enhanced Religiosity: requests religious materials or experiences

Readiness for enhanced Resilience: desire to enhance resilience

Readiness for enhanced Self-Concept: willingness to enhance self-concept

Readiness for enhanced Spiritual well-being: seeking comfort from higher power

Religiosity

Impaired Religiosity (See **Religiosity,** impaired, Section III)

Risk for impaired Religiosity (See **Religiosity,** impaired, risk for, Section III)

Readiness for enhanced Religiosity (See **Religiosity,** readiness for enhanced, Section III)

Religious Concerns

Spiritual distress r/t separation from religious or cultural ties

Risk for impaired Religiosity: Risk factors: ineffective support, coping, caregiving

Risk for Spiritual distress: Risk factors: physical or psychological stress

Readiness for enhanced Spiritual well-being: desire for increased spirituality

Relocation Stress Syndrome

Relocation stress syndrome (See **Relocation** stress syndrome, Section III)

R

Risk for Relocation stress syndrome (See **Relocation** stress syndrome, risk for, Section III)

Renal Failure

Activity intolerance r/t effects of anemia, heart failure

Death Anxiety r/t unknown outcome of disease

Decreased Cardiac output r/t effects of heart failure, elevated potassium levels interfering with conduction system

Impaired Comfort r/t pruritus

Ineffective Coping r/t depression resulting from chronic disease

Fatigue r/t effects of chronic uremia and anemia

Excessive Fluid volume r/t decreased urine output, sodium retention, inappropriate fluid Intake

Ineffective Health management r/t complexity of health care regimen, inadequate number of cues to action, perceived barriers, powerlessness

Imbalanced Nutrition: less than body requirements r/t anorexia, nausea, vomiting, altered taste sensation, dietary restrictions

Impaired Oral Mucous Membrane integrity r/t irritation from nitrogenous waste products

Chronic Sorrow r/t chronic illness

Spiritual distress r/t dealing with chronic illness

Impaired urinary Elimination r/t effects of disease, need for dialysis

Risk for Electrolyte imbalance: Risk factor: renal dysfunction

Risk for Infection: Risk factor: altered immune functioning

Risk for Injury: Risk factors: bone changes, neuropathy, muscle weakness

Risk for impaired Oral Mucous Membrane integrity: Risk factors: dehydration, effects of uremia

Risk for Powerlessness: Risk factor: chronic illness

Risk for Sepsis: Risk factor: infection

Renal Failure Acute/Chronic, Child

Disturbed Body Image r/t growth retardation, bone changes, visibility of dialysis access devices (shunt, fistula), edema

Decreased Diversional acitivity engagement r/t immobility during dialysis

See Child with Chronic Condition; Hospitalized Child

Renal Failure, Nonoliguric

Anxiety r/t change in health status

Risk for deficient Fluid volume: Risk factor: loss of large volumes of urine

See Renal Failure

Respiratory Acidosis

See Acidosis, Respiratory

Respiratory Conditions of the Neonate (Respiratory Distress Syndrome [RDS], Meconium Aspiration, Diaphragmatic Hernia)

Ineffective Airway clearance r/t sequelae of attempts to breathe in utero resulting in meconium aspiration

Fatigue r/t increased energy requirements and metabolic demands

Impaired Gas exchange r/t decreased surfactant, immature lung tissue

Dysfunctional Ventilator weaning response r/t immature respiratory system

Risk for Infection: Risk factors: tissue destruction or irritation as a result of aspiration of meconium fluid

See Bronchopulmonary Dysplasia; Hospitalized Child; Premature Infant, Child

Respiratory Distress

See Dyspnea

Respiratory Distress Syndrome (RDS)

See Respiratory Conditions of the Neonate

Respiratory Infections, Acute Childhood (Croup, Epiglottitis, Pertussis, Pneumonia, Respiratory Syncytial Virus)

Activity intolerance r/t generalized weakness, dyspnea, fatigue, poor oxygenation

Ineffective Airway clearance r/t excess tracheobronchial secretions

Ineffective Breathing pattern r/t inflamed bronchial passages, coughing

Fear r/t oxygen deprivation, difficulty breathing

Deficient Fluid volume r/t insensible losses (fever, diaphoresis), inadequate oral fluid intake

Impaired Gas exchange r/t insufficient oxygenation as a result of inflammation or edema of epiglottis, larynx, bronchial passages

Imbalanced Nutrition: less than body requirements r/t anorexia, fatigue, generalized weakness, poor sucking and breathing coordination, dyspnea

Ineffective Thermoregulation r/t infectious process

Risk for Aspiration: Risk factors: inability to coordinate breathing, coughing, sucking

Risk for Infection: transmission to others: Risk factor: virulent infectious organisms

Risk for Injury (to pregnant others): Risk factors: exposure to aerosolized medications (e.g., ribavirin, pentamidine), resultant potential fetal toxicity

Risk for Suffocation: Risk factors: inflammation of larynx, epiglottis

See Hospitalized Child

Respiratory Syncytial Virus

See Respiratory Infections, Acute Childhood

Restless Leg Syndrome

Disturbed Sleep pattern r/t leg discomfort during sleep relieved by frequent leg movement

Chronic Pain r/t leg discomfort

See Stress

Retinal Detachment

Anxiety r/t change in vision, threat of loss of vision

Deficient Knowledge r/t symptoms, need for early intervention to prevent permanent damage

Vision Loss r/t impaired visual acuity

Risk for impaired Home maintenance: Risk factors: postoperative care, activity limitations, care of affected eye

Risk for impaired Resilience: Risk factor: possible loss of vision

See Vision Impairment

Retinopathy, Diabetic

See Diabetic Retinopathy

Retinopathy of Prematurity (ROP)

Risk for Injury: Risk factors: prolonged mechanical ventilation, ROP secondary to 100% oxygen environment

See Retinal Detachment

Rh Factor Incompatibility

Anxiety r/t unknown outcome of pregnancy

Neonatal Hyperbilirubinemia r/t Rh factor incompatibility

Deficient Knowledge r/t treatment regimen from lack of experience with situation

Powerlessness r/t perceived lack of control over outcome of pregnancy

Risk for Injury: fetal: Risk factors: intrauterine destruction of red blood cells, transfusions

Risk for neonatal Hyperbilirubinemia: Risk factor: Rh factor incompatibility

Readiness for enhanced Health management: prenatal care, compliance with diagnostic and treatment regimen

Rhabdomyolysis

Ineffective Coping r/t seriousness of condition

Impaired physical Mobility r/t myalgia and muscle weakness

Risk for deficient Fluid volume: Risk factor: reduced blood flow to kidneys

Risk for Shock: Risk factor: hypovolemia

Readiness for enhanced Health management: seeks information to avoid condition

See Kidney Failure

Rheumatic Fever

See Endocarditis

Rheumatoid Arthritis (RA)

Imbalanced Nutrition: less than body requirements r/t loss of appetite

Chronic Pain r/t joint inflammation

Disturbed Body Image r/t joint deformity and muscle atrophy

Impaired Physical Mobility r/t pain, impaired joints

Risk for impaired Resilience: Risk factor: chronic, painful, progressive disease

See Arthritis; JRA (Juvenile Rheumatoid Arthritis)

Rib Fracture

Ineffective Breathing pattern r/t fractured ribs

Acute Pain r/t movement, deep breathing

Impaired Gas exchange r/t ventilation-perfusion imbalance, decreased depth of ventilation

Ridicule of Others

Defensive Coping r/t situational crisis, psychological impairment, substance abuse

Risk for Post-Trauma syndrome: Risk factor: perception of event

Ringworm of Body

Impaired Comfort r/t pruritus

Impaired Skin integrity r/t presence of macules associated with fungus

See Itching; Pruritus

Ringworm of Nails

Disturbed Body Image r/t appearance of nails, removed nails

Ringworm of Scalp

Disturbed Body Image r/t possible hair loss (alopecia)

See Itching; Pruritus

Roaches, Invasion of Home with

Impaired Home maintenance r/t lack of knowledge, insufficient finances

See Filthy Home Environment

Role Performance, Altered

Ineffective Role performance (See **Role** performance, ineffective, Section III)

ROP (Retinopathy of Prematurity)

See Retinopathy of Prematurity (ROP)

RSV (Respiratory Syncytial Virus)

See Respiratory Infection, Acute Childhood

Rubella

See Communicable Diseases, Childhood (e.g., Measles, Mumps, Rubella, Chickenpox, Scabies, Lice, Impetigo)

Rubor of Extremities

Ineffective peripheral Tissue Perfusion r/t interruption of arterial flow

See Peripheral Vascular Disease (PVD)

Ruptured Disk

See Low Back Pain

S

SAD (Seasonal Affective Disorder)

Readiness for enhanced Resilience: uses SAD lights during winter months

See Depression (Major Depressive Disorder)

Sadness

Complicated Grieving r/t actual or perceived loss

Impaired Mood regulation r/t chronic illness (See **Mood** regulation, impaired, Section III)

Spiritual distress r/t intense suffering

Risk for Powerlessness: Risk factor: actual or perceived loss

Risk for Spiritual distress: Risk factor: loss of loved one

Readiness for enhanced Communication: willingness to share feelings and thoughts

Readiness for enhanced Spiritual well-being: desire for harmony after actual or perceived loss

See Depression (Major Depressive Disorder); Major Depressive Disorder

Safe Sex

Readiness for enhanced Health management: takes appropriate precautions during sexual activity to keep from contracting sexually transmitted disease

See Sexuality, Adolescent; STD (Sexually Transmitted Disease)

Safety, Childhood

Deficient Knowledge: potential for enhanced health maintenance r/t parental knowledge and skill acquisition regarding appropriate safety measures

Risk for Aspiration (See **Aspiration,** risk for, Section III)

Risk for Injury: Risk factors: developmental age, altered home maintenance

Risk for impaired Parenting: Risk factors: lack of available and effective role model, lack of knowledge, misinformation from other family members (old wives' tales)

Risk for Poisoning: Risk factors: use of lead-based paint; presence of asbestos or radon gas; drugs not locked in cabinet; household products left in accessible area (bleach, detergent, drain cleaners, household cleaners); alcohol and perfume within reach of child; presence of poisonous plants; atmospheric pollutants

Risk for Thermal injury: Risk factor: inadequate supervision

Readiness for enhanced Childbearing process: expresses appropriate knowledge for care of child

Salmonella

Impaired Home maintenance r/t improper preparation or storage of food, lack of safety measures when caring for pet reptile

Risk for Shock: Risk factors: hypovolemia, diarrhea, sepsis

Readiness for enhanced Health management: avoiding improperly prepared or stored food, wearing gloves when handling pet reptiles or their feces

See Gastroenteritis; Gastroenteritis, Child

Salpingectomy

Decisional Conflict r/t sterilization procedure

Grieving r/t possible loss from tubal pregnancy

Risk for impaired Urinary elimination: Risk factor: trauma to ureter during surgery

See Hysterectomy; Surgery, Perioperative Care; Surgery, Postoperative Care; Surgery, Preoperative Care

Sarcoidosis

Anxiety r/t change in health status

Impaired Gas exchange r/t ventilation-perfusion imbalance

Ineffective Health maintenance r/t deficient knowledge regarding home care and medication regimen

Acute Pain r/t possible disease affecting joints

Ineffective Protection r/t immune disorder

Risk for decreased Cardiac tissue perfusion: Risk factor: dysrhythmias

Risk for impaired Skin integrity: Risk factor: immunological disorder

SBE (Self-Breast Examination)

Readiness for enhanced Health management: desires to have information about SBE

Readiness for enhanced Knowledge: SBE

Scabies

See Communicable Diseases, Childhood (e.g., Measles, Mumps, Rubella, Chickenpox, Scabies, Lice, Impetigo)

Scared

Anxiety r/t threat of death, threat to or change in health status

Death Anxiety r/t unresolved issues surrounding end-of-life decisions

Fear r/t hospitalization, real or imagined threat to own well-being

Impaired individual Resilience r/t violence

Readiness for enhanced Communication: willingness to share thoughts and feelings

Schizophrenia

Ineffective Activity planning r/t compromised ability to process information

Anxiety r/t unconscious conflict with reality

Impaired verbal Communication r/t psychosis, disorientation, inaccurate perception, hallucinations, delusions

Ineffective Coping r/t inadequate support systems, unrealistic perceptions, inadequate coping skills, disturbed thought processes, impaired communication

Decreased Diversional activity engagement r/t social isolation, possible regression

Interrupted Family processes r/t inability to express feelings, impaired communication

Fear r/t altered contact with reality

Ineffective Health maintenance r/t cognitive impairment, ineffective individual and family coping, lack of material resources

Ineffective family Health management r/t chronicity and unpredictability of condition

Impaired Home maintenance r/t impaired cognitive or emotional functioning, insufficient finances, inadequate support systems

Hopelessness r/t long-term stress from chronic mental illness

Disturbed personal Identity r/t psychiatric disorder

Impaired Memory r/t psychosocial condition

S

Imbalanced Nutrition: less than body requirements r/t fear of eating, lack of awareness of hunger, disinterest toward food

Impaired individual Resilience r/t psychological disorder

Self-Care deficit: specify r/t loss of contact with reality, impairment of perception

Self-Neglect r/t psychosis

Sleep deprivation r/t intrusive thoughts, nightmares

Impaired Social interaction r/t impaired communication patterns, self-concept disturbance, disturbed thought processes

Social isolation r/t lack of trust, regression, delusional thinking, repressed fears

Chronic Sorrow r/t chronic mental illness

Spiritual distress r/t loneliness, social alienation

Risk for Caregiver Role Strain: Risk factors: bizarre behavior of client, chronicity of condition

Risk for compromised Human Dignity: Risk factor: stigmatizing label

Risk for Loneliness: Risk factor: inability to interact socially

Risk for Post-Trauma syndrome: Risk factor: diminished ego strength

Risk for Powerlessness: Risk factor: intrusive, distorted thinking

Risk for impaired Religiosity: Risk factors: ineffective coping, lack of security

Risk for Suicide: Risk factor: psychiatric illness

Risk for self-directed Violence: Risk factors: lack of trust, panic, hallucinations, delusional thinking

Risk for other-directed Violence: Risk factor: psychotic disorder

Readiness for enhanced Hope: expresses desire to enhance interconnectedness with others and problem-solve to meet goals

Readiness for enhanced Power: expresses willingness to enhance participation in choices for daily living and health and enhance knowledge for participation in change

Sciatica

See Neuropathy, Peripheral

Scoliosis

Risk-prone Health behavior r/t lack of developmental maturity to comprehend long-term consequences of noncompliance with treatment procedures

Disturbed Body Image r/t use of therapeutic braces, postsurgery scars, restricted physical activity

Impaired Comfort r/t altered health status and body image

Impaired Gas exchange r/t restricted lung expansion as a result of severe presurgery curvature of spine, immobilization

Ineffective Health maintenance r/t deficient knowledge regarding treatment modalities, restrictions, home care, postoperative activities

Impaired physical Mobility r/t restricted movement, dyspnea caused by severe curvature of spine

Acute Pain r/t musculoskeletal restrictions, surgery, reambulation with cast or spinal rod

Impaired Skin integrity r/t braces, casts, surgical correction

Chronic Sorrow r/t chronic disability

Risk for Perioperative Positioning injury: Risk factor: prone position

Risk for impaired Resilience: Risk factor: chronic condition

Readiness for enhanced Health management: desires knowledge regarding treatment for condition

See Hospitalized Child; Maturational Issues, Adolescent

Sedentary Lifestyle

Activity intolerance r/t sedentary lifestyle

Sedentary lifestyle (See **Sedentary** lifestyle, Section III)

Obesity (See **Obesity,** Section III)

Overweight (See **Overweight,** Section III)

Risk for Overweight (See **Overweight,** Section III)

Risk for ineffective peripheral Tissue Perfusion: Risk factor: insufficient knowledge of aggravating factors (e.g., immobility, obesity)

Readiness for enhanced Coping: seeking knowledge of new strategies to adjust to sedentary lifestyle

Seizure Disorders, Adult

Acute Confusion r/t postseizure state

Social isolation r/t unpredictability of seizures, community-imposed stigma

Risk for ineffective Airway clearance: Risk factor: accumulation of secretions during seizure

Risk for Falls: Risk factor: uncontrolled seizure activity

Risk for Powerlessness: Risk factor: possible seizure

Risk for impaired Resilience: Risk factor: chronic illness

Readiness for enhanced Knowledge: anticonvulsive therapy

Readiness for enhanced Self-Care: expresses desire to enhance knowledge and responsibility for self-care

See Epilepsy

Seizure Disorders, Childhood (Epilepsy, Febrile Seizures, Infantile Spasms)

Ineffective Health maintenance r/t lack of knowledge regarding anticonvulsive therapy, fever reduction (febrile seizures)

Social isolation r/t unpredictability of seizures, community-imposed stigma

Risk for ineffective Airway clearance: Risk factor: accumulation of secretions during seizure

Risk for delayed Development: Risk factors: effects of seizure disorder, parental overprotection

Risk for Falls: Risk factor: possible seizure

Risk for Injury: Risk factors: uncontrolled movements during seizure, falls, drowsiness caused by anticonvulsants

See Epilepsy

Self-Breast Examination (SBE)

See SBE (Self-Breast Examination)

Self-Care

Readiness for enhanced Self-Care (See **Self-Care,** readiness for enhanced, Section III)

S

Self-Care Deficit, Bathing

Bathing Self-Care deficit (See **Self-Care** deficit, bathing, Section III)

Self-Care Deficit, Dressing

Dressing Self-Care deficit (See **Self-Care** deficit, dressing, Section III)

Self-Care Deficit, Feeding

Feeding Self-Care deficit (See **Self-Care** deficit, feeding, Section III)

Self-Care Deficit, Toileting

Toileting Self-Care deficit (See **Self-Care** deficit, toileting, Section III)

Self-Concept

Readiness for enhanced Self-Concept (See **Self-Concept**, readiness for enhanced, Section III)

Self-Destructive Behavior

Post-Trauma syndrome r/t unresolved feelings from traumatic event

Risk for Self-Mutilation: Risk factors: feelings of depression, rejection, self-hatred, depersonalization; command hallucinations

Risk for Suicide: Risk factor: history of self-destructive behavior

Risk for self-directed Violence: Risk factors: panic state, history of child abuse, toxic reaction to medication

Self-Esteem, Chronic Low

Chronic low Self-Esteem (See **Self-Esteem**, low, chronic, Section III)

Risk for disturbed personal Identity: Risk factor: chronic low self-esteem

Self-Esteem, Situational Low

Situational low Self-Esteem (See **Self-Esteem**, low, situational, Section III)

Risk for situational low Self-Esteem (See **Self-Esteem**, low, situational, risk for, Section III)

Self-Mutilation

Ineffective Impulse control r/t ineffective management of anxiety

Self-Mutilation (See **Self-Mutilation**, Section III)

Risk for Self-Mutilation (See **Self-Mutilation**, risk for, Section III)

Senile Dementia

Ineffective Relationship r/t cognitive changes in one partner

Sedentary lifestyle r/t lack of interest in movement

See Dementia

Separation Anxiety

Ineffective Coping r/t maturational and situational crises, vulnerability related to developmental age, hospitalization, separation from family and familiar surroundings, multiple caregivers

Insomnia r/t separation for significant others

Risk for impaired Attachment: Risk factor: separation

See Hospitalized Child

Sepsis, Child

Impaired Gas exchange r/t pulmonary inflammation associated with disease process

Imbalanced Nutrition: less than body requirements r/t anorexia, generalized weakness, poor sucking reflex

Delayed Surgical recovery r/t presence of infection

Ineffective Thermoregulation r/t infectious process, septic shock

Ineffective peripheral Tissue Perfusion r/t arterial or venous blood flow exchange problems, septic shock

Risk for deficient Fluid volume: Risk factor: inflammation leading to decreased systemic vascular resistance

Risk for impaired Skin integrity: Risk factor: desquamation caused by disseminated intravascular coagulation

See Hospitalized Child; Premature Infant, Child

Septicemia

Imbalanced Nutrition: less than body requirements r/t anorexia, generalized weakness

Ineffective peripheral Tissue Perfusion r/t decreased systemic vascular resistance

Risk for deficient Fluid volume: Risk factors: vasodilation of peripheral vessels, leaking of capillaries

Risk for Shock: Risk factors: hypotension, hypovolemia

Risk for unstable Blood Pressure: Risk factor: hypovolemia

See Sepsis, Child; Shock, Septic

Service Animal

Readiness for enhanced Power: expresses desire to enhance independence with actions for change

Readiness for enhanced Resilience: expresses desire to enhance involvement in activities, desire to enhance environmental safety

Severe Acute Respiratory Syndrome (SARS)

See Pneumonia

Sexual Dysfunction

Sexual Dysfunction r/t insufficient knowledge about sexual function

Ineffective Relationship r/t reported sexual dissatisfaction between partners

Chronic Sorrow r/t loss of ideal sexual experience, altered relationships

Risk for situational low Self-Esteem: Risk factor: alteration in body function

See Erectile Dysfunction (ED)

Sexual Harassment Victim

Anxiety r/t situational crisis

Risk for Compromised Human Dignity: Risk factors: humiliation, dehumanizing treatment

Risk for Post-Trauma syndrome: Risk factors: perceived traumatic event, insufficient social support

Risk for Spiritual Distress: Risk factors: physical, psychological stress

See Assault Victim

Sexuality, Adolescent

Disturbed Body Image r/t anxiety caused by unachieved developmental milestone (puberty) or deficient knowledge regarding reproductive maturation with expressed concerns regarding lack of growth of secondary sex characteristics

Impaired emancipated Decision-Making: sexual activity r/t undefined personal values or beliefs, multiple or divergent sources of information, lack of relevant information

Ineffective Impulse control r/t denial of consequences of actions

Deficient Knowledge: potential for enhanced health maintenance r/t multiple or divergent sources of information or lack of relevant information regarding sexual transmission of disease, contraception, prevention of toxic shock syndrome

See Maturational Issues, Adolescent

Sexuality Pattern, Ineffective

Ineffective Sexuality pattern (See **Sexuality** pattern, ineffective, Section III)

Sexually Transmitted Disease (STD)

See STD (Sexually Transmitted Disease)

Shaken Baby Syndrome

Decreased intracranial Adaptive capacity r/t brain injury

Impaired Parenting r/t stress, history of being abusive

Impaired individual Resilience r/t poor impulse control

Stress overload r/t intense repeated family stressors, family violence

Risk for other-directed Violence: Risk factors: history of violence against others, perinatal complications

See Child Abuse; Suspected Child Abuse and Neglect (SCAN), Child; Suspected Child Abuse and Neglect (SCAN), Parent

Shakiness

Anxiety r/t situational or maturational crisis, threat of death

Shame

Situational low Self-Esteem r/t inability to deal with past traumatic events, blaming of self for events not in one's control

Shingles

Acute Pain r/t vesicular eruption along the nerves

Ineffective Protection r/t abnormal blood profiles

Social isolation r/t altered state of wellness, contagiousness of disease

Risk for Infection: Risk factor: tissue destruction

See Itching

Shivering

Impaired Comfort r/t altered health status

Fear r/t serious threat to health status

Hypothermia r/t exposure to cool environment

Ineffective Thermoregulation r/t serious infectious process resulting in immune response of fever

See Shock, Septic

Shock, Cardiogenic

Decreased Cardiac output r/t decreased myocardial contractility, dysrhythmia

Shock, Hypovolemic

Deficient Fluid volume r/t abnormal loss of fluid, trauma, third spacing

Shock, Septic

Deficient Fluid volume r/t abnormal loss of intravascular fluid, pooling of blood in peripheral circulation, overwhelming inflammatory response

Ineffective Protection r/t inadequately functioning immune system

See Sepsis, Child; Septicemia

Shoulder Repair

Self-Care deficit: bathing, dressing, feeding r/t immobilization of affected shoulder

Risk for Perioperative Positioning injury: Risk factor: immobility

See Surgery, Preoperative Care; Surgery, Perioperative Care; Surgery, Postoperative Care; Total Joint Replacement (Total Hip/Total Knee/Shoulder)

Sickle Cell Anemia/Crisis

Activity intolerance r/t fatigue, effects of chronic anemia

Deficient Fluid volume r/t decreased intake, increased fluid requirements during sickle cell crisis, decreased ability of kidneys to concentrate urine

Impaired physical Mobility r/t pain, fatigue

Acute Pain r/t viscous blood, tissue hypoxia

Ineffective peripheral Tissue Perfusion r/t effects of red cell sickling, infarction of tissues

Risk for decreased Cardiac tissue perfusion: Risk factors: effects of red cell sickling, infarction of tissues

Risk for Infection: Risk factor: alterations in splenic function

Risk for impaired Resilience: Risk factor: chronic illness

Risk for ineffective cerebral Tissue perfusion: Risk factors: effects of red cell sickling, infarction of tissues

See Child with Chronic Condition; Hospitalized Child

SIDS (Sudden Infant Death Syndrome)

Anxiety: parental worry r/t life-threatening event

Interrupted Family processes r/t stress as a result of special care needs of infant with apnea

Grieving r/t potential loss of infant

Insomnia: parental/infant r/t home apnea monitoring

Deficient Knowledge: potential for enhanced health maintenance r/t knowledge or skill acquisition of cardiopulmonary resuscitation and home apnea monitoring

Impaired Resilience r/t sudden loss

S

Risk for Sudden Infant Death (See **Sudden Infant Death**, risk for, Section III)
Risk for Powerlessness: Risk factor: unanticipated life-threatening event
See Terminally Ill Child/Death of Child, Parent

Sitting Problems
Impaired Sitting (See **Sitting,** impaired, Section III)

Situational Crisis
Imbalanced Energy Field r/t hyperactivity of the energy flow
Ineffective Coping r/t situational crisis
Interrupted Family processes r/t situational crisis
Risk for ineffective Activity planning: Risk factor: inability to process information
Risk for disturbed personal Identity: Risk factor: situational crisis
Readiness for enhanced Communication: willingness to share feelings and thoughts
Readiness for enhanced Religiosity: requests religious material and/or experiences
Readiness for enhanced Resilience: desire to enhance resilience
Readiness for enhanced Spiritual well-being: desire for harmony following crisis

SJS (Stevens-Johnson Syndrome)
See Stevens-Johnson Syndrome (SJS)

Skin Cancer
Ineffective Health maintenance r/t deficient knowledge regarding self-care with skin cancer
Ineffective Protection r/t weakened immune system
Impaired Tissue integrity r/t abnormal cell growth in skin, treatment of skin cancer
Readiness for enhanced Health management: follows preventive measures
Readiness for enhanced Knowledge: self-care to prevent and treat skin cancer

Skin Disorders
Impaired Skin integrity (See **Skin** integrity, impaired, Section III)

Skin Turgor, Change in Elasticity
Deficient Fluid volume r/t active fluid loss

Sleep
Readiness for enhanced Sleep (See **Sleep,** readiness for enhanced, Section III)

Sleep Apnea
Ineffective Breathing pattern r/t obesity, substance abuse, enlarged tonsils, smoking, or neurological pathology such as a brain tumor
Impaired Comfort r/t use of bilevel positive airway pressure (BiPAP)/continuous positive airway pressure (CPAP) machine

Sleep Deprivation
Fatigue r/t lack of sleep
Sleep deprivation (See **Sleep** deprivation, Section III)

Sleep Problems
Insomnia (See **Insomnia,** Section III)

Sleep Pattern, Disturbed, Parent/Child
Insomnia: child r/t anxiety or fear
Insomnia: parent r/t parental responsibilities, stress
See Suspected Child Abuse and Neglect (SCAN), Child; Suspected Child Abuse and Neglect (SCAN), Parent

Slurring of Speech
Impaired verbal Communication r/t decrease in circulation to brain, brain tumor, anatomical defect, cleft palate
Situational low Self-Esteem r/t speech impairment
See Communication Problems

Small Bowel Resection
See Abdominal Surgery

Smell, Loss of Ability to
Risk for Injury: Risk factors: inability to detect gas fumes, smoke smells
See Anosmia (Smell, Loss of Ability to)

Smoke Inhalation
Ineffective Airway clearance r/t smoke inhalation
Impaired Gas exchange r/t ventilation-perfusion imbalance
Risk for acute Confusion: Risk factor: decreased oxygen supply
Risk for Infection: Risk factors: inflammation, ineffective airway clearance, pneumonia
Risk for Poisoning: Risk factor: exposure to carbon monoxide
Readiness for enhanced Health management: functioning smoke detectors and carbon monoxide detectors in home and work, escape route planned and reviewed
See Atelectasis; Burns; Pneumonia

Smoking Behavior
Insufficient Breast Milk Production r/t smoking
Risk-prone Health behavior Risk factor: smoking
Ineffective Health maintenance r/t denial of effects of smoking, lack of effective support for smoking withdrawal
Readiness for enhanced Knowledge: expresses interest in smoking cessation
Risk for dry Eye: Risk factor: smoking
Risk for ineffective peripheral Tissue Perfusion: Risk factor: effect of nicotine
Risk for Thermal injury: Risk factor: unsafe smoking behavior
Readiness for enhanced Health literacy: verbalizes desire to enhance understanding of health information to make health care choices

Social Interaction, Impaired
Impaired Social interaction (See **Social** interaction, impaired, Section III)

Social Isolation

Social isolation (See **Social isolation**, Section III)

Sociopathic Personality

See Antisocial Personality Disorder

Sodium, Decrease/Increase

See Hyponatremia; Hypernatremia

Somatization Disorder

Anxiety r/t unresolved conflicts channeled into physical complaints or conditions

Ineffective Coping r/t lack of insight into underlying conflicts

Ineffective Denial r/t displaced psychological stress to physical symptoms

Nausea r/t anxiety

Chronic Pain r/t unexpressed anger, multiple physical disorders, depression

Impaired individual Resilience r/t possible psychological disorders

Sore Nipples, Breastfeeding

Ineffective Breastfeeding r/t deficient knowledge regarding correct feeding procedure

See Painful Breasts, Sore Nipples

Sore Throat

Impaired Comfort r/t sore throat

Deficient Knowledge r/t treatment, relief of discomfort

Impaired Oral Mucous Membrane integrity r/t inflammation or infection of oral cavity

Impaired Swallowing r/t irritation of oropharyngeal cavity

Risk for Dry Mouth: Risk factor: painful swallowing

Sorrow

Grieving r/t loss of significant person, object, or role

Chronic Sorrow (See **Sorrow**, chronic, Section III)

Readiness for enhanced Communication: expresses thoughts and feelings

Readiness for enhanced Spiritual well-being: desire to find purpose and meaning of loss

Spastic Colon

See IBS (Irritable Bowel Syndrome)

Speech Disorders

Anxiety r/t difficulty with communication

Impaired verbal Communication r/t anatomical defect, cleft palate, psychological barriers, decrease in circulation to brain

Spina Bifida

See Neural Tube Defects (Meningocele, Myelomeningocele, Spina Bifida, Anencephaly)

Spinal Cord Injury

Decreased Diversional activity engagement r/t long-term hospitalization, frequent lengthy treatments

Fear r/t powerlessness over loss of body function

Disturbed Body Image r/t alteration in body function

Chronic functional Constipation r/t inhibition of reflex arc

Complicated Grieving r/t loss of usual body function

Ineffective Coping r/t inability to meet basic needs and insufficient sense of control

Sedentary Lifestyle r/t lack of resources or interest

Impaired physical Mobility r/t neuromuscular impairment

Impaired wheelchair Mobility r/t neuromuscular impairment

Impaired Standing r/t spinal cord injury

Urinary Retention r/t inhibition of reflex arc

Risk for Latex Allergy reaction: Risk factor: continuous or intermittent catheterization

Risk for Autonomic Dysreflexia: Risk factors: bladder or bowel distention, skin irritation, deficient knowledge of patient and caregiver

Risk for ineffective Breathing pattern: Risk factor: neuromuscular impairment

Risk for Infection: Risk factors: chronic disease, stasis of body fluids

Risk for Loneliness: Risk factor: physical immobility

Risk for Powerlessness: Risk factor: loss of function

Risk for Pressure ulcer: Risk factor: immobility and decreased sensation

Risk for Thermal Injury: Risk factor: physical immobility

Risk for Venous Thromboembolism: Risk factor: physical immobility

See Child with Chronic Condition; Hospitalized Child; Neural Tube Defects (Meningocele, Myelomeningocele, Spina Bifida, Anencephaly); Paralysis

Spinal Fusion

Impaired bed Mobility r/t impaired ability to turn side to side while keeping spine in proper alignment

Impaired physical Mobility r/t musculoskeletal impairment associated with surgery, possible back brace

Readiness for enhanced Knowledge: expresses interest in information associated with surgery

See Acute Back Pain; Scoliosis; Surgery, Preoperative Care; Surgery, Perioperative Care; Surgery, Postoperative Care

Spiritual Distress

Spiritual distress (See **Spiritual** distress, Section III)

Risk for chronic low Self-Esteem: Risk factor: unresolved spiritual issues

Risk for Spiritual distress (See **Spiritual** distress, risk for, Section III)

Spiritual Well-Being

Readiness for enhanced Spiritual well-being (See **Spiritual** well-being, readiness for enhanced, Section III)

Splenectomy

See Abdominal Surgery

S

Sprains

Acute Pain r/t physical injury

Impaired physical Mobility r/t injury

Impaired Walking r/t injury

Stable Blood Pressure, Risk for Unstable

Deficient Knowledge r/t inconsistency with medication regiment

(See **Unstable Blood Pressure,** Risk for, Section III)

Standing Problems

Impaired Standing (see Impaired **Standing,** Section III)

Stapedectomy

Hearing Loss r/t edema from surgery

Acute Pain r/t headache

Risk for Falls: Risk factor: dizziness

Risk for Infection: Risk factor: invasive procedure

Stasis Ulcer

Impaired Tissue integrity r/t chronic venous congestion

Risk for Infection: Risk factor: open wound

See CHF (Congestive Heart Failure); Varicose Veins

STD (Sexually Transmitted Disease)

Impaired Comfort r/t infection

Fear r/t altered body function, risk for social isolation, fear of incurable illness

Ineffective Health maintenance r/t deficient knowledge regarding transmission, symptoms, treatment of STD

Ineffective Sexuality pattern r/t illness, altered body function, need for abstinence to heal

Social isolation r/t fear of contracting or spreading disease

Risk for Infection: spread of infection: Risk factor: lack of knowledge concerning transmission of disease

Readiness for enhanced Knowledge: seeks information regarding prevention and treatment of STDs

See Maturational Issues, Adolescent; PID (Pelvic Inflammatory Disease)

STEMI (ST-Elevation Myocardial Infarction)

See MI (Myocardial Infarction)

Stent (Coronary Artery Stent)

Risk for Injury: Risk factor: complications associated with stent placement

Risk for decreased Cardiac tissue perfusion: Risk factor: possible restenosis

Risk for Vascular Trauma: Risk factors: insertion site, catheter width

Readiness for enhanced Decision-Making: expresses desire to enhance risk-benefit analysis, understanding and meaning of choices, and decisions regarding treatment

See Angioplasty, Coronary; Cardiac Catheterization

Sterilization Surgery

Decisional Conflict r/t multiple or divergent sources of information, unclear personal values or beliefs

See Surgery, Preoperative Care; Surgery, Perioperative Care; Surgery, Postoperative Care; Tubal Ligation; Vasectomy

Stertorous Respirations

Ineffective Airway clearance r/t pharyngeal obstruction

Stevens-Johnson Syndrome (SJS)

Impaired Oral Mucous Membrane integrity r/t immunocompromised condition associated with allergic medication reaction

Acute Pain r/t painful skin lesions and painful mucosa lesions

Impaired Skin integrity r/t allergic medication reaction

Risk for deficient Fluid volume: Risk factors: factors affecting fluid needs (hypermetabolic state, fever), excessive losses through normal routes (vomiting and diarrhea)

Risk for Infection: Risk factor: sloughing skin

Risk for impaired Liver function: Risk factor: impaired immune response

Stillbirth

See Pregnancy Loss

Stoma

See Colostomy; Ileostomy

Stomatitis

Impaired Oral Mucous Membrane integrity r/t pathological conditions of oral cavity; side effects of chemotherapy

Risk for impaired Oral Mucous Membrane integrity (See impaired **Oral Mucous Membrane** integrity, risk for, Section III)

Stool, Hard/Dry

Chronic functional Constipation r/t inadequate fluid intake, inadequate fiber intake, decreased activity level, decreased gastric motility

Straining with Defecation

Chronic functional Constipation r/t less than adequate fluid intake, less than adequate dietary intake

Risk for decreased Cardiac output: Risk factor: vagal stimulation with dysrhythmia resulting from Valsalva maneuver

Strep Throat

Risk for Infection: Risk factor: exposure to pathogen

See Sore Throat

Stress

Anxiety r/t feelings of helplessness, feelings of being threatened

Ineffective Coping r/t ineffective use of problem-solving process, feelings of apprehension or helplessness

Fear r/t powerlessness over feelings

Stress overload r/t intense or multiple stressors

Readiness for enhanced Communication: shows willingness to share thoughts and feelings

S

Readiness for enhanced Spiritual well-being: expresses desire for harmony and peace in stressful situation
See Anxiety

Stress Urinary Incontinence

Stress urinary Incontinence r/t degenerative change in pelvic muscles

Stridor

Ineffective Airway clearance r/t obstruction, tracheobronchial infection, trauma

Stroke

See CVA (Cerebrovascular Accident)

Stuttering

Anxiety r/t impaired verbal communication

Impaired verbal Communication r/t anxiety, psychological problems

Subarachnoid Hemorrhage

Acute Pain: headache r/t irritation of meninges from blood, increased intracranial pressure

Risk for ineffective Cerebral tissue perfusion: Risk factor: bleeding from cerebral vessel
See Intracranial Pressure, Increased

Substance Abuse

Acute Substance Withdrawal syndrome: Risk factor: developed dependence to alcohol or other addictive substances

Anxiety r/t threat to self-concept, lack of control of drug use

Compromised family Coping r/t codependency issues

Defensive Coping r/t substance abuse

Disabled family Coping r/t differing coping styles between support persons

Ineffective Coping r/t use of substances to cope with life events

Ineffective Denial r/t refusal to acknowledge substance abuse problem

Dysfunctional Family processes r/t substance abuse

Risk-prone Health behavior r/t addiction

Deficient community Health r/t prevention and control of illegal substances in community

Ineffective Impulse control r/t addictive process

Insomnia r/t irritability, nightmares, tremors

Imbalanced Nutrition: less than body requirements r/t poor eating habits

Powerlessness r/t feeling unable to change patterns of drug abuse

Ineffective Relationship r/t inability for well-balanced collaboration between partners

Sexual Dysfunction r/t actions and side effects of drugs

Sleep deprivation r/t prolonged psychological discomfort

Impaired Social interaction r/t disturbed thought processes from drug abuse

Risk for Acute Substance Withdrawal syndrome: Risk factor: developed dependence to alcohol or other addictive substances

Risk for impaired Attachment: Risk factor: substance abuse

Risk for Injury: Risk factors: hallucinations, drug effects

Risk for disturbed personal Identity: Risk factor: ingestion/inhalation of toxic chemicals

Risk for chronic low Self-Esteem: Risk factors: perceived lack of respect from others, repeated failures, repeated negative reinforcement

Risk for Thermal injury: Risk factor: intoxication with drugs or alcohol

Risk for unstable Blood Pressure: Risk factor: vasoconstriction of cardiac arteries

Risk for Vascular Trauma: Risk factor: chemical irritant self injected into veins

Risk for self-directed Violence: Risk factors: reactions to substances used, impulsive behavior, disorientation, impaired judgment

Risk for other-directed Violence: Risk factor: poor impulse control

Readiness for enhanced Coping: seeking social support and knowledge of new strategies

Readiness for enhanced Self-Concept: accepting strengths and limitations
See Alcoholism

Substance Abuse, Adolescent

See Alcoholism; Maturational Issues, Adolescent; Substance Abuse

Substance Abuse in Pregnancy

Ineffective Childbearing process r/t substance abuse

Defensive Coping r/t denial of situation, differing value system

Ineffective Health management r/t addiction

Deficient Knowledge r/t lack of exposure to information regarding effects of substance abuse in pregnancy

Neonatal Abstinence syndrome r/t in utero substance exposure secondary to maternal substance use

Risk for impaired Attachment: Risk factors: substance abuse, inability of parent to meet infant's or own personal needs

Risk for Infection: Risk factors: intravenous drug use, lifestyle

Risk for Injury: fetal: Risk factor: effects of drugs on fetal growth and development

Risk for Injury: maternal: Risk factor: drug or alcohol use

Risk for impaired Parenting: Risk factor: lack of ability to meet infant's needs due to addiction with use of alcohol or drugs
See Alcoholism; Substance Abuse

Substance Withdrawal

See Acute Substance Withdrawal Syndrome

Sucking Reflex

Effective Breastfeeding r/t regular and sustained sucking and swallowing at breast

Sudden Infant Death Syndrome (SIDS)

See SIDS (Sudden Infant Death Syndrome)

Suffocation, Risk for

Risk for Suffocation (See **Suffocation,** risk for, Section III)

S

Suicide Attempt

Risk-prone Health behavior r/t low self-efficacy

Ineffective Coping r/t anger, complicated grieving

Hopelessness r/t perceived or actual loss, substance abuse, low self-concept, inadequate support systems

Ineffective Impulse control r/t inability to modulate stress, anxiety

Post-Trauma syndrome r/t history of traumatic events, abuse, rape, incest, war, torture

Impaired individual Resilience r/t poor impulse control

Situational low Self-Esteem r/t guilt, inability to trust, feelings of worthlessness or rejection

Social isolation r/t inability to engage in satisfying personal relationships

Spiritual distress r/t hopelessness, despair

Risk for Post-Trauma syndrome: Risk factor: survivor's role in suicide attempt

Risk for Suicide (See **Suicide,** risk for, Section III)

Readiness for enhanced Communication: willingness to share thoughts and feelings

Readiness for enhanced Spiritual well-being: desire for harmony and inner strength to help redefine purpose for life

See Violent Behavior

Support System, Inadequate

Readiness for enhanced family Coping: ability to adapt to tasks associated with care, support of significant other during health crisis

Readiness for enhanced Family processes: activities support the growth of family members

Readiness for enhanced Parenting: children or other dependent person(s) expressing satisfaction with home environment

Suppression of Labor

See Preterm Labor

Surgery, Perioperative Care

Risk for imbalanced Fluid volume: Risk factor: surgery

Risk for Perioperative Hypothermia: Risk factors: inadequate covering of client, cold surgical room

Risk for Perioperative Positioning injury: Risk factors: predisposing condition, prolonged surgery

Surgery, Postoperative Care

Activity intolerance r/t pain, surgical procedure

Anxiety r/t change in health status, hospital environment

Deficient Knowledge r/t postoperative expectations, lifestyle changes

Nausea r/t manipulation of gastrointestinal tract, postsurgical anesthesia

Imbalanced Nutrition: less than body requirements r/t anorexia, nausea, vomiting, decreased peristalsis

Ineffective peripheral Tissue Perfusion r/t hypovolemia, circulatory stasis, obesity, prolonged immobility, decreased coughing, decreased deep breathing

Acute Pain r/t inflammation or injury in surgical area

Delayed Surgical recovery r/t extensive surgical procedure, postoperative surgical infection

Urinary retention r/t anesthesia, pain, fear, unfamiliar surroundings, client's position

Risk for Bleeding: Risk factor: surgical procedure

Risk for ineffective Breathing pattern: Risk factors: pain, location of incision, effects of anesthesia or opioids

Risk for Constipation: Risk factors: decreased activity, decreased food or fluid intake, anesthesia, pain medication

Risk for imbalanced Fluid volume: Risk factors: hypermetabolic state, fluid loss during surgery, presence of indwelling tubes, fluids used to distend organ structures being absorbed into body

Risk for Surgical Site Infection: Risk factors: invasive procedure, pain, anesthesia, location of incision, weakened cough as a result of aging

Surgery, Preoperative Care

Anxiety r/t threat to or change in health status, situational crisis, fear of the unknown

Insomnia r/t anxiety about upcoming surgery

Deficient Knowledge r/t preoperative procedures, postoperative expectations

Readiness for enhanced Knowledge: shows understanding of preoperative and postoperative expectations for self-care

Surgical Recovery, Delayed

Delayed Surgical recovery (See **Surgical** recovery, delayed, Section III)

Risk for delayed Surgical recovery (See **Surgical** recovery, delayed, risk for, Section III)

Surgical Site Infection

Anxiety r/t unforeseen result of surgery

Impaired Comfort r/t surgical site pain

Risk for ineffective Thermoregulation: Risk factor: infectious process

Risk for delayed Surgical Recovery: Risk factor: interrupted healing of surgical site

Readiness for enhanced Knowledge: expresses desire for knowledge of prevention and symptoms of infection

Suspected Child Abuse and Neglect (SCAN), Child

Ineffective Activity planning r/t lack of family support

Anxiety: child r/t threat of punishment for perceived wrongdoing

Deficient community Health r/t inadequate reporting and follow-up of SCAN

Disturbed personal Identity r/t dysfunctional family processes

Rape-Trauma syndrome r/t altered lifestyle because of abuse, changes in residence

Risk for impaired Resilience: Risk factor: adverse situation

Readiness for enhanced community Coping: obtaining resources to prevent child abuse, neglect

See Child Abuse; Hospitalized Child; Maturational Issues, Adolescent

Suspected Child Abuse and Neglect (SCAN), Parent

Disabled family Coping r/t dysfunctional family, underdeveloped nurturing parental role, lack of parental support systems or role models

Dysfunctional Family processes r/t inadequate coping skills

Ineffective Health maintenance r/t deficient knowledge of parenting skills as result of unachieved developmental tasks

Impaired Home maintenance r/t disorganization, parental dysfunction, neglect of safe and nurturing environment

Ineffective Impulse control r/t projection of anger, frustration onto child

Impaired Parenting r/t unrealistic expectations of child; lack of effective role model; unmet social, emotional, or maturational needs of parents; interruption in bonding process

Impaired individual Resilience r/t poor impulse control

Chronic low Self-Esteem r/t lack of successful parenting experiences

Risk for other-directed Violence: parent to child: Risk factors: inadequate coping mechanisms, unresolved stressors, unachieved maturational level by parent

Suspicion

Disturbed personal Identity r/t psychiatric disorder

Powerlessness r/t repetitive paranoid thinking

Impaired Social interaction r/t disturbed thought processes, paranoid delusions, hallucinations

Risk for self-directed Violence: Risk factor: inability to trust

Risk for other-directed Violence: Risk factor: impulsiveness

Swallowing Difficulties

Impaired Swallowing (See **Swallowing,** impaired, Section III)

Syncope

Anxiety r/t fear of falling

Impaired physical Mobility r/t fear of falling

Ineffective Health management r/t lack of knowledge in how to prevent syncope

Social isolation r/t fear of falling

Risk for decreased Cardiac output: Risk factor: dysrhythmia

Risk for Falls: Risk factor: syncope

Risk for Injury: Risk factors: altered sensory perception, transient loss of consciousness, risk for falls

Risk for ineffective Cerebral tissue perfusion: Risk factor: interruption of blood flow

Syphilis

See STD (Sexually Transmitted Disease)

Systemic Lupus Erythematosus

See Lupus Erythematosus

T

T & A (Tonsillectomy and Adenoidectomy)

Ineffective Airway clearance r/t hesitation or reluctance to cough because of pain

Deficient Knowledge: potential for enhanced health maintenance r/t insufficient knowledge regarding postoperative nutritional and rest requirements, signs and symptoms of complications, positioning

Nausea r/t gastric irritation, pharmaceuticals, anesthesia

Acute Pain r/t surgical incision

Risk for Aspiration: Risk factors: postoperative drainage and impaired swallowing

Risk for deficient Fluid volume: Risk factors: decreased intake because of painful swallowing, effects of anesthesia (nausea, vomiting), hemorrhage

Risk for imbalanced Nutrition: less than body requirements: Risk factors: hesitation or reluctance to swallow

Tachycardia

See Dysrhythmia

Tachypnea

Ineffective Breathing pattern r/t pain, anxiety, hypoxia

See cause of Tachypnea

Tardive Dyskinesia

Ineffective Health management r/t complexity of therapeutic regimen or medication

Deficient Knowledge r/t cognitive limitation in assimilating information relating to side effects associated with neuroleptic medications

Risk for Injury: Risk factor: drug-induced abnormal body movements

Taste Abnormality

Frail Elderly syndrome r/t chronic illness

TB (Pulmonary Tuberculosis)

Ineffective Airway clearance r/t increased secretions, excessive mucus

Ineffective Breathing pattern r/t decreased energy, fatigue

Fatigue r/t disease state

Impaired Gas exchange r/t disease process

Ineffective Health management r/t deficient knowledge of prevention and treatment regimen

Impaired Home maintenance management r/t client or family member with disease

Ineffective Thermoregulation r/t presence of infection

Risk for Infection: Risk factor: insufficient knowledge regarding avoidance of exposure to pathogens

Readiness for enhanced Health management: takes medications according to prescribed protocol for prevention and treatment

TBI (Traumatic Brain Injury)

Interrupted Family processes r/t traumatic injury to family member

Chronic Sorrow r/t change in health status and functional ability

Risk for Post-Trauma syndrome: Risk factor: perception of event causing TBI

Risk for impaired Religiosity: Risk factor: impaired physical mobility

Risk for impaired Resilience: Risk factor: crisis of injury

See Head Injury; Neurologic Disorders

TD (Traveler's Diarrhea)

See Traveler's Diarrhea

Technology Addiction

Decreased Diversional activity engagement r/t insufficient motivation to separate from electronic devices

Impaired Social interaction r/t lack of desire to engage in personal face-to-face contact with others

Risk for impaired Attachment: Risk factor: preoccupation with electronic devices

Risk for impaired Parenting: Risk factor: insufficient uninterrupted meaningful interaction between parent and child as the result of preoccupation with electronic devices

Risk for ineffective Relationship: Risk factor: ineffective face-to-face communication skills

Temperature, Decreased

Hypothermia r/t exposure to cold environment

Temperature, High

Hyperthermia r/t neurological damage, disease condition with high temperature, excessive heat, inflammatory response

Temperature Regulation, Impaired

Ineffective Thermoregulation r/t trauma, illness, cerebral injury

TEN (Toxic Epidermal Necrolysis)

See Toxic Epidermal Necrolysis (TEN)

TENS Unit (Transcutaneous Electrical Nerve Stimulation)

Risk for unstable Blood Pressure: Risk factor: improper use of TENS unit (front of neck)

Readiness for enhanced Comfort: expresses desire to enhance resolution of complaints

Tension

Anxiety r/t threat to or change in health status, situational crisis

Readiness for enhanced Communication: expresses willingness to share feelings and thoughts

See Stress

Terminally Ill Adult

Death Anxiety r/t unresolved issues relating to death and dying

Imbalanced Energy Field r/t weak energy field patterns

Risk for Spiritual distress: Risk factor: impending death

Readiness for enhanced Religiosity: requests religious material and/or experiences

Readiness for enhanced Spiritual well-being: desire to achieve harmony of mind, body, spirit

See Terminally Ill Child/Death of Child, Parent

Terminally Ill Child, Adolescent

Disturbed Body Image r/t effects of terminal disease, already critical feelings of group identity and self-image

Ineffective Coping r/t inability to establish personal and peer identity because of the threat of being different or not being healthy, inability to achieve maturational tasks

Impaired Social interaction r/t forced separation from peers

See Child with Chronic Condition; Hospitalized Child, Terminally Ill Child/Death of Child, Parent

Terminally Ill Child, Infant/Toddler

Ineffective Coping r/t separation from parents and familiar environment from inability to understand dying process

See Child with Chronic Condition, Terminally Ill Child/Death of Child, Parent

Terminally Ill Child, Preschool Child

Fear r/t perceived punishment, bodily harm, feelings of guilt caused by magical thinking (i.e., believing that thoughts cause events)

See Child with Chronic Condition, Terminally Ill Child/Death of Child, Parent

Terminally Ill Child, School-Age Child/Preadolescent

Fear r/t perceived punishment, body mutilation, feelings of guilt

See Child with Chronic Condition, Terminally Ill Child/Death of Child, Parent

Terminally Ill Child/Death of Child, Parent

Compromised family Coping r/t inability or unwillingness to discuss impending death and feelings with child or support child through terminal stages of illness

Decisional Conflict r/t continuation or discontinuation of treatment, do-not-resuscitate decision, ethical issues regarding organ donation

Ineffective Denial r/t complicated grieving

Interrupted Family processes r/t situational crisis

Grieving r/t death of child

Hopelessness r/t overwhelming stresses caused by terminal illness

Insomnia r/t grieving process

Impaired Parenting r/t risk for overprotection of surviving siblings

Powerlessness r/t inability to alter course of events

Impaired Social interaction r/t complicated grieving

Social isolation: imposed by others r/t feelings of inadequacy in providing support to grieving parents

Social isolation: self-imposed r/t unresolved grief, perceived inadequate parenting skills

Spiritual distress r/t sudden and unexpected death, prolonged suffering before death, questioning the death of youth, questioning the meaning of one's own existence

Risk for complicated Grieving: Risk factors: prolonged, unresolved, obstructed progression through stages of grief and mourning

Risk for impaired Resilience: Risk factor: impending death

Readiness for enhanced family Coping: impact of crisis on family values, priorities, goals, or relationships; expressed interest or desire to attach meaning to child's life and death

T

Tetralogy of Fallot
See Congenital Heart Disease/Cardiac Anomalies

Tetraplegia
Autonomic dysreflexia r/t bladder or bowel distention, skin irritation, infection, deficient knowledge of patient and caregiver

Grieving r/t loss of previous functioning

Powerlessness r/t inability to perform previous activities

Impaired Sitting r/t paralysis of extremities

Impaired spontaneous Ventilation r/t loss of innervation of respiratory muscles, respiratory muscle fatigue

Risk for Aspiration: Risk factor: inadequate ability to protect airway from neurological damage

Risk for Infection: Risk factor: urinary stasis

Risk for impaired Skin integrity: Risk factor: physical immobilization and decreased sensation

Risk for ineffective Thermoregulation: Risk factors: inability to move to increase temperature, possible presence of infection to increase temperature

Thermoregulation, Ineffective
Ineffective Thermoregulation (See **Thermoregulation**, ineffective, Section III)

Risk for Ineffective Thermoregulation, (See **Ineffective Thermoregulation**, risk for, Section III)

Thoracentesis
See Pleural Effusion

Thoracotomy
Activity intolerance r/t pain, imbalance between oxygen supply and demand, presence of chest tubes

Ineffective Airway clearance r/t drowsiness, pain with breathing and coughing

Ineffective Breathing pattern r/t decreased energy, fatigue, pain

Deficient Knowledge r/t self-care, effective breathing exercises, pain relief

Acute Pain r/t surgical procedure, coughing, deep breathing

Risk for Bleeding: Risk factor: surgery

Risk for Surgical Site Infection: Risk factor: invasive procedure

Risk for Injury: Risk factor: disruption of closed-chest drainage system

Risk for Perioperative Positioning injury: Risk factors: lateral positioning, immobility

Risk for Vascular Trauma: Risk factors: chemical irritant; antibiotics

Thought Disorders
See Schizophrenia

Thrombocytopenic Purpura
See ITP (Idiopathic Thrombocytopenic Purpura)

Thrombophlebitis
See Deep Vein Thrombosis (DVT)

Thyroidectomy
Risk for ineffective Airway clearance: Risk factor: edema or hematoma formation, airway obstruction

Risk for impaired verbal Communication: Risk factors: edema, pain, vocal cord or laryngeal nerve damage

Risk for Injury: Risk factor: possible parathyroid damage or removal

See Surgery, Preoperative Care; Surgery, Perioperative Care; Surgery, Postoperative Care

TIA (Transient Ischemic Attack)
Acute Confusion r/t hypoxia

Readiness for enhanced Health management: obtains knowledge regarding treatment prevention of inadequate oxygenation

See Syncope

Tic Disorder
See Tourette's Syndrome (TS)

Tinea Capitis
Impaired Comfort r/t inflammation from skin irritation

See Ringworm of Scalp

Tinea Corporis
See Ringworm of Body

Tinea Cruris
See Jock Itch; Itching; Pruritus

Tinea Pedis
See Athlete's Foot; Itching; Pruritus

Tinea Unguium (Onychomycosis)
See Ringworm of Nails

Tinnitus
Ineffective Health maintenance r/t deficient knowledge regarding self-care with tinnitus

Hearing Loss r/t ringing in ears obscuring hearing

Tissue Damage, Integumentary
Impaired Tissue integrity (See **Tissue** integrity, impaired, Section III)

Risk for impaired Tissue integrity (See **Tissue** integrity, impaired, risk for, Section III)

Tissue Perfusion, Peripheral
Ineffective peripheral Tissue Perfusion (See **Tissue Perfusion**, peripheral, ineffective, Section III)

Risk for ineffective peripheral Tissue Perfusion (See **Tissue Perfusion**, peripheral, ineffective, risk for, Section III)

Toileting Problems
Toileting Self-Care deficit r/t impaired transfer ability, impaired mobility status, intolerance of activity, neuromuscular impairment, cognitive impairment

Impaired Transfer ability r/t neuromuscular deficits

T

Toilet Training

Deficient Knowledge: parent r/t signs of child's readiness for training

Risk for Constipation: Risk factor: withholding stool

Risk for Infection: Risk factor: withholding urination

Tonsillectomy and Adenoidectomy (T & A)

See T & A (Tonsillectomy and Adenoidectomy)

Toothache

Impaired Dentition r/t ineffective oral hygiene, barriers to self-care, economic barriers to professional care, nutritional deficits, lack of knowledge regarding dental health

Acute Pain r/t inflammation, infection

Total Anomalous Pulmonary Venous Return

See Congenital Heart Disease/Cardiac Anomalies

Total Joint Replacement (Total Hip/Total Knee/Shoulder)

Disturbed Body Image r/t large scar, presence of prosthesis

Impaired physical Mobility r/t musculoskeletal impairment, surgery, prosthesis

Risk for Injury: neurovascular: Risk factors: altered peripheral tissue perfusion, impaired mobility, prosthesis

Risk for Peripheral Neurovascular dysfunction: Risk factors: immobilization, surgical procedure

Ineffective peripheral Tissue perfusion r/t surgery

See Surgery, Preoperative Care; Surgery, Perioperative Care; Surgery, Postoperative Care

Total Parenteral Nutrition (TPN)

See TPN (Total Parenteral Nutrition)

Tourette's Syndrome (TS)

Hopelessness r/t inability to control behavior

Impaired individual Resilience r/t uncontrollable behavior

Risk for situational low Self-Esteem: Risk factors: uncontrollable behavior, motor and phonic tics

See Attention Deficit Disorder

Toxemia

See PIH (Pregnancy-Induced Hypertension/Preeclampsia)

Toxic Epidermal Necrolysis (TEN) (Erythema Multiforme)

Death Anxiety r/t uncertainty of prognosis

TPN (Total Parenteral Nutrition)

Imbalanced Nutrition: less than body requirements r/t inability to digest food or absorb nutrients as a result of biological or psychological factors

Risk for Electrolyte imbalance: Risk factor: need for regulation of electrolytes in TPN fluids

Risk for excess Fluid volume: Risk factor: rapid administration of TPN

Risk for unstable blood Glucose level: Risk factor: high glucose levels in TPN to be regulated according to blood glucose levels

Risk for Infection: Risk factors: concentrated glucose solution, invasive administration of fluids

Risk for Vascular Trauma: Risk factors: insertion site, length of treatment time

Tracheoesophageal Fistula

Ineffective Airway clearance r/t aspiration of feeding because of inability to swallow

Imbalanced Nutrition: less than body requirements r/t difficulties swallowing

Risk for Aspiration: Risk factor: common passage of air and food

Risk for Vascular Trauma: Risk factors: venous medications and site

See Respiratory Conditions of the Neonate; Hospitalized Child

Tracheostomy

Ineffective Airway clearance r/t increased secretions, mucous plugs

Anxiety r/t impaired verbal communication, ineffective airway clearance

Disturbed Body Image r/t abnormal opening in neck

Impaired verbal Communication r/t presence of mechanical airway

Deficient Knowledge r/t self-care, home maintenance management

Acute Pain r/t edema, surgical procedure

Risk for Aspiration: Risk factor: presence of tracheostomy

Risk for Bleeding: Risk factor: surgical incision

Risk for Surgical Site Infection: Risk factors: invasive procedure, pooling of secretions

Traction and Casts

Constipation r/t immobility

Decreased Diversional activity engagement r/t immobility

Impaired physical Mobility r/t imposed restrictions on activity because of bone or joint disease injury

Acute Pain r/t immobility, injury, or disease

Self-Care deficit: feeding, dressing, bathing, toileting r/t degree of impaired physical mobility, body area affected by traction or cast

Impaired Transfer ability r/t presence of traction, casts

Risk for Disuse syndrome: Risk factor: mechanical immobilization

See Casts

Transfer Ability

Impaired Transfer ability (See **Transfer** ability, impaired, Section III)

Transient Ischemic Attack (TIA)

See TIA (Transient Ischemic Attack)

Transposition of Great Vessels

See Congenital Heart Disease/Cardiac Anomalies

Transurethral Resection of the Prostate (TURP)

See TURP (Transurethral Resection of the Prostate)

Trauma in Pregnancy

Anxiety r/t threat to self or fetus, unknown outcome

Deficient Knowledge r/t lack of exposure to situation

Acute Pain r/t trauma

Impaired Skin integrity r/t trauma

Risk for Bleeding: Risk factor: trauma

Risk for deficient Fluid volume: Risk factor: fluid loss

Risk for Infection: Risk factor: traumatized tissue

Risk for Injury: fetal: Risk factor: premature separation of placenta

Risk for disturbed Maternal–Fetal dyad: Risk factor: complication of pregnancy

Trauma, Physical, Risk for

Risk for Physical Trauma (See **Physical Trauma,** risk for, Section III)

Traumatic Brain Injury (TBI)

See TBI (Traumatic Brain Injury); Intracranial Pressure, Increased

Traumatic Event

Post-Trauma syndrome r/t previously experienced trauma

Traveler's Diarrhea (TD)

Diarrhea r/t travel with exposure to different bacteria, viruses

Risk for deficient Fluid Volume: Risk factor: excessive loss of fluids

Risk for Infection: Risk factors: insufficient knowledge regarding avoidance of exposure to pathogens (water supply, iced drinks, local cheese, ice cream, undercooked meat, fish and shellfish, uncooked vegetables, unclean eating utensils, improper handwashing

Trembling of Hands

Fear r/t threat to or change in health status, threat of death, situational crisis

Tricuspid Atresia

See Congenital Heart Disease/Cardiac Anomalies

Trigeminal Neuralgia

Ineffective Health management r/t deficient knowledge regarding prevention of stimuli that trigger pain

Imbalanced Nutrition: less than body requirements r/t pain when chewing

Acute Pain r/t irritation of trigeminal nerve

Risk for corneal Injury: Risk factor: possible decreased corneal sensation

Truncus Arteriosus

See Congenital Heart Disease/Cardiac Anomalies

TS (Tourette's Syndrome)

See Tourette's Syndrome (TS)

TSE (Testicular Self-Examination)

Readiness for enhanced Health management: seeks information regarding self-examination

Tubal Ligation

Decisional Conflict r/t tubal sterilization

See Laparoscopy

Tube Feeding

Risk for Aspiration: Risk factors: improper placement of feeding tube, improper positioning of client during and after feeding, excessive residual feeding or lack of digestion, altered gag reflex

Risk for deficient Fluid volume: Risk factor: inadequate water administration with concentrated feeding

Risk for imbalanced Nutrition: less than body requirements: Risk factors: intolerance to tube feeding, inadequate calorie replacement to meet metabolic needs

Tuberculosis (TB)

See TB (Pulmonary Tuberculosis)

TURP (Transurethral Resection of the Prostate)

Deficient Knowledge r/t postoperative self-care, home maintenance management

Acute Pain r/t incision, irritation from catheter, bladder spasms, kidney infection

Urinary retention r/t obstruction of urethra or catheter with clots

Risk for Bleeding: Risk factor: surgery

Risk for deficient Fluid volume: Risk factors: fluid loss, possible bleeding

Risk for urge urinary Incontinence: Risk factor: edema from surgical procedure

Risk for Infection: Risk factors: invasive procedure, route for bacteria entry

U

Ulcer, Peptic (Duodenal or Gastric)

Fatigue r/t loss of blood, chronic illness

Ineffective Health maintenance r/t lack of knowledge regarding health practices to prevent ulcer formation

Nausea r/t gastrointestinal irritation

Acute Pain r/t irritated mucosa from acid secretion

See GI Bleed (Gastrointestinal Bleeding)

Ulcerative Colitis

See Inflammatory Bowel Disease (Child and Adult)

Ulcers, Stasis

See Stasis Ulcer

Unilateral Neglect of One Side of Body

Unilateral Neglect (See **Unilateral Neglect,** Section III)

U

Unsanitary Living Conditions

Impaired Home maintenance r/t impaired cognitive or emotional functioning, lack of knowledge, insufficient finances, addiction

Risk for Allergic reaction: Risk factor: exposure to environmental contaminants

Upper Respiratory Infection

See Cold, Viral

Urgency to Urinate

Urge urinary Incontinence (See **Incontinence,** urinary, urge, Section III)

Risk for urge urinary Incontinence (See **Incontinence,** urinary, urge, risk for, Section III)

Urinary Catheter

Risk for urinary tract Injury: Risk factors: confused client, long-term use of catheter, large retention balloon or catheter, perirectal burn injured client

Urinary Diversion

See Ileal Conduit

Urinary Elimination, Impaired

Impaired Urinary elimination (See **Urinary** elimination, impaired, Section III)

Urinary Incontinence

See Incontinence of Urine

Urinary Retention

Urinary Retention (See **Urinary Retention,** Section III)

Urinary Tract Infection (UTI)

See UTI (Urinary Tract Infection)

Urolithiasis

See Kidney Stone

Uterine Atony in Labor

See Dystocia

Uterine Atony in Postpartum

See Postpartum Hemorrhage

Uterine Bleeding

See Hemorrhage; Postpartum Hemorrhage; Shock, Hypovolemic

UTI (Urinary Tract Infection)

Ineffective Health maintenance r/t deficient knowledge regarding methods to treat and prevent UTIs, prolonged use of indwelling urinary catheter

Acute Pain: dysuria r/t inflammatory process in bladder

Impaired Urinary elimination: frequency r/t urinary tract infection

Risk for acute Confusion: Risk factor: infectious process

Risk for urge urinary Incontinence: Risk factor: hyperreflexia from cystitis

V

VAD (Ventricular Assist Device)

See Ventricular Assist Device (VAD)

Vaginal Hysterectomy

Urinary retention r/t edema at surgical site

Risk for urge urinary Incontinence: Risk factors: edema, congestion of pelvic tissues

Risk for Infection: Risk factor: surgical site

Risk for Perioperative Positioning injury: Risk factor: lithotomy position

Vaginitis

Impaired Comfort r/t pruritus, itching

Ineffective Health maintenance r/t deficient knowledge regarding self-care with vaginitis

Ineffective Sexuality pattern r/t abstinence during acute stage, pain

Vagotomy

See Abdominal Surgery

Value System Conflict

Decisional Conflict r/t unclear personal values or beliefs

Spiritual distress r/t challenged value system

Readiness for enhanced Spiritual well-being: desire for harmony with self, others, higher power, God

Varicose Veins

Ineffective Health maintenance r/t deficient knowledge regarding health care practices, prevention, treatment regimen

Chronic Pain r/t impaired circulation

Ineffective peripheral Tissue Perfusion r/t venous stasis

Risk for impaired Tissue integrity: Risk factor: altered peripheral tissue perfusion

Vascular Dementia (Formerly Called Multi-Infarct Dementia)

See Dementia

Vasectomy

Decisional Conflict r/t surgery as method of permanent sterilization

Venereal Disease

See STD (Sexually Transmitted Disease

Venous Thromboembolism (VTE)

Anxiety r/t lack of circulation to body part

Acute Pain r/t vascular obstruction

Ineffective peripheral Tissue Perfusion r/t interruption of circulatory flow

Risk for Peripheral Neurovascular dysfunction: Risk factor: vascular obstruction

Ventilated Client, Mechanically

Ineffective Airway clearance r/t increased secretions, decreased cough and gag reflex

Ineffective Breathing pattern r/t decreased energy and fatigue as a result of possible altered nutrition: less than body requirements, neurological disease or damage

Impaired verbal Communication r/t presence of endotracheal tube, inability to phonate

Fear r/t inability to breathe on own, difficulty communicating

Impaired Gas exchange r/t ventilation-perfusion imbalance

Powerlessness r/t health treatment regimen

Social isolation r/t impaired mobility, ventilator dependence

Impaired spontaneous Ventilation r/t metabolic factors, respiratory muscle fatigue

Dysfunctional Ventilatory weaning response r/t psychological, situational, physiological factors

Risk for Falls: Risk factors: impaired mobility, decreased muscle strength

Risk for Infection: Risk factors: presence of endotracheal tube, pooled secretions

Risk for pressure Ulcer: Risk factor: decreased mobility

Risk for impaired Resilience: Risk factor: illness

See Child with Chronic Condition; Hospitalized Child; Respiratory Conditions of the Neonate

Ventricular Assist Device (VAD)

Anxiety r/t possible failure of device

Risk for Infection: Risk factor: device insertion site

Risk for Vascular Trauma: Risk factor: insertion site

Readiness for enhanced Decision-Making: expresses desire to enhance the understanding of the meaning of choices regarding implanting a VAD

See Open Heart Surgery

Ventricular Fibrillation

See Dysrhythmia

Veterans

Anxiety r/t possible unmet needs, both physical and psychological

Risk for Post-Trauma Syndrome: Risk factors: witnessing death, survivor role, guilt, environment not conducive to needs

Risk for Suicide: Risk factors: substance abuse, insufficient social support, physical injury, psychiatric disorder

Vertigo

See Syncope

Violent Behavior

Risk for other-directed Violence (See **Violence,** other-directed, risk for, Section III)

Risk for self-directed Violence (See **Violence,** self-directed, risk for, Section III)

Viral Gastroenteritis

Diarrhea r/t infectious process, Norovirus

Deficient Fluid volume r/t vomiting, diarrhea

Ineffective Health management r/t inadequate handwashing

See Gastroenteritis, Child

Vision Impairment

Fear r/t loss of sight

Social isolation r/t altered state of wellness, inability to see

Risk for impaired Resilience: Risk factor: presence of new crisis

See Blindness; Cataracts; Glaucoma

Vomiting

Nausea r/t infectious processes, chemotherapy, postsurgical anesthesia, irritation to the gastrointestinal system, stimulation of neuropharmacological mechanisms

Imbalanced Nutrition: less than body requirements r/t inability to ingest food

Risk for Electrolyte imbalance: Risk factor: vomiting

VTE (Venous Thromboembolism)

See Venous Thromboembolism, Risk for, Section III

W

Walking Impairment

Impaired Walking (See **Walking,** impaired, Section III)

Wandering

Wandering (See **Wandering,** Section III)

Weakness

Fatigue r/t decreased or increased metabolic energy production

Risk for Falls: Risk factor: weakness

Weight Gain

Overweight (See **Overweight,** Section III)

Weight Loss

Imbalanced Nutrition: less than body requirements r/t inability to ingest food because of biological, psychological, economic factors

Wellness-Seeking Behavior

Readiness for enhanced Health management: expresses desire for increased control of health practice

Wernicke-Korsakoff Syndrome

See Korsakoff's Syndrome

West Nile Virus

See Meningitis/Encephalitis

Wheelchair Use Problems

Impaired wheelchair Mobility (See **Mobility,** wheelchair, impaired, Section III)

Wheezing

Ineffective Airway clearance r/t tracheobronchial obstructions, secretions

Wilms' Tumor

Chronic functional Constipation r/t obstruction associated with presence of tumor

Acute Pain r/t pressure from tumor

See Chemotherapy; Hospitalized Child; Radiation Therapy; Surgery, Preoperative Care; Surgery, Perioperative Care; Surgery, Postoperative Care

Withdrawal from Alcohol

See Alcohol Withdrawal

Withdrawal from Drugs

See Acute Substance Withdrawal Syndrome

Wound Debridement

Acute Pain r/t debridement of wound

Impaired Tissue integrity r/t debridement, open wound

Risk for Infection: Risk factors: open wound, presence of bacteria

Wound Dehiscence, Evisceration

Fear r/t client fear of body parts "falling out," surgical procedure not going as planned

Disturbed Body Image r/t change in body structure and wound appearance

Imbalanced Nutrition: less than body requirements r/t inability to digest nutrients, need for increased protein for healing

Risk for deficient Fluid volume: Risk factors: inability to ingest nutrients, obstruction, fluid loss

Risk for Injury: Risk factor: exposed abdominal contents

Risk for delayed Surgical recovery: Risk factors: separation of wound, exposure of abdominal contents

Risk for Surgical Site Infection: Risk factor: open wound after surgical procedure

Wound Infection

Disturbed Body Image r/t open wound

Imbalanced Nutrition: less than body requirements r/t biological factors, infection, fever

Ineffective Thermoregulation r/t infection in wound resulting in fever

Impaired Tissue integrity r/t wound, presence of infection

Risk for imbalanced Fluid volume: Risk factor: increased metabolic rate

Risk for Infection: spread of: Risk factor: imbalanced nutrition: less than body requirements

Risk for delayed Surgical recovery: Risk factor: presence of infection

Wounds, Open

See Lacerations

W

SECTION

III Guide to Planning Care

Section III is a collection of NANDA-I nursing diagnosis care plans. The care plans are arranged alphabetically by diagnostic concept. They contain definitions, defining characteristics, and related factors if appropriate. Risk diagnoses, however, only contain "risk factors." Care plans include suggested outcomes and interventions for all nursing diagnoses.

MAKING AN ACCURATE NURSING DIAGNOSIS

Verify the accuracy of the previously suggested nursing diagnoses (from Section II) or from alphabetized list (front of the book) for the client.

STEPS

- Read the definition for the suggested nursing diagnosis and determine if it is appropriate.
- Compare the Defining Characteristics with the symptoms that were identified from the client data collected.

or

- Compare the Risk Factors with the factors that were identified from the client data collected.

WRITING OUTCOMES STATEMENTS AND NURSING INTERVENTIONS

After selecting the appropriate nursing diagnosis, use this section to write outcomes and interventions.

STEPS

- Use the Client Outcomes/Nursing Interventions as written by the authors and contributors (select ones that are appropriate for your client).

or

- Use the NOC/NIC outcomes and interventions (as appropriate for your client).
- Read the rationales; the majority of rationales are based on nursing or clinical research that validates the efficacy of the interventions. Every attempt has been made to utilize current references; however, some significant research has not been replicated. Important research studies that are older than 5 years are included because they are the only evidence available. They are designated as **CEB** (Classic Evidence-Based).

Following these steps, you will be able to write an evidence-based nursing care plan.

- Follow this care plan to administer nursing care to the client.
- Document all steps and evaluate and update the care plan as needed.

A

Activity intolerance   *Lorraine Duggan, MSN, ACNP-BC*

NANDA-I

Definition

Insufficient physiological or psychological energy to endure or complete required or desired daily activities.

Defining Characteristics

Abnormal blood pressure response to activity; abnormal heart rate response to activity; electrocardiogram (ECG) change; exertional discomfort; exertional dyspnea; fatigue; generalized weakness

Related Factors

Imbalance between oxygen supply/demand; immobility; inexperience with an activity; physical deconditioning; sedentary lifestyle

At-Risk Population

History of previous activity intolerance

Associated Condition

Circulatory problem; respiratory condition

NOC   (Nursing Outcomes Classification)

Suggested NOC Outcomes

Activity Tolerance; Endurance; Energy Conservation; Self-Care: Instrumental Activities of Daily Living (IADLs)

> #### Example NOC Outcome with Indicators
>
> **Activity Tolerance** as evidenced by the following indicators: Oxygen saturation with activity/Pulse rate with activity/Respiratory rate with activity/Blood pressure with activity/Electrocardiogram findings/Skin color/Walking distance. (Rate the outcome and indicators of **Activity Tolerance:** 1 = severely compromised, 2 = substantially compromised, 3 = moderately compromised, 4 = mildly compromised, 5 = not compromised [see Section I].)

Client Outcomes

Client Will (Specify Time Frame)

- Participate in prescribed physical activity with appropriate changes in heart rate, blood pressure, and breathing rate; maintain monitor patterns (rhythm and ST segment) within normal limits
- State symptoms of adverse effects of exercise and report onset of symptoms immediately
- Maintain normal skin color; skin is warm and dry with activity
- Verbalize an understanding of the need to gradually increase activity based on testing, tolerance, and symptoms
- Demonstrate increased tolerance to activity

NIC   (Nursing Interventions Classification)

Suggested NIC Interventions

Activity Therapy; Energy Management; Exercise Therapy: Ambulation

> #### Example NIC Activities—Energy Management
>
> Monitor cardiorespiratory response to activity; Monitor location and nature of discomfort or pain during movement/activity

Nursing Interventions and *Rationales*

- Determine cause of Activity intolerance (see Related Factors) and determine whether cause is physical, psychological, or motivational. **QSEN:** *As nurses we are called on to ensure higher levels of safety and quality*

● = Independent;   ▲ = Collaborative;   EBN = Evidence-Based Nursing;   EB = Evidence-Based

A

for our clients by our governments, professional organizations, and hospital administrations. It is essential that we implement evidence-based nursing care strategies to reduce avoidable errors in care so that clinical outcomes improve (Vollman, 2013).

- If mainly on bed rest, minimize cardiovascular, neuromuscular, and skeletal deconditioning by positioning the client in an upright position several times daily if possible and performing simple range-of-motion (ROM) techniques (passive or active). EB: *Physical inactivity leads to a deconditioning of the skeletal, neuromuscular, and cardiovascular systems. It can lead to impaired quality of life, loss of autonomy, falls, and fractures (Kramer et al, 2017).*

- Assess the client daily for appropriateness of activity and bed rest orders. Mobilize the client as soon as possible. EB: *Mobilization is a cost-effective and simple method of maintaining stable cardiovascular parameters (i.e., blood pressure, heart rate), countering orthostatic intolerance, and reducing the risk of secondary problems in clients during long-term immobilization (Wieser et al., 2014).*

- If the client is mostly immobile, consider use of a transfer chair or a chair that becomes a stretcher. EB: *The use of simple shifting aids can optimize the patient transfer by avoiding heavy lifting situations and possible back injury to the caregivers. It reduces the effort of the caregivers and makes sure that the patient is not hurt during the process of conversion (Ahmed et al, 2015).*

- When appropriate, gradually increase activity, allowing the client to assist with positioning, transferring, and self-care as able. Progress the client from sitting in bed to dangling, to standing, to ambulation. Always have the client dangle at the bedside before standing to evaluate for postural hypotension. EB: *A reduction in plasma volume associated with bed rest impacts the physiological responses of autonomic control of circulation (Dorantes-Mendez et al, 2013; Tibaldi et al, 2014).*

- ▲ When getting a client up, observe for symptoms of intolerance such as nausea, pallor, dizziness, visual dimming, and impaired consciousness, as well as changes in vital signs; manual blood pressure monitoring is best. *When an adult rises to the standing position, blood pools in the lower extremities; symptoms of central nervous system hypoperfusion may occur, including feelings of weakness, nausea, headache, lightheadedness, dizziness, blurred vision, fatigue, tremulousness, palpitations, and impaired cognition.* EB: *Impaired orthostatic blood pressure recovery, delayed recovery, and/or sustained orthostatic hypotension are independent risk factors for future falls, unexplained falls, and injurious falls (Ciaren et al, 2017).*

- If the client has symptoms of postural hypotension, such as dizziness, lightheadedness, or pallor, take precautions, such as dangling the client and applying leg compression stockings before the client stands. EB: *Put graduated compression stockings on the client or use lower limb compression bandaging, if ordered, to return blood to the heart and brain. Have the client dangle at the side of the bed with legs hanging over the edge of the bed, flexing and extending the feet several times after sitting up, then standing slowly with someone holding the client. If the client becomes lightheaded or dizzy, return him or her to bed immediately (Tibaldi et al, 2014).*

- Perform ROM exercises if the client is unable to tolerate activity or is mostly immobile. See care plan for Risk for **Disuse** syndrome.

- Monitor and record the client's ability to tolerate activity: note pulse rate, blood pressure, respiratory pattern, dyspnea, use of accessory muscles, and skin color before, during, and after the activity. If the following signs and symptoms of cardiac decompensation develop, activity should be stopped immediately:
  - ○ Onset of chest discomfort or pain
  - ○ Dyspnea
  - ○ Palpitations
  - ○ Excessive fatigue
  - ○ Lightheadedness, confusion, ataxia, pallor, cyanosis, nausea, or any peripheral circulatory insufficiency
  - ○ Dysrhythmia
  - ○ Exercise hypotension
  - ○ Excessive rise in blood pressure
  - ○ Inappropriate bradycardia
  - ○ Increased heart rate
  - ○ Decreased oxygen saturation

- ▲ Instruct the client to stop the activity immediately and report to the health care provider if the client is experiencing the following symptoms: new or worsened intensity or increased frequency of discomfort; tightness or pressure in chest, back, neck, jaw, shoulders, and/or arms; palpitations; dizziness; weakness; unusual and extreme fatigue; or excessive air hunger. EB: *Cardiovascular deconditioning has long been recognized as a characteristic of the physiological adaptation to long-term bed rest in patients. The process is thought to contribute to orthostatic intolerance and enhance secondary complications in a significant way (Wieser et al, 2014).*

- Observe and document skin integrity several times a day. *Activity intolerance, if resulting in immobility, may lead to pressure ulcers. Mechanical pressure, moisture, friction, and shearing forces all predispose to their development.* Refer to the care plan Risk for impaired **Skin** integrity.
- Assess for constipation. If present, refer to care plan for **Constipation.** *Activity intolerance is associated with increased risk of* **Constipation.**
- ▲ Refer the client to physical therapy to help increase activity levels and strength.
- ▲ Consider a dietitian referral to assess nutritional needs related to **Activity** intolerance; provide nutrition as indicated. If the client is unable to eat food, use enteral or parenteral feedings as needed.
- Recognize that malnutrition causes significant morbidity because of the loss of lean body mass.
- Provide emotional support and encouragement to the client to gradually increase activity. Work with the client to set mutual goals that increase activity levels. Fear of breathlessness, pain, or falling may decrease willingness to increase activity.
- ▲ Observe for pain before activity. If possible, treat pain before activity and ensure that the client is not heavily sedated. *Pain restricts the client from achieving a maximal activity level and is often exacerbated by movement.*
- ▲ Obtain any necessary assistive devices or equipment needed before ambulating the client (e.g., walkers, canes, crutches, portable oxygen).
- ▲ Use a gait-walking belt when ambulating the client. **EBN:** *Use of gait belts is a nurse-driven intervention and encouraged to be used to assist in ambulation and transfer (Walker et al, 2014).*
- ▲ *Use evidence-based practices for safe client handling to reduce the risk of injury for both clients and health care workers (Elnitsky et al, 2014).*

Activity Intolerance Due to Respiratory Disease

- If the client is able to walk and has chronic obstructive pulmonary disease (COPD), use the traditional 6-minute walk distance to evaluate ability to walk.
- ▲ Ensure that the chronic pulmonary client has oxygen saturation testing with exercise. Use supplemental oxygen to keep oxygen saturation 90% or above or as prescribed with activity. **EB:** *Oxygen therapy can prolong life (Apps et al, 2016).*
- Monitor a respiratory client's response to activity by observing for symptoms of respiratory intolerance, such as increased dyspnea, loss of ability to control breathing rhythmically, use of accessory muscles, nasal flaring, appearance of facial distress, and skin tone changes such as pallor and cyanosis.
- Instruct and assist the client with COPD in using conscious, controlled breathing techniques during exercise, including pursed-lip breathing, and inspiratory muscle use.
- ▲ Evaluate the client's nutritional status. Refer to a dietitian if indicated. Use nutritional supplements to increase nutritional level if needed.
- ▲ For the client in the intensive care unit, consider mobilizing the client with passive exercise. **EBN:** *Nurses should consider incorporating at least 20 minutes of passive exercise early in the plan of care for critically ill clients treated with mechanical ventilation so that opportunities to improve client outcomes are not missed (Amidei & Sole, 2013).*
- ▲ *Refer the COPD client to a pulmonary rehabilitation program.* **EB:** *Pulmonary rehabilitation improves patient's functionality and decreases hospital admissions (Apps et al, 2016).*

Activity Intolerance Due to Cardiovascular Disease

- If the client is able to walk and has heart failure, consider use of the 6-minute walk test to determine physical ability.
- Allow for periods of rest before and after planned exertion periods such as meals, baths, treatments, and physical activity.
- ▲ Refer to a heart failure program or cardiac rehabilitation program for education, evaluation, and guided support to increase activity and rebuild life. **EB:** *Exercise training improves functional capacity, the ability to perform activities of daily living (ADLs), and quality of life, and it reduces the risk for subsequent cardiovascular events (Billinger et al, 2014).*
- ▲ Refer to a community support program that includes support of significant others.
- ▲ **EB:** *Contemporary studies now suggest that behavior change and multifactorial risk factor modification—especially smoking cessation and more intensive measures to control hyperlipidemia with diet, drugs, and exercise—may*

● = Independent;   ▲ = Collaborative;   **EBN** = Evidence-Based Nursing;   **EB** = Evidence-Based

slow, halt, or even reverse (albeit modestly) the otherwise inexorable progression of atherosclerotic coronary artery disease (CAD) (Spring, 2013).

- See care plan for Decreased **Cardiac** output for further interventions.

Pediatric

- Focus interview questions toward exercise tolerance specifically including any history of asthma exacerbations. EB: *Cardiopulmonary deconditioning should be considered as an important differential diagnosis for breathlessness among obese adolescents. Some of these children may need pulmonary rehabilitation if difficulty breathing is the perceived reason for not exercising (Shim et al, 2013).*

Geriatric

- Slow the pace of care. Allow the client extra time to perform physical activities. *Slow gait in older adults may be related to fear of falling, decreased strength in muscles, reduced balance or visual acuity, knee flexion contractures, and foot pain.* QSEN: *Older patients with chronic cardiac conditions are more vulnerable to falls and injuries. Cardiovascular conditions, prevalent in older people, are also the frequent cause of potentially harmful fall injuries in this group. The need to identify the fall risk-related factors that cluster with arrhythmia and syncope is relevant, in that it will potentially reduce patients' risk for falls and fall injuries (Belita et al, 2013).*
- Encourage families to help/allow an older client to be independent in whatever activities possible. EB: *Longitudinal observational studies show an association between higher levels of physical activity and a reduced risk of cognitive decline and dementia (Blondell et al, 2014). Older adults can engage in a variety of physical activities to advance health ranging from walking, gardening, to household chores, and/or planned group exercise (World Health Organization, 2017).*
- ▲ Assess for swaying, poor balance, weakness, and fear of falling while older clients stand/walk. Refer to physical therapy if appropriate. EB: *A home exercise program was beneficial to improve the balance of community-dwelling frail older adults (Light et al, 2016).*
- Refer to the care plan for Risk for **Falls** and Impaired **Walking.**
- ▲ Initiate ambulation by simply ambulating a patient a few steps from bed to chair, once a health care provider's out-of-bed order is obtained. EBN: *Lack of ambulation and deconditioning effects of bed rest are one of the most predictable causes of loss of independent ambulation in hospitalized older persons. Nurses have been identified as the professional most capable of promoting walking independence in the hospital setting (Doherty-King & Bowers, 2013).*
- ▲ Evaluate medications the client is taking to see if they could be causing **Activity** intolerance. EB: *Antihypertensive medications were associated with an increased risk of serious fall injuries, particularly among those with previous fall-related injuries. The potential harms versus benefits of antihypertensive medications should be weighed in deciding to continue treatment with antihypertensive medications in older adults with multiple chronic conditions (Tinetti et al, 2014).*
- ▲ If heart disease is causing **Activity** intolerance, refer the client for cardiac rehabilitation.
- ▲ Refer the disabled older client to physical therapy for functional training including gait training, stepping, and sit-to-stand exercises, or for strength training. EBN: *Older adults often experience functional losses during hospitalization. Clinical care activities have been increasingly promoted as a way to help older hospitalized patients offset these losses and recover from acute illness (Casey et al, 2016).*

Home Care

- ▲ Begin discharge planning as soon as possible with the case manager or social worker to assess the need for home support systems and the need for community or home health services. EB: *A structured, moderate-intensity physical activity program compared with a health education program reduced major mobility disability over 2.6 years among older adults at risk for disability. These findings suggest mobility benefit from such a program in vulnerable older adults (Pahor et al, 2014).*
- ▲ Assess the home environment for factors that contribute to decreased activity tolerance such as stairs or distance to the bathroom. Refer the client for occupational therapy, if needed, and to assist the client in restructuring the home and ADL patterns. *During hospitalization, clients and families often estimate energy requirements at home inaccurately because the hospital's availability of staff support distorts the level of care that will be needed.*
- ▲ Refer the client for physical therapy for strength training and possible weight training to regain strength, increase endurance, and improve balance. If the client is homebound, the physical therapist can also initiate

• = Independent; ▲ = Collaborative; EBN = Evidence-Based Nursing; EB = Evidence-Based

A

cardiac rehabilitation. EB: *The older and frailer the individual, the greater the rationale for the addition of progressive resistance and balance training to aerobic exercise programs, given the prevalence of sarcopenia, mobility impairment, and functional dependency in this group. Frailty is not a contraindication to exercise, but conversely, one of the most important reasons to prescribe it (Bauman et al, 2016).*

- Encourage progress with positive feedback. The client's experience should be validated within expected norms. Recognition of progress enhances motivation.
- Teach the client/family the importance of and methods for setting priorities for activities, especially those having a high energy demand (e.g., home/family events). Instruct in realistic expectations.
- Encourage routine low-level exercise periods such as a daily short walk or chair exercises.
- Provide the client/family with resources such as senior centers, exercise classes, educational and recreational programs, and volunteer opportunities that can aid in promoting socialization and appropriate activity. Social isolation can be an outcome of and contribute to **Activity** intolerance.
- Instruct the client and family in the importance of maintaining proper nutrition.
- Instruct the client in use of dietary supplements as indicated. Illness may suppress appetite, leading to inadequate nutrition.
- ▲ Refer to medical social services as necessary to assist the family in adjusting to major changes in patterns of living because of **Activity** intolerance.
- ▲ Assess the need for long-term supports for optimal activity tolerance of priority activities (e.g., assistive devices, oxygen, medication, catheters, massage), especially for a hospice client. Evaluate intermittently.
- ▲ Refer to home health aide services to support the client and family through changing levels of activity tolerance. Introduce aide support early. Instruct the aide to promote independence in activity as tolerated.
- Allow terminally ill clients and their families to guide care. Control by the client or family respects their autonomy and promotes effective coping.
- Provide increased attention to comfort and dignity of the terminally ill client in care planning. *Interventions should be provided as much for psychological effect as for physiological support. For example, oxygen may be more valuable as a support to the client's psychological comfort than as a booster of oxygen saturation.*
- ▲ Institute case management of frail elderly to support continued independent living.

Client/Family Teaching and Discharge Planning

- Instruct the client on techniques for avoiding **Activity** intolerance, such as controlled breathing techniques.
- Teach the client techniques to decrease dizziness from postural hypotension when standing up.
- Help client with energy conservation and work simplification techniques in ADLs.
- Describe to the client the symptoms of **Activity** intolerance, including which symptoms to report to the physician.
- Explain to the client how to use assistive devices, oxygen, or medications before or during activity.
- Help the client set up an activity log to record exercise and exercise tolerance.

REFERENCES

Ahmed, R., Razack, S., Salam, S., et al. (2015). Design and fabrication of pneumatically powered wheel chair-stretcher device. *International Journal of Innovative Research in Science, Engineering and Technology, 4*(10).

Amidei, C., & Sole, M. (2013). Physiological responses to passive exercise in adults receiving mechanical ventilation. *American Journal of Critical Care, 22,* 337–348.

Apps, M., Mukherjee, D., Abbas, S., et al. (2016). A chronic obstructive pulmonary disease service integrating community and hospital services can improve patient care and reduce hospital stays. *American Journal of Respiratory and Critical Care Medicine, 193,* A1523.

Bauman, A., Merom, D., Bull, F., et al. (2016). Updating the evidence for physical activity: Summative reviews of the epidemiological evidence, prevalence, and interventions to promote active aging. *The Gerontologist, 56*(S2), S268–S280.

Belita, L., Ford, P., & Kirkpatrick, H. (2013). The development of an assessment and intervention falls guide for older hospitalized adults with cardiac conditions. *European Journal of Cardiovascular Nursing, 12,* 302–309.

Billinger, S., Arena, R., Bernhardt, J., et al. (2014). Physical activity and exercise recommendations for stroke survivors. *Stroke: A Journal of Cerebral Circulation, 45,* 2532–2553.

Blondell, S., Hammersley-Mather, R., & Veerman, J. (2014). Does physical activity prevent cognitive decline and dementia?: A systematic review and meta-analysis of longitudinal studies. *BMC Public Health, 14,* 510.

Casey, C., Bennett, J., Winters-Stone, K., et al. (2016). Measuring activity levels associated with rehabilitative care in hospitalized older adults. *Geriatric Nursing, 35*(2), S3–S10.

Ciaren, F., O'Connell, M., Donogjue, O., et al. (2017). Impaired orthostatic blood pressure recovery is associated with unexplained and injurious falls. *Journal of the American Geriatrics Society, 65*(3), 474–482.

Doherty-King, B., & Bowers, B. (2013). Attributing the responsibility for ambulating patients: A qualitative study. *International Journal of Nursing Studies, 50,* 1240–1246.

Dorantes-Mendez, G., Baselli, G., Arbeille, P., et al. (2013). Comparison of baroreflex sensitivity gain during mild lower body negative pressure in presence and absence of long duration bed rest. In *Computing in Cardiology Conference* (pp. 763–766). Milan, Italy.

Elnitsky, C. A., et al. (2014). Implications in the use of patient safety in the use of safe patient handling equipment: A national survey. *International Journal of Nursing Studies, 51*(12), 1624–1633.

Kramer, A., Gollhofer, A., Armbrecht, G., et al. (2017). How to prevent the detrimental effects of two months of bed-rest on muscle, bone and cardiovascular system: An RCT. *Scientific Reports, 7*, 13177.

Light, K., Bishop, M., & Wright, T. (2016). Telephone calls make a difference in home balance training outcomes: A randomized trial. *Journal of Geriatric Physical Therapy, 39*(3), 97–101.

Pahor, M., Guralnik, J., Ambrosius, W., et al. (2014). Effect of structured physical activity on prevention of major mobility disability in older adults: The LIFE study randomized clinical trial. *JAMA: The Journal of the American Medical Association, 23*(311), 2387–2396.

Shim, Y., Burnette, A., Lucas, S., et al. (2013). Physical deconditioning as a cause of breathlessness among obese adolescents with a diagnosis of asthma. *PLoS ONE, 8*(4), e61022.

Spring, B. E. (2013). Better population health through behavior change in adults. *Circulation, 128*(19), 2169–2176. Retrieved from https://www.ahajournals.org/doi/pdf/10.1161/01.cir.0000435173.25936.e1.

Tibaldi, M., Brescianini, A., Sciarrillo, I., et al. (2014). Prevalence and clinical implications of orthostatic hypotension in elderly. *Hypertension, 3*, 155.

Tinetti, M., Han, L., Lee, D., et al. (2014). Antihypertensive medications and serious fall injuries in a nationally representative sample of older adults. *JAMA: The Journal of the American Medical Association, 174*(4), 588–595.

Vollman, K. (2013). Interventional patient hygiene: Discussion of the issues and a proposed model for implementation of the nursing care basics. *Intensive and Critical Care Nursing, 29*, 250–255.

Walker, L., O'Connell, M., & Giesler, A., (2014). *Keep a grasp on patient safety.* Lehigh Valley Health Network Scholarly Works. Retrieved from http://scholarlyworks.lvhn.org/patient-care-services-nursing.

Wieser, M., Gisler, S., Sarabadani, A., et al. (2014). Cardiovascular control and stabilization via inclination and mobilization during bed rest. *Medical and Biological Engineering and Computing, 52*(1), 53–64.

World Health Organization (2017) *Physical activity and older adults.* Retrieved from http://www.who.int/dietphysicalactivity/factsheet_olderadults/en/.

A

Risk for Activity intolerance   *Mary Beth Flynn Makic, PhD, RN, CCNS, FAAN, FNAP*

NANDA-I

Definition

Susceptible to experiencing insufficient physiological or psychological energy to endure or complete required or desired daily activities, which may compromise health.

Risk Factors

Imbalance between oxygen supply/demand; immobility; inexperience with an activity; physical deconditioning; sedentary lifestyle

At-Risk Population

History of previous activity intolerance

Associated Condition

Circulatory problem; respiratory condition

NIC, NOC, Client Outcomes, Nursing Interventions and *Rationales,* Client/Family Teaching and Discharge Planning, and References

Refer to care plan for **Activity** intolerance.

Ineffective Activity planning   *Annie Muller, DNP, APRN-BC and Gail B. Ladwig, MSN, RN*

NANDA-I

Definition

Inability to prepare for a set of actions fixed in time and under certain conditions.

Defining Characteristics

Absence of plan; excessive anxiety about a task to be undertaken; fear about task to be undertaken; insufficient organizational skills; insufficient resources; pattern of failure; pattern of procrastination; unmet goals for chosen activity; worried about a task to be undertaken

● = Independent;   ▲ = Collaborative;   EBN = Evidence-Based Nursing;   EB = Evidence-Based

A

Related Factors

Flight behavior when faced with proposed solution; hedonism; insufficient information processing ability; insufficient social support; pattern of procrastination; unrealistic perception of event; unrealistic perception of personal abilities

NOC   Outcomes (Nursing Outcomes Classification)

Suggested NOC Outcomes

Cognition; Cognition Orientation; Concentration; Decision-Making; Information Processing; Memory

> ### Example NOC Outcome with Indicators
>
> **Cognition** as evidenced by the following indicators: Communication clear and appropriate for age/Comprehension of the meaning of situations/Information processing/Alternatives weighed when making decisions. (Rate the outcome and indicators of **Cognition:** 1 = severely compromised, 2 = substantially compromised, 3 = moderately compromised, 4 = mildly compromised, 5 = not compromised [see Section I].)

Patient Outcomes

Patient Will (Specify Time Frame)

- Verbalize need for self-directed activity
- Choose the health care option that fits his or her lifestyle within an appropriate amount of time that allows enactment of the choice
- Describe how the chosen option fits into current lifestyle before or after the decision has been made
- Verbalize the need for a behavioral change to improve physical activity
- Offer alternative options to those with barriers to participating in physical activity

NIC   Interventions (Nursing Interventions Classification)

Suggested NIC Interventions

Activity Therapy; Anxiety Reduction; Behavior Management; Behavior Modification; Calming Technique; Coping Enhancement; Cognitive Restructuring; Decision-Making Support; Life Skills Enhancement

> ### Example NIC Activities—Coping Enhancement
>
> Assist client in developing an objective appraisal of the event; Explore with client previous methods of dealing with life problems

Nursing Interventions and *Rationales*

- Ask clients how they perceive the situation to gather their personal vision of the problem and how they envisage their self-involvement. Specify the goals. *Clients and caregivers may have different priorities on what is important (Junius-Walker et al, 2011).*
  - ○ Identify the informational needs of the client: understanding of the client's state of health, supervision of client's treatment if he or she is receiving treatment, diet, and important telephone numbers. EBN: *This study of clients with stage 4 chronic kidney disease validated the need for an individual assessment to determine the unique informational needs of each person (Lewis et al, 2010).*
  - ○ Tackle the client's fears and worries and encourage him or her to make a cognitive reconstruction. Use "desire thinking." Drill and repeat: "I can change false ideas that make me believe that I am unable to carry out (achieve) my plan." EBN: *Desire thinking is a voluntary cognitive process involving verbal and imaginal elaboration of a desired target. Recent research has highlighted the role of desire thinking in the maintenance of addictive, eating, and impulse control disorders (Caselli & Spada, 2011).*
- Client verbalizes need for behavioral change for improved physical activity. EB: *This study reflects how combining planning and coping planning of a client's self-worth can be beneficial in promoting an exercise program for those individuals who lack self-esteem (Kroon et al, 2014).*
- Encourage clients to verbalize the need for physical activity to help reduce role overload. EB: *This study demonstrated the need for planning activities for those individuals who were experiencing a role overload in life to allow them time for leisure activities (Lovell & Butler, 2015).*

• = Independent;   ▲ = Collaborative;   EBN = Evidence-Based Nursing;   EB = Evidence-Based

▲ Determine as fairly as possible the success factors needed for the planning and success of the project: financial resources; the family situation; prior medical, psychiatric, and psychosocial conditions; material resources; and the ability to manage stress. **EBN:** *Discussions identifying resources help to handle past resources, the functional solutions of everyday life, favorable changes, exceptions and differences in everyday life, the availability of support, and the prospects of future. By noting and providing feedback to families, the nurse offers families a new perspective on themselves (Häggman-Laitila et al, 2010).*

▲ *Older adult patients may be able to delay or prevent problems of chronic diseases by engaging in physical activity (Watson et al, 2016).*

Pediatric

● Begin activity planning in preschool-aged children of working parents. **EB:** *This study focused on the inactivity of migrant workers' preschool-aged children and the need to have a more structured and planned activity for the migrant worker. The focus was on the child because not much is known and very little research has been done. Also, there is a wide disparity of health in this population. The results showed very little physical activity was encouraged by parents and there was a great need for intervention to help with developing a future healthy lifestyle for reducing potential long-term health problems (Grzywacz et al, 2014).*

● Establish a contract. **EBN:** *This study of adolescents with type 1 diabetes indicated that behavioral contracts may be an important adjunct to reduce nagging and improve outcomes with behavioral changes (Carroll et al, 2011).*

● Provide support to the schools for physical activities in all school venues. **EB:** *Depending on the location of the school and the available resources, schools may promote a physical activity program that is beneficial and available to the student. Schools with few resources have limited staff available, which can be a barrier to promoting a healthy lifestyle to the adolescent student (Hobin et al, 2013).*

● Support safe neighborhood activity programs. **EB:** *Children who immigrate to the United States are at higher risk for inactivity than those from the United States. Safety issues in the neighborhoods could be an issue that causes a barrier and prevents them from engaging in outside physical activity (Brewer & Kimbro, 2014).*

Geriatric

● Plan activities for older clients. **EB:** *In a study of stroke clients, it was found that physical activity may improve quality of life, physical function, and self-worth (Walter et al, 2015).*

● Plan activities for older clients with impaired mental function. **EB:** *In this study, it was found that clients with impaired mental function are often limited in their ability to become involved with planned physical activity; therefore staff is needed to intervene and assist with the planned activity (Koring et al, 2012).*

● Community-based activities for older adults. **EB:** *A study for group exercises demonstrated improved mobility of the older adults who attended twice weekly exercises and mobility classes (Brach et al, 2017).*

Multicultural

● Provide literature and information in the appropriate language for the client who speaks little to no English. **EB:** *This study was able to show that those clients who did not speak English fluently were not adequately prepared for or educated on the need for physical activity, and they were not well represented in the study to show that culture was represented in understanding about cognitive health and risks of Alzheimer's disease (Rose et al, 2013).*

● Preplanning educational programs for the culturally diverse population needs to be developed. **EB:** *A low level of preplanning and poor organization of physical activities for the culturally diverse causes a loss of participation by those involved because of a lack of understanding of the concepts involved (Jeong et al, 2015).*

● Education with support from the physician and family to provide teaching on how exercise can help reduce and/or prevent falls of older adults. **EB:** *A study done on how culture influences exercise participation showed cultural values and social support to be positively instrumental in helping to reduce falls in the older population (Jang et al, 2016).*

Home Care

● Have a preplanned activity exercise for the home client with a debilitating musculoskeletal disease to help improve functional status. **EB:** *This study showed an improvement for those clients who were homebound because of a musculoskeletal disorder, which improved their personal commitment to exercise to increase their functional ability by gaining some muscle strength and range of motion (Hideyuki & Hitoshi, 2014).*

● = Independent;   ▲ = Collaborative;   EBN = Evidence-Based Nursing;   EB = Evidence-Based

A

- Assess the home environment for barriers that can impact the client's motivation to be a participant in the activity planned. **EB:** *The research study done on homebound older adults showed that the client knew and understood the need for planned physical activity, but they were not motivated to participate because they thought their age was a barrier. The idea is to teach the older client that although age may be a factor in some types of activity planning or exercise, there are many ways to adapt to the activity that can be accommodating to the client's ability (Burton et al, 2013).*
- Home care for the cardiac rehabilitation patient: **EB:** *Providing a daily exercise plan for the home care cardiac rehabilitation patient did show improvement in the cardiorespiratory function of the patient (Noites et al, 2017).*
- For additional interventions, refer to care plans **Anxiety,** Readiness for enhanced family **Coping,** Readiness for enhanced **Decision-Making, Fear,** Readiness for enhanced **Hope,** Readiness for enhanced **Power,** Readiness for enhanced **Spiritual** well-being, and Readiness for enhanced **Health** management.

REFERENCES

Brach, J. S., Perera, S., Gilmore, S., et al. (2017). Effectiveness of a timing and coordination group exercise program to improve mobility in community-dwelling older adult: A randomized clinical trial. *JAMA Internal Medicine, 177*(10), 1437–1444.

Brewer, M., & Kimbro, R. T. (2014). Neighborhood context and immigrant children's physical activity. *Social Science Medicine, 116,* 1–9.

Burton, E., Lewin, G., & Boldy, D. (2013). Barriers and motivators to being physically active for older home care patients. *Physical & Occupational Therapy in Geriatrics, 31*(1), 21–35.

Carroll, A. E., et al. (2011). Contracting and monitoring relationships for adolescents with type 1 diabetes: A pilot study. *Diabetes Technology & Therapeutics, 13*(5), 543–549.

Caselli, G., & Spada, M. M. (2011). The desire thinking questionnaire: Development and psychometric properties. *Addictive Behaviors, 36*(11), 1061–1067.

Grzywacz, J. G., Suerken, C. K., Zapata-Roblyer, M. I., et al. (2014). Physical activity of preschool-aged Latino children in farm-worker families. *American Journal of Health Behavior, 38*(5), 717–725.

Häggman-Laitila, A., Tanninen, H., & Pietilä, A. (2010). Effectiveness of resource-enhancing family-oriented intervention. *Journal of Clinical Nursing, 19*(17/18), 2500–2510.

Hideyuki, N., & Hitoshi, T. (2014). Effects of home exercise on physical function and activity in home care patients with Parkinson's disease. *Journal of Physical Therapy Science, 26*(11), 1701–1706.

Hobin, E. P., Leatherdale, S., Manske, S., et al. (2013). Are environmental influences on physical activity distinct for urban, suburban, and rural schools? A multilevel study among secondary school students in Ontario, Canada. *Journal of School Health, 83*(5), 357–367.

Jang, H., Clemson, L., Lovarini, M., et al. (2016). Cultural influences on exercise participation and fall prevention: A systematic review and narrative synthesis. *Disability & Rehabilitation, 38*(8), 724–732.

Jeong, S., Ohr, S., Pich, J., et al. (2015). Planning ahead among community-dwelling older people from culturally and linguistically diverse background: A cross-sectional survey. *Journal of Clinical Nursing, 24*(1/2), 244–255.

Junius-Walker, U., Stolberg, D., Steinke, P., et al. (2011). Health and treatment priorities of older patients and their general practitioners: A cross-sectional study. *Quality in Primary Care, 19,* 67–76.

Koring, M., Richert, J., Parchau, L., et al. (2012). A combined planning and self-efficacy intervention to promote physical activity: A multiple mediation analysis. *Psychology, Health & Medicine, 17*(4), 488–498.

Kroon, F. P., van der Burg, L. R., Buchbinder, R., et al. (2014). Self-management education programmes for osteoarthritis. *The Cochrane Database of Systematic Reviews,* (1), CD008963. doi:10.1002/14651858.CD008963.pub2.

Lewis, A. L., Stabler, K. A., & Welch, J. L. (2010). Perceived informational needs, problems, or concerns among patients with stage 4 chronic kidney disease. *Nephrology Nursing Journal: Journal of the American Nephrology Nurses' Association, 37*(2), 143–149.

Lovell, G. P., & Butler, F. R. (2015). Physical activity behavior and role overload in mothers. *Health Care for Women International, 36*(3), 342–355.

Noites, A., Freitas, C. P., Pinto, J., et al. (2017). Effects of a phase IV home-based cardiac rehabilitation program on cardiorespiratory fitness and physical activity. *Heart, Lung, & Circulation, 26*(5), 455–462.

Rose, I. D., Friedman, D. B., Marquez, D. X., et al. (2013). What are older latinos told about physical activity and cognition? A content analysis of a top-circulating magazine. *Journal of Aging & Health, 25*(7), 1143–1158.

Watson, K. B., Carlson, S. A., Gunn, J. P., et al. (2016). Physical activity among adults aged 50 years and older—United States, 2014. *MMWR: Morbidity & Mortality Weekly Report, 65*(36), 954–958.

Walter, T., Hale, L., & Smith, C. (2015). Blue prescription: A single subject design intervention to enable physical therapy for people with stroke. *International Journal of Therapy & Rehabilitation, 22*(2), 87–95.

Risk for Ineffective Activity planning   *Gail B. Ladwig, MSN, RN*

NANDA-I

Definition

Susceptible to an inability to prepare for a set of actions fixed in time and under certain conditions, which may compromise health.

- = Independent;   ▲ = Collaborative;   EBN = Evidence-Based Nursing;   EB = Evidence-Based

Risk Factors

Flight behavior when faced with proposed solution; hedonism; insufficient information processing ability; insufficient social support; pattern of procrastination; unrealistic perception of event; unrealistic perception of personal abilities

NOC, NIC, Client Outcomes, Nursing Interventions and *Rationales,* Client/Family Teaching and Discharge Planning, and References

Refer to ineffective **Activity** planning.

Ineffective Airway clearance   *Debra Siela, PhD, RN, CCNS, ACNS-BC, CCRN-K, CNE, RRT*

NANDA-I

Definition

Inability to clear secretions or obstructions from the respiratory tract to maintain a clear airway.

Defining Characteristics

Absence of cough; adventitious breath sounds; alteration in respiratory pattern; alteration in respiratory rate; cyanosis; difficulty verbalizing; diminished breath sounds; dyspnea; excessive sputum; ineffective cough; orthopnea; restlessness; wide-eyed look

Related Factors

Excessive mucus; exposure to smoke; foreign body in airway; retained secretions; secondhand smoke; smoking

Associated Condition

Airway spasm; allergic airway; asthma; chronic obstructive pulmonary disease; exudate in the alveoli; hyperplasia of the bronchial walls; infection; neuromuscular impairment; presence of artificial airway

NOC   (Nursing Outcomes Classification)

Suggested NOC Outcomes

Aspiration Prevention; Respiratory Status: Airway Patency, Gas Exchange, Ventilation

Example NOC Outcome with Indicators
Respiratory Status: Ventilation as evidenced by the following indicators: Respiratory rate/Respiratory rhythm/Depth of inspiration/Chest expansion symmetrical/Ease of breathing/Tidal volume/Vital capacity. (Rate each indicator of **Respiratory Status: Ventilation:** 1 = severe deviation from normal range, 2 = substantial deviation from normal range, 3 = moderate deviation from normal range, 4 = mild deviation from normal range, 5 = no deviation from normal range [see Section I].)

Client Outcomes

Client Will (Specify Time Frame)

- Demonstrate effective coughing and clear breath sounds
- Maintain a patent airway at all times
- Explain methods useful to enhance secretion removal
- Explain the significance of changes in sputum to include color, character, amount, and odor
- Identify and avoid specific factors that inhibit effective airway clearance

NIC   (Nursing Interventions Classification)

Suggested NIC Interventions

Airway Management; Airway Suctioning; Cough Enhancement

● = Independent;   ▲ = Collaborative;   EBN = Evidence-Based Nursing;   EB = Evidence-Based

A

Instruct how to cough effectively; Auscultate breath sounds, noting areas of decreased or absent ventilation and presence of adventitious sounds

Nursing Interventions and *Rationales*

- Auscultate breath sounds every 1 to 4 hours. The presence of crackles and wheezes may alert the nurse to airway obstruction, which may lead to or exacerbate existing hypoxia. *In severe exacerbations of chronic obstructive pulmonary disease (COPD), lung sounds may be diminished or distant with air trapping (Bickley & Szilagyi, 2017).*
- Monitor respiratory patterns, including rate, depth, and effort. *A normal respiratory rate for an adult without dyspnea is 12 to 16 breaths per minute (Bickley & Szilagyi, 2017). With secretions in the airway, the respiratory rate will increase.*
- Monitor blood gas values and pulse oxygen saturation levels as available. An oxygen saturation of less than 90% (normal: 95%–100%) or a partial pressure of oxygen of less than 80 mm Hg (normal: 80–100 mm Hg) indicates significant oxygenation problems (*Bickley & Szilagyi, 2017; Siela & Kidd, 2017; Lee 2017*).
- ▲ Administer oxygen as ordered. *Oxygen administration has been shown to correct hypoxemia. Administer humidified oxygen through an appropriate device (e.g., nasal cannula or Venturi mask per the health care provider's order); aim for an oxygen (O_2) saturation level of 90% or above. Oxygen should be titrated to target an SpO_2 of 94% to 98%, except with carbon monoxide poisoning (100% oxygen), acute respiratory distress syndrome (ARDS) (88%–95%), those at risk for hypercapnia (88%–92%), and premature infants (88%–94%).*
- Position the client in a semirecumbent position with the head of the bed at a 30- to 45-degree angle to decrease the aspiration of gastric, oral, and nasal secretions (American Association of Critical Care Nurses, 2016, 2017; Grap, 2009; Siela, 2010; Vollman et al, 2017). CEB/EB: *In a mechanically ventilated client, there is a decreased incidence of ventilator-associated pneumonia (VAP)/ventilator-associated event if the client is positioned at a 30- to 45-degree semirecumbent position rather than a supine position (American Association of Critical Care Nurses, 2017; Vollman et al, 2017; Siela, 2010).*
- Help the client deep breathe and perform controlled coughing. Have the client inhale deeply, hold breath for several seconds, and cough two or three times with mouth open while tightening the upper abdominal muscles. CEB: *Controlled coughing uses the diaphragmatic muscles, making the cough more forceful and effective (Gosselink et al, 2008; GOLD, 2017).*
- If the client has obstructive lung disease, such as COPD, cystic fibrosis, or bronchiectasis, consider helping the client use the forced expiratory technique called the "huff cough." The client does a series of coughs while saying the word "huff." *This technique prevents the glottis from closing during the cough and is effective in clearing secretions (Gosselink et al, 2008; GOLD, 2017).*
- ▲ Encourage the client to use an incentive spirometer. Recognize that controlled coughing and deep breathing may be just as effective as incentive spirometry (Gosselink et al, 2008; GOLD, 2017).
- Encourage activity and ambulation as tolerated. If the client cannot be ambulated, turn the client from side to side at least every 2 hours. *Body movement helps mobilize secretions.* (See interventions for impaired **Gas** exchange for further information on positioning a respiratory client.)
- Encourage fluid intake of up to 2500 mL/day within cardiac or renal reserve. *Fluids help minimize mucosal drying and maximize ciliary action to move secretions.*
- ▲ Administer medications such as bronchodilators or inhaled steroids as ordered. Watch for side effects such as tachycardia or anxiety with bronchodilators, or inflamed pharynx with inhaled steroids. *Bronchodilators decrease airway resistance, improve the efficiency of respiratory movements, improve exercise tolerance, and can reduce symptoms of dyspnea on exertion (O'Donnell et al, 2014). Pharmacologic therapy in COPD is used to reduce symptoms, reduce the frequency and severity of exacerbation, and improve health strategies and exercise tolerance (GOLD, 2017).*
- ▲ Provide percussion, vibration, and oscillation as appropriate for individual client needs. *Airway clearance techniques for clients with acute exacerbations of COPD may have a small but important positive effect on the need for and duration of ventilatory assistance, and may reduce hospital length of stay (Osadnik et al, 2013). Mucoregulators such as N-acetylcysteine and carbocysteine are recommended to reduce the frequency of COPD acute exacerbations (GOLD, 2017).*

● = Independent;   ▲ = Collaborative;   EBN = Evidence-Based Nursing;   EB = Evidence-Based

- Observe sputum, noting color, odor, and volume. Normal sputum is clear or gray and minimal, whereas abnormal sputum is green, yellow, or bloody; malodorous; and often copious. The presence of purulent sputum during a COPD exacerbation can be a sufficient indication for starting empirical antibiotic treatment. Notify health care provider of purulent sputum (GOLD, 2017).

Critical Care

▲ In intubated clients, body positioning and mobilization may optimize airway secretion clearance. *Lateral rotational movement provides continuous postural drainage and mobilization of secretions (Wanless & Aldridge, 2011; St. Clair & MacDermott, 2017).* Reposition the client as needed. Use rotational or kinetic bed therapy in clients for whom side-to-side turning is contraindicated or difficult. **EBN:** *Changing position frequently decreases the incidence of atelectasis, pooling of secretions, and resultant pneumonia. Continuous, lateral rotational therapy has been shown to improve oxygenation and decrease the incidence of VAP (St. Clair & MacDermott, 2017; Nino & Makic, 2017).*

- If the client is intubated, consider use of kinetic therapy. Using a kinetic therapy bed slowly moves the client with 40-degree turns. *Kinetic therapy, or rotational therapy, may decrease the incidence of pulmonary complications in high-risk clients with increasing ventilator support requirements who are at risk for VAP, and with clinical indications for acute lung injury or ARDS with worsening Pao_2:Fio_2 ratio, presence of fluffy infiltrates via chest radiograph concomitant with pulmonary edema, and refractory hypoxemia (Bein et al, 2012; St. Clair & MacDermott, 2017; Nino et al, 2017).*

▲ *Early mobility and physical rehabilitation can reduce muscle weakness, mechanical ventilation duration, intensive care unit stay, and hospital stay (Costa et al, 2017; Spruit et al, 2013). The Awakening and Breathing Coordination, Delirium Monitoring and Management, and Early Mobility (ABCDE) bundle has criteria to determine when clients are candidates for early mobility (Balas et al, 2012; Costa et al, 2017).* An early mobility and walking program can promote weaning from ventilator support as a client's overall strength and endurance improve (Gosselink et al, 2008; Perme et al, 2014).

- If the client is intubated and is stable, consider getting the client up to sit at the edge of the bed, transfer to a chair, or walk as appropriate, if an effective interdisciplinary team is developed to keep the client safe (Balas et al, 2012; Costa et al, 2017). *For every week of bed rest, muscle strength can decrease 20%; early ambulation also helped clients develop a positive outlook (Perme et al, 2014).*

- When suctioning an endotracheal tube or tracheostomy tube for a client on a ventilator, do the following:
  ○ Explain the process of suctioning beforehand and ensure the client is not in pain or overly anxious. Suctioning can be a frightening experience; an explanation along with adequate pain relief or needed sedation can reduce stress, anxiety, and pain (Seckel, 2017).
  ○ Hyperoxygenate before and between endotracheal suction sessions. Studies have demonstrated that hyperoxygenation may help prevent oxygen desaturation in a suctioned client (Seckel, 2017; Vollman et al, 2017; Siela, 2010).
  ○ Suction for less than 15 seconds. Studies demonstrated that because of a drop in the partial pressure of oxygen with suctioning preferably there should be no more than 10 seconds of actual suctioning, with the entire procedure taking 15 seconds (Seckel, 2017).
  ○ Use a closed, in-line suction system. Closed in-line suctioning has minimal effects on heart rate, respiratory rate, tidal volume, and oxygen saturation and may reduce contamination (Seckel, 2017).
  ○ Avoid saline instillation during suctioning. **CEBN/EBN:** *Repeated studies have demonstrated that saline instillation before suctioning has an adverse effect on oxygen saturation in both adults and children (Seckel, 2017; Caparros, 2014; Rauen et al, 2008; Siela, 2010).*
  ○ Use of a subglottic suctioning endotracheal tube reduces the incidence of VAP or ventilator-associated complications (Vollman et al, 2017; Haas et al, 2014).
  ○ Use of nonstick endotracheal tubes can reduce the formation of biofilm and hence VAP (Haas et al, 2014).
  ○ Document results of coughing and suctioning, particularly client tolerance and secretion characteristics such as color, odor, and volume (Seckel, 2017).

 Pediatric

- Educate parents about the risk factors for ineffective airway clearance such as foreign body ingestion and passive smoke exposure.
- See the care plan Risk for **Suffocation** for more interventions on choking. **EB:** *Passive smoke exposure significantly increases the risk of asthma and respiratory infections in children (Farber et al, 2016). A recent*

● = Independent; ▲ = Collaborative; **EBN** = Evidence-Based Nursing; **EB** = Evidence-Based

A

study found maternal smoking increased childhood visits to the emergency department for exacerbated respiratory conditions to include asthma (Farber et al, 2016).

- Educate children and parents on the importance of adherence to peak expiratory flow monitoring for asthma self-management.
- Educate parents and other caregivers that cough and cold medication bought over the counter are not safe for a child younger than 2 years unless specifically ordered by a health care provider.

Geriatric

- Encourage ambulation as tolerated without causing exhaustion. Immobility is often harmful to older adults because it decreases ventilation and increases stasis of secretions, leading to atelectasis or pneumonia.
- Actively encourage older adults to deep breathe and cough. Cough reflexes are blunted, and coughing is decreased in older adults.
- Ensure adequate hydration within cardiac and renal reserves. Older adults are prone to dehydration and therefore more viscous secretions because they frequently use diuretics or laxatives and forget to drink adequate amounts of water.

Home Care

- Some of the previously mentioned interventions may be adapted for home care use.
- ▲ Begin discharge planning as soon as possible with the case manager or social worker to assess need for home support systems, assistive devices, and community or home health services.
- Assess home environment for factors that exacerbate airway clearance problems (e.g., presence of allergens, lack of adequate humidity in air, poor air flow, stressful family relationships).
- Assess affective climate within family and family support system. *Problems with respiratory function and resulting anxiety can provoke anger and frustration in the client. Feelings may be displaced onto caregiver and require intervention to ensure continued caregiver support.* Refer to care plan for **Caregiver Role Strain.**
- Refer to GOLD guidelines for management of home care and indications of hospital admission criteria (see http://www.goldcopd.org/).
- When respiratory procedures are being implemented, explain equipment and procedures to family members and caregivers and provide needed emotional support. *Family members assuming responsibility for respiratory monitoring often find this stressful. They may not have been able to assimilate fully any instructions provided by hospital staff.*
- When electrically based equipment for respiratory support is being implemented, evaluate home environment for electrical safety, proper grounding, and so on. Ensure that notification is sent to the local utility company, the emergency medical team, and police and fire departments.
- Provide family with support for care of a client with chronic or terminal illness. *Breathing difficulty can provoke extreme anxiety, which can interfere with the client's ability or willingness to adhere to the treatment plan.*
- Refer to care plan for **Anxiety.** *Witnessing breathing difficulties and facing concerns of dealing with chronic or terminal illness can create fear in the caregiver. Fear inhibits effective coping.* Refer to care plan for **Powerlessness.**
- Instruct the client to avoid exposure to persons with upper respiratory infections, to avoid crowds of people, and wash hands after each exposure to groups of people or public places.
- ▲ Determine client adherence to medical regimen. Instruct the client and family in importance of reporting effectiveness of current medications to health care provider. *Inappropriate use of medications (too much or too little) can influence the amount of respiratory secretions.*
- Teach the client when and how to use inhalant or nebulizer treatments at home.
- Teach the client/family the importance of maintaining regimen and having "as-needed" drugs easily accessible at all times. *Success in avoiding emergency or institutional care may rest solely on medication compliance or availability.*
- Instruct the client and family in the importance of maintaining proper nutrition, adequate fluids, rest, and behavioral pacing for energy conservation and rehabilitation.
- Instruct in use of dietary supplements as indicated. *Illness may suppress appetite, leading to inadequate nutrition. Supplements will allow clients to eat with minimal energy consumption.*
- Identify an emergency plan, including criteria for use. *Ineffective airway clearance can be life-threatening.*

● = Independent;   ▲ = Collaborative;   EBN = Evidence-Based Nursing;   EB = Evidence-Based

A

▲ Refer for home health aide services for assistance with activities of daily living (ADLs). *Clients with decreased oxygenation and copious respiratory secretions are often unable to maintain energy for ADLs.*

▲ Assess family for role changes and coping skills. Refer to medical social services as necessary. *Clients with decreased oxygenation are unable to maintain role activities and therefore experience frustration and anger, which may pose a threat to family integrity. Family counseling to adapt to role changes may be needed.*

▲ For the client dying at home with a terminal illness, if the "death rattle" is present with gurgling, rattling, or crackling sounds in the airway with each breath, recognize that anticholinergic medications can often help control symptoms, if given early in the process. *Anticholinergic medications can help decrease the accumulation of secretions, but do not decrease existing secretions. This medication must be administered early in the process to be effective (Twomey & Dowling, 2013; Fielding & Long, 2014).*

▲ For the client with a death rattle, nursing care includes turning to mobilize secretions, keeping the head of the bed elevated for postural drainage of secretions, and avoiding suctioning. *Suctioning is a distressing and painful event for clients and families, and it is rarely effective in decreasing the death rattle (Twomey & Dowling, 2013; Fielding & Long, 2014).*

 ### Client/Family Teaching and Discharge Planning

▲ Teach the importance of not smoking. Refer to a smoking cessation program, and encourage clients who relapse to keep trying to quit. Ensure that the client receives appropriate medications to support smoking cessation from the primary health care provider. *A Cochrane review found that use of the antidepressant medications increased the rate of smoking withdrawal two to three times more than smoking withdrawal without use of medications (Hughes et al, 2014).*

▲ Teach the client how to use a flutter clearance device if ordered, which vibrates to loosen mucus and gives positive pressure to keep airways open (Gosselink et al, 2008). **CEB:** *A study demonstrated that use of the mucus clearance device had improved exercise performance compared with COPD clients who use a sham device (Osadnik et al, 2013; Morrison & Agnew, 2009).*

▲ Teach the client how to use the peak expiratory flow rate (PEFR) meter if ordered and when to seek medical attention if the PEFR reading drops. Also teach the client how to use metered-dose inhalers and self-administer inhaled corticosteroids as ordered following precautions to decrease side effects.

● Teach the client how to deep breathe and cough effectively. *Controlled coughing uses the diaphragmatic muscles, making the cough more forceful and effective (Gosselink et al, 2008; GOLD, 2017).*

● Teach the client/family to identify and avoid specific factors that exacerbate ineffective airway clearance, including known allergens and especially smoking (if relevant) or exposure to secondhand smoke.

● Educate the client and family about the significance of changes in sputum characteristics, including color, character, amount, and odor. *With this knowledge, the client and family can identify early the signs of infection and seek treatment before acute illness occurs.*

● Teach the client/family the importance of taking antibiotics as prescribed and consuming all tablets until the prescription has run out. *Taking the entire course of antibiotics helps eradicate bacterial infection, which decreases lingering, chronic infection.*

● Teach the family of the dying client in hospice with a death rattle that rarely are clients aware of the fluid that has accumulated, and help them find evidence of comfort in the client's nonverbal behavior (*Twomey & Dowling, 2013; Fielding & Long, 2014*).

REFERENCES

American Association of Critical Care Nurses. (2016). *AACN Practice Alert—Prevention of aspiration in adults.* American Association of Critical Care Nurses. Retrieved from https://www.aacn.org/~/media/aacn-website/clincial-resources/practice-alerts/preventionaspirationpracticealert.pdf. (Accessed 20 February 2018).

American Association of Critical Care Nurses (2017). *AACN Practice Alert—Prevention of ventilator-associated pneumonia in adults.* American Association of Critical Care Nurses. Retrieved from https://www.aacn.org/~/media/aacn-website/clincial-resources/practice-alerts/preventingvapinadults2017.pdf. (Accessed 20 February 2018).

Balas, M. C., Vasilevskis, E. E., Burke, W. J., et al. (2012). Critical care nurses' role in implementing the "ABCDE Bundle" into practice. *Critical Care Nurse, 32*(2), 35–38, 40–48.

Bein, T., Zimmermann, M., Schiewe-Laggartner, F., et al. (2012). Continuous lateral rotation therapy and systematic inflammatory response in posttraumatic acute lung injury: Results from a prospective randomized study. *Injury: International Journal of the Care of the Injured, 43,* 1893–1897.

Bickley, L. S., & Szilagyi, P. (2017). *Bate's guide to physical examination* (12th ed.). Philadelphia, PA: Lippincott, Williams and Wilkins.

Caparros, A. (2014). Mechanical ventilation and the role of saline instillation in suctioning adult intensive care patients. *Dimensions of Critical Care Nursing, 33,* 246–253.

Costa, D. K., White, M. R., Ginier, E., et al. (2017). Identifying barriers to delivering the awakening and breathing coordination, delirium, and early exercise/mobility bundle to minimize adverse outcomes

A

for mechanically ventilated patients: A systemic review. *Chest*, *152*(2), 304–311.

Farber, H. J., Batsell, R. R., Silveira, E. A., et al. (2016). The impact of tobacco smoke exposure on childhood asthma in a medicaid managed care plan. *Chest*, *149*(3), 721–728.

Fielding, F., & Long, C. O. (2014). The death rattle dilemma. *Journal of Hospice and Palliative Nursing*, *16*(8). Retrieved from http://www.medscape.com/viewarticle/834898. (Accessed 22 February 2018).

GOLD. (2017). Global strategy for the diagnosis, management, and prevention of COPD (revised 2017). Global Initiative for Chronic Obstructive Lung Disease. Retrieved from http://www.goldcopd.org. (Accessed 20 February 2018).

Gosselink, R., Bott, J., Johnson, M., et al. (2008). Physiotherapy for adult patients with critical illness: Recommendations of the European Respiratory Society and European Society of Critical Care Medicine task force on physiotherapy for critically ill patients. *Intensive Care Medicine*, *34*(7), 1188–1199.

Grap, M. (2009). Not-so-trivial pursuit: mechanical ventilation risk reduction. *American Journal of Critical Care*, *18*(4), 299–309.

Haas, C. F., Eakin, R. M., Konkle, M. A., et al. (2014). Endotracheal tubes: Old and new. *Respiratory Care*, *59*(6), 933–955.

Hughes, J. R., Stead, L. F., Hartmann-Boyce, J., et al. (2014). Antidepressants for smoking cessation. *Cochrane Database of Systematic Reviews*, (1), CD000031.

Lee, D. (2017). Oxygen saturation monitoring with pulse oximetry. In D. Wiegand (Ed.), *AACN procedure manual for critical care* (7th ed.). Philadelphia: Saunders Elsevier.

Morrison, L., & Agnew, J. (2009). Oscillating devices for airway clearance in people with cystic fibrosis. *Cochrane Database Systematic Review*, (1), CD006842.

Nino, T., & Makic, M. B. F. (2017). Pressure redistribution surfaces: RotoRest™ lateral rotation surface. In D. Wiegand (Ed.), *AACN procedure manual for critical care* (7th ed.). Philadelphia: Saunders Elsevier.

O'Donnell, D., Webb, K., & Mahler, D. (2014). Effect of bronchodilators and inhaled corticosteroids on dyspnea in chronic obstructive pulmonary disease. In D. A. Mahler & D. E. O'Donnell (Eds.),

Dyspnea mechanisms, measurement and management. Boca Raton, FL: CRC Press Taylor & Francis Group.

Osadnik, C., McDonald, C., & Holland, A. (2013). Advances in airway clearance technologies for chronic obstructive pulmonary disease. *Expert Review of Respiratory Medicine*, *7*(6), 673–685.

Perme, C., Nawa, R. K., & Winkelman, C. (2014). A tool to assess mobility status in critically ill patients: The perme intensive care unit mobility score. *Methodist DeBakey Cardiovascular Journal*, *10*(1), 41–49.

Rauen, C. A., Chulay, M., Bridges, E., et al. (2008). Seven evidence-based practice habits: Putting some sacred cows out to pasture. *Critical Care Nurse*, *28*(2), 98–123.

Seckel, M. (2017). Suctioning: Endotracheal tube or tracheostomy tube. In D. Wiegand (Ed.), *AACN procedure manual for critical care* (7th ed.). Philadelphia: Saunders Elsevier.

Siela, D. (2010). Evaluation standards for management of artificial airways. *Critical Care Nurse*, *30*(4), 76–78.

Siela, D., & Kidd, M. (2017). Oxygen requirements for acutely and critically ill patients. *Critical Care Nurse*, *37*(4), 58–70.

Spruit, M. A., Singh, S. J., Garvey, C., et al. (2013). An official American Thoracic Society/European Respiratory Society statement: Key concepts and advances in pulmonary rehabilitation. *American Journal of Respiratory and Critical Care Medicine*, *188*(8), e13–e64.

St. Clair, & MacDermott, J. (2017). Continuous lateral rotation therapy. In D. L. Wiegand (Ed.), *AACN procedure manual for critical care* (7th ed.). Philadelphia: Saunders Elsevier.

Twomey, S., & Dowling, M. (2013). Management of death rattle at end of life. *British Journal of Nursing (Mark Allen Publishing)*, *22*(2), 81–85.

Vollman, K., Sole, M., & Quinn, B. (2017). Endotracheal tube care and oral care practices for ventilated and non-ventilated patients. In D. L. Wiegand (Ed.), *AACN procedure manual for high acuity, progressive, and critical care* (7th ed.). Philadelphia: Saunders Elsevier.

Wanless, S., & Aldridge, M. (2011). Continuous lateral rotation therapy: A review. *Nursing in Critical Care*, *17*, 28–35.

Risk for Allergy reaction   *Julianne E. Doubet, BSN, RN, EMT-B*

NANDA-I

Definition

Susceptible to an exaggerated immune response or reaction to substances, which may compromise health.

Risk Factors

Exposure to allergen; exposure to environmental allergen; exposure to toxic chemical

At-Risk Population

History of food allergy; history of insect sting allergy; repeated exposure to allergen-producing environmental substance

NOC   Outcomes (Nursing Outcomes Classification)

Suggested NOC Outcomes

Allergic Response: Systemic; Immune Hypersensitivity Response; Knowledge: Health Behavior, Risk Control, Risk Detection; Tissue Integrity: Skin and Mucous Membranes

● = Independent;   ▲ = Collaborative;   EBN = Evidence-Based Nursing;   EB = Evidence-Based

> ## Example NOC Outcome with Indicators
>
> **Immune Hypersensitivity Response** as evidenced by the following indicators: Respiratory, cardiac, gastrointestinal, renal and neurological function status IER/Free of allergic reactions. (Rate each indicator of **Immune Hypersensitivity Response:** 1 = not controlled, 2 = slightly controlled, 3 = moderately controlled, 4 = well controlled, 5 = very well controlled [see Section I].)

IER, In expected range.

Client Outcomes

Client Will (Specify Time Frame)

- State risk factors for allergies
- Demonstrate knowledge of plan to treat allergic reaction

NIC   Interventions (Nursing Interventions Classification)

Suggested NIC Interventions

Allergy Management; Environmental Risk Protection

> ## Example NIC Activity
>
> Place an allergy band on client

Nursing Interventions and *Rationales*

- A careful history is important in detecting allergens and avoidance of these allergens. EB: *In a review of the National Institute for Health and Care Excellence (NICE) recommendations, Walsh (2017) agreed that food allergies may be identified by using an "allergy-focused clinical history."*
- Obtain a precise history of allergies, as well as medications taken and foods ingested before surgery. EB: *In their study of perioperative anaphylaxis, Meng et al (2017) confirmed that antibiotics and neuromuscular blocking agents are common producers of anaphylaxis.*
- ▲ Teach the client about the correct use of the injectable epinephrine and have the client do a return demonstration. EB: *Recent research on the correct use of the injectable epinephrine showed that 84% of the patients were unable to do it correctly (Bonds et al, 2015).*
- ▲ Carefully assess the client for allergies. Below is information that is important for clients with allergies. Refer for immediate treatment if anaphylaxis is suspected.

Causes

Common allergens include animal dander; bee stings or stings from other insects; foods, especially nuts, fish, and shellfish; insect bites; medications; plants; pollens

Symptoms

Common symptoms of a mild allergic reaction include hives (especially over the neck and face), itching, nasal congestion, rashes, watery, red eyes

Symptoms of a moderate or severe reaction include cramps or pain in the abdomen; chest discomfort or tightness; diarrhea; difficulty breathing; difficulty swallowing; dizziness or lightheadedness; fear or feeling of apprehension or anxiety; flushing or redness of the face; nausea and vomiting; palpitations; swelling of the face, eyes, or tongue; weakness; wheezing; unconsciousness

First Aid

For a mild to moderate reaction: calm and reassure the person having the reaction because anxiety can worsen symptoms.

1. Try to identify the allergen and have the person avoid further contact with it. If the allergic reaction is from a bee sting, scrape the stinger off the skin with something firm (e.g., fingernail or plastic credit card). Do not use tweezers; squeezing the stinger will release more venom.
2. Apply cool compresses and over-the-counter hydrocortisone cream for itchy rash.
3. Watch for signs of increasing distress.

• = Independent;   ▲ = Collaborative;   EBN = Evidence-Based Nursing;   EB = Evidence-Based

A

4. Get medical help. For a mild reaction, a health care provider may recommend over-the-counter medications (e.g., antihistamines).

For a Severe Allergic Reaction (Anaphylaxis)

1. Check the person's airway, breathing, and circulation (the ABCs of Basic Life Support). A warning sign of dangerous throat swelling is a very hoarse or whispered voice or coarse sounds when the person is breathing in air. If necessary, begin rescue breathing and cardiopulmonary resuscitation.
2. Call 911.
3. Calm and reassure the person.
4. If the allergic reaction is from a bee sting, scrape the stinger off the skin with something firm (e.g., fingernail or plastic credit card). Do not use tweezers; squeezing the stinger will release more venom.
5. If the person has emergency allergy medication on hand, help the person take or inject the medication. Avoid oral medication if the person is having difficulty breathing.
6. Take steps to prevent shock. Have the person lie flat, raise the person's feet about 12 inches, and cover him or her with a coat or blanket. Do NOT place the person in this position if a head, neck, back, or leg injury is suspected or if it causes discomfort.

Do NOT

- Do NOT assume that any allergy shots the person has already received will provide complete protection.
- Do NOT place a pillow under the person's head if he or she is having trouble breathing. This can block the airways.
- Do NOT give the person anything by mouth if the person is having trouble breathing.

When to Contact a Medical Professional

Call for immediate medical emergency assistance if:
- The person is having a severe allergic reaction—always call 911. Do not wait to see if the reaction is getting worse.
- The person has a history of severe allergic reactions (check for a medical ID tag).

Prevention

- Avoid triggers such as foods and medications that have caused an allergic reaction (even a mild one) in the past. Ask detailed questions about ingredients when you are eating away from home. Carefully examine ingredient labels. EB: *Education concerning allergen vulnerability will help patients to prevent most accidental exposures to known allergic triggers (Mahr & Hernandez-Trujillo, 2017).*
- If you have a child who is allergic to certain foods, introduce one new food at a time in limited amounts so you can recognize an allergic reaction. EB: *There is a decrease in the threat for the evolution of food allergies in patients who are at risk with the early introduction of known allergy-producing foods: abstaining from these types of foods, without a clear history of allergic reactions, may increase the chances of developing an allergy (Schroer et al, 2017).*
- People who know that they have had serious allergic reactions should wear a medical ID tag. EBN: *Anaphylaxis is a dangerous, unpredictable, and usually rapid hypersensitivity response to an allergen and is generally caused by a known irritant; it is advised then, that those who have had a severe allergic reaction wear medical alert jewelry (Hunt, 2016).*
- Preoperative patients should be closely assessed for allergies. EB: *According to Kuric et al (2017), general anesthesia may mask the classic, initial signs of allergy, which would be seen in the conscious patient.*
- ▲ If you have a history of serious allergic reactions, carry emergency medications (e.g., a chewable form of diphenhydramine and injectable epinephrine or a bee sting kit) according to your health care provider's instructions. *The initial intervention for anaphylaxis should be epinephrine; medical providers across the board agree that its quick administration is vital to prevent progression of the reaction, improve patient outcomes, and that epinephrine use will contribute to a decrease in hospitalizations and fatalities (Fromer, 2016).*
- Do not give your injectable epinephrine (or any other personal medication), to anyone else. They may have a condition (e.g., a heart problem) that could be negatively affected by this drug. EB: *Negative effects of medicine sharing include adverse events, complications, and a delay in seeking professional help; medicine sharing could also be motivated by ill-advised self-treatment options (Beyene et al, 2014).*

● = Independent;   ▲ = Collaborative;   EBN = Evidence-Based Nursing;   EB = Evidence-Based

▲ Refer the client for skin testing to confirm IgE-mediated allergic response. EB: *Stylianou et al (2016) stated that allergen-specific immunotherapy (SIT) is thought to be the most effective remedy for immunoglobulin E (IgE)-mediated allergies.*

• See care plans for **Latex Allergy** response and Risk for **Latex Allergy** response.

 Pediatric

▲ Teach parents and children with allergies to peanuts and tree nuts to avoid them and to identify them. EBN: *Nut allergies can have an undesirable impact on both the individual and their family; the key responsibilities of the nurse is ongoing support of those affected and to aid in creating a management plan to control allergen response (Proudfoot & Saul, 2016).*

▲ Teach parents and children with asthma about modifiable risk factors, which include allergy triggers. EBN: *Proudfoot & Saul (2016) recommended that those who care for asthmatic children have a "Risk Assessment Management Plan" that includes avoidance of the allergen (nuts, etc.), rescue medication, diabetic referral as needed, and continued support for both child and family.*

▲ Counsel parents to limit infant exposure to traffic and cigarette carbon monoxide pollution. EB: *Early childhood exposure to traffic-related air pollution (TRAP) was linked with the evolution of asthma in childhood (Bowatte et al, 2015).* EBN: *Children exposed to secondhand smoke (SHS) have an elevated rate of respiratory infections, ear infections, SHS-triggered asthma attacks, and sudden infant death syndrome (Kleier et al, 2017).*

▲ Suspect food protein-induced enterocolitis syndrome (FPIES) in formula-fed infants with repetitive emesis, diarrhea, dehydration, and lethargy 1 to 5 hours after ingesting the offending food (the most common are cow's milk, soy, and rice). Remove the offending food. EB: *If FPIES becomes chronic, it may lead to an infant's failure to thrive (Nowak-Wegrzyn et al, 2015).*

▲ Children should be screened for seafood allergies and if an allergy is detected, avoid seafood and any foods containing seafood. EB: *According to a study by Presler (2016), fish and shellfish are powerful allergens that cause grave IgE antibody-mediated untoward reactions in those who are sensitive.*

REFERENCES

Beyene, K., Sheridan, J., & Aspden, T. (2014). Prescription medication sharing: A systematic literature review. *American Journal of Public Health, 104*(4), e15–e26.

Bonds, R. S., Asawa, A., & Ghazi, A. I. (2015). Misuse of medical devices: A persistent problem in self-management of asthma and allergic disease. *Annals of Allergy, Asthma and Immunology, 114*(1), 74–76.e2.

Bowatte, G., Lodge, C., Lowe, A., et al. (2015). The influence of childhood traffic-related air pollution on exposure on asthma, allergy and sensitization: A systematic review and meta-analysis of birth cohort studies. *European Journal of Allergy and Clinical Immunology, 70*(3), 245–256.

Fromer, L. (2016). Prevention of anaphylaxis: The role of epinephrine auto injectors. *Journal of Medicine, 129*(12), 1244–1250.

Hunt, K. (2016). Anaphylaxis. *Practice Nurse, 46*(12), 13–18.

Kleier, J., Mites-Campbell, M., & Henson-Evertz, K. (2017). Children's exposure to secondhand smoke and parental nicotine dependence and motivation to quit smoking. *Pediatric Nursing, 43*(1), 35–39.

Kuric, V., ZaZa, K., & Algazian, S. (2017). Atypical presentation to rocuronium allergy in a 19-year-old patient. *Journal of Clinical Anesthesia, 37,* 163–165.

Mahr, T., & Hernandez-Trujillo, V. (2017). First-ever action plan for epinephrine and anaphylaxis. *Contemporary Pediatrics, 34*(8), 16–42.

Meng, J., Rotiroti, G., Burdett, E., et al. (2017). Anaphylaxis during general anesthesia: Experiences from a drug allergy centre in the UK. *ACTA Anaesthesiologica Scandinavica, 61*(3), 281–289.

Nowak-Wegrzyn, A., Yitzhak, K., Mehr, S., et al. (2015). Non-IgE-mediated gastrointestinal food allergy. *Journal of Allergy and Clinical Immunology, 135*(5), 1114–1124.

Presler, L. (2016). Seafood allergy, toxicity and occupational health, Zagreb, Croatia. *Journal of American College of Nutrition, 35*(3), 271–283.

Proudfoot, C., & Saul, P. (2016). Nut allergy in children: A growing concern. *Practice Nurse, 46*(12), 30–36.

Schroer, B., Bjelac, J., & Leonard, M. (2017). What is new in managing patients with food allergy? Almost everything. *Current Opinion in Pediatrics, 29*(5), 578–583.

Stylianou, E., Ueland, T., Borchsenius, F., et al. (2016). Specific allergen immunotherapy: effects on IgE, IgG4 and chemokines in patients with allergic rhinitis. *Scandinavian Journal of Clinical & Laboratory Investigations, 76*(2), 118–127.

Walsh, J. (2017). NICE food allergy and anaphylaxis quality standards: A review of the 2016 quality standards. *British Journal of General Practice, 67*(656), 138–139. Retrieved from https://doi.org/10.3399/bjgp17x689833.

A

Anxiety   *Gail B. Ladwig, MSN, RN and Julianne E. Doubet, BSN, RN, EMT-B*

NANDA-I

Definition

Vague, uneasy feeling of discomfort or dread accompanied by an autonomic response (the source often nonspecific or unknown to the individual); a feeling of apprehension caused by anticipation of danger. It is an alerting sign that warns of impending danger and enables the individual to take measures to deal with threat.

Defining Characteristics

Behavioral

Decrease in productivity; extraneous movement; fidgeting; glancing about; hypervigilance; insomnia; poor eye contact; restlessness; scanning behavior; worried about change in life event

Affective

Anguish; apprehensiveness; distress; fear; feelings of inadequacy; helplessness; increase in wariness; irritability; nervousness; overexcitement; rattled; regretful; self-focused; uncertainty

Physiological

Facial tension; hand tremors; increase in perspiration; increase in tension; trembling; tremor; voice quivering

Sympathetic

Alteration in respiratory pattern; anorexia; brisk reflexes; cardiovascular excitation; diarrhea; dry mouth; facial flushing; heart palpitations; increase in blood pressure; increase in heart rate; increase in respiratory rate; pupil dilation; superficial vasoconstriction; twitching; weakness

Parasympathetic

Abdominal pain; alteration in sleep pattern; decreased blood pressure; decrease in heart rate; diarrhea; faintness; fatigue; nausea; tingling in extremities; urinary frequency; urinary hesitancy; urinary urgency

Cognitive

Alteration in attention; alteration in concentration; awareness of physiological symptoms; blocking of thoughts; confusion; decrease in perceptual field; diminished ability to learn; diminished ability to problem solve; forgetfulness; fear; preoccupation; rumination; tendency to blame others

Related Factors

Conflict about life goals; interpersonal contagion; interpersonal transmission; stressors; substance misuse; threat of death; threat to current status; unmet needs; value conflict

At-Risk Population

Exposure to toxin; family history of anxiety; heredity; major change; maturational crisis; situational crisis

NOC   (Nursing Outcomes Classification)

Suggested NOC Outcomes

Anxiety Level; Anxiety Self-Control; Coping; Impulse Self-Control Fear level; Fear Self-Control; Mood Equilibrium

---

Example NOC Outcome with Indicators

Anxiety Self-Control as evidenced by the following indicators: Eliminates precursors of anxiety/Monitors physical manifestations of anxiety/Controls anxiety response. (Rate the outcome and indicators of **Anxiety Self-Control:** 1 = never demonstrated, 2 = rarely demonstrated, 3 = sometimes demonstrated, 4 = often demonstrated, 5 = consistently demonstrated [see Section I].)

● = Independent;   ▲ = Collaborative;   EBN = Evidence-Based Nursing;   EB = Evidence-Based

Client Outcomes

Client Will (Specify Time Frame)

- Identify and verbalize symptoms of anxiety
- Identify, verbalize, and demonstrate techniques to control anxiety
- Verbalize absence of or decrease in subjective distress
- Have vital signs that reflect baseline or decreased sympathetic stimulation
- Have posture, facial expressions, gestures, and activity levels that reflect decreased distress
- Demonstrate improved concentration and accuracy of thoughts
- Demonstrate return of basic problem-solving skills
- Demonstrate increased external focus
- Demonstrate some ability to reassure self

NIC   (Nursing Interventions Classification)

Suggested NIC Interventions

Anxiety Reduction; Calming Technique; Coping Enhancement; Impulse Control Training; Relaxation Therapy

Example NIC Activities—Anxiety Reduction

Use calm, reassuring approach; Explain all procedures, including sensations likely to be experienced during the procedure

Nursing Interventions and *Rationales*

- Assess the client's level of anxiety and physical reactions to anxiety (e.g., tachycardia, tachypnea, irritability, restlessness). EBN: *Barley & Lawson (2016) stated in their study of health psychology's effects on common mental disorders that for nurses to deliver holistic care, they must be alert to the possibility that the patient may be undergoing psychological anxiety and then use appropriate communication skills to identify and manage this issue.*
- Rule out withdrawal from alcohol, sedatives, or smoking as the cause of anxiety. EBN: *Signs and symptoms of alcohol withdrawal syndrome (AWS) are many times indistinguishable from other illnesses, especially those seen in the acute care setting (Skinner, 2014).*
- Use empathy to encourage the client to interpret the anxiety symptoms as normal. CEB: *The way a nurse interacts with a client influences his or her quality of life. Providing psychological and social support can reduce the symptoms and problems associated with anxiety (Wagner & Bear, 2009).*
- If irrational thoughts or fears are present, offer the client accurate information and encourage him or her to talk about the meaning of the events contributing to the anxiety. EBN: *In one study providing cancer patients with accurate information about their disease, prognosis and outcomes significantly reduced their anxiety and increased empowerment (Lauzier et al, 2014).*
- Encourage the client to use positive self-talk. EBN: *One research study showed that self-talk strengthens both actual behavior performance and prospective behavioral intentions (Dolcos & Albarracin, 2014).*
- Intervene when possible to remove sources of anxiety. EBN: *Aiding in the reduction of anxiety is an essential nursing intervention in patient care state (Elham et al, 2015).*
- Explain all activities, procedures, and issues that involve the client; use nonmedical terms and calm, slow speech then validate the client's understanding. EBN: *In a study of the needs of anxious and/or depressed patients, Kim (2016) found that nursing care must include patient-centered undertakings to form a bond between patient and nurse, therefore reassuring and empowering these patients.*
- ▲ Use massage therapy to reduce anxiety. EBN: *The use of massage therapy has been shown to markedly reduce psychological stress and anxiety (Kim et al, 2016).*
- ▲ Consider massage therapy for preoperative clients. EBN: *Complementary therapies, including massage, have been shown to aid patient relaxation prior to surgery (Hansen, 2015).*
- Use therapeutic touch and healing touch techniques. EBN: *One study showed that Reiki therapeutic touch reduced anxiety and pain (Sagkal et al, 2013).*
- Use guided imagery to decrease anxiety. EBN: *Guided imagery can be utilized to aid patients in handling undesirable emotions connected with the symptoms of their illness (Nooner et al, 2016).*
- Suggest yoga to the client. EBN: *In a study by Centrella-Negro (2017), it was noted that the practice of yoga was beneficial to the welfare and comfort of cardiac patients.*

● = Independent;   ▲ = Collaborative;   EBN = Evidence-Based Nursing;   EB = Evidence-Based

A

- Provide clients with a means to listen to music of their choice or audiotapes. EBN: *According to Quach (2017), nurses and other providers should recognize the value of music therapies and use them in patient care when appropriate.*

Pediatric

- The previously mentioned interventions may be adapted for the pediatric client.

Geriatric

- ▲ Monitor the client for depression. Use appropriate interventions and referrals. EBN/EB: *Gould et al (2016) stated that "Anxiety disorders are common and debilitating in older individuals" and further noted that simple tests used to recognize anxiety symptoms in the older patient are beneficial because they can begin discussions about current treatments.*
- Observe for adverse changes if antianxiety drugs are taken. EB: *Because of changes in pharmacodynamics and pharmacokinetics in older patients, those who take antianxiety drugs should be watched for potential side effects (Jacobson, 2013).*
- Mindfulness meditation is successful in mediating anxiety. EB: *The use of mindfulness has become an accepted clinical treatment in reducing anxiety and stress (Grecucci et al, 2015).*

Multicultural

- Assess for the presence of culture-bound anxiety states. EBN: *When assessing people with culturally and linguistically diverse (CALD) histories, it is imperative that any special cultural practices, requirements, or beliefs, such as prayers or alternative medicines, are acknowledged and appreciated when planning nursing interventions (Baker et al, 2016).*
- Identify how anxiety is manifested in the culturally diverse client. EB: *People of non-Western ethnocultural origins many times have diverse ideas and contrasting perceptions of mental health and illness as opposed to those from Western societies (Balkir Neftci & Barnow, 2016).*
- For diverse clients experiencing preoperative anxiety, provide music of their choice. EBN: *According to Quach (2017), music, as a complimentary intervention, has been shown to notably improve both patient anxiety and patient physical well-being and should be used in nursing care.*

Home Care

- The previously mentioned interventions may be adapted for home care use.
- ▲ Assess for suicidal ideation. EBN: *Developing a protective setting for patients who are suicidal first necessitates recognizing those patients who are at risk; The Nurses' Global Assessment of Suicide Risk is an assessment tool that is an accepted evidence-based suicide risk evaluation (Adams, 2013).*
- Assess for influence of anxiety on medical regimen. CEB: *Anxiety can affect a patient's ability to complete their medical regimen as prescribed, including taking medications, exercise, diet, and follow-up therapies (Hynninen et al, 2010).*
- Assess for presence of depression. EBN: *Clinician report generally had the most favorable sensitivity and specificity for measuring depressive symptoms and treatment recommendations, respectively (Henry et al, 2014).*
- Assist family to be supportive of the client in the face of anxiety symptoms. EBN: *Vieira et al (2015) surmised in a study that both patient and caregiver/family must realize and accept that medical conditions will bring a change of lifestyle for each and they should adapt as best they can.*
- ▲ Consider referral for the prescription of antianxiety or antidepressant medications for clients who have panic disorder (PD) or other anxiety-related psychiatric disorders. EBN: *Pharmacotherapy is an effective intervention for anxiety disorders because it decreases symptoms and enhances a sense of well-being for the patient (da Cruz et al, 2016).*
- ▲ Assist the client/family to institute the medication regimen appropriately. Instruct in side effects and the importance of taking medications as ordered. EBN: *Instruct the patient and/or caregivers concerning possible drug side effects and interactions that could have detrimental results (sleepiness, nausea, etc.) on the patient and be certain the patient/caregiver understands how the medication is to be given (Creed, 2017).*
- ▲ Refer for psychiatric home health care services. CEB: *Providing home health services for patients with anxiety increases self-efficacy and reduces symptoms of anxiety, stress, and depression (Shelby et al, 2009). EB: A mixture of mental health services is provided in some aging services networks that incorporates screenings, telephone reassurance, individual counseling, and support groups (Roberts et al, 2014).*

● = Independent;   ▲ = Collaborative;   EBN = Evidence-Based Nursing;   EB = Evidence-Based

Client/Family Teaching and Discharge Planning

▲ Teach use of appropriate community resources in emergency situations (e.g., suicidal thoughts), such as hotlines, emergency departments, law enforcement, and judicial systems. **EB:** *Boudreaux et al (2016) suggested that community mental health services, delivered in conjunction with community emergency departments, may improve patient commitment to aftercare and as a result reduce future behavioral health crises as well as decrease return visits to the emergency department.*

• Teach the client/family the symptoms of anxiety.

• Teach the client techniques to self-manage anxiety. **EB:** *Guided Internet-based cognitive-behavioral therapy (ICBT) has been found to be valuable for social anxiety disorder (SAD) by some research groups (Boettcher et al, 2013).*

• Teach the client to visualize or fantasize about the absence of anxiety or pain, successful experience of the situation, resolution of conflict, or outcome of procedure. **EB:** *Guided imagery has been shown to augment comfort and can be used as a psychosupportive intervention (Satija & Bhatnagar, 2017).*

• Teach the relationship between a healthy physical and emotional lifestyle and a realistic mental attitude. **EBN:** *Jiwani (2016) stated that "anxiety leads to physiological and psychological changes in the human body" and can be controlled with various learned self-help techniques.*

REFERENCES

Adams, N. (2013). Developing a suicide precaution procedure. *Medsurg Nursing, 22*(6), 383–386.

Baker, A., Proctor, N., & Ferguson, M. (2016). Engaging with culturally and linguistically diverse communities to reduce the impact of depression and anxiety: A narrative review. *Health and Social Care in the Community, 249*(4), 386–398.

Barley, E., & Lawson, V. (2016). Using health psychology to help patients: Common mental disorders and psychological distress. *British Journal of Nursing, 25*(17), 966–974.

Balkir, N., & Barnow, S. (2016). One size does not fit all in psychotherapy: Understanding depression among patients of Turkish behavior origin in Europe. *Archives of Neuropsychiatry, 53*(1), 72–79.

Boettcher, J., Andersson, G., & Carlbring, P. (2013). Combining attention training with cognitive behavior therapy in internet-based self-help for social anxiety: Study protocol for a randomized controlled trial. *Trials, 14*(1), 68.

Boudreaux, J., Crapanzano, K., Jones, G., et al. (2016). Using mental health outreach teams in the emergency department to improve engagement in treatment. *Community Mental Health Journal, 52*(18), 1009–1014.

Centrella-Negro, A. (2017). Evaluating the edition of hatha yoga in cardiac rehabilitation. *Medsurg Nursing, 26*(1), 39–43.

Creed, S. (2017). Avoiding medication errors in general practice. *Practice Nurse, 47*(2), 24–26.

da Cruz, A., Giacchero, K., do Carmo, M., et al. (2016). Difficulties related to medication therapies for anxiety disorder. *Revista Eletronica de Enfermagem, 18*, 1–10. Retrieved from http://dx.doi.org/10.5216/rec.v18.32741.

Dolcos, S., & Albarracin, D. (2014). The inner speech of behavioral regulation: intentions and task performance strengthen when you talk to yourself as a you. *European Journal of Social Psychology, 44*(6), 636–642.

Elham, H., Hazrat, M., Mommennasab, M., et al. (2015). The effect of need-based spiritual/religious intervention on spiritual well-being and anxiety of elderly. *Holistic Nursing Practice, 29*(3), 136–143.

Gould, C., Beaudreau, S., Gullickson, G., et al. (2016). Implementation of brief anxiety assessment and evaluation in a department of veterans affairs geriatric pulmonary clinic. *Journal of Rehabilitation, Research & Development, 53*(3), 335–344.

Grecucci, A., Pappaianni, E., Siugzdaite, R., et al. (2015). Mindful emotion regulation: Exploring the neurocognitive mechanisms behind mindfulness. *BioMed Research International, 2015*, 1–9.

Hansen, M. (2015). A feasibility pilot study on the use of complimentary therapies delivered via mobile technologies on Icelandic surgical patients reports of anxiety, pain and self-efficacy in healing. *BMC Complimentary and Alternative Medicine, 15*(1), 11–12.

Henry, S. G., Feng, B., Franks, P., et al. (2014). Methods for assessing patient–clinician communication about depression in primary care: What you see depends on how you look. *Health Services Research, 49*(5), 1684–1700.

Hynninen, M., Bjerke, N., Pallesen, S., et al. (2010). A randomized controlled trial of cognitive behavioral therapy for anxiety and depression in COPD. *Respiratory Medicine, 104*(7), 986–994.

Jacobson, S. (2013). Effects of pharmacokinetic and pharmacodynamic changes in the elderly. *Psychiatric Times, 30*(1), 26–29.

Jiwani, K. (2016). Handling challenging emotions in nursing care. *Journal of Nursing, 6*(2), 13–15.

Kim, D., Lee, D., Schreiber, J., et al. (2016). Integrative evaluation of automatic massage combined with thermotherapy: Physical, physiological and psychological viewpoints. *BioMed Research International, 2016*, 1–8.

Kim, J., (2016). Phase II cardiac rehabilitation participants' perception of nurse caring correlated with participants' depression, anxiety, and adherence. *International Journal for Human Caring, 20*(4), 213–219. doi:10.20467/1091-5710-20.4.213.

Lauzier, S., Campbell, H. S., Livingston, P. M., et al. (2014). Indicators for evaluating cancer organizations' support services: Performance and associations with empowerment. *Cancer, 120*(20), 3219–3227.

Nooner, A., Dwyer, K., DeShea, L., et al. (2016). Using relaxation and guided imagery to address pain, fatigue, and sleep disturbances: A pilot study. *Clinical Journal of Oncology Nursing, 20*(5), 547–552.

Quach, J. (2017). Do music therapies reduce depressive symptoms and improve QOL in older adults with chronic disease? *Nursing, 47*(6), 58–63.

Roberts, K., Weaver, R., & Wacker, R. (2014). The health effects of negative social exchanges in later life. *Generations (San Francisco, Calif.), 38*(2), 14–21.

Sagkal, T., Eser, I., & Uyar, M. (2013). The effect of reiki touch therapy on pain and anxiety. *Complementary Medicine, 3*(4), 141–146.

Satija, A., & Bhatnagar, S. (2017). Complimentary therapies for symptom management in cancer patients. *Indian Journal of Palliative Care, 23*(4), 468–479.

Shelby, R., et al. (2009). Pain catastrophizing in patients with noncardiac chest pain: Relationships with pain, anxiety, and disability. *Psychosomatic Medicine, 71*(8), 861–868.

● = Independent; ▲ = Collaborative; EBN = Evidence-Based Nursing; EB = Evidence-Based

A

Skinner, R. (2014). Symptom-triggered vs fixed dosing management of alcohol withdrawal syndrome. *Medsurg Nursing, 23*(5), 307–329.

Vieira, G., Cavalcanti, A., da Silva, S., et al. (2015). Quality of life of caregivers to patients with heart failure: integrative review. *Journal of Nursing UFPE, 9*(2), 750–758. doi:10.5205/reuol.7028-60723-1 -SM.0902201533.

Wagner, D., & Bear, M. (2009). Patient satisfaction with nursing care: a concept analysis within a nursing framework. *Journal of Advanced Nursing, 65*(3), 692–701.

Death Anxiety   *Gail B. Ladwig, MSN, RN and Julianne E. Doubet, BSN, RN, EMT-B*

NANDA-I

Definition

Vague, uneasy feeling of discomfort or dread generated by perceptions of a real or imagined threat to one's existence.

Defining Characteristics

Concern about strain on the caregiver; deep sadness; fear of developing terminal illness; fear of loss of mental abilities when dying; fear of pain related to dying; fear of premature death; fear of prolonged dying process; fear of suffering related to dying; fear of the dying process; negative thoughts related to death and dying; powerlessness; worried about the impact of one's death on significant other

Related Factors

Anticipation of adverse consequences of anesthesia; anticipation of impact of death on others; anticipation of pain; anticipation of suffering; discussions on topic of death; nonacceptance of own mortality; observations related to death; perceived imminence of death; uncertainty about encountering a higher power; uncertainty about life after death; uncertainty about the existence of a higher power; uncertainty of prognosis

At-Risk Population

Discussions on the topic of death; experiencing the dying process; near-death experience; observations related to dying process

NOC   (Nursing Outcomes Classification)

Suggested NOC Outcomes

Acceptance: Health Status; Anxiety Self-Control; Comfort Status: Psychospiritual; Comfortable Death; Coping; Dignified Life Closure; Family Coping; Fear Self-Control; Grief Resolution; Health Beliefs: Perceived Threat: Hope; Personal Resiliency; Psychosocial Adjustment; Life Change; Quality of Life

---

Example NOC Outcome with Indicators

Dignified Life Closure as evidenced by the following indicators: Expresses readiness for death/Resolves important issues/ Shares feelings about dying/Discusses spiritual concerns. (Rate the outcome and indicators of **Dignified Life Closure**: 1 = never demonstrated, 2 = rarely demonstrated, 3 = sometimes demonstrated, 4 = often demonstrated, 5 = consistently demonstrated [see Section I].)

Client Outcomes

Client Will (Specify Time Frame)

- State concerns about impact of death on others
- Express feelings associated with dying
- Seek help in dealing with feelings
- Discuss realistic goals
- Use prayer or other religious practice for comfort

● = Independent;   ▲ = Collaborative;   EBN = Evidence-Based Nursing;   EB = Evidence-Based

NIC (Nursing Interventions Classification)

Suggested NIC Interventions

Active Listening; Animal Assisted Therapy; Anticipatory Guidance; Anxiety Reduction; Aromatherapy; Coping Enhancement; Dying Care; Emotional Support; Grief Work Facilitation; Journaling; Respite Care; Spiritual Support; Support System Enhancement

Example NIC Activities—Dying Care

Communicate willingness to discuss death; Support client and family through stages of grief

Nursing Interventions and *Rationales*

▲ Assess the psychosocial maturity of the individual. EB: *In a large study, females scored higher on death anxiety than males. Additional tests reported that life satisfaction, an altering consciousness coping style, and avoidance coping was significantly related to risk for developing a stress-related illness when faced with the death of a loved one (Moore, 2013).*

▲ Assess clients for pain and provide pain relief measures. EB: *Pain can be a significant problem that has important ramifications on patients' quality of life and the management of pain can be obstructed by poor patient–provider communication (Johnsen et al, 2016).* EBN: *Nurses have a fundamental responsibility for the assessment and alleviation of patient's pain (Brorson et al, 2014).*

● Assess client for fears related to death. EB: *In their study of chronic obstructive pulmonary disease (COPD) patients with end-of-life issues, Stenzel et al (2015) found that patient care should not be limited to managing just the physical manifestation of the disease, but also the need to address psychological anxiety and disease-specific concerns.*

● Assist clients with life planning: consider and redefine main life goals, focus on areas of strength and/or goals that will provide satisfaction, adopt realistic goals, and recognize those that are impossible to achieve. EBN: *Nurses have an obligation in communicating with those under their care, which should include the discussion of life preferences and relating pertinent, personal information (Coyle et al, 2015).*

● Assist clients with life review and reminiscence. EBN: *Chen et al (2017) found in their studies of life review, for those suffering life-threatening illnesses, that this practice aided in diminishing depression and augmenting self-esteem.*

● Provide music of the client's choosing. EB: *There is convincing evidence that music effectively assists those facing end-of-life concerns (Clement-Cortis, 2016).*

● Provide social support for families: understanding what is most important to families who are caring for clients at the end of life. EBN: *Nurses, who deal not only with technical and resuscitative aspects of critical patient care, are now developing their expertise to include "advocating for, communicating with, teaching, and guiding patients and families through end-of-life issues" (Banjar, 2017).*

● Encourage clients to pray. EBN: *The Society of Critical Care Medicine recommends that the spiritual needs of patients facing a critical end-of-life illness should be recognized and managed by the health care team (Fournier, 2017).*

 ### Geriatric

● Carefully assess older adults for issues regarding death anxiety. EB: *This study by Bonnewyn et al (2016) proposed that the way older adults perceive dying, in part, affects whether they have a desire to die: it could be advantageous to explore the subject of death with your patient.*

● Provide back massage for clients who have anxiety regarding issues such as death. EBN: *Back massage significantly reduced anxiety in the study population. Systolic blood pressure (BP) decreased to a greater degree in the male participants, particularly in those with greater levels of anxiety and higher systolic BP (Chen et al, 2013).*

● Refer to care plan for **Grieving.**

 ### Multicultural

● Assist clients to identify with their culture and its values. EBN: *Cultures stand apart in their approach to how death is framed, viewed, and accepted (MacCloud et al, 2016).*

● Refer to care plans for **Anxiety** and **Grieving.**

● = Independent;   ▲ = Collaborative;   EBN = Evidence-Based Nursing;   EB = Evidence-Based

A

Home Care

- The previously mentioned interventions may be adapted for home care.
- Identify times and places when anxiety is greatest. Provide for psychological support at those times, using such strategies as personal contact, telephone contact, diversionary activities, or therapeutic self. **EBN:** *Participants across conditions reported similar levels of anxiety, suggesting that promoting an interest in sustained contact can be accomplished without reducing anxiety, but rather by shielding individuals from the negative effects of anxiety during social interactions (Stern & West, 2014).*
- Support religious beliefs; encourage the client to participate in services and activities of choice. **EBN:** *Enhancing the psychosocial and spiritual well-being of cancer patients can reduce their death anxiety and promote better quality of life (Shukla & Rishi, 2014).*
- ▲ Refer to appropriate medical services, social services, and/or mental health services, as needed. **EBN:** *The union between physical health and mental health needs requires added awareness and acknowledgement in the contemporary nursing care of palliative patients (Hayes, 2017).*
- ▲ Identify the client's preferences for end-of-life care; aid in honoring preferences as much as practicable. **EBN:** *To engage in patient-centered care at end of life requires the entire health care team to enlist patients and families in communication and decision-making, especially about the clients' preferences and decisions concerning the use of life-extending technologies (Nouvet et al, 2016).*
- ▲ Assist the client in making contact with death-related planning organizations, if appropriate, such as the Cremation Society and funeral homes. **EB:** *Advanced care planning is important to older clients. However, when clients are not accepting of death or if death is outside of the client's understanding, it can be difficult to work on advanced care planning. Nurses should explore whether the client accepts dying as a likely outcome and assess the client's fears of dying and need for control before attempting any planning (Piers et al, 2013).*
- Refer to care plan for **Powerlessness.**

Client/Family Teaching and Discharge Planning

- Promote more effective communication to family members engaged in the caregiving role. **CEB:** *Encouraging loved ones to discuss their wishes and areas of concern will assist the family during the grieving process; they will know the wishes of the dying family member and can carry them out as much as possible (Webb & Guarino, 2011).*
- Allow family members to be physically close to their dying loved one, giving them permission, instruction, and opportunities to touch. Keep family members informed. **EBN:** *Dosser & Kennedy (2014) maintained that care giver support is an integral part of nursing care and essential to improved outcomes.*

REFERENCES

Banjar, A. (2017). Till death do us part: The evolution of end-of-life- and death attitudes. *Canadian Journal of Critical Care, 28*(3), 34–40.

Bonnewyn, A., Shah, A., Bruffaerts, R., et al. (2016). Are religiousness and death attitudes associated with the wish to die in older people? *International Psychogeriatrics, 28*(3), 397–404.

Brorson, H., Plymoth, H., Arom, K., et al. (2014). Pain relief at the end-of-life: Nurses' experience regarding end-of-life pain relief in pain relief in patients with dementia. *Pain Management Nursing, 15*(1), 315–323.

Chen, W., Liu, L., Yeh, S., et al. (2013). Effect of back massage intervention on anxiety, comfort, and physiologic responses in patients with congestive heart failure. *The Journal of Alternative and Complementary Medicine, 19*(5), 464–470.

Chen, Y., Xiao, H., Yang, Y., et al. (2017). The effects of life review on psycho-spiritual well-being among patients with life-threatening illness: A systematic review and meta-analysis. *Journal of Advanced Nursing, 73*(7), 1539–1554.

Clement-Cortis, A. (2016). Development and efficacy of music therapy techniques with palliative care. *Complimentary Therapies in Clinical Practice, 23*, 125–129.

Coyle, N., Manna, R., Shen, M., et al. (2015). Discussing death, dying and end-of-life care: A communications skills training module for oncology nurses. *Clinical Journal of Oncology Nursing, 19*(6), 697–702.

Dosser, I., & Kennedy, C. (2014). Improving family carers' experiences of support at the end of life by enhancing communication: An action research study. *International Journal of Palliative Nursing, 20*(12), 608–616.

Fournier, A. (2017). Creating a sacred place in the intensive care unit at the end-of-life. *Dimensions of Critical Care Nursing, 36*(2), 110–115.

Hayes, J. (2017). Specialist palliative care nurses' management of the needs of patients with depression. *International Journal of Palliative Medicine, 23*(6), 298–305.

Johnsen, A., Petersen, M., Snyder, C., et al. (2016). How does pain experience relate to the need for pain relief? A secondary exploratory analysis in a larger sample of cancer patients. *Supportive Care in Cancer, 24*(10), 4187–4195.

MacCloud, R., Crandall, J., Wilson, D., et al. (2016). Death anxiety among New Zealanders: The predictive role of gender and marital status. *Mental Health, Religion & Culture, 19*(4), 339–349.

Moore, G. (2013). *The relationship between religious orientation, coping style, and psychological health on death anxiety and life satisfaction. Bachelor's final year project*, Dublin Business School. Retrieved from http://esource.dbs.ie/handle/10788/1604?show=full.

Nouvet, E., Strachan, P., Kryworuchko, J., et al. (2016). Waiting for the body to fail: Limits to end-of-life communication in Canadian hospitals. *Mortality, 21*(4), 340–346.

● = Independent; ▲ = Collaborative; EBN = Evidence-Based Nursing; EB = Evidence-Based

Piers, R., Eechoud, I., VanCamp, S., et al. (2013). Advance care planning in terminally ill and frail older persons. *Patient Education and Counseling*, 90(3), 323–329.

Shukla, P., & Rishi, P. (2014). A correlational study of psychosocial and spiritual well being and death anxiety among advanced stage cancer patients. *American Journal of Applied Psychology*, 2(3), 59–65.

Stenzel, N. M., Vaske, I., Kühl, K., et al. (2015). Prediction of end-of-life fears in COPD—Hoping for the best but preparing for the worst. *Psychology & Health*, 30(9), 1017–1034.

Stern, C., & West, T. (2014). Circumventing anxiety during interpersonal encounters to promote interest in contact: An implementation intention approach. *Journal of Experimental Psychology*, 50, 82–93.

Webb, J., & Guarino, A. (2011). Life after death of a loved one: Long term distress among surrogate decision makers. *Journal of Hospice & Palliative Nursing*, 13(6), 378–386.

Risk for Aspiration   Debra Siela, PhD, RN, CCNS, ACNS-BC, CCRN-K, CNE, RRT

NANDA-I

Definition

Susceptible to entry of gastrointestinal secretions, oropharyngeal secretions, solids, or fluids to the tracheo-bronchial passages, which may compromise health.

Risk Factors

Barrier to elevating upper body; decrease in gastrointestinal motility; ineffective cough; insufficient knowledge of modifiable factors

Associated Condition

Decrease in level of consciousness; delayed gastric emptying; depressed gag reflex; enteral feedings; facial surgery; facial trauma; impaired ability to swallow; incompetent lower esophageal sphincter; increase in gastric residual; increase in intragastric pressure; neck surgery; neck trauma; oral surgery; oral trauma; presence of oral/nasal tube; treatment regimen; wired jaw

NOC   (Nursing Outcomes Classification)

Suggested NOC Outcomes

Aspiration Prevention; Respiratory Status: Ventilation; Swallowing Status

Example NOC Outcome with Indicators

Aspiration Prevention as evidenced by the following indicators: Avoids risk factors/Maintains oral hygiene/Positions self upright for eating and drinking/Selects foods according to swallowing ability/Selects foods and fluid of proper consistency/Remains upright for 30 minutes after eating. (Rate the outcome and indicators of **Aspiration Prevention:** 1 = never demonstrated, 2 = rarely demonstrated, 3 = sometimes demonstrated, 4 = often demonstrated, 5 = continually demonstrated [see Section I].)

Client Outcomes

Client Will (Specify Time Frame)

- Maintain patent airway and clear lung sounds
- Swallow and digest oral, nasogastric, or gastric feeding without aspiration

NIC   (Nursing Interventions Classification)

Suggested NIC Intervention

Aspiration Precautions

Example NIC Activities—Airway Management

Monitor level of consciousness, cough reflex, gag reflex, and swallowing ability; Check nasogastric or gastrostomy residual before feeding

● = Independent;   ▲ = Collaborative;   EBN = Evidence-Based Nursing;   EB = Evidence-Based

A

Nursing Interventions and *Rationales*

- Monitor respiratory rate, depth, and effort. Note any signs of aspiration such as dyspnea, cough, cyanosis, wheezing, hoarseness, foul-smelling sputum, or fever. If new onset of symptoms, then perform oral suction and notify provider immediately. CEB/EB: *Signs of aspiration should be detected as soon as possible to prevent further aspiration and to initiate treatment that can be lifesaving (Swaminathan et al, 2017). Clients with dysphagia may experience silent aspiration because of laryngeal pooling and residue (Metheny, 2011b).*
- Auscultate lung sounds frequently and before and after feedings; note any new onset of crackles or wheezing. CEB: *With decreased symptoms of pneumonia, an increased respiratory rate and/or crackles may be the first sign of pneumonia (Metheny, 2011b).*
- Take vital signs frequently, noting onset of a fever, increased respiratory rate, and increased heart rate.
- Before initiating oral feeding, check client's gag reflex and ability to swallow by feeling the laryngeal prominence as the client attempts to swallow (Rees, 2013; American Association of Critical Care Nurses, 2016a). If client is having problems swallowing, see nursing interventions for Impaired **Swallowing.**
- If client needs to be fed, feed slowly and allow adequate time for chewing and swallowing. EB: *Slowed feeding allows time for more deliberate swallowing, reducing aspiration (Rees, 2013).*
- When feeding client, watch for signs of impaired swallowing or aspiration, including coughing, choking, and spitting food.
- Have suction machine available when feeding high-risk clients. If aspiration does occur, suction immediately. *A client with aspiration needs immediate suctioning and may need further lifesaving interventions such as intubation and mechanical ventilation (Rees, 2013).*
- Keep the head of the bed (HOB) elevated at 30 to 45 degrees, preferably with the client sitting up in a chair at 90 degrees when feeding. Keep head elevated for an hour after eating. EBP: *Decreased gastric reflux occurs at both 30- and 45-degree HOB elevation. Thus gastric-fed patients should be maintained at the highest HOB elevation that is comfortable to prevent aspiration (Metheny & Frantz, 2013).*
- Note presence of nausea, vomiting, or diarrhea. Treat nausea promptly with antiemetics.
- If the client shows symptoms of nausea and vomiting, position on side. *The side-lying position can help the client expel the vomitus and decrease the risk for aspiration (Chard, 2013).*
- Assess the abdomen and listen to bowel sounds frequently, noting if they are decreased, absent, or hyperactive. *Decreased or absent bowel sounds can indicate an ileus with possible vomiting and aspiration; increased high-pitched bowel sounds can indicate a mechanical bowel obstruction with possible vomiting and aspiration (Kasper et al, 2015).*
- Note new onset of abdominal distention or increased rigidity of abdomen. EB: *Abdominal distention or rigidity can be associated with paralytic or mechanical obstruction and an increased likelihood of vomiting and aspiration (Kasper et al, 2015).*
- If client has a tracheostomy, ask for referral to speech pathologist for swallowing studies before attempting to feed. EB: *There is an increased risk for aspiration when tracheostomy tubes are in place, and inflating the cuff does not prevent aspiration (Rees, 2013).*
- Provide meticulous oral care including brushing of teeth at least two times per day. *Good oral care can prevent bacterial or fungal contamination of the mouth, which can be aspirated (American Association of Critical Care Nurses, 2017a).* EB: *Research has shown that excellent dental care/oral care can be effective in preventing hospital-acquired (or extended care–acquired) pneumonia (Munro, 2014).*
- Sedation agents can reduce cough and gag reflexes as well as interfere with the client's ability to manage oropharyngeal secretions. EB: *Using the smallest effective level of sedation may help reduce risk of aspiration (American Association of Critical Care Nurses, 2016a; Barr et al, 2013).*

Enteral Feedings

▲ Insert nasogastric feeding tube using the internal nares to distal lower esophageal sphincter distance. The ear-to-nose-to-xiphoid-process is often inaccurate. EB: *An integrative review of the evidence found the ear-to-nose-to-xiphoid-process to be less accurate than the method using gender, weight, and nose to the umbilicus with the adult's head flat on the bed (GWNUF) (Santos et al, 2016).*

▲ *Verification of gastric tube placement should initially be obtained by radiography. Other methods of assessing proper gastric tube placement include capnography, aspirate assessment, tube markings, and pH tests. Auscultation should not be used to assess gastric tube placement (American Association of Critical Care Nurses, 2016b; Amirlak et al, 2012; Williams et al, 2014).*

• = Independent;   ▲ = Collaborative;   EBN = Evidence-Based Nursing;   EB = Evidence-Based

A

- Tape the feeding tube securely to the nose using a skin protectant under the tape. CEBN: *A research study found that insertion of the feeding tube into the small intestine and keeping the HOB position elevated to at least 30 degrees reduced the incidence of aspiration and aspiration-related pneumonia drastically in critically ill clients (Metheny et al, 2010). Another study found that aspiration and pneumonia were reduced by feeding the clients in the mid-duodenum or farther in the small intestine (Metheny et al, 2011).*
- Check to make sure the initial nasogastric feeding tube placement was confirmed by x-ray, with the openings of the tube in the stomach, not the esophagus or lungs. This is especially important if a small-bore feeding tube is used, although larger tubes used for feedings or medication administration also should be verified by radiography. *Radiographic verification of placement remains the gold standard for determining safe placement of feeding tubes (American Association of Critical Care Nurses, 2016b; Guenter, 2010; Metheny et al, 2012b; Williams et al, 2014).*
- After radiographic verification of correct placement of the tube in the intestines, mark the tube's exit site clearly with tape or a permanent marker (Simons & Abdallah, 2012).
- Measure and record the length of the tube that is outside of the body at defined intervals to help ensure correct placement. *Note the length of the tube outside of the body; it is possible for a tube to slide out and be in the esophagus, without obvious disruption of the tape (American Association of Critical Care Nurses, 2016b; McClave et al, 2016).*
- Note the placement of the tube on any chest or abdominal radiographs that are obtained for the client. *Acutely ill clients receive frequent x-ray examinations. These are available for the nurse to determine continued correct placement of the nasogastric tube (American Association of Critical Care Nurses, 2016b; McClave et al, 2016; Simons & Abdallah, 2012). When using electromagnetic feed tube placement, radiographic confirmation of tube position is preferred because of the variance of the ability of clinicians to place the tube (Metheny & Meert, 2014).*
- Check the pH of the aspirate. *If the pH reading is 4 or less, the tube is probably in the stomach. Recognize that the pH may not indicate correct placement if the client is receiving continuous tube feedings, is receiving a hydrogen ion blocker or proton pump inhibitor, has blood in the aspirate, or is receiving antacids (American Association of Critical Care Nurses, 2016b; Simons & Abdallah, 2012).*
- Use a number of determinants for verification of correct placement before each feeding or every 4 hours if the client is on continuous feeding. Measure length of tube outside the body, and review recent x-ray results and check pH of the aspirate if relevant and its characteristic appearance. If findings do not ensure correct placement of the tube, obtain a radiograph to verify placement. Do not rely on the air insufflation method to assess correct tube placement. EBN: *The auscultatory air insufflation method is not reliable for differentiating between gastric or respiratory placement; the "whooshing" sound can be heard even if the tube is incorrectly placed in the lung (American Association of Critical Care Nurses, 2016b; Simons & Abdallah, 2012; Williams et al, 2014).*
- *Capnography (CO$_2$ sensor) may be used to assess proper tube placement (American Association of Critical Care Nurses, 2016b; Gilbert & Burns, 2012; Williams et al, 2014).*
- Follow unit policy regarding checking for gastric residual volume during continuous feedings or before feedings, and holding feedings if increased residual is present. CEB/EBN: *There is little evidence to support the use of measuring gastric residual volume, and the practice may or may not be effective in preventing aspiration (Makic et al, 2011; McClave et al, 2016). It is still done at intervals (American Association of Critical Care Nurses, 2016b; Metheny et al, 2012a), especially if there is a question of tube feeding intolerance. The practice of holding tube feedings if there is increased residual reduces the amount of calories given to the client. If the client has a small-bore feeding tube, it is difficult to check gastric residual volume and it may be inaccurate. It is unclear if aspiration for residual volumes helps reduce the risk of aspiration (Metheny et al, 2012a); practice guidelines suggest continuing to feed the client until the residual is greater than 500 mL (Canadian Clinical Practice Guidelines, 2013; Elke et al, 2015).*
- Follow unit protocol regarding returning or discarding gastric residual volume. At this time there is no definitive research base to guide practice. CEBN: *A study of the effectiveness of either returning gastric residual volumes to the client or discarding them resulted in inconclusive findings, and more research is needed in the area (Williams & Leslie, 2010).*
- Do not use glucose testing to determine correct placement of enteral tube or to identify aspirated enteral feeding. *Glucose was found in tracheal secretions of clients who were not receiving enteral feedings (Guenter, 2010).*
- Do not use blue dye to tint enteral feedings (Guenter, 2010). *The presence of blue and green skin and urine and serum discoloration from the use of blue dye has been associated with the death of clients. The US Food*

• = Independent;   ▲ = Collaborative;   EBN = Evidence-Based Nursing;   EB = Evidence-Based

A

and Drug Administration (2009) has reported at least 12 deaths from the use of blue dye in enteral feedings.

- During enteral feedings, position client with HOB elevated 30 to 45 degrees (American Association of Critical Care Nurses, 2016a; Schallom et al, 2015). CEB: *HOB elevation greater than 30 degrees is feasible and preferred to 30 degrees for reducing oral secretion volume, reflux, and aspiration without pressure ulcer development in gastric-fed clients receiving mechanical ventilation (American Association of Critical Care Nurses, 2017b; Schallom et al, 2015). A study of mechanically ventilated clients receiving tube feedings demonstrated that there was an increase of the presence of pepsin (from gastric contents) in pulmonary secretions if the client was in a flat position versus being positioned with the head elevated (Metheny & Frantz, 2013). Generally, do not turn off the tube feeding when repositioning clients. Stopping the tube feeding during repositioning is counterproductive because the client receives less nutrition and the rate of emptying of the stomach is slow. If it is imperative to keep the HOB elevated, consider use of reverse Trendelenburg (head higher than feet) when repositioning (Metheny, 2011a) Precautionary withholding of enteral feedings during repositioning does not reduce the incidence of aspiration in critically ill clients (DiLibero et al, 2015).*
- Take actions to prevent inadvertent misconnections with enteral feeding tubes into intravenous (IV) lines or other harmful connections. Safety actions that should be taken to prevent misconnections include:
  - ○ Trace tubing back to origin. Recheck connections at time of client transfer and at change of shift.
  - ○ Label all tubing.
  - ○ Use oral syringes for medications through the enteral feeding; *do not use IV syringes.*
  - ○ Teach nonprofessional personnel to "do not reconnect" if a line becomes dislodged; rather, find the nurse instead of taking the chance of plugging the tube into the wrong place. *Enteral feeding tube lines have been inadvertently plugged into IV peripheral catheters, peritoneal dialysis catheters, central lines, medical gas tubing, and tracheostomies, resulting in death in some cases (Guenter, 2010).*

Critical Care

- Recognize that critically ill clients are at an increased risk for aspiration because of severe illness and interventions that compromise the gag reflex. *Predisposing causes of aspiration include sedation, endotracheal intubation and mechanical ventilation, neurological disorders, altered level of consciousness, hemodynamic instability, and sepsis (American Association of Critical Care Nurses, 2016a; Makic et al, 2011).*
- Recognize that intolerance to feeding as defined by increased gastric residual is more common early in the feeding process. EB: *A study found that feeding intolerance in critical care clients was common in the first 5 days of feeding, and feeding intolerance was associated with increased length of both critical care and hospital length of stay (O'Connor et al, 2011). For clients receiving gastric tube feedings, assess for gastrointestinal intolerance to the feedings at 4-hour intervals (American Association of Critical Care Nurses, 2016a).*
- *Avoid bolus feedings in tube-fed clients who are at high risk for aspiration (American Association of Critical Care Nurses, 2016a).*
- *Maintain endotracheal cuff pressures at an appropriate level to prevent leakage of secretions around the cuff (American Association of Critical Care Nurses, 2016a).*
- *Pepsin and amylase are biomarkers of microaspiration of gastric contents in tracheal aspirate. Amylase presence is a better biomarker of aspiration of oral contents in the tracheal aspirate. Both pepsin and amylase were present in tracheal aspirate of critically ill clients even with backrest elevation of 30 degrees. HOB elevation is inversely related to the presence of pepsin (Sole et al, 2014). For a desired positive predictive value of 100%, a pH cut point of less than 5.0 provides the best negative predictive values, regardless of gastric acid inhibitor administration and feeding status. The pepsin assay is promising as an additional marker to distinguish gastric from tracheal aspirates (Metheny et al, 2017). Although reflux of gastric juice into the oropharynx must precede its aspiration into the lungs, individual reflux events do not necessarily lead to aspiration. Increased pepsin in oral secretions suggests that the client is at risk for aspiration (Schallom et al, 2013).*

 ### Geriatric

- Carefully check older client's gag reflex and ability to swallow before feeding. *A slowed rate of swallowing is common in older adults (Rees, 2013).*
- Watch for signs of aspiration pneumonia in older adults with cerebrovascular accidents, even if there are no apparent signs of difficulty swallowing or of aspiration. *Bedside evaluation for swallow and aspiration can be inaccurate.* EB: *Silent aspiration can occur in the older population (Metheny, 2011b).*
- Recognize that older adults with aspiration pneumonia have fewer symptoms than younger people; repeat cases of pneumonia in older adults are generally associated with aspiration (Eisenstadt, 2010). *Aspiration*

pneumonia can be undiagnosed in older adults because of decreased symptoms; sometimes the only obvious symptom may be new onset of delirium (Metheny, 2011b).

- Use central nervous system depressants cautiously; older clients may have an increased incidence of aspiration with altered levels of consciousness. *Older clients have altered metabolism, distribution, and excretion of drugs. Many medications can interfere with the swallowing reflex, including antipsychotic drugs, proton pump inhibitors, and angiotensin-converting enzyme inhibitors (van der Maarel-Wierink et al, 2011).*
- Keep older, mostly bedridden clients sitting upright for 45 minutes to 1 hour after meals.
- Recommend to families that enteral feedings may or may not be indicated for clients with advanced dementia. Instead, if possible use hand-feeding assistance, modified food consistency as needed, and feeding favorite foods for comfort (Sorrell, 2010). EB/CEB: *Research has demonstrated that tube feedings in this population do not prevent malnutrition or aspiration, improve survival, reduce infections, or result in other positive outcomes (Teno et al, 2010).*

Home Care

- The previously mentioned interventions may be adapted for home care use.
- For clients at high risk for aspiration, obtain complete information from the discharging institution regarding institutional management.
- Assess the client and family for willingness and cognitive ability to learn and cope with swallowing, feeding, and related disorders.
- Assess caregiver understanding and reinforce teaching regarding positioning and assessment of the client for possible aspiration.
- Provide the client with emotional support in dealing with fears of aspiration. *Fear of choking can provoke extreme anxiety, which can interfere with the client's ability or willingness to adhere to the treatment plan.* Refer to care plan for **Anxiety.**
- Establish emergency and contingency plans for care of the client. *Clinical safety of the client between visits is a primary goal of home care nursing.*
- Have a speech and occupational therapist assess the client's swallowing ability and other physiological factors and recommend strategies for working with the client in the home (e.g., pureeing foods served to the client; providing adequate adaptive equipment for independence in eating). *Successful strategies allow the client to remain part of the family.*
- Obtain suction equipment for the home as necessary.
- Teach caregivers safe, effective use of suctioning devices. Inform the client and family that only individuals instructed in suctioning should perform the procedure.
- Institute case management of frail elderly to support continued independent living.

Client/Family Teaching and Discharge Planning

- Teach the client and family signs of aspiration and precautions to prevent aspiration.
- Teach the client and family how to safely administer tube feeding.
- Teach the family about proper client positioning to facilitate feeding and reduce risk of aspiration.
- Verify client family/caregiver knowledge about feeding, aspiration precautions, and signs of aspiration.

REFERENCES

American Association of Critical Care Nurses. (2016a). *AACN Practice Alert—Prevention of aspiration in adults. American Association of Critical Care Nurses.* Retrieved from https://www.aacn.org/~/media/aacn-website/clincial-resources/practice-alerts/preventionaspirationpracticealert.pdf.

American Association of Critical Care Nurses. (2016b). *AACN Practice Alert—Initial and ongoing verification of feeding tube placement in adults. American Association of Critical Care Nurses.* Retrieved from https://www.aacn.org/~/media/aacn-website/clincial-resources/practice-alerts/feedingtubepa.pdf.

American Association of Critical Care Nurses. (2017a). *AACN Practice Alert—Prevention of ventilator-associated pneumonia in adults. American Association of Critical Care Nurses.* Retrieved from https://www.aacn.org/~/media/aacn-website/clincial-resources/practice-alerts/preventingvapinadults2017.pdf. (Accessed 22 February 2018).

American Association of Critical Care Nurses. (2017b). *AACN Practice Alert—Oral care for acutely and critically ill patients. American Association of Critical Care Nurses.* Retrieved from https://www.aacn.org/~/media/aacn-website/clincial-resources/practice-alerts/oralcarepractalert2017.pdf. (Accessed 22 February 2018).

Amirlak, B., et al. (2012). Pneumothorax following feeding tube placement: Precaution and treatment. *Acta Medica Iranica, 50*(5), 355–358.

Barr, J., Fraser, G. L., Puntillo, K., et al. (2013). Clinical practice guidelines for the management of pain, agitation, and delirium in adult patients in the intensive care unit. *Critical Care Medicine, 41*(1), 263–306.

Canadian Clinical Practice Guidelines (2013). *Strategies to optimize the delivery of EN: Use of and threshold for gastric residual volumes.*

• = Independent;   ▲ = Collaborative;   EBN = Evidence-Based Nursing;   EB = Evidence-Based

Retrieved from http://www.criticalcarenutrition.com/docs/cpgs2012/5.5.pdf. (Accessed 20 February 2018).

Chard, R. (2013). Care of postoperative patients. In D. Ignatavicius & M. L. Workman (Eds.), *Medical-surgical nursing: Patient-centered collaborative care* (7th ed., pp. 284–301). St. Louis: W. B. Saunders Company.

DiLibero, J., Lavieri, M., O'Donoghue, S., et al. (2015). Withholding or continuing enteral feedings during repositioning and the incidence of aspiration. *American Journal of Critical Care, 24*(3), 258–262.

Eisenstadt, E. S. (2010). Dysphagia and aspiration pneumonia in older adults. *Journal of American Academy Nursing Practitioners, 22*(1), 17–22.

Elke, G., Felbinger, T. W., & Heyland, D. K. (2015). Gastric residual volume in critically ill patients: A dead marker or still alive? *Nutrition in Clinical Practice, 30*(1), 59–71.

Gilbert, R. T., & Burns, S. M. (2012). Increasing the safety of blind gastric tube placement in pediatric patients. *Journal of Pediatric Nursing, 27*(5), 528–532.

Guenter, P. (2010). Safe practices for enteral nutrition in critically ill patients. *Critical Care Nurse Clinics of North America, 22*(2), 197–208.

Kasper, D., et al. (2015). *Harrison's principles of internal medicine* (19th ed.). New York: McGraw-Hill.

Makic, M. B. F., VonRueden, K. T., Rauen, C. A., et al. (2011). Evidence-based practice habits: putting more sacred cows out to pasture. *Critical Care Nurse, 31*(2), 38–62.

McClave, S., Taylor, B. E., Martindale, R. G., et al. (2016). Guidelines for the provision and assessment of nutrition support therapy in the adult critically ill patient: Society of Critical Care Medicine (SCCM) and American Society for Parenteral and Enteral Nutrition (A.S.P.E.N.). *Journal of Parenteral and Enteral Nutrition and Critical Care Medicine, 40*(2), 159–211.

Metheny, N. A. (2011a). Turning tube feeding off while repositioning patients in bed: Ask the experts. *Critical Care Nurse, 31*(2), 96–97.

Metheny, N. A. (2011b). Preventing aspiration in older adults with dysphagia. *Med-Surg Matters, 20*(5), 6–7.

Metheny, N. A., Davis-Jackson, J., & Stewart, B. (2010). Effectiveness of an aspiration risk-reduction protocol. *Nursing Research, 59*(1), 18–25.

Metheny, N. A., & Frantz, R. A. (2013). Head-of-bed elevation in critically ill patients: A review. *Critical Care Nurse, 33*(3), 53–67.

Metheny, N. A., & Meert, K. L. (2014). Effectiveness of an electromagnetic feeding tube placement device in detecting inadvertent respiratory placement. *American Journal of Critical Care, 23*(3), 240–248.

Metheny, N. A., Mills, A. C., & Stewart, B. J. (2012a). Monitoring for intolerance to gastric tube feedings: A national survey. *American Journal of Critical Care, 21*(2), e33–e40.

Metheny, N. A., Pawluszka, A., Lulic, M., et al. (2017). Testing placement of gastric feeding tubes in infants. *American Journal of Critical Care, 26*(6), 466–473.

Metheny, N. A., Stewart, B. J., & McClave, S. A. (2011). Relationship between feeding tube site and respiratory outcomes. *Journal of Parenteral and Enteral Nutrition, 35*(3), 346–355.

Metheny, N. A., Stewart, B. J., & Mills, A. C. (2012b). Blind insertion of feeding tubes in intensive care units: A national survey. *American Journal of Critical Care, 21*(5), 352–360.

Munro, C. L. (2014). Oral health: Something to smile about! *American Journal of Critical Care, 23*(4), 282–289.

O'Connor, S., Rivett, J., Deane, A., et al. (2011). Nasogastric feeding intolerance in the critically ill—A prospective observational study. *Australian Critical Care, 24*(1), 22.

Rees, H. C. (2013). Care of patients requiring oxygen therapy or tracheostomy. In D. Ignatavicius & M. L. Workman (Eds.), *Medical-surgical nursing: Patient-centered collaborative care* (7th ed., pp. 562–580). St. Louis: W. B. Saunders Company.

Santos, S. C., Woith, W., deFrietas, M. I. P., et al. (2016). Methods to determine the internal length of nasogastric feeding tubes: An integrative review. *International Journal of Nursing Studies, 61*, 95–103.

Schallom, M., Dykeman, B., Kirby, J., et al. (2015). Head-of-bed elevation and early outcomes of gastric reflux, aspiration, and pressure ulcers: A feasibility study. *American Journal of Critical Care, 24*(1), 57–66.

Schallom, M., Tricomi, S., Chang, Y., et al. (2013). A pilot study of pepsin in tracheal and oral secretions. *American Association of Critical Care Nurses, 22*(5), 408–411.

Simons, S. R., & Abdallah, L. M. (2012). Bedside assessment of enteral tube placement aligning practice with evidence. *American Journal of Nursing, 112*(2), 40–48.

Sole, M. L., Conrad, J., Bennett, M., et al. (2014). Pepsin and amylase in oral and tracheal secretions: A pilot study. *American Journal of Critical Care, 23*(4), 334–338.

Sorrell, J. (2010). Use of feeding tubes in patients with advanced dementia. *Journal of Psychosocial Nursing and Mental Health Services, 48*(5), 15–18.

Swaminathan, A., Stearns, D. A., Varkey, A. B., et al. (2017). Aspiration pneumonitis and pneumonia. *Medscape.* Retrieved from http://emedicine.medscape.com/article/296198-overview#aw2aab6b2. (Accessed 20 February 2018).

Teno, J. M., Mitchell, S. L., Gozalo, P. L., et al. (2010). Hospital characteristics associated with feeding tube placement in nursing home residents with advanced cognitive impairment. *Journal of American Medical Association, 303*, 544–550.

US Food and Drug Administration (USFDA). (2009). *Reports of blue dye discoloration and death in patients receiving enteral feedings tinted with the dye, FD & C Blue no. 1.* FDA Public Health Advisory.

van der Maarel-Wierink, C., Vanobbergen, J. N. O., Bronkhorst, E. M., et al. (2011). Risk factors for aspiration pneumonia in frail older people: A systematic review. *Journal of American Medical Directors Association, 12*(5), 344–354.

Williams, T., & Leslie, G. (2010). Should gastric aspirate be discarded or retained when gastric residual volume is removed from gastric tubes? *Australian Critical Care, 23*(4), 215–217.

Williams, T. A., et al. (2014). Frequency of aspirating gastric tubes for patients receiving enteral nutrition in the ICU: A randomized controlled trial. *JPEN. Journal of Parenteral and Enteral Nutrition, 38*(7), 809–816.

● = Independent;   ▲ = Collaborative;   **EBN** = Evidence-Based Nursing;   **EB** = Evidence-Based

Risk for impaired Attachment

Mary Alice DeWys, RN, BS, CIMI and Margaret Elizabeth Padnos, RN, AB, BSN, MA

NANDA-I

Definition

Susceptible to disruption of the interactive process between parent or significant other and child that fosters the development of a protective and nurturing reciprocal relationship.

Risk Factors

Anxiety; child's illness prevents effective initiation of parental contact; disorganized infant behavior; inability of parent to meet personal needs; insufficient privacy; parental conflict resulting from disorganized infant behavior; parent-child separation; physical barrier; substance misuse

At-Risk Population

Premature infant

NOC (Nursing Outcomes Classification)

Suggested NOC Outcomes

Parent-Infant Attachment; Parenting Performance: Psychosocial Adjustment: Life Change

Example NOC Outcomes with Indicators
Holds infant close, touches, strokes, pats infant, responds to infant cues, holds infant for feeding, vocalizes to infant. (Rate the outcome and indicators of appropriate parent and infant behaviors that demonstrate an enduring affectionate bond: 1 = never demonstrated, 2 = rarely demonstrated, 3 = sometimes demonstrated, 4 = often demonstrated, 5 = consistently demonstrated [see Section I].)

Client Outcomes

Parent(s)/Caregiver(s) Will (Specify Time Frame)

- Be willing to consider pumping breast milk (and storing appropriately) or breastfeeding, if feasible
- Demonstrate behaviors that indicate secure attachment to infant/child
- Provide a safe environment, free of physical hazards
- Provide nurturing environment sensitive to infant/child's need for nutrition/feeding, sleeping, comfort, and social play
- Read and respond contingently to infant/child's distress
- Support infant's self-regulation capabilities, intervening when needed
- Engage in mutually satisfying interactions that provide opportunities for attachment
- Give infant nurturing sensory experiences (e.g., holding, cuddling, stroking, rocking)
- Demonstrate an awareness of developmentally appropriate activities that are pleasurable, emotionally supportive, and growth fostering
- Avoid physical and emotional abuse and/or neglect as retribution for parent's perception of infant/child's misbehavior
- State appropriate community resources and support services

NIC (Nursing Interventions Classification)

Suggested NIC Interventions

Anticipatory Guidance; Attachment Promotion; Coping Enhancement; Counseling; Developmental Enhancement: Infant; Family Involvement Promotion; Parent Education: Infant; Parenting Promotion

Example NIC Activities—Anticipatory Guidance
Instruct about normal development and behavior, as appropriate; Provide a ready reference for the client (e.g., educational materials, pamphlets) as appropriate

● = Independent; ▲ = Collaborative; EBN = Evidence-Based Nursing; EB = Evidence-Based

A   Nursing Interventions and *Rationales*

- Establish a trusting relationship with parent/caregiver. EBN: *"Overall, the research indicates that health care professionals urgently need to address the concerns of parents (N = 600) and their emotional reactions, be positive with communication exchanges, encourage parents to seek help, enhance parents' capability to positively explore the sources of social support and fully mobilize all social forces to ease psychological pressure"* (Kong et al, 2013).

- Support mothers of preterm infants in providing pumped breast milk for their babies until they are ready for oral feedings and transitioning from gavage to breast. EBN: *The Spatz Ten Steps model (Spatz, 2004) is associated with "significant improvements in parents' perception of nurses' support for mothers' efforts to breastfeed and [improvement] in the odds of the VLBW [very-low-birth-weight] infant receiving MOM [mother's own milk] at the time of hospital discharge"* (Fugate et al, 2015).

- Identify factors related to postpartum depression (PPD)/major depression and offer appropriate interventions/referrals. EB: *An Australian study of nulliparous women (N = 1507) highlights the need to "integrate concern for physical health with initiatives to address psychological well-being" for extreme tiredness, lower back pain, breast problems, urinary incontinence, perineal pain, constipation, hemorrhoids, and cesarean wound pain* (Woolhouse et al, 2014). EBN: *Because a mother's unpreparedness for premature childbirth may predispose her to "multiple and continuous waves of emotional responses, which will consequently lead to decline in performance … and mental irritation," more attention should be given to support these mothers as the main caregivers of their infants* (Valizadeh et al, 2014).

- Identify eating disorders/comorbid factors related to depression and offer appropriate interventions/referrals. CEB: *Combined psychological stressors of new motherhood and body image concerns of pregnancy may predispose exacerbation of eating disorder symptoms and development of postpartum mood disorders, in which mothers can be nonresponsive, inconsistent, or rejecting of the infant* (Astrachan-Fletcher et al, 2008). EBN: *Even though they may have prioritized food before their children's need—or in the words of one participant (N = 9), "food comes before anything," overall, mothers juggled the competing demands of their eating disorder with their children's needs"* (Stitt & Reupert, 2014). **Additional relevant research:** (Emerson et al, 2017).

- Nurture parents so that they in turn can nurture their infant/child. EB: *Family-centered developmental care (FCDC) is designed to meet the needs of all babies, healthy newborns as well as hospitalized infants, and the needs of families coping with the crisis of the neonatal intensive care unit (NICU) experience* (Craig et al, 2015).

- Offer parents opportunities to verbalize their childhood fears associated with attachment. CEB: *"Parental lack of resolution concerning loss or trauma has been proposed to result in atypical parenting behaviors, which may have a disorganizing effect on the parent–child relationship"* (Bernier & Meins, 2008).

- Suggest journaling or scrapbooking as a way for parents of hospitalized infants to cope with stress and emotions. EB: *Narrative writing provides opportunities to remember and organize events in a meaningful and sensible manner. It helps create a feeling of problem-solving, stops unpleasant feelings, and gradually leads to the fading of negative experiences* (Kadivar et al, 2015).

- Offer parent-to-parent support to parents of infants in the NICU. EBN: *In one neonatal unit, parent-support volunteers collaborated with staff to create an innovative educational and psychosocial support program specifically targeting teen parents to help them increase engagement with their hospitalized infants and their caregiving confidence* (Walsh & Goser, 2013).

- Encourage parents of hospitalized infants to "personalize the baby" by bringing in clothing, pictures of themselves, toys, and tapes of their voices. CEB: *These actions help parents claim the infant as their own and support families' confidence/competence in caring for their infants at their own pace* (Lawhon, 2002).

- Encourage physical closeness using skin-to-skin experiences as appropriate. EB: *Because kangaroo mother care (KMC) provides proven health benefits to high-risk infants, involves parents in their care, and humanizes the NICU experience/environment, it is a commonly recognized model of care for very preterm (VP) infants as well as infants who "are not so preterm and not so tiny babies who are transferred from or admitted to the NICU"* (Davanzo et al, 2013).

- Plan ways for parents and their support system to interact/assist with infant/child caregiving. EB: *As "full participatory, essential, healing partners with the NICU caregiving team," parents should provide "hands-on care to their baby, including early frequent and prolonged skin-to-skin contact as is medically appropriate, participate in medical rounds and nursing shift change reports, and have full access and input to written and electronic medical records"* (Craig et al, 2015).

● = Independent;   ▲ = Collaborative;   EBN = Evidence-Based Nursing;   EB = Evidence-Based

- Educate parents about the importance of the infant–caregiver relationship as a foundation for the development of the infant's self-regulation capacities. EB: *By showing the "calming and regulating effect" of moderate pressure massage, this study contributes to a greater understanding of the influence of self-regulation on the development of play and playfulness in preterm babies and on mothers' participation in such interventions with their infants (Hendel, 2017).*

- Assist parents in developing new caregiving competencies and/or revising/extending old ones. CEB: *Five caregiving domains are identified: (1) being with infant, (2) knowing infant as a person, (3) giving care, (4) communicating/engaging with others regarding infant/parent needs, (5) problem-solving/decision-making/learning (Pridham et al, 1998). EB: A Canadian study of Family Integrated Care programs in 20 level 3 NICUs gives evidence of parents' empowerment by providing "as much of their infant's care as they are able"; benefits include reduced length of stay, decreased readmission, and improved rate of breastfeeding and weight gain (Lee & O'Brien, 2014).*

- Educate parents in reading/responding sensitively to their infant's unique "body language" (behavior cues), which communicates approach ("I'm ready to play"), avoidance/stress ("I'm unhappy. I need a change."), and self-calming ("I'm helping myself"). CEBN: *Mothers with lower competence and more technology-dependent children may perceive their children as more vulnerable and their cues as harder to read (Holditch-Davis et al, 2011). EB: "Learning the principles of neurodevelopment and understanding the meaning of preterm behavioral cues make it possible for NICU caregivers and parents to provide individualized developmentally appropriate, neuroprotective care to each infant" (Altimier & Phillips, 2016).*

- Educate and support parents' ability to relieve the infant/child's stress/distress/pain. CEBN: *In facilitated tucking by parents (FTP), a parent holds the infant in a side-lying, fetal position and offers skin-to-skin contact (SSC) with the hands during a stressful/painful situation (Axelin et al, 2010). EBN: Various studies demonstrate the efficacy of facilitated tucking as a nonpharmacological pain intervention in premature infants as young as 23 weeks' gestational age during such painful procedures as heel sticks, endotracheal suctioning, and venipuncture (Hartley et al, 2015).*

- Guide parents in adapting their behaviors/activities with infant/child cues and changing needs. EB: *Parents' emotional closeness to their preterm NICU infant "may be crucial to the well-being of the newborn, the development of mutual regulation, the establishment of a functioning parent–infant affective relationship and the parents' confidence in their ability to provide care for their baby" (Stefana & Lavelli, 2017).*

- Attend to both parents and infant/child to strengthen high-quality interactions. CEB: *A mother's behavioral and brain responses to her infant's cues may be important predictors of infant development; in cases of maternal depression or substance abuse, an infant's smiling face may fail to elicit positive caregiving (Strathearn et al, 2008). EBN: NICU fathers of preterm infants have been found to exhibit coping strategies and needs different from NICU mothers. As a result, nursing support and intervention need to be tailored to parents individually to sustain caregiving engagement and the transition to postdischarge parenting (Provenzi & Santoro, 2015).* **Additional relevant research:** *(Strathearn & Kim, 2013).*

- Assist parents with providing pleasurable sensory learning experiences (i.e., sight, sound, movement, touch, body awareness). EB: *Therapeutic use of "parent-preferred lullabies" has been shown to improve feeding behaviors and sucking patterns, may increase prolonged periods of quiet-alert states, and enhance bonding, thus decreasing the stress parents associate with premature infant care" (Loewy et al, 2013).*

- Encourage physical closeness using skin-to-skin experiences as appropriate. EB: *When intermittent KMC is not deemed appropriate, parents must be taught alternative ways to minimize negative effects of separation from their baby (e.g., gentle containing touch, proprioceptive sense stimulation, face-to-face visual contact, talking, reading, singing soothing lullabies, and olfactory stimulation (Davanzo et al, 2013).*

- Encourage parents and caregivers to massage their infants and children. CEB: *Preliminary studies suggest that infant massage combined with kinesthetic stimulation may have positive effects on preterm infants: greater weight gain, improved bone mineralization, earlier hospital discharge, and more optimal behavioral and motor responses compared with controls (Massaro et al, 2009). EB: A study of preterm and low-birth-weight infants who received massage reported greater alert and daytime activity in the first month of life; less awakening during sleep, and less crying in the second and third months; and significantly greater weight gain at 2 and 3 months of age compared with infants who did not receive massage (Karbasi et al, 2014).*

- Identify mothers who may need assistance in enhancing maternal role attainment (MRA). CEBN: *"Mothers with more illness-related distress and less alert infants, and unmarried and less educated mothers may need interventions to enhance MRA" (Miles et al, 2011). EBN: "Peer support and role modeling by NICU-based breastfeeding peer counselors helped mothers throughout every stage of their infants' hospitalizations, from*

A

giving them hope to helping them begin to develop maternal identity, to providing anticipatory guidance about taking their infants home" (Rossman et al, 2015).

- Recognize that fathers, compared with mothers, may have different starting points in the attachment process in the NICU because nurses encourage parents to have early SSC. **CEB:** *One study showed that after giving birth prematurely, mothers felt powerless, experiencing the immediate postnatal period as surreal and strange, whereas fathers experienced the birth as a shock but were ready to become immediately involved (Fegran et al, 2008). Results of this Taiwanese study confirm the positive effects of father–infant SSC "in terms of exploring, talking, touching, and caring" as well as the enhancing of the relationship at 3 days postpartum (Chen et al, 2017).* **Additional relevant research:** (Arockisamy et al, 2008).

Pediatric

- Recognize and support infant/child's capacity for self-regulation and intervene when appropriate. **CEB:** *Infants must learn to take in sensory information while simultaneously managing not to become overaroused and overwhelmed by stimuli (DeGangi & Breinbauer, 1997; Greenspan, 1992).*
- Provide lyrical, soothing music in the nursery and at home that is age appropriate (i.e., corrected, in the case of premature infants) and contingent with state/behavioral cues. **EB:** *A study using pacifier-activated lullabies (PALs) sung by the infants' mothers showed improvement in oral feeding skills in preterm infants, including those with brain injuries (Chorna et al, 2014).*
- Recognize and support infant/child's attention capabilities. **CEB:** *"The ability to take an interest in the sights, sounds, and sensations of the world" is a significant developmental milestone (Greenspan & Wieder, 1998).*
- Encourage opportunities for mutually satisfying interactions between infant and parent. **CEB:** *The process of attachment involves communication and synchronous and rhythmic patterns of interaction (Rossetti, 1999).*
- Encourage opportunities for physical closeness. **CEB:** *Despite overwhelming evidence provided by this comprehensive literature review regarding benefits of infant massage (e.g., increased weight gain and bone density), "preterm infant massage is only practiced in 38% of NICUs (Field et al, 2010).* **EB:** *A study evaluating 11 NICUs in 6 European countries concluded that units providing facilities for parents to stay overnight had a higher level of parental presence, with younger mothers, in particular, staying close to their infants (Raisklia et al, 2017).*

Multicultural

- Provide culturally sensitive parent support to new immigrant families and other non–native-English-speaking mothers and families. **CEBN:** *In a study contrasting NICU norms in Christchurch, New Zealand, and Tokyo, Japan, areas of difference in parental support needs included (1) establishment of oral feeding, (2) nursing care–related decision-making, (3) parental information/involvement early in hospitalization, (4) visiting regulations, and (5) Western-based interventions (Ichijima, 2009; Ichijima et al, 2011).* **EB:** *"Within the premise of providing family-centered care is the concept of honoring cultural, ethnic, and socioeconomic diversity; it is imperative that culturally competent care be considered and implemented as a separate standalone aspect when caring for new immigrant families" (Hendson et al, 2015).*
- Discuss cultural norms with families to provide care that is appropriate for enhancing attachment with the infant/child. **EB:** *It is important to consider factors such as who makes decisions on the child's behalf, how the family prefers to communicate and interact with the medical and nursing team, and roles of family members in the home country (Langer et al, 2015).*
- Promote the attachment process in women who have abused substances by providing a culturally based, women-centered treatment environment. **CEB:** *Pregnant/postpartum Asian/Pacific Islander women identified provisions for the newborn, infant health care, parent education, and infant–mother bonding as conducive to their treatment (Morelli et al, 2001).* **EBN:** *In a study of the experiences of mothers of NICU infants with neonatal abstinence syndrome (NAS), participants said that feeling judged for having used illicit drugs during pregnancy interfered with their ability to trust their nurses; these findings "may lead to more customized nursing care for this high-risk population of mothers and infants" (Cleveland & Bonugli, 2014).*
- Promote attachment process/development of maternal sensitivity in incarcerated women. **CEB:** *By creating a simple and uncomplicated plan for an incarcerated mother to pump and store her breast milk, "nurses have the opportunity to change the mothering experience" as they promote maternal–infant attachment and improve health for mother and infant (Allen & Baker, 2013).*
- Empower family members to draw on personal strengths in which multiple worldviews/values are recognized, incorporated, and negotiated. **CEBN:** *According to a Thai study of NICU parents, the need to be strong, to be there, and to care for infants emerged as main themes in parents' stories (Sitanon, 2009).* **EBN:** *A study*

● = Independent;   ▲ = Collaborative;   EBN = Evidence-Based Nursing;   EB = Evidence-Based

conducted in Taiwan concluded that designing an intervention that provides informational, emotional, instrumental, and esteem support for fathers can empower their parenting abilities as well as reduce their stress (Lee et al, 2013).

- Encourage positive involvement and relationship development between children and fathers. **EB:** *Using the HUG Your Baby DVD and family-friendly instructional programs with NICU fathers increased their knowledge of infant behavior and is likely to boost their confidence, promote the parent–child relationship, and strengthen the family unit (Kadivar & Mozafarinia, 2013).*

 Home Care

- The previously mentioned interventions may be adapted for home care use.
- Assess quality of interaction between parent and infant/child. **CEB:** *In a study examining effectiveness of home visiting by paraprofessionals/nurses, outcomes of nurse visitations in particular included more responsive mother–child interaction, less emotional vulnerability in response to fear stimuli among infants, greater infant emotional vitality in response to joy/anger stimuli, and less likelihood of language delays (Olds et al, 2002).*
- Use "interaction coaching" (i.e., teaching mother to let the infant lead) so that the mother will match her interaction style to the baby's cues. **EB:** *During a feeding interaction, when the infant is thought to have "communicative intent," the focus changes from the volume of milk consumed to a coregulated, cue-based approach through which the infant guides the caregiver (Shaker, 2013).* **EBN:** *The coregulated feeding intervention (CoReg) "aims to prevent stress during the feeing and ease the challenge VP infants experience coordinating breathing and swallowing during the early months" (Thoyre et al, 2016).*
- ▲ Provide supportive care for infants and children whose parents have been deployed during wartime. **CEB:** *Given the stressful task facing returning service members (i.e., reintegrating themselves into families "whose internal rhythms have changed and where children have taken on new roles"), the authors advocate for strengthening community support services and adopting public health education measures that reduce the stigma of seeking treatment for posttraumatic stress disorder (Lester & Flake, 2013).*
- Encourage custodial grandparents to use support groups available for caregivers of children. *Although custodial grandparents are disproportionately poor, female, African American or Latino, and isolated from important resources, a growing body of work on resilience suggests that these grandparents may be supported in successfully coping with the challenges of raising their grandchildren (Dolbin-MacNab & Hayslip, 2014).*

REFERENCES

Allen, D., & Baker, B. (2013). Supporting mothering through breastfeeding for incarcerated women. *Journal of Obstetrical & Gynecological Nursing, 42*(Suppl. 1), S103.

Altimier, L., & Phillips, R. (2016). The neonatal integrative developmental care model: advanced clinical adaptations of the seven core measures for neuroprotective family-centered developmental care. *Newborn and Infant Nursing Reviews, 16*(4), 230–244.

Arockisamy, V., Holsti, L., & Albersheim, S. (2008). Fathers' experience in the neonatal intensive care unit: A search for control. *Pediatrics, 121*(2), e215–e222.

Astrachan-Fletcher, E., Veldhuis, C., Lively, N., et al. (2008). The reciprocal effects of eating disorders and the postpartum period: A review of the literature and recommendations for clinical care. *Journal of Women's Health, 17*(2), 227–239. doi:10.1089/jwh.2007.0550.

Axelin, A., Lehtonen, L., Pelander, T., et al. (2010). Mothers' different styles of involvement in preterm infant pain care. *Journal of Obstetrical & Gynecological Nursing, 39*(4), 415–424. doi:10.1111/j.1552-6909.2010.01150.x.

Bernier, A., & Meins, E. (2008). A threshold approach to understanding the origins of attachment disorganization. *Developmental Psychology, 44*(4), 969–982.

Chen, E. M., Gau, M. L., Liu, C. Y., et al. (2017). Effects of father-neonatal skin-to-skin contact on attachment: A randomized controlled trial. *Nursing Research and Practice*, Article ID 8612024. doi:10.1155/2017/8612024.

Chorna, O. D., Slaughter, J. C., Wang, L., et al. (2014). A pacifier-activated music player with mother's voice improves oral feeding in preterm infants. *Pediatrics, 133*(3), 462–468.

Craig, J. W., Glick, C., Phillips, R., et al. (2015). Recommendations for involving the family in developmental care of the NICU baby. *Journal of Perinatology, 35*, S5–S8. doi:10.1038/jp.2015.142.

Cleveland, L. M., & Bonugli, R. (2014). Experiences of mothers of infants with neonatal abstinence syndrome in the neonatal intensive care unit. *Journal of Obstetric, Gynecologic, & Neonatal Nursing, 43*(3), 318–329. doi:10.1111/1552-6909.12306.

Davanzo, R., Pierpaolo, B., Travan, L., et al. (2013). Intermittent kangaroo mother care: A NICU protocol. *Journal of Human Lactation, 29*(3), 332–338.

DeGangi, G. A., & Breinbauer, C. (1997). The symptomatology of infants and toddlers with regulatory disorders. *Journal of Developmental Learning Disabilities, 1*(1), 183–215.

Dolbin-MacNab, M. L., & Hayslip, B., Jr. (2014). Grandparents raising grandchildren. In J. A. Arditti (Ed.), *Family problems: Stress, risk, and resilience* (p. 133). New York: John Wiley & Sons.

Emerson, J. A., Hurley, K. M., Caulfield, L. E., et al. (2017). Maternal mental health symptoms are positively related to emotional and restrained eating attitudes in a statewide sample of mothers participating in a supplemental nutrition program for women, infants and young children. *Maternal & Child Nutrition, 13*(1), doi:10.1111/mcn.12247.

Fegran, L., Helseth, S., & Fagermoen, M. S. (2008). A comparison of mothers' and fathers' experiences of the attachment process in a neonatal intensive care unit. *Journal of Clinical Nursing, 17*(6), 810–816.

● = Independent;   ▲ = Collaborative;   **EBN** = Evidence-Based Nursing;   **EB** = Evidence-Based

Field, T., Diego, M., & Hernandez-Reif, M. (2010). Preterm infant massage therapy research: A review. *Infant Behavior and Development, 33*(2), 115–124.

Fugate, K., Hernandez, I., Ashmeade, T., et al. (2015). Improving human milk and breastfeeding practices in the NICU. *Journal of Obstetric, Gynecologic, & Neonatal Nursing, 44*(3), 426–438. doi:10.1111/1552-6909.12563.

Greenspan, S. I. (1992). *Infancy and early childhood: The practice of clinical assessment and intervention with emotional and developmental challenges.* Madison, CT: International Universities Press.

Greenspan, S. I., & Wieder, S. (1998). *The child with special needs: Encouraging intellectual and emotional growth.* Reading, MA: Perseus Books.

Hartley, K. A., Miller, C. S., & Gephart, S. M. (2015). Facilitated tucking to reduce pain in neonates: Evidence for best practice. *Advances in Neonatal Care, 15*(3), 201–208. doi:10.1097/ANC .0000000000000193.

Hendel, C. (2017). *The effects of moderate pressure massage on self-regulation and play in preterm babies.* Retrieved from Nova Southeastern University, ProQuest Dissertations Publishing.

Hendson, L., Reis, M. D., & Nicholas, D. B. (2015). Health care providers' perspectives of providing cultural competent care in the NICU. *Journal of Obstetric, Gynecologic, & Neonatal Nursing, 44*(1), 17–27. doi:10.1111/1552-6909.12524.

Holditch-Davis, D., Miles, M. S., Burchinal, M. R., et al. (2011). Maternal role attainment with medically fragile infants: part 2. Relationship to the quality of parenting. *Research Nursing Health, 34*(1), 35–48. doi:10.1002/nur.20418.

Ichijima, E. (2009). *Nursing roles in parental support: A cross-cultural comparison between neonatal intensive care units in New Zealand and Japan.* Canterbury, UK: University of Canterbury.

Ichijima, E., Kirk, R., & Hornblow, A. (2011). Parental support in neonatal intensive care units: A cross-cultural comparison between New Zealand and Japan. *Journal of Pediatric Nursing, 26*(3), 206–215.

Kadivar, M., & Mozafarinia, S. M. (2013). Supporting fathers in a NICU: Effects of the HUG your baby program on fathers' understanding of preterm infant behavior. *Journal of Perinatal Education, 22*(2), 113–119.

Kadivar, M., Seyedfatemi, N., Akbari, N., et al. (2015). The effect of narrative writing on maternal stress in neonatal intensive care settings. *Journal of Maternal-Fetal & Neonatal Medicine, 28*(8), 938–943. doi:10.3109/1467058.2014.937699.

Karbasi, S. S., Golestan, M., & Fallah, R. (2014). Effect of massage therapy on sleep behavior in low birth weight infants. *Iranian Journal of Pediatrics, 24*(S2), S47.

Kong, L.-P., Cui, Y., Qiu, Y.-F., et al. (2013). Anxiety and depression in parents of sick neonates: A hospital-based study. *Journal of Clinical Nursing, 22*, 1163–1172. doi:10.1111/jocn.12090.

Langer, T., Cummings, C. L., & Meyer, E. C. (2015). When worlds intersect: practical and ethical challenges when caring for international patients in the NICU. *Journal of Perinatology, 35*, 982–984.

Lawhon, G. (2002). Integrated nursing care: Vital issues important in the humane care of the newborn. *Seminars in Neonatology, 7*, 441–446.

Lee, T. Y., Wang, M. M., Lin, K. C., et al. (2013). The effectiveness of early intervention on paternal stress for fathers of premature infants admitted to a neonatal intensive care unit. *Journal of Advanced Nursing, 69*(5), 1085–1095. doi:10.1111/j .1365-2648.2012.06097.

Lee, S. K., & O'Brien, K. (2014). Parents as primary caregivers in the neonatal intensive care unit. *Canadian Medical Association Journal, 186*(11), 845–847. doi:10.1503/cmaj.130818.

Lester, P., & Flake, E. (2013). How wartime military service affects children and families. *The Future of Children, 23*(2).

Loewy, J., Stewart, K., Dassler, A. M., et al. (2013). The effects of music therapy on vital signs, feeding, and sleep in premature infants. *Pediatrics, 131*(5), 902–918.

Massaro, A. N., Hammad, T. A., Jazzo, B., et al. (2009). Massage with kinesthetic stimulation improves weight gain in preterm infants. *Journal of Perinatology, 29*(5), 352–357. doi:10.1038/ jp.2008.230.

Miles, M. S., Holditch-Davis, D., Burchinal, M. R., et al. (2011). Maternal role attainment with medically fragile infants: Part 1. Measurement and correlates during the first year of life. *Research in Nursing and Health, 34*(1), 20–34. doi:10.1002/nur.20419.

Morelli, P. T., Fong, R., & Oliveira, J. (2001). Culturally competent substance abuse treatment for Asian/Pacific Islander women. *Journal of Human Behavior in the Social Environment, 3*(3/4), 263.

Olds, D. L., Robinson, J. A., O'Brien, R., et al. (2002). Home visiting by paraprofessionals and by nurses: A randomized, controlled trial. *Pediatrics, 110*(3), 486–496.

Pridham, K. F., Limbo, R., Schroeder, M., et al. (1998). Guided participation and development of care-giving competencies for families of low-birth-weight infants. *Journal of Advanced Nursing, 28*(5), 948–958. doi:10.1046/j.1365-2648.1998.00814.

Provenzi, L., & Santoro, E. (2015). The lived experience of fathers of preterm infants in the neonatal intensive care unit: A systematic review of qualitative studies. *Journal of Clinical Nursing, 24*(13–14), 1784–1794.

Raisklia, S., Axelin, A., Toome, L., et al. (2017). Parents' presence and parent-infant closeness in 11 neonatal intensive car units in six European countries vary between and within the countries. *Acta Paediatrica, 106*(6), 878–888.

Rossetti, L. M. (1999). *Infant-toddler assessment.* Boston: Little, Brown and Company.

Rossman, B., Greene, M. M., & Meier, P. P. (2015). The role of peer support in the development of maternal identity for "NICU moms." *Journal of Obstetric, Gynecologic, & Neonatal Nursing, 44*(1), 3–16.

Shaker, C. S. (2013). Cue-based feeding in the NICU: Using the infant's communication as a guide. *Neonatal Network, 32*(6), 404–408.

Sitanon, T. (2009). *Thai parents' experiences of parenting preterm infants during hospitalization in the neonatal intensive care unit.* Seattle: University of Washington School of Nursing.

Spatz, D. L. (2004). Ten steps for promoting and protecting breastfeeding for vulnerable infants. *Journal of Perinatal & Neonatal Nursing, 18*(4), 385–396.

Stefana, A., & Lavelli, M. (2017). Parental engagement and early interactions with preterm infants during the stay in the neonatal intensive care unit: Protocol of a mixed-method and longitudinal study. *BMJ Open, 7*(2), e013824.

Stitt, N., & Reupert, A. (2014). Mothers with an eating disorder: 'food comes before anything.' *Journal of Psychiatric & Mental Health Nursing, 21*(6), 509–517.

Strathearn, L., & Kim, S. (2013). Mothers' amygdala response to positive or negative infant affect is modulated by personal relevance. *Frontiers in Neuroscience, 7*, 176.

Strathearn, L., Li, J., Fonagy, P., et al. (2008). What's in a smile? Maternal brain responses to infant facial cues. *Pediatrics, 122*(1), 40–51.

Thoyre, S. M., Hubbard, D., Park, J., et al. (2016). Implementing co-regulated feeding with mothers of preterm infants. *MCN, American Journal of Maternal Child Nursing, 41*(4), 204–211.

Valizadeh, L., Zamanzadeh, V., Mohammadi, E., et al. (2014). Continuous and multiple waves of emotional responses: Mother's experience with a premature infant. *Iranian Journal of Nursing and Midwifery Research, 19*(4), 340–348.

● = Independent;   ▲ = Collaborative;   **EBN** = Evidence-Based Nursing;   **EB** = Evidence-Based

Walsh, J., & Goser, L. (2013). Development of an innovative NICU teen parent support program: One unit's experience. *Journal of Perinatal & Neonatal Nursing, 27*(2), 176–183.

Woolhouse, H., Gartland, D., Perlen, S., et al. (2014). Physical health after childbirth and maternal depression in the first 12 months post partum: Results of an Australian nulliparous pregnancy cohort study. *Midwifery, 30*(3), 378–384. doi:10.1016/j.midw.2013.03.006.

Autonomic Dysreflexia *Ellen MacKinnon, MS, RN, CNRN, AGCNS-BC*

NANDA-I

Definition

Life-threatening, uninhibited sympathetic response of the nervous system to a noxious stimulus after a spinal cord injury at the 7th thoracic vertebra (T7) or above.

Defining Characteristics

Blurred vision; bradycardia; chest pain; chilling; conjunctival congestion; diaphoresis above the injury; diffuse pain in different areas of the head; Horner's syndrome; metallic taste in mouth; nasal congestion; pallor below injury; paresthesia; paroxysmal hypertension; pilomotor reflex; red blotches on skin above the injury; tachycardia

Related Factors

Gastrointestinal Stimuli

Constipation; difficult passage of feces; digital stimulation; enemas; fecal impaction; suppositories

Integumentary Stimuli

Cutaneous stimulation; skin irritation

Musculoskeletal-Neurological Stimuli

Irritating stimuli below level of injury; painful stimuli below level of injury; pressure over bony prominence; pressure over genitalia; range of motion exercises; spasm

Regulatory-Situational Stimuli

Constrictive clothing; environmental temperature fluctuations; positioning

Reproductive-Urological Stimuli

Bladder distention; bladder spasm; instrumentation; sexual intercourse

Other

Insufficient caregiver knowledge of disease process; insufficient knowledge of disease process

At-Risk Population

Ejaculation; extremes of environmental temperature; menstruation

Associated Condition

Bowel distention; cystitis; deep vein thrombosis; detrusor sphincter dyssynergia; epididymitis; esophageal reflux disease; fracture; gallstones; gastric ulcer; gastrointestinal system pathology; hemorrhoids; heterotopic bone; labor and delivery period; ovarian cyst; pharmaceutical agent; pregnancy; pulmonary emboli; renal calculi; substance withdrawal; sunburn; surgical procedure; urethritis; urinary catheterization; urinary tract infection; wound

NOC (Nursing Outcomes Classification)

Suggested NOC Outcomes

Neurological Status; Neurological Status: Autonomic; Vital Signs

● = Independent;   ▲ = Collaborative;   EBN = Evidence-Based Nursing;   EB = Evidence-Based

A

Client Outcomes

Client Will (Specify Time Frame)

- Maintain baseline blood pressure
- Remain free of dysreflexia symptoms
- Explain symptoms, treatment, and prevention of dysreflexia

NIC (Nursing Interventions Classification)

Suggested NIC Intervention

Dysreflexia Management

Nursing Interventions and *Rationales*

- Teach spinal cord injury (SCI) patients about potential causes, symptoms, treatment, and prevention of autonomic dysreflexia (AD). EB: *The nurse should inform the individual and his or her family about the signs and symptoms of AD. Written material about AD treatment should be given to the client as well. The nurse should emphasize the importance of keeping a dysreflexia diary and encourage patients to carry an AD card at all times (Vatansever, 2015).*
- Monitor the client for symptoms of dysreflexia, particularly those with high-level and more complete spinal cord injuries. See Defining Characteristics. EB: *This condition most commonly occurs in individuals with lesions at or above the level of sympathetic splanchnic outflow (T6), with incidence increasing with more clinically complete SCI (Solinsky et al, 2016). The most common signs and symptoms of AD are a sudden increase in systolic blood pressure (SBP) of at least 20 mm Hg from baseline, bradycardia, pounding headache, diaphoresis, flushing, and piloerection above the level of injury. Symptoms of AD are observed in about 85% of patients with injuries at T6 and above (Liepvre et al, 2017; Vatansever, 2015).*
- ▲ Collaborate with providers and caregivers to identify the cause of dysreflexia. AD is triggered by a stimulus from below the level of injury, leading to systemic vasoconstriction. The most common triggers are bladder distension, kidney stones, kink in urinary catheter, urinary tract infection, fecal impaction, pressure ulcer, ingrown toenail, menstruation, hemorrhoids, tight clothing, invasive testing, and sexual intercourse (Caruso et al, 2015; Wan & Krassioukov, 2014). EB: *Medical personnel, caregivers, and individuals with SCI should be aware about the timely diagnosis and management of this life-threatening condition that can result in a variety of significant complications including stroke, seizures, myocardial ischemia, and death (Wan & Krassioukov, 2014).*
- If dysreflexia symptoms are present, immediately place client in high Fowler's position, remove all support hoses or binders, loosen clothing, check the urinary catheter for kinks, and attempt to determine the noxious stimulus causing the response. Check the patient's blood pressure every 3 to 5 minutes. If blood pressure cannot be decreased following these initial interventions, notify the provider emergently (i.e., STAT). EB: *Sitting allows some gravitational pooling of blood in the lower extremities. Survey the person for instigating causes beginning with the most common cause, the urinary system. To determine the stimulus for dysreflexia:*
  - ○ First, assess bladder function. Check for distention, and if present catheterize the client using an anesthetic jelly as a lubricant. Do not use the Valsalva maneuver or Crede's method to empty the bladder because this form of reflex voiding could worsen AD. Ensure existing catheter patency and irrigate if necessary. Also assess for signs of urinary tract infection. EB: *Bladder distension or irritation is responsible for up to 90% of AD cases (O'Stephenson & Berliner, 2017; Vatansever, 2015).*

• = Independent;   ▲ = Collaborative;   EBN = Evidence-Based Nursing;   EB = Evidence-Based

○ Second, assess bowel function. Numb the bowel area with a topical anesthetic as ordered and gently check for impaction. **EB:** *Check the rectal vault. Instill lidocaine gel into the rectum, pause 2 minutes, and gently remove any stool (Solinsky et al, 2016). For clients who require manual removal of stool, pretreatment with lidocaine cream may decrease the flow of impulses from the bowel and lower blood pressure during removal (Faaborg et al, 2014).*

○ Third, assess the skin. Look for any pressure points, wounds, and ingrown toenails. **EB:** *Any noxious stimuli can cause AD. Although bladder and intestinal problems are most common, approximately 2% of AD cases are attributed to skin issues (Vatansever, 2015).*

▲ Initiate antihypertensive therapy as soon as ordered and monitor for cardiac dysrhythmias. **EB:** *Because of the large amount of sympathetic discharge following AD, clients in hypertensive crisis are at risk for arrhythmias, myocardial infarction, cerebral hemorrhage, seizures, and death (Furlan, 2013; Wan & Krassioukov, 2014). Antihypertensives should be administered when SBP remains at 150 mm Hg. Nitrates and nifedipine are most commonly used for acute episodes of AD, whereas clonidine is most effective for recurrent AD (Biering-Sorensen et al, 2018; Caruso et al, 2015; O'Stephenson & Berliner, 2017).*

● Monitor vital signs every 3 to 5 minutes during an acute event; continue to monitor vital signs after event is resolved (e.g., symptoms resolve and vital signs return to baseline, usually up to 2 hours postevent). **EB:** *Monitor pulse and blood pressure every 2 to 5 minutes during an episode of AD, keeping in mind that impaired autonomic function can lead to labile blood pressure. Monitor for rebound hypotension following antihypertensive administration (O'Stephenson & Berliner, 2017).*

● Watch for complications of dysreflexia, including signs of cerebral hemorrhage, seizures, cardiac dysfunction, or intraocular hemorrhage. **EB:** *Extremely high blood pressure can cause intracranial hemorrhage, myocardial injury and dysfunction, and death (Wan & Krassioukov, 2014).*

● Accurately and completely record any incidences of dysreflexia; especially note the precipitating stimuli. *It is imperative to determine the noxious stimuli that precipitated AD and whether the condition is recurrent, requiring the client to take medications routinely or to implement different interventions to prevent repeat incidences (Wan & Krassioukov, 2014).*

● Use the following interventions to prevent dysreflexia:
  ○ Ensure catheter patency and empty urinary catheter bags frequently. Assess the client for signs and symptoms of urinary tract infection during every shift. **EB:** *Approximately 90% of AD episodes are caused by genitourinary issues (Vatansever, 2015).*
  ○ Ensure a regular pattern of defecation to prevent fecal impaction. **EB:** *Approximately 8% of AD episodes can be attributed to the gastrointestinal system (Vatansever, 2015). A regular bowel program is essential in preventing constipation, impaction, or ileus. Topical lidocaine is useful in preventing dysreflexia from occurring during a bowel program (O'Stephenson & Berliner, 2017).*
  ○ Frequently change position of client to relieve pressure and prevent formation of pressure injuries. **EB:** *Routine weight shifts while sitting and frequent skin checks are imperative in preventing pressure injury. Any skin breakdown should be addressed by a physician or wound care personnel (O'Stephenson & Berliner, 2017).*

▲ Notify all health care team members of recurrent AD episodes. **EB:** *Recurrent dysreflexia may be caused by an occult or insidious pathophysiological process, which requires a more comprehensive workup (Biering-Sorensen et al, 2018).*

▲ For female clients with SCI, assess the client for AD during menstrual cycle. If the client becomes pregnant, collaborate with obstetrical health care practitioners to monitor for signs and symptoms of dysreflexia. **EB:** *In a recent cohort study, 60% of pregnant women with a spinal cord lesion above T6 experienced AD, with two cases resulting in cerebral hemorrhage during labor. Pregnancy in the female SCI population must be preceded by preconceptional consultation with a multidisciplinary team including both prenatal and neurological specialists (Liepvre et al, 2017).*

Home Care

● The previously mentioned interventions may be adapted for home care use.

● Provide the client and caregiver with written information on common causes of AD and initial treatment. **EB:** *Despite the availability of consensus-based resources, first responders and emergency room (ER) health care professionals (HCPs) have limited knowledge regarding AD (Krassioukov et al, 2016). An AD card is available from the Craig Hospital Autonomic Dysreflexia Resources page (see https://craighospital.org/uploads/Educational-PDFs/624.CRADEnglishWalletID.pdf) as well as from the Christopher and Dana Reeve Foundation*

● = Independent;   ▲ = Collaborative;   **EBN** = Evidence-Based Nursing;   **EB** = Evidence-Based

A

(see https://www.christopherreeve.org/living-with-paralysis/free-resources-and-downloads/wallet-cards) (Craig, 2015; Christopher and Dana Reeve Foundation, 2015).

- Provide resources to clients with any known proclivity toward dysreflexia. Advise them to wear a medical alert bracelet and carry a medical alert wallet card when not accompanied by knowledgeable caregivers. **EB:** *Always keep an AD emergency kit on hand. Include the following items: blood pressure cuff, lubricating jelly (for rectal check), spare urinary catheter and insertion kit, bladder irrigation kit, and prescribed antihypertensives (Craig, 2015).*
- ▲ Establish an emergency plan: maintain a current prescription of antihypertensive medication, and administer antihypertensives when dysreflexia is refractory to nonmedicinal interventions. If SBP remains over 150 mm Hg following the previously mentioned interventions, go to the nearest ER and present the AD wallet card on arrival. **EB:** *A paucity of knowledge regarding AD diagnosis and treatment still exists among ER HCPs; therefore it is important to present the wallet card on arrival to ensure safe and effective care (Krassioukov et al, 2016).*
- When an episode of dysreflexia has resolved, continue to monitor blood pressure every 30 to 60 minutes for the next 2 hours or admit to an institution for observation. **EB:** *AD may resolve following administration of antihypertensive medication; however, if the underlying cause is not corrected, recurrence should be expected (O'Stephenson & Berliner, 2017).*

 Client/Family Teaching and Discharge Planning

- Teach recognition of early dysreflexia symptoms, appropriate interventions, and the need to obtain help immediately. Give client a written card describing signs and symptoms of AD and initial actions. **EB:** *Clients and caregivers at risk for not understanding the key elements of AD occurrence and management are clients with nontraumatic etiologies, those with T5 or lower injuries, those in the youngest age group at injury, and those who had a shorter duration of injury (Schottler et al, 2009). Clients have reported knowledge gaps regarding AD and experiencing symptoms of AD, but not recognizing the condition (McGillivray et al, 2009).*
- Teach steps to prevent dysreflexia episodes: routine bladder and bowel care, pressure injury prevention, and preventing other forms of noxious stimuli (e.g., not wearing clothing that is too tight, nail care). Discuss the potential impact of sexual intercourse and pregnancy on AD. **EB:** *Sperm retrieval methods used in men with SCI lesions at T6 and above can stimulate an episode of AD (Ibrahim et al, 2016).*

REFERENCES

Biering-Sorensen, F., Biering-Sorensen, T., Liu, N., et al. (2018). Alterations in cardiac autonomic control in spinal cord injury. *Autonomic Neuroscience, 209,* 4–18. Retrieved from https://doi.org/10.1016/j.autneu.2017.02.004.

Caruso, D., Gater, D., & Harnish, C. (2015). Prevention of recurrent autonomic dysreflexia: A survey of current practice. *Clinical Autonomic Research, 25,* 293. Retrieved from https://doi-org.aurarialibrary.idm.oclc.org/10.1007/s10286-015-0303-0.

Christopher and Dana Reeve Foundation. *Paralysis Resource Center, AD Card.* Retrieved from http://www.christopherreeve.org/site/c.mtKZKgMWKwG/b.7717499/k.D633/Autonomic_Dysreflexia_AD_Card__Send_to_a_Friend/apps/ka/ecard/choosecard.asp. (Accessed 15 June 2015).

Craig. (2015). *Autonomic Dysreflexia.* Retrieved from https://craighospital.org/resources/disreflexia-autónoma. (Accessed 10 October 2015).

Faaborg, P. M., Christensen, P., Krassioukov, A., et al. (2014). Autonomic Dysreflexia during bowel evacuation procedures and bladder filling in subjects with spinal cord injury. *Spinal Cord, 52,* 494–498.

Furlan, J. C. (2013). Autonomic dysreflexia: A clinical emergency. *The Journal of Trauma and Acute Care Surgery, 75*(3), 496–500.

Ibrahim, E., Lynne, C. M., & Brackett, N. L. (2016). Male fertility following spinal cord injury: An update. *Andrology, 4,* 13–26. doi:10.1111/andr.12119.

Krassioukov, A., Tomasone, J. R., Pak, M., et al. (2016). "The ABCs of AD": A prospective evaluation of the efficacy of an educational

intervention to increase knowledge of autonomic dysreflexia management among emergency health care professionals. *The Journal of Spinal Cord Medicine, 39*(2), 190–196.

Liepvre, H. L., Dinh, A., Chamois, B., et al. (2017). Pregnancy in spinal cord-injured women: A cohort study of 37 pregnancies in 25 women. *Spinal Cord, 55,* 167–171. doi:10.1038/sc.2016.138.

McGillivray, C. F., Hitzig, S. L., Craven, B. C., et al. (2009). Evaluating knowledge of autonomic dysreflexia among individuals with spinal cord injury and their families. *The Journal of Spinal Cord Medicine, 32*(1), 54–62.

O'Stephenson, R., & Berliner, J. (2017). *Autonomic dysreflexia in spinal cord injury.* Retrieved from https://emedicine.medscape.com/article/322809-overview. (Accessed 10 October 2017).

Schottler, J., et al. (2009). Patient and caregiver knowledge of autonomic dysreflexia among youth with spinal cord injury. *Urology, 77*(1), 83–87.

Solinsky, R., Svircev, J. N., James, J. J., et al. (2016). A retrospective review of safety using a nursing driven protocol for autonomic dysreflexia in patients with spinal cord injury. *The Journal of Spinal Cord Medicine, 39*(6), 713–719.

Vatansever, N. (2015). A nursing diagnosis: autonomic dysreflexia. *International Journal of Caring Sciences., 8*(3), 837–842.

Wan, D., & Krassioukov, A. (2014). Life-threatening outcomes associated with autonomic dysreflexia: A clinical review. *The Journal of Spinal Cord Medicine, 37*(1), 2–10.

● = Independent;   ▲ = Collaborative;   EBN = Evidence-Based Nursing;   EB = Evidence-Based

Risk for Autonomic Dysreflexia   *Mary Beth Flynn Makic, PhD, RN, CCNS, FAAN, FNAP*

NANDA-I

Definition

Susceptible to life-threatening, uninhibited response of the sympathetic nervous system post-spinal shock, in an individual with spinal cord injury or lesion at the 6th thoracic vertebra (T6) or above (has been demonstrated in patients with injuries at the 7th thoracic vertebra [T7] and the 8th thoracic vertebra [T8]), which may compromise health.

Risk Factors

Gastrointestinal Stimuli

Bowel distention; constipation; difficult passage of feces; digital stimulation; enemas; fecal impaction; suppositories

Integumentary Stimuli

Cutaneous stimulations; skin irritation; sunburn; wound

Musculoskeletal-Neurological Stimuli

Irritating stimuli below level of injury; painful stimuli below level of injury; pressure over bony prominence; pressure over genitalia; range of motion exercises; spasm

Regulatory-Situational Stimuli

Constrictive clothing; environmental temperature fluctuations; positioning

Reproductive-Urological Stimuli

Bladder distention; bladder spasm; instrumentation; sexual intercourse

Other

Insufficient caregiver knowledge of disease process; insufficient knowledge of disease process

At-Risk Population

Ejaculation; extremes of environmental temperature; menstruation

Associated Condition

Bowel distention; cystitis; deep vein thrombosis; detrusor sphincter dyssynergia; epididymitis; esophageal reflux disease; fracture; gallstones; gastric ulcer; gastrointestinal system pathology; hemorrhoids; heterotopic bone; labor and delivery period; ovarian cyst; pharmaceutical agent; pregnancy; pulmonary emboli; renal calculi; substance withdrawal; sunburn; surgical procedure; urethritis; urinary catheterization; urinary tract infection; wound

NIC, NOC, Client Outcomes, Nursing Interventions and *Rationales,* Client/Family Teaching and Discharge Planning, and References

Refer to care plan for **Autonomic Dysreflexia.**

Risk for Bleeding   *Tara Cuccinelli, RN, MS, ACCNS-BC*

NANDA-I

Definition

Susceptible to a decrease in blood volume, which may compromise health.

Risk Factors

Insufficient knowledge of bleeding precautions

● = Independent;   ▲ = Collaborative;   EBN = Evidence-Based Nursing;   EB = Evidence-Based

B

At-Risk Population

History of falls

Associated Condition

Aneurysm; circumcision; disseminated intravascular coagulopathy; gastrointestinal condition; impaired liver function; inherent coagulopathy; postpartum complication; pregnancy complication; trauma; treatment regimen

NOC   (Nursing Outcomes Classification)

Suggested NOC Outcomes

Blood Coagulation; Blood Loss Severity; Circulation Status; Fall Prevention Behavior; Gastrointestinal Function; Knowledge: Personal Safety, Maternal Status, Physical Injury Severity, Risk Control, Safe Home Environment, Vital Signs

Example NOC Outcome with Indicators

Blood Coagulation as evidenced by the following indicators: Clot formation/International normalized ratio (INR)/Hemoglobin (HGB)/Platelet Count/Bleeding/Bruising/Hematuria/Hematemesis. (Rate the outcome and indicators of **Blood Coagulation:** 1 = severe deviation from normal range, 2 = substantial deviation from normal range, 3 = moderate deviation from normal range, 4 = mild deviation from normal range, 5 = no deviation from normal range.)

Client Outcomes

Client Will (Specify Time Frame)

- Discuss precautions to prevent bleeding complications
- Explain actions that should be taken if bleeding happens
- Maintain adherence to agreed on anticoagulant medication and laboratory work regimens
- Monitor for signs and symptoms of bleeding
- Maintain a mean arterial pressure above 70 mm Hg, a heart rate between 60 and 100 beats per minute with a normal rhythm, and urine output greater than 0.5 mL/kg/hr
- Maintain warm, dry skin

NIC   (Nursing Interventions Classification)

Suggested NIC Interventions

Admission Care; Bleeding Precautions; Bleeding Reduction; Blood Product Administration; Circumcision Care; Fluid Management; Health Screening; Hemorrhage Control; Neurologic Monitoring; Postpartum Care; Risk Identification; Teaching: Disease Process; Teaching: Prescribed Medication; Oxygen Therapy; Shock Prevention; Surveillance; Vital Signs Monitoring

Example NIC Activities—Bleeding Precautions

Monitor the client closely for hemorrhage; Monitor coagulation studies; Monitor orthostatic vital signs, including blood pressure; Instruct the client and/or family on signs of bleeding and appropriate actions in case bleeding occurs

Nursing Interventions and *Rationales*

- Perform admission fall risk assessment. Safety precautions should be implemented for all at-risk clients. EBN: *On client admission to any health care facility, nurses should assess for fall risk factors that could increase the risk of bleeding (Kampfen et al, 2014).*
- Monitor the client closely for hemorrhage, especially in those at increased risk for bleeding. Watch for any signs of bleeding, including bleeding of the gums, nosebleed, blood in sputum, emesis, urine or stool, bleeding from a wound, bleeding into the skin with petechiae, and purpura. EB: *Clients at increased risk for bleeding may include older individuals (>60 years of age) and individuals with active gastroduodenal ulcer, anemia, intrapartum and postpartum women, previous bleeding episode, hypertension, labile INRs or INR greater than 3.0, low platelet count, active malignancy, renal or liver failure, intensive care unit stay,*

● = Independent;   ▲ = Collaborative;   EBN = Evidence-Based Nursing;   EB = Evidence-Based

B

drug or alcohol use, coadministration of antiplatelets and nonsteroidal antiinflammatory drugs (NSAIDs), and antithrombotic and anticoagulant therapies (Hastings-Tolsma et al, 2013; Shoeb & Fang, 2013).

- If bleeding develops, apply pressure over the site or appropriate artery as needed. Apply pressure dressing; if unable to stop the bleeding, then consider a tourniquet if indicated. EB: *Nonpharmacological means, such as application of pressure, may reduce bleeding (Makris et al, 2013; Raval et al, 2017).*

▲ Collaborate on an appropriate bleeding management plan, including nonpharmacological and pharmacological measures to stop bleeding based on the antithrombotic used. EB: *Recommendations for bleeding risk prevention and management carefully weigh the risks and benefits of nonpharmacological and pharmacological interventions (Makris et al, 2013).*

▲ Monitor coagulation studies, including prothrombin time, INR, activated partial thromboplastin time (aPTT), fibrinogen, fibrin degradation/split products, and platelet counts as appropriate. EB: *New direct oral anticoagulants (DOACs) often have no requirement for routine coagulation studies; however, vigilance is still warranted because the risk for bleeding without benefit of reversal agents exists, except for dabigatran (Pradaxa), which can be reversed with intravenous (IV) idarucizumab (Praxbind) (Siegal & Crowther, 2013; Levy, 2014; Burnett et al, 2016; Raval et al, 2017). INR is the preferred method to evaluate warfarin therapy, typically at least 16 hours after the last dose is administered. Dose adjustments will not result in a steady-state INR value for up to 3 weeks (Witt et al, 2016).* CEB: *Assess vital signs at frequent intervals to assess for physiological evidence of bleeding, such as tachycardia, tachypnea, and hypotension. Symptoms may include dizziness, shortness of breath, altered mental status, and fatigue.* EB: *Carefully assess for compensatory changes associated with bleeding, including increased heart rate and respiratory rate. Initially blood pressure may be stable, before beginning to decrease. Assess for orthostatic blood pressure changes (drop in systolic by >20 mm Hg and/or a drop in diastolic by >10 mm Hg in 3 minutes) by taking blood pressure with the client in lying, sitting, and standing positions (Emergency Nurses Association, 2017).*

▲ Monitor all medications for potential to increase bleeding, including antiplatelets, NSAIDs, selective serotonin reuptake inhibitors (SSRIs), and complementary and alternative therapies such as coenzyme Q10 and ginger. EB: *Antiplatelet medications can increase the risk of bleeding in high-risk clients (ginger, when taken with medicines that slow clotting, may increase the chances for bruising and bleeding).* CEB: *There are a multitude of medications including over-the-counter medications and herbs/natural supplements that can interact with anticoagulants. When any of these medications are stopped or started, closer monitoring of INR may be warranted (Burnett et al, 2016; Witt et al, 2016; Harter, Levine, Henderson, 2015).*

Safety Guidelines for Anticoagulant Administration: Joint Commission National Patient Safety Goals

Follow approved protocol for anticoagulant administration:
- Use prepackaged medications and prefilled or premixed parenteral therapy as ordered
- Check laboratory tests (i.e., INR) before administration
- Use programmable pumps when using parenteral administration
- Ensure appropriate education for client/family and all staff concerning anticoagulants used
- Notify dietary services when warfarin is prescribed (to provide consistent vitamin K in diet)
- Monitor for any symptoms of bleeding before administration. EB: *Standard defined protocols can decrease errors in administration (Joint Commission, 2016; Witt et al, 2016).*
- Anticoagulation therapy is complex. EBN: *Nurses have an integral role in medication management through the education of clients.* EB: *Medication reconciliation techniques and predischarge education used by pharmacists in an emergency department setting demonstrated enhanced accuracy of preadmission medication listings, resulting in a reduction in readmission rates (Gardella, Cardwell, & Nnadi, 2012; Nutescu et al, 2013).* CEB: *Risk of bleeding is reduced in clients who receive appropriate education in anticoagulant therapy use (Joint Commission, 2016).*

▲ Before administering anticoagulants, assess the clotting profile of the client. If the client is on warfarin, assess the INR. If the INR is outside of the recommended parameters, then notify the provider. EB: *Target INR for warfarin is between 2 and 3 for nonvalvular atrial fibrillation and between 2.5 and 3.5 for valvular atrial fibrillation. Risk for bleeding is increased when INR is >4 and risk for thromboembolism increases when INR is <1.7. A single slightly out of range INR <0.3 units above or below therapeutic range may just be monitored. It is not recommended to skip or boost doses for a slightly out of range INR in the absence of bleeding (Witt et al, 2016).*

▲ Recognize that vitamin K for vitamin K antagonists (e.g., warfarin, phenprocoumon, Sinthrome, and phenindione) may be given orally or IV as ordered for INR levels greater than 4.5 without signs of

● = Independent; ▲ = Collaborative; EBN = Evidence-Based Nursing; EB = Evidence-Based

B

bleeding. In the case of major bleeding, prohemostatic therapies may be warranted for the rapid reversal of vitamin K antagonists (tranexamic acid, fresh frozen plasma, cryoprecipitate, platelet transfusion, fibrinogen concentrate, factor IV prothrombin complex concentrate [KCentra], and activated prothrombin complex concentrate) (Makris et al, 2013; Witt et al, 2016). EB: *With INR levels above 4.5, it is recommended to give vitamin K rather than withholding the warfarin; administration of vitamin K is by oral or IV route, because subcutaneous and intramuscular routes result in erratic absorption (Christos & Naples, 2016).*

▲ Manage fluid resuscitation and volume expansion as ordered. EB: *A Cochrane systematic review including 86 trials and more than 5000 subjects suggested that there is no evidence that any one colloidal solution is safer or more effective than any other (Bunn & Trivedi, 2012).* CEB: *Blood products (including human albumin), nonblood products, or combinations can be used to restore circulating blood volume in individuals at risk for blood losses from trauma, burns, or surgery. Administration of albumin over normal sterile saline does not alter survival rates (Alderson et al, 2004).*

▲ Consider use of permissive hypotension and restrictive transfusion strategies when treating bleeding episodes. EB: *Hypotensive resuscitation (permissive hypotension), which maintains effective although low mean arterial pressures, may allow adequate perfusion without disruption of coagulation mechanisms, although additional research is warranted (Gourgiotis et al, 2013). A study of 921 subjects with upper gastrointestinal bleeding suggested that restrictive strategies (transfusing when HGB levels fell to below 7 g/dL) improved survival (P = .02) and resulted in fewer adverse events (P = .02) (Villanueva, 2013).*

▲ Consider discussing the coadministration of a proton-pump inhibitor alongside traditional NSAIDs, or with the use of a cyclooxygenase 2 inhibitor with the prescriber. EB: *Risk of NSAID-related bleeding may be reduced with the use of a proton-pump inhibitor or cyclooxygenase 2 inhibitor (Burnett et al, 2016; Witt et al, 2016).*

● Ensure adequate nurse staffing to provide a high level of surveillance capability. EBN/QSEN: *A key component in surveillance is monitoring; additional research is warranted in this area to identify new technologies and processes to optimize surveillance (Gardella et al, 2012).* EB: *The number and skill of nurses staffed in hospitals has been demonstrated to have a direct effect on client outcomes. Lower levels of nurse staffing have been associated with higher rates of poor client outcomes (Cho et al, 2016)*

 Pediatric

▲ Recognize that prophylactic vitamin K administration should be used in neonates for vitamin K deficiency bleeding (VKDB). EB: *A dose of 0.5 to 1 mg vitamin K remains a standard administration for neonates to avoid VKDB and associated problems (Lippi & Franchini, 2011).*

▲ Recognize warning signs of VKDB, including minimal bleeds, evidence of cholestasis (icteric sclera, dark urine, and irritability), and failure to thrive. EB: *Signs of classic VKDB may be mild and include delayed or difficulty feeding or bruising in 24 hours to 1 week, whereas late VKDB associated with breastfeeding may occur at 2 to 12 weeks (Lippi & Franchini, 2011).*

▲ Use caution in administering NSAIDs in children. CEB: *A study of children aged 2 months to 16 years found that although upper gastrointestinal bleeding is rare, one-third of the cases seen were attributable to exposure to NSAIDs at doses used for analgesia or antipyretic purposes.* EB: *A Cochrane review of 15 trials including approximately 1000 children found insufficient evidence to exclude an increase in bleeding risk after using NSAIDs, although the findings supported use of NSAIDs to reduce emesis (Lewis et al, 2013).*

▲ Monitor children and adolescents for potential bleeding after trauma. EB: *Trauma in children aged 1 through 12 years has been associated with early coagulopathy and subsequent bleeding (Christiaans et al, 2014).* CEB: *Children and adolescents who take SSRIs need to be closely monitored because the potential for bleeding exists across age groups (Andrade et al, 2010).*

▲ Closely monitor children after cardiac surgery for excessive blood loss. EB: *In a study of 182 children aged from neonate to older than 3 years, postoperative blood loss was found to be significantly associated with age (P = .003) and the presence of cyanotic disease (P = .01) (Faraoni & Van der Linden, 2014).*

 Client/Family Teaching and Discharge Planning

● Teach client and family or significant others about any anticoagulant medications prescribed, including when to take, how often to have laboratory tests done, signs of bleeding to report, dietary consistency, and need to wear medic alert bracelet and precautions to be followed. Instruct the client to report any adverse side effects to his or her health care provider. *Medication teaching includes the drug name, purpose, administration instructions (e.g., with or without food), necessary laboratory tests, and any side effects. Provision of such information using clear communication principles and an understanding of the client's health literacy*

● = Independent; ▲ = Collaborative; EBN = Evidence-Based Nursing; EB = Evidence-Based

level may facilitate appropriate adherence to the therapeutic regimen by enhancing knowledge base (Joint Commission, 2016; National Institutes of Health [NIH] 2016).

- Instruct the client and family on the disease process and rationale for care. When clients and their family members have sufficient understanding of their disease process they can participate more fully in care and healthy behaviors. Knowledge empowers clients and family members, allowing them to be active participants in their care. **EB/CEBN:** *Use of written, verbal, and/or video education enhances client retention of information needed when managing potent medications. Patients actively engaged in their health care report better experiences, improved outcomes, and lower health care costs (Burnett et al, 2016; Joint Commission, 2016).*

- Provide client and family or significant others with both oral and written educational materials that meet the standards of client education and health literacy. **EB:** *The use of clear communication, materials written at a fifth-grade level, and the teach-back method enhance the client's ability to understand important health-related information and improves self-care safety (Burnett, 2016; NIH, 2016; Hull & Garcia, 2017).*

REFERENCES

Alderson, P., et al. (2004). Human albumin solution for resuscitation and volume expansion in critically ill patients. *Cochrane Database of Systematic Reviews*, (4), CD001208.

Andrade, C., et al. (2010). Serotonin reuptake inhibitor antidepressants and abnormal bleeding: A review for clinicians and a reconsideration of mechanisms. *Journal of Clinical Psychology, 71*, 1565–1575.

Bunn, F., & Trivedi, D. (2012). Colloid solutions for fluid resuscitation. *Cochrane Database of Systematic Reviews*, (7), CD001319. doi:10.1002/14651858.CD001319.pub5.

Burnett, A., Mahan, C., Vazquez, S., et al. (2016). Guidance for the practical management of the direct oral anticoagulants (DOACs) in VTE treatment. *Journal of Thrombosis and Thrombolysis, 41*, 206–232.

Christiaans, S. C., Duhachek-Stapelman, A. L., Russell, R. T., et al. (2014). Coagulopathy after severe pediatric trauma. *Shock (Augusta, Ga.), 41*, 476–490.

Christos, S., & Naples, R. (2016). Anticoagulation reversal and treatment strategies in major bleeding: Update 2016. *The Western Journal of Emergency Medicine, 17*(3), 264–270.

Cho, E., Lee, N. J., Kim, E. Y., et al. (2016). Nurse staffing level and overtime associated with paitent safety, quality of care and care left undone in hospitals: A cross-sectional study. *International Journal of Nursing Studies, 60*, 263–271.

Emergency Nurses Association. (2017). *Emergency nursing core curriculum* (7th ed.). St. Louis: Elsevier.

Faraoni, D., & Van der Linden, P. (2014). Factors affecting postoperative blood loss in children undergoing cardiac surgery. *Journal of Cardiothoracic Surgery, 9*, 32.

Gardella, J. E., Cardwell, T. B., & Nnadi, M. (2012). Improving medication safety with accurate preadmission medication lists and postdischarge education. *Joint Commission Journal on Quality and Patient Safety / Joint Commission Resources, 38*, 452–458.

Gourgiotis, S., Gemenetzis, G., Kocher, H. M., et al. (2013). Permissive hypotension in bleeding trauma patients: Helpful or not and when? *Critical Care Nurse, 33*, 18–25.

Harter, K., Levine, M., & Henderson, S. O. (2015). Anticoagulation drug therapy: A review. *The Western Journal of Emergency Medicine, 16*(1), 11–17.

Hastings-Tolsma, M., Bernard, R., Brody, M., et al. (2013). Chorioamnionitis: Prevention and management. *MCN. The American Journal of Maternal Child Nursing, 38*, 206–212.

Hull, R., & Garcia, D. (2017). *Patient education: Warfarin (Coumadin) (beyond the basics).* Retrieved from https://www.uptodate.com/contents/warfarin-coumadin-beyond-the-basics.

Joint Commission. (2016). *Hospital national patient safety goals.* Retrieved from http://www.jointcommission.org/hap_2016_npsgs/. (Accessed 7 October 2017).

Levy, J. H. (2014). Pharmacology and safety of new oral anticoagulants: The challenge of bleeding persists. *Clinics in Laboratory Medicine, 34*, 443–452.

Lewis, S., Nicholson, A., Cardwell, M. E., et al. (2013). Nonsteroidal anti-inflammatory drugs and perioperative bleeding in paediatric tonsillectomy. *Cochrane Database of Systematic Reviews*.

Lippi, G., & Franchini, M. (2011). Vitamin K in neonates: Facts and myths. *Blood Transfusion, 9*, 4–9.

Kampfen, P., Mean, M., Limacher, A., et al. (2014). Risk of falls and bleeding in elderly patients with acute venous thromboembolism. *Journal of Internal Medicine, 276*, 378–386.

Makris, M., Van Veen, J. J., Tait, C. R., et al. (2013). Guideline on the management of bleeding in patients on antithrombotic agents. *British Journal of Haematology, 160*, 35–46.

National Institutes of Health (NIH). (2016). *Clear communication: An NIH health literacy initiative.* Retrieved from https://www.nih.gov/institutes-nih/nih-office-director/office-communications-public-liaison/clear-communication/clear-simple. (Accessed 15 October 2017).

Nutescu, E. A., Wittkowsky, A. K., Burnett, A., et al. (2013). Delivery of optimized inpatient anticoagulation therapy: Consensus statement from the anticoagulation forum. *The Annals of Pharmacotherapy, 47*, 714–724.

Raval, A., Cigarros, J., Chung, M., et al. (2017). Management of patients on non-vitamin K oral anticoagulants in the acute care and periprocedural setting. *Circulation, 135*, e604–e633.

Siegal, D. M., & Crowther, M. A. (2013). Acute management of bleeding in patients on novel oral anticoagulants. *European Heart Journal, 34*, 489–498b.

Shoeb, M., & Fang, M. (2013). Assessing bleeding risk in patients taking anticoagulants. *Journal of Thrombosis and Thrombolysis, 35*, 312–319.

Villanueva, C., Colomo, A., Bosch, A., et al. (2013). Transfusion strategies for acute upper gastrointestinal bleeding. *The New England Journal of Medicine, 368*, 11–21.

Witt, D. M., Clark, N. P., Kaatz, S., et al. (2016). Guidance for the practical management of warfarin therapy in the treatment of venous thromboembolism. *Journal of Thrombosis and Thrombolysis, 41*, 187–205.

● = Independent;   ▲ = Collaborative;   **EBN** = Evidence-Based Nursing;   **EB** = Evidence-Based

B

Risk for unstable Blood Pressure   *Mary Beth Flynn Makic, PhD, RN, CCNS, FAAN, FNAP*

NANDA-I

Definition

Susceptible to fluctuating forces of blood flowing through arterial vessels, which may compromise health.

Risk Factors

Inconsistency with medication regimen; orthostasis

Associated Condition

Adverse effects of cocaine; adverse effects of nonsteroidal anti-inflammatory drugs (NSAIDs); adverse effects of steroids; cardiac dysrhythmia; Cushing Syndrome; electrolyte imbalance; fluid retention; fluid shifts; hormonal change; hyperosmolar solutions; hyperparathyroidism; hyperthyroidism; hypothyroidism; increased intracranial pressure; rapid absorption and distribution of anti-arrhythmia agent; rapid absorption and distribution of diuretic agent; rapid absorption and distribution of vasodilator agents; sympathetic responses; use of antidepressant agents

NOC   (Nursing Outcomes Classification)

Suggested NOC Outcomes

Fatigue; Arrhythmia; Dizziness; Confusion; Blurred Vision; Circulation Status; Tissue Perfusion: Cardiac; Tissue Perfusion: Cellular; Vital Signs

Example NOC Outcome with Indicators

Tissue Perfusion: Cardiac as evidenced by the following indicators: Heart rate/Arrhythmia/Profuse diaphoresis/Nausea/Vomiting. (Rate the outcome and indicators of **Tissue Perfusion: Cardiac:** 1 = severe, 2 = substantial, 3 = moderate, 4 = mild, 5 = none [see Section I].)

Client Outcomes

Client Will (Specify Time Frame)

- Maintain vital signs within normal range
- Remain asymptomatic with cardiac rhythm (have absence of arrhythmias, tachycardia, or bradycardia)
- Be free from dizziness with changes in positions (lying to standing)
- Deny fatigue, nausea, vomiting
- Deny chest pain

NIC   (Nursing Interventions Classification)

Suggested NIC Interventions

Cardiac Care; Cardiac Precautions; Hypertension Management; Hypotension Management; Dysrhythmia Management; Vital Signs Monitoring

Example NIC Activity—Vital Signs Monitoring

Note trends and wide fluctuations in blood pressure; Monitor blood pressure while client is lying, sitting, and standing before and after position change as appropriate; Monitor blood pressure after patient has taken medications if possible; Monitor for central and peripheral cyanosis

Nursing Interventions and *Rationales*

▲ Hypertension (HTN) is a major risk factor for cardiovascular disease placing the client at increased risk of myocardial infarction and stroke (Whelton et al, 2017). EB: *The 2017 clinical practice guidelines for the management of adults with HTN now defines HTN as a blood pressure above 130/80 mm Hg for anyone at risk of a myocardial infarction or stroke. Significant emphasis is placed on ensuring the client*

• = Independent;   ▲ = Collaborative;   EBN = Evidence-Based Nursing;   EB = Evidence-Based

understands the importance of lifestyle modifications to include regular exercise and dietary changes (Whelton et al, 2017).

- Provide client-specific education about the importance of a healthy lifestyle to reduce complications associated with HTN. EB: *A heart-healthy diet with low-sodium content, maintaining a normal weight, limiting alcohol consumption, and a regular exercise program can lower the client's blood pressure and associated risk of cardiovascular disease (Whelton et al, 2017).*

- Provide drug and client-specific education if medications are prescribed to manage the client's HTN. Blood pressure medications may cause hypotension or secondary complications such as electrolyte imbalances, dehydration, and orthostasis (Whelton et al, 2017).

▲ Screen clients for secondary causes of HTN with abrupt onset or age <30 years. EB: *Secondary HTN should be explored so that the primary cause of the HTN is treated. The client should be evaluated for undetected renal disease, primary aldosteronism, obstructive sleep apnea (OSA), thyroid disease, and alcohol-induced HTN (Grossman & Messerli, 2012; Whelton et al, 2017; Wolf et al, 2018).*

▲ Review the client's past medical history. EB: *Understanding the client's risk for secondary causes of HTN is important to establishing a proper plan of care and follow-up treatments (Wolf et al, 2018).*

- Explore the client's subjective statements concerning poor sleep, report of snoring, and daytime fatigue. EB: *OSA compromises cardiovascular health. Assessment of OSA can be easily incorporated into practice using valid and reliable assessment tools such as STOP Bang (Nagappa et al, 2015; Miller & Berger 2016). If OSA is assessed, the nurse should notify the provider for additional monitoring to address OSA and HTN management.*

- Review the client's history of arrhythmias, especially a history of atrial fibrillation. EB: *Atrial fibrillation alters cardiac output and can cause hypotension and HTN episodes that result in client falls and/or altered mentation, or chest pain (Rapsomaniki et al, 2014).*

- Review the client's current medications both prescribed and over the counter. EB: *Many medications and over-the-counter agents can cause HTN and interfere with antihypertension treatments (Grossman & Messerli, 2012).*

- Steroid agents, administered at higher doses, (e.g., 80–200 mg/day) can trigger HTN (Grossman & Messerli, 2012). Teach the client to monitor blood pressure and report changes to their prescribing provider.

- Ask the client if they are prescribed antidepressant agents. Several antidepressant agents cause an elevation in blood pressure that may be progressively clinically significant if the diastolic blood pressure rises >90 mm Hg (Grossman & Messerli, 2012; Whelton et al, 2017).

- NSAIDs can induce HTN and/or interfere with antihypertensive therapy. EB: *Ask the client if they use NSAIDS to include dose and frequency of consuming these over-the-counter drugs (Grossman & Messerli, 2012; Whelton et al, 2017).*

- Over consumption of caffeine stimulates sympathetic activity, which causes a rise in blood pressure that can be followed by a decrease in blood pressure once the effects of the caffeine have worn off. EB: *Ask the client to describe their caffeine consumption to include frequency, dose, and physical effects when consuming products containing caffeine (Grossman & Messerli, 2012; Turnbull et al, 2017).*

- Licorice consumption may trigger HTN in some patients. EB: *Licorice consumption can prolong cortisol metabolism associated with an 11β-hydroxysteroid dehydrogenase deficiency leading to HTN. Ask the client about typical consumption of licorice (Ferrari, 2010; Grossman & Messerli, 2012).*

- Some herbal products may induce HTN and/or interfere with antihypertensive treatment. EB: *Over-the counter herbal agents are poorly regulated; however, some agents such as arnica, bitter orange, blue-cohosh, dong quai, ephedra, ginkgo, ginseng, guarana, licorice, pennyroyal oil, Scotch broom, senna, southern bayberry, St. John's wort, and yohimbine are known stimulants that may elevate blood pressure (Jalili et al, 2013). Ask the client about herbal agents to include dose, frequency, and reason for taking the herbal agent.*

- Alcohol is known to elevate blood pressure and increases the client's risk of HTN. EB: *Inquire about the client's typical alcohol consumption. Current recommendations suggest men should be limited to no more than two drinks per day and women to no more than one standard alcohol drink per day (Whelton et al, 2017).*

- Blood pressure may be unstable with substance abuse disorders (SUDs). *Certain drugs have specific effects on the cardiovascular system. Clients may experience tachycardia along with severe hypotension or HTN with an overdose of opioid, cocaine, and synthetic cannabinoids (Akerele & Olupona, 2017).*

- Cocaine use causes increased alertness and feelings of euphoria, along with dilated pupils, increased body temperature, tachycardia, and increased blood pressure. Tachyarrhythmias and marked elevated blood pressure can be life-threatening. *Cocaine overdose can present as a myocardial infarction or arterial dissection (Hoffman, 2010; Akerele & Olupona, 2017).*

● = Independent;   ▲ = Collaborative;   EBN = Evidence-Based Nursing;   EB = Evidence-Based

B

- Cocaine overdose is a medical emergency because of the risk of cardiac toxicity. *Treatment is focused on lowering body temperature with external cooling devices and antipyretic medications, administering sedation agents to treat hyperactivity, oxygen to address increased myocardial oxygen needs, and possible administration of antithrombotic agents if a myocardial infarction is suspected (Hoffman, 2010; Akerele & Olupona, 2017).*
- Opioid intoxication results in changes in heart rate, slowed breathing, and decrease in blood pressure leading to loss of alertness. *Opioid intoxication and overdose lead to primarily respiratory arrest with subsequent cardiovascular arrest (Jones et al, 2015; Akerele & Olupona, 2017).*
- Synthetic cannabinoids are man-made, mind-altering chemicals that may be added to foods or inhaled. There is a growing availability of these designer drugs in which adverse effects are not well known. EB: *The primary effect of synthetic cannabinoid intoxication results in severe anxiety, paranoia, nausea, vomiting, and cardiovascular symptoms to include slurred speech, HTN, chest pain, skin pallor, muscle twitches, and hypokalemia that may lead to arrhythmias (Weaver, Hooper, & Gunderson, 2015; Akerele & Olupona, 2017).*

Critical Care

- Monitor the client for symptoms associated with chest pain, myocardial infarction, acute HTN, and hypotension. EB: *Alterations in blood pressure, HTN, and hypotension adversely affect cardiac function and myocardial oxygen consumption that can result in myocardial muscle injury. Nursing interventions to monitor cardiac function and reduce oxygen needs should be implemented along with continuous cardiac function monitoring (Habib, 2018).*
- Clients with hypertensive crisis will require close monitoring for signs and symptoms consistent with acute renal failure, stroke, myocardial infarction, and acute heart failure. *Many conditions may cause hypertensive crisis; however, uncontrolled HTN is the most common cause. Subjective symptoms include severe headache, shortness of breath, faintness, and severe anxiety (Habib, 2018).*
- Myxedema coma is an acute emergency associated with hypothyroidism that manifests with severe hypotension, bradycardia, hypothermia, seizures, and coma. *Treatment focuses on supporting the client's blood pressure and restoring thyroid function by administering levothyroxine as prescribed, and supporting other organ systems (Njoku, 2013).*
- Thyroid storm (thyrotoxicosis) is an acute, life-threatening, hypermetabolic state induced by excessive release of thyroid stimulating hormone (TSH). Symptoms are severe and include fever, tachycardia, HTN, congestive heart failure leading to hypotension and shock, profuse sweating, respiratory distress, nausea and vomiting, diarrhea, abdominal pain, jaundice, anxiety, seizures, and coma. EB: *Nursing care focuses on symptom management to include reducing fever and cardiovascular support (Njoku, 2013).*

 ### Pediatric

- HTN is an underrecognized disease in children. Current recommendations include annual blood pressure monitoring with more focused monitoring in high-risk children. EB: *Blood pressure monitoring should be initiated starting at age 3. Client risk factors that include obesity and inactivity should be addressed during well child visits to reduce the cardiovascular risks associated with childhood HTN (Dionne, 2017).*
- ▲ Secondary causes of HTN should be explored in the absence of childhood obesity, known cardiovascular disease, family history. *Kidney disease should be explored as a possible etiology of unexplained HTN (Dionne, 2017).*
- Normal ranges for child and adolescent blood pressure measurements were recently updated to reflect age, gender, and weight considerations. *Revisions to the blood pressure table are intended to facilitate earlier detection of abnormal blood pressure allowing for earlier intervention to reduce the risk of end-organ injury (Flynn et al, 2017).*

 ### Geriatric

- Risk of cardiac arrhythmias increases with advanced age placing the client at increased risk of HTN and hypotension. EB: *Ask the client about a history of arrhythmias, feeling his or heart "skip beats," history of falls, and lightheadedness (Rapsomaniki et al, 2014).*
- Comorbid cardiovascular disease risks increase with advanced age. EB: *Clients, regardless of age, should be encouraged to engage in daily physical activity, consuming a heart-healthy diet, maintaining ideal body weight, and monitoring effects of prescribed cardiovascular medications (Whelton et al, 2017).*
- Polypharmacy is a risk for both hypotension and HTN in older clients. *Review the client's medications frequently to include prescribed and over-the-counter medications and herbal agents.*

● = Independent;   ▲ = Collaborative;   EBN = Evidence-Based Nursing;   EB = Evidence-Based

Client/Family Teaching and Discharge Planning

- Nutritional education has been found to be an important variable in an individual maintaining cardiovascular health. EB: *Assumptions have been made that individuals understand what a healthy diet means. Current guidelines suggest using props such as a plate and food types/portions along with practicing reading food labels are essential to client nutritional education/learning (Allison, 2017).*
- Teach the client to monitor blood pressure and to report changes in blood pressure to the provider and with each health care visit. EB: *A recent systematic review and meta-analysis found that teaching the client to properly self-monitor blood pressure along with other cardiovascular treatments (i.e., diet, exercise, medications) has been found to clinically lower blood pressure for up to a year (Tucker et al, 2017).*

REFERENCES

Akerele, E., & Olupona, T. (2017). Drugs of abuse. *The Psychiatric Clinics of North America*, 40, 501–517.

Allison, R. L. (2017). Back to basics: The effect of healthy diet and exercise on chronic disease management. *South Dakota Medicine: The Journal of the South Dakota State Medical Association*, 5, 10–18.

Dionne, J. M. (2017). Updated guideline may improve the recognition and diagnosis of hypertension in children and adolescents: Review of the 2017 AAP blood pressure clinical practice guideline. *Current Hypertension Reports*, 19, 84.

Ferrari, P. (2010). The role of 11β-hydroxysteroid dehydrogenase type 2 in human hypertension. *Biochimica et Biophysica Acta*, 1820(12), 1178–1187.

Flynn, J. T., Kaelber, D. C., & Baker-Smith, C. M. (2017). Clinical practice guideline for screening and management of high blood pressure in children and adolescents. *Pediatrics*, 140(3), e20171904.

Grossman, E., & Messerli, F. H. (2012). Drug-induced hypertension: An unappreciated cause of secondary hypertension. *The American Journal of Medicine*, 125, 14–22.

Habib, G. B. (2018). Hypertension. In G. N. Levine (Ed.), *Cardiology secrets* (5th ed., pp. 369–376). St. Louis: Elsevier.

Hoffman, R. S. (2010). Treatment of patients with cocaine-induced arrhythmias: Bringing the bench to the bedside. *British Journal of Clinical Pharmacology*, 69(5), 448–457.

Jalili, J., Askeroglu, U., Alleyne, B., et al. (2013). Herbal products that may contribute to hypertension. *Plastic and Reconstructive Surgery*, 131(1), 168–173.

Jones, C. M., Campopiano, M., Baldwin, G., et al. (2015). National and state treatment need and capacity for opioid agonist medication-assisted treatment. *American Journal of Public Health*, 105(8), E55–E63.

Miller, J. N., & Berger, A. M. (2016). Screening and assessment for obstructive sleep apnea in primary care. *Sleep Medicine Reviews*, 29, 41–51.

Nagappa, M., Liao, P., Wong, J., et al. (2015). Validation of the STOP bang questionnaire as a screening tool for obstructive sleep apnea among different populations: A systematic review and meta-analysis. *PLoS ONE*, 10(12), e014367. doi:10.1371/journal.pone.0143697.

Njoku, M. J. (2013). Patients with chronic endocrine disease. *The Medical Clinics of North America*, 97, 1123–1137.

Rapsomaniki, E., Timmis, A., George, J., et al. (2014). Blood pressure and incidence of twelve cardiovascular diseases: Lifetime risks, healthy life-years lost, and age-specific associations in 1.25 million people. *Lancet*, 383(9932), 1899–1910.

Tucker, K. L., Sheppard, J. P., Stevens, R., et al. (2017). Self-monitoring of blood pressure in hypertension: A systematic review and individual patient data meta-analysis. *PLoS Medicine*, 14(9), e1002389. doi:10.1371/journal.pmed.1002389.

Turnbull, D., Rodricks, J. V., Mariano, G. F., et al. (2017). Caffeine and cardiovascular health. *Regulatory Toxicology and Pharmacology*, 89, 165–185.

Weaver, M. F., Hooper, J. A., & Gunderson, E. W. (2015). Designer drugs 2015: Assessment and management. *Addiction Science & Clinical Practice*, 10(1), 1–9.

Whelton, P. K., Carey, R. M., Aronow, W. S., et al. (2017). ACC/AHA/AAPA/ABC/ACPM/AGS/APha/ASH/ASPC/NMA/PCNA guidelines for the prevention, detection, evaluation, and management of high blood pressure in adults: A report of the American College of Cardiology/American Heart Association Task Forces on Clinical Practice Guidelines. *Journal of the American College of Cardiology*, 71, e127–e248. Retrieved from http://www.onlinejacc.org/content/71/19/e127?_ga=2.66372653.2004839219.1542569578-506177100.1542569578.

Wolf, M., Ewen, S., Mahfoud, F., et al. (2018). Hypertension: History and development of established and novel treatments. *Clinical Research in Cardiology*, 107(Suppl. 2), S16–S29.

Disturbed Body Image   *Gail B. Ladwig, MSN, RN and Marsha McKenzie, MA Ed, BSN, RN*

NANDA-I

Definition

Confusion in mental picture of one's physical self.

Defining Characteristics

Absence of body part; alteration in body function; alteration in body structure; alteration in view of one's body; avoids looking at one's body; avoids touching one's body; behavior of acknowledging one's body; behavior of monitoring one's body; change in ability to estimate spatial relationship of body to environment;

● = Independent;   ▲ = Collaborative;   EBN = Evidence-Based Nursing;   EB = Evidence-Based

B

change in lifestyle; change in social involvement; depersonalization of body part by use of impersonal pronouns; depersonalization of loss by use of impersonal pronouns; emphasis on remaining strengths; extension of body boundary; fear of reaction by others; focus on past appearance; focus on past function; focus on previous strength; heightened achievement; hiding of body part; negative feeling about body; nonverbal response to change in body; nonverbal response to perceived change in body; overexposure of body part; perceptions that reflect an altered view of one's body appearance; personalization of body part by name; personalization of loss by name; preoccupation with change; preoccupation with loss; refusal to acknowledge change; trauma to nonfunctioning body part

Related Factors

Alteration in self-perception; cultural incongruence; spiritual incongruence

At-Risk Population

Developmental transition

Associated Condition

Alteration in body function; alteration in cognitive functioning; illness; impaired psychosocial functioning; injury; surgical procedure; trauma; treatment regimen

NOC   (Nursing Outcomes Classification)

Suggested NOC Outcomes

Body Image; Self-Esteem; Acceptance Health Status: Coping, Personal Identity

Example **NOC Outcome with Indicators**
Body Image as evidenced by the following indicators: Congruence between body reality, body ideal, and body presentation/ Satisfaction with body appearance/Adjustment to changes in physical appearance. (Rate the outcome and indicators of **Body Image:** 1 = never positive, 2 = rarely positive, 3 = sometimes positive, 4 = often positive, 5 = consistently positive [see Section I].)

Client Outcomes

Client Will (Specify Time Frame)

- Demonstrate adaptation to changes in physical appearance or body function as evidenced by adjustment to lifestyle change
- Identify and change irrational beliefs and expectations regarding body size or function
- Recognize health-destructive behaviors and demonstrate willingness to adhere to treatments or methods that will promote health
- Verbalize congruence between body reality and body perception
- Describe, touch, or observe affected body part
- Demonstrate social involvement rather than avoidance and use adaptive coping and/or social skills
- Use cognitive strategies or other coping skills to improve perception of body image and enhance functioning
- Use strategies to enhance appearance (e.g., wig, clothing)

NIC   (Nursing Interventions Classification)

Suggested NIC Interventions

Body Image Enhancement; Counseling; Eating Disorders Management; Referral; Self-Awareness Enhancement; Self-Esteem Enhancement; Support Group; Therapy Group; Weight Gain Assistance

Example **NIC Activities—Body Image Enhancement**
Determine client's body image expectations based on developmental stage; Assist client to identify actions that will enhance appearance

● = Independent;   ▲ = Collaborative;   EBN = Evidence-Based Nursing;   EB = Evidence-Based

Nursing Interventions and *Rationales*

- Incorporate psychosocial questions related to body image as part of nursing assessment to identify clients at risk for body image disturbance.
- Maintain awareness of conditions or changes that are likely to cause a disturbed body image: removal of a body part or change/loss of body function such as blindness or hearing loss, cancer survivors, clients with eating disorders, burns, skin disorders, or those with stomas or other disfiguring conditions, or a loss of perceived attractiveness such as hair loss.
- Be aware of the impact of treatments and surgeries that involve the face and neck and be prepared to address the client's psychosocial needs. **EB:** *A cross-sectional survey of 150 patients with head and neck cancer demonstrated that radical neck surgery has a significant impact on their body image (Tsung-Min et al, 2017)*
- Maintain understanding that age, gender, and other demographic identifiers may be associated with higher degrees of body image disturbance. **EB:** *A study of body image disturbance in clients with stomas was demonstrated to be higher in males, younger adults, and overweight clients (Jayarajah & Samarasekera, 2017).*
- Consideration should be given to providing counseling for women with breast cancer to assist with acceptance of the reality of the disease and to increase their resilience against breast surgery **EB:** *Current research supports previous findings regarding the change in body image satisfaction following breast surgery (Mushtaq & Naz, 2017).*
- Discuss treatment options and outcomes for women diagnosed with breast cancer. Be prepared to explore options of lumpectomy versus mastectomy and the potential for reconstructive surgery. Include cosmetic and appliance options available to mitigate effects of mastectomy and/or chemotherapy, such as wigs and customized mastectomy bras. **EB:** *Disturbance of body image has a relationship to the extent of the surgical procedure and the perceived ability to mitigate these body alterations (Rosenberg et al, 2013).*
- Nurses and other health professionals should support clients with stomas in problem-focused coping strategies. **EBN:** *It is also important for nurses to encourage patients to have contact with their friends and family, as well as stoma support groups (Burch, 2017).*

Pediatric

- Many of the previously mentioned interventions are appropriate for the pediatric client.
- Educate parents on the role their own attitudes play in a child's body perception and acceptance. **EB:** *A recent study confirms previous research demonstrating body dissatisfaction is related to internalization of a socially acceptable body size and the pressure to change body shape among parents. There is an elevated risk that parents can model negative body attitudes to their children (Kościcka et al, 2016).*
- When caring for teenagers, be aware of the impact of acne vulgaris on quality of life. The impact was proportional to the severity of acne. Assess for symptoms of social withdrawal, limited eye contact, and expressions of low self-esteem. Educate teens on skin care and hygiene, and assist with referrals to a dermatologist when needed. **EB:** *Research performed by Tasoula et al (2012) showed that feelings of unworthiness attributable to negative appraisal by peers were present in half of the subjects with acne in their study.*

Geriatric

- Encourage regular exercise for older adults. **EB:** *Research done by Mortensen et al (2012) supports the importance of physical activity to preserve functioning in older adults.*

Multicultural

- Acknowledge that body image disturbances can affect all individuals regardless of culture, race, or ethnicity. Assess for the influence of cultural beliefs, regional norms, and values on the client's body image. **EB:** *A study of Indian college students found that males were slightly more at risk for eating disorders than female students (Chaudhari et al, 2017), and another study found some discrepancies in body image perception correlated to ethnicity (Goldzak-Kunik & Leshem, 2017). A study of Brazilian women found a significant number of those studied reported having a worse quality of life associated with being overweight or underweight (Medeiros De Morais et al, 2017).*

Home Care

- The previously mentioned interventions may be adapted for home care use.
- Assess client's level of social support. Social support is one of the determinants of the client's recovery and emotional health.

● = Independent;   ▲ = Collaborative;   EBN = Evidence-Based Nursing;   EB = Evidence-Based

B

- Assess family/caregiver level of acceptance of the client's body changes.
- Encourage clients to discuss concerns related to sexuality and provide support or information as indicated. Many conditions that affect body image also affect sexuality.
- Teach all aspects of care. Involve clients and caregivers in self-care as soon as possible. Do this in stages if clients still have difficulty looking at or touching a changed body part.

Client/Family Teaching and Discharge Planning

- Advise clients with a stoma about the support available to them. EBN: *Proper discharge preparation for clients with a stoma involves the anticipation of psychological issues and depression and support to manage these issues (Burch, 2017).*

REFERENCES

Burch, J. (2017). Post-discharge care for patients following stoma formation: What the nurse needs to know. *Nursing Standard*, *31*(51), 41. doi:10.7748/ns.2017.e10198.

Chaudhari, B., Tewari, A., Vanka, J., et al. (2017). The relationship of eating disorders risk with body mass index, body image and self-esteem among medical students. *Annals of Medical and Health Sciences Research*, *7*(3), 144–149.

Goldzak-Kunik, G., & Leshem, M. (2017). Body image drawings dissociate ethnic differences and anorexia in adolescent girls. *Child and Adolescent Psychiatry and Mental Health*, 111–116. doi:10.1186/s13034-017-0150-y.

Jayarajah, U., & Samarasekera, D. N. (2017). Psychological adaptation to alteration of body image among stoma patients: A descriptive study. *Indian Journal of Psychological Medicine*, *39*(1), 63–68. doi:10.4103/0253-7176.198944.

Kościcka, K., Czepczor, K., & Brytek-Matera, A. (2016). Body size attitudes and body image perception among preschool children and their parents: A preliminary study. *Archives of Psychiatry and Psychotherapy*, *18*(4), 28–34. doi:10.12740/APP/65192.

Medeiros De Morais, M. S., Andrade Do Nascimento, R., Vieira, M. A., et al. (2017). Does body image perception relate to quality of life in middle-aged women? *PLoS ONE*, *12*(9), 1–12. doi:10.1371/journal.pone.0184031.

Mortensen, S. P., Nyberg, M., Winding, K., et al. (2012). Lifelong physical activity preserves functional sympatholysis and purinergic signalling in the ageing human leg. *The Journal of Physiology*, *590*(Pt. 23), 6227–6236.

Mushtaq, M., & Naz, F. (2017). Body image satisfaction, distress and resilience in women with breast cancer surgery: A within group study. *Journal of Postgraduate Medical Institute*, *31*(1), 39–43.

Rosenberg, S. M., Tamimi, R. M., Gelber, S., et al. (2013). Body image in recently diagnosed young women with early breast cancer. *Psycho-Oncology*, *22*(8), 1849–1855.

Tasoula, E., Gregoriou, S., Chalikias, J., et al. (2012). The impact of acne vulgaris on quality of life and psychic health in young adolescents in Greece. Results of a population survey. *Anais Brasileiros de Dermatologia*, *87*(6), 862–869.

Tsung-Min, H., Ching-Rong, L., Yu-Chun, C., et al. (2017). Body image in head and neck cancer patients treated with radiotherapy: The impact of surgical procedures. *Health and Quality of Life Outcomes.*, 151–157. doi:10.1186/s12955-017-0740-7.

Insufficient Breast Milk production
Kerstin West-Wilson, BS, MS, BSN, RN, IBCLC

NANDA-I

Definition

Inadequate supply of maternal breast milk to support nutritional state of an infant or child.

Defining Characteristics

Absence of milk production with nipple stimulation; breast milk expressed is less than prescribed volume for infant; delay in milk production; infant constipation; infant frequently crying; infant frequently seeks to suckle at breast; infant refuses to suckle at breast; infant voids small amounts of concentrated urine; infant weight gain <500 g in a month; prolonged breastfeeding time; unsustained suckling at breast

Related Factors

Ineffective latching on to breast; ineffective sucking reflex; insufficient opportunity for suckling at the breast; insufficient suckling time at breast; maternal alcohol consumption; maternal insufficient fluid volume; maternal malnutrition; maternal smoking; maternal treatment regimen; rejection of breast

Associated Condition

Pregnancy

● = Independent;   ▲ = Collaborative;   EBN = Evidence-Based Nursing;   EB = Evidence-Based

NOC (Nursing Outcomes Classification)

Suggested NOC Outcomes

Breastfeeding Establishment: Infant, Maternal; Breastfeeding Maintenance; Anxiety Self-Control; Parent-Infant Attachment

Example NOC Outcome with Indicators
Breastfeeding Establishment: as evidenced by the following indicators: Proper alignment/Latch on/Areolar compression/Suck reflex/Nursing minimum of 15 minutes per breast/Urinations and stools appropriate for age/Weight gain appropriated for age. (Rate the outcome and indicators of **Breastfeeding Establishment:** 1 = not adequate, 2 = slightly adequate, 3 = moderately adequate, 4 = substantially adequate, 5 = totally adequate [see Section I].)

Client Outcomes

Client Will (Specify Time Frame)

- State knowledge of indicators of adequate milk supply
- State and demonstrate measures to ensure adequate milk supply

NIC (Nursing Interventions Classification)

Suggested NIC Interventions

Lactation Counseling; Lactation Suppression; Kangaroo Care; Parent Education: Infant

Example NIC Activities—Lactation Counseling
Correct misconceptions, misinformation, and inaccuracies about breastfeeding; Provide educational material, as needed; Encourage attendance at breastfeeding classes and support groups for "perceived insufficient milk supply" (Gatti, 2008)

Nursing Interventions and *Rationales*

- Provide lactation support at all phases of lactation (Neifert & Bunick, 2013; Nielsen et al, 2011).
- *Communicate routine advice to mothers without making them feel pressured or guilty, and nurses should be aware of "how" they give routine instructions (Flaherman et al, 2012).*
- Initiate skin-to-skin contact at birth and undisturbed contact for the first hour following birth; the mother should be encouraged to watch the baby, not the clock. *These behaviors are associated with an abundant milk supply (Noonan, 2011; Parker et al, 2013).*
- Encourage postpartum women to start breastfeeding based on infant need as early as possible and reduce formula use to increase breastfeeding frequency. Use nonnarcotic analgesics as early as possible. EBN: *These interventions are suggested to decrease early weaning in this study of women who had cesarean deliveries and perceived insufficient milk supply (Chantry, 2014; Gatti, 2008; Kent et al, 2013; Lin et al, 2011; Lou et al, 2014; Nielsen et al, 2011).*
- Provide suggestions for mothers on how to increase milk production and how to determine whether there is insufficient milk supply. EBN: *Teach mothers how to determine low intake of breast milk by checking baby's wet diapers (fewer than 6–8) and monitoring the frequency and amount of the baby's bowel movements. Provide suggestions to women on how to increase milk production, such as improving latch-on, increasing frequency of feedings, offering both breasts during each breastfeeding session, and drinking enough fluids (Gatti, 2008; Ndikom et al, 2014; Yen-Ju & McGrath, 2011).*
- Instruct mothers that breastfeeding frequency, sucking times, and amounts are variable and normal. Assist mothers in optimal milk removal frequency. EBN: *Breastfeeding rates may be affected by a maternal perception of insufficient milk production and less than optimal milk removal frequency (Kent et al, 2012, 2013).*
- ▲ Consider the use of medication for mothers of preterm infants with insufficient expressed breast milk. EBN: *Breast milk remains the optimal form of enteral nutrition for term and preterm infants until up to 6 months postnatal age. In these studies there was modest improvement in expressing breast milk (EBM) values with the use of a galactagogue medication (Donovan & Buchanan, 2012).*
- ▲ *Need to be more cautious with recommending galactagogues.*

● = Independent;   ▲ = Collaborative;   EBN = Evidence-Based Nursing;   EB = Evidence-Based

B

▲ *Not in the scope of practice for International Board of Lactation Consultants (IBLC) to recommend galactagogues (Academy of Breastfeeding Medicine Protocol Committee, 2011; Donovan & Buchanan, 2012).*

Pediatric

- Provide individualized follow-up with extra home visits or outpatient visits for teen mothers within the first few days after hospital discharge and encourage schools to be more compatible with breastfeeding. *Adolescent mothers in the United States are much less likely to imitate breastfeeding than older mothers. This study indicated that these interventions may be helpful for teens who desire to breastfeed (Tucker et al, 2011).*

Multicultural

- Provide information and support to mothers on benefits of breastfeeding at antenatal visits. EB: *A study of mothers of infants in Bhaktapur, Nepal, found that, although proper breastfeeding is the most cost-effective intervention for reducing childhood morbidity and mortality, adherence to breastfeeding recommendations in developing countries is not satisfactory. Although many mothers instituted breastfeeding within 1 hour of delivery, continuation for up to 6 months was not common. Very few mothers received any information on breastfeeding during the antenatal visit (Neifert & Bunik, 2013; Sultana et al, 2013; Ulak et al, 2012).*
- Refer to care plans Interrupted **Breastfeeding** and Readiness for enhanced **Breastfeeding** for additional interventions.

REFERENCES

Academy of Breastfeeding Medicine Protocol Committee, ABM Clinical Protocol #9. (2011). Use of galactagogues in initiating or augmenting the rate of maternal milk secretion (first revision January 2011). *Breastfeeding Medicine, 6*(1), 41–49.

Chantry, C. J. (2014). In-hospital formula use increases early breastfeeding cessation among first-time mothers intending to exclusively breastfeed. *The Journal of Pediatrics, 164*(6), 1339–1348.

Donovan, T. J., & Buchanan, K. (2012). Medications for increasing milk supply in mothers expressing breastmilk for their preterm hospitalised infants. *Cochrane Database of Systematic Reviews*, (3), CD005544.

Flaherman, V. J., et al. (2012). Maternal experience of interactions with providers among mothers with milk supply concern. *Clinical Pediatrics, 51*(8), 778–784.

Gatti, L. (2008). Maternal perceptions of insufficient milk supply in breastfeeding. *Journal of Nursing Scholarship, 40*(4), 355–363.

Kent, J., Prime, D., & Garbin, C. (2012). Principles for maintaining or increasing breast milk production. *Journal of Obstetric, Gynecologic, and Neonatal Nursing, 41*(1), 114–121.

Kent, J. C., et al. (2013). Longitudinal changes in breastfeeding patterns from 1 to 6 months of lactation. *Breastfeeding Medicine, 8*(4), 401–407.

Lin, S. Y., et al. (2011). Factors related to milk supply perception in women who underwent cesarean section. *The Journal of Nursing Research, 19*(2), 94–101.

Lou, Z., et al. (2014). Maternal reported indicators and causes of insufficient milk supply. *Journal of Human Lactation* (online publication).

Ndikom, C. M., et al. (2014). Extra fluids for breastfeeding mothers for increasing milk production. *Cochrane Database of Systematic Reviews*, (6).

Neifert, M., & Bunik, M. (2013). Overcoming clinical barriers to exclusive breastfeeding. *Pediatric Clinics of North America, 60*, 115–145.

Nielsen, S., et al. (2011). Adequacy of milk intake during exclusive breastfeeding: A longitudinal study. *Pediatrics, 128*(4), 907–914.

Noonan, M. (2011). Breastfeeding: Is my baby getting enough milk? *British Journal of Midwifery, 19*(2), 82–89.

Parker, L. A., et al. (2013). Strategies for increased milk volume in mothers of VLBW infants. *MCN. The American Journal of Maternal Child Nursing, 38*(6), 385–390.

Sultana, A., et al. (2013). Clinical update and treatment of lactation insufficiency. *Medical Journal of Islamic World Academy of Sciences, 21*(1), 19–28.

Tucker, C. M., Wilson, E. K., & Samandari, G. (2011). Infant feeding experiences among teen mothers in North Carolina: Findings from a mixed-methods study. *International Breastfeeding Journal, 6*, 14.

Ulak, M., et al. (2012). Infant feeding practices in Bhaktapur, Nepal: A cross-sectional, health facility based survey. *International Breastfeeding Journal, 7*(1), 1–8.

Yen-Ju, H., & McGrath, J. (2011). Predicting breastfeeding duration related to maternal attitudes in a Taiwanese sample. *The Journal of Perinatal Education: An ASPO, 20*(4), 188–199.

Ineffective Breastfeeding   *Barbara J. Wheeler, RN, BN, MN, IBCLC*

NANDA-I

Definition

Difficulty feeding milk from the breasts, which may compromise nutritional status of the infant/child.

● = Independent;   ▲ = Collaborative;   EBN = Evidence-Based Nursing;   EB = Evidence-Based

Defining Characteristics

Inadequate infant stooling; infant arching at breast; infant crying at the breast; infant crying within the first hour after breastfeeding; infant fussing within 1 hour of breastfeeding; infant inability to latch on to maternal breast correctly; infant resisting latching on to breast; infant unresponsive to other comfort measures; insufficient emptying of each breast per feeding; insufficient infant weight gain; insufficient signs of oxytocin release; perceived inadequate milk supply; sore nipples persisting beyond first week; sustained infant weight loss; unsustained suckling at the breast

Related Factors

Delayed stage II lactogenesis; inadequate milk supply; insufficient family support; insufficient opportunity for suckling at breast; insufficient parental knowledge regarding breastfeeding techniques; insufficient parental knowledge regarding importance of breastfeeding; interrupted breastfeeding; maternal ambivalence; maternal anxiety; maternal breast anomaly; maternal fatigue; maternal obesity; maternal pain; pacifier use; poor infant sucking reflex; supplemental feedings with artificial nipple

At-Risk Population

Prematurity; previous breast surgery; previous history of breastfeeding failure; short maternity leave

Associated Condition

Oropharyngeal defect

NOC   (Nursing Outcomes Classification)

Suggested NOC Outcomes and Example

Breastfeeding Establishment: Infant/Maternal; Breastfeeding Maintenance; Knowledge: Breastfeeding; Refer to care plan for Readiness for enhanced **Breastfeeding**

Client Outcomes

Client Will (Specify Time Frame)

- Achieve effective milk transfer (dyad)
- Verbalize/demonstrate techniques to manage breastfeeding problems (mother)
- Manifest signs of adequate intake at the breast (infant)
- Manifest positive self-esteem in relation to the infant feeding process (mother)
- Explain alternative method of infant feeding if unable to continue exclusive breastfeeding (mother)

NIC   (Nursing Interventions Classification)

Suggested NIC Interventions

Referral; Lactation Counseling; Teaching Infant Nutrition 0-3 Months

Nursing Interventions and *Rationales*

- Identify women with risk factors for lower breastfeeding initiation and continuation rates, as well as factors contributing to ineffective breastfeeding (see conditions listed in the section Related Factors) as early as possible in the perinatal experience. EB: *Health care professionals are well positioned to identify mothers at risk for breastfeeding challenges, and to provide accurate information and support the development of breastfeeding skills, which facilitates breastfeeding confidence and success (Balogun et al, 2016; Ogbo et al, 2017).*
- Provide time for clients to express expectations and concerns, and provide emotional support as needed. EB: *Lactation consultants, nurses, and peers play a key role in the establishment and continuation of breastfeeding (Balogun et al, 2016; McFadden et al, 2017).*
- Encourage skin-to-skin holding, beginning immediately after delivery. EB: *Skin-to-skin holding is associated with improved milk supply, early initiation of breastfeeding, and improved breastfeeding duration (Moore et al, 2016).*
- Use valid and reliable tools to measure breastfeeding performance and to predict early discontinuance of breastfeeding whenever possible/feasible. EB: *Casal et al (2017) examined the purpose, theoretical*

● = Independent;   ▲ = Collaborative;   EBN = Evidence-Based Nursing;   EB = Evidence-Based

B

underpinnings, and psychometric properties of 16 instruments measuring breastfeeding attitudes, knowledge, and social support. **CEB:** *The Breastfeeding Self-Efficacy Scale (BSES) has been used in many settings and with diverse patient populations, and it has consistently demonstrated an ability to accurately predict breastfeeding success or failure, thus providing opportunity for focused education and support for mothers who need it (Dennis, 2003).*

- Promote comfort and relaxation to reduce pain and anxiety. **EB:** *Discomfort and increased tension are factors associated with reduced likelihood to initiate breastfeeding, reduced let-down reflex, increased use of formula supplements, and premature discontinuance of breastfeeding (Fallon et al, 2016).*
- Avoid supplemental feedings. **EB:** *A correlation exists between formula and/or water supplements and failure to succeed with exclusive breastfeeding (Tarrant et al, 2015).*
- Teach mother to observe for infant behavioral cues and responses to breastfeeding. **EB:** *Providing support and education to mother will build her confidence and knowledge base, and is associated with improved breastfeeding duration and exclusivity (McFadden et al, 2017).*
- ▲ Provide necessary equipment/instruction/assistance for milk expression as needed. **EB:** *Expressing breast milk by hand may be more effective in the removal of milk, particularly in the immediate postpartum period, than the use of electric pumps (Becker et al, 2016).*
- ▲ Provide referrals and resources: lactation consultants, nurse and peer support programs, community organizations, and written and electronic sources of information. **EB:** *Systematic reviews support the use of professionals with special skills in breastfeeding, peer support programs, and written and electronic information to promote continued breastfeeding (McFadden et al, 2017). Novel approaches to education, such as text messages to mothers and interactive online education programs for fathers/partners, have demonstrated improved breastfeeding knowledge base and self-efficacy (Abbass-Dick et al, 2017) and improved breastfeeding exclusivity rates (Harari et al, 2017).*
- See care plan for Readiness for enhanced **Breastfeeding**.

Multicultural

- Assess whether the client's cultural beliefs about breastfeeding are contributing to ineffective breastfeeding. **EB:** *Women from different cultures, such as Chinese, Somali, and Hispanic women, may add formula as a result of concerns that the infant is not getting enough to eat and the perception that "big is healthy" (Kuswara et al, 2016; Waldrop, 2013; Wandel et al, 2016).* **EB:** *Some traditional cultures, including mothers from Asia, Latin America, and sub-Saharan Africa, consider colostrum unsuitable to feed the newborn, thus liquids such as tea, juice, water, or water sweetened with sugar or honey may be given. These feedings may significantly increase the risk of infection, particularly in developing countries in which sanitation may be poor. In addition, failure to empty the breasts regularly in the early hours and days after delivery may result in suboptimal milk supply (Agho et al, 2016).*
- Assess the influence of family support on the decision to continue or discontinue breastfeeding. **EB:** *Family members' impressions and ideas about breastfeeding influence breastfeeding initiation and duration (Lok et al, 2017).*
- See care plan for Readiness for enhanced **Breastfeeding**.

Home Care

- The previously mentioned interventions may be adapted for home care use.
- Provide anticipatory guidance in relation to home management of breastfeeding. **EB:** *The two most common problems experienced by breastfeeding women are nipple and/or breast pain and low (or perceived low) milk supply; these problems may be preventable with anticipatory guidance (Cleugh & Langseth, 2017; Wood & Sanders, 2017). For mothers returning to the workforce, longer maternity leaves and regularly pumping milk during the workday are associated with enhanced work–life balance and longer breastfeeding duration (Jantzer et al, 2017).*
- ▲ Investigate availability of and refer to public health department, hospital home follow-up breastfeeding program, or other postdischarge support. **EBN:** *Postdischarge follow-up has been associated with improved breastfeeding duration (Wood & Sanders, 2017).*
- See care plan for Risk for impaired **Attachment**.

Client/Family Teaching and Discharge Planning

- Instruct the client on maternal breastfeeding behaviors/techniques (preparation for, positioning, initiation of/promoting latch-on, burping, completion of session, and frequency of feeding) using a variety of

B

strategies such as written materials, videos, and online resources. EB: *Assess breastfeeding mothers to determine knowledge deficits and providing individualized teaching facilitates breastfeeding success (Cleugh & Langseth, 2017; Nilsson et al, 2017).*

- Teach the mother self-care measures (e.g., breast care, management of breast/nipple discomfort, nutrition/fluid, rest/activity). EB: *Painful nipples, mastitis, inadequate hydration, and fatigue are some potentially modifiable problems a breastfeeding woman may experience (Cleugh & Langseth, 2017; McFadden et al, 2017).*
- Provide information regarding infant feeding cues and behaviors and appropriate maternal responses, as well as measures of infant feeding adequacy. EB: *Improved knowledge base and ongoing support to learn psychomotor skills facilitates effective breastfeeding (Cleugh & Langseth, 2017; McFadden et al, 2017).*
- Provide education to partner/family/significant others as needed. EB: *Family members' impressions and ideas about breastfeeding influence breastfeeding initiation and duration (Lok et al, 2017).*

REFERENCES

See Readiness for enhanced **Breastfeeding** for additional references.

Abbass-Dick, J., Xie, F., Koroluk, J., et al. (2017). The development and piloting of an eHealth breastfeeding resource targeting fathers and partners as co-parents. *Midwifery, 50*, 139–147.

Agho, K. E., Ogeleka, P., Ogbo, F. A., et al. (2016). Trends and predictors of prelacteal feeding practices in Nigeria (2003–2013). *Nutrients, 8*(8), E462.

Balogun, O. O., O'Sullivan, E. J., McFadden, A., et al. (2016). Interventions for promoting the initiation of breastfeeding. *Cochrane Database Systematic Reviews*, (11), CD001688.

Becker, G. E., Smith, H. A., & Cooney, F. (2016). Methods of milk expression for lactating women. *Cochrane Database Systematic Reviews*, (9), CD006170.

Casal, C. S., Lei, A., Young, S. L., et al. (2017). A critical review of instruments measuring breastfeeding attitudes, knowledge, and social support. *Journal of Human Lactation, 33*(1), 21–47.

Cleugh, F., & Langseth, A. (2017). Fifteen-minute consultation on the healthy child: Breast feeding. *Archives of Disease in Childhood. Education and Practice Edition, 102*, 8–13.

Dennis, C. L. (2003). The breastfeeding self-efficacy scale: Psychometric assessment of the short form. *Journal of Obstetric, Gynecologic, and Neonatal Nursing : JOGNN / NAACOG, 32*(6), 734–744.

Fallon, V., Groves, R., Halford, J. C., et al. (2016). Postpartum anxiety and infant-feeding outcomes. *Journal of Human Lactation, 32*(4), 740–758.

Harari, N., Rosenthal, M. S., Bozzi, V., et al. (2017). Feasibility and acceptability of a text message intervention used as an adjunct tool by WIC breastfeeding peer counselors: The LATCH pilot. *Maternal & Child Nutrition*. doi:10.1111/mcn.12488.

Jantzer, A. M., Anderson, J., & Kuehl, R. A. (2017). Breastfeeding support in the workplace: The relationships among breastfeeding support, work-life balance, and job satisfaction. *Journal of Human Lactation*. doi:10.1177/0890334417707956.

Kuswara, K., Laws, R., Kremer, P., et al. (2016). The infant feeding practices of Chinese immigrant mothers in Australia: A qualitative exploration. *Appetite, 105*, 375–384.

Lok, K. Y. W., Bai, D. L., & Tarrant, M. (2017). Family members' infant feeding preferences, maternal breastfeeding exposures and exclusive breastfeeding intentions. *Midwifery, 53*, 49–54.

McFadden, A., Gavine, A., Renfrew, M. J., et al. (2017). Support for healthy breastfeeding mothers with healthy term babies. *Cochrane Database Systematic Reviews*, (2), CD001141.

Moore, E. R., Bergman, N., Anderson, G. C., et al. (2016). Early skin-to-skin contact for mothers and their healthy newborn infants. *Cochrane Database Systematic Reviews*, (11), CD003519.

Nilsson, I. M. S., Strandberg-Larsen, K., Knight, C. H., et al. (2017). Focused breastfeeding counselling improves short- and long-term success in an early-discharge setting: A cluster-randomized study. *Maternal Child Nutrition, 13*, e12432.

Ogbo, F. A., Eastwood, J., Page, A., et al. (2017). Prevalence and determinants of cessation of exclusive breastfeeding in the early postnatal period in Sydney, Australia. *International Breastfeeding Journal, 12*(16). doi:10.1186/s13006-017-0110-4.

Tarrant, M., Lok, K. Y. W., Fong, D. Y. T., et al. (2015). Effect of a hospital policy of not accepting free infant formula on in-hospital formula supplementation rates and breastfeeding duration. *Public Health Nutrition, 18*(14), 2689–2699.

Waldrop, J. (2013). Exploration of reasons for feeding choices of Hispanic mothers. *MCN. The American Journal of Maternal Child Nursing, 38*(5), 282–288.

Wandel, M., Terragni, L., Nguyen, C., et al. (2016). Breastfeeding among Somali mothers living in Norway: Attitudes, practices and challenges. *Women and Birth: Journal of the Australian College of Midwives, 29*(6), 487–493.

Wood, N. K., & Sanders, K. A. (2017). Mothers with perceived insufficient milk: Preliminary evidence of home interventions to boost mother-infant interactions. *Western Journal of Nursing Research*. doi:10.1177/0193945916687552.

Interrupted Breastfeeding   *Barbara J. Wheeler, RN, BN, MN, IBCLC*

NANDA-I

Definition

Break in the continuity of feeding milk from the breasts, which may compromise breastfeeding success and/or nutritional status of the infant/child.

● = Independent;   ▲ = Collaborative;   EBN = Evidence-Based Nursing;   EB = Evidence-Based

B

Defining Characteristics

Nonexclusive breastfeeding

Related Factors

Maternal employment; maternal-infant separation; needing abruptly to wean infant

At-Risk Population

Hospitalization of child; prematurity

Associated Condition

Contraindications to breastfeeding; infant illness; maternal illness

NOC   (Nursing Outcomes Classification)

Suggested NOC Outcomes

Breastfeeding Maintenance; Knowledge: Breastfeeding; Parent-Infant Attachment

Example NOC Outcome with Indicators
Breastfeeding Maintenance as evidenced by the following indicators: Infant's growth and development in normal range/Ability to safely collect and store breast milk/Awareness that breastfeeding can continue beyond infancy/Knowledge of benefits from continued breastfeeding. (Rate the outcome and indicators of **Breastfeeding Maintenance: Infant:** 1 = not adequate, 2 = slightly adequate, 3 = moderately adequate, 4 = substantially adequate, 5 = totally adequate [see Section I].)

Client Outcomes

Client Will (Specify Time Frame)

Infant
- Receive mother's breast milk if not contraindicated by maternal conditions (e.g., certain drugs, infections) or infant conditions (e.g., galactosemia)

Maternal
- Maintain lactation
- Achieve effective breastfeeding or satisfaction with the breastfeeding experience
- Demonstrate effective methods of breast milk collection and storage

NIC   (Nursing Interventions Classification)

Suggested NIC Interventions

Bottle Feeding; Cup Feeding: Newborn; Emotional Support; Lactation Counseling

Example NIC Activities—Lactation Counseling
Instruct patient to contact health care provider (lactation consultant, nurse, midwife, or physician) to assist in determining status of milk supply (i.e., whether insufficiency is perceived or actual); Encourage employers to provide opportunities and private facilities for lactating mothers to pump and store breast milk during the workday

Nursing Interventions and *Rationales*

- Provide information and support to mother and partner/family regarding mother's desire/intention to begin or resume breastfeeding. EB: *Mothers who perceived that care providers, partners, and other family members favored exclusive breastfeeding achieved significantly higher rates of breastfeeding compared with those who perceived care providers and family were neutral about the method of infant feeding (Lok et al, 2017; Ramakrishnan et al, 2014).*
- Clarify that interruption in breastfeeding is truly necessary. (Expert recommendation): *Mothers are sometimes inappropriately advised to discontinue breastfeeding (ACOG, 2017; CDC, 2016; Ngoh & Ng, 2016).*

● = Independent;   ▲ = Collaborative;   EBN = Evidence-Based Nursing;   EB = Evidence-Based

- Provide anticipatory guidance to the mother/family regarding potential duration of the interruption when possible/feasible, ensuring that measures to sustain or restart lactation and promote parent–infant attachment can make it possible to resume breastfeeding when the condition/situation requiring interruption is resolved. EB: *Mothers who had never breastfed, and those who had stopped, were successful in establishing or reestablishing breastfeeding with the help of a lactation support (Nyati et al, 2014).*
- Reassure the mother/family that the infant will benefit from any amount of breast milk provided. EBN: *One of the most common reasons mothers supplement or stop breastfeeding is their perception of the baby not getting milk and/or enough milk (Wood & Sanders, 2017).*
- Assess mother's concerns, and observe mother performing psychomotor skills (expression, storage, alternative feeding, skin-to-skin care, and/or breastfeeding) and assist as needed. EBN: *Individualized support and instruction improves likelihood of breastfeeding success (Becker et al, 2016; McFadden et al, 2017).*
- Collaborate with mother/family/health care providers (as needed) to develop a plan for skin-to-skin contact. EBN: *Skin-to-skin contact between mothers and newborns results in improved rates of exclusive breastfeeding (McFadden et al, 2017).*
- Collaborate with the mother/family/health care provider/employer (as needed) to develop a plan for expression/pumping of breast milk and/or infant feeding. EB: *Individualized education focused on evidence-based strategies to optimize milk production and extraction enhances milk quality and quantity (Becker et al, 2016)*
- Monitor for signs indicating infant's ability to breastfeed and interest in breastfeeding. EBN: *Teach the mother to recognize and respond to her baby's feeding cues and signs that her breasts are filling (McFadden et al, 2017).*
- ▲ Use supplementation only as medically indicated. EB: *Reducing the number of formula supplements given to infants in the hospital is associated with increased rates of exclusive breastfeeding and breastfeeding duration (Tarrant et al, 2015).*
- Provide anticipatory guidance for common problems associated with interrupted breastfeeding (e.g., incomplete emptying of milk glands, diminishing milk supply, infant difficulty with resuming breastfeeding, or infant refusal of alternative feeding method). EBN and **expert recommendation:** *Emotional support, as well as information regarding how to prevent and respond to breastfeeding problems, contributes to promotion of exclusive breastfeeding (Cleugh & Langseth, 2017; Wood & Sanders, 2017).*
- ▲ Initiate follow-up and make appropriate referrals.
- Assist the client to accept and learn an alternative method of infant feeding if effective breastfeeding is not achieved. CEB: *If it is clear that breastfeeding cannot be achieved after the interruption and an alternative feeding method must be instituted, the mother needs support and education (Mozingo et al, 2000).*
- See care plans for Readiness for enhanced **Breastfeeding** and Ineffective **Breastfeeding.**

Multicultural

- Teach culturally appropriate techniques for maintaining lactation. CEB: *The Oketani method of breast massage is used by Japanese and other Asian women. Oketani breast massage improves the quality of human milk by increasing total solids, lipids, casein concentration, and gross energy (Foda et al, 2004). Some traditional cultures, including Asian, Latin American, and sub-Saharan African, consider colostrum unsuitable to feed the newborn; thus formula is required to prevent hypoglycemia and dehydration, and breast expression/pumping is needed to ensure breasts are regularly emptied, which facilitates an optimal milk supply (Agho et al, 2016).*
- See care plans for Readiness for enhanced **Breastfeeding** and Ineffective **Breastfeeding.**

Home Care

- The previously mentioned interventions may be adapted for home care use.

Client/Family Teaching and Discharge Planning

- Teach mother effective methods to express breast milk. EBN: *Expressing breast milk by hand may be more effective in the removal of milk, particularly in the immediate postpartum period, than the use of electric pumps (Becker et al, 2016).*
- Teach mother/parents about skin-to-skin care. EBN: *Skin-to-skin care promotes attachment, facilitates improved milk production, and contributes to improved rate and duration of breastfeeding (Brown et al, 2014).*

● = Independent;   ▲ = Collaborative;   EBN = Evidence-Based Nursing;   EB = Evidence-Based

B

- Instruct mother on safe breast milk handling techniques. *EB: Breastfeeding mothers can retain the high quality of breast milk and the health of their infant by using safe preparation guidelines and storage methods (CDC, 2017).*
- See care plans for Readiness for enhanced **Breastfeeding** and Ineffective **Breastfeeding.**

REFERENCES

See readiness for enhanced **Breastfeeding** for additional references.

Agho, K. E., Ogeleka, P., Ogbo, F. A., et al. (2016). Trends and predictors of prelacteal feeding practices in Nigeria (2003-2013). *Nutrients, 8*(8), E462.

American College of Obstetricians and Gynecologists (ACOG), Committee of Obstetric Practice. (2017). Guidelines for diagnostic imaging during pregnancy and lactation. *The American College of Obstetricians and Gynecologists, Women's Health Care Physicians, 130*(4), e210–e216.

Becker, G. E., Smith, H. A., & Cooney, F. (2016). Methods of milk expression for lactating women. *Cochrane Database Systematic Reviews,* (9), CD006170.

Brown, P. A., Kaiser, K. L., & Nailon, R. E. (2014). Integrating quality improvement and translational research models to increase exclusive breastfeeding. *Journal of Obstetric, Gynecologic, and Neonatal Nursing, 43,* 545–553.

Centers for Disease Control and Prevention (CDC). (2016). *Breastfeeding: Disease and conditions. When should a mother avoid breastfeeding?* Retrieved from http://www.cdc.gov/breastfeeding/disease/index.htm. (Accessed 31 October 2017).

Centers for Disease Control and Prevention (CDC). (2017). *Proper handling and storage of human milk.* U.S. Department of Health and Human Services, CDC. Retrieved from http://www.cdc.gov/breastfeeding/recommendations/handling_breastmilk.htm. (Accessed 31 October 2017).

Cleugh, F., & Langseth, A. (2017). Fifteen-minute consultation on the healthy child: Breast feeding. *Archives of Disease in Childhood. Education and Practice Edition, 102,* 8–13.

Foda, M. I., et al. (2004). Composition of milk obtained from unmassaged versus massaged breasts of lactating mothers. *Journal of Pediatric Gastroenterology and Nutrition, 38*(5), 484–487.

Lok, K. Y. W., Bai, D. L., & Tarrant, M. (2017). Family members' infant feeding preferences, maternal breastfeeding exposures and exclusive breastfeeding intentions. *Midwifery, 53,* 49–54.

McFadden, A., Gavine, A., Renfrew, M. J., et al. (2017). Support for healthy breastfeeding mothers with healthy term babies. *Cochrane Database Systematic Reviews,* (2), CD001141.

Mozingo, J. N., et al. (2000). "It wasn't working." Women's experiences with short-term breastfeeding. *MCN. The American Journal of Maternal Child Nursing, 25*(3), 120–126.

Ngoh, H. L. S., & Ng, M. C. W. (2016). Vaccination in the primary care setting: When is it safe to proceed? *Singapore Medical Journal, 57*(1), 3–7.

Nyati, M., Kim, H. Y., Goga, A., et al. (2014). Support for relactation among mothers of HIV-infected children: A pilot study in Soweto. *Breastfeeding Medicine.* http://www-ncbi-nlm-nih-gov.proxy2.lib.umanitoba.ca/pubmed/25188674. (Accessed 30 October 2017). [Epub ahead of print].

Ramakrishnan, R., Oberg, C. M., & Kirby, R. S. (2014). The association between maternal perception of obstetric and pediatric care providers' attitudes and exclusive breastfeeding outcomes. *Journal of Human Lactation, 30*(1), 80–87.

Tarrant, M., Lok, K. Y. W., Fong, D. Y. T., et al. (2015). Effect of a hospital policy of not accepting free infant formula on in-hospital formula supplementation rates and breastfeeding duration. *Public Health Nutrition, 18*(14), 2689–2699.

Wood, N. K., & Sanders, K. A. (2017). Mothers with perceived insufficient milk: Preliminary evidence of home interventions to boost mother-infant interactions. *Western Journal of Nursing Research.* doi:10.1177/0193945916687552.

Readiness for enhanced Breastfeeding   *Barbara J. Wheeler, RN, BN, MN, IBCLC*

NANDA-I

Definition

A pattern of providing milk to an infant or young child directly from the breasts, which may be strengthened.

Defining Characteristics

Mother expresses desire to enhance ability to provide breast milk for child's nutritional needs; mother expresses desire to enhance ability to exclusively breastfeed

NOC   (Nursing Outcomes Classification)

Suggested NOC Outcomes

Breastfeeding Establishment: Infant, Maternal; Breastfeeding Maintenance

● = Independent;   ▲ = Collaborative;   EBN = Evidence-Based Nursing;   EB = Evidence-Based

Example NOC Outcome with Indicators
Breastfeeding Establishment: Infant as evidenced by the following indicators: Proper alignment and latch-on/Proper areolar grasp/Effective areolar compression/Correct suck and tongue placement/Audible swallow/Breastfeeding a minimum of 5 to 10 minutes per breast/Minimum eight feedings per day/Urinations per day appropriate for age/Weight gain appropriate for age. (Rate the outcome and indicators of **Breastfeeding Establishment: Infant:** 1 = not adequate, 2 = slightly adequate, 3 = moderately adequate, 4 = substantially adequate, 5 = totally adequate [see Section I].)

Client Outcomes

Client Will (Specify Time Frame)

- Maintain effective breastfeeding
- Maintain normal growth patterns (infant)
- Verbalize satisfaction with breastfeeding process (mother)

NIC (Nursing Interventions Classification)

Suggested NIC Intervention

Lactation Counseling

Example NIC Activities—Lactation Counseling
Provide information about psychological and physiological benefits of breastfeeding; Provide mother the opportunity to breastfeed after birth, when possible

Nursing Interventions and *Rationales*

- Encourage expectant mothers to learn about breastfeeding before and during pregnancy. EB: *Systematic reviews have identified that health education, particularly individualized education, significantly increases breastfeeding initiation rates (Balogun et al, 2016).*
- Encourage and facilitate early skin-to-skin contact. EB: *Skin-to-skin holding is associated with improved milk supply, early initiation of breastfeeding, and improved breastfeeding duration (Moore et al, 2016).*
- Encourage rooming-in and breastfeeding on demand. EBN: *Mothers who room-in with their infants have greater percentages of exclusive breastfeeding when released from the hospital (Neifert & Bunik, 2013).*
- Monitor the breastfeeding process, identify opportunities to enhance knowledge and experience, and provide direction as needed. EB: *Individualized education focused on evidence-based strategies improves breastfeeding duration and exclusivity (McFadden et al, 2017).*
- Give encouragement and positive feedback to mothers as they learn to breastfeed. CEB: *Positive feedback builds confidence. The Breastfeeding Self-Efficacy Scale, which measures maternal breastfeeding confidence, has demonstrated that higher self-efficacy (confidence) is associated with longer duration of breastfeeding (Dennis, 2003).*
- Discuss prevention and treatment of common breastfeeding problems, such as nipple pain and/or trauma. EB & Expert Recommendation: *Common problems experienced by breastfeeding women may be preventable with anticipatory guidance, or successfully managed with prompt assistance from a health care provider (Amir, 2014; Cleugh & Langseth, 2017).*
- Teach mother to observe for infant behavioral cues and responses to breastfeeding. EB & Expert Recommendation: *Awareness and recognition of infant cues facilitate successful breastfeeding (Cleugh & Langseth, 2017; McFadden et al, 2017).*
- Identify current support-person network and opportunities for continued breastfeeding support. EB: *Family members' impressions and ideas about breastfeeding influence breastfeeding initiation and duration (Lok et al, 2017).*
- Use supplementation only as medically indicated, and do not provide samples of formula on discharge from hospital. EB: *Reducing the number of formula supplements given to infants in hospital, and refraining from sending formula samples home, is associated with increased rates of exclusive breastfeeding and increased breastfeeding duration (Tarrant et al, 2015).*
- ▲ Provide follow-up contact; as available provide home visits and/or peer counseling. EB: *Systematic reviews support the use of professionals with special skills in breastfeeding and peer support programs to promote continued breastfeeding (McFadden et al, 2017; Wood & Sanders 2017).*

● = Independent; ▲ = Collaborative; EBN = Evidence-Based Nursing; EB = Evidence-Based

Multicultural

- Assess for the influence of cultural beliefs, norms, and values on current breastfeeding practices. **EB:** *Women from different cultures, such as Chinese, Somali, and Hispanic women, may add formula as a result of concerns that the infant is not getting enough to eat and the perception that "big is healthy" (Kuswara et al, 2016; Waldrop, 2013; Wandel et al, 2016).* **EB:** *Some traditional cultures, including Asian, Latin American, and sub-Saharan African, consider colostrum unsuitable to feed the newborn; thus formula may be required to prevent hypoglycemia and dehydration, and breast expression/pumping is needed to ensure breasts are regularly emptied to facilitate an optimal milk supply (Agho et al, 2016).*

Home Care

- The previously mentioned interventions may be adapted for home care use.

Client/Family Teaching and Discharge Planning

- Include the partner and other family members in education about breastfeeding. **EB:** *Family members' impressions and ideas about breastfeeding influence breastfeeding initiation and duration (Lok et al, 2017).*
- Teach the client the importance of maternal nutrition. **CEB:** *Breastfeeding mothers should consume about 500 calories more per day than nonpregnant, nonnursing women, with a focus on nutrient-dense foods, including 200 to 300 mg docosahexaenoic acid (DHA) (the amount ingested with consumption of one to two portions of fish per week) recommended (AAP, 2012).*
- Teach mother about the infant's subtle hunger cues (e.g., rooting, sucking, mouthing, hand-to-mouth and hand-to-hand activity) and encourage her to breastfeed whenever signs are apparent. **EB:** *Evidence-based practice guidelines support the teaching/reinforcement of these skills as important to effective breastfeeding (McFadden et al, 2017).*
- Review guidelines for frequency (at least every 2–3 hours, or 8–12 feedings per 24 hours) and duration (until suckling and swallowing slow down and satiety is reached) of feeding times. **EB:** *In the first few days, frequent and regular stimulation of the breasts is important to establish an adequate milk supply; after breastfeeding is established, feeding lasts until the breasts are drained (McFadden et al, 2017).*
- Provide information about common infant behaviors related to breastfeeding, and appropriate maternal responses. **EBN:** *Improved knowledge base and ongoing support to learn psychomotor skills facilitates effective breastfeeding (Cleugh & Langseth, 2017; McFadden et al, 2017).*
- ▲ Provide referrals and resources: lactation consultants, nurse and peer support programs, community organizations, and written and electronic sources of information. **EB:** *Systematic reviews support the use of professionals with special skills in breastfeeding, peer support programs, and written and electronic information to promote continued breastfeeding (McFadden et al, 2017).*

REFERENCES

Agho, K. E., Ogeleka, P., Ogbo, F. A., et al. (2016). Trends and predictors of prelacteal feeding practices in Nigeria (2003–2013). *Nutrients, 8*(8), E462.

American Academy of Pediatrics (AAP), Section on Breastfeeding. (2012). Breastfeeding and the use of human milk. *Pediatrics, 129*(3), e827–e841.

Amir, L. H. (2014). Managing common breastfeeding problems in the community. *British Medical Journal, 348,* g2954.

Balogun, O. O., O'Sullivan, E. J., McFadden, A., et al. (2016). Interventions for promoting the initiation of breastfeeding. *Cochrane Database Systematic Reviews,* (11), CD001688.

Cleugh, F., & Langseth, A. (2017). Fifteen-minute consultation on the healthy child: Breast feeding. *Archives of Disease in Childhood. Education and Practice Edition, 102,* 8–13.

Dennis, C. L. (2003). The breastfeeding self-efficacy scale: Psychometric assessment of the short form. *Journal of Obstetric, Gynecologic, and Neonatal Nursing: JOGNN/NAACOG, 32*(6), 734–744.

Kuswara, K., Laws, R., Kremer, P., et al. (2016). The infant feeding practices of Chinese immigrant mothers in Australia: A qualitative exploration. *Appetite, 105,* 375–384.

Lok, K. Y. W., Bai, D. L., & Tarrant, M. (2017). Family members' infant feeding preferences, maternal breastfeeding exposures and exclusive breastfeeding intentions. *Midwifery, 53,* 49–54.

McFadden, A., Gavine, A., Renfrew, M. J., et al. (2017). Support for healthy breastfeeding mothers with healthy term babies. *Cochrane Database Systematic Reviews,* (2), CD001141.

Moore, E. R., Bergman, N., Anderson, G. C., et al. (2016). Early skin-to-skin contact for mothers and their healthy newborn infants. *Cochrane Database Systematic Reviews,* (11), CD003519.

Neifert, M., & Bunik, M. (2013). Overcoming clinical barriers to exclusive breastfeeding. *Pediatric Clinics of North America, 60,* 115–145.

Tarrant, M., Lok, K. Y. W., Fong, D. Y. T., et al. (2015). Effect of a hospital policy of not accepting free infant formula on in-hospital formula supplementation rates and breastfeeding duration. *Public Health Nutrition, 18*(14), 2689–2699.

Waldrop, J. (2013). Exploration of reasons for feeding choices of Hispanic mothers. *MCN. The American Journal of Maternal Child Nursing, 38*(5), 282–288.

● = Independent;   ▲ = Collaborative;   **EBN** = Evidence-Based Nursing;   **EB** = Evidence-Based

Wandel, M., Terragni, L., Nguyen, C., et al. (2016). Breastfeeding among Somali mothers living in Norway: Attitudes, practices and challenges. *Women and Birth: Journal of the Australian College of Midwives*, 29(6), 487–493.

Wood, N. K., & Sanders, K. A. (2017). Mothers with perceived insufficient milk: Preliminary evidence of home interventions to boost mother-infant interactions. *Western Journal of Nursing Research*. doi:10.1177/0193945916687552.

B

Ineffective Breathing pattern   Debra Siela, PhD, RN, CCNS, ACNS-BC, CCRN-K, CNE, RRT

NANDA-I

Definition

Inspiration and/or expiration that does not provide adequate ventilation.

Defining Characteristics

Abnormal breathing pattern; altered chest excursion; bradypnea; decrease in expiratory pressure; decrease in inspiratory pressure; decrease in minute ventilation; decrease in vital capacity; dyspnea; increase in anterior-posterior chest diameter; nasal flaring; orthopnea; prolonged expiration phase; pursed-lip breathing; tachypnea; use of accessory muscles to breathe; use of three-point position

Related Factors

Anxiety; body position that inhibits lung expansion; fatigue; hyperventilation; obesity; pain; respiratory muscle fatigue

Associated Condition

Bony deformity; chest wall deformity; hypoventilation syndrome; musculoskeletal impairment; neurological immaturity; neurological impairment; neuromuscular impairment; spinal cord injury

NOC   (Nursing Outcomes Classification)

Suggested NOC Outcomes

Respiratory Status: Airway Patency, Ventilation; Vital Signs

Example NOC Outcome with Indicators
Respiratory Status: Ventilation as evidenced by the following indicators: Respiratory rate/Moves sputum out of airway/Adventitious breath sounds not present/Shortness of breath not present/Auscultated breath sounds/Auscultated vocalization/Chest x-ray findings. (Rate each indicator of **Respiratory Status: Ventilation:** 1 = severe deviation from normal range, 2 = substantial deviation from normal range, 3 = moderate deviation from normal range, 4 = mild deviation from normal range, 5 = no deviation from normal range [see Section I].)

Client Outcomes

Client Will (Specify Time Frame)

- Demonstrate a breathing pattern that supports blood gas results within the client's normal parameters
- Report ability to breathe comfortably
- Demonstrate ability to perform pursed-lip breathing and controlled breathing
- Identify and avoid specific factors that exacerbate episodes of ineffective breathing patterns

NIC   (Nursing Interventions Classification)

Suggested NIC Interventions

Airway Management; Respiratory Monitoring

Example NIC Activities—Airway Management
Encourage slow, deep breathing, turning, and coughing; Monitor respiratory and oxygenation status as appropriate

● = Independent;   ▲ = Collaborative;   EBN = Evidence-Based Nursing;   EB = Evidence-Based

Nursing Interventions and *Rationales*

- Monitor respiratory rate, depth, and ease of respiration. *Normal respiratory rate is 10 to 20 breaths per minute in the adult (Jarvis, 2015).*
- Note pattern of respiration. If client is dyspneic, note what seems to cause the dyspnea, the way in which the client deals with the condition, and how the dyspnea resolves or gets worse. **EB:** *Ask the client if they are short of breath (Campbell, 2017; Mahler & O'Donnell, 2015). Use dyspnea rating tools such as the dyspnea fatigue index, multidimensional dyspnea profile (Kjellstrom & van der Wal, 2013), or for nonverbal clients the Respiratory Distress Observation Scale is a behavioral scale that can be used to evaluate dyspnea (Campbell, 2017).*
- Note amount of anxiety associated with the dyspnea. **EBN:** *A normal respiratory pattern is regular in a healthy adult. To assess dyspnea, it is important to consider all of its dimensions, including antecedents, mediators, reactions, and outcomes. Dyspnea is a subjective experience of breathing discomfort that is best understood by asking the client about dimensions and triggers of the symptom experience (Campbell, 2017).*
- Attempt to determine if client's dyspnea is physiological or psychological in cause. *The evaluation of a client with dyspnea continues to be dependent on a thorough history and physical examination. In the client with acute worsening of chronic breathlessness, the health care provider must be attuned to the possibility of a new pathophysiological derangement superimposed on a known disorder. Instruments or sections of instruments pertaining to dyspnea should be classified as addressing domains of the sensory-perceptual experience, affective distress, or symptom/disease impact or burden (Kjellstrom & van der Wal, 2013; Mahler & O'Donnell, 2015; Parshall et al, 2012).*
- The rapidity of which the onset of dyspnea is noted is also an indicator of the severity of the pathological condition (Croucher, 2014)

Psychological Dyspnea—Hyperventilation

- Monitor for symptoms of hyperventilation including rapid respiratory rate, sighing breaths, lightheadedness, numbness and tingling of hands and feet, palpitations, and sometimes chest pain (Bickley & Szilagyi, 2016).
- Assess cause of hyperventilation by asking client about current emotions and psychological state.
  - ○ Pulmonary rehabilitation programs that contain elements of behavioral, cognitive, or psychosocial components have been shown to improve dyspnea and reduce anxiety and depression, particularly in clients with chronic obstructive pulmonary disease (COPD) (von Leupoldt et al, 2014).
  - ○ Pharmacological treatment to reduce anxiety and panic that likely increase dyspnea are not recommended for clients with asthma and COPD (von Leupoldt et al, 2014).
- Ask the client to breathe with you to slow down their respiratory rate. *Maintain eye contact and give reassurance. By making the client aware of respirations and giving support, the client may gain control of the breathing rate.*
- ▲ Consider having the client breathe in and out of a paper bag as tolerated. *This simple treatment helps associated symptoms of hyperventilation including helping to retain carbon dioxide, which will decrease associated symptoms of hyperventilation (Bickley & Szilagyi, 2016).*
- ▲ If the client has chronic problems with hyperventilation, numbness and tingling in extremities, dizziness, and other signs of panic attacks, refer for counseling or pulmonary rehabilitation (Lareau et al, 2014).

Physiological Dyspnea

- ▲ Ensure that client in acute dyspneic state has received any ordered medications, oxygen, and any other treatment needed.
- *Determine intensity, unpleasantness, or distress of dyspnea using a rating scale such as an intensity focused modified Borg scale or visual analog scale (Campbell, 2017; Hareendran & Leidy, 2014; Lareau et al, 2014; Parshall and Schwartzstein, 2014; Parshall et al, 2012).*
- *Note client description of the quality of breathing discomfort, such as chest tightness, air hunger, inability to breathe deeply, urge to breathe, starved for air, and feeling of suffocation are different types of dyspnea sensation reported by individuals with breathlessness (Campbell, 2017; Kjellstrom & van der Wal, 2013; Parshall and Schwartzstein, 2014).*
- Acute onset of dyspnea is often accompanied by signs of respiratory distress, which include tachypnea, cough, stridor, wheezing, cyanosis, impaired speech, tachycardia, hypotension, peripheral edema, frothy

• = Independent;   ▲ = Collaborative;   **EBN** = Evidence-Based Nursing;   **EB** = Evidence-Based

sputum, pursed lip breathing, accessory respiratory muscle use, crackles, tripod positioning, and other signs (Croucher, 2014)

- Observe color of tongue, oral mucosa, and skin for signs of cyanosis. *In central cyanosis, both the skin and mucous membranes are affected because of seriously impaired pulmonary function from unventilated or underventilated alveoli. Peripheral cyanosis (skin only) usually indicates vasoconstriction or obstruction to blood flow (Loscalzo, 2013).*

- Auscultate breath sounds, noting decreased or absent sounds, crackles, or wheezes. *These abnormal lung sounds can indicate a respiratory pathology associated with an altered breathing pattern (Croucher, 2014).*

- *Assess for hemodynamic stability for the client with acute dyspnea. Rapid evaluation for impending respiratory failure is essential and includes fragmented speech, tripod positioning, diaphoresis, cyanosis, Pao_2 less than 50 mm Hg, $Paco_2$ greater than 70, and use of accessory muscles. Hypotension along with dyspnea indicates threat of cardiopulmonary collapse (Croucher, 2014).*

- ▲ Monitor oxygen saturation continuously using pulse oximetry. Note blood gas results as available. *An oxygen saturation of less than 90% (normal: 95%–100%) or a partial pressure of oxygen of less than 80 mm Hg (normal: 80–100 mm Hg) indicates significant oxygenation problems.*
  - ○ If a client is both dyspneic and hypoxemic, high-flow oxygen may be more beneficial to relieve the dyspnea. EB: *Significant differences were found between low-flow and high-flow oxygen in reduction of dyspnea perceptions, reduction in respiratory rate, and increase in SaO_2. (Lenglet et al, 2012).*
  - ○ For clients with chronic breathlessness but no hypoxemia, oxygen therapy does not affect the sensation of dyspnea (Siela & Kidd, 2017).

- Using touch on the shoulder, coach the client to slow respiratory rate, demonstrating slower respirations; making eye contact with the client; and communicating in a calm, supportive fashion. *The nurse's presence, reassurance, and help in controlling the client's breathing can be beneficial in decreasing anxiety.* EB: A*nxiety is an important indicator of the severity of the client's COPD (Campbell, 2017).*

- Support the client in using pursed-lip and controlled breathing techniques. *Pursed-lip breathing may relieve dyspnea in advanced COPD (Lareau et al, 2014; Mahler, 2014; Parshall et al, 2012). Pursed-lip breathing results in increased use of intercostal muscles, decreased respiratory rate, increased tidal volume, and improved oxygen saturation levels (Mahler, 2014).*

- If the client is acutely dyspneic, consider having the client lean forward over a bedside table, resting elbows on the table if tolerated (Mahler, 2014). *Leaning forward can help decrease dyspnea, possibly because gastric pressure allows better contraction of the diaphragm (Mahler, 2014). This is called the tripod position and is used during times of distress, including when walking.*

- Position the client in an upright or semi-Fowler's position. *Most clients will have optimal vital capacity, oxygenation, and reduced dyspnea when upright with arms elevated on pillows or a bedside table (Campbell, 2017; Mahler, 2014).* See Nursing Interventions and *Rationales* for Impaired **Gas** exchange for further information on positioning.

- Increased respiratory drive is one of the causes of dyspnea. Pulmonary rehabilitation reduces respiratory drive through endurance exercise training, strength training, restorative therapy with calories and anabolic agents, pacing strategies and pursed lip breathing techniques, and optimizing bronchodilator therapy (Lareau et al, 2014).

- ▲ Administer oxygen as ordered. Supplemental oxygen may not relieve all dyspnea (Parshall et al, 2012). *Supplemental oxygen during exertion can result in marked reductions in exercise-induced breathlessness and improvements in exercise endurance in clients with COPD (Casey & Goldstein, 2014). Palliative oxygen therapy is not superior to medical air for breathlessness in palliative care clients (Casey & Goldstein, 2014). Reducing the effect of impaired ventilatory mechanics through reducing dynamic hyperinflation in COPD and strengthening respiratory muscles can reduce breathlessness. Interventions include exercise training with supplemental oxygen along with bronchodilators and inspiratory muscle training (Lareau et al, 2014).*

- *Mechanical ventilation, invasive or noninvasive, is a reliable means of reducing dyspnea associated with respiratory failure (Campbell, 2017).*

- *Opioids may be used for both acute and terminal dyspnea, considering careful safe dosing for relief and the side effect of constipation (Campbell, 2017; Parshall et al, 2012).*

- Altering the central perception of dyspnea may reduce breathlessness through exercise training, reduction in anxiety and fear of dyspnea, and self-management strategies and promotion of self-efficacy (Lareau et al, 2014).

- Use of music as a distraction may reduce the perception of dyspnea (Mahler, 2014).

● = Independent;   ▲ = Collaborative;   EBN = Evidence-Based Nursing;   EB = Evidence-Based

B

- Inspiratory muscle training likely improves breathlessness during exercise and/or with activities of daily living in clients with COPD and congestive heart failure (CHF) who exhibit inspiratory muscle weakness (Lareau et al, 2014; Mahler, 2014).
- Increase client's activity to walking three times per day as tolerated. Assist the client to use oxygen during activity as needed. See Nursing Interventions and *Rationales* for **Activity** intolerance. Walking 20 minutes per day is recommended for those unable to be in a structured program (GOLD, 2017). *Supervised exercise has been shown to decrease dyspnea and increase tolerance to activity (GOLD, 2017; Lareau et al, 2014).*
- Schedule rest periods before and after activity. *Respiratory clients with dyspnea are easily exhausted and need additional rest. Nurses coordinate all client care and are integral to ensuring spacing of activity to minimize or prevent dyspnea (Campbell, 2017).*
- ▲ Evaluate the client's nutritional status. Refer to a dietitian if needed. Use nutritional supplements to increase nutritional level if needed. *Improved nutrition may help increase inspiratory muscle function and decrease dyspnea.*
- Provide small, frequent feedings. *Small feedings are given to avoid compromising ventilatory effort and to conserve energy. Clients with dyspnea often do not eat sufficient amounts of food because their priority is breathing.*
- Offer a fan to move the air in the environment. CEB/EB: *Handheld fans can significantly reduce dyspnea in clients with chronic breathlessness (Galbraith et al, 2010; Mahler, 2014). A small portable handheld fan provides an effective self-management strategy for clients with dyspnea (Swan & Booth, 2015).*
- Encourage the client to take deep breaths at prescribed intervals and do controlled coughing.
- Help the client with chronic respiratory disease to evaluate dyspnea experience to determine whether previous incidences of dyspnea were similar and to recognize that the client survived those incidences. Encourage the client to be self-reliant if possible, use problem-solving skills, and maximize use of social support. *The focus of attention on sensations of breathlessness has an impact on judgment used to determine the intensity of the sensation (Campbell, 2017).*
- See Ineffective **Airway** clearance if client has a problem with increased respiratory secretions.
- ▲ Refer the client with COPD for pulmonary rehabilitation. EB: *Clients receiving pulmonary rehabilitation have a significant and clinically meaningful improvement in dyspnea discomfort and an impact in improving the effect of dyspnea on activities of daily living and overall quality of life (Lareau et al, 2014). Among the beneficial effects of pulmonary rehabilitation are a reduction in exertional dyspnea during exercise and improved exercise tolerance, as well as decreases in self-reported dyspnea with activity (Parshall et al, 2012). Appropriately resourced home-based exercise training has proven effective in reducing dyspnea and increasing exercise performance activity in the context of pulmonary rehabilitation (Spruit et al, 2013). Pulmonary rehabilitation benefits for COPD clients include reduction of the perceived intensity of breathlessness (GOLD, 2017).*

 Geriatric

- Assess respiratory systems in older adults with the understanding that inspiratory muscles weaken, resulting in a slight barrel chest. Expiratory muscles work harder with the use of accessory muscles (Martin-Plank, 2014).
- Encourage ambulation as tolerated. *Encourage movement because immobility is harmful to older adults and it decreases ventilation and increases stasis of secretions (Frederick, 2017).*
- Encourage older clients to sit upright or stand and to avoid lying down for prolonged periods during the day. *Thoracic aging results in decreased lung expansion; an erect position fosters maximal lung expansion (Frederick, 2017).*

 Home Care

- The previously mentioned interventions may be adapted for home care use.
- Work with the client to determine what strategies are most helpful during times of dyspnea. Provide education to empower the client to self-manage the disease associated with impaired gas exchange.
- Assist the client and family in identifying other factors that precipitate or exacerbate episodes of ineffective breathing patterns (i.e., stress, allergens, stairs, activities that have high energy requirements). *Awareness of precipitating factors helps clients avoid them and decreases the risk of ineffective breathing episodes (Campbell, 2017).*
- Assess client knowledge of and compliance with medication regimen. *Client/family may need repetition of instructions received at hospital discharge and may require reiteration as fear of a recent crisis decreases. Fear interferes with the ability to assimilate new information.*

- = Independent;   ▲ = Collaborative;   EBN = Evidence-Based Nursing;   EB = Evidence-Based

B

▲ Refer the client for telemonitoring with a pulmonologist as appropriate, with use of an electronic spirometer or an electronic peak flowmeter. EB: *A growing body of evidence shows that telemonitoring is both time and cost effective for the provider and client providing more timely continuity of care (Di Cerbo et al, 2015).*

● Teach the client and family the importance of maintaining the therapeutic regimen and having as-needed drugs easily accessible at all times. *Appropriate and timely use of medications can decrease the risk of exacerbating ineffective breathing. The 2017 GOLD Report states that bronchodilator medications are central to management of dyspnea (GOLD, 2017).*

● Provide the client with emotional support in dealing with symptoms of respiratory difficulty. Provide family with support for care of a client with chronic or terminal illness. Refer to care plan for **Anxiety.** Witnessing breathing difficulties and facing concerns of dealing with chronic or terminal illness can create fear in the caregiver. Fear inhibits effective coping (Campbell, 2017).

● When respiratory procedures (e.g., apneic monitoring for an infant) are being implemented, explain equipment and procedures to family members, and provide needed emotional support. *Family members assuming responsibility for respiratory monitoring often find this stressful. They may not have been able to assimilate fully any instructions provided by hospital staff (Martin-Plank, 2014).*

● When electrically based equipment for respiratory support is being implemented, evaluate home environment for electrical safety, such as proper grounding. Ensure that notification is sent to the local utility company, the emergency medical team, and police and fire departments. *Notification is important to provide for priority service.*

● Refer to GOLD guidelines for management of home care and indications of hospital admission criteria.

● Support clients' efforts at self-care. Ensure they have all the information they need to participate in care.

● Identify an emergency plan including when to call your health care provider or 911. *Having a ready emergency plan reassures the client and promotes client safety.*

▲ Refer to occupational therapy for evaluation and teaching of energy conservation techniques.

▲ Refer to home health aide services as needed to support energy conservation. *Energy conservation decreases the risk of exacerbating ineffective breathing.*

▲ Institute case management of frail elderly to support continued independent living (Martin-Plank, 2014).

Client/Family Teaching and Discharge Planning

● Teach pursed-lip and controlled breathing techniques. EB: *Studies have demonstrated that pursed-lip breathing was effective in decreasing breathlessness and improving respiratory function (Lareau et al, 2014; Mahler, 2014). Pursed-lip breathing may relieve dyspnea in advanced COPD (Parshall et al, 2012).*

● Teach about dosage, actions, and side effects of medications. *Inhaled steroids and bronchodilators can have undesirable side effects, especially when taken in inappropriate doses.*

● Teach client progressive muscle relaxation techniques. EB: *Relaxation therapy may help reduce dyspnea and anxiety (von Leupoldt et al, 2014). Benefits of pulmonary rehabilitation include reduction of anxiety and depression associated with COPD (GOLD, 2017).*

● Teach the client to identify and avoid specific factors that exacerbate ineffective breathing patterns, such as exposure to other sources of air pollution, especially smoking. If client smokes, refer to the smoking cessation section in the impaired **Gas** exchange care plan.

REFERENCES

Bickley, L. S., & Szilagyi, P. (2016). *Bate's guide to physical examination* (p. 12). Philadelphia: Lippincott.

Campbell, M. L. (2017). Dyspnea. *Critical Care Nursing Clinics of North America, 29*(4), 461–470.

Casey, D., & Goldstein, R. (2014). Oxygen. In D. A. Mahler & D. E. O'Donnell (Eds.), *Dyspnea mechanisms, measurement and management.* Boca Raton, FL: CRC Press Taylor & Francis Group.

Croucher, B. (2014). The challenge of diagnosing dyspnea. *AACN Advanced Critical Care, 25*(3), 284–290.

Di Cerbo, A., Morales-Medina, J. C., Palmieri, B., et al. (2015). Narrative review of telemedicine consultation in medical practice. *Patient Preference and Adherence, 9*, 65–75.

Frederick, D. E. (2017). Pulmonary issues in the older adult. *Critical Care Nursing Clinics of North America, 29*(4), 91–97.

Galbraith, S., Fagan, P., Perkins, P., et al. (2010). Does the use of a handheld fan improve chronic dyspnea? A randomized controlled crossover trial. *Journal of Pain and Symptom Management, 39*, 831–838.

GOLD Global strategy for the diagnosis, management, and prevention of COPD (revised 2017), Global Initiative for Chronic Obstructive Lung Disease. Retrieved from http://goldcopd.org/wp-content/uploads/2016/12/wms-GOLD-2017-Pocket-Guide.pdf. (Accessed 10 February 2018).

Hareendran, A., & Leidy, N. (2014). Measurement of dyspnea in clinical trials. In D. A. Mahler & D. E. O'Donnell (Eds.), *Dyspnea mechanisms, measurement and management.* Boca Raton, FL: CRC Press Taylor & Francis Group.

● = Independent;   ▲ = Collaborative;   EBN = Evidence-Based Nursing;   EB = Evidence-Based

Jarvis, C. (2015). General survey, measurement, vital signs. In C. Jarvis (Ed.), *Physical examination & health assessment* (7th ed.). St Louis: Saunders Elsevier.

Kjellstrom, B., & van der Wal, M. H. L. (2013). Old and new tools to assess dyspnea in the hospitalized patient. *Current Heart Failure Reports, 10*, 204–211.

Lareau, S., Meek, P., & ZuWallack, R. (2014). Effect of pulmonary rehabilitation on dyspnea. In D. A. Mahler & D. E. O'Donnell (Eds.), *Dyspnea mechanisms, measurement and management*. Boca Raton, FL: CRC Press Taylor & Francis Group.

Lenglet, H., Sztrymf, B., Leroy, C., et al. (2012). Humidified high flow nasal oxygen during respiratory failure in the emergency department: Feasibility and efficacy. *Respiratory Care, 57*(11), 1873–1878.

Loscalzo, J. (2013). Hypoxia and cyanosis. In J. Loscalzo (Ed.), *Harrison's pulmonary and critical care medicine* (2nd ed., pp. 21–25). New York: McGraw-Hill Education Medical.

Mahler, D. (2014). Other treatments for dyspnea. In D. A. Mahler & D. E. O'Donnell (Eds.), *Dyspnea mechanisms, measurement and management*. Boca Raton, FL: CRC Press Taylor & Francis Group.

Mahler, D. A., & O'Donnell, D. E. (2015). Recent advances in dyspnea. *Chest, 147*(1), 232–241.

Martin-Plank, L. (2014). Chest disorders. In L. Kennedy-Malone, K. R. Fletcher, & L. Martin-Plank (Eds.), *Advanced practice nursing in the care of older adults*. Philadelphia: F. A. Davis Company.

Parshall, M. B., & Schwartzstein, R. M. (2014). Domains of dyspnea measurement. In D. A. Mahler & D. E. O'Donnell (Eds.), *Dyspnea mechanisms, measurement and management*. Boca Raton, FL: CRC Press Taylor & Francis Group.

Parshall, M. B., Schwartzstein, R. M., Adams, L., et al. (2012). An official American Thoracic Society statement: Update on the mechanisms, assessment, and management of dyspnea. *American Journal of Respiratory and Critical Care Medicine, 185*(4), 435–452.

Siela, D., & Kidd, M. (2017). Oxygen requirements for acutely and critically ill patients. *Critical Care Nurse, 37*(4), 58–70.

Spruit, M. A., Singh, S. J., Garvey, C., et al. (2013). An official American Thoracic Society/European Respiratory Society Statement: Key concepts and advances in pulmonary rehabilitation. *American Journal of Respiratory and Critical Care Medicine, 188*(8), e13–e64.

Swan, F., & Booth, S. (2015). The role of airflow for the relief of chronic refractory breathlessness. *Current Opinion in Supportive & Palliative Care, 9*(3), 206–211.

von Leupoldt, A., Van den Bergh, O., & Davenport, P. (2014). Anxiety, depression, and panic. In D. A. Mahler & D. E. O'Donnell (Eds.), *Dyspnea mechanisms, measurement and management*. Boca Raton, FL: CRC Press Taylor & Francis Group.

Decreased Cardiac output   *Ann Will Poteet, MS, RN, CNS, AGNP-C*

NANDA-I

Definition

Inadequate blood pumped by the heart to meet the metabolic demands of the body.

Defining Characteristics

Altered Heart Rate/Rhythm

Bradycardia, electrocardiogram (ECG) change; heart palpitations; tachycardia

Altered Preload

Decrease in central venous pressure (CVP); decrease in pulmonary artery wedge pressure (PAWP); edema; fatigue; heart murmur; increase in central venous pressure (CVP); increase in pulmonary artery wedge pressure (PAWP); jugular vein distention; weight gain

Altered Afterload

Abnormal skin color; alteration in blood pressure; clammy skin; decrease in peripheral pulses; decrease in pulmonary vascular resistance (PVR); decrease in systemic vascular resistance (SVR); dyspnea; increase in pulmonary vascular resistance (PVR); increase in systemic vascular resistance (SVR); oliguria; prolonged capillary refill

Altered Contractility

Adventitious breath sounds; coughing; decreased cardiac index; decrease in ejection fraction; decrease in left ventricular stroke work index (LVSWI); decrease in stroke volume index (SVI); orthopnea; paroxysmal nocturnal dyspnea; presence of S3 heart sound; presence of S4 heart sound

Behavioral/Emotional

Anxiety; restlessness

● = Independent;   ▲ = Collaborative;   EBN = Evidence-Based Nursing;   EB = Evidence-Based

Related Factors

To be developed

Associated Condition

Alteration in afterload, alteration in contractility; alteration in heart rate; alteration in heart rhythm; alteration in preload; alteration in stroke volume

NOC (Nursing Outcomes Classification)

Suggested NOC Outcomes

Cardiac Pump Effectiveness; Circulation Status; Tissue Perfusion: Abdominal Organs, Peripheral; Vital Signs

> **Example NOC Outcome with Indicators**
>
> **Cardiac Pump Effectiveness** as evidenced by the following indicators: Blood pressure/Heart rate/Cardiac index/Ejection fraction/Activity tolerance/Peripheral pulses/Neck vein distention not present/Heart rhythm/Heart sounds/Angina not present/Peripheral edema not present/Pulmonary edema not present. (Rate the outcome and indicators of **Cardiac Pump Effectiveness:** 1 = severe deviation from normal range, 2 = substantial deviation from normal range, 3 = moderate deviation from normal range, 4 = mild deviation from normal range, 5 = no deviation from normal range [see Section I].)

Client Outcomes

Client Will (Specify Time Frame)

- Demonstrate adequate cardiac output as evidenced by blood pressure, pulse rate, and rhythm within normal parameters for client; strong peripheral pulses; maintained level of mentation, lack of chest discomfort or dyspnea, and adequate urinary output; an ability to tolerate activity without symptoms of dyspnea, syncope, or chest pain
- Remain free of side effects from the medications used to achieve adequate cardiac output
- Explain actions and precautions to prevent primary or secondary cardiac disease

NIC (Nursing Interventions Classification)

Suggested NIC Interventions

Cardiac Care; Cardiac Care: Acute

> **Example NIC Activities—Cardiac Care**
>
> Evaluate chest pain (e.g., intensity, location, radiation, duration, precipitating and alleviating factors); Document cardiac dysrhythmias

Nursing Interventions and *Rationales*

- Recognize characteristics of decreased cardiac output including, but not limited to, fatigue, dyspnea, edema, orthopnea, paroxysmal nocturnal dyspnea, chest pain, decreased exercise capacity, weight gain, hepatomegaly, jugular venous distension, palpitations, lung rhonchi, cough, clammy skin, skin color changes, dysuria, altered mental status, anemia, and hemodynamic changes.
- Monitor and report presence and degree of symptoms including dyspnea at rest, reduced exercise capacity, difficulty with activities of daily living, orthopnea, paroxysmal nocturnal dyspnea, cough, palpitations, chest pain, distended abdomen, fatigue, presyncope/syncope, or weakness. Monitor and report signs including jugular vein distention, peripheral edema, S3 gallop, rales, positive hepatojugular reflux, ascites, laterally displaced or pronounced point of maximal impact, heart murmur, narrow pulse pressure, cool extremities, tachycardia with pulsus alternans, and irregular heartbeat. EB: *These are symptoms and signs consistent with heart failure (HF) and decreased cardiac output (Yancy et al, 2013).*
- Monitor orthostatic blood pressures, oxygenation, hemodynamic values, and daily weights. EB: *These interventions assess for fluid volume status. Peripheral edema or the lack of peripheral edema is not always indicative of hypervolemia or decreased cardiac output (Yancy et al, 2013).*

● = Independent;   ▲ = Collaborative;   EBN = Evidence-Based Nursing;   EB = Evidence-Based

C

- Recognize that decreased cardiac output can occur in a number of noncardiac disorders such as septic shock and hypovolemia. Expect variation in orders for differential diagnoses related to decreased cardiac output, because orders will be distinct to address the primary cause of the altered cardiac output.
- Obtain a thorough client-specific and familial history. EB: *It is important to assess for cardiac and noncardiac disorders and/or behaviors that might accelerate the progression of HF symptoms, such as high-sodium diet, excess fluid intake, substance abuse, missed medication doses, hypertension, diabetes mellitus, metabolic syndrome, obesity, hyperlipidemia, hormonal abnormalities, genetic disorders, coronary artery disease, sleep disordered breathing, congenital heart disease, cancer, immune disorders, and pregnancy (Bozkurt et al, 2016; Yancy et al, 2013, 2017).*
- ▲ Monitor pulse oximetry and administer oxygen as needed per health care provider's order. Supplemental oxygen increases oxygen availability to the myocardium and can relieve symptoms of hypoxemia. Resting hypoxia or oxygen desaturation may indicate fluid overload or concurrent pulmonary disease.
- Place client in semi-Fowler's or high Fowler's position with legs down or in a position of comfort. Elevating the head of the bed and legs in the down position may decrease the work of breathing and may also decrease venous return and preload.
- During acute events, ensure client remains on short-term bed rest or maintains activity level that does not compromise cardiac output.
- Provide a restful environment by minimizing controllable stressors and unnecessary disturbances. Reducing stressors decreases cardiac workload and oxygen demand.
- ▲ Apply graduated compression stockings or intermittent sequential pneumatic compression (ISPC) leg sleeves as ordered. Ensure proper fit by measuring accurately. Remove stockings at least twice a day, and then reapply. Assess the condition of the extremities frequently. Graduated compression stockings may be contraindicated in clients with peripheral arterial disease (Kahn et al, 2012). EB: *A Cochrane review that assessed use of knee-length graduated compression stockings versus thigh-length graduated compression stockings found no difference in effectiveness. Type of stocking should be determined by client preference, cost, and ease of use (Sajid et al, 2012). EB: Graduated compression stockings, alone or used in conjunction with other prevention modalities, help promote venous return and reduce the risk of deep vein thrombosis in hospitalized clients (Sachdeva et al, 2014).*
- ▲ Check blood pressure, pulse, and condition before administering cardiac medications (e.g., angiotensin-converting enzyme inhibitors, angiotensin receptor blockers, calcium channel blockers, diuretics, digoxin, and beta-blockers). Notify health care provider if heart rate or blood pressure is low before holding medications. It is important that the nurse evaluate how well the client is tolerating current medications before administering cardiac medications; do not hold medications without health care provider input. The health care provider may decide to have medications administered even though the blood pressure or pulse rate has lowered. EB: *Clients with preserved ejection heart failure (HFpEF) or reduced ejection fraction heart failure (HFrEF) and persistent hypertension, and those with HF and increased cardiovascular risk (age >75 years old, established vascular disease, chronic renal disease, or Framingham risk score >15%) should receive guideline-directed medical therapy (GDMT) to maintain a systolic blood pressure less than 130 mm Hg (Yancy et al, 2017).*
- Observe for and report chest pain or discomfort; note location, radiation, severity, quality, duration, and associated manifestations such as nausea, indigestion, or diaphoresis; also note precipitating and relieving factors. Chest pain/discomfort may indicate an inadequate blood supply to the heart, which can further compromise cardiac output. EB: *Clients with decreased cardiac output may present with myocardial ischemia. Those with myocardial ischemia may present with decreased cardiac output and HF (Amsterdam et al, 2014; Yancy et al, 2013).*
- ▲ If chest pain is present, then refer to the interventions in risk for Decreased **Cardiac** tissue perfusion care plan.
- Recognize the effect of sleep-disordered breathing in HF and that sleep disorders are common in clients with HF (Yancy et al, 2013, 2017). EB: *Central sleep apnea is recognized as an independent risk factor for worsening HF and reduced survival in clients with HF. The pathological effects of sleep apnea that contribute to worsening cardiac function include sympathetic nervous system stimulation, systemic inflammation, oxidative stress, and endothelial dysfunction (Costanzo et al, 2015). EB: For obstructive sleep apnea, continuous positive airway pressure (CPAP) can reduce apneic events, improve nocturnal oxygenation, and improve sleep quality (Yancy et al, 2017).*
- Administer CPAP or supplemental oxygen at night as ordered for management of suspected or diagnosed sleep disordered breathing. EB: *Both CPAP and nocturnal oxygen supplementation have been shown to*

• = Independent; ▲ = Collaborative; EBN = Evidence-Based Nursing; EB = Evidence-Based

reduce episodes of sleep apnea, reduce sympathetic nervous system stimulation, and improve cardiac function (Costanzo et al, 2015).

▲ Closely monitor fluid intake, including intravenous lines. Maintain fluid restriction if ordered. In clients with decreased cardiac output, poorly functioning ventricles may not tolerate increased fluid volumes. EB: *Fluid restriction along with sodium restriction can enhance volume management with diuretics, and in some clients can improve outcomes (Yancy et al, 2013).*

● Monitor intake and output (I&O). If client is acutely ill, measure hourly urine output and note decreases in output. Decreased cardiac output results in decreased perfusion of the kidneys, with a resulting decrease in urine output. EB: *Clinical practice guidelines cite that monitoring I&Os is useful for monitoring effects of HF treatment, including diuretic therapy (Yancy et al, 2013).*

▲ Note results of initial diagnostic studies, including electrocardiography, echocardiography, and chest radiography. EB: *Clinical practice guidelines suggest that chest radiography, echocardiography, and electrocardiogram are recommended in the initial assessment of HF (Yancy et al, 2013).*

▲ Note results of further diagnostic imaging studies such as radionuclide imaging, stress echocardiography, cardiac catheterization, or magnetic resonance imaging (MRI). EB: *Clinical practice guidelines state that radionuclide and MRI are useful studies when assessing left ventricular ejection fraction and volume if echocardiography is not sufficient (Yancy et al, 2013).*

▲ Review laboratory data as needed including arterial blood gases, complete blood count, serum electrolytes (sodium, potassium, magnesium, and calcium), blood urea nitrogen, creatinine, iron studies, urinalysis, glucose, fasting lipid profile, liver function tests, thyroid-stimulating hormone, B-type natriuretic peptide (BNP assay), or N-terminal pro-B-type natriuretic peptide (NTpro-BNP). Routine blood work can provide insight into the etiology of HF and extent of decompensation. EB: *Clinical practice guidelines recommend that BNP or NTpro-BNP assay should be measured in clients to determine prognosis or disease severity in chronic or acute decompensated HF, guide treatment during hospitalization, and establish a baseline at time of hospital discharge. BNP can also be evaluated in at-risk clients for prevention in the outpatient setting (Yancy et al, 2017).* EB: *Iron-deficiency anemia is related to decreased exercise capacity, and anemia is a strong indication of HF severity (Yancy et al, 2017).*

● Gradually increase activity when the client's condition is stabilized by encouraging slower paced activities, or shorter periods of activity, with frequent rest periods after exercise prescription; observe for symptoms of intolerance. Take blood pressure and pulse before and after activity and note changes. Activity of the cardiac client should be closely monitored. See **Activity** intolerance.

▲ Encourage a diet that promotes cardiovascular health and reduces risk of hypertension, atherosclerotic disease, renal impairment, insulin resistance, and hypervolemia, within the context of an individual's cultural preferences (Eckel et al, 2013; Van Horn et al, 2016; Whelton et al, 2017). EB: *Reduced sodium intake, weight loss, healthy diet (low sugar, whole grains, fruits and vegetables, low saturated and total fat), and avoidance of excess caloric intake is recommended for individuals with elevated blood pressure and for prevention of cardiovascular disease (Van Horn et al, 2016; Whelton et al, 2017).*

▲ Monitor bowel function. Provide stool softeners as ordered. Caution client not to strain when defecating. Decreased activity, pain medication, and diuretics can cause constipation. EBN: *Clients with HF have autonomic dysfunction, which places them at risk for reduced mean arterial blood pressure and reduced cerebral blood flow. Autonomic challenges, such as the Valsalva maneuver, can put the HF client at risk for hypoperfusion, ischemia, and stroke (Serber et al, 2014).*

● Weigh the client at the same time daily (after voiding). Daily weight is a good indicator of fluid balance. Use the same scale if possible when weighing clients for consistency. Increased weight and severity of symptoms can signal decreased cardiac function with retention of fluids. EB: *Clinical practice guidelines state that weighing at the same time daily is useful to assess effects of diuretic therapy (Yancy et al, 2013).*

▲ Provide influenza and pneumococcal vaccines as needed before client discharge for those who have yet to receive those inoculations (Centers for Disease Control, 2017).

● Assess for presence of depression and/or anxiety and refer for treatment if present. See Nursing Interventions and *Rationales* for **Anxiety** to facilitate reduction of anxiety in clients and family. EB: *Depression is common in clients with HF, and it has been found that individuals with depressive symptoms have poorer quality of life, use health care services more frequently, have poorer self-care, and have worse clinical outcomes (Yancy et al, 2013).*

▲ Refer to a cardiac rehabilitation program for education and monitored exercise. EB: *Exercise training or regular physical activity is recommended for HF clients. Cardiac rehabilitation can improve quality of life and functional capacity, and decrease mortality (Anderson & Taylor, 2014; Yancy et al, 2013). A systematic*

● = Independent; ▲ = Collaborative; EBN = Evidence-Based Nursing; EB = Evidence-Based

C

review of outcomes of exercise-based interventions in clients with systolic HF found that hospitalizations and those for systolic HF were reduced for clients in an exercise program and quality of life was improved (Taylor et al, 2014).

▲ Refer to an HF program for education, evaluation, and guided support to increase activity and rebuild quality of life. Support for the HF client should be client centered, culturally sensitive, and include family and social support. EB: *Multidisciplinary systems of care that are designed to support clients with HF can improve outcomes (Yancy et al, 2013).*

Critically Ill

▲ Observe for symptoms of cardiogenic shock, including impaired mentation, hypotension, decreased peripheral pulses, cold clammy skin, signs of pulmonary congestion, and decreased organ function. If present, notify the health care provider immediately. Cardiogenic shock is a state of circulatory failure from loss of cardiac function associated with inadequate organ perfusion and a high mortality rate. EB: *Critical cardiogenic shock presents with severe hypotension, increasing inotropic and vasopressor support, organ hypoperfusion, and worsening acidosis and lactate levels (Yancy et al, 2013).*

▲ If shock is present, monitor hemodynamic parameters for an increase in pulmonary wedge pressure, an increase in SVR, or a decrease in stroke volume, cardiac output, and cardiac index. EB: *Hemodynamic monitoring with a pulmonary artery catheter can be beneficial in clients with respiratory distress, impaired systemic perfusion, and dependence on intravenous inotropic support, and when clinical assessment is inadequate or severe symptoms persist despite recommended therapies (Yancy et al, 2013).*

▲ Titrate inotropic and vasoactive medications within defined parameters to maintain contractility, preload, and afterload per health care provider's order. By following parameters, the nurse ensures maintenance of a delicate balance of medications that stimulate the heart to increase contractility, while maintaining adequate perfusion of the body. EB: *Clinical practice guidelines recommend that intravenous inotropic drugs might be reasonable for HF clients presenting with low blood pressure and low cardiac output to maintain systemic perfusion and preserve end-organ performance (Yancy et al, 2013).*

▲ Identify significant fluid overload and initiate intravenous diuretics as ordered. Monitor I&Os, daily weight, and vital signs, as well as signs and symptoms of congestion. Watch laboratory data, including serum electrolytes, creatinine, and urea nitrogen. EB: *Intravenous loop diuretics should be initiated in the HF client who presents with significant fluid overload as either intermittent boluses or continuous infusion to reduce morbidity (Yancy et al, 2013).*

▲ When using pulmonary arterial catheter technology, be sure to appropriately level and zero the equipment, use minimal tubing, maintain system patency, perform square wave testing, position the client appropriately, and consider correlation to respiratory and cardiac cycles when assessing waveforms and integrating data into client assessment. EB: *Clinical practice guidelines recommend that invasive hemodynamic monitoring can be useful in acute HF with persistent symptoms when therapy is refractory, fluid status is unclear, systolic pressures are low, renal function is worsening, vasoactive agents are required, or when considering advanced device therapy or transplantation (Yancy et al, 2013).*

▲ Observe for worsening signs and symptoms of respiratory compromise. Recognize that invasive or noninvasive ventilation may be required for clients with acute cardiogenic pulmonary edema. EB: *Clinical practice guidelines for an HF state that CPAP improves daily functional capacity and quality of life for those with HF and obstructive sleep apnea and is reasonable for clients with refractory HF not responding to other medical therapies (Costanzo et al, 2015; Yancy et al, 2013).* EB: *Noninvasive positive pressure ventilation (NPPV), including CPAP and bilevel NPPV, can reduce hospital mortality, intensive care unit (ICU) length of stay, and intubation rate, and result in faster client improvement (Vital et al, 2013).*

▲ Monitor client for signs and symptoms of fluid and electrolyte imbalance when clients are receiving ultrafiltration or continuous renal replacement therapy (CRRT). Clients with refractory HF may have ultrafiltration or CRRT ordered as a mechanical method to remove excess fluid volume. EB: *Clinical practice guidelines cite that ultrafiltration is reasonable for clients with obvious volume overload and congestion, and refractory congestion not responsive to medical therapy (Yancy et al, 2013).*

● Recognize that hypoperfusion from low cardiac output can lead to altered mental status and decreased cognition. CEB: *A study that assessed an association among cardiac index and neuropsychological ischemia found that decreased cardiac function, even with normal cardiac index, was associated with accelerated brain aging (Jefferson et al, 2010).*

● Recognize that clients with severe HF may undergo additional therapies, such as internal pacemaker or defibrillator placement, and/or placement of a ventricular assist device (VAD). EB: *The use of VADs is a*

● = Independent;   ▲ = Collaborative;   EBN = Evidence-Based Nursing;   EB = Evidence-Based

reasonable treatment as a bridge to recovery, transplant, or decision-making in selected HF clients with reduced ejection fraction and profound hemodynamic compromise (Yancy et al, 2013).

Geriatric

- Recognize that older clients may demonstrate fatigue and depression as signs of HF and decreased cardiac output.
- ▲ If the client has heart disease causing activity intolerance, refer for cardiac rehabilitation. EB: *Cardiac rehabilitation can positively affect an individual's quality of life and reduce hospitalizations regardless of age (Anderson & Taylor, 2014; Taylor et al, 2014).*
- ▲ Recognize that edema can present differently in the older population. EB: *In the older population, lower extremity edema is often related to peripheral causes, such as dependency, rather than cardiac causes (Yancy et al, 2013).*
- ▲ Recognize that blood pressure control is beneficial for older clients to reduce the risk of worsening HF. EB: *Hypertension treatment is particularly beneficial in the older population, and control of both systolic and diastolic hypertension has been shown to reduce the risk of incident HF (Yancy et al, 2013). EB: Clients with stage A HF and hypertension, with increased cardiovascular risk (age >75 years old, established vascular disease, chronic renal disease, or Framingham risk score >15%) should have a target systolic blood pressure less than 130 mm Hg (Yancy et al, 2017).*
- ▲ Recognize that renal function is not always accurately represented by serum creatinine in the older population because of less muscle mass (Yancy et al, 2013).
- ▲ Observe for side effects from cardiac medications. Older adults can have difficulty with metabolism and excretion of medications because of decreased function of the liver and kidneys; therefore toxic side effects are more common. EB: *Older adults are at increased risk for digoxin toxicity, especially at larger doses, because of lower body mass and impaired renal function (Yancy et al, 2013).*
- ▲ Older adults may require more frequent visits, closer monitoring of medication dose changes, and more gradual increases in medications, because of changes in the metabolism of medications and impaired renal function (Yancy et al, 2013).
- ▲ As older adults approach end of life, clinicians should help to facilitate a comprehensive plan of care that incorporates the client and family's values, goals, and preferences (Allen et al, 2012; National Consensus Project for Quality Palliative Care, 2013). EB: *For older adults (>65 years old) with multiple comorbidities and limited life expectancy, it is reasonable to use a team-based approach to weigh the risks and benefits of tight blood pressure control and choice of antihypertensive medication (Whelton et al, 2017).*

Home Care

- Some of the previously mentioned interventions may be adapted for home care use. Home care agencies may use specialized staff and methods to care for chronic HF clients. CEB: *A study assessing HF outcomes over a 10-year period between a multidisciplinary home care intervention and usual care found significantly improved survival and prolonged event-free survival and was both cost and time effective (Ingles et al, 2006).*
- Assess for fatigue and weakness frequently. Assess home environment for safety, as well as resources/ obstacles to energy conservation.
- Help family adapt daily living patterns to establish life changes that will maintain improved cardiac functioning in the client. Take the client's perspective into consideration and use a holistic approach in assessing and responding to client planning for the future.
- Assist client to recognize and exercise power in using self-care management to adjust to health change. Refer to care plan for **Powerlessness.**
- ▲ Refer to medical social services, cardiac rehabilitation, telemonitoring, and case management as necessary for assistance with home care, access to resources, and counseling about the impact of severe or chronic cardiac diseases. EB: *Access to systems that promote care coordination is essential for successful care of the HF client. Good communication and documentation between services, health care providers, and transitions of care is essential to ensure improved outcomes in HF clients (Albert et al, 2015; Yancy et al, 2013).*
- ▲ As the client chooses, refer to palliative care for care, which can begin earlier in the care of the HF client. Palliative care can be used to increase comfort and quality of life in the HF client before end-of-life care. EB: *Palliative care should address quality of life, ongoing symptom control, preferences about end of life, psychosocial distress, and caregiver support (National Consensus Project for Quality Palliative Care, 2013; Yancy et al, 2013).*

● = Independent;   ▲ = Collaborative;   EBN = Evidence-Based Nursing;   EB = Evidence-Based

C

▲ If the client's condition warrants, refer to hospice. EB: *The palliative care and HF teams are best suited to determine when end-of-life care is appropriate for the client and family (Yancy et al, 2013).* CEB: *The multidisciplinary hospice team can reduce hospital readmission, increase functional capacity, and improve quality of life in end-stage HF (Coviello et al, 2002).*

 Client/Family Teaching and Discharge Planning

● Begin discharge planning as soon as possible on admission to the emergency department (ED) if appropriate with a case manager or social worker to assess home support systems and the need for community or home health services. EB: *Discharge planning should include adherence to the treatment plan, medication management, follow-up with health care providers and care coordination, dietary and physical activities, cardiac rehabilitation, and secondary prevention recommendations (Albert et al, 2015; Yancy et al, 2013).*

● Discharge education should be comprehensive, evidence based, culturally sensitive, and include both the client and family (Yancy et al, 2013).

● Teach the client about any medications prescribed. Medication teaching includes the drug name; its purpose, administration instructions, such as taking it with or without food; and any side effects. Instruct the client to report any adverse side effects to his or her health care provider.

● Teach the importance of performing and recording daily weights on arising for the day, and to report weight gain. Ask if client has a scale at home; if not, assist in getting one. EB: *Clinical practice guidelines suggest that daily weight monitoring leads to early recognition of excess fluid retention, which, when reported, can be offset with additional medication to avoid hospitalization from HF decompensation (Yancy et al, 2013).*

● Teach the types and progression patterns of worsening HF symptoms, when to call a health care provider for help, and when to go to the hospital for urgent care (Yancy et al, 2013).

● Stress the importance of ceasing tobacco use (Whelton et al, 2017). EB: *Tobacco use can cause or worsen decreased blood flow in the coronaries, as well as cause vasoconstriction, which can lead to atherosclerotic disease. Effects of nicotine include increasing pulse and blood pressure and constricting of blood vessels. Tobacco use is a primary factor in heart disease (American Heart Association, 2014).*

▲ Individuals should be screened for electronic cigarette use (e-cigarette). EB: *Although more studies are needed regarding the health effects of e-cigarette use, the American Heart Association recommends that all health care providers educate their clients regarding the long-term use of e-cigarettes given the known toxicities present in e-cigarettes, as well as the presence of nicotine in most types of e-cigarettes (Bhatnagar et al, 2014).*

● On hospital discharge, educate clients about low-sodium, low–saturated fat diet, with consideration of client education, literacy, and health literacy level.

● Educate clients that comorbidities, including obesity, hypertension, metabolic syndrome, diabetes mellitus, and hyperlipidemia, are common in individuals with HF and can affect clinical outcomes related to HF if not controlled (Bozkurt et al, 2016).

● For clients with diabetes mellitus, educate about the importance of glycemic control. EB: *Individuals with diabetes mellitus are at increased risk for HF, and should be managed according to recommended guidelines. Thiazolidinediones should be avoided in individuals with class III or IV HF because of increased fluid retention (Bozkurt et al, 2016).*

● Instruct client and family on the importance of regular follow-up care with health care providers. EB: *Post discharge support can significantly reduce hospital readmissions and improve health care outcomes, quality of life, and costs (Yancy et al, 2013).*

▲ Teach stress reduction (e.g., meditation, imagery, controlled breathing, muscle relaxation techniques). CEB: *A study that assessed effects of relaxation or exercise in HF clients versus controls found that those who participated in regular relaxation therapy or exercise training reported greater improvements in psychological outcomes, with the relaxation group significantly improving depression and the exercise training group improving fatigue (Yu et al, 2007).* EB: *Meditation is a reasonable adjunct to GDMT for reduction of cardiovascular risk and lifestyle modification (Levine et al, 2017).*

● Discuss advance directives with the HF client, including resuscitation preferences. EB: Evidence suggests that advance directives can help to reduce overall health care costs, reduce in-hospital deaths, and increase hospice use (National Consensus Project for Quality Palliative Care, 2013; Yancy et al, 2013).

● Clients should be provided with education regarding the influenza vaccine and pneumococcal vaccine prior to discharge. EB: *The influenza vaccine is recommended for all adults, and the pneumococcal vaccine is recommended for individuals more than 65 years old and for individuals who are at high risk for cardiovascular disease (Centers for Disease Control, 2017).*

● = Independent;   ▲ = Collaborative;   EBN = Evidence-Based Nursing;   EB = Evidence-Based

- Teach the importance of physical activity as tolerated. EB: *Exercise helps control blood pressure and weight, which are the most important controlled risk factors for cardiovascular disease. Individuals should engage in aerobic physical activity of varying intensity as tolerated and incorporate variable anaerobic activities such as resistance training (Bozkurt et al, 2016; Eckel et al, 2013).* EB: *Exercise is beneficial in the prevention of cardiovascular disease and HF (Bozkurt et al, 2016).* EB: *Clients with arrhythmias or advanced HF may require supervision or monitoring during exercise (Bozkurt et al, 2016).*

C

REFERENCES

Albert, N. M., Barnason, S., Deswal, A., et al. (2015). Transitions of care in heart failure: A scientific statement from the American Heart Association. *Circulation. Heart Failure, 8*, 384–409.

Allen, L. A., Stevenson, L. W., Grady, K. L., et al. (2012). Decision making in advanced heart failure: A scientific statement from the American Heart Association. *Circulation, 125*, 1928–1952.

American Heart Association. (2014). *Smoking & cardiovascular disease (heart disease)*. Retrieved from http://www.heart.org/HEARTORG/HealthyLiving/QuitSmoking/QuittingResources/Smoking-Cardiovascular-Disease_UCM_305187_Article.jsp#.Wm0Ew66nGpo.

Amsterdam, E. A., Wenger, N. K., Brindis, R. G., et al. (2014). AHA/ACC guideline for the management of patients with non-ST elevation acute coronary syndromes: A report of the American College of Cardiology/American Heart Association Task Force on Practice Guidelines. *Circulation, 23*(30), e344–e426.

Anderson, L., & Taylor, R. S. (2014). Cardiac rehabilitation for people with heart disease: An overview of Cochrane systematic reviews. *The Cochrane Library*. Retrieved from http://onlinelibrary.wiley.com.proxy.hsl.ucdenver.edu/doi/10.1002/14651858.CD011273.pub2/full.

Bhatnagar, A., Whitsel, L. P., Ribisl, K. M., et al. (2014). Electronic cigarettes: A policy statement from the American Heart Association. *Circulation, 130*, 1418–1436.

Bozkurt, B., Aguilar, D., Deswal, A., et al. (2016). Contributory risk and management of comorbidities of hypertension, obesity, diabetes mellitus, hyperlipidemia, and metabolic syndrome in chronic heart failure: A scientific statement from the American Heart Association. *Circulation, 134*, e535–e578.

Centers for Disease Control. (Updated 2017). *Adult immunization schedules*. Retrieved from http://www.cdc.gov/vaccines/schedules/hcp/adult.html.

Costanzo, M. R., Khayat, R., Ponikowski, P., et al. (2015). Mechanisms and clinical consequences of untreated central sleep apnea in heart failure. *Journal of American Colleges of Cardiology, 65*(1), 72–84.

Coviello, J. S., Hricz, L., & Masulli, P. S. (2002). Client challenge: Accomplishing quality of life in end-stage heart failure: A hospice multidisciplinary approach. *Home Healthcare Nurse, 20*, 195–198.

Eckel, R. H., Jakicic, J. M., Ard, J. D., et al. (2013). 2013 AHA/ACC guideline on lifestyle management to reduce cardiovascular risk: a report of the American College of Cardiology/American Heart Association Task Force on Practice Guidelines. *Circulation, 129*(Suppl. 2), S76–S99.

Ingles, S. C., et al. (2006). Extending the horizon in chronic heart failure: Effects of multidisciplinary, home-based intervention relative to usual care. *Circulation, 114*(23), 2466–2473.

Jefferson, A. L., et al. (2010). Cardiac index is associated with brain aging: The Framingham Heart Study. *Circulation, 122*(7), 690–697.

Kahn, S., et al. (2012). Antithrombotic therapy and prevention of thrombosis, 9th ed: American College of Chest Physicians evidence-based clinical practice guidelines online only articles. *Chest, 141*(Suppl. 2), e195S–e226S.

Levine, G., Lange, R., & Bairey-Merz, N. (2017). Meditation and cardiovascular risk reduction: A scientific statement from the American Heart Association. *Journal of the American Heart Association, 6*, 1–58.

National Consensus Project for Quality Palliative Care. (2013). *Clinical Practice Guidelines for Quality Palliative Care* (3rd ed.). Retrieved from https://www.nationalcoalitionhpc.org/ncp-guidelines-2013/.

Sachdeva, A., Dalton, M., Amaragiri, S. V., et al. (2014). Graduated compression stockings for prevention of deep vein thrombosis. *The Cochrane Library*, (12). Retrieved from http://onlinelibrary.wiley.com.hsl-ezproxy.ucdenver.edu/doi/10.1002/14651858.CD001484.pub3/abstract.

Sajid, M. S., Desai, M., Morris, R. W., et al. (2012). Knee length versus thigh length graduated compression stockings for prevention of deep vein thrombosis in postoperative surgical patients: Review. *The Cochrane Library*, (5). Retrieved from http://onlinelibrary.wiley.com.hsl-ezproxy.ucdenver.edu/doi/10.1002/14651858.CD007162.pub2/abstract.

Serber, S. L., Rinsky, B., Kumar, R., et al. (2014). Cerebral blood flow velocity and vasomotor reactivity during autonomic challenges in heart failure. *Nursing Research, 63*(3), 194–202.

Taylor, R. S., Sagar, V. A., Davies, E. J., et al. (2014). Exercise based rehabilitation for heart failure. *The Cochrane Library*. Retrieved from http://onlinelibrary.wiley.com.proxy.hsl.ucdenver.edu/doi/10.1002/14651858.CD003331.pub4/full.

Van Horn, L., Carson, J. S., Appel, L. J., et al. (2016). Recommended dietary pattern to achieve adherence to the American Heart Association/American College of Cardiology (AHA/ACC) guidelines: A scientific statement from the American Heart Association. *Circulation, 134*, e505–e529.

Vital, F., Ladeira, M., & Atallah, A. (2013). Non-invasive positive pressure ventilation (CPAP or bilevel NPPV) for cardiogenic pulmonary oedema. *The Cochrane Library*. Retrieved from http://onlinelibrary.wiley.com.proxy.hsl.ucdenver.edu/doi/10.1002/14651858.CD005351.pub3/full.

Whelton, P. K., Carey, R. M., Aronow, W. S., et al. (2017). ACC/AHA/AAPA/ABC/ACPM/AGS/APhA/ASH/ASPC/NMA/PCNA guideline for the prevention, detection, evaluation, and management of high blood pressure in adults; executive summary: A report of the American College of Cardiology/American Heart Association Task Force on Clinical Practice Guidelines. *Hypertension*, 1–401.

Yancy, C. W., Jessup, M., Bozkurt, B., et al. (2013). ACCF/AHA guideline for the management of heart failure: A report of the American College of Cardiology Foundation/American Heart Association Task Force on Practice Guidelines. *Circulation, 128*, e240–e327.

Yancy, C. W., Jessup, M., Bozkurt, B., et al. (2017). ACCF/AHA/HFSA focused update of the 2013 ACCF/AHA guideline for the management of heart failure: A report of the American College of Cardiology Foundation/American Heart Association Task Force on Clinical Practice Guidelines and the Heart Failure Society of America. *Circulation*, 1–75.

Yu, D. S., et al. (2007). Non-pharmacological interventions in older people with heart failure: Effects of exercise training and relaxation therapy. *Gerontology, 53*(2), 74–81.

● = Independent; ▲ = Collaborative; EBN = Evidence-Based Nursing; EB = Evidence-Based

C

Risk for decreased Cardiac output   *Mary Beth Flynn Makic, PhD, RN, CCNS, FAAN, FNAP*

NANDA-I

Definition

Susceptible to inadequate blood pumped by the heart to meet metabolic demands of the body, which may compromise health.

Risk Factors

To be developed

Associated Condition

Alteration in afterload; alteration in contractility; alteration in heart rate; alteration in heart rhythm; alteration in preload; alteration in stroke volume

NIC, NOC, Client Outcomes, Nursing Interventions and *Rationales,* Client/Family Teaching and Discharge Planning, and References

Refer to care plan for Decreased **Cardiac output**.

Risk for decreased Cardiac tissue perfusion   *Ann Will Poteet, MS, RN, CNS, AGNP-C*

NANDA-I

Definition

Susceptible to a decrease in cardiac (coronary) circulation, which may compromise health.

Risk Factors

Insufficient knowledge of modifiable factors; substance misuse

At-Risk Population

Family history of cardiovascular disease

Associated Condition

Cardiac tamponade; cardiovascular surgery; coronary artery spasm; diabetes mellitus; hyperlipidemia; hypertension; hypovolemia; hypoxemia; hypoxia; increase in C-reactive protein; pharmaceutical agent

NOC   (Nursing Outcomes Classification)

Suggested NOC Outcomes

Cardiac Pump Effectiveness; Circulation Status; Tissue Perfusion: Cardiac; Tissue Perfusion: Cellular; Vital Signs

Example NOC Outcome with Indicators
Tissue Perfusion: Cardiac as evidenced by the following indicators: Angina/Arrhythmia/Tachycardia/Bradycardia/Nausea/Vomiting/Profuse diaphoresis. (Rate the outcome and indicators of **Tissue Perfusion: Cardiac:** 1 = severe, 2 = substantial, 3 = moderate, 4 = mild, 5 = none [see Section I].)

Client Outcomes

Client Will (Specify Time Frame)

- Maintain vital signs within normal range
- Retain an asymptomatic cardiac rhythm (have absence of arrhythmias, tachycardia, or bradycardia)

● = Independent;   ▲ = Collaborative;   EBN = Evidence-Based Nursing;   EB = Evidence-Based

- Be free from chest and radiated discomfort as well as associated symptoms related to acute coronary syndromes (ACSs)
- Deny nausea and be free of vomiting
- Have skin that is dry and of normal temperature

NIC (Nursing Interventions Classification)

Suggested NIC Interventions

Cardiac Care; Cardiac Precautions; Embolus Precautions; Dysrhythmia Management; Vital Signs Monitoring; Shock Management: Cardiac

Example NIC Activity—Cardiac Precautions

Avoid causing intense emotional situations; Avoid overheating or chilling the client; Provide small frequent meals; Substitute artificial salt and limit sodium intake if appropriate; Promote effective techniques for reducing stress; Restrict smoking

Nursing Interventions and *Rationales*

- Be aware that the primary cause of ACS, which include unstable angina (UA), non–ST-elevation myocardial infarction (NSTEMI), and ST-elevation myocardial infarction (STEMI), is an imbalance between myocardial oxygen consumption and demand that is associated with partially or fully occlusive thrombus development in coronary arteries (Amsterdam et al, 2014).
- Assess for symptoms of coronary hypoperfusion and possible ACS, including chest discomfort (pressure, tightness, crushing, squeezing, dullness, or achiness), with or without radiation (or originating) in the retrosternum, back, neck, jaw, shoulder, or arm discomfort or numbness; shortness of breath (SOB); associated diaphoresis; abdominal pain; dizziness, lightheadedness, loss of consciousness, or unexplained fatigue; nausea or vomiting with chest discomfort, heartburn, or indigestion; and associated anxiety. **EB:** *These symptoms are signs of decreased cardiac perfusion and ACSs, such as UA, NSTEMI, or STEMI, as well as other cardiovascular disorders such as aortic aneurysm, valve disorders, and pericarditis. A physical assessment will aid in the assessment of the extent, location, and presence of, and complications resulting from a myocardial infarction (MI). It will promote rapid triage and treatment. It is also important to assess whether the client had a prior stroke, heart failure, or other cardiovascular disorder. It is important to note that certain psychiatric disorders (somatoform disorders, panic attack, and anxiety disorders) can mimic ACS, but they are typically noncardiac causes of chest pain (Amsterdam et al, 2014; Mehta et al, 2016).*
- Consider atypical presentations of ACS for women, older adults, and individuals with diabetes mellitus, impaired renal function, and dementia. **EB/CEB:** *Women, older adults, and individuals with diabetes mellitus, impaired renal function, and dementia may present with atypical findings (Amsterdam et al, 2014; McSweeney et al, 2016; Mehta et al, 2016; Mieres et al, 2014). A systematic review of differences showed that women had significantly less chest discomfort and were more likely to present with fatigue, neck pain, syncope, nausea, right arm pain, dizziness, and jaw pain (Coventry et al, 2011). Delaying identification of atypical presentations can have negative effects on timely intervention and management of ACS, resulting in poorer outcomes and higher mortality (Mehta et al, 2016).*
- Review the client's medical, surgical, social, and familial history. **EB:** *A medical history must be concise and detailed to determine the possibility of ACSs and to help determine the possible cause of cardiac symptoms and pathology (Amsterdam et al, 2014).*
- Perform physical assessments for both coronary artery disease (CAD) and noncoronary findings related to decreased coronary perfusion, including vital signs, pulse oximetry, equal blood pressure in both arms, heart rate, respiratory rate, and pulse oximetry. Check bilateral pulses for quality and regularity. Report tachycardia, bradycardia, hypotension or hypertension, pulsus alternans or pulsus paradoxus, tachypnea, or abnormal pulse oximetry reading. Assess cardiac rhythm for arrhythmias; skin and mucous membrane color, temperature, and dryness; and capillary refill. Assess neck veins for elevated central venous pressure, cyanosis, and pericardial or pleural friction rub. Examine client for cardiac S4 gallop, new heart murmur, lung crackles, altered mentation, pain on abdominal palpation, decreased bowel sounds, or decreased urinary output. **EB:** *These indicators help assess for cardiac and noncardiac etiologies of symptoms and differential diagnoses (Amsterdam et al, 2014).*
- ▲ Administer supplemental oxygen as ordered and needed for clients presenting with ACS, respiratory distress, or other high-risk features of hypoxemia to maintain a Po_2 of at least 90%. **EB:** *American Heart*

● = Independent;   ▲ = Collaborative;   EBN = Evidence-Based Nursing;   EB = Evidence-Based

C

Association guidelines for emergency cardiovascular care during ACS recommend administering oxygen for breathlessness, hypoxemia, signs of heart failure, or if signs of shock are present, and the need for oxygen should be guided by noninvasive monitoring of oxygen saturation. There is limited evidence to support or refute the use of high-flow or low-flow supplemental oxygen if a normal oxygen level (>90%) is present, but it is reasonable to withhold supplemental oxygen in normoxic individuals (O'Connor et al, 2015). EB: A Cochrane review found there was limited evidence to support or refute the use of routine supplemental oxygen with acute MI, and that harm from excess supplemental oxygen cannot be ruled out, recommending further studies (Cabello et al, 2016).

▲ Use continuous pulse oximetry as ordered. EB: *Prevention and treatment of hypoxemia includes maintaining arterial oxygen saturation over 90% (Amsterdam et al, 2014).*

▲ Insert one or more large-bore intravenous catheters to keep the vein open. Routinely assess saline locks for patency. Clients who come to the hospital with possible decrease in coronary perfusion or ACS may have intravenous fluids and medications ordered routinely or emergently to maintain or restore adequate cardiac function and rhythm.

▲ Observe the cardiac monitor for hemodynamically significant arrhythmias, ST depressions or elevations, T-wave inversions and/or Q-waves as signs of ischemia or injury. Report abnormal findings. EB: *Arrhythmias and electrocardiogram (ECG) changes indicate myocardial ischemia, injury, and/or infarction. Note that left ventricular hypertrophy, ventricular pacing, and bundle branch blocks can mask signs of ischemia or injury (Amsterdam et al, 2014).*

● Have emergency equipment and defibrillation capability nearby and be prepared to defibrillate immediately if ventricular tachycardia with clinical deterioration or ventricular fibrillation occurs.

▲ Perform a 12-lead ECG as ordered to be interpreted within 10 minutes of emergency department arrival and during episodes of chest discomfort or angina equivalent. EB: *A 12-lead ECG should be performed within 10 minutes of emergency department arrival for all clients who are having chest discomfort. ECGs are used to identify the area of ischemia or injury, such as ST depressions or elevations, new left-bundle branch block, T-wave inversions, and/or Q-waves, and to guide treatment (Amsterdam et al, 2014; O'Gara et al, 2013).*

▲ Administer nonenteric-coated aspirin as ordered, as soon as possible after presentation and for maintenance. EB: *Aspirin has been shown to prevent platelet clumping, aggregation, and activation that leads to thrombus formation, which in coronary arteries leads to ACSs. Contraindications include active peptic ulcer disease, bleeding disorders, and aspirin allergy (Amsterdam et al, 2014; O'Gara et al, 2013).*

▲ Administer nitroglycerin tablets sublingually as ordered, every 5 minutes until the chest pain is resolved while monitoring the blood pressure for hypotension, for a maximum of three doses as ordered. Administer nitroglycerin paste or intravenous preparations as ordered. EB: *Nitroglycerin causes coronary arterial and venous dilation, and at higher doses peripheral arterial dilation, reducing preload and afterload and decreasing myocardial oxygen demand while increasing oxygen delivery (Amsterdam et al, 2014).*

● Do not administer nitroglycerin preparations to individuals with hypotension, or individuals who have received phosphodiesterase type 5 inhibitors, such as sildenafil, tadalafil, or vardenafil, in the last 24 hours (48 hours for long-acting preparations). EB: *Synergistic effect causes marked exaggerated and prolonged vasodilation/hypotension (Amsterdam et al, 2014).*

▲ Administer morphine intravenously as ordered, every 5 to 30 minutes until pain is relieved while monitoring blood pressure when nitroglycerin alone does not relieve chest discomfort. EB: *Morphine has potent analgesic and antianxiolytic effects and causes mild reductions in blood pressure and heart rate that reduce myocardial oxygen consumption. Hypotension and respiratory depression are the most serious complications of morphine use, and naloxone may be administered as ordered for morphine overdose (Amsterdam et al, 2014).*

▲ Assess and report abnormal laboratory work results of cardiac enzymes, specifically troponin I or T, B-type natriuretic peptide, chemistries, hematology, coagulation studies, arterial blood gases, finger stick blood sugar, elevated C-reactive protein, or drug screen. EB: *Abnormalities can identify the cause of the decreased perfusion and identify complications related to the decreased perfusion such as anemia, hypovolemia, coagulopathy, drug abuse, hyperglycemia, kidney (renal) failure, and heart failure. Markedly elevated cardiac enzymes are usually indicative of an MI, and the cardiac enzymes can also help determine short- and long-term prognosis (Amsterdam et al, 2014).*

● Assess for individual risk factors for CAD, such as hypertension, dyslipidemia, cigarette smoking, diabetes mellitus, metabolic syndrome, obesity, or family history of heart disease. Other risk factors including sedentary lifestyle, obesity, or cocaine or amphetamine use. Note age and gender as risk factors. EB:

● = Independent;   ▲ = Collaborative;   EBN = Evidence-Based Nursing;   EB = Evidence-Based

C

Certain conditions place clients at higher risk for decreased cardiac tissue perfusion (Amsterdam et al, 2014; Mehta et al, 2016; Mieres et al, 2014).

▲ Administer additional heart medications as ordered, including beta-blockers, calcium channel blockers, angiotensin-converting enzyme inhibitors, angiotensin II receptor blockers, aldosterone antagonists, antiplatelet agents, and anticoagulants. Always check blood pressure and pulse rate before administering these medications. If the blood pressure or pulse rate is low, contact the health care provider to establish whether the medication should be withheld. Also check platelet counts, renal function, and coagulation studies as ordered to assess proper effects of these agents. EB: *These medications are useful to optimize cardiac and kidney function, including blood pressure, heart rate, myocardial oxygen demand, intravascular fluid volume, and cardiac rhythm (Amsterdam et al, 2014).*

▲ Administer lipid-lowering therapy as ordered. EB: *Use of statin drugs has been shown to reduce an individual's risk of recurrent MI, stroke, and coronary heart disease mortality, especially with high-intensity statins that lower low-density lipoprotein cholesterol levels (Amsterdam et al, 2014; Stone et al, 2013). A systematic review of statin use in primary prevention of cardiovascular disease showed reductions in all-cause mortality, major vascular events, and revascularizations (Taylor et al, 2013).*

▲ Prepare client with education, withholding of meals and/or medications, and intravenous access for early invasive therapy with cardiac catheterization, reperfusion therapy, and possible percutaneous coronary intervention in individuals with refractory angina or hemodynamic or electrical instability, and first medical contact to device time of less than 90 minutes if STEMI is suspected. EB: *First medical contact to device time of less than 90 minutes was associated with improved client outcomes (Amsterdam et al, 2014; O'Gara et al, 2013).*

▲ Prepare clients with education, withholding of meals and/or medications, and intravenous access for noninvasive cardiac diagnostic procedures such as echocardiogram, exercise, or pharmacological stress test, and cardiac computed tomography scan as ordered. EB: *Clients suspected of decreased coronary perfusion should receive these diagnostic procedures as appropriate to evaluate for CAD (Amsterdam et al, 2014; Fletcher et al, 2013; Mieres et al, 2014).*

▲ Request a referral to a cardiac rehabilitation program. EB: *Cardiac rehabilitation programs are designed to limit the physiological and psychological effects of cardiac disease, reduce the risk for sudden cardiac death and reinfarction, control symptoms and stabilize or reverse the process of plaque formation, and enhance psychosocial and vocational status of clients (Amsterdam et al, 2014). EB: Cardiac rehabilitation can improve quality of life and functional capacity, and decrease mortality (Anderson & Taylor, 2014).*

Geriatric

● Consider atypical presentations of possible ACS in older adults. CEB: *Older adults may present with atypical signs and symptoms such as weakness, stroke, syncope, or change in mental status (Amsterdam et al, 2014; McSweeney et al, 2016; Mehta et al, 2016).*

▲ Ask the prescriber about possible reduced dosage of medications for older clients, considering weight, creatinine clearance, and glomerular filtration rate. EB: *Older clients can have reduced pharmacokinetics and pharmacodynamics, including reduced muscle mass, reduced renal and hepatic function, and reduced volume of distribution, which can alter drug dosing, efficacy, and safety, as well as some drug–drug interactions (Amsterdam et al, 2014; Stone et al, 2013).*

● Consider issues such as quality of life, palliative care, end-of-life care, and differences in sociocultural aspects for clients and families when supporting them in decisions regarding aggressiveness of care. Ask about living wills, as well as medical and durable power of attorney. EB: *Management decisions, including decisions regarding invasive treatment, should be client-centered and take into account client preferences and goals, comorbidities, cognitive and functional status, and life expectancy (Amsterdam et al, 2014; McSweeney et al, 2016; Mehta et al, 2016; National Consensus Project for Quality Palliative Care, 2013).*

Client/Family Teaching and Discharge Planning

▲ Client and family education regarding a multidisciplinary plan of care should start early. Special attention to client and family education should occur during transitions of care. EB: *It is important to provide the client and family with a comprehensive plan of care and education materials that are evidence based to assist with client compliance and to potentially reduce hospital readmissions related to ACS. The plan of care should take into consideration the client's psychosocial and socioeconomic status, access to care, risk for depression and/or social isolation, and health care disparities (Amsterdam et al, 2014).*

● = Independent;   ▲ = Collaborative;   EBN = Evidence-Based Nursing;   EB = Evidence-Based

C

- Teach the client and family to call 911 for symptoms of new angina, existing angina unresponsive to rest and sublingual nitroglycerin tablets, or heart attack, or if an individual becomes unresponsive.
- On discharge, instruct clients about symptoms of ischemia, when to cease activity, when to use sublingual nitroglycerin, and when to call 911.
- Teach client about any medications prescribed. Medication teaching includes the drug name, its purpose, administration instructions such as taking it with or without food, and any side effects to be aware of. Instruct the client to report any adverse side effects to the health care provider.
- On hospital discharge, educate clients and significant others about discharge medications, including nitroglycerin sublingual tablets or spray, with written, easy to understand, culturally sensitive information. **EB:** *Clients and significant others need to be prepared to act quickly and decisively to relieve ischemic discomfort (Amsterdam et al, 2014).*
- Provide client education related to risk factors for decreased cardiac tissue perfusion, such as hypertension, hyperlipidemia, metabolic syndrome, diabetes mellitus, tobacco use, obesity, advanced age, and gender (female). **EB:** *Those with two or more risk factors should have a 10-year risk screening for development of symptomatic coronary heart disease. Client education is a vital part of nursing care for the client. Start with the client's base level of understanding and use that as a foundation for further education. It is important to factor in cultural and/or religious beliefs in the education provided (Amsterdam et al, 2014; Barnason et al, 2017; Eckel et al, 2013; Goff et al, 2013).*
- Instruct the client on antiplatelet and anticoagulation therapy, and about signs of bleeding, need for ongoing medication compliance, and international normalized ratio monitoring. **EB:** *Special attention and education should be provided to older individuals, because they are at greater risk for bleeding (Amsterdam et al, 2014).*
- After discharge, continue education and support for client blood pressure and diabetes control, weight management, and resumption of physical activity. **EB:** *Reducing risk factors acts as secondary prevention of CAD (Amsterdam et al, 2014; Eckel et al, 2013).*
- ▲ Clients should be provided with education regarding the influenza vaccine and pneumococcal vaccine before hospital discharge. **EB:** *The influenza vaccine is recommended for all adults, and the pneumococcal vaccine is recommended for individuals older than 65 years and for individuals who are at high risk for cardiovascular disease (Amsterdam et al, 2014; Centers for Disease Control, 2017).*
- ▲ Stress the importance of ceasing tobacco use (Whelton et al, 2017). **EB:** *Tobacco use can cause or worsen decreased blood flow in the coronaries, as well as cause vasoconstriction, which can lead to atherosclerotic disease. Effects of nicotine include increasing pulse and blood pressure and constricting blood vessels. Tobacco use is a primary factor in heart disease (American Heart Association, 2014; Amsterdam et al, 2014).*
- ▲ Individuals should be screened for electronic cigarette use (e-cigarette). **EB:** *Although more studies are needed regarding the health effects of e-cigarette use, the American Heart Association recommends that all health care providers educate their clients regarding the long-term use of e-cigarettes given the known toxicities present in e-cigarettes, as well as the presence of nicotine in most types of e-cigarettes (Bhatnagar et al, 2014).*
- ▲ On hospital discharge, educate clients about a low-sodium, low-saturated fat diet, with consideration to client education, literacy, and health literacy level. **EB:** *Reducing risk factors acts as secondary prevention of CAD (Amsterdam et al, 2014; Eckel et al, 2013).*
- Teach the importance of physical activity as tolerated. **EB:** *Exercise helps control blood pressure and weight, which are the most important controlled risk factors for cardiovascular disease. Individuals should engage in aerobic physical activity of varying intensity as tolerated and incorporate variable anaerobic activities such as resistance training (Amsterdam et al, 2014; Bozkurt et al, 2016; Eckel et al, 2013). **EB:** Exercise is beneficial in the prevention of cardiovascular disease and heart failure (Bozkurt et al, 2016). **EB:** Clients with arrhythmias or advanced heart failure may require supervision or monitoring during exercise (Bozkurt et al, 2016).*

REFERENCES

American Heart Association. (2014). *Smoking & cardiovascular disease (heart disease)*. Retrieved from http://www.heart.org/HEARTORG/HealthyLiving/QuitSmoking/QuittingResources/Smoking-Cardiovascular-Disease_UCM_305187_Article.jsp#.Wm0Ew66nGpo.

Amsterdam, E. A., Wenger, N. K., Brindis, R. G., et al. (2014). AHA/ACC guideline for the management of patients with non-ST elevation acute coronary syndromes: A report of the American

College of Cardiology/American Heart Association Task Force on Practice Guidelines. *Circulation*, 23(30), e344–e426.

Anderson, L., & Taylor, R. S. (2014). Cardiac rehabilitation for people with heart disease: An overview of Cochrane systematic reviews. *The Cochrane Library*. Retrieved from http://onlinelibrary.wiley.com.proxy.hsl.ucdenver.edu/doi/10.1002/14651858.CD011273.pub2/full.

Barnason, S., White-Williams, C., Rossi, L. P., et al. (2017). Evidence for therapeutic patient interventions to promote cardiovascular patient

● = Independent; ▲ = Collaborative; **EBN** = Evidence-Based Nursing; **EB** = Evidence-Based

self-management: A scientific statement for healthcare professionals from the American Heart Association. *Circulation. Cardiovascular Quality and Outcomes, 10,* 1–24.

Bhatnagar, A., Whitsel, L. P., Ribisl, K. M., et al. (2014). Electronic cigarettes: A policy statement from the American Heart Association. *Circulation, 130,* 1418–1436.

Bozkurt, B., Aguilar, D., Deswal, A., et al. (2016). Contributory risk and management of comorbidities of hypertension, obesity, diabetes mellitus, hyperlipidemia, and metabolic syndrome in chronic heart failure: A scientific statement from the American Heart Association. *Circulation, 134,* e535–e578.

Cabello, J. B., Burls, A., Emparanza, J. I., et al. (2016). Oxygen therapy for acute myocardial infarction. *The Cochrane Library.* Retrieved from http://onlinelibrary.wiley.com.proxy.hsl.ucdenver.edu/doi/10.1002/14651858.CD007160.pub4/full.

Centers for Disease Control. (Updated 2017). *Adult immunization schedules.* Retrieved from http://www.cdc.gov/vaccines/schedules/hcp/adult.html.

Coventry, L. L., Finn, J., & Bremner, A. P. (2011). Sex differences in symptom presentation in acute myocardial infarction: A systematic review and meta-analysis. *Heart and Lung: The Journal of Critical Care, 40*(6), 477–491.

Eckel, R. H., Jakicic, J. M., Ard, J. D., et al. (2013). 2013 AHA/ACC guideline on lifestyle management to reduce cardiovascular risk: A report of the American College of Cardiology/American Heart Association Task Force on Practice Guidelines. *Circulation, 129*(Suppl. 2), S76–S99.

Fletcher, G. F., Ades, P. A., Kligfield, P., et al. (2013). Exercise standards for testing and training: A scientific statement from the American Heart Association. *Circulation, 128,* 873–934.

Goff, D. C., Lloyd-Jones, D. M., Bennett, G., et al. (2013). 2013 ACC/AHA guideline on the assessment of cardiovascular risk: A report of American College of Cardiology/American Heart Association Task Force on Practice Guidelines. *Circulation, 129*(Suppl. 2), S49–S73.

McSweeney, J. C., Rosenfeld, A. G., Abel, W. M., et al. (2016). Preventing and experiencing ischemic heart disease as a woman: state of the science: A scientific statement from the American Heart Association. *Circulation, 133,* 1302–1331.

Mehta, L. S., Becki, T. M., DeVon, H. A., et al. (2016). Acute myocardial infarction in women: A scientific statement from the American Heart Association. *Circulation, 133,* 916–947.

Mieres, J. H., Gulati, M., Bairey Merz, N., et al. (2014). Role of noninvasive testing in the clinical evaluation of women with suspected ischemic heart disease: A consensus statement from the American Heart Association. *Circulation, 130,* 350–379.

National Consensus Project for Quality Palliative Care. (2013). *Clinical Practice Guidelines for Quality Palliative Care* (3rd ed.). Retrieved from https://www.nationalcoalitionhpc.org/ncp-guidelines-2013/.

O'Connor, R. E., Al Ali, A. S., Brady, W. J., et al. (2015). Part 9: Acute coronary syndromes: 2015 American Heart Association guidelines update for cardiopulmonary resuscitation and emergency cardiovascular care. *Circulation, 132*(Suppl. 2), S483–S500.

O'Gara, P. T., Kushner, F. G., Ascheim, D. D., et al. (2013). 2013 ACCF/AHA guideline for the management of ST-elevation myocardial infarction: Executive summary: A report of the American College of Cardiology Foundation/American Heart Association Task Force on Practice Guidelines. *Circulation, 127*(4), 529–555.

Stone, N. J., Robinson, J. G., Lichtenstein, A. H., et al. (2013). 2013 ACC/AHA guideline on the treatment of blood cholesterol to reduce atherosclerotic cardiovascular risk in adults: A report of the American College of Cardiology/American Heart Association Task Force on Practice Guidelines. *Circulation, 129*(Suppl. 2), S1–S45.

Taylor, F., Huffman, M. D., Macedo, A. F., et al. (2013). Statins for the primary prevention of cardiovascular disease. *The Cochrane Library.* Retrieved from http://onlinelibrary.wiley.com.proxy.hsl.ucdenver.edu/doi/10.1002/14651858.CD004816.pub5/full.

Whelton, P. K., Carey, R. M., Aronow, W. S., et al. (2017). ACC/AHA/AAPA/ABC/ACPM/AGS/APhA/ASH/ASPC/NMA/PCNA guideline for the prevention, detection, evaluation, and management of high blood pressure in adults; executive summary: A report of the American College of Cardiology/American Heart Association Task Force on Clinical Practice Guidelines. *Hypertension,* 1–401.

Caregiver Role Strain
Barbara A. Given, PhD, RN, FAAN

NANDA-I

Definition

Difficulty in fulfilling care responsibilities, expectations, and/or behaviors for family or significant others.

Defining Characteristics

Caregiving Activities

Apprehensiveness about future ability to provide care; apprehensiveness about the future health of care receiver; apprehensiveness about possible institutionalization of care receiver; apprehensiveness about well-being of care receiver if unable to provide care; difficulty completing required tasks; difficulty performing required tasks; dysfunctional change in caregiving activities; preoccupation with care routine

Caregiver Health Status

Physiological
Fatigue; gastrointestinal distress; headache; hypertension; rash; weight change
Emotional
Alteration in sleep pattern; anger; depression; emotional vacillation; frustration; impatience; ineffective coping strategies; insufficient time to meet personal needs; nervousness; somatization; stressors

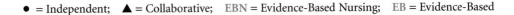
● = Independent; ▲ = Collaborative; EBN = Evidence-Based Nursing; EB = Evidence-Based

C

Socioeconomic

Changes in leisure activities; low work productivity; refusal of career advancement; social isolation

Caregiver-Care Receiver Relationship

Difficulty watching care receiver with illness; grieving of changes in relationship with care recipient; uncertainty about changes in relationship with care receiver

Family Processes

Concerns about family member(s); family conflict

Related Factors

Care Receiver

Condition inhibits conversation; dependency; discharged home with significant needs; increase in care needs; problematic behavior; substance misuse; unpredictability of illness trajectory; unstable health condition

Caregiver

Physical conditions; substance misuse; unrealistic self-expectations; competing role commitments; ineffective coping strategies; inexperience with caregiving; insufficient emotional resilience; insufficient energy; insufficient fulfillment of others' expectations; insufficient fulfillment of self-expectations; insufficient knowledge about community resources; insufficient privacy; insufficient recreation; isolation; not developmentally ready for caregiver role; stressors

Caregiver-Care Receiver Relationship

Abusive relationship; codependency; pattern of ineffective relationships; presence of abuse; conflictual relationships; unrealistic care receiver expectations; violent relationship

Caregiving Activities

Around-the-clock care responsibilities; change in nature care of activities; complexity of care activities; excessive caregiving activities; extended duration of caregiving required; inadequate physical environment for providing care; insufficient assistance; insufficient equipment for providing care; insufficient respite for caregiver; insufficient time; unpredictability of care situation

Family Processes

Family isolation; ineffective family adaptation; pattern of family dysfunction; pattern of family dysfunction prior to the caregiving situation; pattern of ineffective family coping

Socioeconomic

Alienation; difficulty accessing assistance; difficulty accessing community resources; difficulty accessing support; insufficient community resources; insufficient social support; insufficient transportation; social isolation

At-Risk Population

Care receiver's condition inhibits conversation; developmental delay of care receiver; developmental delay of caregiver; exposure to violence; female caregiver; financial crisis; partner as caregiver; prematurity

Associated Condition

Care Receiver

Alteration in cognitive functioning; chronic illness; congenital disorder; illness severity; psychiatric disorder; psychological disorder

Caregiver

Alteration in cognitive functioning; health impairment; psychological disorder

NOC   (Nursing Outcomes Classification)

Suggested NOC Outcomes

Caregiver Adaptation to Patient Institutionalization; Caregiver Emotional Health; Caregiver Home Care Readiness; Caregiver Lifestyle Disruption; Caregiver-Patient Relationship; Caregiver Performance: Direct

● = Independent;   ▲ = Collaborative;   EBN = Evidence-Based Nursing;   EB = Evidence-Based

Care; Caregiver Performance: Indirect Care; Caregiver Physical Health; Caregiver Role Endurance; Caregiver Stressors; Caregiver Well-Being; Family Resiliency; Family Coping

> ### Example NOC Outcome with Indicators
>
> **Caregiver Emotional Health** with plans for a positive future as evidenced by the following indicators: Satisfaction with life/Sense of control/Self-esteem/Certainty about future/Perceived social connectedness/Perceived spiritual well-being/Perceived adequacy of resources. (Rate the outcome and indicators of **Caregiver Emotional Health:** 1 = severely compromised, 2 = substantially compromised, 3 = moderately compromised, 4 = mildly compromised, 5 = not compromised [see Section I].)

Client Outcomes

Throughout the Care Situation, the Caregiver Will

- Be able to express feelings of strain
- Feel supported by health care professionals, family, and friends; feel they have adequate information to provide care
- Report reduced or acceptable feelings of burden or distress
- Take part in self-care activities to maintain own physical and psychological/emotional health; identify resources (family and community) available to help in giving care
- Verbalize mastery of the care activities; feel confident and competent to provide care; have the skills to provide care
- Identify resources to obtain social support
- Ask for help when needed or when feeling comprised in ability to provide care
- Not refuse help when needed and offered; ask for help when needed

Throughout the Care Situation, the Care Recipient Will

- Obtain quality and safe physical care and emotional care
- Be treated with respect and dignity

NIC   (Nursing Interventions Classification)

Suggested NIC Intervention

Caregiver Support

> ### Example NIC Activities—Caregiver Support
>
> Determine caregiver's acceptance of role; Accept expressions of negative emotion

Nursing Interventions and *Rationales*

- Mood management. Regularly monitor signs of depression, anxiety, burden, and deteriorating physical health in the caregiver throughout the care situation if the care demands change frequently, especially if the relationship is poor, the care recipient has cognitive or neuropsychiatric symptoms, there is little social support available, the caregiver becomes enmeshed in the care situation, the caregiver has multiple comorbidities, or has poor preexisting physical or emotional health. Refer to the care plan for **Hopelessness** when appropriate. EBN: *High levels of distress in caregivers are linked to multiple variables (van der Lee et al, 2014) and may include worse quality of life (QoL), sleep disturbance, depressive symptoms, and overall physical health decline (Shaffer et al, 2017; Trevino et al, 2017). Other factors contributing to distress include cognitive and motor function of the care recipient and duration of the disease and caregiving activities (de Wit et al, 2017).* EB: *Caregiving may weaken the immune system and predispose the caregiver to illness (Vitlic et al, 2015). Caregiver depressive symptoms may lead to physical health decline (Shaffer et al, 2017; Trevino et al, 2017).*
- The impact of providing care on the caregiver's emotional health should be assessed at regular intervals using a reliable and valid instrument such as the Caregiver Strain Risk Index (which was validated with caregivers of clients with diagnosed Parkinson's disease), Caregiver Burden Inventory, Caregiver Reaction Assessment, Screen for Caregiver Burden, Subjective and Objective Scale, and Family Caregiver Self Expectations. EBN: *Family caregivers face potential strain in caring for persons with Parkinson's disease and amyotrophic lateral sclerosis (ALS) because of the unpredictability of symptom presentation and*

● = Independent;   ▲ = Collaborative;   EBN = Evidence-Based Nursing;   EB = Evidence-Based

C

greater physical and behavioral impairment (de Wit et al, 2017). The Caregiver Strain Risk Screen (CSRS) was developed and tested for initial validation. The 28-item CSRS demonstrated acceptable validity and reliability in measuring caregiver strain (Abendroth, 2015). Research has validated the effectiveness of a number of evaluation tools for caregiver stress including Caregiver Reaction Assessment (Given et al, 1992), Burden Interview, the Caregiver Strain Index, and the Caregiver Burden Inventory. Caregiver assessment should be done at regular intervals throughout the care trajectory (Adelman et al, 2014) noting changes that require action. Another tool is called the Positive Aspects of Caregiving Questionnaire (Abdollahpour et al, 2017).

- Identify potential caregiver personal resources such as mastery, benefit funding, social support, optimism, and positive aspects of care and resilience. Good outcomes can be achieved through resources (Joling et al, 2017). EB/EBN: *Research has shown that caregivers can have simultaneous positive and negative responses to providing care (Roth et al, 2015). Positive responses may help buffer the negative effects of providing care on caregivers' emotional health and may also increase the effectiveness of interventions to reduce strain. Caregiver resilience can be observed as caregivers feel competent to provide care (Joling et al, 2017).*

- Screen for caregiver role strain at the onset of the care situation, at regular intervals throughout the care situation, at care transitions, and with changes in care recipient status. EB/EBN: *Improvement in patient physical function resulted in both patient and caregiver physical and psychological QoL. Decreases in caregiver burden can be associated with improvement in caregiver physical and psychological QoL (Pucciarelli et al, 2017). Changes in the care recipient's health status necessitate new skills and monitoring from the caregiver and affect the caregiver's ability to continue to provide care and may affect caregiver health (Trevino et al, 2017).*

- Assist the client to identify spiritual beliefs and engage in spiritual practices. EB: *Spiritual beliefs and practices may help caregivers cope because it protects them from depression (Penman, 2017).*

- Regularly monitor social support for the caregiver and help the caregiver identify and use appropriate support systems for varying times in the care situation. EBN: *For heart failure patients Evangelista et al (2016) found in an integrated review that support group interventions affected caregiver burden, depressive symptoms, confidence, and preparedness. Positive effects on empowerment, coping, and resilience can result (Brand et al, 2016; MacCourt et al, 2017).*

- Help the caregiver learn mindfulness stress management techniques, which can reduce psychological distress. EB: *Mindfulness stress reduction interventions can result in improvement in QoL, self-compassion, caregiver burden, and relationship satisfaction (Schellekens et al, 2017).*

- Encourage the caregiver to share feelings, concerns, uncertainties, and fears. Support groups, even Internet-based ones, can be used to gain support. EBN: *For the isolated caregiver support groups can improve feelings of support and self-efficacy.* EB: *Internet social support groups can be an effective form of support (Evangelista et al, 2016; MacCourt et al, 2017; Parker et al, 2017).*

- Observe for any evidence of caregiver or care recipient violence or abuse, particularly verbal abuse and emotional abuse; if evidence is present, identify the conflict and seek help to manage. EB/CEB: *Caregiver abuse is possible, and screening should be done at regular intervals (Hoover & Polson, 2014; Liu et al, 2017).*

- ▲ Encourage regular and open communication with the care recipient and with the health care team. Care transitions are a critical point to ensure that caregivers have adequate information for patient safety and efficient and effective care. EB: *High-quality communication and patient and family engagement facilitate excellent care by families and reduce barriers to care transitions (Scott et al, 2017).*

- Assist caregiver to secure and manage finances to meet care recipient's needs. EB: *Caregivers with financial difficulty were more likely to have depressive symptoms (Nam, 2016).*

- Help the caregiver identify competing occupational demands and potential benefits to maintaining work as a way of providing normalcy. Guide caregivers to seek ways to maintain employment through mechanisms such as working remotely, job sharing, or decreasing hours at work. EB: *Adult children caregivers reported more stress and partner strain, whereas elder caregivers received greater psychological stress. Sandwiched generation caregivers reported poorer overall psychosocial functioning. Adult children female caregivers had more family-to-work conflicts and less partner support than males (de Moor et al, 2017; DePasquale et al, 2017).*

- Help the caregiver problem solve to meet the care recipient's needs. EBN: *Interventions that teach caregivers problem-solving skills have been shown to positively influence caregivers' psychosocial well-being (Cheng et al, 2014).*

● = Independent;   ▲ = Collaborative;   EBN = Evidence-Based Nursing;   EB = Evidence-Based

Geriatric

- Monitor the caregiver for psychological distress and signs of depression, especially if there was an unsatisfactory family relationship before caregiving. **EBN:** *Family caregivers' relationship satisfaction is linked with caregiver role burden, anxiety, and depression (Kruithof et al, 2016).*
- Assess the health of caregivers, particularly their control over chronic diseases and comorbid conditions, at regular intervals. **CEB:** *Caregivers with high levels of depressive symptoms have demonstrated poor health and increased health care utilization and cost (Shaffer et al, 2017; Trevino et al, 2017).*
- Implement a telephone-based collaborative care program to provide support. **EBN:** *Social support has been shown to be an integral part of maintaining caregiver emotional health (Kruithof et al, 2016; Mavandadi et al, 2017).*
- Provide medication management to facilitate safe and effective use of medications for self and care recipient by medication reconciliation and education. **EB:** *Polypharmacy should be avoided and communicated to providers (Koronkowski et al, 2016).*
- To improve the ability to provide safe care: provide skills training related to direct care, perform complex monitoring tasks, supervise and interpret client symptoms, assist with decision-making, assist with medication adherence.
- Provide emotional support and comfort, and coordinate care. Family members need the resources and support to provide care to the care recipient. **CEB:** *Each task demands different skills and knowledge, and caregivers need to be assisted to care (Polenick et al, 2017). Complex tasks are associated with emotional difficulties, thus caregivers need the training to gain the needed skills (Petruzzo et al, 2017; Toye et al, 2016).*
- Insurance authorization: health professionals, such as social workers, assist care recipients to obtain the needed referrals to gain payment for needed health and community services.
- Teach symptom management techniques (assessment, potential causes, aggravating factors, potential alleviating factors, and reassessment), particularly for fatigue, dyspnea, constipation, anorexia, and pain. **EBN:** *Well-prepared caregivers are important for older care recipients. Caregivers require and desire training in care recipient monitoring symptom management and interpretation, and they can benefit from a problem-solving approach (Cheng et al, 2014).*

 Multicultural

- Assess for the influence of cultural beliefs, ethnic and racial norms, and values on the caregiver's ability to provide care as well as the response to care. **EBN:** *What the client considers normal and abnormal may be based on cultural perceptions (Itty et al, 2014).* **EBN:** *Each caregiver should be assessed for the response to care. African American caregivers of dementia patients had decreased positive affect and less physical activity (Cothran et al, 2017). Despite the importance of cultural differences in perceptions of caregiver role strain, there are common characteristics that are distressing to caregivers across multiple cultures and they may experience burden and depression. African American and Hispanic caregivers received less professional intervention support than their white counterparts (Graham-Phillips et al, 2016).* **EBN:** *Social support and care recipients' behavioral differences have been shown to be an important factor in caregiver distress across multiple cultures (Han et al, 2014). Persons with different cultural backgrounds may not perceive the demands of care with equal degrees of distress (Cothran et al, 2017; Graham-Phillips et al, 2016).*
- *Tailoring interventions for caregivers based on racial, ethnic, and cultural characteristics may affect caregiver outcomes (Jessup et al, 2015).*
- Recognize and understand that culture often plays a role in identifying who will be recognized as a family caregiver. **EB:** *In a study of Native Americans, 49% reported stress as a major difficulty; males reported financial difficulty and they desired training in patient care. Gender played a role in differences in activity of caregivers in some tribes (Cordova et al, 2016).*
- Encourage spirituality as a source of support for coping. **EBN:** *Spirituality and spiritual engagement may protect caregiver from depression (Penman, 2017). Spiritual care can reduce care strain in caregivers of elderly patients with Alzheimer's (Mahdavi et al, 2017).*

 Home Care

- Assess the client and caregiver at every visit for the quality of their relationship, and for the quality and safety of the care provided. **EB:** *Quality of the caregiver-care recipient relationship and the impact of the care situation on that relationship can be an important source of distress or support for the caregiver (van*

● = Independent;   ▲ = Collaborative;   **EBN** = Evidence-Based Nursing;   **EB** = Evidence-Based

C

der Lee et al, 2014). Education, social support, and behavioral management are the most effective support for caregivers of dementia patients (Clarkson et al, 2017).

- Encourage use of respite care if it seems appropriate to support the caregiver. Allow the caregiver to gain confidence in the respite provider. EB: *Respite care provides time away from the care situation and may help alleviate some caregiver distress (Vandepitte et al, 2016); others may be too fearful.*
- ▲ Refer the client to home health aide services for assistance with activities of daily living and light housekeeping. Home health aide services can provide physical relief and respite for the caregiver. EB: *Barriers to community social services may be related to minority and ethnic carer satisfaction (Greenwood et al, 2015).*
- Assess preexisting strengths and weaknesses that the caregiver brings to the situation. EB/EBN: *Caregivers' personality type, mastery, self-efficacy, optimism, and social support have all been linked to the amount of distress the caregiver will perceive as a result of providing care (Adelman et al, 2014). Improving caregiver sense of competency to deal with neuropsychiatric symptoms of dementia patients can prevent or reduce caregiver burden (van der Lee et al, 2014).*

 Client/Family Teaching and Discharge Planning

- Identify client and caregiver factors that necessitate the use of formal home care services, that may affect provision of care, or that need to be addressed before the client can be safely discharged from home care. EBN: *Health care practitioners should assess needs for support resources, home care or community assistance prior to discharge, and at routine intervals throughout the care situation.(Greenwood et al, 2015). Interventions to be considered needed at discharge may include medication management, medication reconciliation, symptom monitoring, identification of community-based resources, and specific caregiver concerns about home care. Skills training is needed for many caregiving situations (Mollica et al, 2017).*
- Collaborate with the caregiver and discuss the care needs of the client, disease processes, medications, and what to expect as part of discharge planning and transition care.
  Use a variety of instructional techniques (e.g., explanations, demonstrations, visual aids) until the caregiver is able to express a degree of comfort with needed care. EB: *Knowledge and confidence are separate concepts and both are needed for caregiving. Self-assurance in caregiving will decrease the amount of distress the caregiver perceives as a result of providing care (Jessup et al, 2015; Mollica et al, 2017) and may improve the quality of care provided.*
- Assess family caregiving skill. The identification of caregiver difficulty with any of a core set of processes highlights areas for intervention. EB: *Caregiver skills training has been shown to improve caregiver knowledge and skills (Mollica et al, 2017).*
- Discharge care should be individualized to specific caregiver needs and care situations, and enable them to be prepared. EBN: *Interventions implemented by advance practice nurses have been successful in preventing negative outcomes (Naylor et al, 2017; Stone, 2014; Toles et al, 2017).*
- Assess the caregiver's need for information such as information on symptom management, disease progression, specific skills, and available support. EBN: *Caregiver interventions should be individualized to meet specific caregiver needs (Naylor et al, 2017). Multicomponent strategies to provide education, support, counseling, care continuity, and linkage to community resources to ease transitions can improve caregiver health and coping (Naylor et al, 2017; Ostwald et al, 2014).*
- ▲ Involve the family caregiver in care transitions and discharge from institutions; use a multidisciplinary team to provide medical and social services for detailed instruction and planning specific to the care need. The CARE Act, available in 39 states, requires caregiver instruction at hospital discharge. EB: *Family members need education specific to their situation at discharge, and this educational approach should be based on patient's needs. The postdischarge visit serves as an important vehicle to prevent readmissions and improve quality of care for patients (Rodakowski et al, 2017; Soufer et al, 2017).*
- ▲ Refer to counseling or support groups to assist in adjusting to the caregiver role and periodically evaluate not only the caregiver's emotional response to care but the safety of the care delivered to the care recipient.

REFERENCES

Abdollahpour, I., Nedjat, S., Noroozian, M., et al. (2017). Positive Aspects of Caregiving Questionnaire: A validation study in caregivers of patients with dementia. *Journal of Geriatric Psychiatry Neurology, 30*(2), 77–83. doi:10.1177/0891988716686831.

Abendroth, M. (2015). Development and initial validation of a Parkinson's disease caregiver strain risk screen. *Journal of Nursing Measurement, 23*(1), 4–21.

Adelman, R. D., Tmanova, L. L., Delgado, D., et al. (2014). Caregiver burden: A clinical review. *JAMA: The Journal of the American*

Medical Association, 311(10), 1052–1060. doi:10.1001/jama
.2014.304.

Brand, C., Barry, L., & Gallagher, S. (2016). Social support mediates the
association between benefit finding and quality of life in caregivers.
Journal of Health Psychology, 21(6), 1126–1136. doi:10.1177/
1359105314547244.

Cheng, H. Y., Chair, S. Y., & Chau, J. P. (2014). The effectiveness of
psychosocial interventions for stroke family caregivers and stroke
survivors. *Patient Education and Counseling, 95*(1), 30–44.
doi:10.1016/j.pec.2014.01.005.

Clarkson, P., Davies, L., Jasper, R., et al. (2017). A systematic review of
the economic evidence for home support interventions in dementia.
Value in Health, 20(8), 1198–1209. doi:10.1016/j.jval.2017.04.004.

Cordova, F. M., B Harris, R., Teufel-Shone, N. I., et al. (2016).
Caregiving on the Hopi reservation: Findings from the 2012 Hopi
survey of cancer and chronic disease. *Journal of Community Health,
41*(6), 1177–1186.

Cothran, F. A., Paun, O., Barnes, L. L., et al. (2017). Comparing the
effect of a moderate physical activity intervention on the mental
health outcomes of African American and Caucasian dementia
family caregivers: A secondary data analysis. *Issues in Mental Health
Nursing, 28*, 1–9. doi:10.1080/01612840.2017.1364807.

de Moor, J. S., Dowling, E. C., Ekwueme, D. U., et al. (2017).
Employment implications of informal cancer caregiving. *Journal of
Cancer Survivorship, 11*(1), 48–57. doi:10.1007/s11764-016-0560-5.

DePasquale, N., Polenick, C. A., Davis, K. D., et al. (2017). The
psychosocial implications of managing work and family caregiving
roles: Gender differences among information technology
professionals. *Journal of Family Issues, 38*(11), 1495–1519. doi:
10.1177/0192513X15584680.

de Wit, J., Bakker, L. A., van Groenestijn, A. C., et al. (2017). Caregiver
burden in amyotrophic lateral sclerosis: A systematic review.
Palliative Medicine, Jul 1. doi:10.1177/0269216317709965. [Epub
ahead of print].

Evangelista, L. S., Strömberg, A., & Dionne-Odom, J. N. (2016). An
integrated review of interventions to improve psychological
outcomes in caregivers of patients with heart failure. *Current
Opinion in Supportive and Palliative Care, 10*(1), 24–31.
doi:10.1097/SPC.0000000000000182.

Given, C. W., Given, B., Stommel, M., et al. (1992). The caregiver
reaction assessment (CRA) for caregivers to persons with chronic
physical and mental impairments. *Research in Nursing and Health,
15*(4), 271–283.

Graham-Phillips, A., Roth, D. L., Huang, J., et al. (2016). Racial and
ethnic differences in the delivery of the Resources for Enhancing
Alzheimer's Caregiver Health II intervention. *Journal of the
American Geriatric Society, 64*(8), 1662–1667. doi:10.1111/jgs.14204.

Greenwood, N., Habibi, R., Smith, R., et al. (2015). Barriers to access
and minority ethnic carers' satisfaction with social care services in
the community: A systematic review of qualitative and quantitative
literature. *Health & Social Care in the Community, 23*(1), 64–78.
doi:10.1111/hsc.12116.

Han, Y., Hu, D., Liu, Y., et al. (2014). Coping styles and social support
among depressed Chinese family caregivers of patients with
esophageal cancer. *European Journal of Oncology Nursing, 18*(6),
571–577. doi:10.1016/j.ejon.2014.07.002.

Hoover, R. M., & Polson, M. (2014). Detecting elder abuse and neglect:
Assessment and intervention. *American Family Physician, 89*(6),
453–460.

Itty, T. L., Hodge, F. S., & Martinez, F. (2014). Shared and unshared
barriers to cancer symptom management among urban and rural
American Indians. *The Journal of Rural Health, 30*(2), 206–213.
doi:10.1111/jrh.12045.

Jessup, N. M., Bakas, T., McLennon, S. M., et al. (2015). Are there
gender, racial or relationship differences in caregiver task difficulty,
depressive symptoms and life changes among stroke family
caregivers? *Brain Injury, 29*(1), 17–24. doi:10.3109/02699052.2014
.947631.

Joling, K. J., Windle, G., Dröes, R. M., et al. (2017). What are the
essential features of resilience for informal caregivers of people
living with dementia? A Delphi consensus examination. *Aging &
Mental Health, 21*(5), 509–517. doi:10.1080/13607863.2015
.1124836.

Koronkowski, M., Eisenhower, C., & Marcum, Z. (2016). An update on
geriatric medication safety and challenges specific to the care of
older adults. *Annals of Longterm Care, 24*(3), 37–40.

Kruithof, W. J., Post, M. W., van Mierlo, M. L., et al. (2016). Caregiver
burden and emotional problems in partners of stroke patients at
two months and one year post-stroke: Determinants and
prediction. *Patient Education and Counseling, 99*(10), 1632–1640.
doi:10.1016/j.pec.2016.04.007.

Liu, P. J., Conrad, K. J., Beach, S. R., et al. (2017). The importance
of investigating abuser characteristics in elder emotional/
psychological abuse: Results from adult protective services data.
*The Journals of Gerontology. Series B, Psychological Sciences and
Social Sciences*, May 17. doi:10.1093/geronb/gbx064. [Epub ahead
of print].

MacCourt, P., McLennan, M., Somers, S., et al. (2017). Effectiveness of
a grief intervention for caregivers of people with dementia. *Omega,
75*(3), 230–247. doi:10.1177/0030222816652802.

Mahdavi, B., Fallahi-Khoshknab, M., Mohammadi, F., et al. (2017).
Effects of spiritual group therapy on caregiver strain in home
caregivers of the elderly with Alzheimer's disease. *Archives of
Psychiatric Nursing, 31*(3), 269–273. doi:10.1016/j.apnu.2016.12
.003.

Mavandadi, S., Wright, E. M., Graydon, M. M., et al. (2017). A
randomized pilot trial of a telephone-based collaborative care
management program for caregivers of individuals with dementia.
Psychological Services, 14(1), 102–111. doi:10.1037/ser0000118.

Mollica, M. A., Litzelman, K., Rowland, J. H., et al. (2017). The role of
medical/nursing skills training in caregiver confidence and burden:
A CanCORS study. *Cancer*. doi:10.1002/cncr.30875. [Epub ahead of
print].

Nam, I. (2016). Financial difficulty effects on depressive symptoms
among dementia patient caregivers. *Community Mental Health
Journal, 52*(8), 1093–1097.

Naylor, M. D., Shaid, E. C., Carpenter, D., et al. (2017). Components of
comprehensive and effective transitional care. *Journal of the
American Geriatrics Society, 65*(6), 1119–1125. doi:10.1111/jgs
.14782.

Ostwald, S. K., Godwin, K. M., Cron, S. G., et al. (2014). Home-based
psychoeducational and mailed information programs for
stroke-caregiving dyads post-discharge: A randomized trial.
Disability and Rehabilitation, 36(1), 55–62. doi:10.3109/09638288
.2013.777806.

Parker Oliver, D., Patil, S., Benson, J. J., et al. (2017). The effect of
internet group support for caregivers on social support,
self-efficacy, and caregiver burden: A meta-analysis. *Telemedicine
Journal and E-Health, 23*(8), 621–629. doi:10.1089/tmj.2016
.0183.

Penman, J. (2017). Finding paradise within: How spirituality protects
palliative care clients and caregivers from depression. *Journal of
Holistic Nursing*, Jun 1. [Epub ahead of print].

Petruzzo, A., Paturzo, M., Buck, H. G., et al. (2017). Psychometric
evaluation of the Caregiver Preparedness Scale in caregivers of
adults with heart failure. *Research in Nursing and Health, 40*(5),
470–478. doi:10.1002/nur.21811.

Polenick, C. A., Leggett, A. N., & Kales, H. C. (2017). Medical care
activities among spouses of older adults with functional disability:
Implications for caregiving difficulties and gains. *The American*

C

Journal of Geriatric Psychiatry, 25(10), 1085–1093. doi:10.1016/j.jagp.2017.05.001.

Pucciarelli, G., Vellone, E., Savini, S., et al. (2017). Roles of changing physical function and caregiver burden on quality of life in stroke: A longitudinal dyadic analysis. *Stroke; a Journal of Cerebral Circulation, 48*(3), 733–739. doi:10.1161/STROKEAHA.116.014989.

Rodakowski, J., Rocco, P. B., Ortiz, M., et al. (2017). Caregiver integration during discharge planning for older adults to reduce resource use: A metaanalysis. *Journal of the American Geriatrics Society, 65*(8), 1748–1755. doi:10.1111/jgs.14873.

Roth, D. L., Fredman, L., & Haley, W. E. (2015). Informal caregiving and its impact on health: A reappraisal from population-based studies. *The Gerontologist, 55*(2), 309–319. doi:10.1093/geront/gnu177.

Shaffer, K. M., Kim, Y., Carver, C. S., et al. (2017). Depressive symptoms predict cancer caregivers' physical health decline. *Cancer,* Jun 29. doi:10.1002/cncr.30835 [Epub ahead of print].

Schellekens, M. P. J., van den Hurk, D. G. M., Prins, J. B., et al. (2017). Mindfulness-based stress reduction added to care as usual for lung cancer patients and/or their partners: A multicentre randomized controlled trial. *Psycho-Oncology,* Mar 23. doi:10.1002/pon.4430. [Epub ahead of print].

Scott, A. M., Li, J., Oyewole-Eletu, S., et al. (2017). Understanding facilitators and barriers to care transitions: Insights from Project ACHIEVE site visits. *Joint Commission Journal on Quality and Patient Safety, 43*(9), 433–447. doi:10.1016/j.jcjq.2017.02.012.

Soufer, A., Riello, R. J., Desai, N. R., et al. (2017). A blueprint for the post discharge clinic visit after an admission for heart failure. *Progress in Cardiovascular Diseases, 60*(2), 237–248. doi:10.1016/j.pcad.2017.08.004.

Stone, K. (2014). Enhancing preparedness and satisfaction of caregivers of patients discharged from an inpatient rehabilitation facility using an interactive website. *Rehabilitation Nursing, 39*(2), 76–85. doi:10.1002/rnj.123.

Toles, M., Colón-Emeric, C., Naylor, M. D., et al. (2017). Connect-home: Transitional care of skilled nursing facility patients and their caregivers. *Journal of the American Geriatrics Society, 65*(10), 2322–2328. doi:10.1111/jgs.

Toye, C., Parsons, R., Slatyer, S., et al. (2016). Outcomes for family carers of a nurse-delivered hospital discharge intervention for older people (the Further Enabling Care at Home Program): Single blind randomised controlled trial. *International Journal of Nursing Studies, 64,* 32–41. doi:10.1016/j.ijnurstu.2016.09.012.

Trevino, K. M., Prigerson, H. G., & Maciejewski, P. K. (2017). Advanced cancer caregiving as a risk for major depressive episodes and generalized anxiety disorder. *Psycho-Oncology.* doi:10.1002/pon.4441. [Epub ahead of print].

Vandepitte, S., Van Den Noortgate, N., Putman, K., et al. (2016). Effectiveness of respite care in supporting informal caregivers of persons with dementia: A systematic review. *International Journal of Geriatric Psychiatry, 31*(12), 1277–1288. doi:10.1002/gps.4504.

van der Lee, J., Bakker, T. J., Duivenvoorden, H. J., et al. (2014). Multivariate models of subjective caregiver burden in dementia: A systematic review. *Ageing Research Reviews, 15,* 76–93. doi:10.1016/j.arr.2014.03.003.

Vitlic, A., Lord, J. M., Arlt, W., et al. (2015). T cell immunity and caregiving stress in young and older caregivers. *Healthy Aging Research, 4*(15), 1–3. Retrieved from http://dx.doi.org/10.12715/har.2015.4.15.

Risk for Caregiver Role Strain   *Marina Martinez-Kratz, MS, RN, CNE*

NANDA-I

Definition

Susceptible to difficulty in fulfilling care responsibilities, expectations, and/or behaviors for family or significant others, which may compromise health.

Risk Factors

Care Receiver

Dependency; discharged home with significant needs; increase in care needs; problematic behavior; substance misuse; unpredictability of illness trajectory; unstable health condition

Caregiver

Substance misuse; unrealistic self-expectations; competing role commitments; ineffective coping strategies; inexperience with caregiving; insufficient emotional resilience; insufficient energy; insufficient fulfillment of others' expectations; insufficient fulfillment of self-expectations; insufficient knowledge about community resources; insufficient privacy; insufficient recreation; isolation; not developmentally ready for caregiver role; physical conditions; stressors

Caregiver-Care Receiver Relationship

Abusive relationship; codependency; pattern of ineffective relationships; presence of abuse; unrealistic care receiver expectations; violent relationship

● = Independent;   ▲ = Collaborative;   EBN = Evidence-Based Nursing;   EB = Evidence-Based

Caregiving Activities

Around-the-clock care responsibilities; change in nature of care activities; complexity of care activities; excessive caregiving activities; extended duration of caregiving required; inadequate physical environment for providing care; insufficient assistance; insufficient equipment for providing care; insufficient respite for caregiver; insufficient time; unpredictability of care situation

Family Processes

Family isolation; ineffective family adaptation; pattern of family dysfunction; pattern of family dysfunction prior to the caregiving situation; pattern of ineffective family coping

Socioeconomic

Alienation; difficulty accessing assistance; difficulty accessing community resources; difficulty accessing support; insufficient community resources; insufficient social support; insufficient transportation; social isolation

At-Risk Population

Care receiver's condition inhibits conversation; developmental delay of care receiver; developmental delay of caregiver; exposure to violence; female caregiver; financial crisis; partner as caregiver; prematurity

Associated Condition

Care Receiver

Alteration in cognitive functioning; chronic illness; congenital disorder; illness severity; psychological disorder; psychiatric disorder

Caregiver

Alteration in cognitive functioning; health impairment; psychological disorder

NIC, NOC, Client Outcomes, Nursing Interventions and *Rationales,* Client/Family Teaching, and References

Refer to care plan for **Caregiver Role Strain.**

Risk for ineffective Cerebral tissue perfusion   *Kimberly S. Meyer, PhD, ACNP-BC, CNRN*

NANDA-I

Definition

Susceptible to a decrease in cerebral tissue circulation, which may compromise health.

Risk Factors

Substance misuse

At-Risk Population

Recent myocardial infarction

Associated Condition

Abnormal partial thromboplastin time (PTT); abnormal prothrombin time (PT); akinetic left ventricular wall segment; aortic atherosclerosis; arterial dissection; atrial fibrillation; atrial myxoma; brain injury; brain neoplasm; carotid stenosis; cerebral aneurysm; coagulopathy; dilated cardiomyopathy; disseminated intravascular coagulopathy; embolism; hypercholesterolemia; hypertension; infective endocarditis; mechanical prosthetic valve; mitral stenosis; pharmaceutical agent; sick sinus syndrome; treatment regimen

NOC   (Nursing Outcomes Classification)

Suggested NOC Outcomes

Acute Confusion Level; Tissue Perfusion: Cerebral; Agitation Level; Neurological Status; Cognition; Seizure Control; Motor Strength

● = Independent;   ▲ = Collaborative;   EBN = Evidence-Based Nursing;   EB = Evidence-Based

C

Example NOC Outcome with Indicators

Tissue Perfusion: Cerebral as evidenced by the following indicators: Headache/Restlessness/Listlessness/Agitation/Vomiting/ Fever/Impaired cognition/Decreased level of consciousness/Motor weakness/Dysphagia/Slurred speech. (Rate the outcome and indicators of **Tissue Perfusion: Cerebral:** 1 = severe, 2 = substantial, 3 = moderate, 4 = mild, 5 = none [see Section I].)

Client Outcomes

Client Will (Specify Time Frame)

- State absence of headache
- Demonstrate appropriate orientation to person, place, time, and situation
- Demonstrate ability to follow simple commands
- Demonstrate equal bilateral motor strength
- Demonstrate adequate swallowing ability
- Maintain (or improve) neurological exam

NIC   (Nursing Interventions Classification)

Suggested NIC Interventions

Medication Management; Neurologic Monitoring; Positioning: Neurologic; Cerebral Perfusion Promotion; Fall Prevention; Cognitive Stimulation; Environmental Management: Safety

Example NIC Activities—Neurologic Monitoring

Monitor pupillary size, shape, symmetry, and reactivity; Monitor level of consciousness; Monitor level of orientation; Monitor trend of Glasgow Coma Scale; Monitor facial symmetry; Note complaint of headache; Monitor blood pressure (BP) and heart rate; Monitor respiratory function

Nursing Interventions and *Rationales*

- To decrease risk of reduced cerebral perfusion related to stroke or transient ischemic attack (TIA):
  - Obtain a family history of hypertension, diabetes, and stroke to identify persons who may be at increased risk of stroke. EB: *A positive family history of stroke increases risk of stroke by approximately 30% (Goldstein et al, 2011).*
  - Monitor BP regularly, because hypertension is a major risk factor for both ischemic and hemorrhagic stroke. EB: *Systolic BP should be treated to a goal of less than 140 mm Hg and diastolic BP to less than 90 mm Hg, whereas clients with diabetes or renal disease have a BP goal of less than 130/80 mm Hg (Boan et al, 2014).*
  - Teach hypertensive clients the importance of taking their health care provider-ordered antihypertensive agent to prevent stroke. EB: *Treatment of hypertension in adults with diabetes with a calcium channel blocker may be useful (James et al, 2014).*
  - Stress smoking cessation at every encounter with clients, using multimodal techniques to aid in quitting, such as counseling, nicotine replacement, and oral smoking cessation medications. Provide client and family education to reduce lifestyle-associated risk factors for stroke. EB: *Studies show that a consistent and overwhelming relationship between lifestyle risk factors such as smoking, physical inactivity, and poor diet associated with obesity, increase the client risk of both ischemic and hemorrhagic stroke (Meschia, 2014; Sarikaya et al, 2015).*
  - Teach clients who experience a transient TIA that they are at increased risk for a stroke. EB: *The 90-day risk for stroke after a TIA is as high as 17%, with the greatest risk occurring in the first week (Heron, 2016).*
  - Screen clients 65 years of age and older for atrial fibrillation with pulse assessment. EB: *Atrial fibrillation is associated with a fivefold increase in stroke. Systematic pulse assessment in a primary care setting resulted in a 60% increase in the detection of atrial fibrillation (Proietti et al, 2016; Goldstein et al, 2011; Meschia, 2014).*
  - Call 911 or activate the rapid response team of a hospital immediately when clients display symptoms of stroke as determined by the Cincinnati Stroke Scale (F: facial drooping; A: arm drift on one side; S: speech slurred) being careful to note the time of symptom appearance. Additional symptoms of

• = Independent;   ▲ = Collaborative;   EBN = Evidence-Based Nursing;   EB = Evidence-Based

stroke include sudden numbness/weakness of face, arm, or leg, especially on one side; sudden confusion; trouble speaking or understanding; sudden difficulty seeing with one or both eyes; sudden trouble walking, dizziness, loss of balance, or coordination; or sudden severe headache (Jauch et al, 2013). EB: *The Cincinnati Stroke Scale (derived from the National Institutes of Health [NIH] Stroke Scale) is used to identify clients having a stroke who may be candidates for thrombolytic therapy (Jauch et al, 2013). Emergency medical services (EMS) activation results in faster health care provider assessment, computed tomography, and neurological evaluation, which facilitates administering thrombolytics to eligible stroke victims within the required 3-hour time period (Jauch et al, 2013).*

○ Use clinical practice guidelines for glycemic control and BP targets to guide the care of clients with diabetes who have had a stroke or TIA. EB: *The American Stroke Association recommends that evidence-based guidelines be used in the care of clients with diabetes. Good glycemic control has been associated with decreased incidence of strokes (Meschia, 2014). EB: Hypoglycemia (blood sugar < 60 mg/dL) should be corrected immediately to improve stroke outcomes (Jauch et al, 2013). EB: Persistent hyperglycemia (blood sugar >180 mg/dL) should be avoided because hyperglycemia is associated with worse stroke outcomes (Jauch et al, 2013).*

○ Maintain head of bed less than 30 degrees in the acute phase (<72 hours of symptom onset) of ischemic stroke. EB: *Cortical cerebral blood flow is decreased when head of bed is elevated from 0 to 30 degrees in clients with acute ischemic stroke (Favilla et al, 2014).*

○ Head of bed may be elevated to sitting position without detrimental effect to cerebral blood flow in clients with ischemic stroke or subarachnoid hemorrhagic at 72 hours after symptom onset. EB: *Head of bed elevation of 45 and 70 degrees in the subacute phase of ischemic stroke resulted in minor changes in cerebral blood flow velocities (Aries et al, 2013). EB: Cerebral blood flow had no significant changes in head of bed elevations from 0 to 90 degrees in clients with subarachnoid hemorrhage at days 3, 7, and 10 (Kung et al, 2013).*

○ Administer oral nimodipine as prescribed by the health care provider after subarachnoid hemorrhagic strokes for 21 days. EB: *Nimodipine, a calcium channel blocker, has been shown by multiple randomized clinical trials to improve outcome by limiting delayed cerebral ischemia after subarachnoid hemorrhage strokes (Raya et al, 2014).*

○ Monitor neurological function frequently in the first 2 weeks after subarachnoid hemorrhage because subtle declines may be related to cerebral vasospasm. EB: *Cerebral vasospasm occurs in up to 70% of patients with subarachnoid hemorrhage and can lead to delayed cerebral ischemia (Grasso et al, 2017).*

○ Maintain cerebral perfusion pressure (CPP) 60 to 70 mm Hg in patients with traumatic brain injury. EB: *When injury-related impaired autoregulation is present, CPP less than 60 is associated with worse outcomes (Carney et al, 2016; Guiza et al, 2017).*

▲ To decrease risk of reduced CPP: CPP = Mean arterial pressure − intracranial pressure (CPP = MAP − ICP): See care plan for Decreased **Intracranial** adaptive capacity.

○ Maintain euvolemia. EB: *Infusing isotonic intravenous fluids to sustain normal circulating volume helps maintain normal cerebral blood flow (Hemphill et al, 2015).*

▲ To treat decreased CPP:

○ Clients with subarachnoid hemorrhagic stroke experiencing delayed cerebral ischemia, as evidenced by declining neurological exam, should undergo a trial of induced hypertension. EB: *Medically managed hypertension increased cerebral blood flow and produced neurological improvement in the majority of clients (Raya et al, 2014).*

○ Administer norepinephrine infusion to raise MAP per collaborative protocol. EB: *Patients with delayed cerebral ischemia treated with norepinephrine have better BP augmentation and better clinical outcomes than patients treated with other vasopressors (Roy et al, 2017; Sookplung et al, 2011).*

○ Mobilize patients with subarachnoid hemorrhage as early as 1 day after aneurysm is secured. EB: *Patients undergoing early mobilization are less likely to develop severe cerebral vasospasm (Karic et al, 2017).*

REFERENCES

Aries, M. J., Elting, J. W., Stewart, R., et al. (2013). Cerebral blood flow velocity changes during upright positioning in bed after acute stroke: An observational study. *British Medical Journal Open, 3,* 1–4. Retrieved from http://dx.doi.org/10.1136/bmjopen-2013 -002960.

Boan, A. D., Lackland, D. T., & Ovbiagele, B. (2014). Lowering of blood pressure for recurrent stroke prevention. *Stroke; a Journal of Cerebral Circulation, 45*(8), 2506–2513.

Carney, N., Totten, A. M., O'Reilly, C., et al. (2016). *Guidelines in the management of severe TBI* (4th ed.). Brain Trauma Foundation.

● = Independent;   ▲ = Collaborative;   EBN = Evidence-Based Nursing;   EB = Evidence-Based

C

Favilla, C. G., Mesquita, R. C., Mullen, M., et al. (2014). Optical bedside monitoring of cerebral blood flow in acute ischemic stroke patients during head-of-bed manipulation. *Stroke; a Journal of Cerebral Circulation, 45*, 1269–1274.

Goldstein, L. B., Bushnell, C. D., Adams, R. J., et al. (2011). Guidelines for the primary prevention of stroke: A guideline for healthcare professionals from AHA/ASA. *Stroke; a Journal of Cerebral Circulation, 42*, 517–584.

Grasso, G., Alafac, C., & McDonald, R. L. (2017). Management of SAH: State of the art and future perspectives. *Surgical Neurology International, 8*, 11. doi:10.4103/2152-7806.198738.

Guiza, F., Meyfroidt, G., Piper, I., et al. (2017). Cerebral perfusion pressure insults and associations with outcome in adult traumatic brain injury. *Journal of Neurotrauma, 34*(16), 2425–2431.

Hemphill, J. C., et al. (2015). Guidelines for the management of spontaneous intracerebral hemorrhage. *Stroke; a Journal of Cerebral Circulation, 46*, 2032–2060.

Heron, N. (2016). Optimizing secondary prevention in the acute period following a TIA of ischemic origin. *British Medical Journal, 2*(1). doi:10.1136/bmjsem-2016-000161.

James, P. A., Oparil, S., Carter, B. L., et al. (2014). 2014 Evidence based guidelines for the management of increased blood pressure in adults. *JAMA: The Journal of the American Medical Association, 311*(5), 507–520.

Jauch, E. C., Saver, J. L., Adams, H. P., et al. (2013). Guidelines for the early management of patients with acute ischemic stroke: A guideline for healthcare professionals from the AHA/ASA. *Stroke; a Journal of Cerebral Circulation, 44*, 870–947.

Karic, T., Roe, C., Nordenmark, T. H., et al. (2017). Effect of early mobilization and rehabilitation on complications in aneurysmal subarachnoid hemorrhage. *Journal of Neurosurgery, 126*(2), 518–526.

Kung, D. K., Chalouhi, N., Jabbour, P. M., et al. (2013). Cerebral blood flow dynamics and head-of-bed changes in the setting of subarachnoid hemorrhage. *BioMed Research International, 2013*, 1–4. Retrieved from http://dx.doi.org/10.1155/2013/640638.

Meschia, J. F. (2014). Guidelines for the primary prevention of stroke. *Stroke; a Journal of Cerebral Circulation, 45*, 3754–3832.

Proietti, M., & Lip, G. Y. (2016). Atrial fibrillation and stroke. *Cardiology Clinics, 34*(2), 317–328.

Raya, A. K., & Diringer, M. N. (2014). Treatment of subarachnoid hemorrhage. *Critical Care Clinics, 30*, 719–733.

Roy, B., McCullough, L. D., Dhar, R., et al. (2017). Comparison of initial vasopressors used for delayed cerebral ischemia after subarachnoid hemorrhage. *Cerebrovascular Disease, 43*, 266–271.

Sarikaya, H., Ferro, J., & Arnold, M. (2015). Stroke prevention: Medical and lifestyle measures. *European Neurology, 73*, 150–157.

Sookplung, P., Siriussawakul, A., Malakouti, A., et al. (2011). Vasopressor use and effect on blood pressure after severe adult traumatic brain injury. *Neurocritical Care, 15*(1), 46–54.

Ineffective Childbearing process   Dianne F. Hayward, RN, MSN, WHNP

NANDA-I

Definition

Inability to prepare for and/or maintain a healthy pregnancy, childbirth process, and care of the newborn for ensuring well-being.

Defining Characteristics

During Pregnancy

Inadequate prenatal care; inadequate prenatal lifestyle; inadequate preparation of newborn care items; inadequate preparation of the home environment; ineffective management of unpleasant symptoms in pregnancy; insufficient access of support system; insufficient respect for unborn baby; unrealistic birth plan

During Labor and Delivery

Decrease in proactivity during labor and delivery; inadequate lifestyle for stage of labor; inappropriate response to onset of labor; insufficient access of support system; insufficient attachment behavior

After Birth

Inadequate baby care techniques; inadequate postpartum lifestyle; inappropriate baby feeding techniques; inappropriate breast care; insufficient access of support system; insufficient attachment behavior; unsafe environment for an infant

Related Factors

Domestic violence; inadequate maternal nutrition; inconsistent prenatal health visits; insufficient cognitive readiness for parenting; insufficient knowledge of child-bearing process; insufficient parental role model; insufficient prenatal care; insufficient support system; low maternal confidence; maternal powerlessness; maternal psychological distress; substance misuse; unrealistic birth plan; unsafe environment

● = Independent;   ▲ = Collaborative;   EBN = Evidence-Based Nursing;   EB = Evidence-Based

At-Risk Population

Unplanned pregnancy; unwanted pregnancy

 Nursing Outcomes Classification

Suggested NOC Outcomes

Fetal Status: Antepartum, Intrapartum; Maternal Status: Antepartum, Intrapartum; Depression Level; Family Resiliency; Knowledge: Substance Use Control; Social Support; Spiritual Support

Example NOC Outcome with Indicators
Maternal Status: Antepartum as evidenced by the following indicators: Emotional attachment to fetus/Coping with discomforts of pregnancy/Mood lability/Has realistic birth plan/Has support system. (Rate each indicator of **Maternal Status: Antepartum:** 1 = severe deviation from normal range, 2 = substantial deviation from normal range, 3 = moderate deviation from normal range, 4 = mild deviation from normal range, 5 = no deviation from normal range [see Section I].)

Client Outcomes

Client Will (Specify Time Frame)

Antepartum
- Obtain early prenatal care in the first trimester and maintain regular visits
- Demonstrate appropriate care of oneself during pregnancy including good nutrition and psychological health
- Understand the risks of substance abuse and resources available
- Feel empowered to seek social and spiritual support for emotional well-being during pregnancy
- Prepare home for baby (e.g., crib, diapers, infant car seat, outfits, blankets)
- Use support systems for labor and emotional support
- Develop a realistic birth plan, taking into account any high-risk pregnancy issues
- Understand the labor and delivery process and comfort measures to manage labor pain

Postpartum
- Provide a safe environment for self and infant
- Demonstrate appropriate newborn care and postpartum care of self
- Demonstrate appropriate bonding and parenting skills

NIC **(Nursing Interventions Classification)**

Suggested NIC Interventions

High-Risk Pregnancy Care; Intrapartal Care; Infant Care: Newborn

Example NIC Activities—High-Risk Pregnancy Care
Instruct client in self-care techniques to increase the chance of a healthy outcome (e.g., hydration, diet, activity modifications, importance of regular prenatal checkups, normalization of blood sugars, and sexual precautions, including abstinence).
Monitor physical and psychosocial status closely throughout pregnancy. Refer as appropriate for specific programs (e.g., smoking cessation, substance abuse treatment, diabetes education, preterm birth prevention education, abuse shelter as needed).

Nursing Interventions and *Rationales*

- Encourage early prenatal care and regular prenatal visits. EB: *There are a multitude of comorbidities and prior and current pregnancy complications that may deem a pregnancy high risk (Carter et al, 2016). A small Canadian study of a high-risk obstetric population found that most women who presented with no prenatal care did so late in pregnancy and had high rates of adverse outcomes (Knight et al, 2014). The World Health Organization (WHO) guidelines for antenatal care include a minimum of eight contacts to reduce perinatal mortality and improve women's experience of care, counselling about healthy eating, and keeping physically active during pregnancy (World Health Organization, 2016).*
- ▲ Identify any high-risk factors that may require additional surveillance, such as preterm labor, hypertensive disorders of pregnancy, diabetes, depression, other chronic medical conditions, presence of fetal anomalies,

● = Independent;   ▲ = Collaborative;   EBN = Evidence-Based Nursing;   EB = Evidence-Based

homelessness, or other high-risk factors. **EB:** *Timely and accurate antenatal screening is believed to be an important factor in preventing preterm birth, screening for gestational diabetes, preeclampsia, intrauterine growth restriction, and depression. Finding and treating problems early improves outcome (Beeckman et al, 2013). Health care providers should include disaster preparedness to displaced pregnant women as a part of their care. The displaced women who perceived high levels of social support gave birth to infants with higher birth weights (Sanguanklin et al, 2014).*

▲ Assess and screen for signs and symptoms of depression during pregnancy and in the postpartum period including history of depression or postpartum depression, poor prenatal care, poor weight gain, hygiene issues, sleep problems, substance abuse, and preterm labor. If depression is present, refer for behavioral-cognitive counseling and/or medication. **EB:** *Susser et al (2016) reported that nearly 20% of women in pregnancy and in the postpartum period are affected with depression. There is a high risk of morbidity and mortality when a woman is affected with perinatal depression and this may have long-term consequences on child development. Depression may also affect the maternal infant bond.*

▲ Observe for signs of alcohol use and counsel women to stop drinking during pregnancy. Give appropriate referral for treatment if needed. **EB:** *There is no known safe amount or safe time to drink alcohol during pregnancy or while trying to get pregnant. The sooner a pregnant woman stops drinking, the better it will be for both her baby and herself (Centers for Disease Control and Prevention, 2016).*

▲ Obtain a smoking history and counsel women to stop smoking for the safety of the baby. Give appropriate referral to a smoking cessation program if needed. **EB:** *"Psychosocial interventions to support women to stop smoking in pregnancy can increase the proportion of women who stop smoking in late pregnancy, and reduce low birthweight and preterm births" (Chamberlain et al, 2013).* **EBN:** *A recent study described the development of an iPad application to promote knowledge of tobacco risk and cessation resources for pregnant women and the evaluation of women's acceptance and perceptions regarding the application (Walsh Dotson et al, 2017).*

▲ Monitor for substance abuse with recreational drugs. Refer to a drug treatment program as needed. Refer opiate-dependent women to methadone clinics to improve maternal and fetal pregnancy outcomes. **EBN:** *It is important to involve a pregnant woman in a methadone treatment program because methadone prevents withdrawal symptoms and eliminates drug craving. Methadone blocks the euphoric effects of illegal self-administered narcotics. It also supports stable maternal opioid levels to protect the fetus from repeated occurrences of withdrawal and decreases the risk for sexually transmitted infections by decreasing drug-seeking behaviors such as prostitution. When a woman makes the decision to enroll in a methadone treatment program, she is taking a significant step toward recovery (Maguire, 2014).*

▲ Monitor for psychosocial issues including lack of social support system, loneliness, depression, lack of confidence, maternal powerlessness, and socioeconomic problems. **EBN:** *"To maximize detection of at-risk women, screening must be expanded to include significant risk factors other than depression and anxiety symptoms" (Ruyak et al, 2017).*

▲ Monitor for signs of domestic violence. Refer to a community program for abused women that provides safe shelter as needed. **EB:** *Women who were involved in intimate partner violence were more likely to experience negative outcomes such as preterm delivery and delivery of low-birth-weight infants (Shneyderman & Kiely, 2013).* **EBN:** *The woman who suffers from abuse needs to formulate a safety plan with a professional trained to guide her in the planning The components of a safety plan include: (1) an escape plan; (2) a place for the woman to go should she decide to leave the abuser; (3) a secure place for essential items such as birth certificates, photo identification, welfare card, green card, marriage certificate, custody papers, health insurance, medical prescriptions, bank statements, car titles, deed to the house, or any reports filed to the police; and (4) other items such as extra sets of clothes, an extra set of keys to the house and car, cash, and jewelry. Organizations, such as the Family Violence Prevention Fund, provide information on safety planning that can be shared with women (Bianchi et al, 2016).*

● Provide antenatal education to increase the woman's knowledge needed to make informed choices during pregnancy, labor, and delivery and to promote a healthy lifestyle. **EB:** *Antenatal classes must be interesting enough to maintain attention, relevant to the attendees, and understandable. The parents should feel empowered that the decisions they make about maternity care and parenthood are made with up-to-date evidence-based information and fit into their lifestyle. O'Sullivan et al (2014) found that class sizes tended to be too large to include class participation. They also reported educators sometimes just focused on maternity care and not on parenthood, healthy lifestyle, and changing relationships. Although resources are available, the educators reported their facility had limited educational resources.*

● Encourage expectant parents to prepare a realistic birth plan or "birth preferences" to prepare for the physical and emotional aspects of the birth process and to plan ahead for how they want various situations

● = Independent;   ▲ = Collaborative;   **EBN** = Evidence-Based Nursing;   **EB** = Evidence-Based

handled. EB/EBN: *The birth plan allows the woman to communicate her expectations and needs (Biescas et al, 2017). A flexible approach to the birth plan is necessary, including the consideration of using alternative approaches and allowing for unexpected circumstances (Divall et al, 2017). The term "birth plan" has been considered by some midwives to be inappropriate, especially requests for an intervention-free birth. They suggested that the term "birth preferences" may be a better term. These plans must be flexible or they may lead to disappointment for the woman and her partner when there is a necessary deviation from their birth plan (Welsh & Syman, 2014).*

- Encourage good nutritional intake during pregnancy to facilitate proper growth and development of the fetus. Women should consume an additional 300 calories per day during pregnancy, take a multi-micronutrient supplement containing at least 400 µg folic acid, and achieve a total weight gain of 25 to 30 lb. EB: *A healthy, varied diet (e.g., Choosemyplate.gov) is of vital importance for optimal birth outcome, including taking a multivitamin with folic acid from before conception to at least the twelfth week of pregnancy, as well as a vitamin D supplement throughout pregnancy. Many women are not following the guidelines and there are concerns for these vulnerable groups (US Department of Agriculture, 2014; Williamson & Wyness, 2013). Inadequate levels of key nutrients during crucial periods of fetal development may lead to changes within fetal tissues, predisposing the infant to chronic illnesses and conditions in later life (Procter & Campbell, 2014).*

 Multicultural

- ▲ Provide for a translator if needed. In some cultures a woman prefers to have a female translator. EB: *The health care industry must recognize that providing translators for language assistance is an important tool for improving quality of care, saving lives, and avoiding costly and dangerous medical errors. Although costly, the American health care industry needs to comply with federal and state laws as well as accreditation standards by being prepared to provide care in at least 100 different languages (Rivers & Rivers, 2013). EBN: In the Arab and most Middle Eastern cultures female translators would be necessary because they are reluctant or sometimes forbidden to discuss female concerns with men (Meyer et al, 2016).*
- ▲ Provide depression screening for clients of all ethnicities. EB: *Race and ethnicity are important risk factors for antenatal depression. A 2015 study found that Mexican American women exhibit higher prenatal maternal depressive symptoms relative to the general population. Depressive symptoms increased when the women tried to mesh American and Mexican cultural values, and incorporation of the Anglo value of self-reliance and independence was a risk factor for depression (D'Anna-Hernandez et al, 2015). EB: Santiago and Figueiredo (2015) conducted a systematic literature review to investigate the relationship between sociodemographic characteristics of immigrant women and its impact on factors influencing prenatal and postpartum care and the incidence of postpartum depression. Factors identified were the socioeconomic status of migrant women participants, language barriers, and health care professionals' lack of cultural sensitivity, leading to women's hesitancy in using health services.*
- Perform a cultural assessment and provide obstetrical care that is culturally appropriate to ensure a safe and satisfying childbearing experience. EBN: *Providing nonjudgmental care that promotes equality can be accomplished through the appropriate use of translation services and good communication skills to make certain that women feel heard and have the opportunity to make choices (Rowland-Neve, 2017).*

REFERENCES

Beeckman, K., Louckx, F., Downe, S., et al. (2013). The relationship between antenatal care and preterm birth: The importance of content of care. *European Journal of Public Health*, 23(3), 366–371.

Bianchi, A., Cesario, S. K., & McFarlane, J. (2016). Interrupting intimate partner violence during pregnancy with an effective screening and assessment program. *Journal of Obstetric, Gynecologic, and Neonatal Nursing*, 45, 579–591. Retrieved from http://dx.doi.org/10.1016/j.jogn.2016.02.012.

Biescas, H., Benet, M., Pueyo, M., et al. (2017). A critical review of the birth plan use in Catalonia. *Sexual & Reproductive Healthcare: Official Journal of the Swedish Association of Midwives*, 13, 41–50.

Carter, E. B., Tuuli, M. G., Caughey, A. B., et al. (2016). Number of prenatal visits and pregnancy outcomes in low-risk women. *Journal of Perinatology*, 36, 178–181.

Centers for Disease Control and Prevention. (2016). *Alcohol and pregnancy*. Retrieved from https://www.cdc.gov/vitalsigns/fasd/index.html.

Chamberlain, C., O'Mara-Eves, A., Oliver, S., et al. (2013). Psychosocial interventions for supporting women to stop smoking in pregnancy. *Cochrane Database of Systematic Reviews*, (10), CD001055, Retrieved from http://dx.doi.org.proxy.lib.wayne.edu/10.1002/14651858.CD001055.pub2.

D'Anna-Hernandez, K., Aleman, B., & Flores, A. M. (2015). Acculturative stress negatively impacts maternal depressive symptoms in Mexican-American women during pregnancy. *Journal of Affective Disorders*, 176, 35–42.

Divall, B., Spiby, H., Nolan, M., et al. (2017). Plans, preferences or going with the flow: An online exploration of women's views and experiences of birth plans. *Midwifery*, 54, 29–34. doi:10.1016/

● = Independent;   ▲ = Collaborative;   EBN = Evidence-Based Nursing;   EB = Evidence-Based

j.midw.2017.07.020. Retrieved from http://dx.doi.org/10.1016/j.nwh.2016.08.001.

Knight, E., Morris, M., & Heaman, M. (2014). Descriptive study of women presenting to an obstetric triage unit with no prenatal care. *Journal of Obstetrics and Gynaecology Canada, 36*(3), 216–222.

Maguire, D. (2014). Drug addiction in pregnancy: Disease not moral failure. *Neonatal Network, 33*(1), 11–18.

Meyer, J., Pomeroy, M., Reid, D., et al. (2016). Nursing care of pregnant Muslim women during Ramadan. *Nursing for Women's Health, 20*(5), 456–462.

O'Sullivan, C., O'Connell, R., & Devane, D. (2014). A descriptive survey of the educational preparation and practices of antenatal educators in Ireland. *The Journal of Perinatal Education, 23*(1), 33–40.

Procter, S. B., & Campbell, C. G. (2014). Position of the Academy of Nutrition and Dietetics: Nutrition and lifestyle for a healthy pregnancy outcome. *Journal of the Academy of Nutrition & Dietetics, 114*(7), 1099–1103.

Rivers, K., & Rivers, D. L. (2013). Foreign language difficulties in American healthcare: The challenges of medical translation regulation and remuneration. *National Social Science Proceedings, 52*(1), 150–160.

Rowland-Neve, K. (2017). Seeking asylum while pregnant. *British Journal of Midwifery, 25*(9), 598–602.

Ruyak, S. L., Flores-Montoya, A., & Boursaw, B. (2017). Antepartum services and symptoms of postpartum depression in at-risk women. *Journal of Obstetric, Gynecologic, and Neonatal Nursing, 46*(5), 696–708. Retrieved from http://dx.doi.org/10.1016/j.jogn.2017.07.006.

Sanguanklin, N., McFarin, B. L., Park, C. G., et al. (2014). Effects of the 2011 flood in Thailand on birth outcomes and perceived social support. *Journal of Obstetric, Gynecologic, and Neonatal Nursing, 43*(4), 435–444.

Santiago, M., & Figueiredo, M. (2015). Immigrant women's perspective on prenatal and postpartum care: Systematic review. *Journal of Immigrant & Minority Health, 17*(1), 276–284.

Shneyderman, Y., & Kiely, M. (2013). Intimate partner violence during pregnancy: Victim or perpetrator? Does it make a difference? *BJOG: An International Journal of Obstetrics & Gynaecology, 120*(11), 1375–1385.

Susser, L. C., Sansone, S. A., & Hermann, A. D. (2016). Selective serotonin reuptake inhibitors for depression in pregnancy. *American Journal Obstetrics & Gynecology, 215*(6), 722–730.

US Department of Agriculture (USDA). (2014). *Nutritional needs during pregnancy*. Choosemyplate.gov/pregnancy. Retrieved from http://www.choosemyplate.gov/pregnancy-breastfeeding/pregnancy-nutritional-needs.html.

Walsh Dotson, J., et al. (2017). Development and evaluation of an iPad application to promote knowledge of tobacco use and cessation by pregnant women. *Nursing for Women's Health, 21*, 174–185. doi:10.1016/j.nwh.2017.04.005.

Welsh, J. V., & Symon, A. G. (2014). Unique and proforma birth plans: A qualitative exploration of midwives' experiences. *Midwifery, 30*(7), 885–891. Retrieved from https://doi.org/10.1016/j.midw.2014.03.004.

Williamson, C., & Wyness, L. (2013). Nutritional requirements in pregnancy and use of dietary supplements. *Community Practitioner, 86*(8), 44–47.

World Health Organization. (2016). Retrieved from http://www.who.int/reproductivehealth/news/antenatal-care/en/.

Readiness for enhanced Childbearing process

Gail B. Ladwig, MSN, RN and Dianne F. Hayward, RN, MSN, WHNP

NANDA-I

Definition

A pattern of preparing for and maintaining a healthy pregnancy, childbirth process, and care of newborn for ensuring well-being, which can be strengthened.

Defining Characteristics

During Pregnancy

Expresses desire to enhance knowledge of childbearing process; expresses desire to enhance management of unpleasant pregnancy symptoms; expresses desire to enhance prenatal lifestyle; expresses desire to enhance preparation for newborn

During Labor and Delivery

Expresses desire to enhance lifestyle appropriate for stage of labor; expresses desire to enhance proactivity during labor and delivery

After Birth

Expresses desire to enhance attachment behavior; expresses desire to enhance baby care techniques; expresses desire to enhance baby feeding techniques; expresses desire to enhance breast care; expresses desire to enhance environmental safety for the baby; expresses desire to enhance postpartum lifestyle; expresses desire to enhance use of support system

● = Independent;   ▲ = Collaborative;   EBN = Evidence-Based Nursing;   EB = Evidence-Based

NOC   (Nursing Outcomes Classification)

Suggested NOC Outcomes

Knowledge: Pregnancy; Knowledge: Infant Care; Knowledge: Postpartum Maternal Health; Knowledge: Breastfeeding, Parent-Infant Attachment

---

Example NOC Outcome with Indicators

Knowledge: Pregnancy as evidenced by client conveying understanding of the following indicators: Importance of frequent prenatal care/Importance of prenatal education/Benefits of regular exercise/Healthy nutritional practices/Anatomic and physiological changes of pregnancy/Psychological changes associated with pregnancy/Birthing options/Effective labor techniques/ Signs and symptoms of labor. (Rate the outcome and indicators of **Knowledge: Pregnancy:** 1 = no knowledge, 2 = limited knowledge, 3 = moderate knowledge, 4 = substantial knowledge, 5 = extensive knowledge [see Section I].)

Client Outcomes

Client Will (Specify Time Frame)

During Pregnancy
- Attend all scheduled prenatal visits and attend prenatal education with her significant other or involved family member
- Use appropriate self-care for discomforts of pregnancy
- Make healthy lifestyle choices prenatally: activity and exercise/healthy nutritional practices
- Use strategies to balance activity and rest

During Labor and Delivery
- Demonstrate appropriate lifestyle choices during labor
- State knowledge of birthing options, signs and symptoms of labor
- Demonstrate effective labor techniques

After Birth
- Demonstrate appropriate lifestyle choices postpartum
- Report normal physical sensations after delivery
- State understanding of recommended nutrient intake, strategies to balance activity and rest, appropriate exercise, time frame for resumption of sexual activity, strategies to manage stress
- Demonstrate bonding with infant
- Demonstrate proper handling and positioning of infant/infant safety
- Demonstrate feeding technique and bathing of infant

NIC   (Nursing Interventions Classification)

Suggested NIC Interventions

Prenatal Care; Intrapartal Care; Postpartal Care; Attachment Promotion; Infant Care: Newborn; Lactation Counseling; Family Support

---

Example NIC Activities—Prenatal Care

Encourage prenatal class attendance and encourage involvement of client's partner or involved family member; Discuss nutritional needs and concerns (e.g., balanced diet, folic acid, food safety, and supplements); Discuss activity level with client (e.g., appropriate exercise, activities to avoid, and importance of rest); Discuss importance of participating in prenatal care throughout entire pregnancy

---

Nursing Interventions and *Rationales*

- Refer to care plans Risk for impaired **Attachment;** Readiness for enhanced **Breastfeeding;** Readiness for enhanced family **Coping;** Readiness for enhanced **Family** processes; **Growth;** Readiness for enhanced **Nutrition;** and Readiness for enhanced **Parenting;** Ineffective **Role** performance.

Prenatal Care

▲ Ensure that pregnant clients have an adequate diet and take multimicronutrient supplements containing at least 400 μg of folic acid, especially during early pregnancy. EB: *Cawley et al (2015) recommended*

● = Independent;   ▲ = Collaborative;   EBN = Evidence-Based Nursing;   EB = Evidence-Based

C

taking 400 µg of folic acid 12 weeks before conception, and all childbearing age women should be taking a folic acid supplementation daily to reduce the risk of neural tube defects. EB: *A healthy, varied diet (i.e., Choosemyplate.gov) is of vital importance for optimal birth outcome, and this includes taking a folic acid supplement from before conception to the 12th week of pregnancy, as well as a vitamin D supplement, throughout pregnancy (United States Department of Agriculture [USDA], 2014).* EB: *Fortified cereal is no longer recommended as the only source of folic acid because levels vary by consumption (Viswanathan et al, 2017).*

- Assess smoking status of pregnant clients and offer effective smoking-cessation interventions. EB: *Smoking is the leading cause of preventable death and disease in the United States. Exposure to nicotine during pregnancy adversely affects both maternal and fetal health and contributes to multiple adverse outcomes such as preterm birth and stillbirth and doubles the risk of placenta previa and placenta abruption. When infants are exposed to smoking, either directly or secondhand, their risk for sudden infant death syndrome is increased (United States Department of Health and Human Services [HHS], 2014). "Psychosocial interventions to support women to stop smoking in pregnancy can increase the proportion of women who stop smoking in late pregnancy, and reduce low birthweight and preterm births" (Chamberlain et al, 2013).* EBN: *A recent study described the development of an iPad application to promote knowledge of tobacco risk and cessation resources for pregnant women (Walsh Dotson et al, 2017).*

- See HHS for quitting smoking guidelines (https://betobaccofree.hhs.gov/quit-now/index.html).

- ▲ Assess all pregnant clients for signs of depression and make appropriate referral for inadequate weight gain, underutilization of prenatal care, increased substance abuse, and premature birth. Assess past personal or family history of depression, being single, poor health functioning, and alcohol use. EBN: *Social and emotional health problems associated with depression in the perinatal period can lead to poor outcomes for women, their infants, and their families (Rollans et al, 2013).*

- Discuss breastfeeding with a pregnant client, including all the benefits both to the infant and the mother. EB: *A government-funded nursing study done by Bass, Rodgers, and Baker (2014) placed a lactation consultant in an obstetrics (OB) office providing breastfeeding education throughout pregnancy. This offered the new mothers an opportunity to make an informed decision regarding the feeding choice for their newborns. The theory was that as the mother begins to breastfeed her newborn, her confidence is bolstered. Bass, Rodgers and Baker (2014) found exclusive breastfeeding rates increased from 33% to 60% in 8 months. They proposed that if frontline antenatal, intrapartum, and postpartum nurses begin to increase the mother's breastfeeding knowledge base, and continue to support and promote her feeding efforts, exclusive breastfeeding could increase.*

Intrapartal Care

- Encourage psychosocial support during labor, especially by the father of the baby or the woman's mother if possible. EBN: *When a husband provides continuous support during his wife's labor, his presence is considered effective in reducing her dissatisfaction with the childbirth process. According to de Lacerda, da Silva, and Davim (2014), the ideal companion is someone with whom the client has a bond and is trusted. The father of the child ranked first, followed by the mother of the postpartum woman.* EBN: *The key to promoting a normal birth and reducing medical interventions is high-quality continuous support. This support increases a woman's perception of a positive birth experience, fosters a positive adaptation to motherhood, and reduces the risk for posttraumatic stress disorder and other postpartum mental health problems (Sapkota, Kobayashi, & Takase, 2013; Ross-Davie & Cheyne, 2014).*

- Provide a calm, relaxing, and supportive birth environment. EBN: *The patient's outcome and safety are affected by the birth environment and culture. The care providers, whether midwives, doulas, and/or the nursing staff, must be knowledgeable and committed to providing labor support (Stark, Remynse, & Zwelling, 2016).* EB: *A birth environment that is calming and reduces stress supports physiological birth. Low levels of stress hormones during labor and birth promote uterine blood flow and support neonatal well-being, whereas greater levels of stress hormones can lengthen labor and impede the neonatal transition (Buckley, 2015).*

- Offer the client in labor a clear liquid diet and water if allowed. EB: *There is insufficient evidence to make conclusions about the relationship between fasting times for clear liquids and the risk for emesis, reflux, or pulmonary aspiration during labor. Although there is some disagreement, the majority of experts agree that oral intake of clear liquids during labor does not lead to increased maternal complications (American Congress of Obstetricians and Gynecologists [ACOG], 2013).*

• = Independent;   ▲ = Collaborative;   EBN = Evidence-Based Nursing;   EB = Evidence-Based

Multicultural

Prenatal

▲ Provide for a translator if needed. In some cultures a women prefers to have a female translator. EB: *The health care industry must recognize that providing translators for language assistance is an important tool for improving quality of care, saving lives, and avoiding costly and dangerous medical errors. Although costly, the American health care industry needs to comply with federal and state laws and accreditation standards by being prepared to provide care in at least 100 different languages (Rivers & Rivers, 2013).* EBN: *In the Arab and most Middle Eastern cultures female translators would be necessary because they are reluctant or sometimes forbidden to discuss female concerns with men (Meyer et al, 2016).*

● Assess the client's beliefs and concerns about prenatal care. Provide culturally appropriate prenatal care for clients. EBN: *When caring for a woman of a different culture recognize the danger of making assumptions about the health care needs of the group to which she belongs. Explore the specific needs of the individual. It is fundamental that women need to feel safe and supported, which sometimes involves challenging societal prejudices and providing nonjudgmental care that promotes equality. During this important and vulnerable time, caregivers need to ensure that women feel involved in their care, especially when there are language barriers. This can be accomplished through appropriate use of translation services and good communication skills to make certain that women are listened to and have the opportunity to make choices (Rowland-Neve, 2017).*

▲ Refer the client to a centering pregnancy group (8–10 women of similar gestational age receive group prenatal care after initial obstetrical visit) or group prenatal care. EB: *Group prenatal care appears to have created a benefit to the women, not just with their birth experiences, but also with the psychological and social aspects of this life change (Risisky, Asghar, & Chaffee, 2013).*

Intrapartal

● Assess client's beliefs and concerns about labor. Consider the client's culture when assisting in labor and delivery. EB: *There is a strong need to avert misunderstandings in today's multicultural society, and perhaps harm, through facilitating cultural awareness and competency of care rather than misinterpretations of opposition to care. Religious and traditional beliefs about childbearing practices can be very diverse among women with varied sociocultural backgrounds. Migrating women may not feel comfortable with the highly medicalized maternity care. Adherence to culturally specific traditional belief systems may produce a very different belief about maternity care and health care. They may regard the processes of pregnancy and delivery as normal events; therefore they may not seek maternity care. African women in Australia are not comfortable with pain relief injections. They think that pain relief disrupts normal events and using pain relief interrupts the natural birthing process. They also believe it to be harmful for the baby. Immigrants to a new country are often confronted with language barriers, lack of social supports, and lack of knowledge regarding the availability of conventional and alternative health care service (Higginbottom et al, 2013). According to van Dijk et al (2013) most clients receiving maternity services desired the option of culturally appropriate care but typically did not receive it.*

Postpartal

● Assess client's beliefs and concerns about the postpartum period. Provide culturally appropriate health and nutrition information and guidance on contemporary postpartum practices and take away common misconceptions about traditional dietary and health behaviors (e.g., fruit and vegetables should be restricted because of cold nature). Encourage a balanced diet and discourage unhealthy hygiene taboos. EB: *Many cultures practice food taboos surrounding pregnancy with consequent depletion of vital nutrients, which can be detrimental to both the mother and fetus (Oni & Tukur, 2012).* EBN: *When caring for a woman of a different culture recognize the danger of making assumptions about the health care needs of the group to which she belongs. Explore the specific needs of the individual. It is fundamental that women need to feel safe and supported, which sometimes involves challenging societal prejudices and providing nonjudgmental care that promotes equality (Rowland-Neve, 2017). Our Western ways are not the norm for many other cultures. A new Muslim mother rests for 40 days after giving birth so she may not want to ambulate after giving birth. She also may not want to breastfeed right away. She is considered unclean during this time so others prepare the food and do housework. The new mother in Japan returns to her childhood home to be "mothered" by her mother. There are rules in China that a new mother has to follow to restore balance. The balance of*

● = Independent;   ▲ = Collaborative;   EBN = Evidence-Based Nursing;   EB = Evidence-Based

C

opposites, such as hot and cold, is part of a belief system of many cultural groups such as Filipinos and Hispanics. Many in these groups believe there are natural external factors that must be kept in balance to maintain health (Littleton-Gibbs & Engelbretson, 2013).

Home Care

Prenatal

▲ Involve pregnant drug users in drug treatment programs that include coordinated interventions in several areas, such as drug use, infectious diseases, mental health, personal and social welfare, and gynecological/ obstetric care. EBN: *The drug addict is obsessed by the drug of choice because of a change in the pathophysiology of the brain. Treating addiction as a chronic disease instead of a moral weakness will be more supportive to women who abuse drugs. It is important to involve a pregnant woman in a treatment program such as a methadone clinic to help stabilize the maternal–fetal dyad. Methadone prevents withdrawal symptoms and eliminates drug craving. Methadone blocks the euphoric effects of illegal self-administered narcotics. It also supports stable maternal opioid levels to protect the fetus from repeated occurrences of withdrawal and decreases the risk for sexually transmitted infections (STIs) by decreasing drug-seeking behaviors such as prostitution. When a woman makes the decision to enroll in a methadone treatment program, she is taking a significant step toward recovery (Maguire, 2014).*

Postpartal

● Suggest parenting websites approved by the medical provider to support new parents with postpartum advice, newborn care, and breastfeeding. EBN: *Digital technology is being used to provide innovative family support services via websites. Online family support websites afford parents an alternative, cost-effective service that can be accessed from anywhere, increasing opportunities for parents to become active in their own support. They are, however, largely unfiltered and they raise unique challenges in identifying and managing child safeguarding concerns (Lamberton, Devaney, & Bunting, 2016).*

Client/Family Teaching and Discharge Planning

Prenatal

● Provide dietary and lifestyle counseling as part of prenatal care to pregnant women. EB: *A healthy pre-pregnancy weight, appropriate weight gain, physical activity during pregnancy, intake of a wide variety of foods, appropriate vitamin and mineral supplementation, avoidance of alcohol and other harmful substances, regular prenatal visits, and safe food handling are all components leading to a healthy pregnancy outcome. Pregnancy is a crucial period, and maternal nutrition and lifestyle choices are major influences on mother and infant/child health. Healthy lifestyle changes are the key to the health of the next generation (Procter & Campbell, 2014).*

● Provide group prenatal care to low-risk pregnant women belonging to high-risk demographic groups. EB: *The average pregnant woman who delivers at 40 weeks spends about 2 hours with her health care provider over the course of her entire pregnancy. Women who take part in group care have about 20 hours with their health care provider and have the opportunity to learn and encourage one another. Group prenatal care seems to lead to less low-birth-weight babies and fewer adverse perinatal outcomes compared with women in traditional care. The Carter et al (2017) study findings, together with data from earlier studies, proposed that group prenatal care may be a new and innovative way to provide prenatal care to low-risk individuals belonging to high-risk demographic groups to improve perinatal outcomes (Carter et al, 2017).*

Postpartal

● Encourage physical activity in postpartum women, after being cleared by the health care provider; teach postpartum women that exercise may reduce anxiety and depression, and encourage downloading phone apps that help track exercise like Fitbit or Pedometer Master. EB: *Research on anxiety, depression, and exercise shows that the psychological and physical benefits of exercise can help reduce anxiety and improve mood (Mayo Clinic Staff, 2014).*

▲ Provide breastfeeding mothers contact information for a lactation consultant, phone numbers, and website information for the La Leche League (http://www.lalecheleague.org), and local breastfeeding support groups. EBN: *The Joint Commission in 2014 made the rates of exclusive breastfeeding a perinatal core measure. In 2015 The Association of Women's Health, Obstetric and Neonatal Nurses (AWHONN) published its position statement on breastfeeding: it "supports, protects, and promotes breastfeeding as the ideal and*

● = Independent;   ▲ = Collaborative;   EBN = Evidence-Based Nursing;   EB = Evidence-Based

most normal method for feeding infants" (Henry et al, 2017). EBN: *The World Health Organization (WHO) recommended exclusive breastfeeding for the first 6 months of life for up to 2 years or more. Optimally, breastfeeding should begin within 1 hour of birth even after a C-section; breastfeeding should be "on demand," as often as the infant wants day and night; and bottles or pacifiers should not be used. Breast milk production is essential to long-term breastfeeding, and necessitates early, frequent and successful removal of colostrum. To remove as much milk as possible from the breasts, hand expression is recommended. This is a simple and risk-free method to stimulate milk production and can alleviate the pressure of achieving perfect attachment. The expressed colostrum can be spoonfed or cupfed to the infant. Hand expression and spoon- or cup-feeding also can be used when there is a problem such as sore breasts or difficulty latching. There is a new breastfeeding policy approved by the Centers for Disease Control and Prevention (CDC), United States Breastfeeding Committee (USBC), and the Joint Commission. The policy is called "Ten Steps to Successful Breastfeeding" (Baby-Friendly USA, n.d.). The policy is aimed at the hospital's commitment to breastfeeding and steps to achieve the Baby Friendly Initiative (Morton, Hall, & Pessl, 2014).* EB: *In a French study, polyunsaturated fatty acids (PUFAs) in colostrum and duration of breastfeeding were associated with an increase in children's IQs. The results supported breastfeeding and added evidence for the role of early PUFA exposure on childhood cognition (Bernard et al, 2017).*

- Teach mothers of young children principles of a healthy lifestyle: Substitute foods high in saturated fat with foods moderate in PUFAs such as avocados, tuna, walnuts, and olive oil. Include lean protein, fruits and vegetables, and complex carbohydrates. It is also important to increase physical activity. EB: *In a French study, PUFAs in colostrum and duration of breastfeeding were associated with an increase in children's IQs. The results support breastfeeding and added evidence for the role of early PUFA exposure on childhood cognition (Bernard et al, 2017).* EB: *PUFAs are the chief components of the brain and retina, and are the essential fatty acids with significant physiologically active functions. PUFAs should be provided to children, and they are vital in the brain growth and development for fetuses, newborn infants, and children (Lee, 2013).* EB: *Food preferences are important determinants of children's food intakes. Parental feeding behavior has a significant influence on the development of children's food preferences (Russell, Worsley, & Campbell, 2015).* EBN: *Omega 3 PUFAs are required for very early brain development, and that need continues throughout life. These essential fatty acids are crucial in cell functioning. Humans are not able to synthesize omega 3 PUFAs; therefore they must be included in the daily diet (Helvig & Decker, 2014).*

REFERENCES

American Congress of Obstetricians and Gynecologists (ACOG). ACOG Committee opinion no. 441: Oral intake during labor. (2009 reaffirmed 2013). *Obstetrics & Gynecology, 114*(3), 714.

Baby-Friendly USA. (n.d.). *The ten steps to successful breastfeeding.* Albany, NY: Author. Retrieved from www.babyfriendlyusa.org/about-us/baby-friendly-hospital-initiative/the-ten-steps.

Bass, C., Rodgers, M., & Baker, H. (2014). Can placing a lactation consultant in the obstetric office magically increase exclusive breastfeeding rates? *Journal of Obstetric, Gynecologic, and Neonatal Nursing, 43*(Suppl. 1), S52.

Bernard, J. Y., Armand, M., Peyre, H., et al. (2017). Breastfeeding, polyunsaturated fatty acid levels in colostrum and child intelligence quotient at age 5–6 years. *The Journal of Pediatrics, 183,* 43–50.e3. doi:10.1016/j.jpeds.2016.12.039.

Buckley, S. (2015). *Hormonal physiology of childbearing: Evidence and implications for women, babies, and maternity care.* Washington, DC: National Partnership for Women & Families. Retrieved from http://childbirthconnection.org/pdfs/CC.NPWF.HPoC.Report.2015.pdf.

Carter, E. B., Barbier, K., Sarabia, R., et al. (2017). Group versus traditional prenatal care in low-risk women delivering at term: A retrospective cohort study. *Journal of Perinatology, 37*(7), 769–771. doi:10.1038/jp.2017.33.

Cawley, S., Mullaney, L., McKeating, A., et al. (2015). An analysis of folic acid supplementation in women presenting. *Journal of Public Health, 38*(1), 122–129.

Chamberlain, C., O'Mara-Eves, A., Oliver, S., et al. (2013). Psychosocial interventions for supporting women to stop smoking in pregnancy.

The Cochrane Database of Systematic Reviews, (10), CD001055. doi:10.1002/14651858.CD001055.pub4.

Helvig, A., & Decker, M. (2014). Omega 3 fatty acids and the brain: Implications for nursing practice. *British Journal of Neuroscience Nursing, 10*(1), 29–37.

Henry, L. S., Hansson, M. C., Haughton, V. C., et al. (2017). Application of Kotter's theory of change to achieve baby-friendly designation. *Nursing for Women's Health, 21*(5), 372–382.

Higginbottom, G., Safipour, J., Mumtaz, Z., et al. (2013). "I have to do what I believe": Sudanese women's beliefs and resistance to hegemonic practices at home and during experiences of maternity care in Canada. *BMC Pregnancy and Childbirth, 13,* 51. Retrieved from https://doi.org/10.1186/1471-2393-13-51.

Lamberton, L., Devaney, J., & Bunting, L. (2016). New challenges in family support: The use of digital technology in supporting parents. *Child Abuse Review, 25*(5), 359–372. Retrieved from http://dx.doi.org.proxy.lib.wayne.edu/10.1002/car.2451A.

de Lacerda, A. B., da Silva, R. R., & Davim, R. B. (2014). Women's perception about the companion during labor. *Journal of Nursing UFPE on line, 8*(8), 2710–2715. Available from: CINAHL Complete, Ipswich, MA.

Lee, J.-H. (2013). Polyunsaturated fatty acids in children. *Pediatric Gastroenterology Hepatology Nutrition, 16*(3), 153–161. doi:10.5223/pghn.2013.16.3.153.

Littleton-Gibbs, L. Y., & Engelbretson, J. C. (2013). *Maternity nursing care* (2nd ed.). Clifton Park, NY: Delmar.

Maguire, D. (2014). Drug addiction in pregnancy: Disease not moral failure. *Neonatal Network, 33*(1), 11–18.

● = Independent;   ▲ = Collaborative;   EBN = Evidence-Based Nursing;   EB = Evidence-Based

C

Mayo Clinic Staff. (2014). *Depression and anxiety: Exercise eases symptoms*. Mayo Foundation for Medical Education and Research. Retrieved from http://www.mayoclinic.org/diseases-conditions/depression/in-depth/depression-and-exercise/art-20046495.

Meyer, J., Pomeroy, M., Reid, D., et al. (2016). Nursing care of pregnant Muslim women during Ramadan. *Nursing for Women's Health, 20*(5), 456–462. Retrieved from http://dx.doi.org/10.1016/j.nwh.2016.08.001.

Morton, J., Hall, J. Y., & Pessl, M. (2014). Five steps to improve bedside breastfeeding care. *Nursing for Women's Health, 17*(6), 478–488.

Oni, O. A., & Tukur, J. (2012). Identifying pregnant women who would adhere to food taboos in rural community: A community-based study. *African Journal of Reproductive Health, 16*(3), 68–76.

Procter, S. B., & Campbell, C. G. (2014). Position of the Academy of Nutrition and Dietetics: Nutrition and lifestyle for a healthy pregnancy outcome. *Journal of the Academy of Nutrition & Dietetics, 114*(7), 1099–1103.

Rivers, K., & Rivers, D. L. (2013). Foreign language difficulties in American healthcare: The challenges of medical translation regulation and remuneration. *National Social Science Proceedings, 52*(1), 150–160.

Rollans, M., Schmied, V., Kemp, L., et al. (2013). "We just ask some questions…" the process of antenatal psychosocial assessment by midwives. *Midwifery, 29*(8), 935–942.

Rowland-Neve, K. (2017). Seeking asylum while pregnant. *British Journal of Midwifery, 25*(9), 598–602.

Risisky, D., Asghar, S., & Chaffee, M. (2013). Women's perceptions using the centering pregnancy model of group prenatal care. *The Journal of Perinatal Education, 22*(3), 136–144. doi:10.1891/1058-1243.22.3.136.

Ross-Davie, M., & Cheyne, H. (2014). Intrapartum support: What do women want? A literature review. *Evidence Based Midwifery, 12*(2), 52–58.

Russell, C. G., Worsley, A., & Campbell, K. J. (2015). Strategies used by parents to influence their children's food preferences. *Appetite, 90*,

123–130. Retrieved from http://dx.doi.org.proxy.lib.wayne.edu/10.1016/j.appet.2015.02.038.

Sapkota, S., Kobayashi, T., & Takase, M. (2013). Impact on perceived postnatal support, maternal anxiety and symptoms of depression in new mothers in Nepal when their husbands provide continuous support during labour. *Midwifery, 29*(11), 1264–1271.

Stark, M. A., Remynse, M., & Zwelling, E. (2016). Importance of the birth environment to support physiologic birth. *Journal of Obstetric, Gynecologic, and Neonatal Nursing, 45*(2), 285–294.

US Department of Agriculture (USDA). (2014). *Nutritional needs during pregnancy*. Choosemyplate.gov/pregnancy. Retrieved from http://www.choosemyplate.gov/pregnancy-breastfeeding/pregnancy-nutritional-needs.html.

US Department of Health and Human Services. (2014). *The health consequences of smoking—50 years of progress: A report of the Surgeon General*. Retrieved from https://www.surgeongeneral.gov/library/reports/50-years-of-progress/exec-summary.pdf.

US Department of Health and Human Services. (2017). *Quit smoking guidelines*. https://betobaccofree.hhs.gov/quit-now/index.html.

van Dijk, M., Ruiz, M. J., Letona, D., et al. (2013). Ensuring intercultural maternal health care for Mayan women in Guatemala: A qualitative assessment. *Culture, Health & Sexuality, 15*, S365–S382. doi:10.1080/13691058.2013.779026.

Viswanathan, M., Treiman, K. A., Kish-Doto, J., et al. (2017). Folic acid supplementation for the prevention of neural tube defects: An updated evidence report and systematic review for the US Preventive Services Task Force. *JAMA: The Journal of the American Medical Association, 317*(2), 190–203.

Walsh Dotson, J. A., Pineda, R., Cylkowski, H., et al. (2017). Development and evaluation of an iPad application to promote knowledge of tobacco use and cessation by pregnant women. *Nursing for Women's Health, 21*(3), 174–185.

Risk for ineffective Childbearing process   *Dianne F. Hayward, RN, MSN, WHNP*

NANDA-I

Definition

Susceptible to an inability to prepare for and/or maintain a healthy pregnancy, childbirth process, and care of the newborn for ensuring well-being.

Risk Factors

Domestic violence; inadequate maternal nutrition; inconsistent prenatal health visits; insufficient cognitive readiness for parenting; insufficient knowledge of childbearing process; insufficient parental role model; insufficient prenatal care; insufficient support system; low maternal confidence; maternal powerlessness; maternal psychological distress; substance misuse; unrealistic birth plan; unsafe environment

At-Risk Population

Unplanned pregnancy; unwanted pregnancy

NOC, NIC, Client Outcomes, Nursing Interventions and *Rationales*, Client/Family Teaching, and References

Refer to care plan for Ineffective **Childbearing** process.

● = Independent;   ▲ = Collaborative;   EBN = Evidence-Based Nursing;   EB = Evidence-Based

Impaired Comfort   Gail B. Ladwig, MSN, RN and Julianne E. Doubet, BSN, RN, EMT-B

NANDA-I

Definition

Perceived lack of ease, relief, and transcendence in physical, psychospiritual, environmental, cultural, and/or social dimensions.

Defining Characteristics

Alteration in sleep pattern; anxiety; crying; discontent with situation; distressing symptoms; fear; feeling cold; feeling of discomfort; feeling of hunger; feeling warm; inability to relax; irritability; itching; moaning; restlessness; sighing; uneasy in situation

Related Factors

Insufficient environmental control; insufficient privacy; insufficient resources; insufficient situational control; noxious environmental stimuli

Associated Conditions

Illness-related symptoms; treatment regimen

NOC   (Nursing Outcomes Classification)

Suggested NOC Outcomes

Client Satisfaction; Symptom Control; Comfort Status; Coping; Hope; Pain Control; Anxiety Level Personal Well-Being; Spiritual Health

Example NOC Outcomes with Indicators

Comfort Status as evidenced by the following indicators: Physical and psychological well-being/Symptom control/Enhanced comfort. (Rate the outcome and indicators of **Comfort Status:** 1 = severely compromised, 2 = substantially compromised, 3 = moderately compromised, 4 = mildly compromised, 5 = not compromised [see Section I].)

Client Outcomes

Client Will (Specify Time Frame)

- Provide evidence for improved comfort compared to baseline
- Identify strategies, with or without significant others, to improve and/or maintain acceptable comfort level
- Perform appropriate interventions, with or without significant others, as needed to improve and/or maintain acceptable comfort level
- Evaluate the effectiveness of strategies to maintain/and or reach an acceptable comfort level
- Maintain an acceptable level of comfort when possible

NIC   (Nursing Interventions Classification)

Suggested NIC Interventions

Calming Techniques; Massage; Healing Touch; Heat/Cold Application; Hope Inspiration; Humor; Meditation Facilitation; Music Therapy; Pain Management; Acute/Chronic; Presence; Progressive Muscle Relaxation; Spiritual Growth Facilitation; Distraction

Example NIC Activities—Hope Inspiration

Assist the client/significant others to identify areas of hope in life; Help expand spiritual self; Involve the client actively in own care

Nursing Interventions and *Rationales*

- Assess client's understanding of ranking his or her comfort level. CEB: *Performing accurate comfort measurements is essential for providing evidence about which strategies and interventions are effective (Kolcaba,*

● = Independent;   ▲ = Collaborative;   EBN = Evidence-Based Nursing;   EB = Evidence-Based

C

2003). **EB:** *Teachings are easily understood (as well as patient participation in discussions prior to discharge), which target patient comprehension of instructions, have the potential to increase patient knowledge, and strengthen the ability to self-manage (Flink & Ekstedt, 2016).*

- Ask about client's current level of comfort. This is the first step in helping clients achieve improved comfort. **EBN:** *Sources of assessment data to determine level of comfort can be subjective, objective, primary, or secondary (Kolcaba, 2014).*

- Comfort is a holistic state under which pain management is included. **EBN:** *Nurses, have a responsibility to promote optimal comfort for patients and to intercede in certain situations to protect the patient's level of comfort, including pain (Karabulut et al, 2015).* **EBN:** *One randomized study (N = 53) found that female breast cancer clients undergoing radiation therapy rated their overall comfort as being greater than the sum of the hypothesized components of comfort, which provided evidence for the theory of the holistic nature of comfort (Kolcaba, 2014).*

- Assist clients to understand how to rate their current state of holistic comfort, using the institution's preferred method of documentation. **EBN:** *Documentation of comfort prenursing and postnursing interactions is essential to demonstrate efficacy of nursing activities (Kolcaba, 2014).*

- Enhance feelings of trust between the client and the health care provider. To attain the highest comfort level, clients must be able to trust their nurse. **EBN:** *This randomized design (N = 31) demonstrated the importance of promoting open relationships with clients, which helps to acknowledge their individuality. Knowing the client/significant others is essential in the provision of optimum palliative and terminal care (Kolcaba, 2014).*

- Manipulate the environment as necessary to improve comfort. **CEB:** *Addressing clients' environmental preferences or needs enhances holistic comfort (Kolcaba, 2003).* **EBN:** *The theoretical foundation of holistic comfort, which consists of relief, ease, and transcendence, in the settings of physical, psychological, social, and environmental experiences, enables the nurse to meet the individual comfort needs of a patient (Ng, 2017).*

- Encourage early mobilization and provide routine position changes. Range of motion and weight bearing decrease physical discomforts and disability associated with bed rest. **EBN:** *It has been shown that immobility is linked to many unacceptable patient outcomes in critical care units. Mobility takes many forms (passive and active range of motion exercises, sitting up, dangling legs on side of bed, etc.) along with walking, and these should be included in patient care (Crowe et al, 2017).*

- Provide simple massage. Massage has many therapeutic effects, including improved relaxation, circulation, and well-being. **EBN:** *Several quantitative studies support the efficacy of simple massage for enhancing holistic comfort (Townsend et al, 2014).*

- Provide a healing touch, which is well suited for clients who cannot tolerate more stimulating interventions. **EBN:** *According to Anderson et al (2017), providing nurses with the knowledge of healing touch and demonstrating its use in acute patient care gives the nurse another means of ensuring positive patient outcomes.*

- Encourage clients to use relaxation techniques to reduce pain, anxiety, depression, and fatigue. **EBN:** *In a quantitative study with 22 participants, the effects of traditional massage and cranial still point induction were statistically significant in improving comfort and decreasing chronic pain (Townsend et al, 2014).*

 Geriatric

- Use hand massage for older adults. Most older adults respond well to touch and the health care provider's presence. Lines of communication open naturally during hand massage. **CEB:** *In an experiment (N = 60), the effects of hand massage on the comfort of nursing home residents was found to be significant immediately after the massage compared with residents who did not receive hand massage (Kolcaba, 2014).*

- Discomfort from cold can be treated with warmed blankets. There are physiological dangers associated with hypothermia. **EBN:** *A study (N = 126) found significantly increased comfort and decreased anxiety in clients who used self-controlled warming gowns (Kolcaba, 2014).*

- Use complementary therapies such as doll therapy in clients with dementia to increase comfort and reduce stress. **EBN:** *In a review of the literature, doll therapy reduced panic, anxiety, and aggression while improving the dining experience and social interaction (Mitchell & O'Donnell, 2013).*

- Address any unmet physical, psychological, emotional, spiritual, and environmental needs when attempting to mediate the behavior of an older client with dementia. **EBN:** *As nursing and health care adjust to serve an aging population, there is a renewed interest in providing holistic nursing care appropriate to the patient's mental and physical conditions (Pryor & Clarke, 2017).*

Multicultural

- Identify and clarify cultural language used to describe pain and other discomforts. Expressions of pain and discomfort vary across cultures. CEB: *Clients may interchange words meaning discomfort and pain, may not admit to having pain, may refer to minor discomforts as pain, or may not discuss nonpainful discomforts at all (Kolcaba, 2003).* EBN: *Nurses today are challenged to find means to facilitate culturally harmonious care for all patients: according to Jeffreys and Zoucha (2017), this can be accomplished "through ongoing assessment, education, research, and practice initiatives."*
- Assess skin for ashy or yellow-brown appearance. CEB: *Black skin appears ashy and brown skin appears yellow-brown when clients have pallor sometimes associated with discomfort (Peters, 2007).*
- Use soap sparingly if the skin is dry. Black skin tends to be dry, and soap exacerbates this condition.
- Encourage and allow clients to practice their own cultural beliefs and recognize the impact that diverse cultures have on a client's belief about health care, comforting measures, and decision-making. EBN: *Cultural competence is a necessary element of complete nursing care and is achieved by establishing good communication, having skill in making the correct diagnosis, and by recognition of clients' language and beliefs as it relates to health and illness (Debiasi & Selleck, 2017).*
- Assess for cultural and religious beliefs when providing care. EB: *According to Schweda et al (2017), in their study of cultural stereotyping, it was found that there is not just one perspective on culture and/or religion, but each individual's stance is formed by political, social, and situation beliefs.*

Client/Family Teaching and Discharge Planning

- Teach techniques to use when the client is uncomfortable, including relaxation techniques, guided imagery, hand massage, and music therapy. CEB: *Interventions such as progressive muscle relaxation training, guided imagery, and music therapy can effectively decrease the perception of uncomfortable sensations, including pain (Kolcaba, 2003).* EBN: *Families want to learn how to provide comfort measures to their loved ones who are uncomfortable (Kolcaba, 2014).*
- At end of life, the dying client is comforted by having a companion. EBN: *In a study of literature concerning death and dying while in palliative care, Dobrina et al (2014) found that the nurse's presence alone made the patient's end-of-life journey more comfortable and peaceful.*
- Instruct the client and family about prescribed medications and complementary therapies that improve comfort.
- Teach the client to follow-up with the health care provider if discomfort persists. There are many avenues for enhancing comfort.
- Encourage clients to use the Internet as a means of providing education to complement medical care for those who may be homebound or unable to attend face-to-face education. EB: *Jones et al (2015) surmised that Internet usage by the older population benefits them in many ways (reduces social isolation, access to services, etc.) and especially serves to improve health and give the client a sense of well-being.*

Mental Health

- Encourage clients to use guided imagery techniques. Guided imagery helps distract clients from stressful situations and facilitates relaxation. EBN: *A quasi-experimental study (N = 60) found that clients who listened to a guided imagery compact disk once a day for 10 days had improved comfort and decreased depression, anxiety, and stress over time (Kolcaba, 2014).*
- Provide psychospiritual support and a comforting environment to enhance comfort during emotional crises. EBN: *As health care professionals, nurses should intervene and provide care that recognizes and reduces strain for the patient, caregiver, and family during a mental health crisis (Naseimento et al, 2016).*
- When nurses attend to the comfort of perioperative clients, the clients' sense of hope for a full recovery increases. EBN: *In a quantitative study with 191 participants, direct and significant relationships were observed between comfort and hope (Seyedfatemi et al, 2014).*
- Providing music and verbal relaxation therapy enhances holistic comfort by reducing anxiety. EBN: *In her review of studies using music as a nursing intervention, Eells (2014) found that music is an effective tool in relieving anxiety.*
- Caregivers should not hesitate to use humor when caring for their clients. EB: *Humor is seen as a health-promoting means of handling life's stress (Roaldsen et al, 2015).*

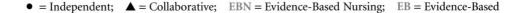

● = Independent;   ▲ = Collaborative;   EBN = Evidence-Based Nursing;   EB = Evidence-Based

C

REFERENCES

Anderson, J., Friesen, M., & Swengros, D. (2017). Examination of the use of healing touch by registered nurses in the acute care setting. *Journal of Holistic Nursing, 35*(1), 97–107.

Crowe, S., Brook, A., & Reynold, J. (2017). You want me to do what? Mobility and continuous renal replacement therapy (CRRT) patients. *The Canadian Journal of Critical Care Nursing, 28*(2), 24–29.

Debiasi, L., & Selleck, C. (2017). Cultural competence training for primary care nurse practioners: An intervention to increase culturally competent care. *Journal of Cultural Diversity, 24*(2), 39–45.

Dobrina, R., Tenze, M., & Palese, A. (2014). An overview of hospice and palliative care nursing models and theories. *International Journal of Palliative Nursing, 20*(2), 75–81.

Eells, K. (2014). The use of music and singing to help manage anxiety in older adults. *Mental Health Practice, 17*(5), 10–17.

Flink, M., & Ekstedt, M. (2016). Prerequisites for patient self-management learning at hospital discharge: An observational multiple case study. *Journal of Integrated Care, 2016*(Suppl. v), 16n6, 1–2.

Jeffreys, M., & Zoucha, R. (2017). Revisiting "The Invisible Culture of the Multiracial Multiethnic Individual": A transcultural imperative. *Journal of Cultural Diversity, 24*(1), 3–5.

Jones, R., Ashurst, E., Atkey, J., et al. (2015). Older people going online: Its value and before-after evaluation of volunteer support. *Journal of Medical Internet Research, 17*(5), e122. Retrieved from doi:10.2196/jmir.3943.

Karabulut, N., Aktas, Y., Gurcayir, D., et al. (2015). Patient satisfaction with their pain management and comfort after open heart surgery. *Australian Journal of Advanced Nursing, 32*(3), 16–24.

Kolcaba, K. (2003). *Comfort theory and practice: A holistic vision for health care.* New York: Springer.

Kolkaba, K., (2014). *TheComfortLine.com.* Retrieved from www.TheComfortLine.com.

Mitchell, G., & O'Donnell, H. (2013). The therapeutic use of doll therapy in dementia. *The British Journal of Nursing, 22*(6), 329–334.

Naseimento, K., Kolhs, M., & Mells, S. (2016). The family challenge in for people suffering from mental disorder. *Journal of Nursing UFPE Online, 10*(3), 940–948. Retrieved from doi:10.5205/reuol.8702 -76273-4-SM.1003201601.

Ng, S. (2017). Application of Kolkaba's Comfort Theory to the management of a patient with heptacellular carcinoma. *Singapore Nursing Journal, 44*(1), 16–23.

Peters, J. (2007). Examining and describing skin conditions. *The Journal of Practical Nursing, 34*(8), 19–40, 43, 45.

Pryor, C., & Clarke, A. (2017). Nursing care for people with delirium superimposed on dementia. *Nursing Older People, 29*(3), 18–21.

Roaldsen, B., Sorlie, T., & Lorem, G. (2015). Cancer survivors' experiences of humour while navigating through challenging landscapes: A socio-narrative report. *Scandinavian Journal of Caring Sciences, 29*(4), 724–733.

Schweda, M., Schicktanz, S., & Raz, A. (2017). Beyond cultural stereotyping: views on end-of-life decision making among religious and secular persons in the USA, Germany, and Israel. *BMC Medical Ethics, 18*, 1–11.

Seyedfatemi, N., Rafi, F., Rezaei, M., et al. (2014). Comfort and hope in the preanesthesia stage in patients undergoing surgery. *Journal of Perianesthesia Nursing, 29*(3), 213–220.

Townsend, C., Bonham, E., Chase, L., et al. (2014). A comparison of still point induction to massage therapy in reducing pain and increasing comfort in chronic pain. *Holistic Nursing Practice, 28*(2), 78–84.

Readiness for enhanced Comfort
Gail B. Ladwig, MSN, RN and Julianne E. Doubet, BSN, RN, EMT-B

NANDA-I

Definition

A pattern of ease, relief, and transcendence in physical, psychospiritual, environmental, and/or social dimensions that is sufficient for well-being and can be strengthened.

Defining Characteristics

Expresses desire to enhance comfort; expresses desire to enhance feelings of contentment; expresses desire to enhance relaxation; expresses desire to enhance resolution of complaints

NOC Outcomes   (Nursing Outcomes Classification)

Suggested NOC Outcomes

Client Satisfaction: Caring; Symptom Control; Comfort Status; Coping; Hope; Motivation; Pain Control; Participation in Health Care Decisions; Spiritual Health

Example NOC Outcomes with Indicators
Comfort Status as evidenced by the following indicators: Physical well-being/Symptom control/Psychological well-being. (Rate the outcome and indicators of **Comfort Level:** I = not at all satisfied, 2 = somewhat satisfied, 3 = moderately satisfied, 4 = very satisfied, 5 = completely satisfied [see Section I].)

● = Independent;   ▲ = Collaborative;   EBN = Evidence-Based Nursing;   EB = Evidence-Based

Client Outcomes

Client Will (Specify Time Frame)

- Assess current level of comfort as acceptable
- Express the need to achieve an enhanced level of comfort
- Identify strategies to enhance comfort
- Perform appropriate interventions as needed for increased comfort
- Evaluate the effectiveness of interventions at regular intervals
- Maintain an enhanced level of comfort when possible

NIC   Interventions (Nursing Interventions Classification)

Suggested NIC Interventions

Calming Technique; Cutaneous Stimulation; Environmental Management: Comfort; Heat/Cold Application; Hope Inspiration; Humor; Meditation Facilitation; Music Therapy; Pain Management: Acute and Chronic; Presence; Guided Imagery; Massage; Relaxation Therapy; Spiritual Growth Facilitation; Therapeutic Play; Therapeutic Touch; Touch; Distraction

Example NIC Activities—Spiritual Growth Facilitation
Assist the client with identifying barriers and attitudes that hinder growth or self-discovery; Assist the client to explore beliefs as related to healing of the body, mind, and spirit; Model healthy relating and reasoning skills

Nursing Interventions and *Rationales*

- Assess clients' comfort needs and current level of comfort in various contexts, as outlined in Kolcaba's (2003) comfort theory and practice: physical, psychospiritual, sociocultural, and environmental. CEB: *Assessing comfort needs helps develop holistic, client-centered comfort interventions, whereas establishing a baseline helps evaluate their effectiveness by comparing comfort levels after each intervention to the previous baseline (Kolcaba, 2003).* EBN: *By using the comfort theory's framework, the nurse can recognize the patient's physical, psychosocial, sociocultural, and environmental needs; bringing these aspects into play will aid in identifying nursing problems and the necessary interventions that can be implemented to enrich the patient's environment (Ng, 2017).*
- Educate clients about the various contexts of comfort and help them understand that enhanced comfort is a desirable, positive, and achievable goal. CEB: *Human beings strive to have their basic comfort needs met, with comfort being more than just the absence of pain (Kolcaba, 2003).* EBN: *According to Silveira Mendes et al (2016), nursing care should incorporate all aspects of the patient's comfort needs and not just the physical, which are both expressed and unexpressed.*
- Enhance feelings of trust between the client and the health care provider to maintain an effective and therapeutic relationship. EBN: *Trust is an essential element in the nurse-client relationship that is fostered through caring attitudes, availability, respect, empathy, sensitivity to client needs, competence, and effective communication (Dinç & Gastmans, 2013).*
- Maintain an open and effective communication with clients and keep them informed about their health, their plan of care, and their environment. EBN: *Communicating to hospitalized cardiothoracic clients the source of sounds heard or expected to be heard around the unit, such as alarms, staff conversations, and rolling carts, alleviated their anxiety and enhanced relaxation (Mackrill et al, 2013), hence, promoting their environmental comfort.*
- Implement comfort rounds that regularly assess for clients' comfort needs. EBN: *Regular 1-hour or 2-hour rounds that address pain, positioning, personal needs, and environment were found to increase client satisfaction, decrease call light usage, and promote safety by decreasing fall rates (Chu, 2014; Ciccu-Moore et al, 2014).*
- Collaborate with other health care professionals, such as health care providers, pharmacists, social workers, chaplains, occupational and physical therapists, and dietitians, among others, in planning interventions that address comfort needs in various contexts: physical, psychospiritual, sociocultural, and environmental. EBN: *Kolcaba's comfort theory can be used as a guide for patient care in offering uncomplicated and holistic standards that assist the nurse in recognizing patient's needs, developing interventions to satisfy those needs, assessing the outcomes of these interventions, and meeting goals of quality patient and family care. These*

● = Independent;   ▲ = Collaborative;   EBN = Evidence-Based Nursing;   EB = Evidence-Based

C

goals may also encompass discharge planning and follow-up with various health and spiritual providers (Boudiab & Kolcaba, 2015).

- Educate clients about and encourage the use of various integrative therapies and modalities to provide options that enhance comfort, beyond the traditional plan of care. Institute of Medicine (IOM) and Pain examples of such modalities are listed below:
  - ○ Therapeutic massage and touch therapy. **EBN:** *Massage and touch therapy have been found to promote comfort in clients with dementia by decreasing anxiety and agitation (Battaglini, 2014). There is evidence to support recommending massage to clients with subacute and chronic back pain, mechanical neck pain, and labor pain, as well as to decrease anxiety and blood pressure and to improve quality of life in clients with HIV/AIDS (D'Arcy, 2014)*
  - ○ Guided imagery. **EBN:** *Guided imagery was also effective in improving chronic tension headaches and body pain, as well as promoting overall mental health and energy level (Read, 2013).*
  - ○ Mindfulness and mindfulness-based interventions such as mindfulness-based stress reduction (MBSR), mantra repetition (silent repetition of a sacred word), mindfulness meditation, and mindful breathing and walking, among others. **EB:** *A study of MBSR in cancer clients concluded that mindfulness promotes a sense of calmness, inner peace, and personal and spiritual growth (Labellea et al, 2014).* **EBN:** *Mantra repetition is found to decrease posttraumatic stress disorder (PTSD) symptoms and increase sense of well-being in veterans when added to their traditional PTSD treatment plan (Bormann et al, 2014).*
  - ○ Energy therapy or biofield therapy such as healing touch, therapeutic touch, and Reiki. Biofield therapy seems to be promising in promoting comfort and relaxation, but more sound and systematic research is needed to build a strong body of evidence. **EBN:** *Healing touch has been found effective as an adjunct therapy in relieving anxiety and depression (Harlow, 2013).* **EBN:** *Biofield therapy strengthens the immune system, decreases stress, and allows the body to heal. It can be integrated in the care of cancer clients in various settings for relaxation and symptom management, as well as in those with musculoskeletal and joint pain, agitation and dementia, and other chronic conditions (Gonella et al, 2014).*
  - ○ Acupuncture and auricular acupuncture. **EBN:** *Faircloth (2015) stated that acupuncture and acupressure have been found to decrease apprehension preoperatively, reduce intraoperative anesthetic requirements, diminish postoperative discomfort, lower the occurrence of postoperative nausea and vomiting, and fortify the treatment of chronic pain management.*
  - ○ Aromatherapy. **EB:** *In their study of individuals exposed to the lemon grass scent, Costa Goes et al (2015) found that there was a reduction in anxiety and subjective stress within minutes of the aroma's administration.*
  - ○ Music. **EBN:** *Music, as a nursing intervention, has been shown to be beneficial in relieving patients' discomfort, apprehension, and distress (Waterworth & Rickson, 2017).*
  - ○ Other mind–body therapies such as meditation, yoga, etc. **EB:** *Meditation is a strategy of self-care that offers potential usefulness in mental health situations, in behavioral self-regulation, and integrative medical care (Burke et al, 2017).*
- Foster and instill hope in clients whenever possible. **EBN:** *A study of clients undergoing surgery in the preanesthesia stage found a strong correlation between hope and comfort (Seyedfatemi et al, 2014). See the care plan for* **Hopelessness.**
- Provide opportunities for and enhance spiritual care activities. **EBN:** *Recognizing and satisfying patients' spiritual needs is essential to nursing care; now, with the acceptance of integrative medicine, nurses play a key role in promoting spiritual comfort for their patients (Chan, 2014).*
- ▲ Enhance social support and family involvement. **EBN:** *In their survey (based on Kolcaba's enhanced comfort theory) addressing family experiences, when a loved one is hospitalized in an intensive care unit, Twohig et al (2015) found that there was an elevated level of satisfaction among family members in all aspects of patient care, including communication and the opportunity to be involved in decision-making.*
- ▲ Promote participation in creative arts and activity programs. **EB:** *Adult education classes in creative arts were found to improve well-being by boosting mood and providing a feeling of belonging. It also supported members in developing self-confidence, in the development of new relationships, and in general it encouraged more active lives (Pearce, 2017).*
- ▲ Encourage clients to use health information technology (HIT) as needed). **EB:** *In a European Union study, Internet users in the United Kingdom validated the concept that the Internet was a good option in gaining knowledge of self-care and care of others and was valuable in positive health care outcomes (Marton, 2015).*
- Evaluate the effectiveness of all comfort interventions at regular intervals and adjust therapies as necessary. **EBN:** *In a study by Coelho et al (2016), patients were asked how they sensed a feeling of comfort, and their responses included: individualized care, symptom containment, need for a comfortable environment, and*

• = Independent; ▲ = Collaborative; **EBN** = Evidence-Based Nursing; **EB** = Evidence-Based

hope and relationships. Recognition of these needs gives the nurse the opportunity to construct personalized interventions that meet these needs as well as to evaluate and revise them as needed.

Geriatric

- Refer to previously mentioned interventions for geriatric interventions.

Pediatric

- Assess and evaluate the child's level of comfort at frequent intervals. With assessment of pain in children, it is best to use input from the parents or a primary care giver. **EBN:** *According to Shaw et al (2017), skillful communication with patients and families is necessary for proficient, personalized comfort care in the pediatric environment.* **EBN:** *Continued research is necessary to establish the most useful and valid methods in assessment of pediatric pain and/or discomfort, and may incorporate technology as a viable assessment tool (Quinn et al, 2014).*
- Skin-to-skin contact (SSC) in the comfort of newborns, especially those at risk. **EBN:** *Newborn SSC practice is natural and instinctive and has been found to have positive effects on health outcomes and comfort, especially for at-risk newborns in low-support environments (Hubbard et al, 2017).*
- Adjust the environment as needed to enhance comfort. **CEB:** *Environmental comfort measures include maintaining orderliness; quiet; minimizing furniture; and special attention to temperature, light and sound, color, and landscape (Kolcaba & DeMarco, 2005).*
- Encourage parental presence whenever possible. **EBN:** *In a study done by Carnevale and Gaudreault (2013) of seriously ill pediatric patients in a university-connected children's hospital, they found that the presence of parents was the most important source of the child's comfort.*
- Promote use of alternative comforting strategies such as positioning, presence, massage, spiritual care, music therapy, art therapy, and story-telling to enhance comfort when needed. **EB:** *In their study of comfort measures and sedation/analgesics used in pediatric intensive care units (PICUs), Guerra et al (2016) found that enhanced comfort care is offered through music, swaddling, pacifiers, television, and sucrose solutions.*
- Support the child's spirituality. **EB:** *A child's spiritual growth is recognized along with moral, mental, and social development as an important part of children's lives and is deserving of preservation and development (Karlsen et al, 2014).*

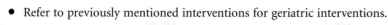
Multicultural

- Identify cultural beliefs, values, lifestyles, practices, and problem-solving strategies when assessing a client's comfort. **EB:** *The responsibility of providing cultural health care to those in our multicultural society continues to prove challenging; it is good to remember that cultural traditions are powerful forces and should not be generalized in caring for clients of diverse cultures (Wiener et al, 2013).*
- Enhance cultural knowledge by actively seeking out information regarding different cultural and ethnic groups **EBN:** *As the multicultural population of the United States continues to expand, there is a growing need for outreach and culturally sensitive education that will better serve these communities (Elminowski, 2015).*
- ▲ Recognize the impact of culture on communication styles and techniques **EBN:** *Livesay et al (2017) surmised that growing diversification of societies places increasing emphasis on the demand for culturally suitable communication, which both addresses the needs of the health care consumer and the provider.*
- Provide culturally competent care to clients from different cultural groups. **EBN:** *It is crucial that nurses, as an important part of the health care team, are cognizant and perceptive concerning the distinctive problems related to providing care and treatment to people from different cultures (Michigan Nurse, 2015).*

Home Care

- The nursing interventions described for Readiness for enhanced **Comfort** may be used with clients in the home care setting. When needed, adaptations can be made to meet the needs of specific clients, families, and communities.
- ▲ Make appropriate referrals to other organizations or health care providers as needed to enhance comfort. **EBN:** *Parker et al (2013) submitted that a palliative care referral that encompasses pain assessment and management, transition and coordination of levels of care, and advanced care planning can enhance outcomes and increase patient satisfaction.* **EBN:** *Unnecessary referrals for older patients may lead to poorer health, decreased feeling of well-being, and magnified confusion (Kihlgren et al, 2016).*

● = Independent; ▲ = Collaborative; EBN = Evidence-Based Nursing; EB = Evidence-Based

C

▲ Promote an interdisciplinary (home care nurses, physicians, pharmacy, etc.) approach to home care. **EBN:** *Imhoff (2016), in his study of nurse-led interdisciplinary team approach to palliative care, found that the nurse specialist was an important player in establishing and sustaining an interdisciplinary complex system of care.*

● Evaluate regularly if enhanced comfort is attainable in the home care setting. **EB:** *A study by Seow et al (2016) found that home care nurses provided comfort and support to cancer patients who wished to die at home and not in the hospital.*

Client/Family Teaching and Discharge Planning

● Teach client how to regularly assess levels of comfort.

● Instruct client that a variety of interventions may be needed at any given time to enhance comfort. **EBN:** *Health care professionals involved in home care should be proficient in medical technology to preserve a feeling of safety and allay fears in both patients and their care givers (Munck & Sandgren, 2017).*

● Help clients understand that enhanced comfort is an achievable goal.

● Teach techniques to enhance comfort as needed.

▲ When needed, empower clients to seek out other health professionals as members of the interdisciplinary team to assist with comforting measures and techniques.

● Encourage self-care activities and continued self-evaluation of achieved comfort levels to ensure enhanced comfort is maintained.

REFERENCES

Battaglini, E. (2014). *Dementia: Massage and touch*. Joanna Briggs Institute [Evidence Summaries]. Retrieved from www.Joannabriggs.org.

Bormann, J. E., Oman, D., Walter, K. H., et al. (2014). Mindful attention increases and mediates psychological outcomes following mantra repetition practice in veterans with posttraumatic stress disorder. *Medical Care*, *52*(12 Suppl. 5), S13–S18.

Boudiab, L., & Kolcaba, K. (2015). Comfort theory: Unraveling the complications of veterans' healthcare needs. *Advances in Nursing Practice*, *38*(4), 270–278.

Burke, A., Lam, C., Stussman, B., et al. (2017). Mind-body therapies. *Journal of the Australian Traditional-Medicine Society, Spring*, *23n.3*, 169–170.

Carnevale, F., & Gaudreault, J. (2013). The experiences of critically ill children: A phenomenological study of discomfort and comfort. *Dynamics (Pembroke, Ont.)*, *24*(1), 19–27.

Chu, V. (2014). *Nursing rounds: Clinician Information*. Joanna Briggs Institute [Evidence Summaries]. Retrieved from www.Joannabriggs.org.

Ciccu-Moore, R., Grant, F., Niven, B., et al. (2014). Care and comfort rounds: Improving standards. *Nursing Management*, *20*(9), 18–23.

Chan, R. (2014). Mantra meditation as a bedside spiritual intervention. *Medsurg Nursing*, *23*(2), 84–100.

Coelho, A., Parola, V., Escobar-Bravo, M., et al. (2016). Comfort experience in palliatie care: A phenomenological study. *BMC Palliative Care*, *15*, 1–8.

Costa Goes, T., Reis Carvalho Ursulino, F., Almeida-Souza, T., et al. (2015). Effect of lemon grass aroma on experimental anxiety in humans. *Journal of Alternative and Complimentary Medicine*, *21*(12), (Article) ISSN, 1075-5535.

D'Arcy, M. (2014). *Massage therapy: various conditions*. Joanna Briggs Institute [Evidence Summaries]. Retrieved from www.Joannabriggs.org.

Dinç, L., & Gastmans, C. (2013). Trust in nurse-patient relationships: A literature review. *Nursing Ethics*, *20*(5), 501–516.

Elminowsky Sanchwz, N. (2015). Developing and implementing a cultural awareness workshop for nurse practitioners. *Journal of Cultural Diversity*, *22*(3), 105–113.

Faircloth, A. (2015). Acupuncture history from the Yellow Emperor to modern anesthesia practice. *AANA Journal*, *83*(4), 289–295.

Gonella, S., Garrino, L., & Dimonte, G. (2014). Biofield therapies and cancer-related symptoms: A review. *Clinical Journal of Oncology Nursing*, *18*(5), 568–576.

Guerra, G., Joffe, A., Cave, D., et al. (2016). Survey of sedation and analgesia practice among Canadian pediatric critical care physicians. *Pediatric Critical Care Medicine*, *17*(9), 823–830.

Harlow, C. R. (2013). *A critical analysis of healing touch for symptoms of depression and anxiety*. (Unpublished doctoral dissertation). University of Arizona, Tucson, AZ.

Hubbard, J., Gattman, K., & Kindsey, R. (2017). Parent-infant skin-to-skin contact following birth: History, benefits, and challenges. *Neonatal Network*, *36*(2), 89–97.

Imhoff, L. (2016). Nurse-led palliatiec care services facilitate an interdisciplinary network of care. *International Journal of Palliative Nursing*, *22*(8), 404–410.

Karlsen, M., Coyle, A., & Williams, E. (2014). "They never listen": towards a grounded theory of the role played by trusted adults in the spiritual levels of children. *Mental Health, Religion & Culture*, *17*(3), 297–312.

Kihlgren, A., Svensson, F., Lovbrand, C., et al. (2016). A decision support system (DDS) for municipal nurses encountering health deterioration among older people. *BMC Nursing*, *15*, 1–10.

Kolcaba, K. (2003). *Comfort theory and practice*. New York: Springer.

Kolcaba, K., & DeMarco, M. (2005). Comfort theory and application to pediatric nursing. *Pediatric Nursing*, *31*(3), 187–194.

Labellea, L. E., Lawlor-Savagea, L., Campbella, T. S., et al. (2014). Does self-report mindfulness mediate the effect of Mindfulness-Based Stress Reduction (MBSR) on spirituality and posttraumatic growth in cancer patients? *The Journal of Positive Psychology*. Retrieved from http://dx.doi.org/10.1080/17439760 .2014.927902.

Livesay, K., Lau, P., McNair, R., et al. (2017). The culturally and linguistically diverse SPs' evaluation of simulation experience. *Clinical Simulation in Nursing*, *13*(5), 228–237.

Mackrill, J., Cain, R., Jennings, P., et al. (2013). Sound source information to improve cardiothoracic patients' comfort. *British Journal of Nursing*, *22*(7), 387–393.

● = Independent;   ▲ = Collaborative;   **EBN** = Evidence-Based Nursing;   **EB** = Evidence-Based

Marton, C. (2015). Understanding the health needs of British internet users seeking healthcare information on line and their perceptions of the quality of the internet as a source of health information. *Journal of Hospital Librarianship, 15*(2), 175–188.

Munck, B., & Sandgren, A. (2017). The impact of medical technology on sense of security in the palliative home care setting. *British Journal of Community Nursing, 22*(3), 130–135.

Ng, S. (2017). Application of Kolcaba's Comfort Theory to the management of a patient with hepatocellular carcinoma. *Singapore Nursing Journal, 44*(1), 16–23.

Michigan Nurse. (2015). Culturally competent nursing care and promoting diversity in our nursing workforce. *The Michigan Nurse, 88*(3), 7–11.

Parker, S., Remington, R., Nannini, A., et al. (2013). Patient outcomes and satisfaction with care following palliative care consultation. *Journal of Hospice & Palliative Nursing, 15*(4), 225–232.

Pearce, E. (2017). Participants' perspective on the social bonding and well-being effects of creative arts adult education classes. *Art & Health: International Journal of Research. Policy & Practice, 9*(1), 42–59.

Quinn, B., Sheldon, L., & Cooley, M. (2014). Pediatric pain assessment by drawn faces scales: A review. *Pain Management Nursing, 15*(4), 909–918.

Read, S. (2013). *Chronic pain: Nursing interventions.* Joanna Briggs Institute [Evidence Summaries]. Retrieved from www.Joannabriggs.org.

Seow, H., Sutradhar, R., McGrail, K., et al. (2016). End of life cancer care: Temperol association between home care nursing and hospitalizations. *Journal of Palliative Medicine, 19*(3), 263–270.

Silveira Mendes, R., Cruz, M., Palva, R., et al. (2016). Comfort Theory as support for a safe clinical nursing care. *Ciencia Cuidado e Saude, 15*(2), 390–395.

Seyedfatemi, N., Rafii, F., Rezaei, M., et al. (2014). Comfort and hope in the preanesthesia stage in patients undergoing surgery. *Journal of Perianesthesia Nursing, 29*(3), 213–220.

Shaw, A., Lind, C., & Ewashen, C. (2017). Harlequin-inspired story based learning: An educational innovation in pediatric nursing. *Journal of Nursing Education, 56*(5), 300–303.

Twohig, B., Manasia, A., Bassily-Marcus, A., et al. (2015). Family experiences survey in the surgical intensive care unit. *Applied Nursing Research, 28*(4), 281–284.

Waterworth, C., & Rickson, D. (2017). Music in nursing. *Kai Tiaki Nursing New Zealand, 23*(7), 28–29.

Wiener, L., McConnell, D., Latella, L., et al. (2013). Cultural and religious considerations in pediatric palliative care. *Palliative and Supportive Care, 11*(1), 47–67.

Readiness for enhanced Communication
Stacey M. Carroll, PhD, APRN-BC and Suzanne White, MSN, RN, PHCNS, BC

NANDA-I

Definition

A pattern of exchanging information and ideas with others, which can be strengthened.

Defining Characteristics

Expresses desire to enhance communication

NOC (Nursing Outcomes Classification)

Suggested NOC Outcomes

Communication; Communication: Expressive, Receptive

> **Example NOC Outcome with Indicators**
>
> **Communication** as evidenced by the following indicators: Use of spoken language/Use of written language/Acknowledgment of messages received/Exchanges messages accurately with others. (Rate the outcome and indicators of **Communication:** 1 = severely compromised, 2 = substantially compromised, 3 = moderately compromised, mildly compromised, 5 = not compromised [see Section I].)

Client Outcomes

Client Will (Specify Time Frame)

- Express willingness to enhance communication
- Demonstrate ability to speak or write a language
- Form words, phrases, and language
- Express thoughts and feelings
- Use and interpret nonverbal cues appropriately
- Express satisfaction with ability to share information and ideas with others

● = Independent; ▲ = Collaborative; EBN = Evidence-Based Nursing; EB = Evidence-Based

C

NIC (Nursing Interventions Classification)

Suggested NIC Interventions

Active Listening; Communication Enhancement: Hearing Deficit; Communication Enhancement: Speech Deficit

Example NIC Activities—Communication Enhancement
Hearing Deficit
Listen attentively; Allow patient adequate time to process communication and respond; Verify what was said or written using patient's response before continuing

Nursing Interventions and *Rationales*

- Establish a therapeutic nurse–client relationship: provide appropriate education for the client, demonstrate caring by being present to the client. **CEB:** *Clients who were nonvocal and ventilated appreciated nursing care that was delivered in an individualized, caring manner (Carroll, 2007).*
- Assess the client's readiness to communicate, using an individualized creative approach, and avoid making assumptions regarding the client's preferred communication method. **EB:** *Creative methodologies such as life history projects, photography, drawing, music, and poetry enhanced communication in those with learning disabilities (Kennedy & Brewer, 2014).*
- Assess the client's literacy level so information can be tailored accordingly. *The Rapid Estimate of Adult Literacy in Medicine–Short Form (REALM-SF) provides a quick valid assessment (Agency for Healthcare Research and Quality, 2014).*
- Use these practical guidelines to assist in communication: Listen attentively and provide a comfortable environment for communicating; slow down and listen to the client's story; use augmentative and alternative communication methods (e.g., lip reading, communication boards, writing, body language, computer/electronic communication devices) as appropriate; repeat instructions if necessary; limit the amount of information given; have the client "teach back" to confirm understanding; avoid asking, "Do you understand?"; and be respectful, caring, and sensitive. **CEB:** *Multiple augmentative and alternative communication methods, applied with an individualized and creative approach, aided in facilitating communication (Radtke et al, 2011).*
- ▲ Use interdisciplinary collaboration to ensure continuity of enhanced communication. **EB:** *Effective interdisciplinary collaboration and follow-up was recommended when working with clients with significant communication impairments after having a stroke (Jones et al, 2013).*
- ▲ Refer couples in maladjusted relationships for psychosocial intervention and social support to strengthen communication; consider nurse specialists. **EB:** *Emotionally focused therapy for couples is an effective evidence-based treatment (Wiebe & Johnson, 2016).*
- Consider using music to enhance communication between a client who is dying and his or her family. **CEB:** *In clients with communication difficulties, music therapy resulted in improvement in communication (Leow et al, 2010).*
- Use social media as a means to facilitate communication. **EB:** *Individuals who use augmentative and alternative communication methods may benefit from integration of social media to further enhance communication (Caron, 2016).*
- Teach clients mindfulness meditation. **EB:** *Mindfulness meditation enhanced language production in clients with aphasia (Dickinson et al, 2017).*
- Use photographs as a communication aid. **EB:** *Use of photographs during conversation resulted in people with aphasia talking more about the topic and staying on that topic (Ulmer, 2017).*
- Encourage clients with aphasia to sing. **EB:** *Participation in a community choir led by a neurologic music therapist resulted in qualitatively identified improvement/changes in communication among clients with aphasia (Tamplin et al, 2013).*
- See care plan for Impaired verbal **Communication.**

 Pediatric

- All individuals involved in the care and everyday life of children with learning difficulties need to have a collaborative approach to communication. **EBN:** *Collaboration in tasks requires the formation of personal relationships based on mutual trust and respect (Callery & Milnes, 2012).*
- See care plan for Impaired verbal **Communication.**

● = Independent; ▲ = Collaborative; **EBN** = Evidence-Based Nursing; **EB** = Evidence-Based

C

 Geriatric

▲ Assess for hearing and vision impairments, and make appropriate referrals for hearing aids. EB: *Healthy People 2020 recommended early identification of people with hearing and vision loss (Healthy People 2020, 2014).*

● Use touch if culturally acceptable when communicating with older clients and their families. CEBN: *Touch has a calming effect on a client who may be frightened because of difficulty with communication (Grossbach et al, 2011).*

● Encourage group singing activities and music therapy interventions in clients with dementia. EB: *"Singing for the Brain" is a group singing activity developed by the Alzheimer's Society and the program resulted in increased social inclusiveness and improvements in relationships (Osman et al, 2016).* EB: *Music therapy with a client with dementia facilitated engagement in communication (Mette Ridder & Gummesen, 2015).*

● Encourage drawing by caregivers of clients with dementia. EBN: *Drawing by caregivers of clients with dementia enhanced the communication experience (McEvoy & Bellass, 2017).*

● See care plan for Impaired verbal **Communication.**

 Multicultural

● See care plan for Impaired verbal **Communication.**

 Home Care

● The interventions described previously may be used in home care.

● See care plan for Impaired verbal **Communication.**

 Client/Family Teaching and Discharge Planning

● See care plan for Impaired verbal **Communication.**

REFERENCES

See impaired verbal **Communication** for additional references.

Agency for Healthcare Research and Quality (AHRQ). (2014). *Health literacy measurement tools.* Retrieved from http://www.ahrq.gov/professionals/quality-patient-safety/quality-resources/tools/literacy/index.html. (Accessed 10 September 2014).

Callery, P., & Milnes, L. (2012). Communication between nurses, children and their parents in asthma review consultations. *Journal of Clinical Nursing, 21*(11/12), 1641–1650.

Carroll, S. M. (2007). Silent, slow lifeworld: The communication experiences of nonvocal ventilated patients. *Qualitative Health Research, 17*(9), 1165–1177.

Caron, J. (2016). Engagement in social media environments for individuals who use augmentative and alternative communication. *Neurorehabilitation, 39*(2016), 499–506.

Dickinson, J., Friary, P., & McCann, C. M. (2017). The influence of mindfulness meditation on communication and anxiety. *Aphasiology, 21*(9), 1044–1058.

Grossbach, I., Stranberg, S., & Chlan, L. (2011). Promoting effective communication for patients receiving mechanical ventilation. *Critical Care Nurse, 31*(3), 46–61.

Healthy People 2020. *Hearing and other sensory or communication disorders.* Retrieved from www.healthypeople.gov/2020/topicsobjectives2020/overviewaspx?topicid=20. (Accessed 12 September 2014).

Jones, C., et al. (2013). Alleviating psychosocial issues for individuals with communication impairments and their families following stroke: A case series of interdisciplinary assessment and intervention. *Neurorehabilitation, 32*(2), 351–358.

Kennedy, L., & Brewer, G. (2014). Creative methodologies to enhance communication. *British Journal of Learning Disabilities, 44*(1), 35–42.

Leow, M., Drury, V., & Hong, P. (2010). The experience and expectations of terminally ill patients receiving music therapy in the palliative setting: A systematic review. *JBI Library of Systematic Reviews, 8*(27), 1088–1111.

Mette Ridder, H., & Gummesen, E. (2015). The use of extemporizing in music therapy to facilitate communication in a person with dementia: An explorative case study. *Australian Journal of Music Therapy, 26*, 6–29.

Osman, S. E., Tischler, V., & Schneider, J. (2016). 'Singing for the Brain': A qualitative study exploring the health and well-being benefits of singing for people with dementia and their carers. *Dementia (Basel, Switzerland), 15*(6), 1326–1339.

McEvoy, P., & Bellass, S. (2017). Using drawings as a reflective tool to enhance communication in dementia care. *Nursing Standard, 31*(19), 46–52.

Radtke, J. V., et al. (2011). Listening to the voiceless patient: Case reports in assisted communication in the intensive care unit. *Journal of Palliative Medicine, 14*(6), 791–795.

Tamplin, J., et al. (2013). 'Stroke a chord': The effect of singing in a community choir on mood and social engagement for people living with aphasia following a stroke. *Neurorehabilitation, 32*(4), 929–941.

Ulmer, E. (2017). Using self-captured photographs to support the expressive communication of people with aphasia. *Aphasiology, 31*(10), 1183–1204.

Wiebe, S. A., & Johnson, S. M. (2016). A review of the research in emotionally focused therapy for couples. *Family Process, 55*(3), 390–407.

● = Independent; ▲ = Collaborative; EBN = Evidence-Based Nursing; EB = Evidence-Based

Impaired verbal Communication
Stacey M. Carroll, PhD, APRN-BC and Suzanne White, MSN, RN, PHCNS, BC

C

NANDA-I

Definition

Decreased, delayed, or absent ability to receive, process, transmit, and/or use a system of symbols.

Defining Characteristics

Absence of eye contact; difficulty comprehending communication; difficulty expressing thoughts verbally; difficulty forming sentences; difficulty forming; difficulty in selective attending; difficulty in use of body expressions; difficulty in use of facial expressions; difficulty maintaining communication; difficulty speaking; difficulty verbalizing; disoriented to person; disoriented to place; disoriented to time; dyspnea; inability to speak; inability to speak language of caregiver; inability to use body expressions; inability to use facial expressions; inappropriate verbalization; partial visual deficit; slurred speech; stuttering; total visual deficit

Related Factors

Alteration in self-concept; cultural incongruence; emotional disturbance; environmental barrier; insufficient information; insufficient stimuli; low self-esteem; vulnerability

At-Risk Population

Absence of significant other

Associated Condition

Alteration in development; alteration in perception; central nervous system impairment; oropharyngeal defect; physical barrier; physiological condition; psychotic disorder; treatment regimen

NOC   (Nursing Outcomes Classification)

Suggested NOC Outcomes

Communication; Communication: Expressive, Receptive

Example NOC Outcome with Indicators

Communication as evidenced by the following indicators: Use of spoken and written language/Acknowledgment of messages received/Exchanges messages accurately with others. (Rate the outcome and indicators of **Communication:** 1 = severely compromised, 2 = substantially compromised, 3 = moderately compromised, 4 = mildly compromised, 5 = not compromised [see Section I].)

Client Outcomes

Client Will (Specify Time Frame)

- Use effective communication techniques
- Use alternative methods of communication effectively
- Demonstrate congruency of verbal and nonverbal behavior
- Demonstrate understanding even if not able to speak
- Express desire for social interactions

NIC   (Nursing Interventions Classification)

Suggested NIC Interventions

Active Listening; Communication Enhancement: Hearing Deficit; Communication Enhancement: Speech Deficit; Presence; Touch

---

● = Independent;   ▲ = Collaborative;   EBN = Evidence-Based Nursing;   EB = Evidence-Based

Example NIC Activities—Communication Enhancement

Hearing Deficit

Listen attentively; Allow client adequate time to process communication and respond; Verify what was said or written using client's response before continuing

C

Nursing Interventions and *Rationales*

- Use a comprehensive nursing assessment to determine the language spoken, cultural considerations, literacy level, cognitive level, and use of glasses and/or hearing aids. EBN: *Language barriers, low literacy, and lack of understanding are barriers to effective communication (Taylor et al, 2013).*
- Determine client's own perception of communication difficulties and potential solutions when possible. CEB: *The Communication Confidence Rating Scale for Aphasia (CCRSA) was found to be an effective tool for assessment of the self-report of communication confidence among clients with aphasia (Babbitt et al, 2011).*
- Involve a familiar person when attempting to communicate with a client who has difficulty with communication, if accepted by the client. EB: *Training communication partners of clients with traumatic brain injury improved the communication experience of the client and family member (Togher et al, 2016).* EB: *Retaining valued relationships facilitated communication in people with dementia (Alsawy et al, 2017).*
- Listen carefully. Validate verbal and nonverbal expressions particularly when dealing with pain and use appropriate scales for pain when appropriate. EBN: *The Critical Care Pain Observation Tool and the Behavioral Pain Scale are valid and reliable options for use in clients who are nonverbal (Makic, 2013).* EB: *The Revised Nonverbal Pain Scale and the Original Nonverbal Pain Scale both demonstrated reliability and validity for assessing pain in clients who are nonverbal and ventilated (Chookalayi et al, 2017).*
- Use appropriate scales to assess communication and behavior in clients who are nonvocal and mechanically ventilated. EBN: *Preliminary research shows that the revised Communication Interaction Behavior Instrument scale has good face validity and shows good interrater reliability for use with older adults who are ventilated and nonvocal (Nilsen et al, 2014).*
- Use therapeutic communication techniques: speak in a well-modulated voice, use simple communication, maintain eye contact at the client's level, get the client's attention before speaking, and show concern for the client. EBN: *Effective communication entails involving clients, being sensitive to client needs, and ensuring client understanding (O'Hagan et al, 2014).*
- Avoid ignoring the client with verbal impairment; be engaged and provide meaningful responses to client concerns. Place call light within reach of client who cannot verbally call for help. EBN: *Ignoring clients was found to be a negative communication strategy (O'Hagan et al, 2014).*
- Validate clients' feelings, focus on their strengths, and assist them in gaining confidence in identifying needs. EBN: *Viewing patients with communicative difficulties in a holistic manner cultivates empowering communication (Parsloe & Carroll, 2018)*
- Use touch as appropriate. EBN: *Gentle touch is a therapeutic communication strategy for clients, such as those with dementia who may be frightened because of difficulty with communication (Veselinova, 2014).*
- Use presence: spend time with the client and allow time for responses. *Client-centered care involves respect, communication, and comfort (Bechtold & Fredericks, 2014).*
- Explain all health care procedures, be persistent in deciphering what the client is saying, and do not pretend to understand when the message is unclear. CEBN: *Persons who were nonvocal and ventilated appreciated persistence on the nurses' part with respect to being understood, found it bothersome when others pretended to understand them, and appreciated explanations from the nurse (Carroll, 2007).*
- Use an individualized and creative multidisciplinary approach to augmentative and alternative communication (AAC) assistance and other communication interventions. *Ensure the choice of AAC is driven by client' communication needs rather than by the device (Light & McNaughton, 2013).* EB: *AAC improved communication among those with intellectual disabilities (Hagan & Thompson, 2014).* EB: *A specialized communication intervention resulted in improved communication between nurses and intensive care unit (ICU) clients who were nonvocal (Happ et al, 2014).*
- Use consistent nursing staff for those with communication impairments. CEBN: *Consistent nursing care increased client–nurse communication and decreased client powerlessness (Carroll, 2007).* EB: *Among linguistically and culturally diverse clients with dementia, other communication methods (body language, etc.) along*

• = Independent;   ▲ = Collaborative;   EBN = Evidence-Based Nursing;   EB = Evidence-Based

C

with spoken language can develop over time, indicating the importance of the continuity of providers (Strandroos & Antelius, 2017).

▲ Consult communication specialists from various disciplines as appropriate. Speech language pathologists, audiologists, and interpreters provide comprehensive communication assistance for those with impaired communication. *Lip reading translators (LRTs) are proficient lip readers who determine what a nonvocal client is mouthing and then verbalize the client's words verbatim to others to facilitate communication (Carroll, 2003).* **CEB:** *Lip reading translators can assist in meeting nonvocal clients' communication needs (Meltzer et al, 2012).*

▲ When the client is having difficulty communicating, assess and refer for audiology consultation for hearing loss. Suspect hearing loss when:
  ○ Client frequently complains that people mumble, claims that others' speech is not clear, or client hears only parts of conversations.
  ○ Client often asks people to repeat what they said.
  ○ Client's friends or relatives state that the client does not seem to hear very well, or plays the television or radio too loudly.
  ○ Client does not laugh at jokes because of missing too much of the story.
  ○ Client needs to ask others about the details of a meeting that the client attended.
  ○ Client cannot hear the doorbell or the telephone.
  ○ Client finds it easier to understand others when facing them, especially in a noisy environment.

● People with hearing loss do not hear sounds clearly. The loss may range from hearing speech sounds faintly or in a distorted way to profound deafness (American Academy of Audiology, 2017).

● When communicating with a client with a hearing loss:
  ○ Obtain client's attention before speaking and face toward his or her unaffected side or better ear while allowing client to see the speaker's face at a reasonably close distance, use gestures as appropriate to aid in communication, do not raise voice or over enunciate, and minimize extraneous noise. *Correct positioning and an optimal listening environment increase the client's awareness of the interaction and enhance the client's ability to communicate (University of California San Francisco, 2017).*
  ○ Provide sufficient light and do not stand in front of a window. *Light illuminates the speaker's face, making expressions and lip movements clearer; standing in front of a window causes glare, which impedes the client's ability to clearly see the speaker (University of California San Francisco, 2017).*
  ○ Remove masks if safe to do so, or use see-through masks. *Removing the mask barrier allows for visibility of the mouth which enhances communication. For information on see-through masks, see* www.amphl .org.
  ○ Avoid making assumptions about the communication choice of those with hearing loss or voice impairments. **CEBN:** *After seeking client input, communication rounds or communication care plans can be completed (Happ et al, 2010).*

 Pediatric

● Observe behavioral communication cues in infants. **EB:** *Reissland et al (2012) studied mothers and infants (N = 50) and found that preverbal infants express pain by crying and with facial and body behaviors, which have to be interpreted by the caregiver.*

● Identify and define at least two new forms of socially acceptable communication alternatives that may be used by children with significant disabilities. **EB:** *Pasco and Tohill (2011) conducted a study of nonverbal children with autism spectrum disorder (N = 23) and found that the Picture Exchange Communication System (PECS) may provide valuable predictive information regarding social communication skills.* **EB:** *Brady et al (2013) investigated a model of language development for nonverbal school-aged children (N = 93) and found the importance of enriching social communication input across home and school environments, as well as assessments of and interventions aimed at improving comprehension, play, visual discrimination, and communication complexity.*

● Teach children with severe disabilities functional communication skills. **EB:** *Allen and Marshall (2011) conducted a study involving parent–child interaction therapy (PCIT) (N = 16) for school-aged children with specific language impairment and found that PCIT offered a single block of therapy in which the parents' communication and interaction skills are developed to provide the child with an appropriate language-rich environment.*

▲ Refer children with primary speech and language delay/disorder for speech and language therapy interventions. **EB:** *Pasco and Tohill (2011) conducted a study of nonverbal children with autism spectrum disorder*

● = Independent;   ▲ = Collaborative;   **EBN** = Evidence-Based Nursing;   **EB** = Evidence-Based

(N = 23) and found the assessment of the developmental level of potential PECS users may provide valuable predictive information for speech-and-language therapists and other professionals in relation to the likely degree of progress and in setting realistic and achievable targets.

Geriatric

- Carefully assess all clients for hearing difficulty using an audiometer. Healthy People 2020 encouraged early identification of people with hearing loss (Healthy People 2020, 2014).
- Avoid use of "elderspeak," which is a speech style similar to baby talk. **EB:** *A brief communication training intervention resulted in lower use of elderspeak by staff and less resistiveness to care among clients with dementia (Williams et al, 2017b).*
- Initiate communication with the client with dementia, and give client time to respond. Use eye contact, gentle touch as appropriate, and shorter sentences. *The responsibility to use a creative approach and take the time to listen and understand clients who have dementia lies with the clinician (Veselinova, 2014).* **EBN:** *The Verbal and Nonverbal Interaction Scale is valid and reliable and can assess sociable and unsociable communication in clients with dementia (Williams et al, 2017a).*
- Encourage the client to wear hearing aids, if appropriate. **EBN:** *Hearing aids assist with communication and hearing aid storage boxes can prevent loss or damage (Holmes, 2014).*
- Facilitate communication through reminiscing with memory boxes that contain objects, photographs, and writings that have meaning for the client. *Reminiscence stimulates memories, thus improving communication (Swann, 2013).* **EB:** *Memory boxes encouraged reminiscence in clients with dementia, facilitating communication (Gulwadi, 2013).*
- Continue to find means to communicate even with those who are completely nonverbal. **EB:** *Spontaneous reciprocal interaction promoted family harmony among nonvocal clients with severe dementia (Walmsley & McCormack, 2014).*

Multicultural

- Attend to the meaning of a culture's nonverbal communication modes, such as eye contact, facial expression, touching, and body language. **EB:** *Attending to nonverbal interactions facilitated communication among culturally and linguistically diverse clients with dementia (Strandroos & Antelius, 2017).*
- Assess for the influence of cultural beliefs, norms, and values on the client's communication process. **EBN:** *Misunderstandings and conflicts can arise when there is a difference in language and/or culture of the provider and client (Crawford et al, 2017).*
- Assess personal space needs, acceptable communication styles, acceptable body language, interpretation of eye contact, perception of touch, and use of paraverbal modes when communicating with the client. **EB:** *When caring for clients of varied ethnicities and languages, nurses used nonverbal means such as pointing, smiling, modeling, and touch to convey information and calm clients in long-term care (Small et al, 2015).*
- Assess how language barriers contribute to health disparities among ethnic and racial minorities. **EBN:** *Language barriers were the main obstacle in eliciting an accurate medical history, explaining and gaining pain scores, communicating reasons for client transport delays, arranging appointments by telephone, explaining medication and side effects, or diagnosing and communicating problems (Taylor et al, 2013).* **EBN:** *Patient safety was compromised when language barriers were present (van Rosse et al, 2016).*
- Although touch is generally beneficial, it is culturally defined and there may be times when it may not be advisable because of cultural considerations. **EB:** *Touch conveys various meanings depending on the client's culture and the situation (Albardiaz, 2014).*
- The Office of Minority Health of the US Department of Health and Human Services national standards on culturally and linguistically appropriate services (CLAS) in health care should be used as needed. **EB:** *These standards aim to improve health care quality and advance health equity by establishing a framework for organizations to serve the nation's increasingly diverse communities (CLAS, 2014).*

Home Care

The interventions described previously may be adapted for home care use.

Client/Family Teaching and Discharge Planning

- ▲ Refer the client to a speech-language pathologist (SLP) or audiologist. Audiological assessment quantifies and qualifies hearing in terms of the degree of hearing loss, the type of hearing loss, and the configuration of the hearing loss. Once a particular hearing loss has been identified, a treatment and management plan

---

● = Independent; ▲ = Collaborative; **EBN** = Evidence-Based Nursing; **EB** = Evidence-Based

C

can be put into place by an SLP. *Audiological services can improve communication in clients with dementia and hearing loss (Mamo et al, 2017). SLPs can provide strategies for communication partners of adults with communication impairments (Ball & Lasker, 2013).*

▲ Teach the client and family techniques to increase communication, including the use of communication devices and tactile touch. Incorporate multidisciplinary recommendations. CEBN: *The nurse plays a critical role in individualized communication assessment as clients transition from hospital to home (Cerantola & Happ, 2012).* CEB: *Clients who are mechanically ventilated at home have a long struggle to find effective communication methods (Laasko et al, 2011).*

REFERENCES

Albardiaz, R. (2014). Teaching non-verbal communication skills: an update on touch. *Education for Primary Care, 25,* 164–170.

Allen, J., & Marshall, C. R. (2011). Parent-Child Interaction Therapy (PCIT) in school-aged children with specific language impairment. *International Journal of Language & Communication Disorders, 46*(4), 397–410.

Alsawy, S., et al. (2017). What is good communication for people living with dementia? A mixed methods systematic review. *International Psychogeriatrics, 29*(11), 1785–1800.

American Academy of Audiology. (2017). *Facts about hearing loss.* Retrieved from https://www.audiology.org/publications-resources/consumer-information/fact-sheets. (Accessed 31 October 2017).

Babbitt, E. M., et al. (2011). Psychometric properties of the Communication Confidence Rating Scale for Aphasia (CCRSA): Phase 2. *Aphasiology, 25*(6/7), 727–735.

Ball, L. J., & Lasker, J. (2013). Teaching partners to support communication for adults with acquired communication impairment. *Perspectives on Augmentative and Alternative Communication, 22*(1), 4–15.

Bechtold, A., & Fredericks, S. (2014). Key concepts in patient-centered care. *American Nurse Today, 9*(7), 35–36.

Brady, N. C., Thiemann-Bourque, K., Fleming, K., et al. (2013). Predicting language outcomes for children learning augmentative and alternative communication: Child and environmental factors. *Journal of Speech, Language, & Hearing Research, 56*(5), 1595–1612.

Carroll, S. M. (2003). Lip-reading translating for non-vocal ventilated patients. *JAMPHL Online, 1*(2). Retrieved from www.amphl.org. (Accessed 26 November 2006).

Carroll, S. M. (2007). Silent, slow lifeworld: The communication experiences of nonvocal ventilated patients. *Qualitative Health Research, 17*(9), 1165–1177.

Cerantola, C., & Happ, M. B. (2012). Transitional care for communication impaired older adults: ICU to home. *Geriatric Nursing, 33*(6), 489–492.

Chookalayi, H., et al. (2017). A study on the psychometric properties of Revised-Nonverbal Pain Scale and Original-Nonverbal Pain Scale in Iranian nonverbal-ventilated patients. *Indian Journal of Critical Care Medicine, 21*(7), 429–435.

CLAS (Culturally and Linguistically Appropriate Services). Retrieved from http://minorityhealth.hhs.gov/omh/browse.aspx?lvl=2&lvlid=53. (Accessed 25 October 2014).

Crawford, T., Candlin, S., & Roger, P. (2017). New perspectives on understanding cultural diversity in nurse-patient communication. *Collegian (Royal College of Nursing, Australia), 24*(1), 63–69.

Gulwadi, G. B. (2013). Establishing continuity of self-memory boxes in dementia facilities for older adults: Their use and usefulness. *Journal of Housing for the Elderly, 27,* 105–119.

Hagan, L., & Thompson, H. (2014). It's good to talk: Developing the communication skills of an adult with intellectual disability through augmentative and alternative communication. *British Journal of Learning Disabilities, 42*(1), 66–73.

Happ, M. B., et al. (2014). Effect of a multi-level intervention on nurse-patient communication in the intensive care unit: Results of the SPEACS trial. *Heart and Lung: The Journal of Critical Care, 43,* 89–98.

Happ, M. B., et al. (2010). SPEACS-2: Intensive care unit "communication rounds" with speech language pathology. *Geriatric Nursing, 31*(3), 170–177.

Healthy People 2020. *Hearing and other sensory or communication disorders.* Retrieved from www.healthypeople.gov/2020/topicsobjectives2020/overviewaspx?topicid=20. (Accessed 12 September 2014).

Holmes, E. (2014). How to address the communication needs of older patients with hearing loss. *Nursing Older People, 26*(6), 27–30.

Laasko, K., et al. (2011). Communication experience of individuals treated with home ventilation. *International Journal of Language and Communication Disorders, 46*(6), 686–699.

Light, J., & McNaughton, D. (2013). Putting people first: Re-thinking the role of technology in augmentative and alternative communication intervention. *Augmentative and Alternative Communication, 29*(4), 299–309.

Makic, M. B. F. (2013). Pain management in the nonverbal critically ill patient. *Journal of Perianesthesia Nursing, 28*(2), 98–101.

Mamo, S. K., Oh, E., & Lin, F. R. (2017). Enhancing communication in adults with dementia and age-related hearing loss. *Seminars in Hearing, 38*(2), 177–183.

Meltzer, E. C., et al. (2012). Lip-reading and the ventilated patient. *Critical Care Medicine, 40*(5), 1529–1531.

Nilsen, M. L., et al. (2014). Adaptation of a communication interaction behavior instrument for use in mechanically ventilated, nonvocal older adults. *Nursing Research, 63*(1), 3–13.

O'Hagan, S., et al. (2014). What counts as effective communication in nursing? Evidence from nurse educators' and clinicians' feedback on nurse interactions with simulated patients. *Journal of Advanced Nursing, 70*(6), 1344–1355.

Pasco, G., & Tohill, C. (2011). Predicting progress in Picture Exchange Communication System (PECS) use by children with autism. *International Journal of Language & Communication Disorders, 46*(1), 120–125.

Parsloe, S., & Carroll, S. M. (2018). Accessibility, acceptance, and equity: Examining disability-linked health disparities as nursing and communication scholars. Nursing communication. *Journal of Psychosocial Nursing and Mental Health Services, 56*(5), 50–55.

Reissland, N., Harvey, H., & Mason, J. (2012). Effects of maternal parity, depression and stress on two-month-old infant expression of pain. *Journal of Reproductive & Infant Psychology, 30*(4), 363–376.

Small, J., et al. (2015). Verbal and nonverbal indicators of quality of communication between care staff and residents in ethnoculturally and linguistically diverse long-term care settings. *Journal of Cross-cultural Gerontology, 30,* 285–304.

Strandroos, L., & Antelius, E. (2017). Interaction and common ground in dementia: Communication across linguistic and cultural

● = Independent;   ▲ = Collaborative;   EBN = Evidence-Based Nursing;   EB = Evidence-Based

diversity in a residential dementia care setting. *Health*, 21(5), 538–554.

Swann, J. I. (2013). Dementia and reminiscence: Not just a focus on the past. *Nursing & Residential Care*, 15(12), 790–795.

Taylor, S. P., Nicolle, C., & Maguire, M. (2013). Cross-cultural communication barriers in health care. *Nursing Standard*, 27(31), 35–43.

Togher, L., et al. (2016). The effectiveness of social communication partner training for adults with severe chronic TBI and their families using a measure of perceived communication ability. *Neurorehabilitation*, 38(2016), 243–255.

University of California San Francisco (UCSF). (2017). *Communicating with people with hearing loss*. Retrieved from https://www.ucsfhealth.org/education/communicating_with_people_with_hearing_loss/.

van Rosse, F., et al. (2016). Language barriers and patient safety risks in hospital care: A mixed methods study. *International Journal of Nursing Studies*, 54(2016), 45–53.

Veselinova, C. (2014). Influencing communication and interactions in dementia. *Nursing & Residential Care*, 16(3), 162–166.

Walmsley, B. D., & McCormack, L. (2014). The dance of communication: Retaining family membership despite severe non-speech dementia. *Dementia (Basel, Switzerland)*, 13(5), 626–641.

Williams, C. L., Newman, D., & Hammar, L. M. (2017a). Preliminary psychometric properties of the Verbal and Nonverbal Interaction Scale: An observational measure for communication in persons with dementia. *Issues in Mental Health Nursing*, 38(5), 381–390.

Williams, K. N., et al. (2017b). A communication intervention to reduce resistiveness in dementia care: A cluster randomized control trial. *The Gerontologist*, 57(4), 707–718.

Acute Confusion   *Kimberly S. Meyer, PhD, ACNP-BC, CNRN*

NANDA-I

Definition

Reversible disturbances of consciousness, attention, cognition, and perception that develop over a short period of time, and which last less than 3 months.

Defining Characteristics

Agitation; alteration in cognitive functioning; alteration in level of consciousness; alteration in psychomotor functioning; hallucinations; inability to initiate goal-directed behavior; inability to initiate purposeful behavior; insufficient follow-through with goal-directed behavior; insufficient follow-through with purposeful behavior; misperception; restlessness

Related Factors

Alteration in sleep-wake cycle; dehydration; impaired mobility, inappropriate use of restraints; malnutrition, pain, sensory deprivation; substance misuse; urinary retention

At-Risk Population

Age ≥60 years; history of cerebral vascular accident; male gender

Associated Condition

Alteration in cognitive functioning; delirium; dementia; impaired metabolic functioning; infection; pharmaceutical agent

NOC   (Nursing Outcomes Classification)

Suggested NOC Outcomes

Improved Cognitive Function; Improved Sensory Perception; Improved Thought Processes

Example NOC Outcome with Indicators
Cognition as evidenced by the following indicators: Communication clear for age/Comprehension of the meaning of situations/Attentiveness/Concentration/Cognitive orientation. (Rate the outcome and indicators of **Cognition:** 1 = severely compromised, 2 = substantially compromised, 3 = moderately compromised, 4 = mildly compromised, 5 = not compromised [see Section I].)

● = Independent;   ▲ = Collaborative;   EBN = Evidence-Based Nursing;   EB = Evidence-Based

C

Client Outcomes

Client Will (Specify Time Frame)

- Demonstrate restoration of cognitive status to baseline
- Be oriented to time, place, and person
- Demonstrate appropriate motor behavior
- Maintain functional capacity
- Remain free from injury

NIC (Nursing Interventions Classification)

Suggested NIC Interventions

Delirium Management; Delusion Management

Example NIC Activities—Delirium Management

Inform client of time, place, and person as needed; Provide information slowly and in small doses with frequent rest periods; Ensure client has appropriate assistive sensory devices (e.g., glasses, hearing aids)

Nursing Interventions and *Rationales*

- Recognize that delirium is characterized by an acute onset, a fluctuating course, inattention, and disordered thinking. EBN: *Delirium is often under recognized and can have significant adverse consequences for clients to include increase in length of hospitalization, cognitive deficits, and increased mortality risk. Common conditions that place clients at risk for delirium include advanced age, pain, dehydration, infections, metabolic disturbances, and surgery. It is important for nurses to assess for delirium and implement interventions. (Faught 2014; Davidson et al, 2015).*
- Identify the three distinct types of delirium: hyperactive (easy to recognize), hypoactive (commonly missed), and mixed (the most commonly occurring) (Downing et al, 2013).
  - Hyperactive: delirium characterized by restlessness, agitation, irritability, hypervigilance, hallucinations, and delusions; client may be combative or may attempt to remove tubes, lines.
  - Hypoactive: delirium characterized by decreased motor activity, decreased vocalization, detachment, apathy, lethargy, somnolence, reduced awareness of surroundings, and confusion.
  - Mixed: delirium characterized by the client fluctuating between periods of hyperactivity and agitation and hypoactivity and sedation. EBN: *Delirium is under recognized by both medical and nursing staff, particularly the hypoactive form (Davidson et al, 2015; Faught 2014).*
- Obtain an accurate history and perform a mental status examination that includes the following assessment:
  - History from a reliable source that documents an acute and fluctuating change in cognitive function, attention, and behavior from baseline.
  - Cognition as evidenced by level of consciousness; orientation to time, person, and place; thought process (thinking may be disorganized, distorted, fragmented, slow, or accelerated with delirium; conversation may be irrelevant or rambling); and content (perceptual disturbances such as visual, auditory, or tactile delusions or hallucinations).
  - Level of attention (may be decreased or may fluctuate with delirium; may be unable to focus, shift, or sustain attention; may be easily distracted or may be hypervigilant).
  - Behavior characteristics and level of psychomotor behavior (activity may be increased or decreased and may include restlessness, finger tapping, picking at bedclothes, changing position frequently, spastic movements or tremors, or decreased psychomotor activity such as sluggishness, staring into space, remaining in the same position for prolonged periods).
  - Level of consciousness (may be easily aroused, lethargic, drowsy, difficult to arouse, unarousable, hyperalert, easily startled, and overly sensitive to stimuli).
  - Mood and affect (may be paranoid or fearful with delirium; may have rapid mood swings).
  - Insight and judgment (may be impaired).
  - Memory (recent and immediate memory is impaired with delirium; unable to register new information).
  - Language (may have rapid, rambling, slurred, incoherent speech).

● = Independent;   ▲ = Collaborative;   EBN = Evidence-Based Nursing;   EB = Evidence-Based

C

○ Altered sleep-wake cycle (insomnia, excessive daytime sleepiness).

○ EB: *Establishing the client's baseline mental status by obtaining an accurate history and performing a brief cognitive assessment observing for key diagnostic criteria are important in the diagnosis of delirium (Davidson et al, 2015; Inouye et al, 2014). Encouraging family to be present will facilitate assessment of subtle changes in cognition (Devlin et al, 2018).*

● Assess the client's behavior and cognition systematically and continually throughout the day and night; use a validated tool to assess presence of delirium, such as the Confusion Assessment Method (CAM) or Delirium Observation Screening Scale (DOS). CEB: *The CAM is accurate, brief, and easy to use (Davidson et al, 2015; Grover & Kate, 2012); the DOS was found to be a useful screening tool in a small study of verbally active palliative care clients (Detroyer et al, 2014).*

● Recognize that delirium may be superimposed on dementia; the nurse must be aware of the client's baseline cognitive function. EB: *Dementia increases the risk and severity of delirium, and current research suggests delirium is an independent risk for subsequent dementia (Fong et al, 2015); delirium superimposed on dementia was a strong predictor of decline in function and resultant institutionalization of older adults admitted to a rehabilitation facility (Morandi et al, 2014).*

● Identify predisposing factors that may precede the development of delirium: dementia, cognitive impairment, functional impairment, visual impairment, alcohol misuse, multiple comorbidities, severe illness, history of transient ischemic attack or stroke, depression, history of delirium, and advanced age (older than 65). EB: *Delirium is a multifactorial syndrome most commonly seen in the intensive care unit (ICU), palliative care, and postoperative settings; identification of risk factors is important for prevention (Inouye et al, 2014; Devlin et al, 2018).*

● Surgical procedures increase the risk of delirium post operatively. EB: *Assess the client for risk factors and implement interventions to re-orient patient post operatively. Effectively treat pain and anxiety with the lowest effective dose. Avoid benzodiazepine agents if possible (Leigh et al, 2016; Devlin et al, 2018).*

● Identify precipitating factors that may precede the development of delirium, especially for individuals with predisposing factors: use of restraints, indwelling bladder catheter, metabolic disturbances, polypharmacy, pain, infection, dehydration, blood loss, constipation, electrolyte imbalances, immobility, general anesthesia, mechanical ventilation, hospital admission for fractures or hip surgery, anticholinergic medications, anxiety, sleep deprivation, lack of use of vision and/or hearing aids, and environmental factors. EB: *Awareness of risk factors for development of delirium helps identify clients at risk for developing delirium (Ahmed et al, 2014). EB: Prevention of delirium needs to remain a high priority in light of frequency of occurrence, high treatment costs, longer hospital length of stay, higher rates of functional decline and resultant institutional care, and greater mortality; delirium may persist and lead to long-term cognitive decline (Davidson et al, 2015; Faught, 2014; Fong et al, 2015). EB: Interventions to prevent or lessen the length and severity of delirium may be developed when early identification of delirium risk is instituted (Davidson et al, 2015).*

● Facilitate appropriate extended visitation for clients at risk of delirium. EB: *Extended visitation is associated with decreased incidence of delirium and shorter length of stay (Rosa et al, 2017).*

▲ Assess for and report possible physiological alterations (e.g., sepsis, hypoglycemia, hypoxia, hypotension, infection, changes in temperature, fluid and electrolyte imbalance, use of medications with known cognitive and psychotropic side effects). EB: *Systemic disturbances, including immunological, metabolic, neuroinflammatory, endocrinological, and neurological factors lead to alterations in neurotransmitter synthesis and availability, which leads to delirium (Maldonado, 2013).*

○ Treat the underlying risk factors or the causes of delirium in collaboration with the health care team: establish/maintain normal fluid and electrolyte balance, normal body temperature, normal oxygenation (if the client experiences low oxygen saturation, deliver supplemental oxygen), normal blood glucose levels, and normal blood pressure, and address malnutrition and anemia. EB: *Early recognition of risk factors may help to prevent the negative sequelae of delirium (Fineberg et al, 2013).*

▲ Conduct a medication review and eliminate unnecessary medications; potentially inappropriate medications for older adults at risk for delirium include anticholinergics, benzodiazepines, corticosteroids, H_2 receptor antagonists, sedative hypnotics, and tricyclic antidepressants (American Geriatrics Society, 2015). EB: *A software-based program that identified potential delirium-causing medications and triggered a medication review and monitoring plan by pharmacists led to a decreased incidence of delirium in long-term care (Clegg et al, 2014); polypharmacy is associated with delirium, and a reduction of polypharmacy improves cognition (van der Cammen et al, 2014).*

○ Communicate client status, cognition, and behavioral manifestations to all necessary health care providers.

● = Independent;   ▲ = Collaborative;   EBN = Evidence-Based Nursing;   EB = Evidence-Based

C

○ Monitor for any trends occurring in these manifestations, including laboratory tests. EB: *Careful monitoring of laboratory tests assessing for metabolic abnormalities is important to identify the potential etiological factors for delirium (Davidson et al, 2015; Faught, 2014).*

- Identify, evaluate, and treat pain quickly and adequately (see care plans for Acute **Pain** or Chronic **Pain**). CEB: *Untreated pain is a potential cause of delirium, as is excessive opioid administration (Clegg & Young, 2011).*

- Facilitate sleep hygiene. Establish day/night routines. EB: *Improved sleep is associated with decreased risk of delirium (Patel et al, 2014; Devlin et al, 2018).*

- Promote regulation of bowel and bladder function; use bladder scanning to identify retention, avoid prolonged insertion of urinary catheters, and remove catheters as soon as possible. EB: *Stool impaction may cause urinary retention, which is associated with delirium (Boddaert et al, 2014).* CEB & EBP: *Constipation may precipitate delirium (O'Mahoney et al, 2011); constipation has been found to be an independent risk factor of delirium with clients who are critically ill and mechanically ventilated (Smonig et al, 2016). Urinary catheterization is associated with delirium (Ahmed et al, 2014).*

- Ensure adequate nutritional and fluid intake. EB: *Malnutrition is significantly associated with delirium (Ahmed et al, 2014); attending to correct levels of B vitamins, antioxidants, glucose, water, and lipids may lead to resolution of delirium (Sanford & Flaherty, 2014).*

- Promote early mobilization and rehabilitation in a progressive manner. EB: *Avoiding immobility and promoting early mobilization postoperatively reduces delirium (Butler et al, 2013).* EBN: *Standardized early mobilization protocols promote functional status, prevent complications associated with functional decline, and contribute to greater well-being and/or decreased length of stay for medical-surgical inpatients (Drolet et al, 2013; Pashikanti & Von Ah, 2012).*

- Promote continuity of care; avoid frequent changes in staff and surroundings. EB: *Changes may contribute to feelings of disorientation and confusion (O'Mahoney et al, 2011).*

- Plan care that allows for an appropriate sleep-wake cycle. Refer to the care plan for **Sleep** deprivation. EB: *Interventions to promote sleep were associated with a decreased incidence of delirium (Patel et al, 2014).*

- Facilitate appropriate sensory input by having clients use aids (e.g., glasses, hearing aids, dentures) as needed; check for impacted ear wax. EB: *Delirium can be addressed with nonpharmacological interventions, such as decreasing sensory impairment (Javedan & Tulebaev, 2014) or avoiding sensory overload for clients with agitation.* EB: *A systematic review of interventions to help reduce delirium risk included multicomponent interventions, such as encouraging use of vision and hearing aids, and may assist in the prevention of delirium in individuals who are not cognitively impaired (Trogrlić et al, 2015).*

- Modulate sensory exposure; eliminate excessive noise, use appropriate lighting based on the time of day, and establish a calm environment. EB: *Noise levels in the hospital, often from staff conversation and other avoidable sources, are higher than recommended and lead to significant sleep loss (Makic et al, 2014).*

- Provide cognitive stimulation through conversation about current events, viewpoints, and relationships and encourage reminiscence or word games. EBN: *Daily cognitive stimulation can prevent cognitive decline and promote cognitive recovery (Trogrlić et al, 2015).*

- Allow appropriate visitation.

- Provide reality orientation, including identifying self by name at each encounter with the client, calling the client by their preferred name, and the gentle use of orientation techniques; when reorientation is not effective, use distraction. EB: *Efforts to reorient may agitate some clients; changing the subject may help calm the client (Davidson et al, 2015; Faught 2014; Trogrlić et al, 2015).*

- Provide clocks and calendars, update dry erase white boards each shift, encourage family to visit regularly and to bring familiar objects from home, such as family photos or an afghan, and gently correct misperceptions. EB: *Persons at risk for delirium should be provided clocks and calendars that are easily visible; family and friends may help with reorientation (O'Mahoney et al, 2011).*

- Use gentle, caring communication; provide reassurance of safety; and give simple explanations of procedures.

- Provide supportive nursing care, including meeting basic needs, such as feeding, regular toileting, and ensuring adequate hydration; closely observe behaviors that provide clues as to what might be distressing the client. Delirious clients are unable to care for themselves because of their confusion (Rubin et al, 2011). EB: *Understanding and anticipating behaviors promotes client comfort and safety (Faught 2014).*

▲ Recognize that delirium is frequently treated with antipsychotic medications or sedatives; if there is no other way to keep the client safe, administer these medications cautiously, as ordered, while monitoring for medication side effects. EB: *Reducing unnecessary medications, pain, stress, sleep deprivation, inflammation,*

● = Independent;   ▲ = Collaborative;   EBN = Evidence-Based Nursing;   EB = Evidence-Based

and other neurological insults is crucial because antipsychotics and sedatives may actually prolong the duration of delirium and worsen outcomes (Inouye et al, 2014).

○ For clients nearing the end of life, for whom delirium may be irreversible, focus on relief of symptoms by increasing supervision, reducing invasive lines and devices that restrict movement, keeping the bed in low position, and placing mats on the floor; support of family, caregivers, and the health care team is also of prime importance. EB: *Nonpharmacological means should always be used to ameliorate delirium and may be used in conjunction with medication; delirium is distressing to those caring for the client (Irwin et al, 2013).*

○ Choose the appropriate medication and consider the type and reversibility of the delirium; titrate the medication to control the symptoms and minimize side effects. EB: *Pharmacological means can be rapid, safe, and effective using the lowest effective dose of the appropriate medication based on the type of delirium (Irwin et al, 2013).*

Critical Care

● Recognize admission risk factors for delirium. EB: *ICU clients are at increased risk for delirium because of greater use of sedatives, analgesics, severity of illness, age, infection, multiorgan failure, sleep deprivation, surgery, fracture, restraint use, immobility, tubes, catheters, hypovolemia, polypharmacy, malnutrition, electrolyte imbalance, and stroke (Barr et al, 2013; Devlin et al, 2018).*

● Obtain an accurate history regarding cognitive impairment and mental health, including history of anxiety and depression, alcohol use, medication use, chronic pain, and use of benzodiazepines. EBN: *An accurate history guides appropriate interventions to maximize neurocognitive status of older adults with complex illnesses in the ICU (Tate & Happ, 2011).*

● Assess level of arousal using the Richmond Agitation Sedation Scale; clients receiving a score of −5 to −4 are comatose and unable to be assessed for delirium. EB: *Establishing level of arousal before using the CAM for the ICU (CAM-ICU) decreases the incidence of inappropriate "unable to assess" (UTA) ratings on the CAM-ICU; it was found that noncomatose clients were inappropriately determined to be UTA (Swan, 2014).*

● Assess for pain every 2 to 3 hours or more frequently as needed with a standardized assessment tool, which includes either a numerical rating scale or one with behavioral indicators, such as the Behavioral Pain Scale (BPS) or Critical Care Pain Observation Tool (CPOT). EB: *The self-report is the gold standard for pain assessment (Barr & Pandharipande, 2013); the BPS and CPOT are the most valid and reliable tools to use for adult ICU clients (excluding brain injured) with intact motor function and observable behaviors who are unable to self-report (Barr et al, 2013).* EBN: *Uncontrolled pain is common in the ICU and can contribute to delirium; routine assessment of pain may decrease duration of ventilation and ICU length of stay and increase client satisfaction (Stites, 2013). Clients are less likely to communicate symptoms such as pain when delirious (Tate et al, 2013).*

▲ Incorporate the Awakening and Breathing Coordination, Delirium Monitoring and Management, and Early Mobility (ABCDE) ICU delirium and weakness prevention bundle in conjunction with the interdisciplinary team. EB: *Interdisciplinary communication and daily rounds and staff education facilitate optimal ABCDE bundle implementation (Balas et al, 2013); bundle implementation leads to less delirium, reduced ventilator time, and more time out of bed (Balas et al, 2014).*

○ Assess safety and implementation of a spontaneous awakening trial (SAT) using an established protocol. EB: *Daily interruption of sedation may be beneficial when it results in a reduced total dose of sedative administered; minimizing the depth and duration of sedation is beneficial for reducing delirium (Reade & Finfer, 2014).*

○ Assess safety and implementation of a spontaneous breathing trial (SBT). EBN: *Implementing SAT/SBT protocols reduces the duration and use of mechanical ventilation, which may lead to decreased complications and does not increase self-extubation (Jones et al, 2014).*

○ Assess sedation and agitation level using a valid and reliable tool; titrate sedation to target sedation level. EB: *Sedatives and analgesics prescribed to improve client–ventilator dyssynchrony and treat anxiety and pain may precipitate delirium (Barr et al, 2013; Davidson et al, 2015); for most clients being ventilated in the ICU, a score of 3 to 4 on the Riker or a score of −2 to 0 on the Richmond are appropriate targets (Reade & Finfer, 2014).*

○ Screen for delirium using a reliable and valid monitoring tool once per shift or more often if delirium is present, and recognize that hypoactive delirium is the form most often present in the ICU; communicate and discuss results with the interdisciplinary team. EB: *The CAM-ICU and the Intensive Care*

● = Independent;   ▲ = Collaborative;   EBN = Evidence-Based Nursing;   EB = Evidence-Based

C

Delirium Screening Checklist are the most valid and reliable tools for adult ICU clients (Barr et al, 2013); staff education, discussion of delirium during bedside rounds, and documentation promote successful screening and treatment (Brummel et al, 2013). EBN: *The hypoactive form of delirium is the most common form seen in the ICU and contributes to the under recognition of delirium by clinicians (Tate et al, 2013).*

- ○ Assess safety to begin mobilization; collaborate with physical therapy (PT), occupational therapy (OT), and respiratory therapy (RT) to implement an early mobility plan using a progressive approach. EB: *Early mobilization of stable ICU clients may significantly reduce the length of delirium and length of stay and prevent other complications related to immobility (Hunter et al, 2014).*
- Encourage visits from families and educate families about delirium if it occurs. EB: *Delirium is distressing to clients and families; providing education can alleviate distress (Irwin et al, 2013).* EBN: *Families are most familiar with the client's baseline behavior, so they can assist in the diagnosis of delirium. Just by their presence, family may help to prevent and ameliorate delirium (Keyser et al, 2012; Devlin et al, 2018).*
- Promote uninterrupted sleep by grouping cares at night to avoid sleep interruption, offering eye mask, soft music, and earplugs; optimizing room temperature; by reducing noise and light after 10 p.m.; and by avoiding excessive daytime napping. EB: *Sleep deprivation and delirium in the ICU may be iatrogenic; engaging clients to keep them more awake during the day may ensure better outcomes (Weinhouse, 2014).* EBN: *Multifaceted approaches are required to promote sleep in the ICU to avoid the negative consequences of disrupted sleep (Kamdar et al, 2014; Patel et al, 2014).*

 Geriatric

- The interventions described previously are relevant to the geriatric client.
- Reorient high-risk clients frequently, answer questions, and discuss concerns; use a white board, clock, watch, and calendar, and encourage family members to bring familiar objects from home such as family photos or afghan to assist with orientation. EB: *Environmental factors may be modified to improve outcomes for clients with delirium (McCusker et al, 2013).*
- Provide cognitive stimulation by discussing current events, reading the newspaper, promoting reminiscence, or using games. EB: *Therapeutic activities can minimize cognitive decline (Zaubler et al, 2013).*
- Promote use of glasses, assistive hearing devices, hearing aids, and dentures. CEB: *Sensory impairment is a modifiable risk factor for delirium.*
- Provide feeding assistance as needed. See care plan for Imbalanced **Nutrition:** less than body requirements.
- ▲ Determine whether the client is adequately nourished; watch for protein–calorie malnutrition. Consult with health care provider or dietitian as needed. EB: *Malnutrition is significantly associated with delirium (Ahmed et al, 2014); attending to correct levels of B vitamins, antioxidants, glucose, water, and lipids may lead to resolution of delirium (Sanford & Flaherty, 2014).*
- Promote adequate hydration; keep a glass of water within easy reach of the client and offer fluids frequently. EB: *Keeping a glass of water within reach abated dehydration and delirium in the long-term care population (McCusker et al, 2013).*
- Avoid use of restraints; remove all nonessential equipment such as telemetry, blood pressure cuffs, catheters, and intravenous lines as soon as possible. CEBN: *In a study of long-term care residents with dementia, the use of physical restraints was the factor most associated with delirium; initiate alternative interventions (Voyer et al, 2011).* EB: *A study that implemented care programs incorporating gentle persuasive approaches in dementia care was found to reduce adverse events in the care of clients with dementia to include fewer violent client interactions, reduced restraint and sitter use, and fewer client safety events (e.g., falls) (Gillies et al, 2015).*
- Consider use of music to decrease the development of delirium, especially in surgical patients. EB: *Listening to music has been found to decrease delirium during acute hospitalization of older clients (Abraha et al, 2015; Cheong et al, 2016).* CEB: *Listening to music before and after surgery has been shown to decrease delirium in geriatric patients undergoing elective surgery (McCaffrey & Locsin, 2004).*
- Evaluate all medications for potential to cause or exacerbate delirium; potentially inappropriate medications for older adults at risk for delirium include tricyclic antidepressants, anticholinergics, antipsychotics, benzodiazepines, corticosteroids, H_2 receptor antagonists, and sedative hypnotics. EB: *To enhance client safety, medications used for older adults should be routinely assessed for inappropriateness (Beers list) (American Geriatrics Society, 2015).*
- Assess pain frequently and treat pain with the lowest dose of regularly scheduled medication as well as with nonpharmacological approaches; use client self-report or a validated behavioral pain scale to assess pain accurately. EB: *Uncontrolled pain can lead to delirium (Stites, 2013).*

● = Independent;   ▲ = Collaborative;   EBN = Evidence-Based Nursing;   EB = Evidence-Based

▲ Assess risk for falls and implement fall prevention strategies. **EB:** *Geriatric syndromes are more common in older adults with delirium discharged to postacute care facilities; proactively addressing risk factors may improve outcomes (Anderson et al, 2012).*

● Recognize that delirium may be superimposed on dementia; determine client's baseline cognitive status. **EB:** *Dementia increases the risk and severity of delirium (Fong et al, 2015); delirium superimposed on dementia was a strong predictor of decline in function and resultant institutionalization of older adults admitted to a rehabilitation facility (Morandi et al, 2014).*

▲ Determine whether the client is nourished; watch for protein–calorie malnutrition. Consult with health care provider or dietitian as needed. **EB:** *Malnutrition is significantly associated with delirium (Ahmed et al, 2014); attending to correct levels of B vitamins, antioxidants, glucose, water, and lipids may lead to resolution of delirium (Sanford & Flaherty, 2014).*

● Explain hospital routines and procedures slowly and in simple terms; repeat information as necessary.

● Provide continuity of care when possible, avoid room changes, and encourage frequent visits from family members or significant others. **EB:** *Frequent changes may contribute to confusion (O'Mahoney et al, 2011).*

● Educate family members about delirium assessment and strategies to use to prevent and lessen delirium; use the Family Confusion Assessment Method (FAM-CAM) assessment tool to solicit accurate information from caregivers regarding the presence of delirium. **EBN:** *A small pilot study found that forming a trusting and respectful partnership with family caregivers in delirium prevention impacts family and nurse satisfaction (Rosenbloom & Fick, 2013). The FAM-CAM is a sensitive screening tool to assist in the early diagnosis of delirium in individuals with preexisting dementia (Steis et al, 2012).*

● If clients know that they are not thinking clearly, acknowledge the concern. Fear is frequently experienced by people with delirium. **EB:** *Confusion is frightening; the memory of the delirium can be distressing to clients and families (Partridge et al, 2013).*

Home Care

● The interventions described previously are relevant to home care use. Assess and monitor for acute changes in cognition and behavior. **EB:** *Delirium has an acute onset and fluctuating course, and it is characterized by disordered thinking and a change in behavior (Downing et al, 2013).*

● Recognize that delirium is reversible but can become chronic if untreated in a multidisciplinary fashion; the client may be discharged from the hospital to home care in a state of undiagnosed delirium. **EB:** *Complete recovery may be possible with appropriate multidisciplinary care (Wakefield et al, 2014).*

● Avoid preconceptions about the source of acute confusion; assess each occurrence on the basis of available evidence.

▲ Institute case management of frail elderly clients to support continued independent living if possible once delirium has resolved.

Client/Family Teaching and Discharge Planning

▲ Teach the family to recognize signs of early confusion and seek medical help.

● Counsel the client and family regarding the management of delirium and its sequelae. Increased care requirements at discharge may be needed for clients who have experienced delirium; frailty and delirium can lead to functional decline and institutionalization (Quinlan et al, 2011).

REFERENCES

Abraha, T. F., Rimland, J. M., Cruz-Jenloft, A., et al. (2015). Efficacy of non-pharmacological intervetnions to prevent and treat delirium in older patients: A systematic overview. *PLoS ONE, 6*, e0123090. doi:10.1371/journal.pone.0123090.

Ahmed, S., Leurent, B., & Sampson, E. L. (2014). Risk factors for incident delirium among older people in acute hospital medical units: A systematic review and meta-analysis. *Age and Ageing, 43*(3), 326–333.

American Geriatrics Society. (2015). Updated Beers criteria for potentially inappropriate medication use in older adults. *Journal of the American Geriatrics Society, 63*(11), 2227–2246. doi:10.1111/jgs.13702.

Anderson, C. P., Ngo, L. H., & Marcantonio, E. R. (2012). Complications in postacute care are associated with persistent delirium. *Journal of the American Geriatrics Society, 60*(6), 1122–1127.

Balas, M. C., Burke, W. J., Gannon, D., et al. (2013). Implementing the awakening and breathing coordination, delirium monitoring/management, and early exercise/mobility bundle into everyday care: opportunities, challenges, and lessons learned for implementing the ICU pain, agitation, and delirium guidelines. *Critical Care Medicine, 41*(9 Suppl. 1), S116–S127.

Balas, M. C., Vasilevskis, E. E., Olsen, K. M., et al. (2014). Effectiveness and safety of the awakening and breathing coordination, delirium monitoring/management, and early exercise/mobility bundle. *Critical Care Medicine, 42*(5), 1024–1036.

Barr, J., & Pandharipande, P. P. (2013). The pain, agitation, and delirium care bundle: Synergistic benefits of implementing the

2013 pain, agitation, and delirium guidelines in an integrated and interdisciplinary fashion. *Critical Care Medicine*, 41(9 Suppl. 1), S99–S115.

Barr, J., Fraser, G. L., Puntillo, K., et al. (2013). Clinical practice guidelines for the management of pain, agitation, and delirium in adult patients in the intensive care unit. *Critical Care Medicine*, 41(1), 263–306.

Boddaert, J., Cohen-Bittan, J., Khiami, F., et al. (2014). Postoperative admission to a dedicated geriatric unit decreases mortality in elderly patients with hip fracture. *PLoS ONE*, 9(1), e83795.

Brummel, N. E., Vasilevskis, E. E., Han, J. H., et al. (2013). Implementing delirium screening in the ICU: Secrets to success. *Critical Care Medicine*, 41(9), 2196–2208.

Butler, I., Sinclair, L., & Tipping, B. (2013). Current concepts in the management of delirium. *Continuing Medical Education*, 31(10), 363–366.

Cheong, C. Y., Tan, J. A., Foong, Y. L., et al. (2016). Creative music therapy in an acute care setting for older patients with delirium and dementia. *Dementia and Geriatric Cognitive Disorders Extra*, 6(2), 268–275. doi:10.1159/000445883.

Clegg, A., & Young, J. B. (2011). Which medications to avoid in people at risk of delirium: A systematic review. *Age and Aging*, 40(1), 23–29.

Clegg, A., Siddiqi, N., Heaven, A., et al. (2014). Interventions for preventing delirium in older people in institutional long-term care. *The Cochrane Database of Systematic Reviews*, (1), CD009537.

Davidson, J. E., Winkelman, C., Gelinas, C., et al. (2015). Pain, agitation, and delirium guidelines: Nurses' involvement in development and implementation. *Critical Care Nurse*, 35(3), 17–31.

Devlin, J. W., Skrobik, Y., Gelinas, C., et al. (2018). Clinical practice guidelines for the prevention and management of pain, agitation/sedation, delirium, immobility, and sleep disruption in adult patients in the ICU. *Critical Care Medicine*, 46(9), e825–e873.

Detroyer, E., Clement, P. M., Baeten, N., et al. (2014). Detection of delirium in palliative care patients: A prospective descriptive study of the Delirium Observation Screening Scale administered by bedside nurses. *Palliative Medicine*, 28(1), 79–86.

Downing, L. J., Caprio, T. V., & Lyness, J. M. (2013). Geriatric psychiatry review: Differential diagnosis and treatment of the 3 D's—delirium, dementia, and depression. *Current Psychiatry Reports*, 15(6), 365.

Drolet, A., DeJuilio, P., Harkless, S., et al. (2013). Move to improve: The feasibility of using an early mobility protocol to increase ambulation in the intensive and intermediate care settings. *Physical Therapy*, 93(2), 197–201. doi:10.2522/ptj.20110400.

Faught, D. D. (2014). Delirium: The nurse's role in prevention, diagnosis, and treatment. *Medsurg Nursing*, 23(5), 301–305.

Fong, T. G., Davis, D., Growdon, M. E., et al. (2015). The interface between delirium and dementia in elderly adults. *The Lancet. Neurology*, 14(8), 823–832. doi:10.1016/S1474-4422(15)00101-5. [Epub 2015 Jun 29].

Fineberg, S. J., Nandyala, S. V., Marquez-Lara, A., et al. (2013). Incidence and risk factors for postoperative delirium after lumbar spine surgery. *Spine (Philadelphia, PA 1976)*, 38(20), 1790–1796.

Gillies, L., Coker, E., Montemuro, M., et al. (2015). Sustainability of an innovation to support and respond to persons with behaviors related to dementia and delirium. *The Journal of Nursing Administration*, 45(2), 70–72.

Grover, S., & Kate, N. (2012). Assessment scales for delirium: A review. *World Journal of Psychiatry*, 2(4), 58–70.

Hunter, A., Johnson, L., & Coustasse, A. (2014). Reduction of intensive care unit length of stay: The case of early mobilization. *The Health Care Manager*, 33(2), 128–135.

Inouye, S. K., Westendorp, R. G., & Saczynski, J. S. (2014). Delirium in elderly people. *Lancet*, 383(9920), 911–922.

Irwin, S. A., Pirrello, R. D., Hirst, J. M., et al. (2013). Clarifying delirium management: Practical, evidenced-based, expert recommendations for clinical practice. *Journal of Palliative Medicine*, 16(4), 423–435.

Javedan, H., & Tulebaev, S. (2014). Management of common postoperative complications: Delirium. *Clinics in Geriatric Medicine*, 30(2), 271–278.

Jones, K., Newhouse, R., Johnson, K., et al. (2014). Achieving quality health outcomes through the implementation of a spontaneous awakening and spontaneous breathing trial protocol. *AACN Advanced Critical Care*, 25(1), 33–42.

Kamdar, B. B., Yang, J., King, L. M., et al. (2014). Developing, implementing, and evaluating a multifaceted quality improvement intervention to promote sleep in an ICU. *American Journal of Medical Quality*, 29(6), 546–554.

Keyser, S. E., Buchanan, D., & Edge, D. (2012). Providing delirium education for family caregivers of older adults. *Journal of Gerontological Nursing*, 38(8), 24–31.

Leigh, V., Tufanaru, C., & Elliott, R. (2016). Effectiveness and harms of pharmacological interventions in the treatment of delirium in adults in intensive care units post cardiac surgery: A systematic review protocol. *JBI Database of Systematic Reviews and Implementation Reports*, 16(5), 1117–1125.

Makic, M. B. F., Rauen, C., Watson, R., et al. (2014). Examining the evidence to guide practice: Challenging practice habits. *Critical Care Nurse*, 34(2), 28–45.

Maldonado, J. R. (2013). Neuropathogenesis of delirium: Review of current etiologic theories and common pathways. *The American Journal of Geriatric Psychiatry*, 21(12), 1190–1222.

McCaffrey, R., & Locsin, R. (2004). The effect of music listening on acute confusion and delirium in elders undergoing elective surgery. *Journal of Clinical Nursing*, 13(s2), 91–96.

McCusker, J., Cole, M. G., Voyer, P., et al. (2013). Environmental factors predict the severity of delirium symptoms in long-term care residents with and without delirium. *Journal of the American Geriatrics Society*, 61(4), 502–511.

Morandi, A., Davis, D., Fick, D. M., et al. (2014). Delirium superimposed on dementia strongly predicts worse outcomes in older rehabilitation inpatients. *Journal of the American Medical Directors Association*, 15(5), 349–354.

O'Mahoney, R., Murthy, L., Akunne, A., et al. (2011). Synopsis of the National Institute for Health and Clinical Excellence guideline for prevention of delirium. *Annals of Internal Medicine*, 154(11), 746–751.

Partridge, J. S., Martin, F. C., Harari, D., et al. (2013). The delirium experience: What is the effect on patients, relatives and staff and what can be done to modify this? *International Journal of Geriatric Psychiatry*, 28(8), 804–812.

Pashikanti, L., & Von Ah, D. (2012). Impact of early mobilization protocol on the medical-surgical inpatient population: An integrated review of literature. *Clinical Nurse Specialist*, 26(2), 87–94.

Patel, J., Baldwin, J., Bunting, P., et al. (2014). The effect of a multicomponent multidisciplinary bundle of interventions on sleep and delirium in medical and surgical intensive care patients. *Anaesthesia*, 69(6), 540–549.

Quinlan, N., Marcantonio, E. R., Inouye, S. K., et al. (2011). Vulnerability: The crossroads of frailty and delirium. *Journal of the American Geriatrics Society*, 59(Suppl. 2), S262–S268.

Reade, M. C., & Finfer, S. (2014). Sedation and delirium in the intensive care unit. *New England Journal of Medicine*, 370(5), 444–454.

Rosa, R. G., Tonietto, T. F., daSilva, D. B., et al. (2017). Effectiveness and safety of an extended ICU visitation model for delirium prevention: A before and after study. *Critical Care Medicine*, 45(10), 1660–1667.

● = Independent; ▲ = Collaborative; EBN = Evidence-Based Nursing; EB = Evidence-Based

Rosenbloom, D. A., & Fick, D. M. (2013). Nurse/family caregiver intervention for delirium increases delirium knowledge and improves attitudes toward partnership. *Geriatric Nursing, 35*(3), 175–181.

Rubin, F. H., Neal, K., Fenlon, K., et al. (2011). Sustainability and scalability of the hospital elder life program at a community hospital. *Journal of the American Geriatrics Society, 59*(2), 359–365.

Sanford, A. M., & Flaherty, J. H. (2014). Do nutrients play a role in delirium? *Current Opinion in Clinical Nutrition and Metabolic Care, 17*(1), 45–50.

Smonig, R., Wallenhorst, T., Bouju, P., et al. (2016). Constipation is independently associated with delirium in critically ill ventilated patients. *Intensive Care Medicine, 42*(1), 126–127. doi:10.1007/s00134-015-4050-4. [Epub 2015 Sep 10].

Steis, M. R., Evans, L., Hirschman, K. B., et al. (2012). Screening for delirium using family caregivers: Convergent validity of the Family Confusion Assessment Method and interviewer-rated Confusion Assessment Method. *Journal of the American Geriatrics Society, 60*(11), 2121–2126.

Stites, M. (2013). Observational pain scales in critically ill adults. *Critical Care Nurse, 33*(3), 68–78.

Swan, J. T. (2014). Decreasing inappropriate unable-to-assess ratings for the confusion assessment method for the intensive care unit. *American Journal of Critical Care, 23*(1), 60–69.

Tate, J. A., & Happ, M. B. (2011). Neurocognitive problems in critically ill older adults: The importance of history. *Geriatric Nursing, 32*(4), 285–287.

Tate, J. A., Sereika, S., Divirgilio, D., et al. (2013). Symptom communication during critical illness: The impact of age, delirium, and delirium presentation. *Journal of Gerontological Nursing, 39*(8), 28–38.

Trogrlić, Z., van der Jagt, M., Bakker, J., et al. (2015). A systematic review of implementation strategies for assessment, prevention, and management of ICU delirium and their effect on clinical outcomes. *Critical Care, 19*(1), 157. doi:10.1186/s13054-015-0886-9. Retrieved from https://www.ncbi.nlm.nih.gov/pmc/articles/PMC4428250/. (Accessed 28 November 2017).

van der Cammen, T. J., Rajkumar, C., Onder, G., et al. (2014). Drug cessation in complex older adults: Time for action. *Age and Ageing, 43*(1), 20–25.

Voyer, P., Richard, S., Doucet, L., et al. (2011). Factors associated with delirium severity among older persons with dementia. *Journal of Neuroscience Nursing, 43*(2), 62–69.

Wakefield, D., Thompson, L., & Bruce, S. (2014). A Lilliputian army under the floorboards: Persistent delirium with complete though prolonged recovery. *BMJ Case Reports*, pii: bcr2013202639.

Weinhouse, G. L. (2014). Delirium and sleep disturbances in the intensive care unit: Can we do better? *Current Opinion in Anaesthesiology, 27*(4), 403–408.

Zaubler, T. S., Murphy, K., Rizzuto, L., et al. (2013). Quality improvement and cost savings with multicomponent delirium interventions: Replication of the Hospital Elder Life Program in a community hospital. *Psychosomatics, 54*(3), 219–226.

Chronic Confusion   *Olga F. Jarrín, PhD, RN*

NANDA-I

Definition

Irreversible, progressive, insidious, and long-term alteration of intellect, behavior, and personality, manifested by impairment in cognitive functions (memory, speech, language, decision making, and executive function), and dependency in execution of daily activities.

Defining Characteristics

Adequate alertness to surroundings; alteration in at least one cognitive function other than memory; alteration in behavior; alteration in long-term memory; alteration in personality; alteration in short-term memory; alteration in short term functioning; inability to perform at least one daily activity; insidious and irreversible onset in cognitive impairment; long-term cognitive impairment; progressive impairment in cognitive functioning

Associated Condition

Cerebrovascular accident; dementia

NOC   (Nursing Outcomes Classification)

Suggested NOC Outcomes

Cognition; Cognitive Orientation; Distorted Thought Self-Control

Example NOC Outcome with Indicators
Cognition as evidenced by the following indicators: Cognitive orientation/Communicates clearly for age/Comprehends the meaning of situations/Attentiveness/Concentration. (Rate the outcome and indicators of **Cognition:** 1 = severely compromised, 2 = substantially compromised, 3 = moderately compromised, 4 = mildly compromised, 5 = not compromised [see Section I].)

● = Independent;   ▲ = Collaborative;   EBN = Evidence-Based Nursing;   EB = Evidence-Based

C

Client Outcomes

Client Will (Specify Time Frame)

- Remain content and free from harm
- Function at maximal cognitive level
- Participate in activities of daily living at the maximum of functional ability
- Have minimal episodes of agitation (agitation occurs in up to 70% of clients with dementia)

NIC (Nursing Interventions Classification)

Suggested NIC Interventions

Dementia Management; Environmental Management; Surveillance: Safety; Validation Therapy

Example **NIC** Activities—Dementia Management
Use distraction rather than confrontation to manage behavior; Give one simple direction at a time

Nursing Interventions and *Rationales*

Note: Nursing science has a rich history of conceptualizing behavioral and psychological symptoms of dementia (including agitation and vocalizations) as expressions of unmet pathophysiological and psychological needs related to environmental and caregiver factors (Kolanowski et al, 2017).

- Assess the client for delirium (physiological causes of delirium include acute hypoxia, pain, medication effects, malnutrition, and infections such as urinary tract infection, fatigue, electrolyte disturbances, constipation, and urinary retention). EB: *Delirium superimposed on dementia (presenting as inattention, and impaired arousal or vigilance) is a common clinical syndrome in hospital and institutional settings that often results in poor outcomes (Morandi et al, 2017).*
- Assess for pain using a method appropriate to the level of cognition. EBN: *Pain assessment should include the use of a valid and reliable observer-rated tool such as the Pain Assessment in Advanced Dementia Scale (PAINAD) (Warden et al, 2003) or Rotterdam Elderly Pain Observation Scale (REPOS) (Masman et al, 2018).*
- Assess the client for signs of depression and anxiety (including sadness, irritability, agitation, somatic complaints, tension, loss of concentration, insomnia, poor appetite, apathy, flat affect, and withdrawn behavior) with an instrument appropriate for the cognitive level. EB: *The Cornell Scale for Depression in Dementia (CSDD) and Hamilton Depression Rating Scale (HDRS) have the highest sensitivity for screening patients with dementia (Goodarzi et al, 2017). The Geriatric Anxiety Inventory (GAI), Hospital Anxiety and Depression Scale (HADS-A), and Rating Anxiety in Dementia (RAID) scale are reliable and valid instruments for identifying and measuring anxiety in dementia (Creighton et al, 2018).*
- Assess the for psychological stressors, including changes in the environment, caregiver, or routine; demands to perform beyond capacity; or multiple competing stimuli, including discomfort; and encourage communication by addressing the client in a calm, gentle tone of voice, using appropriate body language, facial expressions, and gestures. EBN: *Agitated behaviors can be an expression of a need that is not being met; needs assessment is facilitated through methods to enhance communication so that needs may be expressed (Kolanowski et al, 2017).*
- Promote person-centered care through supporting, encouraging, educating, and supervising staff and other caregivers. EBN: *Strong evidence supports person-centered approaches; to improve person-centered care nursing managers should target organizational and environmental factors, including a shared philosophy of care, staff use of time, the physical environment, interprofessional support, and support from leaders and colleagues (Jensen & Padilla, 2017; Sjögren et al, 2017).*
- Begin each interaction with the client by gaining and maintaining eye contact, identifying yourself, and calling the client by name. Approach the client with a caring, accepting, and empathetic attitude, and speak calmly and slowly. CEB: *Specific communication skills training for caregivers improves the well-being and quality of life in individuals with dementia and increases positive interactions (Eggenberger et al, 2013).*
- Enhance communication with a calm approach; avoid distractions; show interest; keep communication simple; give clear choices and one-step instructions; give the client time with word finding; use repetition and rephrasing; and use gestures, prompts, and cues or visual aids. CEB: *These communication*

● = Independent; ▲ = Collaborative; EBN = Evidence-Based Nursing; EB = Evidence-Based

C

techniques assist in focusing attention, incorporate nonverbal means of communication, simplify memory demands, compensate for cognitive slowing, and assist with retrieval and comprehension (Eggenberger et al, 2013).

- Facilitate the use of music therapy; identify the client's music preferences and interview family members if necessary. **EB:** *Music therapy is beneficial and improves behavior disorders, anxiety, depression, and agitation in people living with dementia (Abraha et al, 2017; Gómez-Romero et al, 2017).*
- Promote regular, supervised physical activity and exercise. **EB:** *The beneficial effect of physical activity on cognitive function is driven by interventions that include aerobic exercise, are independent of the clinical diagnosis, and the frequency of the intervention (Groot et al, 2016).* **EB:** *Physical exercise for 1 hour, 2 to 3 days a week improves strength, balance, mobility, and endurance in people with cognitive impairment and dementia (Lam et al, 2018).*
- Facilitate the use of doll therapy for patients with advanced dementia and challenging behaviors. **EB:** *Doll therapy is associated with reducing cognitive, behavioral, and emotional symptoms of dementia; improving overall well-being; and the ability to relate with an external environment (Ng et al, 2017).*
- Obtain information about the client's life history, interests, routines, needs, and preferences from the family or significant others; collaborate with family members to engage in reminiscence. **EBN:** *Understanding the individual's past and sharing memories enhances communication and client and staff satisfaction (Scales et al, 2018).*
- Provide opportunities for contact with nature gardens or nature-based stimuli, such as facilitating time spent outdoors or indoor gardening. **EBN:** *Improvements in mood among clients with dementia were associated with exposures to nature of relatively short duration (Scales et al, 2018; White et al, 2017).*
- Provide animal-assisted activities when possible. **EBN:** *Animal-assisted activities and interventions (including use of centrally located aquariums) showed a strong positive effect on social behaviors, physical activity, and dietary intake in dementia patients and a positive effect on agitation/aggression and quality of life (Scales et al, 2018; Yakimicki et al, 2018).*
- Use individual or group reminiscence therapy. **EBN:** *Reminiscence therapy can positively affect quality of life, attitudes towards old age, and symptoms of depression in elderly adults with cognitive impairment (Scales et al, 2018; Siverova & Buzgova, 2018).*
- Use the Environmental Audit Tool to evaluate and optimize living environment (provide unobtrusive safety features, reduce unnecessary stimulation, enhance useful stimulation, provide for wandering, etc.). **EB:** *Higher quality of life for people living with dementia is associated with a living environment that is familiar and that provides opportunities for engagement with objects and activities, privacy, and social contact, along with the amenities and opportunities to take part in domestic activities (Fleming et al, 2016; Jensen & Padilla, 2017).*
- Use lighting to support regulation of sleep-wake patterns and associated behavioral issues. **EBN:** *An ambient lighting intervention designed to increase daytime circadian stimulation can be used to increase sleep efficiency in persons with dementia and their caregivers (Abraha et al, 2017; Figueiro et al, 2015).*
- Engage volunteers and family caregivers in one-on-one activities with the client, such as folding, sorting, or stacking activities; arranging flowers; or other hobbies or routines the individual enjoyed before the onset of dementia. **EB:** *Volunteers may be trained to engage clients in meaningful individualized activities to enhance quality of life (Van der Ploeg et al, 2014).*
- Provide information to the patient/resident/client and family regarding advance directives, palliative and hospice care options, and discuss/document goals of care. **EB:** *Discussion of delicate and important end-of-life issues should be discussed with patients early in the course of their illness, when analytic capacity is less likely to be impaired, and decisions regarding goals of care may more accurately reflect their true personal preferences (Abu Snineh et al, 2017).* **EBN:** *Advantages of advanced care planning with dementia include increased communication and documentation about end-of-life care preferences; increased concordance between care preferences documented and provided; and lower rates of unwanted, burdensome treatments at end-of-life (Kim et al, 2015).*
- For clients with memory impairment concerns, refer to the Impaired **Memory** care plan.
- For clients who wander, refer to the **Wandering** care plan.
- For care of clients with self-care deficits, see the appropriate care plan (Feeding **Self-Care** deficit; Dressing **Self-Care** deficit; Toileting **Self-Care** deficit; Bathing **Self-Care** deficit, etc.).

 Geriatric

Note: All interventions are appropriate for geriatric clients.

● = Independent;   ▲ = Collaborative;   EBN = Evidence-Based Nursing;   EB = Evidence-Based

Multicultural

- Provide culturally and linguistically appropriate care. EB: *Linguistic and cultural isolation may cause or worsen agitation in people living with dementia (Cooper et al, 2018).*
- Assess for the influence of cultural beliefs, norms, and values on the client and the family's understanding of chronic confusion or dementia; assist the family or caregiver in identifying and accessing available social services or other supportive services. EBN: *In a study of six ethnic groups in the United States, all expressed concern and fear about memory loss, losing independence, and becoming "a burden." American Indians, Chinese Americans, Latinos, and Vietnamese Americans expected memory loss. American Indians, Chinese Americans, and Vietnamese Americans were concerned about the stigma associated with Alzheimer's disease. African Americans, Chinese, and whites expressed concern about genetic risks. African Americans and whites expressed concern about behavior changes (Laditka et al, 2011).* EB: *As in many other cultures, in Eastern Mediterranean countries (i.e., Afghanistan, Bahrain, Egypt, Iran, Iraq, Jordan, Kuwait, Lebanon, Morocco, Pakistan, Saudi Arabia, Somalia, Tunisia, United Arab Emirates, Yemen), the older adult is highly respected, and placement outside of the family home is considered an abandonment of family duty. The term dementia carries stigma, and it is widely believed that dementia is caused by "fate" (Yaghmour et al, in press).*

Home Care

Note: Because community-based care is usually less structured than institutional care, in the home setting the goal of maintaining safety for the client takes on primary importance.

- The interventions described previously may be adapted for home care use.
- Assess the home for safety features and client needs for assistive devices. Refer to the care plans for Feeding **Self-Care** deficit; Dressing **Self-Care** deficit; Toileting **Self-Care** deficit; Bathing **Self-Care** deficit, etc., as needed.
- Provide education and support to the family regarding effective communication, home safety, fall prevention, engagement in meaningful activities, ways to manage cognitive and behavioral changes, and comprehensive health care including screening for depression. Be prepared to offer support and information to family members who also live at a distance. EB: *The need for care, services, and support for individuals in the community with dementia and their caregivers is often unmet; evaluation and diagnosis of dementia, personal and home safety, physical and mental health care, advanced care planning, and legal issues are needs that should be addressed (Poirier et al, 2018; Roberts & Struckmeyer, 2018).*
- Provide information about respite care to family caregivers. EB: *Although many caregivers report that they derive significant emotional and spiritual rewards from their caregiving role, many also experience physical and emotional problems directly related to the stress and demands of daily care. Caregiver resilience can be enhanced through the use of respite programs, including day care, overnight respite, support groups, and counseling services (Roberts & Struckmeyer, 2018).*
- Reinforce the use of therapeutic communication guidelines. *Home-based behavioral management techniques, caregiver-based interventions in communication skills, and person-centered care with supervision during implementation were found to be effective for symptomatic and severe agitation (Abraha et al, 2017).*
- Assess family caregivers for caregiver stress, loneliness, and depression. Refer to the care plan for **Caregiver Role Strain.**

Client/Family Teaching and Discharge Planning

- In the client's early stages of dementia, provide the caregiver with information on illness processes, needed care, available services, role changes, and importance of advance directives discussion; facilitate family cohesion. EBN: *Education provided to caregivers early in the disease trajectory may assist them to anticipate care needs and role changes and to facilitate involving the individual with dementia in care decisions (Abu Snineh et al, 2017; Kim et al, 2015).*
- Provide education and support to the family regarding effective communication, home safety, fall prevention, engagement in meaningful activities, ways to manage cognitive and behavioral changes, and comprehensive health care including screening for depression. Be prepared to offer support and information to family members who also live at a distance. EB: *The need for care, services, and support for individuals in the community with dementia and their caregivers is often unmet; evaluation and diagnosis of dementia, personal and home safety, physical and mental health care, advanced care planning, and legal issues are needs that should be addressed (Poirier et al, 2018; Roberts & Struckmeyer, 2018).*

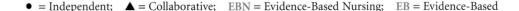

● = Independent;   ▲ = Collaborative;   EBN = Evidence-Based Nursing;   EB = Evidence-Based

REFERENCES

Abraha, I., Rimland, J. M., Trotta, F. M., et al. (2017). Systematic review of systematic reviews of non-pharmacological interventions to treat behavioural disturbances in older patients with dementia. The SENATOR-OnTop series. *BMJ Open*, *7*(3), e012759. doi:10.1136/bmjopen-2016-012759.

Abu Snineh, M., Camicioli, R., & Miyasaki, J. M. (2017). Decisional capacity for advanced care directives in Parkinson's disease with cognitive concerns. *Parkinsonism and Related Disorders*, *39*, 77–79. doi:10.1016/j.parkreldis.2017.03.006.

Cooper, C., Rapaport, P., Robertson, S., et al. (2018). Relationship between speaking English as a second language and agitation in people with dementia living in care homes: Results from the MARQUE (Managing Agitation and Raising Quality of life) English national care home survey. *International Journal of Geriatric Psychiatry*, *33*(3), 504–509. doi:10.1002/gps.4786.

Creighton, A. S., Davison, T. E., & Kissane, D. W. (2018). The psychometric properties, sensitivity and specificity of the geriatric anxiety inventory, hospital anxiety and depression scale, and rating anxiety in dementia scale in aged care residents. *Aging and Mental Health*, 1–10. doi:10.1080/13607863.2018.1439882.

Eggenberger, E., Heimerl, K., & Bennett, M. I. (2013). Communication skills training in dementia care: A systematic review of effectiveness, training content, and didactic methods in different care settings. *International Psychogeriatrics*, *25*(3), 345–358. doi:10.1017/S1041610212001664.

Figueiro, M. G., Hunter, C. M., Higgins, P., et al. (2015). Tailored lighting intervention for persons with dementia and caregivers living at home. *Sleep Health*, *1*(4), 322–330. doi:10.1016/j.sleh.2015.09.003.

Fleming, R., Goodenough, B., Low, L. F., et al. (2016). The relationship between the quality of the built environment and the quality of life of people with dementia in residential care. *Dementia*, *15*(4), 663–680. doi:10.1177/1471301214532460.

Gómez-Romero, M., Jimenez-Palomares, M., Rodriguez-Mansilla, J., et al. (2017). Benefits of music therapy on behaviour disorders in subjects diagnosed with dementia: A systematic review. *Neurologia (Barcelona, Spain)*, *32*(4), 253–263. doi:10.1016/j.nrl.2014.11.001.

Goodarzi, Z. S., Mele, B. S., Roberts, D. J., et al. (2017). Depression case finding in individuals with dementia: A systematic review and meta-analysis. *Journal of the American Geriatrics Society*, *65*(5), 937–948. doi:10.1111/jgs.14713.

Groot, C., Hooghiemstra, A. M., Raijmakers, P. G., et al. (2016). The effect of physical activity on cognitive function in patients with dementia: A meta-analysis of randomized control trials. *Ageing Research Reviews*, *25*, 13–23. doi:10.1016/j.arr.2015.11.005.

Jensen, L., & Padilla, R. (2017). Effectiveness of environment-based interventions that address behavior, perception, and falls in people with Alzheimer's disease and related major neurocognitive disorders: A systematic review. *The American Journal of Occupational Therapy*, *71*(5), 7105180030p7105180031-7105180030p7105180010. doi:10.5014/ajot.2017.027409.

Kim, H., Ersek, M., Bradway, C., et al. (2015). Physician orders for life-sustaining treatment for nursing home residents with dementia. *Journal of the American Association of Nurse Practitioners*, *27*(11), 606–614. doi:10.1002/2327-6924.12258.

Kolanowski, A., Boltz, M., Galik, E., et al. (2017). Determinants of behavioral and psychological symptoms of dementia: A scoping review of the evidence. *Nursing Outlook*, *65*(5), 515–529. doi:10.1016/j.outlook.2017.06.006.

Laditka, J. N., Laditka, S. B., Liu, R. U. I., et al. (2011). Older adults' concerns about cognitive health: Commonalities and differences among six United States ethnic groups. *Ageing and Society*, *31*(07), 1202–1228. doi:10.1017/s0144686x10001273.

Lam, F. M., Huang, M. Z., Liao, L. R., et al. (2018). Physical exercise improves strength, balance, mobility, and endurance in people with cognitive impairment and dementia: A systematic review. *Journal of physiotherapy*, *64*(1), 4–15. doi:10.1016/j.jphys.2017.12.001.

Masman, A. D., van Dijk, M., van Rosmalen, J., et al. (2018). The Rotterdam Elderly Pain Observation Scale (REPOS) is reliable and valid for non-communicative end-of-life patients. *BMC Palliative Care*, *17*(1), 34. doi:10.1186/s12904-018-0280-x.

Morandi, A., Davis, D., Bellelli, G., et al. (2017). The diagnosis of delirium superimposed on dementia: An emerging challenge. *Journal of the American Medical Directors Association*, *18*(1), 12–18. doi:10.1016/j.jamda.2016.07.014.

Ng, Q. X., Ho, C. Y., Koh, S. S., et al. (2017). Doll therapy for dementia sufferers: A systematic review. *Complementary Therapies in Clinical Practice*, *26*, 42–46. doi:10.1016/j.ctcp.2016.11.007.

Poirier, A., Voyer, P., Legare, F., et al. (2018). Caring for seniors living with dementia means caring for their caregivers too. *Canadian Journal of Public Health*, *108*(5–6), 639–642. doi:10.17269/cjph.108.6217.

Roberts, E., & Struckmeyer, K. M. (2018). The impact of respite programming on caregiver resilience in dementia care: A qualitative examination of family caregiver perspectives. *Inquiry: A Journal of Medical Care Organization, Provision and Financing*, *55*, 46958017751507. doi:10.1177/0046958017751507.

Scales, K., Zimmerman, S., & Miller, S. J. (2018). Evidence-based nonpharmacological practices to address behavioral and psychological symptoms of dementia. *The Gerontologist*, *58*(Suppl 1), S88–S102. doi:10.1093/geront/gnx167.

Siverova, J., & Buzgova, R. (2018). The effect of reminiscence therapy on quality of life, attitudes to ageing, and depressive symptoms in institutionalized elderly adults with cognitive impairment: A quasi-experimental study. *International Journal of Mental Health Nursing*, doi:10.1111/inm.12442.

Sjögren, K., Lindkvist, M., Sandman, P. O., et al. (2017). Organisational and environmental characteristics of residential aged care units providing highly person-centred care: A cross sectional study. *BMC Nursing*, *16*, 44. doi:10.1186/s12912-017-0240-4.

Van der Ploeg, E. S., Walker, H., & O'Connor, D. W. (2014). The feasibility of volunteers facilitating personalized activities for nursing home residents with dementia and agitation. *Geriatric Nursing (New York, N.Y.)*, *35*(2), 142–146. doi:10.1016/j.gerinurse.2013.12.003.

Warden, V., Hurley, A. C., & Volicer, L. (2003). Development and psychometric evaluation of the Pain Assessment in Advanced Dementia (PAINAD) scale. *Journal of the American Medical Directors Association*, *4*(1), 9–15. doi:10.1097/01.JAM.0000043422.31640.F7.

White, P. C., Wyatt, J., Chalfont, G., et al. (2017). Exposure to nature gardens has time-dependent associations with mood improvements for people with mid- and late-stage dementia: Innovative practice. *Dementia*, 1471301217723772. doi:10.1177/1471301217723772.

Yaghmour, S. M., Bartlett, R., & Brannelly, T. (In press). Dementia in Eastern Mediterranean countries: A systematic review. *Dementia*. doi:10.1177/1471301217753776.

Yakimicki, M. L., Edwards, N. E., Richards, E., et al. (2018). Animal-assisted intervention and dementia: A systematic review. *Clinical Nursing Research*, *28*(1), 9–29. doi:10.1177/1054773818756987.

C

C

Risk for acute Confusion   Marina Martinez-Kratz, MS, RN, CNE

NANDA-I

Definition

Susceptible to reversible disturbances of consciousness, attention, cognition, and perception that develop over a short period of time, which may compromise health.

Risk Factors

Alteration in sleep-wake cycle; dehydration; impaired mobility; inappropriate use of restraints; malnutrition; pain; sensory deprivation; substance misuse; urinary retention

At-Risk Population

Age ≥60 years; history of cerebral vascular accident; male gender

Associated Condition

Alteration in cognitive functioning; delirium; dementia; impaired metabolic functioning; infection; pharmaceutical agent

NIC, NOC, Client Outcomes, Nursing Interventions and *Rationales,* Client/Family Teaching, and References

Refer to care plan for Acute **Confusion.**

Constipation   Amanda Andrews, BSc (Hons), MA and Bernie St. Aubyn, BSc (Hons), MSc

NANDA-I

Definition

Decrease in normal frequency of defecation accompanied by difficult or incomplete passage of stool and/or passage of excessively hard, dry stool.

Defining Characteristics

Abdominal pain; abdominal tenderness with palpable muscle resistance; abdominal tenderness without palpable muscle resistance; anorexia; atypical presentations in older adults; borborygmi; bright red blood with stool; change in bowel pattern; decrease in stool frequency; decrease in stool volume; distended abdomen; fatigue; hard, formed stool; headache; hyperactive bowel sounds; hypoactive bowl sounds; inability to defecate; increase in intra-abdominal pressure; indigestion; liquid stool; pain with defecation; palpable abdominal mass; palpable rectal mass; percussed abdominal dullness; rectal fullness; rectal pressure; severe flatus; soft, paste-like stool in rectum; straining with defecation; vomiting

Related Factors

Abdominal muscle weakness; average daily physical activity is less than recommended for gender and age; confusion; decrease in gastrointestinal motility; dehydration; depression; eating habit change; emotional disturbance; habitually suppresses urge to defecate; inadequate dietary habits; inadequate oral hygiene; inadequate toileting habits; insufficient fiber intake; insufficient fluid intake; irregular defecation habits; laxative abuse; obesity; recent environmental change

Associated Condition

Electrolyte imbalance; hemorrhoids; Hirschsprung's disease; inadequate dentation; iron salts; neurological impairment; postsurgical bowel obstruction; pregnancy; prostate enlargement; rectal abscess; rectal anal fissure; rectal anal stricture; rectal prolapse; rectal ulcer; rectocele; tumor.

• = Independent;   ▲ = Collaborative;   EBN = Evidence-Based Nursing;   EB = Evidence-Based

NOC (Nursing Outcomes Classification)

Suggested NOC Outcomes

Bowel Elimination; Hydration

> **Example NOC Outcome with Indicators**
>
> **Bowel Elimination** as evidenced by the following indicators: Elimination pattern/Stool soft and formed/Passage of stool without aids/Ease of stool passage. (Rate each indicator of **Bowel Elimination:** 1 = severely compromised, 2 = substantially compromised, 3 = moderately compromised, 4 = mildly compromised, 5 = not compromised [see Section I].)

Client Outcomes

Client Will (Specify Time Frame)

Maintain passage of soft, formed stool every 1 to 3 days without straining; State relief from discomfort of constipation; Identify measures that prevent or treat constipation

NIC (Nursing Interventions Classification)

Suggested NIC Intervention

Constipation/Impaction Management

> **Example NIC Activities—Constipation/Impaction Management**
>
> Identify factors (e.g., medications, bed rest, diet) that may cause or contribute to constipation/impaction; Institute a toileting schedule, as appropriate

Nursing Interventions and *Rationales*

- Introduce yourself to the client and any companions and inform them of your role. Introducing yourself to a client helps establish and develop a therapeutic relationship that recognizes the person within the client and forms the basis for building trust on which to base the provision of care (Howatson-Jones et al, 2012).
- Gain consent to perform care before proceeding further with the assessment. Clients have the right of autonomy both legally and morally and therefore should be fully involved in the decision-making process (Avery, 2013).
- Wash hands using a recognized technique. EB: *Performing strict hand-hygiene regimens significantly reduces the incidence of infection with methicillin-resistant* Staphylococcus aureus *and* Clostridium difficile *infection (Goldberg, 2017).*
- Assess usual pattern of defecation and establish the extent of the constipation problem. EB: *A detailed and accurate assessment of the client enables the nurse to plan interventions, monitor outcomes, and evaluate care, ensuring no unnecessary treatment is rendered (Noiesen et al, 2013).*
- Assess the client's bowel habits:
  - ○ Time of day of bowel evacuation
  - ○ Amount and frequency of stool
  - ○ Consistency of stool (using the Bristol Stool Scale)
  - ○ Bleeding/passing mucus on defecation
  - ○ History of bowel habits and/or laxative use
  Assess usual pattern of defecation, including time of day; amount and frequency of stool; consistency of stool; history of bowel habits or laxative use; and diet, including fiber and fluid intake. A nursing assessment that identifies the client's usual bowel habits will assist in the identification and management of their constipation (Lee, 2015).
- Assess the client's lifestyle factors that may influence constipation:
  - ○ Fiber content in diet
  - ○ Daily fluid intake
  - ○ Exercise patterns
  - ○ Personal remedies for constipation

● = Independent;   ▲ = Collaborative;   EBN = Evidence-Based Nursing;   EB = Evidence-Based

C

❍ Recently stopped smoking
❍ Alcohol consumption/recreational drug use
Assess the client's lifestyle factors that may influence or exacerbate constipation (Lee, 2015).
- Review the client's past medical history:
  ❍ Obstetrical/gynecological/urological history and surgeries
  ❍ Diseases that affect bowel motility
  ❍ Bleeding/passing mucous on defecation
  ❍ Current medications
  Review the client's past medical history for conditions that may contribute to constipation, obstetrical/gynecological history, surgeries, diseases that affect bowel motility, alterations in perianal sensation, and the present bowel regimen. It is imperative to establish a nursing history that identifies the client's bowel habits because this will assist in the identification and management of their constipation (Lee, 2015).
- Assess the client for emotional influences that may be contributing to constipation:
  ❍ Anxiety and depression
  ❍ Long-term defecation issues
  ❍ Stress

Consider emotional influences (e.g., depression and anxiety) on defecation. Emotions influence gastrointestinal function, possibly because control of both emotions and gastrointestinal function is located in the limbic system of the brain. Difficulties with defecation often begin in childhood (e.g., during toilet training), and constipation is also associated with sexual and physical abuse, depression, and anxiety. CEBN: *In a study, clients with functional constipation were compared with normal controls; subjects with functional constipation had significantly higher anxiety and depression scores (Zhou et al, 2010).*
- Complete a physical examination (palpation for abdominal distention, percussion for dullness, and auscultation for bowel sounds). *A physical examination provides positive and negative findings and may provide the diagnosis without the need for further testing. It may also reveal unsuspected findings or confirm normality (Rhoads & Murphy-Jensen, 2014).*
- Encourage the client or family to keep a 7-day diary of bowel habits to include time of day, length of time spent on the toilet, consistency, amount and frequency of stool, and any straining (using the Bristol Stool Scale). EB: *Keeping a diary helps establish a client's bowel pattern and may contribute to the client's adherence to the proposed care plan (Andrews & Morgan, 2013).*
- Encourage the client or family to keep a 7-day diary of lifestyle issues in relation to bowel habits to include fluid consumption, fiber content in diet, usual bowel stimulus, and exercise regimen. EB: *Enabling clients to present their condition in their own words ensures that they feel the health care professionals understand their concerns (Smith, 2012).*
- Use the Bristol Stool Scale to assess stool consistency. *The Bristol Stool Scale is widely used as a more objective measure to describe stool consistency (Tack et al, 2011; DerSarkissian, 2017).*
▲ Review the client's current medications. *A review of current medication should be requested to include recently started medications and any over-the-counter or herbal medications the client is taking. Medications associated with chronic constipation include opioid analgesics, anticholinergics, antipsychotics, antispasmodics, and calcium channel blockers (Joint Formulary Committee, 2016). This baseline information is key to gaining a comprehensive client assessment (Bardsley, 2017).*
- Discuss with clients already taking opioids (temporarily or long term) that constipation is a common side effect. Advise them to contact their health care provider for a prescription of an appropriate laxative. *The thorough and comprehensive assessment of clients on opioids experiencing constipation will also allow for a bowel function approach for laxative prescribing rather than one based on the opioid dose alone (Andrews & Morgan, 2012).*
▲ Recognize that opioids cause constipation. If the client is receiving temporary opioids (e.g., for acute postoperative pain), request an order for routine stool softeners from the primary care provider, monitor bowel movements, and request a laxative for the client if constipation develops. If the client is receiving around-the-clock opiates (e.g., for palliative care), laxatives, then softeners, stimulants, or osmotics should be requested. EB: *Opioids cause constipation because they decrease propulsive movement in the colon and enhance sphincter tone, making it difficult to defecate. Laxatives are the most common first-line management strategy for opioid-induced constipation because they are low cost and high efficacy (Szigethy et al, 2014).*
▲ If the client is terminally ill and is receiving around-the-clock opioids for palliative care, speak with the prescribing health care provider about ordering low-dose naloxone, which is a drug that blocks opioid effects on the gastrointestinal tract without interfering with analgesia *(Sanders et al, 2015).*

● = Independent;   ▲ = Collaborative;   EBN = Evidence-Based Nursing;   EB = Evidence-Based

C

- If new onset of constipation, determine whether the client has recently stopped smoking. CEB/EB: *Constipation is common, but usually transient, when people stop smoking (Wilcox et al, 2010). A recent study surveyed 16,840 individuals between 45 and 75 years of age and found that smoking was associated with abdominal pain, bloating, and constipation (Lundstrome et al, 2016).*
- Palpate for abdominal distention, percuss for dullness, and auscultate bowel sounds. *In clients with constipation the abdomen is often distended and tender, and stool in the colon produces a dull percussion sound; however, bowel sounds will be present.*
- ▲ Check for impaction; if present, then use a combination of oral laxatives and enemas initially to remove fecal loading and impaction (National Institute for Health and Care Excellence, 2015). Clients with neurogenic bowel dysfunction (e.g., spinal cord injury) commonly require manual evacuation of stool (McClurg & Norton, 2016).
- ▲ Advise a fiber intake of 18 to 25 g daily and suggest foodstuffs high in fiber (e.g., prune juice, leafy green vegetables, whole meal bread and pasta). *Fiber creates bulky feces and stretches the bowel wall to stimulate peristalsis, thus shortening bowel transit time (Bardsley, 2017).*
- Add fiber gradually to the diet to decrease bloating and flatus. *Larger stools move through the colon faster than smaller stools, and dietary fiber makes stools bigger because it is undigested in the upper intestinal tract. A study by Lawton et al (2013) looked into whether increasing insoluble fiber improved digestive feelings, well-being, and bowel function. The study found significant improvement in ease of defecation, bloating and digestive discomfort, and the client's perception of general well-being.*
- Provide prunes or prune juice daily. Each 100 g of prunes contains about 6 g of fiber, 15 g of sorbitol, and 184 mg of polyphenol, which all have laxative effects (Attaluri et al, 2011). CEB: *In a randomized study, dried prunes produced significantly more complete spontaneous bowel movements per week than psyllium, and both treatments produced significantly more complete spontaneous bowel movements than at baseline (Attaluri et al, 2011).*
- Advise a fluid intake of 1.5 to 2 L of fluid per day (ideally, 6–8 glasses of water), unless contraindicated by comorbidities, such as kidney or heart disease. *Water passes into the gut to promote the formation of a softer fecal mass and provides lubrication to prevent a blockage of the gut (Boyle, 2013).*
- ▲ If the client is uncomfortable or in pain because of constipation or has acute or chronic constipation that does not respond to increased fiber, fluid, activity, and appropriate toileting, refer the client to the primary care provider for an evaluation of bowel function and health status. *The main aim of referral is to rule out any serious causes of changes in bowel habits, e.g., the presence of tumors, old scarring, and megacolon. The use of red flags (anemia, rectal bleeding, and a family history of bowel cancer or inflammatory bowel disease) are commonly used in general practice to identify the need for further referral (Lee, 2015).*
- Encourage physical activity within the client's current ability to mobilize. Encourage turning and changing position in bed if immobile. For clients with reduced mobility, encourage knee to chest raises, waist twists, and stretching the arms away from the body. For fully mobile clients, encourage walking and swimming. *Physical activity can help stimulate peristaltic waves in the colon and encourage the transit of feces to the rectum (Rogers, 2013).*
- Demonstrate the use of gentle external abdominal massage, using aroma therapy oils, following the direction of colon activity. *Abdominal massage encourages rectal loading by increasing intraabdominal pressure and, in some cases, it may elicit rectal waves, which may stimulate the somatoautonomic reflex and enhance bowel sensation (McClurg et al, 2011).*
- Recommend that clients establish a regular elimination routine. If required assist clients to the bathroom at the same time every day; always be mindful of the need for privacy (closing of bathroom doors). *Establishing a routine allows for the use of the gastrocolic reflex, especially in the morning, which aids defecation (Rogers, 2013).*
- Provide privacy for defecation. If not contraindicated, help the client to the bathroom and close the door. *Bowel elimination is a private act in Western cultures, and a lack of privacy can hinder the defecation urge, thus contributing to constipation.*
- Help clients onto a bedside commode or toilet so they can either squat or lean forward while sitting. Recognize that it is difficult to impossible to defecate in the lying supine position. Sitting upright allows gravity to aid defecation. CEB/EB: *A study of men found that flexing the hip to 90 degrees or more straightens the angle between the anus and the rectum and pulls the anal canal open, decreasing the resistance to the movement of feces from the rectum and the amount of pressure needed to empty the rectum. Hip flexion is greatest when squatting or when leaning forward while sitting (Tagart, 1966; Clark & Currow 2014).*

● = Independent;   ▲ = Collaborative;   EBN = Evidence-Based Nursing;   EB = Evidence-Based

C

- Educate the client about how to adopt the best posture for defecation. Keep knees slightly higher than hips, keep feet flat on the floor, and lean forward putting elbows onto knees. **EB:** *Adopting the correct position to open one's bowels allows the angle of the rectum and anal canal to straighten out. This facilitates an increase in abdominal pressure, which makes defecation more effective (Rogers, 2013).*
- Teach clients about the importance of responding promptly to the urge to defecate. **EB:** *The body's natural "call to stool" should be heeded in that it is a response to the stimulation of nerve endings in the rectum when a stool is present. Ignoring this urge will result in the rectum becoming desensitized to a stool in situ (Coggrave et al, 2014).*
- Consider the use of laxatives, suppositories, enemas, and bowel irrigation as required if other more natural interventions are not effective. *Laxative therapies can be used in conjunction with lifestyle changes (while waiting for the lifestyle changes to take effect or if the change is not sufficient in itself) (Marples, 2011).*
- Discourage the use of long-term laxatives and enemas and advise clients to gradually reduce their use if taken regularly. *Long-term use or overuse of laxatives can cause health problems (e.g., electrolyte imbalance) or hide symptoms that may be from a serious medical condition, such as cardiac arrhythmias (Aschenbrenner, 2014).*

 Geriatric

- Assess older adults for the presence of factors that contribute to constipation, including dietary fiber and fluid intake (less than 1.5 L/day), physical activity, use of constipating medications, and diseases that are associated with constipation.
- Explain the importance of adequate fiber intake, fluid intake, activity, and established toileting routines to ensure soft, formed stool. **EB:** *Strong evidence exists for the efficacy of adequate hydration (Gandell et al, 2013) and dietary fiber (Bardsley, 2017) in the prevention of constipation in older adults. Evidence suggests that the majority of clients would respond to lifestyle modifications reinforced by bowel training measures (De Giorgio et al, 2015).*
- Determine the client's perception of normal bowel elimination and laxative use; promote adherence to a regular schedule. **EB:** *A systematic review on older people's experiences of living with constipation showed that older people had individual and personal strategies relative to their own beliefs. Clients reported bodily experiences of everyday life shadowed by constipation and adverse psychological effects, which need to be explored to prevent and treat constipation (Tvistholm et al, 2017).*
- Explain why straining (Valsalva maneuver) should be avoided. *Excessive straining can cause syncope or cardiac dysrhythmias in susceptible people (Pstras et al, 2016).*
- Respond quickly to the client's call for assistance with toileting.
- Offer food, fluids, activity, and toileting opportunities to older clients who are cognitively impaired. *Even cognitively impaired individuals who are unable to initiate a request for food, fluids, and so forth may respond when opportunities are offered.* **CEB:** *In a randomized controlled trial (RCT) involving nursing home residents, subjects who received the treatment protocol (offering of food, fluid, activity, and toileting opportunities) had significantly more bowel movements than the control group. Both cognitively intact and cognitively impaired subjects benefited from the treatment (Schnelle et al, 2010).*
- Avoid regular use of enemas in older adults. *Enemas can cause fluid and electrolyte imbalances and damage to the colonic mucosa. However, judicious enema use may help prevent impactions (De Giorgio et al, 2015).*
- Advise the client against attempting to remove impacted feces on his or her own. *Older or confused clients in particular may attempt to remove feces and cause rectal damage.*
- ▲ Use opioids cautiously. Opioids cause constipation (Andrews & Morgan, 2013).
- Position the client on the toilet or commode and place a small footstool under the feet. Placing a small footstool helps the client assume a squatting posture to facilitate defecation.

 Home Care

- The interventions described previously may be adapted for home care use.
- Take complaints seriously and evaluate claims of constipation in a matter-of-fact manner. *Continued constipation can lead to bowel obstruction, which is a medical emergency. Use of a matter-of-fact manner will limit positive reinforcement of the behavior if actual constipation does not exist. Refer to the care plan for Perceived* **Constipation***.*
- Assess the self-care management activities the client is already using. **EB:** *Many older adults seek solutions to constipation, with laxative use a frequent remedy that creates its own problems (Tvistholm et al, 2017).*

● = Independent;   ▲ = Collaborative;   **EBN** = Evidence-Based Nursing;   **EB** = Evidence-Based

C

- Offer the following treatment recommendations:
  - ○ Acknowledge the client's lifelong experience of bowel function; respect beliefs, attitudes, and preferences, and avoid patronizing responses.
  - ○ Make available comprehensive, useful written information about constipation and possible solutions.
  - ○ Make available empathetic and accessible professional care to provide treatment and advice; a multi-disciplinary approach (including health care provider, nurse, and pharmacist) should be used.
  - ○ Institute a bowel management program.
  - ○ Consider affordability when suggesting solutions to constipation; discuss cost-effective strategies.
  - ○ Discuss a range of solutions to constipation and allow the client to choose the preferred options.
  - ○ Have orders in place for a suppository and enema as needed. As part of a bowel management program, suppositories or enemas may become necessary.
- Although the use of a bedside commode may be necessitated by the client's condition, allow the client to use the toilet in the bathroom when possible and provide assistance. *Bowel elimination is a private act, and a lack of privacy can contribute to constipation.*
- In older clients, routinely advise consumption of fluids, fruits, and vegetables as part of the diet, and ambulation if the client is able. *Introduce a bowel management program at the first sign of constipation. Constipation is a major problem for terminally ill or hospice clients who may need very high doses of opioids for pain management.*
- ▲ Refer for consideration of the use of polyethylene glycol 3350 (PEG-3350) for constipation. *There is good evidence to support the use of PEG-3350 for both chronic constipation and constipation associated with irritable bowel syndrome (Chapman et al, 2013).*
- When using a bowel program, establish a pattern that is very regular and allows the client to be part of the family unit. *Regularity of the program promotes psychological and/or physiological readiness to evacuate stool. Families of home care clients often cannot proceed with normal daily activities until bowel programs are complete.*

Client/Family Teaching and Discharge Planning

- Instruct the client on normal bowel function and the need for adequate fluid and fiber intake, activity, and a defined toileting pattern in a bowel program.
- Encourage the client to heed defecation warning signs and develop a regular schedule of defecation by using a stimulus such as a warm drink or prune juice. *Most cases of constipation are mechanical and result from habitual neglect of impulses that signal the appropriate time for defecation.*
- Encourage the client to avoid long-term use of laxatives and enemas and to gradually withdraw from their use if they are used regularly. *Use of stimulant laxatives should be avoided; long-term use can result in dependence on laxative for defecation (Roerig et al, 2010).*
- If not contraindicated, teach the client how to do bent-leg sit-ups to increase abdominal tone; also encourage the client to contract the abdominal muscles frequently throughout the day. Help the client develop a daily exercise program to increase peristalsis.
- Provide client with comprehensive written information about constipation and its management. EB: *Providing clients with well-written, evidence-based information about their condition and treatment can have a beneficial effect on the outcomes of treatment. In addition, clients are more likely to retain important information that will assist them in making informed decisions about their care (Coulter, 2011).*
- ▲ Collaborate with members of the interprofessional team to provide treatment and advice to clients and caregivers. *Teamwork is a central process in health care organizations. It increases the capacity of teams to absorb and develop new knowledge, which will improve client health and well-being (Ortega et al, 2013).*
- Formalize all advice by providing a bowel management program reiterating the mechanism of normal bowel function and the need for adequate fluid and fiber intake, physical activity, and a defined toileting pattern in an agreed bowel program. EB: *The implementation of an organized bowel management program is effective and significantly reduces hospital admissions in clients with severe idiopathic constipation (Russell et al, 2013).*
- Document all care and advice given in a factual and comprehensive manner. *Good record keeping is an integral part of nursing practice and is essential to the provision of safe and effective care (St. Aubyn & Andrews, 2015).*

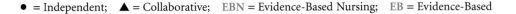

REFERENCES

Andrews, A., & Morgan, G. (2012). Constipation management in palliative care: Treatments and the potential of independent nurse prescribing. *International Journal of Palliative Nursing, 18*(1), 17–22.

Andrews, A., & Morgan, G. (2013). Constipation in palliative care: Treatment options and considerations for individual patient management. *International Journal of Palliative Nursing, 19*(6), 226–273.

Aschenbrenner, D. S. (2014). Overuse of certain OTC laxatives may be dangerous. *American Journal of Nursing, 114*(5), 25.

Attaluri, A., et al. (2011). Randomized clinical trial: Dried plums (prunes) vs psyllium for constipation. *Alimentary Pharmacology and Therapeutics, 33*, 822–828.

Avery, G. (2013). *Law and ethics in nursing and healthcare an introduction.* London: Sage Publications Inc.

Bardsley, A. (2017). Assessment and treatment options for patients with constipation. *The British Journal of Nursing, 26*(6), 312–318.

Boyle, J. (2013). Roughage to regulate. *World of Irish Nursing and Midwifery, 21*(7), 53–55.

Chapman, R. W., et al. (2013). Randomized clinical trial: Macrogol/PEG 3350 plus electrolytes for treatment of patients with constipation associated with irritable bowel syndrome. *The American Journal of Gastroenterology, 108*(9), 1508–1515.

Clark, K., & Currow, D. C. (2014). Advancing research into symptoms of constipation at the end of life. *International Journal of Palliative Nursing, 20*(8), 370–372.

Coggrave, K., Norton, C., & Cody, J. D. (2014). Management of faecal incontinence and constipation in adults with central neurological diseases. *Cochrane Database of Systematic Reviews*, (1), CD002115.

Coulter, A. (2011). *Engaging patients in health care.* Berkshire: McGraw-Hill Open University Press.

De Giorgio, R., et al. (2015). Chronic constipation in the elderly: A primer for the gastroenterologist. *BMC Gastroenterology, 15*, 130.

DerSarkissian, S. (2017). *What kind of poop do I have?* WebMD. Retrieved from https://www.webmd.com/digestive-disorders/poop-chart-bristol-stool-scale. (Accessed 8 March 2018).

Gandell, D., et al. (2013). Treatment of constipation in older people. *The Canadian Medical Association Journal, 185*(8), 663–670.

Goldberg, J. L. (2017). Guideline implementation; hand hygiene. *AORN Journal, 105*(2), 203–212.

Howatson-Jones, L., Standing, M., & Roberts, S. (Eds.), (2012). *Patient assessment and care planning in nursing.* London: Sage Publications Inc.

Joint Formulary Committee. (2016). *British National Formulary 72.* London: BMA/RPS Publishing.

Lawton, C. L., Walton, J., Hoyland, A., et al. (2013). Short term (14 days) consumption of insoluble wheat bran fibre-containing breakfast cereals improves subjective digestive feelings, general wellbeing and bowel function in a dose dependent manner. *Nutrients, 5*(4), 1436–1455. doi:10.3390/nu5041436.

Lee, A. (2015). Combatting the causes of constipation. *Nursing and Residential Care, 117*(6), 327–331.

Lundstrome, O., Manjerb, J., & Ohlssona, B. (2016). Smoking is associated with several functional gastrointestinal symptoms. *Scandinavian Journal of Gastroenterology, 51*(8), 914–922.

Marples, G. (2011). Diagnosis and management of slow transit constipation in adults. *Nursing Standard, 26*(8), 41–48.

McClurg, D., & Norton, C. (2016). What is the best way to manage neurogenic bowel dysfunction? *British Medical Journal, 354*, i3931. doi:10.1136/bmj.i3931.

McClurg, D., Hagen, S., & Dickinson, L. (2011). Abdominal massage for the treatment of constipation (Protocol). *Cochrane Database of Systematic Reviews*, (4), CD009089.

National Institute for Health and Care Excellence. (2015). *Constipation.* Clinical Knowledge summaries. Retrieved from http://cks.nice.org.uk/constipation. (Accessed 18 October 2017).

Noiesen, E., Trosborg, I., Bager, L., et al. (2013). Constipation—Prevalence and incidence among medical patients acutely admitted to hospital with a medical condition. *Journal of Clinical Nursing, 22*(15–16), 2295–2302.

Ortega, A., Sanchez-Manzanares, M., Gil, F., et al. (2013). Enhancing team learning in nursing teams through beliefs about interpersonal contexts. *The Journal of Advanced Nursing, 69*(1), 363–370.

Pstras, L., et al. (2016). The Valsalva manoeuvre: Physiology and clinical examples. *Acta Physiologica, 217*(2), 103–119.

Rhoads, J., & Murphy-Jensen, M. (2014). *Differential diagnoses for the advanced practice nurse.* New York: Springer Publishing Company.

Roerig, J. L., et al. (2010). Laxative abuse: Epidemiology, diagnosis and management. *Drugs, 70*(12), 1487–1503.

Rogers, J. (2013). Management of constipation in the community. *British Journal of Community Nursing, 27*(1), 20–24.

Russell, K. W., et al. (2013). *The implementation of an organized bowel management programme is effective and significantly reduces hospital admissions in patients with severe idiopathic constipation.* Retrieved from https://aap.confex.com/aap/2013/webprogram/Paper21641.html. (Accessed 9 March 2018).

Sanders, M., et al. (2015). New formulation of sustained released naloxone can reverse opioid induced constipation without compromising the desired opioid effects. *Pain Medicine, 16*(8), 1540–1550.

Schnelle, J. F., et al. (2010). A controlled trial of an intervention to improve urinary and fecal incontinence and constipation. *Journal of the American Geriatrics Society, 58*(8), 1504–1511.

Smith, G. D. (2012). Diagnosis and assessment of irritable bowel syndrome: Current perspectives. *Gastrointestinal Nursing, 10*(2), 39.

St. Aubyn, B., & Andrews, A. (2015). If it's not written down it didn't happen. *British Journal of Community Nursing, 29*(5), 20–22.

Szigethy, E., et al. (2014). Narcotic bowel syndrome and opioid induced constipation. *Current Gastroenterology Reports, 16*(10), 410.

Tack, J., et al. (2011). Diagnosis and treatment of chronic constipation—A European perspective. *Neurogastroenterology and Motility, 23*, 697–710.

Tagart, R. E. B. (1966). The anal canal and rectum: their varying relationship and its effect on anal continence. *Diseases of the Colon and Rectum, 9*(6), 449–452.

Tvistholm, N., Munch, L., & Danielsen, A. K. (2017). Constipation is casting a shadow over everyday life—a systematic review of older people's experience living with constipation. *Journal of Clinical Nursing, 26*(7–8), 902–914.

Wilcox, C. S., et al. (2010). An open-label study of naltrexone and bupropion combination therapy for smoking cessation in overweight and obese subjects. *Addictive Behaviors, 35*(3), 229–234.

Zhou, L., et al. (2010). Functional constipation: implications for nursing interventions. *Journal of Clinical Nursing, 19*(13–14), 1838–1843.

● = Independent;   ▲ = Collaborative;   EBN = Evidence-Based Nursing;   EB = Evidence-Based

Risk for Constipation　*Mary Beth Flynn Makic, PhD, RN, CCNS, FAAN, FNAP*

NANDA-I

Definition

Susceptible to a decrease in normal frequency of defecation accompanied by difficult or incomplete passage of stool, which may compromise health.

Risk Factors

Abdominal muscle weakness; average daily physical activity is less than recommended for gender and age; confusion; decrease in gastrointestinal motility; dehydration; depression; eating habit change; emotional disturbance; habitually suppresses urge to defecate; inadequate dietary habits; inadequate oral hygiene; inadequate toileting habits; insufficient fiber intake; insufficient fluid intake; irregular defecation habits; laxative abuse; obesity; recent environmental change

Associated Condition

Electrolyte imbalance; hemorrhoids; Hirschsprung's disease; inadequate dentition; iron salts; neurological impairment; postsurgical obstruction; pregnancy; prostate enlargement; rectal abscess; rectal anal fissure; rectal anal stricture; rectal prolapse; rectal ulcer; rectocele; tumor

NIC, NOC, Client Outcomes, Nursing Interventions and *Rationales,* Client/Family Teaching, and References

Refer to care plan for **Constipation.**

Perceived Constipation　*Amanda Andrews, BSc (Hons), MA and Bernie St. Aubyn, BSc (Hons), MSc*

NANDA-I

Definition

Self-diagnosis of constipation combined with abuse of laxatives, enemas, and/or suppositories to ensure a daily bowel movement.

Defining Characteristics

Enema abuse; expects a daily bowel movement; expects daily bowel movement at same time every day; laxative abuse; suppository abuse

Related Factors

Cultural health beliefs; family health beliefs; impaired thought process

NOC　(Nursing Outcomes Classification)

Suggested NOC Outcomes

Bowel Elimination; Health Beliefs; Health Beliefs: Perceived Threat

Example NOC Outcome with Indicators
Bowel Elimination as evidenced by the following indicators: Elimination pattern/Stool soft and formed/Passage of stool without aids/Ease of stool passage. (Rate each indicator of **Bowel Elimination:** 1 = severely compromised, 2 = substantially compromised, 3 = moderately compromised, 4 = mildly compromised, 5 = not compromised [see Section I].)

● = Independent;　▲ = Collaborative;　EBN = Evidence-Based Nursing;　EB = Evidence-Based

C

Client Outcomes

Client Will (Specify Time Frame)

- Regularly defecate soft, formed stool without use of aids
- Explain the need to decrease or eliminate the use of stimulant laxatives, suppositories, and enemas
- Identify alternatives to stimulant laxatives, enemas, and suppositories for ensuring defecation
- Explain that defecation does not have to occur every day

NIC   (Nursing Interventions Classification)

Suggested NIC Interventions

Bowel Management; Medication Management

Example NIC Activities—Bowel Management
Note preexistent bowel problems, bowel routine, and use of laxatives; Initiate a bowel training program, as appropriate

Nursing Interventions and *Rationales*

- Introduce yourself to the client and any companions, and inform them of your role. *Introducing yourself to a client helps establish and develop a therapeutic relationship that recognizes the person within the client and forms the bases for building trust on which to base the provision of care (Howatson-Jones et al, 2012).*
- Gain consent before proceeding further with the assessment. *Clients have the right of autonomy both legally and morally and therefore should be fully involved in the decision-making process (Avery, 2013).*
- Wash hands using a recognized technique. EB: *Performing strict hand-hygiene regimens significantly reduces the incidence of infection with methicillin-resistant* Staphylococcus aureus *and* Clostridium difficile *infections (Goldberg, 2017).*
- Assess usual pattern of defecation and establish the extent of the perceived constipation problem to include:
- ▲ Assess the client's bowel habits
  - ○ Time of day
  - ○ Amount and frequency of stool
  - ○ Consistency of stool (using the Bristol Stool Scale)
  - ○ Bleeding/passing mucus on defecation
  - ○ Patient history of bowel habits and/or laxative use
  - ○ Family history of bowel habits and/or laxative use

EB: *A detailed and accurate assessment of the patient enables the nurse to plan interventions, monitor outcomes, and evaluate care, ensuring no unnecessary treatment is rendered (Noiesen et al, 2013).*

- ▲ Assess the client's lifestyle that may impact bowel function
  - ○ Fiber content in diet
  - ○ Daily fluid intake
  - ○ Exercise patterns
  - ○ Personal remedies for constipation
  - ○ Cultural remedies for constipation
  - ○ Recently stopped smoking
  - ○ Alcohol consumption/recreational drug use

EB: *One of the key causes of constipation is dehydration of stools. A lack of water in the bowel leads to hard fecal matter, which is difficult to pass (Bardsley, 2017). Alcohol has a dehydrating effect on the body.*

- ▲ Review the client's past medical history
  - ○ Obstetrical/gynecological/urological history and surgeries
  - ○ Diseases that affect bowel motility
  - ○ Bleeding/passing mucus on defecation
  - ○ Current medications

EB: *Review the client's past medical history for conditions that may contribute to constipation, obstetrical/ gynecological history, surgeries, diseases that affect bowel motility, alterations in perianal sensation, and the present bowel regimen (Lee, 2015).*

• = Independent;   ▲ = Collaborative;   EBN = Evidence-Based Nursing;   EB = Evidence-Based

▲ Emotional influences
  ○ Anxiety and depression/psychological disorders
  ○ History of eating disorders
  ○ History of physical/or sexual abuse
  ○ Long-term defecation issues
  ○ Stress

EB: *Clients' psychological reactions to the experience of constipation change over time. Anxiety and fear about the anticipated health-related consequences of constipation are often expressed. The absence of a bowel movement or the failure of constipation treatment can lead to anxiety and depression (Dhingra et al, 2012).* EB: *Stress can alter the mucosal immune function of the central nervous system. This causes afferent signals to the gut to be reduced, causing constipation (Drossman, 2016).*

- Encourage the client or family to keep a 7-day diary of bowel habits to include time of day, length of time spent on the toilet, consistency, amount and frequency of stool, and any straining (using the Bristol Stool Scale). EB: *Keeping a diary helps establish a patient's bowel pattern and may contribute to the patient's adherence to the proposed care plan (Andrews & Morgan, 2013).*

- Encourage the client or family to keep a 7-day diary of lifestyle issues in relation to bowel habits to include fluid consumption, fiber content in diet, usual bowel stimulus, and exercise regimen. EB: *Enabling patients to present their condition in their own words ensures that they feel the health care professionals understand their concerns (Smith, 2012).*

- Educate the client that it is not necessary to have a daily bowel movement. EB: *A healthy bowel function can vary from three stools each day to three stools each week. The criteria of choice used for establishing a diagnosis of constipation are often the Rome IV criteria. The criteria-based definition calls for the presence of two or more of the symptoms for at least 3 months for a definition of constipation (Drossman, 2016).*

- Encourage the client to record use of laxatives, suppositories, or enemas, and suggest replacing them with an increase in fluid and fiber intake. EB: *Overtreatment with laxatives can result in iatrogenic diarrhea, which can lead to dehydration, delirium, and the false-positive labeling and unnecessary treatment of C. difficile carriers. This can result in increased morbidity and mortality, and a longer stay in hospital. By improving the assessment and treatment of constipation, patient outcomes should improve, resulting in significant hospital cost savings (Linton, 2014).*

- Advise a fiber intake of 18 to 30 g daily in adults and suggest foodstuffs high in fiber (e.g., prune juice, leafy green vegetables, whole meal bread and pasta). *Fiber creates bulky feces and stretches the bowel wall to stimulate peristalsis, thus shortening bowel transit time (Bardsley, 2017). For further information on use of fiber, please refer to the care plan for* **Constipation.**

- Advise a fluid intake of 1.5 to 2 L of fluid per day (ideally, 6–8 glasses of water), unless contraindicated by comorbidities, such as kidney or heart disease. *Water passes into the gut to promote the formation of a softer fecal mass and provides lubrication to prevent a blockage of the gut (Boyle, 2013).*

- Obtain a referral to a dietitian for analysis of the client's diet and fluid intake to provide strategies to improve diet and nutrition.

- Encourage physical activity within the client's current ability to mobilize. Encourage turning and changing position in bed if immobile. For clients with reduced mobility, encourage knee to chest raises, waist twists, and stretching the arms away from the body. For fully mobile clients, encourage walking and swimming. *Physical activity can help stimulate peristaltic waves in the colon and encourage the transit of feces to the rectum (Rogers, 2013).*

- Demonstrate the use of gentle external abdominal massage, using aroma therapy oils, following the direction of colon activity. *Abdominal massage encourages rectal loading by increasing intraabdominal pressure and in some cases it may elicit rectal waves, which may stimulate the somatoautonomic reflex and enhance bowel sensation (Turan and Atabek Aşt, 2016).*

- Recommend clients establish a regular elimination routine. If required assist clients to the bathroom at the same time every day being mindful of the need for privacy (closing of bathroom doors). *Establishing a routine allows for the use of the gastrocolic reflex, especially in the morning, which aids in defecation (Rogers, 2013).*

- Observe for the presence of an eating disorder by using laxatives to control or decrease weight; refer for counseling if needed. *People with eating disorders suffer from constipation and other gastrointestinal symptoms, or use laxatives as part of inducing weight loss (Sato & Fukudo, 2015).*

- Observe family cultural patterns related to eating and bowel habits. Cultural patterns may control bowel habits.

C

 Client/Family Teaching and Discharge Planning

- Provide education to the client on ways to adopt the best posture for defecation. Keep knees slightly higher than hips, keep feet flat on the floor and lean forward putting elbows onto knees. *Adopting the correct position to open one's bowels allows the angle of the rectum and anal canal to straighten out. This facilitates an increase in abdominal pressure, which makes defecation more effective (Rogers, 2013).*
- Teach clients the importance of responding promptly to the urge to defecate. EB: *The body's natural "call to stool" should be heeded in that it is a response to the stimulation of nerve endings in the rectum when a stool is present. Ignoring this urge will result in the rectum becoming desensitized to a stool in situ (Coggrave et al, 2014).*
- Discourage the use of long-term laxatives and enemas and explain the potential harmful effects of the continual use of defecation aids such as laxatives and enemas. EB: *"Lazy bowel syndrome" may occur if laxatives are used too frequently, causing the bowel to become dependent on laxatives to stimulate a bowel movement. Overuse of laxatives can also lead to poor absorption of vitamins and other nutrients, and to damage of the gastrointestinal tract (Elran-Barak et al, 2017).*
- Advise clients to gradually reduce their use of laxatives, if taken regularly, which may take months to achieve. *Long-term use or overuse of laxatives can cause health problems (e.g., electrolyte imbalance) or hide symptoms that may be from a serious medical condition, such as cardiac arrhythmias (Aschenbrenner, 2014).*
- Provide client with comprehensive written information about constipation and its management. EB: *Providing patients with well-written, evidence-based information about their condition and treatment can have a beneficial effect on the outcomes of treatment. In addition, patients are more likely to retain important information that will assist them in making informed decisions about their care (Coulter, 2011).*
- Collaborate with members of the interprofessional team to provide treatment and advice to clients and caregivers. *Teamwork is a central process in health care organizations. It increases the capacity of teams to absorb and develop new knowledge, which will improve patient health and well-being (Ortega et al, 2013).*
- Formalize all advice by providing a bowel management program reiterating the mechanism of normal bowel function and the need for adequate fluid and fiber intake, physical activity, and a defined toileting pattern in an agreed bowel program. EB: *The implementation of an organized bowel management program is effective and significantly reduces hospital admissions in patients with severe idiopathic constipation (Russell et al, 2013).*
- Document all care and advice given in a factual and comprehensive manner. *Good record keeping is an integral part of nursing practice and is essential to the provision of safe and effective care (St. Aubyn & Andrews, 2015).*

REFERENCES

Andrews, A., & Morgan, G. (2013). Constipation in palliative care: Treatment options and considerations for individual patient management. *International Journal of Palliative Nursing, 19*(6), 226–273.

Aschenbrenner, D. S. (2014). Overuse of certain OTC laxatives may be dangerous. *American Journal of Nursing, 114*(5), 25.

Avery, G. (2013). *Law and ethics in nursing and healthcare: An introduction.* London: Sage Publications Inc.

Bardsley, A. (2017). Assessment and treatment options for patients with constipation. *The British Journal of Nursing, 26*(6), 312–318.

Boyle, J. (2013). Roughage to regulate. *World of Irish Nursing and Midwifery, 21*(7), 53–55.

Coggrave, K., Norton, C., & Cody, J. D. (2014). Management of faecal incontinence and constipation in adults with central neurological diseases. *Cochrane Database of Systematic Reviews,* (1), CD002115.

Coulter, A. (2011). *Engaging patients in health care.* Berkshire: McGraw-Hill Open University Press.

Dhingra, L., et al. (2012). A qualitative study to explore psychological distress an illness burden associated with opioid induced constipation in cancer patients with advanced disease. *Palliative Medicine, 27*(5).

Drossman, D. A. (2016). Functional gastrointestinal disorders: History, pathophysiology, clinical features and Rome IV. *Gastroenterology, 150*(6), 1262–1279.e2. Retrieved from https://www.ncbi.nlm.nih.gov/pubmed/27144617. (Accessed on 9 March 2018).

Elran-Barak, R., Goldschmidt, A., Scott, J., et al. (2017). Is laxative misuse associated with binge eating? Examination of laxative misuse among individuals seeking treatment for eating disorders. *The International Journal of Eating Disorders, 50*(9), 1114–1118.

Goldberg, J. L. (2017). Guideline implementation; hand hygiene. *AORN Journal, 105*(2), 203–212.

Howatson-Jones, L., Standing, M., & Roberts, S. (Eds.), (2012). *Patient assessment and care planning in nursing.* London: Sage Publications Inc.

Lee, A. (2015). Combatting the causes of constipation. *Nursing and Residential Care, 117*(6), 327–331.

Linton, A. (2014). Improving management of constipation in an inpatient setting using a care bundle. *BMJ Quality Improvement Reports.* Retrieved from http://qir.bmj.com/content/3/1/u201903.w1002.full. (Accessed 9 March 2018).

Noiesen, E., Trosborg, I., Bager, L., et al. (2013). Constipation— Prevalence and incidence among medical patients acutely admitted to hospital with a medical condition. *Journal of Clinical Nursing,* *23*(15–16), 2295–2302.

Ortega, A., Sanchez-Manzanares, M., Gil, F., et al. (2013). Enhancing team learning in nursing teams through beliefs about interpersonal contexts. *The Journal of advanced Nursing, 69*(1), 363–370.

Rogers, J. (2013). Management of constipation in the community. *British Journal of Community Nursing, 27*(1), 20–24.

Russell, K. W., et al. (2013). *The implementation of an organized bowel management programme is effective and significantly reduces hospital admissions in patients with severe idiopathic constipation.* Retrieved from https://aap.confex.com/aap/2013/webprogram/ Paper21641.html. (Accessed 9 March 2018).

Sato, Y., & Fukudo, S. (2015). Gastrointestinal symptoms and disorders in patients with eating disorders. *Clinical Journal of Gastroenterology, 8*(5), 255–263.

Smith, G. D. (2012). Diagnosis and assessment of irritable bowel syndrome: Current perspectives. *Gastrointestinal Nursing, 10*(2), 39.

St. Aubyn, B., & Andrews, A. (2015). If it's not written down it didn't happen. *British Journal of Community Nursing, 29*(5), 20–22.

Turan, N., & Atabek Aşt, T. (2016). The effect of abdominal massage on constipation and quality of life. *Gastroenterology Nursing, 39*(1), 48–59.

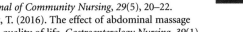

Chronic functional Constipation
Amanda Andrews, BSc (Hons), MA and Bernie St. Aubyn, BSc (Hons), MSc

NANDA-I

Definition

Infrequent or difficult evacuation of feces, which has been present for at least three of the prior 12 months.

Defining Characteristics

Adult: Presence of ≥2 of the following symptoms on Rome III classification system:

Lumpy or hard stools in ≥25% defecations; straining during ≥25% of defecations; sensation of incomplete evacuation for ≥25% of defecations; sensation of anorectal obstruction/blockage for ≥25% of defecations; manual maneuvers to facilitate ≥25% of defecations (digital manipulation, pelvic floor support); ≤3 evacuations per week

Child >4 years; Presence of ≥2 criteria on the Rome III Pediatric classification system for ≥2 months:

≤2 defecations per week; ≥1 episode of fecal incontinence per week; stool retentive posturing; painful or hard bowel movements; presence of large fecal mass in the rectum; large diameter stools that may obstruct the toilet

Child ≤4 years; Presence of ≥2 criteria on the Rome III Pediatric classification system for ≥1 month:

≤2 defecations per week; ≥1 episode of fecal incontinence per week; stool retentive posturing; painful or hard bowel movements; presence of large fecal mass in the rectum; large diameter stools that may obstruct the toilet

General

Distended abdomen; fecal impaction; leakage of stool with digital stimulation; pain with defecation; palpable abdominal mass; positive fecal occult blood test; prolonged straining; type 1 or 2 on Bristol Stool Chart

Related Factors

Decrease in food intake; dehydration; depression; diet disproportionally high in fat; diet disproportionally high in protein; frail elderly syndrome; habitually suppresses urge to defecate; impaired mobility; insufficient dietary intake; insufficient fluid intake; insufficient knowledge of modifiable factors; low caloric intake; low-fiber diet; sedentary lifestyle

Associated Condition

Amyloidosis; anal fissure; anal stricture; autonomic neuropathy; cerebral vascular accident; chronic intestinal pseudoobstruction; chronic renal insufficiency; colorectal cancer; dementia; dermatomyositis; diabetes mellitus; extra intestinal mass; hemorrhoids; Hirschsprung's disease; hypercalcemia; hypothyroidism; inflammatory bowel disease; ischemic stenosis; multiple sclerosis; myotonic dystrophy; panhypopituitarism; paraplegia; Parkinson's disease; pelvic floor dysfunction; perineal damage; pharmaceutical agent; polypharmacy; porphyria;

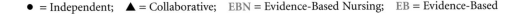

● = Independent;   ▲ = Collaborative;   EBN = Evidence-Based Nursing;   EB = Evidence-Based

C

postinflammatory stenosis; pregnancy; proctitis; scleroderma; slow colon transit time; spinal cord injury; surgical stenosis

NOC   (Nursing Outcomes Classification)

Suggested NOC Outcomes

Bowel Elimination; Symptom Severity

> ### Example NOC Outcome with Indicators
>
> **Bowel Elimination** as evidenced by the following indicators: Elimination pattern/Stool soft and formed/Passage of stool without aids/Ease of stool passage. (Rate each indicator of **Bowel Elimination:** 1 = severely compromised, 2 = substantially compromised, 3 = moderately compromised, 4 = mildly compromised, 5 = not compromised [see Section I].)

Client Outcomes

Client Will (Specify Time Frame)

- Maintain passage of soft, formed stool every 1 to 3 days without straining
- State relief from discomfort of constipation
- Identify measures that prevent or treat constipation

NIC   (Nursing Interventions Classification)

Suggested NIC Intervention

Constipation/Impaction Management

> ### Example NIC Activities—Constipation/Impaction Management
>
> Identify factors (e.g., medications, bed rest, diet) that may cause or contribute to constipation/impaction; Institute a toileting schedule, as appropriate

Nursing Interventions and *Rationales*

All Client Ages

- Introduce yourself to the client and anyone accompanying him or her and inform them of your role. Introducing yourself to a client helps establish and develop a therapeutic relationship that recognizes the person within the client and forms the basis for building trust on which to base the provision of care (Howatson-Jones et al, 2012).
- Gain consent to provide care before proceeding further with the assessment. Clients have the right of autonomy both legally and morally and therefore should be fully involved in the decision-making process (Avery, 2013).
- Wash hands using a recognized technique. Strict hand-hygiene regimens significantly reduce the incidence of methicillin-resistant *Staphylococcus aureus* and *Clostridium difficile* infection (Goldberg, 2017).
- Assess usual pattern of defecation and establish the extent of the constipation problem to include:
▲ Assess bowel habits
  ○ Time of day
  ○ Amount and frequency of stool
  ○ Consistency of stool (using the Bristol Stool Scale)
  ○ Bleeding/passing mucus on defecation
  ○ History of bowel habits and/or laxative use
  ○ Assess children younger than 4 years using the Rome III pediatric classification (for at least 1 month)
  ○ Assess children older than age 4 years using the Rome III pediatric classification (for at least 2 months)
EB: *Assess adults using the Rome IV classification. The Rome Foundation updated the criteria with the release of Rome IV criteria, devised in 2016, which specify that clients must be symptomatic with at least two or more of the criteria that are relevant to their specific age range (Drossman, 2016).*
▲ Assess the client's lifestyle that may impact bowel function
  ○ Fiber content in diet
  ○ Daily fluid intake

● = Independent;   ▲ = Collaborative;   EBN = Evidence-Based Nursing;   EB = Evidence-Based

C

- ○ Exercise patterns
- ○ Personal remedies for constipation
- ○ Recently stopped smoking
- ○ Alcohol consumption/recreational drug use
- ○ Personal habits related to defecation

EB: *Alcohol has a dehydrating effect on the body. One of the key causes of constipation is dehydration of stools. A lack of water in the bowel leads to hard fecal matter, which is difficult to pass (Bardsley, 2017). A detailed and accurate assessment of the patient enables the nurse to plan interventions, monitor outcomes, and evaluate care, ensuring no unnecessary treatment is rendered (Noiesen et al, 2013).*

▲ Review the client's past medical history
- ○ Obstetrical/gynecological/urological history and surgeries
- ○ Existing anatomical anomalies (e.g., anal fissures, anal strictures and hemorrhoids)
- ○ Diseases that affect bowel motility (e.g., colorectal cancer, chronic intestinal pseudoobstruction and Hirschsprung's disease)
- ○ Bleeding/passing mucus on defecation
- ○ Current medications

EB: *Established algorithms and guidelines recommend that secondary pathology and causes of constipation are identified and first excluded before moving on to assessment of diet and lifestyle issues (Tack et al, 2011).*

▲ Emotional influences
- ○ Anxiety and depression
- ○ Long-term defecation issues
- ○ Stress

EB: *A detailed and accurate assessment of the client enables the nurse to plan interventions, monitor outcomes, and evaluate care, ensuring no unnecessary treatment is performed (Noiesen et al, 2013). Stress can alter the mucosal immune function of the central nervous system. This causes afferent signals to the gut to be reduced, causing constipation (Drossman, 2016).*

- ● Complete a physical assessment (palpation for abdominal distention; percussion for dullness; auscultation for bowel sounds; and observation for anal fissures, anal strictures, and hemorrhoids). *A physical examination provides positive and negative findings and may provide the diagnosis without the need for further testing. It may also reveal unsuspected findings or confirm normality (Rhoads & Murphy-Jensen, 2014).*
- ● Encourage the client or family to keep a 7-day diary of bowel habits to include time of day, length of time spent on the toilet, consistency, amount and frequency of stool, and any straining (using the Bristol Stool Scale). *Keeping a diary helps establish a client's bowel pattern and may contribute to the client's adherence to the proposed care plan (Andrews & Morgan, 2013).*
- ● Encourage the client or family to keep a 7-day diary of lifestyle issues in relation to bowel habits to include fluid consumption, fiber content in diet, usual bowel stimulus, and exercise regime. *Enabling clients to present their condition in their own words ensures that they feel the health care professionals understand their concerns (Smith, 2012).*
- ● Actively encourage the use of reward/star charts with children when establishing regular bowel routines. *Research highlights that children respond better to positive enforcement when learning to manage constipation with regular toileting rather than confrontation about the problem (Afzal et al, 2011).*
- ● Discuss with clients already taking opioids (temporarily or long term) that constipation is a common side effect. Advise the client to contact their primary health care provider for a prescription of an appropriate laxative. *The thorough and comprehensive assessment of clients on opioids experiencing constipation will also allow for a bowel function approach for laxative prescribing rather than one based on the opioid dose alone (Andrews & Morgan, 2012).*
- ● Advise a fiber intake of 18 to 30 g of fiber daily in adults and suggest foodstuffs to facilitate this diet (e.g., prune juice, leafy green vegetables, whole meal bread and pasta). *Fiber creates bulky feces and stretches the bowel wall to stimulate peristalsis, thus shortening bowel transit time (Bardsley, 2017).*
- ● Advise a fluid intake of 1.5 to 2 L of fluid per day (ideally, 6–8 glasses of water), unless this is contraindicated by comorbidities such as renal or heart disease. *Water passes into the gut to promote the formation of a softer fecal mass and provides lubrication to prevent a blockage of the gut (Boyle, 2013).*
- ● Encourage physical activity within the client's current ability to mobilize. Encourage turning and changing position in bed if immobile. For reduced mobility clients, encourage knee to chest raises, waist twists, and stretching the arms away from the body. For fully mobile clients, encourage walking and swimming.

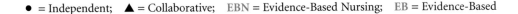

● = Independent; ▲ = Collaborative; EBN = Evidence-Based Nursing; EB = Evidence-Based

C

Physical activity can help stimulate peristaltic waves in the colon and encourage the transit of feces to the rectum (Rogers, 2013).

- Demonstrate the use of gentle external abdominal massage, following the direction of colon activity. EB: *A random control trial established that patients who received abdominal massage experienced reduced symptoms of constipation and an improved quality of life (Turan & Atabek Aşt, 2016).*
- Recommend clients establish a regular elimination routine. If required, assist clients to the bathroom at the same time every day, being mindful of the need for privacy (closing of bathroom doors). *Establishing a routine allows for the use of the gastrocolic reflex, especially in the morning, which aids defecation (Rogers, 2013).*
- Educate the client in how to adopt the best posture for defecation: keep knees slightly higher than hips, keep feet flat on the floor and lean forward, putting elbows onto knees. *Adopting the correct position to open one's bowels allows the angle of the rectum and anal canal to straighten. This facilitates an increase in abdominal pressure, which makes defecation more effective (Rogers, 2013).*
- Consider the teaching of biofeedback therapy to encourage a "new normal" bowel routine for clients to adopt. EB: *A recent literature review concluded that the use of biofeedback therapy in chronic constipation was successful and remains the safest option to successfully manage chronic constipation (Chiarioni, 2016).*
- Teach clients about the need to respond promptly to the defecation urge. EB: *The body's natural "call to stool" should be heeded because it is a response to the stimulation of nerve endings in the rectum when a stool is present. Ignoring this urge results in the rectum becoming desensitized to a stool in situ (Coggrave et al, 2014).*
- Consider the use of laxatives, suppositories, enemas, and bowel irrigation as required when other more natural interventions are not effective. EB: *Laxative therapies can be used in conjunction with lifestyle changes (while waiting for the lifestyle changes to take effect or if the change is not sufficient in itself) (Bardsley, 2017). Bowel irrigation is thought to both stimulate colonic reflex and act as a mechanical bowel washout. It has been acknowledged as a minimally invasive technique with proven clinical benefit to the patient (Holroyd, 2014).*
- Discourage the use of long-term laxatives and enemas and advise clients to gradually reduce their use if taken regularly. *Long-term use or overuse of laxatives can cause health problems (e.g., electrolyte imbalance) or hide symptoms of a serious medical condition, such as cardiac arrhythmias (Aschenbrenner, 2014).*
- Provide client with comprehensive written information about constipation and its management. EB: *Research shows that providing clients with well-written evidence-based information about their condition and treatment can have a beneficial effect on the outcomes of treatment. In addition, clients are more likely to retain important information that will assist them in making informed decisions about their care (Coulter, 2011).*
- Provide written instructions for children about taking their medication and about how the bowel works. *Written clear information provided to children with chronic functional constipation will help them understand and therefore recognize when they are at risk for constipation recurrence (National Institute for Health and Care Excellence, 2017).*
- Liaise with members of the interprofessional team as appropriate to provide treatment and advice to clients and caregivers. *Teamwork is a central process in health care organizations. It increases the capacity of teams to absorb and develop new knowledge, which will improve clients' health and well-being (Ortega et al, 2013).*
- Educate the client on the mechanism of normal bowel function and the need for adequate fluid and fiber intake, physical activity, and a defined toileting pattern in an agreed-on bowel management program. *The implementation of an organized bowel management program is effective and significantly reduces hospital admissions in clients with severe idiopathic constipation (Russell et al, 2013).*
- Document all care and advice given in a factual and comprehensive manner. *Good record keeping is an integral part of nursing practice and is essential to the provision of safe and effective care (St. Aubyn & Andrews, 2015).*

REFERENCES

Andrews, A., & Morgan, G. (2012). Constipation management in palliative care: Treatments and the potential of independent nurse prescribing. *International Journal of Palliative Nursing, 18*(1), 17–22.

Andrews, A., & Morgan, G. (2013). Constipation in palliative care: Treatment options and considerations for individual patient management. *International Journal of Palliative Nursing, 19*(6), 226–273.

● = Independent; ▲ = Collaborative; EBN = Evidence-Based Nursing; EB = Evidence-Based

Aschenbrenner, D. S. (2014). Overuse of certain OTC laxatives may be dangerous. *American Journal of Nursing*, 114(5).

Afzal, N. A., Tighe, M. P., & Thomas, M. A. (2011). *Constipation in children*. Retrieved from http://www.biomedcentral.com/content/pdf/1824-7288-37-28.pdf. (Accessed 9 March 2018).

Avery, G. (2013). *Law and ethics in nursing and healthcare an introduction*. London: Sage Publications Inc.

Bardsley, A. (2017). Assessment and treatment options for patients with constipation. *The British Journal of Nursing*, 26(6), 312–318.

Boyle, J. (2013). Roughage to regulate. *World of Irish Nursing and Midwifery*, 21(7), 53–55.

Chiarioni, G. (2016). Biofeedback treatment of chronic constipation: Myths and misconceptions. *Techniques in Coloproctology*, 20(9), 611–618.

Coggrave, K., Norton, C., & Cody, J. D. (2014). Management of faecal incontinence and constipation in adults with central neurological diseases. *Cochrane Database of Systematic Reviews*, (1), CD002115.

Coulter, A. (2011). *Engaging patients in health care*. Berkshire: McGraw-Hill Open University press.

Drossman, D. A. (2016). Functional gastrointestinal disorders: History, pathophysiology, clinical features and Rome IV. *Gastroenterology*, 150(6), 1262–1279.e2. Retrieved from https://www.ncbi.nlm.nih.gov/pubmed/27144617. (Accessed on 9 March 2018).

Goldberg, J. L. (2017). Guideline implementation; hand hygiene. *AORN Journal*, 105(2), 203–212.

Holroyd, S. (2014). *British Journal of Community Nursing*, 31, 51–56.

Howatson-Jones, L., Standing, M., & Roberts, S. (Eds.). (2012). *Patient assessment and care planning in nursing*. London: Sage Publications Inc.

National Institute for Health and Care Excellence. (2017). *Constipation in children and young people: diagnosis and management*. Retrieved from https://www.nice.org.uk/guidance/cg99. (Accessed on 9 March 2018).

Noiesen, E., Trosborg, I., Bager, L., et al. (2013). Constipation— Prevalence and incidence among medical patients acutely admitted to hospital with a medical condition. *Journal of Clinical Nursing*, 23(15–16), 2295–2302.

Ortega, A., Sanchez-Manzanares, M., Gil, F., et al. (2013). Enhancing team learning in nursing teams through beliefs about interpersonal contexts. *The Journal of advanced Nursing*, 69(1).

Rhoads, J., & Murphy-Jensen, M. (2014). *Differential diagnoses for the advanced practice nurse*. New York: Springer Publishing Company.

Rogers, J. (2013). Management of constipation in the community. *British Journal of Community Nursing*, 27(1), 20–24.

Russell, K. W., Zobell, S., Barnhart, D. C., et al. (2013). The implementation of an organised bowel management programme is effective and significantly reduces hospital admissions in patients with severe idiopathic constipation. Retrieved from https://aap.confex.com/aap/2013/webprogram/Paper21641.html. (Accessed 9 March 2018).

Smith, G. D. (2012). Diagnosis and assessment of irritable bowel syndrome: Current perspectives. *Gastrointestinal Nursing*, 10(2).

St. Aubyn, B., & Andrews, A. (2015). If it's not written down it didn't happen. *British Journal of Community Nursing*, 29(5), 20–22.

Tack, J., Muller–Lissner, S., Stanghellini, V., et al. (2011). Diagnosis and treatment of chronic constipation—A European perspective. *Neurogastroentrology Motility*, 23(8), 697–710.

Turan, N., & Atabek Aşt, T. (2016). The effect of abdominal massage on constipation and quality of life. *Gastroenterology Nursing*, 39(1), 48–59.

Risk for chronic functional Constipation   *Mary Beth Flynn Makic, PhD, RN, CCNS, FAAN, FNAP*

NANDA-I

Definition

Susceptible to infrequent or difficult evacuation of feces, which has been present nearly 3 of the prior 12 months, which may compromise health.

Risk Factors

Decrease in food intake; dehydration; depression; diet proportionally high in fat; diet disproportionally high in protein; frail elderly syndrome; habitually suppresses urge to defecate; impaired mobility; insufficient dietary intake; insufficient fluid intake; insufficient knowledge of modifiable factors; low caloric intake; low-fiber diet; sedentary lifestyle

Associated Condition

Amyloidosis; anal fissure; anal stricture; autonomic neuropathy; cerebral vascular accident; chronic intestinal pseudoobstruction; chronic renal insufficiency; colorectal cancer; dementia; dermatomyositis; diabetes mellitus; extra intestinal mass; hemorrhoids; Hirschsprung's disease; hypercalcemia; hypothyroidism; inflammatory bowel disease; ischemic stenosis; multiple sclerosis; myotonic dystrophy; panhypopituitarism; paraplegia; Parkinson's disease; pelvic floor dysfunction; perineal damage; pharmaceutical agent; polypharmacy; porphyria; postinflammatory stenosis; pregnancy; proctitis; scleroderma; slow colon transit time; spinal cord injury; surgical stenosis

NIC, NOC, Client Outcomes, Nursing Interventions and *Rationales*, Client/Family Teaching and Discharge Planning, and References

Refer to care plan for Chronic functional **Constipation.**

● = Independent;   ▲ = Collaborative;   EBN = Evidence-Based Nursing;   EB = Evidence-Based

Contamination   *Pauline McKinney Green, PhD, RN, CNE*

NANDA-I

C

Definition

Exposure to environmental contaminants in doses sufficient to cause adverse health effects.

Defining Characteristics

Pesticides

Dermatological effects of pesticide exposure; gastrointestinal effects of pesticide exposure; neurological effects of pesticide exposure; pulmonary effects of pesticide exposure; renal effects of pesticide exposure

Chemicals

Dermatological effects of chemical exposure; gastrointestinal effects of chemical exposure; immunological effects of chemical exposure; neurological effects of chemical exposure; pulmonary effects of chemical exposure; renal effects of chemical exposure

Biologics

Dermatological effects of biologic exposure; gastrointestinal effects of biologic exposure; neurological effects of biologic exposure; pulmonary effects of biologic exposure; renal effects of biologic exposure

Pollution

Neurological effects of pollution exposure; pulmonary effects of pollution exposure

Waste

Dermatological effects of waste exposure; gastrointestinal effects of waste exposure; hepatic effects of waste exposure; pulmonary effects of waste exposure

Radiation

Genetic effects of radiation exposure; immunological effects of radiation exposure; neurological effects of radiation exposure; oncological effects of radiation exposure

Related Factors

External

Carpeted flooring; chemical contamination of food; chemical contamination of water; flaking, peeling surface in presence of young children; inadequate breakdown of contaminant; inadequate household hygiene practices; inadequate municipal services; inadequate personal hygiene practices; inadequate protective clothing; inappropriate use of protective clothing; ingestion of contaminated material; playing where environmental contaminants are used; unprotected exposure to chemical; unprotected exposure to heavy metal; unprotected exposure to radioactive material; use of environmental contaminant in the home; use of noxious material in insufficiently ventilated area; use of noxious material without effective protection

Internal

Concomitant exposure; inadequate nutrition; smoking

At-Risk Population

Children <5 years; economically disadvantaged; exposure to areas with high concomitant level; exposure to atmospheric pollutants; exposure to bioterrorism; exposure to disaster; exposure to radiation; female gender; gestational age during exposure; older adults; previous exposure to contaminant

Associated Condition

Pre-existing disease; pregnancy

● = Independent;   ▲ = Collaborative;   EBN = Evidence-Based Nursing;   EB = Evidence-Based

NOC   (Nursing Outcomes Classification)

Suggested NOC Outcomes

Community Health Status; Family Physical Environment; Anxiety Level; Fear Level

> **Example NOC Outcome with Indicators**
>
> **Community Health Status** as evidenced by the following indicators: Evidence of health protection measures/Compliance with environmental health standards/Health status of population. (Rate the outcome and indicators of **Community Health Status:** 1 = poor, 2 = fair, 3 = good, 4 = very good, 5 = excellent [see Section I].)

Client Outcomes

Client Will (Specify Time Frame)

- Have minimal health effects associated with contamination
- Cooperate with appropriate decontamination protocol
- Participate in appropriate isolation precautions

Community Will (Specify Time Frame)

- Use health surveillance data system to monitor for contamination incidents
- Use disaster plan to evacuate and triage affected members
- Have minimal health effects associated with contamination
- Use measures to reduce household environmental risks

NIC   (Nursing Interventions Classification)

Suggested NIC Interventions

Triage: Disaster; Infection Control; Anxiety Reduction; Crisis Intervention; Health Education

> **Example NIC Activities—Triage: Disaster**
>
> Initiate appropriate emergency measures, as indicated; Monitor for and treat life-threatening injuries or acute needs

Nursing Interventions and *Rationales*

▲ Help individuals cope with contamination incident by doing the following:
  - ○ Use groups that have survived terrorist attacks as a useful resource for victims
  - ○ Provide accurate information on risks involved, preventive measures, use of antibiotics and vaccines
  - ○ Assist to deal with feelings of fear, vulnerability, and grief
  - ○ Encourage individuals to talk to others about their fears
  - ○ Assist victims to think positively and to move toward the future
▲ *In a crisis situation, interventions aimed at supporting an individual's cope help the person deal with feelings of fear, helplessness, and loss of control that are normal reactions in a crisis situation.*
- Triage, stabilize, transport, and treat affected community members. EB: *Accurate triage and early treatment provide the best chance of survival to affected persons (Veenema, 2013).*
- Prioritize mental health care for highly vulnerable risk groups or those with special needs (deeply affected groups, women, older persons, children and adolescents, displaced persons—especially those living in shelters, persons with preexisting mental health disorders including those living in institutions) (Pan American Health Organization, 2012).
- Collaborate with members of the health care delivery system and outside agencies (local health department, emergency medical services [EMS], state and federal agencies). *Communication among agencies increases the ability to handle a crisis efficiently (Veenema, 2013; CDC, 2015).*
- Use approved procedures for decontamination of persons, clothing, and equipment. Victims may first require decontamination before entering health facility to receive care to prevent the spread of contamination (US Army Medical Research Institute of Infectious Diseases, 2014).
- Use appropriate isolation precautions: universal, airborne, droplet, and contact isolation to prevent cross-contamination by contaminating agents (US Army Medical Research Institute of Infectious Diseases,

● = Independent;   ▲ = Collaborative;   EBN = Evidence-Based Nursing;   EB = Evidence-Based

C

2014). CEB: *The World Health Organization (WHO) recommends strict guidelines for handwashing at five moments in time: before touching a patient, before clean/aseptic procedures, after body fluid exposure/risk, after touching a patient, and after touching patient surroundings (WHO, 2009).*

- Monitor individuals for therapeutic effects, side effects, and compliance with postexposure drug therapy that may extend over a long period of time and require monitoring for compliance and for therapeutic and side effects (Veenema, 2013; Adalja et al, 2015).
- Perform effective handwashing before and after handling medical charts, entering case notes, touching clients, and performing procedures, especially in intensive care unit environments. EB: *A prospective study to identify and compare the incidence of bacterial contamination of hospital charts found the plastic chart covers to be contaminated (63.5% for general wards and 83.2% for special units); chart covers can act as vectors and potential sources of infection (Chen, Chen, & Wang, 2014).*
- Prevent cross-contamination by systematically disinfecting stethoscopes (diaphragm and tubing) after each use. EB: *A study of the contamination level of health care providers' hands and stethoscopes found that the contamination level of the stethoscope is substantial after a single health care provider examination and is comparable to the contamination of parts of the provider's hand (Longtin, Schneider, & Tschopp, 2014).*
- Minimize occupational exposure to antineoplastic agents by following National Institute of Occupational Safety and Health (NIOSH) guidelines regarding personal protective equipment and correct handling of hazardous drugs. EB: *Nurse safety is directly related to knowledge of hazard assessment, decontamination, and proper use of personal protective equipment (NIOSH, 2009; Crickman & Finnell, 2017).*

 Geriatric

- Help the client identify age-related factors that may affect response to contamination incidents.
- Advise older adults to follow public notices related to drinking water. *Contaminated water can harm the health of older persons and those with chronic conditions (CDC, 2014a).*
- Encourage older adults to receive influenza vaccination when it is available, beginning as early as late August and continuing through the end of February. *Flu vaccination protects against influenza and protects those in proximity who are more vulnerable to serious flu illness (CDC, 2017a).*
- Instruct older adults with special needs or chronic conditions to create and share a plan with family and friends for emergencies and keep medications, prescriptions, and special devices on hand. *Sharing a plan for emergencies helps older adults create a social network that will be available for support and assistance (Federal Emergency Management Agency, 2017).*

 Pediatric

- Provide environmental health hazard information. *Developing children are more vulnerable to environmental toxicants because of greater and longer exposure and particular susceptibility windows (Children's Environmental Health Network, 2017).*
- Reduce risks from exposure to environmental contaminants by identifying the ages and life stages of children. EB: *Coordinate hazard and exposure assessment using children's ages and life stages to accommodate for children's physiology and developmental stage, which contribute to opportunities for environmental exposure and contamination (Hubal, de Wet, & Du Toit, 2014).*
- Screen newly arrived immigrant and refugee children for elevated blood lead levels secondary to lead hazards in older housing. EB: *Resettlement in areas with older housing stock increases risk for lead poisoning (CDC, 2013a).*
- Be aware that the risk for lead exposure is much higher in many countries from which children are adopted than in the United States; screening should then be conducted for those identified from 6 months and up to 16 years of age *(CDC, 2014b).*
- The current reference level of 5 µg/dL is used to identify children and environments associated with lead-exposure hazards. EB: *The Centers for Disease Control and Prevention (CDC) currently recommends using 5 µg/dL as the reference value in place of the previously recommended level of 10 µg/dL; reference values are updated every 4 years based on the most recent population-based blood lead surveys among children (CDC, 2017b).*

 Multicultural

- Ask about use of imported or culture-specific products that contain lead, such as greta and azarcon (Hispanic folk medicine for upset stomach and diarrhea), ghasard (Indian folk medicine tonic), ba-baw-san

● = Independent; ▲ = Collaborative; EBN = Evidence-Based Nursing; EB = Evidence-Based

(Chinese herbal remedy), and daw-tay (Thai and Myanmar remedy). *Immigrant children are at increased risk for contamination, particularly from lead related to exposure to imported culture-specific products (CDC, 2013b).*

- Nurses need to consider the cultural and social factors that impact access to and understanding of the health care system, particularly for groups such as migrant workers who do not have consistent health care providers. EB: *Subtle cultural biases in how nurses approach care can affect outcomes (Holmes, 2012; Hubal, de Wet, & Du Toit, 2014).*

Home Care

- Assess current environmental stressors and identify community resources. *Accessing resources decreases stress and increases ability to cope.*
- Recognize that relocated and unemployed individuals/families are at risk for psychological distress. EB: *People who lose their social network are at a very high risk for postevent psychological distress and require appropriate care (Oyama et al, 2012).*
- Support policy and program initiatives that provide emergency mental health services following large-scale contamination events. EB: *A study of the utilization of mental health services following a major disaster found community mental health service use increased in the period following the event and that brief interventions were more effective than conventional, multisession interventions (Boscarino, Adams, & Figley, 2011).*
- Instruct community members concerned about lead in drinking water from plumbing pipes and fixtures to have the water tested by calling the Environmental Protection Agency (EPA) drinking water hotline at 800-426-4791.
- Educate community members to reduce exposure to lead by inquiring about lead-based paint before buying a home or renting an apartment built before 1978; federal law requires disclosure of known information about lead-based paint *(EPA, 2017).*
- Instruct individuals and families that food contamination occurs through a variety of mechanisms and that food safety is associated with proper washing of hands, surfaces, and utensils; prompt refrigeration of food; and cooking foods at the correct temperature. EB: *Pathogens can be introduced into food from infected humans who handle food without thoroughly washing their hands, from food that touches surfaces or utensils contaminated by pathogens in raw food, and improper refrigeration or heating of food (CDC, 2016).*

Client/Family Teaching and Discharge Planning

- Provide truthful information to the person or family affected.
- Discuss signs and symptoms of contamination.
- Explain decontamination protocols.
- Explain need for isolation procedures.
- *Well-managed efforts at communication of contamination information ensure messages are correctly formulated, transmitted, and received and result in meaningful actions.*
- Emphasize the importance of preexposure and postexposure treatment of contamination. *Early treatment decreases associated complications related to contamination (ATSDR, 2014).*
- Provide parents with actionable information to reduce environmental contamination in the home. EBN: *A randomized educational intervention to reduce contamination in the home demonstrated significant reduction in biomarker levels and improved environmental health self-efficacy and precaution adoption (Butterfield et al, 2011).*

REFERENCES

Adalja, A., Toner, E., & Inglesby, T. V. (2015). Clinical management of bioterrorism-related conditions. *New England Journal of Medicine, 372*(10), 954–962. doi:10.1056/NEJMra409755.

Agency for Toxic Substances and Disease Registry (ATSDR). (2014). *Medical management guideline for parathion.* Retrieved from http://www.atsdr.cdc.gov/MMG/MMG.asp?id=1140&tid=246.

Boscarino, J. A., Adams, R. E., & Figley, C. R. (2011). Mental health service use after the World Trade Center disaster. Utilization trends and comparative effectiveness. *The Journal of Nervous and Mental Diseases, 199,* 91–99.

Butterfield, P. G., Hill, W., Postma, J., et al. (2011). Effectiveness of a household environmental health intervention delivered by rural public health nurses. *American Journal of Public Health, 101*(Suppl. 1), S262–S270. doi:10.2105/AJPH.2011.3001.

Centers for Disease Control & Prevention (CDC). (2013a). *Lead screening during the domestic medical examination for newly arrived refugees.* Retrieved from https://www.cdc.gov/immigrantrefugeehealth/pdf/lead-guidelines.pdf.

Centers for Disease Control & Prevention (CDC). (2013b). *Folk medicine.* Retrieved from https://www.cdc.gov/nceh/lead/tips/folkmedicine.htm.

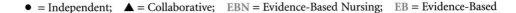

● = Independent; ▲ = Collaborative; EBN = Evidence-Based Nursing; EB = Evidence-Based

Centers for Disease Control & Prevention (CDC). (2014a). *Water-related diseases and contamination in public water systems.* Retrieved from http://www.cdc.gov/healthywater/drinking/public/water_diseases.html.

Centers for Disease Control and Prevention (CDC). (2014b). *International adoption and prevention of lead poisoning.* Retrieved from http://www.cdc.gov/nceh/lead/tips/adoption.htm.

Centers for Disease Control and Prevention (CDC). (2015). *Office of Public Health Preparedness and Response. 2013–2014 national snapshot of public health preparedness.* Retrieved from http://www.cdc.gov/htmllinks/2013/documents/2013_Preparedness _Report_Section3.pdf.

Centers for Disease Control and Prevention (CDC). (2016). *Food safety. Prevention and education.* Retrieved from http://www.cdc.gov/foodsafety/groups/consumers.html.

Centers for Disease Control & Prevention (CDC). (2017a). *What are the benefits of flu vaccination?* Retrieved from http://www.cdc.gov/flu/pdf/protect/keyfacts.htm.

Centers for Disease Control & Prevention (CDC). (2017b). *Blood lead levels in children.* Retrieved from https://www.cdc.gov.nceh/lead/acclpp/lead_levels_in_children_fact_sheet.pdf.

Chen, K. H., Chen, L. R., & Wang, Y. K. (2014). Contamination of medical charts: An important source of potential infection in hospitals. *PLoS ONE*, 9(2), e78512. doi:10.1371/journal.pone .0078512.

Children's Environmental Health Network. (2017). *Children's environmental health 101.* Retrieved from http://www.cehn,org/resources/ceh101.

Crickman, R., & Finnell, D. S. (2017). Chemotherapy safe handling. Limiting nursing exposure with a hazardous drug control program. *Clinical Journal of Oncology Nursing*, 21(1), 73–78. doi:10.1188/17.CJON.73-78.

Environmental Protection Agency (EPA). (2017). *Protect your family from lead in your home.* Retrieved from http://www.epa.gov/lead/protect-your-family-lead-your-home.

Federal Emergency Management Agency (FEMA). (2017). *Individuals with disabilities.* Retrieved from http://www.ready.gov/.

Holmes, S. M. (2012). The clinical gaze in the practice of migrant health: Mexican migrants in the United States. *Social Science and Medicine*, 74(6), 873–881. doi:10.1016/j.socscimed.2011.06.067.

Hubal, E., de Wet, T., & Du Toit, L. (2014). Identifying important life stages for monitoring and assessing risks from exposures to environmental contaminants: Results of a World Health Organization review. *Regulatory Toxicology and Pharmacology*, 69(1), 113–124. doi:10.1016/j.yrtph.2013.09.008.

Longtin, Y., Schneider, A., & Tschopp, C. (2014). Contamination of stethoscopes and physicians' hands after a physical examination. *Mayo Clinic Proceedings*, 89(3), 291–299. doi:10.1016/jmayocp .2013.11.016.

National Institute for Occupational Safety and Health. (2009). *Personal protective equipment for health care workers who work with hazardous drugs.* Retrieved from https://www.cdc.gov/niosh/docs/wp-solutions/2009-106/pdfs/2009-106.pdf.

Oyama, M., Nakamura, K., Suda, Y., et al. (2012). Social network disruption as a major factor associated with psychological distress 3 years after 2004 Niigata-Chuetsu earthquake in Japan. *Environmental Health and Prevention Medicine*, 17(2), 118–123. doi:10.1007/s12199-0225-y.

Pan American Health Organization. (2012). *Mental health and psychosocial support in disaster situations in the Caribbean.* Washington, DC: PAHO.

U.S. Army Medical Research Institute of Infectious Diseases. (2014). *USAMRIID's medical management of biological casualties handbook* (8th ed.). Fort Detrick, MD: Author.

Veenema, T. G. (2013). *Disaster nursing and emergency preparedness for chemical, biological and radiological terrorism and other hazards* (3rd ed.). New York: Springer.

World Health Organization. (2009). *Your 5 moments for hand hygiene.* Retrieved from www.who.int/gpsc/5May/Your_5_Moments_For _Hand_Hygiene_Poster.pdf.

Risk for Contamination   *Mary Beth Flynn Makic, PhD, RN, CCNS, FAAN, FNAP*

NANDA-I

Definition

Susceptible to exposure to environmental contaminants, which may compromise health.

Risk Factors

External

Carpeted flooring; chemical contamination of food; chemical contamination of water; flaking, peeling surface in presence of young children; inadequate breakdown of contaminant; inadequate household hygiene practices; inadequate municipal services; inadequate personal hygiene practices; inadequate protective clothing; inappropriate use of protective clothing; ingestion of contaminated material; playing where environmental contaminants are used; unprotected exposure to chemical; unprotected exposure to heavy metal; unprotected exposure to radioactive material; use of environmental contaminant in the home; use of noxious material in insufficiently ventilated area; use of noxious material without effective protection

Internal

Concomitant exposure; inadequate nutrition; smoking

● = Independent;   ▲ = Collaborative;   EBN = Evidence-Based Nursing;   EB = Evidence-Based

At-Risk Population

Children <5 years; economically disadvantaged; exposure to areas with high contaminant level; exposure to atmospheric pollutants; exposure to bioterrorism; exposure to disaster; exposure to radiation; female gender; gestational age during exposure; older adults; previous exposure to contaminant

Associated Condition

Preexisting disease; pregnancy

NIC, NOC, Client Outcomes, Nursing Interventions and *Rationales,* Client/Family Teaching, and References

Refer to care plan for **Contamination.**

Risk for adverse reaction to iodinated Contrast Media
Pauline McKinney Green, PhD, RN, CNE

NANDA-I

Definition

Susceptible to noxious or unintended reaction associated with the use of iodinated contrast media that can occur within seven days after contrast agent injection, which may compromise health.

Risk Factors

Dehydration; generalized weakness

At-Risk Population

Extremes of age; history of allergy; history of previous adverse effect from iodinated contrast media

Associated Condition

Chronic illness; concurrent use of pharmaceutical agents; contrast media precipitates adverse event; fragile vein; unconsciousness

NOC   (Nursing Outcomes Classification)

Suggested NOC Outcomes

Tissue Perfusion: Renal; Kidney Function

Example NOC Outcome with Indicators

Kidney Function as evidenced by 24-hour intake and output balance/Blood urea nitrogen/Serum creatinine/Urine color/ Serum electrolytes. (Rate the outcome and indicators of **Kidney Function:** I = severely compromised, 2 = substantially compromised, 3 = moderately compromised, 4 = mildly compromised, 5 = not compromised [see Section I].)

Client Outcomes

Client Will (Specify Time Frame)

- Maintain normal blood urea nitrogen and serum creatinine levels
- Maintain urine output of 0.5 mL/kg/hr
- Maintain serum electrolytes (K^+, PO_4, Na^+) within normal limits

NIC   (Nursing Interventions Classification)

Suggested NIC Interventions

Fluid/Electrolyte Management; Laboratory Data Interpretation

● = Independent;   ▲ = Collaborative;   EBN = Evidence-Based Nursing;   EB = Evidence-Based

Example NIC Activities—Fluid/Electrolyte Management
Monitor for serum electrolytes levels, as available; Weigh daily and monitor trends; Monitor vital signs, as appropriate

C

Nursing Interventions and *Rationales*

Recognize that iodinated contrast media can be harmful to clients in a number of ways, including onset of contrast-induced nephropathy (CIN), allergic reactions to the dye, and damage to veins and vascular access devices.

Contrast-Induced Nephropathy

Protect clients from contrast media-induced nephropathy by taking the following actions:

▲ Assess clients for low body mass index (BMI), history of heart failure, or repeated administration of contrast material. *Low BMI and heart failure are risk factors for CIN (Balemans et al, 2012).*

▲ In nondiabetic clients with acute coronary syndrome, assess for presence of hyperglycemia on admission and report to health care provider. *High blood glucose in acute coronary syndrome patients not known to be diabetic is associated with increased incidence of CIN after percutaneous coronary intervention (Islam et al, 2013).*

● Identify clients who have had multiple doses of iodinated contrast media in less than 24 hours and report to health care provider. *Repeat administration of contrast material may be a risk factor for CIN (American College of Radiology, 2017a).*

● Communicate information about at-risk clients to provider and procedure team in the hand-off report and electronic medical record. EBN: *A study of patients undergoing percutaneous coronary interventions with contrast media demonstrated significant reduction in acute kidney injury rates when evidence-based practices in nursing were introduced/standardized (Lambert et al, 2017).*

▲ Ensure that clients having diagnostic testing with contrast are well hydrated with isotonic intravenous (IV) fluids as ordered before and after the examination. EB: *Incidence of CIN is reduced by IV hydration with isotonic fluids (lactated Ringer's or 0.9% normal saline) before and after IV contrast administration (American College of Radiology, 2017a). Low incidence of CIN is associated with the use of hydration (Balemans et al, 2012).*

▲ *Assess patients with symptoms of heart failure on an individual basis to determine tolerance for IV fluids used for hydration in the periprocedure period (Lambert et al, 2017).*

▲ Verify that a baseline serum creatinine has been drawn from clients at risk for CIN. *A baseline value is important for comparison after the contrast injection; estimated glomerular filtration rate is considered a biomarker for CIN risk (American College of Radiology, 2017a).*

● Be vigilant for signs of CIN in clients who have cancer. *Clients with cancer are vulnerable to CIN, especially within 45 days of chemotherapy and in those with hypertension (Cicin et al, 2014).*

▲ Monitor for and report signs of acute kidney injury for 48 hours after iodinated contrast administration in clients at risk: absolute serum creatinine increase ≥0.3 mg/dL, percentage increase in serum creatinine ≥50%, or urine output reduced to ≤0.5 mL/kg/hr for at least 6 hours. (Refer to your institution policy for specific clinical parameters.) *These clinical parameters are suggestive of acute kidney injury (American College of Radiology, 2017a).*

▲ Clients taking metformin may increase client risk of developing lactic acidosis should CIN develop after contrast administration. *Review medications with the provider as metformin may be at the time of the procedure and held for up to 48 hours. Renal function tests should be evaluated prior to restarting metformin (Rose & Choi, 2015).*

Allergic Reaction to Contrast Media

▲ Previous allergic reactions to contrast material, history of asthma, and other allergies are factors that may increase the client's risk of developing an adverse reaction. Discuss premedication with methylprednisolone or diphenhydramine with the provider for clients who have had previous reactions to contrast media or known asthma or allergies. *Premedication may reduce the incidence of allergic reaction in some clients (Rose & Choi, 2015; American College of Radiology, 2017b).*

▲ Monitor carefully for symptoms of a reaction, which can be mild, moderate, or severe. Report all symptoms to the provider because symptoms can advance rapidly from mild to severe.
   ○ *Mild reactions*: Nausea, vomiting, headache, itching, flushing, mild skin rash, or hives
   ○ *Moderate reactions*: Severe skin rash or hives, wheezing, abnormal heart rhythms, high or low blood pressure, shortness of breath, or difficulty breathing

● = Independent;   ▲ = Collaborative;   EBN = Evidence-Based Nursing;   EB = Evidence-Based

○ *Severe reactions*: Difficulty breathing, cardiac arrest, swelling of throat or other parts of the body, convulsion, or profound low blood pressure

○ *Both allergic and allergic-like (anaphylactoid) reactions can occur. Life-threatening events usually occur within 20 minutes after injection. Delayed reactions may occur with rash that appears hours or days afterward (American College of Radiology, 2017b).*

Vein Damage and Damage to Vascular Access Devices

● Recognize that *only* vascular access devices labeled "power injectable" can be used to administer power injected contrast media. These include a power port, a power peripherally inserted central catheter (PICC) line, and a power central venous catheter (*Radiology and Biomedical Imaging, 2017a*). *A regular vascular access device used for administration of contrast media can rupture from the high pressures used to administer the contrast media.* EB: *A retrospective study of the function of 204 power ports found that they are safe for use with power injections of contrast media (Goltz et al, 2012).*

● Reduce the risk of vein and vascular access device damage with the following:
  ○ Maintain constant communication with the client during the injection and monitor client for report of pain or swelling at the injection site. *These are signs of complications that require the injection to be discontinued (American College of Radiology, 2017a).*
  ○ Monitor access site for extravasation during and after the procedure; be vigilant for clients at increased risk of extravasation. *Clients at increased risk include those who cannot communicate such as infants, older adults, or those with altered consciousness; severely ill or debilitated clients; clients with abnormal circulation in the affected limb; clients receiving the injection via a peripheral IV line that has been in place for more than 24 hours or into a vein that has been punctured multiple times; and clients with arterial insufficiency or compromised venous or lymphatic drainage in the affected extremity (American College of Radiology, 2017a).*
  ○ Assess for venous backflow before injecting contrast. *If backflow is not obtained, the catheter may need adjustment (American College of Radiology, 2017a).*
  ○ Directly monitor and palpate the venipuncture site during the first 15 seconds of injection. *A critical step in preventing significant extravasation is direct monitoring of the venipuncture site (American College of Radiology, 2017a).*

Geriatric

● Screen the older client thoroughly before diagnostic testing using contrast media. *Adults over 60 years of age are considered at risk for acute adverse reactions to contrast media (Beckett, Moriority, & Langer, 2015).*

Pediatric

"When the proper technique is used, contrast medium can be safely administered intravenously by power injector at high flow rates of up to 2 mls/second (depending on size of patient). A short peripheral IV catheter in the antecubital or forearm is the preferred route for intravenous contrast administration" (Radiology and Biomedical Imaging, 2017b).

Client/Family Teaching and Discharge Teaching

Provide patient/family teaching on the importance of keeping appointments with provider for monitoring kidney status, reporting symptoms of fluid retention or decrease in urine output, and awareness of increased risk for CIN with repeat exposure to contrast media (Jorgensen, 2013).

REFERENCES

American College of Radiology. (2017a). *ACR manual on contrast media: Version 10.3.* Reston, VA: American College of Radiology.

American College of Radiology. (2017b). *Contrast material. Side effects and allergic reactions.* Retrieved from https://www.radiologyinfo.org/en/info.cfm?pg=safety-side-effects.

Balemans, C. E. A., Reichert, L., van Schelven, B., et al. (2012). Epidemiology of contrast material-induced nephropathy in the era of hydration. *Radiology,* 263(3), 706–713. doi:10.1148/radiol.12111667.

Beckett, K. R., Moriority, A. K., & Langer, J. M. (2015). Safe use of contrast media: What the radiologist needs to know.

Radiographics: A Review Publication of the Radiological Society of North America, Inc, 35, 1738–1750. doi:10.1148/rg.2015150033.

Cicin, I., Erdogan, B., Gulsen, E., et al. (2014). Incidence of contrast-induced nephropathy in hospitalized patients with cancer. *European Radiology,* 24(1), 184–190. doi:10.1007/s00330-013-2996-6.

Goltz, J. P., Noack, C., Petritsch, B., et al. (2012). Totally implantable venous power ports of the forearm and the chest: Initial clinical experience with port devices approved for high-pressure injections. *The British Journal of Radiology,* 85(1019), e966–e972. doi:10.1259/bjr/33224341.

● = Independent;   ▲ = Collaborative;   EBN = Evidence-Based Nursing;   EB = Evidence-Based

Islam, N., Majumder, A., Khalequzzaman, M., et al. (2013). Impact of blood glucose levels on contrast induced nephropathy after percutaneous coronary intervention in patients not known to be diabetic with acute coronary syndrome. *Cardiovascular Journal*, *6*(1), 23–30.

Jorgensen, A. L. (2013). Contrast-induced nephropathy: Pathophysiology and preventive strategies. *Critical Care Nurse*, *33*(1), 37–47. Retrieved from http://dx.doi.org/10.4037/ccn2013680.

Lambert, P., Chaisson, K., Horton, S., et al. (2017). Reducing acute kidney injury due to contrast material: How nurses can improve patient safety. *Critical Care Nurse*, *37*(1), 13–26. Retrieved from https://doi.org/10.4037/ccn2017178.

Radiology and Biomedical Imaging. (2017a). *Vascular access and use of central lines and ports in adults*. University of California San Francisco. Retrieved from http://www.radiology.ucsf.edu/patient-care/patient-safety/contrast/iodinated/vascular-access-adults.

Radiology and Biomedical Imaging. (2017b). *Vascular access and use of central lines and ports in pediatrics*. University of California San Francisco. Retrieved from https://radiology.ucsf.edu/patient-care/patient-safety/contrast/iodinated/vascular-access-pediatrics.

Rose, T. A., & Choi, J. W. (2015). Intravenous imaging contrast media complications: The basics that every clinician needs to know. *The American Journal of Medicine*, *128*(9), 943–949. doi:10.1016/j.amjmed.2015.02.018.

Readiness for enhanced community Coping   *Marina Martinez-Kratz, MS, RN, CNE*

NANDA-I

Definition

A pattern of community activities for adaptation and problem-solving for meeting the demands or needs of the community, which can be strengthened.

Defining Characteristics

Expresses desire to enhance availability of community recreation programs; expresses desire to enhance availability of community relaxation programs; expresses desire to enhance communication among community members; expresses desire to enhance communication between aggregates and larger community; expresses desire to enhance community planning for predictable stressors; expresses desire to enhance community resources for managing stressors; expresses desire to enhance community responsibility for stress management; expresses desire to enhance problem-solving for identified issue

NOC   (Nursing Outcomes Classification)

Suggested NOC Outcomes

Community Competence; Community Health Status

Example NOC Outcome with Indicators
Community Health Status as evidenced by the following indicators: Prevalence of health promotion programs, health status of infants, children, adolescents, adults, elders, participation rates in community health programs. (Rate the outcome and indicators of **Community Health Status:** 1 = poor, 2 = fair, 3 = good, 4 = very good, 5 = excellent [see Section I].)

Community Outcomes

Community Will (Specify Time Frame)

- Develop enhanced coping strategies
- Maintain effective coping strategies for management of stress

NIC   (Nursing Interventions Classification)

Suggested NIC Interventions

Environmental Management: Community; Health Policy Monitoring: Program Development

Example NIC Activities—Program Development
Assist the group or community in identifying significant health needs or problems; Identify alternative approaches to address the need(s) or problem(s)

● = Independent;   ▲ = Collaborative;   EBN = Evidence-Based Nursing;   EB = Evidence-Based

Nursing Interventions and *Rationales*

Note: Interventions depend on the specific aspects of community coping that can be enhanced (e.g., planning for stress management, communication, development of community power, community perceptions of stress, community coping strategies). *Nursing interventions are conducted in collaboration with key members of the community, community/public health nurses, and members of other disciplines (Anderson & McFarlane, 2011).*

▲ Establish a collaborative partnership with the community. EB: *A recent study found that counties whose Area Agencies for the Aging (AAAs) maintained informal partnerships with a broad range of organizations in health care and other sectors had significantly lower hospital readmission rates compared with counties whose AAAs had informal partnerships with fewer types of organizations (Brewster et al, 2018).*

● Assess community needs with the use of concept mapping methodology. EB: *The findings of a recent study showed that an integration of several concept mapping methods into a community engagement process was able to increase the input from a wide range of populations (Velonis et al, 2018).*

● Encourage participation in faith-based organizations that want to improve community stress management. EBN: *A recent study showed that coaching by faith community nurses created an environment of sustained support that promoted improved lifestyles and blood pressure changes over time (Cooper & Zimmerman, 2017).*

▲ Identify the health services and information resources that are currently available in the community through network analysis. EB: *A study found that network analysis served as a useful tool to evaluate community partnerships and facilitate coalition building (Ruopeng et al, 2017).*

● Work with community members to increase problem-solving abilities. EBN: *Problem-solving is essential for effective coping. Findings from a recent study showed positive outcomes from a direct and tailored problem-solving training program (Easom et al, 2018).*

● Provide support to the community and help community members identify and mobilize additional supports. EB: *A community mobilization project demonstrated how cross-sector, coordinated efforts focused on vulnerable populations can leverage local strengths to establish and enhance breastfeeding support services customized to local needs (Colchamiro et al, 2015).*

● Advocate for the community in multiple arenas (e.g., multimedia, social media, and governmental agencies). EB: *A recent study explored how social media can help community organizations engage in advocacy work (Guo et al, 2017).*

● Work with communities to ensure that vulnerable individuals with access and functional needs are included in preparations for, response to, and recovery from disasters. EB: *Analysis of recent disasters has identified that a combination of strategic and operational methods, appropriate planning tools, and planning for the entire community will prevent individuals with access and functional needs from being disproportionately and negatively affected by disasters (Franks & Seaton, 2017).*

● Write grant proposals to help community members obtain funds for programs that reduce stress or improve coping (Anderson & McFarlane, 2011).

● Work with members of the community to identify and develop coping strategies that promote a sense of power (e.g., obtaining sources for funding, collaborating with other communities) (Anderson & McFarlane, 2011).

Pediatric

● Protect children and adolescents from exposure to community violence. EB: *A systematic review found evidence for a positive association between community violence exposure and cardiovascular and sleep problems in children and adolescents (Wright et al, 2017).*

● Assess children and adolescents for the effects of direct and indirect crime exposure rather than only focusing solely on violent victimization. EB: *A study found poor behavioral health outcomes for adolescents with self-reported crime exposure (Grinshteyn et al, 2018).*

Multicultural

● Acknowledge the stressors unique to racial/ethnic communities. EB: *A recent study of Hispanic and African American women found that neighborhood context was an important factor in examining the determinants of health, survivorship, and quality of life outcomes among cancer patients (Wu et al, 2018).*

● Identify community strengths with community members. EBN: *A community-based participatory research approach was used to obtain Native American community input and identify strengths to address youth*

● = Independent;   ▲ = Collaborative;   EBN = Evidence-Based Nursing;   EB = Evidence-Based

C

suicide and substance abuse. The results led to the development of a strengths-based intervention incorporating the Gathering of Native American's curriculum (Holliday et al, 2018).

- Use an empowerment approach to address health behaviors in diverse communities. An empowerment approach includes increasing clients' self-efficacy and capacity to make informed decisions about their health care. **EB:** *A recent study found use of an empowerment approach was effective in changing nonadherent Latinas' breast screening behaviors and promoting them to become agents of change in their communities (Molina et al, 2018). The empowerment intervention has three sessions focused on early detection, sharing information with family/friends, and health volunteerism.*

- Work with members of the community to prioritize and target health goals specific to the community. **EB:** *Recent research found that members of underserved communities, in informed deliberations, prioritized research on quality of life, patient-doctor, special needs, access, and compare approaches (Goold et al, 2017).*

- Establish and sustain partnerships with key individuals within communities when developing and implementing programs. **EB:** *A study of community engagement strategies found the following techniques to be effective: proactively engaging stakeholders in informational meetings, webinars, social media, the promising practice process, and community advisory council meetings (D'Angelo et al, 2017).*

- Use mentoring strategies for community members. **EB:** *A recent study showed parent mentors are highly effective in insuring uninsured Latino children and eliminating disparities (Flores et al, 2018).*

- Use community church settings as a forum for advocacy, teaching, and program implementation. **EBN:** *A recent study found that trust, respect, open dialog with participants, and commitment to address community health needs contributed to successful engagement and recruitment of African American churches to serve as participants in cancer research projects (Slade et al, 2018).*

 Client/Family Teaching and Discharge Planning

- Review coping skills, power for coping, and the use of power resources.

REFERENCES

Anderson, E., & McFarlane, J. (2011). *Community as partner: Theory and practice in nursing* (6th ed.). Philadelphia: Wolters Kluwer/ Lippincott Willams & Wilkins.

Brewster, A. L., et al. (2018). Curry cross-sectoral partnerships by area agencies on aging: Associations with health care use and spending. *Health Affairs*, 37(1), 15–21. Retrieved from http://doi.org.proxy.lib .umich.edu/10.1377/hlthaff.2017.1346.

Colchamiro, R., et al. (2015). Mobilizing community resources to enhance post discharge support for breastfeeding in Massachusetts (USA): Results of a catalyst grant approach. *Journal of Human Lactation*, 31(4), 631–640. Retrieved from http://doi.org.proxy.lib .umich.edu/10.1177/089033441559768.

Cooper, J., & Zimmerman, W. (2017). The effect of a faith community nurse network and public health collaboration on hypertension prevention and control. *Public Health Nursing*, 34(5), 444–453. Retrieved from http://doi.org.proxy.lib.umich.edu/10.1111/ phn.12325.

D'Angelo, G., et al. (2017). Community engagement strategies for implementation of a policy supporting evidence-based practices: A case study of Washington state. *Administration and Policy in Mental Health and Mental Health Services Research*, 44(1), 6–15. Retrieved from http://doi.org.proxy.lib.umich.edu/10.1007/s10488-015 -0664-7.

Easom, L. R., et al. (2018). Operation family caregiver: Problem-solving training for military caregivers in a community setting. *Journal of Clinical Psychology*, 74, 536–553. Retrieved from http://doi.org .proxy.lib.umich.edu/10.1002/jclp.22536.

Flores, G., et al. (2018). Parent mentoring program increases coverage rates for uninsured Latino children. *Health Affairs*, 37(3), 403–412. doi:10.1377/hlthaff.2017.1272.

Franks, S., & Seaton, E. (2017). Utilizing strategic and operational methods for whole-community disaster planning. *Disaster Medicine and Public Health Preparedness*, 11(6), 741–746. doi:10.1017/dmp .2017.6.

Goold, S. D., et al. (2017). Priorities for patient-centered outcomes research: The views of minority and underserved communities. *Health Services Research*, 52(2), 599–615. doi:10.1111/1475-6773 .12505.

Grinshteyn, E. G., et al. (2018). *Community Mental Health Journal*, 54(3), 252–258. Retrieved from http://doi.org.proxy.lib.umich.edu/ 10.1007/s10597-017-0159-y.

Guo, C., et al. (2017). Speaking and being heard: How nonprofit advocacy organizations gain attention on social media. *Nonprofit and Voluntary Sector Quarterly*, 47(1), 5–26. Retrieved from http:// doi.org.proxy.lib.umich.edu/10.1177/0899764017713724.

Holliday, C. E., et al. (2018). A CBPR approach to finding community strengths and challenges to prevent youth suicide and substance abuse. *Journal of Transcultural Nursing*, 29(1), 64–73. Retrieved from http://doi.org.proxy.lib.umich.edu/10.1177/ 1043659616679234.

Molina, Y., et al. (2018). Empowering Latinas to obtain breast cancer screenings: Comparing intervention effects, part 2. *Cancer Epidemiology, Biomarkers & Prevention: A Publication of the American Association for Cancer Research*, 27(3), 353–354. doi:10.1158/1055-9965.EPI-18-0048.

Ruopeng, A., et al. (2017). Assessing the network of agencies in local communities that promote healthy eating and lifestyles among populations with limited resources. *American Journal of Health Behavior*, 41(2), 127–138. doi:10.5993/AJHB.41.2.3.

Slade, J., et al. (2018). Recruitment of African American churches to participate in cancer early detection interventions: A community perspective. *Journal of Religion and Health*, 57(2), 751–761. Retrieved from http://doi.org.proxy.lib.umich.edu/ 10.1007/s10943-018-0586-2.

● = Independent;   ▲ = Collaborative;   **EBN** = Evidence-Based Nursing;   **EB** = Evidence-Based

Velonis, A. J., et al. (2018). "One program that could improve health in this neighbourhood is _?" Using concept mapping to engage communities as part of a health and human services needs assessment. *BMC Health Services Research*, 18(1), 150. Retrieved from http://doi.org.proxy.lib.umich.edu/10.1186/s12913-018-2936-x.

Wright, A. W., et al. (2017). Systematic review: Exposure to community violence and physical health outcomes in youth. *Journal of Pediatric Psychology*, 42(4), 364–378. Retrieved from http://doi.org.proxy.lib.umich.edu/10.1093/jpepsy/jsw088.

Wu, C., et al. (2018). The association of neighborhood context with health outcomes among ethnic minority breast cancer survivors. *Journal of Behavioral Medicine*, 41(1), 52–61. Retrieved from http://doi.org.proxy.lib.umich.edu/10.1007/s10865-017-9875-6.

Defensive Coping   Marina Martinez-Kratz, MS, RN, CNE

NANDA-I

Definition

Repeated projection of falsely positive self-evaluation based on a self-protective pattern that defends against underlying perceived threats to positive self-regard.

Defining Characteristics

Alteration in reality testing; denial of problems; denial of weaknesses; difficulty establishing relationships; difficulty maintaining relationships; grandiosity; hostile laughter; hypersensitivity to a discourtesy; hypersensitivity to criticism; insufficient follow through with treatment; insufficient participation in treatment; projection of blame; projection of responsibility; rationalization of failures; reality distortion; ridicule of others; superior attitude toward others

Related Factors

Conflict between self-perception and value system; fear of failure; fear of humiliation; fear of repercussions; insufficient confidence in others; insufficient resilience; insufficient self-confidence; insufficient support system; uncertainty; unrealistic self-expectations

NOC   (Nursing Outcomes Classification)

Suggested NOC Outcomes

Coping; Decision-Making; Impulse Self-Control; Information Processing

---

Example NOC Outcome with Indicators

Coping as evidenced by the following indicators: Identifies effective and ineffective coping patterns/Modifies lifestyle to reduce stress. (Rate the outcome and indicators of **Coping:** 1 = never demonstrated, 2 = rarely demonstrated, 3 = sometimes demonstrated, 4 = often demonstrated, 5 = consistently demonstrated [see Section I].)

Client Outcomes

Client Will (Specify Time Frame)

- Acknowledge need for change in coping style
- Accept responsibility for own behavior
- Establish realistic goals with validation from caregivers
- Solicit caregiver validation in decision-making

NIC   (Nursing Interventions Classification)

Suggested Nursing Interventions

Body Image Enhancement; Complex Relationship Building; Coping Enhancement; Patient Contracting; Resiliency Promotion; Self-Awareness Enhancement; Self-Esteem Enhancement; Socialization Enhancement; Surveillance

● = Independent;   ▲ = Collaborative;   EBN = Evidence-Based Nursing;   EB = Evidence-Based

Example NIC Activities—Self-Awareness Enhancement
Encourage client to recognize and discuss thoughts and feelings; Assist client in identifying behaviors that are self-destructive

C

Nursing Interventions and *Rationales*

- Assess for possible symptoms associated with defensive coping: depressive symptoms, excessive self-focused attention, negativism and anxiety, hypertension, posttraumatic stress disorder (e.g., exposure to terrorism), substance use symptoms, unjust world beliefs. **EB:** *A study of the features of defensive coping behaviors found that alcohol-dependent women use coping avoidance, impulsive actions, and reactive formations more often than alcohol-dependent men, whereas alcohol-dependent men use intellectualization. Overall, alcohol-dependent men and women express higher levels of aggressive actions, compensation, and substitution (Chkhikvadze et al, 2018).*

- ▲ Use cognitive behavioral interventions. **EBN:** *In a randomized control trial (N = 240), 120 in each group (experimental and control), a nurse-led cognitive behavioral intervention addressed inaccurate thinking and promoted more positive self-regard; the experimental group had improved quality of life, which included physical and psychological health, relief of symptom, and social functioning (Zhuang et al, 2013).*

- Ask appropriate questions to assess whether denial (defensive coping) is being used in association with health problems including alcoholism, myocardial infarction (MI), or rheumatoid arthritis. **EBN:** *In a case-based article, Wilson (2013) demonstrated a nurse-provided approach to screening, brief intervention, and referral to treatment (SBIRT), which is an approach recommended by the Substance Abuse and Mental Health Services Administration (2015), in a client requiring a peripherally inserted central catheter for a man with liver disease caused by alcoholism.* **EB:** *In a 5-year prospective study of adults with rheumatoid arthritis (N = 74), researchers found that defensive coping impacted responses to pain and overall health, leading to poorer outcomes (Goulia et al, 2015).*

- Promote interventions with multisensory stimulation environments. **EB:** *In a review of the literature regarding sharing multisensory body space with others for those with altered bodies, such as amputations or congenital limb absence, researchers concluded that sharing multisensory body space is pertinent and may close the gap between neurology and psychiatry in the treatment of persons with altered bodies (Brugger & Lenggenhager, 2014).*

- Empower the client/caregiver's self-knowledge. **EB:** *In a qualitative study of adults receiving highly active antiretroviral treatment for HIV and methadone maintenance, participants described tension between negative feelings such as denial and positive feelings of empowerment (Batchelder et al, 2013).*

Geriatric

- ▲ Identify problems with alcohol in older adults with the appropriate tools and make suitable referrals. **EB:** *Community-dwelling older adults (N = 370) completed the Drinking Motives Questionnaire (DMQ); findings indicated that the most frequent motivation for drinking was social, with enhancement and coping motives, respectively, as the top three motivations (Gilson et al, 2013).* **CEB:** *Tools such as the Alcohol Use Disorders Identification Test (AUDIT), Michigan Alcohol Screening Test-Geriatric Version (MAST-G), and the Alcohol-Related Problems Survey (ARPS) may have additional use in this population. Brief interventions have been shown to be effective in producing sustained abstinence or reducing levels of consumption, decreasing hazardous and harmful drinking (Culberson, 2006).*

- Encourage exercise for positive coping. **EBN:** *One research group identified that exercise is known to facilitate maintenance of functional abilities in older adults and tested an intervention to encourage older adults (N = 106) to engage in physical activity (PA)/exercise using peer mentors. The researchers found high participation and retention and improved fitness scores in all mentored groups (Dorgo et al, 2013).* **EB:** *Researchers performed a secondary analysis of data to examine the use of PA in middle-aged and older adults during a smoking cessation attempt (N = 799). The researchers found that PA, primarily walking, was used by only a small percentage of participants (11.6%); women were more likely to use PA as a coping strategy than men. The researchers recommended further study and approaches that encourage older adults to engage in PA for general health and quality of life (Treviño et al, 2014).*

- Stimulate individual reminiscence therapy. **EBN:** *Structured reminiscence is an evidence-based, independent nursing intervention that is used with individuals and groups and is used to increase emotional awareness and enhance social interactions in older adults (Stinson & Long, 2014).*

● = Independent;   ▲ = Collaborative;   **EBN** = Evidence-Based Nursing;   **EB** = Evidence-Based

- Stimulate group reminiscence therapy. EBN: *Stinson's structured group reminiscence is a multisession evidence-based approach used with older adults (Stinson & Long, 2014). EB: A multimedia intergenerational reminiscence program was tested in a small (N = 26) group of community-dwelling older adults; qualitative data from stories and focus groups indicated that the intervention showed promise as a group intergenerational intervention (Chonody & Wang, 2013).*

 Multicultural

- Acknowledge racial/ethnic differences at the onset of care. EB: *In a qualitative study of white professionals working with racial minority immigrant clients, researchers found that although some professionals reported being comfortable discussing race and cultural differences, some expressed discomfort and difficulty, and others did not perceive race and culture to be a priority. The researchers recommended further attention to cultural competence training in clinical programs (Singer & Tummala-Narra, 2013).*
- Assess an individual's sociocultural backgrounds in teaching self-management and self-regulation. EBN: *A systematic review of qualitative evidence related to women's coping with type 2 diabetes indicated that in multiple countries self-management is challenged by the complexities of regimens and women's multiple caregiving roles. Researchers recommended recognition of the coping and emotional factors by health care providers, families, and friends; psychoeducation programs for clients and families; and enhanced support of family and friends (Li, Drury, & Taylor, 2014). EB: In a study of the Cellie Coping Kit for Sickle Cell Disease, researchers provided the intervention to 15 black/African American children aged 6 to 14 years and their health care provider. Although the researchers reported strong acceptability, some sociocultural issues like living situation and health literacy did provide challenges to the use of the tool (Marsac et al, 2014).*
- Encourage the client to use spiritual coping mechanisms such as faith and prayer. CEB/EBN: *In a qualitative study of Thai Buddhist and Muslim women's (N = 48) use of religion and spiritual practices related to self-management of type 2 diabetes, researchers found four themes that related to cultural or spiritual practices, including prayer, which helped them cope, despite poor glycemic control (Lundberg & Thrakul, 2013). EB: In a study of religion and coping with racial discrimination among African American (N = 2032) and Caribbean blacks (N = 857), researchers found that both groups were similar in their likelihood of using prayer for coping with discrimination (Hayward & Krause, 2015).*
- Encourage spirituality as a source of support for coping. EBN: *In a small (N = 17) pilot study of African American women with breast cancer, women reported high levels of spiritual and positive religious coping (sense of purpose in life) strategies such as prayer. Researchers recommended that although the findings of the pilot are not generalizable, spirituality and religious coping need to be explored as core coping mechanisms for African American women with breast cancer (Gaston-Johansson et al, 2013).*

 Home Care

- ▲ Refer the client for programs that teach coping skills. EB: *Researchers examining bullying and the association with cultural/family factors, substance use, and depressive symptoms in ninth and tenth grade Hispanic youth (N = 1167) found the stress of acculturation was associated with substance use and depressive symptoms and the need for the development of coping skills in youth. Recommendations included school-based programs to teach coping skills (Forster et al, 2013).*

 Client/Family Teaching and Discharge Planning

- Teach coping skills to clients and caregivers. EBN: *In a trial of a culturally adapted cognitive behavioral therapy intervention to promote coping skills among Chinese Americans with type 2 diabetes, strategies and coping skills that addressed personal, family, and illness-specific topics were included; researchers reported enhanced efficacy for self-management (Chesla et al, 2013).*
- Teach reflexive and expressive writing to address emotions. EBN: *Journaling was used in an intervention study to enhance civility among nursing students; researchers found coping improvements in self-controlling and positive reappraisal (Jenkins et al, 2013). EB: In a randomized trial of expressive writing in the third person, 44 undergraduates wrote about their deepest thoughts and feelings about a traumatic or very stressful life event; findings included less intrusive thinking in both groups, but third-person writers had better outcomes in overall health than did the first-person writers. Researchers recommend third-person expressive writing for those recovering from traumatic or highly stressful events (Andersson & Conley, 2013).*

● = Independent;　▲ = Collaborative;　EBN = Evidence-Based Nursing;　EB = Evidence-Based

REFERENCES

Refer to ineffective **Coping** for additional references.

Andersson, M. A., & Conley, C. S. (2013). Optimizing the perceived benefits and health outcomes of writing about traumatic life events. *Stress and Health: Journal of the International Society for the Investigation of the Stress, 29*, 40–49.

Batchelder, A. W., Brisban, M., Litwin, A. H., et al. (2013). "Damaging what wasn't damaged already": Psychological tension and antiretroviral adherence among HIV-infected methadone-maintained drug users. *AIDS Care, 25*, 1370–1374.

Brugger, P., & Lenggenhager, B. (2014). The bodily self and its disorders: Neurological, psychological, and social aspects. *Current Opinion in Neurology, 27*, 644–652.

Chesla, C. A., Chun, K. M., Kwan, C. M. L., et al. (2013). Testing the efficacy of culturally adapted coping skills training for Chinese American immigrants with type 2 diabetes using community-based participatory research. *Research in Nursing & Health, 36*, 359–372.

Chkhikvadze, T. V., et al. (2018). Peculiarities of coping and mechanisms of psychological defense in persons with alcohol dependence. *Vestnik Rossijskogo Universiteta Družby Narodov: Seriâ Psihologiâ i Pedagogika,* (1), 94–108. doi:10.22363/2313-1683-2018-15-1-94-108.

Chonody, J., & Wang, D. (2013). Connecting older adults to the community through multimedia: An intergenerational reminiscence program. *Activities, Adaptation, & Aging, 37*, 79–93.

Culberson, J. W. (2006). Alcohol use in the elderly: Beyond the CAGE. Part 2: Screening instruments and treatment strategies. *Geriatrics, 61*(11), 20–26.

Dorgo, S., King, G. A., Bader, J. O., et al. (2013). Outcomes of a peer mentor implemented fitness program in older adults: A quasi-randomized controlled trial. *International Journal of Nursing Studies, 50*, 1156–1165.

Forster, M., Dyal, S. R., Baezconde-Garbanati, L., et al. (2013). Bullying victimization as a mediator of associations between cultural/familial variables, substance use, and depressive symptoms among Hispanic youth. *Ethnicity & Health, 18*, 415–432.

Gaston-Johansson, F., Haisfield-Wolfe, M. E., Reddick, B., et al. (2013). The relationships among coping strategies, religious coping, and spirituality in African American women with breast cancer receiving chemotherapy. *Oncology Nursing Forum, 40*, 120–131.

Gilson, K., Bryant, C., Bei, B., et al. (2013). Validation of the drinking motives questionnaire in older adults. *Addictive Behaviors, 38*, 2196–2202.

Goulia, P., Voulgari, P. V., Tsifetaki, N., et al. (2015). Sense of coherence and self-sacrificing defense style as predictors of psychological distress and quality of life in rheumatoid arthritis: A 5-year prospective study. *Rheumatology International, 35*, 691–700.

Hayward, R. D., & Krause, N. (2015). Religion and strategies for coping with racial discrimination among African Americans and Caribbean blacks. *International Journal of Stress Management, 22*, 70–91.

Jenkins, S. D., Kerber, C. S., & Woith, W. M. (2013). An intervention to promote civility among nursing students. *Nursing Education Perspectives, 34*, 95–100.

Li, J., Drury, V., & Taylor, B. (2014). A systematic review of the experience of older women living and coping with type 2 diabetes. *International Journal of Nursing Practice, 20*, 126–134.

Lundberg, P. C., & Thrakul, S. (2013). Religion and self-management of Thai Buddhist and Muslim women with type 2 diabetes. *Journal of Clinical Nursing, 22*, 1907–1916.

Marsac, M. L., Alderfer, M. A., Smith-Whitely, K., et al. (2014). *Clinical Practice in Pediatric Psychology, 2*, 389–399.

Singer, R. R., & Tummala-Narra, P. (2013). White clinicians' perspectives on working with racial minority immigrant clients. *Professional Psychology, Research and Practice, 44*, 290–298.

Stinson, C., & Long, E. M. (2014). Reminiscence: Improving the quality of life for older adults. *Geriatric Nursing, 35*, 399–404.

Substance Abuse and Mental Health Services Administration. (2015). *Screening, brief intervention, and referral to treatment (SBIRT).* Retrieved from http://www.samhsa.gov/sbirt.

Treviño, L. A., Baker, L., McIntosh, S., et al. (2014). Physical activity as a coping strategy for smoking cessation in mid-life and older adults. *Addictive Behaviors, 39*, 885–888.

Wilson, K. M. (2013). Integrating procedural care with addiction support: An example from a PICC nurse. *Medsurg Nursing, 22*, 128–135.

Zhuang, S., An, S., & Zhao, Y. (2013). Effect of cognitive behavioral interventions on the quality of life in Chinese heroin-dependent individuals in detoxification: A randomized controlled trial. *Journal of Clinical Nursing, 23*, 1239–1248.

Ineffective Coping   *Arlene T. Farren, PhD, RN, AOCN, CTN-A, CNE*

NANDA-I

Definition

A pattern of invalid appraisal of stressors, with cognitive and/or behavioral efforts, that fails to manage demands related to well-being.

Defining Characteristics

Alteration in concentration; alteration in sleep pattern; change in communication pattern; destructive behavior toward others; destructive behavior toward self; difficulty organizing information; fatigue; frequent illness; inability to ask for help; inability to attend to information; inability to deal with a situation; inability to meet basic needs; inability to meet role expectation; ineffective coping strategies; insufficient access of social support; insufficient goal directed behavior; insufficient problem resolution; insufficient problem-solving skills; risk taking behavior; substance misuse

● = Independent;   ▲ = Collaborative;   EBN = Evidence-Based Nursing;   EB = Evidence-Based

Related Factors

High degree of threat; inability to conserve adaptive energies; inaccurate threat appraisal; inadequate confidence in ability to deal with a situation; inadequate opportunity to prepare for stressor; inadequate resources; ineffective tension release strategies; insufficient sense of control; insufficient social support

At-Risk Population

Maturational crisis; situational crisis

 (Nursing Outcomes Classification)

Suggested NOC Outcomes

Coping; Decision-Making; Impulse Self-Control; Information Processing

Example NOC Outcome with Indicators
Coping as evidenced by the following indicators: Identifies effective and ineffective coping patterns/Modifies lifestyle to reduce stress. (Rate the outcome and indicators of **Coping:** 1 = never demonstrated, 2 = rarely demonstrated, 3 = sometimes demonstrated, 4 = often demonstrated, 5 = consistently demonstrated [see Section I].)

Client Outcomes

Client Will (Specify Time Frame)

- Use effective coping strategies
- Use behaviors to decrease stress
- Remain free of destructive behavior toward self or others
- Report decrease in physical symptoms of stress
- Report increase in psychological comfort
- Seek help from a health care professional as appropriate

NIC **(Nursing Interventions Classification)**

Suggested NIC Interventions

Coping Enhancement; Decision-Making Support

Example NIC Activities—Coping Enhancement
Assist the client in developing an objective appraisal of the event; Explore with the client previous methods of dealing with life problems

Nursing Interventions and *Rationales*

- Observe for contributing factors of ineffective coping such as poor self-concept, grief, lack of problem-solving skills, lack of support, recent change in life situation, maturational or situational crises. EBN: *Factors predicting maladaptive coping in a small sample of sexual minority men (N = 89) included experiences of intimate partner sexual victimization and intimate partner violence resulting in injury (Goldberg-Looney et al, 2016). EBN: Following infant hospitalization in the neonatal intensive care, researchers identified that mothers experienced greater stress than the fathers with previous miscarriages and the presence of chronic diseases being statistically significant risks for posttraumatic stress disorder in this sample (Aftyka et al, 2017). EB: In a longitudinal study of children and their parents (N = 1064), children living in homes with parental violence were at risk for developing ineffective coping strategies in early adulthood (Jester et al, 2015).*
- Use verbal and nonverbal therapeutic communication approaches including empathy, active listening, and confrontation to encourage the client and family to express emotions such as sadness, guilt, and anger (within appropriate limits); verbalize fears and concerns; and set goals. EBN: *In a qualitative study using focus groups to understand nurses' (N = 27) experiences of presence, researchers found empathy, active listening, and use of silence were among the therapeutic communication approaches that were required to implement presence and improve client outcomes (Stockmann et al, 2016). EB: A survey of people living with*

● = Independent; ▲ = Collaborative; EBN = Evidence-Based Nursing; EB = Evidence-Based

C

spasticity (N = 281) about their experiences and expectations, concluded that there were unmet needs regarding communication and therapeutic relationships with health care providers (Barnes et al, 2017).

- Collaborate with the client to identify strengths such as the ability to relate the facts and to recognize the source of stressors. EBN: *Strength-based nursing (SBN) is a philosophical approach that includes eight values including a collaborative partnership with clients and families (Gottlieb & Gottlieb, 2017).*
- Encourage the client to describe previous stressors and the coping mechanisms used. EB: *A review examining endometriosis and behavioral, cognitive, and emotional coping strategies found that despite mixed results, clinician should engage in an evaluation of women's coping strategies to promote well-being and minimize poor mental health outcomes (Zarbo et al, 2018).*
- Provide opportunities for the client to discuss the meaning the situation might have for the client. EBN: *A qualitative study of the coping experiences of spouses of people with dementia found that spouses search each day for meaning while experiencing stress and using coping strategies (Myhre et al, 2018).* EBN: *A phenomenological study of adults living with diabetes (N = 13) found that the meanings of trigger situations were an opportunity for learning (Kneck et al, 2016).*
- Assist the client to set realistic goals and identify personal skills and knowledge. EBN: *Multiple interviews with 33 nonmetastatic breast cancer clients revealed that some experienced personal goal interference and required goal-based psychosocial support from oncology nurses and other professionals to overcome interference, which can lead to clinical depression (Stefanic et al, 2015).* EBN: *Setting realistic goals is recommended as part of the support needed during weight loss programs (Fruh, 2017).* EB: *In a quantitative study of 272 university students, researchers learned that positive affective states and autonomous goal motivation predicted positive coping (Blouin-Hudon, Gaudreau, & Gareau, 2016).*
- Provide information regarding care before care is given. EBN: *Researchers surveyed 45 family members with a client in the intensive care unit and found that one of the most important needs was related to information about the client and the care provided (Jacob et al, 2016).*
- Discuss changes with the client before making them. EBN: *In a review of evidence about minimally invasive, robotic-assisted cancer surgery, researchers recommended that nursing care should focus on providing information and preparation to patients and families for shorter hospital stays (Sun & Fong, 2017).* EN: *In a study (N = 451) about transfer of patients from an intensive care unit to inpatient unit, researchers learned that informing the client/family in advance about impending transfers would contribute to improving the process (Stelfox et al, 2017).*
- Provide mental and physical activities within the client's ability (e.g., reading, television, radio, crafts, outings, movies, dinners out, social gatherings, exercise, sports, games). EB: *Physical activity contributes indirectly to coping efficacy in middle-aged women (N = 103) experiencing menopausal symptoms (Kishida & Elavsky, 2015).*
- Discuss the power of the client and family to change a situation or the need to accept a situation. EB: *Cox et al (2016) conducted a secondary analysis of data from participants (N = 1189) in the Childhood Cancer Survivor Study to examine selected unmet needs and found that 51% of participants reported unmet information needs related to cancer/treatment.*
- Offer instruction regarding alternative coping strategies. EBN: *Motivational interviewing is a supportive strategy that helps elicit client perspectives and can promote coping (Carr, 2016).* EBN: *Mills, Wong-Anuchit, and Poogpan (2017) conducted a concept analysis of Thum-jai, a Thai coping strategy, and discussed the consequences or outcomes, which include emotional stability, positive thought, and productive change. It is recommended as an alternate coping strategy.*
- Encourage use of spiritual resources as desired. EBN: *Researchers found that in bereaved parents (N = 165) black mothers and Protestant and Catholic parents commonly used religious coping practices, and mothers were more likely to use spiritual and religious coping than fathers (Hawthorne, Youngblut, & Brooten, 2017).* EBN: *Clark and Hunter (2018) conducted a literature review (N = 30) regarding spiritual coping in clients with advanced heart failure and recommend Reed's Theory of Self-Transcendence as a foundation for examining individual's perspectives of their vulnerability and understanding how it affects one's sense of meaning.*
- Encourage use of social support resources. EBN: *Aftyka et al (2017) found mothers (N = 72) of infants in the neonatal intensive care unit (NICU) were more likely than fathers (N = 53) to engage in coping strategies such as venting of emotions and instrumental support.*
- ▲ Refer for additional or more intensive therapies as needed. EB: *More complex interventions are available to assist with coping; for example, a randomized controlled trial of older adults in the community found that mindfulness and a self-compassion program consisting of 10, 2-hour sessions were successful in improving coping strategies (Perez-Blasco et al, 2016).*

● = Independent;   ▲ = Collaborative;   EBN = Evidence-Based Nursing;   EB = Evidence-Based

C

Pediatric

- Monitor the client's risk of harming self or others and intervene appropriately. QSEN: See care plan for Risk for **Suicide**. EBN: *In a study of 140 Taiwanese secondary school students, resourcefulness as a coping strategy was associated with depressive symptoms (r = –0.35, P < .001) and self-harm (r = –0.29, P ≤ .001) (Yang et al, 2017).*
- Monitor adolescents for exposure to community violence. EB: *Researchers found support that active coping mediates exposure to violence and externalizing symptoms in a predominately low-income African American and Latino sample (Carothers et al, 2016). EB: A group intervention (five, 1-hour sessions) modeled after the "Listen to the Children" approach was delivered to 74 African American children and adolescents aged 5 to 19. Chosen discussion topics included bullying, community violence, loss of a loved one, incarceration of a loved one, and conflict. Participants liked the discussion and reported improved feelings, behaviors, and increased hope; parents reported improved behaviors in their children (Allen et al, 2016). EB: In a sample of LGBTQ adolescents aged 13 to 20 attending a HATCH Youth Program, those with longer attendance reported greater social support and improved coping ability. The HATCH program is a series of group sessions. Participants attending 1 to 6 months did have benefits, whereas participants attending 1 month or less did not (Wilkerson et al, 2017).*

Geriatric

- ▲ Assess and report possible physiological alterations (e.g., sepsis, hypoglycemia, hypotension, infection, changes in temperature, fluid and electrolyte imbalances, use of medications with known cognitive and psychotropic side effects). EBN: *Researchers supported the idea that caregivers of older stroke survivors have significant physical and mental comorbidities after conducting a prospective, exploratory study of uncertainty in caregivers of older adults poststroke (Eeseung et al, 2016). EBN: Researchers examined stressful life events in adults aged 55 to 99 and found that health problems were among the most stressful for older adults (Rubio et al, 2016).*
- Screen for elder neglect or other forms of elder mistreatment. EBN/EB: *There is no gold standard for assessment of elder neglect, abuse, or mistreatment. There are several literature reviews exploring best practices for assessment and intervention (Fearing et al, 2017; Hirst et al, 2016; Moore & Browne, 2017) and several studies examining potential screening tools (Cannell et al, 2016; Friedman et al, 2017; Pickering et al, 2017).*
- Encourage the client to make choices (as appropriate) and participate in planning care and scheduled activities. EB: *Researchers found older adults preferred active engagement in making health care decisions, but the preference may be different for those with more comorbidities (four or more) (Chi et al, 2017).*
- Target selected coping mechanisms for older persons based on client features, use, and preferences. EB: *In a small qualitative study of older adults with mild dementia, researchers found three themes related to psychological support, one of which was coping mechanisms. The mechanisms included were asserting control, engaging in new activities, and using humor (Birtwell & Dubrow-Marshal, 2018).*
- Increase and mobilize support available to older persons by encouraging a variety of mechanisms involving family, friends, peers, and health care providers. CEBN: *A trial of a nursing intervention to facilitate older adult access to community resources and remain at home found that the older adults accepted that the intervention had improved health empowerment, purposeful participation in goal attainment, and well-being (Shearer, Fleury, & Belyea, 2010). EB: Families give older adults important psychological support for coping with functional disabilities, pain, and other health issues (Honn Quails, 2016).*
- Actively listen to complaints and concerns. EBN: *During the working phase of Peplau's theory, holistic communication includes the use of active listening to promote the older adult patient's development of a deeper connection with the nurse; active listening and focusing are essential holistic communication skills (Deane & Fain, 2016). EB: A focus on active listening and not interrupting the patient are among key features of patient-centered communication skills (Hashim, 2017).*
- Engage the client in reminiscence. EBN: *A study of older adults with dementia living in a nursing home implemented a combined intervention of music reminiscence therapy with reality orientation techniques. Researchers found positive improvements in depression in the intervention group and recommended further research of the efficacy of the intervention (Onieva-Zafra et al, 2018).*

Multicultural

- Assess for the influence of cultural beliefs, norms, and values on the client's perceptions of effective coping. EB: *Researchers found that in a sample of African American college students (N = 191), a variety of past messages regarding racial socialization may predict race-specific coping in AA college students (Blackmon et al, 2016).*

- Assess for intergenerational family problems that can overwhelm coping abilities. **EBN:** *A study of Chinese family caregivers revealed family expectations to provide care, but family resources contributed to coping, and a sense of self-sacrifice by the caregivers (Qiu, Sit, & Koo, 2018).* **EB:** *A study conducted in South Pacific and Asian cultures found a relationship between problem gambling between parents and participants; the researchers suggested that expectancies and motives about gambling may help to target interventions for offspring of problem gamblers (Dowling et al, 2018).*
- Negotiate with the client regarding aspects of coping behavior that will need to be modified. **QSEN/EBN:** *Adolescents are less likely to engage in help-seeking behaviors, which places them at greater risk for self-harm and suicide; resourcefulness has been found to be negatively and significantly related to self-harm in Taiwanese adolescents (Yang et al, 2017). Likewise, a study of rural American adolescents found that life events and use of positive coping strategies can make a significant difference toward positive outcomes (Rew et al, 2016).*
- Encourage moderate aerobic exercise or other forms of physical activity (as appropriate). **EB:** *Black and Kashikar-Zuck (2017) proposed a novel intervention for juvenile fibromyalgia that combined neuromuscular training and cognitive-behavioral therapy to aid in coping with pain. The training is called the Fibromyalgia Integrative Training for Teens Program or FIT Teens.*
- Identify which family members the client can count on for support. **EBN:** *In Madurai women who underwent hysterectomy (N = 60), researchers found that family support was associated with coping and quality of life and concluded that support from the partner is especially important to both coping and quality of life (Shanthi & Jeyapal, 2016).*
- Support the inner resources that clients use for coping. **EBN:** *Researchers in the United States and Asia have found evidence that supports that self-transcendence is an inner resource for coping and well-being in a variety of populations and situations; the effects of inner resources, such as resilience, self-adjustments, and getting out of oneself for the interest of others, are ways to enhance self-transcendence and meaning in life (Ho et al, 2016; Haase et al, 2017).*
- Use an empowerment framework to redefine coping strategies. **EBN:** *Canadian researchers tested an intervention based on a Caregiver Grief Model that enhanced empowerment and coping in caregivers of people with dementia (MacCourt et al, 2017).*

Home Care

- The interventions described previously may be adapted for home care use.
- ▲ **QSEN:** Assess for suicidal tendencies. Refer for mental health care immediately if indicated.
- ▲ **QSEN:** Identify an emergency plan should the client become suicidal. Ineffective coping can occur in a crisis situation and can lead to suicidal ideation if the client sees no hope for a solution. A suicidal client is not safe in the home environment unless supported by professional help. Refer to the care plan for Risk for **Suicide.**
- Discuss preferred coping strategies of family caregivers. **EBN:** *Coping style and strategies may differ from individual to individual. Gender has been identified as one variant. For example, in family member caregivers (N = 308) of terminally ill cancer patients in Austria, women are more likely to prefer and benefit from adaptive coping strategies that deal with the demands of caregiving and working outside the home (Schrank et al, 2016).*
- Encourage the client to participate knowingly in their care. Refer to the care plan for **Powerlessness.** **EBN:** *Caregivers of school-age female children in Haiti participated in a health patterning modality that included storytelling, goal identification, educational session, and distribution of needed resources to enhance the caregivers' knowing participation in change. The researcher concluded that people can participate knowingly in their care and that knowing participation can be enhanced by relating with clients in a variety of ways (Leveille-Tulce, 2017). EBN: In a study of obstetric nurses, Heelan-Francher (2016) found that power as knowing participation in change had the greatest impact on patient advocacy.*
- ▲ Refer the client and family to support groups. **EB:** *A study of adolescents and adults with neurofibromatosis type 1 (NF1), a genetic, progressive disorder, explored knowledge of the disease, self-esteem, and the impact of support groups. Researchers found that participation in support groups had an influence on self-esteem and recommended that health care professionals inform clients about support groups (Rosnau et al, 2017).*
- ▲ If monitoring medication use, contract with the client or solicit assistance from a responsible caregiver. **EBN:** *Spoelstra et al (2016) have developed a clinical trial to test a multipronged approach to enhance*

adherence to oral anticancer medication regimens for both patients and caregivers; it involves education about self-management and medication teaching, motivational interviewing, and cognitive behavioral approaches.

▲ Institute case management for frail elderly clients to support continued independent living. **EBN:** *Nurse-led community care for the oldest old that includes care coordination and follow-up could preserve functioning in the oldest-old in the community (Bleijenberg et al, 2017).* **EB:** *A study examining tablet and Skype use in a case management program for frail older adults found that the participants had positive experiences with the technology as a means of communicating with case managers (Berner et al, 2016).*

 ### Client/Family Teaching and Discharge Planning

● Teach the client to problem solve. Have the client define the problem and cause, and list the advantages and disadvantages of the options. **EB:** *A problem-solving intervention that included defining the problem and goals, listing multiple solutions, and selecting a solution found improved task-oriented coping, avoidant coping, and generic health-related quality of life (Visser et al, 2016).*

● Teach relaxation techniques. **EBN:** *Nurses in Turkey provided relaxation exercise training to postmenopausal women with insomnia (N = 81 in intervention group and 80 in control group) once per week for 8 weeks in addition to teaching sleep hygiene measures. The researchers concluded that the statistically significant reduction in insomnia suggested that nurses' teaching of progressive relaxation techniques coupled with sleep hygiene training was an effective approach to improving insomnia in postmenopausal women (Duman & Taşhan, 2018).*

● Work closely with the client to develop appropriate educational tools that address individualized needs. **EB:** *A participatory project to develop patient education materials for older adults about lung stereotactic body radiotherapy (SBRT) involved patients at each step of the process. Participants had high health literacy and home Internet access, but researchers found that the participants had a preference for written and verbal teaching about the SBRT procedure (Jewitt et al, 2016).*

▲ Teach the client about available community resources (e.g., therapists, ministers, counselors, self-help groups). **EBN:** *Easom, Cotter, and Ramos (2018) conducted a postparticipation examination of the Resources for Enhancing Alzheimer's Caregiver Health (REACH II) program provided to African American and Caucasian caregivers of people with Alzheimer's disease and found it to be a culturally appropriate and effective program.*

REFERENCES

Aftyka, A., Rybojad, B., Rosa, W., et al. (2017). Risk factors for the development of post-traumatic stress disorder and coping strategies in mothers and fathers following infant hospitalization in neonatal intensive care unit. *Journal of Clinical Nursing, 26*, 4436–4445. doi:10.1111/jocn.13773.

Allen, S. F., Pfefferbaum, B., Nitiema, P., et al. (2016). Resilience and coping intervention with children and adolescents in at risk neighborhoods. *Journal of Loss & Trauma, 21*, 85–98.

Barnes, M., Kocer, S., Murie Fernandez, M., et al. (2017). An international survey of patients living with spasticity. *Disability & Rehabilitation, 39*, 1428–1434. doi:10.1080/09638288.1198432.

Berner, J., Anderberg, P., Rennemark, M., et al. (2016). Case management for frail older adults through tablet computers and Skype. *Informatics for Health & Social Care, 41*, 405–416. doi:10.3109/17538157.2015.1033528.

Birtwell, K., & Dubrow-Marshal, L. (2018). Psychological support for people with dementia: A preliminary study. *Counseling & Psychotherapy Research, 18*(1), 79–88. doi:10.1002/capr.12154.

Black, W. R., & Kashikar-Zuck, S. (2017). Exercise interventions for juvenile fibromyalgia: Current state and recent advancements. *Pain Management, 7*(3), 143–148.

Blackmon, S. M., Coyle, L. D., Davenport, S., et al. (2016). Linking racial-ethnic socialization to culture and race-specific coping among African-American college students. *Journal of Black Psychology, 42*, 549–576. doi:10.1177/0095798415617865.

Bleijenberg, N., Imhof, L., Mahrer-Imhof, R., et al. (2017). Patient characteristics associated with a successful response to nurse-led care programs targeting the oldest-old: A comparison of two RCTs. *Worldviews on Evidence-based Nursing, 14*(3), 210–222.

Blouin-Hudon, E. C., Gaudreau, P., & Gareau, A. (2016). Coping as a building mechanism to explain the unique association of affect and goal motivation with changes in affective states. *Anxiety, Stress, & Coping, 29*, 519–532. Retrieved from http://dx.doi.org/10.108 0/10615806.2015.1100298.

Cannell, M. B., Jetelina, K. K., Zovadsky, M., et al. (2016). Towards the development of a screening tool to enhance detection of elder abuse and neglect by emergency medical technicians. *BMC Emergency Medicine, 16*, 1–10.

Carothers, K. J., Arizaga, J. A., Carter, J. S., et al. (2016). Costs and benefits of active coping for adolescents residing in urban poverty. *Journal of Youth and Adolescence, 45*, 1323–1337. doi:10.1007/s10964-016-0487-1.

Carr, D. D. (2016). Motivational interviewing supports patient centered-care and communication. *Journal of the New York State Nurses Association, 45*(1), 39–43.

Chi, W. C., Wolff, J., Greer, R., et al. (2017). Multimorbidity and decision-making preferences among older adults. *Annals of Family Medicine, 15*, 546–551. doi:10.1370/afm.2106.

Clark, C. C., & Hunter, J. (2018). Spirituality, spiritual well-being, and spiritual coping in advanced heart failure. *Journal of Holistic Nursing*. doi:10.1177/0898010118761401.

Cox, C. L., Zhu, L., Ojha, R. P., et al. (2016). *Journal of Cancer Survivorship, 10*, 743–758. doi:10.1007/s11764-016-0520-0.

Deane, W. H., & Fain, J. A. (2016). Incorporating Peplau's theory of interpersonal relations to promote holistic communication between older adults and nursing students. *Journal of Holistic Nursing, 34*(1), 35–41. doi:10.1177/0898010115577975.

● = Independent;   ▲ = Collaborative;   **EBN** = Evidence-Based Nursing;   **EB** = Evidence-Based

C

Dowling, N. A., Oldenhof, E., Shandley, K., et al. (2018). The intergenerational transmission of problem gambling: The mediating role of offspring gambling expectancies and motives. *Addictive Behaviors*, 77, 16–20. doi:10.1016/j.addbeh.2017.09.003.

Duman, M., & Taşhan, S. T. (2018). The effect of sleep hygiene education and relaxation exercises on insomnia among postmenopausal women: A randomized clinical trial. *International Journal of Nursing Practice*, e12650. doi:10.1111/ijn.12650.

Easom, L., Cotter, E., & Ramos, A. (2018). Comparison of African American and Caucasian caregiver self-efficacy. *Journal of Gerontological Nursing*, 44(3), 16–21. doi:10.3928/00989134 -20171023-01.

Eeseung, B., Riegel, B., Sommers, M., et al. (2016). Caregiving immediately after stroke: A student of uncertainty in caregivers of older adults. *Journal of Neuroscience Nursing*, 48, 343–351. doi:10.1097/JNN.0000000000000238.

Fearing, G., Sheppard, C. L., McDonald, L., et al. (2017). A systematic review on community based interventions for elder abuse and neglect. *Journal of Elder Abuse & Neglect*, 29(2/3), 102–133. doi:10.1080/08946566.2017.1308286.

Friedman, L. S., Avila, S., Liu, E., et al. (2017). Using clinical signs of neglect to identify elder neglect cases. *Journal of Elder Abuse & Neglect*, 29, 270–287. doi:10.1080/08946566.2017.1352551.

Fruh, S. M. (2017). Obesity: Risk factors, complications, and strategies for sustainable long-term weight management. *Journal of the American Association of Nurse Practitioners*, 29, S3–S14. doi:10.1002/2327-6924.12510.

Goldberg-Looney, L. D., Perrin, P. B., Snipes, D. J., et al. (2016). Coping styles used by sexual minority men who experience intimate partner violence. *Journal of Clinical Nursing*, 25, 3687–3696. doi:10.1111/jocn.13388.

Gottlieb, L. N., & Gottlieb, B. (2017). Strengths-based nursing: A process for implementing a philosophy into practice. *Journal of Family Nursing*, 23, 319–340. doi:10.1177/1074840717717731.

Hashim, M. J. (2017). Patient-centered communication: Basic skills. *American Family Physician*, 95(1), 29–34.

Haase, J. E., Kintner, E. K., Robb, S. L., et al. (2017). The resilience in illness model part 2: Confirmatory evaluation in adolescents and young adults with cancer. *Cancer Nursing*, 40, 454–463.

Hawthorne, D. M., Youngblut, J. A., & Brooten, D. (2017). Use of spiritual coping strategies by gender, race/ethnicity, and religion at 1 and 3 months after infant's/child's intensive care unit death. *Journal of the American Association of Nurse Practitioners*, 29, 591–599. doi:10.1002/2327-6924.12498.

Heelan-Francher, L. M. (2016). Patient advocacy in an obstetric setting. *Nursing Science Quarterly*, 29, 3316–3327. doi:10.1177/08943318416660531.

Hirst, S. P., Penney, T., McNeil, S., et al. (2016). Best practice guidelines for prevention of abuse/neglect of older adults. *Canadian Journal on Aging*, 35, 242–260. doi:10.1017/S0714980816000209.

Ho, H., Tseng, Y., Hsin, Y., et al. (2016). Living with illness and self-transcendence: The lived experience of patients with spinal muscular atrophy. *Journal of Advanced Nursing*, 72, 2695–2705. doi:10.1111/jan.13042.

Honn Quails, S. (2016). Caregiving families within the long-term services and support systems for older adults. *American Psychologist*, 71(4), 283–293. doi:10.1037/a0040252.

Jacob, M., Horton, C., Rance-Ashley, S., et al. (2016). Needs of patients' family members in an intensive care unit with continuous visitation. *American Journal of Critical Care*, 25, 118–125. Retrieved from http://dx.doi.org/10.4037/ajcc2016258.

Jester, J. M., Steinberg, D. B., Heitzeg, M. M., et al. (2015). Coping expectancies, not enhancement expectancies mediate trauma experiences effects on problem alcohol use: A prospective study from early childhood to adolescence. *Journal of Studies on Alcohol:*

Quarterly Journal of Studies on Alcohol, 76, 781–789. doi:10.15288/jsad.2015.76.781.

Jewitt, N., Hope, A. J., Milne, R., et al. (2016). Development and evaluation of patient education materials for elderly lung cancer patients. *Journal of Cancer Education*, 31, 70–74. doi:10.1007/s12187-014-0780-1.

Kishida, M., & Elavsky, S. (2015). Daily physical activity enhances resilient resources for symptom management in middle-age women. *Health Psychology*, 34, 756–764. Retrieved from http://dx.doi.org/10.1037/hea0000190.

Kneck, A., Eriksson, L. E., Lundman, B., et al. (2016). Encumbered by vulnerability and temporality-the meanings of trigger situations when learning to live with diabetes. *Journal of Clinical Nursing*, 25, 2874–2883. doi:10.1111/jocn.13339.

Leveille-Tulce, A. M. B. (2017). *A quasi-experimental study of a health patterning modality about childhood vaginitis and power in Haitian primary caregivers.* Unpublished doctoral dissertation.

MacCourt, P., McLennan, M., Somers, S., et al. (2017). Effectivenss of a grief intervention for caregivers of people with dementia. *Omega*, 75(3), 230–247. doi:10.1177/0030222816652802.

Mills, A. C., Wong-Anuchit, C., & Poogpan, J. (2017). A concept analysis of Thum-jai: A Thai coping strategy. *Pacific Rim International Journal of Nursing Research*, 21, 234–243.

Moore, C., & Browne, C. (2017). Elder abuse and neglect: A review of recent developments in the field. *Journal of Family Violence*, 32(4), 383–397.

Myhre, J., Tonga, J. B., Ulstein, I. D., et al. (2018). *Journal of Clinical Nursing*, 27, e495–e502. doi:10.1111/jocn.14047.

Onieva-Zafra, M. D., Hernandez-Garcia, L., Gonzalez-del-Valle, M. T., et al. (2018). Music intervention with reminiscence therapy, and reality orientation for elderly people with Alzheimer's dementia living in a nursing home: A pilot study. *Holistic Nursing Practice*, 32(1), 43–50. doi:10.1097/HNP.0000000000000247.

Perez-Blasco, J., Sales, A., Meléndez, J. C., et al. (2016). The effects of mindfulness and self-compassion on improving the capacity to adapt to stress situations in elderly people living in the community. *Clinical Gerontologist*, 39(2), 90–103. doi:10.1080/07317115.2015 .1120253.

Pickering, C. E. Z., Ridenour, K., Salaysay, Z., et al. (2017). Identifying elder abuse and neglect among family caregiving dyads: A cross-sectional study of psychometric properties of QualCare scale. *International Journal of Nursing Studies*, 69, 41–46. doi:10.1016/j.ijnurstu.2017.01.012.

Qiu, X., Sit, J. W. H., & Koo, F. K. (2018). The influence of Chinese culture on family caregivers of stroke survivors: A qualitative study. *Journal of Clinical Nursing*, 27(1/2), e3090e319.

Rew, L., Young, C., Brown, A., et al. (2016). Suicide ideation and life events in a sample of rural adolescents. *Archives of Psychiatric Nursing*, 30(2), 198–203.

Rosnau, K., Hashmi, S. S., Northrup, H., et al. (2017). Knowledge and self-esteem of individuals with Neurofibromatosis Type 1 (NF1). *Journal of Genetic Counseling*, 26, 620–627. doi:10.1007/s10897 -016-0036-9.

Rubio, L., Dumitrache, C., Cordon-Pozo, E., et al. (2016). Coping: Impact of gender and stressful life events in middle and old age. *Clinical Gerontologist*, 39, 468–488. doi:10.1080/07317115.2015 .1132290.

Schrank, B., Ebert-Vogel, A., Amering, M., et al. (2016). Gender differences in caregiver burden and its determinant in family members of terminally ill cancer patients. *Psycho-Oncology*, 25, 808–814. doi:10.1002/pon.4005.

Shanthi, P., & Jeyapal, M. (2016). Assess the level of coping, family support, and quality of life of women who had undergone hysterectomy in selected hospitals at Madurai. *Asian Journal of Nursing Education and Research*, 6(3), 347–350.

● = Independent;   ▲ = Collaborative;   EBN = Evidence-Based Nursing;   EB = Evidence-Based

Shearer, B. C., Fleury, J. D., & Belyea, M. (2010). Randomized control trial of the health empowerment intervention: Feasibility and impact. *Nursing Research, 59*, 203–211.

Spoelstra, S. L., Burhenn, P. S., DeKoekkoek, T., et al. (2016). A trial examining an advanced practice nurse intervention to promote medication adherence and symptom management in adult cancer patients prescribed oral anti-cancer agents: Study protocol. *Journal of Advanced Nursing, 72*(2), 409–420. doi:10.1111/jan.12828.

Stefanic, N., Caputi, P., Lane, L., et al. (2015). Exploring the nature of situational goal-based coping in early-stage breast cancer patients: A contextual approach. *European Journal of Oncology Nursing, 19*, 604–611. Retrieved from http://dx.doi.org/10.1016/j.ejon.2015.03.008.

Stelfox, H., Leigh, J., Dodek, P., et al. (2017). A multi-center prospective cohort study of patient transfers from the intensive care unit to the hospital ward. *Intensive Care Medicine, 43*, 1485–1494. Retrieved from http://dx.doi.org/10.1007/s00134-017-4910-1.

Stockmann, C., Gabor, O., Divito-Thomas, P., et al. (2016). The use and intended outcomes of presence: A focus group study. *International Journal of Nursing Knowledge, 29*, 59–65.

Sun, V., & Fong, Y. (2017). Minimally invasive cancer surgery: Indications and outcomes. *Seminars in Oncology Nursing, 33*(1), 23–36. doi:10.1016/j.soncn.2016.11.003.

Visser, M. M., Heijenbrok-Kal, M. H., van't Spijker, A., et al. (2016). Problem-solving therapy during outpatient stroke rehabilitation improves coping and health-related quality of life: Randomized controlled trial. *Stroke; a Journal of Cerebral Circulation, 47*, 135–142. doi:10.1161/STROKEAHA.115.010961.

Wilkerson, J. M., Schick, V. R., Romijnders, K. A., et al. (2017). Social support, depression, self-esteem, and coping among LGBTQ adolescents participating in HATCH youth. *Health Promotion Practice, 18*, 358–365. doi:10.1177/1524839916654461.

Yang, F., Lai, C. Y., Yen, C., et al. (2017). The depressive symptoms, resourcefulness, and self-harm behaviors of adolescents. *Journal of Nursing Research, 25*(1), 41–50.

Zarbo, C., Brugnera, A., Friegerio, L., et al. (2018). Behavioral, cognitive, and emotional coping strategies of women with endometriosis: A critical narrative review. *Archives of Women's Mental Health, 21*, 1–13. doi:10.1007/s00737-017-0779-9.

Readiness for enhanced Coping *Marina Martinez-Kratz, MS, RN, CNE*

NANDA-I

Definition

A pattern of valid appraisal of stressors with cognitive and behavioral efforts to manage demands related to well-being, which can be strengthened.

Defining Characteristics

Awareness of possible environmental change; expresses desire to enhance knowledge of stress management strategies; expresses desire to enhance management of stressors; expresses desire to enhance social support; expresses desire to enhance use of emotion-oriented strategies; expresses desire to enhanced use of problem-oriented strategies; expresses desire to enhance use of spiritual resource

NOC (Nursing Outcomes Classification)

Suggested NOC Outcomes

Coping; Personal Well-Being; Social Interaction Skills; Quality of life

---

Example NOC Outcome with Indicators

Coping as evidenced by the following indicators: Identifies effective coping patterns/Uses effective coping strategies. (Rate the outcome and indicators of **Coping:** 1 = never demonstrated, 2 = rarely demonstrated, 3 = sometimes demonstrated, 4 = often demonstrated, 5 = consistently demonstrated [see Section I].)

Client Outcomes

Client Will (Specify Time Frame)

- Acknowledge personal power
- State awareness of possible environmental changes that may contribute to decreased coping
- State that stressors are manageable
- Seek new effective coping strategies
- Seek social support for problems associated with coping
- Demonstrate ability to cope, using a broad range of coping strategies
- Use spiritual support of personal choice

● = Independent;   ▲ = Collaborative;   EBN = Evidence-Based Nursing;   EB = Evidence-Based

C

Suggested NIC Interventions

Coping Enhancement; Health Education; Decision-Making Support

Example NIC Activities—Coping Enhancement

Assist client in developing an objective appraisal of the event; Explore with client previous methods of dealing with life problems

Nursing Interventions and *Rationales*

- Assess and support positive psychological strengths, that is, hope, optimism, self-efficacy, resiliency, and social support. EBN: *Based on a systematic review (N = 57 studies) covering the phases of the cancer experience, researchers found resilience and optimism are protective characteristics that contribute to coping and well-being (Molina et al, 2014).*
- Be physically and emotionally present for the client while using a variety of therapeutic communication techniques. EBN: *A qualitative study using focus groups to understand nurses' (N = 27) experiences of presence, found empathy, active listening, and use of silence were among the therapeutic communication approaches that were required to implement presence and improve client outcomes (Stockmann et al, 2016). EBN: Adult primary care clients (N = 251) receiving early cancer care identified nurses' use of active listening, providing information, and being present for client-centered care as critical behaviors of oncology nurse navigators (Horner et al, 2013).*
- Empower the client to set realistic goals and to engage in problem-solving. EBN: *In a randomized control trial testing the effectiveness of a 16-week Oncology Nurse Navigator (ONN) program compared with standard care to support clients with cancer (N = 251) during early treatment, researchers described the intervention, which included the use of using problem-solving and motivational interviewing in the provision of psychosocial support (Horner et al, 2013).*
- Encourage expression of positive thoughts and emotions. EBN: *In an intervention study of Turkish family caregivers of adults with mental illness, a family-to-family support intervention resulted in improvements in self-confidence and optimism in the experimental group (N = 34) after the intervention from baseline and at 3 months, whereas there was no change in the control group (N = 34) at any measurement period (Bademli & Duman, 2014).*
- Encourage the client to use spiritual coping mechanisms such as faith and prayer. EBN: *In a qualitative study of the lived spiritual experiences of those receiving outpatient surgery, clients (N = 7) described their use of spiritual coping and that spiritual care at a time of vulnerability contributed to their well-being (Griffin, 2013). EBN: Use of spiritual coping such as praying has been associated with increased psychological well-being and decreased psychological distress in samples of Caucasian and African American early breast cancer survivors (Gaston-Johansson et al, 2013b).*
- Help the client with serious and chronic conditions such as depression, cancer diagnosis, and chemotherapy treatment to maintain social support networks or assist in building new ones. EBN: *Women with advanced breast cancer (N = 35) receiving high-dose chemotherapy were treated with a comprehensive coping strategy program that included the use of social support and other coping enhancement skills; the treatment group had improved quality of life at 1 year posttreatment (Gaston-Johansson et al, 2013a).*
- ▲ Refer for cognitive-behavioral therapy (CBT) to enhance coping skills. EBN: *Gaston-Johansson et al (2013a) from the Johns Hopkins School of Nursing conducted an intervention study that included cognitive restructuring as part of a comprehensive coping strategies program and found that women with breast cancer in the intervention group (N = 38) had improved well-being and quality of life compared with the control group (N = 35) at 1 year postintervention. Refer to the care plans for Readiness for enhanced **Communication** and Readiness for enhanced **Spiritual** well-being.*

Pediatric

- Encourage children and adolescents to engage in diversional activities and exercise to promote self-esteem, enhance coping, and prevent behavioral and other physical and psychosocial problems. EBN: *Researchers examining physical activity in children attending school (N = 133) found that enjoyment and self-efficacy were important influences in promoting physical activity in children (Ling et al, 2015). EBN: In a qualitative*

• = Independent; ▲ = Collaborative; EBN = Evidence-Based Nursing; EB = Evidence-Based

study of hospitalized children (N = 10) receiving chemotherapy for cancer, researchers found that engaging children in entertaining activities and having fun were among positive coping strategies (Sposito et al, 2015).

- Provide families of children with chronic illness with education, transitional assistance, and psychosocial support to enhance coping. EBN: *An integrative literature review found that interventions should be directed toward education and psychosocial support for patients and families dealing with a new diagnosis of chronic illnesses (Gunter & Duke, 2018).*

 Geriatric

- Encourage active, meaning-based coping strategies for older adults with chronic illness. EBN: *In a qualitative study of older adults living with HIV (N = 40) residing in an urban environment, researchers uncovered four themes: accessing support, helping one's self and others, and tapping into their own spirituality. These address successful coping for the participants (DeGrezia & Scrandis, 2015).*
- Consider the use of Web-based and technological resources for older adults in the community. EB: *The results of a mixed method systematic review of 112 articles indicated that approximately 24% of the articles addressed Web-based packages and assistive information technology that assists older adults and their family caregivers with health information, resources for performing tasks safely, engaging in self-management, increasing coping strategies, and other types of support; studies indicated client satisfaction as an outcome (Vedel et al, 2013).*
- Refer the older client to self-help support groups that address health, psychosocial, and/or social support. EB: *In a mixed age sample with more than 50% of the participants older than age 50 years (range 19–83 years), Internet-based self-help groups for persons who experienced cancer (N = 350) have been associated with perceived increased coping and improved satisfaction with perceived health status (Seckin, 2013).* EB: *Greysen et al (2013) studied social isolation in older veterans and recommended the use of in-person and Internet-based self-help support groups.*

 Multicultural

- Assess an individual's sociocultural backgrounds to identify factors that support coping. EB: *Researchers found that in a sample of African American college students (N = 191), a variety of past messages regarding racial socialization may predict race-specific coping in AA college students. (Blackmon et al, 2016).* EB: *In a study comparing coping strategies used by Caucasian, Korean, and African American older women (N = 343), researchers found there are differences in preferred coping strategies used by the three ethnic groups; the most common strategy used by all three groups was religious/spiritual belief systems (Lee & Mason, 2013).*
- Encourage spirituality as a source of support for coping. EBN: *Religion and spiritual practices were used by Buddhist and Muslim Thai women to cope with type 2 diabetes self-management (Lundberg & Thrakul, 2013).*
- Facilitate positive ethnocultural identity to enhance coping. EB: *Ojeda and Liang (2014) examined coping in Mexican American adolescent men (N = 93) and found that ethnocultural factors such as positive affirmation and view of one's ethnic identity, as well as culture bound characteristics, such as caballerismo (positive Latino masculinity), was associated with more effective coping strategies, such as positive reframing, planning, and the use of humor.* EB: *In African American women who self-reported experience with trauma (N = 161), higher self-esteem and well-being were associated with more effective, active coping strategies (Stevens-Watkins et al, 2014).*
- Foster family support. EBN: *In Madurai women who underwent hysterectomy (N = 60), researchers found that family support was associated with coping and quality of life and concluded that support from the partner is especially important to both coping and quality of life (Shanthi & Jeyapal, 2016). Refer to the care plan for Ineffective* **Coping.**

 Home Care

- The interventions described previously may be adapted for home care use.
- Engage both clients and their caregivers as a dyad. CEBN: *In a review of a program of research about helping clients and family caregivers cope with cancer, Northouse (2012) related lessons learned about caring for client and family caregiver dyad; recommendations included identifying strengths; three-way, open communication and alliances; and promoting active coping (versus avoidant coping).*
- ▲ Institute case management for frail elderly clients to support continued independent living. EBN: *Nurse-led community care for the oldest-old that includes care coordination and follow-up could preserve functioning*

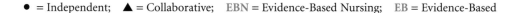

• = Independent; ▲ = Collaborative; EBN = Evidence-Based Nursing; EB = Evidence-Based

C

in the oldest-old in the community (Bleijenberg et al, 2017). EB: A study examining tablet and Skype use in a case management program for frail older adults found that the participants had positive experiences with the technology as a means of communicating with case managers (Berner et al, 2016).

- Refer the client and family to support groups. EB: *A study of adolescents and adults with neurofibromatosis type 1 (NF1), a genetic, progressive disorder, explored knowledge of the disease, self-esteem, and the effect of support groups. Researchers found that participation in support groups had an influence on self-esteem and recommended that health care professionals inform clients about support groups (Rosnau et al, 2017).*
- Refer prostate cancer clients and their spouses to family programs that include family-based interventions of communication, hope, coping, uncertainty, and symptom management. EBN: *Researchers conducted a qualitative study of prostate cancer survivors and their spouses (N = 95) to determine the long-term quality of life effects of treatment at 36 months after treatment; the recommendations included offering counseling to couples after treatment to improve quality of life and assist with managing relationship intimacy (Harden et al, 2013).*
- ▲ Refer military members, veterans, and family members for appropriate health services. EB: *Research found veterans with and without posttraumatic stress disorder (PTSD) enrolled in the Veterans Administration Program of Comprehensive Assistance for Family Caregivers (PCAFC) accessed more mental health, primary, and specialty care services than weighted comparisons (Shepherd-Banigan et al, 2018).*

 Client/Family Teaching and Discharge Planning

- Teach the client about available community resources (e.g., therapists, ministers, counselors, self-help groups, family education groups). EBN: *Easom, Cotter, and Ramos (2018) conducted a postparticipation examination of the Resources for Enhancing Alzheimer's Caregiver Health (REACH II) program provided to African American and Caucasian caregivers of people with Alzheimer's disease and found it to be a culturally appropriate and effective program.*
- Teach caregivers using a variety of interventions that contribute to coping. EBN: *Researchers conducting a systematic review of 17 articles regarding couples-based intervention for coping with cancer recommended interventions that include skills training, psychoeducational interventions, and client/family support (Li & Loke, 2014).*
- Teach expressive writing, journaling, and education about emotions. EBN: *Journaling was one of the components of an intervention study aimed to promote civility among nursing students; there were improvements in coping in the areas of self-controlling, seeking social support, and positive reappraisal after the intervention (Jenkins et al, 2013).*

REFERENCES

Refer to ineffective **Coping** for additional references.

Bademli, K., & Duman, Z. C. (2014). Effects of a family to family support program on mental health and coping strategies of caregivers of adults with mental illness: A randomized control study. *Archives of Psychiatric Nursing, 28,* 392–398.

Berner, J., Anderberg, P., Rennemark, M., et al. (2016). Case management for frail older adults through tablet computers and Skype. *Informatics for Health & Social Care, 41,* 405–416. doi:10.3109/17538157.2015.1033528.

Blackmon, S. M., Coyle, L. D., Davenport, S., et al. (2016). Linking racial-ethnic socialization to culture and race-specific coping among African-American college students. *Journal of Black Psychology, 42,* 549–576. doi:10.1177/0095798415617865.

Bleijenberg, N., Imhof, L., Mahrer-Imhof, R., et al. (2017). Patient characteristics associated with a successful response to nurse-led care programs targeting the oldest-old: A comparison of two RCTs. *Worldviews on Evidence-Based Nursing, 14*(3), 210–222.

DeGrezia, M. G., & Scrandis, D. (2015). Successful coping in urban community-dwelling older adults with HIV. *Journal of the Association of Nurses in Aids Care, 26*(12), 151–163.

Easom, L., Cotter, E., & Ramos, A. (2018). Comparison of African American and Caucasian caregiver self-efficacy. *Journal of Gerontological Nursing, 44*(3), 16–21. doi:10.3928/00989134 -20171023-01.

Gaston-Johansson, F., Fall-Dickson, J., Nanda, J. P., et al. (2013a). Long-term effect of the self-management comprehensive coping strategies program on quality of life in patients with breast cancer treated with high dose chemotherapy. *Psycho-Oncology, 22,* 530–539.

Gaston-Johansson, F., Haisfield-Wolfe, M. E., Reddick, B., et al. (2013b). The relationships among coping strategies, religious coping, and spirituality in African American women with breast cancer receiving chemotherapy. *Oncology Nursing Forum, 40,* 120–131.

Greysen, S. R., Horwitz, L. I., Covinsky, K. E., et al. (2013). Does social isolation predict rehospitalization and mortality among HIV+ and uninfected older veterans? *Journal of the American Geriatric Society, 61,* 1456–1463.

Griffin, A. (2013). The lived spiritual experiences of patients transitioning through outpatient surgery. *AORN Journal, 97,* 243–254.

Gunter, M. D., & Duke, G. (2018). Reducing uncertainty in families dealing with childhood cancers: An integrative literature review. *Pediatric Nursing, 44*(1), 21–37. Retrieved from http://proxy.lib .umich.edu/login?url=https://search-proquest-com.proxy.lib.umich .edu/docview/2006799041?accountid=14667.

Harden, J., Sanda, M. G., Wei, J. T., et al. (2013). Survivorship after prostate cancer treatment: Spouses quality of life at 36 months. *Oncology Nursing Forum, 40,* 567–573.

● = Independent;   ▲ = Collaborative;   EBN = Evidence-Based Nursing;   EB = Evidence-Based

Horner, K., Ludman, E. J., McCorkle, R., et al. (2013). An oncology nurse navigator program designed to eliminate gaps in early cancer care. *Clinical Journal of Oncology Nursing, 17,* 43–48.

Jenkins, S. D., Kerber, C. S., & Woith, W. M. (2013). An intervention to promote civility among nursing students. *Nursing Education Perspective, 34,* 95–100.

Lee, H. S., & Mason, D. (2013). Optimism and coping strategies among Caucasian, Korean, and African American older women. *Healthcare for Women International, 34,* 1084–1096.

Li, Q., & Loke, A. Y. (2014). A systematic review of spousal couple-based intervention studies for couples coping with cancer: Direction for the development of interventions. *Psycho-Oncology, 23,* 731–739.

Ling, J., Robbins, L. B., McCarthy, V. L., et al. (2015). Psychosocial determinants of physical activity in children attending afterschool programs: A path analysis. *Nursing Research, 64,* 190–199.

Lundberg, P. C., & Thrakul, S. (2013). Religion and self-management in Thai Buddhist and Muslim women with type 2 diabetes. *Journal of Clinical Nursing, 22,* 1907–1916.

Molina, Y., Yi, J. C., Martinez-Gutierrez, J., et al. (2014). Resilience among patients across the cancer continuum. *Clinical Journal of Oncology Nursing, 18,* 93–101.

Northouse, L. L. (2012). Helping patients and family caregivers cope with cancer. *Oncology Nursing Forum, 39,* 500–506.

Ojeda, L., & Liang, C. T. (2014). Ethnocultural and gendered determinants of coping in Mexican-American adolescent men. *Psychology of Men and Masculinity, 15,* 296–304.

Rosnau, K., Hashmi, S. S., Northrup, H., et al. (2017). Knowledge and self-esteem of individuals with Neurofibromatosis Type 1 (NF1). *Journal of Genetic Counseling, 26,* 620627. doi:10.1007/s10897-016-0036-9.

Seckin, G. (2013). Satisfaction with health status among cyber patients: Testing a mediation model of electronic coping support. *Behavior and Information Technology, 32,* 91–101.

Shanthi, P., & Jeyapal, M. (2016). Assess the level of coping, family support, and quality of life of women who had undergone hysterectomy in selected hospitals at Madurai. *Asian Journal of Nursing Education and Research, 6*(3), 347–350.

Shepherd-Banigan, M., et al. (2018). The effect of support and training for family members on access to outpatient services for veterans with posttraumatic stress disorder (PTSD). *Administration and Policy in Mental Health,* 1–15. Retrieved from http://doi.org.proxy.lib.umich.edu/10.1007/s10488-017-0844-8.

Sposito, A., Silva-Rodriques, F., Sparapani, V., et al. (2015). Coping strategies used by hospitalized children with cancer undergoing chemotherapy. *Journal of Nursing Scholarship, 47,* 143–151.

Stevens-Watkins, D., Sharma, S., Knighton, J. S., et al. (2014). Examining cultural correlates of active coping among African American female trauma survivors. *Psychological Trauma Theory, Research, Practice, and Policy, 6,* 328–336.

Stockmann, C., Gabor, O., Divito-Thomas, P., et al. (2016). The use and intended outcomes of presence: A focus group study. *International Journal of Nursing Knowledge, 29,* 59–65.

Vedel, I., Akhlaghpour, S., Vaghofi, I., et al. (2013). Health information technology in geriatrics and gerontology: A mixed systematic review. *Journal of American Medical Informatics Association, 20,* 1109–1119.

Wands, L. M. (2011). Caring for veterans returning home from Middle Eastern wars. *Nursing Science Quarterly, 24,* 180–186.

Ineffective community Coping   *Marina Martinez-Kratz, MS, RN, CNE*

NANDA-I

Definition

A pattern of community activities for adaptation and problem-solving that is unsatisfactory for meeting the demands or needs of the community.

Defining Characteristics

Community does not meet expectations of its members; deficient community participation; elevated community illness rate; excessive community conflict; excessive stress; high incidence of community problems; perceived community powerlessness; perceived community vulnerability

Related Factors

Inadequate resources for problem-solving; insufficient community resources; nonexistent community systems

At-Risk Population

Exposure to disaster; history of disaster

NOC   (Nursing Outcomes Classification)

Suggested NOC Outcomes

Community Competence; Community Health Status; Community Violence Level

● = Independent;   ▲ = Collaborative;   EBN = Evidence-Based Nursing;   EB = Evidence-Based

C

Example NOC Outcome with Indicators

Community Competence as evidenced by the following indicators: Participation rates in community activities/ Consideration of common and competing interests among groups when solving community problems/Representation of all segments of the community in problem-solving/Effective use of conflict management strategies. (Rate the outcome and indicators of **Community Competence:** 1 = poor, 2 = fair, 3 = good, 4 = very good, 5 = excellent [see Section I].)

Community Outcomes

A Broad Range of Community Members Will (Specify Time Frame)

- Participate in community actions to improve power resources
- Develop improved communication among community members
- Participate in problem-solving
- Demonstrate cohesiveness in problem-solving
- Develop new strategies for problem-solving
- Express power to deal with change and manage problems

NIC (Nursing Interventions Classification)

Suggested NIC Interventions

Community Health Development; Program Development

Example NIC Activities—Community Health Development

Enhance community support networks; Identify and develop potential community leaders; Unify community members behind a common mission; Ensure that community members maintain control over decision-making

---

Nursing Interventions and *Rationales*

Note: The diagnosis of Ineffective **Coping** does not apply and should not be used when stress is being imposed by external sources or circumstance. If the community is a victim of circumstances, using the nursing diagnosis Ineffective **Coping** is equivalent to blaming the victim. See the care plan for Readiness for enhanced community **Coping.**

▲ Establish a collaborative partnership with the community (see the care plan for Readiness for enhanced community **Coping** for additional references). EB: *A recent study found that counties whose Area Agencies for the Aging (AAAs) maintained informal partnerships with a broad range of organizations in health care and other sectors had significantly lower hospital readmission rates compared with counties whose AAAs had informal partnerships with fewer types of organizations (Brewster et al, 2018).*

● Assess community needs with the use of concept mapping methodology. EB: *The findings of a recent study showed that an integration of several concept mapping methods into a community engagement process was able to increase the input from a wide range of populations (Velonis et al, 2018).*

● Encourage participation in faith-based organizations that want to improve community stress management. EBN: *A recent study showed that coaching by faith community nurses created an environment of sustained support that promoted improved lifestyles and blood pressure changes over time (Cooper & Zimmerman, 2017).*

▲ Identify the health services and information resources that are currently available in the community through network analysis. EB: *A study found that network analysis served as a useful tool to evaluate community partnerships and facilitate coalition building (Ruopeng et al, 2017).*

● Work with community members to increase problem-solving abilities. EBN: *Problem-solving is essential for effective coping. Findings from a recent study showed positive outcomes from a direct and tailored problem-solving training program (Easom et al, 2018).*

● Provide support to the community and help community members identify and mobilize additional supports. EB: *A community mobilization project demonstrated how cross-sector, coordinated efforts focused on vulnerable populations can leverage local strengths to establish and enhance breastfeeding support services customized to local needs (Colchamiro et al, 2015).*

● Advocate for the community in multiple arenas (e.g., multimedia, social media, governmental agencies). EB: *A recent study explored how social media can help community organizations engage in advocacy work (Guo et al, 2017).*

● = Independent;   ▲ = Collaborative;   EBN = Evidence-Based Nursing;   EB = Evidence-Based

- Work with communities to ensure that vulnerable individuals with access and functional needs are included in preparations for, response to, and recovery from disasters. EB: *Analysis of recent disasters has identified that a combination of strategic and operational methods, appropriate planning tools, and planning for the entire community will prevent individuals with access and functional needs from being disproportionately and negatively affected by disasters (Franks & Seaton, 2017).*
- Write grant proposals to help community members obtain funds for programs that reduce stress or improve coping (Anderson & McFarlane, 2011).
- Work with members of the community to identify and develop coping strategies that promote a sense of power (e.g., obtaining sources for funding, collaborating with other communities) (Anderson & McFarlane, 2011).

 Pediatric

- Protect children and adolescents from exposure to community violence. EB: *A systematic review found evidence for a positive association between community violence exposure and cardiovascular and sleep problems in children and adolescents (Wright et al, 2017).*
- Assess children and adolescents for the effects of direct and indirect crime exposure rather than only focusing solely on violent victimization. EB: *A study found poor behavioral health outcomes for adolescents with self-reported crime exposure (Grinshteyn et al, 2018).*

 Multicultural

- Acknowledge the stressors unique to racial/ethnic communities. EB: *A recent study of Hispanic and African American women found that neighborhood context was an important factor in examining the determinants of health, survivorship, and quality of life outcomes among cancer patients (Wu et al, 2018).*
- Identify community strengths with community members. EBN: *A community-based participatory research approach was used to obtain Native American community input and identify strengths to address youth suicide and substance abuse. The results led to the development of a strengths-based intervention incorporating the Gathering of Native American's curriculum (Holliday et al, 2018).*
- Use an empowerment approach to address health behaviors in diverse communities. An empowerment approach includes increasing clients' self-efficacy and capacity to make informed decisions about their health care. EB: *A recent study found use of an empowerment approach was effective in changing nonadherent Latinas' breast screening behaviors and promoting them to become agents of change in their communities (Molina et al, 2018). The empowerment intervention has three sessions focused on early detection, sharing information with family/friends, and health volunteerism.*
- Work with members of the community to prioritize and target health goals specific to the community. EB: *Recent research found that members of underserved communities, in informed deliberations, prioritized research on quality of life, patient-doctor, special needs, access, and compare approaches (Goold et al, 2017).*
- Establish and sustain partnerships with key individuals within communities when developing and implementing programs. EB: *A study of community engagement strategies found the following techniques to be effective: proactively engaging stakeholders in informational meetings, webinars, social media, the promising practice process, and community advisory council meetings (D'Angelo et al, 2017).*
- Use mentoring strategies for community members. EB: *A recent study showed parent mentors are highly effective in insuring uninsured Latino children and eliminating disparities (Flores et al, 2018).*
- Use community church settings as a forum for advocacy, teaching, and program implementation. EBN: *A recent study found that trust, respect, open dialog with participants, and commitment to address community health needs contributed to successful engagement and recruitment of African American churches to serve as participants in cancer research projects (Slade et al, 2018).*

Community Teaching

- Teach strategies for stress management.
- Explain the relationship between enhancing power resources and coping.

REFERENCES

Anderson, E. T., & McFarlane, J. (2011). *Community as partner: Theory and practice in nursing* (6th ed.). Philadelphia: Lippincott Williams & Wilkins.

Brewster, A. L., et al. (2018). Curry cross-sectoral partnerships by area agencies on aging: Associations with health care use and spending.

Health Affairs, 37(1), 15–21. Retrieved from http://doi.org.proxy.lib.umich.edu/10.1377/hlthaff.2017.1346.

Colchamiro, R., et al. (2015). Mobilizing community resources to enhance post discharge support for breastfeeding in Massachusetts (USA): Results of a catalyst grant approach. *Journal of Human*

C

Lactation, 31(4), 631–640. Retrieved from http://doi.org.proxy.lib.umich.edu/10.1177/089033441559768.

Cooper, J., & Zimmerman, W. (2017). The effect of a faith community nurse network and public health collaboration on hypertension prevention and control. *Public Health Nursing, 34*(5), 444–453. Retrieved from http://doi.org.proxy.lib.umich.edu/10.1111/phn.12325.

D'Angelo, G., et al. (2017). Community engagement strategies for implementation of a policy supporting evidence-based practices: A case study of Washington state. *Administration and Policy in Mental Health, 44*(1), 6–15. Retrieved from http://doi.org.proxy.lib.umich.edu/10.1007/s10488-015-0664-7.

Easom, L. R., et al. (2018). Operation family caregiver: Problem-solving training for military caregivers in a community setting. *Journal of Clinical Psychology, 74*, 536–553. Retrieved from http://doi.org.proxy.lib.umich.edu/10.1002/jclp.22536.

Flores, G., et al. (2018). Parent mentoring program increases coverage rates for uninsured Latino children. *Health Affairs, 37*(3), 403–412Q. doi:10.1377/hlthaff.2017.1272.

Franks, S., & Seaton, E. (2017). Utilizing strategic and operational methods for whole-community disaster planning. *Disaster Medicine and Public Health Preparedness, 11*(6), 741–746. doi:10.1017/dmp.2017.6.

Goold, S. D., et al. (2017). Priorities for patient-centered outcomes research: The views of minority and underserved communities. *Health Services Research, 52*(2), 599–615. doi:10.1111/1475-6773.12505.

Grinshteyn, E. G., et al. (2018). *Community Mental Health Journal, 54*(3), 252–258. Retrieved from http://doi.org.proxy.lib.umich.edu/10.1007/s10597-017-0159-y.

Guo, C., et al. (2017). Speaking and being heard: How nonprofit advocacy organizations gain attention on social media. *Nonprofit and Voluntary Sector Quarterly, 47*(1), 5–26. Retrieved from http://doi.org.proxy.lib.umich.edu/10.1177/0899764017713724.

Holliday, C. E., et al. (2018). A CBPR approach to finding community strengths and challenges to prevent youth suicide and substance abuse. *Journal of Transcultural Nursing, 29*(1), 64–73. Retrieved from http://doi.org.proxy.lib.umich.edu/10.1177/1043659616679234.

Molina, Y., et al. (2018). Empowering Latinas to obtain breast cancer screenings: Comparing intervention effects, part 2. *Cancer Epidemiology, Biomarkers & Prevention: A Publication of the American Association for Cancer Research, 27*(3), 353–354. doi:10.1158/1055-9965.EPI-18-0048.

Ruopeng, A., et al. (2017). Assessing the network of agencies in local communities that promote healthy eating and lifestyles among populations with limited resources. *American Journal of Health Behavior, 41*(2), 127–138. doi:10.5993/AJHB.41.2.3.

Slade, J., et al. (2018). Recruitment of African American churches to participate in cancer early detection interventions: A community perspective. *Journal of Religion and Health, 57*(2), 751–761. Retrieved from http://doi.org.proxy.lib.umich.edu/10.1007/s10943-018-0586-2.

Velonis, A. J., et al. (2018). "One program that could improve health in this neighbourhood is _?" Using concept mapping to engage communities as part of a health and human services needs assessment. *BMC Health Services Research, 18*(1), 150. Retrieved from http://doi.org.proxy.lib.umich.edu/10.1186/s12913-018-2936-x.

Wright, A. W., et al. (2017). Systematic review: Exposure to community violence and physical health outcomes in youth. *Journal of Pediatric Psychology, 42*(4), 364–378. Retrieved from http://doi.org.proxy.lib.umich.edu/10.1093/jpepsy/jsw088.

Wu, C., et al. (2018). The association of neighborhood context with health outcomes among ethnic minority breast cancer survivors. *Journal of Behavioral Medicine, 41*(1), 52–61. Retrieved from http://doi.org.proxy.lib.umich.edu/10.1007/s10865-017-9875-6.

Compromised family Coping   Katherina Nikzad-Terhune, PhD, MSW

NANDA-I

Definition

A usually supportive primary person (family member, significant other, or close friend) provides insufficient, ineffective, or compromised support, comfort, assistance, or encouragement that may be needed by the client to manage or master adaptive tasks related to his or her health challenge.

Defining Characteristics

Assistive behaviors by support person produce unsatisfactory results; client complaint about support person's response to health problems; client concern about support person's response to health problem; limitation in communication between support person and client; protective behavior by support person incongruent with client's abilities; protective behavior by support person incongruent with client's need for autonomy; support person reports inadequate understanding that interferes with effective behaviors; support person reports insufficient knowledge that interferes with effective behaviors; support person reports preoccupation with own reaction to client's need; support person withdraws from client

Related Factors

Coexisting situations affecting the support person; exhaustion of support person's capacity; family disorganization; insufficient information available to support person; insufficient reciprocal support; insufficient support given by client to support person; insufficient understanding of information by support person; misinformation obtained by support person; preoccupation by support person with concern outside of family

● = Independent;   ▲ = Collaborative;   EBN = Evidence-Based Nursing;   EB = Evidence-Based

At-Risk Population

Developmental crisis experienced by support person; family role change; prolonged disease that exhausts capacity of support person; situational crisis faced by support person

 (Nursing Outcomes Classification)

C

Suggested NOC Outcomes

Caregiver Emotional Health; Caregiver-Client Relationship; Family Coping; Family Participation in Professional Care; Family Support During Treatment

Example NOC Outcome with Indicators

Family Coping as evidenced by the following indicators: Confronts family problems/Manages family problems/Reports needs for family assistance. (Rate each indicator of **Family Coping:** 1 = never demonstrated, 2 = rarely demonstrated, 3 = sometimes demonstrated, 4 = often demonstrated, 5 = consistently demonstrated [see Section I].)

Client Outcomes

Family/Significant Person Will (Specify Time Frame)

- Verbalize internal resources to help deal with the situation
- Verbalize knowledge and understanding of illness, disability, or disease
- Provide support and assistance as needed
- Identify need for and seek outside support

NIC **(Nursing Interventions Classification)**

Suggested NIC Interventions

Caregiver Support; Coping Enhancement; Family Involvement Promotion; Family Mobilization; Family Support; Mutual Goal Setting; Normalization Promotion; Sibling Support

Example NIC Activities—Family Support

Appraise family's emotional reaction to client's condition; Promote trusting relationship with family

Nursing Interventions and *Rationales*

- Assess the strengths and deficiencies of the family system. Consider using Family Systems Nursing to focus on the entire family as a unit of care. EBN: *A systematic review of the Family Systems Nursing literature found that when the focus was on both the individual and the family as a unit, improvements across cognitive, emotional, and behavioral domains were found, including enhanced understanding and coping, improved emotional well-being for the family and the individual, and improved interactions among family members (Östlund & Persson, 2014).*
- Establish rapport with families by providing accurate communication.
- Assist family members to recognize the need for help and teach them how to ask for it.
- Encourage family members to verbalize feelings. Spend time with them, sit down and make eye contact, and offer coffee and other nourishment.
- Provide family support interventions in situations in which caregiving is involved in the family. EB: *A comprehensive review of caregiving literature in both the fields of aging and developmental disabilities revealed that family-support interventions improved participant well-being, improved service access and satisfaction, reduced caregiver burden, and delayed institutional placement (Heller, Gibbons, & Fisher, 2015).*
- Provide privacy during family visits. If possible, maintain flexible visiting hours to accommodate more frequent family visits. If possible, arrange staff assignments so the same staff members have contact with the family. Familiarize other staff members with the situation in the absence of the usual staff member. Providing privacy, maintaining flexible hours, and arranging consistent staff assignments reduces stress, enhances communication, and facilitates the building of trust.
- Provide education to clients regarding active coping strategies to use in situations involving chronic illnesses. EB: *Mindfulness-based activities and cognitive behavioral therapy strategies can improve emotional, behavioral, and cognitive functioning in individuals experiencing various stressors (Gu et al, 2015).*

● = Independent;   ▲ = Collaborative;   EBN = Evidence-Based Nursing;   EB = Evidence-Based

C

- Provide psychoeducation interventions and support for families providing palliative care to help reduce caregiver stress and burden. **EB:** *Brief psychoeducation interventions helped reduce stress in caregivers caring for a dying relative (Hudson et al, 2015).*
- Refer the family with ill family members to appropriate resources for assistance as indicated (e.g., counseling, psychotherapy, financial assistance, spiritual support).

 Pediatric

- Provide screening for postpartum depression (PPD) during the prenatal period and during the 6-week postpartum checkup to identify symptoms of depression in mothers. **CEB:** *The Edinburgh Postnatal Depression Scale (EPDS) is the most widely used screening tool for detecting PPD and has been shown to be effective both prenatally and postnatally for detecting symptoms of depression in women (Cox, Holden, & Sagovsky, 1987; Zhong et al, 2014).*
- ▲ Consider medication management and psychosocial interventions, including individual therapy, group therapy, support groups, and brief psychotherapy. **EB:** *These are effective treatment strategies for managing PPD (Kleiman & Raskin, 2013; Miniati et al, 2014).*
- ▲ Use preventive strategies, such as screening, psychoeducation, postpartum debriefing, and companionship in the delivery room (e.g., community volunteer). **EBN:** *These strategies play an important role in the prevention of and recovery from PPD (Dennis & Dowswell, 2013).*
- Use technology-based education to help increase knowledge and support for parents performing care procedures for their children. **EBN:** *Research suggests that smartphone-based education should be considered as an effective educational intervention in providing nursing support for parents of children with respiratory disease (Lee, Kim, & Min, 2017).*
- Make communication and environmental adaptations when interacting with children with autism spectrum disorder (ASD) to enhance communication, improve quality of care, and reduce frustration. **EBN:** *Feasible adaptations in communication style can help enhance the nurse–patient relationship with children with ASD. Adaptations include reducing environmental sensory stimuli, recognizing that behavioral outbursts are often a sign of frustration in the child, and allowing for extra time when interacting with children with ASD (Brown & Elder, 2014).*
- Effectively engaging and collaborating with parents is essential for supporting parents of children with long-term health conditions, and it may enhance the parent–professional relationship and communication. **EBN:** *Smith, Swallow, and Coyne (2015) provided a framework for involving parents in the care of a child with long-term health conditions, which includes valuing the parent's knowledge and expertise of their child, supporting parents in their role, establishing rapport, mutually exchanging information with parents, sharing decisions, collaborating during care planning, and designing services around both the needs of the child and the family.*
- Provide evidence-based psychological therapies for parents with children with chronic conditions. **EB:** *Psychological therapies, such as cognitive behavioral therapy, can lead to improvements in mood and behavior in parents of children diagnosed with attention-deficit hyperactivity disorder (ADHD) (Wong et al, 2017).*
- When performing pediatric diabetes care, be attentive to the mother's experience, including burnout experienced as a result of caregiving for the child. **EBN:** *The well-being of the mother has the potential to impact the well-being of the child and the well-being of the family unit. Focusing on the well-being of mothers of children with pediatric diabetes may lead to improvements in overall family functioning, and referrals for appropriate interventions (Lindström et al, 2017).*
- Provide options for home-based interventions when severe childhood illnesses make it difficult for children and families to participate in interventions. In-home visits, assessments, and interventions may help improve self-management among the patient and family, and reduce emergency room (ER) visits and inpatient hospitalizations. **EBN:** *The delivery of a home visit program for pediatric asthma patients enhanced early communication, reduced response time between problem identification and resolution, and reduced inpatient care over the course of 1 year (McClure et al, 2017).*

 Geriatric

- ▲ Perform a holistic assessment of all needs of informal family caregivers. **EB:** *A systematic review of dementia caregivers revealed that caregivers often experience unmet needs regarding their own physical and psychological well-being (McCabe, You, & Tatangelo, 2016).* **EBN:** *Nurse-led caregiver-centered intervention may help prevent decompensation in caregiver well-being. Results from a recent study reveal that caregivers view a*

● = Independent;   ▲ = Collaborative;   **EBN** = Evidence-Based Nursing;   **EB** = Evidence-Based

trusting relationship with mental health nurses as being crucial, and that collaboration with nurses can lead to increased well-being in both care recipients and caregivers (Zegwaard et al, 2017).

▲ Provide caregivers with options for Internet-based support strategies to enhance coping. EB: *Research reveals that more than half of caregivers use the Internet to obtain caregiving information, including conditions or treatments, service availability, and care facilities (Li, 2015).*

● In situations in which familial caregiving is being provided, assess current coping strategies utilized within the family. Provide interventions for family caregivers that are designed specifically to enhance coping skills, including problem-solving strategies and emotional support. EB: *Psychosocial interventions that incorporated problem-solving skills, emotional support, knowledge of dementia, and social resources helped caregivers develop more effective coping strategies, which have the potential to reduce caregiver burden (Chen et al, 2015).*

● Assist informal caregivers with reducing unmet needs by helping them obtain the information and education necessary for caring for an older adult with a chronic health condition. EB: *Internet interventions can help meet the educational and support needs of informal dementia caregivers. Results from a systematic review demonstrate that Internet interventions for informal caregivers of individuals with dementia may lead to improvements in caregiver well-being, including improvements in confidence, depression, and self-efficacy (Boots et al, 2014).*

 Multicultural

● Acknowledge sociocultural differences and health care disparities at the onset of care. EBN: *Consider using Almutairi's critical cultural competence (CCC) model as a comprehensive approach for addressing challenges that may arise from sociocultural and linguistic issues during cross-cultural interactions. Research support use of the Critical Cultural Competence Scale (CCCS) to measure health care providers' perceptions of their CCC (Almutairi, Dahinten, & Rodney, 2015; Almutairi & Dahinten, 2017).*

● Use valid and culturally competent assessment tools and procedures when working with families with different racial/ethnic backgrounds. EBN: *The cultural information in nursing models and assessments should encompass health beliefs and practices, communication styles, religious orientation, and the degree of acculturation among others (Shen, 2015).*

● Assess for the influence of cultural beliefs, norms, and values on the individual/family/community's perceptions of coping. EB: *A comprehensive review of the coping literature reveals that there are culturally preferred coping patterns among acculturating migrants, and that these patterns vary with acculturation levels. Nurses and other health care professionals should educate themselves on their patients' culturally preferred coping patterns (Kuo, 2014).*

● Provide opportunities for families to discuss spirituality. EBN: *African American women with breast cancer use more positive religious coping and experience less distress and greater spiritual well-being (Gaston-Johansson et al, 2013).*

● Ensure culturally responsive approaches to end-of-life care. EBN: *Providing culturally informed nursing care allows elderly immigrants the opportunity to make choices during their end-of-life care that are congruent with their cultural beliefs and expectations (Johnstone et al, 2016).*

 Home Care

● The interventions described previously may be adapted for home care use.

● Assess the reason behind the breakdown of family coping. *Knowledge of the reasons behind compromised coping will assist in identification of appropriate interventions.* Refer to the care plan for **Caregiver Role Strain**.

▲ During the time of compromised coping, increase visits to ensure the safety of the client, support of the family, and reassurance regarding expectations for prognosis as appropriate.

▲ Assess the needs of the caregiver in the home, and intervene to meet needs as appropriate; explore all available resources that may be used to provide adequate home care (e.g., parish nursing as an effective adjunct, home health aide services to relieve the caregiver's fatigue).

▲ Encourage caregivers to attend to their own physical, mental, and spiritual health, and give more specific information about the client's needs and ways to meet them.

▲ Refer the family to medical social services for evaluation and supportive counseling. Serve as an advocate, mentor, and role model for caregiving; provide written information for the care needed by the client.

▲ A positive approach and caring by the nurse and concrete task definition and assignment reinforce positive coping strategies and allow caregivers to feel less guilty when tasks are delegated to multiple caregivers.

● = Independent;   ▲ = Collaborative;   EBN = Evidence-Based Nursing;   EB = Evidence-Based

C

▲ When a terminal illness is the precipitating factor for ineffective coping, offer hospice services and support groups as possible resources. EB: *Research suggests that clients and their families value home hospice care services and report experiencing beneficial outcomes as a result of using hospice services (Ong et al, 2016).*

● Encourage the client and family to discuss changes in daily functioning and routines created by the client's illness, and validate discomfort resulting from changes. *Individuals who live together for a long period tend to become familiar with each other's patterns; for example, meals are expected at certain times or a spouse becomes accustomed to the client's sleep habits.*

● Support positive individual and family coping efforts. *Positive feedback reinforces desired behaviors and supports the family unit.*

● Screen for mental health disorders (MHDs) in the elderly home care population. EBN: *Approximately one-third of elderly patients with MHDs received mental health services during a 60-day home care episode. Regular screening and intervention protocols can improve psychiatric care for the homebound elderly (Wang et al, 2016).*

● During home care visits and assessments, provide individuals and families with information for Internet-based interventions, including information on using social media as a health communications tool. EB: *Social media is now a new dimension to health care that provides a platform for patients and health care providers to communicate about health, and potentially improve health outcomes. A systematic review of the literature revealed various benefits of using social media for health communication, including increased interactions with others, increased accessibility to information, more available shared information, and social support (Moorhead et al, 2013).*

 Client/Family Teaching and Discharge Planning

● Assess grief in parents who have lost a child to help determine parental needs, especially in the first year after the death of a child. EB: *The presentation of grief may differ in mothers and fathers, resulting in different needs during the first year after a child's death (Youngblut et al, 2017).*

▲ Refer women with breast cancer and their family caregivers to support groups (including social network sites and online communities), and to other services that provide assistance with daily coping. EB: *Positive interventions applied to patients and survivors of breast cancer helped enhance quality of life, well-being, feelings of hope, and optimism (Casellas-Grau, Font, & Vives, 2014).*

▲ For families dealing with childhood illnesses or other psychosocial stressors, refer parents to support and education groups to provide opportunities for parents to access support, learn new parenting skills, and obtain additional coping resources. EB: *Childhood cancer support organizations and parent support groups are effective forms of support for families who have children with cancer (Dollman, Bekele, & Watanabe, 2014).* EBN: *Parents report satisfaction with Internet-based peer support, which can be used to supplement support offered by professionals (Niela-Vilén et al, 2014).*

● Provide comprehensive discharge planning for individuals with a mental health diagnosis to help improve quality of life at home. EBN: *During the discharge process, communication between health professionals, patients with a mental health diagnosis, and their families can result in quality of life improvements and reduced hospital readmissions (Nurjannah et al, 2014).*

● Children of parents with dual diagnoses (e.g., psychiatric illness and addiction) require more extensive support and resources. EB: *Preventative support groups for children with parents with comorbidity can help support emotional, social, and cognitive coping skills, and may help reduce the risk of these children developing subsequent problems (van Santvoort et al, 2014a,b).*

● Nurses can help type II diabetes patients with self-management education and support (DSME/S), which includes the facilitation of knowledge, skills, and abilities necessary to manage diabetes, as well as obtaining the support necessary for executing and maintaining the coping and behavioral skills needed for self-management. EB: *Self-management education and support has been shown to improve health outcomes in patients with type II diabetes (Powers et al, 2017).*

● Involve informal caregivers of older adults in the discharge process. EB: *For older adults being discharged to a community setting, integrating informal caregivers into the discharge planning process reduced the risk of hospital readmission (Rodakowski et al, 2017).*

● = Independent;   ▲ = Collaborative;   EBN = Evidence-Based Nursing;   EB = Evidence-Based

REFERENCES

Almutairi, A. F., & Dahinten, V. S. (2017). Construct validity of Almutairi's critical cultural competence scale. *Western Journal of Nursing Research, 39*(6), 784–802.

Almutairi, A. F., Dahinten, V. S., & Rodney, P. (2015). Almutairi's Critical Cultural Competence model for a multicultural healthcare environment. *Nursing Inquiry, 22*(4), 317–325.

Boots, L. M. M., Vugt, M. E., Knippenberg, R. J. M., et al. (2014). A systematic review of Internet-based supportive interventions for caregivers of patients with dementia. *International Journal of Geriatric Psychiatry, 29*(4), 331–344.

Brown, A. B., & Elder, J. H. (2014). Communication in autism spectrum disorder: A guide for pediatric nurses. *Pediatric Nursing, 40*(5), 219.

Casellas-Grau, A., Font, A., & Vives, J. (2014). Positive psychology interventions in breast cancer. A systematic review. *Psycho-Oncology, 23*(1), 9–19.

Chen, H. M., Huang, M. F., Yeh, Y. C., et al. (2015). Effectiveness of coping strategies intervention on caregiver burden among caregivers of elderly patients with dementia. *Psychogeriatrics, 15*(1), 20–25.

Cox, J. L., Holden, J. M., & Sagovsky, R. (1987). Detection of postnatal depression. Development of the 10-item Edinburgh Postnatal Depression Scale. *The British Journal of Psychiatry, 150*(6), 782–786.

Dennis, C. L., & Dowswell, T. (2013). Psychosocial and psychological interventions for preventing postpartum depression. *The Cochrane Database of Systematic Reviews,* (2), CD001134.

Dollman, K., Bekele, W., & Watanabe, K. (2014). Psycho-social aspects/parent support groups. In *Pediatric hematology-oncology in countries with limited resources* (pp. 153–158). New York: Springer.

Gaston-Johansson, F., Haisfield-Wolfe, M. E., Reddick, B., et al. (2013). The relationships among coping strategies, religious coping, and spirituality in African American women with breast cancer receiving chemotherapy. *Oncology Nursing Forum, 40*(2), 120–131.

Gu, J., Strauss, C., Bond, R., et al. (2015). How do mindfulness-based cognitive therapy and mindfulness-based stress reduction improve mental health and wellbeing? A systematic review and meta-analysis of mediation studies. *Clinical Psychology Review, 37,* 1–12.

Heller, T., Gibbons, H. M., & Fisher, D. (2015). Caregiving and family support interventions: Crossing networks of aging and developmental disabilities. *Intellectual and Developmental Disabilities, 53*(5), 329.

Hudson, P., Trauer, T., Kelly, B., et al. (2015). Reducing the psychological distress of family caregivers of home based palliative care patients: Longer term effects from a randomised controlled trial. *Psycho-Oncology, 24*(1), 19–24.

Johnstone, M. J., Hutchinson, A. M., Redley, B., et al. (2016). Nursing roles and strategies in end-of-life decision making concerning elderly immigrants admitted to acute care hospitals: An Australian study. *Journal of Transcultural Nursing, 27*(5), 471–479.

Kleiman, K. R., & Raskin, V. D. (2013). *This isn't what I expected: Overcoming postpartum depression* (2nd ed.). Boston: Da Capo.

Kuo, B. C. (2014). Coping, acculturation, and psychological adaptation among migrants: A theoretical and empirical review and synthesis of the literature. *Health Psychology and Behavioral Medicine: An Open Access Journal, 2*(1), 16–33.

Lee, J. M., Kim, S. J., & Min, H. Y. (2017). The effects of smartphone-based nebulizer therapy education on parents' knowledge and confidence of performance in caring for children with respiratory disease. *Journal of Pediatric Nursing, 36,* 13–19.

Li, H. (2015). Informal caregivers' use of the internet for caregiving information. *Social Work in Health Care, 54*(6), 532–546.

Lindström, C., Åman, J., Norberg, A. L., et al. (2017). "Mission impossible"; the mothering of a child with type 1 diabetes–From the perspective of mothers experiencing burnout. *Journal of Pediatric Nursing, 36,* 149–156.

McCabe, M., You, E., & Tatangelo, G. (2016). Hearing their voice: A systematic review of dementia family caregivers' needs. *The Gerontologist, 56*(5), e70–e88.

McClure, N., Lutenbacher, M., O'Kelley, E., et al. (2017). Enhancing pediatric asthma care and nursing education through an academic practice partnership. *Journal of Pediatric Nursing, 36,* 64–69.

Miniati, M., Callari, A., Calugi, S., et al. (2014). Interpersonal psychotherapy for postpartum depression: A systematic review. *Archives of Women's Mental Health, 17*(4), 257–268.

Moorhead, S. A., Hazlett, D. E., Harrison, L., et al. (2013). A new dimension of health care: Systematic review of the uses, benefits, and limitations of social media for health communication. *Journal of Medical Internet Research, 15*(4).

Niela-Vilén, H., Axelin, A., Salanterä, S., et al. (2014). Internet-based peer support for parents: A systematic integrative review. *International Journal of Nursing Studies, 51*(11), 1524–1537.

Nurjannah, I., Mills, J., Usher, K., et al. (2014). Discharge planning in mental health care: An integrative review of the literature. *Journal of Clinical Nursing, 23*(9–10), 1175–1185.

Ong, J., Brennsteiner, A., Chow, E., et al. (2016). Correlates of family satisfaction with hospice care: General inpatient hospice care versus routine home hospice care. *Journal of Palliative Medicine, 19*(1), 97–100.

Östlund, U., & Persson, C. (2014). Examining family responses to Family Systems Nursing interventions: An integrative review. *Journal of Family Nursing, 20*(3), 259–286.

Powers, M. A., Bardsley, J., Cypress, M., et al. (2017). Diabetes self-management education and support in type 2 diabetes: A joint position statement of the American Diabetes Association, the American Association of Diabetes Educators, and the Academy of Nutrition and Dietetics. *The Diabetes Educator, 43*(1), 40–53.

Rodakowski, J., Rocco, P. B., Ortiz, M., et al. (2017). Caregiver integration during discharge planning for older adults to reduce resource use: A metaanalysis. *Journal of the American Geriatrics Society, 65*(8), 1748–1755.

Shen, Z. (2015). Cultural competence models and cultural competence assessment instruments in nursing: A literature review. *Journal of Transcultural Nursing, 26*(3), 308–321.

Smith, J., Swallow, V., & Coyne, I. (2015). Involving parents in managing their child's long-term condition—A concept synthesis of family-centered care and partnership-in-care. *Journal of Pediatric Nursing, 30*(1), 143–159.

van Santvoort, F., Hosman, C. M., van Doesum, K. T., et al. (2014a). Children of mentally ill parents participating in preventive support groups: Parental diagnoses and child risk. *Journal of Child and Family Studies, 23*(1), 67–75.

van Santvoort, F., Hosman, C. M., van Doesum, K. T., et al. (2014b). Effectiveness of preventive support groups for children of mentally ill or addicted parents: A randomized controlled trial. *European Child & Adolescent Psychiatry, 23*(6), 473–484.

Wang, J., Kearney, J. A., Jia, H., et al. (2016). Mental health disorders in elderly people receiving home care: Prevalence and correlates in the national US population. *Nursing Research, 65*(2), 107–116.

Wong, D. F., Ng, T. K., Ip, P. S., et al. (2017). Evaluating the effectiveness of a group CBT for parents of ADHD children. *Journal of Child and Family Studies,* 1–13.

Youngblut, J. M., Brooten, D., Glaze, J., et al. (2017). Parent grief 1–13 months after death in neonatal and pediatric intensive care units. *Journal of Loss & Trauma, 22*(1), 77–96.

● = Independent;   ▲ = Collaborative;   **EBN** = Evidence-Based Nursing;   **EB** = Evidence-Based

Zegwaard, M. I., Aartsen, M. J., Grypdonck, M. H., et al. (2017). Trust: An essential condition in the application of a caregiver support intervention in nursing practice. *BMC Psychiatry*, *17*(1), 47.

Zhong, Q., Gelaye, B., Rondon, M., et al. (2014). Comparative performance of Patient Health Questionnaire-9 and Edinburgh Postnatal Depression Scale for screening antepartum depression. *Journal of Affective Disorders*, *162*, 1–7.

Disabled family Coping *Marsha McKenzie, MA Ed, BSN, RN*

NANDA-I

Definition

Behavior of primary person (family member, significant other, or close friend) that disables his or her capacities and the client's capacities to effectively address tasks essential to either person's adaptation to the health challenge.

Defining Characteristics

Abandonment; adopts illness symptoms of client; aggression; agitation; client dependence; depression; desertion; disregard for client's needs; distortion of reality about client's health problem; family behaviors detrimental to well-being; hostility; impaired ability to structure a meaningful life; impaired individualization, intolerance; neglect of basic needs of client; neglect of relationship with family member; neglect of treatment regimen; performing routines without regard for client needs; prolonged hyperfocus on client; psychosomatic symptoms; rejection

Related Factors

Ambivalent family relationships; chronically unexpressed feelings by support person; differing coping styles between support person and client; differing coping styles between support persons; inconsistent management of family's resistance to treatment

NOC (Nursing Outcomes Classification)

Suggested NOC Outcomes

Caregiver Well-Being; Family Coping; Family Normalization; Neglect Recovery

> **Example NOC Outcome with Indicators**
>
> **Family Normalization** as evidenced by the following indicators: Adapts family routines to accommodate needs of affected member/Meets physical and psychosocial needs of family members/Provides activities appropriate to age and ability for affected family member/Uses community support groups. (Rate the outcome and indicators of **Family Normalization:** I = never demonstrated, 2 = rarely demonstrated, 3 = sometimes demonstrated, 4 = often demonstrated, 5 = consistently demonstrated [see Section I].)

Client Outcomes

Family/Significant Person Will (Specify Time Frame)

- Identify normal family routines that will need to be adapted
- Participate positively in the client's care within the limits of his or her abilities
- Identify responses that may be harmful
- Acknowledge and accept the need for assistance with circumstances
- Identify appropriate activities for affected family member

NIC (Nursing Interventions Classification)

Suggested NIC Interventions

Family Process Maintenance; Caregiver Support; Family Support; Family Therapy; Respite Care

● = Independent;   ▲ = Collaborative;   EBN = Evidence-Based Nursing;   EB = Evidence-Based

Example NIC Activities—Family Process Maintenance
Determine typical family processes; Minimize family routine disruption by facilitating family routines and rituals such as private meals together or family discussions for communication and decision-making; Design schedules of home care activities that minimize disruption of family routine

C

Nursing Interventions and *Rationales*

- Families dealing with acute trauma are susceptible to mild to very severe levels of anxiety. Support should be offered through necessary channels, which are appropriate to the situation, such as providing frequent information, offering social services, or counseling. EB: *Findings from one study suggest that a large percentage of caregivers of patients with trauma suffered from mild to very severe levels of anxiety (Rahnama et al, 2017).*
- Assess coping strategies of both the patient and the spouse when managing women with breast cancer and men with prostate cancer. EB: *A study conducted by Lambert et al (2012) concluded that coping with prostate cancer was more effective when both the patient and spouse were assisted with management of the illness.*
- Cancer caregiving interventions should include communication skill building, including strategies for self-care. EB: *Findings from this study confirmed that caregiver quality of life is impacted by stress about communication across all domains (Wittenberg et al, 2017).*
- Provide ideas for positive child coping and consider collaboration with mental health providers for children with chronic illnesses who are facing emotional problems. EBN: *One study suggested that negative child coping may have deleterious effects on the family (Woodson et al, 2015).*
- Assess social support of family members caring for survivors of traumatic brain injuries (TBIs). Facilitate realistic expectations about caregiving. EB: *TBI survivors and caregivers had multiple self-reported unaddressed needs after their discharge from facility-based treatment. They expressed the need for further education regarding potential post-TBI challenges and strategies for addressing them, including a need for community and mental health resources (Adams & Dahdah, 2016).*
- Respect and promote the spiritual needs of the client and family. EB: *Spiritual well-being is associated with better mental health and positive coping skills of family caregivers (Kelley & Morrison, 2015).*

 Pediatric

- Assist parents and children suffering from chronic illness to develop accommodative coping skills (adapting to stressors rather than attempting to change the stressors). EB: *Compas et al (2012) found considerable evidence across chronic childhood illnesses and medical conditions that suggests that secondary control coping, or accommodative coping, is related to better adjustment in children and adolescents.*
- Assess educational level of parents of ill children and construct parent teaching to address educational attainment. EB: *Gage-Bouchard, Devine, and Heckler (2013) found programs that address educational gaps and teach caregivers planning and active coping skills may be beneficial for parents with lower educational attainment, particularly men.*

 Geriatric

- Assess the emotional well-being of family members who are caring for clients with long-term illnesses, such as stroke. EB: *A study by Ali and Kausar (2016) studied levels of psychological distress experienced by the caregivers of stroke patients concluding that distress can be reduced by providing greater social support.*
- Be aware of age-related deterioration in coping skills. EB: *Diehl et al (2014) found that the defense mechanisms of doubt, displacement, and regression increased after the age of 65 years. Linear age-related decreases were found for the coping mechanism of ego regression and the defense mechanisms of isolation and rationalization.*

 Multicultural

- Be sensitive to the stigma attached to particular illness in various cultures. EB: *Iseselo, Kajula, and Yahya-Malima (2016) studied families coping with mental illness in Tanzania and concluded that the psychosocial challenges of families and caregivers require a collaborative approach.*

● = Independent;   ▲ = Collaborative;   EBN = Evidence-Based Nursing;   EB = Evidence-Based

Home Care

The interventions described previously may be adapted for home care use:
- Assess for strain in family caregivers.
- Assess for "caregiver fatigue" and provide information related to available respite care.
- Consult social services for available home resources related to the client's age and illness.

Client/Family Teaching and Discharge Planning

- Involve the client and family in the planning of care as often as possible.
- Recognize that family decision makers may need additional psychosocial support services.
- Educate family members regarding stress management techniques including massage and alternative therapies.

REFERENCES

Adams, D., & Dahdah, M. (2016). Coping and adaptive strategies of traumatic brain injury survivors and primary caregivers. *Neurorehabilitation*, 39(2), 223–237. doi:10.3233/NRE-161353.

Ali, N., & Kausar, R. (2016). Social support and coping as predictors of psychological distress in family caregivers of stroke patients. *Pakistan Journal of Psychological Research*, 31(2), 587–608.

Compas, B. E., Jaser, S. S., Dunn, M. J., et al. (2012). Coping with chronic illness in childhood and adolescence. *Annual Review of Clinical Psychology*, 8, 455–480.

Diehl, M., Chui, H., Hay, E. L., et al. (2014). Change in coping and defense mechanisms across adulthood: Longitudinal findings in a European-American sample. *Developmental Psychology*, 50(2), 634–648.

Gage-Bouchard, E. A., Devine, K. A., & Heckler, C. E. (2013). The relationship between socio-demographic characteristics, family environment, and caregiver coping in families of children with cancer. *Journal of Clinical Psychology in Medical Settings*, 20(4), 478–487.

Iseselo, M. K., Kajula, L., & Yahya-Malima, K. I. (2016). The psychosocial problems of families caring for relatives with mental illnesses and their coping strategies: A qualitative urban based study in Dar es Salaam, Tanzania. *BMC Psychiatry*, 161. doi:10.1186/s12888-016-0857-y.

Kelley, A. S., & Morrison, R. S. (2015). Palliative care for the seriously ill. *New England Journal of Medicine*, 373(8), 747–755. doi:10.1056/nejmra140468.

Lambert, S. D., Girgis, A., Turner, J., et al. (2012). A pilot randomized controlled trial of the feasibility of a self-directed coping skills intervention for couples facing prostate cancer: Rationale and design. *Health and Quality of Life Outcomes*, 10, 119.

Rahnama, M., Shahdadi, H., Bagheri, S., et al. (2017). The relationship between anxiety and coping strategies in family caregivers of patients with trauma. *Journal of Clinical & Diagnostic Research*, 11(4), 6–9. doi:10.7860/JCDR/2017/25951.9673.

Wittenberg, E., Borneman, T., Koczywas, M., et al. (2017). Cancer communication and family caregiver quality of life. *Behavioral Sciences*, 7(1). doi:10.3390/bs7010012.

Woodson, K. D., Thakkar, S., Burbage, M., et al. (2015). Children with chronic illnesses: Factors influencing family hardiness. *Issues in Comprehensive Pediatric Nursing*, 38(1), 57–69. doi:10.3109/01460862.2014.988896.

Readiness for enhanced family Coping   Keith A. Anderson, PhD, MSW

NANDA-I

Definition

A pattern of management of adaptive tasks by primary person (family member, significant other, or close friend) involved with the client's health challenge, which can be strengthened.

Defining Characteristics

Expresses desire to acknowledge growth impact of crisis; expresses desire to choose experiences that optimize wellness; expresses desire to enhance connection with others who have experienced a similar situation; expresses desire to enhance enrichment of lifestyle; expresses desire to enhance health promotion

NOC   (Nursing Outcomes Classification)

Suggested NOC Outcomes

Family Coping; Health-Seeking Behavior; Participation in Health Care Decisions

● = Independent;   ▲ = Collaborative;   **EBN** = Evidence-Based Nursing;   **EB** = Evidence-Based

C

Family Coping as evidenced by the following indicators: Confronts and manages family problems/Cares for needs of all family members. (Rate the outcome and indicators of **Family Coping:** 1 = never demonstrated, 2 = rarely demonstrated, 3 = sometimes demonstrated, 4 = often demonstrated, 5 = consistently demonstrated [see Section I].)

Client Outcomes

Client Will (Specify Time Frame)

State a plan indicating coping strengths, abilities, and resources, as well as areas for growth and change; Perform tasks and engage resources needed for growth and change; Evaluate changes and continually reevaluate plan for continued growth

NIC   Interventions (Nursing Interventions Classification)

Suggested NIC Interventions

Family Integration Promotion; Family Involvement Promotion; Family Support; Mutual Goal Setting

Example NIC Activities—Family Coping

Facilitate communication of concerns and feelings between clients and family or among family members; Provide resources that support and encourage adaptive family coping; Respect and support adaptive coping mechanisms used by family

Nursing Interventions and *Rationales*

▲ Assess the structure, resources, and coping abilities of families and use these assessments in selecting interventions and formulating care plans. **EB/EBN:** *It is critical to understand the resiliency and coping capabilities of families; the use of established assessment instruments (e.g., Family Assessment Device, Family Assessment Measure) can provide insight into family dynamics, coping styles, and resources of family systems (Mansfield, Keitner, & Dealy, 2014; Sawin, 2016).*

▲ Acknowledge, assess, and support the spiritual needs and resources of families and clients. **EB/EBN:** *Spirituality has been found to be an important, yet often overlooked, coping resource for families and clients during illness and recovery (O'Brien, 2014; Hodge, 2015; Prouty et al, 2016).*

▲ Establish rapport with families and empower their decision-making through effective communication and patient/family-centered care. **EBN:** *Effective communication and patient/family-centered care approaches can help to establish rapport, personalize treatment plans, and empower families in their caregiving activities and decision-making capacities (Mitchell et al, 2016; Coombs et al, 2017).*

▲ Provide family members with educational and skill-building interventions to alleviate caregiving stress and to facilitate adherence to prescribed plans of care. **EBN:** *The provision of psychoeducational and supportive interventions may enable family members to gain a sense of control in the caregiving role and to become more comfortable in providing care and making informed decisions (Ostlund & Persson, 2014; Dockham et al, 2016).*

▲ Develop, provide, and encourage family members to use counseling services and interventions. **EB/EBN:** *Family-centered counseling interventions have been shown to be effective, particularly in situations regarding serious illness and difficult family decisions (Cheng, Chair, & Chow et al, 2014; Creasy et al, 2015).*

▲ Identify and refer to support programs that discuss experiences and challenges similar to those faced by the family (e.g., cancer support groups). **EB:** *Although there is wide diversity in the format of support programs, couples and family support approaches can be beneficial and enhance coping (Ostlund & Persson, 2014; Inhestern et al, 2016).*

▲ Incorporate the use of emerging technologies to increase the reach of interventions to support family coping. **EBN:** *Emerging computer and Internet-based supportive and educational interventions may hold promise in enhancing family members' well-being and informational needs (Risling, Risling, & Holtslander, 2017; Salem et al, 2017).*

▲ Refer to Compromised family **Coping** for additional interventions.

 Pediatric

▲ Identify and assess the management styles of families and facilitate the use of more effective ways of coping with childhood illness. **EB:** *Understanding the dominant characteristics of each family's coping styles*

• = Independent; ▲ = Collaborative; **EBN** = Evidence-Based Nursing; **EB** = Evidence-Based

C

and resources and helping them to use more effective management styles can result in better family functioning and treatment outcomes (Ketelaar et al, 2016; McCarthy et al, 2016).

▲ Provide educational and supportive interventions for families caring for children with illness and disability. EBN: *Providing information, training parents in care management, and offering supportive programs can reduce stress levels in parents and lead to better outcomes for children (Golfenshtein, Srulovici, & Deatrick, 2016).*

Geriatric

▲ Encourage family caregivers to participate in counseling and support groups. EB/EBN: *Although a wide variety of programs exist, certain counseling and support group programs have been found to be effective in increasing family resourcefulness and lowering caregiver burden, anxiety, depression, and family conflict (Dam et al, 2016; Muller et al, 2017).*

▲ Provide educational and therapeutic interventions to family caregivers that focus on knowledge and skill building. EBN: *Psychoeducational interventions that are accessible and tailored to individual needs can be highly valued and useful to family caregivers (Bakas et al, 2014; Bakas, McCarthy, & Miller, 2017).*

Multicultural

▲ Acknowledge and understand the importance of cultural influences in families and ensure that assessments and assessment tools account for such cultural differences. EB: *Family coping tends to vary across cultures and may affect the fit, reliability, and validity of existing family functioning and coping assessment tools (Desai, Rivera, & Backes, 2016).*

▲ Understand and incorporate cultural differences into interventions to enhance the impact of family interventions. EB/EBN: *Tailoring interventions to the customs, beliefs, preferences, and strengths of specific groups may increase effectiveness (Dayer-Berenson, 2014; McCalman et al, 2017).*

REFERENCES

Bakas, T., Clark, P. C., Kelly-Hayes, M., et al. (2014). Evidence for stroke family caregiver and dyad interventions: A statement for healthcare professionals from the American Heart Association and American Stroke Association. *Stroke; a Journal of Cerebral Circulation, 45*(9), 2836–2852.

Bakas, T., McCarthy, M., & Miller, E. T. (2017). Update on the state of evidence for stroke family caregiver and dyad interventions. *Stroke; a Journal of Cerebral Circulation, 48*(5), e122–e125.

Cheng, H. Y., Chair, S. Y., & Chau, J. P. (2014). The effectiveness of psychosocial interventions for stroke family caregivers and stroke survivors: A systematic review and meta-analysis. *Patient Education and Counseling, 95,* 30–44.

Coombs, M., Puntillo, K. A., Franck, L. S., et al. (2017). Implementing the SCCM Family-Centered Care Guidelines in critical care nursing practice. *AACN Advanced Critical Care, 28*(2), 138–147.

Creasy, K. R., Lutz, B. J., Young, M. E., et al. (2015). Clinical implications of family-centered care in stroke rehabilitation. *Rehabilitation Nursing, 40*(6), 349–359.

Dayer-Berenson, L. (2014). *Cultural competencies for nurses: Impact on health and illness.* Burlington, MA: Jones & Bartlett Learning.

Dam, A. E. H., de Vugt, M. E., Klinkenberg, I. P. M., et al. (2016). A systematic review of social support interventions for caregivers of people with dementia: Are they doing what they promise? *Maturitas, 85,* 117–130.

Desai, P. P., Rivera, A. T., & Backes, E. M. (2016). Latino caregiver coping with children's chronic health conditions: An integrative literature review. *Journal of Pediatric Health Care, 30*(2), 108–120.

Dockham, B., Schafenacker, A., Yoon, H., et al. (2016). Implementation of a psychosocial program for cancer survivors and family caregivers at a cancer support community affiliate: A pilot effectiveness study. *Cancer Nursing, 39*(3), 169–180.

Golfenshtein, N., Srulovici, E., & Deatrick, J. A. (2016). Interventions for reducing parenting stress in families with pediatric conditions:

An integrative review. *Journal of Family Nursing, 22*(4), 460–492.

Hodge, D. R. (2015). Administering a two-stage spiritual assessment in healthcare settings: A necessary component of ethical and effective care. *Journal of Nursing Management, 23*(1), 27–38.

Inhestern, L., Haller, A.-C., Wlodararczyk, O., et al. (2016). Psychosocial interventions for families with parental cancer and barriers and facilitators to implementation and use: A systematic review. *PLoS ONE, 11*(6).

Ketelaar, M., Bogossian, A., Saini, M., et al. (2016). Assessment of the family environment in pediatric neurodisability: A state-of-the-art review. *Developmental Medicine & Child Neurology, 59,* 259–269.

Mansfield, A. K., Keitner, G. I., & Dealy, J. (2014). The Family Assessment Device: An update. *Family Process, 54*(1), 82–93.

McCalman, J., Heyeres, M., Campbell, S., et al. (2017). Family-centred interventions by primary healthcare services for Indigenous early childhood well-being in Australia, Canada, New Zealand, and the United States: A systematic scoping review. *BMC Pregnancy and Childbirth, 17,* 71.

McCarthy, M. C., Wakefield, C. E., DeGraves, S., et al. (2016). Feasibility of clinical psychosocial screening in pediatric oncology: Implementing the PAT2.0. *Journal of Psychosocial Oncology, 34*(5), 363–375.

Mitchell, M. L., Coyer, F., Kean, S., et al. (2016). Patient, family-centred care interventions within the adult ICU setting: An integrative review. *Australian Critical Care, 29*(4), 179–193.

Muller, C., Lautenschlager, S., Meyer, G., et al. (2017). Interventions to support people with dementia and their caregivers during the transition from home care to nursing home care: A systematic review. *International Journal of Nursing Studies, 71,* 139–152.

O'Brien, M. E. (2014). *Spirituality in nursing: Standing on holy ground* (5th ed.). Burlington, MA: Jones & Bartlett Learning.

● = Independent;   ▲ = Collaborative;   EBN = Evidence-Based Nursing;   EB = Evidence-Based

Ostlund, U., & Persson, C. (2014). Examining family responses to family systems nursing interventions: An integrative review. *Journal of Family Nursing, 20,* 259–286.

Prouty, A. M., Fischer, J., Purdom, A., et al. (2016). Spiritual coping: A gateway to enhancing family communication during cancer treatment. *Journal of Religion and Health, 55*(1), 269–287.

Risling, T., Risling, D., & Holtslander, L. (2017). Creating a social media assessment tool for family nursing. *Journal of Family Nursing.* [Epub ahead of print].

Salem, H., Johansen, C., Schmiegelow, K., et al. (2017). FAMily-Oriented Support (FAMOS): Development and feasibility of a psychosocial intervention for families of childhood cancer survivors. *Acta Oncologica, 56*(2), 367–374.

Sawin, K. J. (2016). Measurement in family nursing: Established instruments and new directions. *Journal of Family Nursing, 22*(3), 287–297.

Readiness for enhanced Decision-Making   *Dawn Fairlie, PhD, NP*

NANDA-I

Definition

A pattern of choosing a course of action for meeting short- and long-term health-related goals, which can be strengthened.

Defining Characteristics

Expresses desire to enhance congruency of decisions with sociocultural goal; expresses desire to enhance congruency of decisions with sociocultural value; expresses desire to enhance congruency of decisions with goal; expresses desire to enhance congruency of decisions with values; expresses desire to enhance decision-making; expresses desire to enhance risk-benefit analysis of decisions; expresses desire to enhance understanding of choices for decision-making; expresses desire to enhance understanding of meaning of choices; expresses desire to enhance use of reliable evidence for decisions

NOC   (Nursing Outcomes Classification)

Suggested NOC Outcomes

Decision-Making; Participation in Health Care Decisions; Personal Autonomy

Example NOC Outcome with Indicators

Participation in Health Care Decisions as evidenced by the following indicators: Claims decision-making responsibility/Exhibits self-direction in decision-making/Seeks reputable information/Specifies health outcome preferences. (Rate the outcome and indicators of **Participation in Health Care Decisions:** I = never demonstrated, 2 = rarely demonstrated, 3 = sometimes demonstrated, 4 = often demonstrated, 5 = consistently demonstrated [see Section I].)

Client Outcomes

Client Will (Specify Time Frame)

- Review treatment options with providers
- Ask questions about the benefits and risks of treatment options
- Communicate decisions about treatment options to providers in relation to personal preferences, values, and goals

NIC   (Nursing Interventions Classification)

Suggested NIC Interventions

Decision-Making Support; Mutual Goal Setting; Support System Enhancement; Values Clarification

Example NIC Activities—Decision-Making Support

Help client identify the advantages and disadvantages of each alternative; Facilitate collaborative decision-making; Help client explain decisions to others, as needed

● = Independent;   ▲ = Collaborative;   EBN = Evidence-Based Nursing;   EB = Evidence-Based

D

Nursing Interventions and *Rationales*

- Support and encourage clients and their representatives to engage in health care decisions. **EB:** *Decisional conflict was assessed using the Decisional Conflict Scale among 186 Dutch mental health patients. They concluded that patient participation in decision-making and measuring decisional conflict and knowledge about influencing factors could improve adherence to treatment and clinical outcomes (Metz et al, 2018).* **EBN:** *Decision aids are intended to help people participate in decisions that involve weighing the benefits and harms of treatment options, often with scientific uncertainty. Hart, Tofthagen, and Hsiao-Lan (2016) developed a decision aid that could be adapted and used in a variety of settings with a focus on initiating a conversation between the patient and provider on lung cancer screening. Respect personal preferences, values, needs, and rights.* **EBN:** *"Clarifying values can be a rewarding exercise, as it not only ensures the best possible decision but demonstrates to patients that we are genuinely interested in incorporating their views and how they value the outcomes from screening options" (Lang et al, 2018, p 29).*
- Provide information that is appropriate, relevant, and timely. **EBN:** *Decisional conflict was assessed using the Decisional Conflict Scale (DCS) among surrogate decision-makers to compare end-of-life terminologies "Do Not Resuscitate" (DNR) and "Allow Natural Death" (AND). Findings included that the framing of the decision influenced decision satisfaction and decision-making. Additionally, prior experience with end-of-life decision-making demonstrated lower mean total DCS scores and lower mean subscores, indicating that prior experience is an important aspect of end-of-life decision-making (Fairlie, 2017).*
- Determine the health literacy of clients and their representatives before helping with decision-making. **EB:** *An online decision aid for a low health literacy population will be pilot tested with 30 women diagnosed with early breast cancer with the anticipation that the low health literacy decision aid will be useful and acceptable to young women with low health literacy who have been diagnosed with breast cancer and it will be preferred over the high literacy decision aid (Peate et al, 2017).*
- Tailor information to the specific needs of individual clients, according to principles of health literacy. **EB:** *Altin and Stock (2016) sampled 1125 German adults to examine the contributions of health literacy, shared decision-making, patient-centered communication, and satisfaction with care received by the general practitioner. Respondents with sufficient health literacy skills were 2.06 times as likely to be satisfied with their care.*
- Motivate clients to be as independent as possible in decision-making. **EB:** *A study of shared decision-making and autonomy among patients with multiple sclerosis revealed that patient-centered decision-making was most commonly preferred by study participants, followed by shared decision-making (Cofield et al, 2017).*
- Facilitate communication between the client and family members regarding the final decision; offer support to the person actually making the decision. **EBN:** *A study of surrogate decision-makers' decisional conflict with end-of-life decision-making found that surrogates who had discussed end-of-life preferences with their loved one experienced less decisional conflict than those who had not discussed preferences (Fairlie, 2017).*
- Design educational interventions for decision support. **EBN:** *The goal of patient decision aids is to engage patients in health care decisions by providing evidence-based information in plain language. The goal is to assist patients in understanding the risks and benefits of all available treatment/diagnosis options and engage patients in health care decisions to improve alignment of treatment choices with patients' preferences (Madden & Kleinlugtenbelt, 2017).*

 ### Geriatric

- The previously mentioned interventions may be adapted for geriatric use.
- Facilitate collaborative decision-making. **EB:** *A systematic review of randomized controlled trials evaluating the efficacy of decision aids compared with the usual care for older adults facing treatment, screening, or care decisions found that decision aids improve older adults' knowledge, increase their risk perception, decrease decisional conflict, and seem to enhance participation in shared decision-making (van Weert et al, 2016).*

 ### Multicultural

- Use existing decision aids for particular types of decisions or develop decision aids as indicated. **EB:** *Hoffman et al (2017) measured decisional conflict as a primary measure of decision quality and an intermediate measure in the process of screening uptake in a sample of 88 African American males. The purpose of patient*

● = Independent; ▲ = Collaborative; EBN = Evidence-Based Nursing; EB = Evidence-Based

decision was to prepare patients for a consultation with their doctor. The entertainment–education decision aid significantly improved African American patients' knowledge, reduced their decisional conflict, and increased their sense of self-advocacy regarding colorectal cancer screening.

Home Care

- The previously mentioned interventions may be adapted for home care use.
- Develop clinical practice guidelines that include shared decision-making. **EBN:** *Thoma-Lurken et al (2018) reported that people with dementia who wish to age in place are susceptible to nursing home admission. Nurses can intervene by detecting practical problems people with dementia and caregivers face. They identified three domains, decreased self-reliance, safety-related problems, and informal caregiver/social network-related problems, and proposed addressing these domains to facilitate aging in place.*

Client/Family Teaching and Discharge Planning

- Instruct the client and family members to provide advance directives in the following areas:
  - Person to contact in an emergency
  - Preference (if any) to die at home or in the hospital
  - Desire to initiate advanced directives, such as a living will or medical power of attorney
  - Desire to donate an organ
  - Funeral arrangements (i.e., burial, cremation)
- ▲ **EBN:** *Shared decision-makers experienced less decisional conflict when they had discussed end-of-life preferences with the client (Fairlie, 2017).*

REFERENCES

Altin, S., & Stock, S. (2016). The impact of health literacy, patient-centered communication and shared decision-making on patients' satisfaction with care received in German primary care practices. *BMC Health Services Research, 16*(1), 450.

Cofield, S., Thomas, N., Tyry, T., et al. (2017). Shared decision making and autonomy among US participants with multiple sclerosis in the NARCOMS Registry. *International Journal of MS Care, 19*(6), 303–312.

Fairlie, D. E. (2017). Specific words and experience matter to surrogates when making end of life decisions. *Health Communication, 33*(5), 537–543. doi:10.1080/10410236.2017.1283560.

Hart, K., Tofthagen, C., & Hsiao-Lan, W. (2016). Development and evaluation of a lung cancer screening decision aid. *Clinical Journal of Oncology Nursing, 20*(5), 557–559. doi:10.1188/16.CJON.557-559.

Hoffman, A., Lowenstein, L., Kamath, G., et al. (2017). An entertainment-education colorectal cancer screening decision aid for African American patients: A randomized controlled trial. *Cancer, 123*(8), 1401–1408.

Lang, E., Bell, N., Dickinson, J., et al. (2018). Eliciting patient values and preferences to inform shared decision making in preventive screening. *Canadian Family Physician Medecin De Famille Canadien, 64*(1), 28–31.

Madden, K., & Kleinlugtenbelt, Y. V. (2017). Cochrane in CORR: Decision aids for people facing health treatment or screening decisions. *Clinical Orthopaedics and Related Research, 475*(5), 1298–1304. Retrieved from https://doi.org/10.1007/s11999-017-5254-4.

Metz, M. J., Veerbeek, M. A., van der Feltz-Cornelis, C. M., et al. (2018). *Social Psychiatry and Psychiatric Epidemiology, 53*, 161. Retrieved from https://doi.org/10.1007/s00127-017-1467-9.

Peate, M., Smith, S. K., Pye, V., et al. (2017). Assessing the usefulness and acceptability of a low health literacy online decision aid about reproductive choices for younger women with breast cancer: The aLLIAnCE pilot study protocol. *Pilot and Feasibility Studies, 3*, 31. Retrieved from https://doi.org/10.1186/s40814-017-0144-9.

Thoma-Lurken, T., Bleijlevens, M., Lexis, M., et al. (2018). *Facilitating aging in place: a qualitative study of practical problems preventing people with dementia from living at home. Geriatric Nursing, 39*(1): 29–38.

van Weert, J. C., Van Munster, B. C., Sanders, R., et al. (2016). Decision aids to help older people make health decisions: A systematic review and meta-analysis. *BMC Medical Informatics and Decision Making, 16*(1), 45.

Decisional Conflict   *Dawn Fairlie, PhD, APRN-BC*

NANDA-I

Definition

Uncertainty about course of action to be taken when choice among competing actions involves risk, loss, or challenge to values and beliefs.

Defining Characteristics

Delay in decision-making; distress while attempting a decision; physical sign of distress (e.g., increase in heart rate, restlessness); physical sign of tension; questioning of moral principle while attempting a decision;

● = Independent;   ▲ = Collaborative;   **EBN** = Evidence-Based Nursing;   **EB** = Evidence-Based

D

questioning of moral rule while attempting a decision; questioning of moral values while attempting a decision; questioning of personal beliefs while attempting a decision; questioning of personal values while attempting a decision; recognizes undesired consequences of actions being considered; self-focused; uncertainty about choices; vacillating among choices

Related Factors

Conflict with moral obligation; conflicting information sources; inexperience with decision-making; insufficient information; insufficient support system; interference in making decision-making; moral principle supports mutually inconsistent actions; moral rule supports mutually inconsistent actions; moral value supports mutually inconsistent actions; perceived threat to value system; unclear personal beliefs unclear personal values

NOC (Nursing Outcomes Classification)

Suggested NOC Outcomes

Decision-Making; Information Processing; Participation in Health Care Decisions; Personal Autonomy

> **Example NOC Outcome with Indicators**
>
> **Decision-Making** as evidenced by the following indicators: Identifies relevant information/Identifies alternatives/Identifies potential consequences of each alternative/Identifies needed resources to support each alternative. (Rate the outcome and indicators of **Decision-Making:** 1 = severely compromised, 2 = substantially compromised, 3 = moderately compromised, 4 = mildly compromised, 5 = not compromised [see Section I].)

Client Outcomes

Client Will (Specify Time Frame)

- State the advantages and disadvantages of choices
- Share fears and concerns regarding choices and responses of others
- Seek resources and information necessary for making an informed choice
- Make an informed choice

NIC (Nursing Interventions Classification)

Suggested NIC Intervention

Decision-Making Support

> **Example NIC Activities—Decision-Making Support**
>
> Inform client of alternative views or solutions in a clear and supportive manner; Provide information requested by client

Nursing Interventions and *Rationales*

- Observe for factors causing or contributing to conflict (e.g., value conflicts, fear of outcome, poor problem-solving skills). **EB:** *When studying clients with prostate cancer, Hoffman et al (2018) assessed differences across four treatment groups and asked about decision-making.*
- Decisional conflict was associated with anxiety. Findings suggested a potential role for early use of validated decision aids.
- Provide emotional support. **EB:** *O'Neill et al (2018) assessed the information needs and levels of distress and correlates of this distress of young women with breast cancer. They reported lower distress and significantly lower decisional conflict and greater endorsement of an array of healthy coping strategies and suggested that young adult women have unmet cancer genetic information and support needs.*
- Use decision aids or computer-based decision aids to assist clients in making decisions. **EB:** *Baptista et al (2018) found that Web-based decision aids performed similarly to alternative formats for decision-quality outcomes. Additionally, because of anonymity Web-based decision aids increased access to decision aids that support prostate cancer screening decisions among men. Initiate health teaching and referrals when needed.*

● = Independent; ▲ = Collaborative; EBN = Evidence-Based Nursing; EB = Evidence-Based

EB: *Lopez-Olivo et al (2018) developed and tested multimedia patient education tools (video tools) for patients with knee osteoarthritis (OA), osteoporosis (OP), and rheumatoid arthritis (RA). They found that multimedia educational tools that incorporate videos increase patient understanding and management of their disease.*

- Facilitate communication between the client and family members regarding the final decision; offer support to the person actually making the decision. **EBN:** *A study of surrogate decision makers' decisional conflict with end-of-life decision-making found that surrogates who had discussed end-of-life preferences with their loved ones experienced less decisional conflict than those who had not discussed their preferences (Fairlie, 2018).*

Geriatric

- Carefully assess clients with dementia regarding ability to make decisions. **EBN:** *A study of the shared decision-making process of persons with dementia identified a broad spectrum of the shared decision-making process. Results indicated that not all persons with dementia are excluded from participating in the decision-making process. Loizeau et al (2018) tested the effect of fact box decision support tools on decisional conflict and preferences in advanced dementia. They found that fact boxes reduced decisional conflict, increased knowledge, and promoted preferences to forego antibiotics in advanced dementia in decision makers.*
- Discuss the purpose of advance directives such as a living well or medical power of attorney. **EB:** *Basile et al (2018) studied a Web-based decision aid in patients with severe chronic obstructive pulmonary disease to assist in preparation for decision-making about invasive mechanical ventilation for respiratory failure. Increased knowledge and opportunity to deliberate and discuss treatment choices after using the decision aid improved decision-making at the time of critical illness.*

Multicultural

- Assess for the influence of cultural beliefs, norms, and values on the client's decision-making conflict. **EB:** *A study of couples undergoing genetic counseling found that factors associated with conflict during decision-making included cultural customs, age, emotional state, religious beliefs, and being forced to attend counseling. Provide support for client's decision-making (Schoeffel et al, 2018).*

Home Care

- The interventions described previously may be adapted for home care use.
- ▲ **EB:** *Torke et al (2018) conducted a feasibility study of the Physician Orders for Life-Sustaining Treatment (POLST) with community-dwelling adults aged 65 and older enrolled in a complex care management program. They found that 87.5% of decision makers agreed or strongly agreed that "talking about the (POLST) form helped me think about what I really want."*

Client/Family Teaching and Discharge Planning

- Instruct the client and family members to provide advance directives in the following areas:
  - ○ Person to contact in an emergency
  - ○ Preference (if any) to die at home or in the hospital
  - ○ Desire to initiate advanced directives, such as a living will or medical power of attorney
  - ○ Desire to donate an organ
  - ○ Funeral arrangements (i.e., burial, cremation)
- ▲ **EBN:** *Shared decision makers experienced less decisional conflict when they had discussed the client's preferences with the client (Fairlie, 2018).*
- Inform the family of treatment options; encourage and defend self-determination. **EB:** *Hwang et al (2018) surveyed patients seeking treatment for a lumbar herniated disc and measured decisional conflict using the SURE questionnaire. They found that participants with decisional conflict were less satisfied with their treatment decision and found a high level of decisional conflict when choosing a treatment option. They concluded that there is a need to implement tools and strategies to improve decisional quality, such as decision aids before consultation.*
- Recognize and allow the client to discuss the selection of complementary therapies available, such as spiritual support, relaxation, imagery, exercise, lifestyle changes, diet (e.g., macrobiotic, vegetarian), and nutritional supplementation. **EB:** *Hippman and Balneaves (2018) studied women's decision-making for treatment of depression during pregnancy and found that women require a nonjudgmental environment when choosing between medications, psychotherapy, electroconvulsive therapy, deep brain stimulation, and complementary and alternative medicine options.*

● = Independent; ▲ = Collaborative; EBN = Evidence-Based Nursing; EB = Evidence-Based

▲ Provide the POLST form for clients and families faced with end-of-life choices across the health care continuum. **EB:** *Torke et al (2018) found that a large majority of decision makers agreed or strongly agreed that talking about the (POLST) form helped with decision-making.*

REFERENCES

Baptista, S., Sampaio, E. T., Heleno, B., et al. (2018). Web-based versus usual care and other formats of decision aids to support prostate cancer screening decisions: Systematic review and meta-analysis. *Journal of Medical Internet Research*, 20(6), e228.

Basile, M., Andrews, J., Jacome, S., et al. (2018). A decision aid to support shared decision making about mechanical ventilation in severe chronic obstructive pulmonary disease patients (InformedTogether): Feasibility study. Retrieved from https://jopm.jmir.org/2018/2/e7/. (Accessed 22 January 2018).

Fairlie, D. E. (2018). Specific words and experience matter to surrogates when making end of life decisions. *Health Communication*, 33(5), 537–543.

Hippman, C., & Balneaves, L. G. (2018). Women's decision making about antidepressant use during pregnancy: A narrative review. *Depression and Anxiety*, 35(12), 1158–1167.

Hoffman, R. M., Van Den Eeden, S. K., Davis, K. M., et al. (2018). Decision-making processes among men with low-risk prostate cancer: A survey study. *Psycho-Oncology*, 27(1), 325–332.

Hwang, R., Lambrechts, S., Liu, H., et al. (2018). Decisional conflict among patients considering treatment options for lumbar herniated disc. *World Neurosurgery*, 116, e680–e690.

Lopez-Olivo, M. A., Ingleshwar, A., Volk, R. J., et al. (2018). Development and pilot testing of multimedia patient education tools for patients with knee osteoarthritis, osteoporosis, and rheumatoid arthritis. *Arthritis Care & Research*, 70(2), 213–220.

Loizeau, A. J., Theill, N., Cohen, S. M., et al. (2018). Fact box decision support tools reduce decisional conflict about antibiotics for pneumonia and artificial hydration in advanced dementia: A randomized controlled trial. *Age and Ageing.* doi:10.1093/ageing/afy149. [Epub ahead of print].

O'Neill, S. C., Evans, C., Hamilton, R. J., et al. (2018). Information and support needs of young women regarding breast cancer risk and genetic testing: Adapting effective interventions for a novel population. *Familial Cancer*, 17(3), 351–360.

Schoeffel, K., Veach, P. M., Rubin, K., et al. (2018). Managing couple conflict during prenatal counseling sessions: An investigation of genetic counselor experiences and perceptions. *Journal of Genetic Counseling*, 27(5), 1275–1290.

Torke, A. M., Hickman, S. E., Hammes, B., et al. (2018). POLST facilitation in complex care management: A feasibility study. *American Journal of Hospice and Palliative Medicine®.* doi:10.1177/1049909118797077 [Epub ahead of print].

Impaired emancipated Decision-Making
Ruth A. Wittmann-Price, PhD, RN, CNS, CNE, CHSE, ANEF, FAAN

NANDA-I

Definition

A process of choosing a health care decision that does not include personal knowledge and/or consideration of social norms, or does not occur in a flexible environment, resulting in decisional dissatisfaction.

Defining Characteristics

Delay in enacting chosen health care option; distress when listening to other's opinion; excessive concern about what others think is the best decision; excessive fear of what others think about a decision; feeling constrained in describing own opinion; inability to choose a health care option that best fits current lifestyle; inability to describe how option will fit into current lifestyle; limited verbalization about health care options in others' presence

Related Factors

Decrease in understanding of all available health care options; inability to adequately verbalize perceptions about health care options; inadequate time to discuss health care options; insufficient confidence to openly discuss health care options; insufficient information regarding health care options; insufficient privacy to openly discuss health care options; insufficient self-confidence in decision-making

At-Risk Population

Limited decision-making experience; traditional hierarchical family; traditional hierarchical health care system

● = Independent;   ▲ = Collaborative;   EBN = Evidence-Based Nursing;   EB = Evidence-Based

NOC   Outcomes (Nursing Outcomes Classification)

Suggested NOC Outcomes

Decision-Making; Self-Esteem; Coping; Health Promoting Behavior; Stress Level; Communication; Self-Care Status; Participation in Health Care Decisions; Health-Seeking Processing; Personal Autonomy; Psychosocial Adjustment: Life Change

Example NOC Outcome with Indicators

Participation in Health Care Decisions as evidenced by the following indicator: Claims decision making responsibility. (Rate the outcome and indicators of **Participation in Health Care Decisions:** 1 = never demonstrated, 2 = rarely demonstrated, 3 = sometimes demonstrated, 4 = often demonstrated, 5 = consistently demonstrated [see Section I].)

Client Outcomes

Client Will (Specify Time Frame)

- Verbalize option outcomes freely before making a health care decision
- Freely verbalize own opinion with health care providers before making a health care decision
- Choose the health care option that fits his or her lifestyle within an appropriate amount of time that allows enactment of the choice
- Describe how the chosen option fits into his or her current lifestyle before or after the decision has been made
- Verbalizes appropriate concern about others' opinions before making the health care choice
- Remains stress-free when listening to others' opinions before making the health care choice
- Arrives at a decision in a timely manner

NIC   Interventions (Nursing Interventions Classification)

Suggested NIC Interventions

Decision-Making Support; Health Coaching; Cognitive Restructuring; Self-Awareness Enhancement

Example NIC Activities—Emancipated Decision-Making

Assist client in making an emancipated decision about health care options by discussing social norms with the client; Provide a flexible environment; Encourage the client to use personal knowledge

Nursing Interventions and *Rationales*

- Assess client's readiness to openly discussing the decision-making process. EB: *DenOuden, Vos, and Guy (2017) studied shared decision-making with diabetic patients (N = 72) and found that in a randomized control trial those patients who chose to be involved in the decision-making process achieved better goals (lower A1C levels and lower blood pressures) than those diabetic patients who did not openly participate in health care decision-making.* EB: *Chen (2017) conducted a study with 15 cancer patients about the decision-making process within three stages of cancer treatment and found that different decision-making approaches to provided information was taken by patients and ranged from informed, to paternalistic, to shared. This study demonstrates that increased attention is needed to open a discussion about treatment options and more provider education on the shared decision-making process.*
- Use active listening in a nonjudgmental manner to provide the client with a flexible decision-making environment. EB: *A study done retrospectively with spinal cord injury patients (N = 22) demonstrated that decision-making was easier in the nonacute stage and that the environment affected the patient's decision-making ability. Along with the environment the communication of information was important and assisted patients to "personalize" their decisions (Schelle-Sailer et al, 2017).* EB: *In a randomized control trial, Perestelo-Perez et al (2017) studied patients with depression using a shared decision-making aid (N = 68) with those not using (N = 70) an aid and found that patients using the tool perceived their goals and concerns were better met.*

● = Independent;   ▲ = Collaborative;   EBN = Evidence-Based Nursing;   EB = Evidence-Based

D

- Use anticipatory guidance by proactively providing the client with information. **EB:** *Brom et al (2017) studied shared decision-making with end-of-life patients and found that practitioners need to have ongoing communication to understand patients' expectations and concern to guide patients through the last stages of life.* **CEB:** *Wittmann-Price, Fliszar, and Bhattacharya (2011) found in a mixed method study that the majority of pregnant clients (N = 50) reported they had been provided with information prenatally, but not all clients felt they were given enough information at the time of delivery to make an informed choice.*
- *Establish a purposeful provider–client relationship.* **EB:** *A mixed methods study with Parkinson's patients (N = 65) demonstrated that the provider–patient relationship was important for the patient in the decision-making process. Establishing a relationship affected patients' ability to enact decisions based on their own preference (Zizzo et al, 2017).* **EB:** *In a study involving oncologists it was found that patient preferences (N = 60) were most commonly initiated by the patient and not the provider. The student suggests additional education for providers in eliciting patients' preferences would enhance communication and treatment (Henselmans et al, 2017).*
- ▲ Refer to counseling as needed. **EB:** *Klausen et al (2017) qualitatively studied patients in the outpatient setting (N = 25) who were referred for mental health issues and found four key components to shared decision-making: (1) during admission, (2) in individualized treatment, (3) in different treatment contexts, and (4) in user–professional relationships.* **CEB:** *Wittmann-Price (2006) demonstrated in a quantitative correlational study that women's (N = 97) decision-making was empowered when they were provided resources and information to arrive at an emancipated choice.*
- Provide decision-making support. **EBN:** *A case study of a pregnant patient whose decision-making abilities were deficit highlights the need for ethical consideration of the patient's values in the decision-making process (Mabel, Rose, & Kodish, 2017).* **EBN:** *Lazenby et al (2017) studied 15 physicians and 5 nurses about their involvement in end-of-life conversations and decisions with hemodialysis patients and found that advanced decision-making planning was deficit and needed attention to accommodate patients' wishes.*
- Provide a flexible environment by encouraging others to accept the client's choice. **EBN:** *A qualitative study with 11 women with breast cancer demonstrated that decision-making on treatment was enhanced by practitioners recognizing three aspects of decision-making: (1) issues caused by the health care problem, (2) understanding the societal burden related to gender, and (3) evaluating the patient's support system (Kkotbong & Jinhyang, 2017).* **CEB:** *Wittmann-Price and Bhattacharya (2008) quantitatively studied pain management decisions for clients in labor (N = 92) and found that a flexible environment was needed for the client to make a supported and emancipated decision.*
- Encourage the client to use personal knowledge as part of the decision-making process to increase decisional satisfaction. **CEB:** *Women can make health care decisions that are right for them if they can use personal knowledge to overcome oppressive social forces (Stepanuk et al, 2013).* **CEB:** *Using personal knowledge is the best indicator to making an emancipated decision and correlates strongly and positively with satisfaction with the decision (Wittmann-Price, 2006).*

 Pediatric

- When able, involve the client in health care decision-making when possible. **EBN:** *Adams and Levy (2017) found that a shared decision-making process with families who care for disabled children should include families' values and priorities to make the best decision for the child.* **EBN:** *Craske et al (2017) studied qualitatively how 12 nurses decide on withdrawal of pediatric sedation using vignettes to understand nurses' cognitive process and found in complex pediatric cases that there is a variation in assessing patient behavior and response to treatment. Provide parental information in the decision-making process.* **EBN:** *Delaney et al (2017) studied the use of a tool to assist practitioners to make caring decisions around pediatric end of life and found that it enhanced family empowerment and provided a professional resource.* **EBN:** *Richards et al (2017) performed an integrative review of family-centered behaviors that were experienced in the intensive care unit and found that there were five salient themes needed to engage parents in decision making: (1) sharing information, (2) hearing parental voices, (3) making decisions for or with parents, (4) negotiating roles, and (5) individualizing communication.*
- Enhance client decision-making in critical care setting. **EBN:** *Petrinec (2017) studied the family decision makers (N = 30) for patients in long-term critical care situations and found they had post intensive care syndrome, which warrants nursing awareness and interventions to support family decision makers.* **EBN:** *Stinson (2017) performed a descriptive correlational study with nurses that work in the intensive care unit and compared years of experience with their ability to engage in clinical decision-making. This*

may support separate education for decisional science in nursing education as practitioners and as patient advocates.

Geriatric

- Include geriatric clients in the decisional process. **EB:** *Communication and decision-making go hand-in-hand for end-of-life care. Brooks, Manias, and Nicholson (2017) studied nurses (N = 17) and physicians (N = 11) in an intensive care unit about interprofessional end-of-life care and found that timing and conducting difficult conversations were better implemented with a team approach.* **EB:** *Paillaud et al (2017) studied older (over 70 years) patients' (N = 133) decision-making processes who did and did not have cancer and found that those with cancer had a strong desire for information and to be part of their health care decision-making process.*

D

Multicultural

- Consider cultural influences on decision-making. **EBN:** *A qualitative study of Korean women (N = 32) and their decision to get Pap smears was conducted by Kim et al (2017). The women who made a decision to receive a Pap smear desired to make the decision and were satisfied with their decision.* **EBN:** *Adefris et al (2017) studied women (N = 384) who delayed treatment for uterine prolapse in sub-Saharan Africa and found that it was the "social stigma" within the culture and additional open communication about the problem is needed.*

Home Care

- Use open communication to assist clients to develop health care plans to which they can adhere. **EBN:** *An integrative review of the literature by Bayless et al (2017) found that men who choose active surveillance rather than surgical intervention for prostate cancer take a more active, communicative role in the decision-making process.* **EBN:** *Talley, Davis, and Wyman (2017) presented a case study about ethical decision-making and the concepts that need to be considered in all environments. They used a four-concept approach to decision-making that included health care indications, patient preference, quality of life, and contextual features.*

REFERENCES

Adams, R. C., & Levy, S. E. (2017). Shared decision-making and children with disabilities: Pathways to consensus. *Pediatrics, 139*(6), 1–9. Retrieved from http://dx.doi.org.fmarion.idm.oclc.org/10.1542/peds.2017-0956.

Adefris, M., et al. (2017). Reasons for delay in decision making and reaching health facility among obstetric fistula and pelvic organ prolapse patients in Gondar University hospital, Northwest Ethiopia. *BMC Women's Health, 17*, 1–7. Retrieved from http://dx.doi.org.fmarion.idm.oclc.org/10.1186/s12905-017-0416-9.

Bayless, D. R., Duff, J., Stricker, P., et al. (2017). Decision-making in prostate cancer—Choosing active surveillance over other treatment options: A literature review. *Urologic Nursing, 37*(1), 15–22. Retrieved from http://dx.doi.org.fmarion.idm.oclc.org/10.7257/1053-816X.2017.37.1.15.

Brom, L., et al. (2017). Challenges in shared decision making in advanced cancer care: A qualitative longitudinal observational and interview study. *Health Expectations, 20*(1), 69–84. Retrieved from http://dx.doi.org.fmarion.idm.oclc.org/10.1111/hex.12434.

Brooks, L. A., Manias, E., & Nicholson, P. (2017). Communication and decision-making about end-of-life care in the intensive care unit. *American Journal of Critical Care, 26*(4), 336–341. Retrieved from http://dx.doi.org/10.4037/ajcc2017774.

Chen, S. (2017). Information behaviour and decision-making in patients during their cancer journey. *Electronic Library, 35*(3), 494–506. Retrieved from http://dx.doi.org.fmarion.idm.oclc.org/10.1108/EL-03-2016-0062.

Craske, J., Carter, B., Jarman, I. H., et al. (2017). Nursing judgement and decision-making using the Sedation Withdrawal Score (SWS) in children. *Journal of Advanced Nursing, 73*(10), 2327–2338. Retrieved from http://dx.doi.org.fmarion.idm.oclc.org/10.1111/jan.13305.

Delaney, C., Xafis, V., Gillam, L., et al. (2017). A good resource for parents, but will clinicians use it?: Evaluation of a resource for paediatric end-of-life decision making. *BMC Palliative Care, 16*, 1–10. Retrieved from http://dx.doi.org.fmarion.idm.oclc.org/10.1186/s12904-016-0177-5.

DenOuden, H., Vos, R. C., & Guy, E. H. M. (2017). Effectiveness of shared goal setting and decision making to achieve treatment targets in type 2 diabetes patients: A cluster-randomized trial. *Health Expectations, 20*(5), 1172–1180. Retrieved from http://dx.doi.org/10.1111/hex.12563.

Henselmans, I., Van Laahoven, H. W. M., Van der Vloodt, J., et al. (2017). Shared decision making about palliative chemotherapy: A qualitative observation of talk about patients' preferences. *Palliative Medicine, 31*(7), 625–633. Retrieved from http://dx.doi.org.fmarion.idm.oclc.org/10.1177/0269216316676010.

Kkotbong, K., & Jinhyang, Y. (2017). Decision-making process related to treatment and management in Korean women with breast cancer: finding the right individualized healthcare trajectory. *Applied Nursing Research, 35*, 99–105. Retrieved from http://dx.doi.org.fmarion.idm.oclc.org/10.1016/j.apnr.2017.02.022.

Klausen, R. K., Blix, B. H., Karlsson, M., et al. (2017). Shared decision making from the service users' perspective: A narrative study from community mental health centers in northern Norway. *Social Work in Mental Health, 15*(3), 354–371. Retrieved from http://dx.doi.org.fmarion.idm.oclc.org/10.1080/15332985.2016.1222981.

Lazenby, S., Edwards, A., Samuriwo, R., et al. (2017). End-of-life care decisions for haemodialysis patients—'We only tend to have that discussion with them when they start deteriorating'. *Health Expectations, 20*(2), 260–273. Retrieved from http://dx.doi.org.fmarion.idm.oclc.org/10.1111/hex.12454.

● = Independent;   ▲ = Collaborative;   **EBN** = Evidence-Based Nursing;   **EB** = Evidence-Based

Kim, K., Kim, S., Gallo, J. J., et al. (2017). Decision making about Pap test use among Korean immigrant women: A qualitative study. *Health Expectations*, 20(4), 685–695. Retrieved from http://dx.doi.org/10.1111/hex.12507.

Mabel, H., Rose, S. L., & Kodish, E. (2017). Decision-making for an incapacitated pregnant patient. *Hastings Center Report*, 47(4), 12–15. Retrieved from http://dx.doi.org.fmarion.idm.oclc.org/10.1002/hast.734.

Paillaud, E., et al. (2017). Preferences about information and decision-making among older patients with and without cancer. *Age and Ageing*, 46(4), 665–671. Retrieved from http://dx.doi.org.fmarion.idm.oclc.org/10.1093/ageing/afw256.

Perestelo-Perez, L., et al. (2017). Effectiveness of a decision aid for patients with depression: A randomized controlled trial. *Health Expectations*, 20(5), 1096–1105. Retrieved from http://dx.doi.org.fmarion.idm.oclc.org/10.1111/hex.12553.

Petrinec, A. (2017). Post-intensive care syndrome in family decision makers of long-term acute care hospital patients. *American Journal of Critical Care*, 26(5), 416–422. Retrieved from http://dx.doi.org.fmarion.idm.oclc.org/10.4037/ajcc2017414.

Richards, C. A., Starks, H., O'Connor, M. R., et al. (2017). Elements of family-centered care in the pediatric intensive care unit: An integrative review. *Journal of Hospice & Palliative Nursing*, 19(3), 238–246. Retrieved from http://dx.doi.org.fmarion.idm.oclc.org/10.1097/NJH.0000000000000335.

Schelle-Sailer, A., Post, M. W., Michel, F., et al. (2017). Patients' views on their decision making during inpatient rehabilitation after newly acquired spinal cord injury-A qualitative interview-based study. *Health Expectations*, 20(5), 1133–1142. Retrieved from http://dx.doi.org/10.1111/hex.12559.

Stepanuk, K. M., Fisher, K. M., Wittmann-Price, R., et al. (2013). Women's decision-making regarding medication use in pregnancy for anxiety and/or depression. *Journal of Advanced Nursing*, 69(11), 2470–2480.

Stinson, K. J. (2017). Benner's framework and clinical decision-making in the critical care environment. *Nursing Science Quarterly*, 30(1), 52–57. Retrieved from http://dx.doi.org.fmarion.idm.oclc.org/10.1177/0894318416680536.

Talley, K. M. C., Davis, N. J., & Wyman, J. F. (2017). Determining a treatment plan for urinary incontinence in an older adult: Application of the four-topic approach to an ethical decision-making process. *Urologic Nursing*, 37(4), 181–203. Retrieved from http://dx.doi.org/10.7257/1053-816X.2017.37.4.181.

Wittmann-Price, R. A. (2006). Exploring the subconcepts of the Wittmann-Price theory of emancipated decision-making in women's health care. *Journal of Nursing Scholarship*, 38(4), 377–382.

Wittmann-Price, R. A., & Bhattacharya, A. (2008). Reexploring the subconcepts of the Wittmann-Price theory of emancipated decision-making in women's healthcare. *Advances in Nursing Science*, 31(3), 225–236.

Wittmann-Price, R. A., Fliszar, R., & Bhattacharya, A. (2011). Elective cesarean births: Are women making emancipated decisions? *Applied Nursing Research*, 24, 147–152.

Zizzo, N., Bell, E., LaFontaine, A., et al. (2017). Examining chronic care patient preferences for involvement in health-care decision making: The case of Parkinson's disease patients in a patient-centered clinic. *Health Expectations*, 20(4), 655–664. Retrieved from http://dx.doi.org/10.1111/hex.12497.

Readiness for enhanced emancipated Decision-Making
Ruth A. Wittmann-Price, PhD, RN, CNS, CNE, CHSE, ANEF, FAAN

NANDA-I

Definition

A process of choosing a health care decision that includes personal knowledge and/or consideration of social norms, which can be strengthened.

Defining Characteristics

Expresses desire to enhance ability to choose health care options that best fit current lifestyle; expresses desire to enhance ability to enact chosen health care option; expresses desire to enhance ability to understand all available health care options; expresses desire to enhance ability to verbalize own opinion without constraint; expresses desire to enhance comfort to verbalize health care options in the presence of others; expresses desire to enhance confidence in decision-making; expresses desire to enhance confidence to discuss health care options openly; expresses desire to enhance decision-making; expresses desire to enhance privacy to discuss health care options

NOC   Outcomes (Nursing Outcomes Classification)

Suggested NOC Outcomes

Decision-Making; Self-Esteem; Coping; Health Promotion Behavior; Stress Level; Communication; Self-Care; Participation in Health Care Decisions; Health-Seeking Behavior; Knowledge: Treatment Options; Psychosocial Adjustment

● = Independent;   ▲ = Collaborative;   EBN = Evidence-Based Nursing;   EB = Evidence-Based

> ### Example NOC Outcome with Indicators
>
> **Participation in Health Care Decisions** as evidenced by the following indicator: Claims decision-making responsibility. (Rate the outcome and indicators of **Participation in Health Care Decisions:** 1 = never demonstrated, 2 = rarely demonstrated, 3 = sometimes demonstrated, 4 = often demonstrated, 5 = consistently demonstrated [see Section I].)

Client Outcomes

Client Will (Specify Time Frame)

- Verbalize option of outcomes freely before making a health care decision
- Freely verbalize own opinion with health care providers before making a health care decision
- Choose the health care option that best fits his or her lifestyle within an appropriate amount of time that allows enactment of the choice
- Describe how the chosen option fits into his or her current lifestyle before or after the decision has been made
- Verbalizes appropriate concern about others' opinions before making the health care choice
- Remains stress-free when listening to others' opinions before making the health care choice
- Arrives at a decision in a timely manner

NIC   Interventions (Nursing Interventions Classification)

Suggested NIC Intervention

Decision-Making Support

> ### Example NIC Activities—Emancipated Decision-Making
>
> Assist client in making an emancipated decision about health care options by discussing social norms with the client; Provide a flexible environment; Encourage the client to use personal knowledge

Nursing Interventions and *Rationales*

- Assess client's readiness to choose through active listening. EB: *Hadrych-Rosier (2017) explored the concepts of truly listening to patients by observations of using nonverbal communication, proper eye contact, body language to connect with patients, and avoiding internal thoughts while interacting.* EBN: *Chen et al (2017) applied a home-based, individually tailored intervention, which included nursing education, skills training, listening/counseling, and resources for family caregivers of cognitively impaired individuals. Listening skills and interventions improved caregiving skills and increased the family's quality of life.*
- Use anticipatory guidance by proactively providing the client with information. (Refer to Impaired emancipated **Decision-Making.**)
- Establish a purposeful provider–client relationship. EB: *Researchers examined the quality of the patient–provider relationship and its effect on attachment and self-management of patients with multiple chronic diseases (N =209). The study results demonstrated that patient–provider relationships with attachment and communication provide that patient with information and improve decisions about self-management (Brenk-Franz et al, 2017).* EB: *Chien-Ching et al (2017) studied the relationship of patient–provider communication variable on the physical health quality of life and mental health quality of life of cancer patients (N = 479) and found that reducing communication barriers increased patients' satisfaction in both quality of life indicators. Patients had high mental health quality of life scores if they were comfortable asking their provider questions.*
- ▲ Include interdisciplinary health care professionals as needed to increase knowledge of chosen option. EB: *Researchers designed a pilot study to measure patients' and staffs' perception of teamwork. The results revealed that coordination among nurses scored the highest and were positively correlated with patients' perceptions (Cottingham et al, 2017).* EB: *Wong et al (2017) studied the lived experience of emergency department (ED) staff (N = 31) members caring for agitated patients and found three themes from the focus groups: (1) ED staff provide high-quality care to marginalized patients, (2) teamwork is critical to safely managing patients and hierarchy and professional silos hinder care, and (3) environmental challenges increase threats to staff safety.*
- Provide decision-making support. (Refer to Impaired emancipated **Decision-Making.**)

● = Independent;   ▲ = Collaborative;   EBN = Evidence-Based Nursing;   EB = Evidence-Based

D

- Continue to provide a flexible environment for client to enact choice. EB: *Investigators studied shared decision-making about health care options with spinal cord injury (SCI) patients (N = 22) during the patients' first rehabilitation experience and found using interviews that decision-making capabilities were reduced in the first few days of hospitalizations because of physical, psychological, and environmental factors. Additionally, they stated that understandable, personalized information was necessary to participate in decision-making (Scheek-Sailer et al, 2017).* EB: *Den Ouden, Vos, and Rutten (2017) completed a 5-year clinical trial with type 2 diabetic patients (N = 35) and found that using a shared decision-making model benefited both prioritizing and reaching treatment goals with improved patient outcomes.*
- Encourage the client to use personal knowledge as part of the decision-making process to increase decisional satisfaction. EB: *Hultberg and Rudebeck (2017) explored patient agency and resistance in decision-making about cardiovascular treatments in primary care settings. The study described patient resistance as part of the decision-making process and it can be passive or aggressive. Health care providers need to allow patient agency and open communication to establish a working relationship in shared decision-making.*

Pediatric

- Understand interventions that parents prefer when in the decision-making process. EBN: *Craske et al (2017) studied withdrawal syndrome in children and how nurses (N = 12) make decisions about treatment and qualitatively found each stage of decision-making described as noticing, interpreting, and responding.* EB: *Bekken (2017) explored the distinction that professionals make between difficult and less difficult decisions in pediatric rehabilitation and the child's right to participate in health care decisions concerning their own body and life and found that professional reasoning can work negatively against children's involvement in decisions.*

Multicultural

- Use open communication to assist clients to develop health care plans to which they can adhere. EBN: *Rodrigo, Cais, and Monforte-Rovo (2017) qualitatively studied using grounded theory nurses' participation in decision-making in Spain and found that the health care system still functions mainly from a disease-focused view making it difficult for nurses to take responsibility for decision-making.* EBN: *Kim et al (2017) studied how immigrant women (N = 32) make decisions about Pap tests (screenings) using interviews and found that most women with positive decisions made their own decisions and considered the positive and negative aspects of having a Pap smear. Women who deferred decisions perceived Pap tests as negative and sometimes deferred to the provider or significant other.*

Home Care/Nursing Home Care

- Optimize self-care personal knowledge for home care. EB: *Mariani et al (2017) studied shared decision-making in patients with dementia and allowing the patient to take part in making choices to promote social health and found the following themes: team collaboration and communication skills assisted shared decision-making. Lack of funding and lack of family involvement hindered shared decision-making in nursing home care, but findings can be applicable to home care.* EB: *Reinhardt et al (2017) studied end-of-life care communication between family and providers and found that documentation was in place for nursing home residents and these should be available and done well in advance.*
- Refer to care plan Impaired emancipated **Decision-Making** for additional interventions for pediatric, critical care, geriatric, and multicultural care.

REFERENCES

Bekken, W. (2017). Decision-making in pediatric rehabilitation: Exploring professionals' and children's views on decision-making involvement. *Children & Society, 31*(6), 486–496. Retrieved from http://dx.doi.org/10.1111/chso.12218.

Brenk-Franz, K., Straub, B., Tiesler, F., et al. (2017). Patient-provider relationship as mediator between adult attachment and self-management in primary care patients with multiple chronic conditions. *Journal of Psychosomatic Research, 97*, 131–135. Retrieved from http://dx.doi.org/10.1016/j.jpsychores.2017.04.007.

Chen, M., Chiu, Y., Wei, P., et al. (2017). Reducing the care-related burdens of a family caregiver of a person with mild cognitive impairment: A home-based case management program. *Journal of Nursing, 64*(3), 105–111. Retrieved from http://dx.doi.org/10.6224/JN.000046.

Chien-Ching, L., Matthews, A. K., Dossaji, M., et al. (2017). The relationship of patient-provider communication on quality of life among African-American and White cancer survivors. *Journal of Health Communication, 22*(7), 584–592. Retrieved from http://dx.doi.org/10.1080/10810730.2017.1324540.

Cottingham, A. H., Azar, J. M., Litzelman, D. K., et al. (2017). Evaluation of interprofessional relational coordination and patients' perception of care in outpatient oncology teams. *Journal of Interprofessional Care, 31*(2), 273–276. Retrieved from http://dx.doi.org/10.1080/13561820.2016.1248815.

● = Independent;   ▲ = Collaborative;   EBN = Evidence-Based Nursing;   EB = Evidence-Based

Craske, J., Carter, B., Jarman, I. H., et al. (2017). Nursing judgement and decision-making using the Sedation Withdrawal Score (SWS) in children. *Journal of Advanced Nursing*, 73(10), 2327–2338. Retrieved from http://dx.doi.org/10.1111/jan.13305.

Den Ouden, H., Vos, R. C., & Rutten, G. E. H. M. (2017). Effectiveness of shared goal setting and decision making to achieve treatment targets in type 2 diabetes patients: A cluster-randomized trial. *Health Expectations*, 20(5), 1172–1180. Retrieved from http://dx.doi.org/10.1111/hex.12563.

Hadrych-Rosier, N. (2017). Are we listening? Truly hear your patients' concerns. *ASRT Scanner*, 49(3), 18.

Hultberg, J., & Rudebeck, C. E. (2017). Patient participation in decision-making about cardiovascular preventive drugs—Resistance as agency. *Scandinavian Journal of Primary Health Care*, 35(3), 231–239. Retrieved from http://dx.doi.org/10.1080/02813432.2017.1288814.

Kim, K., Kim, S., Gallo, J. J., et al. (2017). Decision making about Pap test use among Korean immigrant women: A qualitative study. *Health Expectations*, 20(4), 685–695. Retrieved from http://dx.doi.org/10.1111/hex.12507.

Mariani, E., Vernooij-Dassen, M., Koopmans, R., et al. (2017). Shared decision-making in dementia care planning: Barriers and facilitators in two European countries. *Aging & Mental Health*, 21(1), 31–39.

Retrieved from http://dx.doi.org/10.1080/13607863.2016.1255715.

Reinhardt, J. P., Downes, D., Cimarolli, V., et al. (2017). End-of-life conversations and hospice placement: Association with less aggressive care desired in the nursing home. *Journal of Social Work in End-of-Life & Palliative Care*, 13(1), 61–81. Retrieved from http://dx.doi.org/10.1080/15524256.2017.1282919.

Rodrigo, O., Cais, J., & Monforte-Rovo, C. (2017). Professional responsibility and decision-making in the context of a disease-focused model of nursing care: The difficulties experienced by Spanish nurses. *Nursing Inquiry*, 24(4). Retrieved from http://dx.doi.org/10.1111/nin.12202.

Scheek-Sailer, A., Post, M. W., Michel, F., et al. (2017). Patients' views on their decision making during inpatient rehabilitation after newly acquired spinal cord injury—A qualitative interview-based study. *Health Expectations*, 20(5), 1133–1142. Retrieved from http://dx.doi.org/10.1111/hex.12559.

Wong, A. H., Combellick, J., Wispelwey, B. A., et al. (2017). The patient care paradox: An interprofessional qualitative study of agitated patient care in the emergency department. *Academic Emergency Medicine*, 24(2), 226–235. Retrieved from http://dx.doi.org/10.1111/acem.13117.

Risk for impaired emancipated Decision-Making
Ruth A. Wittmann-Price, PhD, RN, CNS, CNE, CHSE, ANEF, FAAN

NANDA-I

Definition

Susceptible to a process of choosing a health care decision that does not include personal knowledge and/or consideration of social norms, or does not occur in a flexible environment, resulting in decisional satisfaction.

Risk Factors

Decrease in understanding of all available health care options; inability to adequately verbalize perceptions about health care options; Inadequate time to discuss health care options; insufficient confidence to openly discuss health care options; insufficient information regarding health care options; insufficient privacy to openly discuss health care options; insufficient self-confidence in decision-making

At-Risk Population

Limited decision-making experience; traditional hierarchical family; traditional hierarchical health care systems

NOC   (Nursing Outcomes Classification)

Suggested NOC Outcomes

Decision-Making; Self-Confidence; Coping; Health Promotion Behavior; Stress Level; Communication; Self-Care; Participation in Health Care Decisions; Health-Seeking Behavior; Knowledge; Treatment Options; Psychosocial Adjustment

Example NOC Outcome with Indicators

Participation in Health Care Decisions as evidenced by the following indicator: Claims decision-making responsibility. (Rate the outcome and indicators of **Participation in Health Care Decisions:** 1 = never demonstrated, 2 = rarely demonstrated, 3 = sometimes demonstrated, 4 = often demonstrated, 5 = consistently demonstrated [see Section I].)

● = Independent;   ▲ = Collaborative;   EBN = Evidence-Based Nursing;   EB = Evidence-Based

D

Client Outcomes

Client Will (Specify Time Frame)

- Verbalize option outcomes freely before making a health care decision in a private setting with in which he or she feels comfortable
- Freely verbalize own opinion with health care providers before making a health care decision
- Discuss how options fit or hinder his or her lifestyle within an appropriate amount of time that allows enactment of the choice
- Discuss concerns about others' opinions before making the health care choice
- Decrease stress about others' opinions by placing options in perspective through informational resources
- Discuss the time frame in which the decision needs to be made

NIC — Interventions (Nursing Interventions Classification)

Suggested NIC Interventions

Establish Rapport; Decision-Making Support

> **Example NIC Activities—Emancipated Decision-Making**
>
> Assist client to verbalize and discuss barriers that she or he perceives in making an emancipated decision about health care options; Acknowledge social norms about decision options; Provide a flexible environment that is safe and private for the discussions; Use empathy to understand the client's personal point of view about the options

Nursing Interventions and *Rationales*

- Assess client's vulnerability for an impaired decision-making process. **EBN:** *Scheepmans et al (2017) studied the decision-making process of placing older adults (N = 5) in restraints at home and found through a cross-sectional survey that the main decision-making variables were safety, keeping the patient home longer, and to provide respite for the caregiver.* **EB:** *Researchers studied the variables related to continuous observation and decisions about safety and privacy in psychiatric patients. Study results indicated that patients struggled with lack of privacy, but they did say they felt safe with the staff. The staff interviewed revealed that decisions were based on patient–staff collaboration (Barnicot et al, 2017).*
- Assess the client's experience with decision-making. **EB:** *Talley (2017) presented a case study regarding the treatment decision-making process for an older adult with urinary incontinence that was dependent on a family caregiver. The study found that care can be complicated by conflicting ethical principles between the patient and caregiver and the principles may account for the decisions made.* **EBN:** *Smith et al (2017) studied cancer patients' (N = 21) perceptions of their involvement in treatment decisions and found that most patients just consented to radiation because of oncologist recommendations. The study recommends that patients be provided with more opportunities to ask questions to be empowered in decisions about their uncertainties and concerns.*
- Recognize the traditional hierarchical family and health care system. **EB:** *Siouta et al (2017) studied how patients with atrial fibrillation were involved in their care and how they were communicated with through a physician perspective. Physician participants revealed that by encouraging patients to be actively involved they increased communication and adherence to treatment options.* **EBN:** *Petrinec (2017) studied the effect of patients' long-term care experiences on the family decision-maker (N = 30) and found, using a qualitative descriptive study method, that family decision-makers need support and often have post intensive care syndrome caused by the stress.*
- Provide privacy to discuss health care options. **EBN:** *Chang et al (2017) studied the decision-making of nurses that triage patients in an emergency department and what factors were considered in their decision-making. The study results indicated that the patients' privacy was an important consideration in choosing care options and prioritizing during a triage situation.* **EB:** *Ng et al (2017) studied patients (N = 11) who use hearing aids and found though qualitative analysis using the constant comparative method that important concepts to the patients were getting to know their clinician and providing privacy when using adaptive smartphones for communication. This study highlighted the concern about privacy in relation to smartphone application and tracking features.*
- Allow the client time to choose. **EB:** *Simmons et al (2017) studied an online decision aid for youth (N = 66) with depression and their ability to make decisions and found that it assisted patients to feel involved in*

● = Independent;   ▲ = Collaborative;   EBN = Evidence-Based Nursing;   EB = Evidence-Based

their decision and providing them with time to make the decision and accessibility. EB: *Researchers studied decision-making and leadership over time and found that participation in decision-making shifts over time, and the value of decision-making is perceived higher earlier in the process (D'Aunno, Alexander, & Lan, 2017).*

▲ Understand the primary care providers' role in the decision-making process. EB: *Hyde et al (2017) did a systematic review about shared decision-making and prescribing analgesia by primary care practitioners for musculoskeletal pain and identified important factors in shared decision-making that mainly focus on patient emotions and conditions that required analgesics.* EB: *Researchers completed a literature review on decision-making by women who had ductal carcinoma in situ breast cancer and found that decisions are influenced by understanding risks, the clinical features of the cancer, and the benefits and harms of treatment. The conclusion was that informed and shared decision-making requires clear communication of and support from clinicians (Wu et al, 2017).*

● Provide informational resources. EBN: *Asiodu et al (2017) completed a critical ethnographic research study to describe breastfeeding perceptions of African American mothers (N = 21) and key themes that were identified about the high percentage of early weaning, which were expressed as guilt and shame for not breastfeeding, stressors, lack of breastfeeding role models, limited experiences, and changes to the family dynamics.* EB: *Paillaud et al (2017) studied older patients (N = 113) with cancer in relation to information, decision-making, and surrogate designation and compared patients with a group without cancer and found increasingly that the cancer patients wanted to receive information and participate in decisions about their care.*

● Provide encouragement so clients increase their confidence in the decision-making process. EB: *Researchers studied patients' (N = 22) perceptions about decision-making involvement and communication with nurses and physicians and found that patients felt involved when obtaining clarifications about their disease and its treatment. Communication with providers built up the patients' confidence in decision-making (Siouta et al, 2017).* EB: *Knox, Douglas, and Bigby (2017) studied how patients with traumatic brain injury (TBI) participated in decision-making and by using grounded theory discovered that self-conceptualization was a theme and that TBI patients wanted a sense of autonomy.*

 Pediatric

● Understand the parent/guardian's vulnerability when making health care decisions for their children. EB: *O'Hare et al (2017) studied a tool to evaluate children and young patient's (N = 151) participation in decision-making. The pilot demonstrated that the reliability and validity of the Child and Adolescent Participation in Decision-Making Questionnaire (CAP-DMQ) showed promise as a useful tool to evaluate decision-making participation, which can assist the family when decisions need to be made.* EB: *Researchers from Johns Hopkins studied sleep-disordered breathing (SDB) in children to understand social and communication factors that influence decision-making for treatment. Researchers surveyed practitioners (N = 10) and found that three main themes were considered during SDB decision-making: (1) approach to treatment and alternatives, (2) communication with families, and (3) sociocultural factors (Boss et al, 2017).*

● Understand the adolescent decision-making processes. EB: *Bernhardt et al (2017) studied impulsive and value-based decision-making in young adults (N = 198) who socially drank alcohol and found that actually chronic alcohol consumption itself is implicated in impulsive behavior rather than innate personality traits.* EB: *Mosner et al (2017) investigated vicarious effort-based decision-making in adolescents (N = 50) with autism spectrum disorders (ASDs) in a comparison study. Group comparisons demonstrated that adolescents with ASD were better choosing for themselves than making choices that involved other people, indicating the participants had decreased sensitivity toward others.*

● Refer to care plan Impaired emancipated **Decision-Making** for additional interventions for critical care, geriatric, multicultural care, and home care.

REFERENCES

Asiodu, I., Waters, C., Dailey, D., et al. (2017). Infant feeding decision-making and the influences of social support persons among first-time African American mothers. *Maternal & Child Health Journal, 21*(4), 863–872. Retrieved from http://dx.doi.org/10.1007/s10995-016-2167-x.

Barnicot, K., Insua-Summerhaves, B., Plummer, E., et al. (2017). Staff and patient experiences of decision-making about continuous observation in psychiatric hospitals. *Social Psychiatry & Psychiatric Epidemiology, 52*(4), 473–483. Retrieved from http://dx.doi.org/10.1007/s00127-017-1338-4.

Bernhardt, N., Nebe, S., Pooseh, S., et al. (2017). Impulsive decision making in young adult social drinkers and detoxified alcohol-dependent patients: A cross-sectional and longitudinal study. *Alcoholism: Clinical & Experimental Research, 41*(10), 1794–1807. Retrieved from http://dx.doi.org/10.1111/acer.13481.

Boss, E. F., Links, A. R., Saxton, R., et al. (2017). Physician perspectives on decision making for treatment of pediatric sleep-disordered breathing. *Clinical Pediatrics, 56*(11), 993–1000. Retrieved from http://dx.doi.org/10.1177/0009922817702939.

● = Independent;   ▲ = Collaborative;   EBN = Evidence-Based Nursing;   EB = Evidence-Based

Chang, W., Liu, H., Goopy, S., et al. (2017). Using the five-level Taiwan triage and acuity scale computerized system: Factors in decision making by emergency department triage nurses. *Clinical Nursing Research*, 26(5), 651–666. Retrieved from http://dx.doi.org/10.1177/1054773816636360.

D'Aunno, T., Alexander, J. A., & Lan, J. (2017). Creating value for participants in multistakeholder alliances: The shifting importance of leadership and collaborative decision-making over time. *Health Care Management Review*, 42(2), 100–111. Retrieved from http://dx.doi.org/10.1097/HMR.0000000000000098.

Hyde, C., Dunn, K. M., Higginbottom, A., et al. (2017). Process and impact of patient involvement in a systematic review of shared decision making in primary care consultations. *Health Expectations*, 20(2), 298–308. Retrieved from http://dx.doi.org/10.1111/hex.12458.

Knox, L., Douglas, J. M., & Bigby, C. (2017). "I've never been a yes person": Decision-making participation and self-conceptualization after severe traumatic brain injury. *Disability & Rehabilitation*, 39(22), 2250–2260. Retrieved from http://dx.doi.org/10.108 0/09638288.2016.1219925.

Mosner, M., Kinard, J., McWeeny, S., et al. (2017). Vicarious effort-based decision-making in autism spectrum disorders. *Journal of Autism & Developmental Disorders*, 47(10), 2992–3006. Retrieved from http://dx.doi.org/10.1007/s10803-017-3220-3.

Ng, S. L., Phelan, S., Leonard, M., et al. (2017). A qualitative case study of smartphone-connected hearing aids: Influences on patients, clinicians, and patient-clinician interactions. *Journal of the American Academy of Audiology*, 28(6), 506–521. Retrieved from http://dx.doi.org/10.3766/jaaa.15153.

O'Hare, L., Santin, O., Winter, K., et al. (2017). The reliability and validity of a child and adolescent participation in decision-making questionnaire. *Child: Care, Health & Development*, 42(5), 692–698. Retrieved from http://dx.doi.org/10.1111/cch.12369.

Paillaud, E., Canoui-Poitrine, F., Varnier, G., et al. (2017). Preferences about information and decision-making among older patients with and without cancer. *Age and Ageing*, 46(4), 665–671. Retrieved from http://dx.doi.org/10.1093/ageing/afw256.

Petrinec, A. (2017). Post-intensive care syndrome in family decision makers of long-term acute care hospital patients. *American Journal of Critical Care*, 26(5), 416–422. Retrieved from http://dx.doi.org/10.4037/ajcc2017414.

Scheepmans, K., Dierckx deCasterle, B., Paquay, L., et al. (2017). Restraint use in older adults receiving home care. *Journal of the American Geriatrics Society*, 65(8), 1769–1776. Retrieved from http://dx.doi.org/10.1111/jgs.14880.

Simmons, M. B., Elmes, A., McKenzie, J. E., et al. (2017). Right choice, right time: Evaluation of an online decision aid for youth depression. *Health Expectations*, 20(4), 714–723. Retrieved from http://dx.doi.org/10.1111/hex.12510.

Siouta, E., Hellstrom, M. U., Hedberg, B., et al. (2017). Patients' experiences of communication and involvement in decision-making about atrial fibrillation treatment in consultations with nurses and physicians. *Scandinavian Journal of Caring Sciences*, 30(3), 535–546. Retrieved from http://dx.doi.org/10.1111/scs.12276.

Smith, S. K., Nathan, D., Taylor, J., et al. (2017). Patients' experience of decision-making and receiving information during radiation therapy: A qualitative study. *European Journal of Oncology Nursing*, 30, 97–106. Retrieved from http://dx.doi.org/10.1016/j.ejon .2017.08.007.

Talley, K. M. C. (2017). Determining a treatment plan for urinary incontinence in an older adult: Application of the four-topic approach to ethical decision-making. *Urologic Nursing*, 37(4), 181–203. Retrieved from http://dx.doi.org/10.7257/105 3-816X.2017.37.4.181.

Wu, J. L., Rutherford, C., Butow, P., et al. (2017). Treatment decision-making in ductal carcinoma in situ: A mixed methods systematic review of women's experiences and information needs. *Patient Education & Counseling*, 100(9), 1654–1666. Retrieved from http://dx.doi.org/10.1016/j.pec.2017.04.009.

Ineffective Denial   *Julianne E. Doubet, BSN, RN, EMT-B*

NANDA-I

Definition

Conscious or unconscious attempt to disavow the knowledge or meaning of an event to reduce anxiety and/or fear, leading to the detriment of health.

Defining Characteristics

Delay in seeking health care; denies fear of death; denies fear of invalidism; displaces fear of impact of the condition; displaces source of symptoms; does not admit impact of disease on life; does not perceive relevance of danger; does not perceive relevance of symptoms; inappropriate affect; minimizes symptoms; refusal of health care; use of dismissive comments when speaking of distressing event; use of dismissive gestures when speaking of distressing event; use of treatment not advised by health care professional

Related Factors

Anxiety; excessive stress; fear of death; fear of losing autonomy; fear of separation; ineffective coping strategies; insufficient emotional support; insufficient sense of control; perceived inadequacy in dealing with strong emotions; threat of unpleasant reality

● = Independent;   ▲ = Collaborative;   **EBN** = Evidence-Based Nursing;   **EB** = Evidence-Based

NOC   (Nursing Outcomes Classification)

Suggested NOC Outcomes

Acceptance: Health Status; Anxiety Self-Control; Health Beliefs: Perceived Threat; Symptom Control

> **Example NOC Outcome with Indicators**
>
> **Anxiety Self-Control** as evidenced by the following indicators: Eliminates precursors of anxiety/Monitors physical manifestations of anxiety/Controls anxiety response. (Rate the outcome and indicators of **Anxiety Self-Control:** 1 = never demonstrated, 2 = rarely demonstrated, 3 = sometimes demonstrated, 4 = often demonstrated, 5 = consistently demonstrated [see Section I].)

Outcomes

Client Will (Specify Time Frame)

- Seek out appropriate health care attention when needed
- Use home remedies only when appropriate
- Display appropriate affect and verbalize fears
- Actively engage in treatment program related to identified "substance" of abuse
- Remain substance free
- Demonstrate alternate adaptive coping mechanism

NIC   (Nursing Interventions Classification)

Suggested NIC Intervention

Anxiety Reduction

> **Example NIC—Activities Anxiety Reduction**
>
> Use a calm, reassuring approach; Stay with the patient to promote safety and reduce fear

Nursing Interventions and *Rationales*

- Assess the client's and family's understanding of the illness, the treatments, and expected outcomes. **CBN:** *Effective communication between client and health care provider in relation to health promotion, disease prevention, and disease management is key to optimal health outcomes (Heinrich & Karner, 2011).*
- Allow client time for adjustment to his or her situation. **EBN:** *Thoughtful contemplation of life expectancy and end-of-life care are vital for clients to ensure their continued optimum quality of life (Walczak et al, 2014).*
- Aid the client in making choices regarding treatment and actively involve him or her in the decision-making process. **EBN:** *Nurses must encourage a client's participation in shared decision-making by providing the client with balanced, evidence-based treatment alternatives, and endeavor to identify what is most important to the client and then support their choices (Stacey & Legare, 2015).*
- Allow the client to express and use denial as a coping mechanism if appropriate to treatment. **EB:** *According to Werner and Steihaug (2017), it is important for the health care provider to respect the client's autonomy and realize that the client has the right to refuse information regarding his or her condition.*
- Support the client's spiritual coping measures. **EBN:** *According to Baldacchino et al (2013), spiritual, although not necessarily religious, coping may enhance adjustment of clients to their chronic illnesses.*
- Develop a trusting, therapeutic relationship with the client/family. **EBN:** *According to Dinc and Gastmans (2013), in their study of the literature focusing on nurse–patient relationships, nurses' professional expertise and interpersonal caring qualities were essential in developing trust.*
- Assist the client in using existing and additional sources of support. **EBN:** *In their study of men with brain tumors who did not access social services, Longbecker, Eckberg, and Yates (2017) opined that there is a divide between patients' needs and utilization of services; this may be a result of the client's expectancy of what the medical system would offer, alternations in standards for well-being, changes in cognition, and difficulties accessing services.*
- Refer to care plans for Defensive **Coping** and Dysfunctional **Family** processes.

● = Independent;   ▲ = Collaborative;   **EBN** = Evidence-Based Nursing;   **EB** = Evidence-Based

Geriatric

- Allow the client to explain his or her concepts of health care needs, and then use reality-focused techniques whenever possible to provide feedback. **EB:** *Clients should be made conscious of the fact that primary medical treatment, even when associated with a positive prognosis, does not in and of itself predict how well clients will fare during their lifetime (Linden et al, 2015).*
- Encourage communication among family members. **EB:** *According to Hays, Maliski, and Warner (2017), family can be the most important means of support for those diagnosed with health problems, if they are made aware of the client's medical issues.*
- Recognize denial and be aware that grieving may prolong denial. **EBN:** *In her study of dying children in palliative care, Smith (2014) stated that denial can be an effective coping technique, and that it allows parents and families the time to gather emotional strength with which to support their child.*

Multicultural

- Assess for the influence of cultural beliefs, norms, and values involved in the client's understanding of and ability to acknowledge health status. **EB:** *Lee and Mason (2014) suggested that health care practitioners should develop programs that include ethnic- and gender-specific components, which, in turn, will aid older adults in coping with the stress caused by illness.*
- Discuss with the client those aspects of his or her health behavior/lifestyle that will remain unchanged by health status and those aspects of health behavior that need to be modified to improve health status. **EBN:** *"Culturally sensitive interventions are required to ensure people of culturally and linguistically diverse backgrounds have the appropriate skills to self-manage their complex medical conditions" (Williams et al, 2015).*
- Assess the role of fatalism in the client's ability to acknowledge health status. **EB:** *Some minorities, because of cultural factors (e.g., fatalism, medical mistrust), have negative attitudes toward health care interventions: targeting these cultural issues may help reduce undertreatment of minorities (Lin et al, 2014).*

Home Care

- Previously mentioned interventions may be adapted for home care utilization.
- Observe family interaction and roles. Refer the client/family for follow-up if prolonged denial is a risk. **EBN:** *Nurses are mentors and guides who can support caregivers of dying family members with coordination of care, symptom management education, and in making referrals to other agencies as needed (Hartnett, Thom, & Kline, 2016).*
Encourage communication between family members, particularly when dealing with the loss of a significant person. **EBN:** *Ineffectual family communication, especially after the loss of a significant loved one, lessens the capacity to cope, leaving those who are grieving more susceptible to complicated grief (Brownhill et al, 2013).*

Client/Family Teaching and Discharge Planning

- Instruct client and family to recognize the signs and symptoms of recurring illness and the appropriate responses to alterations in client's health status. **EBN:** *According to Bagdan and Raines (2016), using interactive communication and literacy screening allows the giver (and receiver) of written and oral discharge instructions to question and strengthen the client's and his or her family's comprehension of vital interventions that may be needed, relieving anxiety related to the client's care.*
- Consider the client's belief in and use of complementary therapies in self-managing his or her disease. **EBN:** *No matter what other care is provided, nurses should support any program type that genuinely makes a difference for the client and his or her family (Madden, 2014).*
- Teach family members that denial may continue throughout the adjustment to treatment and they should not be confrontational. **EB:** *Losses come with progressing years and may dictate interpersonal and selfish readjustments to relationships, occupations, and avocations: the use of denial as a defense mechanism may play a significant role in these situations (Clemens, 2014).*
- ▲ Inform family of available community support resources. **EBN:** *According to study findings by Mendes and Palmer (2016), nurses, especially those involved with the community, can play a pivotal part in aiding caregivers by furnishing useful information, connecting caregivers to community resources, and contributing essential emotional support.*

● = Independent;   ▲ = Collaborative;   EBN = Evidence-Based Nursing;   EB = Evidence-Based

REFERENCES

See defensive **Coping** *for additional references.*

Bagdan, L., & Raines, D. (2016). Reflections of care transitions: A qualitative analysis. *Nursing Research, 65*(2), E49.

Baldacchino, D., Torskenaes, K., Kalfoss, M., et al. (2013). Spiritual coping in rehabilitation—a comparative study: Part 2. *British Journal of Nursing, 11*, 402–408.

Brownhill, S., Chang, E., Bidewell, J., et al. (2013). A decision model for community nurses providing bereavement care. *British Journal of Community Nursing, 18*(3), 133–139.

Clemens, N. A. (2014). On letting go: With age comes renunciation. *Journal of Psychiatric Practice, 20*, 370–372.

Dinc, L., & Gastmans, C. (2013). Trust in nurse-patient relationships: A literature review. *Nursing Ethics, 20*, 501–516.

Hartnett, J., Thom, B., & Kline, N. (2016). Caregiver burden in end stage ovarian. *Clinical Journal of Oncology Nursing, 20*(20), 169–173.

Hays, A., Maliski, R., & Warner, B. (2017). Analyzing the effects of family communication patterns to disclose a health issue to a parent: The benefits of conversation and danger of conformity. *Health Communications, 32*(7), 837–844.

Heinrich, C., & Karner, K. (2011). Ways to optimize understanding health related information: The patients' perspective. *Geriatric Nursing, 32*, 29–38.

Lee, H., & Mason, D. (2014). Cultural and gender differences in coping strategies between Caucasian Americans Korean American older people. *Journal of Cross-Cultural Gerontology, 27*.

Lin, J. J., Mhango, G., Wall, M. M., et al. (2014). Cultural factors associated with disparities in lung cancer care. *Annals of the American Thoracic Society, 11*, 489–495.

Linden, W., MacKenzie, R., Rnic, K., et al. (2015). Emotional adjustment over 1 year post-diagnosis on patients with cancer: Understanding and predicting adjustment trajectories. *Supportive Care in Cancer, 123*(5), 1391–1399.

Longbecker, D., Eckberg, S., & Yates, P. (2017). Don't need help, don't want help, can't get help: How patients with brain tumors account for not using rehabilitation, psychosocial and community services. *Patient Education and Counseling, 100*(7), 1744–1750.

Madden, R. (2014). A nurse's journey into complimentary therapies. *Nursing News, 38*, 5.

Mendes, A., & Palmer, S. (2016). Supporting unpaid carers in the community. *British Journal of Community Nursing, 21*(7), 364.

Smith, H. (2014). Giving hope to families in palliative care and implications for practice. *Nursing Children and Young People, 26*(5), 21–25.

Stacy, D., & Legare, F. (2015). Engaging patients using an interprofessional approach to decision making. *Canadian Oncology Nursing Journal, 25*(4), 455–461.

Walczak, A., Buton, P. N., Clayton, J. M., et al. (2014). Discussing prognosis and end of life care in the final year of life: A randomized trial of nurse-led communication support programme for patients. *BMJ Open, 4*, e005745.

Werner, A., & Steihaug, S. (2017). Conveying hope in consultation with life-threatening diseases: The balance supporting and challenging the patient. *Scandinavian Journal of Primary Health Care, 35*(2), 143–152.

Williams, A., Manias, E., Cross, W., et al. (2015). Motivational interviewing to explore culturally and linguistically diverse people's comorbidity medication self efficacy. *Journal of Clinical Nursing, 24*(9–10):1269–1279.

Impaired Dentition   *Morgan Nestingen, MS, AGCNS, ONS*

NANDA-I

Definition

Disruption in tooth development/eruption pattern or structural integrity of individual teeth.

Defining Characteristics

Absence of teeth; abraded teeth; dental caries; enamel discoloration; erosion of enamel; excessive oral calculus; excessive oral plaque; facial asymmetry; halitosis; incomplete tooth eruption for age; loose tooth; malocclusion; premature loss of primary teeth; root caries; tooth fracture; tooth misalignment; toothache

Related Factors

Barrier to self-care; difficulty accessing dental care; excessive intake of fluoride; excessive use of abrasive oral cleaning agents; habitual use of staining substance; inadequate dietary habits; inadequate oral hygiene; insufficient knowledge of dental health; malnutrition

At-Risk Population

Economically disadvantaged; genetic predisposition

Associated Condition

Bruxism; chronic vomiting; oral temperature sensitivity; pharmaceutical agent

● = Independent;   ▲ = Collaborative;   EBN = Evidence-Based Nursing;   EB = Evidence-Based

D

| **NOC** | (Nursing Outcomes Classification) |

Suggested NOC Outcomes

Oral Health

| **Example NOC Outcome with Indicators** |

Oral Health as evidenced by the following indicators: Cleanliness of teeth/Cleanliness of gums/Cleanliness of dentures/Tongue integrity/Gum integrity. (Rate the outcome and indicators of **Oral Health:** 1 = severely compromised, 2 = substantially compromised, 3 = moderately compromised, 4 = mildly compromised, 5 = not compromised [see Section I].)

Client Outcomes

Client Will (Specify Time Frame)

- Have clean teeth, healthy pink gums
- Be free of halitosis
- Explain and demonstrate how to perform oral care
- Demonstrate ability to masticate foods without difficulty
- State absence of pain in mouth

| **NIC** | (Nursing Interventions Classification) |

Suggested NIC Interventions

Oral Health Maintenance; Oral Health Promotion; Oral Health Restoration

| **Example NIC Activities—Oral Health Maintenance** |

Establish a mouth care routine; Arrange for dental care and check-ups as needed

Nursing Interventions and *Rationales*

▲ Inspect oral cavity/teeth/gingiva at least once daily and note any discoloration, presence of debris, amount of plaque buildup, presence of lesions such as white lesions or patches, edema, or bleeding, and intactness of teeth. Refer to a dentist or periodontist as appropriate. EB: *Inspection is a critical diagnostic tool; observations can identify impending problems. Leukoplakia is the presence of uncharacterized white lesions, which can be a precursor to squamous cell carcinoma. If leukoplakia is observed, prompt referral for diagnosis and potential biopsy is indicated (van Der Waal, 2015; ADA, 2017b).*

- If the client is free of bleeding disorders and able to swallow, encourage toothbrushing with a soft toothbrush using fluoride-containing toothpaste at least two times per day. Do not use foam swabs or lemon glycerin swabs to clean the teeth. EB: *Oral bacteria cause caries and periodontal disease. Plaque is a biofilm of bacteria, which often becomes contaminated with antibiotic-resistant bacteria in the hospitalized client (Olsen, 2015).* CEB/EB: *The toothbrush is the most important tool for oral care. Twice daily mechanical toothbrushing is the most effective method of reducing plaque and controlling periodontal disease (ADA, 2017f). Historically, foam swabs have been found ineffective in the removal of plaque (Pearson & Hutton, 2002). Recently, evidence suggested that with trained technique, foam swabs are equivalent to toothbrushing in the mechanically ventilated patient (Marino et al, 2016). Lemon glycerin swabs dry the oral mucosa and can erode the tooth enamel (Poland, 1987; Meurman et al, 1996; Foss-Durant & McAffee, 1997). Normal gums should be pink and firm. Gingivitis is characterized by changes in gingival tissue including redness, sponginess, bleeding, and changes in contour (Fiorellini & Stathopoulou, 2015).*

- Encourage the client to perform interdental hygiene by flossing or cleaning between teeth with interdental brushes, woodsticks, or oral irrigation at least once per day if free of a bleeding disorder. If the client is unable to floss, assist with flossing or encourage the use of an oral irrigator (i.e., "water flossing"). EB: *A meta-review determined that all forms of interdental cleaning performed in addition to toothbrushing are associated with decreased gingivitis. Interdental cleaning may also be effective at plaque removal, but current findings are inconsistent (Sälzer et al, 2015). Oral irrigators have been shown to be superior to flossing at reducing plaque, but they remain less accepted by users (Stauff et al, 2017).*

● = Independent; ▲ = Collaborative; EBN = Evidence-Based Nursing; EB = Evidence-Based

- Use a rotation-oscillation power toothbrush for removal of dental plaque. EB: *Use of a rotation-oscillation power toothbrush more effectively removes plaque versus manual toothbrushing (Kurtz et al, 2016). Multiple studies have found rotation-oscillation power toothbrushes more effective than ultrasonic power toothbrushes (He et al, 2008; Williams et al, 2008; Grender et al, 2013). Studies have consistently demonstrated that rotation-oscillation powered toothbrushes are safe to use on both hard and soft dental tissues (Robinson, 2011; Dörfer, Staehle, & Wolff, 2016).*
- Determine the client's mental status and manual dexterity; if the client is unable to care for self, nursing personnel must provide dental hygiene. The nursing diagnosis Bathing **Self-Care** deficit is then applicable.
- If the client is unable to brush his or her own teeth, follow this procedure:
  ○ Position the client sitting upright or on side.
  ○ Use a soft bristle baby toothbrush.
  ○ Use fluoride toothpaste and tap water or saline as a solution.
  ○ Brush teeth in an up-and-down manner.
  ○ Suction as needed.

Each client must receive oral care including toothbrushing twice daily to maintain healthy teeth and oral tissues and to prevent complications associated with periodontitis (the advanced form of gum disease that can cause tooth loss), which is associated with health problems such as cardiovascular disease, stroke, and bacterial pneumonia (ADA, 2017f,g).

- Monitor the client's nutritional and fluid status to determine if adequate. Recommend the client eat a balanced diet and limit between-meal snacks. *Poor nutrition predisposes clients to dental disease (Hujoel & Lingström, 2017).*
- Recommend that the client maintain a healthy diet with limited sugar intake; in particular, the client should limit sugary beverages and snacks. *Diets high in sugar are strongly associated with formation of caries (ADA, 2017e).* EB: *A study demonstrated a much higher incidence of caries in children who drank soft drinks and had increased intake of processed foods (Evans et al, 2013).*
- Instruct the client with halitosis to clean the tongue when performing oral hygiene. Brush tongue with a tongue scraper or toothbrush and follow with a mouth rinse. EB: *A Cochrane review found that tongue cleaning was effective for short-term control of halitosis (Mehmet Mustafa, 2015).*
- Determine the client's usual method of oral care. Whenever possible, build on the client's existing knowledge base and current practices to develop an individualized plan of care.
- Instruct the client to use a soft-bristled toothbrush, which should be replaced every 3 to 4 months. Angle the toothbrush at a 45-degree angle to the gums and use short lateral strokes. Brush all surfaces of each tooth. Use short, vertical strokes to clean inner tooth surfaces *(ADA, 2017c).*
- Therapeutic mouthwashes help prevent or reduce periodontal disease symptoms including plaque, gingivitis, and caries. Cosmetic mouthwashes can provide comfort and reduce halitosis, but are otherwise ineffective *(ADA, 2017d).* Avoid the use of hydrogen peroxide, or alcohol-based mouthwashes. CEB/EB: *Hydrogen peroxide can cause mucosal damage and is extremely foul tasting to clients (Tombes & Gallucci, 1993). Use of hydrogen peroxide in mouthwash has been linked with chemical gastritis and colitis (Zanelli, Ragazzi, & De Marco, 2017).*
- ▲ Recommend client see a dentist at prescribed intervals, generally two times per year if teeth are in satisfactory condition. *It is important to see a dentist at regular intervals for preventive dental care and treatment of symptoms (ADA, 2017f).*
- ▲ If there are any signs of bleeding when the teeth are brushed, refer the client to a dentist. If bleeding accompanies apparently inflamed gums, refer client to a periodontist. Bleeding in the presence of halitosis is associated with gingivitis. *Early gingivitis can often be reversed with good oral hygiene. Advanced cases may require treatment by a periodontist.* If platelet numbers are decreased, or if the client is edentulous, use moistened Toothettes or a customized extra soft toothbrush for oral care. *Use of a regular toothbrush can cause soft tissue injury and stimulate bleeding in clients with low platelet counts.*
- Recognize that meticulous dental care/oral care can be effective in preventing hospital-acquired (or extended care-acquired) pneumonia. CEB/EB: *Numerous references have found oral care effective in preventing new-onset pneumonia (Ishikawa et al, 2008; van Der Maarel-Wierink et al, 2013; Quinn et al, 2014).*
- Provide scrupulous dental care to critically ill clients, including ventilated clients to prevent ventilator-associated pneumonia. EB/EBN: *Numerous studies have demonstrated decreased incidence of ventilator-associated pneumonia with good oral care. Germicides (i.e., chlorhexidine gluconate) may further reduce risk of ventilator-associated pneumonia in addition to toothbrushing (Hennequin-Hoenderdos, Slot, & Van Der Weijden, 2016; de Lacerda Vidal et al, 2017).*

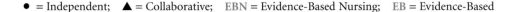

● = Independent;   ▲ = Collaborative;   EBN = Evidence-Based Nursing;   EB = Evidence-Based

D

- If teeth are nonfunctional for chewing, modification of oral intake (e.g., edentulous diet, soft diet) may be necessary. The nursing diagnosis **Imbalanced Nutrition:** less than body requirements may apply.
- If the client is unable to swallow, keep suction nearby when providing oral care.
- See care plan for Impaired **Oral Mucous Membrane.**

Pregnant Client

- Encourage the expectant mother to eat a healthy, balanced diet that is rich in calcium. The teeth usually start to form in the gums during the second trimester of pregnancy. *To encourage the development of good, strong teeth, expectant mothers should eat a healthy, balanced diet that is rich in calcium (ADA, 2017h).*
- Pregnancy is associated with increased risk of oral health complications including gingivitis, caries, erosion, and granulomas. Meticulous, twice daily oral care is critical to maternal health and pregnancy outcomes. Pregnancy complications may be associated with the presence of maternal periodontal disease arising from poor oral hygiene and pregnancy-related hormones (ADA, 2017h).
- Advise the pregnant mother not to smoke. CEB: *Maternal smoking during pregnancy has been associated with increased caries in the teeth of the child (Majorana et al, 2014).*
- Advise the expectant mother to practice good care of her teeth, and to protect her child's teeth once born. Dental caries in children are associated with high levels of Streptococcus mutans. This bacterium is commonly spread from the mother with infected teeth to the infant by tasting of food and sharing of utensils once the child is born (Çolak et al, 2013; Chaffee et al, 2014).

Infant Oral Hygiene

- Gently wipe the infant's gums with a clean washcloth or sterile gauze at least once a day. *Wiping gums prevents bacterial buildup in the mouth.*
- Never allow the infant to fall asleep with a bottle containing milk, formula, fruit juice, or sweetened liquids. If the infant needs a comforter between regular feedings, at night, or during naps, fill a bottle with cool water or provide a clean pacifier recommended by the dentist or health care provider. Never give an infant a pacifier dipped in any sweet liquid. Avoid filling the infant's bottle with liquids such as sugar water and soft drinks. *Decay occurs when sweetened liquids such as milk, formula, and fruit juice are given and are left clinging to an infant's teeth for long periods. Bacteria in the mouth use these sugars as food to produce acids that attack the teeth (Çolak et al, 2013; Majorana et al, 2014).*
- ▲ When multiple teeth appear, brush the child's teeth with a small toothbrush with a small (pea-size) amount of fluoride toothpaste. Application of either a fluoride gel or fluoride varnish is recommended. *Parental toothbrushing and topical fluoride applications (i.e., varnish) have been shown to be effective in reducing the formation of early childhood caries (Jiang et al, 2014).*
- Advise parents to begin dental visits at 1 year of age. *Pediatric periodontal disease has been associated with problems of alignment of permanent teeth; difficulty chewing; and problems speaking, sleeping, concentrating, learning, and with self-esteem (Chaffee et al, 2014).*

Older Children

- ▲ Encourage the family to talk with the dentist about dental sealants, which can help prevent cavities in permanent teeth. EB: *A Cochrane review found that use of dental sealants on the molars of children was effective in preventing caries (Wright et al, 2016).*
- Teach to brush teeth twice a day. EB: *Twice daily tooth brushing is a low-cost, effective strategy to reduce the risk of childhood caries (Huebner & Milgrom, 2015).*
- Recommend the child use dental floss to help prevent gum disease. The dentist will give guidelines on when to start using floss.
- Recommend that parents should not allow the child to smoke or chew tobacco, and stress the importance of setting a good example by not using tobacco products themselves.
- Recommend the child drink fluoridated water when possible. Fluoride in drinking water is one of several available fluoride resources. *The American Dental Association (ADA) strongly endorses use of fluoridated water, based on scientific research that validates the effectiveness in preventing cavities (ADA, 2017a).* EB: *Community water fluoridation remains an effective public health strategy for delivering fluoride to prevent tooth decay and is the most feasible and cost-effective strategy for reaching entire communities (US Department of Health & Human Services Federal Panel on Community Water Fluoridation, 2015).*
- Recommend the child use toothpaste containing fluoride. EB: *Studies demonstrate that fluoride toothpaste is effective in caries prevention and is safe for children of all ages (Wright et al, 2014).*

● = Independent;   ▲ = Collaborative;   EBN = Evidence-Based Nursing;   EB = Evidence-Based

Geriatric

- Provide dentists with accurate medication history to avoid drug interactions and client harm. If the client is taking anticoagulants, laboratory values should be reviewed before providing dental care.
- Help clients brush their own teeth, or provide dental care after breakfast and before bed every day. *If the client lacks dexterity in hands, consider the use of modified dental equipment, including large-handled, powered toothbrushes or interdental cleaning devices (Bissett, 2011; Balzer, 2012).*
- If the client has dementia or delirium and exhibits care-resistant behavior such as fighting, biting, or refusing care, then use the following method:
  - ❍ Ensure client is in a quiet environment such as his or her own bathroom, and sitting or standing at the sink to prime memory for appropriate actions.
  - ❍ Approach the client at eye level within his or her range of vision.
  - ❍ Approach with a smile, and begin conversation with a touch of the hand and gradually move up.
  - ❍ Use mirror–mirror technique, standing behind the client, and brush and floss teeth.
  - ❍ Use respectful adult speech. Do not use "elderspeak," which is a sing-song voice, or diminutive terms such as "deary" or "honey." *Elderspeak is a documented trigger for care-resistant behavior (Williams et al, 2017).*
  - ❍ Promote self-care when client brushes own teeth if possible.
  - ❍ Use distractors when needed: talking, reminiscing, singing.
- ▲ EBN: *Use of specific techniques can decrease resistance to nursing care and increase the effectiveness of nurses providing oral care to clients. Additional research is needed to examine oral care in the client with dementia (Mohammadi, Franks, & Hines, 2015; Rozas, Sadowsky, & Jeter, 2017).*
- ▲ Ensure that dentures are removed and cleaned regularly, after each meal and before bedtime. Brush and rinse dentures to remove debris and soak overnight in a peroxide-based cleaning solution. Dentures left in the mouth at night impede circulation to the palate and predispose the client to oral lesions. EB: *A study found that brushing combined with immersion in a peroxide-based cleaning solution reduce the number of microorganisms surviving on the surface of dentures (Nishi et al, 2014).*
- ▲ Support other caregivers providing oral hygiene. Physical and cognitive impairment in older adults can interfere with the client's ability to perform oral hygiene, and oral hygiene should be provided by a caregiver. If no caregiver is available, the client is prone to dental problems such as dental caries, tooth abscess, tooth fracture, and gingival and periodontal disease.

 Multicultural

- Assess for the influence of cultural beliefs, norms, and values on the client's understanding of dental care. EBN: *What the client considers normal and abnormal dental health and appropriate care may be based on cultural perceptions (Lo & Tan, 2014).*
- Assess for barriers to access to dental care, such as lack of insurance. Minority groups may have limited access to dental care (Da Fonseca & Avenetti, 2017). EB: *Social determinants of health including ethnic minority, low socioeconomic status, impaired family structure, and low health literacy are associated with limited access to care and poor oral health outcomes, including caries and tooth loss (Tellez, Zini, & Estupiñan-Day, 2014; Da Fonseca & Avenetti, 2017).*

 Home Care

- Assess client patterns for daily and professional dental care and related patterns (e.g., smoking, nail biting). Assess for environmental influences on dental status (e.g., fluoride).
- Assess client facilities and financial resources for providing dental care. *Lack of appropriate facilities or financial resources is a barrier to positive dental care patterns. Provision for dental care may be missing from health care plans or unavailable to the uninsured.*
- Request dietary log from the client, adding column for type of food (i.e., soft, pureed, regular).
- Observe a typical meal to assess first-hand the effect of impaired dentition on nutrition. *Clients, especially older adults, are often hesitant to admit nutritional changes that may be embarrassing because of poor dentition.*
- Assist the client with accessing financial or other resources to support optimum dental and nutritional status.

● = Independent;   ▲ = Collaborative;   EBN = Evidence-Based Nursing;   EB = Evidence-Based

D

 Client/Family Teaching and Discharge Planning

- Teach how to inspect the oral cavity and monitor for problems with the teeth and gums.
- Teach how to implement a personal plan of dental hygiene, including appropriate brushing of teeth and tongue and use of dental floss. Use motivational interviewing sessions to facilitate increased compliance in dental care (Stenman et al, 2017). **EB:** *A systematic review demonstrated improved dental hygiene, including interdental cleaning, when motivational interviewing was applied to teaching oral hygiene techniques (Kopp et al, 2017). See Appendix C, Motivational Interviewing, on Evolve.*
- Advise the clients to change their toothbrush every 3 to 4 months, because after that toothbrushes are less effective in removing plaque and are a source of bacterial contamination of the mouth and teeth *(ADA, 2017c).*
- Teach the client the value of having an optimal fluoride concentration in drinking water, and to brush teeth twice daily with toothpaste containing fluoride.
- Teach clients of all ages about the need to decrease intake of sugary foods and to brush teeth regularly.
- Inform individuals who are considering tongue piercing of the potential complications such as chipping and cracking of teeth and possible trauma to the gingiva. If piercing is done, teach the client how to care for the wound and prevent complications. **EB:** *Oral piercings are associated with increased risk of gingival recession and tooth injuries (Hennequin-Hoenderdos, Slot, & Van Der Weijden, 2016).*

REFERENCES

American Dental Association (ADA). (2017a). *ADA fluoridation policy.* Retrieved from http://www.ada.org/en/public-programs/ advocating-for-the-public/fluoride-and-fluoridation/ ada-fluoridation-policy. (Accessed 3 February 2018).

American Dental Association (ADA). (2017b). *Evaluation of potentially malignant disorders in the oral cavity clinical practice guideline.* Retrieved from http://ebd.ada.org/en/evidence/guidelines/ oral-cancer. (Accessed 3 February 2018).

American Dental Association (ADA). (2017c) *Mouth Healthy: Brushing your teeth.* Retrieved from http://www.mouthhealthy.org/en/ az-topics/b/brushing-your-teeth. (Accessed 3 February 2018).

American Dental Association (ADA). (2017d) *Mouth healthy: Mouthwash.* Retrieved from http://www.mouthhealthy.org/en/ az-topics/m/mouthwash. (Accessed 3 February 2018).

American Dental Association (ADA). (2017e) *Mouth healthy: What to eat when you're expecting.* Retrieved from http://www.mouthhealthy .org/en/az-topics/m/mouthwash. (Accessed 3 February 2018).

American Dental Association (ADA). (2017f). *Oral health topics: Home oral care.* Retrieved from http://www.ada.org/en/member-center/ oral-health-topics/home-care. (Accessed 3 February 2018).

American Dental Association (ADA). (2017g). *Oral health topics: Oral-systemic health.* Retrieved from http://www.ada.org/en/ member-center/oral-health-topics/oral-systemic-health. (Accessed 3 February 2018).

American Dental Association (ADA). (2017h). *Oral health topics: pregnancy.* Retrieved from http://www.ada.org/en/member-center/ oral-health-topics/pregnancy. (Accessed 3 February 2018).

Balzer, J. (2012). The use of adaptive oral hygiene devices and orofacial exercise by adults with systemic sclerosis (scleroderma) seems to improve their gingival health. *The Journal of Evidence-Based Dental Practice, 12*(2), 97–98. doi:10.1016/j.jebdp.2012.03.015.

Bissett, S. M. (2011). Guide to providing mouth care for older people. *Nursing Older People, 23*(10), 14–21.

Chaffee, B. W., Gansky, S. A., Weintraub, J. A., et al. (2014). Maternal oral bacterial levels predict early childhood caries development. *Journal of Dental Research, 93*(3), 238–244. doi:10.1177/0022034513517713.

Çolak, H., Dülgergil, Ç., Dalli, M., et al. (2013). Early childhood caries update: A review of causes, diagnoses, and treatments. *Journal of Natural Science, Biology and Medicine, 4*(1), 29–38. doi:10.4103/ 0976-9668.107257.

Da Fonseca, M. A., & Avenetti, D. (2017). Social determinants of pediatric oral health. *Dental Clinics of North America, 61*(3), 519–532. doi:10.1016/j.cden.2017.02.002.

de Lacerda Vidal, C. F., Vidal, A. K. D. L., Monteiro, J. G. D. M., et al. (2017). Impact of oral hygiene involving toothbrushing versus chlorhexidine in the prevention of ventilator-associated pneumonia: A randomized study. *BMC Infectious Diseases, 17*, 112. doi:10.1186/s12879-017-2188-0.

Dörfer, C. E., Staehle, H. J., & Wolff, D. (2016). Three-year randomized study of manual and power toothbrush effects on pre-existing gingival recession. *Journal of Clinical Periodontology, 43*(6), 512. doi:10.1111/jcpe.12518.

Evans, E. W., Hayes, C., Palmer, C. A., et al. (2013). Dietary intake and severe early childhood caries in low-income, young children. *Journal of the Academy of Nutrition and Dietetics, 113*(8), 1057–1061. doi:10.1016/j.jand.2013.03.014.

Fiorellini, J. P., & Stathopoulou, P. G. (2015). Clinical features of gingivitis. In *Carranza's clinical periodontology* (pp. 224–231). Philadelphia: Saunders.

Foss-Durant, A. M., & McAffee, A. (1997). A comparison of three oral care products commonly used in practice. *Clinical Nursing Research, 6*, 1.

Grender, J., Williams, K., Walters, P., et al. (2013). Plaque removal efficacy of oscillating-rotating power toothbrushes: Review of six comparative clinical trials. *American Journal of Dentistry, 26*(2), 68–74.

He, T., et al. (2008). A comparative clinical study of the plaque removal efficacy of an oscillating/rotating power toothbrush and an ultrasonic toothbrush. *The Journal of Clinical Dentistry, 19*(4), 138–142.

Hennequin-Hoenderdos, N. L., Slot, D. E., & Van Der Weijden, G. A. (2016). The incidence of complications associated with lip and/or tongue piercings: A systematic review. *International Journal of Dental Hygiene, 14*(1), 62. doi:10.1111/idh.12118.

Huebner, C., & Milgrom, P. (2015). Evaluation of a parent-designed programme to support tooth brushing of infants and young children. *International Journal of Dental Hygiene, 13*(1), 65–73. (29 ref).

Hujoel, P. P., & Lingström, P. (2017). Nutrition, dental caries and periodontal disease: A narrative review. *Journal of Clinical Periodontology, 44*(S18), S79–S84. doi:10.1111/jcpe.12672.

● = Independent;   ▲ = Collaborative;   EBN = Evidence-Based Nursing;   EB = Evidence-Based

Ishikawa, A., et al. (2008). Professional oral health care reduces the number of oropharyngeal bacteria. *Journal of Dental Research*, *87*(6), 594–598.

Jiang, E. M., Lo, E. C. M., Chu, C. H., et al. (2014). Prevention of early childhood caries (ECC) through parental toothbrushing training and fluoride varnish application: A 24-month randomized controlled trial. *Journal of Dentistry*, *42*(12), 1543–1550. doi:10.1016/j.jdent.2014.10.002.

Kopp, S. L., Ramseier, C. A., Ratka-Krüger, P., et al. (2017). Motivational interviewing as an adjunct to periodontal therapy—A systematic review. *Frontiers in Psychology*, *8*, 279. doi:10.3389/fpsyg.2017.00279.

Kurtz, B., Reise, M., Klukowska, M., et al. (2016). A randomized clinical trial comparing plaque removal efficacy of an oscillating-rotating power toothbrush to a manual toothbrush by multiple examiners. *International Journal of Dental Hygiene*, *14*(4), 278. doi:10.1111/idh.12225.

Lo, E. C. M., & Tan, H. P. (2014). Cultural challenges to oral healthcare implementation in elders. *Gerodontology*, *31*, 72–76. doi:10.1111/ger.12082.

Majorana, A., Cagetti, M. G., Bardellini, E., et al. (2014). Feeding and smoking habits as cumulative risk factors for early childhood caries in toddlers, after adjustment for several behavioral determinants: A retrospective study. *BMC Pediatrics*, *14*, 45. doi:10.1186/1471-2431-14-45.

Marino, P. J., Hannigan, A., Haywood, S., et al. (2016). Comparison of foam swabs and toothbrushes as oral hygiene interventions in mechanically ventilated patients: A randomized split mouth study. *BMJ open respiratory research*, *3*(1), e000150.

Mehmet Mustafa, K. (2015). Current diagnosis and treatment of halitosis. *Duzce Universitesi Tip Fakültesi Dergisi*, *17*(2), 85–88.

Meurman, J. H., et al. (1996). Hospital mouth-cleaning aids may cause dental erosion. *Special Care in Dentistry*, *16*(6), 247–250.

Mohammadi, J. J., Franks, K., & Hines, S. (2015). Effectiveness of professional oral health care intervention on the oral health of residents with dementia in residential aged care facilities: A systematic review protocol. *JBI Database of Systematic Reviews and Implementation Reports*, *13*(10), 110–122. doi:10.11124/jbisrir -2015-2330.

Nishi, Y., Seto, K., Kamashita, Y., et al. (2014). Survival of microorganisms on complete dentures following ultrasonic cleaning combined with immersion in peroxide-based cleanser solution. *Gerodontology*, *31*(3), 202–209. doi:10.1111/ger.12027.

Olsen, I. (2015). Biofilm-specific antibiotic tolerance and resistance. *European Journal of Clinical Microbiology & Infectious Diseases*, *34*(5), 877–886. doi:10.1007/s10096-015-2323-z.

Pearson, L. S., & Hutton, J. L. (2002). A controlled trial to compare the ability of foam swabs and toothbrushes to remove dental plaque. *Journal of Advanced Nursing*, *39*(5), 480.

Poland, J. M. (1987). Comparing Moi-Stir to lemon-glycerin swabs. *The American Journal of Nursing*, *87*(4), 422.

Quinn, B., Baker, D. L., Cohen, S., et al. (2014). Basic nursing care to prevent nonventilator hospital-acquired pneumonia. *Journal of Nursing Scholarship*, *46*(1), 11. doi:10.1111/jnu.12050.

Robinson, P. G. (2011). The safety of oscillating-rotating powered toothbrushes. *Evidence-based Dentistry*, *12*(3), 69.

Rozas, N. S., Sadowsky, J. M., & Jeter, C. B. (2017). Strategies to improve dental health in elderly patients with cognitive

impairment: A systematic review. *The Journal of the American Dental Association*, *148*(4), 236–245.e233. doi:10.1016/j.adaj.2016.12.022.

Sälzer, S., Slot, D. E., Van Der Weijden, F. A., et al. (2015). Efficacy of inter-dental mechanical plaque control in managing gingivitis—A meta-review. *Journal of Clinical Periodontology*, *42*(Suppl. 16), S92. doi:10.1111/jcpe.12363.

Stauff, I., Derman, S., Barbe, A. G., et al. (2017). Efficacy and acceptance of a high-velocity microdroplet device for interdental cleaning in gingivitis patients—A monitored, randomized controlled trial. *International Journal of Dental Hygiene*. doi:10.1111/idh.12292.

Stenman, J., Wennström, J. L., & Abrahamsson, K. H. (2017). A brief motivational interviewing as an adjunct to periodontal therapy—A potential tool to reduce relapse in oral hygiene behaviours. A three-year study. *International Journal of Dental Hygiene*. doi:10.1111/idh.12308.

Tellez, M., Zini, A., & Estupiñan-Day, S. (2014). Social determinants and oral health: An update. *Current Oral Health Reports*, *1*(3), 148–152. doi:10.1007/s40496-014-0019-6.

Tombes, M. B., & Gallucci, B. (1993). The effects of hydrogen peroxide rinses on the normal oral mucosa. *Nursing Research*, *42*, 332.

U.S. Department of Health & Human Services Federal Panel on Community Water Fluoridation (2015). *U.S. Public Health Service Recommendation for Fluoride Concentration in Drinking Water for the Prevention of Dental Caries*. Retrieved from http://www.publichealthreports.org/documents/PHS_2015_Fluoride_Guidelines.pdf. (Accessed 3 February 2018).

van Der Maarel-Wierink, C. D., Vanobbergen, J. N. O., Bronkhorst, E. M., et al. (2013). Oral health care and aspiration pneumonia in frail older people: A systematic literature review. *Gerodontology*, *30*(1), 3. doi:10.1111/j.1741-2358.2012.00637.x.

van Der Waal, I. (2015). Oral leukoplakia, the ongoing discussion on definition and terminology. *Medicina Oral, Patología Oral y Cirugía Bucal*, *20*(6), e685. doi:10.4317/medoral.21007.

Williams, K., et al. (2008). A study comparing the plaque removal efficacy of an advanced rotation-oscillation power toothbrush to a new sonic toothbrush. *The Journal of Clinical Dentistry*, *19*(4), 154–158.

Williams, K., Shaw, C., Lee, A., et al. (2017). Voicing ageism in nursing home dementia care. *Journal of Gerontological Nursing*, *43*(9), 16. doi:10.3928/00989134-20170523-02.

Wright, J. T., Crall, J. J., Fontana, M., et al. (2016). Evidence-based clinical practice guideline for the use of pit-and-fissure sealants: A report of the American Dental Association and the American Academy of Pediatric Dentistry. *The Journal of the American Dental Association*, *147*(8), 672–682.

Wright, J. T., Hanson, N., Ristic, H., et al. (2014). Fluoride toothpaste efficacy and safety in children younger than 6 years: A systematic review. *The Journal of the American Dental Association*, *145*(2), 182–189. doi:10.14219/jada.2013.37.

Zanelli, M., Ragazzi, M., & De Marco, L. (2017). Chemical gastritis and colitis related to hydrogen peroxide mouthwash. *British Journal of Clinical Pharmacology*, *83*(2), 427–428. doi:10.1111/bcp.13100.

● = Independent;   ▲ = Collaborative;   EBN = Evidence-Based Nursing;   EB = Evidence-Based

D

Risk for delayed Development *Marsha McKenzie, MA Ed, BSN, RN*

NANDA-I

Definition

Susceptible to delay of 25% or more in one or more of the areas of social or self-regulatory behavior, or in cognitive, language, gross, or fine motor skills, which may compromise health.

Risk Factors

Inadequate nutrition; presence of abuse; substance misuse; technology dependence

At-Risk Population

Behavioral disorder; economically disadvantaged; exposure to natural disaster; exposure to violence; history of adoption; inadequate maternal nutrition; insufficient parental care; involvement with the foster care system; late-term parental care; maternal age ≤15; maternal age ≥35; maternal function illiteracy; maternal substance misuse; positive drug screen; prematurity; unplanned pregnancy; unwanted pregnancy

Associated Condition

Brain injury; caregiver learning disability; caregiver mental health issue; chronic illness; congenital disorder; endocrine disorder; failure to thrive; genetic disorder; hearing impairment; impaired vision; lead poisoning; parental infection; recurrent otitis media; seizure disorder; treatment regimen

NOC (Nursing Outcomes Classification)

Suggested NOC Outcomes

Abuse Recovery; Child Development: 1 Month, 2 Months, 4 Months, 6 Months, 12 Months, 2 Years, 3 Years, 4 Years, 5 Years, Middle Childhood, Adolescence; Development: Late Adulthood, Middle Adulthood, Young Adulthood; Knowledge: Parenting, Neglect Recovery

Example NOC Outcome with Indicators

Child Development as evidenced by the following indicators: Appropriate milestones of physical, cognitive, and psychosocial age-appropriate progression. (Rate the outcome and indicators of **Child Development:** 1 = never demonstrated, 2 = rarely demonstrated, 3 = sometimes demonstrated, 4 = often demonstrated, 5 = consistently demonstrated [see Section I].)

Client Outcomes

Client/Parents/Primary Caregiver Will (Specify Time Frame)

- Infant/child/adolescent will achieve expected milestones in all areas of development (physical, cognitive, and psychosocial)
- Parent/caregiver will verbalize understanding of potential impediments to normal development and demonstrate actions or environmental/lifestyle changes necessary to provide appropriate care in a safe, nurturing environment

NIC (Nursing Interventions Classification)

Suggested NIC Interventions

Abuse Protection Support: Child; Caregiver Support; Developmental Enhancement: Child/Adolescent; Home Maintenance Assistance; Immunization/Vaccination Management; Infant Care; Kangaroo Care; Lactation Counseling; Learning Facilitation; Newborn Care; Newborn Monitoring; Nonnutritive Sucking; Normalization Promotion; Nutrition Management; Parent Education: Infant/Adolescent/Childbearing Family; Parenting Promotion; Referral; Risk Identification: Childbearing Family; Teaching: (Infant) Nutrition/Safety/Stimulation; (Toddler) Nutrition/Safety; Temperature Regulation (Infant); Therapeutic Play

Example NIC Activities—Parent Education

Instruct parent on normal physiological, emotional, and behavioral characteristics of child

● = Independent; ▲ = Collaborative; EBN = Evidence-Based Nursing; EB = Evidence-Based

Nursing Interventions and *Rationales*

Preconception/Pregnancy

- Assess for alcohol/drug use during pregnancy. Expectant mothers should be instructed that no amount of alcohol consumption is safe during pregnancy. EB: *Alcohol is a well-established teratogen that can cause variable physical and behavioral effects on the fetus. Increased fetal exposure to alcohol and sustained alcohol intake during any trimester of pregnancy is associated with an increased risk of fetal alcohol syndrome (FAS) (Gupta, Gupta, & Shirasaka, 2016).*
- Be aware of state legislation requiring mandatory reporting of maternal prenatal drug use. Be aware that mandatory reporting may further hamper prenatal care in that drug addicted mothers may delay or defer care for fear of legal action. EB: *Wu et al (2013) noted that fear of reporting drug use to authorities can create a "flight from care" environment rather than promote improved prenatal care among drug addicted mothers.*
- Advise expectant mothers to stop smoking and assist with methods of smoking cessation. Smoking is a known precursor to low birth weight and other significant prenatal issues. EB: *Reese et al (2017) noted that pregnant women disproportionately under report smoking and smokers tend to have lower follow-up rates to repeat questionnaires.*
- Recommend that women of childbearing age take 400 μg of folic acid daily to reduce the risk of neural tube defects. CEB: *Taking 400 mcg of folic acid daily, at least 3 months before conception and continuing throughout pregnancy, can prevent as many as 70% of neural tube defects (Greener, 2011).* EB: *Additionally, a comprehensive meta-analysis suggested that maternal use of folic acid supplements during pregnancy could significantly reduce the risk of autism spectrum disorders in children regardless of ethnicity compared with those women who did not supplement with folic acid (Wang et al, 2017).*

Neonate/Infant

- Encourage mother/baby interactions when caring for premature infants.
- Encourage caution regarding use of glucocorticoids in premature and term infants. EB: *Vázquez et al (2012) noted that administration of glucocorticoids in infancy has the potential of causing neurological developmental difficulties, including anxiety and depressive disorders, later in life.*

Toddler/Preschooler/School-Age

- Provide support and education to parents of toddlers with developmental disabilities (i.e., Down's syndrome [DS], cerebral palsy). EB: *A recent study of infants with DS affirmed previous findings showing that the rate of attainment of motor skills is delayed in children with DS compared with children with typical development; however, the developmental sequence is the same. The delayed development is more prominent in more complex skills (Beqaj, Jusaj, & Živković, 2017).*
- Be aware of the role maternal eating disorders plays in childhood development. EB: *Sadeh-Sharvit, Levy-Shiff, and Lock (2016) found that children of mothers with eating disorders showed delayed mental and psychomotor development. Severity of maternal eating disorder symptoms emerged as a significant predictor of child development, but other maternal psychopathology did not. Findings suggest that maternal eating disorder history may play a unique role in the development of neurodevelopmental functions in their children. The children of mothers with eating disorders showed delayed mental and psychomotor development. Severity of maternal eating disorder symptoms appeared as a significant predictor of child development.*
- Encourage parents of toddlers to obtain age-appropriate developmental screenings to detect early problems.
- Toddlers who are underweight should be offered solid foods first rather than juices. *Excessive juice and milk consumption may interfere with nutritional absorption.*
- Teach parents the importance of avoiding lead-based paints in the home and other sources of lead in the environment. EB: *Hou et al (2013) confirmed previous research indicating that when the blood lead level reaches about 50 μg/L in the body of children, it can impair growth, memory, intelligence, and behavior, even when there is no obvious clinical manifestation.*
- Understand the role premature birth plays in the development of speech. EB: *Data suggest that very preterm born children retain atypical bilateral language organization longer than term born controls, which may be explained by a delay in neural language organization caused by very premature birth (Mürner-Lavanchy, 2014).*
- Teach new mothers the importance of breastfeeding. EB: *Moss and Yeaton (2014) found that breastfeeding along with delaying complementary foods yielded consistently and substantially lower the likelihood of obesity and greater probability of healthy weight in infants and toddlers.* EB: *Jäger et al (2014) discovered an inverse association between breastfeeding duration and risk of diabetes.*

● = Independent;   ▲ = Collaborative;   EBN = Evidence-Based Nursing;   EB = Evidence-Based

REFERENCES

Beqaj, S., Jusaj, N., & Živković, V. (2017). Attainment of gross motor milestones in children with Down syndrome in Kosovo-developmental perspective. *Medicinski Glasnik, 14*(2), 189–198. doi:10.17392/917-17.

Greener, M. (2011). The tragedy of congenital abnormalities. *Nurse Prescribing, 9*(3), 117–121.

Gupta, K. K., Gupta, V. K., & Shirasaka, T. (2016). An update on fetal alcohol syndrome—pathogenesis, risks, and treatment. *Alcoholism, Clinical and Experimental Research, 40*, 1594–1602. doi:10.1111/acer.13135.

Hou, S., Yuan, L., Jin, P., et al. (2013). A clinical study of the effects of lead poisoning on the intelligence and neurobehavioral abilities of children. *Theoretical Biology & Medical Modelling, 10*, 13.

Jäger, S., Jacobs, S., Kröger, J., et al. (2014). Breast-feeding and maternal risk of type 2 diabetes: A prospective study and meta-analysis. *Diabetologia, 57*(7), 1355–1365.

Mürner-Lavanchy, I., Steinlin, M., Kiefer, C., et al. (2014). Delayed development of neural language organization in very preterm born children. *Developmental Neuropsychology, 39*(7), 529–542. doi:10.1080/87565641.2014.959173.

Moss, B., & Yeaton, W. (2014). Early childhood healthy and obese weight status: Potentially protective benefits of breastfeeding and delaying solid foods. *Maternal & Child Health Journal, 18*(5), 1224–1232. doi:10.1007/s10995-013-1357-z.

Reese, S. E., Zhao, S., Wu, M. C., et al. (2017). DNA methylation score as a biomarker in newborns for sustained maternal smoking during pregnancy. *Environmental Health Perspectives, 125*(4), 760–766. doi:10.1289/EHP333.

Sadeh-Sharvit, S., Levy-Shiff, R., & Lock, J. D. (2016). Maternal eating disorder history and toddlers' neurodevelopmental outcomes: A brief report. *Eating Disorders, 24*(2), 198–205. doi:10.1080/10640266.2015.1064280.

Vázquez, D. M., Neal, C. R., Patel, P. D., et al. (2012). Regulation of corticoid and serotonin receptor brain system following early life exposure of glucocorticoids: Long term implications for the neurobiology of mood. *Psychoneuroendocrinology, 37*(3), 421–437.

Wang, M., Li, K., Zhao, D., et al. (2017). The association between maternal use of folic acid supplements during pregnancy and risk of autism spectrum disorders in children: A meta-analysis. *Molecular Autism, 8*, 51. doi:10.1186/s13229-017-0170-8.

Wu, M., LaGasse, L. L., Wouldes, T. A., et al. (2013). Predictors of inadequate prenatal care in methamphetamine-using mothers in New Zealand and the United States. *Maternal and Child Health Journal, 17*(3), 566–575.

Diarrhea   *Rosemary Koehl Lee, DNP, ARNP, ACNP-BC, CCNS, CCRN*

NANDA-I

Definition

Passage of loose, unformed stools.

Defining Characteristics

Abdominal pain; bowel urgency; cramping; hyperactive bowel sounds; loose liquid stools, >3 in 24 hours

Related Factors

Anxiety; increase in stress level; laxative abuse; substance misuse

At-Risk Population

Exposure to contaminant; exposure to toxin; exposure to unsanitary food preparation

Associated Condition

Enteral feedings; gastrointestinal inflammation; gastrointestinal irritation; infection; malabsorption; parasite; treatment regimen

NOC   (Nursing Outcomes Classification)

Suggested NOC Outcomes

Bowel Elimination; Electrolyte and Acid-Base Balance; Fluid Balance; Hydration; Risk Control: Environmental Hazards; Community Risk Control: Communicable Disease

Example NOC Outcome with Indicators
Bowel Elimination as evidenced by the following indicators: Elimination pattern/Stool soft and formed/Bowel sounds/Liquid stool. (Rate each indicator of **Bowel Elimination:** 1 = severely compromised, 2 = substantially compromised, 3 = moderately compromised, 4 = mildly compromised, 5 = not compromised [see Section I].)

● = Independent;   ▲ = Collaborative;   EBN = Evidence-Based Nursing;   EB = Evidence-Based

D

Client Outcomes

Client Will (Specify Time Frame)

- Defecate formed, soft stool every 1 to 3 days
- Maintain the perirectal area free of irritation
- State relief from cramping and less or no diarrhea
- Explain cause of diarrhea and rationale for treatment
- Maintain good skin turgor and weight at usual level
- Have negative stool cultures

 NIC (Nursing Interventions Classification)

Suggested NIC Intervention

Diarrhea Management

Example NIC Activities—Diarrhea Management
Evaluate medication profile for gastrointestinal side effects; Suggest trial elimination of foods containing lactose

Nursing Interventions and *Rationales*

- Assess pattern of defecation or have the client keep a diary that includes the following: time of day defecation occurs; usual stimulus for defecation; consistency, amount, and frequency of stool; type of, amount of, and time food consumed; fluid intake; history of bowel habits and laxative use; diet; exercise patterns; obstetrical/gynecological, medical, and surgical histories; medications; alterations in perianal sensations; and present bowel regimen. *Assessment of defecation pattern and factors surrounding diarrhea episode to include changes in diet, medications, exercise, and health history will help direct interventions and treatment (Gale & Wilson, 2016).*
- Recommend use of standardized tool to consistently assess, quantify, and then treat diarrhea. EB: *Stool classification systems include the Hart and Dobb Diarrhea Scale, the Guenther and Sweed Stool Output Assessment Tool, the Bristol Stool Scale, and the Diarrhea Grading Scale (Dag et al, 2015; Ford & Talley, 2016).*
- Inspect, auscultate, palpate, and percuss the abdomen, in that order. *Expect increased frequency of bowel sounds with diarrhea (Lattimer, Chandler, & Borum, 2017).*
- ▲ Use an evidence-based bowel management protocol that includes identifying and treating the cause of the diarrhea, obtaining a stool specimen if infectious etiology is suspected, evaluate current medications and osmolality of enteral feedings, assess and treat hydration status of client, review and stop ordered and/or over-the-counter (OTC) laxatives, assess food preparation practices, assess home environment, provide good skin care and apply barrier creams to prevent skin irritation from diarrhea, and evaluate need for antidiarrheal agents and possible fecal containment device with provider. EB: *The possible cause of the diarrhea needs to be assessed and client hydration and skin protective interventions put into place rapidly to prevent secondary complications associated with the client's diarrhea episodes (DuPont 2016; Gale & Wilson, 2016).*
- ▲ Identify the cause of diarrhea if possible based on history (e.g., infection, gastrointestinal inflammation, medication effect, malnutrition or malabsorption, laxative abuse, osmotic enteral feedings, anxiety, stress). See Related Factors: *Identification of the underlying cause is important, because the treatment is determined based on the cause of diarrhea.*
- ▲ Testing for diarrhea may consist of laboratory work such as a complete blood count with differential and blood cultures if the client is febrile. Also obtain stool specimens as ordered, to either rule out or diagnose an infectious process (e.g., ova and parasites, *Clostridium difficile* infection, bacterial cultures for food poisoning). *Assessing for signs of systemic infection and inflammatory response as well as evaluation of the stool for infection are important first steps in identifying the cause of diarrhea (Schiller & Sellin, 2016).*
- ▲ Consider the possibility of *C. difficile* infection if the client has any of the following: watery diarrhea, low-grade fever, abdominal cramps, history of antibiotic therapy, history of gastrointestinal tract surgery, and if the client is taking medications that reduce gastric acid, including proton-pump inhibitors (PPIs). *Any antibiotic can cause C. difficile infection, but clindamycin, cephalosporins, and fluoroquinolones pose the greatest risk, as do multiple antibiotics and longer duration of antibiotics (Dunne, Hayes, & Marsh, 2016;*

● = Independent; ▲ = Collaborative; EBN = Evidence-Based Nursing; EB = Evidence-Based

D

Schiller & Sellin, 2016; Tariq et al, 2017). **EB:** C. difficile *infections have become increasingly common because of the frequent use of broad-spectrum antibiotics, and now there is a hypervirulent form of* C. difficile *causing increased morbidity and mortality. Antibiotics and gastric acid reducing medications can change normal gut flora, increasing the risk for development of* C. difficile *infection, diarrhea, and colitis) (Dunne, Hays, & Marsh, 2016; Schiller & Sellin, 2016).*

- Use standard precautions when caring for clients with diarrhea to prevent spread of infectious diarrhea; use gloves and handwashing. *C. difficile* and viruses causing diarrhea have been shown to be highly contagious. C. difficile *is difficult to eradicate because of spore formation (Martin et al, 2014).* **EB:** *A review of client care related to* C. difficile *summarizes care to include full contact isolation, soap and water handwashing (alcohol rubs are not effective), use of disposable equipment, and environmental room decontamination (Dubberke et al, 2014; Martin et al, 2014; Centers for Disease Control and Prevention [CDC], 2017).* C. difficile *can survive for at least 24 hours on inanimate surfaces, and spores can survive for months on objects such as toilets, sinks, and bed rails (Martin et al, 2014; CDC, 2017).*

- ▲ Antibiotic stewardship is an important aspect in the prevention of *C. difficile* infections. *Antibiotics should be used judiciously (Vardakas, Trigkidis, & Boukouvala, 2016; CDC, 2017).* If the client has diarrhea associated with antibiotic therapy, consult with the health care provider regarding the use of probiotics, such as yogurt with active cultures, to treat diarrhea, or probiotic dietary supplements, or preferably use probiotics to prevent diarrhea when first beginning antibiotic therapy. **EB:** *Although conclusive evidence on the effectiveness of probiotic in treating and preventing* C. difficile *and diarrhea is lacking, evidence suggests that probiotics may be helpful for some clients. Probiotics may be used in an attempt to balance intestinal flora and restrict the colonization of* C. difficile *(Clauson & Crawford, 2015; Patro-Golab, Shamir, & Szajewska, 2015; Wilkins & Sequoia, 2017).*

- ▲ If a probiotic is ordered, administer it with food. Recommend that it be taken through the antibiotic course and 10 to 14 days afterward. *Food tends to buffer the stomach acids, allowing more of the probiotic ingredients to pass through the stomach for absorption in the intestines. Beginning this therapy early helps prevent antibiotic-associated diarrhea (Clauson & Crawford, 2015).*

- ▲ Recognize that *C. difficile* can commonly recur and that reculturing of stool is often required before initiating retreatment. **EB:** *High reinfection rates have been reported within the first 2 months of initial diagnosis. Repeat courses of antibiotics, usually metronidazole or vancomycin, are necessary to treat repeat* C. difficile *infections. Evidence is evolving to support fecal transplant for clients with severe recurrent* C. difficile *infections (Liubakka & Vaughn, 2016).*

- Have the client complete a diet diary for 7 days and monitor the intake of high fructose corn syrup and fructose sweeteners in relation to onset of diarrhea symptoms. If diarrhea is associated with fructose ingestion, intake should be limited or eliminated. **EB:** *High fructose corn syrup or fructose sweeteners from fruit juices can cause gastrointestinal symptoms of bloating, rumbling, flatulence, and diarrhea at amounts of 25 to 50 g. Malabsorption is demonstrated in clients after 25 g fructose, and most clients develop symptoms with 50 g fructose (Schiller & Sellin, 2016).*

- ▲ If the client has infectious diarrhea, consider avoiding use of medications that slow peristalsis. **EB:** *If an infectious process is occurring, such as* C. difficile *infection or food poisoning, medication to slow peristalsis should generally not be given. The increase in gut motility helps eliminate the causative factor, and use of antidiarrheal medication could result in a toxic megacolon (Schiller & Sellin, 2016).*

- Assess for dehydration by observing skin turgor over sternum and inspecting for longitudinal furrows of the tongue. Watch for excessive thirst, fever, dizziness, lightheadedness, palpitations, excessive cramping, bloody stools, hypotension, and symptoms of shock. *Severe diarrhea can cause deficient fluid volume, electrolyte imbalance, extreme weakness, and a possible shock state (Gale & Wilson, 2016; Schiller & Sellin, 2016).*

- Refer to care plans for Deficient **Fluid** volume and Risk for **Electrolyte** imbalance if appropriate.

- ▲ If the client has frequent or chronic diarrhea, consider suggesting use of dietary fiber after consultation with a nutritionist and/or provider. **EB:** *Use of a fiber supplement decreases the number of incontinent stools and improves stool consistency (Schiller & Sellin, 2016).*

- ▲ If diarrhea is chronic and there is evidence of malnutrition, consult with the provider for a dietary consult and possible nutrition supplementation to maintain nutrition while the gastrointestinal system heals (Schiller & Sellin, 2016).

- Encourage the client to eat small, frequent meals, eating foods that are easy to digest at first (e.g., bananas, crackers, pretzels, rice, potatoes, clear soups, applesauce), but switch to a regular diet as soon as tolerated. Also recommend avoiding milk products, foods high in fiber, and caffeine (dark sodas, tea, coffee, chocolate).

● = Independent;   ▲ = Collaborative;   **EBN** = Evidence-Based Nursing;   **EB** = Evidence-Based

D

The bananas, rice, applesauce, toast (BRAT) diet has been traditionally recommended but may be nutritionally incomplete (International Foundation for Functional Gastrointestinal Disorders, 2014; Schiller, Pardi, & Sellin, 2017).

• Provide a readily available bathroom, commode, or bedpan.

• Thoroughly cleanse and dry the perianal and perineal skin daily as needed using a cleanser capable of stool removal. Apply skin moisture barrier cream as needed. Refer to perirectal skin care in the care plan for Bowel **Incontinence.**

▲ If the client has enteral tube feedings and diarrhea, consider infusion rate; position of feeding tube; tonicity of formula; possible formula contamination; and excessive intake of hyperosmolar medications, such as sorbitol commonly found in the liquid version of medications (Taylor et al, 2016). Consider changing the formula to a lower osmolarity, lactose-free, or high-fiber feeding. *Determination of the cause of diarrhea should include an abdominal examination, fecal leukocytes, quantification of stool, stool culture for C. difficile (and/or toxin assay), serum electrolyte panel, and review of medications (Schiller & Sellin, 2016).*

• Avoid administering bolus enteral feedings into the small bowel. The stomach has a larger capacity for large fluid volumes, whereas the small bowel can usually only tolerate up to 150 mL/hr (Taylor et al, 2016).

▲ Dilute liquid medications before administration through the enteral tube and flush the enteral feeding tube with sufficient water before and after medication administration. *Because many liquid medications contain sorbitol or are hyperosmotic, diluting the medication may help decrease occurrence of diarrhea (Joos et al, 2015).*

• Teach clients with cancer the types of diarrhea they may encounter, emphasizing not only chemotherapy- and radiation-induced diarrhea, but also *C. difficile,* along with associated signs and symptoms, and treatments. EB: *Diarrhea in cancer patients is a common complication that causes dehydration, electrolyte imbalances, nutritional deficits, and hospitalization for treatment. Providing the client education focusing on early recognition of diarrhea necessitating early interventions is important in preventing adverse client outcomes (Tarricone et al, 2016; Escalante et al, 2017; Schiller, Pardi, & Sellin, 2017).*

▲ For chemotherapy-induced diarrhea (CID) and radiation-induced diarrhea (RID), review rationale for pharmacological interventions, along with soluble fiber and probiotic supplements. Consult a registered dietitian to assist with recommendations to alleviate diarrhea, decrease dehydration, and maintain nutritional status. EBN: *Both CID and RID can occur as often as or more than 50% of the time, depending on the chemotherapy regimen or combination with radiation (Escalante et al, 2017; Schiller, Pardi, & Sellin, 2017).*

▲ Acute traveler's diarrhea is the most common illness affecting individuals traveling to, usually, low-income regions of the world. EB: *Improved hygiene and avoidance of foods for which preparation methods are unknown (e.g., street food) can mitigate the severity of gastric distress. Clients should be counseled about precautions they can take while traveling to reduce the severity of the diarrhea, and a self-treatment antibiotic series may be prescribed by the health care provider for at-risk clients (Steffen, Hill, & DuPont, 2015; Porter et al, 2017).*

 Pediatric

▲ Assess for mild or moderate signs of dehydration with both acute and persistent diarrhea: mild (increased thirst and dry mouth or tongue) and moderate (decreased urination; no wet diapers for 3+ hours; feeling of weakness/lightheadedness, irritability, or listlessness; few or no tears when crying) (Gupta, 2016). Refer to primary care provider for treatment.

▲ Recommend that parents give the child oral rehydration fluids to drink in the amounts specified by the health care provider, especially during the first 4 to 6 hours to replace lost fluid. Once the child is rehydrated, an orally administered maintenance solution should be used along with food. Continue even if child vomits. EB: *Treatment with oral rehydration fluids for children is generally as effective as intravenous fluids (Carson, Mudd, & Madati, 2017). Oral rehydration therapy (ORT) is an isoosmolar, glucose-electrolyte solution that has been recognized for more than 40 years to be effective in treating children with dehydration caused by acute infectious diarrhea). Vomiting is not a contraindication to ORT. Adequate ORT is absorbed by most clients during vomiting (Rehydration Project, 2014).*

• Recommend the mother resumes breastfeeding as soon as possible.

• Recommend parents avoid giving the child flat soda, fruit juices, gelatin dessert, or instant fruit drink. *These fluids have a high osmolality from carbohydrate contents and can exacerbate diarrhea. In addition*

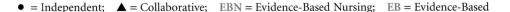

• = Independent; ▲ = Collaborative; EBN = Evidence-Based Nursing; EB = Evidence-Based

they have low sodium concentrations that can aggravate existing hyponatremia (Rehydration Project, 2014).

- Recommend parents give children foods with complex carbohydrates, such as potatoes, rice, bread, cereal, yogurt, fruits, and vegetables. Avoid fatty foods, foods high in simple sugars, and milk products.
- ▲ Recommend rotavirus vaccine within the child's vaccination schedule. **EB:** *Two vaccines, Rotarix and Rotateq, have undergone comprehensive studies with findings that they can significantly prevent severe rotavirus diarrhea and death caused by dehydration in children; (Glass et al, 2014; Mwenda et al, 2017).*

Geriatric

- ▲ Evaluate medications the client is taking. Recognize that many medications can result in diarrhea, including digitalis, propranolol, angiotensin-converting enzyme inhibitors, histamine-receptor antagonists, nonsteroidal antiinflammatory drugs, anticholinergic agents, oral hypoglycemia agents, antibiotics, and so forth. **EB:** *Numerous medications can cause diarrhea. Evaluate changes in the client's medications as a possible cause of the diarrhea (DuPont, 2016; Schiller, Pardi, & Sellin, 2017).*
- ▲ Monitor the client closely to detect whether an impaction is causing diarrhea; remove impaction as ordered. Clients with fecal impaction commonly experience leakage of mucus or liquid stool from the rectum, rectal irritation, distention, and impaired anal sensation (Schiller, Pardi, & Sellin, 2017; Schiller & Sellin, 2016).
- ▲ Seek medical attention if diarrhea is severe or persists for more than 24 hours, or if the client has a history of dehydration or electrolyte disturbances, such as lassitude, weakness, or prostration. *Older adult clients can dehydrate rapidly; especially serious is the development of hypokalemia with dysrhythmias. C. difficile is a common cause of diarrhea in older clients when they have been subjected to long-term antibiotic therapy (Gale & Wilson, 2016; Vardakas, Trigkidis, & Boukouvala, 2016).*
- Provide emotional support for clients who are having trouble controlling unpredictable episodes of diarrhea. Diarrhea can be a great source of embarrassment to older clients and can lead to social isolation and a feeling of powerlessness.

Home Care

Previously mentioned interventions may be adapted for home care use to keep the client well hydrated.

- Assess the home for general sanitation and methods of food preparation. Reinforce principles of sanitation for food handling. *Poor sanitation or mishandling of food may cause bacterial infection or transmission of dangerous organisms from utensils to food.*
- Assess for methods of handling soiled laundry if the client is bed bound or has been incontinent. Instruct or reinforce universal precautions with family and bloodborne pathogen precautions with agency caregivers. *The Bloodborne Pathogen Regulations of the Occupational Safety and Health Administration (OSHA) identify legal guidelines for caregivers.*
- When assessing medication history, include OTC drugs, both general and those currently being used to treat the diarrhea. Instruct clients not to mix OTC medications when self-treating. *Mixing OTC medications can further irritate the gastrointestinal system, intensifying the diarrhea or causing nausea and vomiting.*
- Evaluate current medications for indications that specific interventions are warranted. *Blood levels of medications may increase during prolonged episodes of diarrhea, indicating the need for close monitoring of the client or direct intervention.*
- ▲ Evaluate the need for a home health aide or homemaker service referral. Caregiver may need support for maintaining client cleanliness to prevent skin breakdown.
- Evaluate the need for durable medical equipment in the home. The client may need a bedside commode, call bell, or raised toilet seat to facilitate prompt toileting.

Client/Family Teaching and Discharge Planning

- Encourage avoidance of coffee, spices, milk products, and foods that irritate or stimulate the gastrointestinal tract.
- Teach the appropriate method of taking ordered antidiarrheal medications; explain side effects.
- Explain how to prevent the spread of infectious diarrhea (e.g., careful handwashing, appropriate handling and storage of food, and thoroughly cleaning the bathroom and kitchen). **EB:** *Good hand hygiene has repeatedly been found to be the first step in preventing the spread of infectious diarrhea (Dickinson & Surawicz, 2014; CDC, 2017).*

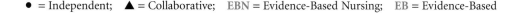

● = Independent; ▲ = Collaborative; **EBN** = Evidence-Based Nursing; **EB** = Evidence-Based

- Help the client to determine stressors and set up an appropriate stress reduction plan, if stress is the cause of diarrhea.
- Teach signs and symptoms of dehydration and electrolyte imbalance.
- Teach perirectal skin care.
- ▲ Consider teaching clients about complementary therapies, such as probiotics, after consultation with primary care provider.

REFERENCES

Carson, R. A., Mudd, S. S., & Madati, P. J. (2017). Evaluation of a nurse-initiated acute gastroenteritis pathway in the pediatric emergency department. *Journal of Emergency Nursing, 43*(5), 406–412. Retrieved from http://dx.doi.org/10.1016/j.jen.2017.01.001.

Centers for Disease Control, and Prevention (2017). *Clostridium difficile*. https://www.cdc.gov/hai/organisms/cdiff/cdiff_clinicians.html. (Accessed 12 November 2017).

Clauson, E. R., & Crawford, P. (2015). What you must know before you recommend a probiotic. *The Journal of Family Practice, 64*(3), 151–155.

Dag, G. S., Dicle, A., Saka, O., et al. (2015). Assessment of the Turkish version of the King's stool chart for evaluating stool output and diarrhea among patients receiving enteral nutrition. *Gastroenterology Nursing, 38*(3), 218–225. doi:10.1097/SGA.0000000000000114.

Dickinson, B., & Surawicz, C. M. (2014). Infectious diarrhea: An overview. *Current Gastroenterology Reports, 16*, 399.

Dubberke, E. R., Carling, P., Carrico, R., et al. (2014). Strategies to prevent *Clostridium difficile* infections in acute care hospitals: 2014 update. *Infection Control and Hospital Epidemiology, 35*(S2), S48–S65.

Dunne, E., Hayes, I., & Marsh, B. (2016). Is prophylaxis for stress ulceration useful? In C. S. Deutschman & P. J. Neligan (Eds.), *Evidence-based practice of critical care* (2nd ed., Chapter 18, pp. 112–116). Philadelphia: Elsevier.

DuPont, H. L. (2016). Persistent diarrhea: A clinical review. *JAMA: The Journal of the American Medical Association, 315*(24), 2712–2723. doi:10.1001/jama.2016.7833.

Escalante, J., McQuade, R. M., Stojanovska, V., et al. (2017). Impact of chemotherapy on gastrointestinal functions and the enteric nervous system. *Maturitas, 105*, 23–29. Retrieved from http://dx.doi.org/10.1016/j.maturitas.2017.04.021.

Ford, A. C., & Talley, N. J. (2016). Irritable bowel syndrome. In M. Feldman, L. Friedman, & L. J. Brandt (Eds.), *Sleisenger and Fordtran's gastrointestinal and liver disease* (10th ed., Chapter 122, pp. 2139–2153). Philadelphia: Elsevier.

Gale, A. R., & Wilson, M. (2016). Diarrhea: Initial evaluation and treatment in the Emergency Department. *Emergency Clinics of North America, 34*, 293–308. Retrieved from http://dx.doi.org/10.1016/j.emc.2015.12.006.

Glass, R. I., Parashar, U., Patel, M., et al. (2014). Rotavirus vaccines: successes and challenges. *Journal of Infection, 68*, S9–S18.

Gupta, R. (2016). Diarrhea. In R. Wyllie, J. S. Hyams & M. Kay (Eds.), *Pediatric gastrointestinal and liver disease* (5th ed., Chapter 9, pp. 104–114). Philadelphia: Elsevier.

International Foundation for Functional Gastrointestinal Disorders (March, 2014). *Nutritional strategies for managing diarrhea*. Retrieved from http://www.iffgd.org/site/gi-disorders/functional-gi-disorders/diarrhea/nutrition. (Accessed 13 April 2015).

Joos, E., Mehuys, E., VanBocxlaer, J., et al. (2015). Drug administration via enteral feeding tubes in residential care facilities for individuals with intellectual disability: An observational study. *Journal of Intellectual Disability Research, 59*(3), 215–225.

Lattimer, L. D. N., Chandler, M., & Borum, M. L. (2017). Chronic diarrhea. In F. J. Domino (Ed.), *The 5-minute clinical consult premium 2018*. Philadelphia: Lippincott Williams & Wilkins.

Liubakka, A., & Vaughn, B. P. (2016). *Clostridium difficile* infection and fecal microbiota transplant. *AACN Advanced Critical Care, 27*(3), 324–337. Retrieved from http://dx.doi.org/10.4037/aacnacc2016703.

Martin, M., Zingg, W., Knoll, E., et al. (2014). National European guidelines for the prevention of *Clostridium difficile* infection: A systematic qualitative review. *Journal of Hospital Infection, 87*, 212e219.

Mwenda, J. M., Burke, R. M., Shaba, K., et al. (2017). Implementation of rotavirus surveillance and vaccine introduction—World Health Organization, 2007–2016. *Morbidity and Mortality Weekly Report., 66*(43), 1192–1196.

Patro-Golab, B., Shamir, R., & Szajewska, H. (2015). Yogurt for treating antibiotic-associated diarrhea: Systematic review and meta-analysis. *Nutrition, 31*, 796–800. Retrieved from http://dx.doi.org/10.1016/j.nut.2014.11.013.

Porter, C. K., Olson, S., Hall, A., et al. (2017). Travelers' diarrhea: An update on the incidence, etiology, and risk in military deployments and similar travel populations. *Military Medicine, 182*(4), 4–10.

Rehydration Project. (2014). Retrieved from http://rehydrate.org/ors/ort.htm. (Accessed 8 January 2018).

Schiller, L. R., Pardi, D. S., & Sellin, J. H. (2017). Chronic diarrhea: diagnosis and management. *Clinical Gastroenterology and Hepatology, 15*, 182–193. Retrieved from http://dx.doi.org/10.1016/j.cgh.2016.07.028.

Schiller, L. R., & Sellin, J. H. (2016). Diarrhea. In M. Feldman, L. Friedman, & L. J. Brandt (Eds.), *Sleisenger and Fordtran's gastrointestinal and liver disease* (10th ed., Chapter 16, pp. 221–241). Philadelphia: Elsevier.

Steffen, R., Hill, D. R., & DuPont, H. L. (2015). Traveler's diarrhea: A clinical review. *JAMA: The Journal of the American Medical Association, 313*(1), 71–80.

Tariq, R., Singh, S., Gupta, A., et al. (2017). Association of gastric acid suppression with recurrent *Clostridium difficile* infection: A systematic review and meta-analysis. *JAMA Internal Medicine, 177*(6), 784–791. doi:10.1001/jamainternmed.2017.0212.

Tarricone, R., Koush, D. A., Nyanzi-Wakholi, B., et al. (2016). A systematic literature review of the economic implications of chemotherapy-induced diarrhea and its impact on quality of life. *Critical Reviews in Oncology/Hematology, 99*, 37–48. Retrieved from http://dx.doi.org/10.1016/j.critrevonc.2015.12.012.

Taylor, B. E., McClave, S. A., Martindale, R. G., et al. (2016). Guidelines for the provision and assessment of nutrition support therapy in the adult critically ill patient: Society of Critical Care Medicine (SCCM) and American Society for Parenteral and Enteral Nutrition (A.S.P.E.N.). *Critical Care Medicine, 44*(2), 390–438. doi:10.1097/CCM.0000000000001525.

Vardakas, K. Z., Trigkidis, K. K., & Boukouvala, E. (2016). *Clostridium difficile* infection following systemic antibiotic administration is randomized controlled trials: A systematic review and meta-analysis. *International Journal of Antimicrobial Agents, 48*, 1–10. Retrieved from http://www.ijaaonline.com/article/S0924-8579(16)30055-3/fulltext.

Wilkins, T., & Sequoia, J. (2017). Probiotics for gastrointestinal conditions: A summary of the evidence. *American Family Physician, 96*(3), 170–178.

● = Independent; ▲ = Collaborative; EBN = Evidence-Based Nursing; EB = Evidence-Based

D

Risk for Disuse syndrome   *Darcy O'Banion, RN, MS, ACCNS-AG*

NANDA-I

Definition

Susceptible to deterioration of body systems as the result of prescribed or unavoidable musculoskeletal inactivity, which may compromise health.

Risk Factors

Pain

Associated Condition

Alteration in level of consciousness; mechanical immobility; paralysis; prescribed immobility

NOC   (Nursing Outcomes Classification)

Suggested NOC Outcomes

Pain Level; Endurance; Immobility Consequences: Physiological; Mobility; Neurological Status: Consciousness; Progressive Mobility

> **Example NOC Outcome with Indicators**
>
> **Immobility Consequences: Physiological** as evidenced by the following indicators: Pressure injury/Constipation/ Compromised nutrition status/Urinary calculi/Compromised muscle strength. (Rate the outcome and indicators of **Immobility Consequences: Physiological:** 1 = severe, 2 = substantial, 3 = moderate, 4 = mild, 5 = none [see Section I].)

Client Outcomes

Client Will (Specify Time Frame)

- Express pain level that is tolerable to allow for desired mobility
- Maintain full range of motion in joints
- Maintain intact skin, good peripheral blood flow, and normal pulmonary function
- Maintain normal bowel and bladder function
- Express feelings about imposed immobility
- Explain methods to prevent complications of immobility

NIC   (Nursing Interventions Classification)

Suggested NIC Interventions

Energy Management; Exercise Therapy: Joint Mobility; Muscle Control; Positioning; Pain management

> **Example NIC Activities—Energy Management**
>
> Determine the client's significant other's perception of causes of fatigue; Use valid instruments to measure fatigue, as indicated

Nursing Interventions and *Rationales*

- Screen for mobility skills in the following order: (1) bed mobility; (2) supported and unsupported sitting; (3) transitional movements such as sit to stand, stand to sit, and transfers to chair from bed, from chair to bed, and so forth; and (4) standing and walking activities. Use a mobility assessment tool such as the Banner Mobility Assessment Tool (Boynton et al, 2014) or the Perme ICU Mobility Score (Perme et al, 2014). EB: *A systematic review showed that early mobilization lead to a greater probability of walking without assistance at time of discharge, and more days alive and out of hospital (Tipping et al, 2017).* EB: *Mobilization of stable, critically ill patients can be done safely with minimal risk (Boynton et al, 2014).*
- Assess the level of assistance needed by the client and express in terms of amount of effort expended by the person assisting the client. The range is as follows: total assist, meaning client performs 0% to 25% of task and, if client requires the help of more than one caregiver, it is referred to as a dependent transfer;

● = Independent;   ▲ = Collaborative;   EBN = Evidence-Based Nursing;   EB = Evidence-Based

maximum assist, meaning client gives 25% of effort while the caregiver performs the majority of the work; moderate assist, meaning client gives 50% of effort; minimal assist, meaning client gives 75% of effort; contact guard assist, meaning no physical assist is given but caregiver is physically touching client for steadying, guiding, or in case of loss of balance; stand by assist, meaning caregiver's hands are up and ready in case needed; supervision, meaning supervision of task is needed even if at a distance; modified independent, meaning client needs assistive device or extra time to accomplish task; and independent, meaning client is able to complete task safely without instruction or assistance. **EB:** Functional status is often based on rating from the Functional Independence Measure, which is an instrument that includes 18 items covering 6 domains of self-care, sphincter control, transfer, locomotion, communication, and social cognition (Graham et al, 2014; Granger, 2015).

▲ Request a referral to a physical therapist (PT) as needed so that client's range of motion, muscle strength, balance, coordination, endurance, and early mobilization can be part of the initial evaluation. The PT may provide the client with bed exercises, including stretching, flexing/extending muscle groups, or using bands to maintain muscle strength and tone. Collaboration with nursing staff, therapy, and respiratory therapy as needed to mobilize patients as early and as safely possible. **EB:** *Muscle atrophy from disuse is associated with disability, functional decline, metabolic derangements, and early mortality (Atherton et al, 2016).*

● Passive range of motion can be done as the client tolerates. **EBN:** *Although there is evidence to support early mobility in reducing complications, recent literature shows that passive range of motion and stretching does not prevent or treat muscle contracture (Prabhu, Swaminathan, & Harvey, 2013; Harvey et al, 2017).*

● Use specialized boots to prevent pressure injury on the heels and foot drop; remove boots twice daily to assess the skin and to provide foot care as needed. Elevate heels off the bed as the client tolerates when boots are not in place. *Boots help keep the foot in normal anatomical alignment to prevent foot drop and off-loading prevents pressure injury formation on the heel.* **EB:** *A Cochrane review found that there is no good evidence base to determine which boots or pressure redistribution system is most effective in preventing heel pressure injury (McInnes et al, 2015).*

● When positioning a client on the side, tilt client 30 degrees or less while lying on the side. *Full (versus tilt) side-lying position places higher pressure on the trochanter, predisposing to skin breakdown; however, more evidence is needed to fully determine the effect of full versus tilted positioning on pressure injury (Gillespie et al, 2014; National Pressure Ulcer Advisory Panel, 2014).*

● Assess skin condition every shift and more frequently if needed. Use a risk assessment tool such the Braden Scale or the Norton Scale to predict the risk of developing pressure ulcers (now referred to as pressure injury). **EBN:** *Use of a risk assessment tool is possibly effective to predict the risk of developing a pressure injury (National Pressure Ulcer Advisory Panel, 2014). Refer to care plan for* risk for Impaired **Skin** integrity.

● Discuss with staff and management a "safe patient handling" policy that may include a "no lift" policy to prevent staff injury. *Lifting equipment can reduce risk of injury; however, the equipment should be an integral part of nursing practice because lifting equipment is not regularly used even when available (Boynton et al, 2014; Lee & Lee, 2017).*

● Turn clients at high risk for pressure/shear/friction frequently. Turn clients at least every 2 to 4 hours on a pressure-reducing mattress and every 2 hours on standard foam mattress. *These are general guidelines for turning, but there is no robust evidence to support frequency of repositioning. Preferably base the turning schedule on close assessment of the client's condition and predisposing conditions (Gillespie et al, 2014; Makic, 2014; National Pressure Ulcer Advisory Panel, 2014).*

● Provide the client with a pressure-relieving horizontal support surface. For further interventions on skin care, refer to the care plan for Impaired **Skin** integrity.

● Help the client out of bed as soon as able. **EB:** *Prolonged immobilization leads to harmful consequences on musculoskeletal, cardiovascular, respiratory, integumentary systems, as well as cognition (Atherton et al, 2016; Parry & Puthucheary, 2015). Early mobilization reduces risk of atelectasis, pneumonia, venous thromboembolism (VTE), and pulmonary embolism, and decreases orthostatic hypotension (Makic, 2014), as well as reducing the risk of skeletal muscle atrophy, joint contractures, insulin resistance, microvascular dysfunction, systemic inflammation, and pressure injury (Parry& Puthucheary, 2015).*

● When getting the client up after bed rest, do so slowly and watch for signs and symptoms of postural (orthostatic) hypotension, including dizziness, tachycardia, nausea, diaphoresis, or syncope. *To assess orthostatic vital signs, take the first blood pressure and heart rate measurements once the client has been lying supine for 5 minutes. Then have the client stand and check blood pressure and heart rate 1 and 3 minutes*

● = Independent;   ▲ = Collaborative;   EBN = Evidence-Based Nursing;   EB = Evidence-Based

D

after standing. A decrease in systolic blood pressure by 20 mm Hg, a decrease in diastolic pressure of 10 mm Hg or more, or an increase in heart rate by 20 beats per minute or more are indicative of intravascular volume loss (Emergency Nurses Association, 2015; CDC, 2017). Compression wraps to abdomen and/or lower limbs can facilitate venous return if hypotension is an issue (Logan et al, 2017).

● Obtain assistive devices such as braces, crutches, or canes to help the client reach and maintain as much mobility as possible. *Assistive devices can help increase mobility (Boynton et al, 2014).*

▲ Apply graduated compression stockings as ordered, if indicated for orthostatic hypotension. Ensure proper fit by measuring accurately. Remove the stockings at least twice a day, in the morning with the bath and in the evening to assess the condition of the extremity, and then reapply. Knee length is preferred rather than thigh length. EB: *The American College of Chest Physicians (AACP, 2016) does not recommend graduated compression stockings to prevent deep vein thrombosis (DVT). Based on recent evidence, compression stockings did not reduce the rate of DVTs. However, intermittent pneumatic compression devices are associated with significantly lower incidences of VTE compared with graduated compression devices (Arabi et al, 2013). Please refer to the ACCP guidelines for use of mechanical prophylaxis for specific client situations.*

● Observe for signs of DVT, including pain, tenderness, redness, and swelling in the calf and thigh. Also observe for signs and symptoms of pulmonary embolism, including sudden onset of dyspnea, chest pain, syncope, dizziness, tachycardia, or tachypnea. *Because of poor specificity of signs and symptoms of VTE, the diagnosis based on clinical manifestation alone is unreliable (Nisio, van Es, & Butler, 2017).*

● Have the client cough and deep breathe or use incentive spirometry every 2 hours while awake. Bed rest compromises breathing and can lead to atelectasis and pneumonia because of decreased chest expansion, decreased cilia activity, pooling of mucus, and the effects of organ shift (such as the diaphragm and heart and pressure on the esophagus when in the supine position) and leads to partial or complete atelectasis usually of the left lower lobe (Parry & Puthucheary, 2015).

● Monitor respiratory functions, noting breath sounds, work of breathing, and respiratory rate. Percuss for new onset of dullness in lungs.

● Note bowel function daily. Provide fluids, fiber, and natural laxatives such as prune juice as needed. Constipation is common in immobilized clients because of decreased activity and reduced fluid and food intake. Refer to care plan for **Constipation.**

● Increase fluid intake to 2000 mL/day within the client's cardiac and renal reserve. Adequate fluids help prevent kidney stones and constipation, both of which are associated with bed rest.

● Encourage intake of a balanced diet with adequate amounts of fiber and protein. Consider recommending Practical Interventions to Achieve Therapeutic Lifestyle Changes (TLC), which includes monounsaturated and polyunsaturated fats, oils, margarines, beans, peas, lentils, soy, skinless poultry, lean fish, trimmed cuts of meat, fat-free and low-fat daily foods, omega-3 polyunsaturated fat sources, and whole grains, including soluble fiber sources such as oats, oat bran, and barley (Osborn et al, 2013).

Critical Care

▲ Recognize that the client who has been in an intensive care environment may develop a neuromuscular dysfunction acquired in the absence of causative factors other than the underlying critical illness and its treatment, resulting in intensive care unit-acquired weakness, with an approximate incidence of 40% requiring more than 1 week of mechanical ventilation (Appleton, Kinsella, & Quasim, 2015). The client may need a workup to determine the cause before satisfactory ambulation can begin. *Critical care clients can develop neuromuscular weakness, polyneuropathy, and delirium (Appleton, Kinsella, & Quasim, 2015; Wintermann et al, 2015).*

▲ Consider the use of a continuous lateral rotation therapy bed. EB: *A systematic review demonstrated limited evidence on the effects of routine lateral repositioning for critically ill patients, although mostly because of poor quality studies (Hewitt, Bucknall, & Faraone, 2016).*

▲ For the stable client in the intensive care unit, consider mobilizing the client in a four-phase method from dangling at the side of the bed to walking if there is sufficient knowledgeable staff available to protect the client from harm. Even intensive care unit clients receiving mechanical ventilation can be mobilized safely if a multidisciplinary team is present to support, protect, and monitor the client for intolerance to activity (Kalisch, Lee, & Dabney, 2013; Boynton et al, 2014; Agency for Healthcare Research and Quality, 2017). EBN: *Critical care clients are at high risk for complications related to immobility such as ventilator-associated pneumonia (VAP), atelectasis, and long-lasting functional limitations. Early mobility has been associated with reduced length of stay and reduced cognitive and physical impairment; therefore once the*

● = Independent;   ▲ = Collaborative;   EBN = Evidence-Based Nursing;   EB = Evidence-Based

client is hemodynamically stable, use progressive mobilization to dangle legs, sit in a chair, stand and bear weight, and walk (Engel et al, 2013; Makic, 2014; Wahab et al, 2016).

Geriatric

- Get the client out of bed as early as possible and ambulate frequently after consultation with the health care provider. *Immobility is a risk factor for VTE; early ambulation can help prevent clot formation (AACP, 2016; Makic, 2014). Functional decline from hospital-associated deconditioning is common in older adults, particularly because they are already more deconditioned and less fit, and early rehabilitation can be effective in preventing this condition in addition to other comorbidities (Menezes et al, 2014; Wood et al, 2014).*
- Consider physical and occupational therapy referrals to guide with environmental safety assessment and home exercise program.
- Monitor nutrition status in the elderly to prevent malnutrition. EB: *Malnutrition related to chronic disease is associated with poor rehabilitation outcomes in hospital-associated deconditioning, and most elderly hospitalized patients with deconditioning are malnourished (Wakabayashi & Sashika, 2014).*
- Monitor for signs of depression: flat affect, poor appetite, insomnia, and many somatic complaints. *Depression can commonly accompany decreased mobility and function in older adults, and mobilization has a positive effect on depressive mood and enhances independence (Kalisch et al, 2013).*
- Keep careful track of bowel function in older adults; do not allow the client to become constipated. *Older adults can easily develop impactions as a result of immobility. Refer to* **Constipation** *care plan.*

Home Care

- Some of the previous interventions may be adapted for home care use.
- ▲ Begin discharge planning at time of admission with case manager or social worker and input from physical and occupational therapy as appropriate to assess need for home support systems and community or home health services.
- ▲ Become oriented to all programs of care for the client before discharge from institutional care.
- ▲ Confirm the immediate availability of all necessary assistive devices for home.
- Perform complete physical assessment and recent history at initial home visit.
- ▲ Refer to physical and occupational therapies for immediate evaluations of the client's potential for independence and functioning in the home setting and for follow-up care.
- Allow the client to have as much input and control of the plan of care as possible. Client perception of control increases self-esteem and motivation to follow medical plan of care.
- Assess knowledge of all care with caregivers. Review as necessary. Having the necessary knowledge and skills to perform care decreases caregiver role strain and supports safety of the client.
- ▲ Support the family of the client in the assumption of caregiver activities. Refer for home health aide services for assistance and respite as appropriate. Refer to medical social services as appropriate.
- ▲ Institute case management of frail elderly to support continued independent living, if possible in the home environment.

Client/Family Teaching and Discharge Planning

- Teach client/family how to perform range-of-motion exercises in bed if not contraindicated; this is referred to as a home exercise program.
- Teach the family how to turn and position the client and provide all care necessary.

Note: Nursing diagnoses that are commonly relevant when the client is on bed rest include **Constipation,** risk for Impaired **Skin** integrity, Disturbed **Sleep** pattern, **Frail Elderly** syndrome, and **Powerlessness.**

REFERENCES

Agency for Healthcare Research and Quality. (2017). *Early mobility guide for reducing ventilator-associated events in mechanically ventilated patients.* Retrieved from https://www.ahrq.gov/sites/default/files/wysiwyg/professionals/quality-patient-safety/hais/tools/mvp/modules/technical/early-mobility-mvpguide.pdf. (Accessed 7 February 2018).

American Association of Chest Physicians (AACP). (2016). *The antithrombotic therapy and prevention of thrombosis, ed 9: American College of Chest Physicians evidence-based clinical practice guidelines.*

Retrieved from http://www.chestnet.org/accp/guidelines/accp-antithrombotic-guidelines-9th-ed-now-available.

Appleton, R., Kinsella, J., & Quasim, T. (2015). The incidence of intensive care unit-acquired weakness syndromes: A systematic review. *Journal of the Intensive Care Society, 16*(2), 126–136.

Arabi, Y. M., Khedr, M., Dara, S. I., et al. (2013). Use of intermittent pneumatic compression and not graduated compression stockings is associated with lower incident VTE in critically ill patients: A

● = Independent;   ▲ = Collaborative;   EBN = Evidence-Based Nursing;   EB = Evidence-Based

D

D

multiple propensity scores adjusted analysis. *CHEST Journal*, *144*(1), 152–159.

Atherton, P. J., Greenhaff, P. L., Phillips, S. M., et al. (2016). Control of skeletal muscle atrophy in response to disuse: Clinical/preclinical contentions and fallacies of evidence. *Am J Pysiolo Endocrinol Metab*, *311*(3), e594–e604. doi:10.1152/ajpendo.00257.2016.

Boynton, T., Kelly, L., Perez, A., et al. (2014). Banner mobility assessment tool for nurses: Instrument validation. *American Journal of Safe Patient Handling & Mobility*, *493*, 86–92.

CDC (2017). *Measuring orthostatic blood pressure*. Retrieved from https://www.cdc.gov/steadi/pdf/measuring_orthostatic_blood _pressure-a.pdf. (Accessed 7 February 2018).

Emergency Nurses Association (2015). *Clinical practice guideline: Orthostatic vital signs*. Retrieved from https://www.ena.org/docs/ default-source/resource-library/practice-resources/cpg/ orthostaticvitalsignscpg.pdf?sfvrsn=c73c24a6_8. (Accessed 7 February 2018).

Engel, H. J., Needham, D. M., Morris, P. E., et al. (2013). ICU early mobilization: From recommendations to implementation at three medical centers. *Critical Care Medicine*, *41*(9), S69–S80.

Gillespie, B. M., Chaboyer, W. P., McInnes, E., et al. (2014). Repositioning for pressure ulcer prevention in adults. *The Cochrane Database of Systematic Reviews*, (4), CD009958. doi:10.1002/ 14651858.CD009958.pub2.

Graham, J. E., Granger, C. V., Karmarkar, A. M., et al. (2014). The Uniform Data System for Medical Rehabilitation: Report of follow-up information on patients discharged from inpatient rehabilitation programs in 2002–2010. *American Journal of Physical Medicine & Rehabilitation*, *93*(3), 231–244.

Granger, C. (2015). *Quality and outcome measure for rehabilitation programs. Medscape*. Retrieved from https://emedicine.medscape .com/article/317865-overview#a2. (Accessed 7 February 2018).

Harvey, L. A., Katalinic, O. M., Herbert, R. D., et al. (2017). Stretch for the treatment and prevention of contracture: An abridged republication of a Cochrane Systematic Review. *Journal of Physiotherapy*, *63*, 67–75.

Hewitt, N., Bucknall, T., & Faraone, N. M. (2016). Lateral positioning for critically ill adult patients. *The Cochrane Database of Systematic Reviews*, (5), CD007205. doi:10.1002/14651858.CD007205.pub2.

Kalisch, B. J., Lee, S., & Dabney, B. W. (2013). Outcomes of inpatient mobilization: A literature review. *Journal of Clinical Nursing*, *23*, 1486–1501.

Lee, S. J., & Lee, J. H. (2017). Safe patient handling behaviors and lift use among hospital nurses: A cross-sectional study. *International Journal of Nursing Studies*, *74*, 53–60.

Logan, A., Marsden, J., Freeman, J., et al. (2017). Effectiveness of non-pharmacological interventions in treating orthostatic hypotension in the elderly and people with a neurological

condition: A systematic review. *JBI Database of Systematic Reviews and Implementation Reports*, *15*(4), 948–960.

Makic, M. B. F. (2014). Preventing postsurgical venous thromboembolism. *Journal of Perianesthesia Nursing*, *29*(4), 317–319.

McInnes, E., Jammali-Blasi, A., Bell-Syer, S., et al. (2015). Support surfaces for pressure ulcer prevention. *Cochrane Database of Systematic Reviews*, (9), CD001735.

Menezes, A. R., Lavie, C. J., Forman, D. E., et al. (2014). Cardiac rehabilitation in the elderly. *Progress in Cardiovascular Disease*, *57*(2), 152–159.

National Pressure Ulcer Advisory Panel. (2014). *Prevention and treatment of pressure ulcers: Quick reference guide*. Retrieved from http://www.npuap.org/wp-content/uploads/2014/08/Updated-10-1 6-14-Quick-Reference-Guide-DIGITAL-NPUAP-EPUAP-PPPIA-1 6Oct2014.pdf. (Accessed 7 February 2018).

Nisio, M. D., van Es, N., & Buller, H. R. (2017). Deep vein thrombosis and pulmonary embolism. *The Lancet*, *388*(10063), 3060–3073.

Osborn, K. S., Wraa, C. E., Watson, A. S., et al. (2013). *Nutrition. Medical-surgical nursing, preparation for practice* (2nd ed.). Upper Saddle River, NJ: Pearson.

Parry, S. M., & Puthucheary, Z. A. (2015). The impact of extended bed rest on the musculoskeletal system in the critical care environment. *Extreme Physiol Med*, *4*, 16. doi:10.1186/s13728-015-0036-7.

Perme, C., Nawa, R. K., Winkelman, C., et al. (2014). A tool to assess mobility status in critically ill patients: The Perme Intensive Care Unit Mobility Score. *Methodist DeBakey Cardiovascular Journal*, *10*(1), 41–49.

Prabhu, R., Swaminathan, N., & Harvey, L. A. (2013). Passive movements for the treatment and prevention of contractures. *Cochrane Database of Systematic Reviews*, (12), CD009331.

Tipping, C. J., Harrold, M., Holland, A., et al. (2017). The effects of active mobilization and rehabilitation in ICU on mortality and function: A systematic review. *Intensive Care Medicine*, *43*(2), 171–183.

Wahab, R., Yip, N. H., Chandra, S., et al. (2016). The implementation of an early rehabilitation program is associated with reduced length of stay: A multi-ICU study. *Journal of Intensive Care Society*, *17*(1), 2–11.

Wakabayashi, H., & Sashika, H. (2014). Malnutrition is associated with poor rehabilitation outcome in elderly inpatients with hospital-associated deconditioning: A prospective cohort study. *Journal of Rehabilitation Medicine*, *46*, 277–282.

Wintermann, G. B., Brunkhorst, F. M., Petrowski, K., et al. (2015). Stress disorders following prolonged critical illness survivors of severe sepsis. *Critical Care Medicine*, *43*(6), 1213–1222.

Wood, W., Tschannen, D., Trotsky, A., et al. (2014). A mobility program for an inpatient acute care medical unit. *The American Journal of Nursing*, *14*(10), 34–40.

Decreased Diversional activity engagement   *Nadia Charania, PhD, RN*

NANDA-I

Definition

Reduceded stimulation, interest, or participation in recreational or leisure activities.

Defining Characteristics

Alteration in mood; boredom; discontent with situation; flat affect; frequent naps; physical deconditioning

● = Independent;   ▲ = Collaborative;   EBN = Evidence-Based Nursing;   EB = Evidence-Based

Related Factors

Current setting does not allow engagement in activity; impaired mobility; environmental barrier; insufficient energy; insufficient motivation; physical discomfort; insufficient diversional activity

At-Risk Population

Extremes of age; prolonged hospitalization; prolonged institutionalization

Associated Condition

Prescribed immobility; psychological stress; therapeutic isolation

NOC (Nursing Outcomes Classification)

Suggested NOC Outcomes

Leisure Participation; Play Participation; Social Involvement

> **Example NOC Outcome with Indicators**
>
> **Leisure Participation** as evidenced by the following indicators: Expresses satisfaction with leisure activities/Feels relaxed from leisure activities/Enjoys leisure activities. (Rate the outcome and indicators of **Leisure Participation:** 1 = never demonstrated, 2 = rarely demonstrated, 3 = sometimes demonstrated, 4 = often demonstrated, 5 = consistently demonstrated [see Section I].)

Client Outcomes

Client Will (Specify Time Frame)

- Engage in personally satisfying diversional activities

NIC (Nursing Interventions Classification)

Suggested NIC Interventions

Recreation Therapy; Self-Responsibility Facilitation

> **Example NIC Activities—Recreation Therapy**
>
> Assist the client to identify meaningful recreational activities; Provide safe recreational equipment

Nursing Interventions and *Rationales*

- Observe ability to engage in activities that require good vision and use of hands. *Diversional activities must be tailored to the client's capabilities.*
- Discuss activities with clients that are interesting and feasible in the present environment.
- Encourage the client to share feelings about situation of inactivity. *Work and hobbies provide structure and continuity to life; the client may feel a sense of loss.*
- Encourage the client to participate in any available social or recreational opportunities in the health care environment. EB: *Social engagement is associated with self-reported physical health in older adults (Cherry et al, 2013).*
- Encourage a mix of physical and mental activities if possible (e.g., crafts, crossword puzzles).
- Provide videos and/or DVDs of movies for recreation and distraction.
- Provide magazines and books of interest.
- Provide books on CD and CD player, and electronic versions of books for listening or reading as available.
- Set up a puzzle in a community space, or provide individual puzzles as desired.
- Provide access to a portable computer so that the client can access email and the Internet. Give client a list of interesting websites, including games and directions on how to perform Web searches if needed.
- Encourage the client to schedule visitors so that they are not all present at once or at inconvenient times. *A schedule prevents the client from becoming exhausted from frequent company.*
- ▲ Request recreational or art therapist to assist with activities. EB: *Art therapy can assist individuals undergoing stroke rehabilitation to reduce anxiety and feelings of isolation (Ali et al, 2014).*

● = Independent;   ▲ = Collaborative;   EBN = Evidence-Based Nursing;   EB = Evidence-Based

▲ Refer to occupational therapy. **EB:** *Occupational therapists are professionals with expertise in the use of activities as therapeutic instruments (Potasz et al, 2014).*

● Provide a change in scenery; get the client out of the room as much as possible. *A lack of sensory stimulation has significant adverse effects on clients.*

● Help the client to experience nature through looking at a nature scene from a window, or walking through a garden if possible. **EB:** *Physical activity in the natural environment can promote emotional well-being (Pasanen, Tyrväinen, & Korpela, 2014).*

● Structure the environment as needed to promote optimal comfort and sensory diversity (e.g., have family bring in posters, banners, or photos; change lighting; change arrangement of furniture). **CEBN:** *For hospitalized clients needing close observation, consider the use of a S.A.F.E. unit that uses trained "diversional partners" rather than sitters; diversional activities were promoted through the use of TVs and VCRs on rolling carts, radios and CD players with music from various genres, movies, rocking chairs, a storage cabinet stocked with games and art supplies, stuffed animals, soft balls, and towels for folding (Nadler-Moodie et al, 2009).*

● Work with family or music therapist to provide music that is enjoyable to the client. **EB:** *Hospitalized patients who received an individualized music therapy session and who were provided with a CD for listening demonstrated marginally better quality of life pain scores after hospitalization and were more likely to recommend the hospital to others (Mandel, Davis, & Secic, 2014).*

● Use art making and music listening. **EBN:** *A randomized trial did not show a significant difference among the control, art making, and diversional music groups in reducing symptoms related to blood and marrow transplantation. It was asserted that art making and music listening are safe and desirable diversional activities for clients undergoing blood and marrow transplant in an outpatient clinic (Lawson et al, 2016).*

● Structure the client's schedule around personal wishes for time of care, relaxation, and participation in fun activities. *Increased client control fosters increased client self-esteem.*

● Spend time with the client when possible, giving the client full attention and being present in the moment, or arrange for a friendly visitor.

● Be creative, for example, use of the activity pillowcases with soft fabric pieces, plastic zipper, and a pouch to hold a picture as a diversional intervention that could be used in inpatient and hospice care settings. **EBN:** *Considered to be helpful aid for adult clients who have intellectual and developmental disabilities and are in need of distraction and sensory input or modulation (Bahle et al, 2016).*

● Engage clients in physical activity or exercise programs as an adjunct treatment modality for a variety of mental illnesses; for example, depression, schizophrenia, anxiety, disorders, posttraumatic stress disorders, and substance abuse. **EB:** *The narrative synthesis of systematic reviews and clinical trials endorsed the integration of physical activity programs as part of the mental health treatment plan (Rosenbaum et al, 2016).*

 Pediatric

▲ Request an order for a child life specialist or, if not available, a play therapist for children. Child life therapists provide opportunities for self-expression and play for hospitalized children and may help to normalize the environment.

● Engage preschool children in play therapy. **EBN:** *The result of a prospective randomized controlled study supported the role of play therapy among preschoolers in promoting their social, emotional, and behavioral skills. Moreover, play therapy might be beneficial in reducing fear and anxiety and promoting communication, coping skills, and self-esteem (Sezici, Ocakci, & Kadioglu, 2017).*

● Engage school-age children in play activities during hospitalization. **EB:** *A randomized control trial results indicated a decrease in cortisol levels after children engaged in play activities (Potasz et al, 2014).*

● Promote a referral to a music therapist. **EBN:** *Music therapy may lead to a decrease in self-reported pain and anxiety in hospitalized children, and it may lead to improved patient and family satisfaction (Colwell et al, 2013).*

● Consider art therapy for children living with chronic illness who have activity restrictions. **CEB:** *In a study of children with persistent asthma, those who engaged in art therapy demonstrated a reduction in anxiety and an improvement in emotional health (Beebe, Gelfand, & Bender, 2010).*

● Provide opportunities for children to connect with family and friends through technology. **EBN:** *Children desire to feel connected to the world outside the hospital environment; technology can reduce isolation as well as support educational needs (Lambert et al, 2014).*

● Provide animal-assisted therapy for hospitalized children. **CEBN:** *Animal-assisted therapy produces a number of therapeutic benefits for hospitalized children, including a reduction in pain (Braun et al, 2009).*

● = Independent;   ▲ = Collaborative;   **EBN** = Evidence-Based Nursing;   **EB** = Evidence-Based

- Provide computer games and virtual reality experiences for children, which can be used as distraction techniques during venipuncture, wound care, or other procedures. **EBN:** *Actively engaging children in serious gaming resulted in lower observed behavioral pain scores and distress for children undergoing wound dressing changes (Nilsson et al, 2013).*

Geriatric

- Assess the interests of older adults and the types of activities that they enjoy; encourage creative expression such as storytelling, drama, dance, art, writing, or music. **EB:** *Art therapy was shown to be effective in reducing anxiety and negative emotions, and improving self-esteem in a group of Korean American older adults (Kim, 2013). Participating in music making with others may improve quality of life, well-being, and physical and mental health in older adults (Creech et al, 2013).*
- If the client is able, arrange for him or her to attend group senior citizen activities. **EB:** *Social connectedness may assist with older adults' perception that they are aging well (Hodge et al, 2013).*
- Promote activity for older adults through the use of exergames (video games combined with exercise). **EB:** *A pilot study demonstrated that Wii interactive videogaming is feasible for use with older adults with mild cognitive impairment. Participants enjoyed physical, mental, and social stimulation from the intervention (Hughes et al, 2014).*
- Encourage involvement in dance. **EB:** *Active participation in dance may enhance healthy aging (Noice, Noice, & Kramer, 2013).*
- Encourage clients to use their ability to help others by volunteering. **EB:** *Volunteering is associated with better self-reported health, fewer functional limitations, reduced depressive symptoms, and lower mortality (Anderson et al, 2014).*
- Provide an environment that promotes activity (e.g., one that has adequate lighting for crafts, large-print books, and adequate acoustics).
- Provide opportunities for storytelling and life review. **EBN:** *Reflection on one's life assists individuals to discover meaning and purpose. A pilot study demonstrated a significant reduction in depressive symptoms after the creation of life story books (Chan et al, 2014).*
- For clients who love gardening but who may have difficulty being outside, bring in seeds, soil, and pots for indoor gardening experiences. Use seeds such as sunflower, pumpkin, and zinnia that grow rapidly. **EB:** *Gardening may foster socialization, fitness, flexibility, cognitive ability, health, and quality of life (Wang & Macmillan, 2013).*
- For hospitalized clients with cognitive impairment, engage the assistance of volunteers to provide diversional activities. **EBN:** *A small pilot study demonstrated that patients, caregivers, staff, and volunteers were satisfied with a volunteer program that engaged hospitalized patients in a variety of activities during hospitalization (Shee, Phillips, & Hill, 2014).*
- For clients in assisted-living facilities, provide leisure educational programs and pleasant dining experiences. **EB:** *Opportunities for social engagement lead to psychological benefits for older adults in assisted living (Jang et al, 2014).*
- For clients who are interested in reading and writing, promote book or writing groups or journaling, and creative or expressive writing. **EB:** *Participation in reading and writing activities positively influenced quality of life in a group of older adults (Sampaio & Ito, 2013).*
- Prescribe activities to engage passive dementia clients based on their former interests and hobbies. **EB:** *Residents of long-term care facilities who have dementia spend the majority of their time engaged in no activity at all, and inactivity has been linked to agitated behavior; stimuli such as looking at and sorting pictures, arranging flowers, folding towels, making puzzles, planting seeds, screwing nuts and bolts together, and listening to and singing along with favorite music led to positive affect and a decrease in agitated behavior (Van der Ploeg et al, 2013).*
- Initiate opportunities for creative expression such as a TimeSlips storytelling group or Memories in the Making project to foster meaningful activities for clients with dementia. **EB:** *A creative storytelling program for clients with dementia, TimeSlips, resulted in increased creativity, quality of life, and involvement in meaningful activity, and positively altered resident behavior while allowing staff to develop a deeper understanding of residents (George & Singer, 2011).*

Home Care

- Many of the previously listed interventions may be administered in the home setting.
- Explore with the client previous interests; consider related activities that are within the client's capabilities.

● = Independent;   ▲ = Collaborative;   **EBN** = Evidence-Based Nursing;   **EB** = Evidence-Based

- ▲ Assess the client for depression. Refer for mental health services as indicated. EB: *Lack of interest in previously enjoyed activities is part of the syndrome of depression (American Psychiatric Association, 2013).*
- ● Assess the family's ability to respond to the client's psychosocial needs for stimulation. Assist as able.
- ▲ Refer to occupational therapy. EB: *Clients with low vision who received adequate training in the use of low vision devices tailored to individual goals were able to improve independence at home (Liu et al, 2013).*
- ● Introduce (or continue) friendly volunteer visitors if the client is willing and able to have the company. If transportation is an issue or if the client does not want visitors in the home, consider alternatives (e.g., telephone contacts, computer messaging).
- ● If the client is approaching the end of life, and is interested, assist in making a videotape, audiotape, or memory book for family members with treasured stories, memoirs, pictures, and video clips. CEB: *Leaving a legacy entails passing on the essence of one's self; passing on values and beliefs is important to older adults (Hunter, 2007–2008).*

 Client/Family Teaching and Discharge Planning

- ● Work with the client and family on learning diversional activities in which the client is interested (e.g., knitting, hooking rugs, writing memoirs).
- ● If the client is in isolation, give the client complete information on why isolation is needed and how it should be accomplished, especially guidelines for visitors; provide diversional activities and encourage visitation. EBN: *Children in isolation feel lonely and bored; access to play, social connections, and education may be helpful (Austin, Prieto, & Rushforth, 2013).*

REFERENCES

Ali, K., Gammidge, T., & Waller, D. (2014). Fight like a ferret: A novel approach of using art therapy to reduce anxiety in stroke patients undergoing a hospital rehabilitation. *Medical Humanities, 40*(1), 56–60.

American Psychiatric Association. (2013). *Diagnostic and statistical manual of mental disorders* (5th ed.). Washington, DC: American Psychiatric Association.

Anderson, N. D., Damianakis, T., Kröger, E., et al. (2014). The benefits associated with volunteering among seniors: A critical review and recommendations for future research. *Psychological Bulletin, 140*(6), 1505–1533.

Austin, D., Prieto, J., & Rushforth, H. (2013). The child's experience of single room isolation: A literature review. *Nursing Children and Young People, 25*(3), 18–24.

Bahle, J., Ludwick, R., Govazzi, G., et al. (2016). Beyond folding washcloths: An innovation for diversional activity. *The American Nurse, 48*(6), 10.

Beebe, A., Gelfand, E. W., & Bender, B. (2010). A randomized trial to test the effectiveness of art therapy for children with asthma. *Journal of Allergy and Clinical Immunology, 126*(2), 263–266.

Braun, C., Stangler, T., Narveson, J., et al. (2009). Animal-assisted therapy as a pain relief intervention for children. *Complementary Therapies in Clinical Practice, 15*(2), 105–109.

Chan, M. F., Leong, K. S., Heng, B. L., et al. (2014). Reducing depression among community-dwelling older adults using life-story review: A pilot study. *Geriatric Nursing, 35*(2), 105–110.

Cherry, K. E., Walker, E. J., Brown, J. S., et al. (2013). Social engagement and health in younger, older, and oldest-old adults in the Louisiana healthy aging study. *Journal of Applied Gerontology, 32*(1), 51–75.

Colwell, C. M., Edwards, R., Hernandez, E., et al. (2013). Impact of music therapy interventions (listening, composition, Orff-based) on the physiological and psychosocial behaviors of hospitalized children: A feasibility study. *Journal of Pediatric Nursing, 28*(3), 249–257.

Creech, A., Hallam, S., Varvarigou, M., et al. (2013). Active music-making: A route to enhanced subjective well-being among older people. *Perspectives in Public Health, 133*(1), 36–43.

George, D. R., & Singer, M. E. (2011). Intergenerational volunteering and quality of life for persons with mild to moderate dementia: Results from a 5-month intervention study in the United States. *American Journal of Geriatric Psychiatry, 19*(4), 392–396.

Hodge, A. M., English, D. R., Giles, G. G., et al. (2013). Social connectedness and predictors of successful ageing. *Maturitas, 75*(4), 361–366.

Hughes, T. F., Flatt, J. D., Fu, B., et al. (2014). Interactive video gaming compared with health education in older adults with mild cognitive impairment: A feasibility study. *International Journal of Geriatric Psychiatry, 29*(9), 890–898.

Hunter, E. G. (2007-2008). Beyond death: Inheriting the past and giving to the future, transmitting the legacy of one's self. *Omega, 56*(4), 313–329.

Jang, Y., Park, N. S., Dominquez, D. D., et al. (2014). Social engagement in older residents of assisted living facilities. *Aging and Mental Health, 18*(5), 642–647.

Kim, S. K. (2013). A randomized, controlled study of the effects of art therapy on older Korean-Americans' healthy aging. *The Arts in Psychotherapy, 40*(1), 158–164.

Lambert, V., Coad, J., Hicks, P., et al. (2014). Social spaces for young children in hospital. *Child: Care, Health & Development, 40*(2), 195–204.

Lawson, L. M., Glennon, C., Fiscus, V., et al. (2016). Effects of making art and listening to music on symptoms related to blood and marrow transplantation. *Oncology Nursing Forum, 43*(2), E56–E63.

Liu, C. J., Brost, M. A., Horton, V. E., et al. (2013). Occupational therapy interventions to improve performance of daily activities at home for older adults with low vision: A systematic review. *American Journal of Occupational Therapy, 67*(3), 279–287.

Mandel, S., Davis, B. A., & Secic, M. (2014). Effects of music therapy on patient satisfaction and health-related quality of life of hospital inpatients. *Hospital Topics, 92*(2), 28–35.

Nadler-Moodie, M., Burnell, L., Fries, J., et al. (2009). A S.A.F.E. alternative to sitters. *Nursing Management, 40*(8), 43–50.

● = Independent;   ▲ = Collaborative;   EBN = Evidence-Based Nursing;   EB = Evidence-Based

Nilsson, S., Enskär, K., Hallqvist, C., et al. (2013). Active and passive distraction in children undergoing wound dressings. *Journal of Pediatric Nursing, 28*(2), 158–166.

Noice, T., Noice, H., & Kramer, A. F. (2013). Participatory arts for older adults: A review of benefits and challenges. *The Gerontologist, 54*(5), 741–753.

Pasanen, T. P., Tyrväinen, L., & Korpela, K. M. (2014). The relationship between perceived health and physical activity indoors, outdoors in built environments, and outdoors in nature. *Applied Psychology: Health and Well Being, 6*(3), 324–346.

Potasz, C., Vilela De Varela, M. J., Coin De Carvalho, L., et al. (2014). Effect of play activities on hospitalized children's stress: A randomized clinical trial. *Scandinavian Journal of Occupational Therapy, 20*(1), 71–79.

Rosenbaum, S., Tiedemann, A., Stanton, R., et al. (2016). Implementing evidence-based physical activity interventions for people with mental illness: An Australian perspective. *Australian Psychiatry, 24*(1), 49–54.

Sampaio, P. Y., & Ito, E. (2013). Activities with higher influence on quality of life in older adults in Japan. *Occupational Therapy International, 20*(1), 1–10.

Sezici, E., Ocakci, A. F., & Kadioglu, K. (2017). Use of play therapy in nursing process: A prospective randomized controlled study. *Journal of Nursing Scholarship, 49*(2), 162–169.

Shee, A. W., Bev Phillips, K., & Hill, K. D. (2014). Feasibility and acceptability of a volunteer-mediated diversional therapy program for older patients with cognitive impairment. *Geriatric Nursing, 35*(5), 300–305.

Van Den Berg, A. E., & Custers, M. H. (2011). Gardening promotes neuroendocrine and affective restoration from stress. *Journal of Health Psychology, 16*(1), 3–11.

Van Der Ploeg, E., Eppingstall, B., Camp, C. J., et al. (2013). A randomized crossover trial to study the effect of personalized, one-to-one interaction using Montessori-based activities on agitation, affect, and engagement in nursing home residents with dementia. *International Psychogeriatrics, 25*(4), 565–575.

Wang, D., & Macmillan, T. (2013). The benefits of gardening for older adults: A systematic review of the literature. *Activities, Adaptation & Aging, 37*(2), 153–181.

E

Ineffective adolescent Eating dynamics   *Marina Martinez-Kratz, MS, RN, CNE*

NANDA-I

Definition

Altered eating attitudes and behaviors resulting in over or under eating patterns that compromise nutritional health.

Defining Characteristics

Avoids participation in regular mealtimes; complains of hunger between meals, food refusal, frequent snacking; frequently eating from fast food restaurants; frequently eating poor quality food; frequently eating processed food; overeating; poor appetite; undereating

Related Factors

Altered family dynamics; anxiety; changes to self-esteem on entering puberty; depression; eating disorder; eating in isolation; excessive family mealtime control; excessive stress; inadequate choice of food; irregular mealtime; media influence on eating behaviors of high caloric unhealthy foods; media influence on knowledge of high caloric unhealthy foods; negative parental influences on eating behaviors; psychological abuse; psychological neglect; stressful mealtimes

Associated Condition

Physical challenge with eating; physical challenge with feeding; physical health issue of parents; psychological health issues of parents

NOC   (Nursing Outcomes Classification)

Suggested NOC Outcomes

Nutritional Status; Nutritional Status: Food and Fluid Intake; Nutrient Intake; Weight Control; Knowledge: Healthy Diet; Knowledge: Weight Management; Eating Disorder Self-Control; Body Image

● = Independent;   ▲ = Collaborative;   EBN = Evidence-Based Nursing;   EB = Evidence-Based

E

Example NOC Outcome with Indicators
Knowledge Healthy Diet as evidenced by the following indicators: Caloric intake appropriate for metabolic needs/ Nutrient intake appropriate for individual needs/Guidelines for food portions/Importance of eating breakfast/Strategies to avoid foods with high caloric value. (Rate the outcome and indicators of **Nutritional Status:** 1 = no knowledge, 2 = limited knowledge, 3 = moderate knowledge, 4 = substantial knowledge, 5 = extensive knowledge [see Section I].)

Client Outcomes

Client Will (Specify Time Frame)

- Maintain weight within normal range for height and age
- Eat breakfast daily
- Participate in meal planning and preparation
- Consume healthy and nutritious foods

NIC (Nursing Interventions Classification)

Suggested NIC Interventions

Nutrition Counseling; Nutrition Monitoring; Family Involvement Promotion; Parenting Promotion

Example NIC Activities—Nutritional Counseling
Establish a therapeutic relationship based on trust and respect; Facilitate identification of eating behaviors to be changed; Discuss the meaning of food to patient

Nursing Interventions and *Rationales*

- Assess for goals and motives related to eating behaviors. EB: *A recent study found that appearance-focused goals and controlled eating regulation were positively related to disordered eating symptoms (Verstuyf et al, 2016).*
- ▲ Assess the adolescent client for comorbid psychological disorders and make appropriate referrals for treatment. EB: *A long-term evolution study's findings suggested a reciprocal relationship between depressive symptoms and unhealthy eating behaviors (Wu et al, 2016). A cross-sectional study found that binge eating was associated with trait anxiety in Korean adolescent girls (Jung et al, 2017).*
- Assess the adolescent for experiences of cyberbullying and the strength of friendship dynamics. EB: *A study found that adolescents who were cyberbullied were almost twice as likely to consider themselves too fat. Stronger friendship dynamics were associated with decreased levels of body dissatisfaction with friendship dynamics partially mediating the relationship between cyberbullying and body dissatisfaction (Kenny et al, 2017).*
- Offer obese or overweight adolescents healthy methods for weight loss. EB: *A recent study showed statistically significant health behavior improvements after implementing a developmentally informed intervention to increase positive health diet and exercise behaviors (Issner et al, 2017).*
- Offer families of obese or overweight children prejudice-free, individually accepting, and supportive interventions to address weight loss. EBN: *Obese children treated with motivational interviewing showed significant improvement in their weight-related behavior and obesity-related anthropometric measures (Wong & Cheng, 2013).*
- Recommend that families eat together for at least one meal per day. EB: *Findings from a review provide clear evidence that family meals (among youth) and shared meals (among adults) are associated with better dietary intake and that these findings transcend the life span (Fulkerson et al, 2014).*
- Recommend involving the adolescents in planning family meals and food preparation. EB: *Results suggested that involving adolescents in food preparation for the family is related to better adolescent dietary quality and eating patterns (Berge et al, 2016).*
- Assist parents at being good role models of healthy eating. EB: *The Healthy Home Offerings via the Mealtime Environment Plus program showed significantly improved parental self-efficacy for identifying appropriate portion sizes (Fulkerson et al, 2018).*
- Recommend that the family try new foods, such as either a new food or recipe every week. EB: *The Healthy Home Offerings via the Mealtime Environment Plus program showed decreasing child neophobia scores over time that were developmentally appropriate (Fulkerson et al, 2018).*

● = Independent;   ▲ = Collaborative;   EBN = Evidence-Based Nursing;   EB = Evidence-Based

- Frame healthy eating as consistent with the adolescent values of autonomy from adult control and the pursuit of social justice. EB: *A study with eighth-graders framed healthy eating as a way to take a stand against manipulative practices of the food industry, such as engineering addictive junk food and marketing to young children. These youth would forgo unhealthy foods for healthier options after associating healthy eating with autonomy-assertive and social justice-oriented behavior (Bryan et al, 2016).*
- Explore the adolescent's friendship dynamics. EB: *Findings from a recent study indicated that adolescent friendships play an integral role in the development of unhealthy weight control and are a useful method to identify adolescents at risk (Simone, Long, & Lockhart, 2018).*

Multicultural

- Assess racial-ethnic minority overweight adolescents for disordered eating behaviors. EB: *A study found that across diverse cultural groups, overweight adolescents are at risk for disordered eating (Rodgers et al, 2017).*
- Assess racial-ethnic minority adolescents for experiences of harassment. EB: *A study found that any type of harassment experienced by racial-ethnic adolescents was significantly associated with poor self-esteem, depressive symptoms, low body satisfaction, substance use, and self-harm behaviors (Bucchianeri et al, 2014).*

Home Care

- The interventions previously described may be adapted for home care use.

Client/Family Teaching and Discharge Planning

▲ Refer the adolescent and family to family treatment-behavior (FT-B) for treatment of eating disorders. EB: *A review found that FT-B is the only well-established treatment for adolescent eating disorders (Lock, 2015).*

▲ Teach the family that hospitalization of the adolescent may be indicated for medical stabilization of serious physical complications and refer as needed. EB: *A study found that inpatient medical stabilization for adolescent eating disorders addresses acute medical complications and also appears to activate the patient and family regarding the need for ongoing treatment (Bravender, Elkus, & Lange, 2017).*

REFERENCES

Berge, J. M., et al. (2016). Family food preparation and its effects on adolescent dietary quality and eating patterns. *Journal of Adolescent Health*, 59(5), 530–536. doi:10.1016/j.jadohealth.2016.06.007.

Bravender, T., Elkus, H., & Lange, H. (2017). Inpatient medical stabilization for adolescents with eating disorders: patient and parent perspectives. *Eating and Weight Disorders—Studies on Anorexia, Bulimia and Obesity*, 22(3), 483–489. doi:10.1007/s40519-016-0270-z.

Bryan, C. J., et al. (2016). Harnessing adolescent values to motivate healthier eating. *Proceedings of the National Academy of Sciences*, 113(39), 10830–10835. doi:10.1073/pnas.1604586113.

Bucchianeri, M. M., et al. (2014). Multiple types of harassment: Associations with emotional well-being and unhealthy behaviors in adolescents. *Journal of Adolescent Health*, 54(6), 724–729. doi:10.1016/j.jadohealth.2013.10.205.

Fulkerson, J. A., et al. (2018). Family home food environment and nutrition-related parent and child personal and behavioral outcomes of the Healthy Home Offerings via the Mealtime Environment (HOME) plus program: A randomized controlled trial. *Journal of the Academy of Nutrition and Dietetics*, 118(2), 240–251. doi:10.1016/j.jand.2017.04.006.

Fulkerson, J. A., et al. (2014). A review of associations between family or shared meal frequency and dietary and weight status outcomes across the lifespan. *Journal of Nutrition Education and Behavior*, 46(1), 2–19. doi:10.1016/j.jneb.2013.07.012.

Issner, J. H., et al. (2017). Increasing positive health behaviors in adolescents with nutritional goals and exercise. *Journal of Child and Family Studies*, 26(2), 548–558. doi:10.1007/s10826-016-0585-4.

Jung, J., et al. (2017). Binge eating is associated with trait anxiety in Korean adolescent girls: a cross sectional study. *BMC Women's Health*, 17(8), 1–7. doi:10.1186/s12905-017-0364-4.

Kenny, U., et al. (2017). The relationship between cyberbullying and friendship dynamics on adolescent body dissatisfaction: A cross-sectional study. *Journal of Health Psychology*, 23(4), 629–639. doi:10.1177/1359105316684939.

Lock, J. (2015). An update on evidence-based psychosocial treatments for eating disorders in children and adolescents. *Journal of Clinical Child & Adolescent Psychology*, 44(5), 707–721. doi:10.1080/15374416.2014.971458.

Rodgers, R. F., et al. (2017). Disordered eating in ethnic minority adolescents with overweight. *International Journal of Eating Disorders*, 50(6), 665–671. doi:10.1002/eat.22652.

Simone, M., Long, E., & Lockhart, G. (2018). The dynamic relationship between unhealthy weight control and adolescent friendships: A social network approach. *Journal of Youth and Adolescence*, 47(7), 1373–1384. doi:10.1007/s10964-017-0796-z.

Verstuyf, J., et al. (2016). Motivational dynamics underlying eating regulation in young and adult female dieters: relationships with healthy eating behaviours and disordered eating symptoms. *Psychology & Health*, 31(6), 711–729. doi:10.1080/08870446.2016.1143942.

Wong, E. M., & Cheng, M. M. (2013). Effects of motivational interviewing to promote weight loss in obese children. *Journal of Clinical Nursing*, 22(17/18), 2519–2530.

Wu, W., et al. (2016). Reciprocal relationship between unhealthy eating behaviours and depressive symptoms from childhood to adolescence: 10-year follow-up of the Child and Adolescent Behaviors in Long-Term Evolution study. *Public Health Nutrition*, 19(9), 1654–1665. doi:10.1017/S1368980015003675.

● = Independent; ▲ = Collaborative; EBN = Evidence-Based Nursing; EB = Evidence-Based

Ineffective child Eating dynamics   *Marina Martinez-Kratz, MS, RN, CNE*

NANDA-I

Definition

Altered attitudes, behaviors, and influences on child eating patterns resulting in compromised nutritional health.

Defining Characteristics

Avoids participation in regular mealtimes; complains of hunger between meals, food refusal, frequent snacking; frequently eating from fast food restaurants; frequently eating poor quality food; frequently eating processed food; overeating; poor appetite; undereating

Related Factors

Eating Habit

Bribing child to eat; consumption of large volumes of food in a short period of time; disordered eating habits; eating in isolation; excessive parental control over child's eating experience; excessive parental control over family mealtime; forcing child to eat; inadequate choice of food; lack of regular mealtimes; limiting child's eating; rewarding child to eat; stressful mealtimes; unpredictable eating patterns; unstructured eating of snacks between meals

Family Process

Abusive relationship; anxious parent–child relationship; disengaged parenting style; hostile parent–child relationship; insecure parent–child relationship; over involved parenting style; tense parent–child relationship; under involved parenting style

Parental

Anorexia; depression; inability to divide eating responsibility between parent and child; inability to divide feeding responsibility between parent and child; inability to support healthy eating patterns; ineffective coping strategies; lack of confidence in child to develop healthy eating habits; lack of confidence in child to grow appropriately; substance misuse

Environmental

Media influence on eating behaviors of high caloric unhealthy foods; media influence on knowledge of high caloric unhealthy foods

At-Risk Population

Economically disadvantaged; homeless; involvement with the foster care system; life transition; parental obesity

Associated Condition

Physical challenge with eating; physical challenge with feeding; physical health issue of parents; psychological health issues of parents

NOC   (Nursing Outcomes Classification)

Suggested NOC Outcomes

Appetite; Parenting Performance; Knowledge: Healthy Diet; Health Beliefs; Nutritional Status

---

Example NOC Outcome with Indicators

Appetite as evidenced by the following indicators: Desire to eat/Food intake/Nutrient intake/Fluid intake/Stimulus to eat. (Rate the outcome and indicators of **Appetite:** 1 = severely compromised, 2 = substantially compromised, 3 = moderately compromised, 4 = mildly compromised, 5 = not compromised [see Section I].)

● = Independent;   ▲ = Collaborative;   EBN = Evidence-Based Nursing;   EB = Evidence-Based

Client Will (Specify Time Frame)

Client Outcomes

- Identify hunger and satiety cues
- Consume healthy and nutritious foods
- Consume adequate calories to support growth and development
- Engage in positive interactions with caregiver during meals

NIC (Nursing Interventions Classification)

Suggested NIC Interventions

Nutrition management; Nutrition Counseling; Nutritional Monitoring

> **Example NIC Activities—Nutritional Counseling**
>
> Establish a therapeutic relationship based on trust and respect; Determine attitudes and beliefs of significant others about food, eating, and the patient's needed nutritional change

Nursing Interventions and *Rationales*

▲ Use a nutritional screening tool designed for nurses such as Subjective Global Nutrition Assessment (SGNA), and refer to a dietician for scores of moderate or severe. **EB:** *A study found that SGNA can be a reliable tool for assessing nutritional status in children (Minocho et al, 2017).*

- Assess parents for food or eating concerns, aberrant feeding behavior, or inappropriate feeding practices. **EB:** *Caregiver concerns about food or child eating warrants additional assessment (Kerzner et al, 2015).*

- Assess child for type of eating difficulty. Children can present with limited appetite, food selectivity, and fear of feeding. **EB:** *Identifying the eating issue will enable appropriate intervention (Kerzner et al, 2015).*

- Assess the caregivers feeding style by asking three questions: How anxious are you about your child's eating? How would you describe what happens during mealtime? What do you do when your child will not eat? **EB:** *Kerzner et al (2015) identify three feeding styles that have negative consequences: neglectful, controlling, and indulgent. Responses from neglectful parents will be vague, and controlling parents will describe pressuring/forcing their child to eat. Indulgent parents will describe pleading, begging, and preparing special foods.*

- Assess the child for persistent picky eating with three questions/answers: Is your child a picky eater? (yes). Does she or he have strong likes with regard to food? (yes). Does your child accept new foods readily? (no). **EB:** *A study found that 3 of 18 feeding behavior questions were significantly associated with persistent picky eaters (Toyama & Agras, 2016). Early identification of picky eating will allow early intervention.*

- Assess child for symptoms of malnutrition including short stature, thin arms and legs, poor condition of skin and hair, visible vertebrae and rib cage, wasted buttocks, wasted facial appearance, lethargy, and in extreme cases, edema.

- Assess weight and height of the child and use a growth chart to help determine growth pattern, which reflects nutrition. Age-related growth charts are available from www.cdc.gov/growthcharts/ (Centers for Disease Control and Prevention, 2016).

- Recommend that families eat together for at least one meal per day. **EB:** *Findings from a review provide unmistakable evidence that family meals (among youth) and shared meals (among adults) are associated with better dietary intake and that these findings transcend the life span (Fulkerson et al, 2014).*

- Encourage parent–child interactions that promote attachment. **EB:** *A study found that insecure attachment was significantly associated with higher body mass index (Maras et al, 2016).*

- Recommend that the child eats an appropriate size breakfast daily. **EB:** *A study of urban children found higher mean body mass index percentiles among children who did not consume any breakfast and those who consumed greater than or equal to three breakfasts daily (Lawman et al, 2014).*

- Recommend involving the family in planning meals and food preparation. Children can learn about nutrition as they help plan and make meals. **EB:** *The Healthy Home Offerings via the Mealtime Environment Plus program showed increased cooking skills among the children participating (Fulkerson et al, 2018).*

● = Independent;   ▲ = Collaborative;   **EBN** = Evidence-Based Nursing;   **EB** = Evidence-Based

E

- Assist parents at being good role models of healthy eating. EB: *The Healthy Home Offerings via the Mealtime Environment Plus program showed significantly improved parental self-efficacy for identifying appropriate portion sizes (Fulkerson et al, 2018).*
- Recommend that the family try new foods, either a new food or recipe every week. EB: *The Healthy Home Offerings via the Mealtime Environment Plus program showed decreasing child neophobia scores over time that were developmentally appropriate (Fulkerson et al, 2018).*
- ▲ Refer children with highly selective food behaviors and sensory food aversion to a nutritional specialist. EB: *Refusal to eat entire categories of foods related to their taste, texture, smell, temperature, and/or appearance can interrupt normal development and have negative health consequences (Kerzner et al, 2015).*
- ▲ Refer children with feeding difficulties caused by a medical condition to the appropriate specialist. EB: *Organic conditions may contribute to feeding difficulties and express as food aversions, fear of feeding, and selective eating (Kerzner et al, 2015).*

 Multicultural

- Assess for the meanings, attitudes, and behaviors related to feeding practices in culturally diverse families. EB: *A qualitative study of Hispanic mothers found feeding attitudes were central to the maternal responsibility of having well-fed children, and feeding practices included the use of coercive/negative reinforcement strategies (Martinez et al, 2015).*
- Assess the feeding styles of Hispanic and African American mothers for congruence with current child feeding recommendations. EB: *A recent study showed that Hispanic and African American mothers seldom spoke to their children about food characteristics, rarely referred to feelings of hunger and fullness, encouraged more eating, and made more attempts to enforce table manners than to teach eating skills (Power et al, 2015).*

 Home Care

- The interventions previously described may be adapted for home care use.

 Client/Family Teaching and Discharge Planning

- Provide parents with the following guidelines: avoid distractions during mealtimes (television, cell phones, etc.), maintain a pleasant neutral attitude throughout meal, feed to encourage appetite, limit meal duration (20–30 minutes), 4 to 6 meals/snacks a day with only water in between, serve age-appropriate foods, systematically introduce new foods (up to 8–15 times), encourage self-feeding, and tolerate age-appropriate mess. EB: *Guidelines will prevent and/or resolve feeding difficulties, whether mild or severe (Kerzner et al, 2015).*
- Teach families to use positive family- and parent-level interpersonal dynamics (i.e., warmth, group enjoyment, parental positive reinforcement) and positive family- and parent-level food-related dynamics (i.e., food warmth, food communication, parental food positive reinforcement) at family meals. EB: *A reduced risk of childhood obesity was significantly associated with positive family- and parent-level interpersonal dynamics and positive family- and parent-level food-related dynamics (Berge et al, 2014).*
- Teach parents to recognize the difference between hunger and satiety in their children. EB: *Parents may misperceive the child's appetite despite normal growth and need encouragement to accept the child's interpretation of their hunger and satiety (Kerzner et al, 2015).*
- Teach parents of children with limited appetites to establish a feeding schedule with a maximum of five meals per day and nothing but water in between. Parents must be taught to model healthy eating, adhere to the established feeding schedule, and set limits/consequences for mealtime behavior. EB: *A feeding schedule will provide adequate nutrition and assist the child with recognizing and responding appropriately to hunger and satiety (Kerzner et al, 2015).*
- Teach parents of children with food selectivity to refrain from coercive and indulgent feeding practices. EB: *Coercive and indulgent feeding practices may create family discord and subsequent child behavioral problems (Kerzner et al, 2015).*
- Teach parents the concept of being a responsive feeder, in which the parent determines where, when, and what the child is fed and the child determines how much to eat. Responsive feeders guide the child's eating, set limits, model appropriate eating, talk positively about food, and respond appropriately to the child's feeding cues. EB: *Research has reported that a responsive feeding style has resulted in children developing a lower risk of being overweight through consumption of more fruits, vegetables, and dairy products and less unhealthy foods (Kerzner et al, 2015).*

● = Independent;   ▲ = Collaborative;   EBN = Evidence-Based Nursing;   EB = Evidence-Based

REFERENCES

Berge, J. M., et al. (2014). Childhood obesity and interpersonal dynamics during family meals. *Pediatrics, 134*(5), 923–932. doi:10.1542/peds.2014-1936.

Centers for Disease Control and Prevention (2016). *National Center for Health Statistics.* Atlanta, GA: Author.

Fulkerson, J. A., et al. (2018). Family home food environment and nutrition-related parent and child personal and behavioral outcomes of the Healthy Home Offerings via the Mealtime Environment (HOME) plus program: A randomized controlled trial. *Journal of the Academy of Nutrition and Dietetics, 118*(2), 240–251. doi:10.1016/j.jand.2017.04.006.

Fulkerson, J. A., et al. (2014). A review of associations between family or shared meal frequency and dietary and weight status outcomes across the lifespan. *Journal of Nutrition Education and Behavior, 46*(1), 2–19. doi:10.1016/j.jneb.2013.07.012.

Kerzner, B., et al. (2015). A practical approach to classifying and managing feeding difficulties. *Pediatrics, 135*(2), 344–353. doi:10.1542/peds.2014-1630.

Lawman, H. G., et al. (2014). Breakfast patterns among low-income, ethnically-diverse 4th–6th grade children in an urban area. *BMC Public Health, 14*(1), 604. doi:10.1186/1471-2458-14-604.

Maras, D., et al. (2016). Attachment style and obesity: Disordered eating behaviors as a mediator in a community sample of Canadian youth. *Journal of Developmental & Behavioral Pediatrics, 37*(9), 762–770. doi:10.1097/DBP.0000000000000361.

Martinez, S. M., et al. (2015). Maternal attitudes and behaviors regarding feeding practices in elementary school–aged Latino children: A pilot qualitative study on the impact of the cultural role of mothers in the US–Mexican border region of San Diego, California. *Journal of the Academy of Nutrition and Dietetics, 115*(5), S34–S41. doi:10.1016/j.jand.2015.02.028.

Minocho, P., et al. (2017). Subjective Global Nutritional Assessment: A reliable screening tool for nutritional assessment in cerebral palsy children. *Indian Journal of Pediatrics, 85*(1), 15–19. doi:10.1007/s12098-017-2501-3.

Power, T. G., et al. (2015). Feeding practices of low-income mothers: how do they compare to current recommendations? *International Journal of Behavioral Nutrition and Physical Activity, 12*(1), 1–11. doi:10.1186/s12966-015-0179-3.

Toyama, H., & Agras, W. S. (2016). A test to identify persistent picky eaters. *Eating Behaviors, 23*, 66–69. doi:10.1016/j.eatbeh.2016.07.003.

Ineffective infant Eating dynamics   *Marina Martinez-Kratz, MS, RN, CNE*

NANDA-I

Definition

Altered parental feeding behaviors resulting in over or under eating patterns.

Defining Characteristics

Food refusal; inappropriate transition to solid foods; overeating; poor appetite; undereating

Related Factors

Abusive relationship; attachment issues; disengaged parenting style; lack of confidence in child to develop healthy eating habits; lack of confidence in child to grow appropriately; lack of knowledge of appropriate methods of feeding infant for each stage of development; lack of knowledge of infant's developmental stages; lack of knowledge of parent's responsibility in infant feeding; media influence on feeding infant high caloric, unhealthy foods; media influence on knowledge of high caloric, unhealthy foods; multiple caregivers; over involved parenting style; under involved parenting style

At-Risk Population

Abandonment; economically disadvantaged; history of unsafe eating and feeding experiences; homeless; involvement with the foster care system; life transition; neonatal intensive care experiences; prematurity; prolonged hospitalization; small for gestational age

Associated Condition

Chromosomal disorders; cleft lip; cleft palate; congenital heart disease; genetic disorder; neural tube defects; physical challenge with eating; physical health issues of parents; prolonged enteral feedings; psychological health issues of parents; sensory integration problems

● = Independent;   ▲ = Collaborative;   **EBN** = Evidence-Based Nursing;   **EB** = Evidence-Based

| NOC | (Nursing Outcomes Classification) |

Suggested NOC Outcomes

Bottle Feeding Establishment: Infant; Bottle Feeding Performance; Breastfeeding Establishment: Infant; Breastfeeding Maintenance; Breastfeeding Weaning; Parenting Performance: Infant; Knowledge: Parenting

Example NOC Outcome with Indicators

Parenting Performance Infant as evidenced by the following indicators: Exhibits a loving relationship/Interacts with infant to promote trust/Provides age-appropriate nutrition/Provides appropriate weaning. (Rate the outcome and indicators of **Nutritional Status:** 1 = never demonstrated, 2 = rarely demonstrated, 3 = sometimes demonstrated, 4 = often demonstrated, 5 = consistently demonstrated [see Section I].)

Client Outcomes

Client Will (Specify Time Frame)

- Infant will consume adequate calories to support growth and development
- Caregiver will follow healthy infant feeding practices
- Caregiver will identify infant behavioral cues related to hunger and satiety
- Caregiver and infant will engage in positive interactions during feeding

| NIC | (Nursing Interventions Classification) |

Suggested NIC Interventions

Infant Care; Bottle Feeding; Teaching: Infant Nutrition

Example NIC Activities—Teaching: Infant Nutrition

Provide parents with written materials appropriate to identified knowledge needs; Instruct parent/caregiver to feed only breast milk or formula for first year (no solids before 4 months)

Nursing Interventions and *Rationales*

- Assess weight and height of the infant and use a growth chart to help determine growth pattern, which reflects nutrition. Age-related growth charts are available from www.cdc.gov/growthcharts/ (Centers for Disease Control and Prevention, 2016).
- Assess mothers for symptoms of postpartum depression. EB: *A study found an association between postpartum depression and poor infant nutritional status (Madeghe et al, 2016).*
- Encourage parent–child interactions that promote attachment. EB: *A study found that insecure attachment was significantly associated with higher body mass index (Maras et al, 2016).*
- Encourage overweight and obese mothers to follow current infant feeding guidelines. EB: *Research indicated that compared with normal weight mothers, overweight/obese mothers were less likely to breastfeed exclusively at infant age 2 months age; they were more likely to breastfeed at low intensity during the first 2 months, and more likely to initiate early introduction of solid foods (Kisantas et al, 2015).*
- Encourage breastfeeding as appropriate. EB: *A study found that adolescents with a history of shorter breastfeeding duration in infancy had poorer satiety response and higher food consumption during an eating in absence of hunger procedure (Reyes et al, 2014).*
- Teach infant caregivers to recognize the following infant communication: infants signal appetite through interest or disinterest in food; infants use rapid and transient facial expressions to signal liking; and they use subtle or potent gestures, body movements, and vocalizations to express wanting. EB: *Research demonstrated the bidirectionality and interdependence of infant communication feeding, with more responsive feeding associated with more proficient communication by the infant (Hetherington, 2017).*
- Provide teaching and resources during pregnancy about recommended infant feeding practices. EB: *The results of a clinical trial testing a prenatal–postpartum individual nutrition/breastfeeding counseling program with follow-up nutrition and parenting support groups showed increased exclusive breastfeeding and reduced complementary foods and liquids in 3-month-old infants (Gross, 2016).*

● = Independent;   ▲ = Collaborative;   EBN = Evidence-Based Nursing;   EB = Evidence-Based

- Provide caregivers of infants with teaching to encourage the early development of healthy eating patterns. EB: *A cross-sectional analysis of 24-hour dietary recall data from the 2008 Feeding Infants and Toddlers Study found that feeding and dietary issues started during infancy continue in toddler and preschool stages (Deming et al, 2014).*
- Provide caregivers of infants with teaching about the strong association between sugar-sweetened beverages, obesity, and related chronic diseases. EB: *A cross-sectional analysis of Special Supplemental Nutrition Program for Women, Infants, and Children (WIC) participants found that compared with nonparticipants, fewer WIC infants were breastfed and consumed any vegetable, but more consumed 100% juice. Fewer WIC toddlers and preschoolers consumed any fruit versus nonparticipants and were more likely to consume sugar-sweetened beverages (Deming et al, 2014).*
- Assist mothers to identify infant engagement and disengagement cues during breastfeeding or formula feeding. EB: *A study found breastfeeding and formula-fed infants exhibited engagement and disengagement during feeding. Supporting a mother's ability to identify engagement and disengagement cues may promote more responsive feeding strategies (Shloim et al, 2017).*
- Provide mothers with unconditional positive regard in their choice of breast, formula, or mixed feeding of their infant. EB: *A study of breastfeeding woman found women experienced feelings of pressure and judgment around their infant feeding decisions (Hunt & Thomson, 2016).*

 ## Multicultural

- Assess for cultural beliefs, values, and practices related to the feeding of infants. EB: *Education and supportive efforts to enhance healthy infant feeding practices should be culturally tailored for success (Fischer & Olson, 2014).*
- Identify the support persons of the infant caregiver and extend healthy infant feeding education and information to those support persons. EB: *A study of first-time African American mothers and breastfeeding indicated that over half of the mothers intended to exclusively breastfeed but were unable to because of life stressors and experiences. An informed support person could promote healthy infant feeding practices (Asiodu et al, 2017).*

 ## Home Care

- The interventions previously described may be adapted for home care use.

 ## Client/Family Teaching and Discharge Planning

- Many of the interventions previously described involve teaching.

REFERENCES

Asiodu, I. V., et al. (2017). Infant feeding decision-making and the influences of social support persons among first-time African American mothers. *Maternal and Child Health Journal, 21*(4), 863–872. doi:10.1007/s10995-016-2167-x.

Centers for Disease Control and Prevention (2016). *National Center for Health Statistics.* Atlanta, GA: Author.

Deming, D. M., et al. (2014). Infant feeding practices and food consumption patterns of children participating in WIC. *Journal of Nutrition Education and Behavior, 46*(3), doi:10.1016/j.jneb .2014.02.020.

Fischer, T. P., & Olson, B. H. (2014). A qualitative study to understand cultural factors affecting a mother's decision to breast or formula feed. *Journal of Human Lactation, 30*(2), 209–216. doi:10.1177/ 0890334413508338.

Gross, R. S., et al. (2016). Randomized controlled trial of a primary care-based child obesity prevention intervention on infant feeding practices. *The Journal of Pediatrics, 174,* 171–177.e2. doi:10.1016/ j.jpeds.2016.03.060.

Hetherington, M. M. (2017). Understanding infant eating behaviour— Lessons learned from observation. *Physiology & Behavior, 176,* 117–124. doi:10.1016/j.physbeh.2017.01.022.

Hunt, L., & Thomson, G. (2016). Pressure and judgement within a dichotomous landscape of infant feeding: A grounded theory study to explore why breastfeeding women do not access peer support provision. *Maternal & Child Nutrition, 13*(2), e12279. doi:10.1111/ mcn.12279.

Kisantas, P., et al. (2015). Nature and nurture in the development of childhood obesity: Early infant feeding practices of overweight/ obese mothers differ compared to mothers of normal body mass index. *The Journal of Maternal-Fetal & Neonatal Medicine, 29*(2), 290–293. doi:10.3109/14767058.2014.999035.

Maras, D., et al. (2016). Attachment style and obesity: Disordered eating behaviors as a mediator in a community sample of Canadian youth. *Journal of Developmental & Behavioral Pediatrics, 37*(9), 762–770. doi:10.1097/DBP.0000000000000361.

Madeghe, B. A., et al. (2016). Postpartum depression and infant feeding practices in a low income urban settlement in Nairobi-Kenya. *BMC Research Notes, 9*(1), 1–9. doi:10.1186/s13104-016-2307-9.

Reyes, M., et al. (2014). Satiety responsiveness and eating behavior among Chilean adolescents and the role of breastfeeding. *International Journal of Obesity, 38*(4), 552–557. doi:10.1038/ ijo.2013.191.

Shloim, N., et al. (2017). Looking for cues—Infant communication of hunger and satiation during milk feeding. *Appetite, 108,* 74–82. doi:10.1016/j.appet.2016.09.020.

• = Independent;   ▲ = Collaborative;   EBN = Evidence-Based Nursing;   EB = Evidence-Based

E

Risk for Electrolyte imbalance   *Susan M. Dirkes, BSN, MSA*

NANDA-I

Definition

Susceptible to changes in serum electrolyte levels, which may compromise health.

Risk Factors

Diarrhea; excessive fluid volume; insufficient fluid volume; insufficient knowledge of modifiable factors; vomiting

Associated Condition

Compromised regulatory mechanism; endocrine regulatory dysfunction; renal dysfunction; treatment regimen

NOC   (Nursing Outcomes Classification)

Suggested NOC Outcomes

Electrolyte and Acid-Base Balance; Fluid Balance; Hydration; Nutritional Status: Biochemical Measures; Nutritional Status: Food and Fluid Intake; Nutritional Status: Nutrient Intake; Kidney Function

Example NOC Outcome with Indicators

Electrolyte and Acid-Base Balance as evidenced by the following indicators: Apical heart rate/Apical heart rhythm/ Serum potassium/Serum sodium/Serum calcium, serum magnesium, serum phosphorus. (Rate the outcome and indicators of **Electrolyte and Acid-Base Balance:** I = severe deviation from normal range, 2 = substantial deviation from normal range, 3 = moderate deviation from normal range, 4 = mild deviation from normal range, 5 = no deviation from normal range [see Section I].)

Client Outcomes

Client Will (Specify Time Frame)

- Maintain a normal sinus heart rhythm with a regular rate
- Have a decrease in edema
- Maintain an absence of muscle cramping
- Maintain normal serum potassium, sodium, calcium, magnesium and phosphorus
- Maintain normal serum pH

NIC   (Nursing Interventions Classification)

Suggested NIC Interventions

Electrolyte Monitoring; Electrolyte Management: Hypokalemia, Hyperkalemia, Hypocalcemia, Hypercalcemia, Hyponatremia, Hypernatremia, Hypomagnesemia, Hypermagnesemia, Hypophosphatemia, and Hyperphosphatemia; Electrolyte Management: Hyponatremia; Fluid/Electrolyte Management; Laboratory Data Interpretation

Example NIC Activities—Electrolyte Monitoring

Identify possible causes of electrolyte imbalances; Monitor the serum level of electrolytes

Nursing Interventions and *Rationales*

▲ Monitor vital signs at least three times a day, or more frequently as needed. Notify health care provider of significant deviation from baseline. *Electrolyte imbalance can lead to clinical manifestations such as respiratory failure, arrhythmias, edema, muscle weakness, and altered mental status (Wagner & Hardin-Pierce, 2014).*

▲ Monitor cardiac rate and rhythm. Report changes to provider. *Hypokalemia and hyperkalemia can result in electrocardiogram (ECG) changes that can lead to cardiac arrest, and ventricular dysrhythmias.* EB:

● = Independent;   ▲ = Collaborative;   EBN = Evidence-Based Nursing;   EB = Evidence-Based

Hypophosphatemia can cause ventricular arrhythmias, derangements of cardiac and respiratory function, and death. It can also cause cardiomyopathy (Ariyoshi et al, 2016; Christopoulou et al, 2017). Magnesium and calcium imbalances also can cause cardiac arrhythmias. Low serum magnesium (≤2 mEq/L) is associated with hypokalemia and ECG changes, and high phosphate may indicate kidney injury (Wagner & Hardin-Pierce, 2014). Low magnesium also may impair respiratory function. It has been associated with higher mortality, the need for mechanical ventilation, and increased length of stay (Upala et al, 2016). Low magnesium also is common in heart failure patients (Gonzales et al, 2013).

- Monitor intake and output and daily weights using a consistent scale. *Weight gain is a sensitive and consistent sign of fluid volume excess (Wagner & Hardin-Pierce, 2014).*
- *Monitor for abdominal distention and discomfort. A focused assessment should be done on any patient presenting with hepatic, gastrointestinal, or pancreatic dysfunction (Wagner & Hardin-Pierce, 2014).* **EB:** *Abdominal distension and intraabdominal swelling can lead to compression of the abdominal contents and acute kidney injury, especially in the postoperative period (Raghavendra et al, 2017).*
- Monitor the client's respiratory status and muscle strength. *Phosphorus is an essential element in cell structure, metabolism, and maintenance of acid-base processes. Consequences of hypophosphatemia include cardiac failure, respiratory failure, and alterations in sensorium (Wagner & Hardin-Pierce, 2014; Diringer, 2017).*
- Assess cardiac status and neurological alterations. **EB:** *Hypophosphatemia can cause myocardial dysfunction, hematological dysfunction, respiratory depression, and neurological changes (Diringer, 2017).*
- *Imbalances of sodium, potassium, calcium, and magnesium all can cause neurological disturbances (Gardner & Gardner, 2014). Hyperphosphatemia is associated with hypocalcemia (because it is inversely related to calcium), causing tetany, muscle spasms, and cardiac arrhythmias, as well as vascular mineralization (Wagner & Hardin-Pierce, 2014; Marcuccilini, Chonchol, & Jovanovich, 2017).*
- ▲ Review laboratory data as ordered and report deviations to provider. *Laboratory studies may include serum electrolytes potassium, chloride, sodium, bicarbonate, magnesium, phosphate, calcium; serum pH; comprehensive metabolic panel; and arterial blood gases.*
- Review the client's medical and surgical history for possible causes of altered electrolytes. *Periods of excess fluid loss can lead to dehydration and resulting loss of electrolytes; fluid can be lost through gastrointestinal illness, renal failure, hyperthermia, blood loss, and perspiration caused by strenuous exercise (Chlibkova et al, 2014; Wagner & Hardin-Pierce, 2014; Hew-Butler et al, 2017). Additional causes of electrolyte imbalances include excessive use of antacids, burns, trauma, sepsis, diabetic ketoacidosis, extensive surgeries, and changes in acid-base balance (Nykamp & Krause, 2013).*
- ▲ Complete pain assessment. Assess and document the onset, intensity, character, location, duration, aggravating factors, and relieving factors. Notify the provider for any increase in pain or discomfort or if comfort measures are not effective. *Symptoms of electrolyte imbalance and dehydration can include muscle cramps, paresthesias, abdominal cramps, skin manifestations, cardiac arrhythmias, and tetany (Wagner & Hardin-Pierce, 2014).*
- ▲ Monitor the effects of ordered medications such as diuretics and heart medications. **EB:** *Medications can have adverse effects on kidney function and electrolyte balance, particularly contrast agents, chemotherapeutic agents, amphotericin B, aminoglycosides, phosphate ingestion, loop diuretics, and vitamin D (Calazza, 2014; Wagner & Hardin-Pierce, 2014).*
- ▲ Administer parenteral fluids as ordered and monitor their effects. *Rapid resuscitation with fluids can cause adverse effects such as electrolyte imbalance, increased bleeding, and coagulopathies (Wang et al, 2014). Administration of fluids should be done to impact the plasma electrolytes and pH and hemodynamic improvement (Vassalos & Rooney, 2013).*

 Geriatric

- Monitor electrolyte levels carefully, including sodium levels and potassium levels, with both increased and decreased levels possible. **EB:** *Older adults are prone to electrolyte abnormalities because of failure of regulatory mechanisms associated with heart and kidney disease, a decrease in the ability to reabsorb sodium, and a loss of diluting capacity in the kidneys (Bolignano, 2014). Dehydration in the elderly is attributable to inadequate water intake caused by dysfunction of the central nervous system controlling thirst. Data also suggest that sodium appetite is reduced in aged rats and therefore also in elderly (Begg, 2017). Many older clients receive selective serotonin reuptake inhibitors for treatment of depression, which can result in hyponatremia (Varela-Piñón & Adán-Manes, 2017).*

E

 Client/Family Teaching and Discharge Planning

- Teach client/family the signs of low potassium and the risk factors. *Signs and symptoms of low potassium include muscle weakness, nausea, vomiting, constipation, and irregular pulse (Wagner & Hardin-Pierce, 2014).*
- Teach client/family the signs of high potassium and the risk factors. *Signs and symptoms of high potassium include restlessness, muscle weakness, slow heart rate, diarrhea, and cramping (Wagner & Hardin-Pierce, 2014).*
- Teach client/family the signs of low sodium and the risk factors. *Early signs of low sodium include nausea, muscle cramps, disorientation, and mental status changes (Wagner & Hardin-Pierce, 2014).*
- Teach client/family the signs of high sodium and the risk factors. *Signs of high sodium include thirst, dry mucous membranes, rapid heartbeat, low blood pressure, and mental status changes; symptoms can progress to confusion, delirium, and seizures (Wagner & Hardin-Pierce, 2014).*
- Teach client/family the importance of hydration during exercise. Dehydration occurs when the amount of water leaving the body is greater than the amount consumed. *The body can lose large amounts of fluid when it tries to cool itself by sweating (Begg, 2017).*
- Teach client/family the warning signs of dehydration. Early signs of dehydration include thirst and decreased urine output. As dehydration increases, symptoms may include dry mouth, muscle cramps, nausea and vomiting, lightheadedness, and orthostatic hypotension. *Severe dehydration can cause confusion, weakness, coma, and organ failure (Wagner & Hardin-Pierce, 2014).*
- Teach client about any medications prescribed. Medication teaching includes the drug name, its purpose, administration instructions such as taking it with or without food, and any side effects. **EB:** *Studies have shown that insufficient and ineffective patient education leading to poor treatment adherence, and suboptimal use of guideline-recommended drug regimens have been identified as contributing factors to patient nonadherence to antiplatelet therapy and high hospital acute coronary syndrome (ACS) readmission rates (Larkin et al, 2017). Patients on a diuretic should understand side effects such as those for low potassium. Diuretic use remains a primary cause of low serum potassium levels (Arampatzis et al, 2013). Patients on warfarin should also be educated on dietary interactions to improve medication efficacy (Jenner et al, 2015).*
- ▲ Instruct the client to report any adverse medication side effects to his or her health care provider. Assessing and instructing clients about medications and focusing on important details can help prevent client medication errors. **EB:** *Pharmacist involvement with patient education can improve medication efficacy and decrease hospital readmissions (Phatak et al, 2016).*

REFERENCES

Arampatzis, B. D., Funk, G. C., Leichtle, A. B., et al. (2013). Impact of diuretic-therapy electrolyte disorders present on admission to the emergency department: a cross-sectional analysis. *BMC Medicine*, *11*, 83.

Ariyoshi, N., Nogi, M., Ando, A., et al. (2016). Hypophosphatemia-induced cardiomyopathy. *The American Journal of the Medical Sciences*, *352*(3), 317–323.

Begg, D. P. (2017). Disturbances of thirst and fluid balance associated with aging. *Physiology & Behavior*, *178*, 28–34. doi:10.1016/j.physbeh.2017.03.003 [Epub 2017 Mar 4].

Bolignano, D., Mattace-Raso, F., Sijbrands, E. J., et al. (2014). The aging kidney revisited: A systematic review. *Ageing Research Reviews*, 65–80.

Calazza, A., Russo, L., Sabbatini, M., et al. (2014). Hemodynamic and tubular changes induced by contrast media. *BioMed Research International*, *2014*, 578974.

Chlibkova, D., Knechtie, B., Roseman, T., et al. (2014). The prevalence of exercise-associated hyponatremia in 24-hour ultra-mountain bikers, 24-hour ultra-runners and multi-stage ultra-mountain bikers in the Czech Republic. *Journal of the International Society of Sports Nutrition*, *11*(1), 3.

Christopoulou, E. C., Fillapatos, T. D., Megapanou, E., et al. (2017). Phosphate imbalance in patients with heart failure. *Heart Failure Reviews*, *22*(3), 349–356.

Diringer, M. (2017). Neurologic manifestations of major electrolyte abnormalities. *Handbook of Clinical Neurology*, *141*, 705–713.

Gardner, J., & Gardner, J. (2014). Neurologic complications of electrolyte disturbances and acid-base balance. In R. V. Biller & J. M. Ferro (Eds.), *Handbook of clinical neurology* (Vol. 119). Amsterdam, Netherlands: Elsevier.

Gonzales, W., Altieri, P. I., Alvarado, S., et al. (2013). Magnesium: The forgotten electrolyte. *Boletín de la Asociación Médica de Puerto Rico*, *105*(3), 17–20.

Hew-Butler, T., Loi, V., Pani, A., et al. (2017). Exercise-associated hyponatremia: 2017 update. *Frontiers in Medicine*, *4*, 21.

Jenner, K. M., Simmons, B. J., Delate, T., et al. (2015). An education program for patient self-management of warfarin. *The Permanente Journal*, *19*(4), 33–38.

Larkin, A., LaCOuture, M., Geissel, K., et al. (2017). Quality improvement in management of acute coronary syndrome: continuing medical education and peer coaching improve antiplatelet medication adherence and reduce hospital readmissions. *Critical Pathways in Cardiology*, *16*(3), 96–101.

Marcuccilini, M., Chonchol, M., & Jovanovich, A. (2017). Phosphate binders and targets over decades: Do we have it right now? *Seminars in Dialysis*, *2*, 134–141.

• = Independent;   ▲ = Collaborative;   **EBN** = Evidence-Based Nursing;   **EB** = Evidence-Based

Nykamp, D., & Kraus, E. J. (2013). Antacid-induced acute pancreatitis. *The Consultant Pharmacist: The Journal of the American Society of Consultant Pharmacists, 28*(4), 247–251.

Phatak, A., Prusi, R., Ward, B., et al. (2016). Impact of pharmacist involvement in the transitional care of high-risk patients through medication reconciliation, medication education, and post-discharge call-backs (IPITCH Study). *Journal of Hospital Medicine, 11*(1), 39–44.

Raghavendra, G., Prasad, J. V., Rao, S., et al. (2017). The role of routine measurement of intra-abdominal pressure in preventing abdominal compartment syndrome. *Journal of Indian Association of Pediatric Surgeons, 22*(3), 134–138.

Rudge, J. E., & Kim, D. (2014). New-onset hyponatraemia after surgery for traumatic hip fracture. *Age and Ageing, 43*(6), 821–826.

Upala, S., Jaruvongvanic, V., Wijarnpreecha, K., et al. (2016). Hypomagnesemia and mortality in patients admitted to intensive

care unit: A systematic review and meta-analysis. *QJM: Monthly Journal of the Association of Physicians, 109*(7), 453–459.

Varela Piñón, M., & Adán-Manes, J. (2017). Selective serotonin reuptake inhibitor-induced hyponatremia: Clinical implications and therapeutic alternatives. *Clinical Neuropharmacology, 40*(4), 177–179.

Vassalos, A., & Rooney, K. (2013). Surviving sepsis guidelines 2012. *Critical Care Medicine, 41*(12), 485–486.

Wagner, K. D., & Hardin-Pierce, M. G. (2014). *High acuity nursing.* (6th ed., pp. 359–629). Boston, MA: Prentice Hall, Inc.

Wang, C. H., Hsieh, W. H., Chou, H. C., et al. (2014). Liberal versus restricted fluid resuscitation strategies in trauma patients: a systematic review and meta-analysis of randomized controlled trials and observational studies. *Critical Care Medicine, 42*(4), 954–961.

E

Imbalanced Energy Field Gail B. Ladwig, MSN, RN, and Julianne E. Doubet, BSN, RN, EMT-B

NANDA-I

Definition

A disruption in the vital flow of human energy that is normally a continuous whole and is unique, dynamic, creative, and nonlinear.

Defining Characteristics

Arrhythmic energy field patterns; blockage of energy flow; congested energy field patterns; congestion of the energy flow; dissonant rhythms of the energy field patterns; energy deficit of the energy flow; expression of the need to regain the experience of the whole; hyperactivity of the energy flow; irregular energy field patterns; magnetic pull to an area of the energy field; pulsating to pounding frequency of the energy field patterns; pulsations sensed in the energy flow; random energy field patterns; rapid energy field patterns; slow energy field patterns; strong energy field patterns; temperature differentials of cold in the energy flow; temperature differentials of heat in the energy flow; tingling sensed in the energy flow; tumultuous energy field patterns; unsynchronized rhythms sensed in the energy flow; weak energy field patterns

Related Factors

Anxiety; discomfort; excessive stress; interventions that disrupt the energetic pattern or flow; pain

At-Risk Population

Crisis states; life transition

Associated Condition

Illness; injury

NOC (Nursing Outcomes Classification)

Suggested NOC Outcomes

Personal Well-Being, Personal Health Status; Psychomotor Energy; Quality of Life

Example NOC Outcome with Indicators
Personal Well-Being as evidenced by the following indicators: Psychological health/Spiritual life/Ability to relax/Level of happiness. (Rate the outcome and indicators of **Personal Well-Being:** 1 = not all satisfied, 2 = somewhat satisfied, 3 = moderately satisfied, 4 = very satisfied, 5 = completely satisfied [see Section I].)

● = Independent; ▲ = Collaborative; EBN = Evidence-Based Nursing; EB = Evidence-Based

E

NIC (Nursing Interventions Classification)

Suggested NIC Interventions

> Therapeutic Touch (TT); Hope Inspiration; Reiki

Nursing Interventions and *Rationales*

- Consider using complimentary health approaches (CHAs)–energy medicine (TT/healing touch, hope inspiration, and reiki) for clients with anxiety, tension, pain, or other conditions that indicate a disruption in the flow of energy. **EBN:** *According to Papathanassoglou (2016), the sense of touch has the potential of evoking and balancing human emotions; interpersonal touch then may perform an influential part in the emotional well-being of the client and family.* **EBN:** *"The goal of Healing Touch is to restore harmony and balance in the energy system, placing the client in a position to self-heal" (Drozdowicz & Dillard, 2014).* **EBN:** *Developing evidence suggested that there is biological support for the lessening of pain and anxiety for patients who receive CHAs in acute care settings (Kramlich, 2017).* **EBN:** *Reiki can contribute to changes in mindfulness from conflict and confusion to harmony and well-being (Jamison & Grohman, 2015).*
- Refer to care plans for **Anxiety,** Acute **Pain,** and Chronic **Pain.**

Guidelines for Complimentary Health Approaches

- CHA may be practiced by anyone with the requisite preparation, desire, and commitment. **EBN:** *Acute and critical care nurses who are certified to practice CHA in the acute care setting must adhere to their scope of practice, be conscious of their role, and recognize their professional boundaries (Kramlich, 2017).*
- Volunteers who are not licensed health care professionals may practice in the home, but not in the health care setting unless they undertake a rigorous training program. **EBN:** *Because patient safety is of utmost concern in the acute and critical care settings, volunteer complimentary health professionals (CHPs) must support infection control, patient privacy, and patient security (Kramlich, 2017).*

 Pediatric

- Consider using CHAs for pediatric clients with adjunct therapies to decrease stress, anxiety, and pain. **EB:** *McClafferty et al (2017) encouraged medical professionals who care for children to foster the utilization of "relevant, safe, effective, and age-appropriate health services and therapies," whether conventional or complementary.* **EB:** *In pediatric cases of pain and chronic conditions, the successful use of complementary alternative medicine (CAM) has markedly increased (Adams et al, 2014).*

 Geriatric

- Consider CHAs for elderly with pain. **EB:** *Overall, CAM therapies are valuable to the geriatric population, especially for those who cope with chronic conditions and suffer from constant pain, therefore enhancing their quality of life. CAM nurtures good health practices and bolsters the body's defenses, its natural healing ability, and promotion of self-care and patient empowerment (Siddiqui et al, 2014).* **EB:** *The use of patient-centered communication about the risks/benefits of CAM is necessary to promote effective management of chronic illnesses and pain among an aging population (Ho et al, 2014).*

 Multicultural

- Assess for the influence of cultural beliefs, norms, and values on the client's use of CAM. **EB:** *CAMs cover a wide range of methodologies (herbal medicine, manual healing techniques, traditional therapies, and mind–body interventions) and are used globally to treat a wide-range of illnesses and to support good health (Mathew et al, 2013).*

 Home Care

- Help the client and family accept CAMS as natural healing interventions. **EB:** *Because homeopathy is one of the most commonly used methods of CAM, Schmacke, Muller, and Stamer (2014), in their survey of homeopathic use, found that the initial homeopathic consultation and the search for appropriate medication was seen by patients as an endorsement of personalized homeopathic treatment.*
- ▲ In the presence of a psychiatric disorder, refer for psychiatric home health care services for client reassurance and implementation of therapeutic regimens. **EB:** *It has been shown that a home visit intervention (HoVI) of psychiatric clients generates positive outcomes shown by the documented decrease in rehospitalization rates and number of days hospitalized, leading to health care cost savings (Chang & Chou, 2015).*

● = Independent;   ▲ = Collaborative;   EBN = Evidence-Based Nursing;   EB = Evidence-Based

Client/Family Teaching and Discharge Planning

- Teach the client how to use guided imagery. EBN: *Urge your client to use guided imagery and relaxation. This nonpharmacological technique has proven valuable in treating sleep deprivation and the promotion of relaxation to reduce pain (Adeola et al, 2015).*
- Consider the use of progressive muscle relaxation, autogenic training, relaxation response, biofeedback, emotional freedom technique, guided imagery, diaphragmatic breathing, transcendental meditation, cognitive behavioral therapy, mindfulness-based stress reduction, and emotional freedom technique. CEB: *These are all evidence-based techniques that are easy to learn and practice and have good results in individuals with good health or with a disease (Varvogli & Darviri, 2011).* EB: *"CAM routines and rituals constitute key elements in cancer patients' regular and satisfied CAM use, and they promote familial strengthening"* (Klafke et al, 2014).

Nurses/Staff

- The practice of CAMs, both giving and receiving, can improve well-being. EBN: *The patient–CAM practitioner connection is vital because it embodies healing intent, which in turn produces substantial influence on positive outcomes (Dunning, 2014).*
- See the EVOLVE website for Weblinks for client education resources.

REFERENCES

Adams, D., Whidden, A., & Honkanea, M. (2014). Complementary and alternative medicine: A survey of its use in pediatric cardiology. *CMAJ Open, 2*(4), E217–E224. doi:10.9778/cmajo.20130075.

Chang, Y., & Chou, F. (2015). Effects of home visit intervention on re-hospitalization rates of psychiatric patients. *Community Mental Health, 51*(5), 598–605. doi:10.1007/s10597-014-9807-7.

Drozdowicz, A., & Dillard, D. (2014). Presence in the neonatal intensive care unit. *International Journal of Childbirth Education, 29*(4), 63–67.

Dunning, T. (2014). Overview of complementary and alternative medicine and diabetes. *Practical Diabetes, 31*(9), 381–386. doi:10.100.2/pdi.1908.

Ho, T., Rowland-Seymour, A., Frankel, E., et al. (2014). Generational differences in complementary and alternative medicine (CAM) use in the context of chronic disease and pain: Baby boomers versus the silent generation. *Journal of the American Board of Family Medicine, 27*(4), 465–473. doi:10.3122/jabfm.2014.04.13023.

Jamison, T., & Grohman, E. (2015). Energy medicine: A complementary modality in nursing. *Quality in Primary Care, 23*(4), 189–191.

Klafke, N., Elliot, J., Oliver, G., et al. (2014). The role of complementary and alternative medicine (CAM) routines and rituals in men with cancer and their significant others (Sos): A qualitative investigation. *Supportive Care in Cancer, 22*(5), 1319–1331. doi:10.1007/s00520-013-2090-2.

Kramlich, D. (2017). Complementary health practitioners in the acute and critical care setting: Nursing considerations. *Critical Care Nursing, 37*(3), 60–65. doi:10.4037/ccn2017181.

Mapes, A., Baird, C., Sands, L., et al. (2015). Active despite pain: Patient experiences with guided imagery with relaxation compared to planned rest. *Clinical Journal of Oncology Nursing, 19*(6), 649–652. doi:10.1188/115.CJON.649-662.

Mathew, E., Muttappallymyalil, J., Sreedharan, J., et al. (2013). Self-reported use of complementary and alternative medicine among health care consumers at a tertiary care center in Ajman, United Arab Emirates. *Annals of Medicine & Health Science Research, 3*(2), 215–219. doi:10.4103/2141-9248.113665.

McClafferty, H., Vohra, S., & Baily, M. (2017). Pediatric integrative medicine. American Academy of Pediatrics Clinical Report. *Pediatrics.* Retrieved from aappublications.org/content/early/2017/08/24/peds.2017-196.

Papathanassoglou, E. (2016). Therapeutic touch in critical care… *WFCCN/ACCN World Congress: The World of Critical Care Nursing, 10*(2), 35.

Schmacke, N., Muller, V., & Stamer, M. (2014). What is it about homeopathy that patients value? And what can family medicine learn from this. *Quality in Primary Care, 22*(1), 17–24.

Siddiqui, M., Min, C., Verma, R., et al. (2014). Role of complementary and alternative medicine in geriatric care: A mini review. *Pharmacology Review, 8*(16), 81–87. doi:10.4103/0973-7847.134230.

Varvogli, L., & Darviri, C. (2011). Stress management techniques: Evidence-based procedures that reduce stress and promote health. *Health Science Journal, 5*(2), 74–89.

Risk for dry Eye   *Mary Beth Flynn Makic, PhD, RN, CCNS, FAAN, FNAP*

NANDA-I

Definition

Susceptible to eye discomfort or damage to the cornea and conjunctiva due to reduced quantity or quality of tears to moisten the eye, which may compromise health.

- = Independent;   ▲ = Collaborative;   EBN = Evidence-Based Nursing;   EB = Evidence-Based

E

Risk Factors

Air conditioning; air pollution; caffeine intake; excessive wind; insufficient knowledge of modifiable factors; low humidity; prolonged reading; smoking; sunlight exposure; vitamin A deficiency

At-Risk Population

Aging; contact lens wearer; female gender; history of allergy

Associated Condition

Autoimmune disease; hormonal change; mechanical ventilation; neurological lesion with sensory or motor reflex loss; ocular surface damage; treatment regime

NOC   (Nursing Outcomes Classification)

Suggested NOC Outcomes (Visual)

Dry Eye Severity; Sensory Function: Vision; Vision Compensation Behavior

Example NOC Outcome with Indicators
Dry Eye Severity as evidenced by the following indicators: Decreased tear production/Redness of conjunctiva/Burning eye sensation/Itchy eye sensation/Eye pain/Excessive watering/Blurred vision. (Rate each indicator of **Dry Eye Severity:** 1 = severe, 2 = substantial, 3 = moderate, 4 = mild, 5 = none [see Section I].)

Client Outcomes

Client Will (Specify Time Frame)

- State eyes are comfortable with no itching, burning, or dryness
- Have corneal surface that is intact and without injury
- Demonstrate self-administration of eye drops if ordered
- State vision is clear

NIC   (Nursing Interventions Classification)

Suggested NIC Interventions

Communication Enhancement: Visual Deficit; Environmental Management

Example NIC Activities—Communication Enhancement: Visual Deficit
Identify yourself when you enter the client's space; Provide adequate room lighting

Nursing Interventions and *Rationales*

- ▲ Assess for symptoms of dry eyes, such as "irritation, tearing, burning, stinging, dry or foreign body sensation, mild itching, photophobia, blurry vision, contact lens intolerance, redness, mucus discharge, increased frequency of blinking, eye fatigue, diurnal fluctuation, symptoms that worsen later in the day" (American Academy of Ophthalmology [AAO], 2015, 2018).
- ▲ If symptoms are present, then refer client to an ophthalmologist for diagnosis and treatment. EB: *Clients with dry eye who are evaluated by nonophthalmologist health care providers should be referred promptly to the ophthalmologist if moderate or severe pain, lack of response to therapy, corneal infiltration or ulceration, or vision loss occurs (AAO, 2018).*
- ▲ Administer ordered eye drops. *As the severity of the dry eye increases, aqueous enhancement of the eye using topical agents is appropriate. Emulsions, gels, and ointments can be used (AAO, 2015, 2018).*
- • Consider use of eyeglass side shields or moisture chambers. EB: *Eyeglass side shields can protect the eyes from drafts. Moisture chambers are a type of eyeglasses that are frequently worn by motorcyclists and mountain climbers and can be purchased at stores or online (AAO, 2015, 2018; American Optometric Association [AOA], 2018).*
- ▲ Watch for symptoms of blepharitis including crusting and irritation at the base of the lashes and adjacent redness of the eyelid, which may accompany dry eye; refer for treatment as needed. EB: *Contributing*

• = Independent;   ▲ = Collaborative;   EBN = Evidence-Based Nursing;   EB = Evidence-Based

ocular factors such as blepharitis should be treated. Particularly effective treatments for evaporative tear deficiency include eyelid therapy for conditions such as blepharitis (AAO, 2015).

▲ Discuss use of caffeine with client's health care provider. **EB:** *Arita et al (2012) and Wachler (2017) found that use of caffeine capsules increased tear volume.*

● Provide education to the client about limiting screen time, computers, smart devices, and television can assist with eyestrain and dry eyes. **EB:** *Eye discomfort is associated with screen time, and digital eyestrain because most people blink less when looking at screens causing eyestrain and dryness (Vimont & Khurana, 2017). Encourage the client to use natural tears if prolonged or frequent digital eye strain is anticipated.*

Geriatric

● Recognize that symptoms of dry eye are more common in menopausal women and geriatric clients. *Hormonal changes after menopause can disrupt tear production. It is estimated that one in three individuals older than 65 years experiences dry eyes (National Health Service [NHS], 2014).*

Critical Care

▲ Provide regular cleaning of the eyes, lubricating eye drops and ointments, and consultation with an ophthalmologist if infection is suspected in clients in the intensive care unit (ICU). *ICU staff may miss ocular complications while caring for life-threatening conditions. Ocular complications can seriously impair vision and quality of life.* **EB:** *"As ICU patients are more susceptible to develop dry eye, keratopathy, and ocular infections, they should be consulted by an ophthalmologist for early diagnosis of ocular surface disorders" (Saritas et al, 2013).*

● Avoid using adhesive tape to keep eyes closed in sedated patients. **EBN:** *In an audit of eye dryness and corneal abrasions of patients in four ICUs in Iran, patients receiving adhesive tape as an eye care method were twice as likely to develop corneal abrasion (Masoudi et al, 2014).*

Client/Family Teaching and Discharge Planning

● Teach client conditions that can exacerbate dry eye symptoms. *Exacerbating conditions include wind, air travel, decreased humidity, air conditioning or heating, and prolonged activities that reduce blink rate such as reading and computer use (AAO, 2015, 2018; AOA, 2018).*

● Teach client good eye hygiene:
  ○ Apply warm compresses for 10-minute intervals using a clean cloth and water that has been boiled and cooled (or sterile water).
  ○ Gently massage around eyelids.
  ○ Gently clean eyelids to remove excess oil, crusts, and bacteria. Use a few drops of baby shampoo in water that has been boiled and cooled, or in sterile water.
  ○ Good hygiene can help improve dry eyes, especially dry eye associated with blepharitis (NHS, 2014).

● Teach clients methods to decrease problems with dry eye including the following:
  ○ Avoid drafty (e.g., ceiling fans) and low-humidity environments.
  ○ Avoid smoking and exposure to secondhand smoke.

▲ Discuss avoidance of offending medications with health care provider.

● Drink plenty of water to keep well hydrated. **EB:** *For patients with a clinical diagnosis of mild dry eye, potentially exacerbating exogenous factors such as antihistamine or diuretic use, cigarette smoking, and exposure to secondhand smoke, and environmental factors such as air drafts and low-humidity environments should be addressed (AAO, 2015, 2018). Symptoms of dry eye may be exacerbated by the use of medications such as diuretics, antihistamines, anticholinergics, antidepressants, and systemic retinoids (AAO, 2015, 2018). Self-care includes drinking plenty of water to stay hydrated (AOA, 2018).*

● Teach client to lower the computer screen to below eye level and to blink more frequently. *Measures such as lowering the computer screen to below eye level to decrease lid aperture, scheduling regular breaks, and increasing blink frequency may decrease the discomfort associated with computer and reading activities (AAO, 2015, 2018).*

▲ Teach client to consult with the health care provider regarding use of omega-3 supplements to decrease dry eye. **EB:** *Omega-3 fatty acid products without ethyl esters may be beneficial in the treatment of dry eye, although they may increase the risk of prostate cancer (AAO, 2015, 2018).*

● Teach client how to self-administer eye drops.

● Warn clients with dry eyes that driving at night can be dangerous. *Clients with dry eyes have light sensitivity and decreased refraction.*

● = Independent; ▲ = Collaborative; **EBN** = Evidence-Based Nursing; **EB** = Evidence-Based

REFERENCES

American Academy of Ophthalmology (AAO). (2015). *Four ways to fight dry eyes*. The Ophthalmic News and Education Network. Retrieved from https://www.aao.org/eye-health/tips-prevention/four-ways-to-fight-dry-eye. (Accessed 10 February 2018).

American Academy of Ophthalmology (AAO). (2018). *Seven tips for battling dry eye*. The Ophthalmic News and Education Network. Retrieved from https://www.aao.org/eye-health/tips-prevention/dry-eye-tips. (Accessed 10 February 2018).

American Optometric Association (AOA). (2018). *Dry eye*. Retrieved from http://www.aoa.org/patients-and-public/eye-and-vision-problems/glossary-of-eye-and-vision-conditions/dry-eye?sso=y>. (Accessed 10 February 2018).

Arita, R., et al. (2012). Caffeine increases tear volume depending on polymorphisms within the adenosine A2a receptor gene and cytochrome P450 1A2. *Ophthalmology, 119*(5), 972–978.

Masoudi, N., et al. (2014). An audit of eye dryness and corneal abrasion in ICU patients in Iran. *Nursing in Critical Care, 19*(2), 73–77.

National Health Service (NHS) England. (2014). *Dry eye syndrome—Self-help*. Retrieved from http://www.nhs.uk/Conditions/Dry-eye-syndrome/Pages/Prevention.aspx.

Saritas, T. B., et al. (2013). Ocular surface disorders in intensive care unit patients. *Scientific World Journal*. Retrieved from http://www.ncbi.nlm.nih.gov/pmc/articles/PMC3830763/.

Vimont, C., & Khurana, R. (2017). *Blue light?* Retrieved from https://www.aao.org/eye-health/tips-prevention/should-you-be-worried-about-blue-light. (Accessed 10 February 2018).

Wachler, B. S. B. (2017). *Caffine and dry eye*. WEBMD. Retrieved from https://www.webmd.com/eye-health/caffeine-dry-eye#1. (Accessed February 10, 2018).

Labile Emotional Control   *Marina Martinez-Kratz, MS, RN, CNE*

NANDA-I

Definition

Uncontrollable outbursts of exaggerated and involuntary emotional expression.

Defining Characteristics

Absence of eye contact; crying; difficulty in use of facial expressions; embarrassment regarding emotional expression; excessive crying without feeling sadness; excessive laughing without feeling happiness; expression of emotion incongruent with triggering factor; involuntary crying; involuntary laughing; uncontrollable crying; uncontrollable laughing; withdrawal from occupational situation; withdrawal from social situation

Related Factors

Alteration in self-esteem; emotional disturbance; fatigue; insufficient knowledge about symptom control; insufficient knowledge of disease; insufficient muscle strength; social distress; stressors; substance misuse

Associated Condition

Brain injury; functional impairment; mood disorder; musculoskeletal impairment; pharmaceutical agent; physical disability; psychiatric disorder

NOC   Outcomes (Nursing Outcomes Classification)

Suggested NOC Outcomes

Coping; Knowledge: Disease Process; Impulse; Self-Control; Self-Esteem; Quality of Life; Personal Well-Being; Stress Level

> ### Example NOC Outcomes with Indicators
>
> **Knowledge: Disease Process** as evidenced by the following indicator: Specific disease process. (Rate the outcome and indicators of **Knowledge: Disease Process:** 1 = no knowledge, 2 = limited knowledge, 3= moderate knowledge, 4 = substantial knowledge, 5 = extensive knowledge [see Section I].)

Client Outcomes

Client Will (Specify Time Frame)

- Improve coping strategies
- Improve knowledge about disease process, signs and symptoms, triggers, symptom control
- Use mechanisms to control impulses and ask for help when feeling impulses

● = Independent;   ▲ = Collaborative;   EBN = Evidence-Based Nursing;   EB = Evidence-Based

- Improve feelings of dignity
- Enhance and improve response to social and environmental stimuli

NIC   Interventions (Nursing Interventions Classification)

Suggested NIC Interventions

Coping Enhancement; Teaching: Disease Process; Enhance Self-Esteem; Improved Quality of Life; Improved Well-Being

> ### Example NIC Activities—Labile Emotional Control
>
> **Coping Enhancement:** Assist the patient to solve problems in a constructive manner; Instruct the patient on the use of relaxation techniques, as needed; Assist the patient to identify positive strategies to deal with limitations and manage needed lifestyle or role changes

Nursing Interventions and *Rationales*

- Identify clients at risk of having labile emotional control. EB: *Clients with traumatic brain injury (TBI), Parkinson's disease (PD), multiple sclerosis (MS), amyotrophic lateral sclerosis (ALS), stroke, and schizophrenia (including schizoaffective and schizophreniform disorders) were most closely associated with pseudobulbar affect (PBA) diagnosis, which is associated with emotional lability (Allen et al, 2017).*
- Assess clients with the Pathological Laughter and Crying Scale (PLACS) to identify pathological laughing and crying or related disorders (e.g., involuntary emotional expression disorder [IEED], PBA). EBN: *PLACS is an interviewer-administered instrument that has been validated in clients with acute stroke. It has shown excellent interrater and test–retest reliability (Ahmed & Simmons, 2013).*
- Assess clients for use of experiential avoidance, which is the process of negatively evaluating, escaping, or avoiding unwanted thoughts, emotions, or sensations. EB: *A recent study found experiential avoidance was associated with both higher levels of negative affect ($P < .001$) and increased emotional lability ($P = .021$) (Gerhart et al, 2018).*
- Offer the client choices when possible in emotional situations. EB: *A study found that choice appears to be a powerful tool that permits regulation of negative emotions in an adaptive fashion (Thuillard & Dan-Glauser, 2017).*
- Provide progressive muscle relaxation (PMR) exercise and guided imagery (GI) techniques. EBN: *A nursing study found that PMR and GI were effective in reducing anxiety and improving mood states in parents of children with malignancy (Tsitsi et al, 2016).*
- Offer instruction regarding alternative coping strategies such as mindfulness and breath awareness. EB: *Increased breath awareness (a fundamental component of mindfulness meditation) has been shown to reduce autonomic and psychological arousal, and this increased capacity to remain calm can help individuals to respond more adaptively to internal and external stressors (Compare et al, 2014).* EB: *Studies have demonstrated the effects of mindfulness and yoga on well-being, somatic effects of stress, immune system, and physical symptoms and chronic conditions (Lazaridou, Philbrook, & Tzika, 2013).*
- Consider using cognitive-behavioral therapy (CBT). EB: *A current study of youth with anxiety disorders found that CBT resulted in decreased sadness and anger dysregulation and increases in adaptive coping with anger (Suveg et al, 2017).*
- Provide music therapy. EB: *The use of music therapy can improve mental well-being, social functioning, quality of life, anxiety, pain, mood, relaxation, and comfort in persons with several disorders/diseases such as cancer, schizophrenia, mood disorders, and autism (Kamioka et al, 2014).*

Pediatric

- Assess adolescents with high emotional dysregulation for substance use disorders. EB: *Study results indicated that adolescents scoring high on emotional dysregulation are at risk for substance dependence because of more externalizing and internalizing symptomatology (Wills et al, 2016).*
- Teach parents that their reactions to their children's emotions play a critical role in teaching children effective emotion regulation. EB: *A recent study suggested that supportive parent emotion socialization practices are associated with parent-rated emotion regulation skills (Breaux et al, 2018).*
- Provide parents with emotion coaching strategies to manage their children's emotional outbursts. Emotion coaching includes fostering parental awareness and acceptance of their children's emotions with behaviors

• = Independent;   ▲ = Collaborative;   EBN = Evidence-Based Nursing;   EB = Evidence-Based

E

that acknowledge their children's emotions, and teaches understanding, coping with, and appropriately expressing emotion. **EB:** *Study results suggested that when children with oppositional defiant disorder (ODD) experience more frequent, intense, and unstable emotions, families are better able to benefit from treatment and reduce children's behavior problems when mothers begin treatment or are already engaging in emotion coaching (Dunsmore et al, 2016).*

▲ Refer adolescent clients to a dialectical behavior therapy (DBT) group. **EB:** *Research shows DBT is an effective means of assisting adolescents to learn to enhance their emotion regulation skills (Gill et al, 2018).*

Geriatric

- Many of the previous interventions may be adapted for geriatric use.
- Evaluate geriatric clients suspected of PBA with the following three-step model: (1) crying inconsistent with environment/stimuli; (2) diagnosis of any of the following neurological disorders, such as TBI, PD, MS, ALS; or (3) at least two of the following disorders, such as stroke, schizophrenia (including schizoaffective and schizophreniform disorders), or documentation of spinal cord injury (SCI) as most closely associated with the PBA diagnosis. **EB:** *Based on analysis, this three-item checklist to facilitate PBA risk assessment in the nursing home setting was developed (Allen et al, 2017).*

Multicultural and Home Care

- The previous interventions may be adapted for multicultural and home care.

Client/Family Teaching and Discharge Planning

- Inform client and family about the emotional lability and talk with them about how to cope with the situation. **EBN:** *Clients and families need more information about this syndrome so they can recognize the signs and symptoms, get a diagnosis, and obtain treatment (Schneider & Schneider, 2017).*
- Use verbal and nonverbal therapeutic communication approaches including empathy, active listening, and confrontation to encourage the client and family to express emotions such as sadness, guilt, and anger (within appropriate limits); verbalize fears and concerns; and set goals. *Solution-focused communication with clients helps focus on goals and helps find solutions*
- Provide psychoeducation for stress-related variables to client and family. **EB:** *Psychoeducation was conducted in seven studies, six of which had positive outcomes on depression, anxiety, or knowledge levels (Bte Iskhandar Shah et al, 2013).*

REFERENCES

Ahmed, A., & Simmons, Z. (2013). Pseudobulbar affect: Prevalence and management. *Therapeutics and Clinical Risk Management, 2013*(9), 483–489.

Allen, C., et al. (2017). Identification of pseudobulbar affect symptoms in the nursing home setting: Development and assessment of a screening tool. *Geriatric Nursing Journal, 39*(1), 54–59. doi:10.1016/j.gerinurse.2017.06.002.

Breaux, R. P., et al. (2018). Longitudinal associations of parental emotion socialization and children's emotion regulation: The moderating role of ADHD symptomatology. *Journal of Abnormal Child Psychology, 46*(4), 671–683. doi:10.1007/s10802-017-0327-0.

Bte Iskhandar Shah, L., Klainin-Yobas, P., Torres, S., et al. (2013). Efficacy of psychoeducation and relaxation interventions on stress-related variables in people with mental disorders: A literature review. *Archives of Psychiatric Nursing, 28*(2), 94–101.

Compare, A., Zarbo, C., Shonin, E., et al. (2014). Emotional regulation and depression: A potential mediator between heart and mind. *Cardiovascular Psychiatry and Neurology, 2014*, 324374.

Dunsmore, J. C., et al. (2016). Emotion socialization in the context of risk and psychopathology: Maternal emotion coaching predicts better treatment outcomes for emotionally labile children with oppositional defiant disorder: Emotion coaching and treatment outcomes for ODD. *Social Development, 25*(1), 8–26. doi:10.1111/sode.12109.

Gerhart, J., et al. (2018). A daily diary study of posttraumatic stress, experiential avoidance, and emotional lability among inpatient nurses. *Psycho-Oncology, 27*(3), 1068–1071. doi:10.1002/pon.4531.

Gill, D., et al. (2018). Group therapy for emotional dysregulation: Treatment for adolescents and their parents. *Child and Adolescent Social Work Journal, 35*(2), 169–180. doi:10.1007/s10560-017-0510-8.

Kamioka, H., Tsutani, K., Yamada, M., et al. (2014). Effectiveness of music therapy: A summary of systematic reviews based on randomized controlled trials of music interventions. *Patient Preference and Adherence, 2014*(8), 727–754.

Lazaridou, A., Philbrook, P., & Tzika, A. (2013). Yoga and mindfulness as therapeutic interventions for stroke rehabilitation: A systematic review. *Evidence-Based Complementary and Alternative Medicine*, doi:10.1155/2013/357108.

Schneider, M. A., & Schneider, D. A. (2017). Pseudobulbar affect: What nurses, stroke survivors, and caregivers need to know. *Journal of Neuroscience Nursing, 49*(2), 114–117.

Suveg, C., et al. (2017). Emotion-focused cognitive-behavioral therapy for youth with anxiety disorders: A randomized trial. *Journal of Abnormal Child Psychology, 46*(3), 569–580. doi:10.1007/s10802-017-0319-0.

Thuillard, S., & Dan-Glauser, E. S. (2017). The regulatory effect of choice in situation selection reduces experiential, exocrine and respiratory arousal for negative emotional stimulations. *Scientific Reports, 7*(12626), 1–14. doi:10.1038/s41598-017-12626-7.

Tsitsi, T., et al. (2016). Effectiveness of a relaxation intervention (progressive muscle relaxation and guided imagery techniques) to reduce anxiety and improve mood of parents of hospitalized children with malignancies: A randomized controlled trial in

● = Independent;   ▲ = Collaborative;   **EBN** = Evidence-Based Nursing;   **EB** = Evidence-Based

Republic of Cyprus and Greece. *European Journal of Oncology Nursing, 26,* 9–18. doi:10.1016/j.ejon.2016.10.007.

Wills, T. A., et al. (2016). Emotional self-control and dysregulation: A dual-process analysis of pathways to externalizing/internalizing symptomatology and positive well-being in younger adolescents. *Drug and Alcohol Dependence, 163*(Suppl. 1), S37–S45. doi:10.1016/j.drugalcdep.2015.08.039.

Risk for Falls   *Sherry A. Greenberg, PhD, RN, GNP-BC*

F

NANDA-I

Definition

Susceptible to increased susceptibility to falling, which may cause physical harm and compromise health.

Risk Factors

Children

Absence of stairway gate; absence of window guard; inadequate supervision; insufficient automobile restraints

Environment

Cluttered environment; exposure to unsafe weather-related condition; insufficient anti-slip material in bathroom; insufficient lighting; unfamiliar setting; use of restraints; use of throw rugs

Physiological

Alteration in blood glucose level; decrease in lower extremity strength; diarrhea; difficulty with gait; faintness when extending neck; faintness when turning neck; impaired mobility; incontinence; sleeplessness; urinary urgency

Other

Alcohol consumption; insufficient knowledge of modifiable factors

At-Risk Population

Age ≥65 years; age ≤2 years; history of falls; living alone; male gender when <1 year of age

Associated Condition

Acute illness; alteration in cognitive functioning; anemia; arthritis; condition affecting the foot; hearing impairment; impaired balance; impaired vision; lower limb prosthesis; neoplasm; neuropathy; orthostatic hypotension; pharmaceutical agent; postoperative recovery period; proprioceptive deficit; use of assistive device; vascular disease

NOC   (Nursing Outcomes Classification)

Suggested NOC Outcomes

Fall Prevention Behavior; Knowledge: Child Physical Safety; Knowledge: Fall Prevention; Risk Control: Falls

Example NOC Outcome with Indicators
Fall Prevention Behavior as evidenced by the following indicators: Uses assistive devices correctly/Eliminates clutter, spills, glare from floors/Uses safe transfer procedures. (Rate each indicator of **Fall Prevention Behavior:** 1 = never demonstrated, 2 = rarely demonstrated, 3 = sometimes demonstrated, 4 = often demonstrated, 5 = consistently demonstrated [see Section I].)

Client Outcomes

Client Will (Specify Time Frame)

- Remain free of falls
- Have a decreased risk of injury if sustains a fall

● = Independent;   ▲ = Collaborative;   **EBN** = Evidence-Based Nursing;   **EB** = Evidence-Based

- Adapt environment to minimize the incidence of falls
- Explain methods to prevent injury

NIC　(Nursing Interventions Classification)

Suggested NIC Interventions

Dementia Management; Fall Prevention; Post-Fall Assessment; Surveillance: Safety

Example NIC Activities—Fall Prevention

Assist unsteady individual with ambulation; Monitor gait, balance, and fatigue level with ambulation

Nursing Interventions and *Rationales*

- Safety Guidelines. Complete a fall-risk assessment for older adults in any health care setting with national guidelines and action plans such as the Falls Free: 2015 National Falls Prevention Action Plan (National Council on Aging, 2015).
- Use a valid and reliable fall risk assessment tool to assess the client risk for falling, for example, in the acute care setting the Hendrich II Model (Hendrich, Bender, & Nyhuis, 2016). Recognize that risk factors for falling include recent history of falls, fear of falling, confusion, depression, altered elimination patterns, cardiovascular/respiratory disease impairing perfusion or oxygenation, postural hypotension, dizziness or vertigo, primary cancer diagnosis, and altered mobility (National Council on Aging, 2015; Gray-Miceli, 2016). EB: *The Hendrich II Fall Risk Model is quick to administer and provides a determination of risk for falling based on gender, mental and emotional status, symptoms of dizziness, and known categories of medications increasing risk (Hendrich, Bender, & Nyhuis, 2016). This tool screens for primary prevention of falls and is integral in a postfall assessment for the secondary prevention of falls (Hendrich, Bender, & Nyhuis, 2016).*
- Screen all clients for balance and mobility skills (i.e., supine to sit, sitting supported and unsupported, sit to stand, standing, walking and turning around, transferring, stooping to floor and recovering, and sitting down). Use tools such as the Balance Scale by Tinetti or the Timed Up & Go Test. CEB/EB: *It is helpful to determine the client's functional abilities and then plan for ways to improve problem areas or determine methods to ensure safety (Podsiadlo & Richardson, 1991; National Council on Aging, 2015; Gray-Miceli, 2016).*
- Carefully assist a mostly immobile client up. Be sure to lock the bed and wheelchair and have sufficient personnel to protect the client from falls. When rising from a lying position, have the client change positions slowly, dangle legs, and stand next to the bed before walking to prevent orthostatic hypotension. *Encourage client engagement in a monitored exercise program that will strengthen core and lower extremities to reduce fall risk (Grabiner, 2013; Hirase et al, 2014; National Institute of Neurological Disorders and Stroke [NINDS], 2018).*
- Use a "high-risk fall" armband/bracelet and fall risk room sign to alert staff for increased vigilance and mobility assistance. *These steps alert the nursing staff of the increased risk of falls (McCarter-Bayer, Bayer, & Hall, 2005; Goodwin et al, 2014).*
- ▲ Evaluate the client's medications to determine whether medications increase the risk of falling. Consult with health care provider regarding the client's need for medication if appropriate. EB: *Polypharmacy, or taking more than four medications, has been associated with increased falls. Medications such as benzodiazepines, as well as antipsychotic and antidepressant medications given to promote sleep, actually increase the rate of falls (Goodwin et al, 2014; National Council on Aging, 2015; The American Geriatrics Society Beers Criteria Update Expert Panel, 2015).* EB: *Short- to intermediate-acting benzodiazepine and tricyclic antidepressants may produce ataxia, impaired psychomotor function, syncope, and additional falls (Greenberg, 2016; The American Geriatrics Society Beers Criteria Update Expert Panel, 2015).*
- Orient the client to the environment. Place the call light within reach and show how to call for assistance; answer call light promptly.
- Use one-fourth to one-half length side rails only, and maintain bed in a low position. Ensure that wheels are locked on the bed and commode. Keep dim light in the room at night. *Use of full side rails can result in the client climbing over the rails, leading with the head, and sustaining a head injury. Side rails with widely spaced vertical bars and side rails not situated flush with the mattress have been associated with asphyxiation deaths because of rail and in-bed entrapment and should not be used (Capezuti, 2004; Goodwin et al, 2014).*

● = Independent;　▲ = Collaborative;　EBN = Evidence-Based Nursing;　EB = Evidence-Based

- *Routinely assist the client with toileting on his or her own schedule. Take the client to the bathroom on awakening and before bedtime (McCarter-Bayer, Bayer, & Hall, 2005; Goodwin et al, 2014).*
- Keep the path to the bathroom clear, label the bathroom, and leave the door open.
- ▲ Avoid use of restraints if possible. Obtain health care provider's order if restraints are deemed necessary, and use the least restrictive device. **EB:** *The use of restraints has been associated with serious injuries including rhabdomyolysis, brachial plexus injury, neuropathy, and dysrhythmias, as well as strangulation, asphyxiation, traumatic brain injuries, and all the consequences of immobility (Evans & Cotter, 2008; Cotter & Evans, 2012).* **CEB:** *A study demonstrated that there was no increase in falls or injuries in a group of clients who were not restrained versus a similar group that was restrained in a nursing home (Capezuti et al, 2004). A study in two acute care hospitals demonstrated that when restraints were not used, there was no increase in client falls, injuries, or therapy disruptions (Mion et al, 2001).*
- In place of restraints, use the following:
  - ○ Well-staffed and educated nursing personnel with frequent client contact with careful consideration during shift changes
  - ○ Nursing units designed to care for clients with cognitive and/or functional impairments
  - ○ Nonskid footwear, sneakers preferable
  - ○ Glasses and/or hearing aids, as needed
  - ○ Adequate lighting, night-light in bathroom
  - ○ Frequent toileting
  - ○ Frequently assess need for invasive devices, tubes, intravenous (IV) access
  - ○ Hide tubes with bandages to prevent pulling of tubes
  - ○ Consider alternative IV placement site to prevent pulling out IV line
  - ○ Alarm systems with ankle, above-the-knee, or wrist sensors
  - ○ Bed or wheelchair alarms
  - ○ Wedge cushions on chairs to prevent slipping
  - ○ Increased observation of the client
  - ○ Locked doors to unit
  - ○ Low or very low height beds
  - ○ Border-defining pillow/mattress to cue the client to stay in bed
- *These alternatives to restraints can be helpful to prevent falls (McCarter-Bayer, Bayer, & Hall, 2005; Cotter & Evans, 2012; Grabiner, 2013).*
- If the client has an acute change in mental status (delirium), recognize that the cause is usually physiological and is a medical emergency. Consider possible causes for delirium. Consult with the health care provider immediately. See interventions for Acute **Confusion.**
- If the client has chronic confusion caused by dementia, implement individualized strategies to enhance communication. *Assessment of specific receptive and expressive language abilities is needed to understand the client's communication difficulties and facilitate communication. See interventions for Chronic* **Confusion.**
- Ask family to stay with the client to assist with activities of daily living and prevent the client from accidentally falling or pulling out tubes.
- ▲ If the client is unsteady on his or her feet, have two nursing staff members alongside when walking the client. Use facility-approved mobility devices to assist with client ambulation (e.g., gait belts, walkers). Consider referral to physical therapy for gait training and strengthening. *The client can walk independently, but the nurse can rapidly ensure safety if the client becomes weak or unsteady. Interprofessional care is most comprehensive and beneficial to the client (Grabiner, 2013).*
- Place a fall-prone client in a room that is near the nurses' station. *Such placement allows more frequent observation of the client.*
- Help clients sit in a stable chair with armrests. Avoid use of wheelchairs except for transportation as needed. *Clients are likely to fall when left in a wheelchair because they may stand up without locking the wheels or removing the footrests.*
- ▲ Refer to physical therapy or other programs for exercise programs that target strength, balance, flexibility, or endurance. **EB:** *Programs with at least two of these components have been shown to decrease the rate of falling and number of people falling (Gillespie et al, 2009; National Council on Aging, 2015).*

 Geriatric

- Assess mobility and gait speed using the Timed Up & Go Test. Ask the client to stand up from a standard arm chair, walk 10 feet (or 3 meters), turn around, walk back to the chair, and sit down (Podsiadlo &

● = Independent; ▲ = Collaborative; **EBN** = Evidence-Based Nursing; **EB** = Evidence-Based

Richardson, 1991). This should be done with the client wearing usual footwear. *Performance on this screening exam demonstrates the client's mobility. If the client completes the test in less than 10 seconds, he or she is considered freely mobile. If completing the test takes 10 to 19 seconds, then the client is considered to be mostly independent in mobility. If the client takes 20 to 29 seconds, then the client is considered to have variable mobility. If the client takes 30 or more seconds, he or she is considered to have impaired mobility, and is more likely to be dependent on others and more likely to sustain a fall (Podsiadlo & Richardson, 1991).*

- ● Complete a fall risk assessment for older adults in acute care using a valid and reliable tool such as the Hendrich II Fall Risk Model. *It is quick to administer and provides a determination of risk for falling based on gender, mental and emotional status, symptoms of dizziness, and known categories of medications increasing risk (Hendrich, Bender, & Nyhuis, 2003; Hendrich, 2016). This tool screens for primary prevention of falls and is integral in a postfall assessment for the secondary prevention of falls (Goodwin et al, 2014; Hendrich, 2016).*

- ▲ If there is new onset of falling, assess for laboratory abnormalities, and signs and symptoms of infection and dehydration, blood glucose level for diabetics, and check blood pressure and pulse rate with client in supine, sitting, and standing positions for hypotension and orthostatic hypotension. If the client has borderline high blood pressure, the risk of falling because of the administration of antihypertensives may outweigh the benefits of the antihypertensive medication. Discuss with the health care provider on a client-to-client basis. *If orthostatic hypotension is present and there is minimal change in the heart rate, most likely the baroreceptors are not working to maintain blood pressure on arising. This is common in older adults and may be caused by hypovolemia resulting from the excessive use of diuretics, vasodilators, or other types of drugs; dehydration; or prolonged bed rest as well as cardiovascular disease, neurological disease, or the adverse effects of another medication (NINDS, 2018). Insertion of a pacemaker can reduce falls in people with frequent falls associated with carotid sinus hypersensitivity, which is a condition that may cause changes in heart rate and blood pressure (Gillespie et al, 2009).*

- ● Complete a fear of falling assessment for older adults. This includes measuring fear of falling, or the level of concern about falling, and falls self-efficacy, which is the degree of confidence a person has in performing common activities of daily living without falling. Fear of falling may be measured by a single-item question asking about the presence of fear of falling or rating severity of fear of falling on a 1 to 4 Likert scale as is commonly done in studies. Falls self-efficacy may be measured using a valid and reliable tool such as the Falls Efficacy Scale-International (Yardley et al, 2005; Greenberg, 2011, 2012; Greenberg et al, 2016).

- ● Encourage the client to wear glasses and use walking aids when ambulating.

- ● If the client experiences dizziness because of orthostatic hypotension when getting up, teach methods to decrease dizziness, such as rising slowly, remaining seated several minutes before standing, flexing feet upward several times while sitting, sitting down immediately if feeling dizzy, and trying to have someone present when standing. **CEB/EB:** *Always have the client dangle at the bedside before standing to evaluate for postural hypotension. Watch the client closely for dizziness during increased activity. Postural hypotension can be detected in up to 30% of older clients. These methods can help prevent falls and maintain adequate fluid intake (Tinetti, 2003; Goodwin et al, 2014).*

- ▲ If the client is experiencing syncope, determine symptoms that occur before syncope, and note medications that the client is taking. Refer for medical care. The circumstances surrounding syncope often suggest the cause. *Use of many medications, including diuretics, antihypertensives, digoxin, beta-blockers, and calcium channel blockers, can cause syncope. Use of the tilt table can be diagnostic in incidences of syncope (Fick & Mion, 2013; Goodwin et al, 2014).*

- ▲ Observe client for signs of anemia, and refer to health care provider for testing if appropriate.

- ● Evaluate client for chronic alcohol intake and mental health and neurological function.

- ▲ Refer to physical therapy for strength training, using free weights or machines, and suggest participation in exercise programs. *Exercise can prevent falls in older people. Greater relative effects are seen in programs that include exercises that challenge balance, use a higher dose of exercise, and do not include a walking program. Service providers can use these findings to design and implement exercise programs for falls prevention (Grabiner, 2013; Hirase et al, 2014; National Council on Aging, 2015).*

- ▲ Evidence-based guidelines for preventing falls in older adults were published by the American Geriatrics Society (AGS) and British Geriatrics Society (BGS) collaboratively and specify recommendations for all clinical settings. These recommendations include screening and assessment and interventions. Examples of interventions include (1) exercise for balance and for gait and strength training, such as tai chi or physical therapy; (2) environmental adaptation to reduce fall risk factors in the home and in daily activities; (3) cataract surgery when indicated; (4) medication reduction with particular attention to medications

● = Independent;   ▲ = Collaborative;   **EBN** = Evidence-Based Nursing;   **EB** = Evidence-Based

that affect the brain such as sleeping medications and antidepressants; (5) assessment and treatment of postural hypotension; (6) identification and appropriate treatment of foot problems; (7) vitamin D supplementation for those with vitamin D deficiency (The American Geriatrics Society [AGS], 2011).

Home Care

- Some of the previously mentioned interventions may be adapted for home care use.
- Implement evidence-based fall prevention practices in community settings and home health care programs for older adults (National Council on Aging, 2015).
- ▲ If delirium is present, assess for cause of delirium and/or falls with the use of an interprofessional team. Consult with the health care provider immediately. Assess and monitor for acute changes in cognition and behavior. *An acute and fluctuating change in cognition and behavior is the classic presentation of delirium. Delirium is reversible and should be considered a medical emergency. Delirium can become chronic if untreated, and clients may be discharged from hospitals to home care in states of undiagnosed delirium.* EB: *Falls may be a precipitating event or an indication of frailty consistent with delirium (Goodwin et al, 2014).*
- Assess home environment for threats to safety including clutter, slippery floors, scatter rugs, and other potential hazards. Additionally, assess external environment (e.g., uneven pavement, unleveled stairs/steps). *Clients suffering from impaired mobility, impaired visual acuity, and neurological dysfunction, including dementia and other cognitive functional deficits, are all at risk for injury from common hazards. These recommendations were shown to be effective to reduce falls (Tinetti, 2003; AGS, 2011; Goodwin et al, 2014; National Council on Aging, 2015).*
- ▲ Institute a home-based, nurse-delivered exercise program to reduce falls or refer to physical therapy services for client and family education of safe transfers and ambulation and for strengthening exercises for the client (Grabiner, 2013; National Council on Aging, 2015).
- ▲ Instruct the client and family or caregivers on how to correct identified hazards for those with visual impairment. Refer to physical and occupational therapy services for assistance if needed. EB: *Interventions to improve home safety were shown to be effective in people at high risk, such as those with severe visual impairment (Gillespie et al, 2009; National Council on Aging, 2015).*
- ▲ Use a multifactorial assessment along with interventions targeted to the identified risk factors. Key components of the interventions include evaluating need for all medications, balance, gait and strength training, use of strategies to deal with postural hypotension if present, home safety evaluation with needed modifications, and any needed cardiovascular treatment. EB: *As people age, they may fall more often for multiple reasons including problems with balance, poor vision, and dementia. Fear of falling can result in self-restricted activity levels (Gillespie et al, 2009; National Council on Aging, 2015).*
- If the client lives alone or spends a great deal of time alone, teach the client what to do if he or she falls and cannot get up, and make sure he or she has a personal emergency response system or a mobile phone that is available from the floor (Tinetti, 2003; AGS, 2011; National Council on Aging, 2015).
- Ensure appropriate nonglare lighting in the home. Ask the client to install indoor strip or "runway" type of lighting to baseboards to help clients balance. Install motion-sensitive lighting that turns on automatically when the client gets out of bed to go to the bathroom.
- Have the client wear supportive, low-heeled shoes with good traction when ambulating. Avoid use of slip-on footwear. Wear appropriate footwear in inclement weather. *Supportive shoes provide the client with better balance and protect the client from instability on uneven surfaces. Anti-slip shoe devices worn in icy conditions have been shown to reduce falls (Gillespie et al, 2009; AGS, 2011; National Council on Aging, 2015).*
- Provide a signaling device for clients who wander or are at risk for falls. *Orienting a vulnerable client to a safety net relieves the anxiety of the client and caregiver and allows for rapid response to a crisis situation.*
- Provide medical identification bracelet for clients at risk for injury from dementia, diabetes, seizures, or other medical disorders.
- Suggest a tai chi class designed for older adults and selected clients who have sufficient balance to participate. EB: *Participation in once per week tai chi classes for 16 weeks can prevent falls in relatively healthy community-dwelling older people (Voukelatos et al, 2007; AGS, 2011).*

Client/Family Teaching and Discharge Planning

- Safety Guidelines. Teach the client and the family about the fall reduction measures that are being used to prevent falls (The Joint Commission, 2017).

● = Independent;   ▲ = Collaborative;   EBN = Evidence-Based Nursing;   EB = Evidence-Based

F

- Teach the client how to safely ambulate at home, including using safety measures such as handrails in bathroom, reaching for items on high shelves, and avoiding carrying things or performing other tasks while walking.
- Teach the client the importance of maintaining a regular exercise program. If the client is afraid of falling while walking outside, suggest that he or she walk the length of a local mall. *Exercise can prevent falls in older people. Greater relative effects are seen in programs that include exercises that challenge balance and use a higher dose of exercise than just walking programs (Sherrington et al, 2008; AGS, 2011; Grabiner, 2013; Hirase et al, 2014).*

REFERENCES

Capezuti, E. (2004). Minimizing the use of restrictive devices in dementia patients at risk for falling. *The Nursing Clinics of North America, 39,* 625.

Cotter, V. T., & Evans, L. (2012). *Try This:® Best practices in nursing care to older adults. Fall risk assessment for older adults: Avoiding restraints in older adults with dementia.* New York: Hartford Institute for Geriatric Nursing and Alzheimer's Association. Retrieved from https://consultgeri.org/try-this/dementia/issue -d1.pdf. (Accessed 29 October 2017).

Evans, L. K., & Cotter, V. T. (2008). Avoiding restraints in patients with dementia: Understanding, prevention, and management are the keys. *The American Journal of Nursing, 108*(3), 40–49.

Fick, D., & Mion, L. (2013). *Try This:® Best practices in nursing care to older adults. Fall risk assessment for older adults: Assessing and managing delirium in older adults with dementia.* New York: Hartford Institute for Geriatric Nursing. Retrieved from https://consultgeri.org/try-this/dementia/issue-d8.pdf. (Accessed 29 October 2017).

Gillespie, L. D., Robertson, M. C., Gillespie, W. J., et al. (2009). Interventions for preventing falls in older people living in the community. *Cochrane Database of Systematic Reviews,* (2), CD007146.

Goodwin, V. A., Abbott, R. A., Whear, R., et al. (2014). Multiple component interventions for preventing falls and fall related injuries among older people: Systematic review and meta-analysis. *BMC Geriatrics, 14,* 15–21.

Grabiner, M. D. (2013). Exercise-based fall prevention programmes decrease fall-related injuries. *Evidence-Based Nursing, 17*(4), 125.

Gray-Miceli, D. (2016). Preventing falls in acute care. In M. Boltz, E. Capezuti, T. Fulmer, et al. (Eds.), *Evidence-based geriatric nursing protocols for best practice* (5th ed.). New York: Springer Publishing Company, LLC.

Greenberg, S. A. (2011). *Try This:® Best practices in nursing care to older adults. Fall risk assessment for older adults: Falls Efficacy Scale-International (FES-I).* New York: Hartford Institute for Geriatric Nursing. Retrieved from https://consultgeri.org/try-this/general-assessment/issue-29. (Accessed 29 October 2017).

Greenberg, S. A. (2012). Analysis of measurement tools of fear of falling among high-risk, community-dwelling older adults. *Clinical Nursing Research, 21*(1), 113–130. doi:10.1177/1054773811433824.

Greenberg, S. A. (2016). *Try This:® Issue 16: The 2015 American Geriatrics Society updated beers criteria for potentially inappropriate medication use in older adults.* New York: Hartford Institute for Geriatric Nursing and The American Geriatrics Society. Retrieved from https://consultgeri.org/try-this/general-assessment/16beers2016-r2.pdf. (Accessed 29 October 2017).

Greenberg, S. A., Sullivan-Marx, E., Sommers, M. S., et al. (2016). Measuring fear of falling among high-risk, urban, community-dwelling older adults. *Geriatric Nursing, 37*(6), 489–495. doi:10.1016/j.gerinurse.2016.08.018.

Hendrich, A. (2016). *Try This:® Best practices in nursing care to older adults. Fall risk assessment for older adults: The Hendrich II Fall Risk Model™.* New York: Hartford Institute for Geriatric Nursing.

Retrieved from https://consultgeri.org/try-this/general-assessment/issue-8.pdf. (Accessed 29 October 2017).

Hendrich, A. L., Bender, P. S., & Nyhuis, A. (2003). Validation of the Hendrich II Fall Risk Model: A large concurrent CASE/control study of hospitalized patients. *Applied Nursing Research, 16*(1), 9–21.

Hirase, T., Inokuchi, S., Matsusaka, N., et al. (2014). A modified fall risk assessment tool that is specific to physical function predicts falls in community-dwelling elderly people. *Journal of Geriatric Physical Therapy (2001), 37,* 159–165.

McCarter-Bayer, A., Bayer, F., & Hall, K. (2005). Preventing falls in acute care: An innovative approach. *Journal of Gerontological Nursing, 31*(3), 25.

Mion, L. C., Fogel, J., Sandhu, S., et al. (2001). Outcomes following physical restraint reduction programs in two acute care hospitals. *The Joint Commission Journal on Quality Improvement, 27*(11), 605–618.

National Council on Aging. (2015). *Falls Free®: 2015 National Falls Prevention Action Plan.* Retrieved from https://www.ncoa.org/resources/2015-falls-free-national-falls-prevention-action-plan/. (Accessed 29 October 2017).

National Institute of Neurological Disorders and Stroke (NINDS). (2018). *Orthostatic hypotension information page.* Retrieved from https://www.ninds.nih.gov/Disorders/All-Disorders/Orthostati c-Hypotension-Information-Page. (Accessed 29 October 2017).

Podsiadlo, D., & Richardson, S. (1991). The timed "Up & Go": A test of basic functional mobility for frail elderly persons. *Journal of the American Geriatrics Society, 39*(2), 142–148.

The American Geriatrics Society (AGS). (2011). 2010 AGS/BGS clinical practice guideline. *Prevention of falls in older persons,* Summary of recommendations. Retrieved from https://hsctc.org/wp-content/uploads/2017/07/2010-American-Geriatrics-Society-Guideli ne_-Prevention-of-Falls-in-Older-Persons.pdf.

The American Geriatrics Society Beers Criteria Update Expert Panel. (2015). American Geriatrics Society 2015 updated beers criteria for potentially inappropriate medication use in older adults. *Journal of the American Geriatrics Society, 63*(11), 2227–2246. doi:10.1111/jgs.13702. Retrieved from http://onlinelibrary.wiley.com/doi/10.1111/jgs.13702/pdf.

The Joint Commission. (2017). *Accreditation program: Home care.* 2017 National Patient Safety Goals. Goal 9. Reduce the risk of falls. Retrieved from https://www.jointcommission.org/assets/1/6/NPSG_Chapter_OME_Jan2017.pdf. (Accessed 8 October 2009).

Tinetti, M. E. (2003). Preventing falls in elderly persons. *The New England Journal of Medicine, 348*(1), 42–49.

Voukelatos, A., Cumming, R. G., Lord, S. R., et al. (2007). A randomized controlled trial of tai chi for the prevention of falls: The Central Sydney tai chi trial. *Journal of the American Geriatrics Society, 55*(8), 1185–1191.

Yardley, L., Beyer, N., Hauer, K., et al. (2005). Development and initial validation of the Falls Efficacy Scale-International (FES-I). *Age and Ageing, 34*(6), 614–619.

● = Independent;   ▲ = Collaborative;   **EBN** = Evidence-Based Nursing;   **EB** = Evidence-Based

Dysfunctional Family processes *Shelley Sadler, BSN, MSN, APRN, WHNP-BC*

NANDA-I

Definition

Family functioning which fails to support the well-being of its members.

Defining Characteristics

Behavioral

Agitation; alteration in concentration; blaming; broken promises; chaos; complicated grieving; conflict avoidance; contradictory communication pattern; controlling communication pattern; criticizing; decrease in physical contact; denial of problems; dependency; difficulty having fun; difficulty with intimate relationships; difficulty with life cycle transitions; disturbances in academic performance in children; enabling substance use pattern; escalating conflict; failure to accomplish developmental tasks; harsh self-judgment; immaturity; inability to accept a wide range of feelings; inability to accept help; inability to adapt to change; inability to deal constructively with traumatic experiences; inability to express wide range of feelings; inability to meet the emotional needs of its members; inability to meet the security needs of its members; inability to meet the spiritual needs of its members; inability to receive help appropriately; inappropriate anger expression; ineffective communication skills; insufficient knowledge about substance abuse; insufficient problem solving skills; lying; manipulation; nicotine addiction; orientation favors tension relief rather than goal attainment; paradoxical communication pattern; power struggles; rationalization; refusal to get help; seeking of affirmation; seeking of approval; self-blame; social isolation; special occasions centered on substance use; stress-related physical illnesses; substance abuse; unreliable behavior; verbal abuse of children; verbal abuse of parent; verbal abuse of partner

Feelings

Abandonment; anger; anxiety; confuses love and pity; confusion; depression; dissatisfaction; distress; embarrassment; emotional isolation; emotionally controlled by others; failure; fear; feeling different from others; feeling misunderstood; feeling unloved; frustration; guilt; hopelessness; hostility; hurt; insecurity; lack of identity; lingering resentment; loneliness; loss; loss of identity; low self-esteem; mistrust; moodiness; powerlessness; rejection; repressed emotions; shame; taking responsibility for substance misuser's behavior; tension; unhappiness; vulnerability; worthlessness

Roles and Relationships

Change in role function; chronic family problems; closed communication systems; conflict between partners; deterioration in family relationships; diminished ability of family members to relate to each other for mutual growth and maturation; disruption in family rituals; disruption in family roles; disturbance in family dynamics; family denial; inconsistent parenting; ineffective communication with partner; insufficient cohesiveness; insufficient family respect for autonomy of its members; insufficient family respect for individuality of its members; insufficient relationship skills; neglect of obligation to family member; pattern of rejection; perceived insufficient parental support; triangulating family relationships

Related Factors

Addictive personality; ineffective coping skills; insufficient problem-solving skills; substance misuse

At-Risk Population

Economically disadvantaged; family history of resistance to treatment; family history of substance misuse; genetic predisposition to substance misuse

NOC (Nursing Outcomes Classification)

Suggested NOC Outcomes

Family Coping; Family Functioning; Family Health Status; Substance Addiction Consequences

● = Independent;   ▲ = Collaborative;   EBN = Evidence-Based Nursing;   EB = Evidence-Based

Example NOC Outcome with Indicators

Family Coping as evidenced by the following indicators: Confronts/manages family problems/Involves family members in decision-making. (Rate the outcome and indicators of **Family Coping:** 1 = never demonstrated, 2 = rarely demonstrated, 3 = sometimes demonstrated, 4 = often demonstrated, 5 = consistently demonstrated [see Section I].)

Client Outcomes

Family/Client Will (Specify Time Frame)

- State one way that alcoholism has affected the health of the family
- Identify three healthy coping behaviors that family members can use to facilitate a shift toward improved family functioning
- Identify one Al-Anon meeting from the Al-Anon meeting schedule that family members express a desire to attend
- Attend different types of meetings (lead, big book, discussion, beginner's meeting) to find a good match and commit to attending that group regularly

NIC   (Nursing Interventions Classification)

Suggested NIC Interventions

Family Process Maintenance; Substance Use Treatment

Example Activities—Family Process Maintenance

Identify effects of role changes on family process; Assist family members to use existing support mechanisms

Nursing Interventions and *Rationales*

- Refer to care plans for Ineffective **Denial** and Defensive **Coping** for additional interventions.
- ▲ Behavioral screening and intervention (BSI) should be integrated into all health care settings. Different terminology has evolved for screening, intervention, and referral for various behavioral issues. The five As—ask, advise, assess, assist, and arrange—apply to tobacco use. Screening, brief intervention, and referral to treatment (SBIRT) pertains to alcohol and drug use. **EB:** *The US Preventive Services Task Force recommends universal screening and intervention for tobacco use, excessive drinking, and depression. These services improve health outcomes, decrease health care costs, enhance public safety, and generate substantial return on investment (Moyer, 2013; Babor, Del Boca, & Bray, 2017).*
- Screen clients for at-risk drinking during routine primary care visits and before surgery using the Alcohol Use Disorders Identification Test (AUDIT). **EB:** *Complications after total joint arthroplasty were significantly related to alcohol misuse in this group of male patients treated at a Veteran Health Administration (VHA) facility. The AUDIT-C has three simple questions that can be incorporated into a preoperative evaluation and can alert the treatment team to patients with increased postoperative risk (Moyer, 2013).*
- Provide brief education and individual counsel as a routine part of primary care. **EB:** *Brief interventions may be effective in helping patients engage in nonharmful drinking. The objective of the current study tested the implementation of a telephone-based brief intervention (telephone care management [TCM]) with heavy drinkers in primary care. The addition of TCM to primary care provider standard care (screening and brief advice) was compared with standard care alone. Both groups significantly decreased their drinking over time, with 40% of participants no longer engaging in heavy drinking at follow-up. Both groups decreased the number of drinking days and the average number of drinks per day over the follow-up period. Participants reported a decrease in alcohol use frequency and alcohol-related problems (Helstrom et al, 2014).*
- Refer for family therapy and other family-oriented resources. **EB:** *Evidence-based interventions targeting affected family members have been shown to improve health outcomes for all family members, result in better addiction treatment outcomes, and prevent adolescent substance use (Ventura & Bagley, 2017).*
- ▲ Refer for possible use of medication-assisted treatment to address substance use. **EB:** *The Food and Drug Administration has approved three medications for treating alcohol dependence. Naltrexone can help people reduce heavy drinking; acamprosate makes it easier to maintain abstinence; and disulfiram blocks the breakdown (metabolism) of alcohol by the body, causing unpleasant symptoms such as nausea and flushing of the skin. Those unpleasant effects can help some people avoid drinking while taking disulfiram. It is important to*

● = Independent;   ▲ = Collaborative;   EBN = Evidence-Based Nursing;   EB = Evidence-Based

remember that not all people will respond to medications, but for a subset of individuals, they can be an important tool in overcoming alcohol dependence (NIH, 2014).

Pediatric

▲ Encourage early intervention. When parental depression, childhood exposure to conflict and violence, and childhood experience with abuse and neglect coexist with parental substance abuse their children are more likely to engage in increased teacher-rated unfavorable student behavioral problems. **EB:** *Early intervention with children of substance abusers (COSA) is necessary to reach children while they are more receptive to treatment (Usher, McShane, & Dwyer, 2015).*

● Encourage parent communication about alcohol use with adolescents. **EB:** *NIH (2017) identified parent–adolescent communication as important in delaying the onset and escalation of alcohol use.*

▲ Consider the Community Reinforcement Approach (CRA), which encourages clients to become progressively involved in alternative non–substance-related pleasant social activities and to work on enhancing the enjoyment they receive within the "community" of their family and job. **EB:** *CRA, originally developed for individuals with alcohol use disorders, has been successfully used to treat a variety of substance use disorders for more than 35 years. Based on operant conditioning, CRA helps adolescents rearrange their lifestyles so that healthy, drug-free living becomes rewarding and thereby competes with alcohol and drug use (Godley et al, 2014).*

▲ Educate family members about available educational and support programs and encourage no/limited alcohol use in the home. **EBN:** *Both individual and multiperson interventions exert an influential role in family-based therapy for treatment of adolescent drug abuse (Gilligan et al, 2016).*

● Encourage adolescents to attend a 12-step program. **EB:** *Wendt et al (2017) demonstrated that adolescents who attend 12-step groups after alcohol and other drug (AOD) treatment are more likely to remain abstinent and to avoid relapse.*

● Provide interactive school-based drug-prevention program to middle school students. **EB:** *A meta-analysis found support for the use of interactive school-based programs to prevent cannabis use among middle school students in North America (Lize et al, 2017).*

Geriatric

● Include the assessment of possible alcohol abuse when assessing older family members. **EB:** *Alcohol abuse and dependence in older people are important problems that frequently remain undetected by health services (Draper et al, 2015). The majority of older alcoholics are married, have low education levels, and do not belong to high social classes (Draper et al, 2015).*

Multicultural

● Acknowledge racial/ethnic differences at the onset of care. **EBN:** *Acknowledgment of race/ethnicity issues will enhance communication, establish rapport, and promote treatment outcomes (Giger & Davidhizar, 2013).*

● Use a family-centered approach when working with Latino, Asian American, African American, and Native American clients. **EBN:** *American Indian families may be extended structures that could exert powerful influences over functioning (George, Duran, & Norris, 2014). Family therapy is important in addressing the needs of Hispanic families with adolescent substance abusers (George, Duran, & Norris, 2014).*

● Some less acculturated Latino families may be unwilling to discuss family issues with health care providers until they perceive a close personal relationship with the provider. **EBN:** *Some Latino families may believe that personal problems should be kept private and may not respond to the health care provider until there is an established personal relationship (George, Duran, & Norris, 2014).*

● Work with families in a way that incorporates cultural elements. **CEB:** *Activities such as tundra walks and time with older adults supported in treatment were used successfully for substance abuse treatment with Yup'ik and Cup'ik Eskimos (Mills, 2003).*

Home Care

Note: In the community setting, alcoholism as a cause of dysfunctional family processes must be considered in two categories: (1) when the client suffers personally from the illness, and (2) when a significant other suffers from the illness, that is, the client is not the active alcoholic but may depend on the alcoholic for caregiving. The following considerations apply to both situations with appropriate adaptation for the circumstances.

● The previous interventions may be adapted for home care use.

● Work with family members to support a sense of valued fit on their part; include them in treatment planning and identify the importance of their roles in the client's care. At the same time, encourage the

● = Independent; ▲ = Collaborative; **EBN** = Evidence-Based Nursing; **EB** = Evidence-Based

pursuit of positive outside activities that enhance their sense of belonging. CEBN: *Sense of belonging (valued fit) has been identified as a buffer to depression among both depressed and nondepressed individuals with a family history of alcoholism. A buffering effect was not found for individuals with a family history of drug abuse (Sargent et al, 2002).*

- Educate client and family regarding the interactions of alcohol use with medications and the therapeutic regimen. *Increased awareness of drug interactions decreases the chance of relapse caused by over-the-counter and other medications (Shapiro, 2015).*
- ▲ Refer for psychiatric home health care services for client reassurance and implementation of therapeutic regimen. CEB: *Twelve studies (five randomized controlled trials, one quasi-experimental study, and six uncontrolled cohort studies) found that home and community-based treatment of psychiatric symptoms of socially isolated older adults with mental illness was associated with improved or maintained psychiatric status. All randomized controlled trials reported improved depressive symptoms, and one reported improved overall psychiatric symptoms (Van Citters & Bartells, 2004).*
- ▲ Consider the use of a smartphone-based intervention for alcohol use disorders. *Participants in a pilot study indicated the smartphone provided numerous features for addressing ongoing drinking, craving, connection with supportive others, managing life problems, high-risk location alerting, and activity scheduling. These intervention modules were helpful in highlighting alcohol use patterns. Tools related to managing alcohol craving, monitoring consumption, and identifying triggers to drink were rated by participants as particularly helpful. Participants also demonstrated significant reductions in hazardous alcohol use while using the system (Dulin, Gonzalez, & Campbell, 2014).*

Client/Family Teaching and Discharge Planning

- Suggest that the client complete a confidential Internet self-screening test for identification of problems and suggestions for treatment if a problem with alcohol is suspected. Many tools are available. *These screenings help individuals to assess their own alcohol consumption patterns to determine whether their drinking is likely harming their health or increasing their risk for future harm. Education and referrals urge those whose drinking is harmful or hazardous to take positive action and informs all adults who consume alcohol about guidelines and caveats for lower risk drinking (Donoghue et al, 2014).*
- Provide education for the family. EB: *Family education facilitates understanding of the disease and its causes, effects, and treatment (US Department of Health and Human Services, 2014).*
- Facilitate participation in mutual help groups (MHGs). EB: *MHGs appear to mobilize the same change processes, such as coping, motivation, and self-efficacy, which are mobilized by many different types of professionally led groups (Kelly et al, 2013).*

REFERENCES

Babor, T. F., Del Boca, F., & Bray, J. W. (2017). Screening, Brief Intervention and Referral to Treatment: Implications of SAMHSA's SBIRT initiative for substance abuse policy and practice. *Addiction (Abingdon, England), 112,* 110–117. doi:10.1111/add.13675.

Donoghue, K., Patton, R., Phillips, T., et al. (2014). The effectiveness of electronic screening and brief intervention for reducing levels of alcohol consumption: A systematic review and meta-analysis. *Journal of Medical Internet Research, 16*(6), E142. doi:10.2196/jmir.3193.

Draper, B., Ridley, N., Johnco, C., et al. (2015). Screening for alcohol and substance use for older people in geriatric hospital and community health settings. *International Psychogeriatrics, 27*(1), 157–166. doi:10.1017/S1041610214002014.

Dulin, P., Gonzalez, V., & Campbell, K. (2014). Results of a pilot test of a self-administered smartphone-based treatment system for alcohol use disorders: Usability and early outcomes. *Substance Abuse, 35*(2), 168–175.

George, S., Duran, N., & Norris, K. (2014). A systematic review of barriers and facilitators to minority research participation among African Americans, Latinos, Asian Americans, and Pacific Islanders. *American Journal of Public Health.* Retrieved from http://

ajph.aphapublications.org/doi/full/10.2105/AJPH.2013.301706. (Accessed 12 February 2018).

Giger, J., & Davidhizar, R. (2013). *Transcultural nursing: Assessment and intervention* (6th ed.). St Louis: Mosby.

Gilligan, C., Wolfenden, L., Foxcroft, D. R., et al. (2016). Family-based prevention programs for alcohol use in young people. *Cochrane Database of Systematic Reviews,* (8), CD012287. doi:10.1002/14651858.CD012287.

Godley, S., Hunter, B., Fernández-Artamendi, S., et al. (2014). A comparison of treatment outcomes for adolescent community reinforcement approach participants with and without co-occurring problems. *Journal of Substance Abuse Treatment, 46*(4), 463–471. Retrieved from https://doi.org/10.1016/j.jsat.2013.10.013.

Helstrom, A., Ingram, E., Wei, W., et al. (2014). Treating heavy drinking in primary care practices: Evaluation of a telephone-based intervention program. *Addictive Disorders & Their Treatment, 13*(3), 101–109.

Kelly, J. F., & Yeterian, J. D. (2013). Mutual-help groups for alcohol and other substance use disorders. In B. S. McCrady & E. E. Epstein (Eds.), *Addictions: A comprehensive guidebook* (pp. 500–525). New York: Oxford University Press.

● = Independent;   ▲ = Collaborative;   EBN = Evidence-Based Nursing;   EB = Evidence-Based

Lize, S. E., et al. (2017). A meta-analysis of the effectiveness of interactive middle school cannabis prevention programs. *Prevention Science, 18*(1), 50–60. doi:10.1007/s11121-016-0723-7.

Mills, P. A. (2003). Incorporating Yup'ik and Cup'ik Eskimo traditions into behavioral health treatment. *Journal of Psychoactive Drugs, 35*(1), 85–88.

Moyer, V. (2013). Screening and behavioral counseling interventions in primary care to reduce alcohol misuse: U.S. Preventative Task Force Recommendation Statement. *Annals of Internal Medicine, 159*(3), 210–218.

NIH, National Institute on Alcohol Abuse and Alcoholism. (2014). *NIH publication no. 14-7974.* Retrieved from http://pubs.niaaa.nih.gov/publications/Treatment/treatment.htm#chapter02. (Accessed 21 January 2018).

NIH, National Institute on Alcohol Abuse and Alcoholism. (2017). *Parenting to prevent childhood alcohol use.* Retrieved from https://pubs.niaaa.nih.gov/publications/adolescentflyer/adolFlyer.pdf. (Accessed 11 February 2018).

Sargent, J., Williams, R. A., Hagerty, B., et al. (2002). Sense of belonging as a buffer against depressive symptoms. *Journal of the American Psychiatric Nurses Association, 8*(4), 120–129.

Shapiro, M. (2015). *8 Medicines that don't mix with alcohol.* Retrieved from https://www.aarp.org/health/healthy-living/info-2015/alcohol-drug-interactions-side-effects.html. (Accessed 12 February 2018).

U.S. Department of Health and Human Services. (2014). *What is substance abuse treatment? A booklet for families.* Retrieved from http://www.samhsa.gov. (Accessed 28 January 2018).

Usher, A., McShane, K., & Dwyer, C. (2015). *A realist review of family-based interventions for children of substance abusing parents.* Retrieved from http://www.ncbi.nlm.nih.gov/pmc/articles/PMC4683863/. (Accessed 1 December 2017).

Van Citters, A. D., & Bartels, S. J. (2004). A systematic review of the effectiveness of community-based mental health outreach services for older adults. *Psychiatric Services: A Journal of the American Psychiatric Association, 55*(11), 1237–1249.

Ventura, A. S., & Bagley, S. M. (2017). To improve substance use disorder prevention, treatment and recovery: Engage the family. *Journal of Addiction Medicine, 11*(5), 339–341. doi:10.1097/ADM.0000000000000331.

Wendt, D. C., Hallgren, K. A., Daley, D. C., et al. (2017). Predictors and outcomes of twelve-step sponsorship of stimulant users: Secondary analyses of a multisite randomized clinical trial. *Journal of Studies on Alcohol and Drugs, 78*(2), 287–295.

F

Interrupted Family processes   *Marina Martinez-Kratz, MS, RN, CNE*

NANDA-I

Definition

Break in the continuity of family functioning which fails to support the well-being of its members.

Defining Characteristics

Change in availability for affective responsiveness; change in family conflict resolution; change in family satisfaction; change in intimacy; change in participation for problem-solving; assigned tasks change; change in communication pattern; change in somatization; change in stress reduction behavior; changes in expressions of conflict with community resources; changes in expressions of isolation from community resources; changes in participation for decision-making; changes in relationship pattern; decrease in available emotional support; decrease in mutual support; ineffective task completion; power alliance change; ritual change

Related Factors

Changes in interaction with community; power shift among family members; shift in family roles

At-Risk Population

Change in family finances; change in family social status; developmental crisis; developmental transition; situational crisis

Associated Condition

Shift in health status of a family member

NOC   (Nursing Outcomes Classification)

Suggested NOC Outcomes

Family Coping; Family Functioning; Family Normalization; Psychosocial Adjustment: Life Change, Role Performance

● = Independent;   ▲ = Collaborative;   EBN = Evidence-Based Nursing;   EB = Evidence-Based

F

Example NOC Outcome with Indicators
Family Coping as evidenced by the following indicators: Confronts/manages family problems/Involves family members in decision-making. (Rate the outcome and indicators of **Family Coping:** 1 = never demonstrated, 2 = rarely demonstrated, 3 = sometimes demonstrated, 4 = often demonstrated, 5 = consistently demonstrated [see Section I].)

Client Outcomes

Family/Client Will (Specify Time Frame)

- Express feelings (family)
- Identify ways to cope effectively and use appropriate support systems (family)
- Treat impaired family member as normally as possible to avoid overdependence (family)
- Meet physical, psychosocial, and spiritual needs of members or seek appropriate assistance (family)
- Demonstrate knowledge of illness or injury, treatment modalities, and prognosis (family)
- Participate in the development of the plan of care to the best of ability (significant person)

NIC   (Nursing Interventions Classification)

Suggested NIC Interventions

Family Integrity Promotion; Family Process Maintenance; Normalization Promotion

Example NIC Activities—Family Integrity Promotion
Collaborate with family in problem-solving and decision-making; Counsel family members on additional effective coping skills for their own use

Nursing Interventions and *Rationales*

- Recognize informal roles in medical decision-making by family members. EBN: *Informal roles emerge in critical situations to help fill the gaps in how family members respond to the challenge of end-of-life decision-making (Connor & Chase, 2015).*
- Acknowledge the range of emotions and feelings that may be experienced when the health status of a family member changes. EBN: *Nurses can better support caregivers regarding their perception of family support and expressive family functioning (Svavarsdottir & Sigurdardottir, 2013).*
- Encourage family members to list their personal strengths and available resources. EBN: *Families provide the main support network, and family strengths are closely associated with the family use of resources (Coym, 2013).*
- Establish relationships among clients, their families, and health care professionals. EBN: *A progressively engaging approach to relationships with clients and their families emphasizes trust and reciprocity, which supports joint decision-making with nurses in acute care settings (Segaric & Hall, 2015).*
- Encourage family to visit the client; adjust visiting hours to accommodate the family's schedule. EBN: *Incorporating visiting family members in the plan of care is complex and requires balancing the visitor's needs for information and access to a loved one with the nurse's need to safely manage the care of a critically ill individual (Alves et al, 2013).*
- Allow and encourage family members to assist in the client's treatment. EBN: *Support for family members is an essential part of quality end-of-life care for residents, and health care facilities should embrace the opportunity to demonstrate the value of family participation in care (Oliver et al, 2014).*
- Support family members during emotional and conflict type situations in the clinical setting. EBN: *A study found that bereaved parents identified nurses as "good" if the nurses looked out for the parents by providing emotional support, comfort, and using presence (Butler et al, 2018).*
- Anticipate and implement family reunification efforts after a disaster. EBN: *Family reunification after disasters should be prioritized and included in plans at all emergency response levels (Chung & Blake, 2014).*
- Refer to the care plan Readiness for enhanced **Family** processes for additional interventions.

 Pediatric

- Carefully assess potential for reunifying children placed in foster care with their birth parents. EB: *Reunifying children placed in foster care with their birth parents is a primary goal of the child welfare system (Orsi et al, 2018).*

● = Independent;   ▲ = Collaborative;   EBN = Evidence-Based Nursing;   EB = Evidence-Based

- Provide prebirth risk assessments to identify prebirth and postbirth supports for high-risk pregnant women. **EB:** *Prebirth risk assessment is a process by which circumstances affecting an unborn child can be identified and support for mother and infant embedded into care (Harnett et al, 2018).*
- Provide parents with both general information and professional support by family-centered early childhood intervention services to their families. **EB:** *Providing families with general information in addition to specialized information about their children is most important to empower parents and increase family resiliency (Frantz et al, 2018).*
- Encourage and support parents/family to assist in client's care. **EBN:** *Parents need to be able to negotiate with health staff as to what this participation will involve and negotiate new roles for themselves in sharing care of their sick child (Kelly & Kelly, 2013).*
- Assess military families for the influence of deployment on family functioning. **EB:** *A study of families with a service member concurrently deployed at the time of a child neglect incident were at higher risk for failure to provide physical needs, lack of supervision, and educational neglect (Cozza et al, 2018).*
- ▲ Refer parents and other primary caregivers to a mindfulness-based stress reduction (MBSR) program. **EBN:** *Community-based MBSR programs can be an effective intervention to reduce stress and improve psychological well-being for parents and caregivers of children, especially those with developmental disabilities (Bazzano et al, 2013).*

Geriatric

- Encourage family members to be involved in the care of relatives who are in residential care settings. **EBN:** *Family involvement in residential long-term care is important especially when preparing for end-of-life care (Oliver et al, 2014).*
- Support group problem-solving among family caregivers and include the older member. **EBN:** *Health personnel must be aware that family caregiving undergoes a transition, shifting both how and when family members mobilize to meet the needs of the older adult (Wongsawang et al, 2013).*
- ▲ Refer family for counseling with a psychotherapist who is knowledgeable about gerontology.
- Refer to care plan for Readiness for Enhanced **Family** processes for additional interventions.

Multicultural

- Motivate family members to speak openly about illnesses, keeping in mind the importance of ethnic origin. **EBN:** *Recognizing ethnic origin to caregivers' open communication can improve the quality of life to allow family members to derive solutions and face challenges (Bachner et al, 2014).*
- Assess LGBTQ youth for factors that contribute to family rejection. **EB:** *A recent study found that poverty and family instability are often precursors to family rejection and ultimately homelessness for LGBTQ youth (Robinson, 2018a).*
- Refer to the care plan Readiness for Enhanced **Family** processes for additional interventions.

Home Care

- The nursing interventions described in the care plan for Compromised family **Coping** should be used in the home environment with adaptations as necessary.
- Encourage family members to find meaning in life with a serious illness. **EB:** *A study found that families dealing with chronic illness move through the process of healing and eventually shift the focus away from illness and toward living (Robinson, 2018b).*

Client/Family Teaching and Discharge Planning

- Refer to Client/Family Teaching and Discharge Planning in Compromised family **Coping** and Readiness for enhanced family **Coping** for suggestions that may be used with minor adaptations.

REFERENCES

Alves, M. V. M. F. F., Cordeiro, J. G., Bronzato Luppi, C. H., et al. (2013). Experience of family members as a result of children's hospitalization at the intensive care unit. *Investigación y Educación en Enfermería*, 31(2), 191–200.

Bachner, G., Yosef-Sela, N., & Carmel, S. (2014). Open communication with terminally ill cancer patients about illness and death. *Cancer Nursing*, 37(1), 50–58.

Bazzano, A., Wolfe, C., Zylowska, L., et al. (2013). Mindfulness based stress reduction (MBSR) for parents and caregivers of individuals with developmental disabilities: A community-based approach. *Journal of Child and Family Studies*, 22(8), 1–11.

Butler, A. E., et al. (2018). "Some were certainly better than others"—Bereaved parents' judgements of healthcare providers in the paediatric intensive care unit: A grounded theory study. *Intensive and Critical Care Nursing, 45,* 18–24. doi:10.1016/j.iccn.2017 .12.003.

Chung, S., & Blake, N. (2014). Family reunification after disasters. *Clinical Pediatric Emergency Medicine, 15*(4), 334–342. doi:10.1016/j.cpem.2014.09.006.

Connor, N. E., & Chase, S. K. (2015). Decisions and caregiving: End of life among blacks from the perspective of informal caregivers and decision makers. *The American Journal of Hospice & Palliative Care, 32*(4), 454–463. doi:10.1177/1049909114529013.

Coym, E. (2013). The strengths and resources used by families of young women with breast cancer. *The Australian Journal of Cancer Nursing, 14*(2), 10–16.

Cozza, S. J., et al. (2018). Deployment status and child neglect types in the U.S. Army. *Child Maltreatment, 23*(1), 25–33. doi:10.1177/1077559517717638.

Frantz, R., et al. (2018). Families as partners: Supporting family resiliency through early intervention. *Infants & Young Children, 31*(1), 3–19.

Harnett, P. H., et al. (2018). Assessing capacity to change in high-risk pregnant women: A pilot study. *Child Abuse Review, 27*(1), 72–84. doi:10.1002/car.2491.

Kelly, P., & Kelly, D. (2013). Childhood cancer-parenting work for British Bangladeshi families during treatment: An ethnographic study. *International Journal of Nursing Studies, 50*(7), 933–944.

Oliver, D. P., Washington, K., Kruse, R. L., et al. (2014). Hospice family members' perceptions of and experiences with end-of-life care in the nursing home. *Journal of the American Medical Directors Association, 15*(10), 744–750.

Orsi, R., et al. (2018). Who's been served and how? Permanency outcomes for children and youth involved in child welfare and youth corrections. *Youth Violence and Juvenile Justice, 16*(1), 3–17. doi:10.1177/1541204017721614.

Robinson, B. A. (2018a). Conditional families and lesbian, gay, bisexual, transgender, and queer youth homelessness: Gender, sexuality, family instability, and rejection. *Journal of Marriage and Family, 80*(2), 383–396. doi:10.1111/jomf.12466.

Robinson, C. A. (2018b). Families living well with chronic illness: The healing process of moving on. *Qualitative Health Research, 27*(4), 447–461.

Segaric, C. A., & Hall, W. A. (2015). Progressively engaging: Constructing nurse, patient, and family relationships in acute care settings. *Journal of Family Nursing, 21*(1), 35–56. doi:10.1177/1074840714564787.

Svavarsdottir, E. K., & Sigurdardottir, A. O. (2013). Benefits of a brief therapeutic conversation intervention for families of children and adolescents in active cancer treatment. *Oncology Nursing Forum, 40*(5), E346–E357.

Wongsawang, N., Lagampan, S., Lapvongwattana, P., et al. (2013). Family caregiving for dependent older adults in Thai families. *Journal of Nursing Scholarship, 45*(4), 336–343.

Readiness for enhanced Family processes   *Kimberly Silvey, MSN, RN, RAC-CT*

NANDA-I

A pattern of family functioning to support the well-being of family members, which can be strengthened.

Defining Characteristics

Expresses desire to enhance balance between autonomy and cohesiveness; expresses desire to enhance communication pattern; expresses desire to enhance energy level of family to support activities of daily living; expresses desire to enhance family adaptation to change; expresses desire to enhance family dynamics; expresses desire to enhance family resilience; expresses desire to enhance growth of family members; expresses desire to enhance interdependence with community; expresses desire to enhance maintenance of boundaries between family members; expresses desire to enhance respect for family members; expresses desire to enhance safety of family members.

NOC   (Nursing Outcomes Classification)

Suggested NOC Outcomes

Family Coping; Health-Promoting Behavior; Health-Seeking Behavior; Parent-Infant Attachment; Parenting Performance

Example NOC Outcome with Indicators

Family Coping as evidenced by the following indicators: Confronts/Manages family problems/Obtains family assistance. (Rate the outcome and indicators of **Family Coping:** 1 = never demonstrated, 2 = rarely demonstrated, 3 = sometimes demonstrated, 4 = often demonstrated, 5 = consistently demonstrated [see Section I].)

Client Outcomes

Family/Client Will (Specify Time Frame)

- Identify ways to cope effectively and use appropriate support systems (family)
- Meet physical, psychosocial, and spiritual needs of members or seek appropriate assistance (family)

● = Independent;   ▲ = Collaborative;   EBN = Evidence-Based Nursing;   EB = Evidence-Based

- Demonstrate knowledge of potential environmental, lifestyle, and genetic risks to health and use appropriate measures to decrease possibility of risk (family)
- Focus on wellness, disease prevention, and maintenance (family and individual)
- Seek balance among exercise, work, leisure, rest, and nutrition (family and individual)

NIC   (Nursing Interventions Classification)

Suggested NIC Interventions

Coping Enhancement; Decision-Making Support; Family Integrity Promotion; Family Involvement Promotion; Family Mobilization; Family Process Maintenance; Parent Education: Adolescent; Childrearing Family; Risk Identification; Role Enhancement

F

Example NIC Activities—Risk Identification

Determine availability and quality of resources (e.g., psychological, financial, education level, family and other social, and community)

Nursing Interventions and *Rationales*

- Assess the family's stress level and coping abilities during the initial nursing assessment. EB: *Assessing parental stress level will help the nurse to plan interventions to better care for the child and their parents (Burke et al, 2014).*
- Consider the use of family-centered theory as the conceptual foundation to help guide interventions. EBN: *Working closely with pediatric patients and their families helps the nurse to plan care with the family in mind (Cady et al, 2015).*
- Use family-centered care and role modeling for holistic care of families. EB: *A holistic approach to care enhances the family's well-being and respects the family's beliefs (Krishna, 2013).*
- Discuss with family members and identify the perceptions of the health care experience. EBN: *Nurses and parents may perceive the care the child receives differently, and it is important to help identify the differences to better care for the child and family (Stuart & Melling, 2014).*
- Support family needs, strengths, and resourcefulness through family interviews. EBN: *Family interviews can give the nurse an understanding of the family's understanding and expectations (Alsem et al, 2014).*
- Spend time with family members; allow them to verbalize their feelings. EB: *Listening to what the family is saying can help the nurse understand how they are feeling (SmithBattle et al, 2013).*
- Encourage family members to find meaning in a serious illness. EBN: *Just because parents have hope for their child does not mean they do not understand their child's prognosis (O'Brien, 2014).*
- Provide family-centered care to explore and use all available resources appropriate for the situation (e.g., counseling, social services, self-help groups, pastoral care). EB: *Family-centered care includes multiple members of the health care team (Hodgetts et al, 2013).*
- Consider focus groups to provide insight into family perceptions of illness and/or disease prevention. EBN: *Focus groups provide insight into the perception of care that is received by the client (Pozzar et al, 2014).*

Pediatric

- Provide a parenting class series based on individual and couple changes in meaning and identity, roles, and relationships and interaction during the transition to parenthood. Address mother and father roles, infant communication abilities, and patterns of the first 3 months of life in a mutually enjoyable, possibility focused manner. EB: *Parenting classes can improve parenting and coping skills to enhance quality of life (Okamoto et al, 2013).*
- Encourage families with children and adolescents to have family meals. EB: *Family meals help strengthen a family and provide structure for better development (Utter et al, 2013). Research found that dinnertime rituals can potentially moderate the effects of parenting stress on child outcomes (Yoon et al, 2015).*

Geriatric

- Carefully listen to residents and family members in the long-term care facility. EBN: *Nurses can improve life and dignity for residents by listening to residents and family members (Nayer et al, 2014).*

• = Independent;   ▲ = Collaborative;   EBN = Evidence-Based Nursing;   EB = Evidence-Based

F

- Support caregivers' awareness of the positive effects of their contribution to the well-being of parents. **EBN:** *Children caring for their elderly parents can have a positive effect on the child and the parent (Lin et al, 2013).*
- Teach family members about the effect of developmental events (e.g., retirement, death, change in health status, and household composition). **EBN:** *Knowledge helps the family to better cope with health care and the care of the client (Nigolian & Miller, 2011).*
- Encourage social networks; social integration; social engagement and Internet social networking with friends, children, and relatives of older adults. **EB:** *Social networking enables older adults to be more engaged (Cornejo et al, 2013).*

 ### Multicultural

- Assess for the influence of cultural beliefs, norms, and values on the family's perceptions of normal functioning. **EBN:** *Cultural beliefs will have a considerable effect on a client's functioning (Mutair et al, 2014).*
- Identify and acknowledge the stresses unique to racial/ethnic families. **EBN:** *Understanding a client's unique racial/ethnic background may help the nurse identify stressors that the client and the family may be experiencing (Balaam et al, 2013).*
- Assess and support spiritual needs of families. **EB:** *Assessing and supporting the spiritual needs of the client and the family can enhance the understanding of the family's perception of care and the care that was actually received (Bernstein et al, 2013).*
- With the client's consent, facilitate a group meeting for family members to discuss how the family is functioning. **EBN:** *Communication with the patient and the family encourages discussion about the wants and needs of each individual and keeps each informed of what is occurring with the patient (Kisvetrová et al, 2016).*
- Facilitate modeling and role playing for the client and family regarding healthy ways to start a discussion about the client's prognosis. **EBN:** *It is helpful to practice communication skills in a safe environment before trying them in a real-life situation (Waite & McKinney 2016).*
- Encourage family mealtimes. **EB:** *Encouraging family mealtimes enhances the health and well-being and can decrease parental stress (Yoon et al, 2015).*

 ### Home Care

- The previous nursing interventions should be used in the home environment with adaptations as necessary.
- ▲ Encourage virtual support groups to family caregivers. **EB:** *Use of online support groups gives the caregiver a forum for giving and receiving guidance and support (Diefenbeck et al, 2014).*

 ### Client/Family Teaching and Discharge Planning

- Refer to Client/Family Teaching and Discharge Planning for readiness for enhanced family **Coping** for suggestions that may be used with minor adaptations.

REFERENCES

Alsem, M. W., Siebes, R. C., et al. (2014). Assessment of family needs in children with physical disabilities: Development of a family needs inventory. *Child: Care, Health and Development, 40*(4), 498–506.

Balaam, M.-C., Akerjordet, K., et al. (2013). A qualitative review of migrant women's perceptions of their needs and experiences related to pregnancy and childbirth. *Journal of Advanced Nursing, 69*(9), 1919–1930.

Bernstein, K., Angelo, L. D., et al. (2013). An exploratory study of HIV+ adolescents' spirituality: Will you pray with me? *Journal of Religion and Health, 52*(4), 1253–1266.

Burke, K., McCarthy, M., et al. (2014). Adapting acceptance and commitment therapy for parents of children with life-threatening illness: Pilot study. *Families, Systems and Health: The Journal of Collaborative Family Healthcare, 32*(1), 122–127.

Cady, R. G., Looman, W. S., Lindeke, L. L., et al. (2015). Pediatric care coordination: Lessons learned and future priorities. *Online Journal of Issues in Nursing, 20*(3), 30.

Cornejo, R., Tentori, M., et al. (2013). Enriching in-person encounters through social media: A study on family connectedness for the elderly. *International Journal of Human-Computer Studies, 71*(9), 889–899.

Diefenbeck, C. A., Klemm, P. R., et al. (2014). Emergence of Yalom's therapeutic factors in a peer-led, asynchronous, online support group for family caregivers. *Issues in Mental Health Nursing, 35*(1), 21–32.

Hodgetts, S., Nicholas, D., et al. (2013). Parents' and professionals' perceptions of family-centered care for children with autism spectrum disorder across service sectors. *Social Science & Medicine, 96*, 138–146.

Kisvetrová, H., Skoloudík, D., Joanovic, E., et al. (2016). Dying care interventions in the intensive care unit. *Journal of Nursing Scholarship, 48*(2), 139.

Krishna, L. (2013). Palliative care imperative: A framework for holistic and inclusive palliative care. *Ethics & Medicine, 29*(1), 41. Retrieved from Questia.

● = Independent;   ▲ = Collaborative;   **EBN** = Evidence-Based Nursing;   **EB** = Evidence-Based

Lin, W., Chen, L., et al. (2013). Adult children's caregiver burden and depression: The moderating roles of parent-child relationship satisfaction and feedback from others. *Journal of Happiness Studies*, 14(2), 673–687.

Mutair, A. S. A., Plummer, V., et al. (2014). Providing culturally congruent care for Saudi patients and their families. *Contemporary Nurse: A Journal for the Australian Nursing Profession*, 46(2), 254–258.

Nayeri, N. D., Mohammadi, S., Razi, S. P., et al. (2014). Investigating the effects of a family-centered care program on stroke patients' adherence to their therapeutic regimens. *Contemporary Nurse: A Journal for the Australian Nursing Profession*, 47(1/2), 88.

Nigolian, C., & Miller, K. L. (2011). Teaching essential skills to family caregivers. *The American Journal of Nursing*, 111(11), 52–58.

O'Brien, R. (2014). Expressions of hope in paediatric intensive care: A reflection on their meaning. *Nursing in Critical Care*, 19(6), 316–321.

Okamoto, M., Ishigami, H., et al. (2013). Early parenting program as intervention strategy for emotional distress in first-time mothers: A propensity score analysis. *Maternal and Child Health Journal*, 17(6), 1059–1070.

Pozzar, R. A., Allen, N. A., et al. (2014). Focusing on feedback: How nurse practitioners can use focus group interviews to build a patient-centered practice. *Journal of the American Association of Nurse Practitioners*, 26(9), 481–487.

SmithBattle, L., Lorenz, R., et al. (2013). Listening with care: Using narrative methods to cultivate nurses' responsive relationships in a home visiting intervention with teen mothers. *Nursing Inquiry*, 20(3), 188–198.

Stuart, M., & Melling, S. (2014). Understanding nurses' and parents' perceptions of family-centred care. *Nursing Children and Young People*, 26(7), 16–20.

Utter, J., Denny, S., et al. (2013). Family meals and the well-being of adolescents. *Journal of Paediatrics and Child Health*, 49(11), 906–911.

Waite, R., & McKinney, N. S. (2016). Capital we must develop: Emotional competence educating pre-licensure nursing students. *Nursing Education Perspectives*, 37(2), 101.

Yoon, Y., Newkirk, K., & Perry-Jenkins, M. (2015). Parenting stress, dinnertime rituals, and child and child well-being in working-class families. *Family Relations*, 64(1), 93.

F

Fatigue   *Barbara A. Given, PhD, RN, FAAN*

NANDA-I

Definition

An overwhelming sustained sense of exhaustion and decreased capacity for physical and mental work at the usual level.

Defining Characteristics

Alteration in concentration; alteration in libido; apathy; disinterest in surroundings; drowsiness; guilt about difficulty maintaining responsibilities; impaired ability to maintain usual physical activity; impaired ability to maintain usual routines; increase in physical symptoms; increase in rest requirement; ineffective role performance; insufficient energy; introspection; lethargy; nonrestorative sleep pattern; tiredness

Related Factors

Anxiety; depression; environmental barrier; increase in physical exertion; malnutrition; nonstimulating lifestyle; demanding occupation; physical deconditioning; sleep deprivation; stressors

At-Risk Population

Demanding occupation; exposure to negative life event

Associated Condition

Anemia; illness; pregnancy

NOC   (Nursing Outcomes Classification)

Suggested NOC Outcomes

Concentration; Endurance; Energy Conservation/Restoration; Nutritional Status; Energy; Vitality

---

Example NOC Outcome with Indicators

Endurance as evidenced by the following indicators: Performance of daily activities/Energy restored after rest/Blood oxygen level with activity/Muscle endurance. (Rate the outcome and indicators of **Endurance:** 1 = severely compromised, 2 = substantially compromised, 3 = moderately compromised, 4 = mildly compromised, 5 = not compromised [see Section I].)

 = Independent;   ▲ = Collaborative;   EBN = Evidence-Based Nursing;   EB = Evidence-Based

F

Client Outcomes

Client Will (Specify Time Frame)

- Identify potential etiology of fatigue
- Identify potential factors that aggravate and relieve fatigue
- Describe ways to assess and track patterns of fatigue over set periods of time (e.g., within a day, a few days, a week, a month)
- Describe ways in which fatigue affects the ability to accomplish activities of daily living (ADLs)
- Verbalize increased energy and improved vitality
- Explain energy conservation plan to offset fatigue
- Explain energy restoration plan to offset fatigue
- Verbalize ability and capacity to concentrate
- Verbalize strategies for restorative activities

NIC   (Nursing Interventions Classification)

Suggested NIC Intervention

Energy management, including both conservation and restoration; conservation interventions are targeted at preserving an individual's energy, whereas restorative interventions are intended to reestablish vitality and energy

Example NIC Activities—Energy Management

Assess client's physiological and psychological status for deficits resulting in fatigue within the context of age, development, and stage of disease or illness; Determine client/significant other's perception of causes of client's fatigue and factors that contribute to the relief. Assessing the pattern within a 24-hour period can be used to recommend usual daily activity.

Nursing Interventions and *Rationales*

- Assess severity of fatigue on a scale of 0 to 10 (average fatigue, worst and best levels); assess frequency of fatigue (number of days per week and time of day), activities and symptoms associated with increased fatigue (e.g., pain), activities that relieve, ability to perform ADLs and instrumental ADLs, interference with social and role function, times of the day for increased energy, ability to concentrate, mood, usual pattern of physical activity, and interference with sleep cycles. Consider use of instruments such as the Profile of Mood State Short Form Fatigue Subscale, the Multidimensional Assessment of Fatigue, the Lee Fatigue Scale, the Multidimensional Fatigue Inventory, the HIV-Related Fatigue Scale, or the Brief Fatigue Inventory, Short Form Vitality Subscale, Piper Fatigue Scale, Chalder Fatigue Scale, or Nottingham of Chronic Illness Therapy Fatigue Scale, and Fatigue Severity Scale. EBN/CEB: *These assessments have all been shown to have good internal reliability. The Fatigue Severity Scale, Fatigue Impact Scale, and Brief Fatigue Inventory are relatively short with good psychometric properties, making them clinically useful. These measures, along with the Multidimensional Assessment of Fatigue, have shown the ability to detect changes in fatigue over time (Whitehead, 2009). The European Organization for Research and Treatment of Cancer Quality of Life Core Questionnaire (EORTC QLQ-FA 13) (Schuler et al, 2016) was proven reliable. Varying populations may respond differently to instruments and there are a number of scales for specific diseases such as stroke, multiple sclerosis, Parkinson's disease, and sleep disorders. The Fatigue Scale for Motor and Cognitive functions and the Unidimensional Fatigue Impact Scale demonstrate good applicability in clients with multiple sclerosis; the Functional Assessment of Chronic Illness Therapy Fatigue subscale and the Fatigue Severity Scale demonstrate good applicability in clients with Parkinson's disease (Elbers, Berendse, & Kwakkel, 2016). Poststroke clients may have severe fatigue without depression (Drummond et al, 2017).*
- Evaluate adequacy of nutrition and sleep hygiene (napping throughout the day, inability to fall asleep or stay asleep). Encourage the client to get adequate rest; limit naps (particularly in the late afternoon or evening); use a routine sleep/wake schedule; plan and prioritize for daily activities as tolerated; allow exposure to sunlight during daytime hours by going outside or opening shades and curtains in the home; use relaxation techniques before bedtime such as meditation, music therapy, or guided imagery (Kwek-keboom & Bratzke, 2016); avoid caffeine in the late afternoon or evening; and eat a well-balanced diet that includes fresh fruits, vegetables, and lean meats. Mindfulness interventions also result in improved sleep quality (Black et al, 2015). Refer to Imbalanced **Nutrition:** less than body requirements or **Insomnia**

● = Independent;   ▲ = Collaborative;   EBN = Evidence-Based Nursing;   EB = Evidence-Based

if appropriate. EBN: *Dysfunction in sleep (too much, too little, or too many interruptions) can aggravate fatigue (Black et al, 2015).*

- Evaluate fluid status and assess for dehydration. Encourage at least eight glasses of water a day. Avoid caffeine, which can cause further dehydration. EB: *Dehydration has been shown to cause fatigue in conditions such as multiple sclerosis (Malkki, 2016). Older adults, and those with other medical conditions, are more susceptible to dehydration often because of symptoms such as diarrhea and vomiting or from treatments such as diuretics.*

▲ Collaborate with the primary care provider to identify physiological and/or psychological causes of fatigue that could be treated, such as anemia, pain, electrolyte imbalance (e.g., altered potassium levels), dehydration, thyroid disorders, anemia, arthritis, depression, anxiety, sleep disturbances (insomnia/sleep deprivation), acute or chronic infection, medication use or side effects, alcohol use/abuse, metabolic disorders (diabetes), or a preexisting comorbidity or disease (multiple sclerosis, cancer or cancer treatment, respiratory disease, fibromyalgia, cardiac disease, renal disease, Parkinson's disease) (Berger et al, 2015). EB/EBN: *If an etiology for fatigue can be determined, the condition should be treated according to the underlying cause. Fatigue is also related to psychological distress, nausea/vomiting (Oh & Seo, 2011), medication side effects, and nutritional deficit (caused by change in taste or cancer affecting swallowing or the digestive tract) (Berger et al, 2015), and from chemotherapy and radiotherapy in cancer (Kolak et al, 2017). Fatigue also negatively affects a client's quality of life (Bower et al, 2014). Tumor necrosis and cytokines, especially proinflammatory ones, have recently been identified (Kolak et al, 2017).*

▲ Work with the primary care provider to determine if the client has chronic fatigue syndrome. *Chronic fatigue syndrome is unexplained fatigue lasting 6 months or longer that is not associated with a diagnosed physical or psychological condition but may include muscle pain, memory problems, headaches, sleep problems, joint pain, and diarrhea (Milrad et al, 2017).* EB: *Proinflammatory cytokines may contribute to these symptoms (Montoya et al, 2017). Studies also suggest there is a genetic component to chronic fatigue syndrome (Pihur, Datta, & Datta, 2011).*

- Encourage the client to express feelings, attribution of cause and behaviors about fatigue, including potential causes of fatigue, and possible interventions to alleviate fatigue. Such interventions could include setting small, easily achieved short-term goals and developing energy management and energy conservation techniques; use active listening techniques to help identify sources of hope. Retroactive activities should be considered. Assess client's level of motivation and willingness to adopt new behaviors that can improve symptoms of fatigue. EBN/EB: *Cognitive behavioral therapy and self-efficacy interventions have been shown to be effective in reducing fatigue (Hoffman et al, 2017). Education, counseling, and expressive therapy have also been shown to be effective for managing fatigue (Bower et al, 2014).*

- Encourage the client to keep a journal of activities (or record using one of the many apps available) that contribute to symptoms of fatigue, patterns of symptoms across days/weeks/months, and feelings, including how fatigue affects the client's normal daily activities and roles. EBN: *Clients may have physical activity promoted by using information and communication technology (Zhang et al, 2017) that results in lower levels of fatigue (Kolak et al, 2017).*

- Help the client identify sources of support and prioritize essential and nonessential tasks to determine which tasks need to be completed and which can be delegated and to whom. Give the client permission to limit or change social and role demands if needed (e.g., switch to part-time employment, give up activities for a short period, hire cleaning service). EBN: *Psychoeducational interventions that include fatigue education, priority setting, self-care, coping techniques, and activity management have been shown to be effective in reducing cancer-related fatigue (Bower et al, 2014). Emotional support has been linked to decreased level of physical symptoms, including fatigue, for heart failure clients (Heo et al, 2017).*

▲ Collaborate with the primary care provider regarding the appropriateness of referrals to physical therapy for carefully monitored aerobic exercise program and possible physical aids, such as a walker or cane if client has a disability. EBN: *Physical activity, exercise, particularly aerobic exercise and yoga, can reduce cancer-related fatigue (Berger et al, 2015).*

- Encourage the client to try complementary and alternative therapy such as guided imagery, massage therapy, relaxation, mediation, mindfulness, and acupressure (Heo et al, 2017). EB: *Mindfulness-cognitive behavioral therapy has exhibited improved outcomes for those experiencing cancer-related fatigue (Berger et al, 2015).*

▲ Refer the client to diagnosis-appropriate support groups such as the National Chronic Fatigue Syndrome Association, National Parkinson Foundation, PatientsLikeMe, Multiple Sclerosis Association, American Cancer Society, or the National Comprehensive Cancer Network.

● = Independent;   ▲ = Collaborative;   EBN = Evidence-Based Nursing;   EB = Evidence-Based

F

▲ For a person with cardiac disease, recognize that fatigue is common with myocardial infarction, congestive heart failure (CHF), or chronic cardiac insufficiency. Refer to cardiac rehabilitation for a carefully prescribed and monitored exercise and rehabilitation program.

● If fatigue is associated with cancer or cancer-related treatment, assess for other symptoms that may enhance fatigue (e.g., pain, insomnia, anemia, emotional distress, electrolyte imbalance [nausea, vomiting, diarrhea], or depression). EBN: *Clients with cancer who reported both pain and fatigue may have more symptoms than clients who reported neither pain nor fatigue (Berger et al, 2015).*

● *Fatigue associated with rheumatoid arthritis can affect a client's quality of life and coping. Group cognitive behavior therapy (CBT) has been shown to be effective in improving fatigue self-management, coping, and fatigue severity. CBT involves using self-management skills such as problem-solving and goal setting to improve self-efficacy while achieving a sense of balance, priority planning, and pacing of activities (Berger et al, 2015).*

▲ Collaborate with the primary care provider to identify attentional fatigue, which may manifest itself as the inability to direct attention necessary to perform usual activities. Attentional fatigue is associated with sleep disturbances, depressive symptoms, anxiety, and psychosocial stressors, which can lead to inability concentrate, inability to plan goals, and inability to control emotions or social interactions. EBN: *A meta-analysis reported that persons with chronic fatigue syndrome had deficits in the areas of attention, memory, and reaction time (Geraghty, Hann, & Kurtez, 2017).*

▲ Collaborate with primary care providers to identify potential pharmacological treatment for fatigue. EBN: *Pharmacological therapy has not been shown to be effective in reducing fatigue, although treatment of comorbidities may be effective (Berger et al, 2015). Psychostimulants, erythropoiesis-stimulating agents (ESAs) for cancer-related fatigue, cytokine blockers, and nutritional supplements have all been shown to have limited improvement of symptoms of fatigue (Berger et al, 2015).*

 ### Geriatric

● Evaluate fatigue in geriatric clients routinely, particularly in clients with limited physical function and lower levels of social support. Chronic conditions related to age can contribute to fatigue in the geriatric client, such as cancer, dyspnea, anemia, multiple medication usage and side effects from medication, depression, insomnia (Keles et al, 2016), nutritional deficiencies, electrolyte imbalance, and comorbidities such as chronic obstructive pulmonary disease (COPD) (Kentson et al, 2016) and cardiac disease (Nasiri et al, 2016). *Older adults report fatigue that limits physical function, sleep, and social ability, which can aggravate comorbid conditions. Fatigue is one of the most common and debilitating symptoms experienced by clients living with chronic conditions.*

● Review medications to determine possible side effects or interaction effects that could cause fatigue. EB: *The aging process changes the way an individual absorbs, metabolizes, and eliminates medications, leaving the geriatric client susceptible to medication side effects and medication-to-medication interactions that can cause fatigue and other conditions.*

● Review comorbid conditions that may contribute to fatigue, such as CHF, pulmonary disease, cardiac disease, multiple sclerosis, arthritis, obesity, anemia, depression, Parkinson's disease, insomnia, and cancer.

● Identify recent losses and even loss of function; monitor for depression or loneliness as a possible contributing factor to fatigue. EB: *There is a strong correlation between depression and fatigue in clients after a stroke (Galligan et al, 2016) and other chronic conditions.*

● Review other symptoms the client may be experiencing. Fatigue is often associated with other symptom clusters such as depression and sleep disturbances *(Mänty et al, 2014; National Comprehensive Cancer Network, 2014).Clusters may be independent of age (Agasi-Idenburg et al, 2017).*

▲ Review medications for side effects. Certain medications (e.g., diuretics with associated loss of potassium, antihypertensives, antihistamines, pain medications [Rich & Nienaber, 2014], anticonvulsants, chemo-therapeutic agents, psychiatric medications, and corticosteroids) may cause fatigue in older adults. Fatigue is a major component of FRAILTY Scales (Gleason et al, 2017).

Home Care

The previously mentioned interventions may be adapted for home care use as well.

● Assess the client's history and current patterns of fatigue as they relate to the home environment and environmental and behavioral triggers of increased fatigue. CEB: *Fatigue may be more pronounced in specific settings for physical, environmental (e.g., stairs required to reach bathroom, patterns of movement around home, cleaning activities that require high energy), or psychological reasons (Wahl et al, 2009). Frailty may be related for the elderly.*

● = Independent; ▲ = Collaborative; EBN = Evidence-Based Nursing; EB = Evidence-Based

▲ Encourage planned exercise regimens or physical activities such as walking or light aerobic exercises. This activity can be organized in the home or in a setting such as senior centers or wellness facilities. **EB:** *Continued physical activity after cancer treatment has been associated with improved functioning in both physical and social realms (Hoffman et al, 2017). After a stroke frail elderly also responded to an individualized exercise program; they also had increased physical endurance and self-efficacy (Liu et al, 2017).*

▲ Refer to occupational and/or physical therapy if substantial intervention is needed to assist the client in adapting to home and daily patterns. **EB:** *Interventions in older adults led by occupational and physical therapists have been associated with less difficulty in ADLs and instrumental ADLs, which may lead to lower levels of fatigue (Murphy & Niemiec, 2014). Occupational and physical therapy rehabilitation have also been shown to decrease fatigue in cancer survivors (Dalzell et al, 2017). Home-based exercise in stage IV lung and colorectal clients has shown improvement in levels of fatigue (Hoffman et al, 2017).*

- For clients receiving chemotherapy, intervene to:
  ○ Relieve symptom distress (anxiety, nausea and vomiting, diarrhea, lack of appetite, emotional distress, difficulty sleeping).
  ○ Encourage as much physical activity as possible with a specific recommendation (Hoffman et al, 2017).
- Teach the client and family the importance of and methods for setting priorities for activities, especially those with high energy demand (e.g., home or family events). Instruct in realistic expectations and behavioral pacing. **EBN:** *Prioritization of activities can be effective in restoring energy (Poort et al, 2017).*
  ○ Identify with the client ways in which he or she continues to be a valued part of his or her social environment.
  ○ Identify with the client ways in which he or she continues to participate in preferred daily activity or social activities.
  ○ Encourage the client to maintain regular family routines (e.g., meals, sleep patterns) as much as possible.

Client/Family Teaching and Discharge Planning

- Help the client to reframe cognitively; share information about fatigue and how to live with it, including need for positive self-talk. **EBN:** *Cognitive behavioral approaches to managing fatigue have been shown to have a positive effect with multiple sclerosis (Wendebourg et al, 2017).*
- Teach strategies for energy conservation (e.g., sitting instead of standing during showering, storing items at waist level). **EB:** *Energy conservation strategies can decrease the amount of energy used (Blikman et al, 2017).*
- Teach the client to carry a pocket calendar, make lists of required activities, and post reminders around the house.
- Teach the importance of following a healthy lifestyle with adequate nutrition, fluids, and rest; pain relief; insomnia correction; and appropriate exercise to decrease fatigue (i.e., energy restoration).
- See **Hopelessness** care plan if appropriate.

REFERENCES

Agasi-Idenburg, S. C., Thong, M. S., Punt, C. J., et al. (2017). Comparison of symptom clusters associated with fatigue in older and younger survivors of colorectal cancer. *Supportive Care in Cancer*, 25(2), 625–632. doi:10.1007/s00520-016-3451-4.

Berger, A. M., Mitchell, S. A., Jacobsen, P. B., et al. (2015). Screening, evaluation, and management of cancer-related fatigue: Ready for implementation to practice? *CA: A Cancer Journal for Clinicians*, 65(3), 190–211. doi:10.3322/caac.21268.

Black, D. S., O'Reilly, G. A., Olmstead, R., et al. (2015). Mindfulness meditation and improvement in sleep quality and daytime impairment among older adults with sleep disturbances: A randomized clinical trial. *JAMA Internal Medicine*, 175(4), 494–501. doi:10.1001/jamainternmed.2014.8081.

Blikman, L. J., van Meeteren, J., Twisk, J. W., et al. (2017). Effectiveness of energy conservation management on fatigue and participation in multiple sclerosis: A randomized controlled trial. *Multiple Sclerosis: Clinical and Laboratory Research*, 23(11), 1527–1541. doi:10.1177/1352458517702751.

Bower, J. E., Bak, K., Berger, A., et al. (2014). Screening, assessment, and management of fatigue in adult survivors of cancer: An American Society of Clinical Oncology clinical practice guideline adaptation. *Journal of Clinical Oncology*, 32(17), 1840–1850. doi:10.1200/JCO.2013.53.4495.

Dalzell, M. A., Smirnow, N., Sateren, W., et al. (2017). Rehabilitation and exercise oncology program: Translating research into a model of care. *Current Oncology*, 24(3), e191–e198. doi:10.3747/co.24.3498.

Drummond, A., Hawkins, L., Sprigg, N., et al. (2017). The Nottingham Fatigue after Stroke (NotFAST) study: Factors associated with severity of fatigue in stroke patients without depression. *Clinical Rehabilitation*, 31(10), 1406–1415. doi:10.1177/0269215517695857.

Elbers, R. G., Berendse, H. W., & Kwakkel, G. (2016). Treatment of fatigue in Parkinson disease. *JAMA: The Journal of the American Medical Association*, 315(21), 2340–2341. doi:10.1001/jama.2016.5260.

Galligan, N. G., Hevey, D., Coen, R. F., et al. (2016). Clarifying the associations between anxiety, depression and fatigue following stroke. *Journal of Health Psychology*, 21(12), 2863–2871.

● = Independent;   ▲ = Collaborative;   **EBN** = Evidence-Based Nursing;   **EB** = Evidence-Based

Geraghty, K., Hann, M., & Kurtev, S. (2017). Myalgic encephalomyelitis/chronic fatigue syndrome patients' reports of symptom changes following cognitive behavioural therapy, graded exercise therapy and pacing treatments: Analysis of a primary survey compared with secondary surveys. *Journal of Health Psychology.* doi:10.1177/1359105317726152. [Epub ahead of print].

Gleason, L. J., Benton, E. A., Alvarez-Nebreda, M. L., et al. (2017). FRAIL questionnaire screening tool and short-term outcomes in geriatric fracture patients. *Journal of the American Medical Directors Association.* doi:10.1016/j.jamda.2017.07.005, pii: S1525-8610(17) 30403-6. [Epub ahead of print].

Heo, S., McSweeney, J., Ounpraseuth, S., et al. (2017). Testing a holistic meditation intervention to address psychosocial distress in patients with heart failure: A pilot study. *The Journal of Cardiovascular Nursing.* doi:10.1097/JCN.0000000000000435. [Epub ahead of print].

Hoffman, A. J., Brintnall, R. A., Given, B. A., et al. (2017). Using perceived self-efficacy to improve fatigue and fatigability in postsurgical lung cancer patients: A pilot randomized controlled trial. *Cancer Nursing,* 40(1), 1–12.

Keles, E., Bayraktar, D., Alpaydin, A. O., et al. (2016). Comparison of physical activity levels and fatigue severity in young and elderly males with COPD. *European Respiratory Journal,* 48, PA1898.

Kentson, M., Tödt, K., Skargren, E., et al. (2016). Factors associated with experience of fatigue, and functional limitations due to fatigue in patients with stable COPD. *Therapeutic Advances in Respiratory Disease,* 10(5), 410–424. doi:10.1177/1753465816661930.

Kolak, A., Kamińska, M., Wysokińska, E., et al. (2017). The problem of fatigue in patients suffering from neoplastic disease. *Contemporary Oncology,* 21(2), 131–135. doi:10.5114/wo.2017.68621.

Kwekkeboom, K. L., & Bratzke, L. C. (2016). A systematic review of relaxation, meditation, and guided imagery strategies for symptom management in heart failure. *The Journal of Cardiovascular Nursing,* 31(5), 457–468. doi:10.1097/JCN.0000000000000274.

Liu, J. Y., Lai, C. K., Siu, P. M., et al. (2017). An individualized exercise programme with and without behavioural change enhancement strategies for managing fatigue among frail older people: A quasi-experimental pilot study. *Clinical Rehabilitation,* 31(4), 521–531. doi:10.1177/0269215516649226.

Malkki, H. (2016). Multiple sclerosis: Dehydration might contribute to fatigue in MS. *Nature Reviews. Neurology,* 12(10), 555. doi:10.1038/nrneurol.2016.139.

Mänty, M., Rantanen, T., Era, P., et al. (2014). Fatigue and depressive symptoms in older people. *Journal of Applied Gerontology,* 33(4), 505–514. doi:10.1177/0733464812454011.

Milrad, S. F., Hall, D. L., Jutagir, D. R., et al. (2017). Depression, evening salivary cortisol and inflammation in chronic fatigue syndrome: A psychoneuroendocrinological structural regression model. *International Journal of Psychophysiology.* doi:10.1016/j.ijpsycho.2017.09.009. [Epub ahead of print].

Montoya, J. G., Holmes, T. H., Anderson, J. N., et al. (2017). Cytokine signature associated with disease severity in chronic fatigue syndrome patients. *Proceedings of the National Academy of Sciences of the United States of America,* 114(34), E7150–E7158. doi:10.1073/pnas.1710519114.

Murphy, S., & Niemiec, S. S. (2014). Aging, fatigue, and fatigability: Implications for occupational and physical therapists. *Current Geriatrics Reports,* 3(3), 135–141.

Nasiri, M., Rahimian, B., Jahanshahi, M., et al. (2016). Study of fatigue and associated factors in patients with chronic heart failure. *Journal of Critical Care Nursing,* 9(3), e8124.

National Comprehensive Cancer Network. (2014). *NCCN Clinical Practice Guidelines in oncology cancer-related fatigue version I.2014.* Retrieved from http://www.nccn.org/professionals/physician_gls/pdf/fatigue.pdf.

Oh, H. S., & Seo, W. S. (2011). Systematic review and meta-analysis of the correlates of cancer-related fatigue. *Worldviews on Evidence -Based Nursing,* 8(4), 191–201. doi:10.1111/j.1741-6787.2011 .00214.x.

Pihur, V., Datta, S., & Datta, S. (2011). Meta analysis of chronic fatigue syndrome through integration of clinical, gene expression, SNP and proteomic data. *Bioinformation,* 6(3), 120–124.

Poort, H., Verhagen, C. A., Peters, M. E., et al. (2017). Study protocol of the TIRED study: A randomised controlled trial comparing either graded exercise therapy for severe fatigue or cognitive behaviour therapy with usual care in patients with incurable cancer. *BMC Cancer,* 17(1), 81. doi:10.1186/s12885-017-3076-0.

Rich, M. W., & Nienaber, W. J. (2014). Polypharmacy and adverse drug reactions in the aging population with heart failure. In B. I. Jugdutt (Ed.), *Aging and heart failure* (pp. 107–116). New York: Springer.

Schuler, M. K., Hornemann, B., Pawandenat, C., et al. (2016). Feasibility of an exercise programme in elderly patients undergoing allogeneic stem cell transplantation—a pilot study. *European Journal of Cancer Care,* 25(5), 839–848. doi:10.1111/ecc.12400.

Wahl, H. W., Fänge, A., Oswald, F., et al. (2009). The home environment and disability-related outcomes in aging individuals: What is the empirical evidence? *The Gerontologist,* 49(3), 355–367. doi:10.1093/geront/gnp056.

Wendebourg, M. J., Heesen, C., Finlayson, M., et al. (2017). Patient education for people with multiple sclerosis-associated fatigue: A systematic review. *PLoS ONE,* 12(3), e0173025. doi:10.1371/journal .pone.0173025.

Whitehead, L. (2009). The measurement of fatigue in chronic illness: A systematic review of unidimensional and multidimensional fatigue measures. *Journal of Pain and Symptom Management,* 37(1), 107–128. doi:10.1016/j.jpainsymman.2007.08.019.

Zhang, Q., Yang, X., Liu, D., et al. (2017). Measurement and assessment of physical activity by information and communication technology. *Biomedical and Environmental Sciences,* 30(6), 465–472. doi:10.3967/bes2017.062.

Fear *Nadia Charania, PhD, RN*

NANDA-I

Definition

Response to perceived threat that is consciously recognized as a danger.

Defining Characteristics

Apprehensiveness; decrease in self-assurance; excitedness; feeling of alarm; feeling of dread; feeling of fear; feeling of panic; feeling of terror; fidgeting; increase in blood pressure; increase in tension; muscle tension; nausea; pallor; pupil dilation; vomiting

● = Independent;   ▲ = Collaborative;   EBN = Evidence-Based Nursing;   EB = Evidence-Based

Cognitive

Decrease in learning ability; decrease in problem-solving ability; decrease in productivity; identifies object of fear; stimulus believed to be a threat

Behaviors

Attack behaviors; avoidance behaviors; focus narrowed to the source of fear; impulsiveness; increase in alertness

Physiological

Anorexia; change in physiological response; diarrhea; dry mouth; dyspnea; fatigue; increase in perspiration

Related Factors

Language barrier; learned response to threat; response to phobic stimulus; separation from support system; unfamiliar setting

NOC   (Nursing Outcomes Classification)

Suggested NOC Outcome

Fear Self-Control

Example NOC Outcome with Indicators

Fear Self-Control as evidenced by the following indicators: Eliminates precursors of fear/Seeks information to reduce fear/Plans coping strategies for fearful situations. (Rate the outcome and indicators of **Fear Self-Control:** 1 = never demonstrated, 2 = rarely demonstrated, 3 = sometimes demonstrated, 4 = often demonstrated, 5 = consistently demonstrated [see Section I].)

Client Outcomes

Client Will (Specify Time Frame)

- Verbalize known fears
- State accurate information about the situation
- Identify, verbalize, and demonstrate those coping behaviors that reduce own fear
- Report and demonstrate reduced fear

NIC   (Nursing Interventions Classification)

Suggested NIC Interventions

Anxiety Reduction; Coping Enhancement; Security Enhancement

Example NIC Activities—Anxiety Reduction

Use a calm, reassuring approach; Stay with the client to promote safety and reduce fear

---

Nursing Interventions and *Rationales*

- Assess source of fear with the client. *Many clients with chronic diseases such as multiple sclerosis or those with mobility issues have a fear of falling (Topuz et al, 2014).*
- Assess for a history of anxiety. EB: *Clients experiencing posttraumatic stress disorder often fear uncertainty, which can exacerbate symptoms (Boswell et al, 2013).*
- Assess for presence of fear avoidance beliefs. EB: *A systematic review found that fear avoidance beliefs were associated with poor treatment outcome in patients with lower back pain of less than 6 months (Wertli et al, 2014).*
- Have the client draw the object of his or her fear. EBN: *In a study of older adults with a fear of falling, a community-based art program helped them overcome fears and anxiety (Beauvais & Beauvais, 2014).*
- Stay with clients when they express fear; provide verbal and nonverbal (touch and hug with permission and if culturally acceptable) reassurances of safety if safety is within control. EBN: *One study in which*

● = Independent;   ▲ = Collaborative;   EBN = Evidence-Based Nursing;   EB = Evidence-Based

nurses stayed with ventilated clients to provide support and reassurance reduced anxiety levels in these clients. Clients' ability to interact with the environment served as a basis for identification and management of anxiety or agitation. Health care providers' attributions about anxiety or agitation, and "knowing the patient," contributed to their assessment of client response (Tate et al, 2013).

- Explore coping skills previously used by the client to deal with fear; reinforce these skills and explore other outlets. Provide backrubs and massage for clients to decrease anxiety. **EB:** *A study of 87 children who received massage prior to a painful treatment had lower levels of fear and anxiety then those who did not receive massage (Celebiogiu et al, 2014). In a group of older adults, those who received massage had less pain after hip or knee surgery (Büyükyılmaz & Aştı, 2013).*
- ▲ Refer for cognitive behavior therapy. **EB:** *Therapeutic touch and harp music reduced fear and anxiety in a group of postoperative clients (Lincoln et al, 2014).*
- ▲ Animal-assisted therapy can be incorporated into the care of clients in hospice situations.
- Encourage clients to express their fears in narrative form. *Refer to care plans for **Anxiety** and Death **Anxiety**.*
- Enhance client's self-efficacy when a client is experiencing initial fear of disease progression. **EBP:** *A research indicated the positive effect of self-efficacy in initial progression of fear of disease progression (Melchior et al, 2013).*
- Engage client in a mindfulness-based stress reduction program. **EBP:** *Mindfulness-based stress reduction significantly reduced fear of illness recurrence and improved physical functioning (Lengacher et al, 2014).*
- Provide brief psychoeducation to client who has fear about surgery. **EBP:** *A randomized trial supported that brief psychoeducation significantly lowered fear scores prior to surgery. Although the exact mechanism of action is not fully known, it could be that brief psychoeducation modifies beliefs (Shahmansouri et al, 2014).*

Pediatric

- Incorporate play therapy as an intervention to reduce fears. **EBN:** *A study concluded that play therapy helped children lower their fear and anxiety levels, improve their communication and coping skills, and promote their self-esteem (Sezici et al, 2014).*

Geriatric

- Provide a protective and safe environment, use consistent caregivers, and maintain the accustomed environmental structure. **CEBN:** *Providing an environment that included safety equipment and balance training reduced the fear of falling among older adults (Gusi et al, 2011).*
- Assess for fear of falls in hospitalized clients with hip fractures to determine risk of poor health outcomes. **EBN:** *Fear of falling can increase risk of depression and isolation, and further decrease physical performance in older clients (Park et al, 2014).*
- Pair cognitive-behavioral strategies with exercises to improve physical skills and mobility to decrease fear of falling. **EBN:** *A study found that the combination of cognitive-behavioral strategies with exercises decreased fear of falling while increasing mobility and muscle strength (Huang et al, 2016).*
- Assist the client in identifying and reducing risk factors for falls, including environmental hazards in and out of the home, the importance of good nutrition and activity, proper footwear, and how to stand up after a fall. **EB:** *Clients receiving education focused on identifying and reducing risk factors for falls were found to have a significant reduction in their fear of falling (Park et al, 2014).*

Multicultural

- Identify what triggers fear response. **EB:** *Culture plays a role in how people perceive themselves in fearful situations. Fear, fatalism, and current and historical relationships influence how people perceive themselves (Somayaji & Cloyes, 2014).*
- Assess for fears of racism in culturally diverse clients.
- Explore client's meaning of illness including a fear of illness. **EBN:** *Research shows that the meaning of illness guides the type of coping strategies used by the client (Obeidat et al, 2013).*
- Provide education, support, and guidance. **EBN:** *Research shows that engagement of the health care providers could help client reframe the negative meaning attached to the fear of an illness to a more positive one (Obeidat et al, 2013).*

Home Care

- The previous interventions may be adapted for home care use.
- Refer to care plan for **Anxiety.**

● = Independent;   ▲ = Collaborative;   **EBN** = Evidence-Based Nursing;   **EB** = Evidence-Based

▲ Encourage the client to seek or continue appropriate counseling to reduce fear associated with stress or resolve alterations in irrational thought processes. *Correcting mistaken beliefs reduces anxiety. Creating a fear appeal that helps the client see that the fear is out of proportion to the situation can reduce fear in some clients (Sandkuhler & Lee, 2013).*

▲ Offer to sit quietly with a terminally ill client as needed by the client or family, or provide hospice volunteers to do the same. EB: *Skill in communicating and being with dying clients and their families is an important aspect of health care (Curtis, Back, & Ford, 2013).*

Client/Family Teaching and Discharge Planning

● Teach the client the difference between warranted and excessive fear. *Different interventions are indicated for rational and irrational fears. Creating a fear appeal that helps the client see that the fear is out of proportion to the situation can reduce fear in some clients (Sandkuhler & Lee, 2013).*

● Teach clients to use guided imagery when they are fearful; have them use all senses to visualize a place that is "comfortable and safe" for them. *Imagery makes use of subjective symbolism, bypassing the rational mind and making the areas "safe" that the client may otherwise be reluctant to face (Milad, Rosenblum, & Simon, 2014).*

● Teach use of appropriate community resources in emergency situations (e.g., hotlines, emergency departments, law enforcement, judicial systems). *Serious emergencies need immediate assistance to ensure the client's safety. Social media has a profound impact on society and affects many aspects of human life. Its applications in combating crises are unanticipated results of social media inventors, and many lessons could be learned from its applications in combating real crises (Chen, Ractham, & Kaewkitipong, 2014).*

● If fear is associated with bioterrorism, provide accurate information and ensure that health care personnel have appropriate training and preparation. *Clear, consistent, accessible, reliable, and redundant information (received from trusted sources) will diminish public uncertainty about the cause of symptoms that might otherwise prompt persons to seek unnecessary treatment. Training for providers is essential.* EB: *Using a diverse group of experts and providing a transparent and open line of communication can reduce fear in communities and the nation regarding bioterrorism (Siegrist & Zingg, 2014).*

REFERENCES

Beauvais, A., & Beauvais, J. (2014). Reducing the fear of falling through a community evidence-based intervention. *Home Healthcare Nurse, 32*(2), 98–105.

Boswell, J., Thompson-Hollands, J., Frachione, T., et al. (2013). Intolerance of uncertainty: A common factor in the treatment of emotional disorders. *Journal of Clinical Psychology, 69*(6), 630–645.

Büyükyılmaz, F., & Aştı, T. (2013). The effect of relaxation techniques and back massage on pain and anxiety in Turkey Total Hip or Knee. *Pain Management Nursing, 14*(3), 143–154.

Celebiogiu, A., Gurol, A., Yildirim, Z. X., et al. (2014). Effects of massage therapy on pain and anxiety arising from interthecal therapy or bone marrow aspiration in children. *International Journal of Nursing Practice*, Published online on April 1, 2014.

Chen, C., Ractham, P., & Kaewkitipong, L. (2014). *The community-based model of using social media to share knowledge to combat crises.* Pacific Asia Conference on Information System. Retrieved from http://aisel.aisnet.org/pacis2014.

Curtis, R., Back, A., & Ford, D. (2013). Effect of communication skills training for residents and nurse practitioners on quality of communication with patients with serious illness. *Journal of the American Medical Association, 310*(21), 2271–2281.

Gusi, N., Adsuar, J., Corzo, H., et al. (2011). Balance training reduces fear of falling and improves dynamic balance and isometric strength in institutionalised older people: A randomised trial. *Journal of Physiotherapy, 58*(2), 97–104.

Huang, T., et al. (2016). Evaluation of a combined cognitive-behavioural and exercise intervention to manage fear of falling among elderly residents in nursing homes. In D. L. Segal, S. H. Qualls, & M. A. Smyer (Eds.), *Aging and mental health* (2nd ed.), *20*(1), 2–12. doi:10.1080/13607863.2015.1020411.

Lengacher, C. A., et al. (2014). Mindfulness based stress reduction (MBSR(BC)) in breast cancer: Evaluating fear of recurrence (FOR) as a mediator of psychological and physical symptoms in a randomized control trial (RCT). *Journal of Behavioral Medicine, 37*, 185–195.

Lincoln, V., Norwak, E., Schommer, B., et al. (2014). Impact of healing touch with healing harp on inpatient acute care pain: A retrospective analysis. *Holistic Nursing Practice, 28*(3), 164–170.

Melchior, H., et al. (2013). Self-efficacy and fear of cancer progression during the year following diagnosis of breast cancer. *Psycho-Oncology, 22*, 39–45. doi:10.1002/pon.2054.

Milad, M., Rosenblum, B., & Simon, N. (2014). Neuroscience of fear extinction: Implications for assessment and treatment of fear-based and anxiety related disorders. *Behaviour Research and Therapy.*

Obeidat, R. F., et al. (2013). Controlling fear: Jordanian women's perceptions of the diagnosis and surgical treatment of early-stage breast cancer. *Cancer Nursing, 36*(6), 484–492.

Park, J., Cho, H., Shin, J., et al. (2014). Relationship among fear of falling, physical performance, and physical characteristics in rural elderly. *American Journal of Physical Medicine and Rehabilitation, 93*(5), 379–386.

Sandkuhler, J., & Lee, J. (2013). How to erase memory traces of pain and fear. *Trends in Neurosciences, 36*(6), 343–352.

Sezici, E., et al. (2014). Use of play therapy in nursing process: A prospective randomized controlled study. *Journal of Nursing Scholarship, 49*(2), 162–169.

Shahmansouri, N., et al. (2014). Effects of a psychoeducation intervention on fear and anxiety about surgery: Randomized trial in patients undergoing coronary artery bypass grafting. *Psychology,*

● = Independent;   ▲ = Collaborative;   EBN = Evidence-Based Nursing;   EB = Evidence-Based

Health & Medicine, 19(4), 375–383. doi:10.1080/13548506.2013 .841966.

Siegrist, M., & Zingg, A. (2014). The role of public trust during pandemics: Implications for crisis communication. *European Psychologist, 19*(1), 23–32.

Somayaji, D., & Cloyes, K. (2014). Cancer, fear and fatalism. *Cancer Nursing, 2014.*

Tate, J., Dabbs, A. D., Hoffman, L., et al. (2013). Anxiety and agitation in mechanically ventilated patients. *Qualitative Health Research, 22*(2), 157–173.

Topuz, S., De Schepper, J., Ulger, O., et al. (2014). Do mobility and life setting affect falling and fear of falling in elderly people. *Topics in Geriatric Rehabilitation, 30*(3), 223–229.

Wertli, M. M., et al. (2014). Fear-avoidance beliefs—a moderator of treatment efficacy in patients with low back pain: A systematic review. *The Spine Journal, 14,* 2658–2678. doi:10.1016/j.spinee.2014.02.033.

F

Ineffective infant Feeding pattern *Shelley Sadler, BSN, MSN, APRN, WHNP-BC*

NANDA-I

Definition

Impaired ability of an infant to suck or coordinate the suck-swallow response resulting in inadequate oral nutrition for metabolic needs.

Defining Characteristics

Inability to coordinate sucking, swallowing, and breathing; inability to initiate an effective suck; inability to sustain an effective suck

Related Factors

Oral hypersensitivity; prolonged nil per os (NPO) status

At-Risk Population

Prematurity

Associated Conditions

Neurological delay; neurological impairment; oral hypersensitivity

NOC   (Nursing Outcomes Classification)

Suggested NOC Outcomes

Bottle Feeding Establishment: Infant; Bottle Feeding Performance; Breastfeeding Establishment: Infant, Maternal; Breastfeeding: Maintenance; Hydration; Nutritional Status: Food and Fluid Intake

> **Example NOC Outcome with Indicators**
>
> **Breastfeeding Establishment: Infant** as evidenced by the following indicators: Proper alignment and latch-on/ Correct suck and tongue placement/Urinations per day appropriate for age/Weight gain appropriate for age. (Rate the outcome and indicators of **Breastfeeding Establishment: Infant:** 1 = not adequate, 2 = slightly adequate, 3 = moderately adequate, 4 = substantially adequate, 5 = totally adequate [see Section I].)

Client Outcomes

Infant Will (Specify Time Frame)

- Consume adequate calories that will result in appropriate weight gain and optimal growth and development
- Have opportunities for skin-to-skin (kangaroo care) experiences
- Have opportunities for "trophic" (i.e., small volume of breast milk/formula) enteral feedings prior to full oral feedings
- Progress to stable, neurobehavioral organization (i.e., motor, state, self-regulation, attention-interaction)
- Demonstrate presence of mature oral reflexes that are necessary for safe feeding

● = Independent;   ▲ = Collaborative;   EBN = Evidence-Based Nursing;   EB = Evidence-Based

- Progress to safe, self-regulated oral feedings
- Coordinate the suck-swallow-breathe sequence while nippling
- Display clear behavioral cues related to hunger and satiety
- Display approach/engagement cues, with minimal avoidance/disengagement cues
- Have opportunities to pace own feeding, taking breaks as needed
- Display evidence of being in the "quiet-alert" state while nippling
- Progress to and engage in mutually positive parent/caregiver–infant/child interactions during feedings

Parent/Family Will (Specify Time Frame)

- Recognize necessity of adequate calories for appropriate weight gain and optimal growth and development
- Learn to read and respond contingently to infant's behavioral cues (e.g., hunger, satiety, approach/engagement, stress/avoidance/disengagement)
- Learn strategies that promote organized infant behavior
- Learn appropriate positioning and handling techniques
- Learn effective ways to relieve stress behaviors during nippling
- Learn ways to help infant coordinate suck-swallow-breathe sequence (i.e., external pacing techniques)
- Engage in mutually positive interactions with infant during feeding
- Recognize ways to facilitate effective feedings: feed in quiet-alert state; keep length of feeding appropriate; burp; prepare/structure environment; recognize signs of sensory overload; encourage self-regulation; respect need for breaks and breathing pauses; avoid pulling and twisting nipple during pauses; allow infant to resume sucking when ready; provide oral support (cheek and/or jaw) as needed; use appropriate nipple hole size and flow rate

NIC (Nursing Interventions Classification)

Suggested NIC Interventions

Bottle Feeding; Fluid Monitoring; Kangaroo Care; Lactation Counseling; Nutritional Monitoring; Teaching: Infant Safety

Example NIC Activities—Lactation Counseling

Provide information about psychological and physiological benefits of breastfeeding; Refer to a lactation consultant

Nursing Interventions and *Rationales*

- Refer to care plans for Disorganized **Infant** behavior, Risk for disorganized **Infant** behavior, Ineffective and Interrupted **Breastfeeding,** and Insufficient **Breast Milk** and assess as needed.
- Interventions follow a sequential pattern of implementation that can be adapted as appropriate.
- Assess coordination of infant's suck, swallow, and gag reflex. EBN: *During this first hour when the infant starts seeking the breast, the rooting reflex becomes successively more mature and distinct (Svensson et al, 2013).*
- ▲ Provide developmentally supportive neonatal intensive care for preterm infants. EBN: *Decrease barriers for mothers to optimize breast milk feedings during infants' first weeks of life (Purdy et al, 2012).*
- Provide opportunities for kangaroo (i.e., skin-to-skin) care. EBN: *Use of kangaroo care increases the interval of breastfeeding and reduces the risk of mortality, infection/sepsis, hypothermia, and length of hospital stay (Gregson & Blacker, 2011).*
- ▲ Before the infant is ready for oral feedings, implement gavage feedings (or other alternative) as ordered, using breast milk whenever possible. EBN: *Gavage feeding is the method used to feed preterm infants or infants with inadequate suck/swallow during feeding (Pineda, 2011).*
- Provide a naturalistic environment for tube feedings (nasoorogastric, gavage, or other) that approximates a pleasurable oral feeding experience: hold infant in semiupright/flexed position; offer nonnutritive sucking; pace feedings; allow for semidemand feedings contingent with infant cues; offer rest breaks; burp, as appropriate. EBN: *Nonnutritive sucking during gavage feeding is comforting for the infant and significantly supports breastfeeding ability (Garpiel, 2012).*
- Foster direct breastfeeding as early as possible and enable the first oral feed to be at the breast in the neonatal intensive care unit (NICU). EBN: *Research demonstrated a link between direct breastfeeding behaviors in the NICU and success with provision of milk at discharge (Pineda, 2011).*

● = Independent; ▲ = Collaborative; EBN = Evidence-Based Nursing; EB = Evidence-Based

F

- Allow parents to feed the infant when possible. EBN: *Parents who feed effectively early on develop positive feeding relationships with their infants and promote infant feeding self-regulation and normative growth patterns (Horodynski et al, 2011).*
- Position infant in semiupright position, with head, shoulders, and hips in a straight line facing the mother with the infant's nose level with the mother's nipple. EBN: *Good positioning of the baby during breastfeeding is crucial to encourage oxytocin and prolactin release (Hughes, 2011).*
- Feed infant in the quiet-alert state. EBN: *Preterm infants who are in awake states at the beginning of nipple feedings are more successful at ingesting their feeding volumes (McCain et al, 2012).*
- Determine the appropriate shape, size, and hole of nipple to provide flow rate for preterm infants. EBN: *The coordination of rhythmic sucking, swallowing, and breathing patterns during feeding is disorganized in preterm infants with bronchopulmonary dysplasia (McCain et al, 2012).*
- Implement pacing for infants having difficulty coordinating breathing with sucking and swallowing. EBN: *Paced feedings decrease risk of fatigue and oxygen desaturation of the infant (McCain et al, 2012).*
- Provide infants with jaw and/or cheek support, as needed. EBN: *Breastfeeding difficulties can be avoided if good attachment and positioning are achieved at the first and early feeds (Goyal et al, 2011).*
- Allow the stable newborn to breastfeed within the first half hour after birth. EBN: *Mothers of infants who were breastfed within 1 to 2 hours were almost three times more likely to experience breastfeeding problems in the postpartum period than those mothers who breastfed within 30 minutes of birth (Demirtas, 2012).*
- Allow appropriate time for nipple feeding to ensure infant's safety, limiting to 15 to 20 minutes for bottle feeding. EBN: *Bottle feeding mothers need to develop responsive behavior to their infants' hunger and satiety cues (Horodynski et al, 2011).*
- Monitor length of breastfeeding so that it does not exceed 30 minutes. Breast milk transfer may last from as little as 5 to 20 minutes during breastfeeding depending on variations in milk supply during a 24-hour day (Flaherman et al, 2012).
- Encourage transitioning from scheduled to semidemand feedings, contingent with infant behavior cues. *Flexible feeding schedules allow infants to feed during awake and alert periods in response to infant's readiness and tolerance of nipple feedings (McCain et al, 2012).*
- ▲ Refer to a multidisciplinary team (e.g., neonatal/pediatric nutritionist, physical or occupational therapist, speech pathologist, lactation specialist) as needed. EB: *Follow-up visits with lactation consultants, nurses, and health care providers are beneficial for breastfeeding mothers (Henry & Britz, 2011).*

Home Care

- The previously mentioned appropriate interventions may be adapted for home care use.
- ▲ Infants with risk factors and clinical indicators of feeding problems present before hospital discharge should be referred to appropriate community early-intervention service providers (e.g., community health nurses, early learning programs [individualized per states], occupational therapy, speech pathologists, feeding specialists) to facilitate adequate weight gain for optimal growth and development. EBN: *Late preterm infants are susceptible to multiple complications including feeding and sucking problems (Henry & Britz, 2011).*

Client/Family Teaching and Discharge Planning

- Provide anticipatory guidance for infant's expected feeding course. *Providing written information and education on breastfeeding with culturally sensitive awareness helps guide parents after early discharge (Wiener & Wiener, 2011).*
- Teach various effective feeding methods and strategies to parents. EBN: *Mothers need to be given evidence-based information and support before discharge, giving mothers a sense of security and providing understanding care (Demirtas, 2015).*
- Teach parents how to read, interpret, and respond contingently to infant cues. EBN: *Parents' ability to recognize and react quickly and consistently to their infant's state or cues leads to parental confidence in providing care, promotes parent–child relationship, and strengthens the family unit (Kadivar & Maryam Mozafarinia, 2013).*
- Help parents identify support systems before hospital discharge. *Nurses need to assess the support system of the family and collaborate with other health care team members to meet the mother's needs for successful breastfeeding (Feldman-Winter, 2013).*
- Provide anticipatory guidance for the infant's discharge. *Providing written information and education on breastfeeding with culturally sensitive awareness helps guide parents after early discharge (Wiener & Wiener, 2011).*

● = Independent;   ▲ = Collaborative;   EBN = Evidence-Based Nursing;   EB = Evidence-Based

REFERENCES

Demirtas, B. (2012). Breastfeeding support received by Turkish first-time mothers. *International Nursing Review, 59*(3), 338–344.

Demirtas, B. (2015). Multiparous mothers: Breastfeeding support provided by nurses. *International Journal of Nursing Practice, 21*(5), 493–504.

Feldman-Winter, L. (2013). Evidence-based interventions to support breastfeeding. *Pediatric Clinics of North America, 60*(1), 169–187.

Flaherman, V. J., Gay, B., Scott, C., et al. (2012). Randomised trial comparing hand expression with breast pumping for mothers of term newborns feeding poorly. *Archives of Disease in Childhood. Fetal and Neonatal Edition, 97*(1), F18–F23.

Garpiel, S. J. (2012). Premature infant transition to effective breastfeeding: A comparison of four supplemental feeding methods. *Journal of Obstetric, Gynecologic, and Neonatal Nursing: JOGNN/NAACOG, 41*, S143.

Goyal, R. C., Banginwar, A. S., Ziyo, F., et al. (2011). Breastfeeding practices: Positioning, attachment (latch-on) and effective suckling—A hospital-based study in Libya. *Journal of Family & Community Medicine, 18*(2), 74–79.

Gregson, S., & Blacker, J. (2011). Kangaroo care in pre-term or low birth weight babies in a postnatal ward. *British Journal of Midwifery, 19*(9), 568–577.

Henry, L., & Britz, S. P. (2011). Breastfeeding the late preterm infant: Hospital-based lactation consultants lead the way. *Journal of Obstetric, Gynecologic, and Neonatal Nursing: JOGNN/NAACOG, 40*, S30–S31.

Horodynski, M. A., Olson, B., Baker, S., et al. (2011). Healthy babies through infant-centered feeding protocol: An intervention targeting early childhood obesity in vulnerable populations. *BMC Public Health, 11*, 868.

Hughes, G. (2011). How to … help with positioning and attachment. *Midwives, 14*(4), 26.

Kadivar, M., & Maryam Mozafarinia, S. (2013). Supporting fathers in a NICU: Effects of the HUG your baby program on fathers' understanding of preterm infant behavior. *The Journal of Perinatal Education, 22*(2), 113–119.

McCain, G. C., Del Moral, T., Duncan, R. C., et al. (2012). Transition from gavage to nipple feeding for preterm infants with bronchopulmonary dysplasia. *Nursing Research, 61*(6), 380–387.

Pineda, R. (2011). Direct breast-feeding in the neonatal intensive care unit: Is it important? *Journal of Perinatology, 31*(8), 540–545.

Purdy, I. B., Singh, N., Le, C., et al. (2012). Biophysiologic and social stress relationships with breast milk feeding pre- and post-discharge from the neonatal intensive care unit. *Journal of Obstetric, Gynecologic, and Neonatal Nursing: JOGNN/NAACOG, 41*(3), 347–357.

Svensson, K. E., Velandia, M. I., Matthiesen, A.-S. T., et al. (2013). Effects of mother-infant skin-to-skin contact on severe latch-on problems in older infants: A randomized trial. *International Breastfeeding Journal, 8*(1), 1.

Wiener, R. C., & Wiener, M. A. (2011). Breastfeeding prevalence and distribution in the USA and Appalachia by rural and urban setting. *Rural and Remote Health, 11*(2), 1–9.

F

Risk for Female Genital Mutilation   *Marina Martinez-Kratz, MS, RN, CNE*

NANDA-I

Definition

Susceptible to full or partial ablation of the female external genitalia and other lesions of the genitalia, whether for cultural, religious, or any other nontherapeutic reasons, which may compromise health.

Risk Factors

Lack of family knowledge about impact of practice on physical health; lack of family knowledge about impact of practice on reproductive health; lack of family knowledge about impact of practice on psychosocial health

At-Risk Population

Residing in country in which the practice is accepted; family leaders belong to ethnic group in which practice is accepted; belonging to family in which any female member has been subjected to the practice; favorable attitude of family toward the practice; female gender; belonging to ethnic group in which the practice is accepted; planning to visit family's country of origin

NOC   (Nursing Outcomes Classification)

Suggested NOC Outcomes

Abuse Cessation; Abuse Protection; Abuse Recovery; Abuse Recovery: Emotional; Abuse Recovery: Physical

Example NOC Outcome with Indicators

Abuse Protection as evidenced by the following indicators: Plan for avoiding abuse/Implementation of plan to avoid abuse/Safety of self/Safety of child/Self-advocacy. (Rate the outcome and indicators of **Abuse Protection:** 1 = not adequate, 2 = slightly adequate, 3 = moderately adequate, 4 = substantially adequate, 5 = totally adequate [see Section I].)

● = Independent;   ▲ = Collaborative;   EBN = Evidence-Based Nursing;   EB = Evidence-Based

Client/Family Outcomes

Client Will (Specify Time Frame)

- Express effects of family/culture on beliefs about female genital mutilation (FGM)
- Demonstrate evidence that FGM has not occurred
- Express/implement a plan for avoiding FGM
- Maintain safety of female children
- Demonstrate the ability to make decisions independent of cultural group
- Demonstrate self-advocacy skills

F

NIC (Nursing Interventions Classification)

Suggested NIC Interventions

Abuse Protection Support; Abuse Protection Support: Child; Abuse Protection Support: Religious

Example NIC Activities—Abuse Protection Support: Child
Identify parents who demonstrate an increased need for parent education; Determine whether a child demonstrates signs of physical abuse; Report suspected abuse or neglect to proper authorities; Refer families to human services and counseling professionals as needed

Nursing Interventions and *Rationales*

- Identify the decision-making process related to the practice of FGM. EB: *The decision to undergo FGM is often a community decision and not an individual or family decision. Some survivors of FGM report that relatives or other community members performed FGM on them without their consent or the consent of their parents (Burrage, 2016).*
- Identify the type of FGM for which the female client is at risk. EB: *The World Health Organization (WHO) classifies types of FGM as follows.* **Type 1:** *Clitoridectomy, which is partial or total removal of the clitoris (a small sensitive and erectile part of the female genitals) and, in rare cases, removal of the prepuce only (the fold of skin surrounding the clitoris).* **Type 2:** *Excision, which is partial or total removal of the clitoris and labia minora with or without removal of the labia majora (the labia are "the lips" that surround the vagina).* **Type 3:** *Infibulation, which is narrowing of the vaginal opening through the creation of a covering seal. The seal is formed by cutting and repositioning the labia minora or majora with or without removal of the clitoris.* **Type 4:** *Other, which includes all other harmful procedures to the genitals for nonmedical reasons, for example, pricking, piercing, incision, scraping, and cauterizing the genital area (WHO, 2016). WHO best practice standards indicated that nurses and health care providers are knowledgeable and aware of the types of FGM (WHO, 2016).*
- Assess and identify geographic, environmental, familial, religious, and/or other cultural factors that increase risk for FGM. EB: *Research indicated that the following are risk factors identified with FGM: older mothers, rural mothers, less educated mothers, maternal fears of social stigma, and mothers who have had FGM (Pashaei et al, 2016). FGM is most common in 30 countries of the western, eastern, and northeastern regions of Africa, in some countries in Asia and the Middle East, and among migrants from these areas. Countries with the highest rates of FGM are Egypt, Ethiopia, and Somalia (WHO, 2016).*
- Encourage the mothers of at-risk daughters to express their beliefs and attitudes toward FGM. EB: *Nurses and health care providers have to first understand the beliefs and attitudes toward FGM before implementing interventions to address the beliefs and attitudes. Among the beliefs for FGM are female cleanliness, beauty, safeguarding virginity, and as a rite of passage to adult womanhood (Pashaei et al, 2016).*
- Assess the mothers of at-risk daughters for positive affect (expression of feelings) and attitudes toward FGM. EB: *A recent Iranian study concluded that mothers' attitudes were the strongest predictor of their intention to allow their daughters to undergo FGM, suggesting that mothers with a more favorable attitude toward FGM are more likely to show the intention of mutilating their daughters (Pashaei et al, 2016).*
- In a respectful and nonjudgmental manner, convey accurate and clear information about FGM, using language and methods that can be readily understood by clients. EB: *Best practices indicated that individuals have the right to be fully informed by appropriately trained personnel with the assistance of an interpreter, if necessary (WHO, 2016).*

● = Independent; ▲ = Collaborative; EBN = Evidence-Based Nursing; EB = Evidence-Based

- In a respectful and nonjudgmental manner, provide the client, client's parents, and family with information that FGM is not a universal practice and that it is an illegal practice in many parts of the world. **EB:** *Women from countries that practice FGM may have inadequate knowledge of their bodies and biological facts and be shocked or angry to learn that FGM is not a universal practice and is illegal in the United States (Costello, 2015).*
- In a respectful and nonjudgmental manner, provide the client, client's parents, and family with health education to address false beliefs about female and clitoral anatomy and the physiology of women. **EB:** *Women from countries that practice FGM may have inadequate knowledge of their bodies and biological facts. Health education needs to convey that there are no known health benefits from FGM, and that women and children who experience FGM have lifelong health complications (WHO, 2016).*
- In a respectful and nonjudgmental manner, provide the client, client's parents, and family with health education to inform about the negative health outcomes associated with FMG. **EB:** *The negative health outcomes are both immediate and long-term. Immediate complications include bleeding, urinary retention, wound infection, sepsis, and death. Long-term complications include dysmenorrhea, dyspareunia, recurrent vaginal and urinary tract infections, infertility, difficult labor and delivery, and sexual dysfunction (Craven et al, 2016).*
- In a respectful and nonjudgmental manner, provide the client, client's parents, and family with health education to inform about the negative birth outcomes associated with mothers who have had FMG. **EB:** *A study found that mothers with FGM experienced the following obstetric complications: increased risk of neonatal resuscitation, low birthrate, stillbirth, and early neonatal death (Reisel & Creighton, 2015).*
- Use therapeutic and culturally competent communication to focus on the current and future safety of the female child at risk for FGM. **EB:** *Therapeutic and culturally competent communication will acknowledge cultural practices without blame or judgment and will leverage parental love and concern to prevent harm to the child (Costello, 2015).*
- Utilize a cultural mediator to interpret cross-cultural norms about FGM. **EB:** *Cultural mediators are community leaders who are respected and known in their community for their opposition to FGM (Costello, 2015).*
- In a respectful and nonjudgmental manner, provide fathers with health education to address beliefs about FGM and provide information about the negative health outcomes associated with FGM. **EB:** *A systematic review found that the level of education of men was one of the most important indicators for men's support for the abandonment of FGM practices (Varol et al, 2015).*
- ▲ Refer families to counseling services **EB:** *Family counseling will ensure that the family understands the reasons for the health care interventions and legislative/legal response and facilitate support of each other through the transition (Costello, 2015).*
- See care plans for **Post-Trauma** syndrome, **Impaired Parenting,** and **Social Isolation.**

 Pediatric

- Identify a system for assessment and referral of female infants at risk of FGM born to mothers who have undergone FGM. **EB:** *A British study assessed the effectiveness of a questionnaire to examine the level of risk of FGM if a girl is born to a mother who has undergone FGM. Study results indicated that the questionnaire formalized the referral process; identified infants at high risk; and helped to stratify risk into low, medium, and high. The questionnaire also indicated the demographics of those at highest risk (Flower et al, 2015).*
- For female children that may be victims of FGM, or are at risk of FGM, notify Child Protective Services and other law enforcement authorities. **EB:** *FGM is child abuse. Nurses are mandated reporters and are legally obligated to report all instances of suspected child abuse and neglect. Notification of Child Protective Services and law enforcement allows appropriate health care intervention and may provide protection for siblings and other girls in the family against FGM (Creighton et al, 2016). All individuals have the right to the highest attainable standard of health and the right to life and physical integrity, including freedom from violence and the right to freedom from torture or cruel, inhumane, or degrading treatment (WHO, 2016).*

REFERENCES

Burrage, H. (2016). *Female mutilation: The truth behind the horrifying global practice of female genital mutilation.* London: New Holland Publishers.

Costello, S. (2015). Female genital mutilation/cutting: Risk management and strategies for social workers and health care professionals. *Risk Management and Healthcare Policy, 8,* 225–233. doi:10.2147/RMHP.S62091.

Craven, S., et al. (2016). Female genital mutilation management in the ambulatory clinic setting: A case study and review of the literature. *Journal of Surgical Case Reports, 2016*(6), 1–3. doi:10.1093/jscr/rjw104.

• = Independent;   ▲ = Collaborative;   EBN = Evidence-Based Nursing;   EB = Evidence-Based

Creighton, S. M., et al. (2016). Multidisciplinary approach to the management of children with female genital mutilation (FGM) or suspected FGM: Service description and case series. *BMJ Open*, 6(2), 1–6. doi:10.1136/bmjopen-2015-010311.

Flower, A., et al. (2015). G48: A system for assessing the risk of female genital mutilation (FGM) for female infants born to mothers who have undergone FGM. *Archives of Disease in Childhood*, 100(S3), A19–A20. doi:10.1136/archdischild-2015-308599.47.

Pashaei, T., et al. (2016). Daughters at risk of female genital mutilation: Examining the determinants of mothers' intentions to allow their daughters to undergo female genital mutilation. *PLoS ONE*, 11(3), 4–12. doi:10.1371/journal.pone.0151630.

Reisel, D., & Creighton, S. M. (2015). Long term health consequences of female genital mutilation (FGM). *Maturitas*, 80(1), 48–51. doi:10.1016/j.maturitas.2014.10.009.

Varol, N., et al. (2015). The role of men in abandonment of female genital mutilation: A systematic review. *BMC Public Health*, 15(1), 1. doi:10.1186/s12889-015-2373-2.

World Health Organization (2016). *WHO guidelines on the management of health complications from female genital mutilation*. Geneva, Switzerland: WHO Press.

F

Risk for imbalanced Fluid volume   *Susan M. Dirkes, BSN, MSA*

NANDA-I

Definition

Susceptible to a decrease, increase, or rapid shift from one to the other of intravascular, interstitial, and/or intracellular fluid, which may compromise health. This refers to body fluid loss, gain, or both.

Risk Factors

To be developed

Associated Condition

Apheresis; ascites; burn injury; intestinal obstruction; pancreatitis; sepsis; trauma; treatment regimen

NOC   (Nursing Outcomes Classification)

Suggested NOC Outcomes

Fluid Balance; Electrolyte and Acid-Base Balance; Hydration

Example NOC Outcome with Indicators
Fluid Balance as evidenced by the following indicators: Blood pressure/Peripheral pulses palpable/Skin turgor/Moist mucous membranes/Serum electrolytes/Hematocrit/Body weight stable/24-hour intake and output balanced/Urine specific gravity. (Rate each indicator of **Fluid Balance:** 1 = severely compromised, 2 = substantially compromised, 3 = moderately compromised, 4 = mildly compromised, 5 = not compromised [see Section I].)

Client Outcomes

- Lung sounds clear, respiratory rate 12 to 20 and free of dyspnea
- Urine output greater than 0.5 mL/kg/hr
- Blood pressure, pulse rate, temperature, and oxygen saturation within expected range
- Laboratory values within expected range, that is, normal serum sodium, hematocrit, and osmolarity
- Extremities and dependent areas free of edema
- Mental orientation appropriate based on previous condition

NIC   (Nursing Interventions Classification)

Suggested NIC Interventions

Autotransfusion; Bleeding Precautions; Bleeding Reduction: Wound; Electrolyte Management; Fluid Management; Fluid Monitoring; Hemodynamic Regulation; Hypervolemia Management; Hypovolemia Management; Intravenous Therapy; Invasive Hemodynamic Monitoring; Shock Management: Volume; Vital Signs Monitoring

● = Independent;   ▲ = Collaborative;   EBN = Evidence-Based Nursing;   EB = Evidence-Based

Example NIC Activities—Fluid Management
Maintain accurate intake and output record; Monitor vital signs

Nursing Interventions and *Rationales*

Surgical Clients

- Monitor the fluid balance. If there are symptoms of hypovolemia, refer to the interventions in the care plan for Deficient **Fluid** volume. If there are symptoms of hypervolemia, refer to the interventions in the care plan for Excess **Fluid** volume.

Preoperative

- Collect a thorough history and perform a preoperative assessment to identify clients with increased risk for hemorrhage or hypovolemia, that is, clients who take herbal supplements, those with recent traumatic injury, abnormal bleeding or altered clotting times, complicated kidney or liver disease, diabetes, cardiovascular disease, major organ transplant, history of aspirin and/or nonsteroidal antiinflammatory drug (NSAID) use, anticoagulant therapy, or history of hemophilia, von Willebrand's disease, or disseminated intravascular coagulation. Assess the client's use of over-the-counter agents to include herbal products. EB: *Use of dietary herbal supplements (DHS) causes the potential for DHS–drug interactions, which may lead to serious adverse events. Although drug-induced adverse events are thought to be responsible for up to 12% of hospitalizations, drug–drug interactions are estimated to be the direct cause of up to 2.8% of hospital admissions. Descriptions of adverse DHS–drug interactions in the surgical setting are found mostly in case reports and animal studies. These interactions mainly affected bleeding tendencies and level of sedation (Levy et al, 2017).*
- Recognize that nothing per mouth (NPO) at midnight may or may not be appropriate for each surgical client. Guidelines from the American Society of Anesthesiologists (2011) recommended that healthy clients having elective surgery should be allowed to have clear liquids up to 2 hours before surgery. CEB: *Research has shown the value of allowing healthy clients to consume clear liquids up to 2 hours before surgery, but the practice is not consistent (Crenshaw, 2011).* EB: *Many clients are unnecessarily dehydrated from lack of fluid for an extended period, which can complicate postoperative recovery. It is important to provide clear communication to the client that only clear liquids can be safely consumed up to 2 hours before surgery (Allison & George, 2014).*
- Determine length of time the client has been without normal intake, been NPO, or experienced fluid loss (e.g., vomiting, diarrhea, bleeding). *The length of time and severity of these factors, along with the presence of a fluid deficit, allow the health care provider to determine a general estimate of preoperative fluid loss, which can affect intraoperative fluid management. However, laboratory testing of hemoglobin, hematocrit, blood urea nitrogen (BUN), and creatinine should be used to corroborate the assessment (Allison & George, 2014).*
- Assess and document the client's mental status. *A baseline assessment is important so that changes in mental status during the postoperative period can be easily identified.*
- Recognize that there is conflicting evidence regarding liberal intraoperative fluid management versus restrictive fluid management. Fluid administration during surgery is more restrictive to prevent pulmonary complications associated with excessive fluid administration (Assaad, Popescu, & Perrino, 2013). CEB: *Hypovolemia and hypervolemia decrease tissue perfusion and may result in organ failure. Measurements to assess volume status include measuring mean arterial pressure (MAP), central venous pressure (CVP), and by observing urine output. However, CVP shows a poor correlation to blood volume, is inadequate to detect hypovolemia reliably, and most notably cannot sense a decreased cardiac output (CO) and tissue oxygen debt in an early state. Furthermore, changes in CVP after volume administration do not allow any conclusions to changes in stroke volume (SV) or CO. Other signs such as hypotension and tachycardia may be more reliable indicators of volume assessment (Strunden et al, 2011). Urine output is a measure of glomerular filtration and can be an effective indicator of fluid status (Macedo et al, 2011; Strunden et al, 2011).*
- *To reduce fluid administration volume, colloids rather than crystalloid fluids may be administered during surgery (Cortes et al, 2015).*
- Recognize that an individualized fluid management plan would be developed incorporating client-specific assessment parameters (e.g., existing comorbid diseases, age) and type of surgical procedure (Allison & George, 2014). EB: *Perioperative hemodynamic and fluid management that is goal directed improved both short- and long-term outcomes and can be achieved easily (Cecconi et al, 2015).*

● = Independent;   ▲ = Collaborative;   EBN = Evidence-Based Nursing;   EB = Evidence-Based

F

- Recognize the effects of general anesthetics, inhalational agents, and regional anesthesia on perfusion in the body and the potential for decreasing the blood pressure. **EB:** *In humans undergoing general anesthesia there is almost no relationship between mean arterial blood pressure and delivery of oxygen (DO$_2$), presumably because of widely varying systemic vascular resistance. Control of blood pressure requires measurement, an algorithm of action, and an intervention, such as medications or fluid administration (Bartels, Esper, & Thiele, 2016).*
- Monitor for signs of intraoperative hypovolemia such as dry skin, dry mucous membranes, tachycardia, decreased urinary output, decreased CVP, hypotension, increased pulse, and/or deep rapid respirations.
- Monitor for signs of intraoperative hypervolemia such as dyspnea, coarse crackles, increased pulse and respirations, decreased oxygenation, and decreased urinary output, all of which could progress to pulmonary edema.
- In the critically ill surgical client a pulmonary artery catheter or other minimally invasive CO monitoring device may be used to determine fluid balance and guide fluid and vasoactive intravenous (IV) drip administration. **EB:** *Devices that directly (pulmonary artery catheter, or arterial liner) or indirectly (minimally or noninvasive such as ongoing blood pressure monitoring) assess the client's cardiac status and fluid volume status may be used to "optimize" cardiac function by allowing better fluid regimens. Fluids must be individually titrated based on each client's changes in monitored variables (Cecconi et al, 2015; Bartels, Esper, & Thiele, 2016).*
- Monitor the client for hyponatremia with symptoms such as headache, anorexia, nausea and vomiting, diarrhea, tachycardia, general malaise, muscle cramps, weakness, lethargy, change in mental status, disorientation, seizures, and death. *Many pathologies can predispose the client to hyponatremia, including adrenal insufficiency, brain tumor, cirrhosis, hypothyroidism, lung cancer, meningitis, renal disease, tuberculosis, use of complementary therapies, and head trauma (Allison & George, 2014).*
- Monitor clients undergoing laparoscopic or hysteroscopic procedures for the development of hyponatremia, hypervolemia, and pulmonary edema when an irrigation fluid is used. **EB:** *Use of local or spinal anesthesia for these operations can cause the client to develop symptoms of hyponatremia and hypervolemia sooner than with other anesthetics (Silva et al, 2013).*
- Monitor clients undergoing transurethral resection of the prostate (TURP) procedures for development of hyponatremia and hypervolemia with symptoms of TURP syndrome including headache, visual changes, agitation, lethargy, vomiting, muscle twitching, bradycardia, diminished pupillary reflexes, hypertension, and respiratory distress. *Considerable fluid absorption occurs during TURP procedures and gynecological procedures, which can result in hyponatremia and/or hypervolemia (Pasha et al, 2015).*
- Measure the irrigation fluid used during urological and gynecological procedures accurately for volume deficit such as amount of irrigation used minus amount of irrigation recovered via suction. *Absorption of large amounts of fluid can cause complications for the client (Silva et al, 2013).*
- Monitor intraoperative intake and output including blood loss, urine output, and third-space losses to provide an estimate of fluid volume. **EBN:** *Weighing used sponges can provide an estimate of blood loss (Blanchard & Burlingam, 2012).* **EB:** *Weighing fluid used and returned provides a more accurate measurement of fluid deficit than measuring the fluids (Silva et al, 2013). The use of balanced electrolyte IV solutions has been shown to be safer than the use of isotonic saline alone (Shaw et al, 2012).*
- Observe the surgical client for hyperkalemia with symptoms including dysrhythmias, heart block, asystole, abdominal distention, and weakness. *Hyperkalemia can occur intraoperatively because of massive blood transfusions, tissue breakdown from surgery, shifting of potassium from the cells into the extracellular fluid, decreased potassium excretion caused by renal failure or hypovolemia, crush injuries, or burns (El-Sharkawy et al, 2014).*
- Maintain the client's core temperature at normal levels, using warming devices as needed. **EB:** Hypothermia (body temperature <36°C) is present in the postoperative period in 26% to 90% of all patients who have undergone elective surgery. The risk of hypothermia is particularly high in patients over 60 years of age with poor nutritional status and preexisting disease, which impairs thermoregulation (e.g., diabetes mellitus with polyneuropathy), and in those who have had major or lengthy surgery. Lower temperatures in the operating room also increase the risk of hypothermia: the lower the temperature, the higher the risk (Torossian et al, 2015).
- Fluids administration during surgery can increase risk of hypothermia. **EB:** *Research has shown that perioperative hypothermia can adversely affect the cardiopulmonary system (Giuliano & Hendricks, 2017).*

• = Independent;   ▲ = Collaborative;   **EBN** = Evidence-Based Nursing;   **EB** = Evidence-Based

Postoperative

- Continue to monitor fluids postoperatively. EB: *Restrictive fluid therapy and liberal conventional therapy were associated with similar rates of overall and cardiopulmonary complications; however, restrictive fluid therapy was associated with a more rapid recovery and a shorter length of hospital stay (Jia et al, 2017). Also, fluid overload is an independent risk factor for the development of acute kidney injury (Salhuddin et al, 2017).*
- Assess the client for development of tissue edema, especially after cataract surgery in patients with comorbidities such as diabetes. EB: *A history of diabetes mellitus has been found to be an independent risk factor for the development of postoperative cystoid macular edema in patients undergoing cataract surgery (Ovewole et al, 2017).*
- Recognize that IV fluid replacement decisions incorporate multiple assessment parameters such as hourly urine output, blood pressure, heart rate, respiratory rate, lung sounds, output from drains, and changes in laboratory results (e.g., hemoglobin/hematocrit, serum electrolytes).

Geriatric

- Check skin turgor of older clients on the forehead, subclavian area, or inner thigh; also look for the presence of longitudinal furrows on the tongue and dry mucous membranes. *Older people commonly have decreased skin turgor from normal age-related loss of elasticity, and checking skin turgor on the arm is not reflective of fluid volume (El-Sharkawy et al, 2014).*
- Closely monitor urine output, concentration of urine, and serum BUN/creatinine results. EB: *Reduced renal perfusion and altered renal function as a normal or abnormal change in physiological aging can compromise the client's fluid volume status (El-Sharkawy et al, 2014).*
- Monitor older clients for excess fluid volume during the treatment of deficient fluid volume: auscultate lung sounds, assess for edema, and trend vital signs.
- Assess the older client's cognitive status. EB: *Cognitive impairment is a risk factor associated with dehydration, especially in the older adult (El-Sharkawy et al, 2014).*

Pediatric

- Assess the pediatric client's weight, length of NPO status, underlying illness, and the surgical procedure to be performed.
- Recognize that newborns require very little fluid replacement when undergoing major surgical procedures during the first few days of life.
- Monitor pediatric surgical clients closely for signs of fluid loss.
- Administer fluids preoperatively until NPO status must be initiated so that fluid deficit is decreased.
- Perform an assessment for signs of fluid responsiveness in the pediatric client. EB: *A systematic review found that respiratory variation was the only assessment parameter to most reliably predict a pediatric client's responsiveness for fluid administration (Gan et al, 2013).* EB: *Rehydration solutions such as low osmolality solutions have been shown to be safe and effective for correcting dehydration in children (Kumar et al, 2015).*

REFERENCES

Allison, J., & George, M. (2014). Using preoperative assessment and patient instruction to improve patient safety. *AORN Journal, 99*(3), 364–375.

American Society of Anesthesiologists. (2011). Practice guidelines for preoperative fasting and the use of pharmacologic agents to reduce the risk of pulmonary aspiration: Application to healthy patients undergoing elective procedures: An updated report by the American Society of Anesthesiologists Committee on Standards and Practice Parameters. *Anesthesiology, 114*(3), 495–511.

Assaad, S., Popescu, W., & Perrino, A. (2013). Fluid management in thoracic surgery. *Current Opinion in Anaesthesiology, 26*, 31–39.

Bartels, K., Esper, S. A., & Thiele, R. H. (2016). Blood pressure monitoring for the anesthesiologist: A practical review. *Anesthesia & Analgesia, 122*(6), 1866–1879.

Blanchard, J., & Burlingam, B. (2012). Perioperative standards and recommended practices. *AORN Journal.*

Cecconi, M., Garcia, M., Romero, M. G., et al. (2015). The use of pulse pressure variation and stroke volume variation in spontaneously breathing patients to assess dynamic arterial elastance and to predict arterial pressure response to fluid administration. *Anesthesia and Analgesia, 210*, 76–84.

Cortes, D. O., Barros, T. G., Njimi, H., et al. (2015). Crystalloids versus colloids: Exploring differences in fluid requirements by systematic review and meta-regression. *Anesthesia and Analgesia, 120*, 398–401.

Crenshaw, J. T. (2011). Preoperative fasting: Will the evidence ever be put into practice? *The American Journal of Nursing, 111*(10), 38–43.

El-Sharkawy, A. M., Sahota, O., Maughan, R. J., et al. (2014). The pathophysiology of fluid and electrolyte balance in the older adult surgical patient. *Clinical Nutrition, 33*, 6–13.

Gan, H., Cannesson, M., Chandler, J. R., et al. (2013). Predicting fluid responsiveness in children: A systematic review. *Anesthesia and Analgesia, 117*, 1380–1392.

● = Independent;   ▲ = Collaborative;   EBN = Evidence-Based Nursing;   EB = Evidence-Based

Giuliano, K. K., & Hendricks, J. (2017). Inadvertent perioperative hypothermia: Current nursing knowledge. *AORN Journal*, 105(5), 453–463.

Jia, F. J., Yan, Q. Y., Sun, Q., et al. (2017). Liberal versus restrictive fluid management in abdominal surgery: A meta-analysis. *Surgery Today*, 47(3), 344–356.

Kumar, R., Kumar, P., Aneja, S., et al. (2015). Safety and efficacy of low-osmolarity ORS vs. modified rehydration solution for malnourished children for treatment of children with severe acute malnutrition and diarrhea: A randomized controlled trial. *Journal of Tropical Pediatrics*, 61(6), 435–441.

Levy, I., Attias, S., Ben-Arye, E., et al. (2017). Perioperative risks of dietary and herbal supplements. *World Journal of Surgery*, 41(4), 927–934.

Macedo, E. 1., Malhotra, R., Bouchard, J., et al. (2011). Oliguria is an early predictor of higher mortality in critically ill patients. *Kidney International*, 80(7), 760–767.

Oyewole, K., Tsogkas, F., Westcott, M., et al. (2017). Benchmarking cataract surgery outcomes in an ethnically diverse and diabetic population: Final post-operative visual acuity and rates of post-operative cystoid macular oedema. *Eye (London, England).* 31(12), 1672–1677.

Pasha, M. T., Khan, M. A., Jamal, Y., et al. (2015). Postoperative complications with glycine and sterile distilled water after transurethral resection of prostate. *Journal of Ayub Medical College, Abbottabad*, 27(1), 135–139.

Salhuddin, N., Sammani, M., Hamdan, A., et al. (2017). Fluid overload is an independent risk factor for acute kidney injury in critically ill patients: Results of a cohort study. *BMC Nephrology*, 18(1), 45.

Shaw, A. D., Bagshaw, S. M., & Goldstein, S. L. (2012). Major complications, mortality, and resource utilization after open abdominal surgery: 0.9% saline compared with Plasma-Lyte. *Annals of Surgery*, 255, 821–829.

Silva, J. M., Jr., Barros, M. A., Chahda, M. A., et al. (2013). Risk factors for perioperative complications in endoscopic surgery with irrigation. *Brazilian Journal of Anesthesiology*, 63(4), 327–333.

Strunden, M. S., Heckel, K., Goetz, A. E., et al. (2011). Perioperative fluid and volume management: Physiological basis, tools and strategies. *Annals of Intensive Care*, 1(1), 2.

Torossian, A., Bräuer, A., Höcker, J., et al. (2015). Preventing inadvertent perioperative hypothermia. *Deutsches Ärzteblatt International*, 112(10), 166–172.

Deficient Fluid volume   *Susan M. Dirkes, RN, MS, CCRN*

NANDA-I

Definition

Decreased intravascular, interstitial, and/or intracellular fluid. This refers to dehydration, water loss alone without change in sodium.

Defining Characteristics

Alteration in mental status; alteration in skin turgor; decrease in blood pressure; decrease in pulse pressure; decrease in pulse volume; decrease in tongue turgor; decrease in urine output; decreased venous filling; dry mucous membranes; dry skin; increase in body temperature; increase in heart rate; increase in hematocrit; increase in urine concentration; sudden weight loss; thirst; weakness

Related Factors

Barrier to accessing fluid; insufficient fluid intake; insufficient knowledge about fluid needs

At-Risk Population

Extremes of age; extremes of weight; factors influencing fluid needs

Associated Condition

Active fluid volume loss; compromised regulatory mechanism; deviations affecting fluid absorption; deviations affecting fluid intake; excessive fluid loss through normal route; fluid loss through abnormal route; pharmaceutical agent

NOC   (Nursing Outcomes Classification)

Suggested NOC Outcomes

Fluid Balance; Hydration; Nutritional Status: Food and Fluid Intake

---

Example NOC Outcome with Indicators

Fluid Balance as evidenced by the following indicators: Elastic skin turgor/Moist mucous membranes/Orthostatic hypotension not present/24-hour intake and output balance/Urine specific gravity. (Rate each indicator of **Fluid Balance:** I = severely compromised, 2 = substantially compromised, 3 = moderately compromised, 4 = mildly compromised, 5 = not compromised [see Section I].)

● = Independent;   ▲ = Collaborative;   EBN = Evidence-Based Nursing;   EB = Evidence-Based

Client Outcomes

Client Will (Specify Time Frame)

- Maintain urine output of 0.5 to 1.5 mL/kg/hr or at least more than 1300 mL/day
- Maintain normal blood pressure, heart rate, and body temperature
- Maintain elastic skin turgor; moist tongue and mucous membranes; and orientation to person, place, and time
- Explain measures that can be taken to treat or prevent fluid volume loss
- Describe symptoms that indicate the need to consult with health care provider

NIC   (Nursing Interventions Classification)

Suggested NIC Interventions

Fluid Management; Hypovolemia Management; Shock Management: Volume

Example NIC Activities—Fluid Management
Monitor hydration status (e.g., moist mucous membranes, adequacy of pulses, and orthostatic blood pressure) as appropriate; Administer intravenous (IV) therapy, as prescribed

Nursing Interventions and *Rationales*

- Watch for early signs of hypovolemia, including thirst, restlessness, headaches, and inability to concentrate. *Thirst is often the first sign of dehydration (Wagner & Hardin-Pierce, 2014).* **EB:** *A study of healthy women showed heart rate was increased by fluid restriction along with increased urine specific gravity, darker urine color, and increased thirst. They also experienced decreased alertness and increased sleepiness, fatigue, and confusion (Pross et al, 2013).*
- Recognize symptoms of cyanosis, cold clammy skin, weak thready pulse, confusion, and oliguria as late signs of hypovolemia. *These symptoms occur after the body has compensated for fluid loss by moving fluid from the interstitial space into the vascular compartment (Wagner & Hardin-Pierce, 2014).*
- Monitor pulse, respiration, and blood pressure of clients with deficient fluid volume every 15 minutes to 1 hour for the unstable client and every 4 hours for the stable client. *Vital sign changes seen with fluid volume deficit include tachycardia, tachypnea, decreased pulse pressure first, then hypotension, decreased pulse volume, and increased or decreased body temperature (Wagner & Hardin-Pierce, 2014).* **CEB:** *A systematic review demonstrated that hypotension and tachycardia, and occasionally fever, are clinical signs of dehydration (Jequier & Constant, 2010).*
- Check orthostatic blood pressures with the client lying, sitting, and standing. *A decrease in systolic blood pressure of 20 mm Hg or a decrease in diastolic blood pressure of 10 mm Hg within 3 minutes of standing when compared with blood pressure from the sitting position is considered orthostatic hypotension. This can occur with dehydration or cardiovascular disorders (Wedro & Stoppler, 2017).*
- Note skin turgor over bony prominences such as the hand or shin.
- Monitor for the existence of factors causing deficient fluid volume (e.g., hypovolemia from vomiting, diarrhea, difficulty maintaining oral intake, fever, uncontrolled type 2 diabetes, diuretic therapy). *Early identification of risk factors and early intervention can decrease the occurrence and severity of complications from deficient fluid volume and acute kidney injury (Ftouh & Lewington, 2014).*
- Observe for dry tongue and mucous membranes, and longitudinal tongue furrows. *These are symptoms of decreased body fluids (Wagner & Hardin-Pierce, 2014).*
- Recognize that checking capillary refill may not be helpful in identifying fluid volume deficit. *Capillary refill can be normal in clients with sepsis because increased body temperature dilates peripheral blood vessels and capillary return may be immediate (Wagner & Hardin-Pierce, 2014). A quick test is compression of the nail bed. If there is good blood flow to the nail bed, a pink color should return in less than 2 seconds after pressure is removed. Slow return to pink color can indicate dehydration (White, 2016).* **CBN:** *Capillary refill has been shown to be a good clinical indicator to detect dehydration with good specificity but poor sensitivity (Shimizu et al, 2012).*
- Weigh client daily and watch for sudden decreases, especially in the presence of decreasing urine output or active fluid loss. *Body weight changes of 1 kg (2.2 pounds) represent a fluid loss of 1 L (Wagner & Hardin-Pierce, 2014).*

● = Independent;   ▲ = Collaborative;   EBN = Evidence-Based Nursing;   EB = Evidence-Based

F

- Monitor total fluid intake and output every 4 hours (or every hour for the unstable client or the client who has urine output equal to or less than 0.5 mL/kg/hr). *Recognize that urine output is an indicator of fluid balance. However, urine output alone does not differentiate between volume-sensitive reductions in glomerular filtration rate and structural kidney injury (Schrezenmeier et al, 2017)*
- A urine output of less than 0.5 mL/kg/hr may be indicative of acute kidney injury (Prowle et al, 2011). Nevertheless, in any condition of hypovolemia, renal perfusion pressure falls. If it falls below the level of autoregulation (blood pressure [BP] <80 mm Hg), then renal blood flow and glomerular filtration will fall (Andeucchi et al, 2017). **EB:** *The RIFLE criteria define oliguria as urine output less than 0.5 mL/kg/hr for each of six or more consecutive hours, which is thought to confer "risk" of kidney injury; when urine output less than 0.5 mL/kg/hr and persists for 12 or more consecutive hours, the kidneys are considered to be "in injury" (James et al, 2016). The Kidney Disease: Improving Global Outcomes (KDIGO) guidelines indicate that acute kidney injury is an increase in creatinine 1.5 to 1.9 times baseline and urine output <0.5 mL/kg/ hr for 6 to 12 hours (Alseiari, 2016).*
- Note the color of urine, urine osmolality, and specific gravity. *Normal urine is straw colored or amber. Dark-colored urine with a specific gravity greater than 1.030 and a high urine osmolality reflects fluid volume deficit (Perrier et al, 2013; Wagner & Hardin-Pierce, 2014). Although these tools for dehydration screening have been advocated for use in the elderly, their diagnostic accuracy is low and may not be useful (Hooper et al, 2016).*
- Provide fresh water and oral fluids preferred by the client (distribute over 24 hours [e.g., 1200 mL during days, 800 mL during evenings, and 200 mL during nights]), provide prescribed diet, offer snacks (e.g., frequent drinks, fresh fruits, fruit juice), and instruct significant other to assist the client with feedings as appropriate. *Distributing the intake over the entire 24-hour period and providing snacks, specifically those with creatine and carnitine, and beverages including caffeine may improve muscular ability, endurance, and alertness (Cherniack, 2012).*
- ▲ Provide oral replacement therapy as ordered and tolerated with a hypotonic glucose-electrolyte solution when the client has acute diarrhea or nausea/vomiting. Provide small, frequent quantities of slightly chilled solutions. *Maintenance of oral intake stabilizes the ability of the intestines to absorb nutrients and promote gastric emptying (Keller & Layer, 2014); glucose-electrolyte solutions increase net fluid absorption while correcting deficient fluid volume. Use diluted carbohydrate-electrolyte solutions, such as sports replacement drinks, and ginger ale (Deshpande, Lever, & Soffer, 2013). The use of diluted oral replacement fluids has been found to reduce the need for IV hydration (Keller & Layer, 2014).*
- ▲ Administer antidiarrheals and antiemetics as ordered and appropriate. Consider what the client is eating to prevent further diarrhea (Bolen, 2018). *The goal is to stop the loss that results from vomiting or diarrhea. Refer to care plan for* **Diarrhea** *or* **Nausea.**
- If the client is on enteral feedings, research has shown either continuous or intermittent feedings had similar results regarding diarrhea and nausea (deAraujo et al, 2014). **EB:** *Evaluate the rate of enteral feeding formula administration and other medications to address diarrhea and nausea (Scott & Bowling, 2015).*
- ▲ Hydrate the client with isotonic IV solutions as prescribed. *For clients with mild to moderate fluid deficit, crystalloids such as 0.9 saline or lactated Ringer's should be used for fluid volume replacement (Peng & Kellum, 2013).*
- Assist with ambulation if the client has postural hypotension. Hypovolemia causes orthostatic hypotension, which can result in syncope when the client goes from a sitting to standing position (Wagner & Hardin-Pierce, 2014).

Critically Ill

- ▲ Monitor stroke volume, passive leg lift, and ultrasound as trends for more accurate fluid volume status. *Hemodynamic pressures such as central venous pressure (CVP) and pulmonary artery pressures have been demonstrated to be less predictive and specific of fluid volume responsiveness (Kalantari et al, 2013), whereas changes in stroke volume measured by a number of noninvasive methods including passive leg lift may more accurately predict fluid volume responsiveness of a client (Marik, Monnet, & Teboul, 2011; Angappan, 2015; Duus et al, 2015).*
- ▲ Monitor serum and urine osmolality blood urea nitrogen (BUN)/creatinine ratio and hematocrit for elevations. *These are all measures of concentration and will be elevated with decreased intravascular volume (Wagner & Hardin-Pierce, 2014).*
- ▲ Insert an indwelling urinary catheter if ordered and measure urine output hourly. Notify health care provider if urine output is less than 0.5 mL/kg/hr. **EB:** *A decrease in urine output is seen with poorly*

• = Independent;   ▲ = Collaborative;   EBN = Evidence-Based Nursing;   EB = Evidence-Based

perfused kidneys and a drop in the glomerular filtration rate in the client with normal kidney function, and action, if taken early, can prevent further deterioration (Zheng et al, 2014). Intensive monitoring of urine output is associated with increased detection of acute kidney injury and improved outcomes (Jin et al, 2017).

▲ When ordered, initiate a fluid challenge of crystalloids (e.g., 0.9% normal saline or lactated Ringer's) for replacement of intravascular volume. EB: *Guidelines for early goal-directed therapy (EGDT) have been developed by the Surviving Sepsis campaign; however, EGDT in one study did not significantly decrease mortality (Zhang et al, 2017).*

▲ Monitor the client's response to prescribed fluid therapy and fluid challenge, especially noting vital signs (mean arterial pressure [MAP] >65 mm Hg in the first 6 hours of treatment, systolic blood pressure >100 mm Hg) (Singer et al, 2016; Rhodes et al, 2017), urine output, blood lactate concentrations, and lung sounds. *A fluid challenge can help the client with deficient fluid volume regain intravascular volume quickly, but the client must be carefully observed to ensure that he or she does not go into fluid volume overload because excess fluid volume can lead to organ edema and increased mortality (Peng & Kellum, 2013; Wang et al, 2014).*

● Position the client flat with legs elevated when hypotensive, if not contraindicated. *This position enhances venous return, and, coupled with stroke volume measurement, is a simple noninvasive technique to determine fluid responsiveness (Assadi, 2017).*

▲ Monitor trends in serum lactic acid levels and base deficit obtained from blood gases as ordered. EB: *A trend of increasing lactic acid levels >2.0 has been shown to increase mortality than levels less than 2.0 (Seymour et al, 2016; Rhodes et al, 2017).*

▲ Consult provider if signs and symptoms of deficient fluid volume persist or worsen. *Prolonged deficient fluid volume increases the risk for development of complications, including decrease in cognitive function, weakness, tachycardia, hemodynamic instability, and kidney injury (Singer et al, 2016).*

 Pediatric

● Monitor the child for signs of deficient fluid volume, including sunken eyes, decreased tears, dry mucous membranes, poor skin turgor, and decreased urine output (Graves, 2013). EB: *These assessment factors are more significant in identifying dehydration, but a combination of physical examination findings is a much better predictor than individual signs (Falszewska, Dziechciarz, & Szajewska, 2014).*

▲ Reinforce the health care provider recommendation for the parents to give the child oral rehydration fluids to drink in the amounts specified, especially during the first 4 to 6 hours to replace fluid losses. Consider using diluted oral rehydration fluids. Once the child is rehydrated, an orally administered maintenance solution should be used along with food. EB: *A study demonstrated that treatment with oral rehydration fluids for children was generally as effective as IV fluids, and IV fluids did not shorten the duration of gastroenteritis and are more likely to cause adverse effects than oral rehydration therapy (Ciccarelli, Stolfi, & Caramia, 2013).* EB: *Many studies have shown that diluted oral replacement fluids and some drugs resulted in reductions in stool output, decreased vomiting, and less need for IV hydration (Ciccarelli, Stolfi, & Caramia, 2013).*

● Recommend that the mother resume breastfeeding as soon as possible.

● Recommend that parents not give the child carbonated soda, fruit juices, gelatin dessert, or instant fruit drink mix; instead, give the child oral rehydration fluids ordered and, when tolerated, food. *Rehydration solutions such as low osmolality solutions have been shown to be safe and effective for correcting dehydration in children (Kumar et al, 2015). Antiemetic, antidiarrheal agents and probiotics have been shown to reduce the duration and severity of infectious diarrhea (Ciccarelli, Stolfi, & Caramia, 2013).*

● Once the child has been rehydrated, begin feeding regular food, but avoid milk products (Guandalini et al, 2017).

 Geriatric

● Monitor older clients for deficient fluid volume carefully, noting new onset of headache, weakness, dizziness, and postural hypotension. *Older people are thought to be at greater risk of dehydration because thirst sensation and urinary concentrating ability frequently decline with age. Many older people use diuretics or laxatives, which encourage fluid loss, and reduced muscle volume leads to a smaller fluid reserve. Oral fluid intake may fall in older people for a variety of reasons including reduced enjoyment of drinks, physical limitations, unmet activities of daily living needs, acute and chronic health problems, and decisions aimed at controlling continence (Oates & Price, 2017). Additionally those with dementia may forget to drink as daily routines are lost and social contact diminishes.*

● = Independent;   ▲ = Collaborative;   EBN = Evidence-Based Nursing;   EB = Evidence-Based

F

- Implement fall precautions for clients experiencing weakness, dizziness, and/or postural hypotension. *Falls are a serious risk in the elderly, especially those with hyponatremia (Kuo, 2017).*
- Evaluate the risk for dehydration using the Dehydration Risk Appraisal Checklist. **CEB:** *A study demonstrated that the checklist has potential to predict the onset of dehydration in nursing home clients (Mentes & Wang, 2011).*
- Check skin turgor of older clients on the forehead and axilla; check for dry mucous membranes and dry tongue. **EB:** *A Cochrane review recommended in clinical practice to avoid the reliance on one clinical symptom as a sign of water-loss dehydration in older people (Hooper et al, 2016a). Older adults are susceptible to dehydration because of acute and chronic health problems, which impair thirst; reduce the ability to drink sufficiently; and/or increase urinary, skin, and respiratory fluid loss (Oates et al, 2017; Hooper et al, 2016b). Older adults present with a constellation of signs and symptoms that need to be further evaluated for connection to dehydration. Signs and symptoms include fatigue, pallor, sunken periorbital area, chapped lips, hypotension, tachycardia, fever, orthostatic blood pressure, weight loss >4%, poor skin turgor over the sternum, and change in mental status (Miller, 2015).*
- Encourage fluid intake by offering fluids regularly to cognitively impaired clients. **EB:** *The single most common risk factor reported associated with dehydration in cognitively impaired clients was a worsening or change in mental state (Oates et al, 2017).*
- Because older clients have low water reserves, they should be encouraged to drink regularly even when not thirsty. Frequent and varied beverage offerings should be made available by hydration assistants to routinely offer increased beverages to clients in extended care. **EB:** *Strategies to improve fluid intake include making healthy drinks and water easily available and accessible at all times and reminding and encouraging older adults to consume these fluids. Older people should not be encouraged to consume large amounts of fluids at once but rather small amounts throughout the day (Oates et al, 2017).*
- Flag the food tray of clients with chronic dehydration to indicate if the client is identified as having chronic dehydration and indicate that they should finish 75% to 100% of their food and fluids. Offering beverages in brightly colored cups may improve fluid intake. *Older clients often have a combination of both malnutrition and fluid deficit and may not have good taste sensation (Hooper et al, 2014).*
- Recognize that lower blood pressures and monitoring of an intake record over 24 hours is recommended to track oral intake and possible dehydration (Oates et al, 2015).
- A higher BUN/creatinine ratio can be significant signs of dehydration in older adults. *Structural changes of the kidney include alterations of renal blood flow of up to 50% from age 20 to 80. As people age, the kidney undergoes age-related changes, which translate in an inexorable and progressive decline in renal function.*
- *In the United States, renal dysfunction has a 15% prevalence in persons older than 70 years (Bolignano et al, 2014).*
- Monitor older clients for excess fluid volume during the treatment of deficient fluid volume: auscultate lung sounds, assess for edema, and note vital signs. *The older client has a decreased ability to adapt to rapid increases in intravascular volume and can quickly develop fluid overload.*

Home Care

- Teach family members how to monitor output in the home (e.g., use of commode "hat" in the toilet, urinal, or bedpan, or use of catheter and closed drainage system). Instruct them to monitor both intake and output. Use common terms such as "cups" or "glasses of water a day" when providing education.
- When weighing the client, use same scale each day. Be sure scale is on a flat, not cushioned, surface. Do not weigh the client with a scale placed on any type of rug because scales provide more accurate readings when used on a hard surface.
- Teach family about complications of deficient fluid volume and when to call the health care provider.
- Teach the family the signs of hypovolemia, especially in older adults, and how to monitor for dizziness or unsteady gait.
- If the client is receiving IV fluids, there must be a responsible caregiver in the home. Teach caregiver about administration of fluids, complications of IV administration (e.g., fluid volume overload, development of phlebitis, speed of medication reactions), and when to call for assistance. Assist caregiver with administration for as long as necessary to maintain client safety. *Administration of IV fluids in the home is a high-technology procedure and requires sufficient professional support to ensure safety of the client.*
- Identify an emergency plan, including when to call 911. *Some complications of deficient fluid volume cannot be reversed in the home and are life-threatening. Clients progressing toward hypovolemic shock will need emergency care.*

● = Independent;   ▲ = Collaborative;   **EBN** = Evidence-Based Nursing;   **EB** = Evidence-Based

- Deficient fluid volume may be a symptom of impending death in terminally ill clients. In palliative care situations, treatment of deficient fluid volume should be determined based on client/family goals. Information and support should be provided to assist the client/family in this decision. Support the family/client in a palliative care situation to decide if it is appropriate to intervene for deficient fluid volume or to allow the client to die without fluids. *Deficient fluid volume may be a symptom of impending death in terminally ill clients. There is no defined gold standard for hydrating dying clients, and hydration and nutrition are considered basic acts for care of a dying client (Ong, Yee, & Lee, 2012).*

Client/Family Teaching and Discharge Planning

- Instruct the client to avoid rapid position changes, especially from supine to sitting or standing.
- Teach the client and family about appropriate diet and fluid intake.
- Teach the client and family how to measure and record intake and output accurately.
- Teach the client and family about measures instituted to treat hypovolemia and to prevent or treat fluid volume loss.
- Instruct the client and family about signs of deficient fluid volume that indicate they should contact health care provider.

REFERENCES

Alseiari, M., Meyer, K. B., & Wong, J. B. (2016). Evidence underlying KDIGO (Kidney Disease: Improving Global Outcomes) guideline recommendations: A systematic review. *American Journal of Kidney Diseases, 67*(3), 417–422.

Andeucchi, M., Faga, T., Pisani, A., et al. (2017). The ischemic/nephrotoxic acute kidney injury and the use of renal biomarkers in clinical practice. *European Journal of Internal Medicine, 39*, 1–8.

Angappan, S., Parida, S., Vasudevan, A., et al. (2015). The comparison of stroke volume variation with central venous pressure in predicting fluid responsiveness in septic patients with acute circulatory failure. *Indian Journal of Critical Care Medicine: Peer-Reviewed, Official Publication of Indian Society of Critical Care Medicine, 19*(7), 394–400.

Assadi, F. (2017). Passive leg raising: Simple and reliable technique to prevent fluid overload in critically ill patients. *International Journal of Preventive Medicine, 8*, 48.

Bolen, B. B. (2018). *What not to eat with diarrhea.* Retrieved from https://www.verywellhealth.com/what-to-eat-for-diarrhea-1944822. (Accessed 8 September 2018).

Bolignano, D., Mattace-Raso, F., Sijbrands, E. J., et al. (2014). The aging kidney revisited: A systematic review. *Ageing Research Reviews*, 65–80.

Cherniack, E. P. (2012). Ergogenic dietary aids for the elderly. *Nutrition (Burbank, Los Angeles County, Calif.), 28*(3), 225–229.

Ciccarelli, S., Stolfi, I., & Caramia, G. (2013). Management strategies in the treatment of neonatal and pediatric gastroenteritis. *Infection and Drug Resistance, 6*, 133–161.

deAraujo, T., Maeve, V., Gomes, P. C., et al. (2014). Enteral nutrition in critical patients; should the administration be continuous or intermittent? *Nutrición Hospitalaria, 29*(5), 563–567.

Deshpande, A., Lever, D. S., & Soffer, E. (2013). *Acute diarrhea.* Cleveland Clinic Continuing Education. Retrieved from http://www.clevelandclinicmeded.com/medicalpubs/diseasemanagement/gastroenterology/acute-diarrhea/. (Accessed 26 January 2018).

Duus, N., Shogilev, D. J., Skibsted, S., et al. (2015). The reliability and validity of passive leg raise and fluid bolus to assess fluid responsiveness in spontaneously breathing emergency department patients. *Journal of Critical Care, 30*(1), 217, e1–e5. doi:10.1016/j.jcrc.2014.07.031.

Falszewska, A., Dziechciarz, P., & Szajewska, H. (2014). The diagnostic accuracy of clinical dehydration scale in identifying children with acute gastroenteritis: A systematic review. *Clinical Pediatrics, 53*(12), 1181–1188.

Ftouh, S., & Lewington, A. (2014). Prevention, detection and management of acute kidney injury: Concise guidelines. *Clinical Medicine (London, England), 14*(1), 61–65.

Graves, N. S. (2013). Acute gastroenteritis. *Primary Care, 40*(3), 727–741.

Guandalini, S., Frye, R. E., Tamer, M. A., et al. (2017). *Diarrhea.* Medscape Reference. Retrieved from https://emedicine.medscape.com/article/928598-overview. (Accessed 6 December 2017).

Hooper, L., Bunn, D. K., Abdelhamid, A., et al. (2016a). Water loss (intracellular) dehydration assessed using urinary tests: How well do they work? Diagnostic accuracy in older people. *The American Journal of Clinical Nutrition, 104*(1), 121–131.

Hooper, L., Bunn, D. K., Downing, A., et al. (2016b). Which frail older people are dehydrated? The UK DRIE Study. *The Journals of Gerontology. Series A, Biological Sciences and Medical Sciences, 71*(10), 1341–1347.

Hooper, L., Bunn, D., Jimoh, F. O., et al. (2014). Water loss dehydration and aging. *Mechanisms of Ageing and Development, 136–137*, 50–58.

James, M. T., Hobson, C. E., Darmon, M., et al. For the Acute Dialysis Quality Initiative (ADQI) Consensus Group. (2016). Applications for detection of acute kidney injury using electronic medical records and clinical information systems: Workgroup statements from the 15th ADQI Consensus Conference. *Canadian Journal of Kidney Health and Disease, 3*, 9. doi:10.1186/s40697-016-0100-2.

Jequier, E., & Constant, F. (2010). Water as an essential nutrient: The physiological basis of hydration. *European Journal of Clinical Nutrition, 64*, 115–123.

Jin, K., Murugan, R., Sileanu, F. E., et al. (2017). Intensive monitoring of urine output is associated with increased detection of acute kidney injury and improved outcomes. *Chest, 152*(5), 972–979.

Kalantari, K., Chang, J. N., Ronco, C., et al. (2013). Assessment of intravascular volume status and volume responsiveness in critically ill patients. *Kidney International, 83*, 1017–1028.

Keller, J., & Layer, P. (2014). The pathophysiology of malabsorption. *Viszeralmedizin, 30*, 150–154. doi:10.1159/000364794.

Kumar, R., Kumar, P., Aneja, S., et al. (2015). Safety and efficacy of low-osmolarity ORS vs. modified rehydration solution for malnourished children for treatment of children with severe acute malnutrition and diarrhea: A randomized controlled trial. *Journal of Tropical Pediatrics, 61*(6), 435–441.

Kuo, S. C. H., Kuo, P. J., Rau, C. S., et al. (2017). Hyponatremia is associated with worse outcomes from fall injuries in the elderly.

International Journal of Environmental Research and Public Health, 26, pii: E460.

Marik, P. E., Monnet, X., & Teboul, J.-L. (2011). Hemodynamic parameters to guide fluid therapy. *Annals of Intensive Care, 1,* 1.

Mentes, J., & Wang, J. (2011). Measuring risk for dehydration in nursing home residents: Evaluation of the dehydration risk appraisal checklist. *Research in Gerontological Nursing, 4*(2), 148–156.

Miller, H. J. (2015). Dehydration in the older adult. *Journal of Gerontological Nursing, 41*(9), 8–13.

Oates, L. L., & Price, C. I. (2017). Clinical assessments and care interventions to promote oral hydration amongst older patients: A narrative systematic review. *BMC Nursing, 16*(4).

Ong, Y. W., Yee, C. M., & Lee, A. (2012). Ethical dilemmas in the care of cancer patients near the end of life. *Singapore Medical Journal, 53*(1), 11–16.

Peng, Z. Y., & Kellum, J. A. (2013). Perioperative fluids: A clear road ahead? *Current Opinion in Critical Care, 19*(4), 353–358.

Perrier, E., Vergne, S., Klein, A., et al. (2013). Hydration biomarkers in free-living adults with different levels of habitual fluid consumption. *The British Journal of Nutrition, 109*(9), 1678–1687.

Pross, N., Demazieres, A., Girard, N., et al. (2013). Influence of progressive fluid restriction on mood and physiological markers of dehydration in women. *The British Journal of Nutrition, 109*(2), 313–321.

Prowle, J. R., Liu, Y. L., Licari, E., et al. (2011). Oliguria as a predictive biomarker of acute kidney injury in critically ill patients. *Critical Care (London, England), 15*(4), R 172.

Rhodes, A., Evans, L. E., Alhazzani, W., et al. (2017). Surviving sepsis campaign: International guidelines for management of sepsis and septic shock: 2016. *Critical Care Medicine, 45*(3), 486–552.

Schrezenmeier, E. V., Barasch, J., Budde, K., et al. (2017). Biomarkers in acute kidney injury—pathophysiological basis and clinical performance. *Acta Physiologica (Oxford, England), 219*(3), 554–572.

Scott, R., & Bowling, T. E. (2015). Enteral tube feeding in adults. *The Journal of the Royal College of Physicians of Edinburgh, 45*(1), 49–54.

Seymour, C. W., Liu, V. S., Iwashyna, T. J., et al. (2016). Assessment of clinical criteria for sepsis: For the Third International Consensus Definitions for Sepsis and Septic Shock (Sepsis-3). *JAMA: The Journal of the American Medical Association, 315*(8), 762–774.

Shimizu, M., Kinoshita, K., Hattori, K., et al. (2012). Physical signs of dehydration in the elderly. *Internal Medicine (Tokyo, Japan), 51*(10), 1207–1210.

Singer, M. (2016). The new sepsis consensus definitions (Sepsis-3): The good, the not-so-bad, and the actually-quite-pretty. *Intensive Care Medicine, 42*(12), 2027–2029.

Wagner, K. D., & Hardin-Pierce, M. G. (2014). *High acuity nursing* (6th ed.). Boston: Prentice Hall, Inc.

Wang, C. H., Hsieh, W. H., Chou, H. C., et al. (2014). Liberal versus restricted fluid resuscitation strategies in trauma patients: A systematic review and meta-analysis of randomized controlled trials and observational studies. *Critical Care Medicine, 42*(4), 954–961.

Wedro, B., & Stoppler, M. C. (2017). *Orthostatic hypotension: Low blood pressure when standing.* Retrieved from http://www.medicinenet.com/orthostatic_hypotension/article.htm. (Accessed 26 January 2018).

White, C. J. (2016). Atherosclerotic peripheral arterial disease. In L. Goldman & A. I. Schafer (Eds.), *Goldman's Cecil machine* (25th ed.). Philadelphia: Elsevier Saunders.

Zhang, Z., Hong, Y., Smischney, N. J., et al. (2017). Early management of sepsis with emphasis on early goal directed therapy: AME evidence series 002. *Journal of Thoracic Disease, 9*(2), 392–405.

Zheng, Z., Xu, X., & Deng, H. (2014). Urine output on ICU entry is associated with hospital mortality in unselected critically ill patients. *Journal of Nephrology, 27*(1), 65–71.

Excess Fluid volume   *Susan M. Dirkes, RN, MS, CCRN*

NANDA-I

Definition

Surplus intake and/or retention of fluid.

Defining Characteristics

Adventitious breath sounds; alteration in blood pressure; alteration in mental status; alteration in pulmonary artery pressure (PAP); alteration in respiratory pattern; alteration in urine specific gravity; anasarca; anxiety; azotemia; decrease in hematocrit; decrease in hemoglobin; dyspnea; edema; electrolyte imbalance; hepatomegaly; increased central venous pressure (CVP); intake exceeds output; jugular vein distention; oliguria; orthopnea; paroxysmal nocturnal dyspnea; pleural effusion; positive hepatojugular reflex; presence of S3 heart sound; pulmonary congestion; restlessness; weight gain over short period of time

Related Factors

Excessive fluid intake; excessive sodium intake

Associated Condition

Compromised regulatory mechanism

● = Independent;   ▲ = Collaborative;   EBN = Evidence-Based Nursing;   EB = Evidence-Based

NOC   (Nursing Outcomes Classification)

Suggested NOC Outcomes

Electrolyte and Acid-Base Balance; Fluid Balance; Fluid Overload Severity; Hydration

> ### Example NOC Outcome with Indicators
>
> **Fluid Balance** as evidenced by the following indicators: Peripheral edema/Neck vein distention/Adventitious breath sounds/ Body weight increase. (Rate each indicator of **Fluid Balance:** 1 = severe, 2 = substantial, 3 = moderate, 4 = mild, 5 = none [see Section I].)

Client Outcomes

Client Will (Specify Time Frame)

- Remain free of edema, effusion, anasarca
- Maintain body weight appropriate for the client
- Maintain clear lung sounds; no evidence of dyspnea or orthopnea
- Remain free of jugular vein distention, positive hepatojugular reflex, and S3 heart sound
- Maintain normal CVP, PAP, cardiac output, and vital signs
- Maintain urine output of 0.5 mL/kg/hr or more with normal urine osmolality and specific gravity
- Explain actions that are needed to treat or prevent excess fluid volume including fluid and dietary restrictions, and medications
- Describe symptoms that indicate the need to consult with health care provider

NIC   (Nursing Interventions Classification)

Suggested NIC Interventions

Fluid Management; Fluid Monitoring

> ### Example NIC Activities—Fluid Monitoring
>
> Monitor weight; Monitor intake and output

Nursing Interventions and *Rationales*

- Monitor location and extent of edema using the 1+ to 4+ scale to quantify edema; also measure the legs using a millimeter tape in the same area at the same time each day. Note differences in measurement between extremities. EBN: *Numerous studies in patients and in experimental models of congestive heart failure (CHF) have established the important role of the renin–angiotensin–aldosterone system (RAAS) and the sympathetic nervous system (SNS) in the progression of cardiovascular and renal dysfunction in CHF. It is now accepted that excessive neurohormonal activation may adversely affect cardiac function and the hemodynamic condition by enhancement of systemic vasoconstriction and promoting salt and water retention by the kidney (Zaher et al, 2017).*
- Monitor daily weight for sudden increases; use same scale and type of clothing at same time each day, preferably before breakfast. *Body weight changes reflect changes in body fluid volume.* EB: *Body weight is commonly used to monitor for fluid overload (Wagner & Hardin-Pierce, 2014).*
- Monitor intake and output; note trends reflecting decreasing urine output in relation to fluid intake. EB: *Abnormally low urine output (oliguria) is a leading indicator of acute kidney injury (AKI), which increases mortality, cost of care, and length of stay (Yong et al, 2013). The volume of all fluids should be measured. If the family is measuring, instruct them on common conversions between household measurements and metric.* EBN: *Chronic heart failure (HF) is characterized by neurohumoral activation and sodium retention that leads to excessive fluid accumulation in the systemic and pulmonary circulations. Lung congestion increases dyspnea and impairs gas transfer (Melenovsky et al, 2015).*
- Chronic HF is characterized by neurohormonal activation and sodium retention that leads to excessive fluid accumulation in the systemic and pulmonary circulations. *Monitor vital signs; note decreasing blood pressure, tachycardia, and tachypnea. Monitor for S3 heart sounds. If signs of HF are present, see the care plan for Decreased **Cardiac** output.*

● = Independent;   ▲ = Collaborative;   EBN = Evidence-Based Nursing;   EB = Evidence-Based

F

- Auscultate lung sounds for crackles, monitor respiration effort, and determine the presence and severity of orthopnea. *The pulmonary system adapts to the increased post CVP, which is believed to be caused by reduced capillary filtration from pulmonary basal membrane thickening, enhanced alveolar fluid clearance, and increased lymphatic drainage (Melenovsky, 2015).*
- Monitor serum and urine osmolality, serum sodium, blood urea nitrogen (BUN)/creatinine ratio, and hematocrit for abnormalities. EB: *Fluid overload is a causative factor for the occurrence of AKI. Volume overload leads to organ congestion and a resultant decrease in renal blood flow (Salahuddin, 2017).*
- BUN and creatinine are monitored currently as biomarkers of kidney injury and failure. EB: *Serum creatinine is an imperfect marker because its levels reflect delayed functional consequences of the injury rather than direct cell injury and is not sensitive and specific in the early diagnosis of AKI (TRIBE-AKI Consortium Investigators, 2017). BUN and creatinine is affected by fluid volume status and medications (Andreucci et al, 2016).*
- With head of bed elevated 30 to 45 degrees, monitor jugular veins for distention with the client in the upright position; assess for positive hepatojugular reflex. *Increased intravascular volume results in jugular vein distention as a result of backflow through the vena cava (Wagner & Hardin-Pierce, 2014).*
- Monitor the client's behavior for restlessness, anxiety, or confusion; use safety precautions if symptoms are present. *When excess fluid volume compromises cardiac output, the client may experience confusion, decreased consciousness, delirium, and HF (Wagner & Hardin-Pierce, 2014).*
- ▲ Monitor for the development of conditions that increase the client's risk for excess fluid volume, including HF, kidney failure, and liver failure, all of which result in decreased glomerular filtration rate and fluid retention. EB: *Other causes are increased intake of oral or intravenous (IV) fluids in excess of the client's cardiac and renal reserve levels, and increased levels of antidiuretic hormone (Ronco et al, 2012). Many clients with fluid overload have AKI, and fluid balance is an important indicator of outcomes. One study of end-stage renal disease patients with chronic fluid overload showed a strong risk factor for death (Zoccali et al, 2017).*
- ▲ Provide a restricted-sodium diet as appropriate if ordered. *Restricting the sodium in the diet will favor the renal excretion of excess fluid. Take care to avoid hyponatremia, which can cause serious complications including nausea, seizures, coma, and death (Rudge & Kim, 2014).*
- ▲ Monitor serum albumin level and provide protein intake as appropriate. *When plasma proteins, especially albumin, no longer sustain sufficient colloid osmotic pressure to counterbalance hydrostatic pressure, edema develops (Wagner & Hardin-Pierce, 2014).*
- ▲ Administer prescribed diuretics as appropriate; ensure adequate blood pressure before administration. If diuretic is administered intravenously, note and record the blood pressure and urine output after the dose. Monitor serum sodium for hyponatremia. EBN: *Increased arginine vasopressin (AVP) levels in HF patients lead to fluid retention by its actions on vasopressin receptors. Hyponatremia is one of the commonly encountered clinical problems among HF patients with a prevalence of about 20% on hospitalization and has been associated with increased length of stay and in-hospital and postdischarge mortality rates. Hyponatremia in HF is mainly dilutional secondary to neurohormonal activation, especially AVP resulting in free water retention and volume overload (Vinod et al, 2017).* EB: *Clinical practice guidelines on HF state that daily weight along with monitoring input and output is useful for monitoring effects of diuretic therapy (Wagner & Hardin-Pierce, 2014).*
- Monitor for side effects of diuretic therapy including orthostatic hypotension (especially if the client is also receiving angiotensin-converting enzyme [ACE] inhibitors), hypovolemia, and electrolyte imbalances (hypokalemia and hyponatremia). *Observe for hyperkalemia in clients receiving a potassium-sparing diuretic and in those on beta-blockers and ACE inhibitors (Rudge & Kim, 2014; Wagner & Hardin-Pierce, 2014).*
- ▲ Implement fluid restriction as ordered, especially when serum sodium is low; include all routes of intake. Schedule limited intake of fluids around the clock, and include the type of fluids preferred by the client. *Fluid restriction may decrease intravascular volume and myocardial workload. Overzealous fluid restriction should not be used because hypovolemia can worsen HF. Client involvement in planning will enhance participation in the necessary fluid restriction.*
- Maintain the rate of all IV infusions, using an IV pump. *This is done to prevent inadvertent exacerbation of excess fluid volume and to more accurately monitor fluid intake.*
- Turn clients with dependent edema at least every 2 hours and monitor for areas that may develop pressure ulcers. *Decreased oncotic pressure caused by low levels of albumin affects distribution of total body fluids. The association between low levels of albumin and increased risk for pressure ulcers may be caused by a change in tissue tolerance, with redistribution of fluid and formation of edema (Serra et al, 2014).*

• = Independent;   ▲ = Collaborative;   EBN = Evidence-Based Nursing;   EB = Evidence-Based

▲ Provide ordered care for edematous extremities including compression, elevation, and muscle exercises. EB: *Treatments for clients with peripheral edema include elevation of the extremities above heart level, use of a specialty bed, and offloading of the extremity by repositioning or the use of pressure-offloading devices (Bly, 2016).*

● Promote a positive body image and good self-esteem. *Visible edema may alter the client's body image.* Refer to the care plan for Disturbed **Body Image.**

▲ Consult with the health care provider if signs and symptoms of excess fluid volume persist or worsen. *Pulmonary edema requires prompt treatment such as preload reducers, afterload reducers, and morphine to relieve anxiety (Mayo Foundation for Medical Education and Research, 2014).*

Critically Ill

● Insert an indwelling urinary catheter if ordered and measure urine output hourly. Notify health care provider if output is less than 0.5 mL/kg/hr. *Urine output of less than 0.5 mL/kg/hr for 6 or more hours is defined as oliguria (Schetz et al, 2017).*

▲ Monitor blood pressure, heart rate, passive leg lift, mean arterial pressure, CVP, PAP, and cardiac output/index; note and report trends of increasing or decreasing pressures over time. *Alterations in these parameters may indicate that the client is going into shock. Hemodynamic criteria for cardiogenic shock are sustained hypotension (systolic blood pressure less than 90 mm Hg for at least 30 minutes) and a reduced cardiac index (less than 2.2 L/min/m^2) in the presence of elevated pulmonary capillary occlusion pressure (greater than 15 mm Hg), pulmonary congestion, dyspnea, and hypoxemia (Wagner & Hardin-Pierce, 2014; Van Diepen et al, 2017).*

▲ Monitor the effects of infusion of diuretic drips. Perform continuous renal replacement therapy (CRRT) as ordered if the client is critically ill and hemodynamically unstable and excessive fluid must be removed. EBN: *CRRT is indicated for hypervolemia, metabolic acidosis, and hyperkalemia (Dirkes, 2014).*

 ### Geriatric

● Recognize that the presence of fluid volume excess is particularly serious in older adults. EB: The kidney undergoes age-related changes that include structural and functional changes, which may increase the incidence of AKI (Bolignano et al, 2014).

● Monitor electrolyte levels carefully, including sodium levels and potassium levels, with both increased and decreased levels possible. *Older adults are prone to electrolyte abnormalities caused by aging, decreased muscle mass, and decreased total body water (Mannesse et al, 2013). Also, the large number of medications that are taken can affect electrolyte levels. Many older clients receive selective serotonin reuptake inhibitors (SSRIs) for treatment of depression, which can result in hyponatremia (Varela Piñón & Adán-Manes, 2017). SSRIs are also known to be responsible for many sexual side effects such as altered libido, erectile dysfunction, vaginal dryness, ejaculatory disorders, and orgasmic problems, which are frequently reported by patients (Reisman, 2017).*

● Refer to the care plan for Risk for **Electrolyte** imbalance and the care plan for **Sexual Dysfunction.**

 ### Home Care

● Assess client and family knowledge of disease processes causing excess fluid volume.

▲ Teach about disease process and complications of excess fluid volume, including when to contact the health care provider.

● Assess client and family knowledge and compliance with medical regimen, including medications, diet, rest, and exercise. Assist family with integrating restrictions into daily living. *Assistance with integration of cultural values, especially those related to foods, with medical regimen promotes compliance and decreased risk of complications.*

▲ Teach and reinforce knowledge of medications. Instruct the client not to use over-the-counter (OTC) medications (e.g., diet medications) without first consulting the provider.

▲ Instruct the client to make the primary health care provider aware of medications ordered by other health care providers.

● Identify emergency plan for rapidly developing or critical levels of excess fluid volume when diuresing is not safe at home. *Excess fluid volume can be life-threatening.*

▲ Teach about signs and symptoms of both excess and deficient fluid volume, such as darker urine, dry mouth, and peripheral edema, and when to call the health care provider. *Urine color may be a simple indicator of hydration (Wagner & Hardin-Pierce, 2014).*

● = Independent;   ▲ = Collaborative;   EBN = Evidence-Based Nursing;   EB = Evidence-Based

Client/Family Teaching and Discharge Planning

- Describe signs and symptoms of excess fluid volume and actions to take if they occur.
- ▲ Teach client on diuretics to weigh self daily in the morning and to notify the health care provider if there is a 2.2 pound (1 kg) or more weight gain (Wagner & Hardin-Pierce, 2014). **EB:** *Clinical practice guidelines on HF suggest that daily weight monitoring leads to early recognition of excess fluid retention, which, when reported, can be offset with additional medication to avoid hospitalization caused by HF decompensation (Wagner & Hardin-Pierce, 2014).*
- ▲ Teach the importance of fluid and sodium restrictions. Help the client and family devise a schedule for intake of fluids throughout the entire day. Refer to a dietitian concerning implementation of a low-sodium diet.
- Teach clients how to measure and document intake and output with common household measurements, such as cups.
- ▲ Teach how to take diuretics correctly: take one dose in the morning and second dose (if taken) no later than 4 p.m. Adjust potassium intake as appropriate for potassium-losing or potassium-sparing diuretics. Note the appearance of side effects such as weakness, muscle cramps, hypertension, or palpitations (Wagner & Hardin-Pierce, 2014).
- For the client undergoing hemodialysis, teach client the required restrictions in dietary electrolytes, protein, and fluid. Spend time with the client to detect any factors that may interfere with the client's compliance with the fluid restriction or restrictive diet. **EBN:** *Nonadherence to fluid restrictions, especially in patients undergoing hemodialysis, has been linked to numerous deleterious outcomes, including patient and provider frustration, treatment failure, illness complications and relapse, and mortality (Howren et al, 2016).*

REFERENCES

Andreucci, M., Faga, T., Pisani, A., et al. (2016). The ischemic/nephrotoxic acute kidney injury and the use of renal biomarkers in clinical practice. *European Journal of Internal Medicine, 39,* 1–8.

Azzam, Z. S., Kinaneh, S., Bahouth, F., et al. (2017). Involvement of cytokines in the pathogenesis of salt and water imbalance in congestive heart failure. *Frontiers in Immunology, 8,* 716.

Bly, D., Schallom, M., Sona, C., et al. (2016). A model of pressure, oxygenation, and perfusion risk factors for pressure ulcers in the intensive care unit. *American Journal of Critical Care, 25*(2), 156–164.

Bolignano, D., Mattace-Raso, F., Sijbrands, E. J., et al. (2014). The aging kidney revisited: A systematic review. *Ageing Research Reviews,* 65–80.

Dirkes, S. (2014). Continuous renal replacement therapy: Dialysis for critically ill patients. *American Nurse Today, 9*(5).

Howren, M. B., Kellerman, Q. D., Hillis, S. L., et al. (2016). Effect of a behavioral self-regulation intervention on patient adherence to fluid-intake restrictions in hemodialysis: A randomized controlled trial. *Annals of Behavioral Medicine: A Publication of the Society of Behavioral Medicine, 50*(2), 167–176.

Mannesse, C. K., Jansen, P. A., Van Marum, R. J., et al. (2013). Characteristics, prevalence, risk factors, and underlying mechanism of hyponatremia in elderly patients treated with antidepressants: A cross-sectional study. *Maturitas, 76*(4), 357–363.

Mayo Foundation for Medical Education and Research (MFMER). (2014). *Diseases and conditions: Pulmonary edema July, 2014.* Retrieved from http://www.mayoclinic.com/health/pulmonary-edema/DS00412/DSECTION=symptoms. (Accessed 18 August 2017).

Melenovsky, V., Andersen, M. J., Andress, K., et al. (2015). Lung congestion in chronic heart failure: Haemodynamic, clinical, and prognostic implications. *European Journal of Heart Failure, 17*(11), 1161–1171.

Reisman, P. (2017). Sexual consequences of post-SSRI syndrome. *Sexual Medicine Reviews. 5*(4), 429–433.

Ronco, C., Kaushik, M., Valle, R., et al. (2012). Diagnosis and management of fluid overload in heart failure and cardio-renal syndrome: The 5B approach. *Seminars in Nephrology, 32*(1), 129–141.

Rudge, J. E., & Kim, D. (2014). New-onset hyponatremia after surgery for traumatic hip fracture. *Age and Ageing, 43*(6), 821–826.

Salahuddin, N., Sammani, M., Hamdan, A., et al. (2017). Fluid overload is an independent risk factor for acute kidney injury in critically ill patients: Results of a cohort study. *BMC Nephrology, 18*(1), 45.

Schetz, M., et al. (2017). Understanding oliguria in the critically ill. *Intensive Care Medicine, 43*(6), 914–916.

Serra, R., Caroleo, S., Buffone, G., et al. (2014). Low serum albumin level as an independent risk factor for the onset of pressure ulcers in intensive care unit patients. *International Wound Journal, 11*(5), 550–553.

TRIBE-AKI Consortium Investigators. (2017). Fluid overload is an independent risk factor for acute kidney injury in critically ill patients: Results of a cohort study. *BMC Nephrology, 18*(1), 218.

Van Diepen, S., Katz, J. N., Albert, N. M., et al. (2017). Contemporary management of cardiogenic shock. *Circulation, 136*(16), E232–E268.

Varela Piñón, M., & Adán-Manes, J. (2017). Selective serotonin reuptake inhibitor-induced hyponatremia: Clinical implications and therapeutic alternatives. *Clinical Neuropharmacology, 40*(4), 177–179.

Vinod, P., Krishnappa, V., Chauvin, A. M., et al. (2017). Cardiorenal syndrome: Role of arginine vasopressin and vaptans in heart failure. *Cardiology Research, 8*(3), 87–95.

Wagner, K. D., & Hardin-Pierce, M. G. (2014). *High acuity nursing* (6th ed.). Boston: Prentice Hall, Inc.

Yong, T. Y., Fok, J. S., Ng, P. Z., et al. (2013). The significance of reduced kidney function among hospitalized acute general medical patients. *QJM: Monthly Journal of the Association of Physicians, 106*(1), 59–65.

Zoccali, C., Moissl, U., Chazot, C., et al. (2017). Chronic fluid overload and mortality in ESRD. *Journal of the American Society of Nephrology, 28*(8), 2491–2497.

● = Independent; ▲ = Collaborative; **EBN** = Evidence-Based Nursing; **EB** = Evidence-Based

Risk for deficient Fluid volume   *Mary Beth Flynn Makic, PhD, RN, CCNS, FAAN, FNAP*

NANDA-I

F

Definition

Susceptible to experiencing decreased intravascular, interstitial, and/or intracellular fluid volumes, which may compromise health.

Risk Factors

Barrier to accessing fluid; insufficient fluid intake; insufficient knowledge about fluid needs

At-Risk Population

Extremes of age; extremes of weight; factors influencing fluid needs

Associated Condition

Active fluid volume loss; compromised regulatory mechanism; deviations affecting fluid absorption; deviations affecting fluid intake; excessive fluid loss through normal route; fluid loss through abnormal route; pharmaceutical agent

NIC, NOC, Client Outcomes, Nursing Interventions and *Rationales,* Client/Family Teaching, and References

Refer to care plan for Deficient **Fluid** volume

Frail Elderly syndrome   *Cynthia DeLeon Thelen, MSN, BSN, RN*

NANDA-I

Definition

Dynamic state of unstable equilibrium that affects the older individual experiencing deterioration in one or more domains of health (physical, functional, psychological, or social) and leads to increased susceptibility to adverse health effects, in particular disability.

Defining Characteristics

Activity intolerance (00092), bathing self-care deficit (00108), decreased cardiac output (00029), fatigue (00093), feeding self-care deficit (00102), hopelessness (00124), imbalanced nutrition: less than body requirements (00002), impaired memory (00131), impaired physical mobility (00085), impaired walking (00088), social isolation (00053), toileting self-care deficit (00110)

Related Factors

Activity intolerance, anxiety, average daily physical activity is less than recommended for gender and age, decrease in energy, decrease in muscle strength, depression, exhaustion, fear of falling, immobility, impaired balance, impaired mobility, insufficient social support, malnutrition, muscle weakness, obesity, sadness, sedentary lifestyle, social isolation

At-Risk Population

Age >70 years, constricted living space, economically disadvantaged, ethnicity other than Caucasian, female gender, history of falls, living alone, low educational level, prolonged hospitalization, social vulnerability

NOC   Outcomes (Nursing Outcomes Classification)

Suggested NOC Outcomes

Activity Tolerance; Balance; Exercise Participation; Hope; Physical Aging; Psychosocial Adjustment: Life Change; Client Satisfaction: Functional Assistance

● = Independent;   ▲ = Collaborative;   EBN = Evidence-Based Nursing;   EB = Evidence-Based

F

Client Outcomes

Client Will (Specify Time Frame)

- Remain living as independently as possible in the home or care setting of his or her choice
- Maintain safety when engaging in activities of daily living and ambulation
- Increase exercise and/or daily physical activity to build muscle strength
- Maintain a healthy weight

NIC   Interventions (Nursing Interventions Classification)

Suggested NIC Interventions

Exercise Promotion; Exercise Promotion: Balance; Exercise Promotion: Strength Training; Hope Inspiration; Nutrition Therapy

Example NIC Activities—Frail Elderly Syndrome
Promote physical activities that build strength and improve balance and endurance

Nursing Interventions and *Rationales*

- Assess frailty with a tool such as the Frailty Index or the Edmonton Frail Scale. EB: *Apóstolo et al (2017) did a systematic review on diagnostic accuracy and predictive ability of frailty measures and found that the Frailty Index had good predictive reliability.* EB: *The Edmonton Frail Scale is a tool designed to identify frail older adults in clinical settings (Perna & Francis, 2017).*
- Recognize that balance and gait impairment are features of frailty and are risk factors for falls. EB: *Cadore et al (2013) did a systematic review of the literature and found that exercise interventions composed of strength, endurance, and balance training improve the rate of falls in frail older adults.* EB: *By reversing frailty through exercise interventions that engender fitness, older adults will remain physically independent longer (Bray et al, 2016).*
- Preserve physical functioning through individualized physical activity plans. EB: *Results from the LIFE-P study found that regular physical activity may reduce frailty, especially in individuals at higher risk of disability (Cesari et al, 2014).* EB: *de Labra et al (2015) did a systematic review of the literature and found that low physical activity has been shown to be one of the most common components of frailty.*
- Assess falls using a falls risk assessment tool such as the Hendrich II Fall Risk Model. EBN: *Falls are an important measure of nursing quality and patient safety (Swartzell, Fulton, & Friesth, 2013).*
- Assess risk of fracture using tools such as the Cardiovascular Health Study (CHS) or Study of Osteoporotic Fracture (SOF) indicators. EBN: *Chen et al (2017) did a systematic review of the literature and in total five studies included 103,783 older people and recorded 2960 fractures.*
- Evaluate the client's medications to determine whether medications increase the risk of frailty and/or are potentially inappropriate mediations (PIM), and if appropriate, consult with the client's health care provider regarding the client's medications. EB: *Polypharmacy is associated with increased risk of mortality in elderly people (Gómez et al, 2015).* EB: *The number of medications prescribed can be useful to help physicians be aware of the high risk for PIM (Tsao et al, 2016).*
- ▲ Refer to a dietitian for an individualized therapeutic diet. EB: *Micronutrient supplementation was associated with a significant increase in the Mini Nutritional Assessment score in persons at risk for malnutrition (von Arnim et al, 2013).* EB: *Malafarina et al (2013) did a systematic review of the literature about nutritional supplements in older adults and found that nutritional supplements are effective in the treatment of muscle mass loss, particularly in conjunction with physical exercise.*
- Refer to care plan for Readiness for enhanced **Nutrition** for additional interventions.

• = Independent;   ▲ = Collaborative;   EBN = Evidence-Based Nursing;   EB = Evidence-Based

- Monitor weight loss. EB: *Weight loss is considered a main component of frailty syndrome (Yannakoulia et al, 2017)*. CEB: *Milne et al (2009) did a systematic literature review and found that when given to older adults, nutritional supplements containing protein and energy result in weight gain.*
- Encourage clients to engage in active lifestyles. CEB: *Peterson et al (2009) studied 2964 older adults for 5 years and found that sedentary older individuals had a greater likelihood of developing frailty than individuals who were engaged in exercise.*
- Provide an exercise-training program. EB: *Physical exercise training leads to improved cognitive functioning as well as psychological well-being in older adults who are frail (Langlois et al, 2013).*
- Promote the benefits of home-based exercise to older clients who are frail. EB: *Clegg et al (2014) conducted a study of 49 frail older adults and found evidence that the deterioration in mobility may be reduced through a 12-week home-based exercise intervention.*
- Use an interprofessional and person-centered approach for supporting frail older adults. EBN: *The focus of caring for frail older adults should not only be on medical problems but also on providing supportive services to help individuals maintain their independence and manage their lives despite frailty (Ebrahimi et al, 2014).* EBN: *Engaging patients, their family members, or care givers in care planning and goal setting during transitions is essential (Jeffs et al, 2017).*
- Develop a trusting and responsive relationship with frail clients. EBN: *Bindels et al (2013) qualitatively interviewed nurses (N = 23) and found that building a trusting relationship, along with competence, responsiveness, and attentiveness were important for providing frail older adults with good care.*

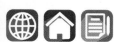

Multicultural, Home Care, and Client/Family Teaching

- The previously mentioned interventions may be adapted for multicultural, home care, and client family teaching.

REFERENCES

Apóstolo, J., Cooke, R., Bobrowicz-Campos, E., et al. (2017). Predicting risk and outcomes for frail older adults: An umbrella review of frailty screening tools. *JBI Database of Systematic Reviews and Implementation Reports, 15*(4), 1154.

Bindels, J., Cox, K., Widdershoven, G., et al. (2013). Care for community-dwelling frail older people: A practice nurse perspective. *Journal of Clinical Nursing.*

Bleijenberg, N., ten Dam, V. H., Drubbel, I., et al. (2013). Development of a proactive care program (U-CARE) to preserve physical functioning of frail older people in primary care. *Journal of Nursing Scholarship, 45*(3), 230–237.

Bray, N. W., Smart, R. R., Jakobi, J. M., et al. (2016). Exercise prescription to reverse frailty. *Applied Physiology, Nutrition, and Metabolism, 41*(10), 1112–1116.

Cadore, E. L., Rodríguez-Mañas, L., Sinclair, A., et al. (2013). Effects of different exercise interventions on risk of falls, gait ability, and balance in physically frail older adults: A systematic review. *Rejuvenation Research, 16*(2), 105–114.

Cesari, M., Vellas, B., Hsu, F. C., et al. (2014). A physical activity intervention to treat the frailty syndrome in older persons—Results from the LIFE-P study. *The Journals of Gerontology. Series A, Biological Sciences and Medical Sciences, 70*(2), 216–222.

Chen, K. W., Chang, S. F., & Lin, P. L. (2017). Frailty as a predictor of future fracture in older adults: A systematic review and meta-analysis. *Worldviews on Evidence-Based Nursing.*

Clegg, A., Barber, S., Young, J., et al. (2014). The home-based older people's exercise (HOPE) trial: A pilot randomised controlled trial of a home-based exercise intervention for older people with frailty. *Age and Ageing, 43*(5), 687–695.

de Labra, C., Guimaraes-Pinheiro, C., Maseda, A., et al. (2015). Effects of physical exercise interventions in frail older adults: A systematic review of randomized controlled trials. *BMC Geriatrics, 15*(1), 154.

Ebrahimi, Z., Dahlin-Ivanoff, S., Eklund, K., et al. (2014). Self-rated health and health-strengthening factors in community-living frail older people. *Journal of Advanced Nursing*, 825–836.

Gómez, C., Vega-Quiroga, S., Bermejo-Pareja, F., et al. (2015). Polypharmacy in the elderly: A marker of increased risk of mortality in a population-based prospective study (NEDICES). *Gerontology, 61*(4), 301–309.

Jeffs, L., Kuluski, K., Law, M., et al. (2017). Identifying effective nurse-led care transition interventions for older adults with complex needs using a structured expert panel. *Worldviews on Evidence-Based Nursing, 14*(2), 136–144.

Langlois, F., Vu, T. T. M., Chassé, K., et al. (2013). Benefits of physical exercise training on cognition and quality of life in frail older adults. *The Journals of Gerontology. Series B, Psychological Sciences and Social Sciences, 68*(3), 400–404.

Malafarina, V., Uriz-Otano, F., Iniesta, R., et al. (2013). Effectiveness of nutritional supplementation on muscle mass in treatment of sarcopenia in old age: A systematic review. *Journal of the American Medical Directors Association, 14*(1), 10–17.

Milne, A. C., Potter, J., Vivanti, A., et al. (2009). Protein and energy supplementation in elderly people at risk for malnutrition. *The Cochrane Database of Systematic Reviews*, (2), CD003288.

Perna, S., Francis, M. D. A., Bologna, C., et al. (2017). Performance of Edmonton Frail Scale on frailty assessment: Its association with multi-dimensional geriatric conditions assessed with specific screening tools. *BMC Geriatrics, 17*(1), 2.

Peterson, M. J., Giuliani, C., Morey, M. C., et al. (2009). Physical activity as a preventative factor for frailty: The health, aging, and body composition study. *The Journals of Gerontology. Series A, Biological Sciences and Medical Sciences, 64*(1), 61–68.

Swartzell, K. L., Fulton, J. S., & Friesth, B. M. (2013). Relationship between occurrence of falls and fall-risk scores in an acute care setting using the Hendrich II fall risk model. *Medsurg Nursing, 22*(3), 180–187.

Tsao, C. H., Tsai, C. F., Lee, Y. T., et al. (2016). Drug prescribing in the elderly receiving home care. *The American Journal of the Medical Sciences, 352*(2), 134–140.

● = Independent;   ▲ = Collaborative;   EBN = Evidence-Based Nursing;   EB = Evidence-Based

von Arnim, C. A., Dismar, S., Ott-Renzer, C. S., et al. (2013). Micronutrients supplementation and nutritional status in cognitively impaired elderly persons: A two-month open label pilot study. *Nutrition Journal, 12*(1), 148.

Yannakoulia, M., Ntanasi, E., Anastasiou, C. A., et al. (2017). Frailty and nutrition: From epidemiological and clinical evidence to potential mechanisms. *Metabolism: Clinical and Experimental, 68*, 64–76.

Risk for Frail Elderly syndrome   Cynthia DeLeon Thelen, MSN, BSN, RN

NANDA-I

Definition

Susceptible to a dynamic of unstable equilibrium that affects the older individual experiencing deterioration in one or more domain of health (physical, functional, psychological, or social) and leads to increased susceptibility to adverse health effects, in particular disability.

Risk Factors

Activity intolerance, anxiety, average daily physical activity is less than recommended for gender and age, decrease in energy, decrease in muscle strength, depression, exhaustion, fear of falling, immobility, impaired balance, impaired mobility, insufficient knowledge of modifiable factors, insufficient social support, malnutrition, muscle weakness, obesity, sadness, sedentary lifestyle, social isolation

At-Risk Population

Age >70 years, contrasted living space, economically disadvantaged, ethnicity other than Caucasian, female gender, history of falls, living alone, low educational level, prolonged hospitalization, social vulnerability

Associated Condition

Alteration in cognitive functioning, altered clotting process, anorexia, chronic illness, decrease in serum 25-hydroxyvitamin D concentration, endocrine, regulatory dysfunction, psychiatric disorder, sarcopenia, sarcopenic obesity, sensory deficit, suppressed inflammatory response, unintentional loss of 25% of body weight over one year, unintentional weight loss >10 pounds (>4.5 kg) in one year, walking 15 feet requires >6 seconds (4 meters > 5 seconds)

NIC, NOC, Client Outcomes, Nursing Interventions and *Rationales,* and References

Refer to care plan for **Frail Elderly** syndrome.

Impaired Gas exchange   Debra Siela, PhD, RN, CCNS, ACNS-BC, CCRN-K, CNE, RRT

NANDA-I

Definition

Excess or deficit in oxygenation and/or carbon dioxide elimination at the alveolar-capillary membrane.

Defining Characteristics

Abnormal arterial blood gases; abnormal arterial pH; abnormal breathing pattern; abnormal skin color; confusion; decrease in carbon dioxide (CO_2) level; diaphoresis; dyspnea; headache on awakening; hypercapnia; hypoxemia; hypoxia; irritability; nasal flaring; restlessness, somnolence; tachycardia; visual disturbances

Related Factors

To be developed

Associated Condition

Alveolar-capillary membrane changes; ventilation-perfusion imbalance

● = Independent;   ▲ = Collaborative;   EBN = Evidence-Based Nursing;   EB = Evidence-Based

NOC   (Nursing Outcomes Classification)

Suggested NOC Outcomes

Respiratory Status: Gas Exchange, Ventilation

Example NOC Outcome with Indicators
Achieves appropriate **Respiratory Status: Gas Exchange** as evidenced by the following indicators: Cognitive status/ Partial pressure of oxygen/Partial pressure of carbon dioxide/Arterial pH/Oxygen saturation. (Rate each indicator of **Respiratory Status: Gas Exchange:** 1 = severe deviation from normal range, 2 = substantial deviation from normal range, 3 = moderate deviation from normal range, 4 = mild deviation from normal range, 5 = no deviation from normal range [see Section I].)

G

Client Outcomes

Client Will (Specify Time Frame)

- Demonstrate improved ventilation and adequate oxygenation as evidenced by blood gas levels within normal parameters for that client
- Maintain clear lung fields and remain free of signs of respiratory distress
- Verbalize understanding of oxygen supplementation and other therapeutic interventions

NIC   (Nursing Interventions Classification)

Suggested NIC Interventions

Acid-Base Management; Airway Management

Example NIC Activities—Acid-Base Management
Monitor for symptoms of respiratory failure (e.g., low PaO_2 and elevated $PaCO_2$ levels and respiratory muscle fatigue); Monitor determinants of tissue oxygen delivery (e.g., PaO_2, SaO_2, and hemoglobin levels, and cardiac output) if available

Nursing Interventions and *Rationales*

- Monitor respiratory rate, depth, and ease of respiration. Watch for use of accessory muscles and nasal flaring. *Normal respiratory rate is 14 to 16 breaths per minute in the adult (Bickley & Szilagyi, 2017). When the respiratory rate exceeds 30 breaths per minute, along with other physiological measures, a significant cardiovascular or respiratory alteration exists.*
- Auscultate breath sounds every 1 to 2 hours. The presence of crackles and wheezes may alert the nurse to airway obstruction, which may lead to or exacerbate existing hypoxia. *In severe exacerbations of chronic obstructive pulmonary disease (COPD), lung sounds may be diminished or distant with air trapping (Bickley & Szilagyi, 2017).*
- The nurse should consider respiratory rate, work of breathing, and lung sounds along with PaO_2 values, arterial oxygen saturation (SaO_2), oxygen saturation continuously using pulse oximetry (SpO_2), patient tidal volume, and minute ventilation. Presence of dyspnea, asynchronous chest and abdominal movements, accessory muscles, and agitation indicate potential oxygenation problems (Barton, Vanderspank-Wright, & Shea, 2016).
- Monitor the client's behavior and mental status for the onset of restlessness, agitation, confusion, and (in the late stages) extreme lethargy. *Changes in behavior and mental status can be early signs of impaired gas exchange. In the late stages the client becomes lethargic and somnolent (Lee, 2017).*
- ▲ Monitor oxygen saturation continuously using pulse oximetry (SpO_2) (Lee, 2017). Note blood gas results as available. *An oxygen saturation of less than 88% (normal is 95%–100%) or a partial pressure of oxygen of less than 55 mm Hg (normal is 80–100 mm Hg) indicates significant oxygenation problems (Bein et al, 2016; Siela & Kidd, 2017). Pulse oximetry is useful for tracking and/or adjusting supplemental oxygen therapy for clients with COPD (GOLD, 2017).*
- Monitor venous oxygen saturation to determine an index of oxygen balance to reflect between oxygen delivery and oxygen consumption (Dirks, 2017).

● = Independent;   ▲ = Collaborative;   EBN = Evidence-Based Nursing;   EB = Evidence-Based

- Measurements of oxygenation supply in the macrocirculation include those made upstream from the tissue level. The parameters measured are arterial partial pressure of oxygen (Pao_2), arterial oxygen content (CaO_2), arterial oxygen saturation (SaO_2) determined on the basis of arterial blood gas (ABG) analysis and pulse oximetry (SpO_2), and ratio of Pao_2 to fraction of inspired oxygen (FiO_2) or the PF ratio. Measurements of oxygenation or oxygen extraction or consumption in the macrocirculation made downstream from tissues include tissue oxygen consumption, mixed venous oxygen saturation (SvO_2) or central venous oxygen saturation ($ScvO_2$), and blood levels of lactate (Siela & Kidd, 2017).
- Observe for cyanosis of the skin, and especially note color of the tongue and oral mucous membranes. EB: *In central cyanosis both the skin and mucous membranes are affected because of seriously impaired pulmonary function from unventilated or underventilated alveoli. Peripheral cyanosis (skin only) usually indicates vasoconstriction or obstruction to blood flow (Loscalzo, 2016). Central cyanosis of the tongue and oral mucosa is indicative of serious hypoxia and is a medical emergency. Peripheral cyanosis in the extremities may be caused by activation of the central nervous system or exposure to cold and may or may not be serious (Bickley & Szilagyi, 2017).*
- Position the client in a semirecumbent position with the head of the bed at a 30- to 45-degree angle to decrease the aspiration of gastric, oral, and nasal secretions (Grap, 2009; Siela, 2010; American Association of Critical Care Nurses, 2016, 2017; Vollman, Dickinson, & Powers, 2017). *Evidence shows that mechanically ventilated clients have a decreased incidence of aspiration pneumonia if the client is placed in a 30- to 45-degree semirecumbent position as opposed to a supine position.*
- If the client has unilateral lung disease, position with head of bed at 30 to 45 degrees with "good lung down" in a side-lying position and affected lung up (Barton, Vanderspank-Wright, & Shea, 2016).
- ▲ If the client is acutely dyspneic, consider having the client lean forward over a bedside table, resting elbows on the table if tolerated. *Leaning forward can help decrease dyspnea, possibly because gastric pressure allows better contraction of the diaphragm (Langer et al, 2009; Mahler, 2014). This is called the tripod position and is used during times of distress, including when walking, leaning forward on the walker.*
- Help the client deep breathe and perform controlled coughing. Have the client inhale deeply, hold the breath for several seconds, and cough two or three times with the mouth open while tightening the upper abdominal muscles as tolerated. *Controlled coughing uses the diaphragmatic muscles, which makes the cough more forceful and effective.* If the client has excessive fluid in the respiratory system, see the interventions for Ineffective **Airway** clearance.
- ▲ Monitor the effects of sedation and analgesics on the client's respiratory pattern; use judiciously (Barton, Vanderspank-Wright, & Shea, 2016). *Both analgesics and medications that cause sedation can depress respiration at times. However, these medications can be very helpful for decreasing the sympathetic nervous system discharge that accompanies hypoxia (Spruit et al, 2013).*
- Schedule nursing care to provide rest and minimize fatigue. *The hypoxic client has limited reserves; inappropriate activity can increase hypoxia (Spruit et al, 2013).*
- ▲ Administer humidified oxygen through an appropriate device (e.g., nasal cannula or Venturi mask per the health care provider's order); aim for an oxygen (O_2) saturation level of 90% or above. Oxygen should be titrated to target an SpO_2 of 94% to 98%, except with carbon monoxide poisoning (100% oxygen), acute respiratory distress syndrome (ARDS) (88%–95%), those at risk for hypercapnia (88%–92%), and premature infants (88%–94%) (Blakeman, 2013). Watch for onset of hypoventilation as evidenced by increased somnolence. *There is a fine line between ideal and excessive oxygen therapy; increasing somnolence is caused by retention of CO_2 leading to CO_2 narcosis (Wong & Elliott, 2009). Promote oxygen therapy during a COPD exacerbation. Supplemental oxygen should be titrated to improve the client's hypoxemia with a target of 88% to 92% (GOLD, 2017).*
- Once oxygen is started, ABGs should be checked 30 to 60 minutes later to ensure satisfactory oxygenation without CO_2 retention or acidosis (GOLD, 2017). EBN: *Use of high-flow nasal cannula oxygen therapy may improve gas exchange and oxygenation in acute hypoxemic respiratory failure (Lenglet et al, 2012; Sztrymf et al, 2012; Rittayamai, Tscheikuna, & Rujiwit, 2014; Siela & Kidd, 2017).*
- *Supplemental oxygen can cause toxicity and should be administered at the lowest level that achieves an arterial saturation appropriate for a given patient (Budinger & Mutlu, 2013; Helmerhorst et al, 2015). Conservative oxygen strategies that target a goal of 88% to 92% SpO_2 levels in patients receiving invasive mechanical ventilation appear justified (Panwar et al, 2016).*
- Assess nutritional status including serum albumin level and body mass index (BMI). *Malnourishment in a client with COPD has a negative effect on the course of the disease; it can result in loss of muscle mass in the respiratory muscles, including the diaphragm, which can lead to respiratory failure (GOLD, 2017).*

● = Independent;   ▲ = Collaborative;   EBN = Evidence-Based Nursing;   EB = Evidence-Based

▲ Assist the client to eat small meals frequently and use dietary supplements as necessary. Engage dietary issues by evaluating and creating an optimal nutrition plan. For some clients, drinking 30 mL of a supplement every hour while awake can be helpful.

● If the client is severely debilitated from chronic respiratory disease, consider the use of a wheeled walker to help in ambulation.

▲ Watch for signs of psychological distress including anxiety, agitation, and insomnia.

▲ Refer the COPD client to a pulmonary rehabilitation program. *Pulmonary rehabilitation is now considered a standard of care for the client with COPD (Nici et al, 2009; Spruit et al, 2013; GOLD, 2017).*

Critical Care

▲ Assess and monitor oxygen indices such as the PF ratio ($FiO_2:Po_2$) and venous oxygen saturation/oxygen consumption (SvO_2 or $ScvO_2$) (Headley & Giuliano, 2011; Dirks, 2017; Siela & Kidd, 2017; Lough, 2018).

▲ Turn the client every 2 hours. Monitor mixed venous oxygen saturation closely after turning. If it drops below 10% or fails to return to baseline promptly, turn the client back into the supine position and evaluate oxygen status. If the client does not tolerate turning, consider use of a kinetic bed that rotates the client from side to side in a turn of at least 40 degrees (St. Clair & MacDermott, 2017).

▲ If the client has ARDS with difficulty maintaining oxygenation, then consider positioning the client prone with the upper thorax and pelvis supported. Monitor oxygen saturation and turn the client back to supine position if desaturation occurs. **EB:** *Oxygenation levels have been shown to improve in the prone position, probably because of decreased shunting and better perfusion of the lungs (Gattinoni et al, 2013; Drahnak & Custer, 2015; Barton, Vanderspank-Wright, & Shea, 2016; Bein et al, 2016; Vollman, Dickinson, & Powers, 2017; Vollman, Sole, Quinn, 2017). Prone ventilation significantly reduced mortality in clients with severe acute hypoxemic respiratory failure, but not in clients with less severe hypoxemia (Sud et al, 2010; Gattinoni et al, 2013). A Pao_2 lower than 150 mm Hg measured on at least 5 cm H_2O positive end-expiratory pressure (PEEP) is a recommended threshold for the application of proning (Gattinoni et al, 2013).* Note: If the client becomes ventilator dependent, see the care plan for Impaired spontaneous **Ventilation.**

▲ High levels of PEEP likely improve oxygenation and gas exchange (Suzumura et al, 2014; Barton, Vanderspank-Wright, & Shea, 2016).

Geriatric

▲ Use central nervous system depressants and other sedating agents carefully to avoid decreasing respiration effort (rate and depth of breathing).

▲ Maintain appropriate levels of supplemental oxygen therapy for clients with impaired gas exchange and hypoxemia (GOLD, 2017).

Home Care

● Work with the client to determine what strategies are most helpful during times of dyspnea. Educate and empower the client to self-manage the disease associated with impaired gas exchange. **EBN/EB:** *A study found that use of oxygen, self-use of medication, and getting some fresh air were most helpful in dealing with dyspnea (Thomas, 2009). Evidence-based reviews have found that self-management offers COPD clients effective options for managing the illness, leading to more positive outcomes (Spruit et al, 2013; GOLD, 2017).*

● Collaborate with health care providers regarding long-term oxygen administration for chronic respiratory failure clients with severe resting hypoxemia. Administer long-term oxygen therapy greater than 15 hours daily for Po_2 less than 55 or SaO_2 at or below 88% (GOLD, 2017).

● Assess the home environment for irritants that impair gas exchange. Help the client adjust the home environment as necessary (e.g., install an air filter to decrease the level of dust).

▲ Refer the client to occupational therapy as necessary to assist the client in adapting to the home and environment and in energy conservation (GOLD, 2017).

● Assist the client with identifying and avoiding situations that exacerbate impairment of gas exchange (e.g., stress-related situations, exposure to pollution of any kind, proximity to noxious gas fumes such as chlorine bleach). *Irritants in the environment decrease the client's effectiveness in accessing oxygen during breathing.*

● Refer to GOLD guidelines for management of home care and indications of hospital admission criteria (GOLD, 2017).

● = Independent;   ▲ = Collaborative;   **EBN** = Evidence-Based Nursing;   **EB** = Evidence-Based

G

- Instruct the client to keep the home temperature above 68°F (20°C) and to avoid cold weather. *Cold air temperatures cause constriction of the blood vessels, which impairs the client's ability to absorb oxygen (Bickley & Szilagyi, 2017).*
- Instruct the client to limit exposure to persons with respiratory infections. *Viruses, bacteria, and environmental pollutants are the main causes of exacerbations of COPD (GOLD, 2017).*
- Instruct the family in the complications of the disease and the importance of maintaining the medical regimen, including when to call a health care provider.
- ▲ Refer the client for home health aide services as necessary for assistance with activities of daily living. *Clients with decreased oxygenation have decreased energy to perform personal and role-related activities.*
- When respiratory procedures are implemented, explain equipment and procedures to family members and provide needed emotional support. *Family members assuming responsibility for respiratory monitoring often find this stressful (Langer et al, 2009).*
- When electrically based equipment for respiratory support is implemented, evaluate home environment for electrical safety, proper grounding, and so on. Ensure that notification is sent to the local utility company, the emergency medical team, and police and fire departments. *Notification is important to provide for priority service.*
- ▲ Assess family role changes and coping ability. Refer the client to medical social services as appropriate for assistance in adjusting to chronic illness. CEB: *Inability to maintain the level of social involvement experienced before illness leads to frustration and anger in the client and may create a threat to the family unit (Langer et al, 2009).*
- Support the family of the client with chronic illness. *Severely compromised respiratory functioning causes fear and anxiety in clients and their families. Reassurance from the nurse can be helpful (Rose et al, 2014).*

Client/Family Teaching and Discharge Planning

- Teach the client how to perform pursed-lip breathing and inspiratory muscle training, and how to use the tripod position. Have the client watch the pulse oximeter to note improvement in oxygenation with these breathing techniques. CEB: *Pursed lip breathing results in increased use of intercostal muscles, decreased respiratory rate, and improved oxygen saturation levels (Mahler, 2014). Pursed-lip breathing may relieve dyspnea in advanced COPD (Mahler, 2014). A systematic review found that inspiratory muscle training was effective in increasing endurance of the client and decreasing dyspnea (Langer et al, 2009). Inspiratory muscle training likely improves breathlessness during exercise and/or with activities of daily living in patients with COPD and congestive heart failure (CHF) who exhibit inspiratory muscle weakness (Mahler, 2014).*
- Teach the client energy conservation techniques and the importance of alternating rest periods with activity. See nursing interventions for **Fatigue.**
- ▲ Teach the importance of not smoking. Refer to smoking cessation programs, and encourage clients who relapse to keep trying to quit. Ensure that clients receive appropriate medications to support smoking cessation from the primary health care provider. EB: *Patients should be referred to a comprehensive smoking cessation program, incorporating behavior change techniques that focus on enhancing patient motivation and confidence, patient education, and pharmacological and nonpharmacological interventions (GOLD, 2017).*
- ▲ Instruct the family regarding home oxygen therapy if ordered (e.g., delivery system, liter flow, safety precautions). *Long-term oxygen therapy can improve survival, exercise ability, sleep, and ability to think in hypoxemic clients. Client education improves compliance with prescribed use of oxygen (GOLD, 2017).*
- ▲ Teach the client the need to receive a yearly influenza vaccine. *Receiving a yearly influenza vaccine is helpful to prevent exacerbations of COPD (GOLD, 2017).*
- Teach the client relaxation techniques to help reduce stress responses and panic attacks resulting from dyspnea. EB: *Relaxation therapy can help reduce dyspnea and anxiety (Langer et al, 2009).*
- Teach the client to use music, along with a rest period, to decrease dyspnea and anxiety (Mahler, 2014; Loscalzo, 2016).

● = Independent; ▲ = Collaborative; EBN = Evidence-Based Nursing; EB = Evidence-Based

REFERENCES

American Association of Critical Care Nurses. (2017). *AACN Practice Alert—Prevention of ventilator-associated pneumonia in adults.* American Association of Critical Care Nurses. Retrieved from https://www.aacn.org/~/media/aacn-website/clincial-resources/practice-alerts/preventingvapinadults2017.pdf.

American Association of Critical Care Nurses. (2016). *AACN Practice Alert—Prevention of aspiration in adults.* American Association of Critical Care Nurses. Retrieved from https://www.aacn.org/~/media/aacn-website/clincial-resources/practice-alerts/preventionaspirationpracticealert.pdf.

Barton, G., Vanderspank-Wright, B., & Shea, J. (2016). Optimizing oxygenation in the mechanically ventilated patient nursing practice implications. *Critical Care Nursing Clinics of North America, 28,* 425–435.

Bein, T., Grassor, S., Moerer, O., et al. (2016). The standard of care of patients with ARDS: Ventilatory settings and rescue therapies for refractory hypoxemia. *Intensive Care Medicine, 42,* 699–711.

Bickley, L. S., & Szilagyi, P. (2017). *Bate's guide to physical examination* (12th ed.). Philadelphia: Lippincott, Williams and Wilkins.

Blakeman, T. (2013). Evidence for oxygen use in the hospitalized patient: Is more really the enemy of good? *Respiratory Care, 58*(10), 1679–1693.

Budinger, G., & Mutlu, G. (2013). Balancing the risks and benefits of oxygen therapy in critically ill adults. *Chest, 143*(4), 1151–1162.

Dirks, J. (2017). Continuous venous oxygen monitoring. In D. L. Wiegand (Ed.), *AACN procedure manual for high acuity, progressive, and critical care* (7th ed.). Philadelphia: Saunders Elsevier.

Drahnak, D., & Custer, N. (2015). Prone positioning of patients with acute respiratory distress syndrome. *Critical Care Nurse, 35*(6), 29–37.

Gattinoni, L., Taccone, P., Carlesso, E., et al. (2013). Prone position in acute respiratory distress syndrome. *American Journal of Respiratory and Critical Care Medicine, 188*(11), 1286–1293.

GOLD. (2017). *Global strategy for the diagnosis, management, and prevention of COPD (revised 2017), Global Initiative for Chronic Obstructive Lung Disease.* Retrieved from http://goldcopd.org/gold-reports-2017/e.

Grap, M. (2009). Not-so-trivial pursuit: Mechanical ventilation risk reduction. *American Journal of Critical Care, 18*(4), 299–309.

Headley, J., & Giuliano, K. (2011). Continuous venous oxygen saturation monitoring. In D. J. Lynn-McHale (Ed.), *AACN procedure manual for critical care* (6th ed.). Philadelphia: Saunders Elsevier.

Helmerhorst, H., Schultz, M., van der Voort, P., et al. (2015). Bench-to-bedside review: The effects of hyperoxia during critical illness. *Critical Care, 19.* doi:10.1186/s13054-015-0996-4.

Langer, D., Hendriks, E., Burtin, C., et al. (2009). A clinical practice guideline for physiotherapists treating patients with chronic obstructive pulmonary disease based on a systematic review of available evidence. *Clinical Rehabilitation, 23*(5), 445–462.

Lee, D. (2017). Oxygen saturation monitoring with pulse oximetry. In D. L. Wiegand (Ed.), *AACN procedure manual for high acuity, progressive, and critical care* (7th ed.). Philadelphia: Saunders Elsevier.

Lenglet, H., Sztrymf, B., Leroy, C., et al. (2012). Humidified high flow nasal oxygen during respiratory failure in the emergency department: Feasibility and efficacy. *Respiratory Care, 57*(11), 1873–1878.

Loscalzo, J. (2016). Hypoxia and cyanosis. In J. Loscalzo (Ed.), *Harrison's pulmonary and critical care medicine* (3rd ed.). New York: McGraw-Hill Education Medical.

Lough, M. (2018). Cardiovascular diagnostic procedures. In L. Urden, K. Stacy, & M. Lough (Eds.), *Critical care nursing diagnosis and management* (8th ed.). Maryland Heights, MO: Elsevier.

Mahler, D. (2014). Other treatments for dyspnea. In D. A. Mahler & D. E. O'Donnell (Eds.), *Dyspnea mechanisms, measurement and management.* Boca Raton: CRC Press Taylor & Francis Group.

Nici, L., Raskin, J., Rochester, C. L., et al. (2009). Pulmonary rehabilitation: What we know and what we need to know. *Journal of Cardiopulmonary Rehabilitation & Prevention, 29*(3), 141–151.

Panwar, R., Hardie, M., Bellomo, R., et al. (2016). Conservative versus liberal oxygenation targets for mechanically ventilated patients. A pilot multicenter randomized controlled trial. *American Journal of Respiratory and Critical Care Medicine, 193*(1), 43–51.

Rittayamai, N., Tscheikuna, J., & Rujiwit, P. (2014). High-flow nasal versus conventional oxygen therapy after endotracheal extubation: A randomized crossover physiologic study. *Respiratory Care, 59*(4), 485–490.

Rose, L., Dainty, K. N., Jordan, J., et al. (2014). Weaning from mechanical ventilation: A scoping review of qualitative studies. *American Journal of Critical Care, 23*(5), e54–e71.

Siela, D., & Kidd, M. (2017). Oxygen requirements for acutely and critically ill patients. *Critical Care Nurse, 37*(4), 58–70.

Siela, D. (2010). Evaluation standards for management of artificial airways. *Critical Care Nurse, 30*(4), 76–78.

Spruit, M. A., Singh, S. J., Garvey, C., et al. (2013). An official American Thoracic Society/European Respiratory Society Statement: Key concepts and advances in pulmonary rehabilitation. *American Journal of Respiratory and Critical Care Medicine, 188*(8), e13–e64.

St. Clair, J., & MacDermott, J. (2017). Continuous lateral rotation therapy. In D. L. Wiegand (Ed.), *AACN procedure manual for critical care* (7th ed.). Philadelphia: Saunders Elsevier.

Sud, S., Friedrich, J., Taccone, P., et al. (2010). Prone ventilation reduces mortality in patients with acute respiratory failure and severe hypoxemia: Systematic review and meta-analysis. *Intensive Care Medicine, 36,* 585–599.

Suzumura, E. A., Figueiro, M., Normilio-Silva, K., et al. (2014). Effects of alveolar recruitment maneuvers on clinical outcomes in patients with acute respiratory distress syndrome: A systematic review and meta-analysis. *Intensive Care Medicine, 40,* 1227–1240.

Sztrymf, B., Messika, J., Mayot, T., et al. (2012). Impact of high-flow nasal cannula oxygen therapy on intensive care unit patients with acute respiratory failure: A prospective observational study. *Journal of Critical Care, 27,* 324.e9–324.e13.

Thomas, L. (2009). Effective dyspnea management strategies identified by elders with end-stage chronic obstructive pulmonary disease. *Applied Nursing Research, 22*(2), 79–85.

Vollman, K., Dickinson, S., & Powers, J. (2017). Pronation therapy. In D. L. Wiegand (Ed.), *AACN procedure manual for high acuity, progressive, and critical care* (7th ed.). Philadelphia: Saunders Elsevier.

Vollman, K., Sole, M., & Quinn, B. (2017). Endotracheal tube care and oral care practices for ventilated and non-ventilated patients. In D. L. Wiegand (Ed.), *AACN procedure manual for high acuity, progressive, and critical care* (7th ed.). Philadelphia: Saunders Elsevier.

Wong, M., & Elliott, M. (2009). The use of medical orders in acute care oxygen therapy. *British Journal of Nursing, 18*(8), 462–464.

● = Independent;   ▲ = Collaborative;   **EBN** = Evidence-Based Nursing;   **EB** = Evidence-Based

Risk for dysfunctional Gastrointestinal motility
Mary Beth Flynn Makic, PhD, RN, CCNS, FAAN, FNAP

NANDA-I

Definition

Susceptible to increased, decreased, ineffective, or lack of peristaltic activity within the gastrointestinal system, which may compromise health.

Risk Factors

Anxiety; change in water source; eating habit change; immobility; malnutrition; sedentary lifestyle; stressors; unsanitary food preparation

At-Risk Population

Aging; ingestion of contaminated material; prematurity

Associated Condition

Decrease in gastrointestinal circulation; diabetes mellitus; enteral feedings; food intolerance; gastroesophageal reflux disease; infection; pharmaceutical agent; treatment regimen

NIC, NOC, Client Outcomes, Nursing Interventions and *Rationales,* Client/Family Teaching and Discharge Planning, and References

Refer to care plan for Dysfunctional **Gastrointestinal** motility.

Dysfunctional Gastrointestinal motility
Rosemary Koehl Lee, DNP, ARNP, ACNP-BC, CCNS, CCRN

NANDA-I

Definition

Increased, decreased, ineffective, or lack of peristaltic activity within the gastrointestinal system.

Defining Characteristics

Abdominal cramping; abdominal pain; absence of flatus; acceleration of gastric emptying; bile-colored gastric residual; change in bowel sounds; diarrhea; difficulty with defecation; distended abdomen; hard, formed stool; increase in gastric residual; nausea; regurgitation; vomiting.

Related Factors

Anxiety; change in water source; eating habit change; immobility; malnutrition; sedentary lifestyle; stressors; unsanitary food preparation

At-Risk Population

Aging; ingestion of contaminated material; prematurity

Associated Condition

Decrease in gastrointestinal circulation; diabetes mellitus; enteral feedings; food intolerance; gastroesophageal reflux disease; infection; pharmaceutical agent; treatment regimen

NOC (Nursing Outcomes Classification)

Suggested NOC Outcomes

Gastrointestinal Function; Electrolyte and Acid-Base Balance; Fluid Balance; Hydration; Nausea and Vomiting Control

● = Independent; ▲ = Collaborative; EBN = Evidence-Based Nursing; EB = Evidence-Based

Example NOC Outcome with Indicators

Gastrointestinal Function as evidenced by the following indicators: Bowel sounds/Stool soft and formed/Appetite present without evidence of reflux, nausea, or vomiting/Reported normal abdominal comfort/Abdomen soft to palpation without evidence of distention. (Rate the outcome and indicators of **Gastrointestinal Function:** I = severely compromised, 2 = substantially compromised, 3 = moderately compromised, 4 = mildly compromised, 5 = not compromised [see Section I].)

Client Outcomes

Client Will (Specify Time Frame)

- Be free of abdominal distention and pain
- Have normal bowel sounds
- Pass flatus rectally at intervals
- Defecate formed, soft stool every day to every third day
- State has an appetite
- Be able to eat food without nausea and vomiting

NIC (Nursing Interventions Classification)

Suggested NIC Intervention

Gastric Motility Management

Example NIC Activities—Gastric Motility Management

Evaluate use of prokinetics for delayed gastric motility; Suggest change in dietary habits to either increase or decrease gastric motility, depending on the presenting complaint

Nursing Interventions and *Rationales*

- Monitor for abdominal distention, and presence of abdominal pain, weight loss, nausea, vomiting, obstipation, or diarrhea. *The acute onset of abdominal distention in conjunction with symptoms of cramping pain, weight loss, nausea, vomiting, constipation, or diarrhea warrants further evaluation for disorders that cause intestinal obstruction (Nagarwala, Dev, & Markin, 2016).*
- Inspect, auscultate for bowel sounds noting characteristics and frequency; palpate and percuss the abdomen. *Hypoactive bowel sounds are found with decreased motility as with peritonitis from paralytic ileus or from late bowel obstruction. Hyperactive bowel sounds are associated with increased motility (Nagarwala, Dev, & Markin, 2016).*
- Review history noting any anorexia or nausea/vomiting. Other symptoms may include relation of symptoms to meals, especially if aggravated by food, satiety, postprandial fullness/bloating, and weight loss or weight loss with severe gastroparesis. *These are signs of abnormal gastric motility (Camilleri, 2016).*
- Monitor for fluid deficits by checking skin turgor and moisture of tongue, daily weights, input and output, and electrolyte values. Refer to care plan for Deficient **Fluid** volume if relevant.
- ▲ Monitor for nutritional deficits by keeping close track of food intake. Review laboratory studies that affirm nutritional deficits, such as decreased albumin and serum protein levels, liver profile, glucose, fecal analysis, and an electrolyte panel. Refer to care plan for Imbalanced **Nutrition:** less than body requirements or Risk for **Electrolyte** imbalance as appropriate.

Slowed Gastric Motility

- *Monitor the client for signs and symptoms of decreased gastric motility, which may include nausea after meals, vomiting, feeling full quickly while eating, abdominal bloating, and abdominal pain (Camilleri, 2016).*
- ▲ Monitor daily laboratory studies and point of care testing blood glucose levels ensuring ordered glucose levels are performed and evaluated. EB: *Elevated blood glucose levels can cause delayed gastric emptying; therefore it is important to normalize blood glucose levels (Wall, 2018).*
- Obtain a thorough gastrointestinal history if the client has diabetes, because he or she is at high risk for gastroparesis and gastric reflux. *Gastroparesis with delayed emptying of the stomach is a well-known complication of diabetes (Camilleri, 2016).*
- ▲ If client has nausea and vomiting, then provide an antiemetic and intravenous fluids as ordered. Offer or perform oral hygiene after vomiting. Refer to the care plan for **Nausea.**

● = Independent;   ▲ = Collaborative;   EBN = Evidence-Based Nursing;   EB = Evidence-Based

▲ Evaluate medications the client is taking. Recognize that vasopressors, opioids, or anticholinergic medications can cause gastric slowing (Magidson & Martinez, 2016).

▲ Review laboratory and other diagnostic tools, including complete blood count, amylase, and thyroid-stimulating hormone level, glucose with other metabolic studies, upper endoscopy, and gastric-emptying scintigraphy. *The diagnosis of diabetic gastroparesis is made when other causes are excluded and postprandial gastric stasis is confirmed by gastric emptying scintigraphy, which is considered the gold standard for diagnosing gastroparesis (Camilleri, 2016).*

▲ Consider abdominal massage for relief of constipation. EB: *Two small randomized controlled studies identified that abdominal massage may relieve constipation and improve quality of life (Kassolik et al, 2015; Turan & Turkinaz, 2016).*

▲ Obtain a nutritional consult, considering a small particle size diet or diets lower or higher in liquids or solids, depending on gastric motility. EB: *A small (N = 45) randomized controlled trial found that diets with smaller particle size reduced the symptoms of gastroparesis in diabetic clients (Olausson et al, 2014).*

▲ If the client is unable to eat or retain food, consult with the registered dietitian and health care provider, considering further nutritional support in the form of enteral or parenteral feedings for the client with gastroparesis. *Some clients require supplementation with either enteral or parenteral nutrition for survival.*

▲ If the client is receiving gastric enteral nutrition, see the care plan Risk for **Aspiration.**

▲ Administer medications that increase gastrointestinal motility as ordered (Nagarwala, Dev, & Markin, 2016).

Postoperative Ileus

● Observe for complications of delayed intestinal motility. Symptoms include vague abdominal pain and distention, nausea, vomiting, anorexia, sometimes bloating, and tympany to percussion. Clients may or may not pass flatus and some stool (Van Bree et al, 2014).

▲ Recommend chewing gum for the abdominal surgery client who is experiencing an ileus, is not at risk for aspiration, and has normal dentition. EB: *Gum chewing may decrease postoperative ileus because it acts as a sham feeding, potentially stimulating gastric and bowel motility. A meta-analysis found that using chewing gum reduces the time of postoperative ileus (Sundsted, Liton, & Bundrick, 2016).*

● Help the client out of bed to walk at least two times per day. Assist client to sit in a rocking chair to rock back and forth. *Exercise may increase gastrointestinal motility.*

▲ If postoperative ileus is associated with opioid pain medication, ensure opioids are decreased or ideally discontinued. Use nonsteroidal antiinflammatory drugs for pain as feasible and if not contraindicated (Cagir, 2016).

▲ Note serum electrolyte levels, especially potassium and magnesium. *A low potassium level decreases the function of intestinal smooth muscle and can result in an ileus. A low magnesium level makes the body refractory to potassium replacement (Viera & Wouk, 2015; Nagarwala, Dev, & Markin, 2016).*

Increased Gastrointestinal Motility

▲ Observe for complications of gastric surgeries such as dumping syndrome. *This syndrome is the effect of changes in size and function of the stomach, with rapid dumping of hyperosmolar food into the intestines (Schattner & Grossman, 2016).*

● Watch for nausea, vomiting, bloating, cramping, diarrhea, dizziness, and fatigue. *These are common signs and symptoms of early rapid gastric emptying (Schattner & Grossman, 2016).*

● Monitor for low blood sugar, weakness, sweating, and dizziness 1 to 3 hours after eating because this is when late rapid gastric emptying may occur. Late rapid gastric emptying is associated with low blood sugar (Schattner & Grossman, 2016).

▲ Order a nutritional consult to discuss diet changes. The diet may vary depending on the kind of surgery causing dumping syndrome. *Encourage small meals that are low in carbohydrates and fats. Space fluids around meal times (Schattner & Grossman, 2016).*

▲ Give intravenous fluids as ordered for the client complaining of diarrhea with weakness and dizziness. Monitor electrolyte panel and acid-base balance. *Severe diarrhea can cause deficient fluid volume with extreme weakness and metabolic acidosis.*

  ❍ Offer bathroom, commode, or bedpan assistance, depending on frequency, amount of diarrhea, and condition of client.

  ❍ Monitor rectal area for decreased skin integrity, and apply barrier creams as needed to protect and treat skin.

● = Independent;   ▲ = Collaborative;   EBN = Evidence-Based Nursing;   EB = Evidence-Based

○ Consider a bowel management system for bed-bound patients with frequent loose stools. This will protect the perineal skin and minimize spread of infection.

- Refer to the care plans for the nursing diagnoses of Deficient **Fluid** volume, **Nausea,** Impaired **Skin** integrity, and **Diarrhea** as relevant.

Pediatric

- Assess infants and children with suspected delayed gastric emptying for fullness and vomiting. Babies and children with delayed gastric emptying take longer to get hungry again and throw up undigested or partially digested food several hours after feeding (Westfal & Goldstein, 2017).
- ▲ Observe for nutritional and fluid deficits with assessment of skin turgor, mucous membranes, fontanels, furrows of the tongue, electrolyte panel, fluid status, input and output, and daily weights (Islam, 2015).
- ▲ Recommend gentle massage for preterm infants as appropriate. EB: *With massage, there was increased vagal activity. This was then associated with increased gastric motility and greater weight gain (Field, Diego, & Hernandez-Reif, 2011).*

Geriatric

- Closely monitor diet and medication use/side effects because they affect the gastrointestinal system. Watch for constipation. *Many gastrointestinal functions are slowed in older adults (Baker & Blakely, 2017).*
- ▲ Watch for symptoms of dysphagia, gastroesophageal reflux disease, dyspepsia, irritable bowel syndrome, maldigestion, and reduced absorption of nutrients. *These are common gastrointestinal disorders in older adults (Baker & Blakely, 2017).*

Client/Family Teaching and Discharge Planning

- Teach the client and caregivers about medications, reinforcing side effects as they relate to gastrointestinal function.
- Teach client and caregivers to report signs and symptoms that may indicate further complications including increased abdominal girth, projectile vomiting, and unrelieved acute cramping pain (bowel obstruction).
- Review signs and symptoms of dehydration with client and caregivers.

REFERENCES

Baker, N. R., & Blakely, K. K. (2017). Gastrointestinal disturbances in the elderly. *Nursing Clinics of North America, 52,* 419–431.

Cagir, B. (2016). *Ileus: Drugs and diseases.* Medscape. Retrieved from https://emedicine.medscape.com/article/2242141-overview. (Accessed 4 November 2017).

Camilleri, M. (2016). Disorders of gastrointestinal motility. In L. Goldman & A. I. Schafer (Eds.), *Goldman-Cecil medicine* (25th ed., Chapter 136, pp. 884–890). Philadelphia: Saunders.

Field, T., Diego, M., & Hernandez-Reif, M. (2011). Potential underlying mechanisms for greater weight gain in massaged preterm infants. *Infant Behavior and Development, 34*(3), 383–389.

Islam, S. (2015). Gastroparesis in children. *Current Opinion in Pediatrics, 27*(3), 377–382.

Kassolik, K., Andrzejewski, W., Wilk, I., et al. (2015). The effectiveness of massage based on the tensegrity principle compared with classical abdominal massage performed on patients with constipation. *Archives of Gerontology & Geriatrics, 61*(2), 202–211.

Magidson, P. D., & Martinez, J. P. (2016). Abdominal pain in the geriatric patient. *Emergency Medical Clinics of North America, 34,* 559–574.

Nagarwala, J., Dev, S., & Markin, A. (2016). The vomiting patient: Small bowel obstruction, cyclic vomiting, and gastroparesis. *Emergency Medical Clinics of North America, 34,* 271–291. Retrieved from http://dx.doi.org/10.1016/j.emc.2015.12.005.

Olausson, E. A., et al. (2014). Small particle size diet reduces upper gastrointestinal symptoms in patients with diabetic gastroparesis: A randomized controlled trial. *The American Journal of Gastroenterology, 109*(3), 375–385.

Schattner, M. A., & Grossman, E. B. (2016). Nutritional management. In M. Feldman, L. Friedman, & L. J. Brandt (Eds.), *Sleisenger and Fordtran's gastrointestinal and liver disease* (10th ed, Chapter 6, pp. 83–101). Philadelphia: Elsevier.

Sundsted, K. K., Liton, S. C., & Bundrick, J. B. (2016). Clinical pearls in perioperative medicine 2016. *Disease-A-Month, 62,* 231–239. Retrieved from http://dx.doi.org/10.1016/j.disamonth.2016.05.005.

Turan, N., & Turkinaz, A. A. (2016). The effect of abdominal massage on constipation and quality of life. *Gastroenterology Nursing, 39*(1), 48–59. doi:10.1097/SGA.0000000000000202.

Van Bree, S. H. J., Bemelman, W. A., Hollman, M. W., et al. (2014). Identification of clinical outcome measures for recovery of gastrointestinal motility in postoperative ileus. *Annals of Surgery, 259*(4), 708–714.

Viera, A. J., & Wouk, N. (2015). Potassium disorders: Hypokalemia and hyperkalemia. *American Family Physician, 92*(6), 487–495.

Wall, R. T. (2018). Endocrine disease. In R. L. Hines & K. E. Marschall (Eds.), *Stoelting's anesthesia and co-existing disease* (7th ed., Chapter 23, pp. 449–475). Philadelphia: Elsevier.

Westfal, M. L., & Goldstein, A. M. (2017). Pediatric enteric neuropathies: Diagnosis and current management. *Current Opinion in Pediatrics, 29*(3), 347–353.

● = Independent;   ▲ = Collaborative;   EBN = Evidence-Based Nursing;   EB = Evidence-Based

Risk for unstable blood Glucose level   *Paula D. Hopper, MSN, RN, CNE*

NANDA-I

Definition

Susceptible to variation in serum levels of glucose from the normal range, which may compromise health.

Risk Factors

Average daily physical activity is less than recommended for gender and age; does not accept diagnosis; excessive stress; excessive weight gain; excessive weight loss; inadequate blood glucose monitoring; ineffective medication management; insufficient diabetes management; insufficient dietary intake; insufficient knowledge of disease management; insufficient knowledge of modifiable factors; nonadherence to diabetes management plan

At-Risk Population

Alteration in mental status; compromised physical health status; delay in cognitive development; rapid growth period

Associated Condition

Pregnancy

NOC   (Nursing Outcomes Classification)

Suggested NOC Outcomes

Compliance Behavior: Prescribed Diet; Compliance Behavior: Prescribed Medication; Coping; Endurance; Knowledge: Diabetes Management; Knowledge: Treatment Regimen; Nutritional Status; Personal Health Status; Self-Management: Diabetes; Weight Maintenance Behavior

Example **NOC** Outcome with Indicators
Blood Glucose Level as evidenced by the following indicators: Blood glucose/Glycosylated hemoglobin/Fructosamine/Urine glucose/Urine ketones. (Rate the outcome and indicators of **Blood Glucose Level:** 1 = severe deviation from normal range, 2 = substantial deviation from normal range, 3 = moderate deviation from normal range, 4 = mild deviation from normal range, 5 = no deviation from normal range [see Section I].)

Client Outcomes

Client Will (Specify Time Frame)

- For most adults, maintain the following glucose targets (American Diabetes Association [ADA], 2017, S52); consult primary care provider for client-specific goals
  - A_{1C} less than 7% (normal level <5.7%)
  - Preprandial blood glucose between 80 and 130 mg/dL
  - Peak postprandial (1–2 hours after beginning of meal) glucose below 180 mg/dL
- For children and adolescents with type 1 diabetes, maintain the following glucose targets (ADA, 2017, S107):
  - A_{1C} less than 7.5%; a goal of less than 7% is appropriate if it can be achieved without excessive hypoglycemia
- Maintain blood glucose for children and adolescents as follows (ADA, 2017, S107):
  - Preprandial between 90 and 130 mg/dL
  - Bedtime/overnight between 90 and 150 mg/dL
- In pregnant women, maintain blood glucose as follows (ADA, 2017, S116):
  - Preprandial ≤95 mg/dL
  - One-hour postprandial level at or below 140 mg/dL
  - Two-hour postprandial at or below 120 mg/dL

● = Independent;   ▲ = Collaborative;   EBN = Evidence-Based Nursing;   EB = Evidence-Based

- In pregnant mothers with preexisting type 1 or 2 diabetes blood glucose as follows (ADA, 2017, S115):
  - Fasting ≤95 mg/dL
  - One-hour postprandial ≤140 mg/dL
  - Two-hour postprandial glucose at ≤120 mg/dL
- In older adults, maintain blood glucose values as follows (ADA, 2017, S101):
  - Healthy older adults: preprandial blood glucose 90 to 130 mg/dL; bedtime 90 to 150 mg/dL
  - Older adults with complex coexisting chronic illness: preprandial blood glucose 90 to 150 mg/dL; bedtime 100 to 180 mg/dL
  - Older adult end-stage chronic illness or moderate to severe cognitive impairment: preprandial blood glucose 100 to 180 mg/dL; bedtime 110 to 200 mg/dL
- Maintain blood glucose in critically ill hospitalized clients between 140 and 180 mg/dL (ADA, 2017, S121)

NIC   (Nursing Interventions Classification)

G

Suggested NIC Interventions

Hypoglycemia Management; Hyperglycemia Management

Example NIC Activities—Hypoglycemia Management
Monitor blood glucose levels, as indicated; Provide simple carbohydrate, as indicated

Nursing Interventions and *Rationales*

▲ Monitor blood glucose in hospitalized patients who are eating, before meals; who are not eating, every 4 to 6 hours; and who are receiving intravenous (IV) insulin, every 30 minutes to 2 hours. **EB:** *Hypoglycemia and hyperglycemia in the hospitalized patient are associated with adverse outcomes, including death (ADA, 2017, S120).*

▲ In patients receiving multiple-dose insulin (MDI) or insulin pump therapy, obtain blood glucose before meals and snacks, at bedtime, occasionally after meals, before exercise or critical tasks such as driving, if low blood glucose is suspected, and after treatment for low blood glucose until normoglycemic. **EB:** *Self-monitoring of blood glucose (SMBG) helps guide treatment and self-management decisions (ADA, 2017, S48).* **EB:** *Evidence supports a correlation between SMBG frequency and lower A_{1C} in patients with type 1 diabetes (ADA, 2017, S48).*

▲ Consider continuous glucose monitoring (CGM) in clients with type 1 diabetes on intensive insulin regimens. **EB:** *"When used properly, continuous glucose monitoring (CGM) in conjunction with intensive insulin regimens is a useful tool to lower A_{1C} in selected adults (aged ≥25 years) with type 1 diabetes" (ADA, 2017).*

▲ Evaluate A_{1C} level for glucose control over previous 3 months. **EB:** *"A_{1C} reflects average glycemia over approximately 3 months and has a strong predictive value for diabetes complications… A reasonable A_{1C} goal for many nonpregnant adults is 7% (53 mmol/mol)" (ADA, 2017, S50).*

▲ Consider monitoring 2 hours after the start of meals in individuals who have premeal glucose values within target but have A_{1C} values above target. **EB:** *"It is clear that postprandial hyperglycemia, like preprandial hyperglycemia, contributes to elevated A_{1C} levels" (ADA, 2017, S52).*

• Monitor for signs and symptoms of hypoglycemia, such as shakiness, dizziness, sweating, hunger, headache, pallor, behavior changes, confusion, or seizures. **EB:** *"Mild hypoglycemia may be inconvenient or frightening to patients with diabetes. Severe hypoglycemia … can progress to loss of consciousness, seizure, coma, or death" (ADA, 2017, S53).*

• If the client is experiencing signs and symptoms of hypoglycemia, test glucose; if the result is below 70 mg/dL, administer 15 to 20 g glucose. Pure glucose is the preferred treatment, but any form of carbohydrate that contains glucose will suffice (a cup of fruit juice or regular [not diet] soda, one cup of milk, a small piece of fruit, or three to four glucose tablets). Avoid treating with foods that contain fat. Repeat test in 15 minutes and repeat treatment if indicated. Once blood glucose returns to normal, the individual should consume a meal or snack to prevent recurrence of hypoglycemia. **EB:** *"Treatment of hypoglycemia (plasma glucose <70 mg/dL) requires ingestion of glucose-containing or carbohydrate-containing foods. The acute glycemic response correlates better with the glucose content than with the carbohydrate content of the food. Although pure glucose is the preferred treatment, any form of carbohydrate that contains glucose will raise blood glucose. Added fat may retard and then prolong the acute glycemic response" (ADA, 2017, S53–S54).*

• = Independent;   ▲ = Collaborative;   **EBN** = Evidence-Based Nursing;   **EB** = Evidence-Based

G

- ▲ Clients who experience asymptomatic hypoglycemia should raise their glucose targets to avoid hypoglycemia for several weeks. **EB:** *"Several weeks of avoidance of hypoglycemia has been demonstrated to improve counterregulation and hypoglycemia awareness in many patients"* (ADA, 2017, S54).
- • Avoid carbohydrate foods that are also high in protein to prevent or treat hypoglycemia. **EB:** *"In individuals with type 2 diabetes, ingested protein appears to increase insulin response without increasing plasma glucose concentrations. Therefore, carbohydrate sources high in protein should not be used to treat or prevent hypoglycemia"* (ADA, 2017, S35).
- • Monitor for signs and symptoms of hyperglycemia, such as increased thirst or urination, or high blood or urine glucose levels. **EB:** *"Better glycemic control is associated with significantly decreased rates of development and progression of microvascular (retinopathy and diabetic kidney disease) and neuropathic complications"* (ADA, 2017, S50).
- ▲ Monitor fluid balance and replace fluids in clients with diabetic ketoacidosis. **EB:** *Prompt rehydration is vital to restore circulating volume and tissue perfusion, clear ketones, and correct electrolyte imbalances … hydration alone restores circulatory volume and tissue perfusion; improves glycaemic control and acid base balance, and reduces counterregulatory hormones"* (Tran et al, 2017).
- ▲ Avoid use of sliding scale insulin alone in hospitalized patients. **EB:** *"An insulin regimen including basal, bolus, and correction (sliding scale) insulin is preferred, to prevent hyperglycemia. Sliding scale insulin only corrects blood sugar that is already high"* (ADA, 2017, S122).
- • Prime IV tubing with 20 mL of diluted insulin solution before initiating insulin drip. **CEB:** *Glucose adsorbs to some IV tubing; priming with 20 mL is enough to minimize this effect* (Goldberg et al, 2006; Zahid et al, 2008).
- ▲ Evaluate the client's medication regimen for medications that can alter blood glucose. Some asthma medications, some antipsychotic and antidepressant agents, thiazide diuretics, and glucocorticoids, among others, can cause hyperglycemia. Aspirin and beta-blockers are among agents that can cause hypoglycemia (National Prescribing Service [NPS], 2017).
- ▲ Refer client to a dietitian for individualized medical nutrition therapy (MNT) instruction. **EB:** *"MNT delivered by a registered dietitian is associated with A_{1C} decreases of 0.3% to 1% for people with type 1 diabetes (38–40) and 0.5% to 2% for people with type 2 diabetes"* (ADA, 2017, S34).
- ▲ Refer people with type 1 diabetes and those with type 2 diabetes who are prescribed a flexible insulin therapy program for education on how to use carbohydrate counting (and in some cases fat and protein gram estimation) to determine mealtime insulin dosing. **EB:** *Education regarding the carbohydrate-counting approach to meal planning can assist with effectively modifying insulin dosing from meal to meal and improve glycemic control* (ADA, 2017, S36).
- ▲ Refer overweight and obese clients with type 2 diabetes for diet, activity, and behavioral therapy. **EB:** *"Modest weight loss, defined as sustained reduction of 5% of initial body weight, has been shown to improve glycemic control and to reduce the need for glucose-lowering medications"* (ADA, 2017, S36). *Structured exercise programs over 8 weeks have been shown to reduce A_{1C} by 0.66%* (ADA, 2017, S37).
- • For interventions regarding foot care, refer to the care plan Ineffective peripheral **Tissue Perfusion.**

Geriatric

- • Watch for age-related cognitive changes that can impair self-management of diabetes. **EBN:** *"Advanced age is associated with higher rates of cognitive dysfunction, causing difficulty in carrying out complex care activities such as glucose monitoring and adjustment of insulin doses"* (Munshi et al, 2016).
- ▲ Consider relaxing glucose targets for older adults. **EB:** *"Hypoglycemia is the leading limiting factor in the glycemic management of type 1 and insulin-treated type 2 diabetes. Multiple factors increase the risk of hypoglycemia in older adults, including impaired renal function, slowed hormonal regulation and counterregulation, variable appetite and nutritional intake, polypharmacy, and slowed intestinal absorption. The strongest predictors of severe hypoglycemia have been found to be advanced age, recent hospitalization, and polypharmacy, all of which are common in the (long term care) population"* (Munshi et al, 2016).
- ▲ In clients with diabetes who require tube feedings, use a diabetes-specific formulation such as Glucerna or Glytrol. **EB:** *"Randomized controlled trials have found diabetes specific formulas for blood glucose management"* (Munshi et al, 2016).

Pediatric

- ▲ Treat hypoglycemia in newborn infants with 0.5 mL/kg oral (buccal) dextrose gel. **EB:** *"Neonatal hypoglycaemia … can be associated with brain injury." "Treatment of infants with neonatal hypoglycaemia with 40% dextrose gel reduces the incidence of mother-infant separation for treatment"* (Weston et al, 2016).

• = Independent;   ▲ = Collaborative;   **EBN** = Evidence-Based Nursing;   **EB** = Evidence-Based

- Teach children and adolescents (and their parents) with type 1 diabetes or on intensive insulin regimens (MDI or insulin pump therapy) to perform SMBG before meals and snacks, occasionally postprandially, at bedtime, before exercise, when they suspect low blood glucose, after treating low blood glucose until they are normoglycemic, and before critical tasks such as driving. EB: *"A database study of almost 27,000 children and adolescents with type 1 diabetes showed that … increased daily frequency of SMBG was significantly associated with lower A_{1C} (−0.2% per additional test per day, leveling off at five tests per day) and with fewer acute complications"* (ADA, 2017, S49).
- Teach parents and children that children and adolescents with type 1 and 2 diabetes should spend 60 minutes daily in moderate to vigorous aerobic activity, and at least 3 days/week in muscle/bone strengthening activity. *"Research is limited on children and activity in diabetes, therefore they should follow general Centers for Disease Control recommendations for children"* (ADA, 2017, S37).

Home Care

▲ Teach family and others having close contact with the person with diabetes how to use an emergency glucagon kit (as prescribed). EB: *If the patient is unable to swallow or is unresponsive, subcutaneous or intramuscular glucagon or intravenous glucose should be given by a trained family member or medical personnel (Handelsman et al, 2015).*

Multicultural

- Provide culturally appropriate diabetes health education. EB: *"Structured interventions that are developed for diverse populations and that integrate culture, language, finance, religion, and literacy and numeracy skills positively influence patient outcomes"* (ADA, 2017, S8).
- Involve community health workers, peers, and lay leaders in diabetes education and support in underserved communities. EB: *"Strong social support leads to improved clinical outcomes, a reduction in psychosocial issues, and adoption of healthier lifestyles"* (ADA, 2017, S8).

Client/Family Teaching and Discharge Planning

- Provide "survival skills" education or review for hospitalized clients, including information about (1) identification of the health care provider who will provide diabetes care after discharge; (2) diagnosis of diabetes, SMBG, explanation of home blood glucose goals, and when to call provider; (3) information on consistent nutrition habits; (4) when and how to take medications including insulin administration; (5) proper use and disposal of needles and syringes if applicable; (6) definition, recognition, treatment, and prevention of hyperglycemia and hypoglycemia; and (7) sick-day management. EB: *Appropriate education at the time of discharge can help prevent a potentially dangerous gap in care (ADA, 2017, S125).*
- Refer clients for individual or group Diabetes Self-Management Education (DSME) and Diabetes Self-Management Support (DSMS) of at least 10 hours' duration. EB: *"Studies have found that DSME is associated with improved diabetes knowledge and self-care behaviors, lower A_{1C}, lower self-reported weight, improved quality of life, healthy coping, and reduced health care costs. Better outcomes were reported for DSME interventions that were over 10 hours in total duration, included follow-up with DSMS, were culturally and age appropriate, were tailored to individual needs and preferences, and addressed psychosocial issues and incorporated behavioral strategies"* (ADA, 2017, S34).
- Evaluate clients' monitoring technique initially and at regular intervals. *Accuracy of SMBG is instrument and user dependent (ADA, 2017, S48).*
- Teach patients with type 2 diabetes the importance of avoiding sedentary behavior, to move around briefly at least every 20 to 30 minutes, and to walk for 15 minutes after meals. EB: *These activities can improve glycemic control (Colberg et al, 2016).*
- Teach clients the importance of at least 150 minutes/week of aerobic physical activity spread over at least 3 days/week. EB: *"In type 1 diabetes, aerobic training increases cardiorespiratory fitness, decreases insulin resistance, and improves lipid levels and endothelial function. In individuals with type 2 diabetes, regular training reduces A_{1C}, triglycerides, blood pressure, and insulin resistance"* (Colberg et al, 2016).
▲ Discuss recommending resistance training with the client's provider. EB: *"Resistance exercise (free weights or weight machines) increases strength in adults with type 2 diabetes by about 50% and improves A_{1C} by 0.57%"* (Colberg et al, 2016).
- Teach clients with type 1 diabetes to test for blood ketones before exercise if they have unexplained hyperglycemia (≥250 mg/dL). EB: *"Exercise should be postponed or suspended if blood ketone levels are*

elevated (≥1.5 mmol/L) as blood glucose levels and ketones may rise further with even mild activity" (Colberg et al, 2016).

▲ Teach clients with type 1 diabetes to check blood glucose prior to exercise. Blood glucose levels prior to exercise should ideally be between 90 and 250 mg/dL (5.0 and 13.9 mmol/L). Discuss carbohydrate use prior to exercise with physician. **EB:** *Exercise can increase risk of hypoglycemia during and for up to 48 hours after exercise (Colberg et al, 2016).*

● Teach clients to use alcohol with caution. **EB:** *Alcohol consumption may place people with diabetes at increased risk for delayed hypoglycemia, especially if taking insulin or insulin secretagogues (ADA, 2017, S35).*

REFERENCES

American Diabetes Association (ADA). (2017). Clinical practice recommendations. *Diabetes Care, 40*(Suppl. 1).

Handelsman, Y., Grunberger, G., Zimmerman, R. S., et al. (2015). *American Association of Clinical Endocrinologists and American College of Endocrinology. Clinical practice guidelines for developing a diabetes mellitus comprehensive care plan 2015.* Retrieved from https://www.aace.com/files/dm-guidelines-ccp.pdf.

Colberg, S. R., SIgal, R. J., Yardley, J. E., et al. (2016). Physical activity/exercise and diabetes: A position statement of the American Diabetes Association. *Diabetes Care, 39*(11), 2065–2079.

Goldberg, P. A., et al. (2006). "Waste not, want not": Determining the optimal priming volume for intravenous insulin infusions. *Diabetes Technology and Therapeutics, 8*(5), 598–601.

Munshi, M. N., Florez, H., Huang, E. S., et al. (2016). Management of diabetes in long-term care and skilled nursing facilities: A position statement of the American Diabetes Association. *Diabetes Care, 39*(2), 308–318.

National Prescribing Service Limited (NPS). (2017). *Medicines that affect blood glucose levels.* Retrieved from https://www.nps.org.au/medical-info/consumer-info/medicines-and-type-2-diabetes.

Tran, T. T. T., Pease, A., Wood, A. J., et al. (2017). Review of evidence for adult diabetic ketoacidosis management protocols. *Frontiers in Endocrinology, 8*, 106. Retrieved from http://doi.org/10.3389/fendo.2017.00106.

Weston, P. J., Harris, D. L., Battin, M., et al. (2016). Oral dextrose gel for the treatment of hypoglycaemia in newborn infants. *Cochrane Database of Systemic Reviews,* (5), CD011027. doi:10.1002/14651858.CD011027.pub2.

Zahid, N., et al. (2008). Adsorption of insulin onto infusion sets used in adult intensive care unit and neonatal care settings. *Diabetes Research and Clinical Practice, 80*(3), e11–e13.

Grieving   *Ruth A. Wittmann-Price, PhD, RN, CNS, CNE, CHSE, ANEF, FAAN*

NANDA-I

Definition

A normal complex process that includes emotional, physical, spiritual, social, and intellectual responses and behaviors by which individuals, families, and communities incorporate an actual, anticipated, or perceived loss into their daily lives.

Defining Characteristics

Alteration in activity level; alteration in dream pattern; alteration in immune functioning; alteration in neuroendocrine functioning; alteration in sleep pattern; anger; blaming; despair; detachment; disorganization; distress; finding meaning in a loss; guilt about feeling relieved; maintaining a connection to the deceased; pain; panic behavior; personal growth; psychological distress

Related Factors

To be developed

At-Risk Population

Anticipatory loss of significant object; anticipatory loss of significant other; death of significant other; loss of significant other

NOC   (Nursing Outcomes Classification)

Suggested NOC Outcomes

Grief Resolution; Dignified Life Closure; Hope; Psychosocial Adjustment: Life Change

● = Independent;   ▲ = Collaborative;   **EBN** = Evidence-Based Nursing;   **EB** = Evidence-Based

Example NOC Outcome with Indicators
Grief Resolution as evidenced by the following indicators: Resolves feelings about the loss/Verbalizes reality and acceptance of loss/Maintains living environment/Seeks social support. (Rate the outcome and indicators of **Grief Resolution:** 1 = never demonstrated, 2 = rarely demonstrated, 3 = sometimes demonstrated, 4 = often demonstrated, 5 = consistently demonstrated [see Section I].)

Client/Family Outcomes

Client/Family Will (Specify Time Frame)

- Discuss meaning of the loss to his or her life and the functioning of the family
- Identify ways to support family members and articulate methods of support he or she requires from family and friends
- Accept assistance in meeting the needs of the family from friends and/or extended family

NIC (Nursing Interventions Classification)

Suggested NIC Interventions

Grief Work Facilitation; Dying Care; Emotional Support: Perinatal Death; Hope Instillation; Support System Enhancement; Family Support; Family Integrity Promotion

Example NIC Activities—Grief Work Facilitation
Identify the loss; Encourage expression of feelings about the loss; Assist to identify personal coping strategies; Identify sources of community support

Nursing Interventions and *Rationales*

Anticipatory Grieving Interventions

- Grieving of a critically ill or dying client and clients' family/relatives for the losses experienced during the deteriorating illness, and the future that will be filled with loss. EBN: *Johnson et al (2017) qualitatively studied anticipatory grieving associated with patients at the end of life and their families and found that less than 50% of the dying patients and their families were given an anticipatory grieving nursing diagnosis and met the nursing outcomes at the time of death (such as the spiritual health outcome), demonstrating that expected outcomes need additional nursing attention.*
- Develop a trusting relationship both with the client and with the family by using presence and therapeutic communication techniques. EB: *Researchers developed a Relationship Tree as an experiential approach to grief counseling. It includes narrative theory and art therapy, and the therapists asked questions that assisted clients in reinterpreting the death experience and grow from it in the future (Peterson & Goldberg, 2016).*
- Keep the family apprised of the client's ongoing condition as much as possible. Consult with the family for decision-making as appropriate. EBN: *Bao-Huan (2016) qualitatively studied anticipatory parents' (N = 19) grieving related to impending loss of school-age children with type I or type II spinal muscular atrophy and found that family members often feel physically and mentally exhausted. The four themes identified in the study included; enduring the helplessness and pressure, suffering caused by the child's rare condition, loss of hope and a reinforcement of the parent–child attachment, and avoiding the pressure of death and enriching the child's life. The study supported nurses recognizing family reactions and in an ongoing fashion to assist them in the grieving process.*
- Keep the family informed of client's needs for physical care and support in symptom control, and inform them about health care options at the end of life, including palliative care, hospice care, and home care. EB: *Brooks (2017) completed an interpretative qualitative study about communication and shared decision-making about end-of-life care in a 24-bed intensive care unit (ICU) using focus groups with 17 nurses and 11 physicians. Findings indicated that improvement was needed in initiating and communicating end-of-life care among health care professionals and with the families. Recommendations include that end-of-life care leaders should be properly introduced and processes clearly followed by all health professionals.*
- Discuss preferred place of death (PPD) with client. EB: *Costa et al (2016) completed a meta-analysis (N = 26 articles) about patients' PPD because many patients express a preference to die at home. The analysis*

● = Independent; ▲ = Collaborative; EBN = Evidence-Based Nursing; EB = Evidence-Based

found that variables that increased the patient being home to die include multidisciplinary home palliative care, preference for home death, cancer diagnoses, early referral to palliative care, not living alone, having a caregiver, and the caregiver's coping skills.

- Ask family members if they are receiving sufficient sleep. If a family member desires to be in the room for sleep, provide a reclining chair or portable bed if possible, and bedding to keep the family member comfortable. If needed, find housing for family member from out of town with the support of a case manager or social worker. **EB:** *Manheim et al (2016) studied family members (N = 8) of patients in a long-term care program until the end of life who were provided community caregivers 24/7. The qualitative study identified the following themes: the program supported families and families as caregivers, the patients' social and cultural needs at the end of life were better met, and the changing needs of the patients and families were addressed.*

- Ask family members about having adequate resources to care for themselves and the critically ill family member. **EBN:** *Eskola et al (2017) used a mixed-method study on parents' experiences and needs during a child's (N = 47) end-of-life care at home and found that parents created a sense of normality for the child, which caused parental exhaustion. Parents needed practical help with housekeeping and dealing with insurance.*

- Listen to the family member's story. **EB:** *Harrop et al (2016) surveyed family caregivers who experienced a loved one in end-of-life care; results included participants sharing feelings of guilt, need for communication and support, and the experience of a "void" created by the withdrawal of professional support after death.*

- Encourage family members to show their caring feelings and talk to the client. **EBN:** *The researchers completed a literature review about using transitional objects with parents for perinatal loss such as taking photographs for parents. The objects provide parents a brief sense of healing, but long-term effects of transitional objects need further investigation (LeDuff et al, 2017).*

- Recognize and respect different feelings and wishes from both the family members and the client. **EBN:** *Chevrier et al (2016) studied the use of multidisciplinary care for end-of-life patients in the ICU environment and found that using the values of holism, patient-centeredness, and healing supports family members in complicated and emotionally challenging situations.*

- If necessary, refer a family member for counseling or to a minister/priest to help him or her cope with the existential questions and current overwhelming reality. **EBN:** *Tan and Cheang (2016) completed a retrospective investigation of interventions provided to patients (N = 50) receiving end-of-life care and their families and found that education of nurses and doctors was needed so that they could identify prompt symptoms of pain and the need for spiritual and religious care and then notify the appropriate ministers.*

- Recognize that one family member may be in a state of caregiver role strain from a long caregiving situation. **EBN:** *Church, Schumacher, and Thompson (2016) completed a mixed-methods study about the strain experienced by family caregivers of nursing home patients. The study results uncovered less recognized sources of caregiver strain including the loss of the older adult's dignity, lack of communication from staff, instances of poor-quality care, residents' symptom distress, and hospice care not offered.*

- Promote mutual goal setting in which decisions are made together that affect the family. **EBN:** *Kim et al (2017) descriptively studied the extent to which the patient caregiver (N = 44) used the advanced directives and agreed on end-of-life care decisions for cancer patient. They found 50% of caregivers did not agree on advanced directives, and the overall recommendation is to better include caregivers in end-of-life decisions to decrease disagreement.*

Grieving Interventions When Death of a Loved One Occurs

Use the following activities when interacting with the bereaved person:
- Be present and attentive, use active empathetic listening. **EBN:** *Rodgers, Calmes, and Grotts (2016) descriptively explored family members' (N = 13) experience of a bathing and honoring practice after a loved one's death in the acute care setting, and all family members stated that the bathing and honoring practice was a positive experience and supported the grieving process.*
- Validate the client's feelings of grief and feeling hurt, stressful, anxious, out of control, and further symptoms of grieving. **EB:** *Vollenbroich et al (2016) retrospectively studied symptom perception by parents (N = 38) and health care professionals for pediatric palliative home care and found that parents who cared for their dying child at home could successfully identify what the child needed by symptoms, and this produced a satisfaction for the parents.*
- Provide time and space for the person to tell their story of loss. **EB:** *Lawrence (2017) completed a case study analysis with individuals that experienced catastrophic events as first responders of lost patients or victims. Telling their story assisted in the grieving process.*

● = Independent;   ▲ = Collaborative;   **EBN** = Evidence-Based Nursing;   **EB** = Evidence-Based

○ *Offer condolences:* "*I am sorry that you lost your husband.*" **EB:** *Librizzi, Isle, and Coyle (2016) investigated how to provide bad news to perinatal patients and what to say, and they found that it is a challenge for health care providers to say "I am sorry" to mothers experiencing a loss. It also shows empathy and does not indicate liability. Explain that feelings will oscillate as the person does grief work, from coping to accepting the loss to coping to build a new life without the loved one.* **EB:** *Levi-Belz (2017) investigated the role of the ongoing relationship with the deceased family member comparing 58 suicide-loss survivors and 48 sudden-death and 53 natural-death bereaved individuals, and the suicide-loss family reported a lower positive ongoing relationship with the deceased.*

○ Intentionally schedule meetings with family members to provide support during grieving. **EB:** *Parravicini (2017) completed a literature review about the protocols for newborns with life-limiting or life-threatening conditions and found a variety of neonatal palliative care programs without standardization. The review concluded that a multidisciplinary team is needed to address the infant's needs, parental grieving process, and providers' distress.*

- Refer to mental health providers as needed. **EBN:** *Palmer, Saviet, and Tourish (2016) explored adolescent and young adults who experienced a loss in their families because it affects social functioning, physical and mental health, and development, and they found that young adults need support and guidance to decrease the intensity of grief and distress. Therefore the recommendations for nurses are to develop individual patient guidance, support, and referrals.*

- Help the client use a method to give voice to his or her unique story of loss. Methods include keeping a personal journal to record feelings and insights; retelling of the loss narrative to a caring person; music therapy techniques with a trained therapist or listening to music that has significance to the relationship; and use of the "virtual dream," which is a dreamlike short story written by the grieving person to tell the narrative of the loss. **EBN:** *Beiermann (2017) studied families' (N = 50) bereavement reactions related to patients dying in the ICU and found that the majority of families responded positively to receiving an ECG Memento, which is a monitor strip of the patients' heart rhythm. Discuss coping methods with the grieving person. Common coping techniques include exercise, telling the story of grief to a caring person, journaling, pets, and developing a legacy for the deceased.* **EB:** *The researchers used kinetic sculpturing as a grief intervention in case studies to create visual examples of family equilibrium before, in the midst of, and after the deaths of family members. Family members found the creative expression beneficial (Brandon & Goldberg, 2017).*

- Encourage the family to create a quiet and comfortable healing environment, and follow comforting grief rituals such as prayer, interacting with nature, or lighting votive candles. **EBN:** *Barrett (2017) reviewed a case study related to how health care professionals provide empathy to grieving parents who lost a child and suggested nursing implications including being present and listening.*

- Refer the family members for spiritual counseling if desired. **EBN:** *Broadhurst and Harrington (2016) completed a literature review to investigate the correlation between transcendent phenomena and peaceful death and identified four themes: spiritual comfort; peaceful, calm death; spiritual transformation; and unfinished business. The results encouraged nurses to recognize the phenomenon and its importance in spiritual care.*

- Help the family determine the best way and place to find social support. Encourage family members to continue to use support for as long as needed. **EB:** *Researchers studied spouses (N = 1224) whose partners died to examine (a) how life satisfaction changed; (b) whether sociodemographic factors and social and health resources moderate effect life satisfaction; and (c) whether anticipation, reaction, and adaptation are related to mortality. Life satisfaction decreases for about 2.5 years and older age was associated with more intense declines (Infurna et al, 2017).*

- Identify available community resources, including bereavement groups at local hospitals and hospice centers. Volunteers who provide bereavement support can also be effective. **EB:** *Gibson (2017) investigated the use of Second Life to symbolically bury and memorialize the real-life biological deaths of people. It was shown to not decrease the loss in real life; instead it provides a method to remember the person.*

- Refer to complicated **Grieving** if grieving fails to follow normative (or cultural) expectations and manifests in functional impairment.

 ### Pediatric/Parent

- Treat the child/parents with respect, give him or her the opportunity to talk about concerns and answer questions honestly. **EB:** *Care providers can give anticipatory guidance to caregivers to support children who are grieving; to assist children to better understand what has happened; and to address any misinformation, misinterpretations, or misconceptions (Schonfeld & Demaria, 2017).*

● = Independent;   ▲ = Collaborative;   **EBN** = Evidence-Based Nursing;   **EB** = Evidence-Based

G

- Listen to the child's expression of grief. **EBN:** *Halliwell and Franken (2016) studied online stories (N = 70) from bereaved siblings about their losses, and discussions supported two main struggles: (1) grieving as deviant behavior versus grieving as a normal process and (2) the deceased as gone forever versus the deceased as still present.*
- Help parents recognize that the grieving child does not have to be "fixed"; instead, they need support going through an experience of grieving just like adults. **EB:** *Templeton et al (2016) studied bereavement in family members who lost a loved one associated with alcohol and/or drugs and found that the stigma associated with the death decreased support for the surviving children and adults. The research uncovered five themes: possibility of death, official processes, stigma, grief, and support. This study demonstrated that this is a marginalized group of bereaved people that includes children that may grieve differently because of lack of social support.*
- Consider the use of art for children in hospice care who are dying or dealing with the death of a parent, sibling, or other family member. **EB:** *Hill and Lineweaver (2016) used art to study the positive and negative affect of grieving children and compared the intervention with another visuospatial task. They found that children who created art individually experienced a significant decrease in negative affect.*
- ▲ Refer grieving children and parents to a program to help facilitate grieving if desired, especially if the death was traumatic. **EB:** *Koblenz (2016) studied adults (N = 19) who were grieving children, and the qualitative descriptions produced five themes: adjustment to catastrophe, support, therapy, continuing a connection with the deceased parent, and reinvestment. The adults stated that these were the most helpful elements in the years after they experienced a death of a loved one.*
- Help the adolescent determine sources of support and how to use them effectively. **EB:** *DeDiego, Wheat, and Fletcher (2017) explored Adventure Based Counseling (ABC) camps for grieving adolescents and children with positive results. This is just one alternative support system for grieving adolescents and children.*
- Encourage grieving parents to take good care of their own health. **EB:** *Albuquerque et al (2017) studied parental relationships (N = 17) after the death of a child by grounded theory method and identified three themes: search for meaning, communication with the partner, and care-in-relation that assisted couples to maintain a healthy relationship.*
- ▲ Encourage grieving parents to seek mental health services as needed. The death of a child is regarded as among the most traumatic, incomprehensible, and devastating of losses, with the potential to precipitate a crisis of meaning for the bereaved parent. **EB:** *Researchers qualitatively studied meaning reconstruction using a life-story interview with a Japanese woman who lost her son to suicide. The analysis revealed three themes: (1) making sense of her son's death and life, (2) relationships with other people, and (3) reconstruction of a bond with the deceased (Daisuke & Kenji, 2017).*
- Recognize that men and women often grieve differently, and explain this to parents if it becomes an issue. **EB:** *Researchers used a mixed-method approach to investigate mothers' (N = 60) grief after losing a child, forgiveness, and posttraumatic growth. There was a negative correlation between forgiveness and grief and a positive correlation between forgiveness and posttraumatic growth (posttraumatic growth was viewed as changes in life) (Martincekova & Klatt, 2017). Steen (2015) studied multicultural perinatal bereavement interventions (N = 59) by using a cross-sectional method and found differences in interventions by nurses/midwives in different countries regarding knowledge, communication skills, and management of personal feelings, indicating that consistent bereavement information is needed.*
- Recognize that mothers who have a miscarriage/stillbirth grieve and experience sorrow because of the loss of the child. **EBN:** *Rocha et al (2017) performed a literature (N = 29) review about prenatal palliative care for parents carrying a fetus with malformations and found no long-term studies about the effects of prenatal palliative care.*

 Geriatric

- Monitor an older adult who has been treated for bereavement-related depression for relapse or recurrence. **EB:** *Tanimukai et al (2017) studied the relationship between depression and insomnia in bereaved families (N = 561) and found that insomnia was highly correlated with depression.*
- Provide support for the family when the loss is associated with dementia of the family member. **EB:** *Researchers studied an intervention with caregivers of veterans with dementia. Caregivers were divided into groups of Internet or telephone intervention and found that in rural populations the Internet was effective if the caregiver was comfortable with technology (Hicken et al, 2017).*
- Determine the social supports of older adults. **EBN:** *Durham, Allmark, and Collins (2017) investigated the experience of cancer pain in elderly patients (N = 9) and by qualitative analysis identified four themes for*

● = Independent;   ▲ = Collaborative;   **EBN** = Evidence-Based Nursing;   **EB** = Evidence-Based

nursing consideration: better to be old than to be dying, maintaining independence, grieving for a former self, and denial of pain.

Multicultural

- See interventions and rationales in care plans for complicated **Grieving** and Chronic **Sorrow.**

Home Care

- The interventions previously described may be adapted for home care use.
- Assessment of activities of daily living (ADLs) and instrumental ADLs is essential as part of comprehensive care after a home care client has suffered the loss of a loved one. **EB:** *Raitio, Kaunonen, and Aho (2017) explored parental grief intervention and its effects on maternal grief with health care provider intervention in one group compared with a control group. Results did not demonstrate a significant difference in the grief reactions between groups and support from the health care professionals was positively correlated with stronger personal growth at 6 months post death.*
- Actively listen as the client grieves for his or her own death or for real or perceived loss. Normalize the client's expressions of grief for self. Demonstrate a caring and hopeful approach. **EB:** *Vergo et al (2017) measured the grief reactions of patients (N = 53) with advanced cancer using the Preparatory Grief in Advanced Cancer (PGAC) instrument and found that preparatory grief was common and 25% of participations had significant grief, and all patients demonstrated distress.*
- ▲ Refer the client to social services as necessary for losses not related to death. Support is helpful to grief work for all types of losses. Social workers can help the client plan for financial changes as a result of job losses and help with community referrals as appropriate. **EB:** *A study by social work researchers about women who experienced a miscarriage, stillbirth, or child's death compared self-esteem to maternal identity and found that stillbirth and death of a child negatively affected self-esteem, and that self-esteem levels were increased by stronger maternal identity (Wonch et al, 2017).*
- ▲ Refer the bereaved to hospice bereavement programs or an Internet self-help group. Relief of the suffering of clients and families (physical, emotional, and spiritual) is the goal of hospice care. **EB:** *A ethnographic study was completed to understand the motivation for grieving mothers to start and maintain a blog. After reviewing 140 blogs the researchers identified themes such as sharing the loss and challenges, creating a network to support and comfort other, guaranteeing a space to express feelings, honoring and perpetuating the image of the child lost, and engaging in social activism (Figueiredo et al, 2017).*

REFERENCES

Albuquerque, S., Ferreira, L., Narciso, I., et al. (2017). Parents' positive interpersonal coping after a child's death. *Journal of Child & Family Studies, 26*(7), 1817–1830. Retrieved from http://dx.doi.org/10.1007/s10826-017-0697-5.

Barrett, M. (2017). 'How would you feel …?' A reflective case study. *British Journal of Cardiac Nursing, 12*(5), 219–222. Retrieved from http://dx.doi.org/10.12968/bjca.2017.12.5.219.

Bao-Huan, Y. (2016). The experiences of families living with the anticipatory loss of a school-age child with spinal muscular atrophy—The parents' perspectives. *Journal of Clinical Nursing, 25*(17/18), 2648–2657. Retrieved from http://dx.doi.org/10.1111/jocn.13312.

Beiermann, M. (2017). Family members' and intensive care unit nurses' response to the ECG Memento© during the bereavement period. *Dimensions of Critical Care Nursing: DCCN, 36*(6), 317–326. Retrieved from http://dx.doi.org/10.1097/DCC.0000000000000269.

Brandon, K. E., & Goldberg, R. M. (2017). A kinetic sculpture intervention for individuals grieving the deaths of family members. *Journal of Creativity in Mental Health, 12*(1), 99–114. Retrieved from http://dx.doi.org/10.1080/15401383.2016.1184114.

Broadhurst, K., & Harrington, A. (2016). A thematic literature review: the importance of providing spiritual care for end-of-life patients who have experienced transcendence phenomena. *American Journal of Hospice & Palliative Medicine, 33*(9), 881–893. Retrieved from http://dx.doi.org/10.1177/1049909115595217.

Brooks, L. A. (2017). Communication and decision-making about end-of-life care in the intensive care unit. *American Journal of Critical Care, 26*(4), 336–341. Retrieved from http://dx.doi.org/10.4037/ajcc2017774.

Chevrier, A., Doucettte, E., Bastarache, S., et al. (2016). Navigating the transition of critical care to end-of-life care using a strengths-based nursing approach…Dynamics of critical care 2016 in Charlottetown, PE, September 25–27, 2016. *Canadian Journal of Critical Care Nursing, 27*(2), 17-17; ISSN:2368-8653.

Church, L. L., Schumacher, K. L., & Thompson, S. A. (2016). Mixed-methods exploration of family caregiver strain in the nursing home. *Journal of Hospice & Palliative Nursing, 18*(1), 46–52. Retrieved from http://dx.doi.org/10.1097/NJH.0000000000000209.

Costa, V., et al. (2016). The determinants of home and nursing home death: a systematic review and meta-analysis. *BMC Palliative Care, 15*, 1–15. Retrieved from http://dx.doi.org/10.1186/s12904-016-0077-8.

Daisuke, K., & Kenji, K. (2017). Meaning reconstruction process after suicide: Life-story of a Japanese woman who lost her son to suicide. *Omega: Journal of Death & Dying, 75*(4), 360–375. Retrieved from http://dx.doi.org/10.1177/0030222816652805.

DeDiego, A. C., Wheat, L. S., & Fletcher, T. B. (2017). Overcoming obstacles: Exploring the use of adventure based counseling in youth grief camps. *Journal of Creativity in Mental Health, 12*(2), 230–241. Retrieved from http://dx.doi.org/10.1080/15401383.2016.1191403.

● = Independent;   ▲ = Collaborative;   **EBN** = Evidence-Based Nursing;   **EB** = Evidence-Based

Durham, M., Allmark, P., & Collins, K. (2017). Older people's experiences of cancer pain: A qualitative study. *Nursing Older People, 29*(6), 28–32. Retrieved from http://dx.doi.org/10.7748/nop.2017.e943.

Eskola, K., Bergstraesser, E., Zimmermann, K., et al. (2017). Maintaining family life balance while facing a child's imminent death—a mixed methods study. *Journal of Advanced Nursing, 73*(10), 2462–2472. Retrieved from http://dx.doi.org/10.1111/jan.13304.

Figueiredo, F., Heloisa, C., Szylit, B. R., et al. (2017). Grieving mothers: design of thematic blogs about loss of a child. *Acta Paulista de Enfermagem, 30*(2), 116–121. Retrieved from http://dx.doi.org/10.1590/1982-0194201700019.

Gibson, M. (2017). Grievable lives: Avatars, memorials, and family 'plots' in Second Life. *Mortality, 22*(3), 224–239. Retrieved from http://dx.doi.org/10.1080/13576275.2016.1263941.

Halliwell, D., & Franken, N. (2016). "He was supposed to be with me for the rest of my life": Meaning-making in bereaved siblings' online stories. *Journal of Family Communication, 16*(4), 337–354. Retrieved from http://dx.doi.org/10.1080/15267431.2016.1194841.

Harrop, E., Morgan, F., Byrne, A., et al. (2016). "It still haunts me whether we did the right thing": A qualitative analysis of free text survey data on the bereavement experiences and support needs of family caregivers. *BMC Palliative Care, 15*, 1–8. Retrieved from http://dx.doi.org/10.1186/s12904-016-0165-9.

Hicken, B. L., Daniel, C., Luptak, M., et al. (2017). Supporting caregivers of rural veterans electronically (SCORE). *Journal of Rural Health, 33*(3), 305–313. Retrieved from http://dx.doi.org/10.1111/jrh.12195.

Hill, K., & Lineweaver, T. T. (2016). Improving the short-term affect of grieving children through art. *Art Therapy: Journal of the American Art Therapy Association, 33*(2), 91–98. Retrieved from http://dx.doi.org/10.1080/07421656.2016.1166414.

Infurna, F. J., et al. (2017). Changes in life satisfaction when losing one's spouse: Individual differences in anticipation, reaction, adaptation and longevity in the German Socio-Economic Panel Study (SOEP). *Ageing & Society, 37*(5), 899–934. Retrieved from http://dx.doi.org/10.1017/S0144686X15001543.

Johnson, J., et al. (2017). Outcomes for end-of-life patients with anticipatory grieving: Insights from practice with standardized nursing terminologies within an interoperable internet-based electronic health record. *Journal of Hospice & Palliative Nursing, 19*(3), 223–231. Retrieved from http://dx.doi.org/10.1097/NJH.0000000000000333.

Kim, S., Koh, S., Park, K., et al. (2017). End-of-life care decisions using a Korean advance directive among cancer patient-caregiver dyads. *Palliative & Supportive Care, 15*(1), 77–87. Retrieved from http://dx.doi.org/10.1017/S1478951516000808.

Koblenz, J. (2016). Growing from grief. *Omega: Journal of Death & Dying, 73*(3), 203–230. Retrieved from http://dx.doi.org/10.1177/0030222815576123.

Lawrence, M. (2017). Near-death and other transpersonal experiences occurring during catastrophic events. *American Journal of Hospice & Palliative Medicine, 34*(5), 486–492. Retrieved from http://dx.doi.org/10.1177/1049909116631298.

LeDuff, L. D., Bradshaw, W. T., Blake, S. M., et al. (2017). Transitional objects to facilitate grieving following perinatal loss. *Advances in Neonatal Care, 17*(5), 347–353. Retrieved from http://dx.doi.org/10.1097/ANC.0000000000000429.

Levi-Belz, Y. (2017). Relationship with the deceased as facilitator of posttraumatic growth among suicide-loss survivors. *Death Studies, 41*(6), 376–384. Retrieved from http://dx.doi.org/10.1080/07481187.2017.1285372.

Librizzi, R. J., Isle, S., & Coyle, A. (2016). What to say and do right when things go wrong. *Contemporary OB/GYN, 61*(11), 22–42.

Manheim, C. E., Haverhals, L. M., Jones, J., et al. (2016). Allowing family to be family: End-of-life care in veterans affairs medical foster homes. *Journal of Social Work in End-of-Life & Palliative Care, 12*(1/2), 104–125. Retrieved from http://dx.doi.org/10.1080/15524256.2016.1156603.

Martincekova, L., & Klatt, J. (2017). Mothers' grief, forgiveness, and posttraumatic growth after the loss of a child. *Omega: Journal of Death & Dying, 75*(3), 248–265. Retrieved from http://dx.doi.org/10.1177/0030222816652803.

Palmer, M., Saviet, M., & Tourish, J. (2016). Understanding and supporting grieving adolescents and young adults. *Pediatric Nursing, 42*(6), 275–281.

Parravicini, E. (2017). Neonatal palliative care. *Current Opinion in Pediatrics, 29*(2), 135–140. Retrieved from http://dx.doi.org/10.1097/MOP.0000000000000464.

Peterson, N. L., & Goldberg, R. M. (2016). Creating relationship trees with grieving clients: An experiential approach to grief counseling. *Journal of Creativity in Mental Health, 11*(2), 198–212. Retrieved from http://dx.doi.org/10.1080/15401383.2016.1181597.

Raitio, K., Kaunonen, M., & Aho, A. L. (2017). Evaluating a bereavement follow-up intervention for grieving mothers after the death of a child. *Scandinavian Journal of Caring Sciences, 29*(3), 510–520. Retrieved from http://dx.doi.org/10.1111/scs.12183.

Rocha, C., et al. (2017). When one knows a fetus is expected to die: Palliative care in the context of prenatal diagnosis of fetal malformations. *Journal of Palliative Medicine, 20*(9), 1020–1031. Retrieved from http://dx.doi.org/10.1089/jpm.2016.0430.

Rodgers, D., Calmes, B., & Grotts, J. (2016). Nursing care at the time of death: A bathing and honoring practice. *Oncology Nursing Forum, 43*(3), 363–371. Retrieved from http://dx.doi.org/10.1188/16.ONF.363-371.

Schonfeld, D. J., & Demaria, T. (2017). Supporting the grieving child and family. *Pediatrics, 138*(3), e1–e12. Retrieved from http://dx.doi.org/10.1542/peds.2016-2147.

Steen, S. E. (2015). Perinatal death: Bereavement interventions used by US and Spanish nurses and midwives. *International Journal of Palliative Nursing, 21*(2), 79–86.

Tan, T., & Cheang, F. (2016). A single-center retrospective analysis of interventions provided to geriatric inpatients receiving end-of-life care. *Progress in Palliative Care, 24*(6), 332–338. Retrieved from http://dx.doi.org/10.1080/09699260.2016.1188521.

Tanimukai, H., et al. (2017). Association between depressive symptoms and changes in sleep condition in the grieving process. *Supportive Care in Cancer, 23*(7), 1925–1931. Retrieved from http://dx.doi.org/10.1007/s00520-014-2548-x.

Templeton, L., et al. (2016). Bereavement through substance use: Findings from an interview study with adults in England and Scotland. *Addiction Research & Theory, 24*(5), 341–354. Retrieved from http://dx.doi.org/10.3109/16066359.2016.1153632.

Vergo, M. T., et al. (2017). Assessing preparatory grief in advanced cancer patients as an independent predictor of distress in an American population. *Journal of Palliative Medicine, 20*(1), 48–52. Retrieved from http://dx.doi.org/10.1089/jpm.2016.0136.

Vollenbroich, R., et al. (2016). Listening to parents: The role of symptom perception in pediatric palliative home care. *Palliative & Supportive Care, 14*(1), 13–19. Retrieved from http://dx.doi.org/10.1017/S1478951515000462.

Wonch, H. P., Cacciatore, J., Shreffler, K. M., et al. (2017). The loss of self: The effect of miscarriage, stillbirth, and child death on maternal self-esteem. *Death Studies, 41*(4), 226–235. Retrieved from http://dx.doi.org/10.1080/07481187.2016.1261204.

● = Independent;   ▲ = Collaborative;   EBN = Evidence-Based Nursing;   EB = Evidence-Based

Complicated Grieving   *Ruth A. Wittmann-Price, PhD, RN, CNS, CNE, CHSE, ANEF, FAAN*

NANDA-I

Definition

A disorder that occurs after the death of a significant other, in which the experience of distress accompanying bereavement fails to follow normative expectations and manifests in functional impairment.

Defining Characteristics

Anger; anxiety; avoidance of grieving; decrease in functioning in life roles; depression; disbelief; distress about the deceased person; excessive stress; experiencing symptoms the deceased experienced; fatigue; feeling dazed; feeling of detachment from others; feeling of emptiness; feeling of shock; feeling stunned; insufficient sense of well-being; longing for the deceased person; low levels of intimacy; mistrust; non-acceptance of a death; persistent painful memories; preoccupation with thoughts about a deceased person; rumination; searching for a deceased person; self-blame; separation distress; traumatic distress

Related Factors

Emotional disturbance; insufficient social support

At-Risk Population

Death of significant other

NOC   (Nursing Outcomes Classification)

Suggested NOC Outcomes

Anxiety Level; Coping; Depression; Grief Resolution; Mood Equilibrium; Personal Well-Being; Psychosocial Adjustment: Life Change; Sleep

Example NOC Outcome with Indicators

See care plan for **Grieving.**

Client Outcomes

Client Will (Specify Time Frame)

- Express appropriate feelings of guilt, fear, anger, or sadness
- Identify somatic distress associated with grief (e.g., anxiety, changes in appetite, insomnia, nightmares, loss of libido, decreased energy, altered activity levels)
- Seek support in dealing with grief-associated issues
- Identify personal strengths and effective coping strategies
- Function at a normal developmental level and begin to successfully and increasingly perform activities of daily living

NIC   (Nursing Interventions Classification)

Suggested NIC Interventions

Grief Work Facilitation; Grief Work Facilitation: Perinatal Death; Guilt Work Facilitation; Hope Installation

Example NIC Activities—Grief Work Facilitation

See care plan for **Grieving.**

Nursing Interventions and *Rationales*

- Assess for signs of complicated grieving that include symptoms that persist at least 6 months after the death and are experienced at least daily or to a disabling degree. Symptoms include feeling emotionally

● = Independent;   ▲ = Collaborative;   EBN = Evidence-Based Nursing;   EB = Evidence-Based

numb, stunned, shocked, and that life is meaningless; dysfunctional thoughts and maladaptive behaviors; experiencing mistrust and estrangement from others; anger and bitterness over the loss; identity confusion; avoidance of the reality of the loss, or excessive proximity seeking to try to feel closer to the deceased, sometimes focused on wishes to die or suicidal statements and behavior; or difficulty moving on with life. *Symptoms must be associated with psychosocial and physical impairments (Kokou-Kpolou et al, 2017).* **EB:** *Brown (2017) studied the recurrent grief in mothers caring for a child with intellectual disability and found that recurrent grief is correlated with coping and challenging behaviors of the child.* **EB:** *Masferrer, Garre-Olmo, and Caparros (2016) studied complicated grief in the substance-abuse population (N = 196) compared with those who did not abuse drugs (N = 100). Complicated grief was significantly higher among the population who abused drugs (34.2% compared with 5% in the control group).*

▲ Determine the client's state of grieving. Use a tool such as the Prolonged Grief Disorder (PGD) scale (Jordan & Litz, 2014), the Grief Support in Health Care Scale (Anderson et al, 2010), the Hogan Grief Reaction Checklist (Hogan, Worden, & Schmidt, 2004), and the Beck Depression Inventory. **EBN:** *Researchers studied the grief of mothers (N = 130) and fathers (N = 52) after infant or child neonatal or pediatric intensive care unit death by completing the Hogan Grief Reaction Checklist at 1, 3, 6, and 13 months post death, and found initial grief reactions decreased from 3 to 13 months for mothers and from 3 to 6 months for fathers (Youngblut et al, 2017).*

▲ Determine whether the client is experiencing depression, suicidal tendencies, or other emotional disorders. Refer the client for counseling or therapy as appropriate. **EB:** *Researchers studied the effect bereavement services have on depression and grief after a person experiences a significant loss, and patients reported that some of the services provided that were most helpful included time alone with the deceased, a quiet room to be alone after the death, sympathy cards from hospital staff, memorial services, chaplain support, an educational grief booklet, grief book recommendations, a check-in phone call, individual counseling, and a relationship-specific support group. The study also found that participants experiencing depression and complicated grief used the services at a more frequent rate than participants who were not clinically depressed (Banyasz et al, 2017).*

● Educate the client and his or her support systems that grief resolution is not a sequential process and that the positive outcome of grief resolution is the integration of the deceased into the ongoing life of the griever. **EB:** *Mowll (2017) studied the ways health care professionals can best support family members (N = 48) who needed to view the body of their relative after a traumatic death, and the study identified qualitative themes. Things that assisted the family members included support during interactions, giving permissions and possibilities, providing information and preparation, being caring, timing experiences appropriately, and tuning into family needs.*

▲ Assess caregivers, particularly younger caregivers, for pessimistic thinking and additional stressful life events. Refer for appropriate support. **EB:** *Researchers studied African American caregivers (family members) (N = 108) of persons with dementia and found that negative thoughts increase depression and physical suffering (Schulz et al, 2017).*

● See the interventions and rationales in the care plans for **Grieving** and Chronic **Sorrow.**

 Pediatric/Parent

▲ Refer grieving children and parents to a program to help facilitate grieving if desired, especially if the death was traumatic. **EB:** *Schreiber, Sands, and Jordan (2017) studied children whose parents died of suicide and found that children felt isolated, abandoned, and responsible. Suggestions for nursing included developmentally appropriate education about suicide grief, depression, and normalizing.*

● Encourage grieving parents to take part in activities that are supportive, such as faith based activities. **EB:** *Nuzum, Meaney, and O'Donoghue (2017) qualitatively studied parents who experienced the loss of a stillborn child, and study results indicated that stillbirth challenges parents' faith, usually one parent more than the other, indicating that all parents should be offered spiritual care after a stillbirth.*

● Encourage grieving parents to seek mental health services as needed. **EBN:** *Morris et al (2017) noted that bereaved parents are an "at-risk" group, and through anecdotal experiences they developed a hospital-wide, preventative model, bereavement program using education, guidance, and support. The model has been received by participants and staff with good results.*

● Help the adolescent determine sources of support and how to use them effectively. If the client is an adolescent exposed to a peer's suicide, watch for symptoms of traumatic grief and posttraumatic stress disorder, which include numbness, preoccupation with the deceased, functional impairment, and poor

G

adjustment to the loss. EB: *Woollett et al (2017) qualitatively studied HIV-positive adolescents in Africa and their ability to disclose the disease and the bereavement process that accompanies the diagnosis. The study found that most participants (N = 25) were orphaned and were really experiencing complicated grief and that was related negatively to mental health and the ability to accept their HIV status and adhere to treatment.*

Geriatric

- Assess for deterioration in bereaved older adults' self-care. EBN: *Skritskaya et al (2017) investigated maladaptive cognitions and their relationship to complicated grief by developing a questionnaire called the Typical Beliefs Questionnaire (TBQ) and piloted the tool on bereaved adults (N = 394) with complicated grief. The new tool was effective in identifying specific maladaptive cognitions related to complicated grief.*
- Those who have lived with older adults with dementia and experienced significant feelings of loss before the loved one's death may be at risk for more intense feelings of grief after the death of the client with dementia. EB: *Berenbaum, Tziraki, and Cohen-Mansfield (2017) studied how people with dementia are told about the death of a peer. Adult daycare staff (N = 52) was qualitatively interviewed and felt that their patients have the emotional capacity to mourn despite their cognitive impairments.*
- Monitor the older client for complicated grieving manifesting in physical and mental health problems. EB: *Boer et al (2017) studied patients with chronic obstructive pulmonary disease (COPD) who have a grieving process because of loss of functioning and found COPD patients experience four stages of grief including denial, resistance, sorrow, and acceptance.*

Multicultural

- Assess for the influence of cultural beliefs, norms, and values on the client's grief and mourning practices. EBN: *Bravo (2017) studied undocumented Latino migrants (N = 12) living in the United States and who have experienced coping with deaths of loved ones in their home countries. The participants experienced sadness and guilt, and communication with those in the home country was an important mechanism for coping.* EB: *Kokou-Kpolou et al (2017) studied European refugees (N = 74) and their experiences of losing a family member to death, which is complicated by immigration status. The study found participants reported a deterioration of their social life and profound feelings of guilt.*
- Encourage discussion of the grief process. EB: *Granek and Peleg-Sagy (2017) completed a literature review about complicated and pathological grief reactions in the US African American population and found 13 articles, but many of the articles were validated using white populations, indicating the need for grief research for African Americans and other ethnic minorities.* EBN: *Mun and Ow (2017) studied the grief process of mothers who lost a child in Singapore and found that qualitatively four themes were identified: (1) meaning to the child's life and death, (2) quality and assurance of an afterlife, (3) the function of crying, and (4) a continuing bond.*
- Identify whether the client had been notified of the health status of the deceased and was able to be present during illness and death. EB: *Young (2017) discussed cases related to people with profound intellectual and multiple disabilities (PIMD) that are bereaved and experience social, emotional, and physical constraints. Young found that people with PIMD are a high-risk group and at greater risk of complicated grieving.*

Home Care

- Consider providing support via the Internet. EB: *Researchers studied an intervention with caregivers of veterans with dementia. Caregivers were divided into groups of Internet or telephone interventions and found that in rural populations the Internet was effective if the caregiver was comfortable with technology (Hicken et al, 2017).*

REFERENCES

Anderson, K., Ewen, H., Miles, E., et al. (2010). The grief support in healthcare scale: Development and testing. *Nursing Research, 59*(6), 372–379.

Banyasz, A., Weikittle, R., Lorenz, A., et al. (2017). Bereavement service preferences of surviving family members: Variation among next of kin with depression and complicated grief. *Journal of Palliative Medicine, 20*(10), 1091–1097. Retrieved from http://dx.doi.org/10.1089/jpm.2016.0235.

Berenbaum, R., Tziraki, C., & Cohen-Mansfield, J. (2017). The right to mourn in dementia: To tell or not to tell when someone dies in dementia day care. *Death Studies, 41*(6), 353–359. doi:10.1080/07481187.2017.1284953.

Bravo, V. (2017). Coping with dying and deaths at home: How undocumented migrants in the United States experience the process of transnational grieving. *Mortality, 22*(1), 33–44. Retrieved from http://dx.doi.org/10.1080/13576275.2016.1192590.

● = Independent; ▲ = Collaborative; EBN = Evidence-Based Nursing; EB = Evidence-Based

Boer, L., Daudey, L., Peters, J., et al. (2017). Assessing the stages of the grieving process in chronic obstructive pulmonary disease (COPD): Validation of the Acceptance of Disease and Impairments Questionnaire (ADIQ). *International Journal of Behavioral Medicine*, 21(3), 561–570. Retrieved from http://dx.doi.org/10.1007/s12529-013-9312-3.

Brown, J. (2017). Recurrent grief in mothering a child with an intellectual disability to adulthood: Grieving is the healing. *Child & Family Social Work*, 21(1), 113–122.

Granek, L., & Peleg-Sagy, T. (2017). The use of pathological grief outcomes in bereavement studies on African Americans. *Transcultural Psychiatry*, 54(3), 384–399. Retrieved from http://dx.doi.org/10.1177/1363461517708121.

Hicken, B. L., Daniel, C., Luptak, M., et al. (2017). Supporting caregivers of rural veterans electronically (SCORE). *Journal of Rural Health*, 33(3), 305–313. Retrieved from http://dx.doi.org/10.1111/jrh.12195.

Hogan, N. S., Worden, J. W., & Schmidt, L. A. (2004). An empirical study of the proposed complicated grief disorder criteria. *Omega*, 48(3), 263–277.

Jordan, A. H., & Litz, B. T. (2014). Prolonged grief disorder: Diagnostic, assessment, and treatment considerations. *Professional Psychology, Research and Practice*, 45(3), 180–187.

Kokou-Kpolou, K., Mbassa, M. D., Moukouta, C. S., et al. (2017). A cross-cultural approach to complicated grief reactions among Togo–Western African immigrants in Europe. *Journal of Cross-Cultural Psychology*, 48(8), 1247–1262. Retrieved from http://dx.doi.org/10.1177/0022022117721972.

Masferrer, L., Garre-Olmo, J., & Caparros, B. (2016). Is complicated grief a risk factor for substance use? A comparison of substance-users and normative grievers. *Addiction Research & Theory*, 25(5), 361–367. Retrieved from http://dx.doi.org/10.1080/16066359.2017.1285912.

Morris, S. E., Dole, O. R., Joselow, M., et al. (2017). The development of a hospital-wide bereavement program: Ensuring bereavement care for all families of pediatric patients. *Journal of Pediatric Healthcare*, 31(1), 88–95. Retrieved from http://dx.doi.org/10.1016/j.pedhc.2016.04.013.

Mowll, J. (2017). Supporting family members to view the body after a violent or sudden death: A role for social work. *Journal of Social Work in End-of-Life & Palliative Care*, 13(2/3), 94–112. Retrieved from http://dx.doi.org/10.1080/15524256.2017.1331182.

Mun, S., & Ow, R. (2017). Death of a child: Perspective of Chinese mothers in Singapore. *Journal of Religion & Spirituality in Social Work*, 36(3), 306–325. Retrieved from http://dx.doi.org/10.1080/15426432.2017.1319781.

Nuzum, D., Meaney, S., & O'Donoghue, K. (2017). The spiritual and theological challenges of stillbirth for bereaved parents. *Journal of Religion & Health*, 56(3), 1081–1095. Retrieved from http://dx.doi.org/10.1007/s10943-017-0365-5.

Schreiber, J. K., Sands, D. C., & Jordan, J. R. (2017). The perceived experience of children bereaved by parental suicide. *Omega: Journal of Death & Dying*, 75(2), 184–206. Retrieved from http://dx.doi.org/10.1177/0030222815612297.

Schulz, R., Savla, J., Czaja, S. J., et al. (2017). The role of compassion, suffering, and intrusive thoughts in dementia caregiver depression. *Aging & Mental Health*, 21(9), 997–1004. Retrieved from http://dx.doi.org/10.1080/13607863.2016.1191057.

Skritskaya, N. A., et al. (2017). Measuring maladaptive cognitions in complicated grief: Introducing the Typical Beliefs Questionnaire. *American Journal of Geriatric Psychiatry*, 25(5), 541–550. Retrieved from http://dx.doi.org/10.1016/j.jagp.2016.09.003.

Woollett, N., Black, V., Cluver, L., et al. (2017). Reticence in disclosure of HIV infection and reasons for bereavement: impact on perinatally infected adolescents' mental health and understanding of HIV treatment and prevention in Johannesburg, South Africa. *African Journal of AIDS Research: AJAR*, 16(2), 175–184. Retrieved from http://dx.doi.org/10.2989/16085906.2017.1337646.

Young, H. (2017). Overcoming barriers to grief: Supporting bereaved people with profound intellectual and multiple disabilities. *International Journal of Developmental Disabilities*, 63(3), 131–137. Retrieved from http://dx.doi.org/10.1080/20473869.2016.1158511.

Youngblut, J. M., Brooten, D., Glaze, J., et al. (2017). Parent grief 1–13 months after death in neonatal and pediatric intensive care units. *Journal of Loss & Trauma*, 22(1), 77–96. Retrieved from http://dx.doi.org/10.1080/15325024.2016.1187049.

Risk for complicated **Grieving**   *Gail B. Ladwig, MSN, RN*

NANDA-I

Definition

Susceptible to a disorder that occurs after death of a significant other in which the experience of distress accompanying bereavement fails to follow normative expectations and manifests in functional impairment, which may compromise health.

Risk Factors

Emotional disturbance; death of a significant other; insufficient social support

At-Risk Population

Death of significant other

NIC, NOC, Client Outcomes, Nursing Interventions and *Rationales,* Client/Family Teaching and Discharge Planning, and References

Refer to care plan for Complicated **Grieving.**

● = Independent;   ▲ = Collaborative;   EBN = Evidence-Based Nursing;   EB = Evidence-Based

Deficient community Health   *Marina Martinez-Kratz, MS, RN, CNE*

NANDA-I

Definition

Presence of one or more health problems or factors that deter wellness or increase the risk of health problems experienced by an aggregate.

Defining Characteristics

Health problem experienced by aggregates or populations; program unavailable to eliminate health problems of an aggregate or population; program unavailable to enhance wellness of an aggregate or population; program unavailable to prevent health problems of an aggregate or population; program unavailable to reduce health problems of an aggregate or population; risk of hospitalization experienced by aggregates or population; risk of physiological states experienced by aggregates or populations; risk of psychological states experienced by aggregates or population

Related Factors

Inadequate consumer satisfaction with program; inadequate program budget; inadequate program evaluation plan; inadequate program outcome data; inadequate social support for program; insufficient access to health care provider; insufficient community experts; insufficient resources; program incompletely addresses health problem

NOC   (Nursing Outcomes Classification)

Suggested NOC Outcomes

Community Grief Response; Community Health Screening Effectiveness; Community Health Status Community Program Effectiveness; Community Resiliency; Community Risk Control: Obesity; Community Risk Control: Unhealthy Cultural Traditions

---

Example NOC Outcome with Indicators

Community Health Status as evidenced by the following indicators: Health status of infants/Children/Adolescents/Adults/Elders/Minority populations/Prevalence of health promotion programs. (Rate the outcome and indicators of **Community Health Status:** 1 = poor, 2 = fair, 3 = good, 4 = very good, 5 = excellent, NA [see Section I].)

Client Outcomes

Community/Adolescents/Minority Clients Will (Specify Time Frame)

- Provide programs for healthy behaviors
- Demonstrate goal setting
- Describe and comply with healthy behaviors
- Describe and demonstrate compliance with hepatitis B virus (HBV) education and testing

NIC   (Nursing Interventions Classification)

Suggested NIC Interventions

Community health development: Identify health concerns, strengths, and priorities with community partners; Assist community members in raising awareness of health problems and concerns

Nursing Interventions and *Rationales*

Refer to care plans: Readiness for Enhanced community **Coping,** Ineffective Community **Coping,** Ineffective **Health** maintenance, Impaired **Home** maintenance, and Risk for other-directed **Violence.**

- Assess for the presence of demographic variables that predict community mortality. EB: *The following demographic variables were associated with increased community mortality: age 65 years or older, poverty, and a high concentration of construction and service workers (Chan et al, 2014).*

● = Independent;   ▲ = Collaborative;   EBN = Evidence-Based Nursing;   EB = Evidence-Based

- Assess for needs related to the community's priority health concerns. EB: *Research results generated from the first study of the National Institutes of Health Sentinel Network identified the top five health concerns of respondents as hypertension, diabetes, cancer, weight, and heart problems (Cottler et al, 2013).*
- Assess patients accessing health services for a history of military service and provide the necessary referrals and information. EBN: *Many veterans eligible for Veteran's Administration (VA) health benefits seek health care from community emergency departments and will benefit from information about VA resources (Merkl et al, 2016).*
- Implement community engagement techniques for collaboration with stakeholders to design, develop, and adapt relevant health interventions. EBN: *In this study's findings, improved nutrition and physical activity behavior were the result of community engagement techniques used to develop culturally relevant obesity prevention interventions for low-income Hispanic mothers with preschool children (Bender, Clark, & Gahagan, 2014).*
- Encourage attendance at community-based exercise programs. EBN: *In this study community-based exercise groups were perceived by pregnant women as a satisfactory and motivating form of exercise engagement (Ette, 2017).*
- Implement community engagement techniques in conjunction with tailored interventions to address health deficiencies. EB: *In this study, community engagement techniques were essential in coordinating interventions and engaging patients, the public, and local practitioners in delivery of mental health care (Lamb et al, 2015).*
- Collaborate with other community-based programs to use the Short Message Service (SMS) to broadcast targeted health messages to reach large numbers of community members. EB: *A study using SMS broadcasting at a metropolitan sexual health clinic to promote the awareness of influenza vaccinations in HIV-positive patients resulted in a significant increase in the number of patients contacted and vaccinated by the clinic (Stowers, Healey, & O'Connor, 2014).*

 Pediatric

▲ Consider use of a clinical-community collaborative to address health deficiencies in underserved populations with children. EB: *A clinical-community collaborative enabled pediatric providers to implement a food insecurity-focused intervention that was associated with improved preventive care outcomes for the infants served (Beck et al, 2014).*
▲ Screen at-risk pediatric populations for lead exposure. EB: *This study showed under testing for lead exposure and no mandatory lead test screening in one-third of eligible children during the study period (Knighton, Payne, & Speedie, 2016).*

 Geriatric

▲ Assess community-dwelling older individuals for cognitive impairment using the Brief Cognitive Assessment Tool-Short Form (BCAT-SF). EBN: *In this study, the BCAT-SF demonstrated sensitivity in differentiating between dementia and nondementia (Mace, Mansbach, & Clark, 2016).*
▲ Assess community-dwelling older individuals with the Identification of Seniors at Risk (ISAR) screening tool when they present for treatment in the emergency department. EBN: *In this study, using the ISAR tool predicted adverse outcomes in elderly patients (Asomaning & Loftus, 2014).*
▲ Screen community-dwelling older individuals for fall risk with the Timed Up and Go Test (TUG) or the Functional Gait Assessment (FGA). EB: *A clinical review of research recommended the use of the TUG and FGA to identify fall risk in community-dwelling older individuals (Lee, Geller, & Strasser, 2013).*

 Multicultural

- Provide culturally and linguistically appropriate risk reduction programs to individuals living in rural and border regions of the country. EBN: *Culturally appropriate risk reduction programs will reduce sexual health disparities (Hernandez et al, 2014).*
- Use decision aids (DAs) (personal counseling, multimedia, and print materials) to facilitate communication between patients and health care providers to determine a plan for health care. EB: *A systematic review found 18 studies illustrating the effectiveness of DAs in improving patient–provider communication and decision quality outcomes in minority populations (Nathan et al, 2016).*

 Home Care and Client/Family Teaching and Discharge Planning

- The previously mentioned interventions may be adapted for home care and client/family teaching.

● = Independent;   ▲ = Collaborative;   EBN = Evidence-Based Nursing;   EB = Evidence-Based

REFERENCES

Asomaning, N., & Loftus, C. (2014). Identification of seniors at risk (ISAR) screening tool in the emergency department: Implementation using the plan-do-study-act model and validation results. *Journal of Emergency Nursing*, 40(4), 357–364. doi:10.1016/j.jen.2013.08.014.

Beck, A. F., Henize, A. W., Kahn, R. S., et al. (2014). Forging a pediatric primary care–community partnership to support food-insecure families. *Pediatrics*, 134(2), e564–e571. doi:10.1542/peds.2013-3845.

Bender, M. S., Clark, M. J., & Gahagan, S. (2014). Community engagement approach: Developing a culturally appropriate intervention for Hispanic mother–child dyads. *Journal of Transcultural Nursing*, 25(4), 373–382.

Chan, K. S., Roberts, E., McCleary, R., et al. (2014). Community characteristics and mortality: The relative strength of association of different community characteristics. *American Journal of Public Health*, 104(9), 1751–1758.

Cottler, L. B., McCloskey, D., Aguilar-Gaxiola, S., et al. (2013). Community needs, concerns, and perceptions about health research: Findings from the clinical and translational science award sentinel network. *American Journal of Public Health*, 103(9), 1685–1692.

Ette, L. (2017). Community-based exercise interventions during pregnancy are perceived as a satisfactory and motivating form of exercise engagement. *Evidence-Based Nursing*, 20, 77–78.

Hernandez, K., Mata, H., Provencio Vasquez, E., et al. (2014). Community outreach along the U.S./Mexico border: Developing HIV health education strategies to engage rural populations. *Online Journal of Rural Nursing & Health Care*, 14(1), 3–17.

Knighton, A. J., Payne, N. R., & Speedie, S. (2016). Lead testing in a pediatric population: Underscreening and problematic repeated tests. *Journal of Public Health Management and Practice*, 22(4), 331–337. doi:10.1097/PHH.0000000000000344.

Lamb, J., Dowrick, C., Burroughs, H., et al. (2015). Community Engagement in a complex intervention to improve access to primary mental health care for hard-to-reach groups. *Health Expectations: An International Journal of Public Participation in Health Care and Health Policy*, 18, 2865–2879. doi:10.1111/hex.12272.

Lee, J., Geller, A. I., Dale, C., et al. (2013). Analytical review: Focus on fall screening assessments. *Physical Medicine & Rehabilitation*, 5(7), 609–621. doi:10.1016/j.pmrj.2013.04.001.

Mace, R. A., Mansbach, W. E., & Clark, K. M. (2016). Rapid cognitive assessment of nursing home residents: A comparison of the Brief Interview for Mental Status (BIMS) and Brief Cognitive Assessment Tool-Short Form (BCAT-SF). *Research in Gerontological Nursing*, 9(1), 35–44. doi:10.3928/19404921-20150522-05.

Merkl, M. A., Tanabe, P., Sverha, J. P., et al. (2016). A quality improvement initiative for designing and implementing a military service screening tool for a community emergency department. *Journal of Emergency Nursing*, 42(5), 400–407. doi:10.1016/j.jen.2015.11.009.

Nathan, A. G., Marshall, I. M., Cooper, J. M., et al. (2016). Use of decision aids with minority patients: A systematic review. *Journal of General Internal Medicine*, 31, 663. doi:10.1007/s11606-016-3609-2.

Stowers, C., Healey, L., & O'Connor, C. C. (2014). Short message service broadcasting to improve the uptake of influenza vaccination in HIV-positive patients at a metropolitan sexual health clinic. *Sexual Health*, 11, 590–591. doi:10.1071/SH14162.

H

Risk-prone Health behavior   *Marina Martinez-Kratz, MS, RN, CNE*

NANDA-I

Definition

Impaired ability to modify lifestyle and/or actions in a manner that improves the level of wellness.

Defining Characteristics

Failure to achieve optimal sense of control; failure to take action that prevents health problem; minimizes health status change; nonacceptance of health status change; smoking; substance misuse

Related Factors

Inadequate comprehension; insufficient social support; low self-efficacy; negative perception of health care provider; negative perception of recommended health care strategy; social anxiety; stressors

At-Risk Population

Family history of alcoholism; economically disadvantaged

NOC   (Nursing Outcomes Classification)

Suggested NOC Outcomes

Participation in Health Care Decisions; Psychosocial Adjustment: Life Change; Risk Detection

● = Independent;   ▲ = Collaborative;   EBN = Evidence-Based Nursing;   EB = Evidence-Based

> ### Example NOC Outcome with Indicators
>
> **Risk Detection** as evidenced by the following indicators: Recognizes signs and symptoms that indicate risks/Identifies potential health risks/Participates in screening at recommended intervals/Obtains information about changes in health recommendations. (Rate the outcome and indicators of **Risk Detection:** 1 = never demonstrated, 2 = rarely demonstrated, 3 = sometimes demonstrated, 4 = often demonstrated, 5 = consistently demonstrated [see Section I].)

Client Outcomes

Client Will (Specify Time Frame)

- State acceptance of change in health status
- Request assistance in altering behaviors to adapt to change
- State personal goals for dealing with change in health status and means to prevent further health problems
- State experience of a period of grief that is proportional to the actual or perceived effect of the loss
- Report and/or demonstrate behavior changes mutually agreed upon with nurse as evidence of positive adaptation

NIC (Nursing Interventions Classification)

Suggested NIC Intervention

Self-Efficacy Enhancement

> ### Example NIC Activities—Self-Efficacy Enhancement
>
> Explore individual's perception of his or her capability to perform the desired behavior; Reinforce confidence in making behavior changes and taking action

Nursing Interventions and *Rationales*

- Assess the client's perceptions of health, wellness, disability, and major barriers to health and wellness. EB: *Understanding the differences in perceptions can direct how a provider talks to clients about their health, but it could also provide insight into how clients value and perceive their own disability and wellness (Morris et al, 2018).*
- Use motivational interviewing to help the client identify and change unhealthy behaviors. EBN: *In these studies, motivational interviewing helped clients identify and examine their high-risk health behaviors (Wong & Cheng, 2013).*
- Encourage mindfulness and meditation to help the client cope with changes in health status. EBN: *Mindfulness and meditation can reduce stress, leading to increased quality of life and self-efficacy (Robins et al, 2014).*
- Allow the client adequate time to express feelings about the change in health status. EB: *A longitudinal study of clients with newly diagnosed diabetes found that there was a perception of time pressure, and considerable time was spent with patients by health professionals repeating information that may not be relevant to patient need (Dowell et al, 2018).*
- Use open-ended questions to allow the client free expression (e.g., "Tell me about your last hospitalization" or "How does this time compare?"). CEB: *Using open-ended questions generates more objective responses with less bias, leading to a more genuine qualitative understanding (Alemi & Harry, 2014).*
- Help the client work through the stages of grief that occur as part of a psychological adaptation to illness or life change. Assess for signs of nonacceptance to illness or change. CEB: *Clients who exhibit nonacceptance are at higher risk for stronger, delayed grief reactions. Identifying these clients and making appropriate referrals for counseling and support groups may prevent future adverse outcomes (Holland et al, 2013).*
- Assess the client for depression and refer for counseling or medical follow-up, as appropriate. CEB: *Depression is often a response to and a comorbid condition of chronic disease. Depression is associated with poorer client outcomes and higher risk behavior (Di Benedetto et al, 2014).*
- Discuss the client's current goals and assist in modification as needed. Use a goal attainment scaling (GAS) approach, which is a therapeutic method that refers to the development of a written follow-up guide between the client and the nurse and is used for monitoring client progress. EB: *A study of clients enrolled*

• = Independent;   ▲ = Collaborative;   EBN = Evidence-Based Nursing;   EB = Evidence-Based

in a geriatric day hospital (GDH) demonstrated short- and long-term effectiveness of GDHs in helping patients achieve individualized outcome measures using GAS (Moorhous et al, 2017).

▲ Encourage participation in appropriate wellness programs associated with health changes. EBN: *Studies of clients with multiple sclerosis and chronic obstructive pulmonary disease found that wellness programs facilitating positive health choices and self-management demonstrated gains in functional status and decreased anxiety and depression (Simpson & Jones, 2013).*

● Give the client positive feedback for accomplishments, no matter how small. Support the client and family and promote their strengths and coping skills. EB: *Support is necessary to help the client and family throughout the illness. Support leads to hopefulness and is associated with improved outcomes (Soundy et al, 2014).*

▲ Promote use of positive spiritual influences, as appropriate. EBN: *Faith- and spiritual-based resources may promote an atmosphere of forgiveness and stress personal resilience. These resources may also provide a sense of community and belonging and provide an additional support network (Brewer-Smith & Koenig, 2014).*

▲ Refer to community resources. Provide general and contact information for ease of use. EBN: *A study of oncology navigators identified that common barriers for clients obtaining assistance included lack of resources (50%), lack of knowledge about resources (46%), and complex/duplicative paperwork (20%) (Spencer et al, 2018).*

 Pediatric

● Include social history in client assessment to help identify past abuse and traumatic experiences. EBN: *A systematic review found that only 28% of abuse or neglect cases identified by researchers are found in clients' files. This information is considered essential for developing comprehensive formulations and effective treatment plans (Read et al, 2018).*

● Encourage parents to process and express grief, uncertainty, and discouragement after learning about their child's diagnosis, prognosis, and treatments. Provide parents with resources and tools to help further their understanding of the illness. EB: *A study assessed the effectiveness of an intervention called the Nurturing Program for Parents and Their Children with Special Needs and Health Challenges (SNHC) and found that after the intervention families showed an increase in empathy toward their children's needs and an increase in empowerment as measured by the family empowerment scale (Burton et al, 2018).*

  ○ Provide parents of critically ill children with individualized coping resources. EBN: *Research findings indicated that a range of diverse coping strategies are used by neonatal intensive care unit parents. The most common are acceptance emotional support, active coping, positive reframing, religion, planning, and instrumental support. Despite this, 91% of participants indicated they would likely attend at least one type of parent support program, if offered according to their preferences (Huenink & Porterfield, 2017).*

● Use distraction with children undergoing procedures or treatment with unpleasant side effects. EB: *This review found that there was strong support for the use of distraction techniques with older children (Ali, McGrath, & Drendel, 2016).*

 Geriatric

▲ Assess for signs of depression resulting from illness-associated changes and make appropriate referrals. EB: *A review of evidence related to depression in older individuals found major depressive disorder (MDD) is less common in late life, but has a more chronic course compared with younger adults with MDD. A significant finding was that older adults with subclinical forms of depression report functional impairment similar to MDD (Haigh et al, 2018).*

● Support activities that promote a sense of purpose for older adults. CEB: *Purpose in life (PIL) is strongly associated with improved mental and physical health outcomes among older adults. Thus interventions to improve and/or maintain higher levels of PIL over time may promote successful aging (Musich et al, 2018).*

  ○ Encourage social support. EB: *In this study, social support was a prerequisite for success of the health-promoting intervention and perceived well-being in older adults (von Berens et al, 2018).*

 Multicultural

● Assess for the influence of cultural beliefs, norms, and values on the client's ability to modify health behavior. CEB: *What the client considers normal and abnormal health behavior may be based on cultural perceptions (Leininger & McFarland, 2002).*

● Assess the role of fatalism on the client's ability to modify health behavior. Fatalistic perspectives, which involve the belief that you cannot control your own fate, may influence health behaviors in some cultures.

● = Independent; ▲ = Collaborative; EBN = Evidence-Based Nursing; EB = Evidence-Based

H

EB: *A study found that patients with type 2 diabetes who exhibited more fatalistic attitudes were younger, of lower education levels, had higher body mass index (BMI), and had fewer diabetes comorbidities. It is crucial for health care practitioners to identify fatalistic patients and to tailor culturally appropriate strategies in diabetes management (Sukkarieh-Haraty et al, 2018).*

- Encourage spirituality as a source of support for coping. **EBN:** *Findings from a study provided data to support an understanding of how African American women define spirituality, the role it plays, the purpose it serves, the function of spirituality in their lives, and the implications for breast health behaviors (Conway-Phillips & Janusek, 2018).*
- Negotiate with the client regarding the aspects of health behavior that will need to be modified. **CEB:** *Give-and-take with the client will lead to culturally congruent care (Leininger & McFarland, 2002).*
- Acknowledge client's identified gender and sexual orientation and refer client and family members to support networks that have experience with lesbian, gay, bisexual, or transgender (LGBT) issues, as appropriate. **EBN:** *Disclosure and support systems are associated with better self-help perception; creating safe and accepting environments for LGBT patients has been shown to improve overall care in this underserved population (Kamen et al, 2015).*

Home Care

- The previously mentioned interventions may be adapted for home care use.
- Take the client's perspective into consideration and use a holistic approach in assessing and responding to client planning for the future. **EB:** *A recent qualitative study described the experience of the client with both type 1 diabetes and an eating disorder and that of their health care providers. Results demonstrated the need for interprofessional, collaborative approaches to treatment (Macdonald et al, 2018).*
- Assist the client/family to adapt to his or her diagnosis and to live with their disease. **EBN:** *Research suggested time-sensitive interventions directed toward education and psychosocial support for all patients and families dealing with a new diagnosis of chronic illnesses are needed (Gunter & Duke, 2018).*
- Ensure that evaluations of the client's ability to perform activities of daily living are age appropriate and consider existing, as well as new, diagnoses. **EB:** *This study used a geriatric-designed functional evaluation that took into account the age-related decrease in flexibility and strength by identifying additional areas for potential loss of function (Adamo, Talley, & Goldberg, 2015).*
- Refer to care plan for **Powerlessness.**

Client/Family Teaching and Discharge Planning

- Assess family/caregivers for coping and teaching/learning styles. **EBN:** *Recommendations for teaching family or caregivers include providing realistic expectations and nurturing psychological safety so caregivers feel comfortable asking questions, expressing their thoughts, and discussing mistakes (Lindauer, Sexson, & Harvath, 2017).*
- Foster communication between the client/family and medical staff. **EBN:** *A study of caregiver communication indicated that oncology nurses must be able to address questions posed by family caregivers and support family communication challenges (Wittenberg et al, 2017).*
- Educate and prepare families regarding the appearance and function of the client and the environment before initial exposure. **EBN:** *A study of mother-caregivers found that health care providers can help anchor family management by recognizing caregiver expectations and facilitating communication about realistic expectations (Barakat et al, 2016).*
- Teach a client and his or her family relaxation techniques (controlled breathing, guided imagery) and help them practice. **EBN:** *Guided imagery with relaxation may be an easy-to-use self-management intervention to improve the quality of life of older adults with osteoarthritis (Helgadottir & Wilson, 2014).*
- Allow the client to proceed at his or her own pace in learning; provide time for return demonstrations (e.g., self-injection of insulin). Tailor teaching and learning materials as appropriate for client and caregiver literacy level. **EBN:** *Use clear and distinct language free of medical jargon and meaningless values. Be sensitive to education levels and cultural environments that may hinder effective communication (Protheroe & Rowlands, 2013).*

● = Independent; ▲ = Collaborative; **EBN** = Evidence-Based Nursing; **EB** = Evidence-Based

REFERENCES

Adamo, D., Talley, S., & Goldberg, A. (2015). Age and task differences in functional fitness in older women: Comparisons with senior fitness test normative and criterion-referenced data. *Journal of Aging and Physical Activity, 23*(1), 47–54.

Alemi, F., & Harry, J. (2014). An alternative to satisfaction surveys: Let the patients talk. *Quality Management in Healthcare, 23*(1), 10–19.

Ali, S., McGrath, T., & Drendel, A. (2016). An evidence-based approach to minimizing acute procedural pain in the emergency department and beyond. *Pediatric Emergency Care, 32*(1), 36–42. doi:10.1097/PEC.0000000000000669.

Barakat, L. P., et al. (2016). Mother-caregiver expectations for function among survivors of childhood brain tumors. *Supportive Care in Cancer, 24*(5), 2147–2154. doi:10.1007/s00520-015-3013-1.

Brewer-Smith, K., & Koenig, H. (2014). Could spirituality and religion promote stress resilience in survivors of childhood trauma? *Issues in Mental Health Nursing, 35*(4), 251–256.

Burton, R. S., et al. (2018). The nurturing program: An intervention for parents of children with special needs. *Journal of Child and Family Studies, 27*(4), 1137–1149. doi:10.1007/s10826-017-0966-3.

Conway-Phillips, R., & Janusek, L. W. (2018). Exploring spirituality among African American women: Implications for promoting breast health behaviors. *Holistic Nursing Practice, 30*(6), 322–329. doi:10.1097/HNP.0000000000000173.

Di Benedetto, M., Lindner, H., Aucote, H., et al. (2014). Co-morbid depression and chronic illness related to coping and physical and mental health status. *Psychology, Health & Medicine, 13*(3), 253–262.

Dowell, A., et al. (2018). A longitudinal study of interactions between health professionals and people with newly diagnosed diabetes. *Annals of Family Medicine, 16*(1), 37–44. doi:10.1370/afm.2144.

Gunter, D. M., & Duke, G. (2018). Reducing uncertainty in families dealing with childhood cancers: An integrative literature review. *Pediatric Nursing, 44*(1), 21–37.

Haigh, E. A. P., et al. (2018). Depression among older adults: A 20-year update on five common myths and misconceptions. *The American Journal of Geriatric Psychiatry, 26*(1), 107–122.

Helgadottir, H., & Wilson, M. (2014). A randomized controlled trial of the effectiveness of educating parents about distraction to decrease postoperative pain in children at home after tonsillectomy. *Pain Management Nursing, 15*(3), 632–640.

Holland, J., Futterman, A., Thompson, L., et al. (2013). Difficulties accepting the loss of a spouse: A precursor for intensified grieving among widowed older adults. *Death Studies, 37*(2), 126–144.

Huenink, E., & Porterfield, S. (2017). Parent support programs and coping mechanisms in NICU parents. *Advances in Neonatal Care, 17*(2), E10–E18. doi:10.1097/ANC.0000000000000359.

Kamen, C., Smith-Stoner, M., Heckler, C., et al. (2015). Social support, self-rated health, and lesbian, gay, bisexual, and transgender identity disclosure to cancer care providers. *Oncology Nursing Forum, 42*(1), 44–51.

Leininger, M., & McFarland, M. (2002). *Transcultural nursing: Concepts, theories, research and practices* (3rd ed.). New York: McGraw-Hill.

Lindauer, A., Sexson, K., & Harvath, T. A. (2017). Teaching caregivers to administer eye drops, transdermal patches, and suppositories. *American Journal of Nursing, 117*(5 Suppl. 1), S11–S16. doi:10.1097/01.NAJ.0000516388.97515.ca.

Macdonald, P., et al. (2018). Eating disorders in people with type 1 diabetes: Experiential perspectives of both clients and healthcare professionals. *Diabetic Medicine, 35*(2), 223–231. doi:10.1111/dme.13555.

Moorhous, P., et al. (2017). Treatment in a geriatric day hospital improve individualized outcome measures using goal attainment scaling. *BMC Geriatrics, 17*(9), 1–7. doi:10.1186/s12877-016-0397-9.

Morris, M. A., et al. (2018). How do patients describe their disabilities? A coding system for categorizing patients' descriptions. *Disability and Health Journal, 11*(2), 310–314. doi:10.1016/j.dhjo.2017.10.006.

Musich, S., et al. (2018). Purpose in life and positive health outcomes among older adults. *Population Health Management, 21*(2), 139–147. doi:10.1089/pop.2017.0063.

Protheroe, J., & Rowlands, G. (2013). Matching clinical information with levels of patient health literacy. *Nursing Management, 20*(3), 20–21.

Read, J., et al. (2018). Do adult mental health services identify child abuse and neglect? A systematic review. *International Journal of Mental Health Nursing, 27*(1), 7–19. doi:10.1111/inm.12369.

Robins, J., Kiken, L., Holt, M., et al. (2014). Mindfulness: An effective coaching tool for improving physical and mental health. *Journal of the American Association of Nurse Practitioners, 26*, 511–518.

Simpson, E., & Jones, M. (2013). An exploration of self-efficacy and self-management in COPD patients. *British Journal of Nursing, 22*(19), 1105–1109.

Soundy, A., Liles, C., Stubbs, B., et al. (2014). Identifying a framework for hope in order to establish the importance of generalised hopes for individuals who have suffered a stroke. *Advances in Medicine*, Article ID 471874. 8 pages.

Spencer, J. C., et al. (2018). Oncology navigators' perceptions of cancer-related financial burden and financial assistance resources. *Supportive Care in Cancer, 26*(4), 1315–1321. doi:10.1007/s00520-017-3958-3.

Sukkarieh-Haraty, O., et al. (2018). Predictors of diabetes fatalism among Arabs: A cross-sectional study of Lebanese adults with type 2 diabetes. *Journal of Religion and Health, 57*(3), 858–868. doi:10.1007/s10943-017-0430-0.

von Berens, A., et al. (2018). "Feeling more self-confident, cheerful and safe." Experiences from a health-promoting intervention in community dwelling older adults—A qualitative study. *The Journal of Nutrition, Health & Aging, 22*(4), 541–548.

Wittenberg, E., et al. (2017). Understanding family caregiver communication to provide family-centered cancer care. *Seminars in Oncology Nursing, 33*(5), 507–516. doi:10.1016/j.soncn.2017.09.001.

Wong, E., & Cheng, M. (2013). Effects of motivational interviewing to promote weight loss in obese children. *Journal of Clinical Nursing, 22*, 2519–2530.

● = Independent; ▲ = Collaborative; **EBN** = Evidence-Based Nursing; **EB** = Evidence-Based

Ineffective Health management   *Ruth A. Wittmann-Price, PhD, RN, CNS, CNE, CHSE, ANEF, FAAN*

NANDA-I

Definition

Pattern of regulating and integrating into daily living a therapeutic regimen for the treatment of illness and its sequelae that is unsatisfactory for meeting specific health goals.

Defining Characteristics

Difficulty with prescribed regimen; failure to include treatment regimen in daily living; failure to take action to reduce risk factor; ineffective choices in daily living for meeting health goal

Related Factors

Decisional conflict; difficulty managing complex treatment regimen; difficulty navigating complex health care systems; excessive demands; family conflict; family pattern of health care; inadequate number of cues to action; insufficient knowledge of therapeutic regimen; insufficient social support; perceived barrier; perceived benefit; perceived seriousness of condition; perceived susceptibility; powerlessness

At-Risk Population

Economically disadvantaged

NOC   (Nursing Outcomes Classification)

Suggested NOC Outcomes

Health Beliefs: Perceived Control, Perceived Threat; Knowledge: Disease Process; Knowledge: Treatment Regimen; Participation in Health Care Decisions

> **Example NOC Outcome with Indicators**
>
> **Knowledge: Treatment Regimen** as evidenced by the following indicators: Extent of understanding of prescribed medication, activity, exercise, and specific disease process. (Rate the outcome and indicators of **Knowledge: Treatment Regimen:** 1 = no knowledge, 2 = limited knowledge, 3 = moderate knowledge, 4 = substantial knowledge, 5 = extensive knowledge [see Section I].)

Client Outcomes

Client Will (Specify Time Frame)

- Describe daily food and fluid intake that meets therapeutic goals
- Describe activity/exercise patterns that meet therapeutic goals
- Describe scheduling of medications that meets therapeutic goals
- Verbalize ability to manage therapeutic regimens
- Collaborate with health professionals to decide on a therapeutic regimen that is congruent with health goals and lifestyle

NIC   (Nursing Interventions Classification)

Suggested NIC Interventions

Adherence Behavior; Health Education; Health System Guidance; Learning Facilitation; Learning Readiness Enhancement; Teaching: Prescribed Diet, Prescribed Exercise, Prescribed Medication

> **Example NIC Activities—Learning Facilitation**
>
> Present the information in a stimulating manner; Encourage the client's active participation

Nursing Interventions and *Rationales*

Note: This diagnosis does not have the same meaning as the diagnosis **Noncompliance.** This diagnosis is made with the client, so if the client does not agree with the diagnosis, it should not be made. The emphasis

● = Independent;   ▲ = Collaborative;   EBN = Evidence-Based Nursing;   EB = Evidence-Based

is on helping the client direct his or her own life and health, not on the client's compliance with the provider's instructions.

- Establish a collaborative partnership with the client for purposes of meeting health-related goals. **EBN:** *Nurse researchers explored ways that nurses and patients can better understand postoperative pain management needs, and the results of a qualitative study revealed the following helpful interventions: (1) communication and knowledge and the patients' ability to communicate, (2) pain assessment using a numerical rating scale, and (3) patient–nurse relationship consisting of frequent and direct contact (Kaptain, Bregnballe, & Dreyer, 2017).* **EBN:** *Bennett (2017) studied patients who experienced a stroke and nurses' roles in the rehabilitation process using an ethnographic approach with 10 cases. Data revealed that the relationships built and sustained between nurses and patients were important in demonstrating caring, which in turn promoted emotional well-being and assisted stroke recovery.*

- Explore the client's perception of their illness experience and identify uncertainties and needs through open-ended questions. **EBN:** *A research team qualitatively explored perceptions and preferences of older adults (N = 13) and their family members about a fall risk assessment system when aging in place and to develop better technology to promote safety. Results demonstrated an acceptance of the technology after participants adapted, and acceptance was a process that grew in stages as the patient became used to technology (Galambos et al, 2017).* **EB:** *Lee and Chen (2017) studied perceptions about smoking after distributing a humorous antitobacco video on health-related social medial. After viewing the video respondents reported a higher level of risk perception of smoking, less positive attitude toward smokers, and a higher level of intention to avoid smoking in the future than others who viewed it on non–health-related social media sites.*

- Assist the client to enhance self-efficacy or confidence in his or her own ability to manage the illness. **EBN:** *Banman and Sawatzky (2017) completed a literature review on cardiovascular disease prevention and uncovered several reasons women are not as active as men in preventative health management: (1) lower self-efficacy beliefs, (2) lack of social support and confidence in their ability to care for themselves, and (3) any findings of depression negatively correlated with women's self-efficacy beliefs related to health behavior.* **EBN:** *Yu-Jie (2017) explored self-efficacy assessment instruments for patients with chronic kidney disease (CKD). Instruments were studied for reliability and validity, and the implication for nursing is the importance of approximately assessing self-efficacy in CKD patients to properly implement health management strategies. Involve family members in knowledge development, planning for self-management, and shared decision-making (SDM).* **EBN:** *Researchers studied the effects of an educational program developed for heart failure patients and their families (N = 100). They compared the results with patients who received the traditional education and found that the patients and families had better self-care maintenance, confidence, and quality of life (QoL) scores (Srisuk et al, 2017).* **EB:** *Adams and Levy (2017) explored the collaboration established by using SDM with children with disabilities and family and found that it promotes discussion of treatment plans, identifying gaps between the values of the child and the family, priorities, and better understanding of patient and family choices.*

- Review factors of the health belief model (HBM) (individual perceptions of seriousness and susceptibility, demographic and other modifying factors, and perceived benefits and barriers) with the client. **EB:** *Vandyke and Shell (2017) explored the role of the HBM in predicting breast cancer screening among women (N = 170) in rural Appalachia and found women perceived mammography more important if they viewed themselves at risk and though the mammogram was easy to obtain. This is consistent with the HBM, but the frequency of obtaining a mammography did not support the HBM.* **EB:** *Researchers studied the variables for nonadherence to immunosuppressive medication of kidney transplant patients (N = 120) based on the HBM. The results were consistent with the HBM because perceived susceptibility to rejection and perceived benefits were variables that predicted better adherence rates (Pen-Chen et al, 2017).*

- Help the client identify and modify barriers to effective self-management. **EB:** *Researchers examined patients (N = 14) with type 2 diabetes and severe mental illness because this group of patients experiences significantly poorer health outcomes than type 2 diabetic patients without diabetes. Participants were aware of the risks and stated that family and health care provider support was important in their self-maintenance (Mulligan et al, 2017).* **EB:** *Bovenkamp and Dwarswaard (2017) performed a qualitative study to gain insight into patients' self-maintenance or self-management practices and found after intervening with patients (N = 20) with chronic conditions that the practice is dependent on personal and social dynamics, patients' ideas of the good life, and their interactions with care professionals.*

- Help the client self-manage his or her own health through education about strategies for changing habits such as overeating, sedentary lifestyle, and smoking. **EB:** *Pappa (2017) investigated the activity behavior and analyzed the message content participants (N = 107,886) in LoseIt (r/loseit), an online weight management*

● = Independent;   ▲ = Collaborative;   **EBN** = Evidence-Based Nursing;   **EB** = Evidence-Based

community of the online social network Reddit, over 30 days and found that the most discussed topics were healthy food, clothing, calorie counting, workouts, looks, habits, support, and unhealthy food. EB: Cruz et al (2017) performed a prospective, cross-sectional, and correlational study with teenagers (N = 150), aged 15 to 17, to determine whether weight, age, and gender have an influence on physical fitness and found that the participants who had normal weight had regular physical fitness and women had more obesity than men.

- Develop a contract with the client to maintain motivation for changes in behavior. *EB: Researchers adapted an existing interprofessional asthma program to fit a smaller practice to promote asthma management and provided a weekly asthma-management clinical for pediatric patients and their families. The results included a 69% and 92% reduction in emergency department (ED)/urgent care visits and hospitalizations, indicating that consistent intervention motivated behavioral changes to improve health (Kwong et al, 2017). EBN: Leine et al (2017) studied patients (N = 6) with chronic obstructive pulmonary disease (COPD) and their understanding and treatment adherence using a partnership-based nursing practice program. Interviews revealed two themes: feeling safe and comforted, and motivation to take better care of themselves.*

- Use focus groups to evaluate the implementation of self-management programs. *EB: Serwe et al (2017) used focus groups (N = 4) to study caregivers' implementation of a telehealth self-maintenance program; the themes suggested that it promoted relationships, promoted positive interactions, and better explained the role.*

- Refer to the care plan Ineffective Family **Health** management.

Geriatric

- Identify the reasons for behaviors that are not therapeutic and discuss alternatives. *EBN: Lee et al (2017) used the Theory of Planned Behavior with older adults to affect diabetes maintenance and found that older adults need adequate social support to sustain diabetes self-management practices. EB: Akmatov et al (2017) studied why patients do not participate in health initiatives. They surveyed participants between 65 and 80 years of age (N = 5582) and found that nonparticipation was associated with a low interest, a preference for less invasive information, and lack of time.*

Multicultural

- Assess the influence of cultural beliefs, norms, and values on the individual's perceptions of the therapeutic regimen. *EBN: Mou (2017) explored traditional Chinese medicine (TCM) as a method for promoting health and found through an online survey in China with 800 responses that cultural orientation and spirituality predicted use of TCM to promote health. EB: Doede et al (2017) studied the increase of noncommunicable diseases (NCDs) in South Africa, and qualitative interviews revealed common themes including resource scarcity, clinic–patient partnerships, management of NCDs, and collaboration between professionals. Discuss all strategies with the client in the context of the client's culture. EB: Bach et al (2017) investigated access to health care for Vietnamese patients (N = 1003) who are on methadone maintenance treatment (MMT) and found that nearly 80% were not currently enrolled in health insurance, participants from rural regions were significantly more likely than urban participants to report poor care access, and 37% of participants reported a lack of information about health insurance and health care options.*

- Provide health information that is consistent with the health literacy of clients. *EB: Sainato et al (2017) studied US adolescents with chronic conditions and found that this high-risk group was twice as likely not to receive routine vaccinations, indicating additional education is needed in families with adolescents 16 to 18 years old with chronic illnesses. EB: Researchers used qualitative methods to study how individuals (N = 26) experienced accessing, understanding, appraising, and applying health information and identified four themes from interviews: using health literacy capacities, psychological and structural factors that affect these capacities, and the relationship quality with the health care providers (McKenna, Sixsmith, & Barry, 2017).*

- Assess for barriers that may interfere with client follow-up of treatment recommendations. *EB: Jena et al (2017) studied the effect of eliminating cost sharing for screening mammography on rates for 53,188 women with individual health insurance compared with those with employer-based health insurance. Findings demonstrated that there was a decline for both groups, indicating that other factors are present that deter health management.*

- Use electronic monitoring and dosing to improve management of medications. *EB: Rogers et al (2017) developed a system and studied individual discharge medication lists for 3 months in an automated medication system to assess errors that effected patients after discharge from the hospital. The most common error was lack of indication for medications; thus the patients did not know why to take them. The system developed reduced errors from 74% to 26%. EBN: Riley and Kruger (2017) examined the use of inhalers in patients with COPD and found that it is imperative to assess and teach patients about using a correct inhalation*

- = Independent; ▲ = Collaborative; EBN = Evidence-Based Nursing; EB = Evidence-Based

technique, assessing adequate dexterity to use the prescribed inhaler, if there is sufficient inspiratory flow rate to achieve adequate lung deposition, and if the inhaler is used by the patient at all.

- Validate the client's feelings regarding the ability to manage his or her own care and the impact on lifestyle. **EBN:** *Lee et al (2017) qualitatively studied patients' perceptions of brisk walking as a method to reduce chronic disease symptomology in the community. Six focus groups were conducted (N = 48) ages 48 to 81, and five themes were identified: (1) health promotion and maintenance, (2) relationship building and social interactions, (3) leaders' enthusiasm and peer pressure, (4) the nature of brisk walking, and (5) becoming part of one's daily life.*

Home Care

- Prepare and instruct clients and family members in the use of a medication box. Set up an appropriate schedule for filling the medication box, and post medication times and doses in an accessible area (e.g., attached by a magnet to the refrigerator). **EBN:** *Milner and Bonaventura (2017) used self-management for patients on anticoagulants at home and it increased patient engagement in anticoagulant management, which resulted in better clinical outcomes.* **EB:** *Flood, Hawkins, and Rohloff (2017) studied diabetes self-management education (DSME) as a home-based intervention in a rural setting with 90 participants implementing six home visits, and hemoglobin (Hb)A1C decreased and systolic blood pressure improved significantly. Monitor self-management of the medical regimen.* **EB:** *Shor et al (2017) studied 1-year medication therapy adherence rates among patients with fibromyalgia (FM) and found that in over 3000 patients 60% did not adhere to their medication regimen, warranting further investigation of intervening factors.*
- Refer to health care professionals for questions and self-care management. **EB:** *Homsted, Magee, and Nesin (2017) studied the use of a comprehensive, medical-home approach to controlling patients' (N = 1300) use of controlled substances. By using a program researchers decreased the use of controlled substances by 67.2% and 65.6%, with fewer patients receiving benzodiazepines.* **EB:** *Researchers studied the effects of a chronic disease self-management program on empowering hemodialysis patients (N = 53) and their QoL. Self-management increased the patients' QoL in 3 months (Ahmadzadeh et al, 2017).*

Client/Family Teaching and Discharge Planning

- Identify the client and/or family's current knowledge and adjust teaching accordingly. Teach the client and family about all aspects of the therapeutic regimen, providing as much knowledge as the client and family will accept, in a culturally congruent manner. **EBN:** *Sugiharto et al (2017) studied the patient outcome of improving nurses' skills and confidence in delivering DSME among type 2 diabetes patients and found that the diabetes training program for community health center nurses increased their skills and confidence in delivering DSME to patients.*
- Teach ways to adjust activities of daily living (ADLs) for inclusion in therapeutic regimens. **EBN:** *Jansons et al (2017) completed a randomized, controlled trial of patients with chronic conditions using a gym-based exercise program for health management and found improved health outcomes in the group that exercised when compared with the control group.* **EBN:** *Nestler et al (2017) performed a literature review (N = 12) related to women's muscle strength and work health issues and found weight training reduced patina and improved outcomes for women working in strenuous and nonstrenuous environments.*
- Teach safety in taking medications. **EB:** *Jones et al (2017) performed a 16-year longitudinal study of patients who were having chronic diseases and had their medication regimen followed and regulated by a specifically designed program. The results show decreased ED use and hospitalization by 18% compared with patients who were not in the program. Teach the client to act as a self-advocate with health providers who prescribe therapeutic regimens.* **EBN:** *Suijn and Hubert (2017) studied three groups with different levels of technology knowledge about accessing personal health information management (PHIM) by online survey and found that advanced PHIM users were significantly more likely to engage in emailing with providers, viewing test results online, and receiving summaries of hospital visits indicating that technology knowledge is important for self-advocating.*

REFERENCES

Adams, R. C., & Levy, S. E. (2017). Shared decision-making and children with disabilities: Pathways to consensus. *Pediatrics, 139*(6), 1–9. doi:10.1542/peds.2017-0956.

Ahmadzadeh, S., Matlabi, H., Allahverdipor, H., et al. (2017). The effectiveness of self-management program on quality of life among

haemodialysis patients. *Progress in Palliative Care, 25*(4), 177–184. doi:10.1080/09699260.2017.1345407.

Akmatov, M. K., Jentsch, L., Riese, P., et al. (2017). Motivations for (non)participation in population-based health studies among the elderly—Comparison of participants and nonparticipants of a

● = Independent;   ▲ = Collaborative;   **EBN** = Evidence-Based Nursing;   **EB** = Evidence-Based

prospective study on influenza vaccination. *BMC Medical Research Methodology, 17,* 1–9. doi:10.1186/s12874-017-0302-z.

Bach, X. T., Boggiano, V., Cuong, T. N., et al. (2017). Barriers to accessing and using health insurance cards among methadone maintenance treatment patients in northern Vietnam. *Substance Abuse Treatment, Prevention & Policy, 12,* 1–9. doi:10.1186/s13011-017-0119-0.

Banman, L., & Sawatzky, J. V. (2017). The role of self-efficacy in cardiovascular disease prevention in women. *Canadian Journal of Cardiovascular Nursing, 27*(3), 11–19. MEDLINE Info: NLM UID: 8913645.

Bennett, B. (2017). A culture of caring: How nurses promote emotional wellbeing and aid recovery following a stroke. *British Journal of Neuroscience Nursing,* S8–S17. ISSN: 1747-0307.

Bovenkamp, H. M., & Dwarswaard, J. (2017). The complexity of shaping self-management in daily practice. *Health Expectations, 20*(5), 952–960. doi:10.1111/hex.12536.

Cruz, E., Tlatempa, F. M., Valdes-Ramos, S. P., et al. (2017). Overweight or obesity, gender, and age influence on high school students of the city of Toluca's physical fitness. *BioMed Research International,* 1–11. doi:10.1155/2017/9546738.

Doede, A. L., Allen, T. E., Gray, J. S., et al. (2017). Community health workers and the management of noncommunicable diseases among rural health clinics in Limpopo Province, South Africa: A pilot study. *Family & Community Health, 40*(4), 338–346. doi:10.1097/FCH.0000000000000158.

Flood, D., Hawkins, J., & Rohloff, P. (2017). A home-based type 2 diabetes self-management intervention in rural Guatemala. *Preventing Chronic Disease, 14,* 1–9. doi:10.5888/pcd14.170052.

Galambos, C., Rantz, M., Back, J., et al. (2017). Older adults' perceptions of and preferences for a fall risk assessment system: Exploring stages of acceptance model. *CIN: Computers, Informatics, Nursing, 35*(7), 331–337. doi:10.1097/CIN.0000000000000330.

Homsted, F. A. E., Magee, C. E., & Nesin, N. (2017). Population health management in a small health system: Impact of controlled substance stewardship in a patient-centered medical home. *American Journal of Health-System Pharmacy, 74*(18), 1468–1475. doi:10.2146/ajhp161032.

Jansons, P., Robins, L., O'Brien, L., et al. (2017). Gym-based exercise and home-based exercise with telephone support have similar outcomes when used as maintenance programs in adults with chronic health conditions: A randomised trial. *Journal of Physiotherapy, 63*(3), 154–160. doi:10.1016/j.jphys.2017.05.018.

Jena, A. B., Huang, J., Fireman, B., et al. (2017). Screening mammography for free: Impact of eliminating cost sharing on cancer screening rates. *Health Services Research, 52*(1), 191–206. doi:10.1111/1475-6773.12486.

Jones, L. K., Greskovic, G., Grassi, D. M., et al. (2017). Medication therapy disease management: Geisinger's approach to population health management. *American Journal of Health-System Pharmacy, 74*(18), 1422–1435. doi:10.2146/ajhp161061.

Kaptain, K., Bregnballe, V., & Dreyer, P. (2017). Patient participation in postoperative pain assessment after spine surgery in a recovery unit. *Journal of Clinical Nursing, 26*(19/20), 2986–2994. doi:10.1111/jocn.13640.

Kwong, K. Y., Redjal, N., Scott, L., et al. (2017). Adaptation of an asthma management program to a small clinic. *American Journal of Managed Care, 23*(7), e231–e237. MEDLINE Info: NLM UID: 9613960.

Lee, L. T., Bowen, P. G., Mosley, M. K., et al. (2017). Theory of Planned Behavior: Social support and diabetes self-management. *Journal for Nurse Practitioners, 13*(4), 265–270. doi:10.1016/j.nurpra.2016.07.013.

Lee, M., & Chen, F. (2017). Circulating humorous antitobacco videos on social media. *Health Promotion Practice, 18*(2), 184–192. doi:10.1177/1524839916677521.

Lee, P., Chuang, Y., Chen, S., et al. (2017). Perspectives of brisk walking among middle-aged and older persons in community: A qualitative study. *Collegian (Royal College of Nursing, Australia), 24*(2), 147–153. doi:10.1016/j.colegn.2015.11.001.

Leine, M., Wahl, A. K., Borge, C. R., et al. (2017). Feeling safe and motivated to achieve better health: Experiences with a partnership-based nursing practice programme for in-home patients with chronic obstructive pulmonary disease. *Journal of Clinical Nursing, 26*(17/18), 2755–2764. doi:10.1111/jocn.13794.

McKenna, V. B., Sixsmith, J., & Barry, M. M. (2017). The relevance of context in understanding health literacy skills: Findings from a qualitative study. *Health Expectations, 20*(5), 1049–1060. doi:10.1111/hex.12547.

Milner, K. A., & Bonaventura, K. R. (2017). Self-management of warfarin: An approach to increase patient engagement in care. *Journal for Nurse Practitioners, 13*(8), e389–e393. doi:10.1016/j.nurpra.2017.06.016.

Mou, Y. (2017). Predicting the use of traditional Chinese medicine health maintenance approach from cultural and spiritual perspectives. *Journal of Religion & Health, 56*(3), 971–985. doi:10.1007/s10943-016-0299-3.

Mulligan, K., McBain, H., Lamontagne Godwin, F., et al. (2017). Barriers and enablers of type 2 diabetes self-management in people with severe mental illness. *Health Expectations, 20*(5), 1020–1030. doi:10.1111/hex.12543.

Nestler, K., Witzki, A., Rohde, U., et al. (2017). Strength training for women as a vehicle for health promotion at work. *Deutsches Aerzteblatt International, 114*(26), 439–446. doi:10.3238/arztebl.2017.0439.

Pappa, G. L. (2017). Factors associated with weight change in online weight management communities: A case study in the LoseIt Reddit community. *Journal of Medical Internet Research, 19*(1), 1–13. doi:10.2196/jmir.5816.

Pen-Chen, K., Mei Chang, Y., Ming-Kuen, L., et al. (2017). Renal transplant recipients: The factors related to immunosuppressive medication adherence based on the Health Belief Model. *Journal of Nursing Research, 25*(5), 392–397. doi:10.1097/jnr.0000000000000181.

Riley, J., & Kruger, P. (2017). Optimising inhaler technique in chronic obstructive pulmonary disease: A complex issue. *British Journal of Nursing, 26*(7), 391–397. MEDLINE Info: NLM UID: 9212059.

Rogers, J., Pai, V., Merandi, J., et al. (2017). Impact of a pharmacy student-driven medication delivery service at hospital discharge. *American Journal of Health-System Pharmacy, 74,* S24–S29. doi:10.2146/ajhp150613.

Sainato, R., Flores, M., Malloy, A., et al. (2017). Health maintenance deficits in a fully insured population of adolescents with chronic medical conditions. *Clinical Pediatrics, 56*(6), 512–518. doi:10.1177/0009922816678183.

Serwe, K. M., Hersh, G. I., Pickens, N. D., et al. (2017). Caregiver perceptions of a telehealth wellness program. *American Journal of Occupational Therapy, 71*(4), 1–5. doi:10.5014/ajot.2017.025619.

Shor, D. B., Weitzman, D., Dahan, S., et al. (2017). Adherence and persistence with drug therapy among fibromyalgia patients: Data from a large health maintenance organization. *Journal of Rheumatology, 44*(10), 1499–1506. doi:10.3899/jrheum.170098.

Srisuk, N., Cameron, J., Ski, C. F., et al. (2017). Randomized controlled trial of family-based education for patients with heart failure and their carers. *Journal of Advanced Nursing, 73*(4), 857–870. doi:10.1111/jan.13192.

Sugiharto, S., Stephenson, M., Yu-Yun, H., et al. (2017). Diabetes self-management education training for community health center nurses in Indonesia: A best practice implementation project. *JBI Database of Systematic Reviews & Implementation Reports, 15*(9), 2390–2397. doi:10.11124/JBISRIR-2016-003329.

● = Independent;   ▲ = Collaborative;   EBN = Evidence-Based Nursing;   EB = Evidence-Based

Suijn, K., & Huber, J. T. (2017). Characteristics of personal health information management groups: Findings from an online survey using Amazon's mTurk. *Journal of the Medical Library Association*, *105*(4), 361–375. doi:10.5195/jmla.2017.312.

Vandyke, S. D., & Shell, M. D. (2017). Health beliefs and breast cancer screening in rural Appalachia: An evaluation of the *Health Belief Model. Journal of Rural Health*, *33*(4), 350–360. doi:10.1111/jrh.12204.

Yu-Jie, G. (2017). Measurements of self-efficacy in patients with chronic kidney disease: A literature review. *Nephrology Nursing Journal*, *44*(2), 159–165. MEDLINE Info: NLM UID: 100909377.

Readiness for enhanced Health management
Ruth A. Wittmann-Price, PhD, RN, CNS, CNE, CHSE, ANEF, FAAN

NANDA-I

H

Definition

A pattern of regulating and integrating into daily living a therapeutic regimen for treatment of illness and its sequelae, which can be strengthened.

Defining Characteristics

Expresses desire to enhance choices of daily living for meeting goals; expresses desire to enhance immunization/vaccination status; expresses desire to enhance management of illness; expresses desire to enhance management of prescribed regimens; expresses desire to enhance management of risk factors; expresses desire to enhance management of symptoms

NOC (Nursing Outcomes Classification)

Suggested NOC Outcomes

Health-Promoting Behavior; Health-Seeking Behavior; Knowledge: Health Behavior; Health Promotion; Health Resources; Illness Care; Medication; Prescribed Activity; Treatment Regimen

Example NOC Outcome with Indicators

Health-Promoting Behavior as evidenced by the following indicators: Monitors personal behavior for risks/Seeks balance activity and rest/Performs healthy behaviors routinely/Uses financial and social support resources to promote health. (Rate each indicator of **Health-Promoting Behavior:** 1 = never demonstrated, 2 = rarely demonstrated, 3 = sometimes demonstrated, 4 = often demonstrated, 5 = consistently demonstrated [see Section I].)

Client Outcomes

Client Will (Specify Time Frame)

- Describe integration of therapeutic regimen into daily living
- Demonstrate continued commitment to integration of therapeutic regimen into daily living routines

NIC (Nursing Interventions Classification)

Suggested NIC Interventions

Anticipatory Guidance; Mutual Goal Setting; Client Contracting; Self-Modification Assistance; Self-Responsibility Facilitation; Support System Enhancement

Example NIC Activities—Mutual Goal Setting

Assist client and significant others to develop realistic expectations of themselves in performance of their roles; Clarify with the client the roles of the health care provider and the client, respectively

Nursing Interventions and *Rationales*

- Acknowledge the expertise that the client and family bring to health management. **EBN:** *nurse researchers compared the perceptions of patients (N = 50) with nurses (N = 100) of hospitalized patient care needs and*

● = Independent;   ▲ = Collaborative;   **EBN** = Evidence-Based Nursing;   **EB** = Evidence-Based

found that surveyed patients and nurses agreed on needed areas such as communication and basic care. Slightly lower agreement scores between nurses and patients were identified for care planning and organization (Fernanades & Galan, 2017). **EBN:** *Jeyathevan, Lemonde, and Cooper (2017) qualitatively explored the role of oncology nurse navigators (ONNs) (N = 4) with adult lung cancer patients (N = 4) in the community, and the results demonstrated that the patients' perceptions of the ONN role was that it assisted with patient-focused care, needs assessments, accessibility, and eliminating care barriers.*

- Review factors that contribute to the likelihood of health promotion and health protection. Use Pender's Health Promotion Model and Becker's Health Belief Model to identify contributing factors (Pender et al, 2015). **EBN:** *Researchers used a quasi-experimental designed study with women (N =108) who were placed in two groups to examine nutritional behavior, and the nurse researchers found that Pender's Health Promotion Model-based nutritional training improved behavior better in the experimental group (Khodaveisi et al, 2017).* **EBN:** *Acikgoz and Kitis (2017) investigated university students' (N = 572) healthy lifestyle behaviors and their health locus of control and health-specific self-efficacy by Internet survey and found that health-specific self-efficacy is an important factor in changing lifestyle behaviors. The health locus of control had varied effects on healthy lifestyle behaviors. The study results supported Pender's model.*

- Further develop and reinforce contributing factors that might change with ongoing management of the therapeutic regimen (e.g., knowledge, self-efficacy, self-esteem, and perceived benefits). **EB:** *Jiao et al (2017) studied the relationship between methadone maintenance treatment patients with mental health illnesses and resilience and found resilience to be negatively correlated with depression and anxiety, indicating that resilience in this population is important for mental health.*

- Review the client's strengths in the management of the therapeutic regimen. **EBN:** *Tao, Chow, and Wong (2017) investigated the effects of a home exercise program on hemodialysis patients' (N = 113) perceptions about exercise and adherence. Patients were divided into two groups, one of which was a nurse-led exercise program. Patients in the nurse-led group did significantly better in meeting their exercise goals then those afforded traditional care modalities.* **EB:** *Researchers studied the results of womens' (N = 4247) glucose challenge tests (GCTs) longitudinally for 9 years and found that 10% of women who had a high-normal result of 126 to 140 mg% had significantly more diabetes than those women whose GCTs were under 125 mg% (Yoles et al, 2017).*

- Collaborate with the client to identify strategies to maintain strengths and develop additional strengths as indicated. **EB:** *Researchers studied patient-centered care (PCC) by surveying and interviewing older patients (N = 56) in relation to being malnourished patients and found themes that effected dietary intake of older adults (>81 years): (1) dietetic follow-up, (2) interdisciplinary coordination, and (3) and high-quality hospital food services. The nutritional recommendations from this study may facilitate evidence-based PCC for older malnourished patients (Hazzard et al, 2017).* **EB:** *Schmidt and Rizzolo (2017) explored the role of health care providers in the health and wellness of transgender and gender-diverse adults by investigating hormone therapy. Better results occurred with the individualization of treatment that was agreed on by the patient.*

- Identify contributing factors that may need to be improved now or in the future. **EB:** *Baill and Castiglioni (2017) examined the screenings women should receive post menopause and found that a woman's cardiovascular risk should be assessed every 5 to 10 years; breast cancer screening every other year; colorectal cancer screening; cervical cancer screening every 3 to 5 years; screening for high-risk women for sexually transmitted infections; and routine screening for depression, alcohol abuse, and intimate partner violence. The authors found that patient education was paramount in follow-through with any or all of the screenings. Provide knowledge as needed related to the pathophysiology of the disease or illness, prescribed activities, prescribed medications, and nutrition.* **EBN:** *Hovsepian, McGah, and O'Brien (2017) studied patient teaching postoperatively and learning retention with postoperative outcomes and found that better outcomes were realized when postoperative teaching was done preoperatively.* **EBN:** *Schneider and Howard (2017) investigated the differences in discharge readiness and postdischarge coping in stroke patients (N = 128) using education provided via a technology package (including patient online portal access, email/secure messaging) compared with current standard discharge teaching methods and found that there was no statistically significant difference between the groups in discharge readiness, but there was a significant increase in coping scores in the technology group.*

- Help the client maintain existing support and seek additional supports as needed. **EBN:** *Westcott and Welding (2017) documented case studies that support continuously reassessing home-bound patients' support surfaces in the house, educating patients, and providing appropriate resources to decrease pressure ulcers in community long-term care patients.* **EB:** *Researchers qualitatively explored the needs of patients (N = 41) who underwent bariatric surgery and found that support was needed from health professionals, significant*

• = Independent;   ▲ = Collaborative;   **EBN** = Evidence-Based Nursing;   **EB** = Evidence-Based

others, peers, and the general community. Lack of support negatively affected surgical outcomes (Sharman et al, 2017).

Geriatric

- Facilitate the client and family to obtain health insurance and drug payment plans whenever needed and possible. **EBN:** *Researchers used an interprofessional approach to explore the needs of geriatric patients (N = 293) and found through surveys and interviews that the patients' needs included guidance around falls prevention, improved nutrition, medication management, referrals to available community, and social service supports (Hansen et al, 2017).* **EBN:** *Lewis, Samperi, and Boyd-Skiner (2017) conducted telephone follow-up calls to elderly patients or bereaved family members after hospital admission, and patients and family reported feeling lonely and isolated. The patients and families were provided with community social support services with good response from patients and families.*

Multicultural

- Assess client's cultural perspectives on health management. **EB:** *Abbasalizad et al (2017) studied the relationship between Mediterranean diets and cardiovascular disease in patients with coronary artery bypass graft (CABG) surgery (N = 454) and found high dietary intakes of saturated fatty acids and cholesterol correlated with lower serum albumin and hemoglobin (Hb) A1C levels.*
- Assess health literacy in clients of diverse backgrounds. **EBN:** *Eun, Hee, and Soondool (2017) investigated the level of health literacy in different age groups of South Koreans (N = 1000) and found that for the 45 through 64 and the 65 and over age groups education was positively associated with health literacy. Additionally, the oldest age group and gender also had a positive association with health literacy. Depression was negatively associated with health literacy.* **EB:** *Almaleh et al (2017) studied the factors that effected inadequate health literacy on patients (N = 805) using outpatient clinics and found that 81% of the patients had limited comprehensive health literacy, 18.9% had sufficient health literacy, and females had lower health literacy than males.*
- Validate the client's feelings regarding the ability to manage his or her own care and the impact on current lifestyle. **EBN:** *Araujo do Reis and de Oliva Menezes (2017) qualitatively studied religiosity and spirituality as a resilience strategy for improved lifestyles and health in aging patients (N = 14) and found those patients who revealed they participated in religious or spiritual habits achieved increased well-being and resiliency and were better able to cope with health and social problems.*
- Facilitate the client and family to obtain financial assistance in the form of health insurance and drug payment plans whenever needed and possible. **EB:** *Tumin et al (2017) studied the change in health insurance after heart transplantation among adolescents (N = 366) and found through statistical analysis that changes in health insurance predicted a greater mortality risk compared with patients with continuous private insurance. Therefore assisting with insurance coverage maintenance may provide better health outcomes.*
- Use electronic monitoring to improve medication adherence. **EB:** *Madrasi et al (2017) studied medication adherence for preexposure prophylaxis for patients (N = 1147) using electronic adherence records recording the date and time of medication bottle cap opening and found that female patients and older patients had better adherence.* **EB:** *Researchers completed a literature review focused on asthma controller medication adherence using electronics including text messaging, smart phone applications, and electronic monitoring devices and found that electronics that remind patients improve adherence controller adherence (Anderson & Anderson, 2017). Discuss with clients their beliefs about medication and treatment to enhance medication and treatment adherence.* **EB:** *Cook et al (2017) studied motivational interviewing (MI) and reminders related to adherence of glaucoma treatment for patients (N = 201), and the results demonstrated that reminder calls increased adherence when compared with usual care, but MI did not increase adherence.* **EBN:** *Low et al (2017) studied medication adherence with post kidney transplantation patients (N = 25) in a descriptive exploratory study, and the themes identified were causes of distress, and coping resources. Researchers concluded that regular reminders, such as alarms to take medications, will reduce the stress of managing a kidney transplant.*

Client/Family Teaching and Discharge Planning

- Review therapeutic regimens and their optimal integration with daily living routines. **EB:** *Zelle et al (2017) studied exercise in patients with chronic kidney disease and found that behavioral approaches need to be better integrated into the care of renal patients along with nutrition to ensure better outcomes and quality of life.* **EBN:** *Nurse researchers evaluated a family-based heart failure education program and performed a*

● = Independent;   ▲ = Collaborative;   **EBN** = Evidence-Based Nursing;   **EB** = Evidence-Based

randomized control trial with patients (N = 50) and caretakers (N = 50) in a rural community and found that patients and family members who received the education program had higher knowledge scores at 3 and 6 months than those who received traditional outpatient education (Srisuk et al, 2017).

- Teach disease processes and therapeutic regimens to clients and peer supporters for management of disease processes. **EB:** *Inauen et al (2017) investigated patients (N = 84) with chronic conditions to assess overall multimedication adherence using self-reporting tools. The researchers recommended further study about multimedication adherence because most reports and tools refer to a single treatment or medication adherence.* **EB:** *Goethals et al (2017) longitudinally studied the role of parental responsiveness and control in relation to treatment adherence in diabetic children (N = 521) and found that lower psychological control and higher parental responsiveness were associated with better treatment adherence.*

REFERENCES

Abbasalizad, F. M., Najafi, M., Asghari, J., et al. (2017). Mediterranean dietary quality index and dietary phytochemical index among patients candidate for coronary artery bypass grafting (CABG) surgery. *BMC Cardiovascular Disorders, 17,* 1–8. doi:10.1186/s12872-017-0544-z.

Acikgoz, C. S., & Kitis, Y. (2017). Relationship between healthy lifestyle behaviors and health locus of control and health-specific self-efficacy in university students. *Japan Journal of Nursing Science, 14*(3), 231–239. doi:10.1111/jjns.12154.

Almaleh, R., Helmy, Y., Farhat, E., et al. (2017). Assessment of health literacy among outpatient clinics attendees at Ain Shams University Hospitals, Egypt: A cross-sectional study. *Public Health, 151,* 137–145. doi:10.1016/j.puhe.2017.06.024.

Anderson, W. C., & Anderson, W. C. (2017). Incorporating technology to advance asthma controller adherence. *Current Opinion in Allergy & Clinical Immunology, 17*(2), 153–159. doi:10.1097/ACI.0000000000000343.

Araujo do Reis, L., & de Oliva Menezes, T. M. (2017). Religiosity and spirituality as resilience strategies among long-living older adults in their daily lives. *Revista Brasileira de Enfermagem, 70*(4), 761–766. doi:10.1590/0034-7167-2016-0630.

Baill, I. C., & Castiglioni, A. (2017). Health maintenance in postmenopausal women. *American Family Physician, 95*(9), 561–570. PMID: 28671391. MEDLINE Info: NLM UID: 1272646.

Cook, P. F., Schmiege, S. J., Mansberger, S. L., et al. (2017). Motivational interviewing or reminders for glaucoma medication adherence: Results of a multi-site randomised controlled trial. *Psychology & Health, 32*(2), 145–165. doi:10.1080/08870446.2016.1244537.

Eun, J. L., Hee, Y. L., & Soondool, C. (2017). Age differences in health literacy: Do younger Korean adults have a higher level of health literacy than older Korean adults? *Health & Social Work, 42*(3), 133–141. doi:10.1093/hsw/hlx026.

Fernanades, M. P., & Galan, P. M. (2017). Care necessities: The view of the patient and nursing team. *Revista Brasileira de Enfermagem, 70*(5), 1026–1032. doi:10.1590/0034-7167-2016-0197.

Goethals, E. R., Oris, L., Berg, C. A., et al. (2017). Parenting and treatment adherence in Type 1 Diabetes throughout adolescence and emerging adulthood. *Journal of Pediatric Psychology, 42*(9), 922–932. doi:10.1093/jpepsy/jsx053.

Hansen, K. T., McDonald, C., O'Hara, S., et al. (2017). A formative evaluation of a nurse practitioner-led interprofessional geriatric outpatient clinic. *Journal of Interprofessional Care, 31*(4), 546–549. doi:10.1080/13561820.2017.1303463.

Hazzard, E., Barone, L., Mason, M., et al. (2017). Patient-centred dietetic care from the perspectives of older malnourished patients. *Journal of Human Nutrition & Dietetics, 30*(5), 574–587. doi:10.1111/jhn.12478.

Hovsepian, J., McGah, C., & O'Brien, C. (2017). Postoperative instructions preoperatively—evaluating the effectiveness of a teaching model on patient satisfaction regarding instructions for home care. *Journal of Perianesthesia Nursing, 32*(3), 231–237. doi:10.1016/j.jopan.2015.12.014.

Inauen, J., Biebauer, W., Luscher, J., et al. (2017). Assessing adherence to multiple medications and in daily life among patients with multimorbidity. *Psychology & Health, 32*(10), 1233–1248. doi:10.1080/08870446.2016.1275632.

Jeyathevan, G., Lemonde, M., & Cooper, B. A. (2017). The role of oncology nurse navigators in facilitating continuity of care within the diagnostic phase for adult patients with lung cancer. *Canadian Oncology Nursing Journal, 27*(1), 74–87. doi:10.5737/236880762717480.

Jiao, M., Gu, J., Xa, H., et al. (2017). Resilience associated with mental health problems among methadone maintenance treatment patients in Guangzhou, China. *AIDS Care, 29*(5), 660–665. doi:10.1080/09540121.2016.1255705.

Khodaveisi, M., Omidi, A., Shima, S., et al. (2017). The effect of Pender's Health Promotion Model in improving the nutritional behavior of overweight and obese women. *International Journal of Community Based Nursing & Midwifery, 5*(2), 165–174. MEDLINE Info: NLM UID: 101615484.

Lewis, E., Samperi, S., & Boyd-Skiner, C. (2017). Telephone follow-up calls for older patients after hospital discharge. *Age and Ageing, 46*(4), 544–546. doi:10.1093/ageing/afw251.

Low, J. K., Crawford, K., Manias, E., et al. (2017). Stressors and coping resources of Australian kidney transplant recipients related to medication taking: A qualitative study. *Journal of Clinical Nursing, 26*(11/12), 1495–1507. doi:10.1111/jocn.13435.

Madrasi, K., Chaturvedula, A., Haberer, J. E., et al. (2017). Markov mixed effects modeling using electronic adherence monitoring records identifies influential covariates to HIV preexposure prophylaxis. *Journal of Clinical Pharmacology, 57*(5), 606–615. doi:10.1002/jcph.843.

Pender, N. J., Murdaugh, C. L., & Parsons, M. A. (2015). *Health promotion in nursing practice* (7th ed.). Upper Saddle River, NJ: Prentice Hall.

Sharman, M., Hensher, M., Wilkinson, S., et al. (2017). What are the support experiences and needs of patients who have received bariatric surgery? *Health Expectations, 20*(1), 35–46. doi:10.1111/hex.12423.

Schmidt, E., & Rizzolo, D. (2017). Disease screening and prevention for transgender and gender-diverse adults. *JAAPA: Journal of the American Academy of Physician Assistants, 30*(10), 11–16. doi:10.1097/01.JAA.0000524709.87224.57.

Schneider, M., & Howard, K. A. (2017). Using technology to enhance discharge teaching and improve coping for patients after stroke. *Journal of Neuroscience Nursing, 49*(3), 152–156. doi:10.1097/JNN.0000000000000275.

Srisuk, N., Caneron, J., Skim, C. F., et al. (2017). Randomized controlled trial of family-based education for patients with heart failure and their carers. *Journal of Advanced Nursing, 73*(4), 857–870. doi:10.1111/jan.13192.

● = Independent;   ▲ = Collaborative;   **EBN** = Evidence-Based Nursing;   **EB** = Evidence-Based

Tao, X., Chow, S. K. Y., & Wong, F. K. Y. (2017). The effects of a nurse-supervised home exercise programme on improving patients' perceptions of the benefits and barriers to exercise: A randomised controlled trial. *Journal of Clinical Nursing*, 26(17/18), 2765–2775. doi:10.1111/jocn.13798.

Tumin, D., Li, S. S., Nandi, D., et al. (2017). Health insurance coverage among young adult survivors of pediatric heart transplantation. *Journal of Pediatrics*, 188, 82–86. doi:10.1016/j.jpeds.2017.06.014.

Yoles, I., Baevsky, T., Rosenberg, R., et al. (2017). High-normal glucose levels in a routine oral 1-hour 50 g glucose challenge test are associated with a poorer glycemic status later in life. *American Journal of Perinatology*, 34(14), 1131–1134. doi:10.1055/s-0037-1604193.

Westcott, S., & Welding, L. (2017). Support surface selection for long-term patients in the community. *Journal of Community Nursing*, 31(4), 36–39. MEDLINE Info: NLM UID: 101090738.

Zelle, D. M., Klaassen, G., van Adrichem, E., et al. (2017). Physical inactivity: A risk factor and target for intervention in renal care. *Nature Reviews. Nephrology*, 13(3), 152–168. doi:10.1038/nrneph.2016.187.

Ineffective family Health management

Gail B. Ladwig, MSN, RN and Julianne E. Doubet, BSN, RN, EMT-B

NANDA-I

Definition

A pattern of regulating and integrating, into family processes a program for the treatment of illness and its sequelae that is unsatisfactory for meeting specific health goals of the family unit.

Defining Characteristics

Acceleration of illness symptoms of a family member; decrease in attention to illness; difficulty with prescribed regimen; failure to take action to reduce risk factors; inappropriate family activities for meeting health goals

Related Factors

Decisional conflict; difficulty managing complex treatment regimen;; difficulty navigating complex of healthcare systems; family conflict

At-Risk Population

Economically disadvantaged

NOC (Nursing Outcomes Classification)

Suggested NOC Outcomes

Family Health-Status; Knowledge: Treatment Regimen; Family Participation in Professional Care

> **Example NOC Outcome with Indicators**
>
> **Knowledge: Treatment Regimen** as evidenced by the following indicator: Understanding conveyed about prescribed medication, activity, exercise, and specific disease process. (Rate the outcome and indicators of **Knowledge: Treatment Regimen:** 1 = no knowledge, 2 = limited knowledge, 3 = moderate knowledge, 4 = substantial knowledge, 5 = extensive knowledge [see Section I].)

Client Outcomes

Client Will (Specify Time Frame)

- Make adjustments in usual activities (e.g., diet, activity, stress management) to incorporate therapeutic regimens of its members
- Reduce illness symptoms of family members
- Desire to manage therapeutic regimens of its members
- Describe a decrease in the difficulties of managing therapeutic regimens
- Describe actions to reduce risk factors

● = Independent;   ▲ = Collaborative;   EBN = Evidence-Based Nursing;   EB = Evidence-Based

NIC   (Nursing Interventions Classification)

Suggested NIC Interventions

Family Involvement Promotion; Family Mobilization; Teaching: Disease Process

Example NIC Activities—Family Involvement Promotion

Identify and respect coping mechanisms used by family members; Provide crucial information to family members about the patient in accordance with client's preference

Nursing Interventions and *Rationales*

- Base family interventions on knowledge of the family, family context, family dynamics, family structure, and family function. **EBN:** *Family research has established that families differ widely from one another, even within cultures (Wright & Leahey, 2013).*
- Use a family approach when helping an individual with a health problem that requires therapeutic management. **EB:** *Cwik et al (2013) suggested that a family meeting, which includes the family member who needs medical accommodation, is the first step in planning coordinated care and its integration into everyday life.*
- Review with family members the congruence and incongruence of family behaviors and health-related goals. **EBN:** *To attain the motivation needed for changes in health habits, family members should understand the relation of daily habits to health-related goals (Wright & Leahey, 2013).*
- Acknowledge the challenge of integrating therapeutic regimens with family behaviors. **EBN:** *Therapeutic regimens require modifications of daily activities that have already been established based on family values and beliefs. Acknowledging the difficulty of changing family habits supports families through the process (Wright & Leahey, 2013).*
- Review the symptoms of specific illnesses and work with the family toward development of greater self-efficacy in relation to these symptoms. **EBN:** *Knowledge of symptoms improves the ability of family members to adjust behaviors to prevent and manage symptoms (Larsen, 2014).*
- Support family decisions to adjust therapeutic regimens as indicated. **EB:** *The National Institute of Neurological Disorders and Stroke (2018) published findings that concluded a woman suffering from epilepsy can have a healthy pregnancy and deliver a healthy child with planned adjustments in medication and the addition of certain supplements.*
- Advocate for the family in negotiating therapeutic regimens with health providers. **CEB:** *Illness regimens generally are neither arbitrary nor absolute; therefore modifications can be discussed as needed to fit with the family lifestyle (Wright & Leahey, 2013).*
- Help the family mobilize social supports. **EBN:** *Nurses in any capacity may detect a family/individual in crisis and will be obliged to provide crisis intervention while connecting the family/individual to other needed support services (Parsons, 2016).*
- Help family members modify perceptions as indicated. **EB:** *Illness perception, family adaptability, and coping mechanisms are key factors for the quality of life of a patient with a chronic disease (Postolica et al, 2017).*
- Use one or more theories of family dynamics to describe, explain, or predict family behaviors (e.g., theories of Bowen, Satir, and Minuchin). **EBN:** *Family systems may not be understood by the nurse without adequate knowledge of family theory (Wright & Leahey, 2013).*
- ▲ Collaborate with expert nurses or other consultants regarding strategies for working with families. **EBN:** *The findings underscore the need for researchers and health care professionals to engage in collaborative discussions and make cooperative efforts to help alleviate treatment burden and tailor treatment regimens to the realities of people's daily lives (Sav et al, 2015).*
- Coaching methods can be used to help families improve their health. **CEB:** *Coaching processes were shown to improve family outcomes related to improved nutrition and physical activity (Heimendinger et al, 2007).* **EB:** *Connecting to Internet sites and online resources that included communication and support from peers; contact with experts, clinicians, and coaches; and those sites offering means of support to the caregiver, improved symptom control in cancer patients (Griffin et al, 2013).*

Pediatric

- Support kangaroo care for infants at risk at birth. Keep infants in an upright position in skin-to-skin contact until they no longer tolerate it. **EBN:** *According to ten Ham-Baloyi, Ricks, and van Rooyen (2017),*

● = Independent;   ▲ = Collaborative;   **EBN** = Evidence-Based Nursing;   **EB** = Evidence-Based

some of the benefits derived from kangaroo mother care (KMC) are improving mother–infant attachment; encouraging the continuance of breastfeeding; and helping to reduce mortality of preterm neonates.

Geriatric

- Recommend that clients use the "Ask Me 3" program when communicating with their health providers (What is my main problem? What do I need to do? Why is it important for me to do this?). **EBN:** *The Ask Me 3 program is an effective means of affirming patients' knowledge and understanding of their conditions and treatments. The program also serves to increase "buy in" to their plan of care, thus promoting healthier outcomes (Marben, 2013).*

Multicultural

- Acknowledge racial and ethnic differences at the onset of care. **CEB:** *Acknowledgment of race and ethnicity issues enhances communication, establishes rapport, and promotes treatment outcomes (Giger & Davidhizar, 2008).*
- Ensure that all strategies for working with the family are congruent with the culture of the family. **CEB:** Many nursing studies among people of a variety of cultures show that cultural variations exist in the management of therapeutic regimens, and these differences should be taken into account when working with families (Hanley, 2008).
- Facilitate modeling and role playing for the family regarding healthy ways to communicate and interact. **EBN:** It is helpful for families and the client to practice communication skills in a safe environment before trying them in a real-life situation (Wright & Leahey, 2013).
- Use the nursing intervention of cultural brokerage to help families deal with the health care system. **CEB:** In a study based on 24 in-depth interviews, four empirical mechanisms of cultural brokerage were identified: translating between health systems, bridging divergent images of medicine, establishing long-term relationships, and working with patients' relational networks (Lo, 2010). **EBN:** Culture brokerage is a type of developing care that can be used in various manners when applied to the community and/or hospital environments. This approach benefits the progression of the nursing discipline (Arias-Murcia & Lopez-Dias, 2013).

Client/Family Teaching and Discharge Planning

- Teach about all aspects of therapeutic regimens. Provide as much knowledge as family members will accept, adjust instruction to account for what the family already knows, and directions provide information in a culturally congruent manner. **EBN:** *Use "tailored to the client" instructions, which may include medical and disease education, skills training, and resource connection (Chin et al, 2017).*
- Teach ways to adjust family behaviors to include therapeutic regimens, such as safety in taking medications and teaching family members to act as self-advocates with health providers who prescribe therapeutic regimens. **EBN:** By using continuous care interventions, a trusting relationship can be established with the family caregiver (Chin et al, 2017).

REFERENCES

Arias-Murcia, S., & Lopez-Diaz, L. (2013). Cultural Brokerage as a form of caring. *Investigecion & Educacion Enfermeria, 31*(3), 441–470.

Chin, M., Chiu, Y., Wei, A., et al. (2017). Reducing the care-related burdens of a family caregiver of a person with mild cognitive impairment: A home-based care management program. *Journal of Nursing, 64*(3), 105–111. doi:10.6224/JN.000046.

Cwik, V., Kennedy, A., Bendett, J., et al. (2013). *MDA ALS Caregiver's Guide, 551*. Retrieved from https://www.mda.org/sites/default/files/publications/ALS_Caregiver'sGuide_P531.pdf.

Giger, J. N., & Davidhizar, R. (2008). *Transcultural nursing: Assessment and intervention* (5th ed.). St Louis: Mosby.

Griffin, J., Meis, L., Carlyle, M., et al. (2013). *Effectiveness of family and caregiver interventions on patient outcomes among adults with cancer or memory-related disorders: a systematic review, VA Evidence- based Synthesis Reports*. Retrieved from https://www.ncbi.nim.nih.gov/pubmedhealth/pmh.

Hanley, K. (2008). Navajos. In J. N. Giger & R. Davidhizar (Eds.), *Transcultural nursing: Assessment and intervention* (5th ed.). St Louis: Mosby.

Heimendinger, J., et al. (2007). Coaching process outcomes of a family visit nutrition and physical activity intervention. *Health Education and Behavior, 34*, 71–89.

Larsen, P. D. (2014). *Lubkin's Chronic illness: Impact and interventions* (9th ed.). Boston: Jones & Bartlett.

Lo, M. C. M. (2010). Cultural brokerage: Creating linkages between voices of lifeworld and medicine in cross-cultural clinical settings. *Health (London, England: 1997), 14*(5), 484–504.

Marben, K. (2013). *Ask Me 3 to enhance high-risk patients knowledge and curiosity of their specific diagnosis and at-home care plans*. Retrieved from https://www.aacpdm.org/userfiles/files/DPSIASKME3_KM-posted.pdf.

National Institute of Neurological Disorders and Strokes. (2018). *The epilepsies and seizures: hope through research*. Retrieved from https://

● = Independent; ▲ = Collaborative; **EBN** = Evidence-Based Nursing; **EB** = Evidence-Based

www.ninds.nih.gov/disorders/patient-caregiver-education/
hope-through-research/epilepsies-and-seizures-hope-through.

Parsons, C. (2016). Evidence-based care of adolescents and families in crisis. *Nursing Clinics*, 51(2), 249–260. doi:10.1016/j.cnurs.2016.01.008.

Postolica, R., Iorga, M., Petrariu, F., et al., (2017). *Cognitive-behavioral coping, illness perception, and family adaptability in oncological patients with a family history of cancer.*

Sav, A., King, M., Whitty, J., et al. (2015). Burden of treatment for chronic illness: A concept analysis and review of the literature.

Health Expectations: An International Journal of Public Participation in Health Care and Health Policy, 18(3), 312–324. doi:10.1111/hex.12046.

ten Ham-Balogi, W., Ricks, E., & van Rooyen, D. (2017). An educational strategy supporting kangaroo mother care: Interviews with health care practitioners. *Africa Journal of Nursing and Midwifery*, 19(3), 1–16. doi:10.25159/2520-5293/1859.

Wright, L. M., & Leahey, M. (2013). *Nurses and families: A guide to family assessment and intervention* (6th ed.). Philadelphia: F. A. Davis.

Ineffective Health maintenance

Kathaleen C. Bloom, PhD, CNM and Lauren McAlister, MSN, FNP, DNP Candidate

NANDA-I

Definition

Inability to identify, manage, and/or seek out help to maintain well-being.

Defining Characteristics

Absence of adaptive behaviors to environmental changes; absence of interest in improving health behaviors; inability to take responsibility for meeting basic health practices; insufficient knowledge about basic health practices; insufficient social support; pattern of lack of health-seeking behavior

Related Factors

Complicated grieving; impaired decision-making; ineffective communication skills; ineffective coping strategies; insufficient resources; spiritual distress

At-Risk Population

Developmental delay

Associated Condition

Alteration in cognitive functioning; decrease in fine motor skills; decrease in gross motor skills; perceptual disorders

NOC   (Nursing Outcomes Classification)

Suggested NOC Outcomes

Health Orientation; Health Beliefs: Perceived Resources; Health-Promoting Behavior; Health-Seeking Behavior

Example NOC Outcome with Indicators
Health-Seeking Behavior as evidenced by the following indicators: Completes health-related tasks/Performs self-screening/Obtains assistance from health professional. (Rate the outcome and indicators of **Health-Seeking Behavior:** 1 = never demonstrated, 2 = rarely demonstrated, 3 = sometimes demonstrated, 4 = often demonstrated, 5 = consistently demonstrated [see Section I].)

Client Outcomes

Client Will (Specify Time Frame)

- Discuss fear of or blocks to implementing health regimen
- Follow mutually agreed on health care maintenance plan
- Meet goals for health care maintenance

● = Independent;   ▲ = Collaborative;   EBN = Evidence-Based Nursing;   EB = Evidence-Based

NIC   (Nursing Interventions Classification)

Suggested NIC Interventions

Health Education; Health System Guidance; Support System Enhancement

Example NIC Activities—Health Education

Prioritize identified learner needs based on client preference, skills of nurse, resources available, and likelihood of successful goal attainment; Emphasize immediate or short-term positive health benefits to be received by positive lifestyle behaviors, rather than long-term benefits or negative effects of noncompliance

Nursing Interventions and *Rationales*

- Assess the client's feelings, values, and reasons for not following the prescribed plan of care. See Related Factors. **EBN:** *A systematic review of 80 studies determined that personal beliefs and values, decisional control preferences, and perception of the decision-making process affect treatment decision-making in older adults diagnosed with cancer (Tariman et al, 2012).*

- Assess for family patterns, economic issues, and spiritual and cultural patterns that influence compliance with a given medical regimen. **CEB:** *A qualitative study (N = 14) found that critical challenges to increasing physical activity among low-income African American women included financial constraints (Harley et al, 2014).*

- Involve the client in shared decision-making regarding health maintenance. **CEB:** *A meta-analysis of 32 clinical trials revealed that assessing client preferences and involving them in shared decision-making had higher adherence, higher satisfaction, and better clinical outcomes (Lindhiem et al, 2014).*

- Show genuine interest in the client's individual needs. **EBN:** *A systematic review of 24 qualitative studies concluded that clients' perceptions of the health care professional's responsiveness, interest in their individual needs, and shared information positively influence self-care for heart failure (Currie et al, 2014).*

- Assist the client in finding methods to reduce stress. **EBN:** *In a survey of 1257 university students, those who had high levels of perceived stress also engaged in high-risk behaviors such as alcohol consumption, unhealthy diet, physical inactivity, and tobacco and drug use (Deasy et al, 2014).*

- Help the client determine how to manage complex medication schedules (e.g., HIV/AIDS regimens or polypharmacy). **EBN:** *In a pilot study with 20 older adults taking an average of 13.2 prescription medications, providing an illustrated daily medication schedule improved both self-efficacy and adherence (Martin, Kripalani, & Durapau, 2012).*

- Identify complementary healing modalities, such as herbal remedies, acupuncture, healing touch, yoga, or cultural shamans that the client uses in addition to or instead of the prescribed allopathic regimen along with the client's perception of the complementary healing modalities. **CEB:** *Use of complementary healing modalities among clients with chronic disease is relatively high. In an exploratory study with 217 Mexican immigrants, a person's beliefs about complementary and alternative therapies may negatively influence medical adherence (Villagran et al, 2012).*

- ▲ Refer the client to appropriate medical and social services as needed, providing adequate information on details about the service, including scheduling. **EBN:** *A metasynthesis of 62 qualitative studies concluded that client participation in services such as cardiac rehabilitation is most strongly associated with perceptions of the nature, suitability, and scheduling, but not the benefits of the rehabilitation program (Clark et al, 2013).*

- Identify support groups related to the disease process. **EBN:** *Individuals who attend support groups demonstrate improved disease management and enhanced quality of life. A systematic review of 84 studies of group visits for chronic illness found client benefits to include greater satisfaction and improved clinical outcomes (Jones et al, 2014).*

- Use social media such as text messaging to remind clients of scheduled appointments. **CEB:** *A Cochrane review of eight randomized controlled trials concluded that text messaging reminders increase attendance at health care appointments similar to telephone reminders but better than no reminders or postal reminders (Gurol-Urganci et al, 2013). Additional relevant research is done by Farmer et al (2014) and McInnes et al (2014).*

- Use telehealth interventions to facilitate self-care. **EBN:** *A systematic review of 14 studies supports telehealth as a positive factor in enabling self-care behaviors related to daily weighing, medication management, exercise adherence, fluid and alcohol restriction, salt restriction, and stress reduction in clients with heart failure (Radhakrishnan & Jacelon, 2012).*

● = Independent;   ▲ = Collaborative;   EBN = Evidence-Based Nursing;   EB = Evidence-Based

H

 Geriatric

- Assess the client's perception of health and health maintenance. **CEB:** *A study of 681 older clients with diabetes or metabolic syndrome found that they often underestimate their cardiovascular risk, with as many as 42% perceiving themselves to be in good or excellent health (Martell-Claros et al, 2013).*
- Assist client to identify both life- and health-related goals. **CEB:** *A study of 308 women demonstrated beginning evidence that when the health goals of older individuals are congruent with their life goals, they are more likely to participate in health-related activities (Saajanaho et al, 2014).*
- Provide information that supports informed decision-making. **CEB:** *In a modified grounded theory study (N = 59), participants endorsed the elements of informed decision-making, including discussion of the role of the client, the clinical issue, the alternatives, and benefits/risks/uncertainties; assessment of client understanding and preference; soliciting input from trusted others; and discussion of the effect on clients' daily lives (Price et al, 2012).*
- Discuss realistic goal setting for changes in health maintenance with the client and support person. **EBN:** *An integrative review of 13 studies revealed that mutual goal-setting between the client and the health care provider improves overall health behaviors and outcomes for older adults with chronic conditions (Anuruang et al, 2014).*
- Educate the client about the symptoms of life-threatening illness, such as myocardial infarction (MI), and the need for timeliness in seeking care. **EBN:** *A qualitative study with 42 persons with an MI found that misinformation regarding the symptoms of MI is common; many believe sudden, intense chest pain is the only indication of MI, resulting in delay in seeking treatment (O'Donnell & Moser, 2012).*

 Multicultural

- Assess influence of cultural beliefs, norms, and values on the client's ability to modify health behavior. **EBN:** *A descriptive qualitative study of 30 Thai Buddhists revealed that understanding the cultural and religious traditions, understanding the influence of family and economics when choosing interventions to help them cope with their illness, and empowering them to control their disease are essential for effective care (Lundberg & Thrakul, 2012).*
- Assess the effect of fatalism on the client's ability to modify health behavior. **CEB:** *A population-based study of 2018 adults found that fatalistic beliefs about cancer may hamper screening and delay help-seeking for symptoms (Beeken et al, 2011).*
- Clarify culturally related health beliefs and practices. **EBN:** *Language, culture, and ethnicity influence the choice of a health care provider and participation in health management strategies. An exploratory descriptive study with 23 women found that health/illness beliefs affect both self-care and care seeking (Hjelm, Berntorp, & Apelqvist, 2012).*
- Provide culturally appropriate education and health care services. **CEB:** *In a randomized controlled trial involving 223 Hispanic women, a culturally tailored lifestyle behavior intervention was shown to significantly influence dietary habits, weight, and waist circumference (Koniak-Griffin et al, 2014). **CEB:** In a systematic review of 28 studies of culturally adapted strategies to improve diet and weight outcomes of African American women, strategies that reflected the group's values and beliefs and that drew from the group's experiences were the most successful (Kong et al, 2014).*

 Home Care

- The interventions described previously may be adapted for home care use.
- ▲ Provide nurse-led case management. **EBN:** *A review of relevant research concluded that individualized, systematic, and guideline-based nurse case management promotes cardiovascular risk reduction in home-based, primary care, and community settings (Berra, 2011).*
- Provide a health promotion focus for the client with disabilities, with the goals of reducing secondary conditions (e.g., obesity, hypertension, pressure sores), maintaining functional independence, providing opportunities for leisure and enjoyment, and enhancing overall quality of life. **CEB:** *A retrospective analysis of data from a national survey comparing the health of adults with and without physical or cognitive disabilities found that individuals living with physical disabilities or cognitive impairment receive fewer preventive services and have higher rates of chronic illness (Reichard, Stolzle, & Fox, 2011). A systematic review of 11 studies found that community-based physical activity and educational programs provide fitness and psychosocial benefits for individuals with intellectual disabilities (Heller et al, 2011).*

● = Independent;   ▲ = Collaborative;   **EBN** = Evidence-Based Nursing;   **EB** = Evidence-Based

- Provide support and individual training for caregivers before the client is discharged from the hospital. EBN: *Caregivers are very interested in receiving instruction and hands-on practice of procedures they would need to perform at home. In a study of hospital-to-home transition of older veterans, caregivers (N = 40) reported increased confidence in their ability to provide such care and to help their loved ones manage symptoms at home (Hendrix et al, 2011).*
- Assist the client to develop confidence in the ability to manage the health condition. CEB: *A clinical trial of self-management education targeted at self-efficacy (N = 57) improved physiological outcomes, enhanced coping techniques, and reduced health care use (Labrecque et al, 2011).*

 ### Client/Family Teaching and Discharge Planning

- Provide the family with credible sources in which information can be obtained from social media. (Most libraries have Internet access with printing capabilities.) CEB: *In an experimental study (N = 197), researchers concluded that websites containing credible and evidence-based medical information positively affected users seeking health information. General, non–evidence-based sites were perceived positively by the user, independent of the site's credibility, often negatively influencing opinions about health practices (Allam, Schulz, & Nakamoto, 2014).*
- ▲ Develop collaborative multidisciplinary partnerships. CEB: *Multidisciplinary and multifactorial interventions are likely to be more effective in achieving desired outcomes. In a quality improvement study of readmission rates for 463 clients with pneumonia, the clients whose in-hospital and postdischarge diagnosis and care were managed by a multidisciplinary team consisting of health care providers, nurses, and social workers had significantly fewer all-cause readmissions and readmissions for pneumonia (Hussein, Golden, & Hahn, 2014).*
- Tailor both the information provided and the method of delivery of information to the specific client and/or family. CEB: *A systematic review of 27 studies related to medication adherence and diabetes outcomes was not able to identify a specific intervention, but it emphasized the need to tailor interventions to optimize management and improve outcomes (Williams et al, 2014).*
- Explain nonthreatening qualities before introducing more anxiety-producing information regarding possible side effects of the disease or medical regimen. EBN: *In a laboratory study of anxiety and task interference (N = 157), anxiety was found to interfere with concentration and the ability to understand and remember (Lachman & Agrigoroaei, 2012).*

REFERENCES

Allam, A., Schulz, P. J., & Nakamoto, K. (2014). The impact of search engine selection and sorting criteria on vaccination beliefs and attitudes: Two experiments manipulating Google output. *Journal of Medical Interest Research, 16,* e100.

Anuruang, S., Hickman, L. D., Jackson, D., et al. (2014). Community-based interventions to promote management for older people: An integrative review. *Journal of Clinical Nursing, 23,* 2110–2120.

Beeken, R. J., Simon, A. E., von Wagner, C., et al. (2011). Cancer fatalism: Deterring early presentation and increasing social inequalities? *Cancer Epidemiology, Biomarkers & Prevention, 20,* 2127–2131.

Berra, K. (2011). Does nurse case management improve implementation of guidelines for cardiovascular disease risk reduction? *Journal of Cardiovascular Nursing, 26,* 145–167.

Clark, A. M., King-Shier, K. M., Spaling, M. A., et al. (2013). Factors influencing participation in cardiac rehabilitation programmes after referral and initial attendance: Qualitative systematic review and meta-synthesis. *Clinical Rehabilitation, 27,* 948–959.

Currie, K., Strachan, P. H., Spaling, M., et al. (2014). The importance of interactions between patients and healthcare professionals for heart failure self-care: A systematic review of qualitative research into patient perspectives. *European Journal of Cardiovascular Nursing,* pii: 1474515114547648.

Deasy, C., Coughlan, B., Pironom, J., et al. (2014). Psychological distress and lifestyle of students: Implications for health promotion. *Health Promotion International,* pii: dau086.

Farmer, T., Brook, G., McSorley, J., et al. (2014). Using short message service text reminders to reduce 'did not attend' rates in sexual health and HIV appointment clinics. *International Journal of STD & AIDS, 25,* 289–293.

Gurol-Urganci, I., de Jongh, T., Vodopivec-Jamsek, V., et al. (2013). Mobile phone messaging reminders for attendance at healthcare appointments. *Cochrane Database of Systematic Reviews,* (12), CD007458.

Harley, A. E., Rice, J., Walker, R., et al. (2014). Physically active, low-income African American women: An exploration of activity maintenance in the context of sociodemographic factors associated with inactivity. *Women and Health, 54,* 354–372.

Heller, T., McCubbin, J. A., Drum, C., et al. (2011). Physical activity and nutrition health promotion interventions: What is working for people with intellectual disabilities? *Intellectual & Developmental Disabilities, 49,* 26–36.

Hendrix, C. C., Hastings, S. N., Van Houtven, C., et al. (2011). Pilot study: Individualized training for caregivers of hospitalized older veterans. *Nursing Research, 60,* 436–441.

Hjelm, K., Berntorp, K., & Apelqvist, J. (2012). Beliefs about health and illness in Swedish and African-born women with gestational diabetes living in Sweden. *Journal of Clinical Nursing, 21,* 1374–1386.

Hussein, H., Golden, M., & Hahn, S. (2014). Multidisciplinary intervention to improve readmission rates of patients discharged with a diagnosis of pneumonia. *Chest, 146,* 905A.

● = Independent;   ▲ = Collaborative;   EBN = Evidence-Based Nursing;   EB = Evidence-Based

Jones, K. R., Kaewluang, N., & Lekhak, N. (2014). Group visits for chronic illness management: Implementation challenges and recommendations. *Nursing Economics, 32*, 118–134, 147.

Kong, A., Tussing-Humphreys, L. M., Odoms-Young, A. M., et al. (2014). Systematic review of behavioural interventions with culturally adapted strategies to improve diet and weight outcomes in African American women. *Obesity Reviews, 4*, 62–92.

Koniak-Griffin, D., Brecht, M. L., Takayanagi, S., et al. (2014). A community health worker-led lifestyle behavior intervention for Latina (Hispanic) women: Feasibility and outcomes of a randomized controlled trial. *International Journal of Nursing Studies*, pii: S0020-7489(14)00253-3.

Labrecque, M., Rabhi, K., Laurin, C., et al. (2011). Can a self-management education program for patients with chronic obstructive pulmonary disease improve quality of life? *Canadian Respiratory Journal, 18*, e77–e81.

Lachman, M. E., & Agrigoroaei, S. (2012). Low perceived control as a risk factor for episodic memory: The mediational role of anxiety and task interference. *Memory & Cognition, 40*, 287–296.

Lindhiem, O., Bennett, C. B., Trentacosta, C. J., et al. (2014). Client preferences affect treatment satisfaction, completion, and clinical outcome: A meta-analysis. *Clinical Psychology Review, 34*, 506–517.

Lundberg, P. C., & Thrakul, S. (2012). Type w diabetes: How do Thai Buddhist people with diabetes practice self-management? *Journal of Advanced Nursing, 68*, 550–558.

Martell-Claros, N., Aranda, P., González-Albarrán, O., et al. (2013). Perception of health and understanding of cardiovascular risk among patients with recently diagnosed diabetes and/or metabolic syndrome. *European Journal of Preventative Cardiology, 20*, 21–28.

Martin, D., Kripalani, S., & Durapau, V. J. (2012). Improving medication management among at-risk older adults. *Journal of Gerontological Nursing, 38*, 24–34.

McInnes, D. K., Sawh, L., Petrakis, B. A., et al. (2014). The potential for health-related uses of mobile phones and internet with homeless veterans: Results from a multisite survey. *Telemedicine Journal and E-Health, 20*, 801–809.

O'Donnell, S., & Moser, D. K. (2012). Slow-onset myocardial infarction and its influence on help-seeking behaviors. *Journal of Cardiovascular Nursing, 27*, 334–344.

Price, E. L., Bereknyei, S., Kuby, A., et al. (2012). New elements for informed decision making: A qualitative study of older adults' views. *Patient Education and Counseling, 86*, 335–341.

Radhakrishnan, K., & Jacelon, C. (2012). Impact of telehealth on patient self-management of heart failure: A review of literature. *Journal of Cardiovascular Nursing, 27*, 33–43.

Reichard, A., Stolzle, H., & Fox, M. H. (2011). Health disparities among adults with physical disabilities or cognitive limitations compared to individuals with no disabilities in the United States. *Disability and Health Journal, 4*, 59–67.

Saajanaho, M., Viljanen, A., Read, S., et al. (2014). Older women's personal goals and exercise activity: An 8-year follow-up. *Journal of Aging and Physical Activity, 22*, 386–392.

Tariman, J. D., Berry, D. L., Cochrane, B., et al. (2012). Physician, patient, and contextual factors affecting treatment decisions in older adults with cancer and models of decision making: A literature review. *Oncology Nursing Forum, 39*, E70–E83.

Villagran, M., Hajek, C., Zhao, X., et al. (2012). Communication and culture: Predictors of treatment adherence among Mexican immigrant patients. *Journal of Health Psychology, 17*, 443–452.

Williams, J. L., Walker, R. J., Smalls, B. L., et al. (2014). Effective interventions to improve medication adherence in Type 2 diabetes: A systematic review. *Diabetes Management, 4*, 29–48.

Impaired Home maintenance

Kathaleen C. Bloom, PhD, CNM and Lauren McAlister, MSN, FNP, DNP Candidate

NANDA-I

Definition

Inability to independently maintain a safe growth-promoting immediate environment.

Defining Characteristics

Difficulty maintaining a comfortable environment; excessive family responsibilities; impaired ability to maintain home; insufficient clothing; insufficient cooking equipment; insufficient equipment for maintaining home; insufficient linen; pattern of disease caused by unhygienic conditions; pattern of infection caused by unhygienic conditions; request for assistance with home maintenance; unsanitary environment

Related Factors

Inadequate role model; insufficient family organization; insufficient family planning; insufficient knowledge of home maintenance; insufficient knowledge of neighborhood resources; insufficient support system

At-Risk Population

Financial crisis

Associated Condition

Alteration in cognitive functioning

● = Independent;   ▲ = Collaborative;   EBN = Evidence-Based Nursing;   EB = Evidence-Based

NOC (Nursing Outcomes Classification)

Suggested NOC Outcomes

Safe Home Environment; Self-Care: Activities of Daily Living (ADLs)

> **Example NOC Outcome with Indicators**
>
> **Safe Home Environment** as evidenced by the following indicators: Elimination of pests/Smoke detector maintenance/ Accessibility of assistive devices/Elimination of tobacco smoke. (Rate the outcome and indicators of **Safe Home Environment:** 1 = not adequate, 2 = slightly adequate, 3 = moderately adequate, 4 = substantially adequate, 5 = totally adequate [see Section I].)

Client Outcomes

Client Will (Specify Time Frame)

- Maintain a healthy home environment
- Use community resources to assist with home care needs
- Maintain a safe home environment

NIC (Nursing Interventions Classification)

Suggested NIC Intervention

Home Maintenance Assistance

> **Example NIC Activities—Home Maintenance Assistance**
>
> Involve client/family in deciding home maintenance requirements; Provide information on how to make home environment safe and clean; Help family use social support network

Nursing Interventions and *Rationales*

- Assess the concerns of family members, especially the primary caregiver, about home care for a long time. **EBN:** *A cross-sectional study of 515 caregiver/client dyads found that caregiver confidence in the ability to contribute to their family member's self-care was a significant determinant of how much they were involved in self-care maintenance and management (Vellone et al, 2014).*
- Provide home safety education and, safety equipment when possible. **CEB:** *A Cochrane review of 98 studies (with meta-analysis of 54 studies) concluded that home safety interventions, especially those delivered in the home, were effective in reducing injury and in increasing uptake of home safety measures, including safe water temperature, functional smoke alarms, a fire escape plan, and storing hazardous items out of reach (Kendrick et al, 2013).*
- ▲ Consider a predischarge home assessment referral to determine the need for accessibility and safety-related environmental changes. **EB:** *A randomized controlled trial (RCT) (N = 842 households, 1848 individual occupants) found significantly fewer falls and fall-related injuries in those households that had specific low-cost home modifications such as alterations in steps inside and outside the house, grab rails and nonslip bath mats in bathrooms, outside lighting, and alterations in carpeting (Keall et al, 2014).*
- Use an assessment tool to identify environmental safety hazards in the home. **EBN:** *In a study of 130 persons receiving discharge teaching, those who received targeted education and practice using a mock-up of their home regarding home safety modifications had significantly fewer overall and in-home falls 1 year after discharge (Kamei et al, 2015).*
- Establish an individualized plan of care for improved home maintenance with the client and family based on the client's needs and the caregiver's capabilities. **EBN:** *In a study involving 116 households with 170 children with asthma, an in-home assessment followed by targeted changes in the home environment resulted in a decrease in all measures of asthma severity and health care utilization (Turcotte et al, 2014).*
- Set up a system of relief for the main caregiver in the home and a plan for sharing household duties and/ or outside assistance. **EBN:** *In a qualitative study, 34 parents providing care to children with disabilities or complex health care needs identified the need for help and support, indicating that respite care was a significant unmet need (Whiting, 2014).*

● = Independent; ▲ = Collaborative; **EBN** = Evidence-Based Nursing; **EB** = Evidence-Based

▲ Provide a multidisciplinary approach to target the home environment and the client's ability to function in the home. **EBN:** *The Community Aging in Place: Advancing Better Living for Elders (CAPABLE), a program involving teams of nurses, occupational therapists, and handymen, targets the home environment and individual physical function (Szanton et al, 2014). An evaluation study of the effectiveness of the program found that 75% of the participants significantly improved their performance of ADLs and had improved ability to do their own shopping and manage their medications (Szanton et al, 2016).*

● Assess the quality of relationships among family members. **CEB:** *In a cross-sectional study of fifth graders (N = 3218), unintentional injuries requiring medical attention were associated with parental marital discord (Schwebel et al, 2012).*

Geriatric

● All of the previously mentioned interventions are applicable for the geriatric population.

● Assess injury prevention knowledge and practices of the client and caregivers and provide information as appropriate. **EBN:** *A survey of 84 older adults showed that only 36% had a working smoke alarm, 22% had a working carbon monoxide alarm, and 36% had water that was hotter than recommended (Shields et al, 2013).*

● Assess functional ability to manage safely after hospital discharge. **EB:** *A validation study of The Assessment of Motor and Process Skills and Cognitive Performance Test were found to reliably predict time to incident of harm post discharge (Douglas et al, 2013).*

● Explore community resources to assist with home maintenance (e.g., senior centers, Department of Aging, hospital case managers, friends and relatives, the Internet, or church parish nurse). **EB:** *In a qualitative study with 43 older adults living at home, participants perceived they were both capable and willing to manage many home maintenance tasks. They reported using compensatory means, such as tools and technologies and to do home maintenance and repairs themselves or hiring someone or having friends, neighbors, or family do the task (Kelly et al, 2014).*

● Provide education related to home modification. **EBN:** *An RCT with 130 community-dwelling older adults found that a home hazard modification program that included education and practice about home safety and specific guidance on how to modify the home to improve safety significantly decreased falls, both indoors and outdoors (Kamei et al, 2015).*

● Focus on the interaction between the older client and the technology, assisting the client to be an active participant in choices of and uses for technology. **EB:** *A qualitative study used focus groups with older adults, care professionals, home care or social work managers, and technology designers and suppliers to identify parameters for technology for aging in place. The researchers found that all groups believed success was enhanced when the older adult's needs and wishes are prioritized and that the technology is accepted by the older adults and perceived as beneficial (Peek et al, 2016).*

● See the care plans for Risk for **Injury** and Risk for **Falls.**

Multicultural

● Acknowledge the stresses unique to racial/ethnic communities. **CEB:** *A systematic review of 57 studies revealed that cultural factors, including distrust of home visits, language barriers and lifestyle, were barriers to home injury prevention interventions (Ingram et al, 2012).*

Home Care

● The previously mentioned interventions incorporate these resources.

● See care plans **Contamination** and Risk for **Contamination.**

Client/Family Teaching and Discharge Planning

● Identify support groups within the community to assist families in the caregiver role. **CEB:** *Community-based participatory research using focus groups with 39 family caregivers found that caregivers are most in need of effective communication, emotional support, education, and advocacy (Macleod, Skinner, & Low, 2012).*

● Provide counseling and support for clients and for caregivers of clients. **EB:** *A systematic review of 28 studies found that education, counseling, and support of caregivers to individuals with disabilities improved the caregivers' quality of life and decreased their perceived stress of the caregivers (Lawang et al, 2013).* Focus teaching on environmental hazards identified in the nursing assessment. Areas may include, but are not limited to the following:

● = Independent;   ▲ = Collaborative;   **EBN** = Evidence-Based Nursing;   **EB** = Evidence-Based

○ **Home Safety.** Identify the need for and use of common safety measures in the home. EB: *An RCT of an injury prevention briefing designed to improve fire safety found numerous risk factors for falls, poisonings, and scalds. Families in the intervention arm were less likely to report match play and more likely to report bedtime fire safety routines (Kendrick et al, 2017).*

○ **Food Safety.** Instruct client to avoid microbial foodborne illness by storing and cooking food at the proper temperature; regularly washing hands, food contact surfaces, and fruits and vegetables; and monitoring expiration dates. EBN: *A qualitative study of 10 households found that all took risks in terms of not following recommended practices with respect to best practices and that the logic behind food practices was often faulty (Dickinson et al, 2014).*

• Teach clients to assess their homes for potential environmental health hazards in the home, including risks related to structure, moisture/mold, fire, pets, electrical, ventilation, pests, and lifestyle. CEB: *The housing-based hazard index (HHI) is a measure of overall home hazards with good reliability and validity and the ability to discriminate between healthy and nonhealthy homes (N = 643) (Nriagu et al, 2012).*

• See care plans **Contamination,** Risk for **Contamination,** Risk for **Falls,** Risk for **Infection,** and Risk for **Injury.**

H

REFERENCES

Dickinson, A., Wills, W., Meah, A., et al. (2014). Food safety and older people: The kitchen life study. *British Journal of Community Nursing, 19,* 226–232. Retrieved from http://dx.doi.org/10.12968/bjcn.2014.19.5.226.

Douglas, A. M., Letts, L. J., Richardson, J. A., et al. (2013). Validity of predischarge measures for predicting time to harm in older adults. *Canadian Journal of Occupational Therapy, 80,* 19–27. Retrieved from http://dx.doi.org/10.1177/0008417412473577.

Ingram, J. C., Deave, T., Towner, E., et al. (2012). Identifying facilitators and barriers for home injury prevention interventions for pre-school children: A systematic review of the quantitative literature. *Health Education Research, 27,* 258–268. Retrieved from http://dx.doi.org/10.1093/her/cyr066.

Kamei, T., Kajii, F., Yamamoto, Y., et al. (2015). Effectiveness of a home hazard modification program for reducing falls in urban community-dwelling older adults: A randomized controlled trial. *Japan Journal of Nursing Science, 12,* 184–197. Retrieved from http://dx.doi.org/10.1111/jjns.12059.

Keall, M. D., Pierse, N., Howden-Chapman, P., et al. (2014). Home modifications to reduce injuries from falls in the Home Injury Prevention Intervention (HIPI) study: A cluster-randomised controlled trial. *Lancet, 385,* 231–238. Retrieved from http://dx.doi.org/10.1016/S0140-6736(14)61006-0.

Kelly, A. J., Fausset, C. B., Rogers, W., et al. (2014). Responding to home maintenance challenge scenarios: The role of selection, optimization, and compensation in aging-in-place. *Journal of Applied Gerontology, 33,* 1018–1042. Retrieved from http://dx.doi.org/10.1177/0733464812456631.

Kendrick, D., Young, B., Mason-Jones, A. J., et al. (2013). Home safety education and provision of safety equipment for injury prevention. *Evidence-based Child Health: A Cochrane Review Journal, 8,* 761–939. Retrieved from http://dx.doi.org/10.1002/ebch.1911.

Kendrick, D., Ablewhite, J., Achana, F., et al. (2017). Keeping Children Safe: A multicentre programme of research to increase the evidence base for preventing unintentional injuries in the home in the under-fives. *NIHR Journals Library, 2017*(7).

Lawang, W., Horey, D., Blackford, J., et al. (2013). Support interventions for caregivers of physically disabled adults: A systematic review. *Nursing & Health Sciences, 15,* 534–545. Retrieved from http://dx.doi.org/10.1111/nhs.12063.

MacLeod, A., Skinner, M. W., & Low, E. (2012). Supporting hospice volunteers and caregivers through community-based participatory research. *Health and Social Care in the Community, 20,* 190–198. Retrieved from http://dx.doi.org/10.1111/j.1365-2524.2011.01030.x.

Nriagu, J., Martin, J., Smith, P., et al. (2012). Residential hazards, high asthma prevalence and multimorbidity among children in Saginaw, Michigan. *Science of the Total Environment, 416,* 53–61. Retrieved from http://dx.doi.org/10.1016/j.scitotenv.2011.10.040.

Peek, S. T., Wouters, E. J., Luijkx, K. G., et al. (2016). What it takes to successfully implement technology for aging in place: Focus groups with stakeholders. *Journal of Medical Internet Research, 18*(5), e98. Retrieved from http://dx.doi.org/10.2196/jmir.5253.

Schwebel, D. C., Roth, D. L., Elliott, M. N., et al. (2012). Marital conflict and fifth-graders' risk for injury. *Accident, Analysis and Prevention, 47,* 30–35. Retrieved from http://dx.doi.org/10.1016/j.aap.2012.01.005.

Shields, W. C., Perry, E. C., Szanton, S. L., et al. (2013). Knowledge and injury prevention practices in homes of older adults. *Geriatric Nursing, 34,* 19–24. Retrieved from http://dx.doi.org/10.1016/j.gerinurse.2012.06.010.

Szanton, S. L., Roth, J., Nkimbeng, M., et al. (2014). Improving unsafe environments to support aging independence with limited resources. *Nursing Clinics of North America, 49,* 133–145. Retrieved from http://dx.doi.org/10.1016/j.cnur.2014.02.002.

Szanton, S. L., Leff, B., Wolff, J. L., et al. (2016). Home-based care program reduces disability and promotes aging in place. *Health Affairs, 35,* 1558–1563. Retrieved from http://dx.doi.org/10.1377/hlthaff.2016.0140.

Turcotte, D. A., Alker, H., Chaves, E., et al. (2014). Healthy homes: In-home environmental asthma intervention in a diverse urban community. *American Journal of Public Health, 104,* 665–671. Retrieved from http://dx.doi.org/10.2105/AJPH.2013.301695.

Vellone, E., D'Agostino, F., Buck, H. G., et al. (2014). The key role of caregiver confidence in the caregiver's contribution to self-care in adults with heart failure. *European Journal of Cardiovascular Nursing, 15,* 372–381. Retrieved from http://dx.doi.org/10.1177/1474515114547649.

Whiting, M. (2014). Support requirements of parents caring for a child with disability and complex health needs. *Nursing Children and Young People, 26*(4), 24–27. Retrieved from http://dx.doi.org/10.7748/ncyp2014.05.26.4.24.e389.

Readiness for enhanced Hope *Marina Martinez-Kratz, MS, RN, CNE*

NANDA-I

Definition

A pattern of expectations and desires for mobilizing energy on one's own behalf, which can be strengthened.

Defining Characteristics

Expresses desire to enhance ability to set achievable goals; expresses desire to enhance belief in possibilities; expresses desire to enhance congruency of expectations with goal; expresses desire to enhance connectedness with others; expresses desire to enhance hope; expresses desire to enhance problem solving to meet goal; expresses desire to enhance sense of meaning in life; expresses desire to enhance spirituality

NOC (Nursing Outcomes Classification)

Suggested NOC Outcomes

Hope; Quality of Life

> **Example NOC Outcome with Indicators**
>
> **Hope** as evidenced by the following indicators: Expresses expectation of a positive future/Expresses faith/Expresses meaning in life/Exhibits a zest for life/Sets goals. (Rate the outcome and indicators of **Hope:** 1 = never demonstrated, 2 = rarely demonstrated, 3 = sometimes demonstrated, 4 = often demonstrated, 5 = consistently demonstrated [see Section I].)

Client Outcomes

Client Will (Specify Time Frame)

- Describe values, expectations, and meanings
- Set achievable goals that are consistent with values
- Design strategies to achieve goals
- Express belief in possibilities

NIC (Nursing Interventions Classification)

Suggested NIC Interventions

Emotional Support; Hope Inspiration; Presence; Support System Enhancement

> **Example NIC Activities—Hope Inspiration**
>
> Assist client and family to identify areas of hope in life; Demonstrate hope by recognizing the client's intrinsic worth; Encourage therapeutic relationships; Help the person expand spiritual self

Nursing Interventions and *Rationales*

- Spend one-on-one time with the client. Use empathy; try to understand what the client is saying and communicate this understanding to the client to create a nonjudgmental trusting environment to develop therapeutic relationships with the client. **EB:** *Patient ratings of the therapeutic relationship predicted social inclusion through hopefulness (Berry & Greenwood, 2015).*
- Assist clients to identify sources of gratitude in their lives using a future-oriented focus. **CEB:** *Research shows that clients with a regulatory focus of promotion were more likely to express gratitude, which inspired them to strengthen their relationships with helpful and responsive partners (Mathews & Shook, 2013).*
- Assist families to identify sources of gratitude in their lives. **CEB:** *Research showed that gratitude fostered all facets of posttraumatic growth, such as relationships, personal strengths, and awareness of meaningful possibilities (Ruini & Vescovelli, 2013).*
- Screen the client for hope using a valid and reliable instrument as indicated. **CEB:** *The HHI is a brief instrument with good psychometric properties that has been developed for clinical use. It has been designed*

• = Independent;   ▲ = Collaborative;   **EBN** = Evidence-Based Nursing;   **EB** = Evidence-Based

to facilitate the examination of hope at various intervals so that changes in levels of hope can be identified (Hunsaker et al, 2016).

- Focus on the positive aspects of hope. EBN: *An integrative study found that when an institution provides a positive context, it promotes hope (e.g., sets goals, generates pathways, sustains motivation) in attaining educational objectives for college students (Griggs, 2017).*
- Assist the client to develop positive expectations outcomes and recognize the pathways to achieve the positive outcomes. EB: *Research findings suggest that lack of positive expectations account for the relationship between hopelessness and future depression and suicidal behavior among adolescents (Horwitz et al, 2017).*
- Explore the meanings, functions, objects, sources, and nature of hope with patients as relates to their current situation. EBN: *A better understanding of the patient's meaning of hope can assist nurses to foster hope and provide better support (Marco, Pérez, & García-Alandete, 2016).*
- Teach individuals how to become aware of attention that is focused on unwanted aspects of life and how to redirect attention toward things that feel more wanted or desired by using a future-directed approach. CEB: *Future-directed therapy is effective at decreasing hopelessness and increases positive future expectations (Vilhauer et al, 2013).*
- Review the client's strengths and resources in conjunction with the client. EBN: *A strengths-based perspective support group intervention reduced the participants' level of depressive symptoms and improved the pathway component of hope (Hou, Ko, & Shu, 2016).*
- Assist the client to consider alternatives and set long- and short-term goals that are important to him or her. EBN: *A mixed-method thematic review found that setting and achieving goals was a theme that increased hope (Broadhurst & Harrington, 2016).*
- Encourage engagement in positive and pleasant events. EB: *This study found that targeting both hopelessness and engagement in pleasant events may be helpful in improving the quality of life of vulnerable, rural, older adults (Scogin et al, 2015).*
- Facilitate sources of the client's resilience. CEB: *Higher levels of resilience were associated with lower levels of hopelessness in children of HIV-positive parents (Mo et al, 2014).*
- Implement social supports and reintegration programs for postdeployment soldiers and veterans in a timely fashion. EB: *Research determined that hopelessness was moderated by timely implementation of postdeployment support and reintegration programs (Martin et al, 2016).*
- Encourage the client to adopt active coping strategies. EB: *In the current study, proactive coping predicted hope regardless of severity of spinal cord injury (Phillips et al, 2016).*
- Identify spiritual beliefs and practices. CEB: *Spirituality was identified as a factor in increasing hope in clients with mental illness (Schrank et al, 2012).*

Home Care

- The previously mentioned interventions may be adapted for home care use.

Client/Family Teaching and Discharge Planning

- Teach alternative coping strategies such as physical activity. CEB: *Clients with severe mental illness showed decreased hopelessness after participation in an adjunct exercise program (Sylvia et al, 2013).*
- ▲ Refer the client to self-help groups. EB: *Support groups provided an experience of community in which hope was encouraged (Behler et al, 2017).*
- Use a family-centered approach to provide information regarding the client's condition, treatment plan, and progress. EBN: *Clients reported increased hope after a planned family-centered discharge process (Ingram et al, 2017).*
- Offer emotional support, active listening, and coping assistance to client families. EBN: *Family hopelessness is addressed when nurses offer emotional support (Coco et al, 2013).*

REFERENCES

Behler, J., Daniels, A., Scott, J., et al. (2017). Depression/bipolar peer support groups: Perceptions of group members about effectiveness and differences from other mental health services. *The Qualitative Report, 22*(1), 213–236. Retrieved from http://proxy.lib.umich.edu/login?url=https://search-proquest-com.proxy.lib.umich.edu/docview/1867929972?accountid=14667.

Berry, C., & Greenwood, K. (2015). Hope-inspiring therapeutic relationships, professional expectations and social inclusion for young people with psychosis. *Schizophrenia Research, 168*(1–2), 153–160. doi:10.1016/j.schres.2015.07.032.

Broadhurst, K., & Harrington, A. (2016). A mixed method thematic review: The importance of hope to the dying patient. *Journal of Advanced Nursing, 72*(1), 18–32. doi:10.1111/jan.12765.

● = Independent; ▲ = Collaborative; EBN = Evidence-Based Nursing; EB = Evidence-Based

Coco, K., Tossavainen, K., Jääskeläinen, J., et al. (2013). The provision of emotional support to the families of traumatic brain injury patients: Perspectives of Finnish nurses. *Journal of Clinical Nursing, 22*(9/10), 1467–1476.

Griggs, S. (2017). Hope and mental health in young adult college students: An integrative review. *Journal of Psychosocial Nursing & Mental Health Services, 55*(2), 28–35. doi:10.3928/02793695 -20170210-04.

Horwitz, A. G., Berona, J., Czyz, E. K., et al. (2017). Positive and negative expectations of hopelessness as longitudinal predictors of depression, suicidal ideation, and suicidal behavior in high-risk adolescents. *Suicide and Life-Threatening Behavior, 47*, 168–176. doi:10.1111/sltb.12273.

Hou, W. L., Ko, N. Y., & Shu, B. C. (2016). Effects of a strengths-based perspective support group among Taiwanese women who left a violent intimate partner relationship. *Journal of Clinical Nursing, 25*, 543–554. doi:10.1111/jocn.13091.

Hunsaker, A. E., Terhorst, L., Gentry, A., et al. (2016). Measuring hope among families impacted by cognitive impairment. *Dementia (Basel, Switzerland), 15*(4), 596–608. doi:10.1177/1471301214531590.

Ingram, J., Redshaw, M., Manns, S., et al. (2017). "Giving us hope": Parent and neonatal staff views and expectations of a planned family-centred discharge process (Train-to-Home). *Health Expectations, 20*, 751–759. doi:10.1111/hex.12514.

Marco, J. H., Pérez, S., & García-Alandete, J. (2016). Meaning in life buffers the association between risk factors for suicide and hopelessness in participants with mental disorders. *Journal of Clinical Psychology, 72*, 689–700. doi:10.1002/jclp.22285.

Martin, R. L., Houtsma, C., Green, B. A., et al. (2016). Support systems: How post-deployment support impacts suicide risk factors in the United States Army National Guard. *Cognitive Therapy and*

Research, 40(14), Retrieved from https://doi-org.proxy.lib .umich.edu/10.1007/s10608-015-9719-z.

Mathews, M. A., & Shook, N. J. (2013). Promoting or preventing thanks: Regulatory focus and its effect on gratitude and indebtedness. *Journal of Research in Personality, 47*, 191–195.

Mo, P. H., Lau, J. F., Yu, X., et al. (2014). The role of social support on resilience, posttraumatic growth, hopelessness, and depression among children of HIV-infected parents in mainland China. *AIDS Care, 26*(12), 1526–1533.

Phillips, B. N., Smedema, S. M., Fleming, A. R., et al. (2016). Mediators of disability and hope for people with spinal cord injury. *Disability and Rehabilitation, 38*(17), 1672–1683. doi:10.3109/09638288.2015. 1107639.

Ruini, C., & Vescovelli, F. (2013). The role of gratitude in breast cancer: Its relationships with post-traumatic growth, psychological well-being and distress. *Journal of Happiness Studies, 14*, 263–274.

Schrank, B., et al. (2012). Determinants, self-management strategies and interventions for hope in people with mental disorders: Systematic search and narrative review. *Social Science and Medicine, 74*(4), 554–564.

Scogin, F., Morthland, M., DiNapoli, E. A., et al. (2015). Pleasant events, hopelessness, and quality of life in rural older adults. *The Journal of Rural Health, 32*, 102–109. doi:10.1111/jrh.12130.

Sylvia, L., Kopeski, L., Brown, C., et al. (2013). An adjunct exercise program for serious mental illness: Who chooses to participate and is it feasible? *Community Mental Health Journal, 49*(2), 213–219.

Vilhauer, J. S., Cortes, J., Moali, N., et al. (2013). Improving quality of life for patients with major depressive disorder by increasing hope and positive expectations with future directed therapy (FDT). *Innovations in Clinical Neuroscience, 10*(3), 12–22.

Hopelessness   *Marina Martinez-Kratz, MS, RN, CNE*

NANDA-I

Definition

Subjective state in which an individual sees limited or no alternatives or personal choices available and is unable to mobilize energy on own behalf.

Defining Characteristics

Alteration in sleep pattern; decrease in affect; decrease in appetite; decrease in initiative; decrease in response to stimuli; decrease in verbalization; despondent verbal cue; inadequate involvement in care; passivity; poor eye contact; shrugging in response to speaker; turning away from speaker

Related Factors

Chronic stress; loss of belief in spiritual power; loss of belief in transcendent values; prolonged activity restriction; social isolation

At-Risk Population

History of abandonment

Associated Condition

Deterioration in physiological condition

• = Independent;   ▲ = Collaborative;   EBN = Evidence-Based Nursing;   EB = Evidence-Based

(Nursing Outcomes Classification)

Suggested NOC Outcomes

Decision-Making; Hope; Mood Equilibrium; Nutritional Status: Food and Fluid Intake; Quality of Life; Sleep

Example NOC Outcome with Indicators
Has a presence of **Hope** as evidenced by the following indicators: Expresses expectation of a positive future/Expresses faith/Expresses will to live. (Rate the outcome and indicators of **Hope:** 1 = never demonstrated, 2 = rarely demonstrated, 3 = sometimes demonstrated, 4 = often demonstrated, 5 = consistently demonstrated [see Section I].)

Client Outcomes

Client Will (Specify Time Frame)

- Verbalize feelings
- Participate in care
- Make positive statements (e.g., "I can" or "I will try")
- Set goals
- Make eye contact, focus on speaker
- Maintain appropriate appetite for age and physical health
- Sleep appropriate length of time for age and physical health
- Express concern for another
- Initiate activity

NIC (Nursing Interventions Classification)

Suggested NIC Intervention

Hope Inspiration

Example NIC Activities—Hope Inspiration
Assist client/family to identify areas of hope in life; Demonstrate hope by recognizing client's intrinsic worth and viewing client's illness as only one facet of the individual; Expand the client's repertoire of coping mechanisms

Nursing Interventions and *Rationales*

- ▲ Assess for, monitor, and document the potential for suicide. (Refer the client for appropriate treatment if a potential for suicide is identified.) Refer to the care plan Risk for **Suicide** for specific interventions. CEB: *In this study of men who had attempted suicide, hopelessness was identified as an important risk factor; thus it is important that it is identified by nurses (Hinkkurinen, Isola, & Kylmä, 2011).*
- ▲ Assess and monitor potential for depression. (Refer the client for appropriate treatment if depression is identified.) CEB: *Hopelessness is a potential predictor for depressive and suicidal symptoms (Wang et al, 2013).*
- ▲ Assess for hopelessness with the modified Beck Hopelessness Scale. CEB: *The modified Beck Hopelessness Scale is a valid and reliable tool to measure hopelessness (Fisher & Overholser, 2013).*
- ● Assess and monitor family caregivers for symptoms of hopelessness. EBN: *Adult daughter caregivers experience hopelessness as part of compassion fatigue (Day, Anderson, & Davis, 2014). Significant correlations were found between hopelessness and coping strategies with a positive correlation between hopelessness and the helpless approaches (Tokem, Ozcelik, & Cicik, 2015).*
- ● Assess for pain and respond with appropriate measures for pain relief. EB: *In the present study, hopelessness played a central role in the relationship between pain and depression with pain intensity positively related to hopelessness (Hülsebusch, Hasenbring, & Rusu, 2016).*
- ● Facilitate sources of the client's resilience. CEB: *Higher levels of resilience were associated with lower levels of hopelessness in children of HIV-positive parents (Mo et al, 2014).*
- ● Assist the adolescent client to develop positive expectations. EB: *Research findings suggest that lack of positive expectations account for the relationship between hopelessness and future depression and suicidal behavior among adolescents (Horwitz et al, 2017).*

● = Independent; ▲ = Collaborative; EBN = Evidence-Based Nursing; EB = Evidence-Based

- Assist the client to explore the meaning of his or her life, satisfaction with his or her life, and life goals. EB: *Research shows that a higher meaning of life buffers the association between suicide risk factors and hopelessness (Marco, Pérez, & García-Alandete, 2016).*
- Encourage adolescent clients to get 9 to 10 hours of sleep nightly. EB: *Research shows that among adolescents, as little as 1 hour less of weekday sleep was associated with significantly greater odds of feeling hopeless (Winsler et al, 2015).*
- Assist the client in looking at alternatives and setting long- and short-term goals that are important to him or her. EBN: *A mixed-method thematic review found that setting and achieving goals was a theme that increased hope (Broadhurst & Harrington, 2016).*
- Explore the meanings, functions, objects, sources, and nature of hope with patients as relates to their current situation. EBN: *A better understanding of the patient's meaning of hope can assist nurses to foster hope and provide better support (Marco et al, 2016).*
- Spend one-on-one time with the client. Use empathy; try to understand what the client is saying and communicate this understanding to the client to create a nonjudgmental trusting environment to develop therapeutic relationships with the client. EB: *Patient ratings of the therapeutic relationship predicted social inclusion through hopefulness (Berry & Greenwood, 2015).*
- Teach alternative coping strategies such as physical activity. CEB: *Clients with severe mental illness showed decreased hopelessness after participation in an adjunct exercise program (Sylvia et al, 2013).*
- Use a future-directed approach that teaches individuals how to become aware of attention that is focused on unwanted aspects of life and how to redirect attention toward things that feel more wanted or desired. CEB: *Future-directed therapy is effective at decreasing hopelessness and increases positive future expectations (Vilhauer et al, 2013).*
- Review the client's strengths and resources in conjunction with the client. EBN: *A strengths-based perspective support group intervention reduced the participants' level of depressive symptoms and improved the pathway component of hope (Hou, Ko, & Shu, 2016).*
- Encourage the client to adopt active coping strategies. EB: *In a current study, proactive coping predicted hope regardless of severity of spinal cord injury (Phillips et al, 2016).*
- Offer emotional support, active listening, and coping assistance to client families. EBN: *Family hopelessness is addressed when nurses offer emotional support (Coco et al, 2013).*
- Implement social supports and reintegration programs for postdeployment soldiers and veterans in a timely fashion. EB: *Research determined that hopelessness was moderated by timely implementation of postdeployment support and reintegration programs (Martin et al, 2016).*
- For additional interventions, see the care plans for Readiness for enhanced **Hope, Spiritual** distress, Readiness for enhanced **Spiritual** well-being, and Disturbed **Sleep** pattern.

Geriatric

- Previous interventions may be adapted for geriatric clients.
- ▲ If depression is suspected, confer with the primary health care provider regarding referral for mental health services. EB: *This study of older adults found that hopelessness was a significant predictor of death ideation (Guidry & Cukrowicz, 2016).*
- Take threats of self-harm or suicide seriously and intervene as needed. EB: *This study of older adults identified hopelessness as a significant predictor of death ideation (Guidry & Cukrowicz, 2016). Older adults have the highest risk of death by suicide in the United States (Fond et al, 2016).*
- Encourage engagement in positive and pleasant events. EB: *This study found that targeting both hopelessness and engagement in pleasant events may be helpful in improving the quality of life of vulnerable, rural older adults (Scogin et al, 2015).*

Multicultural

- Assess for the influence of cultural beliefs, norms, and values on the client's feelings of hopelessness. CEB: *In some Latino cultures, talking about depression (depresión) may be taboo. Hopelessness (desanimo) may be understood differently by clients of various cultural backgrounds and may have a more normative and culturally specific, comfortable sound for clients (Marsiglia et al, 2011).*
- Assess for the effect of fatalism on the client's expression of hopelessness. EBN: *A systemic review of qualitative studies found that fatalistic perspectives were common among the cancer beliefs held by ethnic minority populations (Licqurish et al, 2017).*

● = Independent;   ▲ = Collaborative;   EBN = Evidence-Based Nursing;   EB = Evidence-Based

- Use caution when highlighting health disparities of multicultural populations through public health campaigns and media broadcasts. **EB:** This study found that media campaigns that broadcasted health disparities resulted in the targeted population feeling less hopeful about the future (Lee et al, 2017).
- Encourage spirituality as a source of support for hopelessness. **EB:** Structural equation modeling indicated that Malaysian adolescent students were high in hopelessness and depression, but were also high in spirituality and had less suicidal behavior than others (Talib & Abdollahi, 2017).

Home Care

- Previously mentioned interventions may be adapted for home care use.
- Use in-person problem-solving therapy (PST) to address depressive symptoms and hopelessness. **EB:** In-person PST reduced depressive symptoms and alleviated hopelessness in older homebound adults. PST focused on the participants' appraisal of specific problems, identification of the best possible solutions, and the practical implementation of those solutions (Choi, Marti, & Conwell, 2016).

Client/Family Teaching and Discharge Planning

- Provide information regarding the client's condition, treatment plan, and progress. **EBN:** *Clients reported increased hope after a planned family-centered discharge process(Ingram et al, 2017).*
- ▲ Refer the client to self-help groups. **EB:** *Support groups provided an experience of community in which hope was encouraged (Behler et al, 2017).*

H

REFERENCES

Behler, J., Daniels, A., Scott, J., et al. (2017). Depression/bipolar peer support groups: Perceptions of group members about effectiveness and differences from other mental health services. *The Qualitative Report*, 22(1), 213–236. Retrieved from http://proxy.lib.umich.edu/login?url=https://search-proquest-com.proxy.lib.umich.edu/docview/1867929972?accountid=14667.

Berry, C., & Greenwood, K. (2015). Hope-inspiring therapeutic relationships, professional expectations and social inclusion for young people with psychosis. *Schizophrenia Research*, 168(1–2), 153–160. doi:10.1016/j.schres.2015.07.032.

Broadhurst, K., & Harrington, A. (2016). A mixed method thematic review: The importance of hope to the dying patient. *Journal of Advanced Nursing*, 72(1), 18–32. doi:10.1111/jan.12765.

Choi, N. G., Marti, C. N., & Conwell, Y. (2016). Effect of problem-solving therapy on depressed low-income homebound older adults' death/suicidal ideation and hopelessness. *Suicide Life Threat Behavior*, 46, 323–336. doi:10.1111/sltb.12195.

Coco, K., Tossavainen, K., Jääskeläinen, J., et al. (2013). The provision of emotional support to the families of traumatic brain injury patients: Perspectives of Finnish nurses. *Journal of Clinical Nursing*, 22(9/10), 1467–1476.

Day, J. R., Anderson, R. A., & Davis, L. L. (2014). Compassion fatigue in adult daughter caregivers of a parent with dementia. *Issues in Mental Health Nursing*, 35(10), 796–804.

Fisher, L. B., & Overholser, J. C. (2013). Refining the assessment of hopelessness: An improved way to look to the future. *Death Studies*, 37(3), 212–227.

Fond, G., et al. (2016). Disparities in suicide mortality trends between United States of America and 25 European countries: Retrospective analysis of WHO mortality database. *Scientific Reports*, 6, 20256. doi:10.1038/srep20256.

Guidry, E. T., & Cukrowicz, K. C. (2016). Death ideation in older adults: Psychological symptoms of depression, thwarted belongingness, and perceived burdensomeness. *Aging & Mental Health*, 20(8), 823–830. doi:10.1080/13607863.2015.1040721.

Hinkkurinen, J., Isola, A., & Kylmä, J. (2011). Experiences of self-destruction and related hopelessness in men who have attempted suicide [Finnish]. *Hoitotiede*, 23(3), 230–239.

Horwitz, A. G., Berona, J., Czyz, E. K., et al. (2017). Positive and negative expectations of hopelessness as longitudinal predictors of depression, suicidal ideation, and suicidal behavior in high-risk adolescents. *Suicide and Life-Threatening Behavior*, 47, 168–176. doi:10.1111/sltb.12273.

Hou, W. L., Ko, N. Y., & Shu, B. C. (2016). Effects of a strengths-based perspective support group among Taiwanese women who left a violent intimate partner relationship. *Journal of Clinical Nursing*, 25, 543–554. doi:10.1111/jocn.13091.

Hülsebusch, J., Hasenbring, M. I., & Rusu, A. C. (2016). Understanding pain and depression in back pain: The role of catastrophizing, help-/hopelessness, and thought suppression as potential mediators. *International Journal of Behavavioral Medicine*, 23, 251. doi:10.1007/s12529-015-9522-y.

Ingram, J., Redshaw, M., Manns, S., et al. (2017). "Giving us hope": Parent and neonatal staff views and expectations of a planned family-centred discharge process (Train-to-Home). *Health Expectations*, 20, 751–759. doi:10.1111/hex.12514.

Lee, J. G. L., Landrine, H., Martin, R. J., et al. (2017). Reasons for caution when emphasizing health disparities for sexual and gender minority adults in public health campaigns. *American Journal of Public Health*, 107(8), 1223–1225.

Licqurish, S., Phillipson, L., Chiang, P., et al. (2017). Cancer beliefs in ethnic minority populations: A review and meta-synthesis of qualitative studies. *European Journal of Cancer Care*, 26, e12556. doi:10.1111/ecc.12556.

Marco, J. H., Pérez, S., & García-Alandete, J. (2016). Meaning in life buffers the association between risk factors for suicide and hopelessness in participants with mental disorders. *Journal of Clinical Psychology*, 72, 689–700. doi:10.1002/jclp.22285.

Marsiglia, F. F., Kulis, S., Garcia Perez, H., et al. (2011). Hopelessness, family stress, and depression among Mexican-heritage mothers in the southwest. *Health & Social Work*, 36(1), 7–18. doi:10.1093/hsw/36.1.7.

Martin, R. L., Houtsma, C., Green, B. A., et al. (2016). Support systems: How post-deployment support impacts suicide risk factors in the United States Army National Guard. *Cognitive Therapy and Research*, 40(14). doi:10.1007/s10608-015-9719-z.

Mo, P. H., Lau, J. F., Yu, X., et al. (2014). The role of social support on resilience, posttraumatic growth, hopelessness, and depression among children of HIV-infected parents in mainland China. *AIDS Care*, 26(12), 1526–1533.

● = Independent;   ▲ = Collaborative;   **EBN** = Evidence-Based Nursing;   **EB** = Evidence-Based

Phillips, B. N., Smedema, S. M., Fleming, A. R., et al. (2016). Mediators of disability and hope for people with spinal cord injury. *Disability and Rehabilitation*, 38(17), 1672–1683. doi:10.3109/09638288.2015.1107639.

Scogin, F., Morthland, M., DiNapoli, E. A., et al. (2015). Pleasant events, hopelessness, and quality of life in rural older adults. *The Journal of Rural Health*, 32, 102–109. doi:10.1111/jrh.12130.

Sylvia, L., Kopeski, L., Brown, C., et al. (2013). An adjunct exercise program for serious mental illness: Who chooses to participate and is it feasible? *Community Mental Health Journal*, 49(2), 213–219.

Talib, M. A., & Abdollahi, A. (2017). Spirituality moderates hopelessness, depression, and suicidal behavior among Malaysian adolescents. *Journal of Religion and Health*, 56, 784. doi:10.1007/s10943-015-0133-3.

Tokem, Y., Ozcelik, H., & Cicik, A. (2015). Examination of the relationship between hopelessness levels and coping strategies among the family caregivers of patients with cancer. *Cancer Nursing*, 38, E28–E34. doi:10.1097/NCC.0000000000000189.

Vilhauer, J. S., Cortes, J., Moali, N., et al. (2013). Improving quality of life for patients with major depressive disorder by increasing hope and positive expectations with future directed therapy (FDT). *Innovations In Clinical Neuroscience*, 10(3), 12–22.

Wang, L., Liu, L., Shi, S., et al. (2013). Cognitive trio: Relationship with major depression and clinical predictors in Han Chinese women. *Psychological Medicine*, 43(11), 2265–2275.

Winsler, A., Deutsch, A., Vorona, R. D., et al. (2015). Sleepless in Fairfax: The difference one more hour of sleep can make for teen hopelessness, suicidal ideation, and substance use. *Journal of Youth and Adolescence*, 44, 362. doi:10.1007/s10964-014-0170-3.

H

Risk for compromised Human Dignity
Shari D. Froelich, DNP, MSN, MSBA, ANP-BC, ACHPN, PMHNP-BC

NANDA-I

Definition

Susceptible for perceived loss of respect and honor, which may compromise health.

Risk Factors

Cultural incongruence; dehumanizing treatment; disclosure of confidential information; exposure of the body; humiliation; insufficient comprehension of health information; intrusion by clinician; invasion of privacy; limited decision-making experience; loss of control over body function; stigmatization

NOC   (Nursing Outcomes Classification)

Suggested NOC Outcomes

Health Beliefs: Perceived Control; Decision-Making; Spiritual Control; Perceived Social Support

Example NOC Outcome with Indicators

Health Beliefs: Perceived Control as evidenced by the following indicators: Perceived responsibility for health decisions/Requested involvement in health decisions/Efforts at gathering information/Belief that own decisions control health outcomes/Willingness to designate surrogate decision maker. (Rate the outcome and indicators of **Health Beliefs: Perceived Control:** 1 = very weak, 2 = weak, 3 = moderate, 4 = strong, 5 = very strong [see Section I].)

Client-Based Outcome

Client/Caregiver Will (Specify Time Frame)

- Perceive that dignity is maintained throughout hospitalization/encounter
- Consistently call client by name of choice
- Maintain client's privacy

NIC   (Nursing Interventions Classification)

Suggested NIC Interventions

Presence; Decision-Making Support; Spiritual Support; Hope Instillation

Example NIC Activities—Presence

Demonstrate accepting attitude; Listen to client's concerns

● = Independent;   ▲ = Collaborative;   EBN = Evidence-Based Nursing;   EB = Evidence-Based

Nursing Interventions and *Rationales*

- Be authentically present when with the client, try to limit extraneous thoughts of self or others, and concentrate on the well-being of the client. EBN: *Human presence never leaves one unaffected. Expressed as compassion and caring, it is not only the words that are spoken or the eyes that notice, leading to action (Manookian, Cheraghi, & Nasrabadi, 2014).*
- Enter into and stay within the other's frame of reference. Connect with the inner life world of meaning and spirit of the other. Join in a mutual search for meaning and wholeness of being and becoming to potentiate comfort measures, pain control, a sense of well-being, wholeness, or even spiritual transcendence of suffering. EBN: *Human dignity is a central concept within nursing and the caring professions because it communicates the shared humanity. A shared humanity is evident anywhere in which humans interact, and because nurses are eager to actualize the healing relationship with clients, they have the opportunity to share their humanity (Manookian, Cheraghi, & Nasrabadi, 2014).*
- Determine the client's perspective about his or her health. Example questions include "Tell me about your health." "What is it like to be in your situation?" "Tell me how you perceive yourself in this situation." "What meaning are you giving to this situation?" "Tell me about your health priorities." "Tell me about the harmony you wish to reach." CEB: *Such questions usually contribute to helping people find meaning to the crisis in their life (Watson, 2008).* CEB: *Confirm the person's worthiness and sense of self. A genuine respect for the person as a unique human being, with an inherent desire or right to make choices according to his or her subjective needs, was found to be fundamental in advocating autonomy and integrity. Confirming the person's worthiness and sense of self in this way was identified as crucial in dignity preservation. To preserve personal dignity and reduce the experienced loss of freedom, autonomy, and integrity, going for frequent walks was given high priority (Tranvag, Petersen, & Naden, 2013).*
- Determine the client's preferences for when and how nursing care is needed and follow the client's guidelines if possible. *The client's autonomy must be recognized as part of dignified nursing care.* CEB: *A summary of older adults' perceptions of the most important nurse caring behaviors include knowing what they are doing, know when it's necessary to call the medical provider, treat me as an individual, give my treatments and medications on time, check my condition very closely, give my pain medication on time, know how to handle equipment, keep my family informed of my progress, and don't give up on me when I am difficult to get along with (Marini, 1999).*
- Include the client in all decision-making; if the client does not choose to be part of the decision or is no longer capable of making a decision, then use the named surrogate decision maker. *The Patient Self-Determination Act, effective in 1991, requires that all individuals receiving medical care also receive written information about their right to accept or refuse medical or surgical treatment and their right to initiate advance directives (Dossey & Keegan, 2009).*
- Maintain client's privacy at all times.
- Actively listen to what the client is saying both verbally and nonverbally. CEB: *We must quiet our "inner dialogue" so that we may hear more clearly, allow others to tell the entire story, listen without judgment or advice, and bear witness to the experience. Attentive silence is a communicative act in its own right; it is an act of compassion. It signifies respect, legitimizes what is said, and creates an atmosphere in which self-discovery can occur (Stanley, 2002).*
- Encourage the client to share thoughts about spirituality as desired. CEB: *The care of the soul remains the most powerful aspect of the art of caring in nursing. The caring occasion becomes "transpersonal" when "it allows for the presence of the spirit of both—then the event of the moment expands the limits of openness and has the ability to expand human capabilities" (Watson, 2008).*
- Use interventions to instill increased hope; see the care plan for Readiness for enhanced **Hope.** CEB: *When hope for a cure is no longer possible, help clients recognize that the relationships change between clients, families, and caregivers but do not end. Hope continues, but it has a different focus (Erlen, 2003). Caring does not end but is transformed when intensive treatment ends.*
- For further interventions on spirituality, see the care plan for Readiness for enhanced **Spiritual** well-being.

 Geriatric

- Always ask the client how he or she would like to be addressed. Avoid calling older clients "sweetie," "honey," "Gramps," or other terms that can be demeaning unless this is acceptable in the client's culture or requested by the client. *Appropriate forms of address must be used with older adults to maintain dignity.*

● = Independent;   ▲ = Collaborative;   EBN = Evidence-Based Nursing;   EB = Evidence-Based

CEB: *A respectful form of address has positive effects, whereas overfamiliarity tends to have a negative effect on self-respect, physical and mental health, and recovery from disease, particularly in older adults and those with dementia (Woolhead et al, 2006; Williams et al, 2008).*

- Treat the older client with the utmost respect, even if delirium or dementia is present with confusion. *Confused clients respond positively to caregivers who approach gently, with positive regard, and treat the confused client with respect and dignity.*

Multicultural

- Assess for the influence of cultural beliefs, norms, and values on the client's way of communicating, and follow the client's lead in communicating in matters of eye contact, amount of personal space, voice tones, and amount of touching. If in doubt, ask the client. *What the client considers normal and appropriate communication that maintains and facilitates dignity is based on cultural perceptions.* **CEB:** *Client dignity is promoted when staff provide privacy and use interactions that help clients feel comfortable, in control, and valued. Individual staff behavior has a major effect on whether threats to client dignity actually lead to its loss (Baillie, 2009).*

Home Care

- Most of the interventions described previously may be adapted for home care use.
- Recognize that the client with the caregiver has complete autonomy in the home. *The nurse's role is to provide the care needed and desired. The client and caregiver determine whether the care offered is acceptable.*

Client/Family Teaching and Discharge Planning

- Teach family and caregivers the need for the dignity of the client to be maintained at all times. How an individual cognitively perceives and emotionally deals with the illness can depend on the person's family and social relationships, and ultimately can affect the ability to heal. Note: Caring is integral to maintaining dignity. **CEB:** *According to Watson (2008), a caring occasion is the moment (focal point in space and time) when the nurse and another person come together in such a way that an occasion for human caring is created. Both the one cared for and the one caring can be influenced by the caring moment through the choices and actions decided within the relationship, influencing and becoming part of their own life history.*

REFERENCES

Baillie, L. (2009). Patient dignity in an acute care hospital setting: A case study. *International Journal of Nursing Studies, 46*, 23–37.

Dossey, B., & Keegan, L. (2009). *Holistic nursing: A handbook for practice* (5th ed.). Sudbury, MA: Jones & Bartlett.

Erlen, J. (2003). Caring doesn't end. *Orthopaedic Nursing, 22*(5), 446–449.

Manookian, A., Cheraghi, M. A., & Nasrabadi, A. N. (2014). Factors influencing patients' dignity: A qualitative study. *Nursing Ethics, 21*(3), 323–334.

Marini, B. (1999). Institutionalized older adults' perception of nursing caring behaviors: A pilot study. *Journal of Gerontological Nursing, 25*(5), 10–16.

Stanley, K. (2002). The healing power of presence: Respite from the fear of abandonment. *Oncology Nursing Forum, 39*(6), 935–940.

Tranvag, O., Petersen, K. A., & Naden, D. (2013). Dignity-preserving dementia care: A metasynthesis. *Nursing Ethics, 20*(8), 861–880.

Watson, J. (2008). *Nursing: The philosophy and science of caring.* Boulder: University Press of Colorado.

Williams, K., et al. (2008). Elderspeak communication: Impact on dementia care. *American Journal of Alzheimer's Disease and Other Dementias, 24*(1), 11–20.

Woolhead, G., et al. (2006). "Tu" or "vous"? A European qualitative study of dignity and communication with older people in health and social care settings. *Patient Education and Counseling, 61*(3), 363–371.

Neonatal Hyperbilirubinemia
Original author David Wilson, MS, RNC; revised by Barbara J. Wheeler, RN, BN, MN, IBCLC

NANDA-I

Definition

The accumulation of unconjugated bilirubin in the circulation (<15 mL/dL; <257 µmol/L) that occurs after 24 hours of life.

- = Independent; ▲ = Collaborative; EBN = Evidence-Based Nursing; EB = Evidence-Based

Defining Characteristics

Abnormal blood profile; bruised skin; yellow mucous membranes; yellow sclera; yellow-orange skin color

Related Factors

Deficient feeding pattern; delay in meconium passage; infants with inadequate nutrition

At-Risk Population

ABO incompatibility; age ≤7 days; American Indian ethnicity; blood type incompatibility between mother and infant; East Asian ethnicity; infant who is breastfed; infant with low birthweight; maternal diabetes mellitus; population living at high altitudes; premature infant; previous sibling with jaundice; rhesus (Rh) incompatibility; significant bruising during birth

Associated Condition

Bacterial infection; infant with liver malfunction; infant with enzyme deficiency; internal bleeding; prenatal infection; sepsis; viral infection

H

NOC   (Nursing Outcomes Classification)

Suggested NOC Outcomes

Breastfeeding Establishment: Infant; Breastfeeding Maintenance; Bowel Elimination; Parent: Knowledge: Parenting/Infant Care; Risk Detection/Control

Example NOC Outcome with Indicators
Breastfeeding Establishment: Infant as evidenced by the following indicators: Proper alignment and latch-on/Proper areolar grasp/Proper areolar compression/Correct suck and tongue placement/Audible swallow/Minimum eight feedings per day/ Urinations per day appropriate for age/Weight gain appropriate for age. (Rate the outcome and indicators of **Breastfeeding Establishment: Infant:** 1 = not adequate, 2 = slightly adequate, 3 = moderately adequate, 4 = substantially adequate, 5 = totally adequate [see Section I].)

Client Outcomes

Client (Infant) Will (Specify Time Frame)

- Establish effective feeding pattern (breast or bottle)
- Receive bilirubin assessment and screening within the first few days of life to identify potentially harmful levels of serum bilirubin
- Receive appropriate therapy to enhance indirect bilirubin excretion
- Receive nursing assessments to determine risk for severity of jaundice
- Maintain hydration: moist buccal membranes, four to six wet diapers in a 24-hour period, weight loss no greater than 10% of birth weight
- Evacuate stool within 48 hours of birth, and pass three or four stools per 24 hours by day 4 of life

Client (Parent[s]) Will (Specify Time Frame)

- Receive information on neonatal jaundice prior to discharge from birth hospital
- Verbalize understanding of physical signs of jaundice prior to discharge
- Verbalize signs requiring immediate health practitioner notification: sleepy infant who does not awaken easily for feedings, fewer than four to six wet diapers in 24-hour period by day 4, fewer than three to four stools in 24 hours by day 4, breastfeeds fewer than eight times per day
- Demonstrate ability to operate home phototherapy unit if prescribed

NIC   (Nursing Interventions Classification)

Suggested NIC Interventions

Parent Education: Infant; Phototherapy: Neonate

• = Independent;   ▲ = Collaborative;   EBN = Evidence-Based Nursing;   EB = Evidence-Based

Review maternal and infant history for risk factors for hyperbilirubinemia (e.g., Rh or ABO incompatibility, polycythemia, sepsis, prematurity, malpresentation); Observe for signs of jaundice

Nursing Interventions and *Rationales*

- Evaluate maternal and delivery history for risk factors for neonatal jaundice (RhD, ABO, G6PD deficiency, direct Coombs). **EB:** *Assessment of maternal and neonatal risk factors that may cause jaundice is important in the detection of neonatal jaundice (Barrington & Sankaran, 2018).*
- Perform neonatal gestational age assessment once the newborn has had an initial period of interaction with mother and father. **EB:** *Infants who are born late preterm (34 to 36⁶⁄₇ weeks at birth) and early term (37 and 38⁶⁄₇ weeks at birth) are at significantly increased risk for problems related to hyperbilirubinemia, feeding problems, and hospital readmission (Reichman et al, 2015).*
- Encourage breastfeeding within the first hour of the neonate's life. **EB:** *Early feedings increase neonatal intestinal activity, and infant begins establishing intestinal flora; in addition, early breastfeeding promotes enhanced maternal confidence in breastfeeding (Flaherman & Maisels, 2017).*
- Encourage skin-to-skin mother–newborn contact shortly after delivery. **EB:** *Early skin-to-skin mother–baby contact helps promote maternal confidence in nurturing abilities, and it is correlated with improved milk supply and milk transfer (Flaherman & Maisels, 2017).*
- Assess infant's skin color at birth and every 8 hours thereafter until birth hospital discharge for the appearance of jaundice. **EB:** *Initial and ongoing neonatal skin assessment is important in the detection of jaundice (Hockenberry, Wilson, & Rodgers, 2017).* **CEB:** *Jaundice is visible when bilirubin levels reach 5 to 6 mg/dL (Blackburn, 2013), and it appears first on the face and head, then slowly advances to the trunk, arms, and lower extremities.* **CEB:** *Skin color alone is not a reliable assessment for neonatal jaundice; therefore it is important that such assessments are supported with empirical serum bilirubin measurements or trans-cutaneous bilirubin measurements when jaundice is suspected (American Academy of Pediatrics, 2004).*
- Encourage and assist mother with frequent breastfeeding. **EB:** *Increased frequency of* breastfeeding *accelerates weight gain and increases defecation frequency, reducing the severity of neonatal* hyperbilirubinemia *(Hassan, Zakerihamidi, & Boskabadi, 2018). Exclusive breastfeeding is recommended for neonatal feedings yet is associated with the development of hyperbilirubinemia and not directly as a result of the feeding substrate; perhaps, it is caused by decreased caloric intake in the first week of life and a substance in breast milk that may interfere with bilirubin excretion (Flaherman & Miasels, 2017).*
- Assist parents who choose to bottle feed their neonate. **EB:** *Adequate caloric intake is essential for the promotion of stooling and the subsequent elimination of bilirubin from the intestine; bottle-feeding parents must be helped to optimize feedings (Hockenberry & Wilson, 2015).*
- Avoid feeding supplements such as water, dextrose water, or any other milk substitutes in breastfeeding neonate. **EB:** *Supplements may act to decrease the effective establishment of breastfeeding (Flaherman & Maisels, 2017).*
- Assess neonate's stooling pattern in first 48 hours of life. *Delayed stooling may indicate inadequate breast milk intake and may further increase reabsorption of bilirubin from neonate's intestine (Hockenberry, Wilson, & Rodgers, 2017).*
- ▲ Collect and evaluate laboratory blood specimens as prescribed or per unit protocol. **EB:** *Because visual assessments of skin color alone are inadequate to determine rising levels of bilirubin, serum bilirubin measurement may be gathered to evaluate risk for pathology (Hockenberry, Wilson, & Rodgers, 2017). The purpose of monitoring, evaluating, and implementing treatment in moderate to severe cases of neonatal hyperbilirubinemia is to prevent acute bilirubin encephalopathy, which is an early acute central nervous system bilirubin toxicity that is related to the amount of unbound (indirect) bilirubin. Kernicterus describes the yellow staining of brain cells and subsequent necrosis that occurs secondary to exposure to high levels of unconjugated (indirect) bilirubin; kernicterus involves long-term, permanent central nervous system changes (Hockenberry, Wilson, & Rodgers, 2017).* **CEB:** *Bilirubin-induced neurologic dysfunction is a term used to describe the spectrum of symptoms associated with acute bilirubin encephalopathy and kernicterus (Johnson & Bhutani, 2011).*
- ▲ Monitor transcutaneous bilirubin level in jaundiced neonate per unit protocol. **EB:** *Noninvasive bilirubin monitoring is a safe and effective means for monitoring bilirubin levels and determining risk for increasing serum bilirubin levels in infants who are NOT treated with phototherapy (van den Esker-Jonker et al, 2016; Jain et al, 2017).*

• = Independent;   ▲ = Collaborative;   **EBN** = Evidence-Based Nursing;   **EB** = Evidence-Based

H

- Perform hour-specific total serum bilirubin (TSB) risk assessment before discharge from hospital or birth center and document the results. **CEB:** *The use of an hour-specific nomogram for designation of risk in healthy, late preterm, early term, and term infants, as well as clinical risk factors, may be used to determine the relative risk of rapidly increasing bilirubin levels requiring medical intervention such as phototherapy (American Academy of Pediatrics, 2004; Maisels et al, 2009). The hour-specific nomogram estimates the TSB in one of four risk zones: low risk, low intermediate risk, high intermediate risk (75th to 94th percentile), and high risk (95th percentile or greater). Infants with TSB values at or above the 75th percentile in addition to risk factors, such as preterm birth, may require medical intervention such as phototherapy (Maisels et al, 2009).*

- Monitor newborn for signs of inadequate breast milk or formula intake: dry oral mucous membranes, fewer than 4 to 6 wet diapers per 24 hours, no stool in 24 hours, and body weight loss greater than 10%. **EB:** Inadequate intake of breast milk or formula in the neonatal period has been identified as a risk factor for the development of hyperbilirubinemia (Flaherman & Maisels, 2017).

- Assess late preterm infant (born between 34 weeks and 36⅞ weeks' gestation) for ability to breastfeed successfully and adequate intake of breast milk. **EB:** Late preterm infants are at higher risk for difficulty breastfeeding and suboptimal milk intake caused by physiological immaturity; thus such infants are also at a much higher risk for severe jaundice than term counterparts (Reichman et al, 2015; Barrington & Sakaran, 2018).

- Assist mother with breastfeeding and assess latch-on. **EB:** Successful breastfeeding in the first few weeks of life is associated with decreased levels of serum bilirubin (Flaherman & Maisels, 2017).

- Encourage alternate methods for providing expressed breast milk if maternal health status is compromised, and assist mother with collection of breast milk via use of breast pump or hand expression. **EB:** Alternate feeding methods for the ingestion of breast milk may be used to enhance milk intake necessary to promote stooling and enhance bilirubin excretion (Flaherman & Maisels, 2017).

- Encourage father's participation in newborn care by changing diapers, helping position newborn for breastfeeding, and holding newborn while mother rests. **EB:** Paternal involvement in the care of the newborn helps solidify the father's role as a parent and strengthens the paternal–infant attachment process; paternal participation also helps the mother rest during the recovery from labor and delivery (Hockenberry & Wilson, 2015).

- Weigh newborn daily. **EB:** Daily weights assist in the detection of excess weight loss, which is often indicative of inadequate caloric intake (Flaherman & Maisels, 2017).

- ▲ When phototherapy is ordered, place seminude infant (diaper only) under prescribed amount of phototherapy lights. **EB:** *Phototherapy is the primary therapy used to treat mild to moderate neonatal indirect (unconjugated) hyperbilirubinemia; the infant must have a large skin surface area exposed to the light source for optimal effectiveness (Stokowski, 2011; Hockenberry, Wilson, & Rodgers, 2017).* **CEB:** *Turning the infant periodically has not been shown to reduce circulating bilirubin levels (Stokowski, 2011).*

- Protect infant's eyes from phototherapy light source with eye shields; remove eye shields periodically when infant is removed from light source for feeding and parent–infant interaction. **EB:** *Retinal damage may occur from light exposure (Bhutani, Committee on Fetus and Newborn, & American Academy of Pediatrics, 2014; Hockenberry, Wilson, & Rodgers, 2017); however, there is no evidence that removing the infant for parent–infant interaction during feedings and for brief caregiving activities prevents the effectiveness of phototherapy when the infant has mild to moderate hyperbilirubinemia (Hockenberry, Wilson, & Rodgers, 2017).*

- Monitor infant's hydration status, fluid intake, skin status, and body temperature while undergoing phototherapy. **EB:** *Transient side effects of phototherapy include increased body temperature, increased insensible water loss, increased gastrointestinal water loss (loose stools), lethargy, irritability, and poor feeding (Hockenberry, Wilson, & Rodgers, 2017).*

- ▲ Collect and evaluate laboratory blood specimens (TSB) while infant is undergoing phototherapy. **CEB:** *Transcutaneous bilirubin measurements do not provide an adequate estimate of serum bilirubin level and are not effective once phototherapy has been initiated (American Academy of Pediatrics, 2004; Hockenberry, Wilson, & Rodgers, 2017).*

- Encourage continuation of breastfeeding and brief infant care activities such as changing diapers while the infant is being treated with phototherapy; phototherapy may be interrupted for breastfeeding. **EB:** *In most cases breastfeeding is not interrupted for phototherapy; the benefits of breastfeeding exceed any potential harm (Muchowski, 2014). If the infant's oral intake with breastfeeding is inadequate, supplementation with expressed breast milk or infant formula may be recommended (Flaherman & Maisels, 2017).*

● = Independent;　▲ = Collaborative;　**EBN** = Evidence-Based Nursing;　**EB** = Evidence-Based

- Provide emotional support for parents of infants undergoing phototherapy. EB: *Separation of the infant from the mother for phototherapy disrupts parent–infant interaction and may promote parental stress and decrease the effective establishment of breastfeeding (Hockenberry, Wilson, & Rodgers, 2017).*

H

Multicultural

- Assess infants of Asian or American Indian ethnicity for early rising bilirubin levels, especially when breastfeeding. EB: *Studies have shown Asian and American Indian newborns to have higher peak serum bilirubin levels than Caucasian and African American newborns (Hockenberry, Wilson, & Rodgers, 2017).*
- Encourage early and exclusive breastfeeding among Asian and American Indian newborns. EB: *Early and exclusive breastfeeding may increase elimination of bilirubin in stool (Flaherman & Maisels, 2017).*

Client/Family Teaching and Discharge Planning

- Teach the breastfeeding mother and support persons about the appearance of jaundice (yellow or orange color of skin) after hospital or birth center discharge, and provide health care resource telephone number for parents to call for concerns related to newborn's care. CEB: *Follow-up for evaluation of jaundice and feeding may be recommended as early as within the first 48 hours of discharge, depending on newborn's age at discharge and individual risk assessment (Maisels et al, 2009).*
- Teach parents the signs of inadequate milk intake: fewer than three to four stools per day by day 4, fewer than four to six wet diapers in 24 hours, and dry oral mucous membranes; additional danger signs include a sleepy baby that does not awaken for breastfeeding or appears lethargic (decreased activity level from usual newborn pattern). EB: *Providing information about jaundice and effective breastfeeding may serve to decrease risk factors associated with increasing bilirubin levels (Flaherman & Maisels, 2017).*
- ▲ Teach parents about the importance of medical follow-up in the first several days of life for the evaluation of jaundice. CEB: *With early postpartum hospital discharge, follow-up visits may be needed as early as 48 hours post discharge for the evaluation of breastfeeding, stooling and voiding pattern (hydration), and jaundice (American Academy of Pediatrics, 2004).*
- Teach parents about the use of phototherapy (hospital or home, as prescribed), the proper use of the phototherapy equipment; feedings; and assessment of hydration, body temperature, skin status, and urine and stool output. *Provide information to the parents of the infant undergoing phototherapy to prevent misinformation about the infant's condition and treatment and to decrease parental anxiety and stress (Hockenberry & Wilson, 2015).*

Quality and Safety in Nursing

- **Client safety:** Minimizes risk of harm to client
- Knowledge: Nurses continually assess newborns for risk factors associated with the development of jaundice
- Skills: Nurses use transcutaneous and serum bilirubin measurements to determine the newborn's bilirubin risk according to the hour-specific nomogram
- Attitudes: Nurses appreciate their role as one of promoting safety for the newborn at risk for developing jaundice
- Knowledge: Nurses implement client-focused strategies to promote serum bilirubin reduction; these include but are not limited to placing the newborn to mother's breast in first hours of life and encouraging frequent breastfeeding of no less than 10 to 12 feedings per 24 hours
- Skills: Nurses identify individual clinical risk factors in the neonate that place him or her at risk for jaundice
- Attitudes: Nurses value their role as a health care team member to promote the safe care of the newborn at discharge from the birth center and beyond
- Knowledge: Nurses understand use of phototherapy to reduce levels of indirect bilirubin
- Skills: Nurses use phototherapy lights appropriately
- Skills: Nurses assess infant for untoward effects of phototherapy
- Attitudes: Nurses appreciate the role of phototherapy as a treatment
- Attitudes: Nurses value their role in the promotion of safety with the use of phototherapy
- Quality and safety education for nurses at www.qsen.org

● = Independent;　▲ = Collaborative;　EBN = Evidence-Based Nursing;　EB = Evidence-Based

REFERENCES

American Academy of Pediatrics. (2004). Management of hyperbilirubinemia in the newborn infant 35 or more weeks of gestation. *Pediatrics, 114*(1), 297–316.

Barrington, K. J., & Sankaran, K. (2018). *The Canadian Paediatric Society Position Statement:* Guidelines for detection, management and prevention of hyperbilirubinemia in term and late preterm newborn infants. Retrieved from https://www.cps.ca/en/documents/position/hyperbilirubinemia-newborn. (Accessed 14 May 2018).

Bhutani, V. K., & Committee on Fetus and Newborn, & American Academy of Pediatrics. (2014). Phototherapy to prevent severe neonatal hyperbilirubinemia in the newborn infant 35 or more weeks of gestation. *Pediatrics, 128*(4), e1046–e1052. Reaffirmed *134*(3), e920.

Blackburn, S. T. (2013). *Maternal, fetal, & neonatal physiology: A clinical perspective* (4th ed.). St Louis: Elsevier.

Flaherman, V. J., & Maisels, M. J. (2017). Academy of Breastfeeding Medicine clinical protocol #22: Guidelines for management of jaundice in the breastfeeding infant 35 weeks or more of gestation. *Breastfeeding Medicine, 12*(5). doi:10.1089/bfm.2017.29042.vjf.

Hassan, B., Zakerihamidi, M., & Boskabadi, H. (2018). The correlation between frequency and duration of breastfeeding and the severity of neonatal hyperbilirubinemia. *Journal of Maternal-Fetal & Neonatal Medicine, 31*(4), 457–463.

Hockenberry, M. J., & Wilson, D. (2015). *Wong's nursing care of infants and children* (10th ed.). St. Louis: Elsevier.

Hockenberry, M. J., Wilson, D., & Rodgers, C. C. (2017). *Wong's essentials of pediatric nursing* (10th ed.). St. Louis: Elsevier.

Jain, M., Bang, A., Tiwari, A., et al. (2017). Prediction of significant hyperbilirubinemia in term neonates by early non-invasive bilirubin measurement. *World J Pediatrics, 13*(3), 222–227.

Johnson, L., & Bhutani, V. K. (2011). The clinical syndrome of bilirubin-induced neurologic dysfunction. *Seminars in Perinatology, 35*(3), 101–113.

Maisels, M. J., et al. (2009). Hyperbilirubinemia in the newborn infant ≥35 weeks' gestation: An update with clarifications. *Pediatrics, 124*(4), 1193–1198.

Muchowski, K. E. (2014). Evaluation and treatment of neonatal hyperbilirubinemia. *American Family Physician, 89*(11), 873–878.

Reichman, N. E., Teitler, J. O., Moullin, S., et al. (2015). Late-preterm birth and neonatal morbidities: Population-level and within-family estimates. *Annals of Epidemiology, 25*(2), 126–132.

Stokowski, L. A. (2011). Fundamentals of phototherapy for neonatal jaundice. *Advances in Neonatal Care, 11*(5S), S10–S21.

Van den Esker-Jonker, B., den Boer, L., Pepping, R. M., et al. (2016). Transcutaneous bilirubinometry in jaundiced neonates: A randomized controlled trial. *Pediatrics, 138*(6), pii:e20162414.

H

Risk for neonatal Hyperbilirubinemia

Original author David Wilson, MS, RNC; revised by Barbara. J. Wheeler, RN, BN, MN, IBCLC

NANDA-I

Definition

Susceptible to the accumulation of unconjugated bilirubin in the circulation (less than 15 mL/dL; less than 257 μmol/L) that occurs after 24 hours of life, which may compromise health.

Risk Factors

Deficient feeding pattern; delay in meconium passage; infants with inadequate nutrition

At-Risk Population

ABO incompatibility; age ≤7 days; American Indian ethnicity; blood type incompatibility between mother and infant; East Asian ethnicity; infant who is breastfed; infant with low birthweight; maternal diabetes mellitus; population living at high altitudes; premature infant; previous sibling with jaundice; rhesus (Rh) incompatibility; significant bruising during birth

Associated Condition

Bacterial infection; infant with liver malfunction; infant with enzyme deficiency; internal bleeding; prenatal infection; sepsis; viral infection

NOC   (Nursing Outcomes Classification)

See care plan for Neonatal **Hyperbilirubinemia** for suggested NOC outcomes.

Client Outcomes

- Neonatal total serum bilirubin (TSB) will be monitored and there will be no undetected TSB values in the high-risk (95th percentile or greater) or high-intermediate risk (75th to 94th percentile) zones (as determined by the hour-specific nomogram)

• = Independent;   ▲ = Collaborative;   EBN = Evidence-Based Nursing;   EB = Evidence-Based

- Newborn will receive appropriate therapies to enhance bilirubin excretion
- Newborn will remain free of undetected signs of acute bilirubin neurotoxicity
- Establish effective feeding pattern (breast or bottle)
- Receive bilirubin assessment and screening within the first few days of life to detect increasing levels of serum bilirubin
- Receive nursing assessments to determine risk for severity of jaundice prior to discharge from birth hospital
- Maintain hydration: moist buccal membranes, four to six wet diapers in a 24-hour period, weight loss no greater than 10% of birth weight
- Evacuate stool within 48 hours of birth, and pass three to four stools per 24 hours by day 4 of life

NIC   (Nursing Interventions Classification)

See the care plan for Neonatal **Hyperbilirubinemia** for suggested NIC interventions.

Nursing Interventions and *Rationales*

- Identify clinical risk factors that place the infant at greater risk for development of neonatal jaundice: exclusive breastfeeding, isoimmune or hemolytic disease, preterm birth 38⁶⁄₇ weeks' gestation or less), weight loss of 10% or more from birth weight, maternal diabetes, maternal obesity, previous sibling with jaundice, East Asian ethnicity, and significant bruising or cephalhematoma. **EB:** *Exclusive breastfeeding that is not going well (suboptimal intake) and preterm birth have been identified as the most predictive of neonatal jaundice (Flaherman & Maisels, 2017). The other risk factors listed may also play a significant role in the development of neonatal jaundice and should be considered in the overall assessment.*
- Measure transcutaneous bilirubin (TcB) of all newborns in the first 24 to 48 hours of life, using a noninvasive transcutaneous bilirubinometer. Plot TcB on a nomogram standardized for the appropriate patient population; determine newborn's risk of subsequent significant hyperbilirubinemia. **EB:** *Transcutaneous measurement of bilirubin, in conjunction with use of a nomogram standardized for the appropriate patient population, has been demonstrated to be an accurate predictor of subsequent hyperbilirubinemia (Jain et al, 2017). The use of TcB in jaundiced neonates is safe and results in a significant reduction of phlebotomy for serum bilirubin measurement (van den Esker-Jonker et al, 2016).*

Refer to care plan for Neonatal **Hyperbilirubinemia** for additional interventions for multicultural and discharge planning.

 ## Client/Family Teaching and Discharge Planning

▲ Teach parents about the importance of medical follow-up in the first several days of life for the evaluation of jaundice, especially in the late preterm infant. **EB:** *Late preterm infants (34–36 weeks' gestation) are at much greater risk for hyperbilirubinemia than infants born at term (37–41 weeks' gestation) and should be followed closely in the first few weeks of life (Reichman et al, 2015).*

Refer to care plan for Neonatal **Hyperbilirubinemia** for additional interventions.

 ## Quality and Safety in Nursing

Refer to care plan for Neonatal **Hyperbilirubinemia** for additional interventions.

REFERENCES

Flaherman, V. J., & Maisels, M. J. (2017). Academy of Breastfeeding Medicine clinical protocol #22: Guidelines for management of jaundice in the breastfeeding infant 35 weeks or more of gestation. *Breastfeeding Medicine, 12*(5). doi:10.1089/bfm.2017.29042.vjf.

Jain, M., Bang, A., Tiwari, A., et al. (2017). Prediction of significant hyperbilirubinemia in term neonates by early non-invasive bilirubin measurement. *World J Pediatrics, 13*(3), 222–227.

Reichman, N. E., Teitler, J. O., Moullin, S., et al. (2015). Late-preterm birth and neonatal morbidities: Population-level and with-in family estimates. *Annals of Epidemiology, 25*(2), 126–132.

van den Esker-Jonker, B., den Boer, L., Pepping, R. M., et al. (2016). Transcutaneous bilirubinometry in jaundiced neonates: A randomized controlled trial. *Pediatrics, 138*(6). doi:10.1542/peds.2016-2414.

● = Independent;   ▲ = Collaborative;   **EBN** = Evidence-Based Nursing;   **EB** = Evidence-Based

Hyperthermia   *Rosemary Timmerman, DNP, APRN, CCNS, CCRN-CSC-CMC*

NANDA-I

Definition

Core body temperature above the normal diurnal range due to failure of thermoregulation.

Defining Characteristics

Abnormal posturing; apnea; coma; flushed skin; hypotension; infant does not maintain suck; irritability; lethargy; seizure; skin warm to touch; stupor; tachycardia; tachypnea; vasodilation

Related Factors

Dehydration; inappropriate clothing; increase in metabolic rate; vigorous activity

At-Risk Population

Exposure to high environmental temperature

Associated Condition

Decrease in sweat response; illness; ischemia; pharmaceutical agent; sepsis; trauma

NOC   (Nursing Outcomes Classification)

Suggested NOC Outcomes

Thermoregulation; Thermoregulation: Newborn

Example NOC Outcome with Indicators
Thermoregulation as evidenced by the following indicators: Increased skin temperature/Decreased skin temperature/Skin color changes/Dehydration/Hyperthermia. (Rate the outcome and indicators of **Thermoregulation:** 1 = severe, 2 = substantial, 3 = moderate, 4 = mild, 5 = none [see Section I].)

Client Outcomes

Client Will (Specify Time Frame)

- Maintain core body temperature within adaptive levels (less than 104°F, 40°C)
- Remain free of complications of malignant hyperthermia
- Remain free of complication of neuroleptic malignant syndrome
- Remain free of dehydration
- Remain free from infection
- Verbalize signs and symptoms of heat stroke and actions to prevent heat stroke
- Verbalize personal risks for malignant hyperthermia and neuroleptic malignant syndrome to be reported during health history reviews to all health care professionals, including pharmacists

NIC   (Nursing Interventions Classification)

Suggested NIC Interventions

Fever Treatment; Malignant Hyperthermia Precautions; Temperature Regulation

Example NIC Activities—Hyperthermia Treatment
Monitor core body temperature using appropriate device; Monitor for abnormalities in mental status

Nursing Interventions and *Rationales*

Temperature Measurement

- Recognize that hyperthermia is a rise in body temperature above 40°C (104°F) that is not regulated by the hypothalamus, resulting in an uncontrolled increase in body temperature exceeding the body's ability to lose heat. It is a medical emergency (Leon & Bouchama, 2015; Gaudio & Grissom, 2016).

• = Independent;   ▲ = Collaborative;   EBN = Evidence-Based Nursing;   EB = Evidence-Based

H

- Continually measure a client's core temperature with a distal esophageal probe or obtain near core body temperature measurements with a rectal or bladder temperature probe and verify with a second method. **EBN:** *Obtaining an accurate core body temperature is essential for detecting heat stroke and monitoring the client's response to treatment; if a core temperature reading is not available or practical, a rectal or bladder temperature measurement provides a closer approximation of the core body temperature than temporal, axillary, oral, aural, or skin measurements (Lipman et al, 2013; Leon & Bouchama, 2015).* **CEB:** *Research is limited on the accuracy of temporal artery measurements outside normal ranges; axillary temperature is accurate in neonates but is not well supported in adults, and tympanic membrane measurements and chemical dot thermometers are least accurate and should be avoided in caring for the acutely ill adult client (Hooper et al, 2010; Makic et al, 2011).*
- Use the same site and method (device) for temperature measurement for a given client so that temperature trends are assessed accurately; record site of temperature measurement. **EBN/CEB:** *There are differences in temperature depending on the site from which temperature measurement is obtained; however, differences between sites should not be greater than 0.3°C to 0.5°C (Bridges & Thomas, 2009; Makic et al, 2011).*
- ▲ Work with the health care provider to help determine the cause of the temperature increase (hyperthermia), which will often help direct appropriate treatment. *It is important to treat the underlying cause of the temperature to preserve neurologic function of the client as well as implement interventions to rapidly lower the core temperature (Bohman & Levine, 2014; Gaudio & Grissom, 2016).*
- Refer to care plan for Ineffective **Thermoregulation** for interventions managing fever (pyrexia).

Heat Stroke

- Recognize that heat stroke may be separated into two categories: classic and exertional. *Classic heat stroke usually involves the very young and older client during environmental heat waves. Exertional heat stroke occurs in young adults performing strenuous physical activity in hot climates (Leon & Bouchama, 2015; Gaudio & Grissom, 2016).*
- Watch for risk factors for classic heat stroke, which include (Leon & Bouchama, 2015; Gaudio & Grissom, 2016):
  - Medications, especially diuretics, anticholinergic agents, beta-blockers, anti-Parkinson's medications, antidepressants, and antihistamines
  - Alcoholism
  - Mental illness
  - Obesity
  - Heart disease
- ▲ **EB:** *Physiologic effects of aging include lower onset of sweating and rate of sweating needed to help with dissipation of body heat; medications can dehydrate the client and blunt the physiologic responses necessary to assist with heat dissipation, increasing the risk of heat stroke in older clients (Leon & Bouchama, 2015; Gaudio & Grissom, 2016).*
- Risk factors of exertional heat stroke include (Gaudio & Grissom, 2016; Lipman et al, 2013):
  - Preexisting illness
  - Drug use (e.g., alcohol, amphetamines, ecstasy)
  - Wearing protective clothing (uniforms and athletic gear) that limits heat dissipation
- Recognize signs and symptoms of hyperthermia: core body temperature greater than 40°C (104°F), exercise-associated muscle cramps, tachycardia, tachypnea, orthostatic dizziness, weakness, vomiting, headache, confusion, delirium, seizures, coma, acute kidney injury (rhabdomyolysis), and hot dry skin (classic heat stroke) (Pryor et al, 2013; Gaudio & Grissom, 2016).
- Recognize that antipyretic agents are of little use in treatment of hyperthermia. **EB:** *Because the cause of the hyperthermia does not involve the hypothalamus, antipyretic agents are ineffective and not indicated in treatment of clients with hyperthermia (Lipman et al, 2013; Gaudio & Grissom, 2016).*
- ▲ Assess fluid loss and facilitate oral intake or administer intravenous fluids as ordered to accomplish fluid replacement and support the cardiovascular system. *Increased metabolic rate, diuresis, and diaphoresis-associated exertional hyperthermia cause loss of body fluids (Lipman et al, 2013; Leon & Bouchama, 2015).* Refer to the care plan for Deficient **Fluid** volume.
- ▲ Recognize use of alpha-adrenergic agents should be avoided if possible. *Alpha-adrenergic agonist agents cause cutaneous vasoconstriction, which impairs cooling (Gaudio & Grissom, 2016).*
- Remove clothing and immerse young and healthy clients who have suffered exertional heat stroke in a cold water bath ensuring the head does not go underwater, or continuously douse the client with cold

• = Independent;   ▲ = Collaborative;   **EBN** = Evidence-Based Nursing;   **EB** = Evidence-Based

water. EB: *Cold water immersion rapidly cools the core temperature because of the high thermal conductivity of water but may not be practical because of client agitation and limited access for cardiovascular monitoring (Leon & Bouchama, 2015; Gaudio & Grissom, 2016).* For clients with classic heat stroke, remove clothes and spray or douse the skin with water and provide continual airflow over the body with a fan. EB: *Wetting the skin and directing airflow over the body promotes evaporative and convective cooling; this method is less effective for clients with exertional heat stroke (Leon & Bouchama, 2015; Gaudio & Grissom, 2016).*

▲ Recognize adjunctive cooling measures include administering cold (4°C) intravenous fluids, water circulating hydrogel coated pads placed over the chest and legs, ice packs over the entire body, intravascular cooling catheter, and cooling blankets. EB: *There is insufficient evidence to recommend using adjunctive measures as a primary cooling method (Leon & Bouchama, 2015; Gaudio & Grissom, 2016).*

▲ Continuously monitor the effects of cooling measures, stop cooling interventions once the body temperature is less than 39°C, and benzodiazepines may be administered to control shivering. EB/EBN: *Hyperthermia must be treated aggressively to lower the body temperature; however, overshooting of the cooling process with resultant hypothermia must be prevented and avoidance of shivering is essential because of the associated increase in heat production, oxygen consumption, and cardiorespiratory effort (Leon & Bouchama, 2015; Gaudio & Grissom, 2016).*

▲ Continually assess the client's neurologic and other organ function, especially kidney function (i.e., signs of rhabdomyolysis), for signs of injury from hyperthermia. EB/EBN: *Hyperthermia can cause permanent neurologic injury, acute kidney injury, electrolyte imbalances, and coagulation disorders so continuous assessment of neurologic and other organ function is essential (Leon & Bouchama, 2015; Gaudio & Grissom, 2016).*

Malignant Hyperthermia

▲ If the client has just received general anesthesia, especially halothane, sevoflurane, desflurane, enflurane, isoflurane, or succinylcholine, recognize that the hyperthermia may be caused by malignant hyperthermia and requires immediate treatment to prevent death. *Malignant hyperthermia is often a fatal disease and must be treated promptly with rapid administration of the medication dantrolene, increasing oxygenation, assisting ventilation, initiating external cooling measures, and treating acid-base (e.g., metabolic acidosis) and electrolyte disorders (Rosenberg et al, 2015; Safety Committee of Japanese Society of Anesthesiologists [SCJSA], 2017).*

● Monitor core temperature for all clients receiving general anesthetic agents for longer than 30 minutes. EB/EBN: *Hyperthermia typically occurs 30 minutes after induction of anesthesia and is associated with a higher mortality rate (Larach et al, 2014; Rosenberg et al, 2015).*

● Recognize that signs and symptoms of malignant hyperthermia typically occur suddenly after exposure to the anesthetic agent and include rapid rise in core body temperature, hypercarbia (increase in end tidal carbon dioxide), muscle rigidity, masseter muscle spasm, dysrhythmias, tachycardia, tachypnea, rhabdomyolysis, acute kidney injury, and elevated serum calcium and potassium, progressing to disseminated intravascular coagulation and cardiac arrest (Rosenberg et al, 2015; SCJSA, 2017).

▲ If the client has malignant hyperthermia, begin treatment as ordered, including cessation of the anesthetic agent and intravenous administration of dantrolene sodium, STAT, along with cooling measures, hyperventilation with 100% oxygen, antidysrhythmics, and continued support of the cardiovascular system. *Dantrolene helps decrease the increased muscle activity associated with malignant hyperthermia and can be life-saving (Rosenberg et al, 2015; SCJSA, 2017).*

▲ Recognize that dysrhythmias must not be treated with calcium channel blockers (e.g., verapamil) when the client has malignant hyperthermia. *Calcium channel blockers in combination with dantrolene can lead to cardiac arrest (Rosenberg et al, 2015; SCJSA, 2017).*

● Provide client and family education when malignant hyperthermia occurs because it is an inherited muscle disorder. *Obtaining a thorough health history to include family history of adverse experiences with anesthesia or muscle disorders is important in identifying clients at risk for malignant hyperthermia. Genetic counseling may also be indicated (Malignant Hyperthermia Association of the United States [MHAUS], 2015).*

Neuroleptic Malignant Syndrome

▲ Recognize that neuroleptic malignant syndrome is a rare condition associated with clients who are taking typical and atypical antipsychotic agents or after abrupt discontinuation of dopaminergic agonist agents

● = Independent;   ▲ = Collaborative;   EBN = Evidence-Based Nursing;   EB = Evidence-Based

used for Parkinson's disorder (Paden, Franjic, & Halcomb, 2013; Pileggi & Cook, 2016). **EB/EBN:** *The most common agents associated with the condition are dopamine-2 inhibiting antipsychotic agents (e.g., haloperidol, fluphenazine, chlorpromazine, quetiapine, risperidone, olanzapine) and dopamine antagonists (e.g., metoclopramide, promethazine, prochlorperazine, droperidol); sudden cessation of dopamine agonists (amantadine, levodopa, lithium, and bromocriptine) have also been associated with neuroleptic malignant syndrome (Paden, Franjic, & Halcomb, 2013; Pileggi & Cook, 2016).*

- Watch for signs and symptoms that can range from mild to severe and include a sudden change in mental status, rapid rise in body temperature, muscle rigidity, tachycardia, tachypnea, elevated or labile blood pressure, diaphoresis, rhabdomyolysis, and acute kidney injury (Paden, Franjic, & Halcomb, 2013; Pileggi & Cook, 2016).
- ▲ Begin treatment when diagnosed, including cessation of the neuroleptic or dopamine antagonist agent or resumption of dopamine agonist agent that may have been abruptly discontinued; order administration of dantrolene, bromocriptine, amantadine, or benzodiazepine; and continue support of the cardiovascular, pulmonary, and renal systems (Paden, Franjic, & Halcomb, 2013; Pileggi & Cook, 2016).
- A client health history that reports extrapyramidal reaction to any medication should be further explored for risk of neuroleptic malignant syndrome because this syndrome can occur at any time during a client's treatment with typical and atypical antipsychotic agents (Paden, Franjic, & Halcomb, 2013; Pileggi & Cook, 2016).
- Recognize that clients receiving rapid dose escalation of antipsychotic agents (e.g., haloperidol) intramuscularly for acute treatment of delirium may be at increased risk for neuroleptic malignant syndrome (Paden, Franjic, & Halcomb, 2013; Pileggi & Cook, 2016).

Pediatric

- Assess risk factors of malignant hyperthermia including a personal or family history of anesthesia-related complications or death or a history of muscle disorders. *There is an increased prevalence of malignant hyperthermia in the pediatric population, and the administration of inhalation anesthesia and succinylcholine is common in this age group (MHAUS, 2015; Pileggi & Cook, 2016).*
- ▲ Administer dantrolene, provide oxygen and assist with ventilation, monitor heart rate and rhythm, and treat electrolyte and acid-base disorders (i.e., metabolic acidosis) as ordered if malignant hyperthermia is present. *Dantrolene and airway management/support are necessary during emergent treatment of malignant hyperthermia (Nelson & Litman, 2014).*

Geriatric

- Help the client seek medical attention immediately if elevated core temperature is present. To diagnose the hyperthermia, assess for possible precipitating factors, including changes in medication, environmental changes, and recent medical interventions or infectious exposures. *Older adults are more susceptible to environmentally and medication-induced hyperthermia, because of the greater incidence of underlying chronic medical conditions that impair thermal regulation or prevent removal from a hot environment (Leon & Bouchama, 2015).*
- In hot weather, encourage the client to wear lightweight cotton clothing (Leon & Bouchama, 2015).
- Provide education on the importance of drinking eight glasses of fluid per day (within their cardiac and renal reserves) regardless of whether they are thirsty and wearing appropriate clothing for the environmental temperature; assess for the need for and presence of fans or air conditioning. *Older adults are more susceptible to a hot environment than younger adults because of a decreased sensitivity to heat, decreased sweat gland function, decreased thirst, and decreased mobility (Leon & Bouchama, 2015).*
- In hot weather, monitor the older client for signs of heat stroke such as rising temperature, orthostatic blood pressure drop, weakness, restlessness, mental status changes, faintness, thirst, nausea, and vomiting. If signs are present, move the client to a cool place, have the client lie down, give sips of water, check orthostatic blood pressure, spray with lukewarm water, cool with a fan, and seek medical assistance immediately. *Older adults are predisposed to heat exhaustion and should be watched carefully for occurrence; if present, it should be treated promptly (Leon & Bouchama, 2015).*
- During warm weather, help the client obtain a fan or an air conditioner to increase evaporation, as needed. Help the older client locate a cool environment to which they can go for safety in hot weather.
- Take the temperature of the older client in hot weather. *Older clients may not be able to tell that they are hot because of decreased sensation.*

● = Independent;   ▲ = Collaborative;   **EBN** = Evidence-Based Nursing;   **EB** = Evidence-Based

Home Care

- Some of the interventions described previously may be adapted for home care use.
- Determine whether the client or family has a functioning thermometer, and know how to use it. Refer to the previous interventions on taking a temperature.
- Help the client and caregivers prevent and monitor for heat stroke/hyperthermia during times of high outdoor temperatures. *Preventive measures include minimizing time spent outdoors, use of air conditioning or fans, increasing fluid intake, and taking frequent rest periods (Centers for Disease Control and Prevention [CDC], 2017).*
- To prevent heat-related injury in athletes, laborers, and military personnel, instruct them to acclimate gradually to the higher temperatures, increase fluid intake, wear vapor-permeable clothing, and take frequent rests (Leon & Bouchama, 2015; CDC, 2017).
- In the event of temperature elevation above the adaptive range, institute measures to decrease temperature (e.g., get the client out of the sun and into a cool place, remove excess clothing, have the client drink fluids, spray the client with lukewarm water, fan with cool air, initiate emergency transport). *Hyperthermia is an acute and possibly life-threatening situation (Kerr et al, 2014; CDC, 2017).*

 Client/Family Teaching and Discharge Planning

- ▲ Instruct to increase fluids to prevent heat-induced hyperthermia and dehydration in the presence of fever. *Liberal fluid intake replaces fluid lost through perspiration and respiration (Lipman et al, 2013).*
- Teach the client to stay in a cooler environment during periods of excessive outdoor heat or humidity. If the client does go out, instruct him or her to avoid vigorous physical activity; wear lightweight, loose-fitting clothing; and wear a hat to minimize sun exposure. *Such methods reduce exposure to high environmental temperatures, which can cause heat stroke and hyperthermia (Kerr et al, 2014; CDC, 2017).*

REFERENCES

Bohman, L. E., & Levine, J. M. (2014). Fever and therapeutic normothermia in severe brain injury: An update. *Current Opinion in Critical Care, 20*, 182–188. doi:10.1097/MCC.0000000000000070.

Bridges, E., & Thomas, K. (2009). Noninvasive measurement of body temperature in critically ill patients. *Critical Care Nurse, 29*(3), 94–97. doi:10.4037/ccn2009132.

Centers for Disease Control and Prevention (CDC). (2017). *Heat stress. NIOSH workplace safety and health tips.* Retrieved from https://www.cdc.gov/niosh/topics/heatstress/. (Accessed 24 August 2017).

Gaudio, F. G., & Grissom, C. K. (2016). Cooling methods in heat stroke. *The Journal of Emergency Medicine, 50*, 607–616. doi:10.1016/j.jemermed.2015.09.014.

Hooper, V. D., et al. (2010). ASPAN's evidence-based clinical practice guideline for the promotion of perioperative normothermia: second edition. *Journal of Perianesthesia Nursing, 25*, 346–365. doi:10.1016/j.jopan.2010.10.006.

Kerr, Z. Y., Marshall, S. W., Cornstock, D., et al. (2014). Exertional heat stroke management strategies in United States high school football. *The American Journal of Sports Medicine, 42*(1), 70–81. doi:10.1177/0363546513502940.

Larach, M. G., Brandom, B. W., Allen, G. C., et al. (2014). Malignant hyperthermia deaths related to inadequate temperature monitoring, 2007-2012: A report from the North American Malignant Hyperthermia Registry of the Malignant Hyperthermia Association of the United States. *Anesthesia and Analgesia, 119*, 1359–1366. doi:10.1213/ANE.0000000000000421.

Leon, L. R., & Bouchama, A. (2015). Heat stroke. *Comprehensive Physiology, 5*, 611–647. doi:10.1002/cphy.c140017.

Lipman, G. S., Eifling, K. P., Ellis, M. A., et al. (2013). Wilderness Medical Society practice guidelines for the prevention and treatment of heat-related illness. *Wilderness & Environmental Medicine, 24*, 351–361. doi:10.1016/j.wem.2014.07.017.

Makic, M. B. F., et al. (2011). Evidence-based practice habits: Putting more sacred cows out to pasture. *Critical Care Nurse, 31*, 38–62. doi:10.4037/ccn2011908.

Malignant Hyperthermia Association of the United States (MHAUS). (2015). *Website.* Retrieved from http://www.mhaus.org/. (Accessed 23 August 2017).

Nelson, P., & Litman, R. S. (2014). Malignant hyperthermia in children: An analysis of the North American Malignant Hyperthermia Registry. *Anesthesia and Analgesia, 118*, 369–374. doi:10.1213/ANE.0b013e3182a8fad0.

Paden, M. S., Franjic, L., & Halcomb, E. (2013). Hyperthermia caused by drug interactions and adverse reaction. *Emergency Medicine Clinics of North America, 31*, 1035–1044. doi:10.1016/j.emc.2013.07.003.

Pileggi, D. J., & Cook, A. M. (2016). Neuroleptic malignant syndrome: Focus on treatment and rechallenge. *The Annals of Pharmacotherapy, 50*, 973–981. doi:10.1177/1060028016657553.

Pryor, R. R., Casa, D. J., Holschen, J. C., et al. (2013). Exertional heat stroke: Strategies for prevention and treatment from the sports field to the emergency department. *Clinical Ped Emergency Medicine, 14*(4), 267–278.

Rosenberg, H., Pollock, N., Schiemann, A., et al. (2015). *Orphanet Journal of Rare Diseases, 10*, 93. doi:10.1186/s13023-015-0310-1.

Safety Committee of Japanese Society of Anesthesiologists (SCJSA). (2017). JSA guideline for the management of malignant hyperthermia crisis 2016. *Journal of Anesthesia, 31*, 307–317. doi:10.1007/s00540-016-2305-z.

● = Independent;   ▲ = Collaborative;   EBN = Evidence-Based Nursing;   EB = Evidence-Based

Hypothermia   *Rosemary Timmerman, DNP, APRN, CCNS, CCRN-CSC-CMC*

NANDA-I

Definition

Core body temperature below normal diurnal range due to failure of thermoregulation.

Defining Characteristics

Acrocyanosis; bradycardia; cyanotic nail beds; decrease in blood glucose level; decrease in ventilation; hypertension; hypoglycemia; hypoxia; increase in metabolic rate; increase in oxygen consumption; peripheral vasoconstriction; piloerection; shivering; skin cool to touch; slow capillary refill; tachycardia

Neonates

Infant with insufficient energy to maintain sucking; infant with insufficient weight gain (<30 g/day); irritability; jaundice; metabolic acidosis; pallor; respiratory distress

Related Factors

Alcohol consumption; decrease in metabolic rate; excessive conductive heat transfer; excessive convective heat transfer; excessive evaporative heat transfer; excessive radiative heat transfer; inactivity; insufficient caregiver knowledge of hypothermia prevention; insufficient clothing; low environmental temperature; malnutrition

Neonates

Delay in breastfeeding; early bathing of newborn; increase in oxygen demand

At-Risk Population

Economically disadvantaged; extremes of age; extremes of weight; high-risk out-of- hospital birth; increased body surface area to weight ratio; insufficient supply of subcutaneous fat; unplanned out-of-hospital birth

Associated Condition

Damage to hypothalamus; immature stratum corneum; increase in pulmonary vascular resistance (PVR); ineffective vascular control; inefficient nonshivering thermogenesis; pharmaceutical agent; radiation therapy; trauma

NOC   (Nursing Outcomes Classification)

Suggested NOC Outcomes

Thermoregulation; Thermoregulation: Newborn

Example **NOC Outcome with Indicators**
Thermoregulation as evidenced by the following indicators: Increased skin temperature/Decreased skin temperature/Skin color changes/Dehydration/Hypothermia. (Rate the outcome and indicators of **Thermoregulation:** 1 = severe, 2 = substantial, 3 = moderate, 4 = mild, 5 = none [see Section I].)

Client Outcomes

Client Will (Specify Time Frame)

- Maintain body temperature within normal range
- Identify risk factors of hypothermia
- State measures to prevent hypothermia
- Identify symptoms of hypothermia and actions to take when hypothermia is present
- If hypothermia is medically induced client/family will state goals for hypothermia treatment

● = Independent;   ▲ = Collaborative;   EBN = Evidence-Based Nursing;   EB = Evidence-Based

NIC (Nursing Interventions Classification)

Suggested NIC Interventions

Hypothermia Treatment; Temperature Regulation; Temperature Regulation: Intraoperative; Vital Signs Monitoring

Example NIC Activities—Temperature Regulation
Institute use of a continuous core temperature-monitoring device, as appropriate; Promote adequate fluid and nutritional intake

Nursing Interventions and *Rationales*

Temperature Measurement

- Recognize hypothermia as a drop in core body temperature below 35°C (95°F) (Paal et al, 2016; Zafren, 2017).
- Measure and record the client's temperature hourly, or if the client's temperature is less than 35°C (95°F), continuously. EB: *Ongoing temperature measurements are needed for timely treatment decisions (Paal et al, 2016; Zafren, 2017).*
- Select a core or a near core measurement site based on the clinical situation and ability to obtain an accurate measurement; verify the temperature reading with a second monitoring device as needed. EB: *Hypothermia can be a life-threatening crisis and obtaining an accurate temperature measurement is essential for detecting hypothermia and monitoring the client's response to treatment. A core temperature measurement from a pulmonary artery catheter is considered the gold standard, but it is often not practical and may precipitate dysrhythmias in hypothermic clients. A probe placed in the distal esophagus correlates with the pulmonary artery temperature and can be used when the client has a decreased level of consciousness and the upper airway is secured. An indwelling urinary catheter with a temperature probe allows for simultaneous measurement of bladder temperatures and urine output but may not be accurate with a low urine output. Rectal and bladder probes provide near core temperature readings but may lag behind core temperatures during rapid cooling and rewarming. Tympanic measurements may give falsely low readings in clients with unstable or absent circulation; oral, skin, and temporal artery temperatures are inaccurate in hypothermic states (Soreide, 2014; Paal et al, 2016; Zafren, 2017).*
- Use the same site and method (device) for a given client so that temperature trends are accurately assessed. CEB: *There are differences in temperature measurements depending on the site from which the temperature measurement is obtained; however, differences between sites should not be more than 0.3°C to 0.5°C (Makic et al, 2011).*
- See the care plan for Ineffective **Thermoregulation** as appropriate.

Accidental Hypothermia

- Recognize that there are three types of accidental hypothermia (environmental causes):
  - Acute hypothermia, also called immersion hypothermia, often from sudden exposure to cold through immersion in cold water or snow
  - Exhaustion hypothermia, caused by exposure to cold in association with lack of food and exhaustion
  - Chronic hypothermia that occurs over days or weeks and primarily affects older adults (Petrone, 2014)
- Remove the client from the cause of the hypothermic episode (e.g., cold environment, cold or wet clothing), bring into a warm environment, cover the client with warm blankets, and apply a covering to the head and neck to conserve body heat. *Layering of dry clothing, including wearing a hat, can be effective in warming a client with mild hypothermia; the goal is also to prevent any further heat loss (Soreide, 2014; Rischall & Rowland-Fisher, 2016; Zafren, 2017).*
- Keep the moderately and severely hypothermic client horizontal and handle gently during movements. EB: *Because cold myocardial tissue is irritable, rough or sudden movements of hypothermic clients can precipitate lethal ventricular dysrhythmias; a vertical position may cause severe cardiovascular stress (Paal et al, 2016; Zafren, 2017).*
- Monitor the client for signs of hypothermia: shivering, slurred speech, confusion, clumsy movements, fatigue progressing to a further decrease in level of consciousness, bradycardia, hypoventilation, hypotension, ventricular fibrillation, and asystole (*Rischall & Rowland-Fisher, 2016; Zafren, 2017*). Hypothermic patients have decreased oxygen needs and generally do not need supplemental oxygen (Zafren & Giesbrecht, 2014).

● = Independent; ▲ = Collaborative; EBN = Evidence-Based Nursing; EB = Evidence-Based

H

- Monitor the client's vital signs every hour and as appropriate, noting changes associated with hypothermia, such as increased pulse rate, respiratory rate, and blood pressure, as well as diuresis with mild hypothermia, progressing to a decreased pulse rate, respiratory rate and blood pressure, and oliguria with moderate to severe hypothermia. EB: *With mild hypothermia, the sympathetic nervous system is activated, which increases the heart rate and respiratory rate; as hypothermia progresses, decreased circulating volume develops, which results in decreased cardiac output and decreased oxygen delivery. Hypoxia, metabolic acidosis, and intrinsic irritability of a cold myocardium result in dysrhythmias (Petrone, 2014; Zafren, 2017).*
- ▲ Attach electrodes and a cardiac monitor and monitor for dysrhythmias. EB: *With hypothermia, the client is prone to dysrhythmias because of the cold myocardium; dysrhythmias may include atrial fibrillation, ventricular fibrillation, or asystole (Paal et al, 2016; Zafren, 2017).*
- ▲ Recognize that clients with a core temperature less than 30°C are at a higher risk for cardiac arrest; if the client arrests:
  - ❍ Check the pulse for up to 1 minute because the pulse may be slow and weak.
  - ❍ Provide chest compressions and ventilations at the same rate as for a normothermic client.
  - ❍ Limit defibrillations to one attempt at maximal power for clients with ventricular fibrillation or pulseless ventricular tachycardia until the client's core temperature is at least 30°C.
  - ❍ Medications may be withheld until the client has a core temperature greater than 30°C; double the interval between doses once the temperature is above 30°C; resume normal doses of medications once the temperature reaches 35°C.
  - ❍ Recognize prolonged cardiopulmonary resuscitation may be necessary as the client is rewarmed.
  - ❍ EB: *Defibrillation and medications are less effective in the moderately or severely hypothermic client (Zafren & Griesbrecht, 2014).*
- ▲ Monitor for signs of coagulopathy (e.g., oozing of blood from any open areas or from intravascular catheter sites or mucous membranes) and note the results of clotting studies as available. EB: *Coagulopathy is a common occurrence during hypothermia because of reduced platelet function and coagulation enzymatic activity (Paal et al, 2016; Rischall & Rowland-Fisher, 2016).*
- For mild hypothermia (core temperature of 32.2°C–35°C [90°F–95°F]), rewarm client passively:
  - ❍ Set room temperature to 21°C to 24°C (70°F–75°F).
  - ❍ Keep the client dry; remove any damp or wet clothing.
  - ❍ Layer clothing and blankets and cover the client's head.
  - ❍ Offer warm fluids, particularly beverages high in carbohydrates for clients who are shivering and able to safely swallow; avoid alcohol or caffeine (Zafren & Giesbrecht, 2014; Zafren, 2017).
- For mild hypothermia, allow the client to rewarm at his or her own pace as heat is generated through the normal metabolism; warm fluids help reduce further heat loss and carbohydrates help fuel metabolic processes (Rischall & Rowland-Fisher, 2016; Zafren, 2017).
- ▲ For moderate hypothermia (core temperature 28°C–32.1°C [82.4°F–90°F]) or any client with a decreased level of consciousness, use active external rewarming methods, not exceeding an increase of more than 0.5°C to 1°C (1.8°F) per hour. EB: *Passive rewarming is not recommended for clients with temperatures lower than 32.2°C (90°F) because it is a slow process, requires sufficient glycogen stores to be used by the client's body, and may increase oxygen consumption, increasing the risk of adverse cardiac events (Rischall & Rowland-Fisher, 2016; Zafren, 2017).*
- Methods to rewarm the client include the following (Paal et al, 2016; Zafren, 2017):
  - ❍ Forced-air warming blankets
  - ❍ Circulation of warm water through external pads
  - ❍ Heated and humidified oxygen (42°C–46°C) through the ventilator circuit as ordered
  - ❍ Warmed (40°C–42°C) intravenous (IV) fluids and blood products using a commercial IV fluid warmer
  - ❍ Radiant heat sources
- ▲ For severe hypothermia (core temperature below 28°C [82.4°F]), use active core rewarming techniques as ordered (Paal et al, 2016; Rischall & Rowland-Fisher, 2016):
  - ❍ Hemodialysis
  - ❍ Intravascular temperature management catheter
  - ❍ Body cavity (thorax, peritoneal, stomach, and bladder) lavage with warmed fluid
  - ❍ Recognize that warming by extracorporeal life support (ECLS) using venoarterial extracorporeal membrane oxygenation (ECMO) or cardiopulmonary bypass is essential for clients experiencing hemodynamic instability or hypothermic cardiac arrest

• = Independent;   ▲ = Collaborative;   EBN = Evidence-Based Nursing;   EB = Evidence-Based

- Rewarm clients slowly, generally at a rate of 0.5°C to 1°C every hour. EB: *Slow rewarming helps prevent a phenomenon called "afterdrop," in which cold, hyperkalemic blood from the periphery returns to the heart, resulting in a biochemical injury, leading to dysrhythmias and severe hypotension (Rischall & Rowland-Fisher, 2016; Zafren, 2017).*
- Measure the blood pressure frequently when rewarming and monitor for hypotension. EB: *As the body warms, formerly vasoconstricted vessels dilate, resulting in hypotension; dehydration from cold diuresis worsens hypotension (Petrone, 2014; Zafren, 2017).*
- ▲ Administer isotonic IV fluids warmed to 40°C to 42°C as prescribed. EB: *Significant amounts of IV fluids are often needed to maintain adequate perfusion to vital tissues and organs because of hypovolemia from cold diuresis and vasodilation from rewarming; warmed IV fluid does not significantly raise the body temperature but does help prevent further heat loss (Rischall & Rowland-Fisher, 2016; Zafren, 2017).*
- Place a barrier between the patient and the heating blanket and monitor the client's skin. EB: *Cold skin is susceptible to pressure and thermal injury (Rischall & Rowland-Fisher, 2016; Zafren, 2017).*
- Determine the factors leading to the hypothermic episode, particularly if the client fails to rewarm, and treat the underlying condition; see Related Factors. *It is important to assess risk factors and precipitating events to prevent another incident of hypothermia and detect and treat underlying disease processes that impede thermoregulation (Rischall & Rowland-Fisher, 2016).*
- ▲ Request a social service referral to help the client obtain the heat, shelter, and food needed to maintain body temperature. *A preventive approach that includes adequate food and fluid intake, shelter, heat, and clothing decreases the risk of hypothermia.*
- ▲ Encourage proper nutrition and hydration. *Request a referral to a dietitian to identify appropriate dietary needs; insufficient calorie and fluid intake predisposes the client to hypothermia, especially in older adults (Rischall & Rowland-Fisher, 2016).*

Targeted Temperature Hypothermia

- Recognize that targeted temperature management, also called therapeutic hypothermia, is the active lowering of the client's body temperature, in a controlled manner, to preserve neurological function after a cardiac arrest; targeted temperature management may also be considered for clients who have refractory intracranial hypertension. EB: *In the event the client is successfully resuscitated after a cardiac arrest, recognize that medically induced targeted temperature management has been shown to provide neurological protection against ischemic neuronal injury after cardiac arrest (Donnino et al, 2016; Cook, 2017).*
- Recognize that controlled cooling of clients should be considered for all unconscious survivors of in-hospital or out-of-hospital cardiac arrest with an initial shockable (ventricular fibrillation or pulseless ventricular tachycardia) or nonshockable (asystole or pulseless electrical activity) rhythm; achieve and maintain a constant target temperature between 32°C and 36°C for at least 24 hours. EB: *The American Heart Association and the International Liaison Committee on Resuscitation have included therapeutic hypothermia as an intervention to be considered in the management of cardiac arrest patients to optimize neurological outcomes after return of spontaneous circulation (Donnino et al, 2016; Geocadin et al, 2017).*
- Monitor core or near core temperatures continuously using two methods of temperature monitoring. *To ensure that the targeted temperature is achieved and maintained closely within the prescribed temperature range, two methods of core or near core temperature monitoring are recommended (Avery et al, 2015; Cook, 2017).*
- Recognize that cooling may be achieved noninvasively, using fluid-filled cooling pads, or invasively, with an intravascular cooling catheter. EB/EBN: *Invasive cooling and surface cooling pads provide a more predictable and rapid cooling, minimizing adverse electrolyte shifts and shivering. Less optimal methods of cooling include the use of fans, ice packs, or blankets, which do not provide temperature regulation feedback between the machine and client (Olson & Hoffman, 2016; Wilson & Penna, 2016).*
- Monitor for signs of infection and implement measures to prevent hospital-acquired infections. *Hypothermia places the client at higher risk for infection because of immunosuppression (Beseda, Smith, & Veenstra, 2014; Cook, 2017).*
- Obtain vital signs hourly (or via continuous monitoring) to include continuous electrocardiogram monitoring, and observe for signs of hypotension, bradycardia, and dysrhythmias. Mechanical ventilation is required to protect the client's airway and breathing during treatment. EB: *Diuresis is more pronounced during the induction of hypothermia; hypotension may be more prominent as the client is rewarmed because of vasodilatation, requiring close monitoring and interventions to support blood pressure. Bradycardia associated with hypothermia is often not responsive to atropine but does not need to be treated unless the client is*

● = Independent;   ▲ = Collaborative;   EBN = Evidence-Based Nursing;   EB = Evidence-Based

hemodynamically unstable. If the client is overcooled (temperature drops below 32°C), the risk of dysrhythmias will increase and ventricular fibrillation refractory to defibrillation may occur at temperatures below 30°C (Olson & Hoffman, 2016; Cook, 2017).

▲ Observe for shivering and implement skin counterwarming with blankets; administer sedatives, opioids, neuromuscular blocking agents, buspirone, acetaminophen, or magnesium sulfate as prescribed. EB: *Shivering typically occurs as the client transitions between 37°C and 35°C and significantly increases the body's metabolic rate and oxygen consumption (Nakajima, 2016; Cook, 2017).*

▲ Closely inspect the skin before and throughout the cooling intervention and implement frequent turning and other pressure reduction interventions as indicated. *Lowering the body temperature causes vasoconstriction and can compromise perfusion to the skin, increasing the client's risk of skin breakdown and impaired wound healing (Olson & Hoffman, 2016; Cook, 2017).*

▲ Monitor and treat serum electrolytes (e.g., potassium, magnesium, calcium, phosphorus) and serum glucose closely during targeted hypothermia and during rewarming of the client; electrolytes will fluctuate as the client is rewarmed. EB/EBN: *Hypokalemia can occur during the induction phase of targeted temperature management as potassium moves intracellularly and is also lost through diuresis; as the client is rewarmed, electrolyte replacements, especially potassium replacements, should be closely monitored to prevent rebound hyperkalemia that may occur as the body temperature rises (Petrone, 2014; Cook, 2017).*

▲ Monitor blood cell counts and observe for signs and symptoms of coagulopathy during targeted hypothermia treatment. EB: *For every 1°C decline in temperature, the hematocrit may increase by approximately 2%, requiring monitoring but not treatment. Platelet counts decrease during hypothermic states, but research has not found a significant risk of bleeding during targeted hypothermia treatment (Petrone, 2014; Olson & Hoffman, 2016).*

● Rewarming should occur in a controlled manner, with a rise in body temperature of 0.25°C to 0.5°C per hour and a targeted goal of normothermia, 37°C for 36 hours. EB: *Aggressive rewarming may cause rebound hyperthermia, cerebral edema, seizures, hypotension, and ventricular fibrillation; hyperthermia during the 36 hours after a cardiac arrest is associated with worse neurological outcomes and a higher mortality rate (Beseda et al, 2014; Kim, Bravo, & Nichol, 2015).*

▲ Neurological and cognitive function should be assessed during targeted temperature treatment and after rewarming. EB: *The goal of targeted temperature treatment is neurological protection; close monitoring of neurological function after intervention and serial assessments are indicated (Donnino et al, 2016; Geocadin et al, 2017).*

Pediatric

● Recognize that pediatric clients have a decreased ability to adapt to temperature extremes; take the following actions to maintain body temperature in the infant/child:
  ○ Keep the head covered.
  ○ Use blankets to keep the client warm.
  ○ Keep the client covered during procedures, transport, and diagnostic testing.
  ○ Keep the room temperature at 22.2°C (72°F).

● *The combination of a relatively smaller body surface area, smaller body fluid volume, less well-developed temperature control mechanisms, and smaller amount of protective body fat limits the infant's and child's ability to maintain normal temperatures (Wyckoff, 2014).*

● For the preterm or low-birth-weight newborn, set the room temperature to 25°C (77°F) before the delivery; cover the infant's head with a wool or polyethylene cap; and use specially designed bags, skin-to-skin care, transwarmer mattresses, radiant warmers, and thermal blankets to keep the infant warm. EB/EBN: *These methods can help keep the vulnerable newborn warm in the delivery room (Wyckoff, 2014; Hsu et al, 2015).*

● Avoid bathing neonates for at least 6 hours after birth or until physiological stability is achieved; avoid removing the vernix caseosa and allow it to wear off with normal activity and handling; grossly contaminated vernix caseosa may be gently removed. EBN: *Early bathing of a neonate can result in hypothermia; the vernix caseosa protects and moisturizes the skin (Colwell, 2015).*

● Targeted hypothermia to 34°C for 72 hours may be implemented in the treatment of neonates with hypoxic-ischemic encephalopathy (HIE). EB: *Cooling may be achieved by selective head cooling or passively, to the entire body, by withholding external heat sources, which requires frequent monitoring of the neonate's temperature to prevent severe hypothermia (Wyckoff, 2014; Douglas-Escobar & Weiss, 2015).*

● = Independent; ▲ = Collaborative; EBN = Evidence-Based Nursing; EB = Evidence-Based

- Measure the temperature of the neonate undergoing therapeutic hypothermia for HIE with a rectal or nasopharyngeal probe. **EB:** *Although rectal and nasopharyngeal temperature accurately reflect the core body temperature of neonates undergoing targeted hypothermia, axillary temperature measurements do not (Landry et al, 2013; Hine et al, 2017).*

Geriatric

- Normal aging often includes changes in touch-related sensations, making it harder to differentiate cool and cold. *Decreased temperature sensitivity increases the risk of hypothermia in the older adult (Martin, 2016).*
- Recognize that older adults can develop hypothermia even from exposure to mildly cold temperatures of 60°F to 65°F (15.5°C–18.3°C). *Clients present with vague complaints of mental and/or other skill deterioration (Hypothermia and Older Adults, 2016).*
  - ○ Set the room temperature to 68°C to 70°C (20°C–21.1°C).
  - ○ Instruct client to wear warm clothes as appropriate (long underwear, socks, slippers, and a cap or hat) and to use a blanket to keep shoulders and legs warm while indoors.
  - ○ Instruct client to dress in layers and wear a hat, scarf, and gloves or mittens when going outside during cold weather.
  - ○ Instruct client to maintain adequate calorie intake.
- Assess neurological signs frequently, watching for confusion and decreased level of consciousness. **CEB:** *Mechanisms to control body temperature decrease with age, coupled with a slower counterregulatory response, lower rate of metabolism, and less effective vascular response, making hypothermia less obvious (Danzl et al, 2011).*

Home Care

- Hypothermia is not a symptom that appears in the normal course of home care, but when it occurs it is a clinical emergency, and the client/family should access emergency medical services immediately.
- Some of the interventions described earlier may be adapted for home care use.
- Before a medical crisis occurs, confirm that the client or family has a thermometer that registers accurately and the client or family can read it.
- Instruct the client or family to take the temperature when the client displays cyanosis, pallor, or shivering.
- ▲ Monitor temperature every hour, as noted previously; if the temperature of the client begins dropping below the normal range, apply layers of clothing or blankets, or adjust environmental heat to the comfort level, being careful to not overheat the client. *Passive rewarming is the only method of rewarming that is appropriate for home care under normal circumstances.*
- ▲ If temperature continues to drop, activate the emergency system and notify a health care provider. *Hypothermia is a clinically acute condition that cannot be managed safely in the home.*
- ▲ If the client is in hospice care or is terminally ill, follow advance directives, client wishes, and the health care provider's orders; keep the client free of pain. *The goal of terminal care is to provide dignity and comfort during the dying process.*

Client/Family Teaching and Discharge Planning

- Teach the client and family signs of hypothermia and the method of taking the temperature (age appropriate).
- Teach the client methods to prevent hypothermia: wearing adequate clothing, including a hat and mittens; heating the environment to a minimum of 20°C (68°F); and ingesting adequate food and fluid. *Simple measures such as layering clothes, wearing a hat, and avoiding extremes in temperature prevent significant heat loss (Petrone, 2014).*
- Teach clients who engage in cold weather outdoor activities the importance of appropriate clothing, survival skills, and emergency planning.
- ▲ Teach the client and family about medications such as sedatives, opioids, and anxiolytics that predispose the client to hypothermia (as appropriate). *If the client has had hypothermia in the past, using alternative medications is an option if there is no contraindication (Danzl et al, 2011).*

REFERENCES

Avery, K. R., O'Brien, M., Pierce, C. D., et al. (2015). Use of a nursing checklist to facilitate implementation of a therapeutic hypothermia after cardiac arrest. *Critical Care Nurse, 35*(1), 29–38. doi:10.4037/ccn2015937.

Beseda, R., Smith, S., & Veenstra, A. (2014). Therapeutic hypothermia after cardiac arrest and return of spontaneous circulation: It's complicated. *Critical Care Nursing Clinics of North America, 26,* 511–524. doi:10.1016/j.ccell.2014.08.001.

Colwell, A. (2015). To bathe or not to bathe: The neonatal question. *Neonatal Network, 34,* 216–219. doi:10.1891/0730-0832.34.4.216.

Cook, C. J. (2017). Induced hypothermia in neurocritical care: A review. *Journal of Neuroscience Nursing, 49*(1), 5–11. doi:10.1097/JNN.0000000000000215.

Danzl, D. F., et al. (2011). Hypothermia and frostbite. In A. S. Fauci (Ed.), *Harrison's principles of internal medicine* (18th ed.). New York: McGraw-Hill.

Donnino, M. W., Andersen, L. W., Berg, K. M., et al. the ILCOR ALS Task Force. (2016). Temperature management after cardiac arrest: An advisory statement by the Advanced Life Support Task Force of the International Liaison Committee on Resuscitation and the American Heart Association Emergency Cardiovascular Care Committee and the Council on Cardiopulmonary, Critical Care, Perioperative and Resuscitation. *Resuscitation, 98,* 97–104. doi:10.1016/j.resuscitation.2015.09.396.

Douglas-Escobar, M., & Weiss, M. D. (2015). Hypoxic-ischemic encephalopathy: A review for the clinician. *JAMA Pediatrics, 169,* 397–403. doi:10.1001/jamapediatrics.2014.3269.

Geocadin, R. G., Armstrong, M. J., Damian, M., et al. (2017). Practice guideline summary: Reducing brain injury following cardiopulmonary resuscitation: Report of the Guideline Development, Dissemination, and Implementation Subcommittee of the American Academy of Neurology. *Neurology, 88,* 214–2149. doi:10.1212/WNL.0000000000003966.

Hine, K., Hosono, S., Kawabata, K., et al. (2017). Nasopharynx is well-suited for core temperature measurement during hypothermia therapy. *Pediatrics International, 59,* 29–33. doi:10.1111/ped.13046.

Hsu, K., Chiang, M., Lin, S., et al. (2015). Thermal blanket to improve thermoregulation in preterm infants: A randomized controlled trial. *Pediatric Critical Care Medicine, 16,* 637–643. doi:10.1097/PCC.0000000000000447.

Hypothermia and older adults. (2016). *Home Healthcare Now, 34*(1), 9.

Kim, F., Bravo, P. E., & Nichol, G. (2015). What is the use of hypothermia for neuroprotection after out-of-hospital cardiac arrest? *Stroke: A Journal of Cerebral Circulation, 46,* 592–597. doi:10.1161/STROKEAHA.114.006975.

Landry, M., Doyle, L. W., Lee, K., et al. (2013). Axillary temperature measurement during hypothermic treatment for neonatal hypoxic-ischaemic encephalopathy. *Archives of Disease in Childhood. Fetal and Neonatal Edition, 98*(1), F54–F58. doi:10.1136/archdischild-2011-301066.

Makic, M. B. F., et al. (2011). Evidence-based practice habits: Putting more sacred cows out to pasture. *Critical Care Nurse, 31,* 38–62. doi:10.4037/ccn2011908.

Martin, J. (2016). Aging changes in the senses. In *MedlinePlus medical encyclopedia, U.S. National Library of Medicine.* Retrieved from https://medlineplus.gov/ency/article/004013.htm.

Nakajima, Y. (2016). Controversies in the temperature management of critically ill patients. *Journal of Anesthesia, 30,* 873–883. doi:10.1007/s00540-016-2200-7.

Olson, D. M., & Hoffman, J. (2016). Approaches for therapeutic temperature management. *Journal of Infusion Nursing, 39*(1), 26–29. doi:10.1097/NAN.0000000000000146.

Paal, P., Gordon, L., Strapazzon, G., et al. (2016). Accidental hypothermia—An update: The content of this review is endorsed by the International Commission for Mountain Emergency Medicine (ICAR MEDCOM). *Scandinavian Journal of Trauma, Resuscitation and Emergency Medicine, 24,* 111. doi:10.1186/s13049-016-0303-7.

Petrone, P. (2014). Management of accidental hypothermia and cold injury. *Current Problems in Surgery, 51*(10), 417–431. doi:10.1067/j.cpsurg.2014.07.004.

Rischall, M. L., & Rowland-Fisher, A. (2016). Evidence-based management of accidental hypothermia in the emergency department. *Emergency Medicine Practice, 18*(1), 1–18.

Soreide, K. (2014). Clinical and translational aspects of hypothermia in major trauma patients: From pathophysiology to prevention, prognosis and potential preservation. *Injury. Circulation, 45,* 647–654. doi:10.1161/CIRCULATIONAHA.111.076851.

Wilson, M., & Penna, A. D. (2016). Targeted temperature modulation in the neuroscience patient. *Critical Care Nursing Clinics of North America, 28,* 125–136. doi:10.1016/j.cnc.2015.10.006.

Wyckoff, M. H. (2014). Initial resuscitation and stabilization of the periviable neonate: The golden-hour approach. *Seminars in Perinatology, 38,* 12–16.

Zafren, K. (2017). Out-of-hospital evaluation and treatment of accidental hypothermia. *Emergency Medicine Clinics of North America, 35,* 261–279. doi:10.1016/j.emc.2017.01.003.

Zafren, K., & Griesbrecht, G. (2014). *State of Alaska: Cold injuries guidelines.* Retrieved from http://dhss.alaska.gov/dph/Emergency/Documents/ems/documents/Alaska%20DHSS%20EMS%20Cold%20Injuries%20Guidelines%20June%202014.pdf.

Risk for Hypothermia   *Rosemary Timmerman, DNP, APRN, CCNS, CCRN-CSC-CMC*

NANDA-I

Definition

Susceptible to a failure of thermoregulation that may result in a core body temperature below the normal diurnal range, which may compromise health.

Risk Factors

Alcohol consumption; excessive conductive heat transfer, excessive convective heat transfer; excessive evaporative heat transfer; excessive radiative heat transfer; inactivity; insufficient caregiver knowledge of hypothermia prevention; insufficient clothing; low environmental temperature; malnutrition

● = Independent;   ▲ = Collaborative;   **EBN** = Evidence-Based Nursing;   **EB** = Evidence-Based

Neonates

Decrease in metabolic rate; delay in breastfeeding; early bathing of newborn; increase in oxygen demand

At-Risk Population

Economically disadvantaged; extremes of age; extremes of weight; high-risk out-of-hospital birth; increased body surface area to weight ratio; insufficient supply of subcutaneous fat; unplanned out-of-hospital birth

Associated Condition

Damage to hypothalamus; immature stratum corneum; increased in pulmonary vascular resistance (PVR); ineffective vascular control; inefficient nonshivering thermogenesis; pharmaceutical agent; radiation therapy; trauma

NIC, NOC, Client Outcomes, Nursing Interventions and *Rationales,* Client/Family Teaching and Discharge Planning, and References

Refer to care plan for **Hypothermia**

H

Risk for Perioperative Hypothermia
Catherine Kleiner, PhD, MSN, BSN

NANDA-I

Definition

Susceptible to an inadvertent drop in core body temperature below 36°C/96.8°F occurring one hour before to 24 hours after surgery, which may compromise health.

Risk Factors

Excessive conductive heat transfer; excessive convective heat transfer; excessive radiative heat transfer; low environmental temperature

At-Risk Population

American Society of Anesthesiologist (ASA) Physical Status classification score >1; low body weight; low preoperative temperature (<36°C/96.8°F)

Associated Condition

Cardiovascular complications; combined regional and general anesthesia; diabetic neuropathy; surgical procedure

NOC (Nursing Outcomes Classification)

Suggested NOC Outcomes

Thermoregulation

Example NOC Outcome with Indicators
Thermoregulation as evidenced by the following indicators: Increased skin temperature/Decreased skin temperature/Skin color changes/Dehydration/Hypothermia. (Rate the outcome and indicators of Thermoregulation: 1 = severe, 2 = substantial, 3 = moderate, 4 = mild, 5 = none [see Section I].)

Client Outcomes

Client Will (Specify Time Frame)

- Maintain body temperature within normal range
- Identify risk factors of hypothermia
- State measures to prevent hypothermia

● = Independent;   ▲ = Collaborative;   EBN = Evidence-Based Nursing;   EB = Evidence-Based

- Identify symptoms of hypothermia and actions to take when hypothermia is present
- Client will be free of surgical site infection

NIC   (Nursing Interventions Classification)

Suggested NIC Interventions

Hypothermia Treatment; Temperature Regulation; Temperature Regulation: Intraoperative; Vital Signs Monitoring

Example NIC Activities—Temperature Regulation

Institute use of a continuous core temperature-monitoring device, as appropriate; Promote adequate fluid and nutritional intake

Nursing Interventions and *Rationales*

Temperature Measurement

- Recognize perioperative hypothermia as a drop in core body temperature below 36°C (96.8°F) (Campbell et al, 2015; Centers for Disease Control and Prevention [CDC], 2018).
- Measure the client's temperature frequently, at least every 15 minutes, while the patient is undergoing general anesthesia and with changes in client condition (e.g., chills, change in mental status); if more than mild hypothermia is present (temperature lower than 36°C/96.85°F), use a continuous temperature-monitoring device. Two modes of temperature monitoring may be indicated. Continuous temperature monitoring using an indwelling method of temperature measurement is usually indicated to monitor effectiveness of treating body alterations in core body temperature. EBN: *Hypothermia can be a life-threatening crisis that requires accurate temperature measurement. Core temperature is obtained by a pulmonary artery catheter or less invasive from sublingual, the distal esophagus, nasopharyngeal, or direct tympanic sites (Torossian et al, 2016). Near core temperature measurement sites include oral, bladder, rectal, and temporal artery, and peripheral measurements are obtained by skin surface measurements and in the axilla (Barnason et al, 2012). Research is limited on the accuracy of temporal artery, carotid artery, and "zero heat flux" measurements outside normal ranges; however, recent research is demonstrating improved accuracy and reliability (Iden et al, 2015; Imani et al, 2016; Evron et al, 2017). Axillary temperature is accurate in neonates, but it is not well supported in adults; tympanic membrane measurements and chemical dot thermometers are least accurate and should be avoided in caring for the acutely ill adult client (Barnason et al, 2012; Winslow et al, 2012). As technology improves the accuracy and reliability of noninvasive temperature monitoring will make the use of these measures an acceptable choice.*
- Use the same site and method (device) for temperature measurement for a given client so that temperature trends are assessed accurately, and record site of temperature measurement. EB: *There are differences in temperature depending on the site (esophageal, oral, bladder, rectal, axillary, or temporal artery); however, differences should not be greater than 0.3°C to 0.5°C (Barnason et al, 2012; Torossian et al, 2016).*
- Bladder temperature may be used because an indwelling urinary catheter is often inserted in the management of hypothermia to monitor diuresis. EBN: *Bladder temperature probes have been shown to be accurate during states of increased diuresis, but measurements may be less accurate when urine volume is low (low rate of diuresis). Temperatures obtained by this method may lag up to 20 minutes during targeted temperature hypothermia interventions (Burlingame & Conner, 2015).*

Unintentional Perioperative Hypothermia

- Keep the client warm throughout the perioperative period (preoperative, intraoperatively, and postoperatively) to prevent unintentional perioperative hypothermia. EB: *Initiating warming interventions preoperatively has been found to assist with normothermia and client comfort (Horosz & Malec-Milewska, 2014).*
- Factors that increase the risk of perioperative hypothermia include anesthetic agents, ambient room air temperature, intravenous (IV) fluid infusion, cavity solution irrigation, blood product administration, duration and type of surgical procedure, anemia, extremes of age, neurological disorders, cachexia, and preexisting conditions (e.g., peripheral vascular disease, endocrine disease, pregnancy, burns, open wounds) (Billeter et al, 2014; American Society of PeriAnesthesia Nurses [ASPAN], 2015).
- Closely monitoring and preventing unintentional perioperative hypothermia is necessary to prevent adverse patient outcomes. CEB: *Adverse outcomes include client discomfort, shivering, cardiac events (e.g., arrhythmias), increased catecholamine release, impaired coagulation, altered drug metabolism, impaired wound healing,*

• = Independent;   ▲ = Collaborative;   EBN = Evidence-Based Nursing;   EB = Evidence-Based

and impaired immune function *(Winslow et al, 2012; Horosz & Malec-Milewska, 2014; Kuchena, Merkel, & Hutches, 2014; ASPAN, 2015).*

- Several interventions should be implemented to prevent unintentional perioperative hypothermia:
  - Use warming booties perioperatively
  - Use warming blankets over and under the client perioperatively
  - Use warming blankets under the client on the operating table
  - Use of reflective blankets
  - Adjust environmental room controls to maintain ambient room temperature between 68°F and 77°F
  - Use humidified heated breathing circuit
  - Use warmed forced-air blankets preoperatively, during surgery, and in the postanesthesia care unit
  - Use circulating-water mattress
  - Use warmed IV fluids and irrigation solutions
  - Designate responsibility and accountability for thermoregulation

▲ EBN/EB: *Maintaining the client's temperature during the surgical procedure has been found to be essential in preventing surgical complications, especially surgical site infections. Maintaining normothermia also enhances client comfort (Institute for Healthcare Improvement [IHI], 2012a; ASPAN, 2015; CDC, 2018). Preoperative warming should be initiated for any patient with a core temperature below 36°C prior to induction of anesthesia, whereas preoperative warming for at least 10 minutes for any patient may prevent the patient from developing hypothermia (Horn et al, 2016; Wetz et al, 2016; Connelly et al, 2017). One study found that clients who experienced unintentional perioperative hypothermia during elective operations experienced a fourfold increase in mortality and stroke (Billeter et al, 2014).*

- Using warmed IV fluids and irrigation solutions during the operative period may assist with reducing the client's risk of unintentional perioperative hypothermia. EB: *Researchers found that warmed IV fluids and irrigation solutions kept the core temperatures of study participants warmer than those in clients receiving room temperature fluids (Campbell et al, 2015; Torossian et al, 2016).*

- Active warming interventions include the use of warm blankets and forced-air warming devices. EBN: *Blankets used for warming clients quickly lose heat. To prevent rapid heat loss from blankets, warming cabinets should be set at 200°F, and reapply blankets frequently (Kelly et al, 2013).* EBN: *Actively warming clients with forced-air warming is the most effective method to prevent hypothermia and offers a clinically important reduction in time to achieve normothermia in postoperative clients (Warttig et al, 2014; Connelly et al, 2017).*
  - A heated humidified breathing circuit can be used intraoperatively to decrease hypothermia. EB: *Heated humidified breathing circuits have decreased the severity of hypothermia in patients undergoing thyroid surgery (Park et al, 2017).*

- Watch the client for signs of hypothermia: shivering, slurred speech, confusion, clumsy movements, fatigue, and dehydration. Shivering increases oxygen consumption by about 40%. As hypothermia progresses, the skin becomes pale, muscles are tense, fatigue and weakness progress, breathing is decreased, and pulmonary congestion is present, compromising oxygenation. Pulses are decreased and blood pressure and heart rate decrease, progressing to lethal arrhythmias (e.g., ventricular fibrillation) (Danzl, 2012; Petrone, 2014; Torossian et al, 2016).

▲ Administer oxygen as ordered. Oxygenation is hampered by the change in the oxyhemoglobin curve caused by hypothermia (Danzl, 2012).

▲ Attach electrodes and a cardiac monitor. Watch for dysrhythmias. With hypothermia, the client is prone to dysrhythmias because of the cold myocardium; dysrhythmias may include atrial fibrillation, ventricular fibrillation, or asystole (Danzl, 2012; Petrone, 2014).

▲ Monitor for signs of coagulopathy (e.g., oozing of blood from any open areas or from intravascular catheter sites or mucous membranes). Also note results of clotting studies as available. Coagulopathy is a common occurrence during hypothermia (Petrone, 2014; Soreide, 2014; ASPAN, 2015).

▲ Monitor for signs of surgical site infection (e.g., increased incisional pain, drainage, poor healing, poor incision approximation). Unintentional perioperative hypothermia has been associated with increased risk of surgical site infections (IHI, 2012a; ASPAN, 2015; CDC, 2018).

- See care plans for **Ineffective Thermoregulation** and **Hypothermia** as appropriate.

Pediatric

- Interventions implemented in the care of adult clients are similar when providing care to pediatric clients to prevent hypothermia. EB: *Keep the head covered, use warm blankets, or force warm air to keep the client warm; maintain normal ambient room temperature in the perioperative units and use warmed IV fluids*

H

(IHI, 2012b). EBN: *Children with a lower preoperative body temperature are more likely to develop hypothermia during the intraoperative and postoperative period (Beedle et al, 2017).*

Home Care

▲ Hypothermia is not a symptom that appears in the normal course of postoperative home care. If the client continues to complain of chills or feeling cold after discharge home from a surgical procedure, provide the client with warm blankets and if the client is allowed to drink, provide warm fluids by mouth.

▲ Monitor temperature every hour, as noted previously. If the temperature of the client begins dropping below the normal range, apply layers of clothing or blankets, or adjust environmental heat to the comfort level. Do not overheat. Contact a health care provider. Passive rewarming is the only method of rewarming that is appropriate for home care under normal circumstances.

▲ If temperature continues to drop, activate the emergency system and notify a health care provider. Hypothermia is a clinically acute condition that cannot be managed safely in the home.

Client/Family Teaching and Discharge Planning

• Teach the client/family signs of hypothermia and the method of taking the temperature (age appropriate).

▲ Teach the client and family about medications such as sedatives, opioids, and anxiolytics that predispose the client to hypothermia (as appropriate). If the client has had hypothermia in the past, using alternative medications is an option if there is no contraindication (Danzl, 2012).

REFERENCES

American Society of PeriAnesthesia Nurses (ASPAN). (2015). *Normothermia clinical guideline.* Retrieved from http://www.aspan.org/Clinical-Practice/Clinical-Guidelines/Normothermia. (Accessed 9 January 2018).

Barnason, S., et al. (2012). Emergency nursing resource: Non-invasive temperature measurement in the emergency department. *Journal of Emergency Nursing, 38,* 523–530.

Beedle, S. E., Phillips, A., Wiggins, S., et al. (2017). Preventing unplanned perioperative hypothermia in children. *AORN Journal, 105*(2), 170–183. doi:10.1016/j.aorn.2016.12.002.

Billeter, A. T., Hohmann, S. F., Dren, D., et al. (2014). Unintentional perioperative hypothermia is associated with severe complications and high mortality in elective operations. *Surgery, 156,* 1245–1252.

Burlingame, B. L., & Conner, R. (2015). Guideline for the prevention of unplanned patient hypothermia. In R. Conner (Ed.), *Guidelines for perioperative practice* (2017 ed., pp. 567–590). Denver, CO: AORN.

Campbell, G., Alderson, P., Smith, A. F., et al. (2015). Warming of intravenous and irrigation fluids for preventing inadvertent perioperative hypothermia (Review). *The Cochrane Collaboration,* (4), CD009891.

Centers for Disease Control and Prevention (2018). *Surgical site infection event.* Retrieved from https://www.cdc.gov/nhsn/PDFs/pscManual/9pscSSIcurrent.pdf. (Accessed 9 January 2018).

Connelly, L., Cramer, E., DeMott, Q., et al. (2017). The optimal time and method for surgical prewarming: A comprehensive review of the literature. *Journal of Perianesthesia Nursing, 32*(3), 199–209. doi:10.1016/j.jopan.2015.11.010.

Danzl, D. F. (2012). Hypothermia and frostbite. In A. S. Fauci (Ed.), *Harrison's principles of internal medicine* (18th ed.). New York: McGraw-Hill.

Evron, S., Weissman, A., Toivis, V., et al. (2017). Evaluation of the temple touch pro, a novel noninvasive core-temperature monitoring system. *Anesthesia & Analgesia, 125*(1), 103–109. doi:10.1213/ane.0000000000001695.

Horn, E. P., Bein, B., Broch, O., et al. (2016). Warming before and after epidural block before general anaesthesia for major abdominal surgery prevents perioperative hypothermia: A randomised controlled trial. *European Journal of Anaesthesiology, 33*(5), 334–340. doi:10.1097/EJA.0000000000000369.

Horosz, B., & Malec-Milewska, M. M. (2014). Methods to prevent intraoperative hypothermia. *Anaesthesiology Intensive Therapy, 46*(2), 96–100.

Iden, T., Horn, E. P., Bein, B., et al. (2015). Intraoperative temperature monitoring with zero heat flux technology (3M SpotOn sensor) in comparison with sublingual and nasopharyngeal temperature: An observational study. *European Journal of Anaesthesiology, 32*(6), 387–391. doi:10.1097/EJA.0000000000000232.

Imani, F., Karimi Rouzbahani, H. R., Goudarzi, M., et al. (2016). Skin temperature over the carotid artery, an accurate non-invasive estimation of near core temperature. *Anesthesiology and Pain Medicine, 6*(1), e31046. doi:10.5812/aapm.31046.

Institute for Healthcare Improvement. (2012a). *How-to-guide: Prevent surgical site infections.* Cambridge, MA: Institute for Healthcare Improvement. Retrieved from www.ihi.org. (Accessed 9 January 2018).

Institute for Healthcare Improvement. (2012b). *How-to guide: Prevent surgical site infections, pediatric supplement.* Cambridge, MA: Institute for Healthcare Improvement. Retrieved from www.ihi.org. (Accessed 9 January 2018).

Kelly, P. A., Cooper, S. K., Krogh, M. L., et al. (2013). Thermal comfort and safety of cotton blankets warmed at 130°F and 200°F. *Journal of Perianesthesia Nursing, 28*(6), 337–346.

Kuchena, A., Merkel, M. J., & Hutches, M. P. (2014). Postcardiac arrest temperature management: Infectious risks. *Current Opinion in Critical Care, 20,* 507–515.

Park, H. J., Moon, H. S., Moon, S. H., et al. (2017). The effect of humidified heated breathing circuit on core body temperature in perioperative hypothermia during thyroid surgery. *International Journal of Medical Sciences, 14*(8), 791–797. doi:10.7150/ijms.19318.

Petrone, P. (2014). Management of accidental hypothermia and cold injury. *Current Problems in Surgery, 51*(10), 417–431.

Soreide, K. (2014). Clinical and translational aspects of hypothermia in major trauma patients: From pathophysiology to prevention, prognosis and potential preservation. *Injury-International Journal of the Care of the Injured, 45,* 647–654.

• = Independent;   ▲ = Collaborative;   EBN = Evidence-Based Nursing;   EB = Evidence-Based

Torossian, A., Van Gerven, E., Geertsen, K., et al. (2016). Active perioperative patient warming using a self-warming blanket (BARRIER EasyWarm) is superior to passive thermal insulation: A multinational, multicenter, randomized trial. *Journal of Clinical Anesthesia, 34*, 547–554. doi:10.1016/j.jclinane.2016.06.030.

Wetz, A. J., Perl, T., Brandes, I. F., et al. (2016). Unexpectedly high incidence of hypothermia before induction of anesthesia in elective surgical patients. *Journal of Clinical Anesthesia, 34*, 282–289. doi:10.1016/j.jclinane.2016.03.065.

Warttig, S., Alderson, P., Campbell, G., et al. (2014). Interventions for treating inadvertent postoperative hypothermia (review). *The Cochrane Collaboration*, (11), CD009892.

Winslow, E. H., Cooper, S. K., Hawas, D. M., et al. (2012). Unplanned perioperative hypothermia and agreement between oral, temporal artery, and bladder temperatures in adult major surgery patients. *Journal of Perianesthesia Nursing, 27*(3), 165–180.

Disturbed personal Identity   *Ruth A. Wittmann-Price, PhD, RN, CNS, CNE, CHSE, ANEF, FAAN*

NANDA-I

Definition

Inability to maintain an integrated and complete perception of self.

Defining Characteristics

Alteration in body image; confusion about cultural values; confusion about goals; confusion about ideological values; delusional description of self; feeling of emptiness; feeling of strangeness; fluctuating feelings about self; gender confusion; inability to distinguish between internal and external stimuli; inconsistent behavior; ineffective coping strategies; ineffective relationships; ineffective role performance

Related Factors

Alteration in social role; cult indoctrination; cultural incongruence; discrimination; dysfunctional family processes; low self-esteem; manic states; perceived prejudice; stages of growth

At-Risk Population

Developmental transition; situational crisis; exposure to toxic chemical

Associated Condition

Dissociative identity disorder; organic brain disorder; pharmaceutical agent; psychiatric disorder

NOC   (Nursing Outcomes Classification)

Suggested NOC Outcomes

Anxiety Self-Control; Abuse Recovery (Emotional, Physical, Sexual); Body Image; Decision-Making; Distorted Thought Self-Control; Identity; Mutilation; Suicide/Self-Restraint

> **Example NOC Outcome with Indicators**
>
> **Identity** as evidenced by the following indicators: Verbalizes affirmations of personal identity/Exhibits congruent verbal and nonverbal behavior about self/Differentiates self from environment and other human beings. (Rate the outcome and indicators of **Identity:** 1 = never demonstrated, 2 = rarely demonstrated, 3 = sometimes demonstrated, 4 = often demonstrated, 5 = consistently demonstrated [see Section I].)

Client Outcomes

Client Will (Specify Time Frame)

- Demonstrate new purposes for life
- Show interests in surroundings
- Perform self-care and self-control activities appropriate for age
- Acknowledge personal strengths
- Engage in interpersonal relationships

● = Independent;   ▲ = Collaborative;   EBN = Evidence-Based Nursing;   EB = Evidence-Based

| NIC | (Nursing Interventions Classification) |

Suggested NIC Interventions

Decision-Making Support; Mutual Goal Setting; Self-Awareness Enhancement; Self-Esteem Enhancement; Sexual Counseling; Substance Use Prevention

| Example **NIC** Activities—Self-Esteem Enhancement |

Monitor client's statements of self-worth; Encourage client to identify strengths

Nursing Interventions and *Rationales*

- Assess and support family strengths of commitment, appreciation, and affection toward each other; positive communication; time together; a sense of spiritual well-being; and the ability to cope with stress and crisis. EB: *Hayes, Maliski, and Warner (2017) discovered through a qualitative study that family is an important support for patients, but found that patients are less likely to disclose sensitive health issues when family members are present.* EB: *Hoffman et al (2017) studied African American youths (N = 380) longitudinally over 7 years and found that racial identity grew over time and was influenced in a positive way by their mothers.*
- ▲ Assess for suicidal ideation and make appropriate referral for clients dealing with diversity or mental or chronic somatic illness. EB: *Lesbian, gay, and bisexual (LGB) individuals (N = 356) were studied for their mechanisms of coping with discrimination and researchers found that the combination of education and advocacy predicted self-awareness and personal growth for LGB people (Szymanski, Mikorski, & Carretta, 2017).* EB: *Dutta et al (2017) completed a large quantitative study about the genetics of suicidal ideation with twins (N = 3906 twins) and nontwins (N = 2016) and found that suicidal ideation was 13.0% for men, 21.8% for women, and no difference between twins and nontwins.*
- ▲ Assess clients with mood disorders and make appropriate referrals for treatment. EB: *Verhoeven et al (2017) compared the Mini International Neuropsychiatric Interview (MINI) with clinical diagnosis for mood disorders and anxiety differentiation and found that agreement between the MINI and clinical diagnoses was moderate but increased for patients with just one diagnosis.* EB: *A study using cognitive behavior therapy (CBT) and an active social control (befriending) on depression and anxiety symptoms in people (N = 110) with chronic obstructive pulmonary disease (COPD) demonstrated improvement in anxiety and depression for the befriending group and improved depression for the CBT group (Doyle et al, 2017), indicating that telephone contact is useful.*
- ▲ Assess and make appropriate referrals for clients with physical or mental disabilities. EB: *Gonzalez-Garcia et al (2017) used a sample of children 6 to 18 years old (N = 1216) in residential care and found that 4 of 10 children identified as within the clinical range of abnormal child behavior were not receiving any kind of treatment.* EB: *A study compared mental health and physical health participants (N = 701) attending an exercise referral program over a 12-month period and found that mental health participants were more likely to drop out than those with physical health problems, indicating that better referral decisions can be made (Tobi, Kemp, & Schmidt, 2017).*
- ▲ Assess clients for substance abuse and make appropriate referrals. EB: *Nandrino and Gandolphe (2017) studied patients with alcohol disorder (N = 27), and their self-defining memories (SDMs) and their relationship to personal identity disrupts positive memories and negatively effects personal identity and personal goals.* EB: *Moshtagh et al (2017) completed 31 in-depth interviews with women who were sexually addicted and found that painful emotional experiences created an inner conflict and disrupted their personal identity.*
- Use empathetic communication and encourage the client and family to verbalize fears, express emotions, and set goals. EBN: *Families (N = 612) were provided interventions with emphasis on five positive psychology themes, such as gratitude, flow, happiness, health, and savoring, in a "kitchen project" and results demonstrated that family communication time and frequency of family meal preparation increased with sustainable effects (Ho et al, 2017).* EBN: *Nurse researchers studied mothers and children with HIV (N = 102 pairs) and found the relationship between parenting stress and child perceptions of family functioning demonstrated greater maternal parenting stress associated with poorer family functioning outcomes (reported by both the child and the mother) (Schulte et al, 2017).*
- Be present for clients physically or by telephone. EBN: *Barrett (2017) completed a grounded theory study about the use of teleconsultation by nurses (N = 17) using video in health care and found that nursing presence*

● = Independent;   ▲ = Collaborative;   EBN = Evidence-Based Nursing;   EB = Evidence-Based

was the core category identified and subcategories of nursing presence were operational, clinical, therapeutic, and social, indicating that nurses provided presence during teleconsultation.

▲ EBN: *A qualitative study by Costello (2017) looked at what patients perceived as qualities that increased nurses' presence and identified the following four characteristics: looking for commonalities, sharing personal experiences, use of humor, and caring for spiritual needs.*

• Encourage expression of positive thoughts and emotions. EB: *Researchers studied discrimination of lesbian, gay, bisexual, transgender, and queer (LGBTQ) students and its negative affect on academic performance and personal identity development and identified three major themes: (1) the need for programs to better promote LGBTQ identity, (2) a lack of LGBTQ content in curriculums, and (3) lack of support in schools (Craig et al, 2017). EBN: Hughes, Williams, and Shaw (2017) did a literature review (N = 6) about psychological issues faced by teenagers and young adults during cancer treatment, and analysis identified the following themes: anxieties about treatment, concerns regarding the impact on life (feeling restricted and different, the benefits of being sick, facing uncertainty), and coping strategies (positive thinking and problem-solving, support).*

• Encourage the client to use coping mechanisms. EBN: *Nursing researchers used a cross-sectional study to better understand family satisfaction with health care of their child by measuring support, family quality of life, expressive family functioning, coping strategies, and health care satisfaction in parents (159 mothers and 60 fathers). Results for mothers demonstrated that satisfaction with health care was predicted by family support and their coping strategies, whereas for fathers, satisfaction was predicted by perceived family support, family quality of life, and whether the child had been hospitalized before (Sigurdardottir, Garwick, & Svavarsdottir, 2017). EBN: Rossman et al (2017) completed a narrative qualitative study to understand maternal role attainment of mothers with neonatal intensive care unit (NICU) infants. They found resilience in advocating for their infants, and NICU nurses can assist mothers' health-promoting strengths with resources and coping strategies to decrease their stress.*

• Help clients with serious and chronic conditions to maintain social support networks or assist in building new ones. EB: *A mixed-method (qualitative and quantitative) study was done to evaluate person-centered care for skilled nursing patients (N = 40). The person-centered care included (1) biweekly interdisciplinary care plan meetings with the patient, (2) patient selection of health-related goals that guide team discussions, (3) use of lay language, (4) team accountability to the patient, and (5) monthly care-team meetings. A significant (P < .01) improvement was noted on the Care for Chronic Conditions and Patient Activation Measure surveys. Members viewed the person-centered care experience positively (Abrahamson, Myers, & Nazir, 2017). EBN: Hagedoom et al (2017) descriptively studied family caregiving of elderly patients (N = 62) with one or more chronic conditions, and themes identified were addressing the patients' social network, which included "social network structure" and "social network support," and addressing coordination of care issues.*

▲ Refer women facing diagnostic and curative breast cancer surgery for psychosocial support. EBN: *Wilson (2017) studied exercise for quality of life improvement for breast cancer patients postsurgery and found that it decreased the side effects of surgery. EB: Literature review (N = 190) about breast cancer treatment for African women found that breast tumors are diagnosed at earlier ages and later stages than in high-income countries, and there is a higher prevalence of triple-negative cancers. Lack of nursing care, inadequate access to radiotherapy and surgery, and poor availability of systemic therapies produces poor survival rates (Vanderpuve et al, 2017).*

• Refer for CBT. EBN: *Burn and Lee (2017) used CBT in palliative care (PC) and demonstrated that the CBT tools increased nurses' knowledge and confidence in caring for patients. EBN: Choi, Lee, and Cho (2017) used CBT with patients (N = 76) who had panic disorder and found it useful and produced greater positive effects in the acute treatment phase than those they experience when receiving only routine treatment.*

▲ Refer clients with borderline personality disorder (BPD) and dual-diagnosed BPD and substance-dependent female clients for dialectical behavior therapy (DBT) and psychoanalytical-orientated day-hospital therapy. EB: *Perry, Bond, and Bekes (2017) followed patients with BPD (N = 16) and 35 with non-BPD for 3 to 5 years and found psychotherapy did not always provide faster rates of improvement of the condition. EB: Stepp and Lazarus (2017) did a study to identify dimensions of children (N = 2450) with temperament and psychopathology symptoms that predict future BPD. Researchers found that parent and teacher ratings of emotionality predicted BPD; therefore early detection may increase care for children with BPD.*

▲ Refer to the care plans for Readiness for enhanced **Communication** and Readiness for enhanced **Spiritual** well-being.

• = Independent;　　▲ = Collaborative;　　EBN = Evidence-Based Nursing;　　EB = Evidence-Based

Pediatric

- Encourage adolescents to promote positive self-esteem, to enhance coping, and to prevent behavioral and psychological problems. **EB:** *Thomas et al (2017) studied group identification (N = 369) longitudinally related to sports teams and found three motivators: (1) individuals' personal feelings of self-esteem, (2) social identity, and (3) one collective identity motive. All of these helped meet personal needs.* **EBN:** *Ruhl and Lordly (2017) found that students who are a part of a competitive educational program display a negative effect on personal identity, learning motivation, student collaboration, participation in academic opportunities, and student relationships with faculty.*
- Evaluate and refer children and adolescents for eating disorder prevention programs to include medical care, nutritional intervention, and mental health treatment and care coordination. **EBN:** *Kendal et al (2017) qualitatively studied eating disorders and social media (400 messages) and found the following online discussion themes: taking on the role of mentor, the online discussion forum as a safe space, friendship within the online forum, flexible help, and peer support for recovery and relapse prevention.* **EB:** *Darrow et al (2017) studied the family types of children (N = 123) with eating disorders and categorized them into types that assisted the child to get treatment: (1) control-oriented, (2) system maintenance-oriented, and (3) conflict-oriented.*
- Use computer-mediated support groups to enhance identity formation. **EBN:** *Jackson and Mixer (2017) used Apple iPads in a pilot study for pediatric patients and families who spoke Spanish and found it assisted in bedside communication, and the results assisted in developing a larger scale communication interface.* **EB:** *Sundstrom, Blankers, and Khadjesari (2017) studied computer-based alcohol interventions by completing a systematic review and found supporting evidence for continuing their use.*

Geriatric

- Evaluate the effectiveness of nursing interventions used to promote positive self-identify in older adults. **EBN:** *A descriptive study about applying a therapeutic relationship to people (N = 112) with a common mental disorder and the results were gathered using frequency statistics and found that the nursing therapeutic relationship in mental health transcends the area of specialty and builds patient coping strategies and helps them make changes in daily life (Nobrega et al, 2017).* **EB:** *Researchers used the international classification of functioning, disability, and health to develop a tool to assess functioning in elderly patients (N = 251). The tool was reliable in assessing the needs of elderly patients and can be studied further for use and to devise care (Ahsberg et al, 2017).*
- Encourage clients to discuss their "life histories." Life history-based interventions and self-esteem and life-satisfaction questionnaires may be used to reinforce personal identity and foster hope. **EBN:** *Tamura-Lis (2017) used reminiscing as an effective evidence-based tool in understanding and treating older adults. Reminiscing has demonstrated that it improves communication and socialization.* **EB:** *Researchers found that health care providers can better understand the needs of PC patients by using storytelling. Storytelling was described in two themes, the living–dying dialect and the practicing–advocating dialog. Understanding the perspective of PC patients can assist caregivers in providing better communication and end-of-life care (Omilion-Hodges & Swords, 2017).*
- ▲ Refer the older client to self-help support groups. **EB:** *Ilha et al (2017) completed a qualitative study of elderly people (N = 13) with Alzheimer's disease and their caregivers participating in support groups and found the experience positively influenced education by building knowledge that was applied in practice.* **EB:** *Canata et al (2017) studied telephone support for diabetic control in elderly patients compared with patients in a group with written materials and found the telephone group had better metabolic results in glucose level and blood pressure.*
- ▲ Refer the client with Alzheimer's disease who is terminally ill to hospice. **EBN:** *Schaustz, Chaves, and Serejo (2017) studied overload in caregivers (N = 53) of the elderly and found that 45.3% of the caregivers presented moderate overload, 13.2% presented with moderate to severe overload, 3.8% presented with severe overload, and 32.1% presented with no overload, indicating the need for supportive care.* **EBN:** *Goldsborough and Matzo (2017) discussed the need for PC based on experience and observation within the acute care setting and promoting education of acute care nurses to understand the implications of end-of-life care for elderly patients.*

Multicultural

- Assess an individual's sociocultural background in teaching self-management and self-regulation as a means of supporting hope and coping. **EB:** *Meca et al (2017) qualitatively studied recent Hispanic adolescent*

● = Independent;   ▲ = Collaborative;   **EBN** = Evidence-Based Nursing;   **EB** = Evidence-Based

immigrants (N = 302) in the United States and found that personal identity associated with the US-predicted positivism and decreased antisocial behavior. EB: *Sica et al (2017) studied the identity formation of Italian university students through narrative accounts of five identify dimensions: achievement, foreclosure, moratorium, diffused diffusion, carefree diffusion, and undifferentiated. The connections between dimensions reflected a particular personal identity.* EB: *Ozer et al (2017) qualitatively studied the globalization-based acculturation process of Ladakhi youth (N = 8) and found participants reported negotiating their cultural identity through discussion of culture, religion, and social issues within social constraints and that researchers found that the acculturation process is complex and ongoing for the young participants.*

- Decrease discrimination to promote positive ethnic identity. EB: *Baldwin-White et al (2017) studied the relationship among acculturation, discrimination, and ethnic–racial identity (ERI) in Latino youths (N = 830) and found higher levels of acculturation were associated with lower levels of searching and affirmation, and higher perceived discrimination was associated with higher affirmation.* EB: *Researchers studied ethnic identity development of East Asian adolescents (N = 13) and found that five themes emerged in their qualitative study: ethnic/cultural identity and socialization, bicultural living, racial context-racism and stereotypes, family context-parental expectation, and peer context-friendship/dating. Participants' experienced hurtful racial discrimination, but experienced ethnic identity at home (Eunju et al, 2017).*
- Refer to care plan for Ineffective **Coping.**

Home Care

- The interventions described previously may be adapted for home care use.
- Provide an Internet-based health coach to encourage self-management for clients with chronic conditions such as depression, impaired mobility, and chronic pain. Use computer-mediated support groups to enhance identify formation. EB: *Phelan et al (2017) tested using the Internet for women receiving the Special Supplemental Nutrition Program for Women, Infants, and Children (WIC) postpartum (N = 371) compared with a nonintervention group. The intervention group lost more weight in 12 months.* EB: *Researchers studied using the Internet to treat social anxiety disorder (SAD) in participants (N = 42) randomized into two groups. One group had therapy support. Both groups decreased symptoms of SAD, and the group with the therapist interventions had a lower attrition rate (Gershkovich et al, 2017).*
- ▲ Refer the client to mutual health support groups. Participating in mutual health support groups led to enhanced coping by improving psychological and social functioning. EB: *Urbanoski, Mierlo, and Cunningham (2017) used social network analysis to examine online support groups for patients with drinking addictions (N = 711) and found active members were older and after 5 years the online support group was cohesive and stable.* EB: *Bossy et al (2017) studied self-management of patients (N = 16) with type 2 diabetes who participated in a support group, and the findings supported group-based self-management support assisted with decreasing self-blame and assisted identity building.*
- ▲ Refer cancer clients and their spouses to family programs that include family-based interventions for communication, hope, coping, uncertainty, and symptom management. EB: *A qualitative study explored the role of family members (N = 41) with cancer patients in the communication process, and all patients and family members preferred open communication with physicians. The study discussed the importance of family for physical and psychological care and discovered that there needed to be a balance between patient autonomy and relative's desire to be protective (Datta et al, 2017).* EB: *Prioli et al (2017) evaluated the direct costs and effectiveness of the mindfulness-based art therapy (MBAT) compared with the cost and effectiveness of a breast cancer support group (BCSG); both methods worked effectively, but BCSG was more cost-efficient than MBAT.*
- Refer combat veterans and service members directly involved in combat, as well as those providing support to combatants, including nurses, for mental health services. EB: *Stana, Flynn, and Almeida (2017) conducted a thematic analysis of 466 Internet discussion posts by veterans (N = 623) and partners to understand the type of social support that was available, and most was informational support and network/ community support. There was little emotional support.* EB: *Gould et al (2017) developed a telephone-based program for older veterans to reduce loneliness and qualitatively found that it benefited socialization, which included connectedness, learning from others, being active despite limitations, and distraction from limitations.*

Client/Family Teaching and Discharge Planning

- Teach the client about available community resources (e.g., therapists, ministers, counselors, self-help groups, family education groups). EB: *A 5-year longitudinal study compared participation in pleasant*

● = Independent;   ▲ = Collaborative;   EBN = Evidence-Based Nursing;   EB = Evidence-Based

leisure activities and blood pressure in caregivers of Alzheimer's patients (N = 126) and found that greater engagement in pleasant leisure reduced mean arterial blood pressure (Mausbach et al, 2017). **EBN:** *Kangovi et al (2017) examined if community health worker (CHW) interventions improved outcomes in a low-income population (N = 302) with multiple chronic conditions. They found that using a standardized intervention improved chronic disease control, mental health, and quality of care.*

- Teach coping skills to family caregivers of cancer clients. **EB:** *Blanco et al (2017) studied family environment (N = 50) in relation to childhood and found that families with obese children had higher trait anxiety, criticism and overprotectiveness, and maladaptive coping skills.* **EB:** *Takizawa et al (2017) evaluated the job stress and coping style of caregivers (N = 134) of dementia patients before and after they have completed training. They found that educating caregivers increases coping skills.*

- Refer to Ineffective **Coping** for additional references.

REFERENCES

Abrahamson, K., Myers, J., & Nazir, A. (2017). Implementation of a person-centered medical care model in a skilled nursing facility: A pilot evaluation. *Journal of the American Medical Directors Association*, 18(6), 539–543. Retrieved from http://dx.doi.org/10.1016/j.jamda.2017.03.001.

Ahsberg, E., Fahlstrom, G., Ronnback, E., et al. (2017). Development of an instrument for assessing elder care needs. *Research on Social Work Practice*, 27(3), 291–306. Retrieved from http://dx.doi.org/10.1177/1049731515572913.

Baldwin-White, A. J. M., Kiehne, E., Umana-Taylor, A., et al. (2017). In pursuit of belonging: Acculturation, perceived discrimination, and ethnic–racial identity among Latino youths. *Social Work Research*, 41(1), 43–52. Retrieved from http://dx.doi.org/10.1093/swr/svw029.

Barrett, D. (2017). Rethinking presence: A grounded theory of nurses and teleconsultation. *Journal of Clinical Nursing*, 26(19/20), 3088–3098. Retrieved from http://dx.doi.org/10.1111/jocn.13656.

Blanco, M., et al. (2017). Examining maternal psychopathology, family functioning and coping skills in childhood obesity: A case-control study. *European Eating Disorders Review*, 25(5), 359–365. Retrieved from http://dx.doi.org/10.1002/erv.2527.

Bossy, D., Knutsen, I. R., Rogers, A., et al. (2017). Group affiliation in self-management: Support or threat to identity? *Health Expectations*, 20(1), 159–170. Retrieved from http://dx.doi.org/10.1111/hex.12448.

Burn, K., & Lee, L. (2017). Cognitive behavioural therapy in palliative care: Evaluation of staff following a foundation level course. *International Journal of Palliative Nursing*, 23(6), 270–278. Retrieved from http://dx.doi.org/10.12968/ijpn.2017.23.6.270.

Canata, B. T. A., et al. (2017). Effects of supportive telephone counseling in the metabolic control of elderly people with diabetes mellitus. *Revista Brasileira de Enfermagem*, 70(4), 704–710. Retrieved from http://dx.doi.org/10.1590/0034-7167-2017-0089.

Choi, Y. S., Lee, E. J., & Cho, Y. (2017). The effect of Korean-group cognitive behavioural therapy among patients with panic disorder in clinic settings. *Journal of Psychiatric & Mental Health Nursing*, 24(1), 28–40. Retrieved from http://dx.doi.org/10.1111/jpm.12337.

Costello, M. (2017). Nurses' self-identified characteristics and behaviors contributing to patients' positive perceptions of their nursing care. *Journal of Holistic Nursing*, 35(1), 62–66. Retrieved from http://dx.doi.org/10.1177/0898010116643835.

Craig, S. L., Iacono, G., Paceley, M. S., et al. (2017). Intersecting sexual, gender, and professional identities among social work students: The importance of identity integration. *Journal of Social Work Education*, 53(3), 466–479. Retrieved from http://dx.doi.org/10.1080/10437797.2016.1272516.

Darrow, S. M., Accurso, E. C., Nauman, E. R., et al. (2017). Exploring types of family environments in youth with eating disorders. *European Eating Disorders Review*, 25(5), 389–396. Retrieved from http://dx.doi.org/10.1002/erv.2531.

Datta, S. S., et al. (2017). Pivotal role of families in doctor-patient communication in oncology: A qualitative study of patients, their relatives and cancer clinicians. *European Journal of Cancer Care*, 26(5), 1–8. Retrieved from http://dx.doi.org/10.1111/ecc.12543.

Doyle, C., Bhar, S., Fearn, M., et al. (2017). The impact of telephone-delivered cognitive behaviour therapy and befriending on mood disorders in people with chronic obstructive pulmonary disease: A randomized controlled trial. *British Journal of Health Psychology*, 22(3), 542–556. Retrieved from http://dx.doi.org/10.1111/bjhp.12245.

Dutta, R., Ball, H. A., Siribaddana, S. H., et al. (2017). Genetic and other risk factors for suicidal ideation and the relationship with depression. *Psychological Medicine*, 47(14), 2438–2449. Retrieved from http://dx.doi.org/10.1017/S0033291717000940.

Eunju, Y., Adams, K., Clawson, A., et al. (2017). *Journal of Counseling Psychology*, 64(1), 65–79. Retrieved from http://dx.doi.org/10.1037/cou0000181.

Gershkovich, M., Herbert, J. D., Forman, E. M., et al. (2017). Internet-delivered acceptance-based cognitive-behavioral intervention for social anxiety Disorder with and without therapist support: A randomized trial. *Behavior Modification*, 41(5), 583–608. Retrieved from http://dx.doi.org/10.1177/0145445517694457.

Goldsborough, J. L., & Matzo, M. (2017). Palliative care in the acute care setting. *AJN American Journal of Nursing*, 117(9), 64–67. MEDLINE Info: *NLM UID*: 0372646.

Gonzalez-Garcia, C., Bravo, A., Arruabarrena, I., et al. (2017). Emotional and behavioral problems of children in residential care: Screening detection and referrals to mental health services. *Children & Youth Services Review*, 73, 100–106. Retrieved from http://dx.doi.org/10.1016/j.childyouth.2016.12.011.

Gould, C., et al. (2017). RESOLV: Development of a telephone-based program designed to increase socialization in older veterans. *Educational Gerontology*, 43(8), 379–392. Retrieved from http://dx.doi.org/10.1080/03601277.2017.1299522.

Hagedoom, E. I., Paans, W., Jaarsma, T., et al. (2017). Aspects of family caregiving as addressed in planned discussions between nurses, patients with chronic diseases and family caregivers: A qualitative content analysis. *BMC Nursing*, 16, 1–10. Retrieved from http://dx.doi.org/10.1186/s12912-017-0231-5.

Hayes, A., Maliski, R., & Warner, B. (2017). Analyzing the effects of family communication patterns on the decision to disclose a health issue to a parent: The benefits of conversation and dangers of conformity. *Health Communication*, 32(7), 837–844. Retrieved from http://dx.doi.org/10.1080/10410236.2016.1177898.

Ho, H., et al. (2017). Happy family kitchen: Behavioral outcomes of a brief community-based family intervention in Hong Kong. *Journal of Child & Family Studies*, 26(10), 2852–2864. Retrieved from http://dx.doi.org/10.1007/s10826-017-0788-3.

● = Independent;   ▲ = Collaborative;   **EBN** = Evidence-Based Nursing;   **EB** = Evidence-Based

Hoffman, A. J., Kurtz-Costes, B., Rowley, S. J., et al. (2017). Bidirectional influence between African American mothers' and children's racial centrality from elementary through high school. *Developmental Psychology*, 53(6), 1130–1141. Retrieved from http://dx.doi.org/10.1037/dev0000307.

Hughes, N., Williams, J., & Shaw, C. (2017). Supporting the psychological needs of teenagers and young adults during cancer treatment: A literature review. *British Journal of Nursing*, 26(4), S4–S10. NLM UID: 9212059.

Ilha, S., et al. (2017). Complex educational and care (geron) technology for elderly individuals/families experiencing Alzheimer's disease. *Revista Brasileira de Enfermagem*, 70(4), 726–732. Retrieved from http://dx.doi.org/10.1590/0034-7167-2016-0687.

Jackson, K. H., & Mixer, S. J. (2017). Using an iPad for basic communication between Spanish-speaking families and nurses in pediatric acute care: A feasibility pilot study. *Computers, Informatics, Nursing*, 35(8), 401–407. Retrieved from http://dx.doi.org/10.1097/CIN.0000000000000354.

Kangovi, S., Mitra, N., Grande, D., et al. (2017). Community health worker support for disadvantaged patients with multiple chronic diseases: A randomized clinical trial. *American Journal of Public Health*, 107(10), 1660–1667. Retrieved from http://dx.doi.org/10.2105/AJPH.2017.303985.

Kendal, S., Kirk, S., Elvey, R., et al. (2017). How a moderated online discussion forum facilitates support for young people with eating disorders. *Health Expectations*, 20(1), 98–111. Retrieved from http://dx.doi.org/10.1111/hex.12439.

Mausbach, B. T., et al. (2017). Engagement in pleasant leisure activities and blood pressure: A 5-year longitudinal study in Alzheimer caregivers. *Psychosomatic Medicine*, 79(7), 735–741. Retrieved from http://dx.doi.org/10.1097/PSY.0000000000000497.

Meca, A., et al. (2017). Personal and cultural identity development in recently immigrated Hispanic adolescents: Links with psychosocial functioning. *Cultural Diversity & Ethnic Minority Psychology*, 23(3), 348–361. Retrieved from http://dx.doi.org/10.1037/cdp0000129.

Moshtagh, M., Mirlashari, J., Rafiey, H., et al. (2017). Human identity versus gender identity: The perception of sexual addiction among Iranian women. *Health Care for Women International*, 38(7), 732–752. Retrieved from http://dx.doi.org/10.1080/07399332.2017.1322594.

Nandrino, J., & Gandolphe, M. (2017). Characterization of self-defining memories in individuals with severe alcohol use disorders after mid-term abstinence: The impact of the emotional valence of memories. *Alcoholism, Clinical and Experimental Research*, 41(8), 1484–1491. Retrieved from http://dx.doi.org/10.1111/acer.13424.

Nobrega, S., Perpetuo, M., Fernandes, T., et al. (2017). Application of the therapeutic relationship to people with common mental disorder. *Revista Gaucha de Enfermagem*, 38(1), 1–8. Retrieved from http://dx.doi.org/10.1590/1983-1447.2017.01.63562.

Omilion-Hodges, L. M., & Swords, N. M. (2017). The Grim Reaper, Hounds of Hell, and Dr. Death: The role of storytelling for palliative care in competing medical meaning systems. *Health Communication*, 32(10), 1272–1283. Retrieved from http://dx.doi.org/10.1080/10410236.2016.1219928.

Ozer, S., Bertelsen, P., Singla, R., et al. (2017). "Grab your culture and walk with the global": Ladakhi students' negotiation of cultural identity in the context of globalization-based acculturation. *Journal of Cross-Cultural Psychology*, 48(3), 294–318. Retrieved from http://dx.doi.org/10.1177/0022022116687394.

Perry, J. C., Bond, M., & Bekes, V. (2017). The rate of improvement in long-term dynamic psychotherapy for borderline personality disorder. *Journal of Nervous & Mental Disease*, 205(7), 517–524. Retrieved from http://dx.doi.org/10.1097/NMD.0000000000000697.

Phelan, S., et al. (2017). Effect of an internet-based [rogram on weight loss for low-income postpartum women: A randomized clinical trial.

JAMA: Journal of the American Medical Association, 317(23), 2381–2391. Retrieved from http://dx.doi.org/10.1001/jama.2017.7119.

Prioli, K. M., et al. (2017). Costs and effectiveness of mindfulness-based art therapy versus standard breast cancer support group for women with cancer. *American Health & Drug Benefits*, 10(6), 288–294. ISSN:1942-2962.

Rossman, B., Greene, M. M., Kratovil, A. L., et al. (2017). Resilience in mothers of very-low-birth-weight infants hospitalized in the NICU. *JOGNN: Journal of Obstetric, Gynecologic & Neonatal Nursing*, 46(3), 434–445. Retrieved from http://dx.doi.org/10.1016/j.jogn.2016.11.016.

Ruhl, I., & Lordly, D. (2017). The nature of competition in dietetics education: A narrative review. *Canadian Journal of Dietetic Practice & Research*, 78(3), 129–136. Retrieved from http://dx.doi.org/10.3148/cjdpr-2017-004.

Schaustz, B. F., Chaves, S. S. P., & Serejo, C. R. (2017). Overload in caregivers of the elderly. *Journal of Nursing UFPE*, 11(1), 160–164. Retrieved from http://dx.doi.org/10.5205/reuol.9978-88449-6-1101201719.

Schulte, M. T., et al. (2017). Maternal parenting stress and child perception of family functioning among families affected by HIV. *JANAC: Journal of the Association of Nurses in AIDS Care*, 28(5), 784–794. Retrieved from http://dx.doi.org/10.1016/j.jana.2017.05.004.

Sica, L., Luyckx, K., Goossens, L., et al. (2017). Identity statuses and event-focused narratives at university starting point in Italy. *Journal of Adult Development*, 24(2), 89–108. Retrieved from http://dx.doi.org/10.1007/s10804-016-9249-2.

Sigurdardottir, A. O., Garwick, A. W., & Svavarsdottir, E. K. (2017). The importance of family support in pediatrics and its impact on healthcare satisfaction. *Scandinavian Journal of Caring Sciences*, 31(2), 241–252. Retrieved from http://dx.doi.org/10.1111/scs.12336.

Stana, A., Flynn, M. A., & Almeida, E. (2017). Battling the stigma: Combat veterans' use of social support in an online PTSD forum. *International Journal of Men's Health*, 16(1), 20–36. Retrieved from http://dx.doi.org/10.3149/jmh.1601.20.

Stepp, S. D., & Lazarus, S. A. (2017). Identifying a borderline personality disorder prodrome: Implications for community screening. *Personality & Mental Health*, 11(3), 195–205. Retrieved from http://dx.doi.org/10.1002/pmh.1389.

Sundstrom, C., Blankers, M., & Khadjesari, Z. (2017). Computer-based interventions for problematic alcohol use: A review of systematic reviews. *International Journal of Behavioral Medicine*, 24(5), 646–658. Retrieved from http://dx.doi.org/10.1007/s12529-016-9601-8.

Szymanski, D. M., Mikorski, R., & Carretta, R. F. (2017). Heterosexism and LGB positive identity: Roles of coping and personal growth initiative. *Counseling Psychologist*, 45(2), 294–319. Retrieved from http://dx.doi.org/10.1177/0011000017697195.

Takizawa, T., Takahashi, M., Takai, M., et al. (2017). Changes in job stress and coping skills among caregivers after dementia care practitioner training. *Psychogeriatrics*, 17(1), 52–60. Retrieved from http://dx.doi.org/10.1111/psyg.12188.

Tamura-Lis, W. (2017). Reminiscing—A tool for excellent elder care and improved quality of life. *Urologic Nursing*, 37(3), 151–156, 142. Retrieved from http://dx.doi.org/10.7257/1053-816X.2017.37.3.151.

Thomas, W. E., et al. (2017). Social identification in sports teams: The role of personal, social, and collective identity motives. *Personality & Social Psychology Bulletin*, 43(4), 508–523. Retrieved from http://dx.doi.org/10.1177/0146167216689051.

Tobi, P., Kemp, P., & Schmidt, E. (2017). Cohort differences in exercise adherence among primary care patients referred for mental health versus physical health conditions. *Primary Health Care Research & Development*, 18(5), 463–471. Retrieved from http://dx.doi.org/10.1017/S1463423617000214.

Urbanoski, K., Mierlo, T., & Cunningham, J. (2017). Investigating patterns of participation in an online support group for problem drinking: A social network analysis. *International Journal of*

● = Independent;   ▲ = Collaborative;   **EBN** = Evidence-Based Nursing;   **EB** = Evidence-Based

Behavioral Medicine, 24(5), 703–712. Retrieved from http://dx.doi.org/10.1007/s12529-016-9591-6.

Vanderpuye, V., et al. (2017). An update on the management of breast cancer in Africa. *Infectious Agents & Cancer, 12*, 1–12. Retrieved from http://dx.doi.org/10.1186/s13027-017-0124-y.

Verhoeven, F. E. A., et al. (2017). Agreement between clinical and MINI diagnoses in outpatients with mood and anxiety disorders. *Journal of Affective Disorders, 221*, 268–274. Retrieved from http://dx.doi.org/10.1016/j.jad.2017.06.041.

Wilson, D. (2017). Exercise for the patient after breast cancer surgery. *Seminars in Oncology Nursing, 33*(1), 98–105. Retrieved from http://dx.doi.org/10.1016/j.soncn.2016.11.010.

Risk for disturbed personal Identity   *Marina Martinez-Kratz, MS, RN, CNE*

NANDA-I

Definition

Susceptible to the inability to maintain an integrated and complete perception of self, which may compromise health.

Risk Factors

Alteration in social role; cult indoctrination; cultural incongruence; discrimination; dysfunctional family processes; low self-esteem; manic states; perceived prejudice; stages of growth

At-Risk Population

Developmental transition; exposure to toxic chemical; situational crisis

Associated Condition

Dissociative identity disorder; organic brain disorder; pharmaceutical agent; psychiatric disorder

NOC, NIC, Client Outcomes, Nursing Interventions and *Rationales,* Client/Family Teaching and Discharge Planning, and References

Refer to care plan for Disturbed personal **Identity.**

Risk for complicated Immigration Transition
Nadia Charania, PhD, RN

NANDA-I

Definition

Susceptibility to experiencing negative feelings (loneliness, fear, anxiety) in response to unsatisfactory consequences and cultural barriers to one's immigration transition, which may compromise health.

Related Factors

Available work is below educational preparation; cultural barriers in host country; unsanitary housing; insufficient knowledge about the process to access resources in the host country; insufficient social support in host country; language barriers in host country; multiple nonrelated persons in household; overcrowded housing; overt discrimination; parent–child conflicts related to enculturation in the host country; and abusive landlord

At-Risk Population

Forced migration; hazardous work conditions with inadequate training; illegal status in host country; labor exploitation; precarious economic situation; separation from family in home country; separation from friends in home country; unfulfilled expectations of immigration

NOC   (Nursing Outcomes Classification)

Suggested NOC Outcomes

Relocation Adaptation, Anxiety Level; Fear Level; Loneliness Severity; Coping

● = Independent;   ▲ = Collaborative;   EBN = Evidence-Based Nursing;   EB = Evidence-Based

---

> ### Example NOC Outcome with Indicators
>
> **Relocation Adaptation** as evidenced by the following indicators: Participates in decision-making in new environment/Expresses satisfaction with daily routine/Fear/Loneliness/Anxiety/. (Rate the outcome and indicators of **Relocation Adaptation**: 1 = never demonstrated; 2 = rarely demonstrated, 3 = sometimes demonstrated, 4 = often demonstrated, 5 = consistently demonstrated [see Section I].)

Client Outcomes

Client Will (Specify Time Frame)

- Participates in community activities
- State satisfaction with social relationships, living arrangements, and social integration
- State satisfaction with health status and access to health care
- Demonstrate actions that are congruent with expressed feelings and thoughts
- State sense of belonging
- Accept strengths and limitations of new environment

NIC   (Nursing Interventions Classification)

Suggested NIC Interventions

Support System Enhancement; Socialization Enhancement; Values Clarification

> ### Example NIC Activities—Risk for Complicated Immigration Transition
>
> Encourage patience in developing relationships; Encourage social and community activities

Nursing Interventions and *Rationales*

- Understand immigrants' personal perspectives/stories about their health maintenance and illness management. CEBN: *Nurses are concerned with the life experiences of people and how these life experiences may affect their health and responses to illness. Furthermore, to diagnose and treat immigrants who are ill, we must be able to put their responses within the context of their lives; otherwise, our understanding and interpretation of their responses to illness will be limited (Meleis, 2010).*
- Focus on providing holistic (physical, emotional, psychological, social, and spiritual) care while caring for immigrants. When appropriate, integrate use of spirituality and connection with ethnic faith institutions. CEB: Ethnic faith institutions could be a valuable resource for immigrants and their families because these institutions provide support and relevant services to help immigrants balance their transition, such as providing a valuable link to the home culture and values, providing services in the areas of language acquisition, job training, and child care services (Slessarev-Jamir, 2008).
- Acknowledge the reciprocal relationship of immigrant and his and her cultural context. EB: Cultural context shapes the ways in which immigrants conceptualize, express, and cope with distress, resilience, and help-seeking (American Psychological Association [APA], 2013).
- Identify immigrant's sociocultural context, particularly to identify his or her unique perspectives with respect to cultural assimilation and cultural distinctiveness and whether or not he or she considers there is a possibility of combining both perspectives. EB: Recognize the role of sociocultural context and assist in providing ethical and appropriate care. Use an approach of combining both perspectives of cultural assimilation and cultural distinctiveness, in which an immigrant preserves his or her cultural distinctiveness yet simultaneously works toward developing a shared identity with those who were born in the country to which the individual immigrated (APA, 2013).
- Consider exploring the following factors in planning and providing care to immigrants: (1) premigration factors; (2) migration experience; (3) reception into new environment and trauma; (4) language/communication; (5) symptom expression; (6) changes in gender roles and intergenerational issues, economic stress, and marginalization; (7) resilience; and (8) multiplicity of identity need. EB: The understanding of such factors and how they interact in promoting or preventing the immigrant's health assists in providing culturally competent care (APA, 2013).
- Ensure that immigrants' cultural identities, rights, and needs are respected in the delivery of health care. CEBN: Sensitivity in integrating cultural safety when caring for a socially disadvantaged cultural

● = Independent;   ▲ = Collaborative;   EBN = Evidence-Based Nursing;   EB = Evidence-Based

minority group is imperative because cultural safety affects how health care is delivered to them (Baker, 2007).

- Assist immigrants in their transition toward health and a perception of well-being. CEBN: Nurses are an integral part of the health care team working with the immigrant population because nurses have a unique perspective on transition, which focuses on facilitating transitions to enhance a sense of well-being (Meleis & Trangestein, 2010).
- Be aware of the benefits and risks of involving an interpreter in providing care to immigrants. EBN: In a qualitative research study, nurses shared their perceptions of working with immigrant patients and interpreters and indicated that the interpreter supports the communication between the nurse and the patient but also increases the amount of work undertaken by nurses, complicates the nurse–patient relationship, and/or creates ethical problems (Eklöf, Hupli, & Leino-Kilpi, 2014).

Pediatric

- Explore current barriers and facilitators that are faced by children of immigrants to assimilate into the immigrated country's educational system. EB: *Such knowledge plays a significant role in the future of the immigrants' children on many fronts, including addressing barriers to seeking health care and acculturation (APA, 2013).*
- Invest effort in understanding the unique experiences of immigrant children, their health insurance status, and access to care. CEB: *The value of such understanding is critical in planning and promoting health care of immigrant children. Low rates of health insurance and limited access to care compounds the risk for deteriorating health (Perreira & Ornelas, 2011).*
- Explore the actual or perceived discrimination experienced by immigrant youth. CEB: *Evidence supports the relationship between racial discrimination and health such that they report more anxiety, depression, and risky health behaviors; low levels of self-esteem; and decreased academic motivation and expectations (Gonzales, Fabrett, & Knight, 2009).*
- Health care providers and school personnel need to encourage involvement of immigrant parents in their children's school-based activities. EB: *Parents involvement in school-based activities affects behavioral well-being of children of immigrants. Understanding parents' perceptions of parental involvement is important because parent involvement may mean something different in different cultures (Beauregard, Petrakos, & Dupont, 2014).*
- Identify the dynamics between immigrant children and their parents, including intergenerational conflict. EB: *Evidence supports that intergenerational conflict (a differing degree of acculturation between parents and children) contributes to acculturative stress (Rogers-Sirin, Ryce, & Sirin, 2014).*
- Encourage children to verbalize their understanding of being separated from their parent(s) or loved ones because of migration. CEB: *The process family or loved ones uses to prepare the child for separation plays a central role in how the child makes meaning of and responds to the challenge of separation, for example, feeling abandoned when separation is not framed as temporary and needed versus feeling resilient when separation is framed otherwise (Suarez-Orozco, Todorova, & Louie, 2002).*
- Explore acculturation process-related stress, social support, and ethnic identity of youth. EB: *Evidence supports that the increase in acculturative stress over time increases the internalizing of mental health symptoms; however, the presence of social support and ethnic identity plays a protective role against acculturative stress among youth and prevents the internalizing of mental health symptoms (Rogers-Sirin, Ryce, & Sirin, 2014).*
- Focus on assisting adolescent immigrants in their transition to developing bicultural competencies. CEB: *Bicultural competencies serve as a protective factor in lowering the chances of developing problematic mental health symptoms in adolescents (Smokowski, Chapman, & Bacallao, 2007).*

Geriatric

Note: All interventions are relevant and appropriate for geriatric immigrants.

Multicultural

Note: All interventions are relevant and appropriate for geriatric immigrants.

Home Care

- Encourage family members of immigrants to engage in home care tasks. Cultures with collective societal values are strongly expected to participate in the meeting of home care tasks for the elderly and needy.

CEB: *Elderly who reside with relatives and family members usually fulfill home care tasks. At the same time, there is a strong expectation, for example, within the Chinese community, that children or the younger generation are meeting the elderly's daily needs (Lai, 2004).*

- Educate and encourage immigrants' family members to use available home care-specific support services as needed. EB: It is critical to recognize that the immigrated family is faced with both health care system barriers (e.g., discrimination within the health care system and complex bureaucracies) and individual barriers (e.g., limited communication ability, lack of financial resources, and the experience of shame or stigma) when in need of accessing care (Hacker, Anies, Folb, & Zallman, 2015).

REFERENCES

American Psychological Association. (2013). *Working with immigrant-origin clients: An update for mental health professionals.* Based on Crossroads: The Psychology of Immigration in the New Century the Report of the APA Presidential Task Force on Immigration. Retrieved from http://www.apa.org/topics/immigration/immigration-report-professionals.pdf.

Baker, C. (2007). Globalization and the cultural safety of an immigrant Muslim community. *Journal of Advanced Nursing, 57*(3), 296–305. doi:10.1111/j.1365-2648.2006.04104.x.

Beauregard, F., Petrakos, H., & Dupont, A. (2014). Family-school partnership: Practices of immigrant parents in Quebec, Canada. *School Community Journal, 24*(1), 177–210.

Eklöf, N., Hupli, M., & Leino-Kilpi, H. (2014). Nurses' perceptions of working with immigrant patients and interpreters in Finland. *Public Health Nursing, 32*(2), 143–150.

Gonzales, N. A., Fabrett, F. C., & Knight, G. P. (2009). Acculturation, enculturation, and the psychosocial adaptation of Latino youth. In F. A. Villarruel, G. Carlo, J. M. Grau, et al. (Eds.), *Handbook of U.S. Latino psychology: Developmental and community-based perspectives* (pp. 115–134). Thousand Oaks, CA: Sage Publications, Inc.

Hacker, K., Anies, M., Folb, B. L., et al. (2015). Barriers to health care for undocumented immigrants: A literature review. *Risk Management and Healthcare Policy, 8*, 175–183.

Lai, D. W. L. (2004). Use of home care services by elderly Chinese immigrants. *Home Health Care Services Quarterly, 23*(3), 41–56. doi:10.1300/J027v23n03_03.

Meleis, A. I. (2010). Immigrant transitions and health care: An action plan. In A. I. Meleis (Ed.), *Transition theory* (pp. 241–242). New York: Springer.

Meleis, A. I., & Trangestein, P. A. (2010). Facilitating transitions: Redefinition of the nursing mission. In A. I. Meleis (Ed.), *Transition theory* (pp. 65–72). New York: Springer.

Perreira, K. M., & Ornelas, I. J. (2011). The physical and psychological well-being of immigrant children. *The Future of Children, 21*(1), 195–218. doi.org/10.1353/foc.2011.0002.

Rogers-Sirin, L., Ryce, P., & Sirin, S. R. (2014). Acculturation, acculturative stress, and cultural mismatch and their influences on immigrant children and adolescents' well-being. In R. Dimitrova, M. Bender, & F. van de Vijver (Eds.), *Global perspectives on well-being in immigrant families: Advances in immigrant family research.* New York: Springer.

Slessarev-Jamir, H. (2008). Immigrant faith institutions: Supporting and strengthening vulnerable families. *Zero to Three, 28*(3), 23–28.

Smokowski, P. R., Chapman, M. V., & Bacallao, M. L. (2007). Acculturation risk and protective factors and mental health symptoms in immigrant Latino adolescents. *Journal of Human Behavior in the Social Environment, 16*(3), 33–55. doi:10.1080/10911350802107710.

Suarez-Orozco, C., Todorova, I. L. G., & Louie, J. (2002). Making up for lost time: The experience of separation and reunification among immigrant families. *Family Process, 41*(4), 625–643.

Ineffective Impulse control   Marina Martinez-Kratz, MS, RN, CNE

NANDA-I

Definition

A pattern of performing rapid, unplanned reactions to internal or external stimuli without regard for the negative consequences of these reactions to the impulsive individual or to others.

Defining Characteristics

Acting without thinking; asking personal questions despite the discomfort of others; gambling addiction; inability to save money or regulate finances; inappropriate sharing of personal details; irritability; overly familiar with strangers; sensation seeking; sexual promiscuity; temper outbursts; violent behavior

Related Factors

Hopelessness; mood disorder; smoking; substance misuse

Associated Condition

Alteration in cognitive functioning; alteration in development; organic brain disorder; personality disorder

- = Independent;   ▲ = Collaborative;   EBN = Evidence-Based Nursing;   EB = Evidence-Based

NOC (Nursing Outcomes Classification)

Suggested NOC Outcome

Impulse Self-Control

Example NOC Outcome with Indicators

Impulse Self-Control as evidenced by the following indicators: Identifies harmful impulsive behaviors/Identifies feelings that lead to impulsive actions/Avoids high-risk situations/Controls impulses/Maintains self-control without supervision. (Rate the outcome and indicators of **Impulse Self-Control:** 1 = never demonstrated, 2 = rarely demonstrated, 3 = sometimes demonstrated, 4 = often demonstrated, 5 = continually demonstrated [see Section I].)

Client Outcomes

Client Will (Specify Time Frame)

- Be free from harm
- Cooperate with behavioral modification plan
- Verbalize adaptive ways to cope with stress by means other than impulsive behaviors
- Delay gratification and use adaptive coping strategies in response to stress
- Verbalize understanding that behavior is unacceptable
- Accept responsibility for own behavior

NIC (Nursing Interventions Classification)

Suggested NIC Intervention

Impulse Control Training

Example NIC Activities—Impulse Control Training

Use a behavior modification plan, as appropriate, to reinforce the problem-solving strategy that is being taught; Teach client to cue himself/herself to "stop and think" before acting impulsively

---

Nursing Interventions and *Rationales*

- Refer to mental health treatment for cognitive behavioral therapy (CBT). **EB:** *CBT has been beneficial in treating substance use disorders and impulse control disorders (Okai et al, 2013).*
- Assess the circumstances that led the client to seek help for their impulse control disorder. **EB:** *Clients may seek help because they continue to struggle with the desire to engage in the behavior because of the impact of their mounting social, occupational, financial, or legal problems (Grant, Schreiber, & Odlaug, 2013).*
- Assess individuals with impulsive behaviors for exposure to trauma and referral for mental health evaluation. **EB:** *Research indicates that impulsivity is associated with trauma exposure and posttraumatic stress disorder (PTSD) (Netto et al, 2016).*
- Implement motivational interviewing for clients with impulse control disorders. **EB:** *This research review found motivational interviewing helps individuals with gambling addictions work through ambivalence and commit to change (Choi et al, 2017).*
- Teach client mindfulness meditation techniques. Mindfulness meditation includes observing experiences in the present moment, describing those experiences without judgments or evaluations, and participating fully in one's current context. **EB:** *This study showed developing mindfulness was an effective way of diminishing binge eating, eating psychopathology, and depression, and increasing quality of life in women with obesity (Pinto-Gouveia et al, 2016).*
- Refer to self-help groups such as Gambler's Anonymous. **EB:** *This research review found that Gambler's Anonymous is helpful as an adjunct therapy for individuals with gambling addictions (Choi et al, 2017).*
- Use a brief intervention model to screen and provide information and referral to services for clients that may experience at-risk gambling. **EB:** *A pilot study found that when trained, primary care staff were able to screen clients at routine visits for at-risk gambling behavior by using the brief intervention model (Nehlin et al, 2016).*

● = Independent;   ▲ = Collaborative;   **EBN** = Evidence-Based Nursing;   **EB** = Evidence-Based

- Teach clients to use urge surfing techniques when impulses or urges are triggered. EB: *This study demonstrated that the mindfulness coping skill of urge surfing was an effective intervention when used by teens experiencing urges to use alcohol (Harris, Stewart, & Stanton, 2017).*
- Teach client to use cue avoidance techniques to reduce impulsive behaviors. EB: *This study shows that cue avoidance techniques were successful in reducing alcohol consumption (Di Lemma & Field, 2017).*
- Implement strategies to engage a high-level construal mindset by asking "why" abstaining from the targeted behavior will benefit the client. EB: *Questions of why are effective in priming a high-level construal mindset, which then is effective at reducing the targeted behavior (Chiou et al, 2013).*

Pediatric

- Assess children for environmental lead exposure. EB: *This research shows that a 1-μg/dL increase in average childhood blood lead level significantly predicts a 0.37 (95% confidence interval [CI] = 0.11, 0.64) point increase in adolescent impulsivity (Winter & Sampson, 2017).*
- Assess the risk-taking and impulsive behaviors of the peer group. EB: *Research found an increase in impulsivity in the presence of peers (Weigard et al, 2014).*
- Refer to mental health treatment for CBT. EB: *CBT has been beneficial in treating impulse control disorders in pediatric populations (Farrell et al, 2016).*

Geriatric

- Assess for impulsive symptoms and maintain increased surveillance of the client whenever the use of dopamine agonists has been initiated. EB: *Dopamine agonist therapy is related to the development of impulse control disorders in clients with Parkinson's disease (Voon et al, 2017).*
- Implement fall risk screening and precautions for geriatric clients with inattention and impulse control symptoms. EBN: *The Marianjoy Fall Risk Assessment tool has internal validity and reliability and includes impulsive behavior as one of the fall risk indicators (Ruroede, Pilkington, & Guernon, 2016).*
- Monitor caregivers for evidence of caregiver burden. EB: *Recent research shows that significantly greater burden was seen in caregivers of Parkinson's disease clients with impulse control disorders (Marechal et al, 2014).*

Client/Family Teaching and Discharge Planning

- Families should be encouraged to use practical measures to manage behavior such as limiting access to credit cards and restricting and monitoring Internet access gambling and casino websites, checking medication compliance, reporting behavior typical of impulse control disorders (ICDs), and transferring control of financial affairs to a partner or other family members. EB: *This recent review showed effective management of impulsive behaviors through patient and caregiver education (Zhang et al, 2016).*

REFERENCES

Chiou, W., Wu, W., & Chang, M. (2013). Think abstractly, smoke less: A brief construal-level intervention can promote self-control, leading to reduced cigarette consumption among current smokers. *Addiction (Abingdon, England)*, 108(5), 985–992.

Choi, S. W., Shin, Y. C., Kim, D. J., et al. (2017). Treatment modalities for patients with gambling disorder. *Annals of General Psychiatry*, 16, 23. Retrieved from https://doi-org.proxy.lib.umich.edu/10.1186/s12991-017-0146-2.

Di Lemma, L. C. G., & Field, M. (2017). Cue avoidance training and inhibitory control training for the reduction of alcohol consumption: A comparison of effectiveness and investigation of their mechanisms of action. *Psychopharmacology*, 234(16), 2489–2498. Retrieved from https://doi-org.proxy.lib.umich.edu/10.1007/s00213-017-4639-0.

Farrell, L. J., et al. (2016). Brief intensive CBT for pediatric OCD with E-therapy maintenance. *Journal of Anxiety Disorders*, 42, 85–94. Retrieved from https://doi.org/10.1016/j.janxdis.2016.06.005.

Grant, J., Schreiber, L., & Odlaug, B. (2013). Phenomenology and treatment of behavioural addictions. *Canadian Journal of Psychiatry*, 58(5), 252–259.

Harris, J. S., Stewart, D. G., & Stanton, B. C. (2017). Urge surfing as aftercare in adolescent alcohol use: A randomized control trial. *Mindfulness*, 8(1), 144–149. Retrieved from https://doi-org.proxy.lib.umich.edu/10.1007/s12671-016-0588-7.

Marechal, E., Denoiseux, B., Thys, E., et al. (2014). Caregiver burden in impulse control disorders in Parkinson's disease. *Movement Disorders: Official Journal of the Movement Disorder Society*, 29.

Netto, L. R., et al. (2016). Impulsivity is relevant for trauma exposure and PTSD symptoms in a non-clinical population. *Psychiatry Research*, 239, 204–211.

Nehlin, C., Nyberg, F., & Jess, K. (2016). Brief intervention within primary care for at-risk gambling: A pilot study. *Journal of Gambling Studies*, 32, 1327–1335. Retrieved from https://doi-org.proxy.lib.umich.edu/10.1007/s10899-016-9610-1.

Okai, D., Askey-Jones, S., Samuel, M., et al. (2013). Trial of CBT for impulse control behaviors affecting Parkinson patients and their caregivers. *Neurology*, 80(9), 792–799.

Pinto-Gouveia, J., Carvalho, S. A., Palmeira, L., et al. (2016). BEfree: A new psychological program for binge eating that integrates psychoeducation, mindfulness, and compassion. *Clinical Psychology* and *Psychotherapy, 24*, 1090–1098. Retrieved from https://doi-org. proxy.lib.umich.edu/10.1002/cpp.2072.

Ruroede, K., Pilkington, D., & Guernon, A. (2016). Validation study of the Marianjoy Fall Risk Assessment Tool. *Journal of Nursing Care Quality, 31*(2), 146–152.

Voon, V., et al. (2017). Impulse control disorders and levodopa-induced dyskinesias in Parkinson's disease: An update. *The Lancet. Neurology, 16*(3), 238–250. Retrieved from https://doi.org/10.1016/S1474-4422(17)30004-2.

Weigard, A., Chein, J., Albert, D., et al. (2014). Effects of anonymous peer observation on adolescents' preference for immediate rewards. *Developmental Science, 17*, 71–78. doi:10.1111/desc.12099.

Winter, A. S., & Sampson, R. J. (2017). From lead exposure in early childhood to adolescent health: A Chicago birth cohort. *American Journal of Public Health, 107*(9), 1496–1501. Retrieved from http://dx.doi.org.proxy.lib.umich.edu/10.2105/AJPH.2017.303903.

Zhang, S., Dissanayaka, N. N., Dawson, A., et al. (2016). Management of impulse control disorders in parkinson's disease. *International Psychogeriatrics, 28*(10), 1597–1614. Retrieved from http://dx.doi.org.proxy.lib.umich.edu/10.1017/S104161021600096X.

Functional urinary Incontinence

Amanda Andrews, BSc (Hons), MA and Bernie St. Aubyn, BSc (hons), MSc

NANDA-I

Definition

Inability of a usually continent person to reach the toilet in time to avoid unintentional loss of urine.

Defining Characteristics

Completely empties bladder; early morning urinary incontinence; sensation of need to void; time required to reach toilet is too long after sensation of urge; voiding prior to reaching toilet

Related Factors

Alteration in environmental factor; weakened supporting pelvic structure

Associated Condition

Alteration in cognitive functioning; impaired vision; neuromuscular impairment; psychological disorder

NOC (Nursing Outcomes Classification)

Suggested NOC Outcomes

Urinary Continence; Urinary Elimination

> **Example NOC Outcome with Indicators**
>
> **Urinary Continence** as evidenced by the following indicators: Recognizes urge to void/Responds to urge in timely manner/Voids in appropriate receptacle/Underclothing remains dry during day/Underclothing or bedding remains dry during night. (Rate the outcome and indicators of **Urinary Continence:** 1 = never demonstrated, 2 = rarely demonstrated, 3 = sometimes demonstrated, 4 = often demonstrated, 5 = consistently demonstrated [see Section I].)

Client Outcomes

Client Will (Specify Time Frame)

- Eliminate or reduce incontinent episodes
- Eliminate or overcome environmental barriers to toileting
- Use adaptive equipment to reduce or eliminate incontinence related to impaired mobility or dexterity
- Use portable urinary collection devices or urine containment devices when access to the toilet is not feasible

NIC (Nursing Interventions Classification)

Suggested NIC Interventions

Urinary Habit Training; Urinary Incontinence Care

• = Independent;   ▲ = Collaborative;   EBN = Evidence-Based Nursing;   EB = Evidence-Based

Example NIC Activities—Urinary Habit Training
Keep a continence-specification record for 3 days to establish voiding pattern; Establish interval for toileting of preferably not less than 2 hours

Nursing Interventions and *Rationales*

- Introduce yourself to the client and anyone accompanying him or her and inform them of your role. *Introducing yourself to a client helps establish and develop a therapeutic relationship that recognizes the person within the client and forms the bases for building trust on which to base the provision of care (Howatson-Jones, Standing, & Roberts, 2012).*
- Gain consent to provide care before proceeding further with the assessment. For clients unable to give consent, discuss permission with relevant health care professionals and/or family members. *Clients have the right of autonomy both legally and morally; therefore they should be fully involved in the decision-making process (Avery, 2013).*
- Wash hands using a recognized technique. *Evidence shows that strict hand hygiene regimens significantly reduce the incidence of methicillin-resistant Staphylococcus aureus and Clostridium difficile infection (Goldberg, 2017).*
- Assess usual pattern of bladder management and establish the extent of the problem to include a detailed and accurate assessment of the client. *This assessment enables the nurse to plan interventions, monitor outcomes, and evaluate care, ensuring no unnecessary treatment is implemented (NICE, 2015).*
- Evaluate the client's bladder habits:
  - Episodes of incontinence during the day and night
  - Alleviating and aggravating factors
  - Current management strategies to include containing/collection devices, restriction of fluid intake, and avoidance of fluid/food groups that cause bladder irritation
- Complete a Lifestyle and Risk Assessment: Toilet facility access and ability to use, including:
  - Distance of the toilet from the bed, chair, and living quarters
  - Characteristics of the bed, including presence of side rails and distance of the bed from the floor
  - Characteristics of the pathway to the toilet, including barriers such as stairs, loose rugs on the floor, and inadequate lighting
  - Characteristics of the bathroom, including patterns of use, lighting, height of the toilet from the floor, the presence of handrails to assist transfers to the toilet, and breadth of the door and its accessibility for a wheelchair, walker, or other assistive device

For older adults who may have limited mobility, the nurse must assess environmental barriers that may restrict access to the toilet (Nazarko, 2013).

- Assess the client's physical and mental abilities:
  - Ability to rise from chair and bed, transfer to the toilet, and ambulate, and the need for physical assistive devices such as a cane, walker, or wheelchair. *Urinary incontinence can occur as a direct consequence of the inability to reach and use the toilet either independently or with the assistance of aids or caregivers (Ostaszkiewicz et al, 2013).*
  - Ability to manipulate buttons, hooks, snaps, loop and pile closures, and zippers as needed to remove clothing. *Functional continence requires the ability to remove clothing to urinate; individuals with compromised visual acuity, dexterity, and mobility will need specific interventions to assist with these challenges to continence (Abrams, Andersson, & Birder, 2010).*
  - Functional and cognitive status assessment should be done using a tool such as the Mini Mental Status Examination for the older client with functional incontinence. *A dementia diagnosis (or severe cognitive impairment) is associated with a higher prevalence of incontinence compared with people without such a diagnosis (Gove et al, 2017). An association has also been observed between incontinence and more severe cognitive impairment and mobility problems (Jerez-Roig et al, 2016).*
  - Daily fluid intake included amount of types of fluids drank.
  - Risk of falls caused by dizziness, impaired vision, and hearing.
  - Functional ability declines secondary to comorbidities (cerebral vascular incidents, amputation).
- Discuss quality of life issues relating to socialization and family events. A comprehensive assessment enables the problem to be identified, generating a baseline of information from which to accurately diagnose and plan treatment and care (Reid, 2014).

● = Independent;   ▲ = Collaborative;   EBN = Evidence-Based Nursing;   EB = Evidence-Based

I

- Review the client's past medical history:
  - ○ Obstetrical/gynecological/urological history and surgeries
  - ○ Relevant comorbidities such as cardiac, respiratory, renal, or neurological
  - ○ Recurrent urinary tract infections

  Reviewing the client's past medical history to identify conditions that may affect an individual's ability to maintain continence is an important step in assessing the client's primary problem (Nazarko, 2013).
- Teach the client, the client's care providers, or the family to complete a bladder diary. Each 24-hour period should be subdivided into 1- to 2-hour periods and include number of urinations occurring in the toilet, actual episodes of incontinence and amount of urine leaked, reasons for episode of incontinence, type and amount of liquid intake, number of bowel movements, and incontinence pads or other products used. **EB:** *Bladder diaries provide accurate data and are more reliable than patients' recollections of symptoms. In addition to being inexpensive and low risk, patients view diaries as easy to complete and helpful for their care (Dixon & Nakib, 2016).*
- Consult with the health care provider and complete a medication review relating to side effects and contraindications. NICE (2015) recommended that a holistic continence assessment should include a medication history to ascertain whether side effects of the medication are contributing to the continence issues.
- Ensure that an appropriate, safe urinary receptacle such as a three-in-one commode, female or male handheld urinal, no-spill urinal, or containment device when toileting access is limited by immobility or environmental barriers is available to assist the client with elimination needs while other interventions are being implemented. **EB:** Toileting aids should be generally considered as a short-term strategy and/ or an addition to ongoing treatment. It is recommended that long-term management with such items should only be considered when all other options have been excluded (NICE, 2015).
- ▲ Refer to occupational therapy for help in obtaining assistive devices and adapting the home for optimal toilet accessibility. *Occupational therapists are needed to assist patients with dexterity and mobility issues that may be contributing to incontinence (Spencer, McManus, & Sabourin, 2017).*
- Provide advice to clients relating to loose-fitting clothing with stretch waistbands rather than buttoned or zippered waist; minimize buttons, snaps, and multilayered clothing; and substitute a loop-and-pile closure or other easily loosened systems such as Velcro for buttons, hooks, and zippers in existing clothing. *Clients with impaired dexterity or weakness may benefit from clothing that has been modified or is without buttons and zippers (Leaver, 2017).*
- Work with the client on retraining the bladder by regular timed toileting regimens (every 2 hours). For the older client in the home or a long-term care facility who has functional incontinence and dementia:
  - ○ Determine the frequency of current urination using an alarm system or check-and-change device.
  - ○ Record urinary elimination and incontinent patterns in a bladder log to use as a baseline for assessment and evaluation of treatment efficacy.
  - ○ Begin a prompted toileting program based on the results of this program; toileting frequency may vary from every 1.5 to 2 hours to every 4 hours.
  - ○ Provide positive reinforcement.

  EB: *Based on a systematic review of 14 clinical trials, prompted voiding has been shown to improve daytime incontinence and the percentage of appropriate toileting episodes in clients with dementia and functional incontinence (Flanagan et al, 2012).*
- Monitor older clients in a long-term care facility, acute care facility, or home for dehydration. **EB:** *Dehydration can exacerbate urine loss, and it is essential to consider it a factor when managing incontinence, particularly in care home settings (Flanagan et al, 2014).*
- Inspect the perineal and perianal skin for evidence of incontinence-associated dermatitis, including inflammation, vesicles in skin exposed to urinary leakage, and especially skinfolds or denudation of the skin, particularly when incontinence is managed by absorptive pads or containment briefs. **EB:** *Skinfolds and the perineal skin are at risk for dermatitis and fungal or bacterial infections (Beeckman, 2017).*
- Begin a preventive skin care regimen for all clients with urinary incontinence and treat clients with incontinence-associated dermatitis or related skin damage. **EB:** *Minimizing exposure to urine; gentle cleansing; moisture protection, preferably with an emollient; and application of a skin protectant are the necessary components of a skin protection program (Beekman, 2017).*
- Advise the client about the advantages of using disposable or reusable insert pads, pad-pant systems, or replacement briefs specifically designed for urinary incontinence as indicated for short-term/long-term use, including social events. *A systematic review identified that the use of incontinence pads are the main*

● = Independent;   ▲ = Collaborative;   **EBN** = Evidence-Based Nursing;   **EB** = Evidence-Based

conservative behavioral approach to managing continence. They are preferred to invasive management strategies (e.g., catheterization) (Roe, Flanagan, & Maden 2015).

- Consider the use of an indwelling catheter for continuous drainage in the client who is both homebound and bedbound and is receiving palliative or end-of-life care (requires a health care provider's order). **EB:** *Indwelling catheters may be used for clients who are at the end of life, when repositioning adds to discomfort or pain (Talley et al, 2014).*

- When an indwelling urinary catheter is in place, follow prescribed maintenance protocols for managing the catheter, taping and replacing the catheter, the drainage bag, and care of perineal skin and urethral meatus. Teach infection control measures adapted to the home care setting. *Proper care reduces the risk of catheter-associated urinary tract infection (Centers for Disease Control and Prevention, 2018).*

- Assist the client in adapting to the catheter. Encourage discussion of the client's response to the catheter. *Research has consistently shown that indwelling catheter users need to be given more information, but some patients still feel poorly informed. Nurses are in a good position to find out what people know, what they need, and to ensure that patients have contact phone numbers for further information and details of reliable websites and support organizations (Prinjha et al, 2016).*

- Provide client with comprehensive written information about bladder care. *Providing clients with well-written, evidence-based information about their condition and treatment can have a beneficial effect on the outcomes of treatment. In addition, clients are more likely to retain important information that will assist them in making informed decisions about their care (Coulter, 2011).*

- Document all care and advice given in a factual and comprehensive manner. *Good record keeping is an integral part of nursing practice and is essential to the provision of safe and effective care (St. Aubyn & Andrews, 2015).*

I

REFERENCES

Avery, G. (2013). *Law and ethics in nursing and healthcare: an introduction.* London: Sage Publications Inc.

Abrams, P., Andersson, K. E., & Birder, L. (2010). Fourth International Consultation on Incontinence recommendations of the international scientific committee: Evaluations and treatment of urinary incontinence, pelvic organ prolapse, and fecal incontinence. *Neurourol Urodynam, 29*(1), 213–240.

Beeckman, D. (2017). A decade of research on Incontinence-Associated Dermatitis (IAD): Evidence, knowledge gaps and next steps. *Journal of Tissue Viability, 26*(1), 47–56. doi:10.1016/j.jtv.2016.02.004.

Centers for Disease Control and Prevention. *Urinary Tract Infection (Catheter-Associated Urinary Tract Infection [CAUTI] and Non-Catheter-Associated Urinary Tract Infection [UTI]) and Other Urinary System Infection [USI]) Events.* Retrieved from http://www.cdc.gov/nhsn/PDFs/pscManual/7pscCAUTIcurrent.pdf. (Accessed 9 March 2018).

Coulter, A. (2011). *Engaging patients in health care.* Berkshire: McGraw-Hill Open University Press.

Dixon, C. A., & Nakib, N. A. (2016). Are bladder diaries helpful in management of overactive bladder? *Current bladder dysfunction reports, 11*(1), 14–17.

Flanagan, L., Roe, B., Jack, B., et al. (2012). A systematic review of care intervention studies for the management of incontinence and promotion of continence in older people in care homes with urinary incontinence as the primary focus. *Geriatrics and Gerontology International, 12*(4), 600–611.

Flanagan, L., Roe, B., Jack, B., et al. (2014). Factors with the management of incontinence and promotion of continence in older people in care homes. *Journal of Advanced Nursing, 70*(3), 476–496.

Gove, D., Scerri, A., Georges, J., et al. (2017). Continence care for people with dementia living at home in Europe: A review of literature with a focus on problems and challenges. *Journal of Clinical Nursing, 26*(3), 356–365.

Goldberg, J. L. (2017). Guideline implementation; hand hygiene. *The AORN Journal, 105*(2), 203–212.

Howatson-Jones, L., Standing, M., & Roberts, S. (Eds.), (2012). *Patient assessment and care planning in nursing.* London: Sage Publications Inc.

Jerez-Roig, J., et al. (2016). Prevalence of urinary incontinence and associated factors in nursing home residents. *Neurourology and Urodynamics, 35*(1), 102–107.

Leaver, R. (2017). Assessing Patients with urinary incontinence: The basics. *Journal of Community Nursing., 31*(1), 40–46.

Nazarko, L. (2013). Continence series 4: The importance of assessment. *British Journal of HCA, 7*(3), 118–124.

NICE. (2015). *Urinary Incontinence in women: Management clinical guideline CG171* Retrieved from https://www.nice.org.uk/guidance/cg171. (Accessed 1 November 2017).

Ostaszkiewicz, J., Eustice, S., Roe, B., et al. (2013). *Toileting assistance programmes for the management of urinary incontinence in adults.* Cochrane Incontinence Group. Retrieved from http://www.cochrane.org/CD010589/INCONT_toileting-assistance-programmes-for-the-management-of-urinary-incontinence-in-adults. (Accessed 8 March 2018).

Prinjha, S., Chapple, A., Feneley, R., et al. (2016). Exploring the information needs of people living with a long-term indwelling urinary catheter: A qualitative study. *Journal of Advanced Nursing, 72*(6), 1335–1346.

Reid, J. (2014). Managing urinary incontinence: Guidelines for community nurses. *Journal of Christian Nursing, 28*(6), 20–26.

Roe, B., Flanagan, L., & Maden, M. (2015). Systematic review of systematic reviews for the management of urinary incontinence and promotion of continence using conservative behavioural approaches in older people in care homes. *Journal of Advanced Nursing, 71*(7), 1464–1483.

Spencer, M., McManus, K., & Sabourin, J. (2017). Incontinence in the older adult: The role of the geriatric multidisciplinary team. *The British Columbia Medical Journal, 59*(2), 99–105.

St. Aubyn, B., & Andrews, A. (2015). If it's not written down—It didn't happen. *Journal of Community Nursing, 29*(5), 20–22.

Talley, K. M., Wyam, J. F., Bronas, U. G., et al. (2014). Factors associated with toileting disability in older adults without dementia living in residential care facilities. *Nursing Research, 63*(2), 94–104.

Overflow urinary Incontinence   *Gail Ladwig, RN, MSN*

NANDA-I

Definition

Involuntary loss of urine associated with overdistention of the bladder.

Defining Characteristics

Bladder distention; high postvoid residual volume; involuntary leakage of small volume of urine; nocturia

Related Factors

Fecal impaction

Associated Condition

Bladder outlet obstruction; detrusor external sphincter dyssynergia; detrusor hypocontractility; severe pelvic organ prolapse; treatment regimen; urethral obstruction

NOC, NIC, Client Outcomes, Nursing Interventions and *Rationales,* Client/Family Teaching and Discharge Planning, and References

Refer to care plan for **Urinary Retention.**

Reflex urinary Incontinence
Amanda Andrews, BSc (Hons), MA and Bernie St. Aubyn, BSc (hons), MSc

NANDA-I

Definition

Involuntary loss of urine at somewhat predictable intervals when a specific bladder volume is reached.

Defining Characteristics

Absence of voiding sensation; absence of urge to void; inability to voluntarily inhibit voiding; inability to voluntarily initiate voiding; incomplete emptying of bladder with lesion above pontine micturition center; predictable pattern of voiding; sensation of urgency to void without voluntary inhibition of bladder contraction; sensations associated with full bladder

Related Factors

To be developed

Associated Condition

Neurological impairment above level of pontine micturition center; neurological impairment above level of sacral micturition center; tissue damage

NOC   (Nursing Outcomes Classification)

Suggested NOC Outcomes

Urinary Continence; Urinary Elimination

● = Independent;   ▲ = Collaborative;   EBN = Evidence-Based Nursing;   EB = Evidence-Based

Urinary Continence as evidenced by the following indicators: Absence of urinary leakage between catheterizations or containment of micturition by condom catheter and drainage bag/Absence of symptomatic urinary tract infection (absence of leukocytes and absence of bacterial growth or >100,000 colony-forming units/mL)/Underclothing dry during day/Underclothing or bedding dry during night. (Rate the outcome and indicators of **Urinary Continence:** 1 = never demonstrated, 2 = rarely demonstrated, 3 = sometimes demonstrated, 4 = often demonstrated, 5 = consistently demonstrated [see Section I].)

Client Outcomes

Client Will (Specify Time Frame)

- Follow prescribed schedule for bladder emptying
- Have intact perineal skin
- Remain clear of symptomatic urinary tract infection
- Demonstrate how to apply containment device or insert intermittent catheter or be able to provide caregiver with instructions for performing these procedures

NIC (Nursing Interventions Classification)

Suggested NIC Interventions

Urinary Catheterization: Intermittent; Urinary Elimination Management; Urinary Incontinence Care

Example NIC Activities—Urinary Elimination Management

Monitor urinary elimination including frequency, consistency, odor, volume, and color as appropriate; Teach client signs and symptoms of urinary tract infection

Nursing Interventions and *Rationales*

- Introduce yourself to the client and anyone accompanying him or her and inform them of your role. *Introducing yourself to a client helps establish and develop a therapeutic relationship that recognizes the person within the client and forms the bases for building trust on which to base the provision of care (Howatson-Jones, Standing, & Roberts, 2012).*
- Gain consent to provide care before proceeding further with the assessment. *Clients have the right of autonomy both legally and morally; therefore they should be fully involved in the decision-making process (Avery, 2013).*
- Wash hands using a recognized technique. EB: *Evidence shows that strict hand hygiene regimens significantly reduce the incidence of methicillin-resistant* Staphylococcus aureus *and* Clostridium difficile *infection (Goldberg, 2017).*
- Assess the usual pattern of bladder management and establish the extent of the problem. EB: *A detailed and accurate assessment of the client enables the nurse to plan interventions, monitor outcomes, and evaluate care, ensuring no unnecessary treatment is performed (NICE, 2015) (refer to Functional urinary* **Incontinence** *care plan).*
- Ask the client to complete a bladder diary/log to determine the pattern of urine elimination, any incontinence episodes, and current bladder management program. An electronic voiding diary may be kept whenever feasible. EB: *Bladder diaries provide accurate data and are more reliable than clients' recollections of symptoms. In addition to being inexpensive and low risk, clients view diaries as easy to complete and helpful for their care (Dixon & Nakib, 2016).*
- ▲ Consult with the health care provider concerning current bladder function and the potential of the bladder to produce hydronephrosis, vesicoureteral reflux, febrile urinary tract infection, or compromised renal function. *Whether the client has urinary retention directs the method of urine management to prevent damage to the renal system from unrelieved obstruction (Dorsher & McIntosh, 2012).*
- ▲ Consult with the health care provider and physical therapist concerning the neuromuscular ability to perform bladder management. The type of neurological disorder, as well as the level of neurological impairment and the ability to use the hands effectively, determines the method of urine management in reflex incontinence. *Continence assessment needs to be an active process and as such should be undertaken as often as the client's progressive neurological condition dictates (Mangnall, 2011).*

● = Independent;   ▲ = Collaborative;   EBN = Evidence-Based Nursing;   EB = Evidence-Based

- Inspect the perineal and perigenital skin for signs of incontinence-associated dermatitis and pressure ulcers (Beeckman, 2017). **EB:** *Standardizing skin care routines and making them an integrated part of essential care for incontinence clients will improve client care in specialized areas, which helps reduce the incidence of incontinence-associated dermatitis.*
- ▲ In consultation with the rehabilitation team, counsel the client and family concerning the merits and potential risks associated with each possible bladder management program, including spontaneous voiding, intermittent self-catheterization (ISC), and reflex voiding with condom catheter containment and in some cases, indwelling suprapubic catheterization. *All bladder management programs carry some risk of urinary incontinence or serious urinary system complications (Newman & Willson, 2011).* **CEB:** *Spontaneous voiding and intermittent catheterization carry greater risk of urine loss than condom catheter containment or indwelling catheter. A study demonstrated increased rates of complications and a high rate of infection with indwelling catheter use compared with other modes of management (Singh et al, 2011). Some studies support the use of suprapubic catheters for long-term treatment of reflex incontinence in spinal cord injury clients (Colli & Lloyd, 2011; Böthig, Hirschfeld, & Thietje, 2012).*

Intermittent Self-Catheterization

- Begin intermittent catheterization as ordered using sterile technique; the client may be taught to use clean technique in the home situation. **EB:** *Intermittent catheterization is considered the preferred long-term management for a neurogenic bladder. Sterile intermittent catheterization should be used in hospitals, rehabilitation centers, and extended care facilities (Newman & Willson, 2011). There is an associated risk of urinary tract infection with any type of bladder management; however, by performing ISC the risk of urinary tract infections is reduced because the residual volume in the bladder is resolved (Winder, 2012).*
- Schedule the frequency of intermittent catheterization based on the frequency/volume records of previous catheterizations, functional bladder capacity, and the impact of catheterization on the quality of the client's life. *Bladder volumes must be kept lower to prevent development of urinary tract infection from retention of urine, and draining the urine regularly helps prevent movement of bacteria into the bladder long enough to produce symptomatic infection (Newman & Willson, 2011; Dorsher & McIntosh, 2012).*
- Teach the client to recognize signs of symptomatic urinary tract infection and to seek care promptly when these signs occur. The signs of symptomatic infection include the following:
  - Discomfort over the bladder or during urination
  - Acute onset of urinary incontinence
  - Fever
  - Markedly increased spasticity of muscles below the level of the spinal lesion
  - Malaise, lethargy
  - Hematuria
  - Autonomic dysreflexia (hyperreflexia) symptoms

Signs of symptomatic urinary tract infection as indicated previously should be treated promptly with antimicrobial therapy, whereas asymptomatic bacteriuria should not generally be treated (Matthews, 2011).

- Recognize that intermittent catheterization is typically associated with asymptomatic bacteriuria, and the indwelling catheter is routinely associated with asymptomatic colonization. **EB:** *There is a clinical need to refine the management of asymptomatic infection in association with bacteriuria. Effective strategies should include minimizing inappropriate antimicrobial use unless a symptomatic infection is detected (Nicolle, 2016).*
- Teach intermittent catheterization as the client approaches discharge as per operational guidelines and best practice. Instruct the client and at least one family member in the performance of catheterization. Teach the client with quadriplegia how to instruct others to perform this procedure. **EB:** *Intermittent catheterization is a safe and effective bladder management strategy for persons with reflex urinary incontinence. More and more patients are advised to perform intermittent catheterization. Quality-of-life studies show that intermittent catheterization has a great impact on daily life (Cobussen-Boekhorst et al, 2016).*
- Teach the client managed by intermittent catheterization to self-administer antispasmodic (parasympatholytic) medications as prescribed by the consulting health care provider and to recognize and manage potential side effects as needed. Antimuscarinic medications should be considered in patients when urodynamic investigations show impaired bladder storage. It is important to consider the potential central nervous system-related side effects when prescribing to clients with multiple sclerosis (e.g., confusion). Clients also should be aware of the increased risk of constipation with the use of these medications (NICE, 2012).

• = Independent;   ▲ = Collaborative;   **EBN** = Evidence-Based Nursing;   **EB** = Evidence-Based

Condom Catheter/Sheath System

- For a male client with reflex incontinence who does not have urinary retention and cannot manage the condition effectively with spontaneous voiding, who does not choose to perform intermittent catheterization, or who cannot perform catheterization, teach the client and his family to obtain, select, and apply an external collective device and urinary drainage system. Assist the client and family to choose a product that adheres to the glans penis or penile shaft without allowing seepage of urine onto surrounding skin or clothing, which avoids provoking hypersensitivity reactions on the skin, and that includes a urinary drainage reservoir that is easily concealed under the clothing and does not cause irritation to the skin of the thigh. EB: *When considering the use of an external continence device it is vital that the correct size is measured and fitted to eliminate many of the problems associated with leakage and the sheath falling off (Woodward, 2015). National Institute for Health and Care Excellence (NICE) guidance (NICE, 2012) advocates that all risks and benefits are discussed relating to the available sheath system options.*
- Teach the client whose incontinence is managed by a condom catheter to routinely inspect the skin with each catheter change for evidence of lesions caused by pressure from the containment device or by exposure to urine, to cleanse the penis thoroughly, and to reapply a new device daily or every other day. EB: *A well fitted sheath reduces the risk of skin irritation or ulceration. The sheath should always be fitted leaving a space between the tip of the penis and the shaft allowing urine to flow without the sheath "ballooning" (Woodward, 2015).*
- Ensure the client is aware of when and how to report any problems and/or complications of reflex incontinence care when at home. *Early detection allows for rapid diagnosis and treatment. Information about this should be individually presented to the clients and specifically tailored to their physical condition and cognitive abilities to encourage self-management (Swain, 2012).*
- Encourage a program of self-care management. EB: *Addressing self-care activities through exercise, diet, fluid intake, and protective devices helps the client to exercise control over incontinence and may reduce the substantial burden affecting a significant proportion of spouse, partner, or familial care providers.*
- Assist the family with arranging care in a way that allows the client to participate in family or favorite activities without embarrassment. Elicit discussion of the client's concerns about the social or emotional burden of incontinence. EB: *Urinary incontinence has a substantial negative effect on the quality of life for clients, both socially and financially. Further studies are needed to determine the true extent of the problem and to address it (Tapia et al, 2013).*
- Teach the client to ensure good hydration. Total daily fluid intake should be approximately 2.7 L/day for women and 3.7 L/day for men. *Adequate fluid helps wash out bacteria from the urethra to prevent urinary tract infections, helps prevent kidney stones, and potentially protects the client from development of cancer of the bladder from exposure to carcinogens concentrated in the urine (Newman & Willson, 2011).*
- Teach the client with a spinal injury the signs of autonomic dysreflexia, its relationship to bladder fullness, and management of the condition. Refer to the care plan for **Autonomic Dysreflexia.**
- Provide the client with comprehensive written information about bladder care. EB: *Providing clients with well-written, evidence-based information about their condition and treatment can have a beneficial effect on the outcomes of treatment. In addition, clients are more likely to retain important information that will assist them in making informed decisions about their care (Coulter, 2011).*
- Document all care and advice given in a factual and comprehensive manner. *Good record keeping is an integral part of nursing practice and is essential to the provision of safe and effective care (St. Aubyn & Andrews, 2015).*

REFERENCES

Avery, G. (2013). *Law and ethics in nursing and healthcare an introduction.* London: Sage Publications Inc.

Beeckman, D. (2017). A decade of research on Incontinence-Associated Dermatitis (IAD): Evidence, knowledge gaps and next steps. *Journal of Tissue Viability, 26*(1), 47–56. doi:10.1016/j.jtv.2016.02.004.

Böthig, R., Hirschfeld, S., & Thietje, R. (2012). Quality of life and urological morbidity in tetraplegics with artificial ventilation managed with suprapubic or intermittent catheterization. *Spinal Cord, 50*(3), 247–251.

Cobussen-Boekhorst, H., Hermeling, E., Heesakkers, J., et al. (2016). Patients' experience with intermittent catheterisation in everyday life. *Journal of Clinical Nursing, 25*(9/10), 1253–1261.

Colli, J., & Lloyd, K. (2011). Bladder neck closure and suprapubic catheter placement as definitive management of neurogenic bladder. *The Journal of Spinal Cord Medicine, 34*(3), 273–277.

Coulter, A. (2011). *Engaging patients in health care.* Berkshire: McGraw-Hill Open University Press.

Dixon, C. A., & Nakib, N. A. (2016). Are bladder diaries helpful in management of overactive bladder? *Current bladder dysfunction reports, 11*(1), 14–17.

Dorsher, P., & McIntosh, P. (2012). Neurogenic bladder. *Advances in Urology, 2012,* 816274.

Goldberg, J. L. (2017). Guideline implementation; hand hygiene. *The AORN Journal, 105*(2), 203–212.

● = Independent; ▲ = Collaborative; EBN = Evidence-Based Nursing; EB = Evidence-Based

Howatson-Jones, L., Standing, M., & Roberts, S. (Eds.), (2012). *Patient assessment and care planning in nursing*. London: Sage Publications Inc.

Mangnall, J. (2011). Continence during progressive neurological disease. *Nursing and Residential Care, 13*(12), 582.

Matthews, E. (2011). *Nursing care planning*. London: Lippincott Williams & Wilkins.

Newman, D., & Willson, M. (2011). Review of intermittent catheterization and current best practices. *Urologic Nursing, 31*(1), 12–48.

NICE. (2012). *Urinary Incontinence in neurological disease: Management of lower urinary tract dysfunction in neurological disease*. NICE guidance CG128. Retrieved from http://www.nice.org.uk/guidance/CG148/chapter/4-Research-recommendations. (Accessed 8 March 2018).

NICE. (2015). *Urinary Incontinence in women: Management clinical guideline CG171*. Retrieved from https://www.nice.org.uk/guidance/cg171. (Accessed 8 March 2018).

Nicolle, L. (2016). Asymptomatic bacteriuria in older adults. *Current geriatrics reports, 5*(1), 1–8.

Singh, R., et al. (2011). Bladder management methods and urological complications in spinal cord injury patients. *Indian Journal of Orthopaedics, 45*(2), 141–147.

St. Aubyn, B., & Andrews, A. (2015). If it's not written down—It didn't happen. *Journal of Community Nursing., 29*(5), 20–22.

Swain, S. (2012). *Urinary Incontinence in neurological disease: management of lower urinary tract dysfunction in neurological disease: summary of NICE guidance*. Retrieved from http://www.bmj.com/content/345/bmj.e5074. (Accessed 8 March 2018).

Tapia, C., Khalaf, K., Berenson, K., et al. (2013). Health-related quality of life and economic impact of urinary incontinence due to detrusor overactivity associated with a neurological condition: A systematic review. *Health & Quality of Life Outcomes*. Retrieved from http://www.biomedcentral.com/content/pdf/1477-7525-11-13.pdf. (Accessed 8 March 2018).

Winder, A. (2012). Good practice in catheter care. *Journal of Community Nursing, 26*(6), 15–20.

Woodward, J. (2015). Selecting and fitting a penile sheath. *British Journal of Nursing, 25*(5), 290–292.

I

Stress urinary Incontinence
Amanda Andrews, BSc (Hons), MA and Bernie St. Aubyn, BSc (hons), MSc

NANDA-I

Definition

Sudden leakage of urine with activities that increase intra-abdominal pressure.

Defining Characteristics

Involuntary leakage of small volume of urine; involuntary leakage of small volume of urine in the absence of detrusor contraction; involuntary leakage of small volume of urine in the absence of overdistended bladder

Related Factors

Weak pelvic floor muscles

Associated Condition

Degenerative changes in pelvic floor muscles; increase in intra-abdominal pressure; intrinsic urethral sphincter deficiency

NOC   (Nursing Outcomes Classification)

Suggested NOC Outcomes

Urinary Continence; Urinary Elimination

> ### Example NOC Outcome with Indicators
>
> **Urinary Continence** as evidenced by the following indicators: Experiences no urine leakage with increased abdominal pressure (e.g., sneezing, laughing, lifting)/Voids in appropriate receptacle/Able to move to toilet after strong desire to urinate is perceived/Underclothing remains dry during day/Underclothing or bedding remains dry during night. (Rate the outcome and indicators of **Urinary Continence:** 1 = never demonstrated, 2 = rarely demonstrated, 3 = sometimes demonstrated, 4 = often demonstrated, 5 = consistently demonstrated [see Section I].)

Client Outcomes

Client Will (Specify Time Frame)

- Report fewer stress incontinence episodes and/or a decrease in the severity of urine loss

● = Independent;   ▲ = Collaborative;   EBN = Evidence-Based Nursing;   EB = Evidence-Based

- Experience reduction in frequency of urinary incontinence episodes as recorded on voiding diary (bladder log)
- Identify containment devices that assist in management of stress incontinence

NIC (Nursing Interventions Classification)

Suggested NIC Interventions

Pelvic Muscle Exercises; Urinary Incontinence Care

Example NIC Activities—Urinary Incontinence Care

Explain etiology of problem and rationale for actions; Modify clothing and environment to provide easy access to toilet

Nursing Interventions and *Rationales*

- Introduce yourself to the client and anyone accompanying him or her and inform them of your role. *Introducing yourself to a client helps establish and develop a therapeutic relationship that recognizes the person within the client and forms the bases for building trust on which to base the provision of care (Howatson-Jones, Standing, & Roberts, 2012).*
- Gain consent to provide care before proceeding further with the assessment. In clients unable to give consent, discuss permission with relevant health care professionals and/or family members. *Clients have the right of autonomy both legally and morally; therefore they should be fully involved in the decision-making process (Avery, 2013).*
- Wash hands using a recognized technique. *Evidence shows that strict hand hygiene regimens significantly reduce the incidence of methicillin-resistant* Staphylococcus aureus *and* Clostridium difficile *infection (Goldberg, 2017).*
- Assess usual pattern of bladder management to understand the extent of the problem and establish pattern of bladder management. EB: *A detailed and accurate assessment of the client enables the nurse to plan interventions, monitor outcomes, and evaluate care, ensuring no unnecessary treatment is performed (NICE, 2015). Refer to the Functional urinary* **Incontinence** *care plan.*
  - Review the client's past medical history to identify possible risk factors for stress incontinence (i.e., pregnancy, parity, large babies, forceps or breech deliveries, obesity, chronic cough, physical activity, previous urinary tract or gynecological surgery, smoking history). *Nazarko (2013) identified the importance of considering other conditions that will affect an individual's ability to maintain continence.* EB: *The most common types of urinary incontinence in adult women are stress, urge, or a combination of both (Knarr et al, 2014). Many women are reluctant to initiate a discussion regarding incontinence; identifying women at risk is essential for effective screening (Keyock & Newman, 2011).*
  - Review the client's medication list (e.g., diuretics, lithium, adrenergic blockers, diabetes medications) to see what may exacerbate the client's urinary urgency.
- *Stress urinary incontinence may be caused by anatomical defects in the supporting structures of the bladder and the urethra. This results in suboptimal positioning of these structures leading to involuntary urine leakage on physical exertion (Dumoulin, Hay-Smith, & Mac Habbe-Seguin, 2014).*
- Review the client's bladder habits:
  - Onset and duration of urinary leakage
  - Related lower urinary tract symptoms, including voiding frequency (day/night) and urgency, severity (small, moderate, large amounts) of urinary leakage
  - Factors provoking urine loss (diuretics, bladder irritants, alcohol), focusing on the differential diagnosis of stress, urge or mixed stress, and urge urinary symptoms; consider using a symptom questionnaire that elicits relevant lower urinary tract symptoms and provides differentiation between stress and urge incontinence symptoms
- Stress urinary incontinence is more common in young and middle-aged women, is characterized by incontinence in small amounts (drops, spurts), no nocturia or incontinence at night, and incontinence without sensation of urine loss (Strothers & Friedman, 2011).
- Assess for mixed urinary incontinence (a combination of stress and urge incontinence) by asking the client:
  - Can you delay urination for a 2-hour movie or car ride?
  - How often do you wake/arise at night to urinate?
  - When you have the urge to urinate, can you reach the toilet without leaking?

● = Independent; ▲ = Collaborative; EBN = Evidence-Based Nursing; EB = Evidence-Based

I

EB: *Farrell et al (2013) established that by using a questionnaire for urinary tract diagnosis, the client's ability to assess their own incontinence type was improved. To further enhance this assessment the questionnaire needs to be a validated incontinence-specific quality of life questionnaire (Bardsley, 2016).*

- Complete a lifestyle assessment to understand the effect of stress urinary incontinence on an individual's lifestyle. Inquire about incontinence pad use and change in daily, social, or recreational activities, as well as emotional impact. **EB:** *The impact of urinary incontinence on the quality of life is well recognized and includes a negative effect on psychological well-being, social interactions and activities, and sexual and interpersonal relationships (Minassian et al, 2015).*

- Inspect the perineal skin for evidence of incontinence-associated dermatitis, including inflammation, vesicles in skin exposed to urinary leakage, and especially skinfolds or denudation of the skin, particularly when incontinence is managed by absorptive pads or containment briefs. **CEB/EB:** Ammonia produced from the breakdown of urea in urine causes an increase in skin pH, which increases the permeability of the skin; excess moisture and damage to the acid mantle further increases permeability and vulnerability to bacterial and fungal infections (Langemo et al, 2011; Beeckman, 2017). Skin exposed to urine or stool will become bright red, and the surface may appear shiny because of serous exudate; inflamed areas of individuals with darker skin tones may be a duller red or hypopigmented when compared with adjacent skin. Inspect the skin for a maculopapular red rash typical of candidiasis (Gray, 2010; Beeckman, 2017).

- ▲ Refer client for specific testing to confirm etiology of incontinence etiology and diagnosis. If trained to do so, perform the cough stress test, and request 24-hour pad test (if appropriate) and urodynamic studies (to include urine speed and flow, postvoid residual measurement, leak point pressure, and pressure flow study). **EB:** *A greater agreement rating was found between cough stress test and urodynamics than between 24-hour pad test and urodynamics in the assessment of stress incontinence (Price & Noblett, 2012; Minassian, et al, 2015).*

- Establish with the client the current use of containment devices; evaluate the devices for their ability to adequately contain urine loss, protect clothing, and control odor. Assist the client in identifying containment devices specifically designed to contain urinary leakage. **EB:** *Recommend that the client buy incontinent products specifically designed to contain urine using hydrogel to contain fluid, and to not use sanitary pads. Using a combination of products may be more effective and economical (Roem Flanagan, & Maden, 2014).* **EB:** *Recognize that incontinence products may present a significant financial burden to clients. Chong, Khan, and Anger (2011) reported that approximately 70% of expenditures attributed to containment devices, laundry, and dry cleaning expenses were paid by the clients themselves.*

- Teach the client to complete a bladder diary by recording voiding frequency, the frequency and degree of urinary incontinence episodes, association with urgency (a sudden and strong desire to urinate that is difficult to defer), fluid intake, and pad usage over a 3- to 7-day period. An electronic voiding diary may be kept whenever feasible. **EB:** *Use of a bladder diary may reduce client discrepancies in recall and is a valuable tool for assessment; the short (24-hour) duration of the bladder diary may yield inadequate data, and excessive diary duration reduces compliance (Dixon and Nakib, 2016).*

- ▲ With the client and in close consultation with the health care provider, review treatment options, including behavioral management; drug therapy; use of a pessary, vaginal device, or urethral insert; and surgery. Outline the potential benefits, efficacy, and side effects of each treatment option. **CEB:** *A 10-year review of the literature identified that there are two common conservative treatments recommended to treat stress urinary incontinence in women: strengthening pelvic floor muscles including biofeedback and weighted vaginal cones, and the use of intravaginal devices such as pessaries (McIntosh, Andersen, & Reekie, 2015).*

- Teach the client undergoing pelvic floor muscle training to identify, contract, and relax the pelvic floor muscles without contracting distal muscle groups (e.g., abdominal muscles or gluteus muscles) using verbal feedback based on vaginal or anal palpation, biofeedback, or electrical stimulation and the assistance of an incontinence specialist or health care provider as necessary. **EB:** *Pelvic floor muscle training is effective in the treatment of stress, urge, and mixed urinary incontinence; participation in a supervised program for at least 3 months may yield improved outcomes (Dumoulin, Hay-Smith, & Mac Habbe-Seguin, 2014).*

- **CEB:** To find the proper muscles, the client may be instructed to think about trying to control the urge to pass gas; women will feel a lifting sensation in the vaginal area and a pulling in of the rectum (Keyock & Newman, 2011). When learning to control pelvic floor muscles, clients may recruit other muscles such as the rectus abdominis or gluteal muscles, which may be counterproductive; these muscles must be relaxed to avoid increasing pressure on the bladder or pelvic floor (Burgio et al, 2009).

- Incorporate principles of exercise physiology into a pelvic muscle training program using the following strategies:

● = Independent;   ▲ = Collaborative;   **EBN** = Evidence-Based Nursing;   **EB** = Evidence-Based

❍ Begin a graded exercise program, usually starting with 5 to 10 repetitions and advancing gradually to no more than 35 to 50 repetitions every day or every other day based on baseline and ongoing evaluation of maximal strength and endurance.

❍ Continue exercise sessions over a period of 3 to 6 months.

❍ Integrate muscle training into activities of daily living.

❍ Assess progress every 2 weeks during the first month and every 4 to 6 weeks thereafter.

CEB/EB: *Pelvic floor muscle training strengthens urethral sphincter tone (Chong, Khan, & Anger, 2011) and is the first-line conservative approach for all types of incontinence and in particular for stress and mixed urinary incontinence. Women report an improvement in symptoms and quality of life after undergoing this training (Dumoulin, Hay-Smith, & Mac Habbe-Seguin, 2014).*

• Implement a bladder training program with the client. Assist the client in completing a bladder diary over a period of a minimum of 3 days or up to 7 days.

❍ Review the results of the diary with the client, determining typical voiding frequency and establishing goals for voiding frequency.

❍ Using baseline voiding frequency, as determined by the diary, teach the client to urinate by the clock when awake, typically every 30 to 120 minutes.

❍ Encourage adherence to the program with timing devices, as well as verbal encouragement and support, and address individual reasons for schedule interruption.

❍ Gradually increase the time between urinations to the negotiated goal. Time intervals between voiding are typically increased in increments of 15 to 30 minutes for clients with a baseline frequency of less than every 60 minutes and increments of 25 to 30 minutes for clients with a baseline frequency of more than every 60 minutes.

EB: *Bladder training reduces the frequency and severity of urinary leakage in women with stress incontinence, urge incontinence, and mixed incontinence.*

• Combining pelvic floor muscle training with bladder training is more effective than bladder training alone in the short term for treating stress urinary incontinence (Kaya et al, 2015).

▲ Teach the client to self-administer duloxetine and imipramine as ordered by the consulting health care provider, and to monitor for adverse side effects. **CEB/EB:** *There are no prescriptive drugs approved for use in stress urinary incontinence in the United States. Nevertheless, several agents are sometimes prescribed to highly selected clients with stress urinary incontinence. They include duloxetine (Schagen van Leeuwen et al, 2008) and imipramine (Andersson, 2000). A systematic review and meta-analysis (Li et al, 2013) concluded that duloxetine decreased incontinence episodes by 50% in more than 56% of clients; however, adverse effects were experienced by 83% of the subjects.*

▲ Teach the client to self-administer topical (vaginal) estrogens as directed, and to monitor for adverse side effects. **EB:** *Intravaginal estrogen has an effect on the bladder and urethral epithelium and can help to relieve symptoms of urinary frequency, particularly in postmenopausal women with vaginal atrophy (Panay et al, 2013).*

• Refer the female client with stress urinary incontinence and pelvic organ prolapse who wishes to use a pessary to manage stress incontinence to a nurse specialist or gynecologist with expertise in the placement and maintenance of these devices. **CEB:** *The use of pessaries can help resolve stress urinary incontinence, with the common types being the dish or the ring. These differ from other pessaries because the ring or dish is placed at the level of the urethral vesical junction to provide additional support to the urethra (Keyock and Newman, 2011).*

• Discuss potentially reversible or controllable risk factors, such as weight loss, with the client with stress incontinence, and assist the client to formulate a strategy to eliminate these conditions. *Although research supports a strong familial predisposition to stress incontinence among women, other risk factors, including obesity, smoking, and chronic coughing from smoking, are reversible.* **CEB:** *Being obese may increase pressure on the pelvic floor and doubles the risk for incontinence (Strothers & Friedman, 2011).*

• Provide information about support resources such as the National Association for Continence, the Simon Foundation for Continence, or the Total Control Program.

• Refer the client with persistent stress incontinence to a continence service, health care provider, or nurse who specializes in the management of this condition. *All clients presenting with incontinence should be offered an initial assessment by an individual who specializes in management of continence disorders.*

• Teach the client to ensure good hydration. Total daily fluid intake should be approximately 2.7 L/day for women and 3.7 L/day for men. **EB:** *Adequate fluid helps wash out bacteria from the urethra to prevent*

• = Independent; ▲ = Collaborative; **EBN** = Evidence-Based Nursing; **EB** = Evidence-Based

I

urinary tract infections, helps prevent kidney stones, and potentially protects the client from development of cancer of the bladder from exposure to carcinogens concentrated in the urine (Newman & Willson, 2011).

- Provide client with comprehensive written information about bladder care. **EB:** *Providing clients with well-written, evidence-based information about their condition and treatment can have a beneficial effect on the outcomes of treatment. In addition, clients are more likely to retain important information that will assist them in making informed decisions about their care (Coulter, 2011).*

- Encourage a program of self-care management. Addressing self-care activities through exercise, diet, fluid intake, and protective devices helps the client exercise control over incontinence and may reduce the substantial care provider burden affecting a significant proportion of spouse, partner, or familial care providers.

- Assist the family with arranging care in a way that allows the client to participate in family or favorite activities without embarrassment. Elicit discussion of the client's concerns about the social or emotional burden of incontinence. **EB:** Urinary incontinence has a substantial negative effect on the quality of life for clients, both socially and financially. Further studies are needed to determine the true extent of the problem and to address it (Tapia et al, 2013).

- Document all care and advice given in a factual and comprehensive manner. Good record keeping is an integral part of nursing practice and is essential to the provision of safe and effective care (St. Aubyn and Andrews, 2015).

REFERENCES

Andersson, K. E. (2000). Drug therapy for urinary incontinence. *Bailliere's Best Practice and Research. Clinical Obstetrics and Gynaecology, 14*(2), 291.

Avery, G. (2013). *Law and ethics in nursing and healthcare: an introduction.* London: Sage Publications Inc.

Bardsley, A. (2016). An overview of urinary incontinence. *British Journal of Nursing, 25*(18), s14–s21.

Beeckman, D. (2017). A decade of research on Incontinence-Associated Dermatitis (IAD): Evidence, knowledge gaps and next steps. *Journal of Tissue Viability, 26*(1), 47–56. doi:10.1016/j.jtv.2016.02.004.

Burgio, K. L., et al. (2009). Behavioral treatment of urinary incontinence, voiding dysfunction, and overactive bladder. *Obstetrics and Gynecology Clinics of North America, 36*(3), 475–491.

Chong, E. C., Khan, A. A., & Anger, J. T. (2011). The financial burden of stress urinary incontinence among women in the United States. *Current Urology Reports, 12*(5), 358–362.

Coulter, A. (2011). *Engaging patients in health care.* Berkshire: McGraw-Hill Open University Press.

Dixon, C. A., & Nakib, N. A. (2016). Are bladder diaries helpful in management of overactive bladder? *Current bladder dysfunction reports, 11*(1), 14–17.

Dumoulin, C., Hay-Smith, J., & Habbe-Seguin, G. (2014). Pelvic floor muscle training versus no treatment, or interactive control treatments, for urinary incontinence in women. *The Cochrane Library.* doi:10.1002/14651858.CD005654.pub3.

Farrell, S. A., Bent, A., Amir-Khalkhali, B., et al. (2013). Women's ability to assess their own urinary incontinence type using the QUID as an educational tool. *International Urogynaecology Journal, 24*(5), 759–762.

Goldberg, J. L. (2017). Guideline implementation; hand hygiene. *AORN Journal, 105*(2), 203–212.

Gray, M. (2010). Optimal management of incontinence-associated dermatitis in the elderly. *American Journal of Clinical Dermatology, 11*(3), 201–210.

Howatson-Jones, L., Standing, M., & Roberts, S. (Eds.), (2012). *Patient assessment and care planning in nursing.* London: Sage Publications Inc.

Kaya, S., Turkan, A., Ceren, G., et al. (2015). Short-term effect of adding pelvic floor muscle training to bladder training for female

urinary incontinence: A randomized controlled trial. *The International Urogynacological Journal, 26*(2), 285–293.

Keyock, K., & Newman, D. (2011). Understanding stress urinary incontinence. *The Nurse Practitioner, 36*(10), 24–36.

Knarr, J., Musil, C., Warner, C., et al. (2014). Female stress urinary incontinence: An evidence based case study approach in. *Urologic Nursing, 34*(3), 143–151.

Langemo, D., et al. (2011). Incontinence and incontinence-associated dermatitis. *Advances in Skin and Wound Care, 24*(3), 126–140.

Li, J., Yang, L., Pu, C., et al. (2013). The role of duloxetine in stress urinary incontinence systematic review and meta-analysis. *The International Journal of Urology and nephrology, 145*(3), 679–686.

McIntosh, L., Andersen, E., & Reekie, M. (2015). Conservative treatment of stress urinary incontinence in women: A ten year (2004–2013) scoping review of the literature. *Urologic Nursing, 35*(4), 179–186.

Minassian, V. A., Sun, H. Y., Clerk, D. N., et al. (2015). The interaction of stress and urgency urinary incontinence and its effect on quality of life. *The International Urogynecology Journal, 26*(2), 269–276.

Nazarko, L. (2013). Continence series 4: The importance of assessment. *British Journal of HCA, 7*(3), 118–124.

Newman, D., & Willson, M. (2011). Review of intermittent catheterization and current best practices. *Urologic Nursing, 31*(1), 12–48.

NICE. (2015). *Urinary Incontinence in women: Management clinical guideline CG171.* Retrieved from https://www.nice.org.uk/guidance/cg171. (Accessed 1 November 2017).

Panay, N., Hamoda, H., Arya, R., et al. (2013). The 2013 British Menopause Society and Women's Health Concern recommendations on hormone replacement therapy. *Menopause International Journal, 19*(2), 59–68.

Price, D. M., & Noblett, K. (2012). Comparison of the cough stress test and 24 hour pad test in the assessment of stress urinary incontinence. *International Urogynecology Journal, 23*(4), 429–433.

Roe, B., Flanagan, L., & Maden, M. (2014). Systematic review of systematic reviews for the management of urinary incontinence and promotion of continence using conservative behavioural approaches in older people in care homes. *The Journal of Advanced Nursing, 71*(7), 1464–1483.

● = Independent; ▲ = Collaborative; **EBN** = Evidence-Based Nursing; **EB** = Evidence-Based

Schagen van Leeuwen, J. H., et al. (2008). Efficacy and safety of duloxetine in elderly women with stress urinary incontinence or stress-predominant mixed urinary incontinence. *Maturitas, 60*(2), 138–147.

St.Aubyn, B., & Andrews, A. (2015). If it's not written down—It didn't happen. *Journal of Community Nursing., 29*(5), 20–22.

Strothers, L., & Friedman, B. (2011). Risk factors for the development of stress urinary incontinence in women. *Current Urology Reports, 12*, 363–369.

Tapia, C., Khalaf, K., Berenson, K., et al. (2013). Health-related quality of life and economic impact of urinary incontinence due to detrusor overactivity associated with a neurological condition: A systematic review. *Health & Quality of Life Outcomes.* Retrieved from http://www.biomedcentral.com/content/pdf/1477-7525-11-13.pdf. (Accessed 3 March 2018).

Urge urinary Incontinence
Amanda Andrews, BSc (Hons), MA and Bernie St. Aubyn, BSc (hons), MSc

NANDA-I

Definition

Involuntary passage of urine occurring soon after a strong sensation or urgency to void.

Defining Characteristics

Inability to reach toilet in time to avoid urine loss; involuntary loss of urine with bladder contractions; involuntary loss of urine with bladder spasms; urinary urgency

Related Factors

Alcohol consumption; caffeine intake; fecal impaction; ineffective toileting habits; involuntary sphincter relaxation

Associated Condition

Atrophic urethritis; atrophic vaginitis; bladder infection; decrease in bladder capacity; detrusor hyperactivity with impaired bladder contractility; impaired bladder contractility; treatment regimen

NOC   (Nursing Outcomes Classification)

Suggested NOC Outcomes

Tissue Integrity: Skin and Mucous Membranes; Urinary Continence; Urinary Elimination

Example NOC Outcome with Indicators

Urinary Continence as evidenced by the following indicators: Responds in timely manner to urge/Voids in appropriate receptacle/Has adequate time to reach toilet between urge and evacuation of urine/Underclothing remains dry during day/Underclothing or bedding remains dry during night. (Rate the outcome and indicators of **Urinary Continence:** 1 = never demonstrated, 2 = rarely demonstrated, 3 = sometimes demonstrated, 4 = often demonstrated, 5 = consistently demonstrated [see Section I].)

Client Outcomes

Client Will (Specify Time Frame)

- Report relief from urge urinary incontinence or a decrease in the frequency of incontinent episodes
- Identify containment devices that assist in the management of urge urinary incontinence

NIC   (Nursing Interventions Classification)

Suggested NIC Interventions

Urinary Habit Training; Urinary Incontinence Care

● = Independent;   ▲ = Collaborative;   EBN = Evidence-Based Nursing;   EB = Evidence-Based

Example NIC Activities—Urinary Habit Training
Keep a continence specification record for 3 days to establish voiding pattern; Establish interval for toileting of preferably not less than 2 hours

Nursing Interventions and *Rationales*

- Introduce yourself to the client and anyone accompanying him or her and inform them of your role. *Introducing yourself to a client helps establish and develop a therapeutic relationship that recognizes the person within the client and forms the bases for building trust on which to base the provision of care (Howatson-Jones, Standing, & Roberts, 2012).*
- Gain consent to perform care before proceeding further with the assessment. *Clients have the right to autonomy both legally and morally; therefore should be fully involved in the decision-making process (Avery, 2013).*
- Wash hands using a recognized technique. *Evidence shows that strict hand hygiene regimens significantly reduce the incidence of methicillin-resistant* Staphylococcus aureus *and* Clostridium difficile *infection (Goldberg, 2017).*
- Assess the usual pattern of bladder management and establish the pattern of bladder management and extent of the problem. *A detailed and accurate assessment of the client enables the nurse to plan interventions, monitor outcomes, and evaluate care, ensuring no unnecessary treatment is performed (Matthews, 2011).* Refer to Functional urinary **Incontinence** care plan.
- Assess bladder habits and quality of life issues:
  - ○ Diurnal frequency (voiding more than once every 2 hours while awake)
  - ○ Urgency, daytime frequency and nocturia
  - ○ Involuntary leakage and leakage accompanied by or preceded by urgency
  - ○ Amount of urine loss, moderate or large volume
  - ○ Severity of symptoms
  - ○ Alleviating and aggravating factors
  - ○ Effect on quality of life
- ▲ **EB:** *Incontinence is distressing and may contribute to decreased quality of life. This includes a negative effect on psychological well-being, social interactions and activities, and sexual and interpersonal relationships (Minassian et al, 2015).*
- ▲ Urge urinary incontinence occurs when involuntary leakage of urine is accompanied by or immediately preceded by urgency; overactive bladder is characterized by the storage symptoms of urgency with or without incontinence and is usually accompanied by frequency and nocturia (Abrams et al, 2010).
- Ask specific questions relating to urge presentation:
  - ○ Can you delay urination for a 2-hour movie or car ride?
  - ○ How often do you wake at night to urinate?
  - ○ When you have the urge to urinate, can you reach the toilet without leaking?
- ▲ **EB:** *A history of urine loss associated with urgency is the most helpful criterion for diagnosing urge urinary incontinence (Holroyd-Leduc et al, 2011). To further enhance this assessment the questionnaire needs to be a validated incontinence-specific quality of life questionnaire (Bardsley, 2016).*
- ▲ In close consultation with a health care practitioner or advanced practice nurse, consider administering a symptom questionnaire that elicits relevant lower urinary tract symptoms and differentiates stress and urge incontinence symptoms. **CEB:** *The Urogenital Distress Inventory short form (UDI-6) is a reliable and valid tool for identifying types of urinary incontinence (Dowling-Castronovo, 2008).*
- Assess the severity of incontinence and the effect on the individual's lifestyle; inquire about incontinence pad use and change in daily, social, or recreational activities, and emotional impact. **EB:** *Incontinence is distressing and may contribute to decreased quality of life, especially for women with mixed incontinence (Bardsley, 2016).*
- ▲ Perform a focused physical assessment, in close consultation with a health care practitioner or advanced practice nurse including:
  - ○ Bladder palpation after voiding to check for retention
  - ○ Bladder scanning for postvoid residual
  - ○ Inspection of the perineal skin
  - ○ Vaginal examination to determine hypoestrogenic changes in the mucosa (may contribute to urge incontinence)

● = Independent;   ▲ = Collaborative;   **EBN** = Evidence-Based Nursing;   **EB** = Evidence-Based

❍ Pelvic examination to determine the presence, location, and severity of vaginal wall prolapse, and reproduction of stress urinary incontinence with the cough test

- Anal tone and constipation should be assessed. *A thorough abdominal and pelvic examination must be completed to accurately assess incontinence. Identification of "red flag" symptoms (e.g., nocturia, hematuria) needs referral to the appropriate consultant (NICE, 2015).*
- Inspect the perineal and perianal skin for evidence of incontinence-associated dermatitis, including inflammation, vesicles in skin exposed to urinary leakage, and especially skinfolds or denudation of the skin, particularly when incontinence is managed by absorptive pads or containment briefs. **EB:** *Ammonia produced from the breakdown of urea in urine causes an increase in skin pH, which increases the permeability of the skin; excess moisture and damage to the acid mantle further increases permeability and vulnerability to bacterial and fungal infections (Beeckman, 2017). Skin exposed to urine or stool will become bright red, and the surface may appear shiny because of serous exudate; inflamed areas of individuals with darker skin tones may be a duller red or hypopigmented when compared with adjacent skin. Inspect the skin for a maculopapular red rash typical of candidiasis (Beeckman, 2017).*
- Teach the client to complete a bladder diary by recording voiding frequency, the frequency and degree of urinary incontinence episodes, their association with urgency (a sudden and strong desire to urinate that is difficult to defer), fluid intake, and pad usage over a 3- to 7-day period. An electronic voiding diary may be kept whenever feasible. In addition to these parameters, the client may be asked to record voided volume and fluid intake. **EB:** *Use of a bladder diary may reduce client discrepancies in recall and is a valuable tool for assessment; short (24-hour) duration of the bladder diary may yield inadequate data, and excessive diary duration reduces compliance (Dixon & Nakib, 2016).*
- Review all medications the client is receiving, paying particular attention to sedatives, opioid analgesics, diuretics, antidepressants, psychotropic drugs, and cholinergics. Consult the health care practitioner or nurse practitioner about altering or eliminating these medications if they are suspected of affecting incontinence. **EB:** *All medications should be reviewed to determine whether they are contributing to incontinence (Abrams et al, 2010).*
- Assess the client for urinary retention (see the care plan for **Urinary Retention**).
- Assess the client for functional limitations (environmental barriers, limited mobility or dexterity, and impaired cognitive function). Clients with impaired dexterity or weakness may benefit from clothing that has been modified or is without buttons and zippers (Leaver, 2017). Refer to the care plan for Functional urinary **Incontinence.**
- Consult the health care practitioner concerning diabetic management or pharmacotherapy for urinary tract infection when indicated. In specific cases, urgency and an increased risk of urge incontinence may be related to bacteriuria or urinary tract infection (Gupta & Trautner, 2011).
- ▲ Assess for signs and symptoms of atrophic vaginal changes in the perimenopausal or postmenopausal woman, including vaginal dryness, tenderness to touch, mucosal dryness, friability, and discomfort with gentle palpation. Specifically query the woman with atrophic vaginitis concerning associated lower urinary tract symptoms (usually voiding frequency, urgency, and dysuria). Refer the woman with atrophic vaginal changes and bothersome lower urinary tract symptoms to a gynecologist, urologist, or women's health nurse practitioner for further evaluation and management. *Vaginal topical estrogens may reduce urge incontinence, prevent urogenital atrophy, and prevent recurrent urinary tract infections. Intravaginal estrogen has an effect on the bladder and urethral epithelium and can help to relieve symptoms of urinary frequency, particularly in postmenopausal women with vaginal atrophy (Panay et al, 2013).*

Pelvic Floor Training Program

- Pelvic floor muscle training is effective in the treatment of stress, urge, and mixed urinary incontinence; participation in a supervised program for at least 3 months may yield improved outcomes (Dumoulin, Hay-Smith, & Mac Habbe-Seguin, 2014).
- Teach the client undergoing pelvic floor muscle training to identify, contract, and relax the pelvic floor muscles without contracting distal muscle groups (e.g., abdominal muscles or gluteus muscles) using verbal feedback based on vaginal or anal palpation, biofeedback, or electrical stimulation, using the assistance of an incontinence specialist or health care provider as necessary. **EB:** *To find the proper muscles, the client may be instructed to think about trying to control the urge to pass gas; women will feel a lifting sensation in the vaginal area and a pulling in of the rectum (Keyock & Newman, 2011).* **CEB:** *When learning to control pelvic floor muscles, clients may recruit other muscles such as the rectus abdominis or gluteal muscles,*

● = Independent; ▲ = Collaborative; **EBN** = Evidence-Based Nursing; **EB** = Evidence-Based

which may be counterproductive; these muscles must be relaxed to avoid increasing pressure on the bladder or pelvic floor (Burgio, 2009; Burgio et al., 2010).

- Incorporate principles of exercise physiology into a pelvic muscle training program using the following strategies:
  - Begin a graded exercise program, usually starting with 5 to 10 repetitions and advancing gradually to no more than 35 to 50 repetitions every day or every other day based on baseline and ongoing evaluation of maximal strength and endurance.
  - Continue exercise sessions over a period of 3 to 6 months.
  - Integrate muscle training into activities of daily living.
  - Assess progress every 2 weeks during the first month and every 4 to 6 weeks thereafter.

Pelvic floor muscle training strengthens urethral sphincter tone (Chong, Khan, & Anger, 2011) and is the first-line conservative approach for all types of incontinence, particularly for stress and mixed urinary incontinence; women report an improvement in symptoms and quality of life after undergoing this training (Dumoulin, Hay-Smith, & Mac Habbe Seguin, 2014).

Bladder Training Program

- Assist the client in completing a voiding diary over a period of a minimum of 3 days or up to 7 days.
- Review the results with the client, determining typical voiding frequency and establishing goals for voiding frequency based on the longest time interval between voids that is comfortable for the client.
- Using baseline voiding frequency, as determined by the diary, teach the client to void first thing in the morning, every time the predetermined voiding interval passes, and before going to bed at night.
- Encourage adherence to the program with timing devices and verbal encouragement and support, and address individual reasons for schedule interruption.
- Teach distraction and urge suppression techniques (see later discussion) to control urgency while the client postpones urination.
- Gradually increase the time between urinations to the negotiated goal. Time intervals between voiding are typically increased in increments of 15 to 30 minutes for clients with a baseline frequency of less than every 60 minutes and increments of 25 to 30 minutes for clients with a baseline frequency of more than every 60 minutes. The voiding interval should be increased by 15 to 30 minutes each week (based on the client's tolerance) until a voiding interval of 3 to 4 hours is achieved. Use a bladder diary to monitor progress. **EB:** *Bladder training involves adjusting your habits and developing a schedule to void even if the client does not have an urge to void. Gradually increase the time intervals between urination allowing the bladder to fill more fully and providing more control over the urge to urinate (Mayo Clinic, 2017).*
- Review with the client the types of beverages consumed, focusing on the intake of caffeine, which is associated with a transient effect on lower urinary tract symptoms. Advise all clients to reduce or eliminate intake of caffeinated beverages or over-the-counter medications of dietary aids containing caffeine. Identify and counsel the client to eliminate other bladder irritants that may exacerbate incontinence, such as smoking, carbonated beverages, citrus, sugar substitutes, and tomato products. **CEB/EB:** *Caffeine is a diuretic, a bladder irritant, increases detrusor pressure, and is a risk factor for detrusor instability; reducing caffeine may decrease both stress and urge incontinence. Decrease caffeine gradually to avoid caffeine withdrawal. Carbonated beverages, citrus fruits, sugar substitutes, and tomato products may be bladder irritants (Burgio, 2009; Mayo Clinic, 2017).*
- Review with the client the volume of fluids consumed; fluids may be reduced with caution, *particularly in clients who do not drink more than 1500 mL during the day*, to alleviate urinary frequency, especially in the evening after 6 p.m. or 3 to 4 hours before bedtime to reduce nocturia. **EB:** *Be aware that adequate fluid intake is essential; six 8-ounce glasses per 24 hours, 1500 mL, or 30 mL/kg body weight is recommended. The type and amount of fluid intake is associated with frequency and urge urinary incontinence (Segal, Saks, & Arya, 2011).*
- Teach the client methods to avoid constipation such as increasing dietary fiber, moderately increasing fluid intake, exercising, and establishing a routine defecation schedule.
- Refer to **Constipation** care plans.

Urge Suppression

- *Urge suppression skills are essential in helping clients learn a new way of responding to the sense of urgency. Rushing to the toilet increases physical pressure on the bladder, enhances the sensation of fullness, exposes the client to visual cues that can trigger incontinence, and exacerbates urgency (Burgio, 2009).*

- Teach the client the following techniques:
  - ○ When a strong or precipitous urge to urinate is perceived, teach the client to avoid running to the toilet.
  - ○ Pause, sit down, and relax the entire body.
  - ○ Perform repeated, rapid pelvic muscle contractions until the urge is relieved.
  - ○ Use distraction: count backward from 100 by sevens; recite a poem; write a letter; balance a checkbook; do handwork such as knitting; and take five deep breaths, focusing on breathing.
  - ○ Relief is followed by micturition within 5 to 15 minutes, using nonhurried movements when locating a toilet and voiding.
  - ○ Use urge suppression strategies on waking during the night. If the urge subsides, the client should be encouraged to go back to sleep. If after a minute or two the urge does not subside, clients should be instructed to get up to void to avoid sleep interruption. EB: *Behavioral training for urge incontinence can reduce nocturia (Burgio, 2009).*
- Teach the client to self-administer antimuscarinic (anticholinergic) drugs as directed. Teach dosage side effects and administration of the medication and the importance of combining pharmacotherapy with scheduled voiding, adequate fluid intake, restriction of bladder irritants, and urge suppression techniques. EB: *Antimuscarinic drugs increase bladder capacity, reduce the frequency of incontinence episodes, and diminish voiding frequency. However, they do not cure bladder dysfunction or reduce the time between perception of a strong urge and onset of an overactive detrusor contraction. Approximately two-thirds of clients treated with antimuscarinic medication discontinue use within 3 to 4 months; the efficacy of pharmacotherapy for urge incontinence is enhanced when combined with behavioral interventions (Burgio et al, 2010).*
- Assist the client in selecting, obtaining, and applying a containment device for urine loss as indicated. *The use of containment devices can be useful as "stop gap" strategies used alongside long-term management options (Reid, 2014).*
- Provide the client with information about incontinence support groups such as the National Association for Continence and the Simon Foundation for Continence. A helpful website titled Total Control (http://www.totalcontrolprogram.com/Pelvic+Health/Bladder+Health) can be accessed to give support and information to women with incontinence. EB: *Knowledge contributes to effective self-management; women with incontinence often do not seek help from others and prefer to self-manage their incontinence (Holroyd-Leduc et al, 2011).*
- Assess the functional and cognitive status of all clients with urge incontinence; use interventions to improve mobility. EB: *Clients with severe cognitive impairments (dementia) and functional mobility problems have an increased likelihood of developing urge incontinence (Jerez-Roig, 2016).*
- Refer client for occupational therapy for help in obtaining assistive devices and adapting the home for optimal toilet accessibility. *Occupational therapists are needed to assist patients with dexterity and mobility issues that may be contributing to incontinence (Spencer, McManus, & Sabourin, 2017).*
- Encourage the client to develop an action plan for self-care management of incontinence. *Making an action plan facilitates behavior change*
- Provide client with comprehensive written information about bladder care. EB: *Providing clients with well-written, evidence-based information about their condition and treatment can have a beneficial effect on the outcomes of treatment. In addition, clients are more likely to retain important information that will assist them in making informed decisions about their care (Coulter, 2011).*
- Document all care and advice given in a factual and comprehensive manner. *Good record keeping is an integral part of nursing practice and is essential to the provision of safe and effective care (St. Aubyn & Andrews, 2015).*

REFERENCES

Abrams, P., et al. (2010). The standardization of terminology of lower urinary tract function: Report from the standardization sub-committee of the international continence society. *American Journal of Obstetrics and Gynecology, 187*(1), 116–126.

Avery, G. (2013). *Law and ethics in nursing and healthcare: an introduction.* London: Sage Publications Inc.

Bardsley, A. (2016). An overview of urinary incontinence. *British Journal of Nursing (Urology Supplement), 25*(18), s14–s21.

Beeckman, D. (2017). A decade of research on Incontinence-Associated Dermatitis (IAD): Evidence, knowledge gaps and next steps. *Journal of Tissue Viability, 26*(1), 47–56. doi:10.1016/j.jtv.2016.02.004.

Burgio, K. L. (2009). Behavioral treatment of urinary incontinence, voiding dysfunction, and overactive bladder. *Obstetrics and Gynecology Clinics of North America, 36*(3), 475–491.

Burgio, K. L., et al. (2010). The effects of drug and behavior therapy on urgency and voiding frequency. *International Urogynecology Journal, 21*(6), 711–719.

● = Independent;　▲ = Collaborative;　EBN = Evidence-Based Nursing;　EB = Evidence-Based

Chong, E. C., Khan, A. A., & Anger, J. T. (2011). The financial burden of stress urinary incontinence among women in the United States. *Current Urology Reports, 12*(5), 358–362.

Coulter, A. (2011). *Engaging patients in health care.* Berkshire: McGraw-Hill Open University Press.

Dixon, C. A., & Nakib, N. A. (2016). Are bladder diaries helpful in management of overactive bladder? *Current bladder dysfunction reports, 11*(Iss 1), 14–17.

Dowling-Castronovo, A. (2008). *Urinary incontinence assessment in older adults: Part II—Established urinary incontinence.* From Try This: Best Practices in Nursing Care to Older Adults, Hartford Institute for Geriatric Nursing, New York University, College of Nursing. Retrieved from http://consultgerirn.org/uploads/File/trythis/try_this_11_2.pdf. (accessed March 8, 2018).

Dumoulin, C., Hay-Smith, J., & Mac Habbe-Seguin, G. (2014). Pelvic floor muscle training versus no treatment, or interactive control treatments, for urinary incontinence in women. *The Cochrane Library.* doi:10.1002/14651858.CD005654.pub3.

Goldberg, J. L. (2017). Guideline implementation; hand hygiene. *AORN Journal, 105*(2), 203–212.

Gupta, K., & Trautner, B. (2011). Urinary tract infections, pyelonephritis and prostatitis. In D. L. Longo, et al. (Eds.), *Harrison's principles of internal medicine* (18th ed.). New York: McGraw-Hill.

Holroyd-Leduc, J. M., et al. (2011). Translation of evidence into a self-management tool for use by women with urinary incontinence. *Age and Ageing, 40*(2), 227–233.

Howatson-Jones, L., Standing, M., & Roberts, S. (Eds.), (2012). *Patient assessment and care planning in nursing.* London: Sage Publications Inc.

Jerez-Roig, J., et al. (2016). Prevalence of urinary incontinence and associated factors in nursing home residents. *Neurourology and Urodynamics, 35*(2), 102–107.

Keyock, K., & Newman, D. (2011). Understanding stress urinary incontinence. *The Nurse Practitioner, 36*(10), 24–36.

Leaver, R. (2017). Assessing Patients with urinary incontinence: The basics. *Journal of Community Nursing., 31*(1), 40–46.

Matthews, E. (2011). *Nursing care planning.* London: Lippincott Williams & Wilkins.

Mayo Clinic (2017). *Bladder control: Lifestyle strategies ease problems.* Retrieved from https://www.mayoclinic.org/diseases-conditions/urinary-incontinence/in-depth/bladder-control-problem/ART-20046597?p=1. (Accessed 9 March 2018).

Minassian, V. A., Sun, H. Y., Clerk, D. N., et al. (2015). The interaction of stress and urgency urinary incontinence and its effect on quality of life. *The International Urogynecology Journal, 26*(2), 269–276.

NICE. (2015). *Suspected cancer: recognition and referral.* Retrieved from https://www.nice.org.uk/guidance/ng12. (Accessed 3 November 2017).

Panay, N., Hamoda, H., Arya, R., et al. (2013). The 2013 British menopause society and women's health concern recommendations on hormone replacement therapy. *Menopause International Journal, 19*(2), 59–68.

Reid, J. (2014). Managing urinary incontinence: Guidelines for community nurses. *Journal of Christian Nursing, 28*(6), 20–26.

Segal, S., Saks, E. K., & Arya, L. A. (2011). Self-assessment of fluid intake behavior and the relationship to lower urinary tract symptoms in women with urinary incontinence. *Journal of Women's Health, 20*, 1–5.

Spencer, M., McManus, K., & Sabourin, J. (2017). Incontinence in the older adult: The role of the geriatric multidisciplinary team. *The British Columbia Medical Journal, 59*(2), 99–105.

St.Aubyn, B., & Andrews, A. (2015). If it's not written down—It didn't happen. *Journal of Community Nursing., 29*(5), 20–22.

Risk for urge urinary Incontinence   *Mary Beth Flynn Makic, PhD, RN, CCNS, FAAN*

NANDA-I

Definition

Susceptible to involuntary passage of urine occurring soon after a strong sensation or urgency to void, which may compromise health.

Risk Factors

Alcohol consumption; caffeine intake; fecal impaction; ineffective toileting habits; involuntary sphincter relaxation

Associated Condition

Atrophic urethritis; atrophic vaginitis; bladder infection; decrease in bladder capacity; detrusor hyperactivity with impaired bladder contractility; impaired bladder contractility; treatment regimen

NIC, NOC, Client Outcomes, Nursing Interventions and *Rationales,* Client/Family Teaching and Discharge Planning, and References

Refer to care plan for Urge urinary **Incontinence.**

Bowel Incontinence   *Kim L. Paxton, DNP, APRN, ANP-BC, LHIT-C*

NANDA-I

Definition

Involuntary passage of stool.

Defining Characteristics

Bowel urgency; constant passage of soft stool; does not recognize urge to defecate; fecal staining; inability to delay defecation; inability to expel formed stool despite recognition of rectal fullness; inability to recognize rectal fullness; inattentive to urge to defecate

Related Factors

Difficulty with toileting self-care; environmental factor; generalized decline in muscle tone; immobility; inadequate dietary habits; incomplete emptying of bowel; laxative abuse; stressors

Associated Condition

Abnormal increase in abdominal pressure; abnormal increase in intestinal pressure; alteration in cognitive functioning; chronic diarrhea; colorectal lesion; dysfunctional rectal sphincter; impaction; impaired reservoir capacity; lower motor nerve damage; pharmaceutical agent; rectal sphincter abnormality; upper motor nerve damage

NOC   (Nursing Outcomes Classification)

Suggested NOC Outcomes

Bowel Continence; Bowel Elimination

> **Example NOC Outcome with Indicators**
>
> **Bowel Continence** as evidenced by the following indicators: Maintains predictable pattern of stool evacuation/Maintains control of stool passage/Evacuates stool at least every 3 days. (Rate the outcome and indicators of **Bowel Continence:** 1 = never demonstrated, 2 = rarely demonstrated, 3 = sometimes demonstrated, 4 = often demonstrated, 5 = consistently demonstrated [see Section I].)

Client Outcomes

Client Will (Specify Time Frame)

- Have regular, complete evacuation of fecal contents from the rectal vault (pattern may vary from every day to every 3 days)
- Have regulation of stool consistency (soft, formed stools)
- Reduce or eliminate frequency of incontinent episodes
- Exhibit intact skin in the perianal/perineal area
- Demonstrate the ability to isolate, contract, and relax pelvic muscles (when incontinence related to sphincter incompetence or high-tone pelvic floor dysfunction)
- Increase pelvic muscle strength (when incontinence related to sphincter incompetence)
- Identify triggers that precipitate change in bowel continence

NIC   (Nursing Interventions Classification)

Suggested NIC Interventions

Bowel Incontinence Care; Bowel Incontinence Care: Encopresis; Bowel Training

> **Example NIC Interventions—Bowel Incontinence Care**
>
> Determine physical or psychological cause of fecal incontinence; Instruct client/family to record fecal output, as appropriate

● = Independent;   ▲ = Collaborative;   EBN = Evidence-Based Nursing;   EB = Evidence-Based

Nursing Interventions and *Rationales*

I

- In a private setting, directly question client about the presence of fecal incontinence. If the client reports altered bowel elimination patterns, problems with bowel control, or "uncontrollable diarrhea," complete a focused nursing history including previous and present bowel elimination routines, dietary history, frequency and volume of uncontrolled stool loss, and aggravating and alleviating factors. EB: *Unless questioned directly or the client is experiencing bothersome fecal incontinence, clients are often hesitant to report the presence of fecal incontinence (Spiegel et al, 2014). The nursing history determines the patterns of stool elimination, to characterize involuntary stool loss and the likely etiology of the incontinence (Willson et al, 2014).*
- Recognize that risk factors for fecal incontinence include older individuals, female sex, impaired mobility, cognitive impairment, obesity, individuals who have undergone pelvic surgery, diabetes, and structural or functional impairment of bowel function (Ditah et al, 2014; Willson et al, 2014, Young et al, 2017). *Although fecal incontinence is more common in women, it is also a problem for men and should not be overlooked when obtaining a health history (Young et al, 2017). Physiological changes of the female pelvis that occur with aging, along with those that occur with childbirth increase the risk of elimination problems, both constipation and incontinence (Mannella et al, 2013; Young et al, 2017).* EBN: *The prevalence of double incontinence, defined as urinary and fecal incontinence, is nationally estimated to be 10.6% for noninstitutionalized persons 65 and over who reported an occurrence of urinary leakage along with accidental bowel leakage as recorded from the face-to-face National Health and Nutrition Examination Survey (2007–2010) (Gorina et al, 2014).*
- Recognize that additional risk factors for bowel incontinence in hospitalized clients include antibiotic therapy, medications, enteral feeding, indwelling urinary catheter placement, immobility, inability to communicate elimination needs, acute disease processes and procedures (e.g., cancer, abdominal surgery), sedation, and mechanical ventilation (Chang & Huang, 2013; Gorina et al, 2014; Eman & Lohrmann, 2015).
- ▲ Conduct a health history assessment that includes a review of current bowel patterns/habits to include constipation and use of laxatives; diarrhea; pelvic floor injury with childbirth; acute trauma to organs, muscles, or nerves involved in defecation; gastrointestinal inflammatory disorders; functional disability; and medications (Kaiser et al, 2014; Whitehead, Palsson, & Simren, 2016).
- ▲ Closely inspect the perineal skin and skinfolds for evidence of skin breakdown in clients with incontinence. EBN: *An expert consensus statement defined moisture-associated skin damage as inflammation and erosion of the skin caused by prolonged exposure to various sources of moisture (Coyer, Gardner, & Doubrovsky, 2017). Incontinence-associated dermatitis (IAD) is a form of skin irritation that develops from chronic exposure to urine or liquid stool (Bliss et al, 2015; Coyer, Gardner, & Doubrovsky, 2017). A recent meta-analysis found a strong association between IAD and a client developing a pressure ulcer (Beeckman et al, 2014).*
- ▲ Use a validated tool that focuses on bowel elimination patterns to help provide a clearer understanding of the client's individual challenges and perceptions of symptoms associated with fecal incontinence (Gillibrand, 2012; Jelovsek et al, 2014).
- ▲ Complete a focused physical assessment, including inspection of perineal skin, pelvic muscle strength assessment, digital examination of the rectum for the presence of impaction and anal sphincter strength, and evaluation of functional status (mobility, dexterity, and visual acuity).
- Complete an assessment of cognitive function; explore for a history of dementia, delirium, or acute confusion (Bliss et al, 2015; Drennan, Greenwood, & Cole, 2014). EBN: *A study found that critically ill clients who were less cognitively aware were 50% more likely to develop IAD than clients who were more cognitively aware (Bliss et al, 2015).*
- Document patterns of stool elimination and incontinent episodes through a bowel record, including frequency of bowel movements, stool consistency, frequency and severity of incontinent episodes, precipitating factors, and dietary and fluid intake. *Documented patterns of elimination are used to narrow the likely etiology of stool incontinence and serve as a baseline to evaluate treatment efficacy (Willson et al, 2014; Rao et al, 2016).*
- Assess stool consistency and its influence on risk for stool loss. *Several classification systems for stool exist and may assist the nurse and client to differentiate among normal soft, formed stool, hardened stools associated with constipation, and liquid stools associated with diarrhea.* EBN: *A study of stool consistency found good reliability when evaluated by nurses and clients. Word-only descriptors yielded equivocal consistency when assessed by subjects, as did tools that combined words with illustrations of various stool consistencies (Bliss*

• = Independent;   ▲ = Collaborative;   EBN = Evidence-Based Nursing;   EB = Evidence-Based

et al, 2015). Less well-formed (loose or liquid) stool is associated with an increased severity and frequency of fecal incontinence episodes and potential for compromised skin integrity (Bliss et al, 2015; Willson et al, 2014; Beeckman, 2017; Coyer, Gardner, & Doubrovsky, 2017).

- Identify conditions contributing to or causing fecal incontinence. *Fecal incontinence is frequently multifactorial. Accurate assessment of the probable etiology of fecal incontinence is necessary to select a treatment plan likely to control or eliminate the condition (Unger, Goldman, & Jelovesk, 2014; Willson et al, 2014).*
- Improve access to toileting:
  - ○ Identify usual toileting patterns and plan opportunities for toileting accordingly.
  - ○ Provide assistance with toileting for clients with limited access or impaired functional status (mobility, dexterity, and access).
  - ○ Institute a prompted toileting program for persons with impaired cognitive status.
  - ○ Provide adequate privacy for toileting.
  - ○ Respond promptly to requests for assistance with toileting.
- ▲ **EB:** *Acute or transient fecal incontinence frequently occurs in the acute care or long-term care facility secondary to mentation changes associated with environment change, inadequate access to toileting facilities, insufficient assistance with toileting, or inadequate privacy when attempting to toilet (Jelovsek et al, 2014; Park & Kim, 2014; Blekken et al, 2016).*
- Review the client's nutritional history and evaluate methods to normalize stool consistency with dietary adjustments (e.g., avoiding high-fat content foods) and use of fiber along with assessing for use of caffeine, lactose, and sugar replacements (*International Foundation for Functional Gastrointestinal Disorders [IFFGD], 2018; Willson et al, 2014; Paquette et al, 2017*). **EB:** *Diet modifications have been found to be helpful in the management of fecal incontinence, including restrictions of some foods, adding fiber to the diet, and establishing consistent eating patterns (National Institute for Diabetes and Digestive and Kidney Diseases, 2013; Willson et al, 2014).*
- Encourage the client to keep a nutrition log to track foods that irritate the bowel *(Paquette et al, 2017).*
- For hospitalized clients with tube feeding–associated fecal incontinence, involve the nutrition specialist to evaluate the formula composition, osmolality, and fiber content.
- For the client with intermittent episodes of fecal incontinence related to acute changes in stool consistency, begin a bowel reeducation program consisting of the following:
  - ○ Cleansing the bowel of impacted stool if indicated
  - ○ Normalizing stool consistency by adequate intake of fluids (30 mL/kg of body weight per day) and dietary or supplemental fiber
  - ○ Establishing a regular routine of fecal elimination based on established patterns of bowel elimination (patterns established before onset of incontinence)

Education on bowel patterns and strategies to establish normal defecation patterns and stool consistency to reduce or eliminate the risk of recurring fecal incontinence have been found to be beneficial in controlling fecal incontinence associated with changes in stool consistency (IFFGD, 2018; NHS *Choices Information, 2018).*

- ▲ Implement a scheduled stimulation defecation program for persons with neurological conditions causing fecal incontinence:
  - ○ Cleanse the bowel of impacted fecal material before beginning the program.
  - ○ Implement strategies to normalize stool consistency, including adequate intake of fluid and fiber and avoidance of foods associated with diarrhea.
  - ○ Determine a regular schedule for bowel elimination (typically every day or every other day) based on prior patterns of bowel elimination.
  - ○ Provide a stimulus before assisting the client to a position on the toilet; digital stimulation, a stimulating suppository, "mini-enema," or pulsed evacuation enema may be used for stimulation.

The scheduled, stimulated program relies on consistency of stool and a mechanical or chemical stimulus to produce a bolus contraction of the rectum with evacuation of fecal material (Duelund-Jakobsen et al, 2016; Paquette et al, 2017).

- ▲ Begin a reeducation or pelvic floor muscle exercise program for the person with sphincter incompetence or high-tone pelvic floor muscle dysfunction of the pelvic muscles, or refer persons with fecal incontinence related to sphincter dysfunction to a nurse specialist or other therapist with clinical expertise in these techniques of care. **EB:** *Although evidence of overall effectiveness of pelvic floor muscle exercise programs is inconclusive as a treatment strategy for fecal incontinence, the programs are not harmful (Mannella et al, 2013; Unger, Goldman, & Jelovesk, 2014).*

● = Independent;   ▲ = Collaborative;   EBN = Evidence-Based Nursing;   EB = Evidence-Based

▲ Consider a sacral nerve stimulation program in clients with urgency to defecate and fecal incontinence related to weakened sphincter muscles or sphincter defect. **EB:** *Sacral nerve stimulation has been found to significantly reduce incontinence for some clients (Van Koughnett & Wexner, 2013; Kaiser et al, 2014).*

● Institute a structured skin care regimen that incorporates three essential steps: cleanse, moisturize, and protect:
  ○ Select a cleanser with a pH range comparable to that of normal skin (usually labeled "pH balanced").
  ○ Moisturize with an emollient to replace lipids removed with cleansing and protect with a skin. Products containing petrolatum, dimethicone, or zinc oxide base or a no-sting skin barrier should be used.
  ○ Routine incontinence care should include daily perineal skin cleansing and after each episode of incontinence.
  ○ When feasible, select a product that combines two or all three of these processes into a single step. Ensure that products are available at the bedside when caring for a client with total incontinence in an inpatient facility.

▲ Use of absorptive pads or adult containment briefs that are applied next to the client's skin increases the risk of IAD. Absorbent underpads that wick moisture away from skin may be used with immobile clients. **EBN:** *A structured skin care regimen based on a three-step process (cleanse, moisturize, and protect) is effective for the prevention of IAD (Willson et al, 2014; Gray, McNickol, & Nix, 2016; Beeckman, 2017; Beeckman et al, 2014; Coyer, Gardner, & Doubrovsky, 2017).*

▲ Consult the provider if a fungal infection is suspected. An antifungal cream or powder beneath a protective ointment may be indicated (*Willson et al, 2014;Gray, McNickol, & Nix et al., 2016; Coyer, Gardner, & Doubrovsky, 2017*).

● Assist the client to select and apply a containment device for occasional episodes of fecal incontinence. A fecal containment device will prevent soiling of clothing and reduce odors in the client with uncontrolled stool loss. **EBN:** *A study of community persons with fecal incontinence who used an absorptive dressing to contain mucus and stool leakage after surgery revealed that the device was preferred over traditional pads in 92% (Bliss et al, 2015).*

● In the client with frequent episodes of fecal incontinence and limited mobility, monitor the sacrum and perineal area for pressure ulcerations. **EBN:** *Limited mobility, particularly when combined with fecal incontinence and increased moisture, increases the risk of pressure ulceration. Routine cleansing, pressure reduction techniques, and management of fecal and urinary incontinence reduce this risk (Beeckman et al, 2014; Willson et al, 2014; Beeckman, 2017).*

● With acutely ill clients, anticipate and evaluate the cause of acute diarrhea. Anticipate diarrhea associated with treatment or specific interventions (e.g., medications, initiation of tube feedings). *Interventions to manage acute diarrhea include use of absorbent pads and skin protectant moisturizers or fecal collector/pouch (Willson et al, 2014; Beeckman, 2017; Pather et al, 2017).*

▲ Consult a provider about insertion of a bowel management system (BMS) in the critically ill client when conservative measures have failed and fecal incontinence is excessive and/or produces perianal skin injury or IAD. *Indwelling BMSs, also called fecal management systems (FMSs), are commercially available and designed to direct, collect, and contain liquid stool in immobile clients. BMS devices are approved by the Food and Drug Administration for up to 29 days for management of liquid stool.(Whitely et al., 2014)* **EBN:** *Devices other than BMSs should not be used for indwelling bowel/feces diversion (Munhall & Jindal, 2013; Whitely et al, 2014; Willson et al, 2014).*

 Geriatric

● Evaluate all older clients for established or acute fecal incontinence when the older client enters the acute or long-term care facility and intervene as indicated. **EB:** *Fecal incontinence often coexists with urinary incontinence, necessitating evidence-based interventions to prevent skin breakdown and/or pressure ulcer development in the older client (National Pressure Ulcer Advisory Panel, 2014; Willson et al, 2014; Shahin & Lohrmann, 2015).*

● Determine the client's cognitive level using a screening tool such as the Mini-Mental State Exam (MMSE), Montreal Cognitive Assessment (MoCA), the Confusion Assessment Method (CAM), or Mini-Cog. **EB:** *Use of a standard evaluation tool such as the MMSE or MoCA can help determine the client's abilities and assist in planning appropriate nursing interventions. Acute or established dementias increase the risk of fecal incontinence among older adults (Jerez-Roig et al, 2015; Trzepacz et al, 2015).*

● = Independent;   ▲ = Collaborative;   **EBN** = Evidence-Based Nursing;   **EB** = Evidence-Based

❍ Teach nursing colleagues, nonprofessional care providers, family, and clients the importance of providing toileting opportunities and adequate privacy for the client in an acute or long-term care facility.

 Home Care

- The preceding interventions may be adapted for home care use.
- Assess and teach a bowel management program to support continence. Address timing, diet, fluids, and actions taken independently to deal with bowel incontinence. *Identifying factors that change level of incontinence may guide interventions. If the client has been taking over-the-counter medications or home remedies, it is important to consider their influence.*
- Instruct the caregiver to provide clothing that is nonrestrictive, can be manipulated easily for toileting, and can be changed with ease. *Avoidance of complicated maneuvers increases the chance of success in toileting programs and decreases the client's risk for embarrassing incontinent episodes.*
- Evaluate self-care strategies of community-dwelling older adults, strengthen adaptive behaviors, and counsel older adults about altering strategies that compromise general health.
- Assist the family in arranging care in a way that allows the client to participate in family or favorite activities without embarrassment. *Careful planning can both help the client retain dignity and maintain integrity of family patterns.*
- ▲ If the client is limited to bed (or bed and chair), provide a commode or bedpan that can be easily accessed. Involve occupational and physical therapy services as indicated to promote safe transfers.
- ▲ If the client is frequently incontinent, refer for home health aide services to assist with hygiene and skin care.
- ▲ Refer the family to support services to assist with in-home management of fecal incontinence as indicated.

Note: Refer to nursing diagnoses **Diarrhea** and **Constipation** for detailed management of these related conditions.

REFERENCES

Beeckman, D. (2017). A decade of research on Incontinence-Associated Dermatitis (IAD): Evidence, knowledge gaps and next steps. *Journal of Tissue Viability*, 26(1), 47–56. doi:10.1016/j.jtv.2016 .02.004.

Beeckman, D., VanLancker, A., VanHecke, A., et al. (2014). A systematic review and meta-analysis of incontinence-associated dermatitis, incontinence, and moisture as risk factors for pressure ulcer development. *Research in Nursing & Health*, 37, 201–218.

Blekken, L. E., Vinsnes, A. G., Gjeilo, K. H., et al. (2016). Exploring faecal incontinence in nursing home patients: A cross-sectional study of prevalence and associations derived from the Residents Assessment Instrument for Long Term Care Facilities. *Journal of Advanced Nursing*, 72(7), 1579–1591. doi:10.1111/ jan.1293.

Bliss, D. Z., Funk, T., Jacobson, M., et al. (2015). Incidence and characteristics of Incontinence-Associated dermatitis in Community-Dwelling persons with fecal incontinence. *Journal of Wound Ostomy Continence Nursing*, 42(5), 525–530. doi:10.1097/WON.0000000000000159.

Chang, S. J., & Huang, H. H. (2013). Diarrhea in enterally fed patients: Blame the diet? *Current Opinion in Clinical Nutrition and Metabolic Care*, 2013(16), 588–594.

Coyer, F., Gardner, A., & Doubrovsky, A. (2017). An interventional skin care protocol (InSPiRE) to reduce incontinence-associated dermatitis in critically ill patients in the intensive care unit: A before and after study. *Intensive and Critical Care Nursing*, 40, 1–10. Retrieved from http://doi.org/10.1016/j.iccn.2016.12.001.

Ditah, I., Devaki, P., Luma, H. N., et al. (2014). Prevalence, trends, and risk factors for fecal incontinence in United States adults, 2005–2010. *Clinical Gastroenterology and Hepatology*, 12(4).

Drennan, V. M., Greenwood, N., & Cole, L. (2014). Continence care for people with dementia at home. *Nursing Times*, 110(9), 19.

Duelund-Jakobsen, J., Worsoe, J., Lundby, L., et al. (2016). Management of patients with faecal incontinence. *Therapeutic Advances in Gastroenterology*, 9(1), 86–97. Retrieved from http://doi.org/10.1177 /1756283X15614516.

Eman, S. M., & Lohrmann, C. (2015). Prevalence of fecal and double fecal and urinary incontinence in hospitalized patients. *Journal of Wound, Ostomy & Continence Nursing*, 42(1), 89–93. doi:10.1097/ WON.0000000000000082.

Gillibrand, W. (2012). Faecal incontinence in the elderly: Issues and interventions in the home. *British Journal of Community Nursing*, 17(8), 364–368.

Gorina, Y., Schappert, S., Bercovitz, A., et al. (2014). Prevalence of incontinence among older adults. *Vital and Health Statistics [DHHS Publication no. 2014-1420]*, 3(36), 1–33.

Gray, M., McNickol, L., & Nix, D. (2016). Incontinence-associated dermatitis progress, promises, and ongoing challenges. *Journal of Wound, Ostomy, and Continence Nursing*, 43(2), 188–192. doi:10.1097/WON.0000000000000217.

International Foundation for Functional Gastrointestinal Disorders. (October 2018). *Nutritional strategies for managing diarrhea.* Retrieved from https://www.iffgd.org/lower-gi-disorders/diarrhea/ nutrition-strategies.html.

Jelovsek, J. E., Chen, Z., Markland, A. D., et al. (2014). Minimum important differences for scales assessing symptom severity and quality of life in patients with fecal incontinence. *Female Pelvic Medical Reconstructive Surgery*, 20(6), 342–348. doi:10.1097/ SPV.0000000000000078.

Jerez-Roig, J., Souza, D., Amaral, F., et al. (2015). Prevalence of fecal incontinence (FI) and associated factors in institutionalized older adults. *Archives of Gerontology and Geriatrics*, 60(3), 425–430. Retrieved from doi.org/10.1016/j.archger.2015.02.003.

● = Independent;   ▲ = Collaborative;   EBN = Evidence-Based Nursing;   EB = Evidence-Based

Kaiser, A. M., Orangio, G. R., Zutshi, M., et al. (2014). Current status: New technologies for the treatment of patients with fecal incontinence. *Surgical Endoscopy*, 28, 2277–2301.

Mannella, P., Palla, G., Bellini, M., et al. (2013). The female pelvic floor through midlife and aging. *Maturitas*, 76, 230–234.

Munhall, A. M., & Jindal, S. K. (2013). Massive gastrointestinal hemorrhage as a complication of the flexi-seal fecal management system. *American Journal of Critical Care*, 22(6), 537–543.

NHS Choices Information. (2018). *Bowel incontinence-treatment*. Retrieved from http://www.nhs.uk/Conditions/Incontinence-bowel/Pages/Treatment.aspx.

National Institute for Diabetes and Digestive and Kidney Diseases (2013). *Fecal incontinence*. Retrieved from http://www.niddk.nih.gov/health-information/health-topics/digestive-diseases/fecal-incontinence/Pages/facts.aspx#eating.

National Pressure Ulcer Advisory Panel (2014). *Prevention and Treatment of pressure ulcers: quick reference guide*. Cambridge Media. Retrieved from http://www.npuap.org/wp-content/uploads/2014/08/Updated-10-16-14-Quick-Reference-Guide-DIGITAL-NPUAP-EPUAP-PPPIA-16Oct2014.pdf.

Paquette, I. M., Varma, M. G., Kaiser, A. M., et al. (2017). The American Society of Colon and Rectal Surgeons' clinical practice guideline for the treatment of fecal incontinence. *Diseases of the Colon and Rectum*, 58(7), 623–636. doi:10.1097/DCR.0000000000000397.

Park, K. H., & Kim, K. S. (2014). Effect of a structured skin care regimen on patients with fecal incontinence: A comparison cohort study. *Journal of Wound, Ostomy, and Continence Nursing*, 41(2), 161–167.

Pather, P., Hines, S., Kynoch, K., et al. (2017). Effectiveness of topical skin products in the treatment and prevention of incontinence-associated dermatitis: A systematic review. *JBI Database of Systematic Reviews and Implementation Reports*, 15(5), 1473–1496. doi:10.11124/JBISRIR-2016-003015.

Rao, S. C., Bharucha, A. E., Chiarioni, G., et al. (2016). Anorectal disorders. *Gastroenterology*, 150(6), 1430–1442. doi:10.1053/j.gastro.2016.02.009.

Shahin, E. S. M., & Lohrmann, C. (2015). Prevalence of fecal and double fecal and urinary incontinence in hospitalized patients. *Journal of Wound, Ostomy, and Continence Nursing*, 42(1), 89–93.

Spiegel, B. M. R., Hays, R. D., Bolus, R., et al. (2014). Development of the NIH Patient-reported outcomes measurement information system (PROMIS) gastrointestinal symptom scales. *The American Journal of Gastroenterology*, 109(11), 1804–1814.

Trzepacz, P. T., Hochstetler, H., Wong, S., et al. (2015). Relationship between the Montreal Cognitive Assessment and Mini-mental State Examination for assessment of mild cognitive impairment in older adults. *BMC Geriatrics*, 15(107), 1–9. doi:10.1186/s12877-015-0103-3.

Unger, C. A., Goldman, H. B., & Jelovesk, J. E. (2014). Fecal incontinence: The role of the urologist. *Current Urology Reports*, 15, 388–398.

Van Koughnett, J. A., & Wexner, S. D. (2013). Current management of fecal incontinence: Choosing amongst treatment options to optimize outcomes. *World Journal of Gastroenterology*, 19(48), 9216–9230.

Whitely, I., Sinclair, G., Comm, M., et al. (2014). A retrospective review of outcomes using a fecal management system in acute care patients. *Ostomy/Wound Management*, 60(12), 37–43.

Willson, M. M., Angyus, M., Beals, D., et al. (2014). Executive summary: A quick reference guide for managing fecal incontinence. *Journal of Wound, Ostomy, and Continence Nursing*, 41(1), 61–69.

Whitehead, W. E., Palsson, O. S., & Simren, M. (2016). Treating fecal incontinence: An unmet need in primary care medicine. *North Carolina Medical Journal*, 77(3), 211–215.

Young, C. J., Zahid, A., Koh, C. E., et al. (2017). Hypothesized summative anal physiology score correlates but poorly predicts incontinence severity. *World Journal of Gastroenterology*, 59(2), 99–105.

Disorganized Infant behavior

Mary Alice DeWys, RN, BS, CIMI and Margaret Elizabeth Padnos, RN, AB, BSN, MA

NANDA-I

Definition

Disintegration of the physiological and neurobehavioral systems of functioning.

Defining Characteristics

Attention-Interaction System

Impaired response to sensory stimuli

Motor System

Alteration in primitive reflexes; exaggerated startle response; fidgeting; finger splaying; fisting; hands to face; hyperextension of extremities; impaired motor tone; tremor; twitching; uncoordinated movement

Physiological

Abnormal skin color; arrhythmia; bradycardia; feeding intolerance; oxygen desaturation; tachycardia; time-out signals

Regulatory Problems

Inability to inhibit startle reflex; irritability

● = Independent;   ▲ = Collaborative;   EBN = Evidence-Based Nursing;   EB = Evidence-Based

State-Organization System

Active-awake; diffuse alpha electroencephalogram (EEG) activity with eyes closed; irritable crying; quiet-awake; state oscillation

Related Factors

Caregiver cue misreading; environmental overstimulation; feeding intolerance; inadequate physical environment; infant malnutrition; insufficient caregiver knowledge of behavioral cures; insufficient containment within environment; insufficient environmental sensory stimulation; pain; sensory deprivation; sensory overstimulation

At-Risk Population

Low postconceptual age; prematurity; parental exposure to teratogen

Associated Condition

Congenital disorder; genetic disorder; infant illness; immature neurological functioning; impaired infant motor functioning; invasive procedure; infant oral impairment

I

NOC   (Nursing Outcomes Classification)

Suggested NOC Outcomes

Child Development; Neurological Status; Newborn Adaptation; Preterm Infant Organization; Sleep; Thermoregulation: Newborn; Infant Nutritional Status

Example NOC Outcome with Indicators
Preterm Infant Organization as evidenced by the following indicators: O_2 saturation >85%/Thermoregulation/ Sleep-awake state organization/Smooth transition between states/Ability to attend to visual and auditory stimuli/Habituation. (Rate the outcome and indicators of **Preterm Infant Organization:** 1 = severely compromised, 2 = substantially compromised, 3 = moderately compromised, 4 = mildly compromised, 5 = not compromised [see Section I].)

Client Outcomes

Client Will (Specify Time Frame)

Infant/Child
- Display physiological/autonomic stability: cardiopulmonary, digestive functioning
- Display signs of organized motor system (Wyngarden, DeWys, & Padnos, 1999)
- Display signs of organized state system: ability to achieve and maintain a state, and transition smoothly between states (Wyngarden, DeWys, & Padnos, 1999)
- Demonstrate progress toward effective self-regulation (Wyngarden, DeWys, & Padnos, 1999)
- Demonstrate progress toward or ability to maintain calm attention
- Demonstrate progress or ability to engage in positive interactions
- Demonstrate ability to respond to sensory information (visual, auditory, tactile) in an adaptive way

Parent/Significant Other
- Recognize infant/child behaviors as a complex communication system that expresses specific needs and wants (e.g., hunger, pain, stress, desire to engage or disengage)
- Educate parents/caregivers to recognize infant's avenues of neurobehavioral communication: autonomic/ physiological, motor, state, attention/interaction
- Recognize how infants respond to environmental sensory input through stress/avoidance and approach/ engagement behaviors
- Recognize and support infant's self-regulatory, coping behaviors used to regain or maintain homeostasis
- Teach parents to "tune in" to their own interactive style and how that affects their infant's behavior
- Teach parents ways to adapt their interactive style in response to infant's style of communication appropriate for developmental stage and gestational age
- Identify appropriate positioning and handling techniques that will enhance normal motor development (Wyngarden, DeWys, & Padnos, 1999)
- Promote infant/child's attention capabilities that support visual and auditory development (Wyngarden, DeWys, & Padnos, 1999)

● = Independent;   ▲ = Collaborative;   EBN = Evidence-Based Nursing;   EB = Evidence-Based

- Engage parents in pleasurable parent–infant interactions that encourage bonding and attachment (Wyngarden, DeWys, & Padnos, 1999)
- Structure and modify the environment in response to infant/child's behavior and personal needs; personalize their bed space (Wyngarden, DeWys, & Padnos, 1999)
- Identify available community resources that provide early intervention services, emotional support, community health nursing, and parenting classes (Wyngarden, DeWys, & Padnos, 1999)
- Communicate the infant's medical, nursing and developmental needs to the family in a culturally sensitive and appropriate way that is understandable (DeWys et al, 2016)

NIC   (Nursing Interventions Classification)

Suggested NIC Interventions

Physiological and Autonomic Stability; Developmental Enhancement; Infant Care; Environmental Management; Kangaroo Care; Nonnutritive Sucking; Parent Education: Infant; Positioning and Handling; Sleep and Awake Stability; Teaching: Infant Stimulation 0-4 months; Bonding and Attachment

Example NIC Activities—Developmental Enhancement, Infant

Provide information to parent about child development and child rearing; Promote and facilitate family bonding and attachment with infant

Nursing Interventions and *Rationales*

- Sensitive nursing care must be implemented at the infant's admission to the neonatal intensive care unit (NICU), continued stay, and continue past discharge as the family adjusts to transitioning home and into the community. EBN: *"Learning the principles of neurodevelopment and understanding the meaning of preterm behavioral cues make it possible for NICU caregivers and parents to provide individualized developmentally appropriate, neuroprotective care to each infant" (Altimier & Phillips, 2016).*
- Recognize the neurobehavior systems through which infants communicate organized and/or disorganized/ stress behaviors within the subsystems of functioning (i.e., physiological/autonomic, motor, states, attention/interactional, self-regulatory). CEB: The Assessment of Preterm Infants' Behavior (APIB) is based on the theory that each subsystem functions independently and interactively with the other subsystems. Infant's physiological/autonomic subsystem has to be stable/organized, enabling infant to attend and/or interact with animate and inanimate environment (Als et al, 2005).
- Recognize and educate parents to recognize the behavior cues infants use to communicate stress/avoidance and approach/engagement. CEB: The neurobehavior system theory provides a framework for reading, interpreting, and responding to cues that value the infant's importance and ability to affect the environment (Als et al, 2005).
- Provide high-quality individualized developmental care for low-birth-weight preterm infants in a family-centered care environment that promotes normal neurological, physical, and emotional developmental and prevents disabilities. EBN: A study focused on changing NICU "to family-integrated care where parents are intimately involved in baby's care for as many hours a day" and changed the unit's name to newborn intensive parenting unit (NIPU), leading to improved outcomes for NIPU babies (Hall et al, 2017).
- Identify and manage pain using appropriate pain management techniques during invasive procedures (e.g., tube insertion, heel sticks, intravenous lines). EB: A combination of oral sucrose and nonnutritive sucking reduces pain during procedures (Liu et al, 2017). EB: Kangaroo care is an effective way parents can decrease infant pain during invasive procedures (Bailey & Committee on Fetus and Newborn, 2015). EBN: The skin-to-skin method reduces procedural pain (Johnson et al, 2017). EB: Odor of breast milk has an analgesic effect and can be used as a safe method for pain relief and calming (Karbandi et al, 2015).
- Provide developmentally correct positioning and handling to facilitate optimal tone, normal neurodevelopmental outcomes that promote physiological stability, and sleep, and to reduce stress (King & Norton, 2017). Availability of positioning tool at bedside (integrated practice assessment tool [IPAT]) for nurses and parent education are important (Spilker, Hill, & Rosenblum, 2016).
- Provide care that supports development state organization, such as the ability to achieve and maintain quiet sleep and awake states and transition smoothly between states. EBN: Promote sleep by timing care and avoiding unnecessary procedures that disrupts sleep (Altimier & Phillips, 2016). EB: Recommended

---

• = Independent;   ▲ = Collaborative;   EBN = Evidence-Based Nursing;   EB = Evidence-Based

NICU noise level between 44 and 45 decibels (Bonan et al, 2014). EBN: A study found methods to reduce NICU noise are necessary and achievable (Reeves-Messner & Spilker, 2017).

- EB: Supine swaddling decreases restlessness and promotes quiet for sleep for NICU infants (Pease et al, 2016).
- Encourage parents to speak slowly and/or sing to their babies during visits EB: Maternal voice demonstrates increased stability in preterm infants (Filippa et al, 2017).
- Provide infants several opportunities for nonnutritive sucking (NNS). EB: Infants receiving NNS during tube feedings showed reduced time transitioning to full oral feedings and decreased the length of hospital stay (Foster, Psaila, & Patterson, 2016).
- Provide parents opportunities to experience physical closeness through loving touch, massage, cuddling, and skin-to-skin (kangaroo care), which enhances parent–infant attachment EBN: Kangaroo care positively affects mother–infant relationship, sleep, and brain maturation (Ludington-Hoe, 2013).
- Provide an environment that helps infants learn to self-regulate by encouraging self-calming behaviors (e.g., curing up, sucking fingers/fists). A study found that teaching parents ways to calm fussy infants and support good sleep patterns decreased regulatory problems at 12 months of age (Sidor et al, 2013).
- Parental engagement and early interactions in the NICU set the foundation for parent–infant attachment and social relationships. EB: Parents emotional closeness to NICU infants may be crucial for developing an affective parent–infant relationship (Stefana & Lavelli, 2017).
- Support effective and pleasurable feeding practices, such as breast, bottle, or combination, as essential for healthy nutrition/calories, for mother-baby bonding and attachment, and for setting the foundation for successful feeding/eating patterns. EBN: Support breastfeeding for successful oral feedings (Altimier & Phillips, 2016). EB: Full or partial breastfeeding for the first few months lowers sudden infant death syndrome (SIDS) risk (National Institutes of Health, US National Library of Medicine, 2017).
- Provide infants with positive sensory experiences (i.e., visual, auditory, tactile, olfactory, vestibular, proprioceptive) to enhance development of sensory pathways and avoid overstimulation of sensory systems. **Auditory EB:** Music as medicine by Novotney (2013) showed that the maternal voice demonstrates increased physiological stability in preterm infants (Filippa et al, 2017). **Gustatory EBN:** Position infant allowing finger/fist sucking. **Tactile EBN:** Skin-to-skin is a positive sensory experience for both mothers and babies (Baily et al, 2015). **Olfactory EB:** Exposure of breast milk odor can reduce need for O2 therapy (Karbandi et al, 2015). **Visual EBN:** Provide stable lighting, shield eyes from bright lights, and monitor visual stimulation until 37 weeks' gestation (Altimier & Phillips, 2016). **Vestibular EBN:** Change position every 4 hours (Altimier & Phillips, 2016).
- Incorporate parents as coparticipants of infant care by communicating daily progress of their infants' condition. EBN: Parents would rather speak with a physician or nurse they are already familiar with versus outside sources for education and support (Wigert & Bry, 2017). EB: Parents are an integral partner in the NICU staff (Altimier & Phillips, 2016).

EBN: "*The ultimate goal of NICU nurses is to provide caring environment for parents that supports infant development, and physical and emotional closeness (Freeley et al, 2016).*

- Provide social support to parents including all members of the family. EB: *Implement parent-to-parent support as an effective way for NICU parents to gain confidence, improve mental health, and prepare for discharge (Hall et al, 2017).*

Multicultural

- Identify cultural beliefs, norms, and values of family's perceptions of infant/child behavior.
- EB: *Health care providers need to deliver appropriate care that supports the culture of American Indian mothers and their premature infants (Brooks et al, 2016).*
- Recognize and support positive mother–infant interactive behaviors and be sensitive to cultural and ethnic backgrounds. CBN: *A study identified similar and yet different mother–infant interactive behaviors between American Indian and African American mother–infant dyads. It is important for nurses who work with different ethnic groups to know the different interactive behaviors (Brooks et al, 2013).*

Client/Family Teaching and Discharge Planning

- ▲ Provide information or refer to community-based follow-up programs for preterm/at-risk infants and their families. EB: "*Working together, the care teams can help families build bridges from NICU to community*" (Purdy, Craig, & Zennah, 2015). CEB: *Request that parents ask the primary health care provider to implement*

Ages & Stages Questionnaires (ASQ) at regular follow-up visits to monitor developmental milestones (Bricker & Squires, 2009). **EB:** *Parents of late-term premature infants are recommended to have developmental monitoring for their babies (Tripathni & Dusing, 2015).*

- Educate parents on safe "back-to-sleep" practice before NICU discharge. **EB:** *Studies found educating parents before NICU discharge on safe-to-sleep practices improved parental compliance of supine positioning from 39% to 83% (Gelfer et al, 2013).*
- Educate and demonstrate to parents prior to NICU discharge a variety of development positions and handling that encourages free body movement, hand-to-mouth and eye–hand coordination, visual scanning, and auditory localizing, and to avoid overuse of infant swings/carriers/bouncy seats. **CEB:** *Support parent education using a variety of different positions during play that increase free movement and tummy time and engage promoting pleasurable parent–infant interaction (Waitzman, 2007).*

 Home Care

- NICU discharge is a vulnerable time for parents, and nurses have a key role in increasing parents' confidence by listening to fears, answering questions, and giving time to practice new skills before discharge. **EB:** *"To make parents confident and prepared for taking their infant home, giving tailored information, guidance and hands-on experience caring for their infant before discharge is crucial" (Aagaard et al, 2015).*
- Encourage parents to use home visitation whenever possible because it enhances neonatal progress and parental support. **EB:** *Home visitation is effective for education and support for infant and families after NICU discharge (Parker, Warmuskerken, & Sinclair, 2015).*
- Encourage families to teach extended family and support persons to recognize and respond appropriately to the infant's behavioral cues; supportive help may be most appreciated doing physical tasks. **CEB:** *A study found families need to feel comfortable with persons supporting them and need to communicate what support they needed (Als et al, 2005).*
- Provide education on positioning and handling that supports optimal infant growth and development. **EB:** *Encourage the importance of tummy time when awake and supervised (National Institute of Child Health and Development, 2017).* **CEB:** *Support developmental play activities (Waitzman, 2007).*
- Home visitors to need to recognize maternal depression resulting from the NICU experience. **EB:** *A study found maternal depression can have a negative effect on infant health and development (Laszewski et al, 2016). Infant mental health services should be infused with at-risk families struggling with a multitude of factors (Tomlin, Deloian, & Woolesen, 2016).* **EB:** *Home visitation by trained paraprofessionals and nurses is cost-effective and can benefit low-resource mothers by improving the language, behavior, and attention of their children (Olds et al, 2014).*
- Provide families with information about community resources, developmental follow-up services, parent-to-parent support programs, and request primary health care providers to follow developmental progress with parent friendly developmental questionnaires. **EB:** *The ASQ can detect severe developmental delay in preterm children regardless of maternal education. Researchers found that successful follow-up programs included mental health services (Tomlin, Veihweg, & Weatherston, 2016). The newly validated "Premature and Young Infant Development Assessment Tool (PYIDAT)" is designed for premature infants from 34 weeks' gestation to 5 months adjusted age, and is a validated tool that offers a comprehensive assessment of premature infants (DeWys et al, 2016).*

REFERENCES

Aagaard, H., Uhrenfeldt, L., Spliid, M., et al. (2015). Parents' experiences of transition when their infants are discharged from the Neonatal Intensive Care Unit: A systematic review protocol. *JBI Database of Systematic Reviews and Implementation Reports, 13*(10), 123–132. doi:10.11124/jbisrir-2015-2287.

Altimier, L., & Phillips, R. (2016). The neonatal integrative developmental care model: Advance clinical applications of the seven core measures for neuroprotective family-centered developmental care. *Newborn & Infant Nursing Reviews, 16*(4), 230–244.

Als, H., et al. (2005). The assessment of preterm infants' behavior (APIB): Furthering the understanding and measurement of neurodevelopmental competence in preterm and full-term infants. *Mental Retardation and Developmental Disabilities Research Reviews, 11*(1), 94–102.

Bailey, J., & Committee on Fetus and Newborn. (2015). Skin-to-skin care for term and preterm infants in the neonatal NICU. *Pediatrics, 136*, 596–599.

Bonan, K., Filho, J., Tristo, R. M., et al. (2014). Sleep deprivation, pain and prematurity: A review study. *Arquivos de Neuro-Psiquiatria, 73*(2), 147–154. doi:10.1590/0004-282X20140214.

Bricker, D., & Squires, J. (2009). Ages and Stages Questionnaire (ASQ-3). In *Parent completed child monitoring system*. Baltimore, MD: Paul Brookes Publishing.

Brooks, J. L., Holditch-Davis, D., & Landerman, L. R. (2013). Interactive behaviors of ethnic minority mothers and their premature infants. *Journal of Obstetric, Gynecologic, & Neonatal Nursing, 42*(3), 357–368.

● = Independent;   ▲ = Collaborative;   EBN = Evidence-Based Nursing;   EB = Evidence-Based

Brooks, J. L., Holditch-Davis, D., Sharron, L., et al. (2016). Birthing and parenting a premature infant in a cultural context. *Qualitative Health Research*, 26(3), 387–398.

DeWys, M., Mlynarczyk, S., Anderson, K., et al. (2016) *Reliability and validity of the Premature & Young Infant Assessment Tool (PYIDAT)*. Grand Valley State University, presentation, 40 Annual, Midwest Nursing Research Conference, Milwaukee, WI.

Filippa, M., Panza, C., Ferrari, F., et al. (2017). Systematic review of maternal voice interventions demonstrates increased stability in preterm infants. *Acta Paediatrica*, 106(8), 1220–1229. doi:10.1111/apa.13832.

Foster, J. P., Psaila, K., & Patterson, T. (2016). Non-nutritive sucking for increasing physiologic stability and nutrition in preterm infants. *The Cochrane Database of Systematic Reviews*, (10), CD001071.

Freeley, N., Genest, C., Niela-Vilen, H., et al. (2016). Parents and nurses balancing parent-closeness and separation: A qualitative study of NICU nurses'perseptions. *BMI Pediatric*, 16, 134. doi:10.1186/s12887-016-0663-1.

Gelfer, P., Cameron, R., Masters, K., et al. (2013). Integrating "Back to Sleep" recommendations into neonatal ICU practice. *Pediatrics*, 131(4), 1264–1270.

Hall, S. L., et al. (2017). The neonatal intensive parenting unit: An introduction. *Journal of Perinatology*, 37(12), 1259–1264. doi:10.1038/jp.2017.108.

Johnson, C., et al. (2017). Skin-to-skin care with newborns cuts down procedural pain. *Cochrane Database of Systematic Reviews, Neonatal Group* doi:10.1002/14651858.CD008435.pub3. Retrieved from http://neonatal.cochran.org.

Karbandi, S., Dehghanian, S. N., Pourarian, S., et al. (2015). The effect of breast milk odor on concentration percent of oxygen saturation and respiratory rate in premature infants. *Evidenced Based Care Journal*, 5(1), 25–34.

King, C., & Norton, D. (2017). *Does therapeutic positioning preterm infants impact upon optimal health outcomes? A literature review*, Retrieved from https://doi.org/10.1016/jnn.2017.03.004.

Laszewski, A., Wichman, C. L., Doering, J. J., et al. (2016). Perinatal dealgorithm: A home visitor step-by-step guide for advanced management of perinatal depression symptoms. *Zero to Three*, 36, 2–9.

Liu, L., Huang, X., Luo, B., et al. (2017). Effects of combined oral sucrose and nonnutritive sucking (NNS) on procedural pain of NICU newborns, 2001 to 2016. *Medicine*, 96(6), e6108.

Ludington-Hoe, S. M. (2013). Kangaroo care as neonatal therapy. *Newborn and Infant Nursing Reviews*, 3(2), 73–75.

National Institute of Child Health and Human Development. (2017). Retrieved from www.nichd.nih.gov/sts/pages/tummytime.aspx. Also in Spanish.

National Institutes of Health, US National Library of Medicine. (2017). *Even partial breast-feeding for first few months lowers SIDS risk*. Retrieved from https://medlineplus.gov.

Novotney, A. (2013). Music as medicine. *American Psychological Association*, 44(10), 46.

Olds, D. L., et al. (2014). Effects of home visits by paraprofessionals and by nurses on children: Follow-up a randomized trial at ages 6 and 9 years. *JAMA Pediatrics*, 168(2), 114–121.

Parker, C., Warmuskerken, G., & Sinclair, L. (2015). Enhancing neonatal wellness with home visitation. *Nurs Womens Health*, 19, 37–41.

Pease, A. C., et al. (2016). Swaddling and the risk of sudden death: Meta-analysis. *Pediatrics, AAP News & Journals, Gateway*.

Purdy, I. B., Craig, J. W., & Zennah, P. (2015). NICU discharge planning and beyond: Recommendations for parent psychosocial support. *J Perinatology*, 35, 24–28.

Reeves-Messner, T., & Spilker, A. (2017). Shh…Babies growing: A clinical practice guideline for reducing noise level in the neonatal intensive care unit. *Journal of Neonatal Nursing*, 23(4), 199–203.

Sidor, A., Fischer, C., Eickhorst, A., et al. (2013). Influence of early regulatory in infants on their development at 12 months: A longitudinal study in a high-risk sample. *Child and Adolescent Psychiatry and Mental Health*. Retrieved from https://doi.org/10.1186/1753-2000-7-35.

Spilker, A., Hill, C., & Rosenblum, R. (2016). The effectiveness of a standardized positioning tool and bedside education on the developmental positioning proficiency of NICU nurses. In *Intensive and critical care nursing* (Vol. 35, pp. 10–15). St Louis: Elsevier.

Stefana, A., & Manuela, L., (2017). Parental engagement and early interactions with preterm infants during the stay in the neonatal intensive care unit: Protocol of a mixed-method and longitudinal study. doi:10.1136/bmjopen-2016-013824.

Tomlin, A. M., Deloian, B., & Wollesen, L., (2016) *Infant/early childhood mental health and collaborative partnerships beyond the NICU*. Retrieved from http://dxdoi/10.1053/j.nainr.2016.09.025.309-315.

Tomlin, A. M., Viehweg, S. A., & Weatherston, D. (2016) *Tackling the Tough Stuff: a home visitor's Guide to Supporting Families at Risk*. Brooks Baltimore.

Tripathni, T., & Dusing, S. (2015). Long term neuro neurodevelopmental outcomes of infants born late preterm: A systematic review. *Res Rep Neurology*, 5, 91–111.

Waitzman, K. A. (2007). The importance of the near-term infant for sleep, play, and development. *Newborn & Nursing Reviewers*, 7(2), 76–81.

Wigert, H., & Bry, K. (2017). Dealing with parents'existential issues in neonatal intensive care. *J. of Neonatal Nursing*. Retrieved from http://doi.org/10.1016/jnn.2017.09.002.

Wyngarden, K., DeWys, M., & Padnos, P. (1999). *Learnings from the field: The impact of using two new nursing diagnoses, organized infant behavior and disorganized infant behavior [abstract]*. Classification of Nursing Diagnoses: Proceedings of the Thirteenth Conference, NANDA.

I

Readiness for enhanced organized Infant behavior   *Gail B. Ladwig, MSN, RN*

NANDA-I

Definition

An integrated pattern of modulation of the physiological and neurobehavioral systems of functioning, which can be strengthened.

Defining Characteristics

Parent expresses desire to enhance cue recognition; parent expresses desire to enhance environmental conditions; parent expresses desire to enhance recognition of infant's self-regulatory behaviors

● = Independent;   ▲ = Collaborative;   EBN = Evidence-Based Nursing;   EB = Evidence-Based

NOC, NIC, Client Outcomes, Nursing Interventions and *Rationales,* Client/Family Teaching and Discharge Planning and References

Refer to care plans for Disorganized **Infant** behavior and Risk for disorganized **Infant** behavior.

Risk for disorganized Infant behavior   *Gail B. Ladwig, MSN, RN*

NANDA-I

Definition

Susceptible to disintegration in the pattern of modulation of the physiological and neurobehavioral systems of functioning, which may compromise health.

Risk Factors

Caregiver cue misreading; environmental overstimulation; feeding intolerance; inadequate physical environment; infant malnutrition; insufficient caregiver knowledge of behavioral cues; insufficient containment within environment; insufficient environmental sensory stimulation; pain; sensory deprivation; sensory overstimulation

At-Risk Population

Low postconceptual age; prematurity; prenatal exposure to teratogen

Associated Condition

Congenital disorder; genetic disorder; infant illness; immature neurological functioning; impaired infant motor functioning; invasive procedure; infant oral impairment

NOC, NIC, Client Outcomes, Nursing Interventions and *Rationales,* Client/Family Teaching and Discharge Planning, and References

Refer to Disorganized **Infant** behavior.

Risk for Infection   *Ruth M. Curchoe, RN, BSN, MSN, CIC*

NANDA-I

Definition

Susceptible to invasion and multiplication of pathogenic organisms, which may compromise health.

Risk Factors

Alteration in peristalsis; alteration in skin integrity; inadequate vaccination; insufficient knowledge to avoid exposure to pathogens; malnutrition; obesity; smoking; stasis of body fluid

At-Risk Population

Exposure to disease outbreak

Associated Condition

Alteration in pH of secretion; chronic illness; decrease in ciliary action; decrease in hemoglobin; immunosuppression; invasive procedure; leukopenia; premature rupture of amniotic membrane; prolonged rupture of amniotic membrane; suppressed inflammatory response

NOC   (Nursing Outcomes Classification)

Suggested NOC Outcomes

Risk Control: Infectious Process; Immune Status

• = Independent;   ▲ = Collaborative;   EBN = Evidence-Based Nursing;   EB = Evidence-Based

Client Outcomes

Client Will (Specify Time Frame)

- Remain free from symptoms of infection during contact with health care providers
- State symptoms of infection before initiating a health care–related procedure
- Demonstrate appropriate care of infection-prone sites within 48 hours of instruction
- Maintain white blood cell count and differential within normal limits within 48 hours of treatment initiation
- Demonstrate appropriate hygienic measures such as handwashing, oral care, and perineal care within 24 hours of instruction

NIC (Nursing Interventions Classification)

Suggested NIC Interventions

Immunization/Vaccination Management; Infection Control; Infection Protection

Nursing Interventions and *Rationales*

- Implement targeted surveillance for methicillin-resistant *Staphylococcus aureus* (MRSA) (screen clients at risk for MRSA on admission) and other multidrug-resistant organisms (MDROs). **EB:** *Universal screening for MRSA increased screenings and costs but resulted in few additional cases being detected. Where MRSA is endemic, targeted screening remains the most efficient strategy for early identification of MRSA-positive clients (National Strategy for Combating Antibiotic-Resistant Bacteria, 2014).*
- Obtain a travel history from clients presenting to the health care site (e.g., emergency department, clinic). **EB:** *Outbreaks, such as Ebola and avian flu identified in foreign countries, often present with fever and flu-like symptoms (Centers for Disease Control and Prevention [CDC], 2014a).*
- Observe and report as redness, warmth, discharge, and increased body temperature. **CEB:** *Change in mental status, fever, shaking, chills, and hypotension are indicators of sepsis (Perry, Potter, & Ostendurr, 2014).*
- Assess temperature of neutropenic clients; report a single temperature of greater than 100.5°F. **CEB:** *Fever is often the first sign of an infection (National Guideline Clearing House [NGC], 2015; Klastersky et al, 2016).* **CEBN:** *The immunocompromised host may present with a very different clinical picture compared with an immunocompetent host. The progress of the infection may be more rapid, and the infection may quickly become life-threatening; repeat temperature measurement if significant changes occur and report temperature changes from baseline (EB Medicine, 2013).*
- Oral, rectal, tympanic, temporal artery, or axillary thermometers may be used to assess temperature in adults and infants. **EBN:** *The use of axillary in addition to oral, tympanic, and temporal artery temperature measurement is supported (Bland, Conner, & Messenger, 2017) Rectal and oral temperature measurements are more accurate than other methods of temperature measurement, such as temporal or axillary measurement (Bland, Conner, and Messenger, 2017).*
- ▲ Note and report laboratory values (e.g., white blood cell count and differential, serum protein, serum albumin, cultures). **EBN:** *Although the white blood cell count may be in the normal range, an increased number of immature bands may be present (Versalovic et al, 2011).* **CEBN:** *A neutropenic client with fever represents an absolute medical emergency (EB Medicine, 2013).*
- Assess skin for color, moisture, texture, and turgor (elasticity). Keep accurate, ongoing documentation of changes. **EB:** *A number of instruments have been developed to assess for risk of pressure ulcers, including the*

● = Independent;   ▲ = Collaborative;   EBN = Evidence-Based Nursing;   EB = Evidence-Based

Braden, Norton, and Waterlow scales. All three scales include items related to activity mobility, nutritional status, incontinence, and cognition (Balzar & Kottner, 2015; Goldberg, 2015).

- Carefully wash and pat dry skin, including skinfold areas. Use hydration and moisturization on all at-risk surfaces. EBN: *Moisturizers result in an increase of skin hydration and restoration of the skin barrier function and play a prominent role in the long-term management of atopic dermatitis (Healthbeat, 2016).* EB: *Application of moisturizers containing humectants is clearly effective in enhancing skin barrier function (Kottner, Lichterfelo, & Blume-Peytavi, 2013).*
- Refer to care plan for Risk for impaired **Skin** integrity.
- ▲ Monitor client's vitamin D level. EB: *Vitamin D deficiency has been correlated with increased risk and greater severity of infection, particularly of the respiratory tract. Vitamin D influences the body's immune system by influencing the production of endogenous antimicrobial peptides and regulating the inflammatory cascade (Dankers et al, 2016).*
- Refer to care plan Readiness for enhanced **Nutrition** for additional interventions.
- Use strategies to prevent health care–acquired pneumonia, assess lung sounds and sputum color and characteristics, provide daily oral care with chlorhexidine, use sterile technique when suctioning, suction secretions above tracheal tube before suctioning, drain accumulated condensation in ventilator tubing into a fluid trap or other collection device before repositioning the client, assess patency and placement of nasogastric tubes, and elevate the client's head to 30 degrees or higher to prevent gastric reflux of organisms in the lung (Peyrani, 2014). EB: *Hospital mortality of ventilated clients who develop ventilator-associated pneumonia (VAP) is 46% compared with 32% of those ventilated clients without VAP. VAP also adds an estimated cost of $40,000 to a typical hospital admission (CDC, 2005, updated 2014).*
- Encourage fluid intake. EB: *Fluid intake helps thin secretions and replace fluid lost during fever (Ackley & Ladwig, 2014; Mayo Clinic Staff, 2016).*
- Use appropriate hand hygiene (i.e., handwashing or use of alcohol-based hand rubs). EBN: *Meticulous infection prevention precautions are required to prevent health care–associated infection, with particular attention to hand hygiene and standard precautions (CDC, 2011a).* EB: *Handwashing is currently the recommended strategy for reducing transmission of* Clostridium difficile. *Alcohol gels do not inactivate C. difficile spores (World Health Organization [WHO], 2009; Edmonds et al, 2013).*
- When using an alcohol-based hand rub, apply an ample amount of product to the palm of one hand and rub hands together, covering all surfaces of hands and fingers, until hands are dry. Note that the volume needed to reduce the number of bacteria on hands varies by product. EBN: *Adequate hand antisepsis reduces infection rates. The use of alcohol-based hand rubs is particularly effective; in contrast to handwashing, hand rubs kill susceptible bacteria more rapidly and to a greater extent, and are less time-consuming. Also, skin health is better preserved when moisturizers are added (Hass, 2014).*
- Follow standard precautions and wear gloves during any contact with blood, mucous membranes, nonintact skin, or any body substance except sweat. Use goggles and gowns when appropriate. Standard precautions apply to all clients. You must assume all clients are carrying blood-borne pathogens (CDC, 2007). EBN: *Hands of health care workers are the most common cause of health care–associated infections (Hass, 2014).*
- Implement respiratory hygiene/cough etiquette. CEB: *Providing control measures (tissues and masks) and accessibility to hand hygiene materials reduces risks of transmission of respiratory illness (CDC, 2007).*
- Follow transmission-based precautions for airborne-, droplet-, and contact-transmitted microorganisms:
  - **Airborne:** Isolate the client in a room with monitored negative air pressure, with the room door closed and the client remaining in the room. Always wear appropriate respiratory protection when you enter the room. Limit the movement and transport of the client from the room to essential purposes only. Have the client wear a surgical mask during transport.
  - **Droplet:** Keep the client in a private room, if possible. If not possible, maintain a spatial separation of 3 feet from other beds or visitors. The door may remain open. Wear a surgical mask when you must come within 3 feet of the client. Some hospitals may choose to implement a mask requirement for droplet precautions for anyone entering the room. Limit transport to essential purposes and have the client wear a mask, if possible.
  - **Contact:** Place the client in a private room, if possible, or with someone (cohorting) who has an active infection from the same microorganism. Wear clean, nonsterile gloves when entering the room. When providing care, change gloves after contact with any infective material such as wound drainage. Remove the gloves and clean your hands before leaving the room and take care not to touch any potentially infectious items or surfaces on the way out. Wear a gown if you anticipate your clothing may have

● = Independent;   ▲ = Collaborative;   EBN = Evidence-Based Nursing;   EB = Evidence-Based

substantial contact with the client or other potentially infectious items. Remove the gown before leaving the room. Limit transport of the client to essential purposes and take care that the client does not contact other environmental surfaces along the way. Dedicate the use of noncritical client care equipment to a single client. **CEB:** *If use of common equipment is unavoidable, adequately clean and disinfect equipment before use with other clients (CDC, 2007).*

▲ Use alternatives to indwelling catheters whenever possible (external catheters, incontinence pads, and bladder control techniques). **EB:** *It is estimated that catheter-associated urinary tract infections (CAUTIs) increase length of stay by 0.5 to 1 day and increase costs between $1200 and $4700 (2009 dollars) (Brusch et al, 2015).*

● If a urinary catheter is necessary, follow catheter management practices. All indwelling catheters should be connected to a sterile, closed drainage system (i.e., not broken), except for good clinical reasons. Cleanse the perineum and meatus twice daily using soap and water. **EBN:** *A nurse-driven protocol achieved a 27.7% reduction in the use of catheters (mean dwell time was 3.46 days) and a CAUTI rate of 0.35% (Mori, 2014).* **EB:** *Significant rates of inappropriate urinary catheter use underscore the importance of establishing guidelines and implementing policy for appropriate use of urinary catheters (Agency for Healthcare Quality and Research [AHRQ], 2015).*

● Use evidence-based practices and educate personnel in care of peripheral catheters: use aseptic technique for insertion and care, label insertion sites and all tubing with date and time of insertion, inspect every 8 hours for signs of infection, record, and report. **EB:** *Use of chlorhexidine gluconate for vascular catheter site care reduces catheter-related bloodstream infections and catheter colonization (CDC, 2011b).*

● Use sterile technique wherever there is a loss of skin integrity. **EBN:** *Skin and soft tissue infections arise when skin integrity is broken by treatments associated with trauma, surgery, burns, and so forth (Apisarnthanara & Mundy, 2014).*

● Ensure the client's appropriate hygienic care with handwashing; bathing; oral care; and hair, nail, and perineal care performed by either the nurse or the client. **CEBN:** *Daily showers or baths can help to reduce the number of bacteria on the client's skin. The oral cavity is a common site for infection (Perry, Potter, & Ostendurr, 2014).*

● Recommend responsible use of antibiotics; use antibiotics sparingly. **EB:** *Use and misuse of antibiotics diminishes their therapeutic benefit and facilitates the development of MDROs and C. difficile-associated disease, and increases health care costs. Antibiotic stewardship is essential in reducing current and future resistance in bacteria (CDC, 2017).* **EB:** *The rate of damage to the fallopian tubes increases with subsequent pelvic inflammatory disease episodes, from 34% for the first episode to 54% in women with second and third episodes (Puscheck, Scott-Lucidi, & Woodard, 2013).*

Pediatric

Note: Many of the preceding interventions are appropriate for the pediatric client.

● Follow meticulous hand hygiene when working with children. **EB:** *Keep nails short; prohibit false fingernails, and limit wearing jewelry because it interferes with effective hand hygiene (AAPeds, 2016). Parents recognize the importance of hand hygiene, but in a study only 67% would definitely remind health care workers of its importance (Buser et al, 2012; James, Nelson, & Ashwill, 2014).*

● Cluster nursing procedures to decrease number of contacts with infants, allowing time for appropriate hand hygiene. **EBN:** *Audit programs to track compliance with hand hygiene identified a drop in the incidence of health care–associated infections in very low-birth-weight infants in the neonatal intensive care unit (Mendicino, Morrell, & Hernandez, 2014).*

● Avoid the prophylactic use of topical cream in premature infants. **CEB:** *Prophylactic application of topical ointment increases the risk of coagulase-negative staphylococcal infection and any health care–acquired infection. A trend toward increased risk of any bacterial infection was noted in infants treated prophylactically (Ackley & Ladwig, 2014).*

● Encourage early enteral feeding with human milk. *Human milk enhances immune defenses of the infant (Praveen et al, 2015).*

▲ Monitor recurrent antibiotic use in children.

● Instruct parents on appropriate indicators for medical visits and the risks associated with overuse of antibiotics. **EB:** *Guidelines addressing treatment of asthma in children state that antibiotics should not be used as part of chronic asthma therapy or for acute exacerbations, with the exception of clients with comorbid bacterial infections such as pneumonia or sinusitis (Leung, Szefler, & Akdis, 2015).*

● = Independent;   ▲ = Collaborative;   **EBN** = Evidence-Based Nursing;   **EB** = Evidence-Based

I

Geriatric

▲ Suspect pneumonia when the client has symptoms of lethargy or confusion. Assess response to treatment, especially antibiotic therapy. EB: *Leading causes of illness and death among older adults are both community and health care–associated respiratory infections. In long-term care facilities, the risk for pneumonia ranges from 0.3 to 2.5 events per 1000 resident-days (Montoya & Moody, 2011).*

● Most clients develop health care–associated pneumonia (HCAP) by either aspirating contaminated substances or inhaling airborne particles. Refer to care plan for Risk for **Aspiration.**

▲ *Carefully screen older women with incontinence for urinary tract infections.* CEB: *Consider alternatives to chronic indwelling catheters, such as intermittent catheterization. CAUTI has been associated with increased morbidity, mortality, hospital cost, and length of stay (CDC, 2009).*

● Observe and report if the client has a low-grade fever or new onset of confusion. EB: *Those caring for older clients must be alerted to the potential presence of infection when even low-grade temperature elevations appear for short periods (Arinzon et al, 2012).*

● Recommend that the geriatric client receive an annual influenza immunization and one-time pneumococcal vaccine. EB: *Immunization against influenza is an effective intervention that reduces serologically confirmed cases (CDC, 2014b,c).*

● Recognize that chronically ill geriatric clients have an increased susceptibility to *C. difficile* infection; practice meticulous hand hygiene and monitor antibiotic response to antibiotics. EB: *The incidence of* C. difficile *illness (CDI) is increasing with the greatest impact in persons older than 65 years. More than 90% of deaths from CDI have occurred in this population (CDC, 2012; Kelly & LaMont, 2013; CDC, 2017).*

Home Care

● Adapt the previously mentioned interventions for home care as needed.

● Assess and treat wounds in the home. EBN: *Promotion of wound healing is a nursing priority. Specific wound care regimens administered depend on the type, size, and location of the wound and overall treatment goals (Colwell, 2013).*

● Review standards for surveillance of infections in home care. EB: *Challenges to surveillance in the home care setting include loss of clients to follow-up, lack of laboratory data, and difficulty in obtaining accurate numerator and denominator data (Yeung, 2014).*

● Maintain infection-prevention policies. EBN: *The complexity of clients' conditions is frequently high because the incidence of chronic disease and MDROs is increasing (Yeung, 2014).*

● Refer for nutritional evaluation; implement dietary changes to support recovery and maintain health. EB: *Medical nutrition therapy (MNT) is important in preventing diabetes; managing existing diabetes; and preventing, or at least slowing, the rate of development of diabetes complications. Therefore it is important at all levels of diabetes prevention. MNT is also an integral component of diabetes self-management education (or training) Administration on Aging [AOA], 2012).*

Client/Family Teaching and Discharge Planning

● Teach the client risk factors contributing to surgical wound infection. EB: *The risk of infection is influenced by characteristics of the client such as age, obesity, and nutritional status (Murphy, 2014).*

● Teach the client and family the importance of hand hygiene in preventing postoperative infections. EB: *Two-thirds of wound infections occur after discharge. Using good hand hygiene practices is effective for preventing these infections (CDC, 2011a).*

▲ Encourage high-risk persons, including health care workers, to get vaccinated (CDC, 2011c).

▲ Influenza: Teach symptoms of influenza and the importance of vaccination for influenza. EB: *Everyone 6 months of age and older should get the flu vaccine. Seasonal flu vaccine is effective and has a very good safety track record (CDC, 2014b,c).* Teach the client and family how to take a temperature. Encourage the family to take the client's temperature between 4 p.m. and 10 p.m. at least once daily. CEBN: *The lowest body temperature usually occurs between 4 a.m. and 5 a.m., with highest readings recorded between 4 p.m. and 8 p.m. (Peate & Wild, 2012).*

REFERENCES

AAPeds, et al. (2016). Infection control. In L. E. Riley & A. R. Stark (Eds.), *Guidelines for perinatal care*. Elk Grove Village, IL: American Academy of Pediatrics.

Ackley, B. J., & Ladwig, G. B., (2014). *Nursing diagnosis handbook*. (10th ed.). Retrieved from http://evolve.elsevier.com.

Administration on Aging (AOA). (2012). *A profile of older Americans*. Retrieved from www.aoa.gov/AoARoot/Aging_Statistics/Profile/2012/3.aspx.

Agency for Healthcare Quality and Research (AHRQ). (2015). *Toolkit for reducing catheter-associated urinary tract infections in hospital units: implementation guide. Appendix M*.

Apisaranthanara, A., & Mundy, L. (2014). Skin and soft tissue infections. In *APIC test of infection control and epidemiology* (4th ed.). Washington, DC: Association for Professionals in Infection Control and Epidemiology. (Accessed 20 August 2017; last revised 6 June 2014).

Arinzon, Z., Shabat, S., Peisakh, A., et al. (2012). Clinical presentation of urinary tract infection (UTI) differs with aging women. *Archives of Gerontology and Geriatrics*, 55(1), 145–147.

Bland, W., Conner, H. M., & Messenger, D. (2017). *Fever temperatures: accuracy and comparison*. Retrieved from https://www.ghc.org. (Accessed 22 August 2017).

Brusch, J. L., Bronze, M. S., et al. (2015). Catheter-related urinary tract infection. *Medscape*, 18, 2015.

Buser, G. L., Fisher, B. T., Shea, J. A., et al. (2012). Parent willingness to remind health care workers to perform hand hygiene. *American Journal of Infection Control*, 41(6), 492–496.

Centers for Disease Control and Prevention (CDC). (2005, updated 2014). *Guideline for the management of adults with health care acquired ventilator associated pneumonia*. Retrieved from http://cdc.gov/hicpac/pdf (Accessed 2 October 2017).

Centers for Disease Control and Prevention (CDC). (2007). *Healthcare Infection Control Practices Advisory Committee: guideline for isolation precautions: preventing transmission of infectious agents in healthcare settings*. Retrieved from http://www.cdc.gov/ncidad/dh9p/pdf/guidelines/isolation2007.pdf. (updated 2014, (Accessed 6 September 2017).

Centers for Disease Control and Prevention (CDC). (2009). *Healthcare Infection Control Practices Advisory Committee: guideline for prevention of catheter-associated urinary tract infections*. Retrieved from http://www.cdc.gov/hicpac/pdf/CAUTI/CAUTIguideline2009final.pdf. (Accessed 8 August 2014).

Centers for Disease Control and Prevention (CDC). (2011a). Guideline for hand hygiene in health-care settings. Recommendations of the Healthcare Infection Control Practices Advisory Committee and the HICPAC/SHEA/APIC/IDSA Hand Hygiene Task Force. *MMWR. Recommendations and Reports: Morbidity and Mortality Weekly Report. Recommendations and Reports*, 51(RR–16), 1–45. Retrieved from http://www.cdc.gov/handhygiene/Guidelines.html. (Accessed 14 August 2017; updated 2014).

Centers for Disease Control and Prevention (CDC). (2011b). *Guideline for the prevention of intravascular catheter related infections*. Retrieved from http://www.cdc.gov/hicpac. (Accessed 5 August 2017).

Centers for Disease Control and Prevention (CDC). (2011c). Prevention and control of influenza: recommendations of the Advisory Committee on Immunization Practices (ACIP). *MMWR. Morbidity and Mortality Weekly Report, Recommendations and Reports*, 60(33), 1128–1132.

Centers for Disease Control and Prevention (CDC). (2012). Vital signs: preventing *Clostridium difficile* infections. *MMWR. Morbidity and Mortality Weekly Report*, 61(9), 157–162.

Centers for Disease Control and Prevention (CDC). (2014a). *Ebola (Ebola Virus Disease), Interim Guidance for Monitoring and Movement of Person with Ebola Virus Disease Exposure*. Retrieved from http://www.cdc.gov/vhf/ebola/hcp/monitoring-and-movement-of-persons-with-exposure.html. (Accessed 15 August 2017).

Centers for Disease Control and Prevention (CDC). (2014b). *Preventing seasonal flu with vaccination*. Retrieved from www.CDC.gov/flu/protect/vaccine. (Accessed 12 August 2014).

Centers for Disease Control and Prevention (CDC). (2014c). *Vaccine information statement (VIS): Influenza*.

Centers for Disease Control and Prevention (CDC). (2017). *Core elements of hospital antibiotic stewardship programs. CDC/IHI* antibiotic stewardship drivers and change package.

Colwell, J. (2013). Skin integrity and wound care. In *Potter, Perry fundamentals of nursing* (8th ed.). St. Louis: Elsevier.

Dankers, W., Colin, E. M., van Hamburg, J. P., et al. (2016). Vitamin D in autoimmunity: Molecular mechanisms and therapeutic potential. *Frontiers in Immunology*, 7, 697.

EB Medicine. (2013). *Oncologic emergencies*. Retrieved from https://www.ebmedicine.net. (Accessed 17 August 2017).

Edmonds, S. L., Zapka, C., Kaspar, D., et al. (2013). Effectiveness of hand hygiene for removal of *Clostridium difficile* spores from hands. *Infection Control and Hospital Epidemiology*, 34, 302–306.

Goldberg, M. (2015). *Preventive skin care guideline. National Pressure Ulcer Advisory Panel.(NPUAP)* Retrieved from https://www.npuap.org. (Accessed 23 August 2017).

Hass, J. (2014). Hand hygiene. In *APIC test of infection control and epidemiology* (4th ed.). Washington, DC: Association for Professionals in Infection Control and Epidemiology. (Accessed 4 September 2017; last revised 6 June 2014).

Healthbeat. (2016). *How to moisturize your skin. Harvard Health Publications*. Retrieved from https://www.harvardhealth.com. (Accessed 21 September 2017).

James, S. R., Nelson, K., & Ashwill, J. (2014). *Nursing care of children. E Book: principles and practices* (4th ed.). Retrieved from https://www.amazon.com. (Accessed 12 September 2017).

Kelly, C. P., & LaMont, J. T. (2013). *Clostridium difficile* in adults: treatment. *UpToDate*. Retrieved from: http://www.update.com/contents/clostridium-difficile-in-adults-treatment.

Klastersky, J., deNaurois, K., et al. (2016). Management of febrile neutropenia: ESMO clinical practice guidelines. *Annals of Oncology: Official Journal of the European Society for Medical Oncology / ESMO*, 27(Suppl. 5), V111–V118.

Kottner, J., Lichterfelo, A., & Blume-Peytavi, U. (2013). Maintaining skin integrity in the aged. *The British Journalof Dermatology*, 169(3), 528–542.

Leung, D. Y., Szefler, S., & Akdis, C., (2015) *Pediatric allergy: Principles and practices* (p. 283). Retrieved from https://books.google.com.

Mayo Clinic Staff. (2016). *Dehydration: self management*. Retrieved from www.mayoclinic.org/diseases-conditions/dehydration/manage/ptc-202.6/161. (Accessed 2 October 2017).

Mendicino, N., Morrell, G., & Hernandez, S. L. (2014). Neonates. In *APIC test of infection control and epidemiology* (4th ed.). Washington, DC: Association for Professionals in Infection Control and Epidemiology. (Accessed 28 September 2017; last revised 6 June 2014).

Montoya, A., & Moody, L. (2011). Common infections in nursing homes: A review of current issues and challenges. *Aging Health*, 7(6), 689–699.

Mori, C. (2014). A-voiding catastrophe: implementing a nurse-driven protocol. *Medsurg Nursing*, 23(1), 15–21.

Murphy, R. (2014). Surgical services. In *APIC test of infection control and epidemiology* (4th ed.). Washington, DC: Association for Professionals in Infection Control and Epidemiology. (Accessed 21 September 2017; last revised 6 June 2014).

I

● = Independent;   ▲ = Collaborative;   **EBN** = Evidence-Based Nursing;   **EB** = Evidence-Based

National Guideline Clearing House (NGC). (2015). *Approach to fever assessment in ambulatory cancer patients receiving chemotherapy.* Rockville, MD: Agency for Healthcare Research and Quality (AHRQ). Retrieved from https://www.guideline.gov. (Accessed 17 August 2017).

National strategy for combating antibiotic resistant bacteria. (2014). Retrieved from https://www.cdc.gov/drugresistance/pdf/carb_national_strategy.pdf. (Accessed 3 September 2017).

Peate, I., & Wild, K. (2012). Clinical observations 1/6: assessing body temperature. *British Journal of Healthcare Assistants, 6*(5), 215–219.

Perry, A., Potter, P., & Ostendurr, W. (2014). Measuring body temperature. In *Clinical nursing skills and techniques* (9th ed.). Retrieved from https://www.elsevier.com. (Accessed 21 August 2017).

Peyrani, P. (2014). Pneumonia. In *APIC test of infection control and epidemiology* (4th ed.). Washington, DC: Association for Professionals in Infection Control and Epidemiology. (Accessed 14 September 2017; last revised 6 June 2014).

Praveen, P., Jordon, F., Priami, C., et al., (2015) *The role of breast-feeding in infant immune system: a systems perspective on the intestinal microbiome.* Retrieved from https://www.doi.org. (Accessed 2 October 2017).

Puscheck, E. E., Scott-Lucidi, R., & Woodard, T. L. (2013). *Infertility, 013.* Retrieved from www.emedicine.medscape.com. (Accessed 5 September 2017).

World Health Organization (WHO). (2009) Guide to appropriate hand hygiene in connection with clostridium difficile spread. WHO Appendix 2. Retrieved from https://www.ncbi..nim.nih.gov. (Accessed 3 September 2017).

Versalovic, J., Carroll, K. C., Funke, G., et al. (2011). *Manual of clinical microbiology* (10th ed.). VI. Washington, DC: ASM Press.

Yeung, C. (2014). Home care. In *APIC test of infection control and epidemiology* (4th ed.). Washington, DC: Association for Professionals in Infection Control and Epidemiology. (Accessed 22 September 2017; last revised 6 June 2014).

Risk for surgical site Infection   *Teri Hulett, RN, BSN, CIC, FAPIC*

NANDA-I

Definition

Susceptible to invasion of pathogenic organisms at surgical site, which may compromise health.

Risk Factors

Alcoholism, Obesity, Smoking

At-Risk Population

Cold temperature of operating room; excessive number of personnel present during the surgical procedure; increased environmental exposure to pathogens; sub-optimal American Society of Anesthesiologists (ASA) physical health status score; surgical wound contamination

Associated Condition

Comorbidity; Diabetes mellitus; duration of surgery; hypertension; immunosuppression; inadequate antibiotic prophylaxis; ineffective antibiotic prophylaxis; infections at other surgical sites; invasive procedure; post-traumatic osteoarthritis; Rheumatoid arthritis; type of anesthesia; type of surgical procedure; use of implants and/or prostheses

NOC   (Nursing Outcomes Classification)

Suggested NOC Outcomes

Risk Control: Infectious Process, Immune Status

Example NOC Outcome with Indicators
Risk Control: Infectious Process. Personal actions to understand, prevent, eliminate, or reduce the threat of acquiring an infection as evidenced by client demonstrating the following indicators: Identifies risk factors for infection/Acknowledges personal risk factors for infection/Acknowledges behaviors associated with risk for infection/Monitors personal behaviors for factors associated with infection/Maintains a clean environment/Practices hand sanitization. (Rate the outcome and indicators of **Risk Control: Infectious Process:** I = never demonstrated, 2 = rarely demonstrated, 3 = sometimes demonstrated, 4 = often demonstrated, 5 = consistently demonstrated [see Section I].)

● = Independent;   ▲ = Collaborative;   EBN = Evidence-Based Nursing;   EB = Evidence-Based

Client Outcomes

Client Will (Specify Time Frame)

- Remain free from symptoms of surgical site infections (SSIs)
- Identify personal risk factors associated with increased SSI risk
- Modify personal behaviors that increase SSI risk
- Demonstrate appropriate hygienic practices to reduce infection risk such as handwashing

NIC   (Nursing Interventions Classification)

Infection Control, Infection Control: Intraoperative, Infection Protection, Teaching: Individual, Preoperative

Example NIC—Risk for Surgical Site Infection

Verify that prophylactic antibiotics have been ordered and administered as appropriate; Monitor and maintain client normothermia (temperature of 35.5°C [95.9°F] or above) during the perioperative period

Nursing Interventions and *Rationales*

- ▲ The number of surgical procedures performed in the United States continues to rise, and surgical clients often have comorbidities that increase the complexity. It is estimated that approximately half of SSIs are deemed preventable using evidence-based strategies (World Health Organization [WHO], 2017). SSIs are a complication of surgical care and are associated with significant morbidity, mortality, and cost (Preas, O'Hara, & Thom, 2017).
- ▲ Optimizing the client's medical condition prior to surgery and eliminating or even diminishing modifiable risk factors for infection can lower the risk of SSIs (Hutzler & Williams, 2017). EB: *Modifiable risk factors include current or history of orthopedic infection, rheumatoid arthritis, poor oral health, urinary tract infection, obesity, methicillin-resistant* Staphylococcus aureus *(MRSA), preoperative and anticipated postoperative anemia, smoking, malnutrition, diabetes, and HIV (Hutzler & Williams, 2017).* The American College of Surgeons (ACS) identifies additional modifiable risk factors as poor glycemic control and diabetic status, dyspnea, alcohol and smoking history, preoperative albumin level (<3.5 mg/dL), total bilirubin >1.0 mg/dL, obesity, and immunosuppression (Ban et al, 2016).
- ▲ SSI prevention, known as surgical care bundles, are evidence-based interventions that when implemented together can reduce the risk of infection. There are different surgical care bundles for specific high-risk surgical procedures, for example, colorectal surgery bundle, pediatric spinal surgery bundle, total joint arthroplasty surgery bundle, and cardiothoracic surgery bundle. EB: *Aspects of each surgical care bundle that are universal for all surgical procedures include: prehospital preoperative bathing, smoking cessation, and glucose control. Hospital-focused bundle interventions include perioperative blood glucose monitoring, surgical site hair-removal technique, surgical site skin preparation, surgical hand scrub, antibiotic prophylaxis, intraoperative normothermia, and supplemental oxygen delivery for patients undergoing general anesthesia (intubated patients) (Ban et al, 2016).*
- ▲ SSIs can occur because of either client-related (endogenous) or procedure-related (exogenous) risk factors. Risk factors are further stratified into preoperative, intraoperative, and postoperative risk.
- • Endogenous client-related risk factors: EBN: *Review client history with client prior to surgical procedure to identify modifiable risk factors that can be addressed preoperatively (Smith & Dahlen, 2013).*

Compromised Host Defenses

- • Age: Extremes of ages and advanced age increase client risk. EB: *Relationship to increased risk of SSI may be secondary to comorbidities or immunosenescence associated with age (Smith & Dahlen, 2013; Singh, Singla, & Chaudhary, 2014).*
- • Wound: A wound classification scoring system is used to identify the degree of surgical site skin integrity at the time of surgery. Assess and document skin integrity during the preoperative period to identify classification of surgical site. EB: The Centers for Disease Control and Prevention (CDC) recommends assessing surgical wounds and determining the probability of SSI by using a classification that consists of four types of surgical wounds: clean (sterile body site), clean-contaminated, contaminated, and dirty (heavily contaminated site) wounds (Smith & Dahlen, 2013). EB: The method of wound classification has been adopted by the ACS and has been effectively used for more than 40 years to stratify the client's

• = Independent;   ▲ = Collaborative;   EBN = Evidence-Based Nursing;   EB = Evidence-Based

risk for SSI. The traditional wound classification system of categorizing procedures into risk groups is based on the degree of microbial contamination (Allen, Apisarnthanarak, & Archer, 2017).

- Smoking: The nicotine in tobacco products results in microvascular vasoconstriction, in addition to tissue hypoxia, which can contribute to the development of SSI (Smith & Dahlen, 2013). **EB:** The increased risk of SSI in clients who smoke is partially related to vasoconstriction of vessels in the surgical bed, which leads to tissue hypovolemia and hypoxia. Poor tissue perfusion affects the transport of nutrients and alters the immune response, which affects healing (Ban et al, 2016).
- ▲ Assess client's smoking status and offer smoking cessation information to the receptive client. Seek nicotine patch order for client use during hospital admission.
- ▲ Educate the client on smoking risks using the CDC Fact Sheet on Health Effects of Cigarette Smoking (CDC, 2018).
- Nutrition status: Assess the client's nutrition status. Preoperative risk factors include albumin <3.5 mg/dL or total bilirubin >1.0 mg/dL (Ban et al, 2016). Malnutrition leads to less competent immune response and increased risk of acquiring infections (Singh, Singla, & Chaudhary, 2014). **EBN:** *Clients who are malnourished and have low albumin levels are more likely to develop SSIs (Smith & Dahlen, 2013). Review preoperative laboratory tests and monitor postoperative laboratory values to assess for malnourishment. Provide nutritional consult and support as needed. Anticipate the malnourished client to receive total parenteral nutrition (TPN) in addition to oral nutrition during the initial postoperative period. Consider the administration of oral nutritional supplements (i.e., protein shakes, high-protein snacks) as recommended by the registered dietician after dietary consult.*
- Immunocompromised/immunosuppression: Clients who are immunocompromised or who have immunosuppression are at increased risk of developing infection because of their weakened immune system and inability to mount a defense against pathogenic organisms. Clients who may be immunocompromised or immunosuppressed are clients receiving cancer treatment, organ transplant recipients, clients taking steroids, and clients with HIV. **EBN:** *Determine the use of chronic medications such as steroids and immunosuppressives. These medications have been shown to increase SSI rates and negatively affect wound healing. There is no recommendation to taper or discontinue systemic steroid use (when medically permissible) before elective surgery (Smith & Dahlen, 2013).*
- Review the client's medical history and current medications. Medications that compromise the client's immune response may increase the risk of SSI.
- Diabetes mellitus: Monitor blood glucose levels with the goal to maintain normoglycemia in the perioperative period. Educate the client of the increased risk for SSI with episodes of hyperglycemia. When available, coordinate referral to a diabetic educator as part of the discharge education. **EB:** *Clients with diabetes have a 2.7-fold increase in the risk of developing a wound infection. Postoperative hyperglycemia and previously undiagnosed diabetes are associated with SSIs among cardiothoracic, general, and vascular surgery patients. Hyperglycemia in the postoperative period was identified as an independent risk factor for developing infection that correlated with a 30% increased risk of infection for every 40 mg/dL increase in postoperative glucose level. Improved glycemic management can restore white blood cell function and reduce risk of infection (Shaw, Saleem, & Gahtan, 2014).*
- Preexisting infection: Be aware of all preoperative laboratory work, positive cultures, and actions taken to treat the infection (i.e., was the client started on oral antibiotics). **EBN:** *Remote infections should be identified and treated following evidence-based guidelines prior to surgical procedure (Smith & Dahlen, 2013).*
- Obesity: Obesity is defined as a body mass index (BMI) >30 kg/m^2. Obese clients are at a significant risk factor for SSI, more surgical blood loss, and experience a longer operation time. **EB:** *Obese clients have excessive subcutaneous fat tissue, which predisposes these clients to impaired healing, low regional perfusion, and low oxygen tension at the surgical site. Longer operation times and increased blood loss >1 L are significant predictors of postoperative wound infections. The obese client is also likely to have more comorbidities, such as diabetes, than nonobese clients, increasing the risk of SSI (Tjeertes et al, 2015). Provide discharge teaching for signs and symptoms of poor wound healing and SSI.*

Procedure-Related Risk Factors—Exogenous

- Observe clients identified as being at increased risk for SSI because of modifiable risk factors for signs and/or symptoms of postoperative SSI (Smith & Dahlen, 2013).
- Extended procedure time. **EB:** Prolonged operations that increase the length of time that tissues are exposed increases the risk of exogenous contamination of the surgical site (Smith & Dahlen, 2013; Singh, Singla, & Chaudhary, 2014; Ban et al, 2016).

● = Independent;   ▲ = Collaborative;   **EBN** = Evidence-Based Nursing;   **EB** = Evidence-Based

- Estimated blood loss greater than 1 L requiring blood transfusion increases the risk of SSI **EB:** *Blood transfusions increase the risk of SSI by decreasing macrophage function (Anderson et al, 2014). The use of allogenic(donor) blood transfusions is associated with increased length of stay and induces immunomodulation that can lead to increased risk for infection at the surgical site (Huntzler & William, 2017).*

- Suboptimal timing of prophylactic antibiotic places the client at increased risk of SSI. **EB:** Administer preoperative prophylactic antimicrobial agent(s) as prescribed (*Berríos-Torres et al, 2017*). *Surgical antibiotic prophylaxis (SAP) should be administered within 1 hour before incision or within 2 hours for vancomycin or fluoroquinolones. This allows for maximal antibiotic concentration circulating in the blood serum and tissue at the time of surgical incision (Ban et al, 2016). Evidence shows that the administration of SAP after the incision causes a significant increase of SSI risk compared with administration of the SAP prior to incision (WHO, 2016).*

- Preoperative infections place the client at increased risk of SSI prior to elective surgery. **EB:** Identify and treat infections (i.e., urinary tract infection) prior to surgical procedure. Do not routinely treat urinary tract colonization or contamination in the absence of clinical urinary tract infection symptoms (urgency, costovertebral angle [CVA] pain, flank pain, pain with urination, and fever) (Anderson et al, 2014).

- Preoperative interventions: Establish a protocol for procedure-specific preoperative testing to detect medical conditions that increase the risk of SSI. The protocol should focus on nutritional counseling, smoking cessation, preadmission infections, and reconciling mediations with adjustments prior to surgery as indicated (Anderson et al, 2014).
  - Identify high-risk clients: Clients at high risk for developing SSIs have diabetics, history of transplant, are receiving chemotherapy, are immunosuppressed and immunocompromised, are elderly, have poor dentition, are obese, and are malnourished. Clients having a high-risk procedure with an extended surgical procedure time (i.e., cardiac surgery, joint replacement, major abdominal surgery) are at increased risk of SSI. **EB:** *Identifying high-risk patients through screening and electronic medical record alerts should be used to inform all members of the perioperative team of the client's high-risk condition(s) (Anderson et al, 2014).*
  - Maintain glycemic control for both diabetic and nondiabetic clients. **EB:** *Elevated blood glucose levels >200 mg/dl cause the release of proinflammatory cytokines that depress the immune system, increasing susceptibility to SSIs (Singh, Singla, & Chaudhary, 2014). Hyperglycemia in the immediate preoperative period is associated with an increased risk of SSI (Ban et al, 2016).*
  - Staphylococcus aureus (SA) is the most common pathogen causing SSIs. Colonization with SA, primarily in the nares, occurs in roughly one in four persons and increases the risk of SSI by 2- to 14-fold. Perform SA intranasal decolonization by using cotton-tipped applicators to apply a 2% mupirocin ointment in each nostril for up to 5 days prior to surgery, when appropriate and according to evidence-based guidelines (Bratzler et al, 2013). **EB:** *Screen for SA (methicillin-sensitive SA [MSSA] and MRSA) colonization and decolonize surgical patients prior to high-risk procedures, including some orthopedic and cardiothoracic procedures (Anderson et al, 2014).*
  - Provide education on preoperative bathing with soap (antimicrobial or nonantimicrobial) or an antiseptic agent on at least the night before and morning of the day of surgical intervention. **EB:** *It is good clinical practice for the client to bathe or shower before surgery to ensure that the skin is as clean as possible and to reduce the bacterial load, especially at the site of incision (WHO, 2016). Instruct the client to bathe, at a minimum, the night before and morning of the surgical procedure using liquid soap, clean washcloth, and clean towel each time. Instruct the client to wear freshly laundered pajamas after showering the night before the surgical procedure, and freshly laundered clothes the morning of the procedure. This process of using liquid soap and clean washcloths, towels, and clothes prevents recontamination with shed epithelial cells from previously used bar soap, washcloths/towels, and clothes.*
  - Address preexisting dental and nutritional status. **EBN:** *Preoperative dental screenings are needed to evaluate for the presence of tooth decay, inflammatory gum disease/gingivitis, periodontitis, or dental abscesses, which lead to seeding of bacteria and a deep joint infection (Smith & Dahlen, 2013). Educate the client on the need for good oral hygiene to decrease the risk of developing SSI. Provide the client with oral hygiene products while in the hospital. Perform oral hygiene for the client if unable to perform independently.*
  - Nutrition consult as needed.
  - Prepare the surgical site using an alcohol-based antiseptic agent unless contraindicated to reduce SSI risk. **EB:** *Alcohol-based antiseptic solutions for surgical site skin preparation are more effective compared with aqueous solutions in reducing SSIs (WHO, 2016; Berríos-Torres et al, 2017).* **EB:** *Overall, there is*

● = Independent;   ▲ = Collaborative;   EBN = Evidence-Based Nursing;   EB = Evidence-Based

evidence that alcohol-based preparations are more effective in reducing SSIs than aqueous preparations and should be used unless contraindications exist (Ban et al, 2016).

- ○ Proper hair removal: When hair removal at the operative site is necessary, removal should be done using clippers. EB: *Do not remove hair at the operative site unless the presence of hair will interfere with the operation. Do not use razors. If hair removal is necessary, remove hair outside the operating room using clippers or a depilatory agent (Anderson et al, 2014). Shaving causes microscopic cuts and abrasions, resulting in disruption of the skin's barrier defense against microorganisms (Ban et al, 2016).*

- If possible, educate the client preoperatively on the risk of shaving the surgical site, or the area near in which the surgical incision will be, because of the risk for microscopic cuts and abrasions. These cuts and abrasions increase the risk of developing an SSI. For example, for breast surgery, instruct the client not to shave underarms because the underarm is potentially in close proximity to the surgical site. Another example is instructing the client having a total knee replacement not to shave the leg involved in the surgery.

- Intraoperative interventions:
  - ○ Maintain glycemic control: EB: *Implement perioperative glycemic control and use blood glucose target levels <200 mg/dL in diabetic and nondiabetic clients (Berríos-Torres et al, 2017). Short-term glucose control can be more impactful in decreasing SSIs than long-term control of hemoglobin (Hgb) A1C (Ban et al, 2016).*
  - ○ Maintain normothermia (temperature of 35.5°C [95.9°F] or above) during the perioperative period in surgical clients who have an anesthesia duration of at least 60 minutes (Anderson et al, 2014). WHO defines hypothermia as a core temperature <36°C (WHO, 2016). EB: *Hypothermia can trigger subcutaneous vasoconstriction and subsequent tissue hypoxia and increase blood loss that may lead to wound hematomas or need for transfusion, both of which can increase SSI rates (Anderson et al, 2014).*
  - ○ Provide supplemental oxygenation, during surgery for intubated clients and in the immediate postoperative period for 2 to 6 hours via a nonrebreathing mask for procedures performed under general anesthesia to ensure a Hgb saturation of >95% is maintained. EB: *Studies have found that perioperative hyper-oxygenation led to a 25% decrease in SSIs (Anderson et al, 2014; WHO, 2016).* EB: *For patients with normal pulmonary function undergoing general anesthesia with endotracheal intubation, administer increased FiO_2 intraoperatively and postextubation in the immediate postoperative period (Berríos-Torres et al, 2017). The administration of supplemental oxygen is recommended in the immediate postoperative period after surgery performed under general anesthesia (Ban et al, 2016).*

- Postoperative interventions:
  - ○ Discharge instructions: Teach the client postoperative self-care after discharge. Provide written instructions that include information on how and when to contact the provider, date and time for the scheduled follow-up visit, and signs and symptoms of infection. EB: *Educational materials should be provided in multiple languages based on the population served (Anderson et al, 2014).*
  - ○ Wound care: Wound care instructions will be based on the type of surgical wound closure. EB: *Protect primarily closed incisions with a sterile dressing for 24 to 48 hours postoperatively (Berríos-Torres et al, 2017). Instruct the client to keep their surgical wound clean and dry. Teach the client signs and symptoms that would indicate an SSI, such as fever, redness, drainage, swelling, pain, and foul odor at the surgical site. Stress to the client and family that any of these signs and symptoms should be promptly reported to their provider. Assess whether the client and family know how to read a thermometer and provide instructions as necessary. Provide written wound care instructions on the prevention of SSI.*
  - ○ Nutrition follow-up: For the malnourished and obese clients, provide written dietary instructions by the registered dietician, if appropriate. Encourage a diet that supports wound healing (high protein) and glycemic control. If appropriate, provide written information on community nutrition support group options and contact information.
  - ○ Bathing/showering instructions: Review instructions with client and family on timing to shower and if/when the client can take a bath. Explain to the client that taking a bath is generally discouraged, at a minimum, for the first week after surgery. Submerging a fresh surgical wound in warm bath water and allowing it to soak is not advised because this provides an environment that potentially exposes the surgical wound to pathogenic organisms, increasing the risk for surgical wound infection.
  - ○ Physical therapy (PT): For clients prescribed PT after discharge, review options to access services, provide contact phone numbers to call and schedule therapy, and review options for transportation to PT appointments (e.g., spouse, family, friend, senior center transport, cab, Uber, Lyft). Work with the discharge coordinator for client assistance with transport options as needed.

● = Independent;   ▲ = Collaborative;   EBN = Evidence-Based Nursing;   EB = Evidence-Based

○ Medications: Review discharge medication prescription(s). Provide written instructions on medication(s) ordered, how often to take them, and side effects of the prescribed medication(s). Reinforce with client and family that client should not be driving if taking prescription narcotic medications. Review with client and family pain relief expectations, explaining that 100% postoperative pain relief is not realistic, but adequate pain relief should allow the client to function, to ambulate, and to perform activities of daily living (ADLs) with minimal pain.

Pediatric

SSI prevention measures deemed effective in adults are also indicated in the pediatric surgical population (Berríos-Torres et al, 2017).

Geriatric

- The most common cause of postoperative complication in the frail elderly is delirium (Ersan & Schwer, 2015). *Delirium will affect the ability to provide postoperative education in this population.*
- For the frail, elder client who lived independently in a private home prior to surgical procedure, work with the discharge coordinator to assess appropriate client placement in the immediate postoperative period. Explore independent living, acute rehabilitation facility, or skilled nursing facility.
- For the cognitively impaired client being discharged back to independent living (private home or home with a family member), identify a key contact person who will participate in discharge education. Assess for any need of community services (food assistance, meal prep, transport, home health care, etc.) at time of discharge.
- Nutritional deficiencies can be common in elderly clients. Monitor laboratory tests; an albumin <3.2 mg/dL and a cholesterol level of <160mg/dL in the frail elderly are indicators for increased mortality. A BMI of <20 kg/m² is a marker for increased risk of wound healing. A dietary consult should be initiated, and nutritional supplements should be provided (Ersan & Schwer. 2015).
- As part of the discharge process, ask the client how they will be obtaining groceries: Will they be cooking? Will they need assistance with meal prep? Do they have someone (friend or family member) who can come into the home to assist with cooking? Does the client need to have a food service (i.e., Meals on Wheels) set up for the immediate postdischarge period? Refer client to community services as necessary.

Multicultural

- Consider race and ethnicity as a key factor when developing the client's plan of care. EBN: *Nurses should use culturally competent verbal and nonverbal communication skills to identify clients' values, beliefs, practices, perceptions, and unique health care needs. Effective cultural communication demonstrates respect, dignity, and the preservation of human rights.*
- In the case of a language barrier, use a qualified interpreter rather than family members, unless as a last resort, to communicate with the non–English-speaking client. The use of family members to translate health care-specific information may risk patient privacy issues and interpretation bias. Nurses must be attentive to nonverbal cues, such as effective listening, attentive body language, and use of eye contact.
- Cultural nonverbal communication may also include values of modesty, touch, silence, and provider gender (Douglas et al, 2014). Identify the need for an interpreter at time of admission and schedule an interpreter to be available, either by phone or in person, for discussions with providers and for education sessions.
- Identify and accommodate the client that prefers same-gender providers. Effective communication may be affected in the client assigned opposite-gender caregivers, which may negatively affect recovery.

Home Care

- Previously listed interventions appropriately pertain to the home care.
- Coordinate with discharge planner, as necessary, for assessment of the client's home care situation that suggests potential safety and mobility concerns.
- Clients discharged back to independent living with new use of walker, crutches, wheelchair, oxygen, and so forth, should have egress access evaluated, and bathing/showering options and potential need for grab bars.

● = Independent;   ▲ = Collaborative;   EBN = Evidence-Based Nursing;   EB = Evidence-Based

REFERENCES

Allen, V., Apisarnthanarak, A., & Archer, J., (2017). *APIC Text of infection control and epidemiology.* [Online Version]. Retrieved from http://text.apic.org/. (Accessed 25 February 2018).

Anderson, D. J., Podgorny, K., Berrios-Torres, S. I., et al. (2014). Strategies to prevent surgical site infections in acute care hospitals: 2014 update. *Infection Control and Hospital Epidemiology, 35*(6), 605–627.

Ban, K. A., Minei, J. P., Laronga, C., et al. (2016). American College of Surgeons and Surgical Infection Society: Surgical site infection guidelines, 2016 update. *Journal of the American College of Surgeons, 22*(1), 59–74.

Berríos-Torres, S. I., Umscheid, C. A., Bratzler, D. W., et al. (2017). Healthcare Infection Control Practices Advisory Committee. Centers for Disease Control and Prevention guideline for prevention of surgical site infection, 2017. *JAMA Surgery, 152*(8), 784–791.

Bratzler, D. W., Dellinger, E. P., Olsen, M. K., et al. (2013). Clinical practice guidelines for antimicrobial prophylaxis in surgery. *American Journal Health-System Pharmacists, 70,* 195–283.

Centers for Disease Control and Prevention. (2018). *Health effects of cigarette smoking.* Retrieved from https://www.cdc.gov/tobacco/data_statistics/fact_sheets/health_effects/effects_cig_smoking/index.htm. (Accessed 11 November 2018).

Douglas, M. K., Rosenkoetter, M., Pacquiao, D. F., et al. (2014). Guidelines for implementing culturally competent nursing care. *Journal of Transcultural Nursing, 25*(2), 109–121.

Ersan, T., & Schwer, W. A. (2015) *Perioperative management of the geriatric patient.* Retrieved from https://emedicine.medscape.com/article/285433-overview#a2. (Accessed 17 February 2018).

Hutzler, L., & Williams, J. (2017). Decreasing the incidence of surgical site infections following joint replacement surgery. *Bulletin of the Hospital for Joint Diseases, 75*(4), 268–273.

Preas, M. A., O'Hara, L., & Thom, K. (2017). *2017 HICPAC-CDC Guideline for prevention of surgical site infection: What the infection preventionist needs to know. Fall 2017 APIC Prevention strategist.* Retrieved from https://apic.org/Resource_/TinyMceFileManager/Periodical_images/SSI_2017_Fall_PS.pdf. (Accessed 23 January 2018).

Shaw, P., Saleem, T., & Gahtan, V. (2014). Correlation of hemoglobin A1C level with surgical outcomes: Can tight perioperative glucose control reduce infection and cardiac events? *Seminars in Vascular Surgery, 27,* 156–161.

Singh, R., Singla, P., & Chaudhary, U. (2014). Surgical site infections: Classification, risk factors, pathogenesis and preventive management. *International Journal of Pharma Research and Health Sciences, 2*(3), 203–214.

Smith, M. A., & Dahlen, N. R. (2013). Clinical practice guideline surgical site infection prevention. *Journal of Orthopaedic Nursing., 32*(5), 242–248.

Tjeertes, E. K. M., Hoeks, S. E., Beks, S. B. J. C., et al. (2015). Obesity—A risk factor for postoperative complications in general surgery? *BMC Anesthesiology, 15,* 112.

World Health Organization. (2016). *Global guidelines for the prevention of surgical site infection.* Geneva, Switzerland: WHO Press. Retrieved from http://www.who.int/gpsc/ssi-guidelines/en/.

Risk for Injury   *Julianne E. Doubet, BSN, RN, EMT-B*

NANDA-I

Definition

Susceptible to physical damage due to environmental conditions interacting with the individual's adaptive and defensive resources, which may compromise health.

Risk Factors

Compromised nutritional source; exposure to pathogen; exposure to toxic chemical; immunization level with community; insufficient knowledge of modifiable factors; malnutrition; nosocomial agent; physical barrier; unsafe mode of transport

At-Risk Population

Extremes of age; impaired primary defense mechanisms

Associated Condition

Abnormal blood profile; alteration in cognitive functioning; alteration in psychomotor functioning; alteration in sensation; autoimmune dysfunction; biochemical dysfunction; effector dysfunction; immune dysfunction; sensory integration dysfunction; tissue hypoxia

NOC   (Nursing Outcomes Classification)

Suggested NOC Outcomes

Personal Safety Behavior; Risk Control; Safe Home Environment; Knowledge: Fall Prevention

● = Independent;   ▲ = Collaborative;   EBN = Evidence-Based Nursing;   EB = Evidence-Based

Example NOC Outcome with Indicators
Risk Control as evidenced by the following indicators: Monitors environmental risk factors/Develops effective risk control strategies/Follows selected risk control strategies. (Rate the outcome and indicators of **Risk Control:** 1 = never demonstrated, 2 = rarely demonstrated, 3 = sometimes demonstrated, 4 = often demonstrated, 5 = consistently demonstrated [see Section I].)

Client Outcomes

Client Will (Specify Time Frame)

- Remain free of injuries
- Explain methods to prevent injuries
- Demonstrate behaviors that decrease the risk for injury

NOC (Nursing Outcomes Classification)

Suggested NOC Outcomes

Health Education; Environmental Management; Fall Prevention

Example NIC Activities—Health Education
Identify internal or external factors that may enhance or reduce motivation for healthy behavior; Determine current health knowledge and lifestyle behaviors of individual, family, or target group

Nursing Interventions and *Rationales*

Prevent iatrogenic harm to the hospitalized client by following the National Patient Safety goals.
- Accuracy of Client Identification:
  - Use at least two methods (e.g., client's name and medical record number or birth date) to identify the client on initial entrance to a client's room and before administering medications, blood products, treatments, or procedures.
  - Before beginning any invasive or surgical procedure, have a final verification to confirm the correct client, the correct procedure, and the correct site for the procedure using active communication techniques.
  - Label containers used for blood and other specimens in the presence of the client.
- Effectiveness of Communication Among Care Staff:
  - Verbal or telephone orders should be written and then read back for verification to the individual giving the order. Avoid verbal or telephone orders whenever possible.
  - Standardize use of abbreviations, acronyms, symbols, and dose designations that are used in the institution.
  - Ensure that critical test results and values are recorded and reported in a timely manner.
  - Use a standardized approach of "handing off" communications, including opportunities to ask and answer questions.
  - Use only approved abbreviations.
  - Staff should always wear hospital nametags.
- Medication Safety:
  - Standardize and limit the number of drug concentrations used by the institution (e.g., concentrations of medications such as morphine in client-controlled analgesia pumps).
  - Label all medications and medication containers (e.g., syringes, medication cups, or other solutions on or off the surgical field).
  - Identify all of the client's current medications on admission to a health care facility, and ensure that all health care staff has access to the information.
  - Ensure that accurate medicine information is sent with the client throughout their care.
  - Reconcile all medication at admission and discharge, and provide list to the client.
  - Improve the effectiveness of alarm systems in the clinical area.
  - Standardize a list of medications that look alike or sound alike. This list needs to be updated yearly.
  - Identify and take extra care with clients who are on anticoagulants.

● = Independent;   ▲ = Collaborative;   EBN = Evidence-Based Nursing;   EB = Evidence-Based

- Infection Control:
  - ○ Reduce the risk of infections by following Centers for Disease Control and Prevention (CDC, 2017) hand hygiene guidelines.
  - ○ Document clearly when clients obtain injuries or die of infectious disease.
  - ○ Use proven guidelines to prevent infections that are difficult to treat.
  - ○ Use proven guidelines to prevent infection of the blood from central lines.
  - ○ Use safe practices to treat the surgical site of the client.
  - ○ Use proven guidelines to prevent catheter-associated urinary tract infections.
- Fall Prevention:
  - ○ Evaluate all clients for fall risk daily and take appropriate actions to prevent falls.
- Client Involvement in Care:
  - ○ Educate the client and family on how to recognize and report concerns about safety issues.
- Identify Clients with Safety Risks:
  - ○ Identify which clients are at risk for harming themselves.
- Identify Clients Who Are Susceptible to Changes in Health Status:
  - ○ Educate staff on how to recognize changes in client condition, how to respond quickly, and how to alert specially trained staff to intervene if needed.
  - ○ Prevent errors in surgery by following established protocols. Update protocols yearly.
  - ○ Standardize steps to educate staff so documents for surgery are ready before surgery.
  - ○ Educate staff to mark the body part scheduled for surgery and engage the client in this process as well.

These actions have been shown to increase client safety and are required actions for accreditation by The Joint Commission (2017).

- See care plan for Risk for **Falls.**
- Avoid use of physical and chemical restraints, if at all possible. Restraint free is now the standard of care for hospitals and long-term care facilities. Obtain a health care provider's order if restraints are necessary. EBN: *The use of restraints has been associated with serious patient injuries and at present there is no satisfactory evidence to confirm that the use of restraints is beneficial in reducing falls and preventing injuries (Park & Tang, 2007; Rahn et al, 2017).* EBN: *Along with physical restraints, other nonpharmaceutical measures can be used to promote safe mobility in client-centered care (Gulpers et al, 2013).*
- Consider providing individualized music of the client's choice if a client is agitated. EBN: *Blackburn and Bradshaw (2014) found that music therapy is not only promising in the reduction of agitation in older adults with dementia, but it also helps lessen anxiety and depression, while seemingly improving cognitive function.*
- Review drug profile for potential side effects and interactions that may increase risk of injury. EB: *The use of polypharmacy, as prescribed to older adults, is the most significant factor in risk injury in those same adults (Scott et al, 2014).*
- Provide a safe environment:
  - ○ Use one-fourth– to one-half–length side rails only, and maintain bed in a low position. Ensure that wheels are locked on bed and commode. Keep dim light in room at night.
  - ○ Remove all possible hazards in environment such as razors, medications, room clutter, wet floors, and matches.
- Place an "at risk for injury" client in a room that is near the nurse's station. EBN: *According to Wang et al (2014), when clients' safety culture is improved, there is a decrease in client adverse events.*
  - ○ If the client has a new onset of confusion (delirium), refer to the care plan for Acute **Confusion.** If the client has chronic confusion, see the care plan for Chronic **Confusion.**
- Involve family in helping to provide a culture of safety. EBN: *A client-centered approach to care should include the family, in both planning and decision-making (Wrobleski et al, 2014).*
- Refer the client for physical therapy for strengthening as needed.
- ▲ Use nonphysical forms of behavior management for the agitated psychotic client. EB: *Okumura, Togo, and Fujita (2014) stated that there is a call for approaches to client agitation that focus on psychosocial interventions, antipsychotic withdrawal, and the need to moderate the overall incidence of antipsychotics use.*

 Pediatric

- Teach parents the need for close supervision of young children playing near water. EB: *Semple-Hess and Campwala (2014) stated that drowning and submersion injuries are one of the most common, yet avoidable, causes of childhood mortality and morbidity.*

● = Independent;   ▲ = Collaborative;   EBN = Evidence-Based Nursing;   EB = Evidence-Based

- If the child has an underlying medical problem that puts him or her at risk for drowning, it is recommended that the child be given showers, not tub baths. No unsupervised swimming is ever allowed. EB: *Caregivers should understand the necessity for constant supervision while children are bathing, especially if the child has an underlying condition such as epilepsy (Bamber et al, 2014).*
- Assess the client's socioeconomic status because financial hardship may correlate with increased rates of injury. EB: *According to Anderson, Pomerantz, and Gittelman (2014), there may be a relationship between intentional injury rates and those children in families living below poverty level and experiencing financial hardship.*
- Never leave young children unsupervised around cooking or open flames. EB: *Risks for children's thermal injuries can be modified by caregiver awareness of hazards (Jamshidi & Sato, 2013).*
- Teach parents and children the need to maintain safety for the exercising child, including wearing helmets when biking. EB: *Parents should be educated in the use of bicycle helmets for their children and set a good example by wearing helmets themselves (Baeseman & Corden, 2014).* EB: *It has been proven that the use of bicycle helmets helps prevent or reduce severe head injuries in bicycle riders (Basch et al, 2014).*
- Encourage parents to insist on safety precautions in all phases of participation sports involving children. EB: *Parents and youth athletes should be aware that there are increased risks of injury caused by sports specialization and the intense volume of participation the child is subject to when involved in many sports (Post et al, 2017).*
- Provide parents of children with traumatic brain injury with written instruction and emergency phone numbers. Ensure that instructions are understood before the child is discharged from a health care setting. Instruct parents to observe for the following symptoms: nausea, mild headache, dizziness, irritability, lethargy, poor concentration, loss of appetite, and insomnia.
- ▲ EBN: *The nurse plays a pivotal part in educating the patient, family, school, and perhaps coaches on the necessity of lifestyle modifications based on the patient's condition (Gillooly, 2016).*
- Teach both parents and children the need for gun safety; refer to hunting safety courses. EBN: *Barton and Kologi (2014), in their study, found that thousands of children are killed or injured every year in the United States because of access to loaded and not safely stored firearms.*
- Educate parents regarding proper car safety seat use. EB: *Deaths among children, who are occupants in automobiles, has decreased over the last 10 years, but many more could be prevented with the consistent use of child safety restraints (Sauber-Schatz et al, 2014).*

 Geriatric

- Encourage the client to wear glasses and hearing aids and to use walking aids, including nonslip footwear when ambulating. EB: *It has been observed that gait and balance problems lead to falls and injuries in older people; the use of walking aids is meant to augment gait safety and prevent falls (Hardi et al, 2014).*
- Assess for orthostatic hypotension when getting up, teach methods to decrease dizziness, such as rising slowly, remaining seated several minutes before standing, flexing feet upward several times while sitting, sitting down immediately if feeling dizzy, and trying to have someone present when standing. EBN: *In a study by Nazarko (2015), it was found that addressing physiological risk factors for falls improves functional capability, a feeling of well-being, and improvement in the quality of life.*
- Discourage driving at night. EB: *Older adult drivers who drive at night are at heightened risk for injury because of age-related changes in the amount of light reaching the retina, weaker contrast sensitivity, and variations in dark and light adaptation (Boot, Stothart, & Charness, 2014).*

 Multicultural

- Acknowledge racial/ethnic differences at the onset of care. EBN: *Alpers and Hanssen (2014) noted that experience in and of itself does not provide nurses with sufficient knowledge for intercultural symptom assessment and culturally competent treatment and care; access to appropriate information is needed along with their perception of clinical practice.*
- Evaluate the influence of culture on the client's perceptions of risk for injury. EB: *More African American and Hispanic children, compared with Caucasian children, are dying in automobile crashes because they are unrestrained; effective interventions and education would increase proper restraint use (Sauber-Schatz et al, 2014).*
- Evaluate whether exposure to community violence is a contributor to a client's risk for injury. EB: *Exposure to violence can result in many negative consequences for youth, including use of tobacco, alcohol, marijuana, and persistence in neighborhood violence (Fagan, Wright, & Pinchevsky, 2014).*

● = Independent; ▲ = Collaborative; EBN = Evidence-Based Nursing; EB = Evidence-Based

- Use culturally relevant injury prevention programs when possible. Validate the client's feelings and concerns related to environmental risks. **EB:** *According to research supported by the findings of Richardson, Van Brakle, and St. Vil (2014), parents of adolescent African American males are tested daily in attempting to keep their children safe in high-risk neighborhoods.*

Home Care and Client/Family Teaching and Discharge Planning

- See Risk for **Trauma** for Nursing Interventions and *Rationales*.

REFERENCES

Alpers, L. M., & Hanssen, I. (2014). Caring for ethnic minority patients: A mixed method study of nurses' self-assessment of cultural competency. *Nursing Education Today, 34*, 999–1004.

Anderson, B. L., Pomerantz, W. J., & Gittelman, M. A. (2014). Intentional injuries in young Ohio children: Is there an urban/rural variation. *The Journal of Trauma and Acute Care Surgery, 77*, 538–540.

Baeseman, Z. J., & Corden, T. E. (2014). A social-ecologic framework for improving bicycle helmet use by children. *Wisconsin Medical Journal, 113*, 49–51.

Bamber, A. R., Pryce, J. W., Ashworth, M. T., et al. (2014). Immersion-related deaths in infants and children: Autopsy experience from a specialist center. *Forensic Science, Medicine, and Pathology, 10*, 363–370.

Barton, B. K., & Kologi, S. M. (2014). Why do you keep them there: A qualitative assessment of firearms storage practices. *Journal of Pediatric Nursing, 10*.

Basch, C., Ethan, D., Rajan, S., et al. (2014). Helmet use among users of the Citi Bike bicycle-sharing program: A pilot study in New York City. *Journal of Community Health, 39*, 503–507.

Blackburn, R., & Bradshaw, T. (2014). Music therapy for service users with dementia: A critical review of the literature. *Journal of Psychiatric and Mental Health Nursing, 10*, 879–888.

Boot, W. R., Stothart, C., & Charness, N. (2014). Improving the safety of aging road users: A mini-review. *Gerontology, 100*, 90–96.

Centers for Disease Control and Prevention. (2017). *Hand hygiene guideline.* Retrieved from https://www.cdc.gov/handhygiene/providers/guideline.html. (Accessed 15 October 2017).

Fagan, A. A., Wright, E. M., & Pinchevsky, G. M. (2014). The protective effects of neighborhood collective efficacy on adolescent substance use and violence following exposure to violence. *Journal of Youth and Adolescence, 43*, 1408–1512.

Gillooly, D. (2016). Current recommendations on management of pediatric concussions. *Pediatric Nursing, 42*(5), 217–220.

Gulpers, M. J., Bleijlevens, M. H., Ambergen, T., et al. (2013). Reduction of belt restraint use: Long term effects of EXBELT intervention. *Journal of the American Geriatric Society, 61*, 107–112.

Hardi, I., Bridenbaugh, S. A., Gschwind, Y. J., et al. (2014). The effect of walking aids on spatio-temporal parameters in community dwelling older adults. *Aging Clinical and Experimental Research, 26*, 221–228.

Jamshidi, R., & Sato, T. T. (2013). Initial assessment and management of thermal burn injuries in children. *Pediatrics in Review, 24*, 395–404.

Nazarko, L. (2015). Modifiable risk factors for falls and minimizing the risk of harm. *Nurse Prescribing, 13*(4), 192–198.

Okumura, Y., Togo, T., & Fujita, J. (2014). Trends in use of psychotropic medications among patients treated with cholinesterase inhibitors in Japan from 2002 to 2010. *International Psychogeriatrics, 12*, 1–9.

Park, M., & Tang, J. H. (2007). Evidence-based guideline-changing the practice of physical restraint use in acute care. *Journal of Gerontological Nursing, 33*, 9–16.

Post, E., Trigsted, S., Bell, D., et al. (2017). The association of sport specialization and training volume with injury history in youth athletes. *American Journal of Sports Medicine, 45*(6), 1405–1412.

Rahn, A., Behncke, A., Buhl, A., et al. (2017). Implementation of guideline-bases programme on physical restraint reduction in home care and nursing homes in northern Germany-multi-centre before-after study. *BMC Nursing, 16*, 4–11.

Richardson, J. B., Jr., Van Brakle, M., & St Vil, C. (2014). Taking boys out of the hood: Exile as a parenting strategy for African American male youth. *New Directions for Child and Adolescent Development, 14*, 11–21.

Sauber-Schatz, E. K., West, B. A., & Bergen, G. (2014). Vital signs: Restraint use and motor vehicle occupant death rates among children aged 0–2 years—United States, 2002–2011. *Morbidity and Mortality Weekly Report, Centers for Disease Control, 63*, 113–116.

Semple-Hess, J., & Campwala, R. (2014). Pediatric submersion injuries and emergency care and resuscitation. *Pediatric Emergency Medicine, 11*, 1–21.

Scott, A., Anderson, K., Freeman, C. R., et al. (2014). First do no harm: a real need to deprescribe in older patients. *Medical Journal of Australia, 201*, 390–392.

The Joint Commission (2017). *National patient safety goals.* Retrieved from http://www.jointcommission.org/PatientSafety/NationalPatientSafetyGoals/07_npsg_facts.htm. (Accessed 15 December 2017).

Wang, X., Liu, K., You, L. M., et al. (2014). The relationship between patient safety culture and adverse events: A questionnaire survey. *The International Journal of Nursing Studies, 51*, 1114–1122.

Wrobleski, D. M. S., Joswiak, M. E., Dunn, D. F., et al. (2014). Discharge planning rounds to the bedside: A patient and family-centered approach. *Medsurg Nursing, 23*, 111–116.

Risk for corneal injury   Michelle Acorn, DNP, NP PHC/Adult, BA, BScN/PHCNP, MN/ACNP, GNC(C), CGP

NANDA-I

Definition

Susceptible to infection or inflammatory lesion in the corneal tissue that can affect superficial or deep layers, which may compromise visual health.

● = Independent;   ▲ = Collaborative;   **EBN** = Evidence-Based Nursing;   **EB** = Evidence-Based

Risk Factors

Exposure of the eyeball; insufficient knowledge of modifiable factors

At-Risk Population

Prolonged hospitalization

Associated Condition

Blinking <5 times per minute; Glasgow Coma Scale score <6; intubation; mechanical ventilation; oxygen therapy; periorbital edema; pharmaceutical agent; tracheostomy

NOC   (Nursing Outcomes Classification)

Suggested NOC Outcomes (Visual)

Sensory Function: Vision; Vision Compensation Behavior

Example NOC Outcome with Indicators
Vision Compensation Behavior as evidenced by the following indicators: Wears protective eye wear for prevention/ Eye discomfort improves daily with healing. (Rate each indicator of **Vision Compensation Behavior:** 1 = never demonstrated, 2 = rarely demonstrated, 3 = sometimes demonstrated, 4 = often demonstrated, 5 = consistently demonstrated [see Section I].)

Client Outcomes

Client Will (Specify Time Frame)

- Demonstrate relaxed facial expressions and grimacing reduction
- Remain as independent as possible
- Remain free of physical harm resulting from vision injury risk
- Demonstrate improvement in visual acuity

NIC   (Nursing Interventions Classification)

Suggested NIC Interventions

Visual Deficit; Environmental Management

Example NIC Activities—Communication Enhancement: Visual Deficit
Clearly identify yourself when you enter the client's space; Build on client's remaining vision, as appropriate

Nursing Interventions and *Rationales*

Emergency Department Visits or Primary Care Office Visit

- ▲ Perform a standard ophthalmic exam or examine eye with a slit lamp using fluorescein stain to optimize visualization of the abrasion injury if available.
- Attempt visual acuity measuring using the Snellen eye chart (corrected with glasses).
- Ensure immunization status is current, namely tetanus-diphtheria-pertussis status (every 10 years).
- Teach the client that fingernail-induced corneal abrasions are one of the most common eye injuries and are at risk for complications (Lin & Gardiner, 2014). EB: *The Cochrane systematic review of 12 randomized controlled trials (RCTs) with 1080 participants suggested that treating simple corneal abrasions with a patch may not improve healing or reduce pain. This is important because patching the eye probably does not speed up healing and may not have an important effect on pain relief. Furthermore, people receiving an eye patch may be less likely to have a healed corneal abrasion after 24 to 72 hours. Additionally, corneal abrasions in people patched probably take slightly longer to heal. Last, using eye patches may lead to more pain at 24 hours (Lim, Turner, & Lim, 2016).*
- Provide analgesia as needed. Clients with all but the most minor abrasions usually require a strong oral narcotic analgesic initially (Verma & Khan, 2014).

● = Independent;   ▲ = Collaborative;   EBN = Evidence-Based Nursing;   EB = Evidence-Based

- EB: *According to the Cochrane systematic review of nine RCTs with 637 participants. The findings of the studies do not provide strong evidence to support the use of topical nonsteroidal antiinflammatory drugs (NSAIDS) in traumatic corneal abrasions. This is important because NSAIDS are associated with higher costs compared with oral analgesia (Wakai et al, 2017).*
- Injuries that penetrate the cornea are more serious. The outcome depends on the specific injury. Corneal abrasions usually heal quickly and without vision concerns. Even after the original injury is healed, however, the surface of the cornea is sometimes not as smooth as before. *Clients who have had a corneal abrasion may notice that the eye feels irritated for a while after the abrasion heals (Cleveland Clinic, 2015).*

Hospitalization

- Traumatic corneal abrasions are very common ophthalmic injuries accounting for 6% of emergency department visits and 65% trauma related of which 24% were corneal abrasions (Wakai et al, 2017; Menghini et al, 2013).
- Perioperative corneal abrasions typically heal within 72 hours. Risk factors include advanced age, prominent eyes (proptosis, exophthalmos), ocular surface abnormalities (dry eye, recurrent erosion syndrome), surgery greater than 60 to 90 minutes, prone/lateral and Trendelenburg positions, operations on the head and neck body regions, intraoperative hypotension, and preoperative anemia. Potential sources of corneal injury in the surgical patient are after induction (laryngoscope, name badge, watch band), before incision (surgical preparation, gauze/sponges/drapes), during the procedure (instruments, chemical solutions, heat sources, pressure on globe, eye shields), and awakening/recovery (oxygen face mask, fingernails) (Segal et al, 2014; Malafa et al, 2016).
- ▲ All surgical patients should have eyelids secured in the closed position immediately after induction. A strip of tape is generally sufficient; however, in high-risk cases with Trendelenburg position patients may benefit from use of transparent biooclusive dressing, which can span the entire lid and provide strong uniform closure, minimizing tear evaporation and acting as a barrier to trauma (Malafa et al, 2016). EB: *Clients receiving adhesive tape as an eye care method were twice as likely to develop corneal abrasions (Masoudi et al, 2013).*
- Ocular lubricants support surface moisture, but studies comparing different types of lubricants fail to demonstrate differences in efficacy. However, preservative-free methylcellulose-based ointments are preferred because they are retained in the eye longer than aqueous solutions. Paraffin-based (petroleum) ointments disrupt tear film stability, carrying a higher risk of eye irritation, and are flammable (Malafa, 2016).
- Assess for corneal abrasion and eye dryness, which are common problems in clients in the intensive care unit. Eye dryness is the main risk factor for the development of corneal abrasions. EB: *Sedated clients or clients in induced comas may experience ineffective eye closure, presenting higher risk for corneal injury (Werli-Alvarenga et al, 2013). Consider a humidity chamber with polyethylene fill for best practice (Werli-Alvarenga et al, 2013).*
- EBN: *Eye care and eye assessment should be essential parts of nursing care for clients in intensive care. To prevent corneal abrasions, use eye lubricants, which are more effective than closing eyes by adhesive tapes (Masoudi et al, 2013).*

Client/Family Teaching and Discharge Planning

- ▲ First-aid principles should be reinforced in the event of an eye injury. Clients should not attempt to remove any object in the eye; reserve this for the provider. A referral to an ophthalmologist may be required (Jacobs, 2017).
- Teach clients to use caution when using household cleaners. Many household products contain strong acids, alkalis, or other chemicals. Drain and oven cleaners are particularly dangerous, and can lead to blindness if not used correctly (Vorvick, 2014).
- If chemical exposure has occurred, flush the eye immediately with clean water for 10 minutes. Seek prompt health care attention.
- Wear safety goggles at all times when using hand or power tools or chemicals, during high-impact sports, or in other situations when eye injury is more likely.
- Wear sunglasses that screen ultraviolet light when outdoors, even in winter.
- Pain is usually improved within 3 days. If pain becomes intolerable, an analgesic may be prescribed short term. Seek medical attention if pain is not resolving.
- Driving should be restricted for safety until client's visual acuity is evaluated.

● = Independent; ▲ = Collaborative; **EBN** = Evidence-Based Nursing; **EB** = Evidence-Based

REFERENCES

Cleveland Clinic. (2015). *Corneal abrasion*. Retrieved from http://my.clevelandclinic.org/services/cole-eye/diseases-conditions/hic-corneal-abrasion. (Accessed 31 October 2017).

Jacobs, D. S. (2017). *Corneal abrasions and injury*. Retrieved from http://www.uptodate.com/contents/corneal-abrasions-and-corneal-foreign-bodies-management?source=see_link. (Accessed 31 October 2017).

Lim, C. H., Turner, A., & Lim, B. X. (2016). Patching for corneal abrasion. *The Cochrane Database of Systematic Reviews*, (7), CD004764.

Lin, Y. B., & Gardiner, M. F. (2014). Fingernail-induced corneal abrasions: Case series from an ophthalmology emergency department. I. *Cornea*, *33*(7), 691–695.

Masoudi, A. N., Sharifitabar, Z., Shaeri, M., et al. (2013). An audit of eye dryness and corneal abrasion in ICU patients in Iran. *British Association of Critical Care Nurses*, *19*(2), 73–77.

Menghini, M., Knecht, P. B., Kaufmann, C., et al. (2013). Treatment of traumatic corneal abrasion: A three-arm prospective randomized study. *Ophthalmic Research*, *50*(1), 13–18.

Malafa, M., Coleman, E., Bowman, R., et al. (2016). Perioperative corneal abrasion: Updated guidelines for prevention and management. *American Society of Plastic Surgeons*, *137*, 790e.

Segal, K. L., Fleischut, P. M., Kim, C., et al. (2014). Evaluation and treatment of perioperative corneal abrasions. *Journal of Ophthalmology*, 320–326. Retrieved from http://dx.doi.org/10.1155/2014/901901. (Accessed 31 October 2017).

Werli-Alvarenga, A., Ercole, F. F., Herdman, T. H., et al. (2013). Nursing interventions for adult intensive care patients with risk for corneal injury: A systemic review. *International Journal of Nursing Knowledge*, *24*(1), 25–29.

Wakai, A., Lawrenson, J. G., Lawrenson, A. L., et al. (2017). Topical non-steroidal anti-inflammatory drugs for analgesia in traumatic corneal abrasion. *The Cochrane Database of Systematic Reviews*, (5), CD009781.

Verma, A., & Khan, H. R. (2014). *Corneal abrasion*. Retrieved from http://emedicine.medscape.com/article/1195402-overview. (Accessed 31 October 2017).

Vorvick, L. J. (2014). *Corneal injury*. Retrieved from http://umm.edu/health/medical/ency/articles/corneal-injury. (Accessed 31 October 2017).

Risk for occupational Injury   *Kathleen Buckheit, MPH, BSN, RN, CEN, COHN-S/CM, CCM, FAAOHN*

NANDA-I

Definition

Susceptible to sustain a work-related accident or illness, which may compromise health.

Risk Factors

Individual

Excessive stress; improper use of personal protective equipment; inadequate role performance; inadequate time management; ineffective coping strategies; insufficient knowledge; misinterpretation of information; psychological distress; unsafe acts of overconfidence; unsafe acts of unhealthy negative habits

Environmental

Distraction from social relationships; exposure to biological agents; exposure to chemical agents; exposure to extremes of temperature; exposure to noise; exposure to radiation; exposure to teratogenic agents; exposure to vibration; inadequate physical environment; labor relationships; lack of personal protective equipment; night shift work rotating to day shift work; occupational burnout; physical workload; shift work

NOC   (Nursing Outcomes Classification)

Suggested NOC Outcomes

Personal Health and Safety Behaviors; Risk Control; Adequate Training

Example NOC Outcome with Indicators
Occupational Health as evidence by Knowledge and compliance with health and safety policies and procedures/Demonstration of personal health-promoting behaviors/Knowledge and self-management of a healthy lifestyle. (Rate the outcome and indicators of **Occupational Health:** 1 = never demonstrated, 2 = rarely demonstrated, 3 = sometimes demonstrated, 4 = often demonstrated, 5 = consistently demonstrated [see Section I].)

● = Independent;   ▲ = Collaborative;   EBN = Evidence-Based Nursing;   EB = Evidence-Based

Client Outcomes

Client Will (Specify Time Frame)

- Attend and participate in all required health and safety training activities
- Demonstrate safe and healthy work behaviors to reduce the risk of occupational injuries and illnesses
- Comply with the organization's health and safety policies and procedures
- Inspect all equipment and tools before use
- Report to management any work hazards, such as facility, tools, and equipment that needs to be repaired
- Demonstrate healthy personal habits, such as healthy nutritional choices, regular exercise, smoking cessation, and effective sleep patterns

NIC   (Nursing Interventions Classification)

Suggested NIC Interventions

Health Coaching; Health Education; Health Screening; Risk Identification

Example NIC Activities—Risk for Occupational Injury

Encourage early reporting of signs and symptoms related to health and safety hazard exposures

Nursing Interventions and *Rationales*

- Interventions to reduce the risks of occupational injury focus on providing resources for safe work and education to the individual to know safety rules and procedures. Occupational safety requires the individual to engage in safe acts, proper use of equipment to include personal protective equipment (PPE), cognitive focus during work, and self-identification of stressors that may adversely impact the individual's personal safety during work.
- Environmental risks that need to be addressed to ensure a safe work environment focus on elements such as excessive noise, poorly maintained equipment or lack of PPE, uneven or poorly designed work spaces, inadequate lighting, and lack of safety training.
- Alternating shift work or night shift work provides an additional risk related to reduced strength and chronic fatigue. EB: *A study looked at nurses' strength and fatigue relative to day or night shift work. A compressed nursing work schedule was found to result in decreased strength and fatigue placing the individual at increased risk for occupational injury (Thompson, Stock, & Banuelas, 2017). A study by Larsen et al (2017) found that individuals exposed to night work were more likely to have accidental injuries compared with nonnight shift workers.*
- Assist the client in reduction of personal and work stress and distractions to increase coping skills, improve interpersonal relationships, and increase personal job performance and satisfaction. Emphasize paying attention to work activities and environment in hazardous and normal work situations. EB: *A variety of studies have examined the relationship between job stress and job performance. Job performance has been viewed as an activity in which an individual is able to successfully accomplish the tasks assigned, dependent on the normal constraints of reasonable utilization of the available resources. According to a study by Dar (2011), job stress had a negative relationship with job performance so that when stress occurs it negatively effects the employee's performance, and when stress is lowered, the performance increases.*
- The stress in the work environment negatively effects the intention of employees to perform better in their jobs. EB: *When considering work stress, evidence showed that job stress results in employees feeling undervalued and workplace victimization/bullying, unclear role/errands, and fear of joblessness increases. Recommendations included that organizations should reduce psychological strain, work overload, and role ambiguity through the adoption of job redesign techniques and organizational support of counseling and stress reduction workshops (Dar, 2011).*
- Maintaining good interpersonal relationships and communications with management and coworkers can be achieved by leaders who encourage high-quality relationships among employees in the workplace. Strong interpersonal relationships assist in developing trust, respect, and a willingness to share information, resources, and perspectives (Phillips, Rothbard, & Dumas, 2009).
- Cognitive distractions tend to decrease productivity and increase the number of errors workers make (Ratwani, Trafton, & Myers, 2006). CEB: *Disruptive behaviors, interruptions, and nonoccupational activities,*

● = Independent;   ▲ = Collaborative;   EBN = Evidence-Based Nursing;   EB = Evidence-Based

such as use of cell phones and radio headsets, might need to be prohibited while on duty to reduce distractions (Ratwani, Trafton, & Myers, 2006).

- Visual deprivation occurs when pedestrians elect to look at the cell phone screen, reducing the available skills necessary to see features in the walking environment. **EB:** *The Ohio State University reports that an estimate of more than 1500 pedestrians were treated in emergency rooms in 2010 for injuries related to using a cell phone while walking, which is more than double the number of cases seen in 2005, according to their nationwide study. According to the researcher, "The role of cell phones in distracted driving injuries and deaths gets a lot of attention and rightly so, but we need to also consider the danger cell phone use poses to pedestrians." The study found that those ages 16 to 25 were most likely to be injured as distracted pedestrians, and most were hurt while talking rather than texting* (Nasar & Troyer, 2013).

- Assist in the integration of personal health behaviors that promote total worker health and safety for the employee, which translates to a more productive worker generating better quality products, resulting in less occupational injuries and illnesses for the workers**. EB:** *Studies have shown that health education activities and materials should address prevention topics for modifiable behaviors observed to be injury risk factors, such as overuse of alcohol and drugs, stress, tobacco use, and poor sleep habits* (Schuh-Renner et al, 2017).

- A community-based study found that gender, young age, regular psychotropic drug use, and diseases influence the occupational injuries. Smokers, overweight subjects, and excess alcohol use also had increased risk for occupational injury. **CEB:** *Preventive measures concerning work conditions, risk assessment, and job knowledge should be conducted. A campaign should be implemented to address concerns with this group of workers that are exposed to higher risk to prevent occupational injury* (Bhattacherjee et al, 2003).

- Sleep is an active process enabling the body to restore and regenerate. Adequate sleep is essential to health and cognitive function. It is critical for cell repair, immune system health, and regulation of hormones, and it critically aids in learning, memory, and emotion. **EB:** *Long-term inadequate sleep can result in many chronic health and mental conditions. The two common sleep disorders affecting the workplace are insomnia and obstructive sleep apnea, which can negatively affect quality of life and increase work-related injuries* (Judd, 2017).

- Maintaining good sleep hygiene promotes alertness and results in decreased occupational injuries and illnesses. However, good sleep hygiene may be difficult in employees without consistent sleep patterns. **CEB:** *A study by Dembe et al (2005) found that working schedules routinely involving overtime work or extended hours increased the risk of injury or illness. Overtime schedules had the greatest relative risk, followed by long daily shifts (>12 hours) or long work weeks (>60 hours). These results indicate that long working hours indirectly precipitate workplace accidents from fatigue or stress* (Dembe et al, 2005).

- Sensory deprivation, also called environmental isolation, occurs when the use of cell phones and other electronics results in limited hearing and peripheral vision. **EB:** *When pedestrians are wearing headphones or are engaged in conversation on a cell phone, the inability to hear sounds emanating from the local surroundings may present unique problems in walking environments in which auditory cues can be more important than visual ones, such as around trains* (Lichenstein et al, 2012).

- Fatigue has been associated with negative safety outcomes. Poor-quality or decreased sleep has been associated with obesity (higher body mass index [BMI]), and higher BMI rates are related to increased injury risk. Sleep is an active process; the body undergoes restoration and regeneration. According to Judd (2017), adequate sleep is essential to health and cognitive function. Sleep is critical for cell repair, a healthy immune system, and hormonal regulation, and aids in the process of learning, memory, and emotion. Inadequate sleep can lead to multiple chronic health and mental conditions over time. The occupational health nurse can be instrumental in screening for two of the most common sleep disorders, insomnia and obstructive sleep apnea, by asking workers key questions and using simple screening tools to prevent the negative effects of sleep disorders on quality of life and increase in work-related injuries (Judd, 2017). **EB:** *Results from a large sample of US workers found an increase in injury risk for reduced sleep habits, regardless of body mass, but also shows an increase in injury risk for higher BMI, regardless of usual daily sleep duration* (Lombardi et al, 2012).

- When the Occupational Safety and Health Administration (OSHA) professionals understand potential interruptions and adopt a task-design–oriented approach founded in ergonomics and human factors principles and methods, they can focus on aspects of the work environment that can be observed, measured, and controlled. **EB:** *Using signs, a no-interruptions zone, personal electronics policies, and available technologies to promote attention-keeping and interruption recovery can be implemented by organizations to maintain safe environments* (Cohen, LaRue, & Cohen, 2017).

● = Independent;   ▲ = Collaborative;   **EBN** = Evidence-Based Nursing;   **EB** = Evidence-Based

- Provide medical screening, surveillance, and postexposure testing for symptomatic employees to identify and provide the focus on the exposure to control effects that can lead to illness and injury. **EB:** *OSHA requires that exposures to specific hazards require a medical surveillance program to identify adverse effects related to those exposures. OSHA Standards provide the opportunity to monitor exposure to health hazards from inhalation, ingestion, or skin absorption from chemical, biological agent, or radiological exposures. The fundamental purpose of screening is early diagnosis and treatment with a clinical focus, whereas surveillance is to detect and eliminate the underlying causes providing a prevention focus. Although both contribute to worksite health and safety programs, OSHA "medical surveillance" is generally clinically focused to include medical and work histories, physical assessment, and biological testing, which is used in the monitoring and analysis elements of medical surveillance (United States Department of Labor, OSHA, 2000). According to OSHA, "Medical surveillance is the analysis of health information to look for problems that may be occurring in the workplace that require targeted prevention. Thus, surveillance serves as a feedback loop to the employer. OSHA Surveillance may be based on a single case or sentinel event, but more typically uses screening results from the group of employees being evaluated to look for abnormal trends in health status" (United States Department of Labor, OSHA, 2000).*
- Although compliance with health and safety policies and procedures must be encouraged and enforced, when the employee becomes ill or injured, the occupational health nurse must provide assessment and treatment. **EB:** *Occupational health nursing focuses on promotion and restoration of health, prevention of illness and injury, protection from work-related and environmental hazards, and corporate profitability (McCullagh & Berry, 2015). The roles of today's occupational health nurses are diverse, and their position responsibilities cover an ever-expanding range of tasks. Occupational health nurses can assist employers in controlling their health care costs and maintaining business health by developing, implementing, and evaluating health promotion and disease and injury prevention programs and services for specific workers (Thompson & Wachs, 2012).*
- Many workers have comorbidities (e.g., hypertension, diabetes, hyperlipidemia, asthma), some of which are related to lifestyle choices or the environment. **EB:** *In a study by Duffy et al (2011) operating engineers were found to have many health behavior risk factors, including smoking, drinking alcohol, diet, exercise, sleep, and sun exposure.*
- Implementing programs that assist overweight and obese workers to increase both strengthening and cardiovascular exercise can result in weight loss and also reduce employees' risk of injury and chronic diseases and improve their mobility and quality of life. Health coaching is the use of evidence-based skillful conversation, clinical strategies, and interventions to actively and safely engage clients in health behavior change to better self-manage their health, health risk(s), and acute or chronic health conditions, resulting in optimal wellness, improved health outcomes, lowered health risk, and decreased health care costs (Huffman, 2016). **EB:** *Rather than focusing on health education, nurses and other health care professionals are now using health coaching based on motivational interviewing to assist workers in changing health-related behaviors (Huffman, 2016).*
- Encourage early reporting of signs and symptoms related to health hazard exposures to provide early recognition and treatment, which is aimed at reducing disability, pain, and workers' compensation costs; absence; and retraining and replacement workers. *Work accommodations may be necessary to keep the employee working.*
- Case management to ensure appropriate referrals and communication is necessary to achieve safe work environment goals and include follow-up assessment to ensure that the worker is not further injured or ill by the accommodated work situation. *Providing appropriate medical referrals and interdisciplinary collaboration can reduce occupational risks to health and safety.*
- OSHA requires a mechanism that identifies to whom the employees report injuries and illnesses and that they are encouraged to do so as early as possible. One of OSHA's strategies is to be proactive and reduce injuries and illnesses by implementing a reporting system that would develop and communicate a simple procedure for workers to report any injuries, illnesses, incidents (including near misses/close calls), hazards, or safety and health concerns without fear of retaliation. This also includes an option for reporting hazards or concerns anonymously (United States Department of Labor, OSHA, 2016a). *Educating the employees on the signs and symptoms of occupational disease is critical to stop and reverse the process before disability results. Early reporting of signs and symptoms related to health hazard exposures provides for the best outcomes of treatment (United States Department of Labor, OSHA, 2016a).*
- Occupational back pain is a multifactorial condition commonly encountered in the workforce. It is very costly for the health care system and industry but can be prevented or limited in its severity. **EB:** *Discouraging*

● = Independent;   ▲ = Collaborative;   **EBN** = Evidence-Based Nursing;   **EB** = Evidence-Based

bed rest and promoting early return to work with modified job tasks in which accommodations avoid back injury risk factors, individualized interventions, and with follow-up monitoring for assurance is encouraged as part of the rehabilitation program (Al-Otaibi, 2015).

- Enforce compliance with organizational and regulatory health and safety policies and procedures, demonstrating at least adequate training and the proper use of appropriate tools, equipment, and PPE to reduce risk of injury and illness and ensure that the client receives appropriate training and education on occupational tasks and equipment. *Health education activities and materials should address prevention topics for modifiable behaviors observed to be injury risk factors, such as overuse of alcohol and drugs, stress, tobacco use, and poor sleep habits (Farnacio et al, 2017).*

- *Ensuring that workers are following policies can reduce exposure and illness when exposed to chemicals.* EB: *Studies have been done focusing on chemical exposures among agricultural workers and their families, using community-based participatory research methods to work with vulnerable, difficult to access working populations. Research has documented the effects of low levels of pesticide exposures on neurobehavioral performance in adults and children of agricultural workers (McCauley, 2012).*

- Ensure workers have access to and wear PPE to reduce noise exposure. Engineering and administrative controls should be considered before the use of PPE. EB: *A United Auto Workers–General Motors–funded study assessed the effects of noise on blood pressure and heart rate that demonstrated a significant positive relationship between acute noise exposure and both diastolic and systolic blood pressure and heart rate. In assessing the effect of chronic noise exposure, workers who used hearing protection had lower blood pressure and heart rate than workers without hearing protection (McCauley, 2012).*

- A critical component in safety risk management is to adequately identify hazards and mitigate its associated risk using safety program elements (Yorio & Wachter, 2014). EB: *An American Society of Safety Engineers (ASSE) published a study identifying quality measures of occupational health and safety management system (OHSMS) activities as important performance variables. Quality measures to consider include safety training test scores, correction rates of inspection nonconformance findings, and perception survey results on the state of the organizational culture and its conduciveness to safe operations (Haight et al, 2014).*

- Employees are at risk when exposed to welding fumes, dust, or chemicals. Continued exposure to these substances can place employees at risk for permanent lung changes. EB: *Research illustrates that the health of workers is affected by continued exposure to welding fumes released by the cutting or connecting of metal using a welding technique (Roach, 2017). Exposure to welding fumes is completely preventable. Provide resources to the client to guide ways to address organizational policies and procedures to prevent exposure to fumes during welding work (United States Department of Labor, OSHA, 2016b).*

- Noise in health care varies according to the type of facility and patient care rendered. Mechanical noise from equipment (i.e., from alarms, monitors) can be disruptive to concentration, especially if it is loud and unexpected; patient vocalization depending on the cause (i.e., from pain, fear, disorientation) and amount, volume, and length of time can be considered another type of stressor. Published studies indicate that noise levels in hospitals, particularly in intensive care units (ICUs), are above those recommended by OSHA and have been measured at 90 dB-A, the Action level of the OSHA Noise Standard. Staff exposed to excessive noise experience anxiety and stress and can cause other psychological effects associated with annoyance. The Joint Commission on Accreditation of Healthcare Organizations has identified noise as a potential risk factor for medical and nursing errors, stating that ambient sound should not exceed the level that would prohibit clinicians from clearly understanding each other, so that nurses are not at risk of error when the noise level is 40 dB-A or greater. EB: *In a study by Kol et al (2015), rearranging the nurses' station and treatment area, providing staff education, displaying a sign to remind staff and visitors that noise is constantly monitored in the ICU setting, and implementing repairs to ICU equipment were effective noise reduction measures that resulted in a statistically significant decrease (P < .05) in noise levels (Kol et al, 2015).*

- Ensure that infection prevention and control policies and procedures are enforced. Blood-borne pathogen risks are inherent when providing nursing care in health care facilities of for injured or ill employees, and appropriate measures must be taken to avoid contact with and spread of infectious organisms.

- Ensure appropriate protection is initiated when workers are exposed to those considered contagious through airborne exposure. Respiratory protection is required when airborne or droplet exposure to disease agents is suspected. Appropriate selection, training, and fit-testing is required before use of respirators is allowed.

- Provide resources to assist with smoking/vaping cessation. According to the American Lung Association (2018), smoking is the leading cause of preventable death in the United States, causing more than 438,000

● = Independent;   ▲ = Collaborative;   EBN = Evidence-Based Nursing;   EB = Evidence-Based

deaths per year, and worsening preexisting conditions including cardiovascular disease. Cigars have many of the same health risks as cigarettes, including causing certain cancers. Marijuana smoke contains many of the same toxins, irritants, and carcinogens as tobacco smoke. Smokeless tobacco products are a known cause of cancer and are not a safe alternative to cigarettes. Secondhand smoke is a serious health hazard for people of all ages, causing more than 41,000 deaths each year (American Lung Association, 2018). Electronic cigarettes are a new tobacco product, and the potential health consequences and safety of these products are unknown. The process of using an e-cigarette is called "vaping" rather than smoking. The US Food and Drug Administration (FDA) describes an e-cigarette as a battery-operated device that turns nicotine, formaldehyde, flavorings (diacetyl that causes popcorn lung), and other chemicals into a vapor that can be inhaled. WebMD.com (2018) provides information about smoking and smoking cessation programs that can be helpful when counseling employees as to the adverse effects of smoking (https://www.webmd.com/smoking-cessation/default.htm).

- Provide interdisciplinary collaboration to reduce occupational risks to health and safety. According to Wachs (2005), teamwork is beneficial to American business and industry because of its strength through diversity when a variety of interdisciplinary health and safety professionals offer solutions to complex problems. Teamwork among occupational health and safety professionals, management, and employees is vital to solving complex problems cost-effectively. No single discipline can meet all the needs of workers and the workplace (Wachs, 2005). OSHA has identified that an effective occupational safety and health program involves many components and recommended practices (United States Department of Labor, OSHA, 2016a).
- Maintain a drug-free workplace through the identification of abuse of prescription and illegal drugs, which includes any substance that inhibits the mental, emotional, and physical functioning of the worker.
- Provide accurate and legal documentation for medical and exposure records with adverse health effects from health and safety exposures, maintaining confidentiality of personal medical issues. Legal requirements for documentation ensure correct communication of all aspects of the injury or illness and protects the nurse in case of litigation.
- Documentation communicates information about the employee and confirms that care was provided using the NANDA nursing diagnoses, the NIC, and the NOC as the basis for documentation. **EB:** *All charting should be accurate, complete, objective, and timely. There are several charting guidelines related to vocabulary, descriptions, legibility, errors, and omissions to ensure that charting meets legal requirements and provides an accurate unbiased record of client care. There are many different types of documentation and very little consistency from one organization to another. Each state has its own Nurse Practice Act, but all establish guidelines for documentation and accountability. These include the nursing process of assessment, diagnosis, planning, implementation, and evaluation. The Nurse Practice Act provides for standardized vocabulary, a list of approved abbreviations and symbols, and using legible writing in blue or black ink. Errors require a line to delete with "Error" and a signature; errors cannot be erased, whited-out, or otherwise made illegible (Lockwood, 2017).*
- OSHA *documentation specifics* include medical, exposure, and training records that must be retained for a period of time, usually at least 30 years. The documentation provides a history of the employee's exposure to hazards, assessment and treatment received, and any worksite hazard abatements or reduction to exposures, and any outcomes of exposure and treatments (United States Department of Labor, OSHA, 2011).
- The Health Insurance Portability and Accountability Act (HIPAA) and Privacy Rule provide the right of privacy to the client, and this extends to all forms of documentation related to the client. *HIPAA of 1996 documents the rights of the individual in relation to privacy regarding health information. The final Privacy Rule, issued in 2000 and modified in 2002, provides for the right to decide who can have access to private health information and requires health care providers to provide confidentiality. Personal employee information is considered protected health information (PHI), which includes any identifying or personal information about the health history, condition, or treatments in any form, including electronic, verbal, or written documentation. Some areas provide extra confidentiality, including assessment and treatment of HIV, substance abuse, rape, pregnancy, and psychiatric disorders (Lockwood, 2017; United States Department of Labor, OSHA, 2013).*
- Considerations for nursing practice include the following:
  - Identify high-risk work areas and processes for developing occupational injuries and illnesses through (1) auditing of injury and illness reports and insurance claims and (2) conducting periodic walkthroughs of the workplace for unsafe acts and conditions.

● = Independent; ▲ = Collaborative; **EBN** = Evidence-Based Nursing; **EB** = Evidence-Based

○ Encourage employee compliance with safety policies and procedures to reduce the opportunity for (1) slips, trips, and falls; (2) breaks in skin integrity through chemical exposure, mechanical means (trauma, friction, pressure), physical exposure (heat, cold, radiation), and exposure to biological elements (viruses, bacteria, fungi); (3) musculoskeletal injuries; and (4) misuse of equipment and tools.

○ Ensure appropriate training through medical, exposure, and training records and notify management to correct when necessary.

○ Ensure employee availability and understanding of accurate and current Safety Data Sheets for all personnel.

○ Encourage early reporting of signs and symptoms related to health and safety hazard exposures.

○ Provide appropriate primary, secondary, and tertiary prevention strategies to ensure the health and safety of the workforce.

○ For adverse effects of workplace exposures, counsel employees, notify management, and follow OSHA standards (and other regulatory requirements) and company policies and procedures to reduce exposure and reverse the adverse effects to workers.

○ Promote and assist employees in integrating personal health behaviors that lead to total worker health and safety, such as not smoking or using vapes; exercise; weight loss; stress reduction; hypertension reduction; drug and alcohol-controlled use; and managing personal health issues, such as blood sugar levels.

○ Monitor employees for an adverse health status through medical surveillance and physical assessment examinations required for workplace exposures, such as chemicals, noise, ergonomic issues, pulmonary stressors, and radiation.

○ Provide employee counseling specific to employee, health status, and work processes.

○ Encourage compliance with health and safety policies and procedures that reduces opportunity exposure to health hazards from inhalation; ingestion; or skin absorption from chemical, biological agent, or radiological exposure.

○ Encourage early reporting of signs and symptoms related to health hazard exposures.

○ Provide postexposure testing for symptomatic employees or per specific organizational policies and procedures.

○ Provide interdisciplinary collaboration to reduce occupational risks to health and safety.

○ Provide appropriate medical referrals as needed.

○ Provide accurate and legal documentation for medical and exposure records with adverse health effects from health and safety exposures.

○ Maintain confidentiality of personal medical issues.

Geriatric

• Consider the physiological changes in the aging population. *The aging workforce typically has experienced changes in their physical systems that require attention to physical needs. These changes may include slower reaction times, predisposing factors to developing musculoskeletal disorders, a compromised cardiovascular system, less acute hearing and vision, and impaired cognition (Algarni et al, 2015).*

• Although older clients may experience less occupational injuries and illnesses, the aging workforce may take longer to heal injuries and return to work and normal functioning. EB: *A review of current best practices by Delloiacono (2015) found that the extent of age-related physical changes in older workers is significantly influenced by chronic illnesses. However, improving lifestyles could reduce organizational costs, and reducing costs is important because although older worker statistics report lower work-related injury rates, their recovery is slower and lost work time is longer. Also, identifying ergonomic risk factors will assist in workplace design improvements in workplace to reduce risks of musculoskeletal disorders for the aging population (Delloiacono, 2015).*

Multicultural

• Address differences in cultures that affect attitudes toward health care professionals and treatment modalities. *Understanding the written and verbal language can significantly affect the instructions and training given to workers.*

• According to the Centers for Disease Control and Prevention (CDC, 2018), young workers have high rates of job-related injury. These injuries are often the result of the many hazards present in the places they typically work, such as sharp knives and slippery floors in restaurants. Limited or no prior work experience and a lack of safety training also contribute to high injury rates. Middle and high school

• = Independent; ▲ = Collaborative; EBN = Evidence-Based Nursing; EB = Evidence-Based

I

workers may be at increased risk for injury because they may not have the strength or cognitive ability needed to perform certain job duties. *In 2016, there were about 19.3 million workers under the age of 24. These workers represented 13% of the total workforce, and in 2015, 403 workers under the age of 24 died from work-related injuries (CDC, 2018).*

- The US workforce is becoming more diverse (National Center for Public Policy Research, 2005). Baby boomers are remaining in the workforce past traditional retirement age because their health is better, and they need or want additional income (Bureau of Labor Statistics, 2008). Physical changes occur with the aging workforce that need to be addressed, such as decreased visual acuity that requires increased lighting, decreased hearing from presbycusis, difficulty with balance, and increase in healing time from musculoskeletal injuries. **EB:** *According to a study by Loeppke et al (2013), issues were explored related to the aging workforce, including barriers to integrating health promotion and protection programs to provide recommendations for best practices to maximize contributions of that worker population. Reducing injury costs is important because although older worker statistics report lower work-related injury rates, their recovery is slower and lost work time is longer. The conclusion was a national dialog on this topic was needed, and the result will be that workers will benefit from improved health and job performance, employers will have more productive and engaged workers, and the United States will have a more competitive workforce (Loeppke et al, 2013).*

- The size of the minority workforce is growing, and more women are entering the workforce (Thompson and Wachs, 2012). There is greater diversity in the workplace, and people from different backgrounds and cultures are working alongside each other, often speaking different languages with different educational and literacy backgrounds. **EB:** *As the minority workforce continues to grow, especially the Hispanic workforce, businesses must recognize the unique needs and contributions of this workforce in terms of language, customs, culture, and values (Thompson and Wachs, 2012). According to Burgel, Nelson, and White (2015), results of a study on Latino day workers add to the growing body of research documenting the higher prevalence of work-related health complaints or injuries among those workers with work-related health complaints or injuries who were older, reporting poor or fair general physical and mental health, and more likely than those without health complaints or injury, to work in pain during the prior work week without work breaks. Most health complaints or injuries were unreported. Those that occurred within the prior year experienced a higher prevalence of depression and arthritis compared with their counterparts without work-related health complaints or injuries in the prior year. Recommendations were that occupational health nurses should promote the health of and prevent injuries among this group of vulnerable workers at both the individual and system levels.*

- Depending on the setting, comprehensive health care, including, for example, smoking cessation and early diagnosis and treatment of depression, could be provided to this high-risk population using culturally sensitive outreach and motivational interviewing strategies. **EB:** *Because of underreporting, active case findings for occupational injuries are needed when day laborers access any health care system. To ensure the provision of health and safety training and PPE for day laborers at the system level, occupational health nurses can advocate for comprehensive occupational health and safety legal protections for all contingent workers. Reporting health complaints and injuries, in addition to providing rest breaks, deserves further study in this population. In addition to targeted hearing conservation and respiratory protection programs for this high-risk group, the risk of falls from heights is a serious hazard facing day laborers, and this phenomenon also deserves further investigation (Burgel, Nelson, & White, 2015).*

- As women continue to earn significantly less than their male counterparts, they may believe that they need to work harder to prove themselves to earn the promotions and higher pay scales. *The nurse may recognize these situational stressors and need to refer female employees more than the male employees for counseling, such as initiating assistance offered by employee assistance programs or community resources for family support.*

- The Americans with Disabilities Act (ADA) requires that public buildings be designed to accommodate wheelchairs and other accommodations and that jobs be modified if accommodation is reasonable, so more challenged individuals gain access to buildings and jobs (see https://www.ada.gov/ada_req_ta.htm [ADA]).

● = Independent;   ▲ = Collaborative;   **EBN** = Evidence-Based Nursing;   **EB** = Evidence-Based

REFERENCES

Algarni, F. S., Gross, D. P., Senthilselvan, A., et al. (2015). Ageing workers with work-related musculoskeletal injuries. *Occupational Medicine, 65*(3), 229–237.

Al-Otaibi, S. T. (2015). Prevention of occupational back pain. *Journal of Family Community Medicine, 22*(2), 73–77.

American Lung Association. *Smoking Facts*. Retrieved from http://www.lung.org/stop-smoking/smoking-facts/. (Accessed 12 April 2018).

Americans with Disabilities Act. *ADA requirements and technical assistance*. Retrieved from https://www.ada.gov/ada_req_ta.htm. (Accessed 2 January 2018).

Bhattacherjee, A., Chau, N., Sierro, C. O., et al. (2003). Relationships of job and some individual characteristics to occupational injuries in employed people: A community-based study. *Journal of Occupational Health, 45*(6), 382–391.

Bureau of Labor Statistics. (2008). *More seniors working fulltime*. Retrieved from https://www.bls.gov/opub/ted/2008/aug/wk1/art03.htm. (Accessed 2 January 2018).

Burgel, B., Nelson, R. W., Jr., & White, M. C. (2015). Work-related health complaints and injuries, and health and safety perceptions of Latino day laborers. *Workplace Health & Safety., 63*(8), 350–361.

Centers for Disease Control and Prevention (CDC), (2018). *Workplace safety and health*. Retrieved from https://www.cdc.gov/niosh/injury/data.html. (Accessed 1 May 2018).

Cohen, J., LaRue, C., & Cohen, H. H. (2017). Attention interrupted - cognitive distraction & workplace safety. *Professional Safety, 2017*(11), 28–34. Retrieved from http://www.safetybok.org/assets/1/7/F1_1117.pdf. (Accessed 1 December 2017).

Dar, L., Akmal, A., Naseem, M. A., et al. (2011). Impact of stress on employees job performance in business sector of Pakistan. *Global Journal of Management and Business Research, 11*(6). Retrieved from https://globaljournals.org/GJMBR_Volume11/1-Impact-of-Stress-on-Employees-Job-Performance.pdf. (Accessed 12 December 2017).

Delloiacono, N. (2015). Musculoskeletal safety for older adults in the workplace review of current best practice evidence. *Workplace Health & Safety, 63*(2), 48–53.

Dembe, A. E., Erickson, J. B., Delbos, R. G., et al. (2005). The impact of overtime and long work hours on occupational injuries and illnesses: New evidence from the United States. *Occupational and Environmental Medicine, 47*(62), 588–597.

Duffy, S. A., Missel, A. L., Waltje, A. H., et al. (2011). Health behaviors of operating engineers. *AAOHN Journal, 59*(7), 293–301.

Farnacio, Y., Pratt, M. E., Marshall, E. G., et al. (2017). Are workplace psychosocial factors associated with work-related injury in the US workforce?: National Health Interview Survey, 2010. *Journal of Occupational and Environmental Medicine, 59*(10), 164–171.

Haight, J. M., Yorio, P., Rost, K. A., et al. (2014). Safety management systems comparing content & impact. *ASSE Professional Safety, May 2014*, 44–51. Retrieved from https://www.asse.org/assets/1/7/PSJ_Haight_Safety_Management_Systems.pdf. (Accessed 4 January 2018).

Huffman, M. (2016). Advancing the practice of health coaching —Differentiation from wellness coaching. *Workplace Health & Safety., 64*(9), 400–403.

Judd, S. R. (2017). Uncovering common sleep disorders and their impacts on occupational performance. *Workplace Health and Safety, 65*(5), 232.

Kol, E., Demircan, A., Erdogn, A., et al. (2015). The effectiveness of measures aimed at noise reduction in an intensive care unit. *Workplace Health and Safety, 63*(12), 539–545.

Larsen, A. D., Hannerz, H. M., Dyreborg, S. V., et al. (2017). Night work, long work weeks, and risk of accidental injuries: A register-based study. *Scandinavian Journal of Work, Environment, & Health, 43*(6), 578–586.

Lichenstein, R., Smith, D. C., Ambrose, J. L., et al. (2012). Headphone use and pedestrian injury and death in the U.S.: 2004–2011. *Injury Prevention, 2012*(18), 287–290.

Lockwood, W. (2017). *Documentation: Accurate and legal. WWW. RN.ORG®*. Retrieved from http://www.rn.org/courses/coursematerial-66.pdf. (Accessed 2 January 2018).

Lombardi, D. A., Wirtz, A., Willetts, J. L., et al. (2012). Independent effects of sleep duration and body mass index on the risk of a work-related injury: Evidence from the US National Health Interview Survey (2004–2010). *Chronobiology International, 29*(5), 556–564.

Loeppke, R. R., Schill, A. L., Chosewood, L. C., et al. (2013). Advancing workplace health protection and promotion for an aging workforce. *Journal of Occupational and Environmental Medicine, 55*(5), 500–506.

McCauley, L. A. (2012). Research to practice in occupational health nursing. *Workplace Health and Safety, 60*(4), 183–190.

McCullagh, M. C., & Berry, P. (2015). A safe and healthful work environment. *Workplace Health and Safety, 63*(8), 328–332.

Phillips, K. W., Rothbard, N. P., & Dumas, T. L. (2009). To disclose or not disclose: Status distance and self-disclosure in diverse environments. *Academy of Management Journal, 2009*(34), 710–732.

Nasar, J. L., & Troyer, D. (2013). Pedestrian injuries due to mobile phone use in public places. *Accident; Analysis and Prevention, 57*(8), 91–95.

National Center for Public Policy Research. (2005). *Income of U.S. workforce projected to decline if education doesn't improve*. Retrieved from http://www.highereducation.org/reports/pa_decline/index.shtml. (Accessed 12 April 2018).

Ratwani, R. M., Trafton, J. G., & Myers, C. (2006). *Helpful or harmful? Examining the effects of interruptions on task performance*. Proceedings of the Human Factors and Ergonomics Society 50th Annual Meeting (pp. 372–375).

Roach, L. L. (2017). The relationship of welding fume exposure, smoking, and pulmonary function in welders. *Workplace Health and Safety, 66*(1), 34–40.

Schuh-Renner, A., Canham-Chervak, M., Hearn, D. W., et al. (2017). Factors associated with injury among employees at a U.S. army hospital. *Workplace Health & Safety, 62*(12). Retrieved from https://doi.org/10.1177/2165079917736069. (Accessed 14 December 2017).

Thompson, M. C., & Wachs, J. E. (2012). Occupational health nursing in the United States. *Workplace Health and Safety, 60*(3), 127–133.

Thompson, B. J., Stock, M. S., & Banuelas, V. K. (2017). Effects of accumulating work shifts on performance-based fatigue using multiple strength measurements tin day and night shift nurses and aides. *The Journal of Human Factors and Ergonomics Society, 59*(3), 346–356.

United States Department of Labor, Occupational Safety and Health Administration (OSHA). (2000). *Medical screening and surveillance*. Retrieved from https://www.osha.gov/SLTC/medicalsurveillance/index.html. (Accessed 10 December 2017).

United States Department of Labor, Occupational Safety and Health Administration (OSHA). (2011). *Access to medical and exposure records*. Retrieved from https://www.osha.gov/Publications/osha3110.pdf. (Accessed 10 December 2017).

United States Department of Labor, Occupational Safety and Health Administration (OSHA). (2013). *Facts about hospital worker safety*. Retrieved from https://www.osha.gov/dsg/hospitals/documents/1.2_Factbook_508.pdf. (Accessed 10 December 2017).

United States Department of Labor, Occupational Safety and Health Administration (OSHA). (2016a). *Recommended practices for safety and health programs*. Retrieved from https://www.osha.gov/shpguidelines/docs/OSHA_SHP_Recommended_Practices.pdf. (Accessed 4 January 2018).

I

● = Independent;   ▲ = Collaborative;   **EBN** = Evidence-Based Nursing;   **EB** = Evidence-Based

United States Department of Labor, Occupational Safety and Health Administration. (2016b). *Welding OSHA fact sheet*. Retrieved from https://www.osha.gov/Publications/OSHA_FS-3647_Welding.pdf. (Accessed 4 January 2018).

Wachs, J. (2005). Building the occupational health team keys to successful interdisciplinary collaboration. *Workplace Health and Safety*, 53(4), 166–171.

WebMD.com. (2018). *Smoking cessation health center*. Retrieved from https://www.webmd.com/smoking-cessation/default.htm. (Accessed 11 November 2018).

Yorio, P. L., & Wachter, J. K. (2014). Safety-and-health-specific high-performance work practices & occupational injury and illness prevention: The mediating role of task & team safety proficiency behaviors. *ASSE Journal of Safety, Health & Environmental Research*, 10(1), 123–134.

Risk for urinary tract Injury　*Tammy Spencer, DNP, RN, CNE, AGCNS-BC, CCNS*

NANDA-I

Definition

Susceptible to damage of the urinary tract structures from use of catheters, which may compromise health.

Risk Factors

Confusion; deficient patient or caregiver knowledge regarding care of urinary catheter; obesity

At-Risk Population

Extremes of age

Associated Condition

Anatomical variation in the pelvic organs; condition preventing ability to secure catheter; detrusor sphincter dyssynergia; impaired cognition; latex allergy; long-term use of urinary catheter; medullary injury; multiple catheterizations; retention balloon inflated to ≥30 mL; use of large caliber urinary catheter

NOC　(Nursing Outcomes Classification)

Suggested NOC Outcomes

Urinary Elimination; Knowledge: Infection Management; Treatment Regimen; Treatment Procedure, Tissue Integrity: Skin and Mucous Membranes, Risk Control: Infectious Process, Risk Detection

> **Example NOC Outcome with Indicators**
>
> **Urinary Elimination** as evidenced by the following indicators: Urine clarity/Urine odor, Urine volume, fluid intake, pain with urination. (Rate the outcome and indicators of **Urinary Elimination:** 1 = severely compromised 2 = substantially compromised, 3 = moderately compromised, 4 = mildly compromised, 5 = not compromised [see Section I].)

Client Outcomes

Client Will (Specify Time Frame)

- Remain free of urinary tract injury
- State absence of pain with catheter care and during urination
- Experience unobstructed urination after removal of catheter
- Identify interventions to prevent catheter-associated urinary tract infection (CAUTI)
- Maintain adequate urine volume (0.5–1.0 mL/kg/hr for adult); urine without odor; urine clear
- Maintain adequate fluid intake considering client age and comorbidities

NIC　(Nursing Interventions Classification)

Suggested NIC Intervention

Urinary Elimination Management

● = Independent;　▲ = Collaborative;　EBN = Evidence-Based Nursing;　EB = Evidence-Based

Example NIC Activities—Urinary Elimination Management
Monitor urinary elimination, including frequency, consistency, odor, volume, and color, as appropriate; Assess client for pain and increased temperature associated with catheter

Nursing Interventions and *Rationales*

- Monitor urinary elimination, including frequency, consistency, odor, volume, and color, as appropriate.
- Teach the client and caregiver signs and symptoms of urinary tract infection and CAUTI. *Clients may be asymptomatic or have a range of symptoms that may include a persistent urge to urinate, burning sensation during urination, cloudy and/or strong-smelling urine, blood tinged urine, and fatigue.*
- Assess for appropriate use of an indwelling urinary catheter. Insert urinary catheters only when indicated and leave in only as long as clinically necessary. **EB:** *To prevent trauma to the urinary tract structure as well as infections (e.g., CAUTI and urosepsis), use urinary catheters only as indicated (Yokoe et al, 2014; Centers for Disease Control and Prevention [CDC], 2017). Approximately 80% of all health care–associated urinary tract infections are caused by urinary catheterization; infection represents the most significant adverse event following urinary catheter use (Lo et al, 2014; CDC, 2017). CAUTIs are linked to increased mortality, morbidity, hospital cost, antibiotic use, and length of stay (CDC, 2017). Health care providers need to have written guidelines for the use, insertion, and maintenance of urinary catheters (Lo et al, 2014; Yokoe et al, 2014).*
- ▲ To prevent injury, educate the client and family and/or caregiver regarding the use of an indwelling urinary catheter (Lo et al, 2014; Scott et al, 2014). **EB:** *Accidental or improper removal of catheter can cause urethral injury. Urinary catheters are used in up to 16% of adult hospital inpatients (Lo et al, 2014).*
- Assess clinical indication for urinary catheter daily. **EB:** *Studies found that 21% to 63% of all indwelling urinary catheters are inappropriately placed and are not medically indicated (Meddings et al, 2014). Minimize urinary catheter use in all clients, especially those at risk for CAUTI such as women, the elderly, and immunocompromised clients (Lo et al, 2014; CDC, 2017). Urinary catheter use is inappropriate when used as a substitute for nursing care of the incontinent client, when obtaining a urine culture for the client who can void, and for prolonged periods after surgery without appropriate indications (CDC, 2017). There is a 3% to 7% daily risk of bacteriuria when an indwelling urinary catheter remains in place (Lo et al, 2014). Decreasing the number of days the catheter is in place and avoiding unnecessary catheterization are the primary interventions to decrease CAUTI and unintended client harm (Lo et al, 2014; Meddings et al, 2014).*
- To avoid catheterizations, evaluate alternative strategies for managing urine output for the client. **EB:** *Developing toileting schedules, providing assistance with toileting, and incorporating toileting activities into frequent, scheduled nursing staff rounding can reduce urgency and incontinence episodes. For clients with limited mobility, use a bedside commode with a toileting schedule (Uberoi et al, 2013). Use moisture wicking incontinence pads to reduce moisture-associated skin injury (Oman et al, 2012). Consider using external catheters or intermittent catheterization in appropriate clients (CDC, 2017; Yokoe et al, 2014).*
- If an indwelling urinary catheter is determined to be clinically indicated in the care of a client, proper selection of the right catheter, technique during insertion, and evidence-based care management are needed to reduce infection and injury to the urinary tract structures.
  - ○ Perform hand hygiene and use Standard Precautions before and after insertion of the urinary catheter and any time the catheter, catheter site, or collection system is accessed (Yokoe et al, 2014; CDC, 2017).
  - ○ Ensure that only properly trained personnel familiar with appropriate catheter care techniques are used for inserting and maintaining the catheter (Yokoe et al, 2014; CDC, 2017). *Periodic in-service training helps personnel to maintain proper catheter care techniques (CDC, 2017).*
- Selecting the smallest catheter size (e.g., smaller than 18 French) reduces irritation and inflammation of the urethra and reduces infection risk (Yokoe et al, 2014; CDC, 2017).
- Insert the catheter using aseptic technique in the acute care setting. Wash hands and use sterile technique when opening the catheterization kit and cleansing the urethral meatus and perineal area with an antiseptic solution. Insert the catheter using a no-touch technique (Yokoe et al, 2014; CDC, 2017). In the nonacute care setting, nonsterile technique may be used for intermittent catheterization (CDC, 2017). *Using a no-touch technique may reduce the risk of infection.*
- Provide routine hygiene care; once a urinary catheter is placed, optimal management includes care of the urethral meatus according to "routine hygiene" (e.g., daily cleansing of the meatal surface during

● = Independent;　▲ = Collaborative;　EBN = Evidence-Based Nursing;　EB = Evidence-Based

bathing with soap and water and as needed, such as following a bowel movement) (Yokoe et al, 2014; CDC, 2017). Do not clean the periurethral area with antiseptics while the catheter is in place (CDC, 2017).

- Secure the catheter after placement to reduce friction and pain from movement (Clarke et al, 2013; Yokoe et al, 2014).
  - ❍ Disruptions in aseptic technique, disconnection, or leakage require the catheter and collection system to be replaced using aseptic technique and sterile equipment(Yokoe et al, 2014; CDC, 2017). *Risk factors for CAUTI include not maintaining a closed drainage system (Lo et al, 2014).*
  - ❍ Maintain unobstructed urine flow; maintain the catheter and collecting tube below the level of the bladder and free of kinks. Do not rest the collection bag on the floor. *Keeping the collection bag off the floor prevents contamination. Maintaining the urine collection bag below the level of the bladder and the catheter without kinks minimizes reflux into the catheter itself, preventing retrograde flow of urine and risk for infection (Lo et al, 2014; CDC, 2017).*
- Establish workflow protocols to routinely empty the drainage bag frequently and before transport to reduce urine reflux and opportunities for infection. *Use a separate, clean collecting container for each client when emptying the collection bag; avoid splashing, and prevent contact of the drainage spout with a nonsterile container (Lo et al, 2014; CDC, 2017). The collection bag of a bacteriuric client is a reservoir for organisms that may be transmitted by the hands of health care personnel to other clients (Lo et al, 2014).*
- Change urinary catheters and drainage systems based on clinical indications such as infection, obstruction, or when the drainage system is not adequately maintained. Changing indwelling catheters or drainage bags at a routine time interval is not recommended because it opens a closed drainage system and predisposes the client to infection (Lo et al, 2014; CDC, 2017).
- Monitor the client with an indwelling urinary catheter for increased temperature (>38°C), suprapubic pain, frequency, urgency, and flank pain; monitor the skin around the catheter for redness, drainage, or swelling. **EB:** The most common clinical presentation for CAUTI is fever with a positive urine culture (Lo et al, 2014). **EBN:** Monitor the client for CAUTI symptoms caused by localized or systemic inflammatory response (Blodgett et al, 2015).
- Consider an ultrasound scanner for clients who require intermittent catheterization to assess urine volume and reduce unnecessary catheter insertion (CDC, 2017).
- ▲ Implement systemwide quality improvement programs to include the following interventions to decrease CAUTI:
  - ❍ Establish health care provider alerts or reminders for all clients with catheters regarding the need for continued catheterization. **EB/EBN:** *Healthcare providers frequently forget that the catheter is in place, increasing the risk for CAUTI. Studies have shown the rate of CAUTI was decreased with the use of daily checklists, catheter reminders, and stop orders (Halm & O'Connor, 2014; CDC, 2017).*
  - ❍ Provide performance feedback and education to personnel responsible for catheter care (CDC 2017; Yokoe et al, 2014).
  - ❍ Establish evidence-based "bladder bundles" as part of a multimodal approach to preventing CAUTI. "Bladder bundles" may include educational interventions aimed at health care providers for appropriate use of urinary catheters, use of appropriately trained personnel to insert and care for the catheter, catheter restriction and removal protocols, and the use of bladder ultrasound to assess urine volume (Lo et al, 2014; Meddings et al, 2014). **EB/EBN:** *Evidence-based "bundles" of interventions, when implemented simultaneously, decrease the risk of CAUTI (**EB:** Lo et al, 2014; **EBN:** Halm & O'Connor, 2014).*

Home Care and Client/Family Teaching and Discharge Planning

- Teach the client and family discharged with an indwelling urinary catheter or performing intermittent catheterization at home techniques for care of urinary catheter and collection bag using the interventions listed above. (Clarke et al, 2013; Yokoe et al, 2014; CDC, 2017)
- Ensure client has adequate supplies at home for catheter insertion and care.
- Teach the client and family to contact the health care provider regarding symptoms of CAUTI including increased temperature (>38°C), suprapubic pain, frequency, urgency, and flank pain; no drainage of urine in the collection bag; and foul smelling, cloudy, or bloody urine (Medline Plus, 2017).
- Teach the client and family methods to keep the urinary tract healthy. Refer to Client/Family Teaching in the care plan for Readiness for enhanced **Urinary** elimination.

• = Independent;   ▲ = Collaborative;   EBN = Evidence-Based Nursing;   EB = Evidence-Based

REFERENCES

Blodgett, T. J., Gardner, S. E., Blodgett, N. P., et al. (2015). A tool to assess the signs and symptoms of catheter associated urinary tract infection: Development and reliability. *Clinical Nursing Research*, 24(4), 341–356.

Centers for Disease Control and Prevention. (2017). *Guidelines for prevention of catheter-associated urinary tract infections*. Retrieved from https://www.cdc.gov/infectioncontrol/pdf/guidelines/cauti-guidelines.pdf. (Accessed 30 October 2017).

Clarke, K., Tong, D., Pan, Y., et al. (2013). Reduction in catheter-associated urinary tract infections by bundling interventions. *International Journal for Quality Health Care*, 25(1), 43–49.

Halm, M. A., & O'Connor, N. (2014). Do systems-based interventions affect catheter-associated urinary tract infection? *American Journal of Critical Care Nurse*, 23, 505–509.

Lo, E., Nicolle, L. E., Coffin, S. E., et al. (2014). Strategies to prevent catheter-associated urinary tract infections in acute care hospitals: 2014 update. *Infection Control and Hospital Epidemiology*, 35(Suppl. 2), S32–S47. doi:10.1086/675718.

Meddings, J., Rogers, M. A. M., Krein, S. L., et al. (2014). Reducing unnecessary urinary catheter use and other strategies to prevent catheter-associated urinary tract infection: An integrative review. *BMJ Quality & Safety*, 23(4), 277–289.

Medline Plus. (2017). *Indwelling catheter care*. Retrieved from https://medlineplus.gov/ency/patientinstructions/000140.htm. (Accessed 31 October 2017).

Oman, K. S., Makic, M. B. F. M., Fink, R., et al. (2012). Nurse-directed interventions to reduce catheter-associated urinary tract infections. *American Journal of Infection Control*, 40, 548–553.

Scott, R. A., Oman, K. S., Makic, M. B. F., et al. (2014). Reducing indwelling urinary catheter use in the emergency department: A successful quality-improvement initiative. *Journal of Emergency Nursing*, 40, 237–240.

Uberoi, V., Calixte, N., Coronel, V. R., et al. (2013). Reducing urinary catheter days. *Nursing*, 43(1), 16–20.

Yokoe, D. S., Anderson, D. J., Berenholtz, S. M., et al. (2014). A compendium of strategies to prevent healthcare- associated infections in the acute care hospitals: 2014 updates. *Infection Control and Hospital Epidemiology*, 35(8), 967–977.

Insomnia *Judith Ann Floyd, PhD, RN, FNAP, FAAN*

NANDA-I

Definition

A disruption in amount and quality of sleep that impairs functioning.

Defining Characteristics

Alteration in affect; alteration in concentration; alteration in mood; alteration in sleep pattern; compromised health status; decrease in quality of life; difficulty initiating sleep; difficulty maintaining sleep state; dissatisfaction with sleep; early awakening; increase in absenteeism; increase in accidents; insufficient energy; nonrestorative sleep pattern; sleep disturbance producing next-day consequences

Related Factors

Alcohol consumption; anxiety, average daily physical activity is less than recommended for gender and age; depression; environmental barrier; fear; frequent naps; grieving; inadequate sleep hygiene; physical discomfort; stressors

Associated Condition

Hormonal change; pharmaceutical agent

NOC (Nursing Outcomes Classification)

Suggested NOC Outcomes

Comfort Level; Pain Level; Personal Well-Being; Psychosocial Adjustment: Life Change; Quality of Life; Rest; Sleep

Example NOC Outcome with Indicators

Sleep as evidenced by the following indicators: Hours of sleep/Sleep pattern/Sleep quality/Sleep efficiency/Feels rejuvenated after sleep/Sleeps consistently through the night. (Rate the outcome and indicators of **Sleep:** 1 = severely compromised, 2 = substantially compromised, 3 = moderately compromised, 4 = mildly compromised, 5 = not compromised [see Section I].)

● = Independent; ▲ = Collaborative; EBN = Evidence-Based Nursing; EB = Evidence-Based

Client Outcomes

Client Will (Specify Time Frame)

- Verbalize plan to implement sleep-promoting routines
- Fall asleep with less difficulty a minimum of four nights out of seven
- Wake up less frequently during night a minimum of four nights out of seven
- Sleep a minimum of 6 hours most nights and more if needed to meet next stated outcome
- Awaken refreshed and not be fatigued during day most of the time

NIC (Nursing Interventions Classification)

Suggested NIC Intervention

Sleep Enhancement

Example NIC Activities—Sleep Enhancement
Monitor/record client's sleep pattern and number of sleep hours; Encourage client to establish a bedtime routine to facilitate transition from wakefulness to sleep

Nursing Interventions and *Rationales*

- Obtain a sleep history including amount of time needed to initiate sleep, duration of any awakenings after sleep onset, total nighttime sleep amounts, and dissatisfaction with daytime energy levels and alertness. *Inability to drift off to sleep at bedtime or during the night if awakened can lead to short sleep and poor daytime functioning, as well as negatively affect physical and mental health (Khurshid, 2015).*
- From the history, assess client's current ability to initiate and maintain sleep and the short-term versus chronic nature of inability to initiate and maintain sleep. *Adults can be considered to have insomnia if their daytime tiredness and sleepiness is accompanied by shortened nighttime caused by (1) inability to initiate sleep and/or (2) awakening during the night with inability to reinitiate sleep 3+ nights/week. Insomnia is considered chronic if the inability to initiate sleep continues beyond three months (Khurshid, 2015).*

For short-term insomnia:

- For clients historically able to initiate and maintain sleep, but unable to do so in the current situation (1) minimize sleep disruptions (see Nursing Interventions and *Rationales* for Disturbed **Sleep** pattern), and (2) promote sleep hygiene practices (see Nursing Interventions and *Rationales* for Readiness for enhanced **Sleep**). *Inability to initiate and maintain sleep is common in new sleep environments, especially during times of stress or worry (Dambrosio & Maxanec, 2013).*
- Also attend to the following factors often associated with short-term insomnia:
  - ❍ Assess pain medication use and, when feasible, advocate for pain medications that promote rather than interfere with sleep. (See Nursing Interventions and *Rationales* for Acute **Pain** and Chronic **Pain.**) *Some pain medications also promote sleep, whereas others promote alertness and thus interfere with falling and staying asleep (Laudon & Frydman-Marom, 2014).*
  - ❍ Assess level of tension and encourage use of relaxation techniques as needed. **EBN:** *A review of evidence from nine intervention studies suggested relaxation, meditation, guided imagery, or combinations of these strategies resulted in better sleep and less fatigue in heart-failure patients (Kwekkeboom & Bratzke, 2016).* **EBN:** *A well-controlled clinical pilot study (N = 12) found that patient-controlled relaxation and/or imagery interventions may improve sleep for hospitalized patients (Nooneret et al, 2016).*
  - ❍ Assess level of distress and use therapeutic communication to increase comfort. (See further Nursing Interventions and *Rationales* for Readiness for Enhanced **Comfort.**) **EBN:** *A qualitative study of 10 patients' experiences with sleep during hospitalization identified several themes that promote patients' comfort, increase patients' ability to initiate and maintain sleep and support the nurse's ability to co-create a safe sleep environment with the patient (Gellerstedt, Medin, & Karlsson, 2014).* **EBN:** *A qualitative study of how experienced nurses promote sleep in hospitals (N = 8) identified caring conversation as one of four sleep-promoting nursing strategies (Salzmann-Erikson, Lagerqvist, & Pousette, 2016).*
  - ❍ Assess for signs of overactive bladder. **EB:** *A descriptive study (N = 24) found subjects with overactive bladder syndrome (OAB), but no formal insomnia diagnosis, awakened during sleep as often as insomniacs;*

• = Independent;   ▲ = Collaborative;   **EBN** = Evidence-Based Nursing;   **EB** = Evidence-Based

however, waking durations were shorter in OAB subjects than those with diagnosed insomnia (Preud'homme et al, 2013).

For chronic insomnia:

▲ Rule-out/address any disorders and syndromes associated with chronic insomnia (e.g., addiction to alcohol or other psychoactive substances, anxiety and depressive disorders, chronic pain syndrome, restless leg syndrome, or other sleep disorders). *Coexisting medical conditions, mental disorders, and sleep disorders are interactive and bidirectional (Khurshid, 2015). EB: In a study of 39 older insomnia patients, those with higher anxiety and depression responded better to treatments for chronic insomnia when anxiety and depression were also treated (Troxel et al, 2013).*

● Encourage practices that calm the mind and body prior to bedtime.
  ○ Introduce music into bedtime routines if client finds music relaxing. EB: *A meta-analysis of six experimental studies showed that listening to music led to insomnia patients reporting better sleep, although no objective evidence was found of shorter sleep latencies, less waking after sleep onset, or increased total sleep time (Jespersen et al, 2015).*
  ○ Teach progressive muscle relaxation as a way to relax at bedtime. EB: *An experimental study found that multicomponent treatment programs that included progressive muscle relaxation were effective for decreasing insomnia patients' reports of insomnia severity and increasing self-reported sleep quality (Pech & O'Kearney, 2013).*
  ○ Support client's meditation or prayer practices as part of bedtime rituals if client finds them relaxing. EB: *A 7-week randomized controlled trial of 54 adults with chronic insomnia that used a treatment of mindfulness meditation reported that improved sleep was found, especially at the 3-month follow-up on both objective and subjective measures of sleep (Ong et al, 2014).*

● Encourage use of the following stimulus control strategies in addition to relaxation and sleep hygiene interventions recommended for short-term insomnia; (1) if feasible, have client arise from bed to participate in calming activities whenever anxious about failure to fall asleep; (2) if not feasible for client to get out of bed when unable to sleep, encourage sitting up in bed to engage in calming activities or simply resting in bed without attempting to fall asleep; (3) avoid a focus on what time it is and subsequent worry about amount of sleep time lost to sleeplessness; and (4) distract from sleeplessness with a focus on positive aspects of life. EB: *A meta-analysis of 37 comparative effectiveness studies found medium to large improvements in the ability to initiate and maintain sleep when a combination of stimulus control, relaxation, and sleep hygiene strategies were used to treat insomnia in patients with comorbid medical and psychiatric conditions (Wu et al, 2015).*

● Consider use of foot baths. CEB: *Small manipulations of core body and skin temperature were found to affect sleep onset in adults, including normal older sleepers and older insomniacs (Raymann & Van Someren, 2008). EBN: A review of evidence from 31 papers found that passive body heating via foot baths often relaxed and improved quality of sleep in insomnia patients (Talebi, Heydari-Gorji, & Hadinejad, 2016).*

● Be aware that clients diagnosed with chronic insomnia may have a low pain threshold. CEB: *In a laboratory study (N = 34), subjects with shortened sleep caused by chronic insomnia, were twice as likely to report experiencing spontaneous pain as healthy controls with no sleep loss; they also had lower pain thresholds during applications of heat and pressure than healthy controls (Haack et al, 2012).*

● For clients whose chronic inability to initiate and maintain sleep has led to sleep deprivation, see Nursing Interventions and *Rationales* for **Sleep** deprivation.

▲ For clients with unremitting chronic insomnia, refer to a nurse practitioner trained in cognitive behavioral therapies for insomnia (CBT-I). EB: *A meta-analysis of 37 comparative effectiveness studies found chronic insomnia patients with comorbid medical and psychiatric conditions improved their ability to initiate and maintain sleep after completion of multicomponent CBT-I programs (Wu et al, 2015).*

▲ Assist clients diagnosed with chronic insomnia who have been treated with CBT-I to limit use of sleeping agents and to select intermittent nights for sleeping pill use if complete discontinuance of sleeping pills is not feasible. *One option to reduce the risk of habituation or dependence on sleeping medication is to adopt an intermittent dosing approach in which patients are given 10 to 15 tablets for the entire month and are allowed to use them on an as-needed basis (Gooneratne & Vitiello, 2014). EB: An updated review of evidence supported the ability of patients treated with CBT-I to reduce or even eliminate their dependence on sleeping pills (Bonnet & Arand, 2017).*

● Supplement other interventions with teaching about sleep and sleep promotion. (See further Nursing Interventions and *Rationales* for Readiness for enhanced **Sleep.**)

● = Independent;   ▲ = Collaborative;   EBN = Evidence-Based Nursing;   EB = Evidence-Based

Geriatric

- Most interventions discussed previously may be used with geriatric clients. In addition, see the Geriatric section of Nursing Interventions and *Rationales* for (1) Readiness for enhanced **Sleep** and (2) Disturbed **Sleep,** and **Sleep** deprivation**.**
- Especially helpful for the elderly client is routine exercise unless contraindicated. **EB:** *In an evidence review of 34 research reports, exercise increased sleep efficiency and duration in healthy older adults regardless of the mode and intensity of activity, and even more so in the elderly with sleep disorders (Dolezal et al, 2017).*
- ▲ Monitor for uncomfortable sensations in legs and involuntary leg movements during sleep. **EB:** *An observational study of 2872 older community-dwelling men, using home polysomnography, reported that periodic limb movements were common in this population and resulted in more fragmented sleep (Claman et al, 2013).*

Home Care

- Assessments and interventions discussed previously can all be adapted for use in home care.
- In addition, see the Home Care section of Nursing Interventions and *Rationales* for Readiness for enhanced **Sleep.**

Client/Family Teaching

- Teach family about normal sleep and promote adoption of behaviors that enhance it. See Nursing Interventions and *Rationales* for Readiness for enhanced **Sleep.**
- Teach family about sleep deprivation and how to avoid it. See Nursing Interventions and *Rationales* for **Sleep** deprivation.
- Advise family of importance of not disrupting sleep of others unnecessarily. See Nursing Interventions and *Rationales* for Disturbed **Sleep** pattern.
- Advise family of importance of minimizing noise and light, including light from electronic devices in the sleep environment. See Nursing Interventions and *Rationales* for Disturbed **Sleep** pattern.
- Help family members understand the difference between insomnia and externally caused sleep disruption/resultant sleep deprivation. *Insomnia is generally a stress-related, medication-related, or disease-related psychophysiological activation that interferes with the person's ability to calm the mind and body adequately for initiation and maintenance of sleep (Gooneratne & Vitiello, 2014).*

REFERENCES

Bonnet, M. H., & Arand, D. L. (2017). *Treatment of insomnia. UpToDate, Topic 7691, Version 59.0.* Retrieved from https://www.uptodate.com/contents/treatment-of-insomnia-in-adults. (Accessed 1 November 2017).

Claman, D. M., Ewing, S. K., Redline, S., et al. (2013). Study of osteoporotic fractures research group periodic leg movements are associated with reduced sleep quality in older men: The MrOS sleep study. *Journal of Clinical Sleep Medicine: JCSM: Official Publication of the American Academy of Sleep Medicine, 9*(11), 1109–1117. doi:10.5664/jcsm.3146.

Dambrosio, N. M., & Maxanec, P. (2013). "Nurse, I can't sleep!": Approaches to management of insomnia in oncology patients. *Journal of Hospice & Palliative Nursing, 15*(5), 267–275. doi:10.1097/NJH.0b013e318296839b.

Dolezal, B. A., Neufeld, E. V., Boland, D. M., et al. (2017). Interrelationship between sleep and exercise: A systematic review. *Advances in Preventive Medicine, 2017,* 14. Retrieved from https://doi.org/10.1155/2017/1364387. (Accessed 29 January 2018).

Gellerstedt, L., Medin, J., & Karlsson, M. R. (2014). Patients' experiences of sleep in hospital: A qualitative interview study. *Journal of Research in Nursing, 19*(3), 176–188. doi:10.1177/1744987113490415.

Gooneratne, N. S., & Vitiello, M. V. (2014). Sleep in older adults: Normative changes, sleep disorders, and treatment options. *Clinics in Geriatric Medicine, 30*(3), 591–627. doi:10.1016/j.cger.2014.04.007.

Haack, M., Scott-Sutherland, J., Santangelo, G., et al. (2012). Pain sensitivity and modulation in primary insomnia. *European Journal of Pain, 16*(4), 522–533. doi:10.1016/j.ejpain.2011.07.007.

Kwekkeboom, K., & Bratzke, L. C. (2016). A systematic review of relaxation, meditation, and guided imagery strategies for symptom management in heart failure. *Journal of Cardiovascular Nursing, 31*(5), 457–468. doi:10.1097/JCN.0000000000000274.

Khurshid, K. A. (2015). A review of changes in DSM-5 sleep-wake disorders. *Psychiatric Times, 32*(9), 1–3. doi:10.1016/j.patbio.2014.07.002.

Jespersen, K. V., Koenig, J., Jennum, P., et al. (2015). Music for insomnia in adults. *The Cochrane Database of Systematic Reviews,* (8), CD010459, N.PAG-N.PAG (1p).

Laudon, M., & Frydman-Marom, A. (2014). Therapeutic effects of melatonin receptor agonists on sleep and comorbid disorders. *International Journal of Molecular Sciences, 15,* 15924–15950. doi:10.3390/ijms150915924.

Nooner, A. K., Dwyer, K., DeShea, L., et al. (2016). Using relaxation and guided imagery to address pain, fatigue, and sleep disturbances: A pilot study. *Clinical Journal of Oncology Nursing, 20*(5), 547–552. doi:10.1188/16.CJON.547-552.

Ong, J. C., Manber, R., Segal, Z., et al. (2014). A randomized controlled trial of mindfulness meditation for chronic insomnia. *Sleep, 37*(9), 1553–1563.

Pech, M., & O'Kearney, R. (2013). A randomized controlled trial of problem-solving therapy compared to cognitive therapy for the

● = Independent;   ▲ = Collaborative;   **EBN** = Evidence-Based Nursing;   **EB** = Evidence-Based

treatment of insomnia in adults. *Sleep, 36*(5), 739–749. doi:10.5665/sleep.2640.

Preud'homme, X. A., Amundsen, C. L., Webster, G. D., et al. (2013). Comparison of diary-derived bladder and sleep measurements across OAB individuals, primary insomniacs, and healthy controls. *International Urogynecological Journal, 24*, 501–508. 10.1007/s00192-012-1890-0.

Raymann, R. J., & Van Someren, E. J. (2008). Diminished capability to recognize the optimal temperature for sleep initiation may contribute to poor sleep in elderly people. *Sleep, 31*(9), 1301–1309.

Salzmann-Erikson, M., Lagerqvist, L., & Pousette, S. (2016). Keep calm and have a good night: Nurses' strategies to promote inpatients' sleep in the hospital environment. *Scandinavian Journal of Caring Science, 30*, 356–364. doi:10.1111/scs.12255.

Talebi, H., Heydari-Gorji, M. A., & Hadinejad, Z. (2016). The impact of passive body heating on quality of sleep: A review study. *Journal of Sleep Science, 1*(4), 176–181.

Troxel, W. M., Conrad, T. S., Germain, A., et al. (2013). Predictors of treatment response to brief behavioral treatment of insomnia (BBTI) in older adults. *Journal of Clinical Sleep Medicine: JCSM: Official Publication of the American Academy of Sleep Medicine, 9*(12), 1281–1289. doi:10.5664/jcsm.3270.

Wu, J. Q., Appleman, E. R., Salazar, R. D., et al. (2015). Cognitive behavioral therapy for insomnia co-morbid with psychiatric and medical conditions: A meta-analysis. *JAMA Internal Medicine, 175*(9), 1461–1472. 10.1001/jamainternmed.2015.3006.

Decreased Intracranial adaptive capacity   Kimberly Meyer, PhD, ACNP-BC, CNRN

NANDA-I

Definition

Compromise in intracranial fluid dynamic mechanisms that normally compensate for increases in intracranial volumes, resulting in repeated disproportionate increases in intracranial pressure (ICP) in response to a variety of noxious and nonnoxious stimuli.

Defining Characteristics

Baseline intracranial pressure (ICP) ≥10 mm Hg; disproportionate increase in intracranial pressure (ICP) following stimuli; elevated tidal wave intracranial pressure (P2 ICP) waveform; repeated increase in intracranial pressure (ICP) ≥10 mm Hg for ≥5 minutes following external stimuli; volume-pressure response test variation (volume: pressure ratio 2, pressure-volume index <10); wide-amplitude intracranial pressure (ICP) waveform

Related Factors

To be developed

Associated Condition

Brain injury; decrease in cerebral perfusion ≤50 to 60 mm Hg; sustained increase in intracranial pressure (ICP) of 10 to 15 mm Hg; systemic hypotension with intracranial hypertension

NOC   (Nursing Outcomes Classification)

Suggested NOC Outcomes

Neurological Status; Neurological Status: Consciousness

> **Example NOC Outcome with Indicators**
>
> **Neurological Status** as evidenced by the following indicators: Consciousness/Intracranial pressure/Vital signs/Central motor control/Cranial sensory-motor function/Spinal sensory-motor function. (Rate the outcome and indicators of **Neurological Status:** 1 = severely compromised, 2 = substantially compromised, 3 = moderately compromised, 4 = mildly compromised, 5 = not compromised [see Section I].)

Client Outcomes

Client Will (Specify Time Frame)

- Experience fewer than five episodes of DIICP in 24 hours
- Avoid neurological status changes that are triggered by episodes of disproportionate increases in intracranial pressure (DIICP)
- Have cerebral perfusion pressure (CPP) remaining greater than 60 to 70 mm Hg in adults

● = Independent;   ▲ = Collaborative;   EBN = Evidence-Based Nursing;   EB = Evidence-Based

---

NIC	(Nursing Interventions Classification)

Suggested NIC Interventions

Cerebral Edema Management; Cerebral Perfusion Promotion; Intracranial Pressure Monitoring; Neurological Monitoring

Example NIC Activities—Cerebral Edema Management

Monitor for confusion, changes in mentation, complaints of dizziness, syncope; Allow ICP to return to baseline between nursing activities

Nursing Interventions and *Rationales*

▲ To assess ICP and CPP effectively:
  ○ Monitor and display ICP and CPP in clients with severe traumatic brain injury (TBI) and spontaneous intracranial hemorrhage (ICH). **EB:** *Lack of ICP/CPP monitoring in severe TBI increases mortality (Heck 2016; Carney et al, 2017).*
  ○ Maintain systolic blood pressure (SBP) >110 mm Hg in patients 15 to 49 years of age or over 70 years of age and SBP >100 mm Hg in patients 50 to 69 years of age to improve outcomes. **EB:** *Targeted blood pressure supports adequate CPP, especially in cases of elevated ICP (Carney et al, 2017).*
  ○ Monitor jugular bulb oxygenation (SjO_2) in select patients with severe TBI. **EB:** *SjO_2 monitoring may provide information for management decisions that can reduce morbidity and mortality associated with elevated ICP (Carney et al, 2017).*
  ○ Maintain ICP less than 22 mm Hg and CPP greater than 60 mm Hg. **EB:** *The Guidelines for the Management of Severe Brain Injury established the treatment threshold for ICP as greater than 22 mm Hg and CPP less than 60 mm Hg (Carney et al, 2017).*
  ○ Monitor neurological status frequently (hourly in acute situations) determining both pupillary size and reaction to light and the Glasgow Coma Scale (GCS) score, noting changes in eye opening; motor response to painful stimuli; and awareness of self, time, and place. **EB:** *The combination of a GCS score and the pupil size and reactivity are predictive of outcome and aid in discussions of prognosis with family (Hoffmann et al, 2012).* **EB:** *Research exploring the reliability of automated pupillometers may help reduce the subjective error of estimating client pupil size, allowing for more accurate trending of ICP concerns (Olson et al, 2017).*
  ○ Monitor brain tissue oxygen ($PbtO_2$). **CEB/EB:** *Low brain $PbtO_2$ is predictive of increased mortality in clients with severe TBI and worse 6-month outcomes (Bohman et al, 2011; Eriksson et al, 2012; Okonkwo et al, 2017).*
▲ To prevent harmful increases in ICP:
  ○ Elevate head of bed 30 to 45 degrees with head in midline position. **CEB/EB:** *Elevating the head of the bed allows for increased venous drainage that decreases ICP (Fan, 2004; Ledwith et al, 2010; McNett & Olson, 2013).* **EB:** *If client is suffering acute stroke, CPP may be compromised with head elevation during the first 72 hours after injury (Favilla et al, 2014). See care plan for Risk for ineffective **Cerebral** tissue perfusion.*
  ○ Administer sedation per collaborative protocol. **EB:** *Sedatives including propofol, morphine, and midazolam are effective in controlling ICP (Carney et al, 2017). Sedation was effective in 66% of episodes of decreased $PbtO_2$ (Bohman et al, 2011).*
  ○ Maintain glycemic control per collaborative protocol. **CEB:** *Maintain glucose levels between 110 and 180 mg/dL using insulin therapy in critically ill brain-injured clients (Kramer, Roberts, & Zygun, 2012).*
  ○ Maintain optimal oxygenation and ventilation, applying positive end-expiratory pressure (PEEP) as needed and avoiding hyperventilation. **CEB/EB:** *PEEP levels of 10 cm H_2O have been found to produce no significant changes in ICP, especially when combined with head of bed elevation of 30 degrees. Hyperventilation has been found to worsen outcomes in TBI clients and should be avoided, especially in the first 24 hours after injury (Videtta et al, 2002; Carney et al, 2017).*
  ○ Provide hyperbaric oxygen/normobaric hyperoxia if available during the acute phase of severe TBI. **EB:** *Sixty minutes of hyperbaric oxygen at 1.5 ATA followed by 3 hours of an FiO_2 of 100% every 24 hours during the first 72 hours of severe TBI lowered ICP for the entire 3-day study period in severe TBI clients (Rockswold et al, 2013).*

● = Independent;   ▲ = Collaborative;   EBN = Evidence-Based Nursing;   EB = Evidence-Based

▲ To prevent and treat harmful decreases in CPP:
- ○ See care plan for Risk for ineffective **Cerebral** tissue perfusion.

▲ To treat sustained ICP (>22 mm Hg):
- ○ Remove or loosen rigid cervical collars. CEB/EB: *Loosening or removing these collars allows for unrestricted venous drainage that lowers ICP (Mobbs, Stoodley, & Fuller, 2002; McNett & Olson, 2013).*
- ○ Administer hypertonic saline (bolus or continuous infusion) per collaborative protocol. EB: *Hyperosmolar therapy reduces brain water content. A comparison of mannitol and hypertonic saline found that multiple studies, including randomized controlled trials (RCTs), demonstrated superior effectiveness of hypertonic saline in decreasing ICP (Mortazavi et al, 2012). Alternatively, administer mannitol boluses for increased ICP. EB: Mannitol controls elevated ICP when given in bolus doses of 0.25 to 1 g/kg as long as hypotension is avoided (Carney et al, 2017).*
- ○ Drain cerebrospinal fluid (CSF) from an intraventricular catheter system per collaborative protocol. EB: *CSF drainage has been found to be effective in decreasing ICP (Bhargava et al, 2013; Srinivasan et al, 2014).*
- ○ Use targeted temperature management to facilitate control of ICP. EB: *Target temperatures vary according to intracranial pathology with temperatures 35°C to 37°C associated with lower ICP and temperatures as low as 32°C offering neuroprotection after cardiac arrest (Cariou et al, 2017).*

I

REFERENCES

Bhargava, D., Alalade, A., Ellamushi, H., et al. (2013). Mitigating effects of external ventricular drain usage in the management of severe head injury. *Acta Neurochirurgica, 155*(11), 2129–2132.

Bohman, L., Heuer, G. G., Macyszyn, L., et al. (2011). Medical management of compromised brain oxygen in patients with severe traumatic brain injury. *Neurocritical Care, 14,* 361–369.

Cariou, A., Payen, J.-F., Asehnoune, K., et al. for the Société de Réanimation de Langue Française (SRLF) and the Société Française d'Anesthésie et de Réanimation (SFAR) In conjunction with the Association de Neuro Anesthésie Réanimation de Langue Française (ANARLF), the Groupe Francophone de Réanimation et Urgences Pédiatriques (GFRUP), the Société Française de Médecine d'Urgence (SFMU), and the Société Française Neuro-Vasculaire (SFNV). (2017). Targeted temperature management in the ICU: Guidelines from a French expert panel. *Annals of Intensive Care, 7,* 70. Retrieved from http://doi.org/10.1186/s13613-017-0294-1.

Carney, N., Totten, A. M., O'Reilly, C., et al. (2017). Guidelines for the management of severe traumatic brain injury. *Neurosurgery, 80*(1), 6–15.

Eriksson, E. A., Barletta, J. F., Figueroa, B. E., et al. (2012). The first 72 hours of brain tissue oxygenation predicts patient survival with traumatic brain injury. *The Journal of Trauma and Acute Care Surgery, 72,* 1345–1349.

Fan, J. (2004). Effect of backrest position on intracranial pressure and cerebral perfusion pressure in individuals with brain injury: A systematic review. *Journal of Neuroscience Nursing, 36*(5), 278–288.

Favilla, C. G., Mesquita, R. C., Mullen, M., et al. (2014). Optical bedside monitoring of cerebral blood flow in acute ischemic stroke patients during head-of-bed manipulation. *Stroke; a Journal of Cerebral Circulation, 45,* 1269–1274.

Heck, C. (2016). Invasive neuromonitoring. *Critical Care Nursing Clinics of North America, 28*(1), 77–86.

Hoffmann, M., Lefering, R., Rueger, J. M., et al. (2012). Pupil evaluation in addition to glasgow coma scale components in prediction of traumatic brain injury mortality. *The British Journal of Surgery, 99*(Suppl. 1), 122–130.

Kramer, A. H., Roberts, D. J., & Zygun, D. A. (2012). Optimal glycemic control in neurocritical care patients: A systematic review and meta-analysis. *Critical Care: The Official Journal of the Critical Care Forum, 16.* Retrieved from http://ccforum.com/content/16/5/R203. (Accessed 10 February 2018).

Ledwith, B., Blood, S., Maloney-Wilensky, E., et al. (2010). Effect of body position on cerebral oxygenation and physiological parameters in patients with acute neurological conditions. *Journal of Neuroscience Nursing, 42*(5), 280–287.

McNett, M. M., & Olson, D. M. (2013). Evidence to guide nursing interventions for critically ill neurologically impaired patients with ICP monitoring. *J NeuroScience Nurs, 45*(3), 120–123.

Mobbs, R., Stoodley, M., & Fuller, J. (2002). Effect of cervical hard collar on intracranial pressure after head injury. *ANZ Journal of Surgery, 72*(6), 389–391.

Mortazavi, M. M., Romeo, A. K., Deep, A., et al. (2012). Hypertonic saline for treating raised intracranial pressure: Literature review with meta-analysis. *Journal of Neurosurgery, 116,* 210–221.

Okonkwo, D. O., Shutter, L. A., Moore, C., et al. (2017). Brain oxygen optimization in severe traumatic brain injury phase-II: A phase II randomized trial. *Critical Care Medicine, 45,* 1907–1914.

Olson, D. M., Stutzman, S. E., Atem, F., et al. (2017). Establishing normative data for pupillometer assessment in neuroscience intensive care: The "END-PANIC" registry. *Journal of Neuroscience Nursing, 49*(4), 251–254.

Rockswold, S. B., Rockswold, G. L., Zaun, D. A., et al. (2013). A prospective, randomized Phase II clinical trial to evaluate the effect of combined hyperbaric and normobaric hyperoxia on cerebral metabolism, intracranial pressure, oxygen toxicity, and clinical outcome in severe traumatic brain injury. *Journal of Neurosurgery, 118,* 1317–1328.

Srinivasan, V. M., O'Neill, B. R., Jho, D., et al. (2014). The history of external ventricular drainage. *Journal of Neurosurgery, 120,* 228–236.

Videtta, W., Villarejo, F., Cohen, M., et al. (2002). Effects of positive end-expiratory pressure on intracranial pressure and cerebral perfusion pressure. *Intracranial Pressure and Brain Biochemical Monitoring Acta Neurochirurgica Supplements, 81,* 93–97.

● = Independent;   ▲ = Collaborative;   EBN = Evidence-Based Nursing;   EB = Evidence-Based

Deficient Knowledge   *Lauren McAlister, MSN, FNP, DNP Candidate and Kathaleen C. Bloom, PhD, CNM*

NANDA-I

Definition

Absence or deficiency of cognitive information related to a specific topic or its acquisition.

Defining Characteristics

Inaccurate follow-through of instruction; inaccurate performance on a test; inappropriate behavior; insufficient knowledge

Related Factors

Insufficient information; insufficient interest in learning; insufficient knowledge of resources; misinformation presented by others

Associated Condition

Alteration in cognitive functioning; alteration in memory

NOC   (Nursing Outcomes Classification)

K

Suggested NOC Outcomes

Knowledge: Disease Process; Energy Conservation; Health Behavior; Health Resources; Healthy Diet; Infection Management; Medication; Personal Safety; Prescribed Activity; Substance Use Control; Treatment Procedure(s); Treatment Regimen

> **Example NOC Outcome with Indicators**
>
> **Knowledge: Health Behavior** as evidenced by the following indicators: Healthy nutritional practices/Benefits of regular exercise/Safe use of prescribed and nonprescribed medication. (Rate the outcome and indicators of **Knowledge: Health Behavior:** 1 = no knowledge, 2 = limited knowledge, 3 = moderate knowledge, 4 = substantial knowledge, 5 = extensive knowledge [see Section I].)

Client Outcomes

Client Will (Specify Time Frame)

- Explain disease state, recognize need for medications, and understand treatments
- Describe the rationale for therapy/treatment options
- Incorporate knowledge of health regimen into lifestyle
- State confidence in one's ability to manage health situation and remain in control of life
- Demonstrate how to perform health-related procedure(s) satisfactorily
- Identify resources that can be used for more information or support after discharge

NIC   (Nursing Interventions Classification)

Suggested NIC Interventions

Teaching: Disease Process, Individual; Learning Facilitation

> **Example NIC Activities—Teaching: Disease Process**
>
> Discuss therapy/treatment options; Describe rationale behind management/therapy/treatment recommendations

Nursing Interventions and *Rationales*

- Consider the health literacy and the readiness to learn for all clients and caregivers (e.g., mental acuity, ability to see or hear, existing pain, emotional readiness, motivation, previous knowledge). EBN: *A new study looking at a new tool, the Newest Vital Sign (NVS), was used to measure the patient's health literacy.*

● = Independent;   ▲ = Collaborative;   EBN = Evidence-Based Nursing;   EB = Evidence-Based

Findings showed that this tool is efficient to administer and could help identify low health literacy patients (McCune, Hynha, & Pohl, 2016).

- Focus on the nature of spoken and written communication when teaching clients and caregivers, especially those who may have health literacy needs. **EBN:** *Lambert and Keogh (2014) provided an overview of tools for effective teaching communication including providing feedback, actively seeking questions, using a teach-back method, and providing age-appropriate client education materials that are in are written in everyday layman's language.* **EBN:** *A recent qualitative study explored the relationship between health literacy and effective communication. One of the overarching themes was that building trust and relationships with the older adults to achieve effective communication can then be applied to meet the individual health literacy needs of the patient (Brooks et al, 2017).*

- Consider the context, timing, and order of how information is presented. **CEB:** *A systematic review of 56 studies on educational interventions found that presenting the most important information first and the use of simplifying, "chunking," and grouping information presented in short sessions were effective (Berkman et al, 2011).*

- Use client-centered approaches that engage clients and caregivers as active versus passive learners. **EB:** *A systematic review of 38 trials with clients with asthma found that using empathy-building strategies within a framework of person-centered counseling would maximize the effectiveness of self-care interventions for those with poorly controlled asthma (Denford et al, 2014).*

- Reinforce learning through frequent repetition and follow-up sessions. **EBN:** *A systematic review of six studies found that frequent and regular educational sessions, including "boost" sessions, improved medication and self-care management outcomes for those with a chronic condition, including stroke clients (Chapman & Bogle, 2014).* **EBN:** *In a qualitative study with semistructured interviews, it was discovered that patients who were in the intensive care unit (ICU) and who attended a follow-up session were better able to process their feelings and emotions. The findings from this study supported the hypothesis that the follow-up session for an ICU patient can aid in processing the illness after the fact (Haraldsson et al, 2015).*

- Use electronic methods for delivery of information when appropriate. **EB:** *A Cochrane review of 24 studies with 8112 participants found that the use of multimedia education (video, audio, and self-paced computer programs) as an adjunct with current programs was most effective (Ciciriello et al, 2013).* **EB:** *In a Cochrane review of 16 trials with 3478 participants, the use of computer programs and the use of mobile phone interventions helped clients with diabetes type 2 improve blood glucose control, although not all clients have access (Pal et al, 2013).*

- Help the client and caregivers locate appropriate postdischarge groups and resources. **EBN:** *A recent systematic review concluded that the utilization of postdischarge support for patients with chronic obstructive pulmonary disease (COPD) significantly reduced the readmission rates within 30 days and had an effect up to 180 days (Pedersen et al, 2017).*

- Encourage clients and caregivers to maintain and/or expand supportive social networks as self-care learning resources when appropriate. **EB:** *In a longitudinal study of 300 patients with long-term chronic health conditions, those who had sustained or expanded community networks were more likely to sustain self-care management, maintain behavioral change and treatment regimens, and access voluntary caregiving over formal caregiving (Reeves et al, 2014).*

 Pediatric

- Use family-centered approaches when teaching children and adolescents. **EBN:** *According to Manente (2017), when families are educated about the patient and know what to expect during the transition out of the ICU, their fears and anxieties are decreased, which can promote healing for the patient.*

- Guide children and adolescents to credible information about their condition. **EBN:** *A recent mixed methods study showed that the best way to inform adolescents about HIV and sexual/reproductive health is via the radio, television, mass media, and social media (Adams et al, 2017).*

 Geriatric

- Educate all older clients on safety issues, including fall prevention and medication management. **QSEN:** *In a meta-analysis of 19 studies, clients receiving targeted fall prevention education face to face or through multimedia methods had decrease in falls from those either receiving no formal education or written education (Lee et al, 2014).*

- Use multidisciplinary teams to enhance patient education. **EBN:** *A qualitative study exploring medication management in people with dementia showed potential positive benefits of a community pharmacist working*

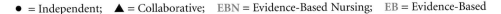

● = Independent;   ▲ = Collaborative;   EBN = Evidence-Based Nursing;   EB = Evidence-Based

in a multidisciplinary environment outside the pharmacy and can improve medication management (Maidment et al, 2016).

- Consider using teaching methods and materials appropriate for older adults, especially those with cognitive challenges. **EBN:** *A recent study concluded that screening for cognitive impairment in the elderly population and including the family and caregivers in the discharge education has the potential to minimize the risk of readmission (Agarwal et al, 2016).*
- Assess readiness of older adults for use of technological resources. **EBN:** *Health care providers need to assess the experience and willingness of older adults to use the Internet as a source of health information, and Internet sites need to be assessed for readability, large fonts, and simple structure (Chang & Im, 2014).*

 Multicultural

- Use educational interventions that are culturally tailored to the health literacy needs of the client. A Cochrane review of 33 randomized controlled trials focusing on diabetes type 2 found that culturally appropriate health education improved blood sugar control among participants, compared with those receiving the "usual" care, at 3, 6, 12, and 24 months after the intervention (Attridge et al, 2014).
- Assess for cultural/ethnic self-care practices. **CEB:** *The knowledge of patients' cultural practices can be used by health care providers to help design more culturally competent care for the patient (Theroux, Klar, & Messenger, 2013).*
- Consider the potential influence of medical interpreters in information sharing and decision-making and of the possible difficulties for clients when using medical interpreters. **EBN:** *The use of medical interpreters can help bridge the culture and language gap, allowing patients to feel more comfortable expressing themselves (Rorie, 2015).*
- Consider involving bilingual members of a community who are considered outside the traditional health care system who may assist in the teaching of community health issues. **EBN:** *A recent cross-sectional design study examined challenges associated with migrant and English-speaking cancer patients and found that the majority of participants in all migrant groups reported difficulty communicating with the health care providers and team in English (Hyatt et al, 2016).*

 HomeCare

- All of the previously mentioned interventions are applicable to the home setting.
- Use telehealth and technology-enhanced practices as appropriate. **EBN:** *Findings from a literature review of 48 papers supported previous findings that technology is desired by consumers and can be effective, but the appropriateness for use should take into consideration the abilities of the clients, as well as the credibility of software applications and the accessibility of the type of technology, including computers and mobile devices (Fitzner & Moss, 2013).* **EBN:** *A recent review of 11 studies looking at the role of telehealth in diabetic foot ulcer management found that telehealth was well received by patients and providers; assessments via the telehealth modalities were congruent with face-to-face assessment (Singh et al, 2016).*

REFERENCES

Adams, R. M., Riess, H., Massey, P. M., et al. (2017). Understanding where and why Senegalese adolescents and young adults access health information: A mixed methods study examining contextual and personal influences on health information seeking. *Journal of Communication in Healthcare, 10,* 116–148. Retrieved from http://dx.doi.org/10.1080/17538068.2017.1313627.

Agarwal, K. S., Kazim, R., Xu, J., et al. (2016). Unrecognized cognitive impairment and its effect on heart failure readmissions of elderly adults. *Journal of the American Geriatrics Society, 64,* 2296–2301. Retrieved from http://dx.doi.org/10.1111/jgs.14471.

Attridge, M., Creamer, J., Ramsden, M., et al. (2014). Culturally appropriate health education for people in ethnic minority groups with type 2 diabetes mellitus. *Cochrane Database of Systematic Reviews, 2014*(9), 1–591. Retrieved from http://dx.doi.org/10.1002/14651858.CD006424.pub3.

Berkman, N. D., Sheridan, S. L., Donahue, K. E., et al. (2011). *Health literacy interventions and outcomes: An updated systematic review.*

(evidence report/technology assessment no. 199). Rockville, MD: Agency for Healthcare Research and Quality. (Prepared by RTI International–University of North Carolina Evidence-Based Practice Center under contract no. 290-2007-10056-I. AHRQ Publication Number E006.)

Brooks, C., Ballinger, C., Nutbeam, D., et al. (2017). The importance of building trust and tailoring interactions when meeting older adults' health literacy needs. *Disability and Rehabilitation, 39,* 2428–2435. Retrieved from http://dx.doi.org/10.1080/09638288.2016.1231849.

Chang, S. U., & Im, E. O. (2014). A path analysis of internet health information seeking behavior among older adults. *Geriatric Nursing, 35,* 137–141. Retrieved from http://dx.doi.org/10.1016/j.gerinurse.2013.11.005.

Chapman, B., & Bogle, V. (2014). Adherence to medication and self-management in stroke patients. *The British Journal of Nursing, 23,* 158–166. Retrieved from http://dx.doi.org/10.12968/bjnn.2014.10.Sup2.32.

Ciciriello, S., Johnston, R. V., Osborne, R. H., et al. (2013). Multimedia educational interventions for consumers about prescribed and over-the-counter medications. *Cochrane Database of Systematic Reviews, 2013*(4), 1–242. Retrieved from http://dx.doi.org/10.1002/14651858.CD008416.pub2.

Denford, S., Taylor, R. S., Campbell, J. L., et al. (2014). Effective behavior change techniques in asthma self-care interventions: Systematic review and meta-regression. *Health Psychology, 33,* 577–587. Retrieved from http://dx.doi.org/10.1037/a0033080.

Fitzner, K., & Moss, G. (2013). Telehealth—An effective delivery method for diabetes self-management education? *Population Health Management, 16,* 169–177. Retrieved from http://dx.doi.org/10.1089/pop.2012.0054.

Haraldsson, L., Christensson, L., Conlon, L., et al. (2015). The experiences of ICU patients during follow up sessions—a qualitative study. *Intensive and Critical Care Nursing, 31,* 223–231. Retrieved from http://dx.doi.org/10.1016/j.iccn.2015.01.002.

Hyatt, A., Lipson-Smith, R., Schofield, P., et al. (2016). Communication challenges experienced by migrants with cancer: A comparison of migrant and English-speaking Australian-born cancer patients. *Health Expectations: An International Journal of Public Participation in Health Care and Health Policy, 20,* 886–895. Retrieved from http://dx.doi.org/10.1111/hex.12529.

Lambert, V., & Keogh, D. (2014). Health literacy and its importance for effective communication. Part 2. *Nursing Children and Young People, 26*(4), 32–36. Retrieved from http://dx.doi.org/10.7748/ncyp2014.05.26.4.32.e387.

Lee, D., Pritchard, E., McDermott, F., et al. (2014). Falls prevention education for older adults during and after hospitalization: A systematic review and meta-analysis. *Health Education Journal, 73,* 530–544. Retrieved from http://dx.doi.org/10.1177/0017896913499266.

Maidment, I. D., Aston, L., Moutela, T., et al. (2016). A qualitative study exploring medication management in people with dementia living in the community and the potential role of the community pharmacist. *Health Expectations: An International Journal of Public Participation in Health Care and Health Policy, 20,* 929–942. Retrieved from http://dx.doi.org/10.1111/hex.12534.

Manente, L. (2017). Transitioning patients from the intensive care unit to the general pediatric unit: A piece of the puzzle in family centered care. *Pediatric Nursing, 43*(2), 77–95.

McCune, R. L., Hyunhaw, L., & Pohl, J. M. (2016). Assessing health literacy in safety net primary care practices. *Applied Nursing Research, 29,* 188–194. Retrieved from http://dx.doi.org/10.1016/j.apnr.2015.04.004.

Pal, K., Eastwood, S. V., Michie, S., et al. (2013). Computer-based diabetes self-management interventions for adults with type 2 diabetes mellitus. *Cochrane Database of Systematic Reviews, 2013*(3), 1–148. Retrieved from http://dx.doi.org/10.1002/14651858.CD008776.pub2.

Pedersen, P. U., Ersgard, K. B., Soerensen, T. B., et al. (2017). Effectiveness of structured planned post discharge support to patients with chronic obstructive pulmonary disease for reducing readmission rates: A systematic review. *JBI Database of Systematic Reviews and Implementation Reports, 15,* 2060–2086. Retrieved from http://dx.doi.org/10.11124/JBISRIR-2016-003045.

Reeves, D., Blickem, C., Vassilev, I., et al. (2014). The contribution of social networks to the health and self-management of patients with long-term conditions: A longitudinal study. *PLoS ONE, 9*(6), e98340. Retrieved from http://dx.doi.org/10.1371/journal.pone.0098340.

Rorie, S. (2015). Using medical interpreters to provide culturally competent care. *AORN Journal, 101*(2), P7–P9. Retrieved from https://doi.org/10.1016/S0001-2092(14)01420-3.

Singh, T. P., Vangaveti, V. N., Kennedy, R. L., et al. (2016). Role of telehealth in diabetic foot ulcer management: A systematic review. *The Australian Journal of Rural Health, 24,* 224–229. Retrieved from http://dx.doi.org/10.1111/ajr.12284.

Theroux, R., Klar, R., & Messenger, L. (2013). Working hard: Women's self-care practices in Ghana. *Health Care for Women International, 34,* 651–673. Retrieved from http://dx.doi.org/10.1080/07399332.2012.736574.

Readiness for enhanced Knowledge

Lauren McAlister, MSN, FNP, DNP Candidate and Kathaleen C. Bloom, PhD, CNM

NANDA-I

Definition

A pattern of cognitive information related to a specific topic or its acquisition, which can be strengthened.

Defining Characteristics

Expresses desire to enhance learning

NOC   (Nursing Outcomes Classification)

Suggested NOC Outcome

Knowledge: Health Promotion

Example NOC Outcome with Indicators
Knowledge: Health Promotion as evidenced by the following indicators: Behaviors that promote health/Reputable health care resources. (Rate the outcome and indicators of **Knowledge: Health Promotion:** 1 = no knowledge, 2 = limited knowledge, 3 = moderate knowledge, 4 = substantial knowledge, 5 = extensive knowledge [see Section I].)

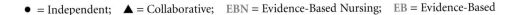

● = Independent;   ▲ = Collaborative;   EBN = Evidence-Based Nursing;   EB = Evidence-Based

Client Outcomes

Client Will (Specify Time Frame)

- Meet personal health-related goals
- Explain how to incorporate new health regimen into lifestyle
- List sources to obtain information

NIC (Nursing Interventions Classification)

Suggested NIC Interventions

Health Education; Health System Guidance

Example NIC Activities—Health Education
Prioritize identified learner needs based on client preference, skills of nurse, resources available, and likelihood of successful goal attainment

Nursing Interventions and *Rationales*

- Assume a facilitator role versus authority role when engaging clients seeking health-related knowledge. EBN: *According to Stacey and Legare (2015), by assuming a facilitator role, nurses are able to provide balanced evidence on options, understand what is most important to the patient, and advocate for the patient's preferences. All of this facilitates shared decision-making and enables the opportunity to determine best practice.* EBN: *A descriptive survey (N = 312) found that nurses may make inaccurate assumptions about the willingness and abilities of clients to become engaged in self-care learning (Wu et al, 2014).*
- Consider "health coaching" and motivational interviewing techniques when focusing on health-related goals, priorities, and preferences. EBN: *In a randomized controlled trial (RCT) by Benzo et al (2017), health coaching, using motivational interviewing, significantly improved disease-specific quality of life compared with the control group.*
- Seek teachable moments for those with chronic conditions to enhance their knowledge of health promotion. EB: *Findings from a recent study indicated that using cancer diagnosis as the teachable moment for health promotion efforts should be tailored and targeted at specific comorbidities (Highland et al, 2015).*
- ▲ Refer clients to lifestyle and health promotion resources delivered in the workplace or community sites outside traditional health care environments. EB: *In a compilation of literature addressing the outcomes of workplace health promotion programs (WHPPs), Goetzel et al (2014) found success in programs focusing on areas of wellness, especially in organizations that had a "culture of health."* EB: *A meta-analysis of 18 studies found that WHPPs with younger populations and that had weekly contacts were the most effective. Positive effects were seen in self-perceived health and in absences caused by illness (Rongen et al, 2013).*
- Refer clients to interactive and Web-based technological resources as appropriate. EB: *In a recent qualitative study by van der Gugten et al (2016), 70% of adults report that they seek health-related information through Internet resources.*
- Refer to Deficient **Knowledge** care plan.

 Pediatric

- Consider the use of mobile text messaging as a resource for delivery of health promotion information. EB: *A systematic review of 16 studies indicated that the use of multimedia technologies and mobile messaging are viable adjuncts that can help engage adolescents in disease prevention and health promotion (Geckle, 2016).*
- Incorporate health promotion education that reflects the unique cultural interests and values of diverse groups. EB: *In a systematic review of 80 papers, Suarez-Balcazar, Friesema, and Lukyanova (2013) found that adapting physical activities, ethnic dancing, and playing games that are culturally relevant were most effective for promoting health and addressing obesity in African American and Latino youth.*
- Involve children and especially adolescents in designing health promotion programs and teaching methods. EBN: *In a recent systematic review of eight qualitative studies, when the health care professional ensures children receive education and information appropriate to their health literacy, children are apt to be more involved in their decision-making (Davies & Randall, 2015).*

● = Independent; ▲ = Collaborative; EBN = Evidence-Based Nursing; EB = Evidence-Based

- Consider settings outside traditional health care centers and interdisciplinary approaches for engaging children and adolescents in preventive health care. **EB:** *A systematic review of 55 studies found that schools may be the best place to implement health-related prevention programs to reduce health risk because of the accessibility of youth and the importance of school and peer learning (Hale, Fitzgerald-Yau, & Viner, 2014).*
- Refer to Deficient **Knowledge** care plan.

 Geriatric

- Discuss healthy lifestyle changes that promote safety, health promotion, and health maintenance for older clients. **EB:** *A recent study by Hsu et al (2016) indicated that the elderly individuals with poor health status were more apt to receive a health examination for their diseases. Early detection via health promotion and disease prevention of the potential health risks would reduce the severity of diseases in the prognosis.*
- Consider involving bilingual members of a community who are considered outside the traditional health care system who may assist in the teaching of community health issues. **EB:** *A systematic review of 39 studies found that the use of multicultural health care workers improved chronic disease prevention and self-management (Goris et al, 2013).*

 Multicultural

- Refer to Geriatric.
- Refer to Deficient **Knowledge** care plan.

REFERENCES

Benzo, R., et al. (2017). Health coaching in severe COPD after a hospitalization: A qualitative analysis of a large randomized study. *Respiratory Care, 62*(11), 1403–1411. doi:10.4187/respcare.05574.

Davies, A., & Randall, D. (2015). Perceptions of children's participation in their healthcare: A critical review. *Issues in Comprehensive Pediatric Nursing, 38,* 202–221. Retrieved from http://dx.doi.org/10.3109/01460862.2015.1063740.

Geckle, J. (2016). Use of multimedia or mobile devices by adolescents for health promotion and disease prevention: A literature review. *Pediatric Nursing, 42,* 163–167.

Goetzel, R. Z., Henke, R. M., Tabrizi, M., et al. (2014). Do workplace health promotion (wellness) programs work? *Journal of Occupational and Environmental Medicine / American College of Occupational and Environmental Medicine, 56,* 927–934. Retrieved from http://dx.doi.org/10.1097/JOM.0000000000000276.

Goris, J., Komaric, N., Guandalini, A., et al. (2013). Effectiveness of multicultural health workers in chronic disease prevention and self-management in culturally and linguistically diverse populations: a systematic literature review. *Australian Journal of Primary Health, 19,* 14–37. Retrieved from http://dx.doi.org/10.1071/PY11130.

Hale, D. R., Fitzgerald-Yau, N., & Viner, R. (2014). A systematic review of effective interventions for reducing multiple health risk behaviors in adolescence. *American Journal of Public Health, 104*(5), e19–e41. Retrieved from http://dx.doi.org/10.2105/AJPH.2014.301874.

Highland, K. B., Hurtado-de-Mendoza, A., Stanton, C. A., et al. (2015). Risk-reduction opportunities in breast cancer survivors: Capitalizing on teachable moments. *Supportive Care in Cancer, 23,* 933–941. Retrieved from http://dx.doi.org/10.1007/s00520-014-2441-7.

Hsu, H. C., Chang, W. C., Luh, D. L., et al. (2016). Health, healthy lifestyles, and health examinations among the older people in Taiwan. *Australasian Journal on Ageing, 35,* 161–166. Retrieved from http://dx.doi.org/10.1111/ajag.12249.

Rongen, A., Robroek, S. J., van Lenthe, F. J., et al. (2013). Workplace health promotion: A meta-analysis of effectiveness. *American Journal of Preventive Medicine, 44,* 406–415. Retrieved from http://dx.doi.org/10.1016/j.amepre.2012.12.007.

Suarez-Balcazar, Y., Friesema, J., & Lukyanova, V. (2013). Culturally competent interventions to address obesity among African American and Latino children and youth. *Occupational Therapy in Health Care, 27,* 113–128. Retrieved from http://dx.doi.org/10.3109/07380577.2013.785644.

Stacey, D., & Legare, F. (2015). Engaging patients using an interprofessional approach to shared decision making. *Canadian Oncology Nursing Journal, 25,* 455–461.

Van der Gugten, A. C., de Leeuw, R. J. R. J., Verheij, T. J. M., et al. (2016). E-health and health care behaviour of parents of young children: A qualitative study. *Scandinavian Journal of Primary Health Care, 34*(2), 135–142. Retrieved from http://doi.org/10.3109/02813432.2016.1160627.

Wu, S., Tung, H., Liang, S., et al. (2014). Differences in the perceptions of self-care, health education barriers and educational needs between diabetes patients and nurses. *Contemporary Nurse, 46,* 187–196. Retrieved from http://dx.doi.org/10.5172/conu.2013.2767.

Latex Allergy reaction   *Gail B. Ladwig, MSN, RN and Julianne E. Doubet, BSN, RN, EMT-A*

NANDA-I

Definition

A hypersensitive reaction to natural latex rubber products.

Defining Characteristics

Life-Threatening Reactions Within 1 Hour of Exposure

Bronchospasm; chest tightness; contact urticaria progressing to generalized symptoms; dyspnea; edema; hypotension; myocardial infraction; respiratory arrest; syncope; wheezing

Type IV Reactions Occurring ≥ 1 Hour After Exposure

Discomfort reaction to additives; eczema; skin irritation; skin redness

Generalized Characteristics

Generalized discomfort; generalized edema; reports total body warmth; restlessness; skin flushing

Gastrointestinal Characteristics

Abdominal pain; nausea

Orofacial Characteristics

Erythema; itching; nasal congestion; periorbital edema; rhinorrhea; tearing of the eyes

Related Factors

To be developed

At-Risk Population

Frequent exposure to latex product; history of allergy; history of asthma; history of food allergy; history of latex reaction; history of poinsettia plant allergy; history of surgery during infancy

Associated Condition

Hypersensitivity to natural latex rubber protein; multiple surgical procedures

NOC   (Nursing Outcomes Classification)

Suggested NOC Outcomes

Allergic Response: Localized, Systemic; Immune Hypersensitivity Response; Symptom Severity; Tissue Integrity: Skin and Mucous Membranes

Example NOC Outcome with Indicators
Immune Hypersensitivity Response as evidenced by the following indicators: Respiratory, cardiac, gastrointestinal, renal, and neurological function status IER/Free of allergic reactions. (Rate the outcome indicators of **Immune Hypersensitivity Response:** 1 = severely compromised, 2 = substantially compromised, 3 = moderately compromised, 4 = mildly compromised, 5 = not compromised [see Section I].)

IER, In expected range.

Client Outcomes

Client Will (Specify Time Frame)

* Identify presence of natural rubber latex (NRL) allergy
* List history of risk factors
* Identify type of reaction
* State reasons not to use or to have anyone use latex products
* Experience a latex-safe environment for all health care procedures

● = Independent; ▲ = Collaborative; EBN = Evidence-Based Nursing; EB = Evidence-Based

- Avoid areas in which there is powder from NRL gloves
- State the importance of wearing a medical alert bracelet and wear one
- State the importance of carrying an emergency kit with a supply of nonlatex gloves, antihistamines, and an autoinjectable epinephrine syringe (EpiPen), and carry one

NIC (Nursing Interventions Classification)

Suggested NIC Interventions

Allergy Management; Latex Precautions

Example NIC Activities—Latex Precautions
Question client or appropriate other about history of systemic reaction or sensitization to NRL (e.g., facial or scleral edema, tearing eyes, urticaria, rhinitis, and wheezing); Place an allergy band on client

Nursing Interventions and *Rationales*

- Identify clients at risk as those persons who are most likely to exhibit sensitivity to NRL, which may result in varying degrees of reactivity. Consider the following client groups:
- Persons with neural tube defects including spina bifida and myelomeningocele/meningocele. **EB:** *In their research, Moroz, Flanagan, and Zaretsky (2017) found that as many as 50% of those who have spina bifida may have a latex allergy, which is probably caused by their multiple surgeries, intermittent catheterization, and condition-related susceptibility.*
- Children with spinal cord injuries. **CEB:** *The frequency of daily bladder catheterizations with latex catheters has been correlated with latex sensitivity (Venkata & Lerman, 2011).*
  - Clients with a history of multiple surgeries or other latex-exposing procedures. **EB:** *Patients who have experienced multiple surgeries have an elevated risk for latex allergy (Werfel et al, 2015).*
  - Children who have experienced three or more surgeries, particularly as neonates. **CEB:** *A significant correlation between the total number of surgeries, particularly during the first year of life, and degree of sensitization has been established (Venkata & Lerman, 2011).*
- Atopic individuals (persons with a tendency to have multiple allergic conditions including allergies to certain food products). **EB:** *A report by Werfel et al (2015) stated that 86% of patients with a positive history of fruit allergy, but having no risk factors for latex sensitization, showed latex-specific IgE antibodies.*
- Persons who have an ongoing occupational exposure to NRL, including health care workers, rubber industry workers, bakers, laboratory personnel, food handlers, hairdressers, janitors, policemen, and firefighters. **EB:** *Products manufactured with latex and the environmental allergen exposure that occurs in the work place are risk factors for the development of occupational latex allergy, especially among health care workers, followed by hairdressers, cleaners, food handlers, and those producing NRL (Caballero & Quirce, 2015).*
  - Latex sensitization is also prevalent in older adults, but they are often overlooked as a high-risk population. **EB:** *Latex allergy has not been studied extensively among older adults, but a recent study demonstrated that approximately 11.4% of the older adults in the study had latex sensitization (Grieco et al, 2014).*
- Take a thorough history of the client at risk. **EB:** *It is of immense importance to recognize allergic disorders in their primary phase so that avoidance and treatment plans can be implemented (Caballero & Quirce, 2015).*
- Have management protocols in place for treating anaphylaxis. **EB:** *Prompt initial treatment is essential in anaphylaxis because a few minutes' delay can lead to hypoxic-ischemic brain damage or death (Simons et al, 2013).* **EB:** *A report from the World Allergy Organization (Kowalski et al, 2016) advised that safety measures such as continuous supervision, specific emergency equipment, and quick access to emergency services should be readily available during at-risk testing procedures.*
- Question the client about associated symptoms of itching, swelling, and redness after contact with rubber products such as rubber gloves, balloons, and barrier contraceptives, or swelling of the tongue and lips after dental examinations. **EB:** *Latex allergy is an IgE-mediated hypersensitivity to NRL and can feasibly cause symptoms in a sensitized person ranging from urticaria to anaphylaxis (German, 2016).* **CEB:** *The range of clinical allergy-induced symptoms may include localized or generalized urticaria, rhinitis, conjunctivitis, bronchospasm, laryngospasm, hypotension, and full-blown anaphylaxis (Behrman, 2013).*
- Consider a blood test to measure serum IgE levels. **CEB:** *In theory, allergy blood testing may be safer because it does not expose the client to any allergens (Siles & Hsieh, 2011).*

● = Independent; ▲ = Collaborative; **EBN** = Evidence-Based Nursing; **EB** = Evidence-Based

- All latex-sensitive clients are treated as if they have NRL allergy. EB: *The prevention of further episodes of untoward reactions to the allergen is based on the client's removal from exposure (Siracusa et al, 2014).*
- Clients with spina bifida and others with a positive history of NRL sensitivity or NRL allergy should have all medical/surgical/dental procedures performed in a latex-controlled environment. EB: *The institution of primary and secondary prevention latex-safety policies has contributed to the decrease in latex allergy reactions (Mertes et al, 2016).* CEB: *Clients who are latex allergic should have a surgical procedure performed as the first case in the morning, when the levels of latex aeroallergens in the environment are the lowest (Siles & Hsieh, 2011).*
- In select high-risk atopic individuals, a specific immunotherapy regimen should be discussed with their health care provider. EB: *The initiation of a molecular-based diagnosis supports a continuing focus on allergen immune therapy (AIT) (Passalacqua & Canonica, 2016).* EB: *Raulf (2016) stated that molecular allergy diagnosis based on the discovery and quantity of specific IgE to single allergens is quickly developing in importance.*
- ▲ The most effective approach to preventing NRL anaphylaxis is complete latex avoidance. EB: *According to Quirce and Fladur (2016), the client must be removed from exposure to a known allergen to avert another reactive event.*
- ▲ Materials and items that contain NRL must be identified and latex-free alternatives must be found. EBN: *It is of upmost importance for patient safety to create a latex-free environment for those sensitive to the allergen (Doenges, Moorhouse, & Murr, 2016).* EB: *The substitution of nonlatex materials and the identification of latex-derived products are valuable in the successful control of health risks linked to NRL (Quirce & Fladur, 2016).*
- ▲ If latex gloves are chosen for protection from blood or body fluids, a reduced-protein, powder-free glove should be selected. EB: *According to a study by Baid and Agarwal (2017), powdered gloves have been shown to have greater NRL proteins compared with nonpowdered gloves: these substances could cause life-threatening reactions in sensitized patients and present a risk to health care workers.*

Home Care

- Assess the home environment for presence of NRL products (e.g., balloons, condoms, gloves, and products of related allergies, such as bananas, avocados, and poinsettia plants). EB: *According to Wu et al (2016), latex-derived products are still in use universally and latex allergy remains a widespread health risk for many occupations and for the general populace.*
- At onset of care, assess client history and status of NRL allergy response. EBN: *A meticulous history must be taken to ascertain the origin and effects of the client's exposure to NRL (Doenges et al, 2016).*
- ▲ Seek medical care as necessary.
- Assist the client in identifying and obtaining alternatives to NRL products. EBN: *If possible, provide a list of latex-free products to the client/caregiver (Doenges et al, 2016).*

Client/Family Teaching and Discharge Planning

- Provide written information about NRL allergy and sensitivity. EB: *Clients at risk for a severe allergic reaction/anaphylaxis should be provided with a written action plan that includes education concerning the avoidance of allergic triggers and the self-administration of epinephrine when needed (Lieberman et al, 2015).*
- ▲ Instruct the client to inform health care professionals if he or she has an NRL allergy, particularly if the client is scheduled for surgery. EB: *Anaphylaxis caused by an allergic response in the course of general anesthesia (GA) is uncommon, but it is a life-threatening event that may lead to cardiorespiratory compromise (Krishna et al, 2014).*
- Teach the client what products contain NRL and to avoid direct contact with all latex products and foods that trigger allergic reactions. EB: *Patients who are affected by a latex allergy could also develop allergies to avocados, bananas, kiwifruit, chestnuts, and other foods (Werfel et al, 2015).*
- Teach the client to avoid areas in which powdered latex gloves are used and in which latex balloons are inflated or deflated. CEB: *Powdered gloves have been shown to increase airborne NRL antigens compared with nonpowdered gloves (Palosuo et al, 2011).*
- Instruct the client with an NRL allergy to wear a medical identification bracelet and/or carry a medical identification card. EB: *ID jewelry, such as those provided by Medic Alert, should be suggested (Lieberman et al, 2015).*
- Instruct the client to carry an emergency kit with a supply of nonlatex gloves, antihistamines, and an autoinjectable epinephrine syringe (EpiPen). EB: *Clients at risk for a severe allergic reaction/anaphylaxis should be provided with a written action plan that includes education concerning the avoidance of allergic triggers and the self-administration of epinephrine when needed (Lieberman et al, 2015).*

● = Independent; ▲ = Collaborative; EBN = Evidence-Based Nursing; EB = Evidence-Based

REFERENCES

Baid, R., & Agarwal, R. (2017). Powdered gloves: Time to bid adieu. *Journal of Postgraduate Medicine, 63*(3), 206. Retrieved from http://www.jpgonline.com/text.asp?2017/63/3/206/210068).

Behrman, A. (2013). *Latex allergy.* Retrieved from http://emedicine.medscape.com/article/756632-overview. (Accessed 14 September 2014).

Caballero, M., & Quirce, S. (2015). Identification and practical management of latex allergy in occupational settings. *Expert Review of Clinical Immunology, 11*(9), 977–992. Retrieved from http://dx.doi.org/10.1586/1744666x.2015.1059754.

Doenges, M., Moorhouse, M., & Murr, A. (2016). *Nurse's pocket guide: Diagnoses, prioritized interventions, and healthcare rationales* (14th ed., pp. 512–518). Philadelphia: E. A. Davis.

German, D. (2016). Latex Allergy. In M. Mahmoudi (Ed.), *Allergy and asthma* (pp. 397–405). Cham: Springer. Retrieved from http://dx.doi.org/10.1007/978-3-319-30835-7_26.

Grieco, T., Faina, V., Dies, L., et al. (2014). Latex sensitization in elderly: Allergological study and diagnostic protocol. *Immunity and Ageing, (7)*, 11.

Kowalski, M., Ansotegui, I., Aberer, W., et al. (2016). Risk and safety requirements for diagnostic and therapeutic procedures in allergology. World Allergy Organization statement. *World Allergy Association Journal, 9*(33). Retrieved from http://dx.doi.org/10.1186/s40413-016-0122-3.

Krishna, M., York, M., Chin, T., et al. (2014). Multi-centre retrospective analysis of anaphylaxis during general anaesthesia in the United Kingdom: Aetiology and diagnostic performance of acute serum tryptase. *Clinical and Experimental Immunology, 178*(2), 399–404. doi:10.1111/cei.12424.

Lieberman, P., Nicklas, R., Randolph, C., et al. (2015). Anaphylaxis—A practice parameter update 2015. *Annals of Allergy, Asthma and Immunology, 115*(5), 341–384. Retrieved from http://dx.doi.org/10.1016/j.anal.2015.07.019.

Mertes, P., Volcheck, G., Garvey, L., et al. (2016). Epidemiology of perioperative anaphylaxis. *La Presse Medicale, 45*(9), 758–767. Retrieved from http://dx.doi.org/10.1016/j.lpm.2016.02.024.

Moroz, A., Flanagan, S., & Zaretsky, N. (2017). *Medical aspects of disability: a handbook for the rehabilitation professional* (5th ed., p. 327). New York: Springer Publishing.

Palosuo, T., et al. (2011). Latex medical gloves: Time for a reappraisal. *International Archives of Allergy and Immunology, 156*(3), 234–246.

Passalacqua, G., & Canonica, G. (2016). Allergan immune therapy: History and future developments. *Immunology & Allergy Clinics, 36*(1), 1–12. Retrieved from http://dx.doi.org/10.1016/iac2015.08.001.

Quirce, S., & Fladur, A. (2016). How should occupational anaphylaxis be investigated and managed. *Current Opinion in Allergy and Clinical Immunology, 16*(2), 86–92. Retrieved from http://dx.doi.org/10.1097/ACI.0000000000000241.

Raulf, M. (2016). Allergen component analysis as a tool in the diagnosis of occupational allergy. *Current Opinion in Allergy and Clinical Immunology, 16*(2), 93–100. Retrieved from http://dx.doi.org/10.1097/ACL.0000000000000246.

Siles, R. I., & Hsieh, F. H. (2011). Allergy blood testing: A practical guide for clinicians. *Cleveland Clinic Journal of Medicine, 78*(9), 585–592.

Simons, F. E., Ardusso, L. R., Dimov, V., et al. (2013). World Allergy Organization anaphylaxis guidelines: 2013 update of the evidence base. *International Archives of Allergy and Immunology, 162*, 193–204.

Siracusa, A., Follett, R., van, Wijk, M., et al. (2014). Occupational anaphylaxis—An EAACI task force consensus statement. *European Journal of Allergy and Clinical Immunology, 70*(2), 141–152. Retrieved from http://dx.doi.org/10.1111/all.12541.

Venkata, S., & Lerman, J. (2011). Case scenario: Perioperative latex allergy in children. *Anesthesiology, 114*(3), 673–680.

Werfel, T., Asero, B., Ballman-Weber, B., et al. (2015). Position paper of EAACI: Food allergy due to immunological cross-reactions with common inhalant allergies. *European Journal of Allergy and Clinical Immunology, 70*(9), 1079–1090. Retrieved from http://dx.doi.org/10.1111/all.12666.

Wu, M., McIntosh, J., & Liu, J. (2016). Current prevalence rate of latex allergy: Why it remains a problem. *Journal of Occupational Health, 58*(2), 138–144. doi:10.1539/joh.15-0275-RA.

L

Risk for Latex Allergy reaction   *Gail B. Ladwig, MSN, RN and Julianne E. Doubet, BSN, RN, EMT-A*

NANDA-I

Definition

Susceptible to a hypersensitive reaction to natural latex rubber products, which may compromise health.

Risk Factors

To be developed

At-Risk Population

Frequent exposure to latex product; history of allergy; history of asthma; history of food allergy; history of latex reaction; history of poinsettia plant allergy; history of surgery during infancy

Associated Condition

Hypersensitivity to natural latex rubber protein; multiple surgical procedures

● = Independent;   ▲ = Collaborative;   EBN = Evidence-Based Nursing;   EB = Evidence-Based

NOC (Nursing Outcomes Classification)

Suggested NOC Outcomes

Allergic Response: Systemic; Immune Hypersensitivity Response; Risk Control; Risk Detection; Tissue Integrity: Skin and Mucous Membranes

> #### Example NOC Outcome with Indicators
>
> **Immune Hypersensitivity Response** as evidenced by the following indicators: Respiratory, cardiac, gastrointestinal, renal, and neurological function status IER/Free of allergic reactions. (Rate the outcome and indicators of **Immune Hypersensitivity Response:** 1 = not controlled, 2 = slightly controlled, 3 = moderately controlled, 4 = well controlled, 5 = very well controlled [see Section I].)

IER, In expected range.

Client Outcomes

Client Will (Specify Time Frame)

- State risk factors for natural rubber latex (NRL) allergy
- Request latex-free environment
- Demonstrate knowledge of plan to treat NRL allergic reaction

L NIC Interventions (Nursing Interventions Classification)

Suggested NIC Interventions

Allergy Management; Latex Precautions; Environmental Risk Protection

> #### Example NIC Activities—Latex Precautions
>
> Question client or appropriate other about history of systemic reaction to NRL (e.g., facial or scleral edema, tearing eyes, urticaria, rhinitis, and wheezing); Place an allergy band on client

Nursing Interventions and *Rationales*

- Clients at high-risk for NRL allergy need to be identified. **EB:** *Products manufactured with latex and the environmental allergen exposure that occurs in the work place are risk factors for the development of occupational latex allergy; especially among health care workers, followed by hairdressers, cleaners, food handlers, and those making NRL (Caballero & Quirce, 2015).*
- Clients with spina bifida are a high-risk group for NRL allergy and should remain latex free from the first day of life. **EB:** *In their research, Moroz et al (2017) found that as many as 50% of those who have spina bifida may have a latex allergy probably caused by their multiple surgeries, intermittent catheterization, and condition-related susceptibility.*
- Children who require regular medical treatments at home (e.g., catheterization, home ventilation) should be assessed for NRL allergy. **CEB:** *The frequency of daily bladder catheterizations with latex catheters has been correlated with latex sensitivity (Venkata & Lerman, 2011).*
- Assess for NRL allergy in clients who are exposed to "hidden" latex. **EB:** *According to Wu, McIntosh, and Liu (2016), latex-derived products are still in use universally and latex allergy remains a widespread health risk for many occupations and for the general populace as well.*
- See care plan for **Latex Allergy** reaction.

 Home Care

- Ensure that the client has a medical plan if a response develops. **EB:** *Prompt treatment of anaphylactic symptoms decreases the probability of a life-threatening situation. Authors of this report (Sicherer & Simons, 2017) stress the importance of patient, family, and community education in the recognition and immediate management of anaphylaxis.*
- See care plan for **Latex Allergy** reaction. Note client history and environmental assessment.

● = Independent;   ▲ = Collaborative;   EBN = Evidence-Based Nursing;   EB = Evidence-Based

Client/Family Teaching and Discharge Planning

▲ A client who has had symptoms of NRL allergy or who suspects he or she is allergic to latex needs to give this information to health care providers. **EB:** *Clients should be made aware of any agents that would place them at risk for a serious reaction/anaphylaxis (Liebermann et al, 2015).*

● Provide written information about latex allergy and sensitivity. **EB:** *Client's at risk for a severe allergic reaction/anaphylaxis should be provided with a written action plan that includes education concerning the avoidance of allergic triggers and the self-administration of epinephrine when needed; ID jewelry, such as those provided by Medic Alert, could also be suggested (Liebermann et al, 2015).*

● Health care workers should avoid the use of latex gloves and seek alternatives such as unpowdered gloves made from nitrile. **EB:** *According to a study by Baid and Agarwal (2017), powdered gloves have been shown to have greater NRL proteins in contrast to unpowdered gloves: these substances could cause life-threatening reactions in sensitized patients and they present a risk to health care workers a well.*

● Health care institutions should develop prevention programs and establish latex-safe areas in their facilities. **EBN:** *According to Doenges, Moorhouse, and Murr (2016), the creation of latex-free environments will support client and staff safety.*

● Institute measures that reduce or completely avoid any latex exposure to clients. **EB:** *It is of immense importance to recognize allergic disorders in their primary phase to implement avoidance plans (Cabellero & Quirce, 2015).*

REFERENCES

Baid, R., & Agarwal, R. (2017). Powdered gloves: Time to bid adieu. *Journal of Postgraduate Medicine, 63*(3), 206. Retrieved from https//www.jpgonline.com/text.asp?2017/63/3/206/210068.

Caballero, M. L., & Quirce, S. (2015). Identification and practical management of latex allergy in occupational settings. *Expert Review of Clinical Immunology, 11*(9), 977–992. doi:10.1586/1744666x.2015.1059754.

Doenges, M., Moorhouse, M., & Murr, A. (2016). *Nurse's pocket guide: Diagnoses, prioritized interventions, and healthcare rationales* (14th ed., pp. 512–518). Philadelphia: E. A. Davis.

Liebermann, P., Nicklas, R., Randolph, C., et al. (2015). Anaphylaxis—A practice parameter update 2015. *Annals of Allergy, Asthma & Immunology, 115*(5), 341–384. doi:10.1016/janl.2015.07.019.

Moroz, A., Flannagon, S., & Zaretsky, N. (2017). *Medical aspects of disability: A handbook for the rehabilitation professional* (5th ed., p. 327). New York: Springer Publishing.

Sicherer, S., & Simons, F. E. (2017). Epinephrine for first-aid management of anaphylaxis. *American Academy of Pediatrics, 139*(3), doi:10.1542/peds.2016-4006.

Venkata, S., & Lerman, J. (2011). Case scenario: Perioperative latex allergy in children. *Anesthesiology, 114*(3), 673–680.

Wu, M., McIntosh, J., & Liu, J. (2016). Current prevalence rate of latex allergy: Why it remains a problem. *Journal of Occupational Health, 58*(2), 138–144. doi:10.1539/joh.15-0275-RA.

L

Readiness for enhanced health Literacy   *Kathaleen C. Bloom, PhD, CNM*

NANDA-I

Definition

A pattern of using and developing a set of skills and competencies (literacy, knowledge, motivation, culture, and language) to find, comprehend, evaluate and use health information and concepts to make daily health decisions to promote and maintain health, decrease health risks, and improve overall quality of life, which can be strengthened.

Defining Characteristics

Expresses desire to enhance ability to read, write, speak, and interpret numbers for every day health needs; expresses desire to enhance awareness of civic and/or government processes that impact public health; expresses desire to enhance health communication with health care providers; expresses desire to enhance knowledge of current determinants of health on social and physical environments; expresses desire to enhance personal health care decision-making; expresses desire to enhance social support for health; expresses desire to enhance understanding of customs and beliefs to make health care decisions; expresses desire to enhance understanding of health information to make health care choices; expresses desire to obtain sufficient information to navigate the health care system

● = Independent;   ▲ = Collaborative;   EBN = Evidence-Based Nursing;   EB = Evidence-Based

NOC   (Nursing Outcomes Classification)

Suggested NOC Outcomes

Health Beliefs: Perceived Resources; Health-Promoting Behavior; Health-Seeking Behavior

> ### Example NOC Outcome with Indicators
>
> **Health-Seeking Behavior** as evidenced by the following indicators: Completes health-related tasks/Performs self-screening/ Obtains assistance from health professional/Uses reputable heath information. (Rate the outcome and indicators of **Health-Seeking Behavior:** 1 = never demonstrated, 2 = rarely demonstrated, 3 = sometimes demonstrated, 4 = often demonstrated, 5 = consistently demonstrated [see Section I].)

Client Outcomes

Client Will (Specify Time Frame)

- Use reputable information sources
- Seek information from health care providers
- Communicate with health care provider about understanding of information provided

NIC   (Nursing Interventions Classification)

Suggested NIC Interventions

Health Literacy Enhancement; Health Education; Health System Guidance

> ### Example NIC Activities—Health Literacy Enhancement
>
> Create a health care environment in which a patient with impaired literacy can seek help without feeling ashamed or stigmatized; Provide understandable health information; Use strategies to enhance understanding

Nursing Interventions and *Rationales*

- Use a standard tool to identify the level of health literacy. *A variety of tools have been developed to measure individuals' health-related reading comprehension (Health Literacy Measurement Tools, 2016).*
- Identify and take into consideration factors affecting health literacy such as age, ethnicity, education, and cognitive function EBN: *Improved health literacy is associated with positive outcomes including decreased recidivism (Cloonan, Wood, & Riley, 2013), increased patient satisfaction with nurse communication (Stikes, Arterberry, & Logsdon, 2015), and increased health promotion (Chahardah-Cherik et al, 2018).*
- Implement health literacy universal precautions: assume that all patients may have difficulty understanding health information. *Less than 15% of adults possess the level of health literacy needed to navigate the health care system (AHRQ Health Literacy Toolkit, 2017). All patients need health information that is accurate, accessible, and understandable (French, 2015).*
- Determine readiness for increased health literacy. EB: *Assessing motivation and readiness to learn and change has the potential to allow identification of obstacles and overcoming resistance (Ceccarini et al, 2015).*
- Tailor health teaching and educational materials to accommodate the needs of those with low health literacy. EBN: *A systematic review and meta-analysis of diabetes self-management interventions (N = 13 studies) found that health literacy–sensitive interventions focused on communication (both written and spoken) and empowerment in the context of language and cultural considerations were the most effective for self-care and health outcomes, including reduction of hemoglobin (Hb)A1C (Kim & Lee, 2016).*
- Modify health teaching and educational materials to patient preferences. EB: *Individuals who have lower health literacy prefer, understand, and correctly interpret pictures and icons that are familiar, contextual, and less complex (van Beusekom et al, 2015, 2017; Arcia et al, 2016).*
- Use empowerment to enhance health literacy and improve patient outcomes. EBN: *A study with 295 individuals with type 2 diabetes found empowerment directly leading to health literacy, which then influenced self-efficacy, self-care behaviors, and finally HbA1C levels (Lee et al, 2016).*
- Use individual or group interventions as preferred by the patient and appropriate to the topic. EB: *A systematic review of 52 studies of interventions examining health literacy and smoking, nutrition, alcohol,*

● = Independent;   ▲ = Collaborative;   EBN = Evidence-Based Nursing;   EB = Evidence-Based

physical activity, and/or weight found 73% of the studies with positive associations between improved health literacy and improved outcome (Taggart et al, 2012).

Geriatric

- The above interventions may be adapted for geriatric use.
- Use simple educational materials targeted at health-promoting behaviors. EB: *Older adults with good health literacy are more likely to have mammography, to exercise, and to eat nutritiously and are less likely to perform monthly breast exams or to smoke (Fernandez, Larson, & Zikmund-Fisher, 2016; Geboers et al, 2016).*

Multicultural

- Take the patient's culture into account when designing teaching and education materials. EB: *Higher levels of health literacy challenge are associated with being from a culturally diverse background and/or not speaking English (Jessup et al, 2017).* EB: *A scoping review of 27 studies revealed three consistent barriers to health care services access: cultural differences between providers and patients, language barriers, and information barriers (Kalich, Heinemann, & Ghahari, 2016).*

Client/Family Teaching and Discharge Planning

- Promote shared decision-making. EB: *A systematic review of 19 studies revealed that shared decision-making strategies targeted to low-literacy individuals increased knowledge, informed choice, and participation in decision-making (Durand et al, 2014).*

REFERENCES

AHRQ health literacy universal precautions toolkit (2nd ed.). (2017). Rockville, MD: Agency for Healthcare Research and Quality. Retrieved from http://www.ahrq.gov/professionals/quality -patient-safety/quality-resources/tools/literacy-toolkit/index.html.

Arcia, A., Suero-Tejeda, N., Bales, M. E., et al. (2016). Sometimes more is more: Iterative participatory design of infographics for engagement of community members with varying levels of health literacy. *Journal of the American Medical Informatics Association, 23*, 174–183. Retrieved from http://dx.doi.org/10.1093/jamia/ocv079.

Ceccarini, M., Borrello, M., Pietrabissa, G., et al. (2015). Assessing motivation and readiness to change for weight management and control: An in-depth evaluation of three sets of instruments. *Frontiers in Psychology, 6*, 511. Retrieved from http:// dx.doi.org/10.3389/fpsyg.2015.00511.

Chahardah-Cherik, S., Gheibizadeh, M., Jahani, S., et al. (2018). The relationship between health literacy and health promoting behaviors in patients with type 2 diabetes. *International Journal of Community Based Nursing and Midwifery, 6*, 65–75. Retrieved from http://ijcbnm.sums.ac.ir.

Cloonan, P., Wood, J., & Riley, J. B. (2013). Reducing 30-day readmissions: Health literacy strategies. *Journal of Nursing Administration, 43*, 382–387. Retrieved from http:// dx.doi.org/10.1097/NNA.0b013e31829d6082.

Durand, M. A., Carpenter, L., Dolan, H., et al. (2014). Do interventions designed to support shared decision-making reduce health inequalities? A systematic review and meta-analysis. *PLoS ONE, 9*(4), e94670. Retrieved from http://dx.doi.org/10.1371/journal.pone.0094670.

Fernandez, D. M., Larson, J. L., & Zikmund-Fisher, B. J. (2016). Associations between health literacy and preventive health behaviors among older adults: Findings from the health and retirement study. *BMC Public Health, 16*, 596. Retrieved from http://dx.doi.org/10.1186/s12889-016-3267-7.

French, K. S. (2015). Transforming nursing care through health literacy ACTS. *Nursing Clinics of North America, 50*, 87–98. Retrieved from http://dx.doi.org/10.1016/j.cnur.2014.10.007.

Geboers, B., Reijneveld, S. A., Jansen, C. J., et al. (2016). Health literacy is associated with health behaviors and social factors among older adults: Results from the LifeLines Cohort Study. *Journal of Health Communication, 21*(Suppl. 2), 45–53. Retrieved from http:// www.tandfonline.com/loi/uhcm20.

Health literacy measurement tools (revised). (2016). Rockville, MD: Agency for Healthcare Research and Quality. Retrieved from http:// www.ahrq.gov/professionals/quality-patient-safety/ quality-resources/tools/literacy/index.html.

Jessup, R. L., Osborne, R. H., Beauchamp, A., et al. (2017). Health literacy of recently hospitalised patients: A cross-sectional survey using the Health Literacy Questionnaire (HLQ). *BMC Health Services Research, 17*, 52. Retrieved from http://dx.doi.org/10.1186/ s12913-016-1973-6.

Kalich, A., Heinemann, L., & Ghahari, S. (2016). A scoping review of immigrant experience of health care access barriers in Canada. *Journal of Immigration and Minority Health, 18*, 697–709. Retrieved from http://dx.doi.org/10.1007/s10903-015-0237-6.

Kim, S. H., & Lee, A. (2016). Health-literacy-sensitive diabetes self-management interventions: A systematic review and meta-analysis. *Worldviews on Evidence-based Nursing, 13*, 324–333. Retrieved from http://dx.doi.org/10.1111/wvn.12157.

Lee, Y. J., Shin, S. J., Wang, R. H., et al. (2016). Pathways of empowerment perceptions, health literacy, self-efficacy, and self-care behaviors to glycemic control in patients with type 2 diabetes mellitus. *Patient Education and Counseling, 99*, 287–294. Retrieved from http://dx.doi.org/10.1016/j.pec.2015.08.021.

Stikes, R., Arterberry, K., & Logsdon, M. C. (2015). A nurse leadership project to improve health literacy on a maternal-infant unit. *Journal of Obstetric, Gynecologic, and Neonatal Nursing, 44*, 665–676. Retrieved from http://dx.doi.org/10.1111/1552-6909.12742.

Taggart, J., Williams, A., Dennis, S., et al. (2012). A systematic review of interventions in primary care to improve health literacy for chronic disease behavioral risk factors. *BMC Family Practice, 13*, 49. Retrieved from http://dx.doi.org/10.1186/1471-2296-13-49.

van Beusekom, M., Bos, M., Wolterbeek, R., et al. (2015). Patients' preferences for visuals: differences in the preferred level of detail, type of background and type of frame of icons depicting organs between literate and low-literate people. *Patient Education and*

L

● = Independent;   ▲ = Collaborative;   EBN = Evidence-Based Nursing;   EB = Evidence-Based

Counseling, 98, 226–233. Retrieved from http://dx.doi.org/10.1016/j.pec.2014.10.023.

van Beusekom, M. M., Land-Zandstra, A. M., Bos, M. J. W., et al. (2017). Pharmaceutical pictograms for low-literate patients:

understanding, risk of false confidence, and evidence-based design strategies. *Patient Education and Counseling, 100*, 966–973. Retrieved from http://dx.doi.org/10.1016/j.pec.2016.12.015.

Risk for impaired Liver function   *Janelle M. Tipton, MSN, RN, AOCN*

NANDA-I

Definition

Susceptible to a decrease in liver function, which may compromise health.

Risk Factors

Substance misuse

Associated Condition

Human immunodeficiency virus (HIV) coinfection; pharmaceutical agent; viral infection

NOC   (Nursing Outcomes Classification)

Suggested NOC Outcome

Knowledge: Health Behavior; Liver Function

> **Example NOC Outcome with Indicators**
>
> **Knowledge: Health Behavior** as evidenced by the following indicators: Safe use of prescription drugs/Adverse health effects of alcohol misuse/Adverse health effects of recreational drug use/Healthy nutritional practices/Self-screening techniques. (Rate the outcome and indicators of **Knowledge: Health Behavior:** 1 = no knowledge, 2 = limited knowledge, 3 = moderate knowledge, 4 = substantial knowledge, 5 = extensive knowledge [see Section I].)

Client Outcomes

Client Will (Specify Time Frame)

- State the upper limit of the amount of acetaminophen safely taken per day
- Verbalize understanding that over-the-counter (OTC) medications may contain acetaminophen (e.g., OTC cold medicines)
- Have normal liver enzymes, serum and urinary bilirubin levels, white blood cell count, and red blood cell count
- Be free of unexplained weight loss, jaundice, pruritus, bruising, petechiae, gastrointestinal bleeding, and hemorrhage
- Be free of abdominal tenderness/pain, increased abdominal girth, and have normal-colored stool and urine
- Be able to eat frequent small meals per day without nausea and/or vomiting
- If alcohol abuse is factor, state relationship between abuse and worsening gastrointestinal and liver disease

NIC   (Nursing Interventions Classification)

Suggested NIC Interventions

Teaching: Disease Process; Substance Use Treatment

> **Example NIC Activities—Teaching Disease Process**
>
> Appraise the client's current level of knowledge related to specific disease process; Discuss lifestyle changes that may be required to prevent future complications and/or control the disease process

● = Independent;   ▲ = Collaborative;   EBN = Evidence-Based Nursing;   EB = Evidence-Based

Nursing Interventions and *Rationales*

▲ Assess for signs of liver dysfunction including fatigue, nausea, jaundice of the eyes or skin, pruritus, gastrointestinal bleeding, coagulopathy, infections, increasing abdominal girth, fluid overload, shortness of breath, mental status changes, light-colored stools, dark urine, and increased serum and urinary bilirubin levels. *These are symptoms and laboratory results associated with liver disorders (Ghany et al, 2015; Lee, Divens, & Fowler, 2017).*

▲ Evaluate liver function tests. Standard liver panels include the serum enzymes aspartate transaminase (AST), alanine transaminase (ALT), alkaline phosphatase, and γ-glutamyl transferase; total, direct, and indirect serum bilirubin; and serum albumin. **EB:** *Hepatitis C is often asymptomatic early in the disease state (Kwo, Cohen, & Lim, 2017) and may be found during a routine examination when liver function test results are elevated (Ferguson, 2014).*

▲ Discuss with the client/family preparations for other diagnostic studies, such as ultrasound, computed tomography, and magnetic resonance imaging (MRI) exams. *Although costly, MRI has the best quantification of steatosis (Cassard, Gerard, & Perlemuter, 2017).*

▲ Evaluate coagulation studies such as international normalized ratio, prothrombin time, and partial thromboplastin time, especially when there is bleeding of the mouth or gums. *Prolonged prothrombin time and decreased production of clotting factors can result in bleeding.*

● Monitor for signs of hemorrhage, especially in the upper gastrointestinal tract, because it is the most frequent site. *Synthesis of coagulation factors is affected with liver impairment (Lopez & Hendrickson, 2014).*

● Obtain a list of all medications, including OTC nonsteroidal antiinflammatory drugs, acetaminophen, herbal remedies, and dietary supplements. Review risk of drug-induced liver disease. The list includes some antibiotics, anticonvulsants, antidepressants, antiinflammatory drugs, antiplatelets, antihypertensives, calcium channel blockers, cyclosporine, lipid-lowering drugs, chemotherapy drugs, oral hypoglycemics, proton pump inhibitors, inhaled anesthetics, and tranquilizers, among others (Hamilton, Collins-Yoder, & Collins, 2016). If client is taking either OTC medications or herbals, discuss signs and symptoms of toxic hepatitis. *Toxic hepatitis is caused by direct toxins, drugs, herbs, and industrial chemicals. The risk of toxicity with aspirin, ibuprofen, naproxen sodium, and acetaminophen increases with frequency and in combination with use of alcohol (Lopez & Hendrickson, 2014).*

▲ For clients receiving drugs associated with liver injury, review risk factors to prevent potentially severe drug reactions. *Drug-induced liver disease accounts for about 50% of hepatitis cases. The most common risk factors are advanced age, female gender, alcohol use with associated infection, and genetic predisposition (Hamilton, Collins-Yoder, & Collins, 2016).*

▲ Determine the total amount of acetaminophen the client is taking per day. The amount of acetaminophen ingested should not exceed 3.25 g/day, or even lower in the client with chronic alcohol intake (Hamilton, Collins-Yoder, & Collins, 2016). *It is common for clients to take multiple pain medications, all containing acetaminophen. Acetaminophen is the most common cause of drug-induced liver injury, and approximately 46% of all people with acute liver failure in the United States have liver damage caused by acetaminophen (Ortega-Alonso et al, 2016).*

▲ Evaluation of acetaminophen-associated drug-induced liver injury is done by patient history of ingestion, time, and doses of the medication per weight calculation and serum level of acetaminophen. **EB:** *One of the tools most commonly used for decision-making in the use of N-acetylcysteine is the Rumack-Matthew nomogram for drug overdose. Prompt intervention with N-acetylcysteine has reduced mortality to 0.7% for those patients who overdosed on acetaminophen (Hamilton, Collins-Yoder, & Collins, 2016).*

▲ If the client is on statin medications, ensure that liver enzyme testing is done at intervals. Liver enzymes can become elevated from taking statin medications; it is rare, but possible for statins to cause actual liver damage (Hamilton, Collins-Yoder, & Collins, 2016).

▲ If the client is an alcoholic, refer to a cessation program. It is essential the client stop drinking as soon as possible to allow the liver to heal. Alcoholism is associated with malnutrition, which is harmful to the liver (Fabrellas, 2017). Alcoholism is also associated with increased plasma endotoxins and disruption of the gut barrier, which cause inflammation and resultant damage to the liver (Cassard, Gerard, & Perlemuter, 2017). See care plans for Ineffective **Denial** and Dysfunctional **Family** processes.

▲ Provide frequent smaller meals for easier digestion. Provide diet with optimal carbohydrates, proteins, and fats. Consult with a registered dietitian to discuss best nutritional support. *Proteins can be increased as tolerated and serum protein, albumin levels, and bilirubin levels indicate improved liver function. The goals of nutrition therapy are to provide adequate nutrition, support growth, preserve lean body mass, and prevent micronutrient deficiencies (Leon & Lerret, 2017).*

● = Independent;   ▲ = Collaborative;   **EBN** = Evidence-Based Nursing;   **EB** = Evidence-Based

L

▲ Recognize that severe malnutrition may result in acute liver failure, which is reversible with improved nutrition.

▲ Review medical history with the client, recognizing that obesity and type 2 diabetes, along with hyper-triglyceridemia and polycystic ovarian syndrome, are major risk factors in the development of liver disease, specifically nonalcoholic fatty liver disease. *For those clients showing signs of fatty liver involvement, sound nutritional support can reduce the severity and mitigate the already existing secondary malnutrition (Kunutsor et al, 2014).*

• Encourage vaccinations for hepatitis A and B for all ages. *Hepatitis A can affect anyone in the United States. Vaccination can prevent hepatitis A and B, which at times can cause liver failure (Centers for Disease Control and Prevention [CDC], 2016).*

• Measure abdominal girth if individual presents with abdominal distention and pain. *Increasing abdominal distention and pain are signs of impending portal hypertension with the presence of fluid shifts, resulting in ascites (Ghany et al, 2015).*

• Assess for tenderness and/or pain level in the right upper quadrant. Tenderness in this area is a symptom of biliary, liver, and/or pancreatic problems. *This pain, along with a palpable mass and weight loss, are a classic triad for malignancies (Ferguson 2014; Kunutsor et al, 2014).*

• Use standard precautions for handling of blood and body fluids. Review sterile techniques when giving intravenous solution and/or medications. **EB:** *This is imperative to decrease the incidence of infection with hepatitis B and hepatitis C viruses. The viruses have been spread in health care settings when injection equipment and intravenous solutions were mishandled and became contaminated (CDC, 2016).*

▲ Observe for signs and symptoms of mental status changes such as confusion from encephalopathy. *The symptoms can fluctuate in severity within hours. Blood concentration of ammonia is not correlated with the severity of hepatic encephalopathy. The most commonly used medical treatment is lactulose because it has a prebiotic effect, lowers the pH in the colon, binds to ammonia, and excretion is promoted by this laxative effect (Bager, 2017).*

 Pediatric/Parents

▲ Prescreen pregnant women for hepatitis B surface antigens. If found, recommend nursing case management during pregnancy. **EB:** *Despite advances in prevention of hepatitis B transmission, approximately half of the infections are caused by mother-to-child transmission. Efforts to prevent transmission are an essential element of perinatal maternal and infant care (Ma et al, 2014).*

▲ Recommend implementation of postexposure prophylaxis, including the hepatitis B virus vaccine for an infant born to a hepatitis B surface antigen–positive woman (CDC, 2016).

• Encourage vaccinations for hepatitis A and B for all ages. *Children should be vaccinated between ages 12 and 23 months for hepatitis A (CDC, 2016).*

▲ Recognize that children can develop fatty liver disease, which can result in liver failure. Most children are asymptomatic, but others complain of malaise, fatigue, or vague recurrent abdominal pain (Marzuillo, del Guidice, & Santoro, 2014).

▲ During a well-baby visit, assess for signs of potential liver problems. Observe for prolonged jaundice, pale stools, and urine that is anything other than colorless. Consult with health care provider to order a split bilirubin as needed (CDC, 2016).

 Home Care

• Encourage rest, optimal nutrition (high carbohydrates, sufficient protein, and essential vitamins and minerals) during initial inflammatory processes of the liver.

 Client/Family Teaching and Discharge Planning

• Teach the client and family to examine all medications the client is taking, looking for acetaminophen as an ingredient, and reinforce the 3.25-g upper limit of intake of acetaminophen to protect liver function (Hamilton, Collins-Yoder, & Collins, 2016).

• For the caregiver or client with hepatitis A, B, or C, teach the need for careful handwashing, use of gloves, and other precautions to prevent spread of any of these diseases.

• Teach avoidance of high-risk behaviors that cause hepatitis and ways to avoid those behaviors.

• Educate clients and their caregivers about treatment options and interventions for hepatitis. Recommend other informational support: risk factors, side effects of the different treatment options, and dietary advice.

• = Independent;   ▲ = Collaborative;   **EBN** = Evidence-Based Nursing;   **EB** = Evidence-Based

- Recommend psychological support if possible during education sessions. **EBN:** *Hepatitis can result in liver inflammation and chronic liver disease and is a common reason for a liver transplant. The client may not have an understanding of liver disease or its complications, may be elderly, or may have mental health issues or additions that affect the need for nursing intervention. Developing a plan and/or services to support and to give patient-centered care can provide better support to the client in dealing with liver disease (Greenslade, 2017).*

- Assess for adherence to antiviral therapies for the treatment of hepatitis and institute nursing interventions such as client education, communication, and reminder tools to assist patients in medication adherence. *Adherence to antiviral therapies is imperative to help suppress viral load and to reduce progressive liver disease (Polis et al, 2017).*

- For those clients with mental health problems, collaborate with outreach programs to teach signs/symptoms of hepatitis, risk factors, and factors that increase transmission. **EBN:** *These clients have higher potential for substance use and injected-drug use, and increased chances of transmission because of homelessness and living conditions in night shelters. Protocols have proven to be successful in developing an effective approach to meeting the needs of clients with or at risk for infection with hepatitis A, B, and C virus and severe mental health problems. Culturally sensitive, nurse-led interventions, such as counseling and bringing vaccinations to the community through mobile services, are valuable health promotion strategies in high-risk populations (Nyamathi et al, 2015; Fabrellas, 2017).*

REFERENCES

Bager, P. (2017). The assessment and care of patients with hepatic encephalopathy. *British Journal of Nursing, 26*(13), 724–729.

Cassard, A. M., Gerard, P., & Perlemuter, G. (2017). Microbiota, liver diseases, and alcohol. *Microbiology Spectrum, 5*(4), 1–19.

Centers for Disease Control and Prevention (CDC). (2016). *The ABCs of hepatitis.* Retrieved from https://www.cdc.gov/hepatitis/resources/professionals/pdfs/abctable.pdf. (Accessed 21 January 2018).

Fabrellas, N. (2017). Research about nursing care for persons with liver disease: A step in the right direction. *Nursing Research, 66*(6), 419–420.

Ferguson, L. A. (2014). Autoimmune hepatitis: A noninfectious killer. *Journal of the American Association of Nurse Practitioners, 26*, 13–18.

Ghany, M., Hoofnagle, J., et al. (2015). Approach to the patient with liver disease. In D. Kasper, A. Fauci, S. Houser, et al. (Eds.), *Harrison's principles of internal medicine* (19th ed.). New York: McGraw-Hill.

Greenslade, L. (2017). Providing high-quality care for patients with liver disease. *British Journal of Nursing, 26*(13), 739.

Hamilton, L. A., Collins-Yoder, A., & Collins, R. E. (2016). Drug-induced liver injury. *AACN Critical Care, 27*(4), 430–440.

Kunutsor, S. K., Apekey, T. A., Seddoh, D., et al. (2014). Liver enzymes and risk of all cause mortality in general populations: A systematic review and meta-analysis. *International Journal of Epidemiology, 43*, 187–201.

Kwo, P. Y., Cohen, S. M., & Lim, J. K. (2017). ACG clinical guideline: evaluation of abnormal liver chemistries. *The American Journal of Gastroenterology, 112*, 18–35.

Lee, S., Divens, L., & Fowler, L. H. (2017). The role of liver function in the setting of cirrhosis with chronic infection and critical illness. *Critical Care Nursing Clinics of North America, 29*, 37–50.

Leon, C. D. G., & Lerret, S. M. (2017). Role of nutrition and feeding for the chronically ill pediatric liver patient awaiting liver transplant. *Gastroenterology Nursing, 40*(2), 109–116.

Lopez, A. M., & Hendrickson, R. G. (2014). Toxin induced hepatic injury. *Emergency Medicine Clinics of North America, 32*, 103–125.

Ma, L., Alla, N. R., Li, X., et al. (2014). Mother to child transmission of HBV: Review of current clinical management and prevention strategies. *Reviews in Medical Virology, 24*, 396–406.

Marzuillo, P., del Guidice, E. M., & Santoro, N. (2014). Pediatric fatty liver disease: Role of ethnicity and genetics. *World Journal of Gastroenterology, 20*(23), 7347–7355.

Nyamathi, A., Salem, B. E., Zhang, S., et al. (2015). Nursing case management, peer coaching, and hepatitis A and B vaccine completion among homeless men and recently released on parole: Randomized clinical trial. *Nursing Research, 64*, 177–189.

Ortega-Alonso, A., Stephens, C., Lucena, M. I., et al. (2016). Case characterization, clinical features and risk factors in drug-induced liver injury. *International Journal of Molecular Science, 17*(5), 714.

Polis, S., Zablotska-Manos, I., Zekry, A., et al. (2017). Adherence to hepatitis B antiviral therapy: A qualitative study. *Gastroenterology Nursing, 40*(3), 239–246.

Risk for Loneliness   Julianne E. Doubet, BSN, RN, EMT-B

NANDA-I

Definition

Susceptible to experiencing discomfort associated with a desire or need for more contact with others, which may compromise health.

Risk Factors

Affectional deprivation; emotional deprivation; physical isolation; social isolation

● = Independent;   ▲ = Collaborative;   **EBN** = Evidence-Based Nursing;   **EB** = Evidence-Based

NOC (Nursing Outcomes Classification)

Suggested NOC Outcomes

Loneliness Severity; Social Interaction Skills; Social Involvement; Social Support

> **Example NOC Outcome with Indicators**
>
> **Loneliness Severity** as evidenced by the following indicators: Sense of social isolation/Difficulty in establishing contact with others. (Rate the outcome and indicators of **Loneliness Severity:** 1 = severe, 2 = substantial, 3 = moderate, 4 = mild, 5 = none [see Section I].)

Client Outcomes

Client Will (Specify Time Frame)

- Maintain one or more meaningful relationships (growth-enhancing versus codependent or abusive in nature)
- Sustain relationships that allow self-disclosure and demonstrate a balance between emotional dependence and independence
- Participate in personally meaningful activities and interactions that are ongoing, positive, and relevant socially
- Demonstrate positive use of time alone when socialization is not possible

NIC (Nursing Interventions Classification)

Suggested NIC Interventions

Family Integrity Promotion; Socialization Enhancement; Visitation Facilitation

> **Example NIC Activities—Socialization Enhancement**
>
> Encourage enhanced involvement in already established relationships; Help client increase awareness of strengths and limitations in communicating with others

Nursing Interventions and *Rationales*

- Assess the client's perception of loneliness. (Is the person alone by choice, or are there other factors that contribute to the feelings of loneliness? Is the client in one of the at-risk populations for loneliness?) EBN: *Nyatanga (2017) stated that loneliness can be a consequence of hardship, discrimination, inequality, loss of control, decrease in independence, and lack of options.*
- Use active listening skills. Establish a therapeutic relationship and spend quality time with the client. EB: *In their study of clients and families involved in palliative health care, Ciemins et al (2014) found that one of the client's expectations of health care providers included skillful listening abilities.*
- Assess how unmet needs challenge the client. Note: See care plan for Disturbed **Body Image** if loneliness is associated with chronic illness and/or afflictions (e.g., multiple sclerosis, skin disturbance, mental illness). EB: *Unmet needs may exceed what is customary for those clients who are minority, low-income community residents; caregivers with lower education; clients with early-stage dementia; and those with depression (Black et al, 2013).*
- ▲ Assess the bereaved client for risk of suicide and make appropriate referrals as necessary. EB: *A study by Stickley and Koyanago (2016) found that there is a connection between loneliness and suicidal ideation; therefore efforts to reduce loneliness may play a significant part in decreasing its detrimental effects on the client's health and well-being.*
- Assess the client who is alone for substance abuse and make appropriate referrals. EBN: *Murdoch's (2014) article emphasized that all health care professionals are responsible for raising the issue of substance misuse/abuse and referring the client to specialized services if needed.*
- Evaluate the client's desire for social interaction. EB: *Nurses and other health professionals must have an awareness of the client's social disconnectedness so that they can offer assistance in making and perpetuating social connections (Dinkins, 2017).*

● = Independent;   ▲ = Collaborative;   EBN = Evidence-Based Nursing;   EB = Evidence-Based

- Assess the client for feelings of loneliness. **EB:** *According to Pikhartova, Bowling, and Victor (2014), the report of loneliness is contingent on sociodemographic factors, such as gender, household income, household living arrangements, and health status.*
- Explore ways to increase the client's support systems. **EBN:** *Nurses must recognize those who need help in dealing with their loneliness and provide direction and support (Kirkevoid et al, 2013).*
- Show respect for the client's personal attributes. **EB:** *Grover (2014) characterized respect as an expression of trust that another person has value.*

Adolescents

- Assess the client's social support system. **EB:** *According to Rowe et al (2014), relationship impediments and a lack of knowledge about where to go for support may hold back an adolescent from seeking help.*
- Evaluate the family stability of adolescent clients. **EBN:** *In their review of literature, Kao, Luplya, and Clemen-Stone (2014) found that family efficacy, characterized as a family's confidence in its ability to manage varied situations and to realize a desired outcome, is associated with the decreased likelihood of adolescents engaging in risky health behaviors.*
- Evaluate peer relationships. **EB:** *Peer relationships have been shown to play a significant role in self-esteem development across adolescence and also to remain influential throughout adulthood (Gruenenfelder-Steiger, Harris, & Fend, 2016).*
- **EBN:** *Encourage social support for clients with disabilities.* **EB:** *In their revisit of a 2006 study involving young adults who suffer from chronic health disorders, Sattoe et al (2014) found that social participation was strongly connected to the client's feelings of independence and self-efficacy.*
- Encourage relationships with peers and involvement with groups and organizations. **EB:** *According to Choukas-Bradley et al (2015), researchers have reported that peer influence is not intrinsically detrimental and that attempts to fashion one's own attitude to match that of peers could be seen as a healthy, constructive growth pattern.*

 ### Geriatric

- Evaluate the client for any health deviations that may limit or decrease his or her ability to interact with others. **EB:** *A study by Kvaal, Halding, and Kvigne (2014) made the point that loneliness is extensive among older people suffering from chronic physical illness.*
- Assess family caregivers of older persons with chronic conditions for depression related to loneliness. **EBN:** *Caregivers of loved ones many times are subjected to physical, psychological, emotional, social, and financial effects that can be called "caregiver burden" (Sorrell, 2014).*
- Identify support systems for older adults. **EB:** *Senior centers are ideal settings for providing evidence-based health programs to the fast-growing population of older adults and to help facilitate their continued good health and independence (Felix et al, 2014).*
- When relocation is necessary for older adults, evaluate relocation stress as a contributing factor to loneliness. **EB:** *A preliminary study by Theurer et al (2014) suggested that mutual support groups have the potential to offset loneliness, helplessness, and depression among clients in extended care facilities.* **EBN:** *(Sprinks, 2014).*
- Identify risk factors for loneliness in older persons. **EB:** *In their study of aging and loneliness, Brittain et al (2017) stated that recognized risks factors for loneliness include widowhood, living alone, depression, and being female.*
- Encourage support for the client when the decision to stop driving must be made. **EB:** *The nurse should direct the client toward community support systems and alternate methods of transportation when it is no longer feasible for them to continue driving (Pachana, 2015).*
- Provide activities that are pleasurable to the client. **EB:** *In their review of one of the results of the English Longitudinal Study on Aging, Gale et al (2014) found that older people who take pleasure in life tend to live longer, indicating that psychological well-being could be a promising resource for healthier aging. Refer to the care plan for* **Social** *isolation for additional interventions.*

 ### Multicultural

- Refer to the care plan for **Social** isolation.

 ### Home Care

- ▲ The preceding interventions may be adapted for home care use.
- ▲ Assess for depression with the lonely older client and make appropriate referrals. **EBN:** *The heightened prevalence of depressive symptoms and their relationship to the associated factors (gender, age group, schooling,*

● = Independent;   ▲ = Collaborative;   **EBN** = Evidence-Based Nursing;   **EB** = Evidence-Based

marital status, and place of residence) of depression in the elderly affirm the necessity to implement means for the advancement of public policies and prioritize strategies that can best guarantee health care for the elderly population (Cambo Leal et al, 2015).

- If the client has unexplained somatic complaints, evaluate these complaints to ensure that his or her physical needs are being met, and assess for a possible relationship between somatic complaints and loneliness. **EB:** *"Our bodies manifest emotions physically when we cannot effectively express them" (Spencer, 2016).* **EBN:** *In their study, Zimmerman et al (2016) confirmed that the nurse can, in collaboration with the client's physician, competently support self-management of patients with psychosomatic symptoms and their psychosocial needs.*
- Evaluate alternatives to being alone. **EB:** *O'Connor, Arizmendi, and Kaszniak (2014) conducted a preliminary study of an online support group for those isolated while caring for clients with dementia; the study established the viability of interactive groups in virtual environments to connect members in significant interaction.*
- Refer to the care plan for **Social** isolation.

 ### Client/Family Teaching and Discharge Planning

- Identify the type of loneliness that the client is experiencing as emotional and/or social. **EB:** *If both emotional and social loneliness are to be reduced in older people, strategies should be directed to widening the ranges of interventions (Dahlberg & McKee, 2014).*
- Encourage family members' involvement, if possible, in helping alleviate client's loneliness. **EBN:** *Decreased satisfaction with family support was one of the important predictors of depression levels in older people: this is a factor that should be considered when planning care (Tanner, Martinez, & Harris, 2014).*
- Include the family, if possible, in all client-teaching activities, and give them accurate information. **EBN:** *One of the nurse's central roles is to ensure continuity of care applied to all the client's health care settings; therefore patient and family education is of utmost importance (Marshall et al, 2015).*
- Provide appropriate education for clients and their support persons about disease transmission and treatment if applicable. **EBN:** *Home health patients are cared for in a totally unconstrained environment innate with infection possibilities, so concluded Pandur (2015) in her study of infections in home care settings.*
- Refer to the care plan for **Social** isolation for additional interventions.

REFERENCES

Black, B. S., Johnston, D., Rabins, P. V., et al. (2013). Unmet needs of community-residing persons with dementia and their informal caregivers: Findings from the Maximizing Independence at Home Study. *Journal of the American Geriatrics Society, 61,* 2087–2095.

Brittain, K., Kingston, A., Davis, K., et al. (2017). An investigation into patterns of loneliness and loss in the oldest old—Newcastle 85+ study. *Ageing and Society, 37*(1), 39–62.

Choukas-Bradley, S., Giletta, M., Cohen, G., et al. (2015). Peer influence, peer status, and prosocial behavior: An experimental investigation of peer socialization and adolescents' intentions to volunteer. *Journal of Youth and Adolescence, 44*(12), 2197–2210.

Ciemins, F. L., Brant, J., Kersten, D., et al. (2014). A qualitative analysis of patient and family perspectives on palliative care. *Journal of Palliative Medicine, 9.*

Cambo Leal, M., Apostolo, J., Mendes, A., et al. (2015). Depression among elderly in the community, and age care centers, and geriatric homes. *Journal of Nursing UFPE Online, 9*(4), 7383–7390. Retrieved from http://dx.doi.org/10.5205/reuol.7275-62744-1-SM-09904201525.

Dahlberg, L., & McKee, K. J. (2014). Correlates of social and emotional loneliness in older people: evidence from an English community study. *Aging and Mental Health, 18,* 504–514.

Dinkins, C. (2017). Seeing oneself in the face of the other: The value and challenge of human connectedness for older adults. *Journal of Psychosocial Nursing & Mental Health, 55*(7), 13–17.

Felix, H. C., Adams, B., Cornnell, E., et al. (2014). Barriers and facilitators to senior center participating in translational research. *Research on Aging, 36,* 22–39.

Gale, C. R., Cooper, C., Deary, U., et al. (2014). Psychological well-being and incident frailty in men and women: The English longitudinal study of aging. *Psychological Medicine, 44,* 697–708.

Grover, S. L. (2014). Unraveling respect in organization studies. *Human Relations, 67,* 27–51.

Gruenenfelder-Steiger, A., Harris, M., & Fend, H. (2016). Subjective and objective peer approval evaluation and self esteem development: A test of reciprocal, prospective, and long term effects. *Developmental Psychology, 52*(10), 1563–1577.

Kao, T. S., Luplya, C. M., & Clemen-Stone, S. (2014). Family efficacy as a protective factor against immigrant adolescent risky behavior: A literature review. *Journal of Holistic Nursing, 32,* 202–216.

Kirkevold, M., Moyle, W., Wilkinson, C., et al. (2013). Facing the challenge of adopting a life "alone": The influences of losses. *Journal of Advanced Nursing, 69,* 394–403.

Kvaal, K., Halding, A. G., & Kvigne, K. (2014). Social provision and loneliness among older people suffering from chronic physical illness: A mixed-methods approach. *Scandinavian Journal of Caring Solutions, 28,* 104–111.

Murdoch, J. (2014). Alcohol misuse: assessment, treatment and aftercare. *Nursing Older People, 28,* 18–24.

Marshall, L., Dall'Oglio, I., Davis, D., et al. (2015). Nurses as educators within health systems…Chapter from mastering patient and family education STTI book. *Reflections on Nursing Leadership, 41*(4), 1–17.

Nyatanga, B. (2017). Being lonely and isolated: Challenges for palliative care. *British Journal of Community Nursing, 22*(7), 360.

O'Connor, M. F., Arizmendi, B. J., & Kaszniak, A. W. (2014). Virtually supportive: A feasibility pilot study of an on line support group for dementia caregivers in a 3D virtual environment. *Journal of Aging Studies, 30,* 87–93.

Pikhartova, J., Bowling, A., & Victor, C. (2014). Does owning a pet protect older people against loneliness? *BMC Geriatrics, 14,* 106.

Pachana, N. (2015). Driving, space, and access to activity. *The Journal of Gerontology: Series B: Psychological Sciences & Social Sciences, 71*(1), 69–70.

Pandur, R. (2015). Infection surveillance in the home health care setting. *Australian Nursing and Midwifery Journal, 23*(3), 43.

Rowe, S. L., French, R. S., Henderson, C., et al. (2014). Help-seeking behaviour and adolescent self-harm: A systematic review. *Australian and New Zealand Journal of Psychiatry, 21.*

Sattoe, J. N. T., Hilberink, S. R., van Staa, A., et al. (2014). Lagging behind or not? Four distinct social participation patterns among young adults with chronic conditions. *Journal of Adolescent Health, 54,* 397–403.

Sorrell, J. M. (2014). Moving beyond caregiver burden: Identifying helpful interventions for family caregivers. *Journal of Psychosocial Nursing and Mental Health Services, 52,* 15–18.

Spencer, D., (2016). *Managing psychosomatic symptoms.* Retrieved from: http://dx.doi.org/10.1002/cbl.30142.

Sprinks, J. (2014). Social engagement crucial to tackling loneliness in old age. *Nursing Older People, 26,* 8–9.

Stickley, A., & Koyanago, A. (2016). Loneliness, common mental disorders and suicidal behavior: Findings from a general population survey. *Journal of Affective Disorders, 197,* 81–87.

Tanner, E. F., Martinez, I. L., & Harris, M. (2014). Examining functional and social detriments of depression in community-dwelling older adults: Implications for practice. *Geriatric Nursing, 35,* 236–240.

Theurer, K., Walter, A., Chaudhury, H., et al. (2014). The development and evaluation of mutual support groups in long-term care homes. *Journal of Applied Gerontology, 33,* 387–415.

Zimmerman, T., Puschmann, E., van den Bussche, H., et al. (2016). Collaborative nurse-led self management support of primary care patients with anxiety, depression or somatic problems: Cluster-randomized controlled trial (findings of SMADS study). *International Journal of Nursing Studies, 63,* 101–111.

Risk for disturbed Maternal–Fetal dyad *Dianne F. Hayward, RN, MSN, WHNP*

NANDA-I

M

Definition

Susceptible to a disruption of the mother-fetal relationship as a result of comorbid or pregnancy-related conditions, which may compromise health.

Risk Factors

Inadequate prenatal care; presence of abuse; substance misuse

Associated Condition

Alteration in glucose metabolism; compromised fetal oxygen transport; pregnancy complication; treatment regimen

NOC (Nursing Outcomes Classification)

Suggested NOC Outcomes

Fetal Status: Antepartum; Maternal Status: Antepartum, Intrapartum; Depression Level; Blood Glucose Level; Family Resiliency; Knowledge: Self-Management; Nausea and Vomiting Severity; Social Support; Spiritual Support, Parent-Infant Attachment

Example NOC Outcome with Indicators
Maternal Status: Antepartum as evidenced by the following indicators: Emotional attachment to fetus/Coping with discomforts of pregnancy/Mood lability/Blood pressure/Blood glucose/Hemoglobin. (Rate the outcome and indicators of **Maternal Status: Antepartum:** 1 = Severe deviation from normal range, 2 = Substantial deviation from normal range, 3 = Moderate deviation from normal range, 4 = Mild deviation from normal range, 5 = No deviation from normal range [see Section I].)

Client Outcomes

Client Will (Specify Time Frame)

- Cope with discomforts of high-risk pregnancy until delivery of baby
- Demonstrate emotional attachment to fetus
- Adhere to prescribed regimens to maintain homeostasis during pregnancy

● = Independent; ▲ = Collaborative; EBN = Evidence-Based Nursing; EB = Evidence-Based

NIC	(Nursing Interventions Classification)

Suggested NIC Interventions

High-Risk Pregnancy Care; Intrapartal Care: High-Risk Delivery

Example NIC Activities—High-Risk Pregnancy Care
Determine the presence of medical factors that are related to poor pregnancy outcome (e.g., diabetes, hypertension, lupus erythematosus, herpes, hepatitis, HIV, multiple gestation, substance abuse, epilepsy); Provide educational materials that address the risk factors and usual surveillance tests and procedures

Nursing Interventions and *Rationales*

- Standardize internal and external transport forms using the situation, background, assessment, and recommendation (SBAR) format to provide safe and efficient care of a high-risk pregnant client. **EBN:** *SBAR is a powerful tool that is used to improve the effectiveness of communication between individuals. It is an easy-to-use protocol that provides a concise and prioritized structure, which supports consistent, comprehensive, and client-centered reports (Cornell et al, 2013).*
- Assess the antenatal client for fear related to high-risk pregnancy and fetal outcomes. Encourage verbalization of feelings, beliefs, and concerns about fetal well-being, maternal health, and family functioning. Include family when possible. Refer for treatment as needed. **EBN:** *An Istanbul study found that pregnant women with a poor level of psychosocial adaptation showed more depressive manifestations (Fiskin, Kaydirak, & Oskay, 2017).* **EB:** *When a pregnant woman exhibits symptoms of anxiety, she might need counseling and/ or treatment to decrease her anxiety (Rubertsson et al, 2014).*
- Assess antepartum clients for depression using a culturally competent tool that evaluates the bio-psycho-social-spiritual dimensions. **EBN:** *Screening and appropriate management is essential to prevent adverse consequences to both the woman and her unborn infant (Anderson & Lieser, 2015).*
- Offer flexible visiting hours, private space for families, and nursing support for management of family stressors; provide distractors such as music, TV, and laptops with Internet access during hospitalization for high-risk pregnancy. **EB:** *Assisting high-risk antepartum hospitalized women should include a focus on family function, liberal visiting hours, a "child-friendly" family visitation room, and education. Understanding the situation can help women accept the responsibility of remaining pregnant and in labor and delivery (Lederman et al, 2013).*
- Focus on the abilities of a pregnant woman with disabilities by encouraging identification of support systems, resources, and need for environmental modification. **EBN:** *In a recent study of pregnant women with disabilities, the women reported a lack of knowledge, awareness, sensitivity, and respect, as well as stereotyping, as issues that contributed to compromised perinatal care (Smeltzer et al, 2016).*
- Assess for lack of social support system, loneliness, depression, lack of confidence, maternal powerlessness, domestic violence, and socioeconomic problems. **EBN:** *Screening should include significant risk factors to detect at-risk women (Ruyak, Flores-Montoya, & Boursaw, 2017).*
- Recognize patterns of physical abuse in all pregnant and postpartum women, regardless of age, race, and socioeconomic status. **EBN:** *Abuse during pregnancy can result in poor maternal, neonatal, and early childhood outcomes; routine screening and assessment may interrupt further abuse and promote positive outcomes (Bianchi, Cesario, & McFarlane, 2016).*
- Perform accurate blood pressure readings at each client's clinic encounter. **EB:** *Elevated blood pressure during pregnancy, regardless of etiology or known risk factors, indicates high risk for preeclampsia and for later cardiovascular disease, chronic kidney disease, and diabetes mellitus (Mannisto et al, 2013).*
- Provide educational materials and support for personal autonomy about genetic counseling and testing options before pregnancy with preimplantation genetic testing or during pregnancy with fetal nuchal translucency ultrasound, quadruple screen, and cystic fibrosis screening. **EBN:** *Health care providers are presented with several challenges now that consumers have direct access to genetic tests that they may not fully comprehend, which may lead them to act on the results inappropriately (Beery, 2014). Nurses can advocate, understand the perceptions of, and assist patients in their reproductive decision-making (Shiroff & Nemeth, 2015).*
- Identify adherence barriers and assist with meal selections to maintain optimal nutrition and safe pregnancy weight gain (25–35 pounds; 15–25 pounds if overweight). Identify cultural beliefs and nutritional patterns.

● = Independent;   ▲ = Collaborative;   **EBN** = Evidence-Based Nursing;   **EB** = Evidence-Based

A prenatal vitamin with 400 mcg of folate should also be strongly recommended. **EB:** *A British task force showed that many women are not following nutritional guidelines. Pregnancy provides an opportunity for health care professionals to encourage women to make dietary improvements (e.g., following "myplate.com") because they tend to be more motivated to change aspects of their diet and lifestyle during this time (Williamson & Wyness, 2013). All women in the reproductive years should consume at least 400 mcg of folic acid per day to reduce risk for neural tube defects (Littleton-Gibbs & Engebretson, 2013).*

- Teach pregnant women diagnosed with gestational diabetes about management and treatment. **EBN:** *To reduce morbidity related to gestational diabetes, clients need education to manage blood glucose levels during pregnancy. When diet and exercise are not enough to control blood glucose levels, drug therapy is the next option. Although insulin remains the treatment of choice, insulin therapy requires sufficient education and skills on the part of the woman with gestational diabetes to be properly managed and may cause hypoglycemia, fear, and anxiety (Mnatsakanyan, Rosario-Sim, & Caboral-Stevens, 2014). Good control of blood glucose is important during delivery to reduce the risk of neonatal hypoglycemia (King, 2017).*

- Assess use of tobacco and, if positive for use, offer a tobacco cessation program and explain the health risks to the unborn fetus and mother. **EB:** *Depressive symptoms were a predictor of tobacco consumption but not of spontaneous quitting; spontaneous quitting was better predicted by anxiety symptoms. Therefore anxious symptoms should be targeted in interventions for smoking cessation during pregnancy (Miguez, Pereira, & Figueiredo, 2017). See US Department of Health and Human Services (USDHHS, 2017) for quitting smoking guidelines at https://betobaccofree.hhs.gov/quit-now/index.html.*

- Assess for alcohol use and counsel women to stop drinking during pregnancy. Give appropriate referral for treatment if needed. **EB:** *There is no known safe amount or safe time to drink alcohol during pregnancy. Drinking alcohol during pregnancy can cause miscarriage; stillbirth; and a range of permanent physical, behavioral, and fetal alcohol spectrum disorders (FASDs) (Centers for Disease Control and Prevention, 2016).*

- Screen for current illicit drug use. Emphasize the risks or drug exposure to the fetus/newborn and the potential for withdrawal. Offer nonjudgmental compassionate care. **EBN:** *"All nurses, regardless of their beliefs about perinatal addiction, must provide nonjudgmental compassionate care that is person-centered" (McKeever, Spaeth-Brayton, & Sheerin, 2014).*

- Refer clients who self-report drug abuse or have positive toxicology screens to a comprehensive addiction program designed for the pregnant woman. Children born to addicted mothers often have poor neonatal outcomes. **EBN:** *It is important to involve a pregnant woman in treatment programs like methadone clinics to stabilize the maternal–fetal dyad. When a woman makes the decision to enroll in a methadone treatment program, she is taking a significant step toward recovery (Maguire, 2014).*

- Encourage pregnant women to use digital resources, such as Text4Baby (see https://www.text4baby.org) or https://www.whattoexpect.com, to track pregnancy progress and provide education and motivation to make healthy lifestyle choices (abstinence from poor nutrition, smoking, and alcohol). **EBN:** *A recent study described the development of an iPad application to promote knowledge of tobacco risk and cessation resources for pregnant women and the evaluation of women's acceptance and perceptions regarding the application (Walsh Dotson et al, 2017).*

REFERENCES

Anderson, C. A., & Lieser, C. (2015). Prenatal depression: Early intervention. *Nurse Practitioner, 40*(7), 38–46.

Beery, T. A. (2014). Genetic and genomic testing in clinical practice: What you need to know. *Rehabilitation Nursing, 39*(2), 70–75.

Bianchi, A. L., Cesario, S. K., & McFarlane, J. (2016). Interrupting intimate partner violence during pregnancy with an effective screening and assessment program. *Journal of Obstetric Gynecological and Neonatal Nursing, 45*(4), 579–591.

Centers for Disease Control and Prevention. (2016). *Alcohol and pregnancy.* Retrieved from https://www.cdc.gov/vitalsigns/fasd/index.html.

Cornell, P., Gervis, M. T., Yates, L., et al. (2013). Improving shift report focus and consistency with the situation, background, assessment, recommendation protocol. *Journal of Nursing Administration, 43*(7/8), 422–428.

Fiskin, F., Kaydirak, M. M., & Oskay, U. Y. (2017). Psychosocial adaptation and depressive manifestations in high-risk pregnant women: Implications for clinical practice. *Worldviews on Evidence-based Nursing, 14*(1), 55–64.

King, P. (2017). Gestational diabetes: A practical guide. *Journal of Diabetes Nursing, 21*(3), 84–89.

Lederman, R. P., Boyd, E., Pitts, K., et al. (2013). Maternal development experiences of women hospitalized to prevent preterm birth. *Sexual and Reproductive Healthcare, 4*(4), 133–138.

Littleton-Gibbs, L., & Englebretson, J. (2013). *Maternity nursing care.* Clifton Park, NY: Delmar.

Maguire, D. (2014). Drug addiction in pregnancy: Disease not moral failure. *Neonatal Network, 33*(1), 11–18.

Mannisto, T., Mendola, P., Vaarasmaki, M., et al. (2013). Elevated blood pressure in pregnancy and subsequent chronic disease risk. *National Institute of Health: Circulation, 127*(6), 681–690.

McKeever, A. E., Spaeth-Brayton, S., & Sheerin, S. (2014). The role of nurses in comprehensive care management of pregnant women with drug addiction. *Nursing for Women's Health, 18*(4), 284–293.

● = Independent;   ▲ = Collaborative;   **EBN** = Evidence-Based Nursing;   **EB** = Evidence-Based

Miguez, M. C., Pereira, B., & Figueiredo, B. (2017). Tobacco consumption and spontaneous quitting at the first trimester of pregnancy. *Addictive Behaviors, 64,* 111–117.

Mnatsakanyan, K., Rosario-Sim, M., & Caboral-Stevens, M. (2014). A review of the treatment options for gestational diabetes: The evidence base. *Journal of Diabetes Nursing, 18*(4), 156–161.

Rubertsson, C., Hellström, J., Cross, M., et al. (2014). Anxiety in early pregnancy: Prevalence and contributing factors. *Archives of Women's Mental Health, 17*(3), 221–228.

Ruyak, S. L., Flores-Montoya, A., & Boursaw, B. (2017). Antepartum services and symptoms of postpartum depression in at-risk women. *Journal of Obstetric, Gynecological, & Neonatal Nursing, 46*(5), 696–708. Retrieved from http://dx.doi.org/10.1016/j.jogn.2017.07.006.

Shiroff, J. J., & Nemeth, L. S. (2015). Public perceptions of recessive carrier testing in the preconception and prenatal periods. *Journal of Gynecological and Neonatal Nurses, 44*(6), 717–725.

Smeltzer, S. C., Mitra, M., Iezzoni, L. I., et al. (2016). Perinatal experiences of women with physical disabilities and their recommendations for clinicians. *Journal of Gynecological and Neonatal Nurses, 45*(6), 781–789.

US Department of Health & Human Services USDHHS (2017). *Quit now.* Retrieved from https://betobaccofree.hhs.gov/quit-now/index.html. (Accessed 10 February 2018).

Walsh Dotson, J. A., Pineda, R., Cylkowski, H., et al. (2017). Development and evaluation of an iPad application to promote knowledge of tobacco use and cessation by pregnant women. *Nursing for Women's Health, 21*(3), 174–185.

Williamson, C., & Wyness, L. (2013). Nutritional requirements in pregnancy and use of dietary supplements. *Community Practitioner: The Journal of the Community Practitioners' and Health Visitors' Association, 86*(8), 44–47.

Impaired Memory   *Olga F. Jarrín, PhD, RN*

NANDA-I

M

Definition

Persistent inability to remember or recall bits of information or skills.

Defining Characteristics

Consistently forgets to perform a behavior at the scheduled time; persistent forgetfulness; persistent inability to learn a new skill; persistent inability to learn new information; persistent inability to perform a previously learned skill; persistent inability to recall factual information or events; persistent inability to recall familiar names, words, or objects; persistent inability to recall if a behavior was performed; persistent inability to retain a new skill; persistent inability to retain new information; preserved capacity to perform daily activities independently

Related Factors

Alterations in fluid volume

Associated Condition

Anemia; brain injury; decrease in cardiac output; electrolyte imbalance; hypoxia; mild cognitive impairment; neurological impairment; Parkinson's disease

NOC   Outcomes (Nursing Outcomes Classification)

Suggested NOC Outcomes

Cognitive Orientation; Memory; Neurological Status: Consciousness

> **Example NOC Outcome with Indicators**
>
> **Memory** as evidenced by the following indicators: Recalls immediate information accurately/Recalls recent information accurately/Recalls remote information accurately. (Rate each indicator of **Memory:** 1 = severely compromised, 2 = substantially compromised, 3 = moderately compromised, 4 = mildly compromised, 5 = not compromised [see Section I].)

Client Outcomes

Client Will (Specify Time Frame)

- Demonstrate use of techniques to help with memory loss
- State he or she has improved memory for everyday concerns

● = Independent;   ▲ = Collaborative;   EBN = Evidence-Based Nursing;   EB = Evidence-Based

NIC	Interventions (Nursing Interventions Classification)

Suggested NIC Interventions

Memory Training; Dementia Management; Reality Orientation

> **Example NIC Activities—Memory Training**
>
> Discuss with patient/family any practical memory problems experienced; Implement appropriate memory techniques, such as visual imagery, mnemonic devices, memory games, memory cues, association techniques, making lists, using computers, using name tags, or rehearsing information; Structure the teaching methods according to patient's organization of information; Refer to occupational therapy, as appropriate; Monitor changes in memory with training

Nursing Interventions and *Rationales*

- Determine whether onset of memory loss is gradual or sudden. **EB:** *Acute onset of memory loss may be associated with neurological disease, medication effect, electrolyte disturbances, hypoxia, hypothyroidism, mental illness, posttraumatic stress disorder, drug addiction, or many other physiological factors (Schwabe, Nader, & Pruessner, 2014).*
- Assess overall cognitive function and memory. A brief screening instrument such as the Montreal Cognitive Assessment (s-MoCA) is useful as a first level of evaluation. **EB:** *The s-MoCA is valid across neurological disorders and can be administered in approximately 5 minutes to determine whether the client has cognitive impairment and needs to be referred for further evaluation and treatment (Roalf et al, 2016, 2017).*
- Assess risk of malnutrition, including risk for thiamine (B_1) associated with chronic alcohol abuse, cancer, bariatric surgery, and risk of vitamin D deficiency–associated history of inadequate exposure to sunlight. **EB:** *Wernicke–Korsakoff syndrome is a disorder of the brain that is the result of vitamin B_1 deficiency associated with chronic abuse of alcohol, cancer, and bariatric surgery (Manzo et al, 2014). Vitamin D insufficiency is associated with cognitive impairment (Goodwill & Szoeke, 2017).*
- Determine the client's sleep quality and patterns. If sleep quantity and quality are insufficient, or symptoms of obstructive sleep apnea are reported, refer to the care plan for Disturbed **Sleep** pattern. **EB:** *Sleep disordered breathing is associated with an increased risk of cognitive impairment and a small worsening of executive function (Leng et al, 2017).*
- Teach clients, including those with cognitive disorders, to use memory techniques such as concentrating and attending, repeating information, making mental associations, and placing items in strategic places so that they will not be forgotten. **EBN:** *A meta-analysis of memory-focused interventions found they effectively improved memory-related performance in people with cognitive disorders (Yang et al, 2017).*
- Encourage the client to participate in a multicomponent cognitive rehabilitation program that includes stress and relaxation training, physical activity, structured learning, and social interaction. **EB:** *Mind–body practice, arts-based activities, structured arithmetic, reading aloud, and writing have been shown to improve working memory and cognitive function (Kawashima et al, 2015; Young, Camic, & Tischler, 2016; Chan et al, 2017a,b).*
- Encourage the client to develop an aerobic exercise program. **EB:** *Reviews demonstrated that diet and lifestyle may prevent the onset of age-related problems and can lead to improvements in cognition and memory (Meeusen, 2014; Wang et al, 2014).*
- For clients with memory impairments associated with dementia, also see care plan for Chronic **Confusion**.

 Geriatric

- Assess for signs and symptoms of depression. **EBN:** *Depression is often associated with memory loss in older adults; however, cognitive behavior therapy, competitive memory training, reminiscence group therapy, problem-adaptation therapy, and problem-solving therapy are all effective interventions to reduce depressive symptoms (Apóstolo et al, 2016).*
- Teach older adults that they can improve their memory and learn strategies to compensate for memory loss. **EBN:** *Octogenarians were able to improve their memory performance when they challenged their limits, used appropriate strategies, practiced yoga, and invested the energy and time in learning novel memory techniques (McDougall et al, 2015).*

● = Independent;   ▲ = Collaborative;   **EBN** = Evidence-Based Nursing;   **EB** = Evidence-Based

▲ Refer the client for cognitive training. **EB:** *Cognition training has been shown to improve verbal recall, face–name memory, and processing speed (Tak & Hong, 2014; Chan et al, 2016).*

Multicultural

- When using cognitive assessments that have been translated into other languages, refer to translation-specific scoring instructions and any recommended adjustment for low-levels of education. **EB:** *Although cognitive assessments like the MoCA and Mini-Mental State Examination (MMSE) have been translated and validated in many languages, there is wide variation in published cutoff scores, and not correcting for educational bias may result in inappropriate referral or diagnosis (Rosli et al, 2016; Delgado, Araneda, & Behrens, 2017).*
- Assess for the influence of cultural beliefs, norms, and values on the family or caregiver's understanding of impaired memory. **CEB:** American Indians, Chinese Americans, Latino Americans, and Vietnamese Americans may believe serious cognitive decline is a normal part of aging. American Indian, Chinese, and Vietnamese older adults may have great concerns about stigma associated with cognitive impairment (Laditka et al, 2011).
- Visitation facilitation: stigma may result in social isolation, and older adults with memory impairment may need assistance to rebuild and strengthen their social network. **EB:** *Social network quality and emotional closeness are positively associated with cognitive functioning among older Chinese adults (Li & Dong, 2017).*

Home Care

- The previously mentioned interventions may be adapted for home care use.
- Assist clients to select and use cuing strategies or assistive technology, such as a smart watch, smart phone, pill box, calendar, alarm clock, microwave oven, whistling tea kettle, sign, or written list to cue behaviors at designated times. **EB:** *Cues and assistive technology are positively associated with individuals' abilities to perform daily tasks regardless of age or cognitive disease (Leopold et al, 2015).*

Client/Family Teaching and Discharge Planning

- When teaching the client, determine what the client knows about memory techniques and then build on that knowledge. **EBN:** *New material is organized in terms of what knowledge already exists, and efficient teaching should attempt to take advantage of what is already known to graft on new material (McDougall et al, 2014).*
- When teaching a skill to the client, set up a series of practice attempts that will enhance motivation. Begin with simple tasks so the client can be positively reinforced and progress to more difficult concepts. **EB:** *Distributed practice with correct recall attempts can be a very effective teaching strategy, especially when used over time (Gross et al, 2014).*
- ▲ Refer for care coordination if family caregiver is unavailable or unable to assist. **EB:** *Home-based dementia care coordination delivered by nonclinical community workers trained and overseen by geriatric clinicians reduced unmet needs, improved self-reported quality of life, and led to delays in nursing home admission (Samus et al, 2014).*

REFERENCES

Apóstolo, J., Bobrowicz-Campos, E., Rodrigues, M., et al. (2016). The effectiveness of non-pharmacological interventions in older adults with depressive disorders: a systematic review. *International Journal of Nursing Studies*, 58, 59–70. doi:10.1016/j.ijnurstu.2016.02.006.

Chan, M. Y., Haber, S., Drew, L. M., et al. (2016). Training older adults to use tablet computers: Does it enhance cognitive function? *The Gerontologist*, 56(3), 475–484. doi:10.1093/geront/gnu057.

Chan, A. S., Cheung, W. K., Yeung, M. K., et al. (2017a). A Chinese Chan-based Mind-Body Intervention improves memory of older adults. *Front Aging Neurosci*, 9, 190. doi:10.3389/fnagi.2017.00190.

Chan, S. C. C., Chan, C. C. H., Derbie, A. Y., et al. (2017b). Chinese calligraphy writing for augmenting attentional control and working memory of older adults at risk of mild cognitive impairment: A randomized controlled trial. *Journal of Alzheimer's Disease*, 58(3), 735–746. doi:10.3233/JAD-170024.

Delgado, C., Araneda, A., & Behrens, M. I. (2017). Validation of the Spanish-language version of the Montreal Cognitive Assessment test in adults older than 60 years. *Neurologia (Barcelona, Spain)*. doi:10.1016/j.nrl.2017.01.013.

Goodwill, A. M., & Szoeke, C. (2017). A systematic review and meta-analysis of the effect of low vitamin D on cognition. *Journal of the American Geriatrics Society*, 65(10), 2161–2168. doi:10.1111/jgs.15012.

Gross, A. L., Brandt, J., Bandeen-Roche, K., et al. (2014). Do older adults use the method of loci? Results from the ACTIVE study. *Experimental Aging Research*, 40(2), 140–163. doi:10.1080/0361073X.2014.882204.

Kawashima, R., Hiller, D. L., Sereda, S. L., et al. (2015). SAIDO learning as a cognitive intervention for dementia care: A preliminary study. *Journal of the American Medical Directors Association*, 16(1), 56–62. doi:10.1016/j.jamda.2014.10.021.

● = Independent;   ▲ = Collaborative;   **EBN** = Evidence-Based Nursing;   **EB** = Evidence-Based

Laditka, J. N., Laditka, S. B., Liu, R. U. I., et al. (2011). Older adults' concerns about cognitive health: Commonalities and differences among six United States ethnic groups. *Ageing and Society, 31*(07), 1202–1228. doi:10.1017/s0144686x10001273.

Leng, Y., McEvoy, C. T., Allen, I. E., et al. (2017). Association of sleep-disordered breathing with cognitive function and risk of cognitive impairment: A systematic review and meta-analysis. *JAMA Neurol, 74*(10), 1237–1245. doi:10.1001/jamaneurol.2017.2180.

Li, M., & Dong, X. (2017). Is social network a protective factor for cognitive impairment in US Chinese older adults? Findings from the PINE study. *Gerontology.* doi:10.1159/000485616. [Epub ahead of print].

Leopold, A., Lourie, A., Petras, H., et al. (2015). The use of assistive technology for cognition to support the performance of daily activities for individuals with cognitive disabilities due to traumatic brain injury: The current state of the research. *Neurorehabilitation, 37*(3), 359–378. doi:10.3233/NRE-151267.

Manzo, G., De Gennaro, A., Cozzolino, A., et al. (2014). MR imaging findings in alcoholic and nonalcoholic acute Wernicke's encephalopathy: A review. *BioMed Research International, 2014*, 503596. doi:10.1155/2014/503596.

McDougall, G. J., Pituch, K. A., Stanton, M. P., et al. (2014). Memory performance and affect: Are there gender differences in community-residing older adults? *Issues in Mental Health Nursing, 35*(8), 620–627. doi:10.3109/01612840.2014.895071.

McDougall, G. J., Jr., Vance, D. E., Wayde, E., et al. (2015). Memory training plus yoga for older adults. *The Journal of Neuroscience Nursing: Journal of the American Association of Neuroscience Nurses, 47*(3), 178–188. doi:10.1097/JNN.0000000000000133.

Meeusen, R. (2014). Exercise, nutrition and the brain. *Sports Medicine (Auckland, N.Z.), 44*(Suppl. 1), S47–S56. doi:10.1007/s40279-014-0150-5.

Roalf, D. R., Moore, T. M., Mechanic-Hamilton, D., et al. (2017). Bridging cognitive screening tests in neurologic disorders: A crosswalk between the short Montreal Cognitive Assessment and Mini-Mental State Examination. *Alzheimer's & Dementia, 13*(8), 947–952. doi:10.1016/j.jalz.2017.01.015.

Roalf, D. R., Moore, T. M., Wolk, D. A., et al. (2016). Defining and validating a short form Montreal Cognitive Assessment (s-MoCA) for use in neurodegenerative disease. *Journal of Neurology, Neurosurgery, and Psychiatry, 87*(12), 1303–1310. doi:10.1136/jnnp-2015-312723.

Rosli, R., Tan, M. P., Gray, W. K., et al. (2016). Cognitive assessment tools in Asia: A systematic review. *International Psychogeriatrics, 28*(2), 189–210. doi:10.1017/S1041610215001635.

Samus, Q. M., et al. (2014). A multidimensional home-based care coordination intervention for elders with memory disorders: The Maximizing Independence at Home (MIND) pilot randomized trial. *American Journal of Geriatric Psychiatry, 22*, 398–414. doi:10.1016/j.jagp.2013.12.175.

Schwabe, L., Nader, K., & Pruessner, J. C. (2014). Reconsolidation of human memory: Brain mechanisms and clinical relevance. *Biological Psychiatry, 76*(4), 274–280. doi:10.1016/j.biopsych.2014.03.008.

Tak, S. H., & Hong, S. H. (2014). Face-name memory in Alzheimer's disease. *Geriatric Nursing, 35*, 290–294. doi:10.1016/j.gerinurse.2014.03.004.

Wang, C., Yu, J. T., Wang, H. F., et al. (2014). Non-pharmacological interventions for patients with mild cognitive impairment: A meta-analysis of randomized controlled trials of cognition-based and exercise interventions. *Journal of Alzheimer's Disease, 42*(2), 663–678. doi:10.3233/JAD-140660.

Yang, H. L., Chan, P. T., Chang, P. C., et al. (2017). Memory-focused interventions for people with cognitive disorders: A systematic review and meta-analysis of randomized controlled studies. *International Journal of Nursing Studies.* doi:10.1016/j.ijnurstu.2017.08.005.

Young, R., Camic, P. M., & Tischler, V. (2016). The impact of community-based arts and health interventions on cognition in people with dementia: A systematic literature review. *Aging and Mental Health, 20*(4), 337–351. doi:10.1080/13607863.2015.1011080.

Risk for Metabolic Imbalance syndrome *Marina Martinez-Kratz, MS, RN, CNE*

NANDA-I

Definition

Susceptible to a toxic cluster of biochemical and physiological factors associated with the development of cardiovascular disease arising from obesity and type 2 diabetes, which may compromise health.

Risk Factors

Ineffective health maintenance (00099), obesity (00232), overweight (00233), risk for unstable blood glucose level (00179), risk-prone health behavior (00188), sedentary lifestyle (00168), stress overload (00177)

At-Risk Population

Age >30 years, family history of diabetes mellitus, family history of dyslipidemia, family history of hypertension, family history of obesity

Associated Condition

Excessive endogenous or exogenous glucocorticoids >25 g/dL, microalbuminuria >30 mg/dL, polycystic ovary syndrome, unstable blood pressure, uric acid >7 mg/dL

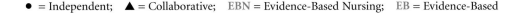

● = Independent; ▲ = Collaborative; EBN = Evidence-Based Nursing; EB = Evidence-Based

(Nursing Outcomes Classification)

Suggested NOC Outcomes

Weight Loss Behavior; Blood Glucose Level; Circulation Status; Exercise Participation; Hypertension Severity; Knowledge: Lipid Disorder Management; Knowledge: Hypertension Management; Knowledge: Prescribed Diet; Knowledge: Prescribed Activity; Knowledge: Weight Management; Metabolic Function; Nutritional Status: Nutrient Intake; Risk Control: Obesity; Risk Control: Lipid Disorder; Risk Control: Hypertension

Example NOC Outcome with Indicators

Risk Control: Lipid Disorder as evidenced by the following indicators: Seeks current information about lipid disorders/ Identifies risk factors for lipid disorders/Modifies lifestyle to reduce risk/Develops effective risk control strategies/Maintains recommended body weight. (Rate the outcome and indicators of **Risk Control: Lipid Disorder**: 1 = severe deviation from normal range, 2 = substantial deviation from normal range, 3 = moderate deviation from normal range, 4 = mild deviation from normal range, 5 = no deviation from normal range [see Section I].)

Client Outcomes

Client Will (Specify Time Frame)

- Maintain blood glucose within normal limits
- Explain actions and precautions to decrease cardiovascular risk
- Maintain waist circumference of less than 102 cm/40 inches in men, or less than 88 cm/35 inches in women
- Explain the risk factors associated with lipid disorders
- Maintain normal laboratory results, specifically high-sensitivity C-reactive protein, triglycerides, fasting blood glucose, and high-density lipoprotein (HDL) cholesterol
- Design lifestyle modifications to meet individual long-term goal of health, using effective risk control strategies
- Maintain weight within normal range for height and age
- Develop a system of self-management, for improved dietary intake and physical activity

NIC **(Nursing Interventions Classification)**

Suggested NIC Interventions

Cardiac Risk Management; Exercise Promotion; Health Screening; Hyperglycemia Management; Hyperlipidemia Management; Nutritional Counseling; Teaching: Disease Process

Example NIC Activities—Cardiac Risk Management

Screen patient for risk behaviors associated with adverse cardiac events; Prioritize areas for risk reduction in collaboration with patient and family

Nursing Interventions and *Rationales*

- Assess for risk factors associated with metabolic syndrome. Risk factors for metabolic syndrome include central obesity, dyslipidemia, insulin resistance, and increased blood pressure. CEB: *Metabolic syndrome is a clustering of metabolic abnormalities associated with subsequent cardiovascular disease and mortality (Grundy et al, 2005).*
- Assess clients for elevated waist circumference measures; greater than 102 cm/40 inches or more in men, or greater than 88 cm/35 inches or more in women. EB: *An elevated waist circumference reflects central obesity and metabolic syndrome screening is recommended in the effort to combat cardiovascular disease and type II diabetes mellitus (Cheong et al, 2015).*
- Examine the client's skin for acanthosis nigricans, acrochordons, keratosis pilaris, hyperandrogenism, and hirsutism, which are skin diseases associated with insulin resistance and obesity. EB: *Early recognition of insulin resistance and obesity-associated skin diseases may facilitate an earlier metabolic syndrome diagnoses and therapy initiation (Uzuncakmak et al, 2018).*

• = Independent;   ▲ = Collaborative;   EBN = Evidence-Based Nursing;   EB = Evidence-Based

- Assess the effect of psychosocial risk factors on cardiovascular risk. EBN: *A study found that metabolic syndrome among blue collar workers is closely related to psychosocial factors, such as job stress, social support, and risk perception, with the effect of job stress a point of difference between men and women (Hwang & Lee, 2014).*

- Assess and report abnormal laboratory results, specifically high-sensitivity C-reactive protein, triglycerides, fasting blood glucose, and HDL cholesterol. EB: *A recent study found that high-sensitivity C-reactive protein, triglycerides, fasting blood glucose, and HDL cholesterol were factors associated with metabolic syndrome (Tayefi et al, 2018).*

- Screen clients who are prescribed antipsychotic medications for metabolic syndrome during routine health treatment. EBN: *A recent study found that despite an increased awareness of comorbid physical health issues among mental health consumers, guidelines and policy directives to clinical practice to address this disparity remains low (Ward et al, 2018).*

- Screen clients with a family history of polycystic ovary syndrome for metabolic syndrome. EB: *A recent meta-analysis suggests that mothers, fathers, sisters, and brothers of women with polycystic ovary syndrome have an increased risk of metabolic syndrome, hypertension, and dyslipidemia when compared with parents and siblings of women without polycystic ovary syndrome (Yilmaz et al, 2018).*

- Assist obese clients to develop a system of self-management, which may include self-monitoring of weight, body mass index (BMI), realistic goal setting, planning, and action planning for improved dietary intake and physical activity; problem-solving; and tracking dietary intake and exercise. EB: *A key component of successful weight loss and maintenance is regular self-monitoring (Thomason et al, 2016).*

- Encourage strength training for the client to address modifiable risk factors of metabolic syndrome. EBN: *A recent study of a 12-week strength training protocol demonstrated a significant reduction in C-reactive protein level, a positive trend in other biomarkers, and increased functional outcomes of premenopausal women with moderate cardiovascular risk (Flandez et al, 2017).*

- Provide nutritional teaching targeted at reducing daily energy, fat intakes, sugar intakes, and increasing the frequency of eating two portions of vegetables during each meal. EB: *A randomized controlled trial demonstrated a reduction in metabolic syndrome risk factors after the implementation of lifestyle modifications focused on dietary intake and physical activity (Watanabe et al, 2016). A study of clients with metabolic syndrome showed that consumption of added sugar decreased after 1 year with American Heart Association dietary counselling (Zhang et al, 2018).*

- Encourage the client to engage in vigorous-intensity physical activity for at least 150 minutes weekly or moderate-intensity physical activity for at least 300 minutes weekly to improve cardiorespiratory fitness and influence body shape and weight. EB: *A recent study indicated that being highly fit increased the likelihood of lower metabolic risk approximately 2 and 2.5 times independently of central adiposity compared with average and low fitness, respectively (Lätt et al, 2018).*

- Counsel clients to slow the pace of their eating during meals. EB: *A Japanese study found that a fast eating speed was associated with obesity and future prevalence of metabolic syndrome (Yamaji et al, 2018).*

- Provide teaching about reducing intake of ultra-processed foods and increasing intake of minimally processed foods. EB: *A study divided foods into ultra-processed, processed, and minimally processed. Ultra-processed foods consisted mainly of fast foods, snacks, sausage, nuts, sweets, and liquor, whereas minimally processed foods consisted mostly of fruits, vegetables, legumes, breads, cheeses, and eggs. Participants in the highest quartile of the "minimally processed/processed" pattern had significantly lower odds for metabolic syndrome (Nasreddine et al, 2018).*

- Encourage once or more weekly consumption of lean fish. EB: *A Norwegian study found lean fish consumption once a week or more was significantly associated with decreased future metabolic score, decreased triglycerides, and increased HDL cholesterol in both men and women. In addition, men also showed decreased waist circumference and decreased blood pressure (Torris et al, 2017).*

- Use social media for communication with clients to implement social support and share information about lifestyle modifications. EB: *A study using social media to augment the delivery of, and provide support for, a weight management program delivered to overweight and obese individuals during a 24-week intervention found the Facebook group reported a 4.8% reduction in initial weight and numerically greater improvements in BMI, waist circumference, fat mass, lean mass, and energy intake (Monica et al, 2017).*

- Refer clients with Class II and III obesity and diabetes for bariatric surgery consideration. EB: *A recent review found that metabolic surgery is highly effective in obtaining significant and durable weight loss, enhancing glycemic control, and achieving diabetes remission (Pareek et al, 2018).*

● = Independent;   ▲ = Collaborative;   EBN = Evidence-Based Nursing;   EB = Evidence-Based

Pediatric

- Assess adolescent clients for vitamin D deficiency with additional screening for prediabetes if deficiencies are found. EBN: *A recent study found an association of vitamin D deficiency with an increased risk of elevated fasting blood glucose levels (Kim et al, 2018).*
- Provide preventive interventions for obesity during early childhood. EBN: A meta-analysis found that overweight or obesity in early childhood was associated with a higher risk of adult metabolic syndrome compared with the controls (Kim et al, 2017).

Geriatric

Note: Many of the preceding interventions also apply.

- Encourage strength training for older women. EB: *A recent study found that women who participated in a 12-week resistance training program showed decreased C-reactive protein concentrations, reduced blood glucose levels, decreased waist circumference, and lowered systolic blood pressure regardless of diet (Tomeleri et al, 2018).*
- Encourage Tai chi training for older adults. EB: *Recent research found that the practice of Tai chi exercise was associated with a statistically significant decrease in hemoglobin (Hb)A1C concentration and oxidative stress score in a group of older adults (Mendoza-Núñez et al, 2018).*

Multicultural

- Use criteria in addition to overweight and obesity when screening for cardiometabolic abnormalities in racial/ethnic minority populations. EB: *A cross-sectional study with participants from several US racial/ethnic groups found that nearly a third of the participants with normal weight had cardiometabolic abnormalities (Gujral et al, 2017).*
- Provide African American women with community-based prevention education targeted toward improving knowledge, reducing clinical risk profiles, adoption of heart-healthy lifestyles, reducing inflammatory burden, and decreasing cardiometabolic risk. EB: *A 4-month precardiovascular/postcardiovascular disease preventive educational intervention found that compared with baseline, there was a 60% reduction (P < 0.05) in the number of participants who met diagnostic criteria for metabolic syndrome (Villablanca et al, 2016).*

Home Care

- Previously discussed interventions may be adapted for home care use.

Client/Family Teaching and Discharge Planning

- Many of the preceding interventions involve teaching.
- Work with the family members regarding information on how to identify and reduce risk factors related to metabolic syndrome.

REFERENCES

Cheong, K. C., et al. (2015). The discriminative ability of waist circumference, body mass index and waist-to-hip ratio in identifying metabolic syndrome: Variations by age, sex and race. *Diabetes & Metabolic Syndrome: Clinical Research & Reviews, 9*(2), 74–78. doi:10.1016/j.dsx.2015.02.006.

Flandez, J., et al. (2017). Metabolic and functional profile of premenopausal women with metabolic syndrome after training with elastics as compared to free weights. *Biological Research for Nursing, 19*(2), 190–197. doi:10.1177/1099800416674307.

Grundy, S. M., et al. (2005). Diagnosis and management of the metabolic syndrome: An American Heart Association/National Heart, Lung, and Blood Institute scientific statement. *Circulation, 112*, 2735–2752. doi:10.1161/CIRCULATIONAHA.105.169404.

Gujral, U. P., et al. (2017). Cardiometabolic abnormalities among normal-weight persons from five racial/ethnic groups in the United States: A cross-sectional analysis of two cohort studies. *Annals of Internal Medicine, 166*, 628–636. doi:10.7326/M16-1895.

Hwang, W. J., & Lee, C. Y. (2014). Effect of psychosocial factors on metabolic syndrome in male and female blue-collar workers. *Japan*

Journal of Nursing Science, 11(1), 23–34. doi:10.1111/j.1742-7924.2012.00226.x.

Kim, Y., et al. (2018). The association between vitamin D deficiency and metabolic syndrome in Korean adolescents. *Journal of Pediatric Nursing, 38*, e7–e11. doi:10.1016/j.pedn.2017.11.005.

Kim, J., et al. (2017). Overweight or obesity in children aged 0 to 6 and the risk of adult metabolic syndrome: A systematic review and meta-analysis. *Journal of Clinical Nursing, 26*(23–24), 3869–3880. doi:10.1111/jocn.13802.

Lätt, E., et al. (2018). Low fitness is associated with metabolic risk independently of central adiposity in a cohort of 18-year-olds. *Scandinavian Journal of Medicine & Science in Sports, 28*(3), 1084–1091. doi:10.1111/sms.13002.

Mendoza-Núñez, V. M., et al. (2018). Hypoglycemic and antioxidant effect of Tai chi exercise training in older adults with metabolic syndrome. *Clinical Interventions in Aging, 13*, 523–531. doi:10.2147/CIA.S157584.

Monica, J., et al. (2017). Effects of a weight management program delivered by social media on weight and metabolic syndrome risk

● = Independent;   ▲ = Collaborative;   EBN = Evidence-Based Nursing;   EB = Evidence-Based

factors in overweight and obese adults: A randomised controlled trial. *PLoS ONE, 12*(6), 1–20. doi:10.1371/journal.pone.0178326.

Nasreddine, L., et al. (2018). A minimally processed dietary pattern is associated with lower odds of metabolic syndrome among Lebanese adults. *Public Health Nutrition, 21*(1), 160–171. doi:10.1017/S1368980017002130.

Pareek, M., et al. (2018). Metabolic surgery: Weight loss, diabetes, and beyond. *Journal of the American College of Cardiology, 71*(6), 670–687. doi:10.1016/j.jacc.2017.12.014.

Tayefi, M., et al. (2018). Evaluating of associated risk factors of metabolic syndrome by using decision tree. *Comprehensive Clinical Pathology, 27*(1), 215–223. doi:10.1007/s00580-017-2580-6.

Thomason, D. L., et al. (2016). A systematic review of adolescent self-management and weight loss. *Journal of Pediatric Health Care, 30*(6), 569–582. doi:10.1016/j.pedhc.2015.11.016.

Tomeleri, C. M., et al. (2018). Resistance training reduces metabolic syndrome and inflammatory markers in older women: A randomized controlled trial. *Journal of Diabetes, 10*, 328–337. doi:10.1111/1753-0407.12614.

Torris, C., et al. (2017). Lean fish consumption is associated with beneficial changes in the metabolic syndrome components: A 13-year follow-up study from the Norwegian Tromsø Study. *Nutrients, 9*(3), 1–19. doi:10.3390/nu9030247.

Uzuncakmak, T. K., et al. (2018). Cutaneous manifestations of obesity and the metabolic syndrome. *Clinics in Dermatology, 36*(1), 81–88. doi:10.1016/j.clindermatol.2017.09.014.

Villablanca, A. C., et al. (2016). Inflammation and cardiometabolic risk in African American women is reduced by a pilot community-based educational intervention. *Journal of Women's Health, 25*(2), 188–199. doi:10.1089/jwh.2014.5109.

Ward, T., et al. (2018). Who is responsible for metabolic screening for mental health clients taking antipsychotic medications? *International Journal of Mental Health Nursing, 27*(1), 196–203. doi:10.1111/inm.12309.

Watanabe, M., et al. (2016). Effects of a lifestyle modification programme to reduce the number of risk factors for metabolic syndrome: A randomized controlled trial. *Public Health Nutrition, 20*(1), 142–153. doi:10.1017/S1368980016001920.

Yamaji, T., et al. (2018). Does eating fast cause obesity and metabolic syndrome? *Journal of the American College of Cardiology, 71*(11), A1846. doi:10.1016/S0735-1097(18)32387-8.

Yilmaz, B., et al. (2018). Metabolic syndrome, hypertension, and hyperlipidemia in mothers, fathers, sisters, and brothers of women with polycystic ovary syndrome: A systematic review and meta-analysis. *Fertility and Sterility, 109*(2), 356–364, e32. doi:10.1016/j.fertnstert.2017.10.018.

Zhang, L., et al. (2018). Effect of AHA dietary counselling on added sugar intake among participants with metabolic syndrome. *European Journal of Nutrition, 57*(3), 1073–1082. doi:10.1007/s00394-017-1390-6.

Impaired bed Mobility   Wendie A. Howland, MN, RN-BC, CRRN, CCM, CNLCP, LNCC

NANDA-I

Definition

Limitation of independent movement from one bed position to another.

Defining Characteristics

Impaired ability to move between long sitting and supine positions; impaired ability to move between prone and supine positions; impaired ability to move between sitting and supine positions; impaired ability to reposition self in bed; impaired ability to turn from side to side

Related Factors

Environmental barrier; insufficient knowledge of mobility strategies; insufficient muscle strength; obesity; pain; physical deconditioning

Associated Condition

Alteration in cognitive functioning; musculoskeletal impairment; neuromuscular impairment; pharmaceutical agent

NOC   Outcomes (Nursing Outcomes Classification)

Suggested NOC Outcomes

Immobility Consequences: Physiological; Mobility; Self-Care: Activities of Daily Living (ADLs)

Example NOC Outcome with Indicators

Immobility Consequences: Physiological as evidenced by the following indicators: Pressure sores/Constipation/Hypoactive bowel/Paralytic ileus/Urinary calculi/Contracted joints/Venous thrombosis/Pneumonia. (Rate the outcome and indicators of **Immobility Consequences: Physiological:** 1 = severely compromised, 2 = substantially compromised, 3 = moderately compromised, 4 = mildly compromised, 5 = not compromised [see Section I].)

● = Independent;   ▲ = Collaborative;   EBN = Evidence-Based Nursing;   EB = Evidence-Based

Client Outcomes

Client Will (Specify Time Frame)

- Demonstrate optimal independence in positioning, exercising, and performing functional activities in bed
- Demonstrate ability to direct others on how to do bed positioning, exercising, and functional activities

NIC	Interventions (Nursing Interventions Classification)

Suggested NIC Intervention

Bed Rest Care

Example NIC Activities—Best Rest Care
Position in proper body alignment; Teach bed exercises, as appropriate

Nursing Interventions and *Rationales*

- ▲ Recognize that components of normal bed mobility include rolling, bridging, scooting, long sitting, and sitting upright. Activity starts with the client supine, flat in bed, and promotes normal movements that are bilateral, segmental, well timed, and involve set positions such as weight bearing and trunk centering. Refer to a physical therapist (PT) for individualized instructions and mobility strategies.
- Choose therapeutic beds and positions based on client's history and risk profile.
  - ❍ Advocate for specialty beds for bedbound patients incorporating low-airloss pressure relief, shear-reduction with position changes, and turn assist.
  - ❍ Use devices such as a trapeze, friction-reducing slide sheets, mechanical lateral transfer aids, and ceiling-mounted or floor lifts to move (rather than drag) clients in bed to prevent injury to staff.
  - ❍ Use special beds and equipment to move clients, such as mattress overlay, sliding/roller board, trapeze, stirrup, and pulley attached to overhead traction system (holds one leg up during pericare).
- Place clients in free-standing or ceiling-mounted lifts with padded slings while changing bed linen. EB: *Turn-assist features in beds greatly decreased spine loading and pull forces for nurses turning and lateral repositioning in patients of both normal and obese weight, thus decreasing injury potential to staff (Wiggerman, 2016; D'Arcy, Sasai, & Stearns, 2012). Staff should use lifting/transfer equipment and devices, ergonomic assessments, no-lift policies, and education to decrease risk of injury (Choi and Brings, 2016). Only about one-third of nurses with available lifting equipment use it (Lee et al, 2017). A sliding sheet is preferable over a regular cotton sheet to decrease musculoskeletal load for caregivers (Weiner et al, 2016).*
- All patients can benefit from a high sitting position to potentially minimize orthostatic intolerance (Khan et al, 2002).
- Assess to determine whether positioning for one condition may negatively affect another; use critical thinking skills for risk–benefit analysis. EB: *Elevation of head of bed (HOB) to a semirecumbent position (at least 30 degrees) is an effective, low-cost, and low-risk intervention associated with a decreased incidence of aspiration and ventilator-associated pneumonia (Agency for Healthcare Research and Quality [AHRQ], 2017). Use critical thinking to determine when specialty bed surfaces will help protect patients from tissue injury if frequent turning is contraindicated by patient instability.*
- Elevate HOB to 30 to 45 degrees unless contraindicated, and elevate HOB to 90 degrees during oral intake of fluids, solids, and oral medications.
- Raise HOB to 30 degrees for clients with acute increased intracranial pressure and brain injury. Refer to care plan for Decreased **Intracranial** adaptive capacity.
- ▲ Consult health care provider for HOB elevation for acute stroke and monitor response. Refer to care plan for Decreased **Intracranial** adaptive capacity.
- Raise HOB as close to 45 degrees as possible for critically ill ventilated clients to prevent pneumonia (this height may place clients at higher risk for pressure ulcers). Elevating the HOB decreases regurgitation and risk for aspiration of gastric contents.
- Assist client with dysphagia to sit as upright as possible for oral intake, including solids, fluids, and oral medications. Refer to care plan for Impaired **Swallowing**.
- Periodically sit client upright as tolerated in bed; dangle client, if vital signs and oxygen saturation levels remain stable. *Placing a client who is generally immobilized in an upright position is beneficial, using adaptive*

• = Independent;   ▲ = Collaborative;   EBN = Evidence-Based Nursing;   EB = Evidence-Based

equipment if necessary (Green et al, 2016). Being vertical has many physiological and psychological benefits (Green et al, 2016)

- To decrease risk of pressure injury, maintain HOB at lowest elevation that is medically possible and raise the foot of the bed to prevent shear-related injury. Assess the client's sacrum, ischial tuberosities, and heels at least every 2 hours. **EB:** *Shear results when external friction stretches the top layers of the skin as it slides against underlying layers and as internal tissues slide over deeper muscle and bone. These forces increase over the ischial tuberosities and sacrum when the backrest of the bed is elevated and result in tissue damage. Raising the foot of the bed in proportion to the HOB to distribute weight brings the body into maximum contact with the supporting surface, helping to eliminate shear. Placing a client who is generally immobilized in a recliner is a good alternative to the bed only if shear- and pressure-reducing bed surfaces cannot be obtained (Guerin et al, 2013; Martin et al, 2017). Use critical thinking and consult with nurse specialist in pressure injury harm reduction to determine when advocating for specialty bed surfaces will help protect patients from tissue injury.*

- Try periods of prone positioning for clients and monitor their tolerance/response. **EB/CEB:** *Prone positioning after both above the knee and below the knee amputations promotes extension, preventing flexor contractions in lower extremity residual joints (Wright & Flynn, 2011; Gattinoni et al, 2013; Gosselin & Smith, 2014).*

- Assess client's risk for falls using a valid fall risk assessment tool, such as the Morse Fall Scale (Morse, Tylko, & Dixon, 1987) and implement specific measures to mitigate identified risk factors. **CEB:** *Establish individualized fall prevention strategies and perform postfall assessment to further refine fall prevention interventions.*

- Beds should be kept locked and in the lowest position when occupied. Specialty low beds in which mattresses are approximately 8 to 12 inches from the floor are helpful for clients at risk for falls. Cushioned mats, 2 to 3 inches thick, with beveled edges lined with reflective tape and covered by a rubberized material are also helpful. *Mats seemed to provide "a protective effect" for the pelvis during head-first falls and for the thorax during feet-first falls (Hill & Fauerbach, 2014).*

- ▲ Bed rails and restraints must be prescribed by a health care provider.

- ▲ While placing all four bed rails up is considered a form of restraint and requires a health care provider's prescription, two and even three rails up can be a support for bed mobility. *Nursing staff can work with physical and occupational therapists to determine the most effective techniques for bed mobility, including recommendations on the number of bedrails (Hill & Fauerbach, 2014).*

- Place frequently used items within client's reach; demonstrate use of call bell (Hill & Fauerbach, 2014).

- Use a formalized screening tool to identify clients who are at high risk for deep venous thrombosis (e.g., obesity, cancer diagnosis, pelvic surgery, immobility, prior history of deep vein thrombosis [DVT]). **EB:** *Best clinical practice encourages the use of a clinical decision tool that determines deep venous thrombosis risk based on predisposing factors and certain clinical signs and symptoms (Anthony, 2013).*

- ▲ Assess for injury associated with thromboembolism prophylaxis and other prescribed treatment (e.g., anticoagulants, compression stockings, elastic leg wraps, sequential compression devices, feet/ankle exercises, and hydration). Refer to care plan for Ineffective peripheral **Tissue Perfusion.**

- Use a valid and reliable tool to assess a client's risk for pressure injury. **EB:** *Routine assessment of risk factors is crucial in planning individualized interventions to diminish the risk of hospital-acquired pressure injury occurrences (Braden and Bergstrom, 1989; Moyses et al, 2017).*

- Implement the following interventions to prevent pressure ulcers and complications of immobility:
  - ○ Position sitting clients with special attention to the individual's anatomy, postural alignment, distribution of weight, and foot support.
  - ○ Use static/dynamic bed surfaces and assess for "bottoming out" under susceptible bony areas (body sinks into mattress, thus the recommended 1 inch between mattress/bones is absent). Refer to care plan for Risk for impaired **Skin** integrity.
  - ○ Use heel protection devices that completely float or offload heels (National Pressure Ulcer Advisory Panel et al, 2014).
  - ○ Implement a 2-hour on/off schedule for heel protector boots or high-top tennis shoes with socks underneath in clients with paralyzed feet, and check condition of heels when removed.
  - ○ Strictly maintain leg abduction in persons with a surgical hip pinning or replacement by placing an abductor splint/pillow between legs if prescribed.
  - ○ Place bariatric beds along a corner wall, which helps keep the bed from moving during repositioning.

- Identify/modify hospital beds with large gaps between bed rail/mattress that create an entrapment hazard. Ensure that mattresses fit the bed; install gap fillers/rail inserts, then monitor effectiveness.

M

- Apply elbow pads to comatose and/or restrained clients and to those who use their elbows to prop or scoot up in bed. Apply nocturnal elbow splint as prescribed if ulnar nerve palsy exists or if painful elbow with paresthesia in ulnar side of fourth/fifth fingers develops. Reassess sensation every 2 to 4 hours. *The use of pads assists with preventing prolonged compression or flexion pressure on the ulnar nerve, causing neuropathy/nerve damage. Consider obtaining prescription for an enclosure bed for agitated clients to alleviate restraints, preventing arm abrasions, nerve damage, and pain.*
- Explain importance of exhaling versus holding one's breath (Valsalva maneuver) and straining during bed activities.
- Reassess pain level, especially before movement and/or exercising, and accept clients' pain ratings and levels they think is appropriate for comfort. Administer analgesics based on clients' pain rating. Refer to Acute **Pain** or Chronic **Pain.**

Exercise

- Test strength in bilateral grips, arms at elbow flexion and extension, bilateral arm abduction and adduction, bilateral leg or thigh raise (one at a time in bed or chair), and quadriceps and hamstring strength to extend and flex at knee to assess baseline and interval strength gains.
- Perform passive range of motion (ROM) of three repetitions, at least twice a day, to immobile joints. *Perform ROM slowly and rhythmically. Do not range beyond point of pain. Range only to point of resistance in those with loss of sensation and mentation. Fast, jerky ROM increases pain and tone. Slow, rhythmical movements relax/lengthen spastic muscles so they can be ranged further. For clients with neuromuscular conditions, consult with physical therapy for ROM exercises.*
- Range or move a hemiplegic arm with the shoulder slightly externally rotated (hand up).
- ▲ Encourage client's practice of exercises taught by therapists (muscle setting, strengthening, contraction against resistance, and weight lifting). *Exercises and weight lifting help maintain muscle tone, strength, and lengthening.*

Bed Positioning

- Incorporate the following measures to promote normal tone and prevent complications in clients with neurological impairment:
  ❍ Use a flat head pillow when clients are supine. Use a small pillow behind the head and/or between shoulder blades if neck extension occurs to prevent contractures of the cervical spine and abnormal tone of the neck.
  ❍ Abduct the shoulders of clients with high paraplegia or quadriplegia horizontally to 90 degrees briefly two to three times a day while client is supine.
  ❍ Position a hemiplegic shoulder fairly close to the client's body.
- Tilt hemiplegics onto both unaffected and affected sides with the affected shoulder slightly forward (e.g., move/lift the affected shoulder, not the forearm/hand).
- ▲ Elevate a client's paralyzed forearms on a pillow when client is supine. Elevate edematous legs on a pillow supporting the knees to prevent hyperextension. Apply resting wrist, hand, and foot/ankle splints and pressure garments or other devices as prescribed. Range joints before applying splints. Adhere to on/off schedule as prescribed by the PT. Remove splints and compression garments or devices to check *underlying tissues for signs of pressure/poor circulation every 2 hours or more often if client resists or manipulates them.*

Geriatric

- Assess caregiver's strength, health history, and cognitive status to predict ability/risk for assisting bedbound clients at home. *Explore alternatives if risk is too high. Caregivers are often frail older adults with chronic health problems who cannot physically help loved ones.* Refer to care plan for **Caregiver Role Strain.**
- Assess the client's stamina and energy level during bed activities/exercises; if limited, spread out activities and allow rest breaks.

Home Care

- ▲ Collaborate with nurse case managers, care coordinators, social workers, and physical/occupational therapists to assess home support systems and needs, and to provide for home modifications, durable medical equipment, assistive technology, and home health services.
- Encourage use of the client's own bed unless contraindicated. Raise HOB with commercial blocks or grooved-out pieces of wood under legs; set bed against walls in a corner. Emotionally, clients may benefit from sleeping in their own beds with familiar partners.

● = Independent; ▲ = Collaborative; **EBN** = Evidence-Based Nursing; **EB** = Evidence-Based

M

- Stress psychological/physical benefits of clients being as self-sufficient as possible with bed mobility/care even though it may be time-consuming. Allowing independence and autonomy may help prevent disuse syndromes and feelings of helplessness and low self-esteem.
- Offer emotional support and help client identify usual coping responses to help with adjustment and loss issues. The home environment may trigger the reality of lost function and disability.
- Discuss support systems available for caregivers to help them cope. Refer to care plan for **Caregiver Role Strain.**
- ▲ In the presence of medical disorders, institute case management for frail older adults to support continued independent living as much as possible or desired by the client.
- Refer to the home care interventions in the care plan for Impaired physical **Mobility.**

 ### Client/Family Teaching and Discharge Planning

- Use various sensory modalities to teach client/caregivers correct ROM, exercises, positioning, self-care activities, and use of devices. Readiness and learning styles vary but may be enhanced with visual/auditory/tactile/cognitive stimulus as follows:
    - ❍ Provide demonstrations, sketches, instructional videos, and written directions/schedules, notes.
    - ❍ Provide verbal instructions, recorded audiotapes, timers, reading aloud written directions, and self-talk during activities.
    - ❍ Use motor task practice/repetition, return demonstrations, note taking, manual guidance, or staff's hand-on-client's-hand technique.
- ▲ Schedule time with family/caregivers for education and practice for nursing, physical therapy, and occupational therapy. Suggest family come prepared with questions and wear comfortable, safe clothing/shoes. Practice provides opportunity for learning; repetition helps memory retention.
- ▲ Implement safe approaches for caregivers/home care staff and reinforce an adequate number of people and handling equipment (e.g., friction pads, slide boards, lifts) during bed mobility, exercise, toileting, and bathing to decrease risk of injury.
- ▲ Coordinate evaluations for bariatric equipment for home use before discharge, including a weight-rated bed, a wheelchair or mobility device (scooter), and lift device. Doorways may need to be widened, floors reinforced, and ramps added for safety.

M

REFERENCES

Agency for Healthcare Research and Quaity (AHRQ). (2017). *Head of bed elevation or semirecumbent positioning literature review.* Content last reviewed January 2017. Rockville, MD: Agency for Healthcare Research and Quality. Retrieved from http://www.ahrq.gov/professionals/quality-patient-safety/hais/tools/mvp/modules/technical/head-bed-elevation-litreview.html. (Accessed 1 November 2017).

Anthony, M. (2013). Nursing assessment of deep vein thrombosis. *Medsurg Nursing, 22*(2), 95–98.

Braden, B. J., & Bergstrom, N. (1989). Clinical utility of the Braden scale for predicting pressure sore risk. *Decubitus, 2*(3), 44–51. Retrieved from http://www.ncbi.nlm.nih.gov/pubmed/2775473.

Choi, S. D., & Brings, K. (2016). Work-related musculoskeletal risks associated with nurses and nursing assistants handling overweight and obese patients. *Work (Reading, MA), 53*(2), 439–448.

D'Arcy, L. P., Sasai, Y., & Stearns, S. C. (2012). Do assistive devices, training, and workload affect injury incidence? Prevention efforts by nursing homes and back injuries among nursing assistants. *Journal of Advanced Nursing, 68*(4), 836–845.

Gattinoni, L., Taccone, P., Carlesso, E., et al. (2013). Prone position in acute respiratory distress syndrome: Rationale, indications, and limits. *American Journal of Respiratory and Critical Care Medicine, 188*(11), 1286–1293.

Gosselin, R. A., & Smith, R. G. (2014). Amputations. In M. Foltz, R. A. Gosselin, & R. G. Smith (Eds.), *Global orthopedics* (Chapter 43). New York: Springer Science + Business Media.

Green, M., Marzano, V., et al. (2016). Mobilization of intensive care patients: A multidisciplinary practical guide for clinicians. *Journal of Multidisciplinary Healthcare, 9,* 247–256.

Guerin, C., Reigneir, J., Richard, J.-C., et al. (2013). In cases of severe ARDS, early prone-positioning sessions significantly decreased 28- and 90-day mortality. *The New England Journal of Medicine, 368,* 2159–2168.

Hill, E., & Fauerbach, L. A. (2014). Falls and fall prevention in older adults. *Journal of Legal Nurse Consulting, 25*(2), 24–29.

Khan, M. H., Kunselman, A. R., et al. (2002). Attenuated sympathetic nerve responses after 24 hours of bed rest. *American Journal of Physiology, Heart and Circulatory Physiology, 282*(6), H2210–H2215.

Lee, S.-J., et al. (2017). Safe patient handling behaviors and lift use among hospital nurses: A cross-sectional study. *International Journal of Nursing Studies, 74,* 53–60.

Martin, D., Albensi, L., et al. (2017). Healthy skin wins: A glowing pressure ulcer prevention program that can guide evidence-based practice. *Worldviews on Evidence-based Nursing, 14*(6), 473–483.

Moyse, T., Bates, J., et al. (2017). Validation of a model for predicting pressure injury risk in patients with vascular diseases. *Journal of Wound, Ostomy & Continence Nursing, 44*(2), 118–122.

Morse, J. M., Tylko, S. J., & Dixon, H. A. (1987). Characteristics of the fall-prone patient. *The Gerontologist, 27*(4), 516–522.

National Pressure Ulcer Advisory Panel, European Pressure Ulcer Advisory Panel and Pan Pacific Pressure Injury Alliance. (2014). In: E. Haesler (Ed.), *Prevention and treatment of pressure ulcers: clinical practice guideline.* Osborne Park, Australia: Cambridge Media.

Weiner, C., Kalichman, L., et al. (2016). Repositioning a passive patient in bed: choosing an ergonomically advantageous assistive device. *Applied Ergonomics, 60*: 22–29.

● = Independent;   ▲ = Collaborative;   EBN = Evidence-Based Nursing;   EB = Evidence-Based

Wiggerman, N. (2016). Biomechanical evaluation of a bed feature to assist in turning and laterally repositioning patients. *Human Factors*, 58, 748–757. Retrieved from https://doi.org/10.1177/0018720815612625.

Wright, A. D., & Flynn, M. (2011). Using the prone position for ventilated patients with respiratory failure: A review. *Nursing in Critical Care*, 16(1), 19–27.

Impaired physical Mobility   *Wendie A. Howland, MN, RN-BC, CRRN, CCM, CNLCP, LNCC*

NANDA-I

Definition

Limitation in independent, purposeful physical movement of the body or of one or more extremities.

Defining Characteristics

Alteration in gait; decrease in fine motor skills; decrease in gross motor skills; decrease in range of motion; decrease in reaction time; difficulty turning; discomfort; engages in substitutions for movement; exertional dyspnea; movement-induced tremor; postural instability; slowed movement; spastic movement; uncoordinated movement

Related Factors

Activity intolerance; anxiety; body mass index (BMI) >75th percentile appropriate for age and gender; cultural belief regarding acceptable activity; decrease in endurance; decrease in muscle control; decrease in muscle mass; decrease in muscle strength; depression; disuse; insufficient environmental support; insufficient knowledge of value of physical activity; joint stiffness; malnutrition; pain; physical deconditioning; reluctance to initiate movement; sedentary lifestyle

Associated Condition

Alteration in bone structure integrity; alteration in cognitive functioning; alteration in metabolism; contractures; developmental delay; musculoskeletal impairment; neuromuscular impairment; pharmaceutical agent; prescribed movement restrictions; sensory-perceptual impairment

NOC   (Nursing Outcomes Classification)

Suggested NOC Outcomes

Ambulation; Ambulation: Wheelchair; Mobility; Self-Care: Activities of Daily Living (ADLs); Instrumental Activities of Daily Living (IADLs); Transfer Performance

---

Example NOC Outcome with Indicators

Ambulation as evidenced by the following indicators: Walks with effective gait/Walks at moderate pace/Walks up and down steps/Walks moderate distance. (Rate the outcome and indicators of **Ambulation:** 1 = severely compromised, 2 = substantially compromised, 3 = moderately compromised, 4 = mildly compromised, 5 = not compromised [see Section I].)

Client Outcomes

Client Will (Specify Time Frame)

- Meet mutually defined goals of increased ambulation and exercise that include individual choice, preference, and enjoyment in the exercise prescription
- Describe feeling stronger and more mobile
- Describe less fear of falling and pain with physical activity
- Demonstrate use of adaptive equipment (e.g., wheelchairs, walkers, gait belts, weighted walking vests) to increase mobility
- Increase exercise to 20 minutes/day for those who were previously sedentary (less than 150 minutes/week). Note: Light to moderate intensity exercise may be beneficial in deconditioned persons. In very deconditioned individuals exercise bouts of less than 10 minutes are beneficial

● = Independent;   ▲ = Collaborative;   EBN = Evidence-Based Nursing;   EB = Evidence-Based

- Increase pedometer step counts by 1000 steps per day every 2 weeks to reach a daily step count of at least 7000 steps per day, with a daily goal for most healthy adults of 10,000 steps per day (approximately 5 miles)
- Perform resistance exercises that involve all major muscle groups (legs, hips, back, chest, abdomen, shoulders, and arms) performed 2 or 3 days/week
- Perform flexibility exercise (stretching) for each of the major muscle-tendon groups 2 days/week for 10 to 60 seconds to improve joint range of motion (ROM); greatest gains occur with daily exercise
- Engage in neuromotor exercise 20 to 30 minutes/day including motor skills (e.g., balance, agility, coordination, gait), proprioceptive exercise training, and multifaceted activities (e.g., Tai chi, yoga) to improve and maintain physical function and reduce falls in those at risk for falling (older persons)
- Engage in purposeful moderate-intensity cardiorespiratory (aerobic) exercise for 30 to 60 minutes/day at least 5 days/week for a total of 2 hours and 30 minutes (150 minutes) per week

NIC   (Nursing Interventions Classification)

Suggested NIC Interventions

Exercise Therapy: Ambulation; Joint Mobility; Positioning

Example NIC Activities—Exercise Therapy
Assist the client to use footwear that facilitates walking and prevents injury; Instruct in use of assistive devices, if appropriate

Nursing Interventions and *Rationales*

- Adults with disabilities should follow the adult guidelines. If this is not possible, they should be as physically active as their abilities allow and avoid inactivity (US Department of Labor, 2008). Use "start low and go slow" approach for intensity and duration of physical activity if client is highly deconditioned, functionally limited, or has chronic conditions affecting performance of physical tasks. When progressing client's activities, use an individualized and tailored approach based on client's tolerance and preferences (Riebe et al, 2015).
- Assess for fear of falling. EBN: *Self-reported fear of falling has been shown to be a significantly more sensitive predictor for fall risk than the STRATIFY fall risk assessment tool (Strupeit, Buss, & Wolf-Ostermann, 2016).*
- Screen for mobility skills in the following order: (1) bed mobility; (2) dangling and supported and unsupported sitting; (3) weight-bearing for sit to stand, transfer to chair; (4) standing and walking with assistance; and (5) walking independently. EBN: *Use a structured tool to assess and determine the patient's highest activity level and guide planning exercise progression toward independence (Jackman et al, 2016).*
- Assess muscle strength and other factors affecting balance, mobility, and endurance. Immobility can affect tissue perfusion and increase risk of postural hypotension; shortness of breath decreases endurance and increases fear; bowel or bladder incontinence can decrease motivation to be mobile; cognitive and neuromuscular deficits, including side effects of medication, can affect balance, coordination, and movement; and pain, fear, or sick role expectations can decrease willingness to be mobile. EBN: *Assess for mobility impairment, hazards of limited mobility, and plan care to mitigate complications (Crawford and Harris, 2016).*
- Refer to care plans for Risk for **Falls,** Acute **Pain,** Chronic **Pain,** Ineffective **Coping,** or **Hopelessness.**
- Increase activity tolerance with graded increases in self-care (function-focused care [FFC]), such as bathing, walking to the bathroom instead of using a bedpan/urinal, and ROM. EBN: *A study of FFC in older adults hospitalized after trauma found greater improvement in function, less fear of falling, and better physical resilience than controls at discharge and 30 days after (Resnick, Galik, & Vigne 2016).*
- Consider patient's self-reported fear of falling. EBN: *Self-reported fear of falling has been shown to be a sensitive predictor for fall risk (Strupeit, Buss, & Wolf-Ostermann, 2016).*
- ▲ Before activity, observe for and, if possible, treat pain with massage, heat pack to affected area, or medication. Ensure that the client is not oversedated. *Pain limits mobility and if exacerbated by specific movements should be temporarily avoided (American College of Sports Medicine [ACSM], 2018).*
- Obtain any assistive devices needed for activity, such as gait belt, weighted vest, walker, cane, crutches, or wheelchair, ergonomic shower chairs; ceiling and floor-based lifts; and air-assisted lateral transfer devices.
- Monitor and record the client's response to activity, such as pulse rate, blood pressure, dyspnea, skin color, subjective report. Refer to the care plan for **Activity** intolerance. EB: *Use valid and reliable screening*

M

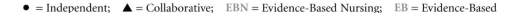

● = Independent;   ▲ = Collaborative;   EBN = Evidence-Based Nursing;   EB = Evidence-Based

procedures and tools to assess the client's preparticipation in exercise health screening and risk stratification for exercise testing (low, moderate, or high risk) (ACSM, 2018).

Special Considerations: Immobility

- Perform passive ROM exercises at least twice a day unless contraindicated; repeat each maneuver three times. **EB:** *Physical rehabilitation interventions were found to be safe, reduced disability, and resulted in few adverse events (Crocker et al, 2013).*
- ▲ Consult with health care provider for a safety evaluation before beginning an exercise program; if program is approved, begin with the following exercises:
  - ○ Active ROM exercises using both upper and lower extremities (e.g., flexing and extending at ankles, knees, hips)
  - ○ Chin-ups and pull-ups using a trapeze in bed (may be contraindicated in clients with cardiac conditions)
  - ○ Strengthening exercises such as gluteal or quadriceps sitting exercises
- Use assistive technology for mobilizing bedbound patients. Refer to the care plan for Impaired bed **Mobility**.
- Help the client achieve mobility and start walking as soon as possible if not contraindicated. **EBN:** *To prevent hospital-acquired disability, organizational values should consider both safety (e.g., fall prevention) and injury protection in concert with a philosophy that enables older adults to be self-directed and independent (Boltz et al, 2014).* **EB:** *Early mobilization after hip replacement surgery resulted in decreased time until readiness for discharge (Okamoto et al, 2016).*
- Initiate a "no lift" policy where appropriate assistive devices are used for manual lifting. **EBN:** *Relevance of manual client handling policies that may promote overuse of equipment should be openly discussed among nurse managers and direct care providers to avoid hospital-related loss of mobility among clients (Kneafsey, Clifford, & Greenfield, 2015).* See care plan for Impaired bed **Mobility**.

Other Clinical Conditions:

- ▲ If the client has osteoarthritis or rheumatoid arthritis, consult with a physical therapist to on ways to integrate aerobic exercise, resistance exercise, and flexibility exercise (stretching) into care.
- ▲ If client has had a cerebrovascular accident (CVA) with hemiparesis, consult with physical therapist on constraint-induced movement therapy, in which the functional extremity is purposely constrained and the client is forced to use the involved extremity. **EB:** *Use of this therapeutic approach produced significant positive effects in improving arm function after stroke (Wattchow, McDonnell, & Hillier, 2018).*
- If the client does not feed or groom self, sit side by side with the client, put your hand over the client's hand, support the client's elbow with your other hand, and help the client feed self; use the same technique to help the client comb hair. **EBN:** *Hospitalized older adults who received a family-centered intervention to promote functional and cognitive recovery (family-centered FFC) had improved ADLs and walking ability and less severe and shorter duration of delirium (Boltz et al, 2014).*

 ### Geriatric

- Assess ability to move using valid and reliable criterion-referenced standards for fitness testing that can predict the level of capacity associated with maintaining physical independence into later years of life (e.g., Get Up and Go test).
- Help the mostly immobile client achieve mobility as soon as possible, depending on physical condition. **EB:** *A meta-analysis found exercise beneficial in increasing gait speed and improving balance and ADL performance (Lipardo et al, 2017). Mobilization should occur at least three times daily, mobilization should be progressive and scaled, and assessment should take place within 24 hours of admission (Liu et al, 2017).*
- Use the FFC rehabilitative philosophy of care in older adults to prevent avoidable functional decline. **EBN:** Mood, satisfaction with staff and activities, and social support for exercise were directly associated with time spent in physical activity (Holmes, Galik, & Resnick, 2017; Resnick & Galik, 2013).
- If the client is scheduled for an elective surgery that will result in admission into the intensive care unit and immobility, or recovery from a joint replacement, for example, initiate a prehabilitation program that includes warm-up, aerobic activity, strength, flexibility, neuromotor, and functional task work. **EBN:** The risk of declines in functional status when older adults are hospitalized requires using evidence-based strategies to reduce the incidence and effect of decreased mobility, pressure ulcers, pain, dehydration, malnutrition, and sequelae of invasive treatments (Resnick et al, 2016).

● = Independent;   ▲ = Collaborative;   EBN = Evidence-Based Nursing;   EB = Evidence-Based

- Use gestures and nonverbal cues when helping clients move if they are anxious or have difficulty understanding and following verbal instructions. Nonverbal gestures are part of a universal language that can be understood when the client is having difficulty with communication.
- Recognize that wheelchairs are not a good mobility device and often serve as a mobility restraint.
- Ensure that chairs fit clients. Chair seat should be 3 inches above the height of the knee. Provide a raised toilet seat if needed. Raising the height of a chair can dramatically improve the ability of many older clients to stand up. Low, deep, soft seats with armrests that are far apart reduce a person's ability to get up and down without help.
- If the client is mainly immobile, provide opportunities for socialization and sensory stimulation (e.g., television and visits). Refer to the care plan for Deficient **Diversional** activity.
- Recognize that immobility and a lack of social support and sensory input may result in confusion or depression in older adults. Refer to nursing interventions for Acute **Confusion** or **Hopelessness** as appropriate.

Home Care

- The preceding interventions may be adapted for home care use.
- ▲ Begin discharge planning as soon as possible with a personal health navigator (e.g., nurse care coordinator or case manager) to assess need for and arrange home support systems, assistive devices, and community or home health services. Nurses are often the first health care providers to assess the patient on admission; this creates the opportunity for early discharge planning (McNeil, 2016).
- ▲ Assess home environment for factors that create barriers to physical mobility. Refer to occupational therapy services if needed to assist the client in restructuring home environment and daily living patterns. EB: *Use the Home Safety Self-Assessment Tool to identify fall risk, prevent falls, and improve mobility and function (Horowitz, Almonte, & Vasil, 2016).*
- ▲ Refer to home health aide services to support the client and family through changing levels of mobility. Reinforce need to promote independence in mobility as tolerated. *Providing unnecessary assistance with transfers, bathing, and dressing activities may promote dependence and a loss of mobility rather than optimizing a person's underlying physical capability. Such attentive care may actually prevent older adults from using their remaining abilities (Resnick et al, 2016).*
- ▲ Refer to physical therapy for gait training, strengthening, and balance training. Physical therapists can provide direct interventions and assess need for assistive devices (e.g., cane, walker) (Miller, Sabol, & Pastva, 2017).
- Assess skin condition at every visit. Establish a skin care program that enhances circulation and maximizes position changes. *Impaired mobility decreases circulation to dependent areas. Decreased circulation and shearing place the client at risk for skin breakdown.*
- Once the client is able to walk independently, suggest that the client enter an exercise program, or walk with a friend. CEB: *Nurse practitioners providing primary care should prescribe regular physical activity to minimize progressive impaired mobility (Miller, Sabol, & Pastva, 2017).*
- Provide support to the client and family/caregivers during long-term impaired mobility. *Long-term impaired mobility may necessitate role changes within the family and precipitate caregiver stress.* Refer to the care plan for **Caregiver Role Strain.**

Client/Family Teaching and Discharge Planning

- Consider using motivational interviewing techniques when working with both children and adult clients to increase their activity. Refer to the care plan for **Sedentary** lifestyle or *Rationales* for motivational interviewing.
- Teach the client and caregivers processes and tools used during care to use at home to assess fall risk and promote progressive mobility. Involve them in planning for these activities at home. EBN: *Few studies have investigated the point of view of older patients on prevention of this decline. Within the framework of a descriptive qualitative study, the perceptions of 30 hospitalized older adults were collected regarding their personal prevention strategies, the barriers to implementing these, and nursing staff interventions deemed useful. Results show that participants are sensitive to the risk of functional decline and use various preventive strategies particularly to maintain their physical abilities, maintain good spirits, keep a clear mind, and foster nutrition and sleep. Their strategies are difficult to implement because of internal and external barriers. Nursing interventions deemed useful are good relational approach, strong basic care, appropriate assessment, and respect for level of autonomy. The study underscores that older hospitalized patients are applying strategies to prevent functional decline, but some nursing interventions may thwart their efforts (Lafreniere et al, 2017).*

● = Independent;   ▲ = Collaborative;   EBN = Evidence-Based Nursing;   EB = Evidence-Based

M

REFERENCES

American College of Sports Medicine (ACSM). (2018). *American College of Sports Medicine's guidelines for exercise testing and prescription* (10th ed.). Philadelphia: Lippincott Williams & Wilkins.

Boltz, M., Resnick, B., Chippendale, T., et al. (2014). Testing a family-centered intervention to promote functional and cognitive recovery in hospitalized older adults. *Journal of American Geriatrics Society*, 62, 2398–2407.

Crawford, A., & Harris, H. (2016). Caring for adults with impaired physical mobility. *Nursing*, 46, 36–41.

Crocker, T., Forster, A., Young, J., et al. (2013). Physical rehabilitation for older people in long-term care. *Cochrane Database of Systematic Reviews*, (2), CD004294. doi:10.1002/14651858.CD004294.pub3.

Holmes, S., Galik, E., & Resnick, B. (2017). Factors that influence physical activity among residents in assisted living. *Journal of Gerontological Social Work*, 60(2), 120–137.

Horowitz, B., Almonte, T., & Vasil, A. (2016). Use of the Home Safety Self-Assessment Tool (HSSAT) within community health education to improve home safety. *Occupational Therapy In Health Care*, 30(4), 356–372.

Jackman, C., Gammon, H., Kane, P., et al. (2016). A reliable mobility assessment tool for multidisciplinary use. *Journal of Physical Medicine, Rehabilitation & Disabilities*, 2: 009.

Kneafsey, R., Clifford, C., & Greenfield, S. (2015). Perceptions of hospital manual handling policy and impact on nursing team involvement in promoting patients' mobility. *Journal of Clinical Nursing*, 24, 289–299.

Lafreniere, S., Folch, N., Dubois, S., et al. (2017). Strategies used by older patients to prevent functional decline during hospitalization. *Clinical Nursing Research*, 26(1), 6–26.

Lipardo, D., Aseron, A., Kwan, M., et al. (2017). Effect of exercise and cognitive training on falls and fall-related factors in older adults with mild cognitive impairment: A systematic review. *Archives of Physical Medicine and Rehabilitation*, 98(10), 2079–2096.

Liu, B., Moore, J., Khan, S., et al. (2017). Sustainability and spread of Move On: A mobilization initiative two years after implementation. *Innovation in Aging*, 1(Suppl. 1), 652–653.

McNeil, A. (2016). Using evidence to structure discharge planning. *Nursing Management*, 47(5), 22–23.

Miller, J., Sabol, V., & Pastva, A. (2017). Promoting older adult physical activity throughout care transitions using and interprofessional approach. *The Journal for Nurse Practitioners*, 13(1), 64–71.

Okamoto, T., Ridley, R., Edmonston, S., et al. (2016). Day-of-surgery mobilization reduces the length of stay after elective hip arthroplasty. *The Journal of Arthroplasty*, 31(10), 2227–2230.

Riebe, D., Franklin, B., et al. (2015). Updating American College of Sports Medicine's recommendations for exercise preparticipation health screening. *Medicine & Science in Sports & Exercise*, 47(11), 2473–2479. doi:10.1249/MSS.0000000000000664.

Resnick, B., & Galik, E. (2013). Using function-focused care to increase physical activity among older adults. *Annual Review of Nursing Research*, 31, 175–208.

Resnick, B., Wells, C., et al. (2016). Feasibility and efficacy of function-focused care for orthopedic trauma patients. *Journal of Trauma Nursing*, 23(3), 144–155.

Resnick, R., Galik, E., Vigne, E., et al. (2016). Dissemination and implementation of function focused care for assisted living. *Health Education and Behavior*, 43(3), 296–304.

Strupeit, S., Buss, A., & Wolf-Ostermann, K. (2016) Assessing risk of falling: A comparison of three different methods. *Sigma Theta Tau International Nursing Research Congress*. Retrieved from http://www.nursinglibrary.org/vhl/handle/10755/617041. (Accessed 2 November 2017).

U.S. Department of Labor. (2008). *Americans With Disabilities Act*. Retrieved from https://www.dol.gov/general/topic/disability/ada. (Accessed 8 November 2018).

Wattchow, K., McDonnell, M., & Hillier, S. (2018). Rehabilitation interventions for upper limb function in the first four weeks following stroke: A systematic review and meta-analysis of the evidence. *Archives of Physical Medicine and Rehabilitation*, 99(2), 367–382. doi:10.1016/j.apmr.2017.06.014.

Impaired wheelchair Mobility   *Wendie A. Howland, MN, RN-BC, CRRN, CCM, CNLCP, LNCC*

NANDA-I

Definition

Limitation of independent operation of wheelchair within environment.

Defining Characteristics

Impaired ability to operate power wheelchair on a decline; impaired ability to operate power wheelchair on an incline; impaired ability to operative power wheelchair on curbs; impaired ability to operative power wheelchair on even surface; impaired ability to operate power wheelchair on uneven surface; impaired ability to operate wheelchair on a decline; impaired ability to operate wheelchair on an incline; impaired ability to operate wheelchair on curbs; impaired ability to operate wheelchair on even surface; impaired ability to operate wheelchair on uneven surface

Related Factors

Alteration in mood; decrease in endurance; environmental barrier; insufficient knowledge of wheelchair use; insufficient muscle strength; obesity; pain; physical deconditioning

• = Independent;   ▲ = Collaborative;   EBN = Evidence-Based Nursing;   EB = Evidence-Based

Associated Condition

Alteration in cognitive functioning; impaired vision; musculoskeletal impairment; neuromuscular impairment

NOC   (Nursing Outcomes Classification)

Suggested NOC Outcome

Ambulation: Wheelchair

> **Example NOC Outcome with Indicators**
>
> **Ambulation: Wheelchair** as evidenced by the following indicators: Propels wheelchair safely/Transfers to and from wheelchair/ Maneuvers curbs, doorways, ramps. (Rate the outcome and indicators of **Ambulation: Wheelchair:** 1 = severely compromised, 2 = substantially compromised, 3 = moderately compromised, 4 = mildly compromised, 5 = not compromised [see Section I].)

Client Outcomes

Client Will (Specify Time Frame)

- Demonstrate independence in operating and moving a wheelchair or other wheeled device
- Demonstrate ability to direct others in operating and moving a wheelchair or other device
- Demonstrate therapeutic positioning, pressure relief, and safety principles while operating and moving a wheelchair or other wheeled device

NIC   (Nursing Interventions Classification)

Suggested NIC Interventions

Exercise Therapy: Muscle Control; Positioning: Wheelchair

> **Example NIC Activities—Positioning**
>
> Wheelchair
>
> Collaborate with occupational therapist [OT]/physical therapist [PT] to select the appropriate wheelchair for the client: standard adult, semireclining, fully reclining, amputees; Monitor client's ability to maintain correct positioning in wheelchair

Nursing Interventions and *Rationales*

- ▲ Refer to physical and occupational therapy or wheelchair seating clinic. *Seating for wheelchair-dependent clients should be assessed by health care specialists in conjunction with client/caregiver education on weight shift maneuvers (Sprigle & Sonenblum, 2011).*
- ▲ Recognize that support surfaces on chairs and beds redistribute pressure and should be used for at-risk clients as an adjunct to reduce risk of pressure injury (Sprigle & Sonenblum, 2011; Requejo, Furumasu, & Mulroy, 2015). EB: *Sitting-acquired pressure injuries occur primarily over the ischial tuberosities; sacral injuries primarily result from shear and excessive loading in bed (Gefen, Farid, & Shaywitz, 2013; Agency for Healthcare Research and Quality [AHRQ], 2014). Foam cushions increased pressure in seating and should not be relied on for pressure relief (Slayton, Morris, & Brinkley, 2017). There are many pressure-relieving cushions. Several that are commonly used are the ROHO cushion, Varilite Evolution, and Invacare Matrix cushions.* Refer to care plan for Risk for **Pressure Ulcer.**
- Optimize nutrition and hydration for skin and tissue health.
- Intervene to maintain continence or use absorbent underpads or diapers to help prevent skin breakdown caused by excessive moisture and macerated skin. Some wheelchair cushions have moisture-wicking characteristics. *Use air-permeable underpads to decrease maceration (National Pressure Ulcer Advisory Panel, 2014).*
- Assess client's sitting posture frequently and reposition for alignment. Document specific measures to allow for reproducibility. EB: *Pressure mapping alone insufficiently describes tissue health (National Pressure Ulcer Advisory Panel, 2014).*
- Implement use of friction-coated projection hand rims and leather gloves for clients to propel manual wheelchairs. *Friction-coated projection rims are less invasive and slippery than aluminum rims; gloves absorb forces of propulsion and help prevent nerve damage/carpal tunnel injury.*

- = Independent;   ▲ = Collaborative;   EBN = Evidence-Based Nursing;   EB = Evidence-Based

- Manually guide or explain to the client to push forward on both wheel rims to move ahead, push the right rim to turn left and vice versa, and pull backward on both wheel rims to back up.
- Recommend that clients back wheelchair into an elevator. If entering face first, instruct them to turn chairs around to face the elevator doors and controls.
- ▲ In conjunction with physical therapy for teaching and assessment, reinforce principle of descending a curb backward ("popping a wheelie") if balance, trunk control, strength, and timing are adequate. *Backward descent carries less risk of clients losing control and falling forward out of the wheelchair.*
- Ascend curbs in a forward position by popping a wheelie or having someone aid in tilting the chair back, place front wheels over curb, and roll chair up. If surface is muddy or sandy, ascend backward. *Front casters will not roll on soft surfaces; a backward approach requires less energy and prevents getting stuck or falling forward.*
- During assisted wheelies, helper must hold wheelchair until all four wheels are back on the ground and client has control of wheelchair. *Releasing one's grip too soon may alter client's balance and cause injury.*
- ▲ Follow therapist's recommendations for how clients should propel manual wheelchairs to prevent upper extremity pain and joint degeneration.
- Recognize that ultra-lightweight, push rim–activated, power-assisted, or powered wheelchairs may be indicated. Striking the balance between optimum independence and preventing injury (e.g., rotator cuff injury from years of manual propulsion) is a consideration. *Consider push rim–activated power-assisted wheelchairs (manual wheelchairs with a motor linked to the push rim in each rear hub) because they reduce energy needed for propulsion and reserve energy for uneven terrain or obstacle negotiation. Recommend antirollback devices for inclined planes to decrease stress on shoulders.* EB: *Full-time manual wheelchair users are at high risk for developing shoulder injury (Rice and Rice, 2017). If the client does not have sufficient strength or motor control of the extremities to propel a standard wheelchair, then the client should be evaluated for a power chair.*
- ▲ Reduce floor clutter and establish safety rules for drivers of electric/power mobility devices; make referrals to physical or occupational therapy for driver reevaluations if accidents occur or client's health deteriorates.
- Request and receive client's permission before moving an unoccupied wheelchair in the room or out to hallway. *Wheelchair-dependent clients may view the chair as part of their identity and independence.*
- Reinforce compensatory strategies for unilateral neglect and agnosia (e.g., visual scanning, self-talk, self-questioning as to what could be wrong) as clients propel wheelchair through doorways and around obstacles. *Too often nurses physically move the wheelchair or obstacle instead of cueing the client to detect and solve problems.* Refer to care plan for **Unilateral Neglect.**
- Offer support to help clients cope with issues related to physical disability. *Depression and anxiety may occur with physical loss.* Refer to care plan for Ineffective **Role** performance.
- Provide information on support group and reliable Internet resource options.
- Provide information about advocacy, accessibility, assistive technology, and issues under the Americans with Disabilities Act as Amended (2008) (Jackson, 2017).
- ▲ Make social service or wheelchair clinic referral to educate clients on financial coverage/regulations of third-party payers and Health Care Financing Association for wheelchairs. *It is wise to recognize cost, advantages, and durability of different wheelchair models before purchasing one.*
- Recommend that clients test-drive wheelchairs and try out cushions/postural supports with the advice of a qualified seating professional, not a vendor, before purchasing. If a specialty chair is indicated, for example, for sports or outdoor use, having clients test-drive the wheelchair is especially important. *Equipment is expensive, and different models have different advantages and disadvantages.*

Pediatric

- ▲ EB: *Consult physical or occupational therapist for special considerations for wheelchair fitting and positioning for pediatric client. In children with cerebral palsy, poor trunk control can lead to spinal deformity and pulmonary compromise. Evidence links posture and pulmonary function; special techniques for measuring these may be necessary (Barks & Shaw, 2011).*
- ▲ Help client/family transition from a manual to a powered wheelchair/scooter if disability is severe. EB: *Wheelchairs are essential for maximizing mobility and function. Power wheelchairs can enhance independence for children who are able to use them with hand, head, or mouth mechanisms (Hoon & Tolley, 2013).*

Geriatric

- Avoid using restraints on fidgeting clients who slide down in a wheelchair. Instead, assess for deformities; spinal curvatures; abnormal tone; limited joint range; discomfort from clothing, pressure, or constriction areas; social isolation, and toileting needs.

● = Independent; ▲ = Collaborative; EBN = Evidence-Based Nursing; EB = Evidence-Based

- Ensure proper seat depth/leg positioning and use custom footrests (not elevated leg rests) to prevent older adults from sliding down in wheelchairs.
- ▲ Assess for side effects of medications and potential need for dosage readjustments to increase wheelchair tolerance. Give prescribed hydration and medications to treat orthostatic hypotension. Consider leg wraps. Assist client to perform warm-up bed exercises if possible. *Cerebral hypoperfusion and prolonged bedrest are common causes of orthostatic intolerance and hypotension; see care plan for Impaired Bed Mobility.*
- Allow client to control speed to propel wheelchair independently if possible. *Older adults may move slowly because of diminished range of motion/strength, stiff/sore joints, and cardiopulmonary compromise. Observe carefully for fatigue, shoulder pain, or other signs of activity intolerance.*
- Assess the client's ability to safely maneuver independently using a wheelchair. **EB:** *Use an evidence-based tool to assess the client's skill and physical ability to safely use a wheelchair (AHRQ, 2017).*

Home Care

- ▲ Establish a support system for emergency and contingency care (e.g., remote monitoring, emergency call system, alert local emergency medical system). *Wheelchair dependence may be life-threatening during a crisis (e.g., fall, fire, or other environmental emergency).*
- Recommend the following changes to the home to accommodate the use of a wheelchair:
  - ○ Arrange traffic patterns so they are wide enough to maneuver a wheelchair.
  - ○ Recognize that a 5-foot turning space is necessary to maneuver wheelchairs, doorways need to have 32 to 36 inches clear width, and entrance ramps/path slope should be assessed before permanent ramps are installed because standardized slopes may not be appropriate. Temporary ramps are cost-effective and easier to adjust (Sofka, 2011).
  - ○ Replace door hardware with fold-back hinges, remove doorway encasements (if too narrow), remove/replace thresholds (if too high), hang wall-mounted sinks/handrails, grade floors in showers for roll-in chairs, and use nonskid/nonslip floor coverings (e.g., nonwaxed wood, linoleum, or Berber carpet).
  - ○ Rearrange room functions, furniture, and storage so that toileting, sleeping, bathing, and preparing/eating meals can safely take place on one level of the home.
  - ○ *Refer to the Easter Seals Summary on Home Accessibility for further details* (see http://www.easterseals.com/shared-components/document-library/easy_access_housing.pdf).
- ▲ Request physical and occupational therapy referrals to evaluate wheelchair fitting, skills, safety, and maintenance. Suggest community resources for servicing and tuning up wheelchairs and/or locating parts so clients can service their own chairs; an annual tune-up is recommended.

Client/Family Teaching and Discharge Planning

- ▲ Assess pain levels of long-term wheelchair users and make referrals to therapists or wheelchair clinics for modifications as needed.
- Instruct and have client return demonstrate reinflation of pneumatic tires; encourage client to monitor tire pressure every 2 to 3 weeks.
- Instruct family/clients to remove large wheelchair parts (leg rests, armrests) when lifting wheelchair into car for transport; when reassembling, check that all parts are fastened securely and temperature is tepid. *This reduces weight that needs to be lifted; locked parts and a safe temperature prevent injury/thermal injury.*
- Teach the critical importance of using seatbelts and secure chair tie-downs when riding in motor vehicles in a wheelchair. Never transport a client in an unsecured wheelchair in any kind of vehicle.
- For further information, refer to care plan for Impaired **Transfer** ability.

REFERENCES

AHRQ (2014). *Quality indicators tool kit: Preventing pressure ulcers in hospitals: a tool kit for improving quality of care.* Retrieved from https://www.ahrq.gov/professionals/systems/hospital/pressureulcertoolkit/index.html (Accessed 29 January 2018).

AHRQ (2017). *Wheelchair seating assessment.* Rockville, MD: Agency for Healthcare Research and Quality. Retrieved from https://www.ahrq.gov/professionals/systems/long-term-care/resources/injuries/fallspx/fallspxmanapb4.html. (Accessed 29 January 2018).

Barks, L., & Shaw, P. (2011). Wheelchair positioning and breathing in children with cerebral palsy: Study methods and lessons learned. *Rehabilitation Nursing, 36,* 146–152.

Gefen, A., Farid, K. J., & Shaywitz, I. (2013). A review of deep tissue injury development, detection and prevention: Shear savvy. *Ostomy/Wound Management, 59*(2), 26–35.

Hoon, A., & Tolley, F. (2013). Cerebral palsy. In M. L. Batshaw, N. J. Roizen, & G. R. Lotrecchiano (Eds.), *Children with disabilities.* Baltimore, MD: Paul H. Brookes Publishing Co.

● = Independent;   ▲ = Collaborative;   EBN = Evidence-Based Nursing;   EB = Evidence-Based

Jackson, R. (2017). ADA case review. *Journal of Legal Nurse Consulting, 28*(4).

National Pressure Ulcer Advisory Panel. (2014). *Prevention and treatment of pressure ulcers: Quick reference guide* (2nd ed.). Cambridge, United Kingdom: Cambridge Media.

Requejo, P. S., Furumasu, J., & Mulroy, S. J. (2015). Evidence-based strategies for preserving mobility for elders and aging manual wheelchair users. *Topics in Geriatric Rehabilitation, 31*(1), 26–41.

Rice, L., & Rice, I. (2017). Evidenced-based education interventions to preserve upper limb function among full time manual wheelchair users. *Medical Research Archives, 5*(3). Retrieved from http://

www.journals.ke-i.org/index.php/mra/article/view/1038/792. (Accessed 28 January 2018).

Slayton, S., Morris, P., & Brinkley, J. (2017). Pressure mapping of a standard hospital recliner and select cushions with healthy adults: A comparative study. *Journal of Wound Ostomy & Continence Nursing, 44*(3), 228–235.

Sofka, K. (2011). *Technology corner: It's all downhill ramps, part 1, JNLCP XI.3:438 ff and part 2, JNLCP XI.4: 476 ff.*

Sprigle, S., & Sonenblum, S. (2011). Assessing evidence supporting redistribution of pressure for pressure ulcer prevention: A review. *Journal of Rehabilitation Research and Development, 48*(3), 203–214.

Impaired Mood regulation

Wolter Paans, MSc, PhD, Anna van der Woude, BSN, Carolien van der Velde, Marloes Harkema, BA, and Milou Zemering, BN

NANDA-I

Definition

A mental state characterized by shifts in mood or affect, which is comprised of a constellation of affective, cognitive, somatic, and/or physiological manifestations varying from mild to severe.

Defining Characteristics

Change in verbal behavior; disinhibition; dysphoria; excessive guilt; excessive self-awareness; excessive self-blame; flight of thoughts; hopelessness; impaired concentration; influenced self-esteem; irritability; psychomotor agitation; psychomotor retardation; sad affect; withdrawal

Related Factors

Alteration in sleep pattern; anxiety; appetite change; hypervigilance; impaired social functioning; loneliness; pain; recurrent thoughts of death; recurrent thoughts of suicide; social isolation; substance misuse; weight change

Associated Condition

Chronic illness; functional impairment; psychosis

NOC   (Nursing Outcomes Classification)

Suggested NOC Outcomes

Agitation Level; Hope; Symptom Control; Mood Equilibrium; Comfort Status: Psychospiritual; Concentration; Symptom Severity; Self-Esteem

Example **NOC** Outcome with Indicators
Mood Equilibrium as evidenced by the following indicators: Exhibits affect that fits situation/Exhibits impulse control/ Shows interest in surroundings. (Rate the outcome and indicators of **Mood Equilibrium:** 1 = never demonstrated, 2 = rarely demonstrated, 3 = sometimes demonstrated, 4 = often demonstrated, 5 = consistently demonstrated [see Section I].)

Client Outcomes

Client Will (Specify Time Frame)

- State feelings related to changes in mood
- Eat appropriate diet for height and weight
- Follow exercise plan
- Have no attempts at self-harm
- Attention during activities

● = Independent;   ▲ = Collaborative;   EBN = Evidence-Based Nursing;   EB = Evidence-Based

NIC   (Nursing Interventions Classification)

Suggested NIC Interventions

Activity Therapy; Aromatherapy; Art Therapy; Cognitive Restructuring; Emotional Support; Environmental Management; Forgiveness Facilitation; Hope Inspiration; Milieu Therapy; Presence; Mood Management; Suicide Prevention; Exercise Promotion; Health Education

Nursing Interventions and *Rationales*

- Provide nutritional intake for a client who is unable to feed self. EB: *This study aimed to define the role of nutritional interventions in the prevention and treatment of malnutrition in head and neck cancer clients undergoing chemoradiotherapy (CRT) and their effect on CRT-related toxicity and survival. Head and neck cancer clients are frequently malnourished at the time of diagnosis and prior to the beginning of treatment. In addition, CRT causes or exacerbates symptoms, such as alteration or loss of taste, mucositis, xerostomia, fatigue, and nausea and vomiting, with consequent worsening of malnutrition. Nutritional counseling and oral nutritional supplements should be used to increase dietary intake and prevent therapy-associated weight loss and interruption of radiation therapy (Bossola, 2015). Some of the symptoms (e.g., fatigue, loss of taste) are also present in clients with the diagnostic concept "impaired mood regulation." This study clearly demonstrates that nutritional counseling should be used to increase dietary intake and to prevent weight loss.*
- Encourage regular physical exercise to maintain or advance to a higher level of fitness and health. EB: Negative affective states such as anxiety, depression, and stress are significant risk factors for cardiovascular disease, particularly in cardiac and postcardiac rehabilitation populations. In this study, yoga is used as physical exercise. Breathing control and meditation can reduce psychosocial symptoms and improve cardiovascular and cognitive function (Yeung et al, 2014). This study showed the interest of physical exercise to advance a higher level of health.
- This intervention can be substantiated by Brett, Traynor, and Stapley (2016) and Carter et al (2016).
- Reduce the risk of self-inflicted harm for a client in crisis or severe depression with a planned treatment program. CEB/EBN: This study is about childhood suicidal behavior. This is a complex symptom that requires a carefully planned treatment program that includes multiple modalities of care. Treatment requires a long-term approach that constantly reassesses potential for serious suicidal risk. Psychiatric hospitalization may be required to protect the child from self-inflicted harm and to allow evaluation and appropriate intervention (Pfeffer, 1984). This study is not recent, but it confirms that the risk of self-inflicted harm for a client in crisis should be reduced.
- Advise the client to listen to music in a negative mood (Gold, 2013; Aalbers et al, 2017).
- Try to perceive possible suicidal thoughts on time (Sohn et al, 2017).
- Enable the client to express his or her feelings and try to support the client emotionally if necessary (Kim et al, 2017).
- When possible, use (aromatherapy) massage when in a negative mood (Babaee et al, 2012; Ho et al, 2017).
- Consider recommending cognitive behavior therapy (Whitten & Stanik-Huff, 2011; Cajanding, 2016; Andersen et al, 2017).
- Consider recommending psychotherapy (Szczepanska-Gieracha et al, 2013).
- Give the client hope, for example, about regaining his or her health (Svensson, Nilsson, & Svantesson, 2016).
- If necessary, emphasize the importance of daily activity and routine (Crowe, Beaglehole, & Inder, 2016).
- Signal and treat pain on time (Husebo et al, 2014).
- Promote the self-efficacy of the client (Madueno Caro et al, 2017).
- In case of a persistent negative mood, recommend meditation to theclient (Yuichi et al, 2015).
- The use of a doll in people with dementia can contribute to a better mood (Shin, 2015).

 Client Family Teaching and Discharge Planning

- Provide a treatment involving the cooperation of several aid workers in neighborhood teams and providing customized treatment at the place in which the client resides. EB/EBN: *The use of teams is a well-known approach in a variety of settings, including health care, in both developed and developing countries. Team performance comprises teamwork and task work, and ascertaining whether a team is performing as expected to achieve the desired outcome has rarely been done in health care settings in resource-limited countries (Yeboah-Antwi et al, 2013). This article shows that this intervention is still used.*

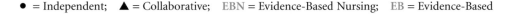

● = Independent;   ▲ = Collaborative;   EBN = Evidence-Based Nursing;   EB = Evidence-Based

REFERENCES

Aalbers, S., Fusar-Poli, L., Freeman, R. E., et al. (2017). Music therapy for depression. *Cochrane Library*, (11), CD004517. doi:10.1002/14651858.CD004517.pub3.

Andersen, L. S., Magidson, J. F., O'Cleirigh, C., et al. (2017). A pilot study of a nurse-delivered cognitive behavioral therapy intervention (Ziphamandla) for adherence and depression in HIV in South Africa. *Journal of Health Psychology*, 23(6), 776–787.

Babaee, S., Shafiei, Z., Sadeghi, M. M., et al. (2012). Effectiveness of massage therapy on the mood of patients after open-heart surgery. *Iranian Journal Nursing Midwifery Research*, 17(2 Suppl 1), S120–S124.

Bossola, M. (2015). Nutritional interventions in head and neck cancer patients undergoing chemoradiotherapy: A narrative review. *Nutrients*, 7(1), 265–276.

Brett, L., Traynor, V., & Stapley, P. (2016). Effects of physical exercise on health and well-being of individuals living with a dementia in nursing homes: A systematic review. *Journal of the American Medical Directors Association*, 17(2), 104–116.

Cajanding, R. J. M. (2016). The effectiveness of a nurse-led cognitive-behavioral therapy on the quality of life, self-esteem and mood among Filipino patients living with heart failure: A randomized controlled trial. *Elsevier*, 31, 86–93.

Carter, T., Morres, I., Repper, J., et al. (2016). Exercise for adolescents with depression: Valued aspects and perceived change. *Journal of Psychiatric and Mental Health Nursing*, 23, 37–44. doi:10.1111/jpm.12261.

Crowe, M., Beaglehole, B., & Inder, M. (2016). Social rhythm interventions for bipolar disorder: A systematic review and rationale for practice. *Journal of Psychiatric and Mental Health Nursing*, 23, 3–11. doi:10.1111/jpm.12271.

Gold, K. (2013). But does it do any good? Measuring the impact of music therapy on people with advanced dementia. *Dementia (Basel, Switzerland)*, 13(2), 258–264. doi:10.1177/1471301213494512.

Ho, S. S. M., Kwong, A. N. L., Wan, K. W. S., et al. (2017). Experiences of aromatherapy massage among adult female cancer patients: A qualitative study. *Journal of Clinical Nursing*, 26(23–24), 4519–4526. doi:10.1111/jocn.13784.

Husebo, B. S., Ballard, C., Fritze, F., et al. (2014). Efficacy of pain treatment on mood syndrome in patients with dementia: A randomized clinical trial. *Geriatric Psychiatry*, 29, 828–836.

Kim, Y. H., Choi, K. S., Han, K., et al. (2017). A psychological intervention programme for patients with breast cancer under chemotherapy and at a high risk of depression: A randomised clinical trial. *Journal of Clinical Nursing*, 27(3–4), 572–581. doi:10.1111/jocn.13910.

Madueno Caro, A. J., Mellado Fernández, M. L., Delgado Pacheco, J., et al. (2017). Perceived self-efficacy, personality and bioethics before a heart rehabilitation programme in primary health care. *Enfermeria Clinica*, 27(6), 346–351.

Pfeffer, C. (1984). Modalities of treatment for suicidal children: An overview of the literature on current practice. *American Journal of Psychotherapy*, 38(3), 364–372.

Shin, J. H. (2015). Doll therapy: An intervention for nursing home residents with dementia. *Journal of Psychosocial Nursing and Mental Health Services*, 53(1), 13–18. doi:10.3928/02793695-20141218-03.

Sohn, M., Heymin, O. H., Lee, S., et al. (2017). Suicidal ideation and related factors among Korean high school students: A focus on cyber addiction and school bullying. *The Journal of School Nursing*, 34(4), 310–318. doi:10.1177/1059840517734290.

Svensson, M., Nilsson, U., & Svantesson, M. (2016). Patients' experience of mood while waiting for day surgery. *Journal of Clinical Nursing*, 25, 2600–2608. doi:10.1111/jocn.13304.

Szczepanska-Gieracha, J., Kowalska, J., Pawik, M., et al. (2013). Evaluation of a short-term group psychotherapy used as part of the rehabilitation process in nursing home patients. *Disability and Rehabilitation: An International, Multidisciplinary Journal*, 1–6. doi:10.3109/09638288.2013.825331.

Whitten, S. K., & Stanik-Hutt, J. (2011). Group cognitive behavioral therapy to improve the quality of care to opioid-treated patients with chronic noncancer pain: A practice improvement project. *Journal of the American Association of Nurse Practitioners*, 25, 368–376. doi:10.1111/j.1745-7599.2012.00800.x.

Yeboah-Antwi, K., Snetro-Plewman, G., Waltensperger, K., et al. (2013). Measuring teamwork and taskwork of community-based "teams" delivering life-saving health interventions in rural Zambia: A qualitative study. *BMC Medical Research Methodology*, 13, 84.

Yeung, A., Kiat, H., Denniss, A., et al. (2014). Randomised controlled trial of a 12 week yoga intervention on negative affective states, cardiovascular and cognitive function in post-cardiac rehabilitation patients. *BMC Complementary and Alternative Medicine*, 14, 411.

Yuichi, K., Toshihiko, S., Thein, A. K., et al. (2015). Psychological effects of meditation at a Buddhist monastery in Myanmar. *Journal of Mental Health*, 26(1), 4–7. doi:10.3109/09638237.2015.1124405.

Moral Distress   *Ruth A. Wittmann-Price, PhD, RN, CNS, CNE, CHSE, ANEF, FAAN*

NANDA-I

Definition

Response to the inability to carry out one's chosen ethical or moral decision and/or action.

Defining Characteristics

Anguish about acting on one's moral choice

Related Factors

Conflict among decision makers; conflicting information available for ethical decision-making; conflicting information available for moral decision-making; cultural incongruence; difficulty reaching end of life decisions; difficulty reaching treatment decision; time constraint for decision-making

● = Independent;   ▲ = Collaborative;   EBN = Evidence-Based Nursing;   EB = Evidence-Based

At-Risk Population

Loss of autonomy; physical distance of decision maker

NOC (Nursing Outcomes Classification)

Suggested NOC Outcomes

Personal Autonomy; Client Satisfaction; Protection of Rights

Example NOC Outcomes with Indicators
Client Satisfaction: Protection of Rights as evidenced by the following indicators: Requests respected/Included in decisions about care/Care consistent with religious and spiritual needs. (Rate the outcome and indicators of **Client Satisfaction: Protection of Rights**: 1 = not at all satisfied, 2 = somewhat satisfied, 3 = moderately satisfied, 4 = very satisfied, 5 = completely satisfied [see Section I].)

Client Outcomes

Client Will (Specify Time Frame)

- Be able to act in accordance with values, goals, and beliefs
- Regain confidence in the ability to make decisions and/or act in accord with values, goals, and beliefs
- Express satisfaction with the ability to make decisions consistent with values, goals, and beliefs
- Have choices respected

NIC (Nursing Interventions Classification)

Suggested NIC Interventions

Patient Rights Protection; Emotional Support

Example NIC Activities—Patient Rights Protection
Provide environment conducive for private conversations between client, family, and health care professionals

Nursing Interventions and *Rationales*

- Assess if moral distress is present and its relationship to intrinsic or extrinsic factors. EB: *Researchers investigated the role of intrinsic motivation (IM) in regimen adherence and glycemic control in type 1 diabetic youths (N = 51) using a new tool to measure IM and found that higher IM was positively correlated with better glycemic control. The 12-item tool is called the Intrinsic Motivation Inventory for Diabetes Management (IMI-DM) (Delamater et al, 2017).* EB: *Cannizzaro et al (2017) studied patients' readiness to change by using the Treatment Motivation Questionnaire in substance-abusing patients (N = 145) to examine intrinsic and extrinsic motivation, and results supported that intrinsic and extrinsic motivation can be used to predict treatment outcome. Additionally, extrinsic motivation might play an important role in the initial stages of treatment, whereas IM plays a role in the later stages of treatment.*
- Affirm the distress, commitment "to take care of yourself," and your obligations. Validate feelings and perceptions with others. EB: *Hjelle et al (2017) qualitatively studied reablement (a home-based, intensive, goal-oriented rehabilitation intervention for older adults) using semistructured interviews with eight patients, and four main themes emerged: "My willpower is needed," "Being with my stuff and my people," "The home-trainers are essential," and "'Training is physical exercises, not everyday activities."* EB: *Blank et al (2017) reviewed research that supports exercise as an IM for adolescents to quit smoking.*
- Implement strategies to change situations causing moral distress. EB: *Sabin (2017) studied moral distress in organizations and deduced moral distress in individuals can be reduced when their reports are given attention and crucial data are extracted on an organization level. Individuals must be able to articulate their concerns without fear of retribution, and leaders must be committed to quality improvement.* EBN: *Karagozoglu et al (2017) studied the use of a moral distress tool in another country to evaluate the moral distress of nurses (N = 200) in an intensive care unit (ICU) by descriptive and cross-sectional design. The results concluded that the tool was reliable and valid, and the study identified communication as key to decreasing moral distress.*

● = Independent;   ▲ = Collaborative;   EBN = Evidence-Based Nursing;   EB = Evidence-Based

- Assess sources and severity of distress. EBN: *Henrich et al (2017) qualitatively examined the effects of moral distress in ICUs using focus groups and found that frustration was the most common emotion associated with moral distress. Specific adverse patient care incidences were also correlated with moral distress.* EBN: *Young, Froggatt, & Brearley (2017) studied moral distress in nursing home clinicians (N = 16) with patients who are near the end of life using an interpretive descriptive design and found participants described holding "good dying" values, which influenced their practice including advocating, caring, communicating, and relating with residents and were found to influence interactions with residents, relatives, general practitioners, and colleagues. Moral distress was described when the right thing could not be done and a "bad death" incurred because of a feeling of powerlessness.*
- Give voice/recognition to moral distress and express concerns about constraints to supportive individuals. EBN: *Schroter (2017) discussed the differences between moral distress and moral resiliency and advocates assisting others to turn negatives into solutions and positive future outlooks to decrease moral distress.* EBN: *Researchers explored moral distress in Chief Nursing Officers (CNOs) (N = 20) using interviews and found six themes emerged including lacking psychological safety, feeling a sense of powerlessness, seeking to maintain moral compass, drawing strength from networking, moral residue, and living with the consequences. This research demonstrated that CNOs experience moral distress but are pressed to show moral courage (Prestia, Sherman, & Demezier, 2017).*
- Engage in healthy problem-solving. EBN: *Authors studied strategies to decrease nurses' moral distress and provide better patient care and strategies including legitimizing the experience, mentoring and empowering one another, allocating a safe haven, and improving the ethical climate of organizations (Forozeiya et al, 2017).* EBN: *Lachance (2017) completed a review of moral courage and how it emerges to offset moral distress and found that it encompasses building safe, collaborative patient- and family-centered teams. Engage in interdisciplinary problem-solving forums including family meeting and/or interdisciplinary rounds.* EB: *Researchers studied the Family Group Decision Making (FGDM) as a strategy to involve family members and social services to make decisions for children and families and found that family participation in family meetings predict planning to ensure services are obtained and reaching family goals (Xu, Ahn, & Bright, 2017).* EBN: *Anderson and Puntillo (2017) studied the integration of palliative care in ICUs and provided nurses (N = 428) with professional development, which resulted in increased communication skills and better provision of palliative care needs to patients and families.*
- Identify/use a support system. EBN: *Ramdinmawii (2017) completed a descriptive study to understand the level of stress, social support, and life satisfaction among parents (N = 60) who have a child with autism spectrum disorder (ASD). Results showed that parents have moderate stress, moderate social support, and a neutral life satisfaction, and social support is correlated inversely to stress and positively with life satisfaction.* EB: *Barimani et al (2017) qualitatively studied the transition to parenthood to discover, describe, and understand transitional conditions that parents perceive as facilitating and inhibiting during the transition to parenthood and to use that knowledge to develop recommendations for professional interventions that support and facilitate the transition to parenthood. The elements that helped the transition to parenthood included perceiving parenthood as normal, enjoying the child's growth, being prepared, having knowledge, and having social support. Initiate an ethics consult or ethics committee review.* EBN: *Kuis & Goossensen (2017) investigated whether the emotional touchpoint method (significant moments when patients were effected physically or emotionally by care) interviews of patients (N = 31) met appropriate ethical standards when used for evaluating care. The study results demonstrated that the touchpoint method was ethical and valuable in evaluating patient care.* EBN: *Crigger et al (2017) used qualitative research to understand the basic process of ethics consultation services by investigating perceptions of health care professionals and found three stages, moral questioning, seeing the big picture, and coming together, which assisted professionals in ethical decision-making.*

 Pediatric

- Consider the developmental age of children when evaluating decisions and conflict. EB: *Malas et al (2017) studied somatic symptom disorder (SSD) in children who present disproportionate or inconsistent physical manifestations with history, physical examination, laboratory, and other assessment findings and made recommendations on how to evaluate and assist parents and children who exhibit manifestations and their underlying cause.* EB: *Wocial et al (2017) completed a pilot project that included formal weekly discussions about prolonged-stay pediatric ICU (PICU) patients to reduce health care providers' moral distress and decrease length of stay (LOS) and found that the intervention had a positive effect on some factors that contribute to moral distress and shortened the LOS for some patients.*

● = Independent;   ▲ = Collaborative;   EBN = Evidence-Based Nursing;   EB = Evidence-Based

Multicultural

- Acknowledge and understand cultural differences that may influence a client's moral choices. EBN: *Bressler, Hanna, and Smith (2017) qualitatively studied moral distress in a nursing care unit with elderly Orthodox Jewish patients at the end of life to better understand the cultural complexity and differences in expectations for patient care between nurses and families. Interviews revealed the incongruence of perspectives indicating there is needed educational strategies, clinical interventions, and research to address moral distress and cultural complexity.* EB: *Howe (2017) discussed observations related to moral distress not only among professionals but also patients and families with a professional-cultural view to view moral distress as a challenge to provide better care.*

Geriatric and Home Care

- Previous interventions may be adapted for geriatric or home care use. EB: *Harigane et al (2017) explored the relationship between psychological distress and degree of functional independence among elderly adults (N = 20,282) and found that psychological distress was significantly associated with decreased independence in all activities of daily living.* EB: *Knight and Alarie (2017) studied the outcomes of a 10-week multimodal mental health day treatment program for elderly patients (N = 255) with mood and anxiety disorders and found that the program improved anxiety and depression.*

REFERENCES

Anderson, W. G., & Puntillo, K. (2017). Palliative care professional development for critical care nurses: A multicenter program. *American Journal of Critical Care, 26*(5), 361–371. Retrieved from http://dx.doi.org.fmarion.idm.oclc.org/10.4037/ajcc2017336.

Barimani, M., Vikstom, A., Rosander, M., et al. (2017). Facilitating and inhibiting factors in transition to parenthood—Ways in which health professionals can support parents. *Scandinavian Journal of Caring Sciences, 31*(3), 537–546. Retrieved from http://dx.doi.org.fmarion.idm.oclc.org/10.1111/scs.12367.

Blank, M. D., Ferris, K. A., Metzger, A., et al. (2017). Physical activity and quit motivation moderators of adolescent smoking reduction. *American Journal of Health Behavior, 41*(4), 419–427. Retrieved from http://dx.doi.org.fmarion.idm.oclc.org/10.5993/AJHB.41.4.6.

Bressler, T., Hanna, D. R., & Smith, E. (2017). Making sense of moral distress within cultural complexity. *Journal of Hospice & Palliative Nursing, 19*(1), 7–16. Retrieved from http://dx.doi.org.fmarion.idm.oclc.org/10.1097/NJH.0000000000000308.

Cannizzaro, D., Stohl, M., Hasin, D., et al. (2017). Intrinsic and extrinsic motivation predict treatment outcome in a sample of HIV+ drug users. *Drug & Alcohol Dependence, 171*, e34. Retrieved from http://dx.doi.org.fmarion.idm.oclc.org/10.1016/j.drugalcdep.2016.08.106.

Crigger, N., Fox, M., Rosell, T., et al. (2017). Moving it along: A study of healthcare professionals' experience with ethics consultations. *Nursing Ethics, 24*(3), 279–291. Retrieved from http://dx.doi.org.fmarion.idm.oclc.org/10.1177/0969733015597571.

Delamater, A. M., Daigre, A. L., Marchante, A. N., et al. (2017). Intrinsic motivation in ethnic minority youth with type 1 diabetes. *Children's Health Care, 46*(3), 215–229. Retrieved from http://dx.doi.org.fmarion.idm.oclc.org/10.1080/02739615.2015.1124777.

Forozeiya, D., Vanderspank-Wright, B., Fothergill-Bourbonnais, F., et al. (2017). Searching for answers: Strategies for supporting nurses who experience moral distress. *Canadian Journal of Critical Care Nursing, 28*(2), 34–35.

Henrich, N. J., Dodek, P. M., Gladstone, E., et al. (2017). Consequences of moral distress in the intensive care unit: A qualitative study. *American Journal of Critical Care, 26*(4), e48–e57. Retrieved from http://dx.doi.org.fmarion.idm.oclc.org/10.4037/ajcc2017786.

Hjelle, K. M., Tuntland, H., Forland, O., et al. (2017). Driving forces for home-based reablement; A qualitative study of older adults' experiences. *Health & Social Care in the Community, 25*(5), 1581–1589. Retrieved from http://dx.doi.org.fmarion.idm.oclc.org/10.1111/hsc.12324.

Howe, E. G. (2017). Fourteen important concepts regarding moral distress. *Journal of Clinical Ethics, 28*(1), 3–14.

Karagozoglu, S., Yildirim, G., Ozden, D., et al. (2017). Moral distress in Turkish intensive care nurses. *Nursing Ethics, 24*(2), 209–221. Retrieved from http://dx.doi.org.fmarion.idm.oclc.org/10.1177/0969733015593408.

Knight, C. A., & Alarie, R. M. (2017). Improving mental health in the community: Outcome evaluation of a geriatric mental health day treatment service. *Clinical Gerontologist, 40*(2), 77–87. Retrieved from http://dx.doi.org.fmarion.idm.oclc.org/10.1080/07317115.2016.1263709.

Kuis, E. E., & Goossensen, A. (2017). Evaluating care from a care ethical perspective: A pilot study. *Nursing Ethics, 24*(5), 569–582. Retrieved from http://dx.doi.org.fmarion.idm.oclc.org/10.1177/0969733015620939.

Lachance, C. (2017). Tough decisions, lots of uncertainties: Moral courage as a strategy to ease moral distress. *Canadian Journal of Critical Care Nursing, 28*(2), 37.

Malas, N., Ortiz-Aguayo, R., Giles, L., et al. (2017). Pediatric somatic symptom disorders. *Current Psychiatry Reports, 19*(2), 1–11. Retrieved from http://dx.doi.org.fmarion.idm.oclc.org/10.1007/s11920-017-0760-3.

Harigane, M., Suzuki, Y., Yasumura, S., et al. (2017). The relationship between functional independence and psychological distress in elderly adults following the Fukushima Daiichi nuclear power plant accident: The Fukushima health management survey. *Asia-Pacific Journal of Public Health, 29*, 120S–130S. Retrieved from http://dx.doi.org.fmarion.idm.oclc.org/10.1177/1010539516683498.

Prestia, A. S., Sherman, R. O., & Demezier, C. (2017). Chief nursing officers' experiences with moral distress. *Journal of Nursing Administration, 47*(2), 101–107. Retrieved from http://dx.doi.org.fmarion.idm.oclc.org/10.1097/NNA.0000000000000447.

Ramdinmawii, K. R. (2017). A descriptive study to assess the level of stress, social support and life satisfaction among parents of children with autism spectrum disorder at selected centres in Delhi. *International Journal of Nursing Education, 9*(2), 172–177. Retrieved from http://dx.doi.org.fmarion.idm.oclc.org/10.5958/0974-9357.2017.00058.7.

Sabin, J. E. (2017). Using moral distress for organizational improvement. *Journal of Clinical Ethics, 28*(1), 33–36.

Schroter, K. (2017). Ethics in practice: from moral distress to moral resilience. *Journal of Trauma Nursing, 24*(5), 290–291. Retrieved

M

from http://dx.doi.org.fmarion.idm.oclc.org/10.1097/JTN
.0000000000000317.

Wocial, L., Acjkerman, V., Leland, B., et al. (2017). Pediatric Ethics and Communication Excellence (PEACE) rounds: Decreasing moral distress and patient length of stay in the PICU. *HEC Forum: An Interdisciplinary Journal on Hospitals' Ethical and Legal Issues, 29*(1), 75–91. Retrieved from http://dx.doi.org.fmarion.idm.oclc.org/10 .1007/s10730-016-9313-0.

Xu, Y., Ahn, H., & Bright, C. L. (2017). Family involvement meetings: Engagement, facilitation, and child and family goals. *Children &*

Youth Services Review, 79, 37–43. Retrieved from http:// dx.doi.org.fmarion.idm.oclc.org/10.1016/j.childyouth.2017.05.026.

Young, A., Froggatt, K., & Brearley, S. G. (2017). Powerlessness' or 'doing the right thing'—Moral distress among nursing home staff caring for residents at the end of life: An interpretive descriptive study. *Palliative Medicine, 31*(9), 853–860. Retrieved from http:// dx.doi.org.fmarion.idm.oclc.org/10.1177/0269216316682894.

Risk for dry Mouth   Katherine Foss, MSN, RN

NANDA-I

Definition

Susceptible to discomfort or damage to the oral mucosa due to reduced quality or quality of saliva to moisten the mucosa, which may compromise health.

Risk Factors

Dehydration; depression; excessive stress; excitement; smoking

Associated Condition

Chemotherapy; fluid restriction; inability to feed orally; oxygen therapy; pharmaceutical agent; pregnancy; radiation therapy to the head and neck; systemic diseases

NOC   (Nursing Outcomes Classification)

Suggested NOC Outcomes

Oral Health; Self-Care: Oral Hygiene; Tissue Integrity: Skin and Mucous Membranes

Example **NOC** Outcome with Indicators
Oral Health as evidenced by the following indicators: Cleanliness of mouth and teeth/Moisture of oral mucosa and tongue/Color of mucous membranes/Oral mucosa/Tongue/Gum integrity. (Rate the outcome and indicators of **Oral Health:** 1 = severely compromised, 2 = substantially compromised, 3 = moderately compromised, 4 = mildly compromised, 5 = not compromised [see Section I].)

Client Outcomes

Client Will (Specify Time Frame)

- Maintain intact, moist oral mucous membranes that are free of ulceration, inflammation, infection, and debris
- Demonstrate measures to maintain or regain oral health
- Demonstrate oral hygiene knowledge and skills to maintain moisture within the mouth
- Be free of halitosis and oral discomfort
- State tolerable to no changes in taste sensation (dysgeusia)

NIC   (Nursing Interventions Classification)

Suggested NIC Intervention

Oral Health Restoration

Example **NIC** Activities—Oral Health Restoration
Monitor condition of client's mouth including character of abnormalities; Instruct client to perform regular oral hygiene measures

● = Independent;   ▲ = Collaborative;   EBN = Evidence-Based Nursing;   EB = Evidence-Based

Nursing Interventions and *Rationales*

- Perform a comprehensive extraoral and intraoral examination for associated conditions and risk factors that reduce quantity or quality of saliva and patient complaints of oral dryness and difficulty speaking, eating, or swallowing. *Inspection is a critical assessment and diagnostic tool that can lead to identification of current oral health and impending problems (van Der Waal, 2015).*
- Assess for symptoms of dry mouth. EB: Observe for atrophic and erythematous oral mucosa, loss of papillae on the tongue, and lips that peel and crack. Traumatic lesions may be visible on the buccal mucosa and the lateral borders of the tongue (American Dental Association [ADA], 2015).
- Inspect and palpate major salivary glands and lymph nodes for masses, enlargement, tenderness, purulent discharge, or absence of salivary pooling/secretions are components of a comprehensive head and neck examination to differentiate between salivary and nonsalivary causes of dry mouth (ADA, 2015).
- Inspect nasal turbinates for enlargement, swelling, polyps, and nasal flow because nasal blockages increase mouth breathing, which may exacerbate oral dryness symptoms.
- Assess patient for oral candidiasis, dental caries, and gingival recession (ADA, 2015). Oral candidiasis may suggest the client is immunocompromised or on treatment that increases the risk of fungal infection, which can lead to additional health care concerns.
- Assess patient for dental caries and gingival recession because clinical signs of hyposalivation also include increased incidence of tooth decay at the gingival margin and nonspecific gingival inflammation (Plemons, Al-Hashimi, & Marek, 2014; ADA, 2015).
- Assess patient for difficulty chewing, swallowing (dysphagia), or speaking. Dry mouth may cause difficulties with chewing and swallowing, which may place the client at risk of choking and or malnutrition (ADA, 2015; American Academy of Oral Medicine [AAOM], 2016).
- Assess patient for mouth breathing caused by functional impairment of the upper airway and/or presence of nasal, endotracheal, or orogastric tubes that may prevent mouth closure or irritate oral mucosa, which may contribute to an increase in dry mouth symptoms experienced by clients.

- Assess patient hydration status. EB: A dry tongue and mucous membranes are symptoms of decreased hydration status (Wagner & Hardin-Pierce, 2014). Decreased hydration status can worsen symptom of dry mouth.
- Assess fluid status because dehydration will also affect salivary flow (Plemons, Al-Hashimi, & Marek, 2014). Consider fluid loss associated with fever, cachexia, vomiting, or diarrhea. Recognize that dehydration is prevalent in older adults and may affect salivary flow (ADA, 2015).
- ▲ Dry mouth, mouth dryness, or oral dryness (xerostomia) is a dryness of the oral cavity resulting from insufficient or complete lack of saliva secretion. Although dry mouth is a common symptom of salivary gland hyposecretion, there is a distinction between dryness caused by malfunction of the salivary glands and the patient's subjective report of oral dryness despite normal salivary gland function (Tanasiewicz, Hildebrandt, & Obersztyn, 2016). EB: *In a review summary of 90 articles, clinical application to the etiology, diagnosis, and treatment of dry mouth requires an interdisciplinary approach to symptom assessment, clinical examination, functional and cognitive assessment, and identifying goals of care. The management of dry mouth begins with a thorough history of symptoms; review of medical, dental, and medication use history; clinical exam; salivary flow rate measurements; salivary imaging studies; and biopsies and laboratory analysis (Han, Suarez-Durall, & Mulligan, 2015).* CEB: *In a literature review of dry mouth diagnosis and treatment, measurement of salivary output is required to differentiate between salivary and nonsalivary causes of xerostomia (Napeñas, Brennan, & Fox, 2009).*
- ▲ The client may require a dental referral to evaluate salivary flow rate as a tool to monitor dry mouth symptoms (Plemons, Al-Hashimi, & Marek, 2014; ADA, 2015).
- ▲ Consider use of oral screening, patient self-report tool, and/or subjective questioning regarding dry mouth symptoms to assess client oral health and to predict need for dental intervention and degree of salivary hypofunction. EB: *One validated screening tool, for use by nondental professionals, to assess client oral health and identification of need for a dental exam is the Oral Health Assessment Tool (OHAT) and can be used to monitor client progress during an oral hygiene plan of care (Australian Department of Health and Aging, 2009).*
- ▲ Use client self-report to measure symptoms of dry mouth. EB: *The Xerostomia Inventory (XI) questionnaire, developed in Australia during the 1990s and validated in international studies, provided a summative rating of client's xerostomia symptoms (Thomson, 2015). EB: A Cochrane review found that a change in XI core of 6 or more points is likely to be meaningful, and the tools measure the severity of dry mouth and act as a responsive measure to interventions for dry mouth (Furness et al. 2013).*

• = Independent;   ▲ = Collaborative;   EBN = Evidence-Based Nursing;   EB = Evidence-Based

- Ask the client about symptoms of hyposalivation. CEB/EB: *A study of subjective oral dryness compared with salivary flow reports that certain complaints were highly predictive of impaired salivary flow. Positive responses to any of the following complaints are associated with significant hyposalivation: oral dryness when eating, need to sip fluids to swallow dry foods, difficulty swallowing, and the perception of too little saliva (Fox, Busch, & Baum, 1987; Napeñas, Brennan, & Fox, 2009).*
- ▲ Review client medication usage for dry mouth as a side effect of medication. If symptoms are present consult with provider, or refer client to see a dentist or specialist. EB: *Assess the client's use of xerostomic medications or medications that are known to directly inhibit saliva flow (ADA, 2015). Anticholinergic and antihypertensive drugs (angiotensin-converting enzyme inhibitors, angiotensin receptor blockers, α- and β-adrenergic blockers, and diuretics) antihistamines, opioids, antidepressants, immunostimulants, and antipsychotic and skeletal muscle relaxant drugs are identified as common causes of dry mouth.* EBN: *Consult with a pharmacist regarding timing of medications and possible drug substitutions. Most medications do not cause damage to salivary glands but can reduce salivary flow (Plemons, Al-Hashimi, & Marek, 2014; Tanasiewicz, Hildebrandt, & Oberształyn, 2016).*
- ▲ Administer pilocarpine and cevimeline as prescribed because these medications are considered first-line therapy in Sjögren's syndrome and head and neck cancer clients with radiotherapy-induced dry mouth and hyposalivation. EB: *A systematic review and meta-analysis of 1732 patients in 20 studies indicated that both cevimeline and pilocarpine can reduce dry mouth symptoms and increase salivary flow compared with placebo (Mercadante et al, 2017).*
- ▲ ADA council on scientific affairs report identifies that pilocarpine and cevimeline have US Food and Drug Administration approval for treating dry mouth caused by Sjögren's syndrome or radiation therapy (ADA, 2015).
- ▲ Administer amifostine as prescribed to reduce the incidence of acute and late xerostomia for clients treated with standard fractionated radiation and gland-sparing radiation technique to the head and neck. EB: *A systematic review of the cytoprotectant amifostine has been shown to reduce the acute and late incidence of xerostomia in head and neck cancer patients treated with conventional radiation therapy (Shiboski et al, 2007).*
- Teach clients about conditions that can exacerbate dry mouth symptoms, including:
  - ○ Avoidance of low-humidity environments
  - ○ Avoidance of oral irritants: acidic fluids such as carbonated beverages and juices, caffeine, alcohol, tobacco
  - ○ Avoidance of salty, spicy, acidic, or high-sucrose content foods
  - ○ Avoidance of dry, hard, and sticky foods
  - ○ Referral of patient to smoking and/or alcohol cessation program

EB: *Avoiding conditions that can worsen dry mouth can facilitate client self-management of the symptom severity (ADA, 2015; Agency for Healthcare Research and Quality [AHRQ], 2016).*

- Teach the client good oral hygiene:
  - ○ Twice daily toothbrushing with regular topical fluoride toothpaste.
  - ○ Use of soft bristle toothbrush. EB: *Twice daily use of a soft bristle toothbrush is an accepted standard of care by the ADA to maintain and promote oral health and dentition (ADA, 2017a).*
  - ○ Daily use of dental floss or another interdental cleaner. EB: *Daily use of dental floss or interdental cleaner is an accepted standard of care to maintain and promote oral health and dentition (ADA, 2017a).*
  - ○ Daily use of alcohol-free mouth rinse. EB: *Systematic review by an expert panel recommends regular use of fluoride toothpastes or mouth rinses as highly effective in preventing caries in dry mouth (Zero et al, 2016).*
  - ○ Recommend use of prescription-strength fluoride toothpastes for severe salivary hypofunction. EB: *The use of 1.1% neutral sodium fluoride, or fluoride gel in custom-fit oral tray, or 0.09% fluoride mouth rinse daily (Plemons, Al-Hashimi, & Marek, 2014; ADA, 2017b).*
- Provide instruction regarding cleaning, and assist with care of dental prosthesis as needed. Daily cleansing of a dental prosthetic is an accepted standard of care to maintain and promote oral health and dentition (ADA, 2017a).
- ▲ Provide instruction on candidiasis prevention and control. Administer antifungal topical treatments as prescribed using available suspensions, pastilles, and lozenges for uncomplicated oral candidiasis. Systemic antifungal agents may be prescribed for complicated candidiasis mucosal infection (Baer et al, 2017).
- ▲ Soak partial or complete dental prosthesis overnight in 0.2% chlorhexidine HCL. EB: *A literature review of treatment of dry mouth and other nonocular sicca symptoms in Sjögren's syndrome identified that oral*

● = Independent;   ▲ = Collaborative;   EBN = Evidence-Based Nursing;   EB = Evidence-Based

candidiasis mucosal infection is common in clients with salivary gland hypofunction. Administer prescribed antifungal rinses, ointments, or lozenges. Include daily partial or complete denture antifungal treatment; soak dentures overnight in 0.2% chlorhexidine HCL (Baer et al, 2017).

▲ Recommend professional dental oral examination every 3 to 6 months. Recommend professional teeth cleaning at least every 6 months. **EB:** *ADA Council of Scientific Affairs identifies preventative oral health care for patients with hyposalivation as essential. This includes more frequent dental visits and associated management of secondary infections (ADA, 2015).*

• Discuss selection and use of salivary substitutes with patient and health care provider to assist in maintaining mouth moisture. **EB:** *A Cochrane review of nonpharmacological topical treatments for dry mouth that included salivary substitutes of sugar-free gums, mints, lozenges, sprays, gels, oils, and toothpastes indicated lack of strong evidence that topical therapies are effective in improving salivary flow. Many saliva substitutes are available without prescription and contain a mix of components such as carboxymethylcellulose, polyethylene glycol, sorbitol, and electrolytes. These products typically provide more viscosity and lubrication than water. A saliva spray that contains oxygenated glycerol trimester (OGT) is more effective than a water-based electrolyte spray (McMillan, 2016).*

• Teach the client that any topical product that is acidic or contains sugar, or noted as sugarless with high fructose, should be avoided. **EB:** *Citrus-flavored sugar-free tablets or oral drops with malic acid may stimulate salivary flow. Additional nonpharmacological management of dry mouth using gel-releasing devices worn in the mouth requires more research. Patient preference also appears to have significant affect in the acceptance and attribution of topical agent efficacy (Furness et al, 2011; Treister, Villa, & Thompson, 2017).* **EB:** *A predesign and postdesign study of 118 elderly patients using an edible oral moisturizing jelly (OMJ) examined the efficacy of OMJ with results of reduced symptoms of dry mouth and prevention of decline of saliva pH, but further study is needed with a larger population and randomized-controlled study design (Dalodom et al, 2016).*

• Encourage the client to try several products, based on client preference, to find a suitable saliva substitute. Clients reported that use of saliva substitutes may be more helpful before sleep because of diurnal variation on reduction in salivary flow at night. It is also suggested that patients mix and match salivary agents based on their daily schedules or activities such as eating or public speaking (Baer et al, 2017). **CEB/EB:** *A literature review through September 2017 of treatment of dry mouth and other nonocular sicca symptoms in Sjögren's syndrome that use saliva substitutes is supported by several randomized trials and studies that show benefit when compared with placebo in relieving symptoms of dry mouth, burning tongue, and difficulties with chewing and swallowing (Wu, 2008; National Institute of Dental and Craniofacial Research, 2016).*

• Lubricate lips every 2 hours, while awake, and as needed. Apply moisturizer (e.g., lanolin) to dry lips every 2 hours, as needed to assist with dryness.

• Teach patients preventative measures to reduce oral dryness:
  ○ Maintain adequate oral hydration by sipping water regularly and/or sucking on ice chips (AAOM, 2016)
  ○ While eating, drink fluids carefully.
  ○ Maintain an oral intake log.
  ○ Rinse with normal saline or clean water as a part of daily oral care to prevent dry mouth, or sodium bicarbonate solution (1 teaspoon salt and 1 teaspoon baking soda to 1 L of water). **EB:** *Oral rinses with clean water or normal saline every 2 hours while awake promote a moist oral mucosa, neutralize oral pH, and are readily available with minimal side effects and are inexpensive (AAOM, 2016; ADA, 2017).*

• Encourage the client to use sugar-free gum or sugar-free candy to promote salivary flow. **EB:** *A Cochrane review of nonpharmacological topical treatments for dry mouth included salivary substitutes of sugar-free gum and candy. Although mastication increases saliva production, the evidence is not conclusive that sugar-free chewing gum is better or worse than other saliva substitutes for symptom management of dry mouth, but the use of these interventions also was supported by extensive clinical experience (Furness et al, 2011).*

• Encourage the client to use saline nasal sprays to maintain open nasal passages. *Maintenance of open nasal passage to avoid mouth breathing include saline nasal sprays or gentle nasal lavage to remove dried secretions (AAOM, 2016; Baer, 2017).*

• The client may find the use of a humidifier during sleep at night helpful in reducing symptoms.

▲ Discuss with the client the use of acupuncture, electrical nerve stimulation, and powered versus manual toothbrushes to assist in maintaining mouth moisture. **EB:** *In a systematic review, nonpharmacological therapies using acupuncture, transcutaneous electrical nerve stimulation, and powered versus manual*

M

• = Independent;   ▲ = Collaborative;   **EBN** = Evidence-Based Nursing;   **EB** = Evidence-Based

toothbrushing were reported as insufficient or low-quality evidence to determine effects of these interventions on dry mouth or saliva production but continued to be studied as alternatives for symptom relief (Simcock et al, 2012; Furness et al, 2013).

▲ Encourage the client to discuss the use of emerging preventative treatments with the health care provider such as gene therapy, tissue engineering, stem cell therapy, and growth factors for etiologies associated with dry mouth. EB: *Current research of Sjögren syndrome and head and neck radiation etiologies associated with salivary hypofunction reported that future approaches to treatment and/or prevention of the feeling of dry mouth includes gene therapy, stem cell therapy, and tissue engineering (Quock, 2016).* EB: *In a review of 90 articles with clinical application, there are emerging therapies for radiation-induced salivary hypofunction, but the most efficacious with cost-effectiveness are not identified (Han, Suarez-Durall, & Mulligan, 2015).*

▲ Discuss use of Bethanechol HCL saliva stimulant in head and neck cancer patients with radiotherapy-induced dry mouth and hyposalivation with the client and health care provider. EB: *Clinical application of Bethanechol HCL to treat dry mouth in clients with radiation therapy-induced dry mouth and salivation is not supported because further research is needed to determine optimal dosing, frequency of use, long-term efficacy, and safety (Han, Suarez-Durall, & Mulligan, 2015; McMillan, 2016).*

Geriatric

- Recognize that symptoms of dry mouth are more common in menopausal women and geriatric patients. *Symptoms of dry mouth are more common in menopausal women and almost 50% of the elderly population because of an age-related increase of systemic disease occurrence and disease treatment, including medications (Turner & Ship, 2007; Thompson, 2015; Dalodom, 2016).*

- Age-associated increase of systemic disease and subsequent disease treatment is the primary cause of dry mouth. EB: *Systematic review of the literature from 1980 to 2010 indicates a high prevalence of xerostomia and salivary gland hypofunction in the very elderly population with associated factors of polypharmacy, poor general health, and old age (Liu et al, 2012).*

- Older adults are at risk of xerostomia from a variety of etiologies. EB: *In a narrative review of systemic disease in older adults and review of the literature of xerostomia caused by various etiologies, it is recommended to assess the patient for dehydration, nutritional alteration manifested by weight loss, decreased appetite, increased thirst, and any changes in food or beverage preferences. Oral symptoms of malnutrition, such as sore tongue, burning mouth, and gingivitis, may be caused by iron, vitamin B_1, B_2, B_6, and B_{12} or vitamin C deficiencies (Tanasiewicz, Hildebrandt, & Obersztyn, 2016; Critchlow, 2017).*

- Review client medication list routinely. EB: *In a cross-sectional study to examine the relationship between nutrition, oral health, and drug use among adults aged 75 and older, it was found that excessive polypharmacy, the use of particular drug groups, and depressive symptoms were associated with xerostomia, supporting the need for a multidisciplinary approach to care (Thompson 2015; Viljakainen et al, 2016).*

Multicultural and Home Care Considerations

- The previously mentioned nursing interventions and client teaching may be adapted for multicultural and home care considerations. See care plan on Impaired **Oral Mucous Membrane** integrity.

REFERENCES

Agency for Healthcare Research and Quality. (2016). *American Cancer Society Head and Neck Survivorship Care Guidelines.* Retrieved from https://www.guideline.gov/summaries/summary/51021/america n-cancer-society-head-and-neck-cancer-survivorship-care-guideline ?q=dry+mouth. (Accessed 26 February 2018).

American Academy of Oral Medicine. (2016). AAOM Clinical Practice Statement. Subject: clinical management of cancer therapy-induced salivary gland hypofunction and xerostomia. *Oral Surgery, Oral Medicine, Oral Pathology, Oral Radiology,* 122(3), 310–312. Retrieved from http://dx/doi/10.1016/j.oooo.2016.04.015.

American Dental Association (2015). *Managing xerostomia and salivary gland hypofunction: A report on the ADA Council of Scientific Affairs.* Retrieved from http://jada.ada.org/content/145/8/867.abstract.

American Dental Association. (2017a). *Home oral care.* Retrieved from http://www.ada.org/en/member-center/oral-health-topics/ home-care. (Accessed 26 February 2018).

American Dental Association. (2017b). *Xerostomia (dry mouth).* Retrieved from http://www.ada.org/en/member-center/ oral-health-topics/xerostomia. (Accessed 26 February 2018).

Australian Department of Health and Aging. 2009. *Trial of the draft national framework for documentation care in residential aged care services.* Retrieved from https://www.aihw.gov.au/reports/aged-care/ caring-for-oral-health-in-australian-residential-c/contents/ table-of-contents. (Accessed 26 February 2018).

Baer, A. N. (2017). *Treatment of dry mouth and other non-ocular sicca symptoms in Sjögren's syndrome.* Retrieved from https://www

● = Independent;   ▲ = Collaborative;   EBN = Evidence-Based Nursing;   EB = Evidence-Based

-uptodate-com.proxy.hsl.ucdenver.edu/contents/treatment-of-dry-mouth-and-other-non-ocular-sicca-symptoms-in-sjogrens-syndrome/print?source=search_result&search=xerostomia%20treatment&selectedTitle=1~150.

Critchlow, D. (2017). Part 3: Impact of systemic conditions and medication on oral health. *British Journal of Community Nursing*, 22(4), 181–190.

Dalodom, S., Jeanmaneechotechai, S., Intachai, W., et al. (2016). Influence of oral moisturizing jelly as a saliva substitute for the relief of xerostomia in elderly patients with hypertension and diabetes mellitus. *Geriatric Nursing*, 37, 101–109. Retrieved from http://dx.doi.org/10.106/j.gerinurse.2015.10.014.

Fox, P. C., Busch, K. A., & Baum, B. J. (1987). Subjective reports of xerostomia and objective measures of salivary gland performance. *Journal of the American Dental Association*, 115, 581–584.

Furness, S., Worthington, H. V., Bryan, G., et al. (2011). Interventions for the management of dry mouth: Topical therapies. *Cochrane Database of Systematic Reviews*, (12), CD008934. doi:10.1002/14651858.CD008934.pub2.

Furness, S., Bryan, G., McMillan, R., et al. (2013). Interventions for the management of dry mouth: Non-pharmacological interventions. *Cochrane Database of Systematic Reviews*, (9), CD009603. doi:10.1002/14651858.CD009603.pub3.

Han, P., Suarez-Durall, P., & Mulligan, R. (2015). Dry mouth: A critical topic for older adult patients. *Journal of Prosthodontic Research*, 59, 6–19. Retrieved from https://dx.doi.org/10.1016/j.jpor.2014.11.001.

Liu, B., Dion, M., Jurasic, M. M., et al. (2012). Xerostomia and salivary hypofunction in vulnerable elders: Prevalence and etiology. *Oral Surgery, Oral Medicine, Oral Pathology, Oral Radiology*, 114(1), 52–60.

McMillan, R., Forssell, H., Buchanan, J. A. G., et al. (2016). Interventions for treating burning mouth syndrome. *Cochrane Database of Systematic Reviews*, (11), CD002779. doi:10.1002/14651858.CD002779.pub3.

Mercadante, V., Al Hamad, A., Lodi, G., et al. (2017). Interventions for the management of radiotherapy-induced xerostomia and hyposalivation: A systematic review and meta-analysis. *Oral Oncology*, 66, 64–74. Retrieved from https://www.ncbi.nlm.nih.ov/pubmed/28249650.1.

Napeñas, J., Brennan, M. T., & Fox, P. C. (2009). Diagnosis and treatment of xerostomia (dry mouth). *Odontology/The Society of the Nippon Dental University*, 97, 76–83. doi:10.1007/s10266-008-0099-7.

National Institute of Dental and Craniofacial Research. (2016). *Dry mouth*. Retrieved from https://www.nidcr.nih.gov/OralHealth/Topics/DryMouth/DryMouth.htm#. (Accessed 26 February 2018).

Plemons, J. M., Al-Hashimi, I., & Marek, C. (2014). Managing xerostomia and salivary gland hypofunction. *The Journal of the American Dental Association*, 145(8), 867–873. Retrieved from https://dx.doi.org/10.14219/jada.archive.2007.0358.

Quock, R. (2016). Xerostomia: current streams of investigation. *Oral Surgery, Oral Medicine, Oral Pathology, Oral Radiology*, 122, 53–60. Retrieved from https://doi.org/10.1016/j.oooo.2016.03.002.

Shiboski, C. H., Hodgson, T. A., Ship, J. A., et al. (2007). Management of salivary hypofunction during and after radiotherapy. *Oral Surgery, Oral Medicine, Oral Pathology. Oral Radiology, Endondontic*, 103(Suppl. 1), S66.e1–S66.e19. doi:10.1016/j.tripleo.2016.11.013.

Simcock, R., Fallowfield, L., Monson, K., on behalf of the ARIX Steering Committee, et al. (2012). ARIX: A randomised trial of acupuncture v oral care sessions in patients with chronic xerostomia following treatment of head and neck cancer. *Annals of Oncology*, 24(3), 776–783. Retrieved from https://doi-org.proxy.hsl.ucdenver.edu/10.1093/annonc/mds515.

Tanasiewicz, M., & Hildebrandt, T. (2016). Xerostomia of various etiologies: A review of the literature. *Advanced Clinical Exploratory Medicine*, 25(1), 199–206. doi:10.17219/acem/29375.

Thomson, W. M. (2015). Dry mouth and older people. *Australian Dental Journal*, 60(1 Suppl.), 54–63. doi:10.1111/adj.12284.

Treister, N. S., Villa, A., & Thompson, L. (2017). *Palliative care: Overview of mouth care at the end of life*. Retrieved from https://www.uptodate-com.proxy.hsl.ucdenver.edu/contents/palliative-care-overview-of-mouth-care-at-the-end-of-life/print?source=search_result&search=xerostomia&selectedTitle=3~150.

Turner, M. D., & Ship, J. (2007). Dry mouth and its effects on the oral health of elderly people. *Journal of the American Dental Association*, 138, 15S–20S.

van Der Waal, I. (2015). Oral leukoplakia: The ongoing discussion on definition and terminology. *Medicina Oral, Patología Oral y Cirugía Bucal*, 20(6), e685. doi:10.4317/medoral.21007.

Viljakainen, S., Nykänen, I., Ahonen, R., et al. (2016). Xerostomia among older home care clients. *Community Dentistry and Oral Epidemiology*, 44, 232–238. doi:10.1111/cdoe.12210.

Wagner, K. D., & Hardin-Pierce, M. G. (2014). *High acuity nursing* (6th ed.). Boston: Prentice Hall, Inc.

Wu, A. J. (2008). Optimizing dry mouth treatment for individuals with Sjögren's syndrome. *Rheumatic Disease Clinics of North America*, 34, 1001–1010.

Zero, D. T., Brennan, M. T., Daniels, T. E., et al. (2016). Clinical practice guidelines for oral management of Sjögren disease: Dental caries prevention. *Journal of the American Dental Association*, 147, 295.

N

Nausea   *Janelle M. Tipton, MSN, RN, AOCN*

NANDA-I

Definition

A subjective, phenomenon of an unpleasant feeling in the back of the throat and stomach, which may or may not result in vomiting.

Defining Characteristics

Aversion toward food; gagging sensation; increase in salivation; increase in swallowing; sour taste

Related Factors

Anxiety; exposure to toxin; fear; noxious environmental stimuli; noxious taste; unpleasant visual stimuli

● = Independent;   ▲ = Collaborative;   EBN = Evidence-Based Nursing;   EB = Evidence-Based

Associated Condition

Biochemical dysfunction; esophageal disease; gastric distention; gastrointestinal irritation; increase in intra-cranial pressure (ICP); intra-abdominal tumors; labyrinthitis; liver capsule stretch; localized tumors; Ménière's disease; meningitis; motion sickness; pancreatic disease; pregnancy; psychological disorder; splenetic capsule stretch; treatment regimen

NOC   (Nursing Outcomes Classification)

Suggested NOC Outcomes

Comfort Level; Hydration; Nausea and Vomiting Severity; Nutritional Status: Food and Fluid Intake; Nutrient Intake

> **Example NOC Outcome with Indicators**
>
> **Nausea and Vomiting Severity** as evidenced by the following indicators: Frequency of nausea/Intensity of nausea/Distress of nausea. (Rate the outcome and indicators of **Nausea and Vomiting Severity:** I = severe, 2 = substantial, 3 = moderate, 4 = mild, 5 = none [see Section I].)

Client Outcomes

Client Will (Specify Time Frame)

- State relief of nausea
- Explain methods clients can use to decrease nausea and vomiting (N&V)

NIC   (Nursing Interventions Classification)

Suggested NIC Interventions

Distraction; Medication Administration; Progressive Muscle Relaxation; Simple Guided Imagery; Therapeutic Touch

> **Example NIC Activities—Distraction**
>
> Encourage the individual to choose the distraction techniques desired, such as music, engaging in conversation or telling a detailed account of event or story, guided imagery, or humor; Advise client to practice the distraction technique before the time needed, if possible

Nursing Interventions and *Rationales*

▲ Determine cause or risk for N&V (e.g., medication effects, infectious causes [viral and bacterial gastro-enteritis], disorders of the gut and peritoneum [mechanical obstruction, motility disorders, or other intraabdominal causes], central nervous system causes [including anxiety], endocrine and metabolic causes [including pregnancy], postoperative-related status). *Because N&V are clinically identifiable symptoms, it is important for the cause to be determined and appropriate plan and interventions to be developed. Review the client's medication record, alcohol history, and electrolytes as appropriate for early identification of cause of nausea (Goel & Wilkinson, 2013; Koth & Kolesar, 2017).* **EB:** *Prophylactic interventions given before chemotherapy have proven to be most successful in preventing N&V. Client expectancy of nausea after che-motherapy is predictive of that treatment-related side effect (Kamen et al, 2014; Oncology Nursing Society, 2017).*

▲ Evaluate and document the client's history of N&V, with attention to onset, duration, timing, volume of emesis, frequency of pattern, setting, associated factors, aggravating factors, and past medical and social histories. *The onset and duration of N&V may be distinctly associated with specific events and may be treated differently (Irwin & Johnson, 2014; Tipton, 2014).*

- Document each episode of nausea and/or vomiting separately and the effectiveness of interventions. Consider an assessment tool for consistency of evaluation. **EB:** *A systematic approach can provide consistency, accuracy, and measurement needed to direct care. It is important to recognize that nausea is a subjective experience (Irwin & Johnson, 2014).*

• = Independent;   ▲ = Collaborative;   EBN = Evidence-Based Nursing;   EB = Evidence-Based

- Identify and eliminate contributing causative factors. This may include eliminating unpleasant odors or medications that may be contributing to nausea. *These interventions are theory based; however, there is no research evidence to support these interventions outside of expert opinion.*

▲ Implement appropriate dietary measures such as nothing by mouth (NPO) status as appropriate; small, frequent meals; and low-fat meals. It may be helpful to avoid foods that are spicy, fatty, or highly salty. Reverting to previous practices when ill in the past and consuming "comfort foods" may also be helpful at this time. *Expert opinion consensus recommends these interventions, with no research data available (Irwin & Johnson, 2014).*

▲ Recognize and implement interventions and monitor complications associated with N&V. This may include administration of intravenous fluids and electrolytes. *Recognition of complications of N&V is critical to prevent and manage complications of dehydration, electrolyte imbalance, and malnourishment. Adequate hydration corrects imbalances and reduces further emesis (Gan et al, 2014).*

▲ Administer appropriate antiemetics, according to emetic cause, by most effective route, considering the side effects of the medication, with attention to and coverage for the time frames in which the nausea is anticipated. EB: *Antiemetic medications are effective at different receptor sites and treat different causes of N&V. A combination of agents may be more effective than single agents (Jordan et al, 2014; Koth & Kolesar, 2017).*

- Consider nonpharmacological interventions such as acupressure, acupuncture, music therapy, distraction, and slow, deliberate movements. EB: *Nonpharmacological interventions can augment pharmacological interventions because they predominantly affect the higher cortical centers that trigger N&V. Nonpharmacological interventions are often low cost, relatively easy to use, and have few adverse events. The nonpharmacological interventions most likely to be effective include progressive muscle relaxation, hypnosis for anticipatory chemotherapy-induced N&V (CINV), and managing client expectations. Effectiveness has not been established for several other nonpharmacological interventions, primarily because of study limitations, lack of effect in small studies, and inconsistent results (Irwin & Johnson, 2014; Oncology Nursing Society, 2017).*

- Provide oral care after the client vomits. Oral care helps remove the taste and smell of vomitus, reducing the stimulus for further vomiting.

Nausea in Pregnancy

- Early recognition and conservative measures are recommended to successfully manage nausea in pregnancy, and to prevent progression to hyperemesis gravidarum. Dietary and lifestyle modifications should be implemented before pharmacological interventions. Avoidance of any aversive odors or foods is recommended. Eating multiple small meals per day is also recommended to have some food in the stomach at all times, avoiding hypoglycemia and gastric overdistention. Foods with higher protein (before bedtime) and carbohydrate and lower fat content are helpful (between meals and before getting out of bed early in the morning). Drinking smaller volumes of liquids at multiple times throughout the day is recommended. *These are traditional strategies for alleviating nausea during pregnancy, and there is limited evidence supporting the effectiveness of dietary changes on minimizing N&V with pregnancy symptoms (Clark, Dutta, & Hankins, 2014; Campbell et al, 2016; Argenbright, 2017).*

▲ Because of the high incidence of coexisting gastroesophageal reflux disease (GERD), it is important to assess and manage these symptoms of heartburn, belching, and indigestion. EB: *Dietary and lifestyle factors are recommended first, with the use of calcium or aluminum-containing antacids. H_2 receptor blockers or proton pump inhibitors (PPIs) may be needed if antacids have failed (Clark, Dutta, & Hankins, 2014).*

▲ It is well-established that *Helicobacter pylori* infection is associated with hyperemesis gravidarum. *It may also be recommended to test for* H. pylori *if there are persistent symptoms of nausea with pregnancy, prolonged symptoms of GERD, or a previous history of* H. pylori *infection.* H. pylori *is an independent risk factor for vomiting in pregnancy, and in women with daily vomiting, there is an association of adverse birth outcomes such as reduced birth weight (Clark, Dutta, & Hankins, 2014; Grooten et al, 2017).*

▲ Coexisting psychosocial factors may also influence the severity of N&V with pregnancy. Symptoms of anxiety and depression can occur in early pregnancy, especially when N&V is severe and can make the treatment of the N&V more challenging and even ineffective. *Timely diagnosis and treatment is recommended (Clark, Dutta, & Hankins, 2014).*

▲ The American College of Obstetricians and Gynecologists (ACOG) currently recommends converting the prenatal vitamin to folic acid only if nausea persists. Pharmacological options include a combination of oral pyridoxine hydrochloride (vitamin B_6, 10–25 mg) and doxylamine succinate (antihistamine 12.5 mg) to be used three to four times a day as first-line treatment for N&V of pregnancy after failure of pyridoxine

● = Independent;　▲ = Collaborative;　EBN = Evidence-Based Nursing;　EB = Evidence-Based

alone. This combination agent of pyridoxine and doxylamine (Diclegis) is the only US Food and Drug Administration pregnancy Category A approved therapy for N&V of pregnancy. There are, however, several pharmacological treatments outlined by the ACOG. *A stepwise, cost-effective strategy may be helpful in approaching N&V. Considerable N&V with associated dehydration may require intravenous antiemetics, hydration, and/or parenteral nutrition (Clark, Dutta, & Hankins, 2014; Campbell et al, 2016; ACOG, 2018).*

▲ Nonpharmacological interventions that are recommended include P6 acupressure with wrist bands and ginger capsules, 250 mg four times a day. EB: *These interventions have been shown to be safe and beneficial for the treatment of N&V with pregnancy (Campbell et al, 2016; ACOG, 2018). Mindfulness-based cognitive therapy may also be a helpful adjunct to pyridoxine therapy (Campbell et al, 2016).*

Nausea After Surgery

▲ Evaluate for risk factors for postoperative N&V (PONV). EB: *Strong evidence suggests that client-related risk factors such as female gender, age group (<50 years), history of PONV, history of motion sickness, nonsmoking behavior, and environmental risk factors such as postoperative opioid use, emetogenic surgery (type and duration), and volatile anesthetics may increase the risk for PONV. It is important to determine this risk in the preoperative period to better plan strategies to reduce baseline risk (Kovac, 2013; Gan et al, 2014; Smith & Ruth-Sahd, 2016). Childhood risk factors include surgery duration of more than 30 minutes, age older than 3 years, strabismus surgery, and a history of postoperative vomiting or a relative with PONV (Gan, 2014). PONV in children is twice as common as it is in adults, with the occurrence of 13% to 42% in all pediatric cases (Matthews, 2017).*

▲ Reduction of risk factors associated with PONV is beneficial for both adults and children. EB: *Avoidance of the use of general anesthesia by the use of regional anesthesia has been associated with a decreased incidence of PONV. The avoidance of both nitrous oxide and volatile anesthetics has also minimized PONV. Decreased and minimal use of intraoperative and postoperative opioids has demonstrated reduction in PONV. Adequate hydration is also an intervention to decrease the risk of PONV (Gan et al, 2014; Skolnik & Gan, 2014; Matthews, 2017).*

▲ Medicate the client prophylactically for nausea as ordered, throughout the period of risk. EB: *Antiemetic medications can reduce the incidence of PONV and use of combination treatment such as 5-HT3 antagonist plus dexamethasone is more effective than monotherapy. This recommendation is for clients at moderate or high risk for PONV. Other antiemetics, such as the neurokinin (NK-1) receptor antagonists, may have a role, particularly in preventing vomiting and severity 24 to 48 hours after surgery (Kovac, 2013; Gan et al, 2014). Antihistamines may be helpful in those with previous motion sickness or after ear surgery (Matthews, 2017).*

▲ Alleviate postoperative pain using ordered analgesic agents (refer to care plan for Acute **Pain**). *Pain is known to be a factor in the development of PONV (Bruderer et al, 2017).*

● Consider the use of nonpharmacological techniques, such as P6 acupoint stimulation, as an adjunct for controlling PONV, which has been shown to be effective in reducing PONV by 30%. Acupoint pressure is noninvasive, inexpensive, and has no side effects; thus it is part of a combined approach with antiemetic medication. EB: *Acupuncture and acustimulation have been studied with the most consistent results, similarly effective across methods of stimulation (acupuncture or acupressure or wristlike electrical stimulation) (Gan et al, 2014; Matthews, 2017).*

● Include client education on the management of PONV for all outpatients and discuss key assessment criteria (Odom-Forren et al, 2014).

Nausea After Chemotherapy

● Perform risk assessment before chemotherapy administration. Risk factors include female gender, younger age, history of low alcohol consumption, history of morning sickness during pregnancy, anxiety, previous history of chemotherapy, client expectancy of nausea, and emetic potential of the regimen. *It is important to recognize the many risk factors individual clients may have and tailor the antiemetic strategy accordingly. N&V continues to be among the most feared side effects of cancer treatment and can significantly affect quality of life and other complications. Poor control of N&V also has an economic impact, with increased costs related to increased emergency room visits, hospitalizations, and outpatient visits (Koth & Kolesar, 2017).*

▲ Initiate antiemetic strategy prophylactically or when N&V occurs in accordance with evidence-based guidelines. *Preventing N&V is important; one failure in antiemetic therapy can result in anticipatory nausea for the remainder of the client's treatments, and interventions are less likely to be effective (Tageja & Groninger, 2016).*

● = Independent; ▲ = Collaborative; EBN = Evidence-Based Nursing; EB = Evidence-Based

▲ Drug classes that are recommended for practice include the serotonin receptor antagonists, the NK-1 receptor antagonists, and cannabinoids. *Triple-drug regimens including serotonin receptor antagonists, NK-1 receptor antagonists, and dexamethasone are recommended for adults receiving highly emetogenic chemotherapy (Tageja & Groninger, 2016; Koth & Kolesar, 2017).*

▲ Consider the use of the following integrative therapies that are likely to be effective in reducing N&V: hypnosis with anticipatory N&V, and progressive muscle relaxation and guided imagery with antiemetics. **EB:** *There has been benefit associated with these interventions; however, further data are warranted (Irwin & Johnson, 2014; Oncology Nursing Society, 2017).*

● Consider managing client expectations about CINV. **EBN:** *Education and discussion are interventions that may minimize negative expectations. This intervention is based on the idea that if a patient expects to experience a problem, he or she is more likely to do so. If a patient believes that an intervention will be effective for symptoms, it is more likely to be effective (Irwin & Johnson, 2014; Oncology Nursing Society, 2017).*

Geriatric

● There are no specific guidelines that address the prophylaxis of CINV specifically in older adults. Risk still needs to be assessed, although many older clients are often treated with less emetic chemotherapy. Chemotherapy, however, can cause increased toxicity caused by age-related decreases in organ function, comorbidities, and drug–drug interactions secondary to polypharmacy. Additionally, adherence may be an issue because of cognitive decline, impaired senses, and economic issues. *Increased caution is warranted in this population because of increased safety concerns (Naeim et al, 2014).*

Pediatric

● Interventions for CINV should be implemented before and after chemotherapy. *Despite the extensive use of antiemetics, it is estimated that nausea occurs 40% to 70% in children treated for cancer (Hockenberry & Rodgers, 2015).*

● Relatively few systematic reviews exist examining the antiemetic medications used for CINV in children. It appears that 5-HT3 antagonists, with palonosetron preferred, combined with dexamethasone and aprepitant (in children 6 months of age or older) are recommended in children receiving highly emetogenic chemotherapy (Dupuis et al, 2017; Patel et al, 2017).

● Integrative therapies for control of nausea in children with cancer have not yet been studied as adequately as they have with adults. Some integrative therapies with potential include cognitive distraction, hypnosis, and acupressure (Momani & Berry, 2017).

Home Care

● Previously mentioned interventions may be adapted for home care use.

▲ In hospice care clients, N&V is common, and can considerably affect quality of life. Assessment is relevant in the management of N&V, and should include history, physical exam, and evaluation of reversible causes. *There can be multiple causes of nausea in clients with advanced cancer, and the causes may be treatment related, or nontreatment related. The causes may be obstructive; examples include increased ICP and bowel obstruction. Metabolic causes may be related to hypercalcemia, hyponatremia, or opioids (Walsh et al, 2017).* **EBN:** *Nausea can effectively be controlled if a cause can be identified. An N&V protocol (e.g., Horvitz Center for Palliative Medicine N&V Protocol) can be used to identify and resolve any reversible causes of nausea, such as metabolic abnormalities or medications (Gupta et al, 2013). If none are found and symptoms persist, a flat-plate radiograph of the abdomen is done to evaluate for obstruction or constipation. Appropriate medications can then be used to treat central nervous system causes and obstructive or nonobstructive causes (Gordon, LeGrand, & Walsh, 2014).*

● Assist the client and family with identifying and avoiding irritants in the home that exacerbate nausea (e.g., strong odors from food, plants, perfume, and room deodorizers). All medications except antiemetics should be given after meals to minimize the risk of nausea. **EB:** *Nausea triggered by odors is related to altered chemoreceptors and pathology (Tipton, 2014).*

Client/Family Teaching and Discharge Planning

● Teach the client techniques to use before and after chemotherapy, including antiemetics/medication management schedules and dietary approaches, such as eating smaller meals, avoiding spicy and fatty foods, and avoiding an empty stomach before chemotherapy (Irwin & Johnson, 2014).

● = Independent;   ▲ = Collaborative;   **EBN** = Evidence-Based Nursing;   **EB** = Evidence-Based

REFERENCES

American College of Obstetricians and Gynecologists. (2018). Clinical management guidelines for obstetrician-gynecologists: Nausea and vomiting of pregnancy. *ACOG Practice Bulletin, 131*(1), 190–193.

Argenbright, C. A. (2017). Complementary approaches to pregnancy induced nausea and vomiting. *International Journal of Childbirth Education, 32*(1), 6–9.

Bruderer, U., Fisler, A., Steurer, P., et al. (2017). Post-discharge nausea and vomiting after total intravenous anaesthesia and standardized PONV prophylaxis for ambulatory surgery. *Acta Anaesthesiologica Scandinavica, 61*, 758–766.

Campbell, K., Rowe, H., Azzam, H., et al. (2016). The management of nausea and vomiting of pregnancy. *Journal of Obstetrics and Gynaecology of Canada, 339*, 1127–1137.

Clark, S. M., Dutta, E., & Hankins, G. D. (2014). The outpatient management and special considerations of nausea and vomiting in pregnancy. *Seminars in Perinatology, 38*(8), 496–502. Retrieved from http://dx.doi.org/10.1053/j.semperi.2014.08.014.

Dupuis, L. L., Sung, L., Molassiotis, A., et al. (2017). 2016 updated MASCC/ESMO consensus recommendations: Prevention of acute chemotherapy-induced nausea and vomiting in children. *Supportive Care in Cancer, 25*, 323–331.

Gan, T. J., Diemunsch, P., Habib, A. S., et al. (2014). Consensus guidelines for the management of postoperative nausea and vomiting. *Anesthesia & Analgesia, 118*(1), 85–113.

Goel, R., & Wilkinson, M. (2013). Recommended assessment and treatment of nausea and vomiting. *Prescriber, 5*, 23–27.

Gordon, P., LeGrand, S. B., & Walsh, D. (2014). Nausea and vomiting in advanced cancer. *European Journal of Pharmacology, 722*, 187–191.

Grooten, I. J., Den Hollander, W. J., Roseboom, T. J., et al. (2017). *Helicobacter pylori* infection: A predictor of vomiting severity in pregnancy and adverse birth outcome. *American Journal of Obstetrics & Gynecology, 216*, 512e1–512e9.

Gupta, M., Davis, M., LeGrand, S., et al. (2013). Nausea and vomiting in advanced cancer: The Cleveland Clinic protocol. *The Journal of Supportive Oncology, 11*(1), 8–13.

Hockenberry, M. J., & Rodgers, C. C. (2015). Nausea, vomiting, anorexia, and fatigue. In L. S. Wiener, M. Pao, A. E. Kazak, et al. (Eds.), *Pediatric psycho-oncology: A quick reference on psychosocial dimensions of cancer symptom management* (pp. 79–104). New York: Oxford University Press.

Irwin, M., & Johnson, L. A. (2014). *Putting evidence into practice: A pocket guide to cancer symptom management*. Pittsburgh: Oncology Nursing Society.

Jordan, K., Gralla, R., Jahn, F., et al. (2014). International antiemetic guidelines on chemotherapy induced nausea and vomiting (CINV): Content and implementation in daily routine practice. *European Journal of Pharmacology, 722*, 197–202.

Kamen, C., Tejani, M., Chandwani, K., et al. (2014). Anticipatory nausea and vomiting due to chemotherapy. *European Journal of Pharmacology, 722*, 172–179.

Koth, S. M., & Kolesar, J. (2017). New options and controversies in the management of chemotherapy-induced nausea and vomiting. *American Journal of Health-System Pharmacists, 74*, 812–819.

Kovac, A. L. (2013). Update on the management of postoperative nausea and vomiting. *Drugs, 73*, 1525–1547.

Matthews, C. (2017). A review of nausea and vomiting in the anaesthetic and post anaesthetic environment. *Journal of Perioperative Practice, 27*(10), 224–227.

Momani, T. G., & Berry, D. L. (2017). Integrative therapeutic approaches for the management and control of nausea in children undergoing cancer treatment: A systematic review. *Journal of Pediatric Oncology Nursing, 34*(3), 173–184.

Naeim, A., Aapro, M., Subbarao, R., et al. (2014). Supportive care considerations for older adults with cancer. *Journal of Clinical Oncology, 32*(24), 2627–2632.

Odom-Forren, J., Hooper, V., Moser, D. K., et al. (2014). Postdischarge nausea and vomiting: management strategies and outcomes over 7 days. *Journal of Perianesthesia Nursing, 29*(4), 275–284.

Oncology Nursing Society. (2017). *Putting evidence into practice for chemotherapy-induced nausea and vomiting—Adult*. Retrieved from https://www.ons.org/practice-resources/pep/chemotherapy-induced-nausea-and-vomiting/chemotherapy-induced-nausea-and. (Accessed 21 January 2018).

Patel, P., Robinson, P. D., Thackray, J., et al. (2017). Guideline for the prevention of acute chemotherapy-induced nausea and vomiting in pediatric cancer patients: A focused update. *Pediatric Blood & Cancer, 64*, e26542. Retrieved from https://doi.org/10.1002/pbc.26542.

Skolnik, A., & Gan, T. J. (2014). Update on the management of postoperative nausea and vomiting. *Current Opinion in Anaesthesiology, 27*(6), 605–609.

Smith, C. A., & Ruth-Sahd, L. (2016). Reducing the incidence of postoperative nausea and vomiting begins with risk screening: An evaluation of the evidence. *Journal of Perianesthesia Nursing, 31*(2), 158–171.

Tageja, N., & Groninger, H. (2016). Chemotherapy-induced nausea and vomiting: An overview and comparison of three consensus guidelines. *Postgraduate Medicine, 92*, 34–40.

Tipton, J. M. (2014). Nausea and vomiting. In C. H. Yarbro, D. Wujcik, & B. H. Gobel (Eds.), *Cancer symptom management* (pp. 213–233). Burlington, MA: Jones & Bartlett.

Walsh, D., Davis, M., Ripamonti, C., et al. (2017). 2016 Updated MASCC/ESMO consensus recommendations: Management of nausea and vomiting in advanced cancer. *Supportive Care in Cancer, 25*, 333–340.

Neonatal Abstinence syndrome   *Patricia Hindin, PhD, CNM*

NANDA-I

Definition

A constellation of withdrawal symptoms observed in newborns as a result of in-utero exposure to addicting substances, or as a consequence of postnatal pharmacological pain management.

● = Independent;   ▲ = Collaborative;   EBN = Evidence-Based Nursing;   EB = Evidence-Based

Defining Characteristics

Diarrhea (00013); disorganized infant behavior (00116); disturbed sleep pattern (00198); impaired comfort (00214); ineffective feeding pattern (00107); neurobehavioral stress; risk for aspiration (00039); risk for imbalanced body temperature (00005); risk for impaired attachment (00058); risk for impaired skin integrity (00047); risk for injury (00035)

Related Factors

To be developed

At-Risk Population

Iatrogenic substance exposure for pain control following a critical illness or surgery; in utero substance exposure secondary to material substance use

NOC   Outcomes (Nursing Outcomes Classification)

Suggested NOC Outcomes

Comfort Status: Physical; Breastfeeding Establishment: Infant; Bottle Feeding Establishment: Infant; Parent-Infant Attachment; Stress Level; Sleep; Thermoregulation: Newborn; Tissue Integrity: Skin and Mucous Membranes; Newborn Adaptation; Risk Control; Bowel Elimination; Risk Control: Aspiration

---

Example NOC Outcome with Indicators

Parent-Infant Attachment as evidenced by the following indicators: Holds infant close/Uses eye contact/Infant looks at parent/Consoles infant/Responds to infant cues. (Rate the outcome and indicators of **Parent-Infant Attachment:** 1 = never demonstrated, 2 = rarely demonstrated, 3 = sometimes demonstrated, 4 = often demonstrated, 5 = consistently demonstrated range [see Section I].)

N

Client Outcomes

Client Will (Specify Time Frame)

- Tolerate small frequent formula feedings or frequent breast feedings
- Maintain weight and readjust feedings frequency as necessary for appropriate growth
- Provide calorie-dense formula, which is appropriate for weight gain
- Maintain proper hydration with elastic skin turgor and moist mucus membranes
- Maintain adequate nutrition which will promote adequate growth
- Preserve skin integrity in perianal area

NIC   Intervention (Nursing Interventions Classification)

Suggested NIC Interventions

Diarrhea Management; Bottle Feeding; Infant Care: Newborn; Developmental Enhancement: Infant; Feeding

---

Example NIC Activities—Diarrhea Management

Monitor for signs and symptoms of diarrhea; Observe skin turgor regularly; Monitor skin in perianal area for irritation and ulceration, weigh patient regularly

---

Nursing Interventions and *Rationales*

- Provide supportive nonpharmacological care with formula feeding as prescribed. EBN: *A randomized controlled trial (N = 49) assessed the early initiation of feeding infants with a high-calorie formula compared with feeding with standard-calorie formula. The authors concluded that high-calorie feeding might be advantageous for weight gain (Bogen et al, 2018).*
- Encourage breastfeeding for nutrition and nonpharmacological supportive care. EB: *A retrospective cohort study of neonatal abstinence syndrome (NAS) neonates (N = 3725) indicated that there is an association between breastfeeding and a 9.4% decrease in length of stay when compared with nonbreastfed neonates*

● = Independent;   ▲ = Collaborative;   EBN = Evidence-Based Nursing;   EB = Evidence-Based

(Short, Gannon, & Abatemarco, 2016). **EB:** *Breastfeeding may decrease the incidence of NAS and the need for pharmacological treatment while reducing the hospital length of stay (Kocherlakota, 2014).*

- Use nursing skills to provide supportive nonpharmacological care. **EBN:** *An ethnographic study described the culture of care provided by 12 full-time registered nurses to infants with NAS in an intensive care unit (ICU). The six themes point to the direction for the culture of care practice: learn the baby, team relationships, role satisfaction, grief, making a difference, and educate and care for the mother (Nelson, 2016).*

- Use vibrotactile stimulation (VS) as a nonpharmacological supportive care option. **EB:** *A prospective study was conducted on 26 opioid-exposed newborns to determine whether exposure to a specially constructed mattress that delivered a dose of stochastic (randomly determined) VS would affect symptoms. The results indicated a 35% reduction in movement with a significant increase in normal breathing and heart rate (Zuzarte et al, 2017).*

- Practice supportive nursing interventions with an understanding of the levels of evidence. **EB:** *Ryan et al (2018) reviewed research papers on NAS from the years 2000 and 2017. The author's goal was to substantiate the efficacy of supportive interventions for the treatment of NAS. The authors determined that level I to III evidence (experimental studies) exists for breastfeeding, swaddling, rooming-in, skin to skin, and environmental control for NAS infants.* **EBN:** *A systematic review performed by MacMullen, Dulski, and Blobaum (2014) evaluated supportive nursing care with NAS infants. The authors found level IV evidence (expert opinion, case reports, and descriptive studies) for interventions such as swaddling, gentle awaking, quiet environment, and nonnutritive sucking.*

- Provide pharmacological treatment as indicated for symptoms. **EB:** *A double-blind, randomized control trial assigned term infants who had been exposed to opioids in utero to either a sublingual buprenorphine treatment group or an oral morphine treatment group. The authors noted that the infants treated with sublingual buprenorphine experienced a shorter duration of treatment (15 days versus 28 days) and a shorter length of hospital stay (21 days versus 33 days) (Kraft et al, 2017).* **EB:** *Streetz, Gildon, and Thompson (2016) engaged in a systematic review of clonidine as treatment for NAS. There is limited evidence that clonidine as a single therapy or in combination with other therapies can be effective with limited adverse reactions and a shorter treatment time.*

- Use of nonpharmacological and complementary therapy to comfort infants and provide relief of symptoms. **EB:** *A prospective, cohort, pilot study was conducted with a sample of infants who were given a one-dose, 30-minute Reiki massage session. The authors found the treatment to be safe for the infants and acceptable to the mothers (Radziewicz et al, 2018).*

- Use of rooming-in and promotion of maternal–infant bonding for mother–infant dyad. **EB:** *A systematic review and meta-analysis were conducted on 549 infants with NAS. MacMillan et al (2018) concluded that rooming-in was associated with a reduction in pharmacological treatment and earlier discharge when compared with infants treated in the ICU.* **EB:** *Schiff et al (2017) performed a retrospective, single cohort study with 86 mother–infant dyads. Infants with NAS were treated with pharmacological modalities and the rooming-in model of care. The presence of the parents was associated with decreased NAS scores and reduction in opioid treatment days.* **EB:** *Boucher (2017) reviewed eight studies on the rooming-in model of care and the use of acupuncture for NAS infants. The author established that the rooming-in model might decrease use of opioids and length of stay, and that acupuncture is safe for infants.*

- Provide compassionate care, free of judgement to substance-abusing mothers. **EBN:** *A qualitative study was conducted with 15 mothers with substance abuse disorders. The judgmental attitudes and behaviors of health care professionals served to retraumatize them during their hospitalization. The importance of nursing care with the empathic approach is essential in the care of these women (Cleveland, Bonugli, & McGlothen, 2016).* **EBN:** *The use of a structured communication tool based on the organization of the concepts of knowledge creates circumstances for reflection, teaching, and support (ACTS) script. The ACTS was an implementation to assist neonatal ICU (NICU) nurses in developing positive strategies to change negative attitudes among their peer toward substance-abusing mothers (Marcellus & Poag, 2016).*

Pediatric

- When available consider professional, supportive programs for infants with a history of NAS. **EB:** *Beckwith and Burke (2015) followed the development of 28 infants exposed to prenatal drugs over a 3-year period and determined the exposed infants have a limitation in language and cognition.*

Multicultural

- Specific rural areas are high risk for NAS. **EB:** *Brown, Goodin, and Talbert (2018) reviewed data in Kentucky and determined that rural Appalachian counties in Kentucky experienced NAS rate per 1000 births that are*

● = Independent; ▲ = Collaborative; **EBN** = Evidence-Based Nursing; **EB** = Evidence-Based

2 to 2.5 times greater than urban and non-Appalachian counties in the state. EB: The authors evaluated NAS admissions from the Uniform Billing data form the West Virginia Health Care Authority. They found the NAS rate in rural West Virginia increased from 7.74 to 31.5 per live births per year, indicating an increased need for services for this growing health problem (Stabler et al, 2017).

Home Care

- Consider alternative models of care for treatment for infants with NAS. **EB:** *Smirk et al (2014) reviewed the treatment of 118 infants with NAS. Thirty-eight infants were managed at home and compared with the rest of the infant population treated in the hospital. The authors found home-based detoxification care reduced length of hospital stay and increased breastfeeding.* **EB:** *Seventy-five patients were weaned from methadone in the hospital, and 46 were treated as outpatients. The combined in-hospital and outpatient management of methadone treatment decreased length of hospital stay and reduced cost. There was more breastfeeding (24 versus 8% P < .05) in the combined group (Backes et al, 2012).* **EP:** *Belcher et al (2005) reported on three community programs implemented in Baltimore to provide services to substance-abusing mothers and their infants. The Early Transition Center provided 24-hour on-call services for newly discharged mother and infant dyads. The Home-U-Go-Safely program used community nurses to provide supportive care, health monitoring of the infant, and education to mothers.*

REFERENCES

Backes, C. H., Backes, C. R., Gardner, D., et al. (2012). Neonatal abstinence syndrome: Transitioning methadone-treated infants from an inpatient to an outpatient setting. *Journal of Perinatology*, 32(6), 425–430. doi:10.1038/jp.2011.114.

Beckwith, A. M., & Burke, S. A. (2015). Identification of early developmental deficit in infants with prenatal heroin, methadone, and other opioid exposure. *Clinical Pediatrics*, 54(4), 328–335. doi:10.1177/0009922814549545.

Belcher, H. E., Butz, A. M., Wallace, P., et al. (2005). Spectrum of early intervention services for children with intrauterine drug exposure. *Infants & Young Children*, 18(1), 2–15.

Bogen, D. L., et al. (2018). Randomized clinical trial of standard- versus high-calorie formula for methadone-exposed infants: A feasibility study. *Hospital Pediatrics*, 8(1), 7–14. doi:10.1542/hpeds.2017-0114.

Boucher, A. M. (2017). Nonopioid management of neonatal abstinence syndrome. *Advanced Neonatal Care*, 17(2), 84–90. doi:10.1097/anc.0000000000000371.

Brown, J. D., Goodin, A. J., & Talbert, J. C. (2018). Rural and Appalachian disparities in neonatal abstinence syndrome incidence and access to opioid abuse treatment. *Journal of Rural Health*, 34(1), 6–13.

Cleveland, L. M., Bonugli, R. J., & McGlothen, K. S. (2016). The mothering experiences of women with substance use disorders. *Advances in Nursing Science*, 39(2), 119–129. doi:10.1097/ANS.0000000000000118.

Kocherlakota, P. (2014). Neonatal abstinence syndrome. *Pediatrics*, 134, e547–e561. doi:10.1542/peds.2013-3524.

Kraft, W. K., Adeniyi-Jones, S. C., Chervoneva, I., et al. (2017). Buprenorphine for the treatment of the neonatal abstinence syndrome. *The New England Journal of Medicine*, 376(24), 2341–2348. doi:10.1056/NEJMoa1614835.

Marcellus, L., & Poag, E. (2016). Adding to our practice toolkit: Using the ACTS script to address stigmatizing peer behaviors in the context of maternal substance use. *Neonatal Network*, 35(5), 327–331. doi:10.1891/0730-0832.35.5.327.

MacMullen, N. J., Dulski, L. A., & Blobaum, P. (2014). Evidenced-based interventions for neonatal abstinence syndrome. *Pediatric Nursing*, 40(4), 165–172.

McMillan, K. D., Rendon, C. P., Verma, K., et al. (2018). Association of rooming-in with outcomes for neonatal abstinence syndrome: A systematic review and meta-analysis. *JAMA Pediatrics*. doi:10.1001/jamapediatrics.2017.5195.

Nelson, M. M. (2016). NICU culture of care for infants with neonatal abstinence syndrome: A focused ethnography. *Neonatal Network*, 35(5), 287–296. doi:10.1891/0730-0832.35.5.287.

Radziewicz, R. M., Wright-Esber, S., Zupancic, J., et al. (2018). Safety of Reiki therapy for newborns at risk for neonatal abstinence syndrome. *Holistic Nursing Practice*, 32(2), 63–70. doi:10.1097/HNP.0000000000000251.

Ryan, G., Dooley, J., Finn, G., et al. (2018). Nonpharmacological management of neonatal abstinence syndrome: A review of the literature. *Journal of Maternal and Fetal Neonatal Medicine*, 8, 1–6. doi:10.1080/14767058.2017.1414180.

Schiff, D. M., Penwill, N., Si, W., et al. (2017). Impact of parental presence at infants' bedside on neonatal abstinence syndrome. *Hospital Pediatrics*, 7(2), 63–69. doi:10.1542/hpeds.2016-0147.

Short, V. L., Gannon, M., & Abatemarco, D. J. (2016). The association between breastfeeding and length of stay among infants diagnosed with neonatal abstinence syndrome: A population-based study of in-hospital births. *Breastfeeding Medicine*, 11, 343–349. doi:10.1089/bfm.2016.0084.

Smirk, C. L., Bowman, E., Doyle, L. W., et al. (2014). Home-based detoxification for neonatal abstinence syndrome reduces length of hospital admission without prolonged treatment. *Acta Paediatrica*, 103(6), 601–604. doi:10.1111/apa.12603.

Stabler, M. E., Long, D., Chetok, I. R., et al. (2017). Neonatal abstinence syndrome in West Virginia substate regions, 2007–2013. *Journal of Rural Health*, 33(1), 92–101.

Streetz, V. N., Gildon, B. L., & Thompson, D. F. (2016). Role of clonidine in neonatal abstinence syndrome: A systematic review. *The Annals of Pharmacotherapy*, 50(4), 301–310. doi:10.1177/1060028015626438.

Zuzarte, I., Indic, P., Barton, B., et al. (2017). Vibrotactile stimulation: A non-pharmacological intervention for opioid-exposed newborns. *PLoS ONE*, 12(4), e0175981. doi:10.1371/journal.pone.0175981.

N

● = Independent; ▲ = Collaborative; **EBN** = Evidence-Based Nursing; **EB** = Evidence-Based

Readiness for enhanced Nutrition   *Marina Martinez-Kratz, MS, RN, CNE*

NANDA-I

Definition

A pattern of nutrient intake, which can be strengthened.

Defining Characteristics

Expresses desire to enhance nutrition

NOC   (Nursing Outcomes Classification)

Suggested NOC Outcomes

Nutritional Status; Nutritional Status: Food and Fluid Intake; Nutrient Intake; Weight Control

Example NOC Outcome with Indicators
Nutritional Status as evidenced by the following indicators: Food and fluid intake/Hydration/Body mass index/Weight-height ratio/Hematocrit. (Rate the outcome and indicators of **Nutritional Status:** I = severe deviation from normal range, 2 = substantial deviation from normal range, 3 = moderate deviation from normal range, 4 = mild deviation from normal range, 5 = no deviation from normal range [see Section I].)

Client Outcomes

Client Will (Specify Time Frame)

- Explain how to eat according to the US Dietary Guidelines
- Design dietary modifications to meet individual long-term goal of health, using principles of variety, balance, and moderation
- Maintain weight within normal range for height and age

NIC   (Nursing Interventions Classification)

Suggested NIC Interventions

Nutrition Management; Nutritional Counseling; Weight Reduction Assistance

Example NIC Activities—Nutrition Management
Determine the client's motivation for changing eating habits; Develop with the client a method to keep a daily record of intake

Nursing Interventions and *Rationales*

- Assess the meaning and importance of food in the client's life. EB: *Recent research found strong associations between the different domains of food meanings and behavioral outcomes (Arbit et al, 2017).*
- Assess client readiness to determine whether he or she is ready to discuss enhanced nutrition and/or would like nutrition information. EB: *Client motivation is a key component of success in a weight loss program and a prerequisite for weight loss therapy (Raynor & Champagne, 2016).*
- Use a motivational interviewing technique when working with clients to promote healthy eating and improved nutrition. EB: *Research shows significant weight loss for clients when motivational interviewing techniques were used (Barnes et al, 2018).*
- Counsel the client to measure regularly consumed foods periodically. Help the client learn usual portion sizes. Measuring food alerts the client to normal portion sizes. Estimating amounts can be extremely inaccurate. EB: *A randomized controlled trial of 278 overweight and obese participants was conducted to increase portion size awareness with results that demonstrated that the intervention improved portion control behavior and in turn influenced body mass index (BMI) (Poelman et al, 2015).*
- Assist the client to develop a system of self-management, which may include self-monitoring of weight and BMI; realistic goal setting, planning, and action planning for improved dietary intake and physical

• = Independent;   ▲ = Collaborative;   EBN = Evidence-Based Nursing;   EB = Evidence-Based

activity; problem-solving; and tracking dietary intake and exercise. EB: *A key component of successful weight loss and maintenance is regular self-monitoring (Thomason et al, 2016).*

- Document the client's height and weight and teach the significance of his or her BMI in relation to current nutritional health. Use a chart or a website such as http://www.cdc.gov/healthyweight/assessing/bmi/index.html (Centers for Disease Control and Prevention [CDC], 2015). EB: *Successful enhancement of nutrition in adults requires adoption and maintenance of effective self-monitoring (Raynor & Champagne, 2016).*
- Encourage the client to engage in vigorous-intensity physical activity for at least 150 minutes weekly or moderate-intensity physical activity for at least 300 minutes weekly. EB: *Research evidence suggests that regular physical activity is critical for weight maintenance (Ostendorf et al, 2018).*
- Recommend that the client avoids eating in fast-food restaurants. CEB: *A 15-year study demonstrated that people who frequently eat fast foods gain an average of 10 pounds more than those who eat fast food less often, and were two times more likely to develop insulin resistance, which can lead to diabetes (Pereira et al, 2005).*
- Assist the client to reframe slips in nutrition or physical activity behavior as lapses that are a single event and not a full return to previous unhealthy behaviors. Relapse prevention strategies include managing lapses in healthy behavior, identifying high-risk situations for relapses, self-monitoring, providing social support, enhancing skills for coping, and increasing self-efficacy for avoiding relapse. EB: *A study of a weight maintenance intervention, delivered primarily by telephone, modestly slowed the rate of weight regain (Voils et al, 2017).*
- Assist clients to engage their social support systems either digitally or face to face in ways that facilitate healthy eating and physical activity behavior change. EB: *Significant others, family, friends, and coworkers can facilitate or hinder weight loss success (Romo, 2018).*
- Assist the client to implement informal and formal mindfulness-based interventions (MBIs). Informal MBIs include mindful eating, increasing awareness of hunger and satiety cues, taste satisfaction, and decreasing impulsive tendencies to overeat when experiencing negative emotions. Meditation practice is a formal MBI. EB: *Results of a research review suggest that a combination of formal and informal MBIs are effective in reducing weight and improving obesity-related eating behaviors among individuals with overweight and obesity (Carrière et al, 2018).*
- Assist the client to develop stimulus control techniques designed to reduce environmental cues associated with eating behaviors. Specifically clients should be taught to limit the presence of high-calorie/high-fat foods in the home; to reduce the visibility of unhealthy food choices in the home; to limit where and when they eat; to avoid distractions like reading, using the computer, or watching television when eating; and to eat more slowly. EB: *Stimulus control strategies are the keys to healthy eating (Butryn et al, 2017).*
- Encourage 7.5 to 8.5 hours of sleep nightly. EB: *Recent evidence suggests weight management is hindered when attempted in the context of sleep restriction because there is an upregulation of reward, pleasure, and salience networks in response to food stimuli (St-Onge, 2017).*
- Recommend that clients use dietary supplements such as vitamins and minerals after consulting with their primary health care provider. EB: *Research shows micronutrient deficits are prevalent in weight-loss plans, especially vitamin B_{12}, calcium, and vitamin D (Engel et al, 2018).*
- Incorporate the following recommendations from the Academy of Nutrition and Dietetics: Interventions for the Treatment of Overweight and Obesity in Adults (Raynor & Champagne, 2016):
  - Assess food and nutrition-related history; anthropometric measures; biochemical data, medical tests, and procedures; nutrition-focused physical findings; and client history.
  - Assess the energy intake and nutrient content of the diet.
  - Use height and weight to calculate BMI, and waist circumference to determine risk of cardiovascular disease (CVD), type 2 diabetes, and all-cause mortality.
  - Use a measured resting metabolic rate (RMR) to determine energy needs.
  - Set a realistic weight-loss goal, such as one of the following: up to 2 pounds/week, up to 10% of baseline body weight, or a total of 3% to 5% of baseline weight if cardiovascular risk factors (hypertension, hyperlipidemia, and hyperglycemia) are present.
  - To achieve weight loss, use an individualized diet, including patient preferences and health status, to achieve and maintain nutrient adequacy and reduce caloric intake, based on one of the following caloric reduction strategies: 1200 to 1500 kcal/day for women and 1500 to 1800 kcal/day for men, with an energy deficit of approximately 500 kcal/day or 750 kcal/day.

• = Independent;   ▲ = Collaborative;   EBN = Evidence-Based Nursing;   EB = Evidence-Based

Pediatric

- Offer obese or overweight adolescents healthy methods for weight loss. EB: *A recent study showed statistically significant health behavior improvements after implementing a developmentally informed intervention to increase positive health diet and exercise behaviors (Issner et al, 2017).*
- Offer families of obese or overweight children prejudice-free, individually accepting, and supportive interventions to address weight loss. EBN: *Obese children treated with motivational interviewing showed significant improvement in their weight-related behavior and obesity-related anthropometric measures (Wong & Cheng, 2013).*
- Recommend that families eat together for at least one meal per day. EB: *Findings from a review provide clear evidence that family meals (among youth) and shared meals (among adults) are associated with better dietary intake and that these findings transcend the life span (Fulkerson et al, 2014).*
- Recommend involving the family in planning meals and food preparation. Children can learn about nutrition as they help plan and make meals. EB: *The Healthy Home Offerings via the Mealtime Environment Plus program showed increased cooking skills among the children participating (Fulkerson et al, 2018).*
- Assist parents at being good role models of healthy eating. EB: *The Healthy Home Offerings via the Mealtime Environment Plus program showed significantly improved parental self-efficacy for identifying appropriate portion sizes (Fulkerson et al, 2018).*
- Recommend that the family try new foods, either a new food or recipe every week. EB: *The Healthy Home Offerings via the Mealtime Environment Plus program showed decreasing child neophobia scores over time that were developmentally appropriate (Fulkerson et al, 2018).*

Geriatric

- Determine the risks and benefits of weight loss in the older client. A BMI greater than 30 in the older client suggests a moderate weight loss approach. EB: *Recommendations for treating obesity in the elderly include ensuring a balanced and appropriately distributed intake of high-quality nutrients, particularly of high-quality protein (i.e., 1.2 to 1.5 g/kg of body weight), limiting the intake of simple carbohydrates and saturated fats, and providing sufficient intake of calcium and vitamin D_3 (Blaz, 2016).*
- Observe for social, psychological, and economic factors that influence diet quality. EB: *An exploratory study of diet quality influences in community-dwelling older individuals revealed the following influences: food experiences, retirement, bereavement, medical conditions, food environment, food-related habits, social engagement, personal/psychological factors, and transportation (Bloom et al, 2017).*

Multicultural

- Tailor nutritional interventions to be consistent with cultural beliefs, norms, and values. EB: *A systemic review of culturally tailored interventions for Hispanic women included literacy modification, Hispanic foods/ recipes, cultural diabetes beliefs, family/friend participation, structured community input, and innovative experiential learning (McCurley et al, 2016).*
- Offer tailored lifestyle counseling via the telephone. EBN: *Investigators have included biweekly and/or monthly health coach calls for African American participants with significant weight gain prevention (Goode et al, 2017).*
- Integrate weight loss and weight maintenance interventions with church faith-based concepts for cultural congruence with African American clients. EB: *Recent research suggested that integrating faith themes into a weight loss maintenance program may increase its long-term effect on participants' health behavior change (Seale et al, 2013).*

Client/Family Teaching and Discharge Planning

- The majority of the preceding interventions involve teaching.
- Work with the family members regarding information on how to support and promote enhanced nutritional choices and healthy intakes.

REFERENCES

Arbit, N., et al. (2017). Development and validation of the meaning of food in life questionnaire (MFLQ): Evidence for a new construct to explain eating behavior. *Food Quality and Preference, 59,* 35–45. doi:10.1016/j.foodqual.2017.02.002.

Barnes, R. D., et al. (2018). Examining motivational interviewing plus nutrition psychoeducation for weight loss in primary care. *Journal of Psychosomatic Research, 104,* 101–107. doi:10.1016/j.jpsychores .2017.11.013.

● = Independent;   ▲ = Collaborative;   EBN = Evidence-Based Nursing;   EB = Evidence-Based

Blaz, M. K. (2016). Obesity in the elderly, weight loss yes or no? *Clinical Nutrition ESPEN, 14*, 56. doi:10.1016/j.clnesp.2016.04.025.

Bloom, I., et al. (2017). What influences diet quality in older people? A qualitative study among community-dwelling older adults from the Hertfordshire Cohort Study, UK. *Public Health Nutrition, 20*(15), 2685–2693. doi:10.1017/S1368980017001203.

Butryn, M. L., et al. (2017). Efficacy of environmental and acceptance-based enhancements to behavioral weight loss treatment: The ENACT trial. *Obesity, 25*(5), 866–872. doi:10.1002/oby.21813.

Carrière, K., et al. (2018). Mindfulness-based interventions for weight loss: A systematic review and meta-analysis. *Obesity Reviews, 19*(2), 164–177. doi:10.1111/obr.12623.

Centers for Disease Control and Prevention. (2015). *Healthy weight—It's not a diet, it's a lifestyle!* Retrieved from http://www.cdc.gov/healthyweight/assessing/bmi/index.html. (Accessed 25 March 2018).

Engel, M. G., et al. (2018). Micronutrient gaps in three commercial weight-loss diet plans. *Nutrients, 10*(1), 108. doi:10.3390/nu10010108.

Fulkerson, J. A., et al. (2018). Family home food environment and nutrition-related parent and child personal and behavioral outcomes of the Healthy Home Offerings via the Mealtime Environment (HOME) Plus program: A randomized controlled trial. *Journal of the Academy of Nutrition and Dietetics, 118*(2), 240–251. doi:10.1016/j.jand.2017.04.006.

Fulkerson, J. A., et al. (2014). A review of associations between family or shared meal frequency and dietary and weight status outcomes across the lifespan. *Journal of Nutrition Education and Behavior, 46*(1), 2–19. doi:10.1016/j.jneb.2013.07.012.

Goode, R. W., et al. (2017). African Americans in standard behavioral treatment for obesity, 2001–2015: What have we learned? *Western Journal of Nursing Research, 39*(8), 1045–1069. doi:10.1177/0193945917692115.

Issner, J. H., et al. (2017). Increasing positive health behaviors in adolescents with nutritional goals and exercise. *Journal of Child and Family Studies, 26*(2), 548–558. doi:10.1007/s10826-016-0585-4.

McCurley, J. L., et al. (2016). Diabetes prevention in U.S. Hispanic adults: A systematic review of culturally tailored interventions.

American Journal of Preventive Medicine, 52(4), 519–529. doi:10.1016/j.amepre.2016.10.028.

Ostendorf, D. M., et al. (2018). Objectively measured physical activity and sedentary behavior in successful weight loss maintainers. *Obesity, 26*(1), 53–60. doi:10.1002/oby.22052.

Pereira, M., et al. (2005). Fast-food habits, weight gain, and insulin resistance (the CARDIA study): 15-Year prospective analysis. *Lancet, 365*(9453), 36–42.

Poelman, M. P., et al. (2015). PortionControl@HOME: Results of a randomized controlled trial evaluating the effect of a multi-component portion size intervention on portion control behavior and body mass index. *Annals of Behavioral Medicine, 49*(1), 18–28. doi:10.1007/s12160-014-9637-4.

Raynor, H. A., & Champagne, C. M. (2016). Position of the Academy of Nutrition and Dietetics: Interventions for the treatment of overweight and obesity in adults. *Journal of the Academy of Nutrition and Dietetics, 116*(1), 129–147.

Romo, L. K. (2018). An examination of how people who have lost weight communicatively negotiate interpersonal challenges to weight management, health communication. *Health Communication, 33*(4), 469–477. doi:10.1080/10410236.2016.1278497.

Seale, J. P., Fifield, J., Davis-Smith, Y. M., et al. (2013). Developing culturally congruent weight maintenance programs for African American church members. *Ethnicity & Health, 18*(2), 152–167.

St-Onge, M. P. (2017). Sleep-obesity relation: Underlying mechanisms and consequences for treatment. *Obesity Reviews, 18*(S1), 34–39. doi:10.1111/obr.12499.

Thomason, D. L., et al. (2016). A systematic review of adolescent self-management and weight loss. *Journal of Pediatric Health Care, 30*(6), 569–582. doi:10.1016/j.pedhc.2015.11.016.

Voils, C. I., et al. (2017). Maintenance of weight loss after initiation of nutrition training: A randomized trial. *Annals of Internal Medicine, 166*(7), 463–471. doi:10.7326/M16-2160.

Wong, E. M., & Cheng, M. M. (2013). Effects of motivational interviewing to promote weight loss in obese children. *Journal of Clinical Nursing, 22*(17/18), 2519–2530.

N

Imbalanced Nutrition: less than body requirements

Jacqueline A. Hogan, RD, CSO, LD

NANDA-I

Definition

Intake of nutrients insufficient to meet metabolic needs.

Defining Characteristics

Abdominal cramping; abdominal pain; alteration in taste sensation; body weight 20% or more below ideal weight range; capillary fragility; diarrhea; excessive hair loss; food aversion; food intake less than recommended daily allowance (RDA); hyperactive bowel sounds; insufficient information; insufficient interest in food; insufficient muscle tone; misinformation; misperception; pale mucous membranes; perceived inability to ingest food; satiety immediately on ingesting food; sore buccal cavity; weakness of muscles required for mastication; weakness of muscles required for swallowing; weight loss with adequate food intake

Related Factors

Insufficient dietary intake

● = Independent; ▲ = Collaborative;   EBN = Evidence-Based Nursing;   EB = Evidence-Based

At-Risk Population

Biological factors; economically disadvantaged

Associated Condition

Inability to absorb nutrients; inability to digest food; inability to ingest food; psychological disorder

NOC   (Nursing Outcomes Classification)

Suggested NOC Outcomes

Nutritional Status; Food and Fluid Intake; Nutrient Intake; Weight Control

Example NOC Outcome with Indicators
Nutritional Status as evidenced by the following indicators: Food and fluid intake/Body mass index/Weight-height ratio/Hematocrit. (Rate the outcome and indicators of **Nutritional Status:** 1 = severe deviation from normal range, 2 = substantial deviation from normal range, 3 = moderate deviation from normal range, 4 = mild deviation from normal range, 5 = no deviation from normal range [see Section I].)

Client Outcomes

Client Will (Specify Time Frame)

- Progressively gain weight toward desired goal
- Weigh within normal range for height and age
- Recognize factors contributing to being underweight
- Identify nutritional requirements
- Consume adequate nourishment
- Be free of signs of malnutrition

NIC   (Nursing Interventions Classification)

Suggested NIC Interventions

Feeding; Nutrition Management; Nutrition Therapy; Weight Gain Assistance

Example NIC Activities—Nutrition Management
Ascertain the client's food preferences; Provide the client with high-protein, high-calorie, nutritious finger foods and drinks that can be readily consumed, as appropriate

Nursing Interventions and *Rationales*

- Conduct a nutrition screen on all clients within 24 hours of admission and refer to a dietitian as deemed necessary. EB: *A study showed that malnutrition at admission and poor food intake early during hospitalization were associated with prolonged length of stay (LOS), suggesting that prompt nutrition intervention and monitoring should be performed when patients are admitted to the hospital (Allard et al, 2016).*
- The screening tool should be based on the client population and the validity and reliability of the screening tool. The Malnutrition Universal Screening Tool (MUST), for example, is considered a quick easy-to-use tool to assess body mass index (BMI), unintentional weight loss, acuity of illness, and nutritional intake. EB: *A study demonstrated the validity of MUST compared with a reference nutrition assessment using a patient-generated subjective global assessment-(PG-SGA) in elderly acutely unwell patients. The MUST tool was shown to be reasonably effective in identifying patients at risk of malnutrition when compared with PG-SGA with a sensitivity of 69.7% (Sharma et al, 2017).*
- Recognize the importance of rescreening and monitoring oral intake in hospitalized individuals to help facilitate the early identification and prevention of nutritional decline.
- Recognize the characteristics that classify individuals as malnourished and refer to a dietitian for a complex nutritional assessment and intervention. CEB: *According to the Academy of Nutrition and Dietetics and the American Society of Parenteral and Enteral Nutrition, two or more of the following characteristics are*

● = Independent;   ▲ = Collaborative;   EBN = Evidence-Based Nursing;   EB = Evidence-Based

recommended to support the diagnosis of malnutrition: insufficient energy intake, weight loss, loss of muscle mass, loss of subcutaneous fat, localized or generalized fluid accumulation, and/or decreased functional status (White, Guenter, & Gordon, 2012).

- Recognize clients who are likely to experience malnutrition in the context of social or environmental circumstances, characterized by pure chronic starvation and anorexia nervosa without the presence of an inflammatory process (White, Guenter, & Gordon, 2012).
  - ○ Chronic disease-related malnutrition: those with organ failure, pancreatic cancer, rheumatoid arthritis, sarcopenic obesity
  - ○ Acute disease or injury-related malnutrition: those with major infection, burns, trauma, closed-head injuries accompanied by a marked inflammatory response (White, Guenter, & Gordon, 2012)
- ▲ Note laboratory values cautiously; decrease in albumin and prealbumin may be indicators of the inflammatory response that often accompanies acute malnutrition, but it should not be used to diagnose malnutrition. Other potential indicators of inflammatory response include C-reactive protein, white blood cell count, and blood glucose values.
- Weigh the client daily in acute care and weekly to monthly in extended care at the same time (usually before breakfast) with same amount of clothing.
- Observe for potential barriers to eating such as willingness, ability, and appetite. EB: *Depression, impaired function, and poor oral intake are associated with increased likelihood of weight loss, low BMI, and poor nutrition in nursing home residents (Tamura et al, 2013).*

Note: If the client is unable to feed self, refer to Nursing Interventions for Feeding **Self-Care** deficit. If the client has difficulty swallowing, refer to Nursing Interventions for Impaired **Swallowing.** If the client is receiving tube feedings, refer to the Nursing Interventions for Risk for **Aspiration.**

- Advocate for the implementation of a feeding protocol, if not already in place, to avoid unnecessary and/or prolonged nothing by mouth (mouth)/clear liquid diet (NPO/CLD) status in hospitalized clients. EB: *A study found that on average, patients with unjustified NPO or CLD orders spent 3 days on an NPO or CLD diet, which corresponded to a mean of 10 missed meals (Gallinger et al, 2017).*
- For the client with anorexia nervosa, consider offering high-calorie foods and snacks often. EB: *A study found that higher calorie diets led to faster weight gain in hospitalized adolescents with anorexia nervosa compared with lower calorie diets (Garber et al, 2013).*
- For the client who is able to eat but has a decreased appetite, try the following activities:
  - ○ Offer oral nutritional supplements (ONS) early after admission and continue to encourage intake of ONS throughout the hospital stay. EB: *A study found that use of ONS in the inpatient population decreased LOS, episode cost, and 30-day readmission risk (Philipson et al, 2013). A meta-analysis found that use of ONS significantly reduced hospital readmissions, particularly in older adults (Stratton, Hebuterne, & Elia, 2013).*
  - ○ Avoid interruptions during mealtimes and offer companionship; meals should be eaten in a calm and peaceful environment. EB: *A study found that the implementation of protected mealtimes and use of additional assistant-in-nursing assistance alone and in combination improved nutritional intake of hospitalized clients (Young et al, 2013).*
  - ○ Allow for access to meals or snacks during "off times" if the client is not available at time of meal delivery, monitor food and ONS intake, and communicate with dietitian/health care provider. EB: *The Alliance Nutrition Care Recommendations include a multidisciplinary approach to address adult hospital malnutrition, which included the rapid implementation of nutrition intervention and continued monitoring (Tappenden et al, 2013).*
  - ○ If the client lacks endurance, schedule rest periods before meals, and open packages and cut up food for the client. *Nursing assistance will conserve the client's energy for eating.*
- Vitamin D deficiency has been shown to be associated with greater risk of falls and fractures in older people. For the client with fracture caused by a fall, consider the need for vitamin D supplementation. EB: *A study found that vitamin D without exercise was associated with less injurious falls (Uusi-Rasi et al, 2017).*
- For the client who has had a stroke, repeat nutritional screenings weekly and provide timely interventions for those at risk or who may already be malnourished. EB: *According to a recent study, the prevalence of malnutrition and risk of malnutrition in clients with acute stroke increases significantly during the first 10 days of admission (Mosselman et al, 2013). A separate study found that stroke patients identified as having a risk of malnutrition using the nutrition screening tool MUST had a highly significant increase in mortality (Gomes et al, 2016).*

● = Independent;   ▲ = Collaborative;   EBN = Evidence-Based Nursing;   EB = Evidence-Based

- Recognize the importance of offering high-protein foods and beverages to most hospitalized individuals (use caution with those with compromised renal/liver function). EB: *A study found that maintaining adequate dietary protein aids in muscle mass preservation during periods of muscle disuse. Such strategies are of particular relevance to the older patient who is at risk of developing sarcopenia (Wall & van Loon, 2013).*
- Monitor state of oral cavity (gums, tongue, mucosa, and teeth). Provide good oral hygiene before each meal. *Good oral hygiene enhances appetite; the condition of the oral mucosa is critical to the ability to eat. The oral mucosa must be moist, with adequate saliva production to facilitate and aid in the digestion of food.*
- ▲ Administer antiemetics and pain medications as ordered and needed before meals. *The presence of nausea or pain decreases the appetite.*
- If client is nauseated, remove cover of food tray before bringing it into the client's room. *The sudden, concentrated food odors that come when the cover is removed in front of the client can trigger nausea.*
- Work with the client to develop a plan for increased activity. *Immobility leads to negative nitrogen balance, which fosters anorexia.*

Critical Care

- Recognize the need to begin enteral feeding within 24 to 48 hours of admission to the critical care environment, once the client is free of hemodynamic compromise, if the client is unable to eat. CEB: *The guidelines for the provision and assessment of nutrition support therapy in the adult critically ill client call for early enteral feeding (McClave et al, 2009).* EB: *Per a meta-analysis of randomized controlled trials, provision of early enteral nutrition was associated with a significant reduction in mortality and infectious morbidity, compared with withholding early enteral nutrition (delayed enteral nutrition or standard therapy) (McClave et al, 2016).*
- Recognize that it is important to administer feedings to the client and that frequently checking for gastric residual and fasting clients for procedures can be a limiting factor to adequate nutrition in the tube-fed client. EBN: *A study found that implementing a protocol for managing gastric residual volumes, not fasting clients for procedures, and reducing fasting times when weaning clients for extubation reduced the number of interruptions to enteral feeding (Williams et al, 2013). Refer to care plan for Risk for* **Aspiration.**

Pediatric

- ▲ Use a nutritional screening tool designed for nurses such as the Subjective Global Nutrition Assessment (SGNA), and if the child's malnutrition is identified as moderate or severe, refer to a dietitian. EB: *A study found that SGNA can be a reliable tool for assessing the nutritional status in children (Minocho et al, 2018).*
- Watch for symptoms of malnutrition in the child including short stature; thin arms and legs; poor condition of skin and hair; visible vertebrae and rib cage; wasted buttocks; wasted facial appearance; lethargy; and in extreme cases, edema.
- Weigh and measure the length (height) of the child and use a growth chart to help determine growth pattern, which reflects nutrition. *Age-related growth charts are available from* www.cdc.gov/growthcharts/.
- ▲ Refer to a health care provider and a dietitian a child who is underweight for any reason. *Good nutrition is extremely important for children to ensure sufficient growth and development of all body systems.*
- Work with the child and parent to develop an appropriate weight gain plan. *The goal for a child is sometimes to maintain existing weight as the body grows taller.*
- Recognize that a large percentage of girls and teenagers are dieting, which can result in nutritional problems.

Geriatric

- Screen for malnutrition in older clients. EB: *A study found that the following screening tools were accurate in identifying malnutrition and can be recommended for use in the older adults who are hospitalized: the Malnutrition Screening Tool (MST), the Mini Nutritional Assessment–Short Form (MNA-SF), MUST, the Short Nutritional Assessment Questionnaire (SNAQ), and the Simplified Nutritional Appetite Questionnaire (Young et al, 2013).*
- Screen for dysphagia in all older clients. EB: *A study found that prevalence of dysphagia was higher than malnutrition in older patients. Dysphagia was also an independent risk factor for malnutrition and both conditions were related to poor outcomes (Carron et al, 2015). See care plan for Impaired* **Swallowing.**

● = Independent;   ▲ = Collaborative;   EBN = Evidence-Based Nursing;   EB = Evidence-Based

N

- Recognize that geriatric clients with moderate or severe cognition impairment have a significant risk for developing malnutrition. EBN: *Dementia is one of the factors most consistently associated with poor nutrition (Tamura et al, 2013).*
- ▲ Interpret laboratory findings cautiously. Watch the color of urine for an indication of fluid balance; darker urine demonstrates dehydration. Low axillary moisture could indicate mild to moderate dehydration. CEB/EB: *Because urine color is correlated with urine specific gravity and urine osmolality, observing urine color is a low-cost method of monitoring dehydration (Wakefield et al, 2002). Compromised kidney function makes reliance on blood and urine samples for nutrient analyses less reliable in older adults than in younger persons. Findings of a small pilot study suggest that measuring the axillary moisture of older adults has the potential as a simple tool for detecting dehydration at home and in nursing homes (Kinoshita et al, 2013).*
- Consider using dining assistants and trained nonnursing staff, to provide feeding assistance care in extended care facilities to ensure adequate time for feeding clients as needed. EB: *A study found that when trained volunteers were able to deliver mealtime assistance on a large scale nursing staff could complete clinical tasks (Roberts et al, 2017).*
- Consider offering healthy snacks such as yogurt, which is a good source of protein, calcium, zinc, B vitamins, and probiotics. EB: *Observational studies suggest that yogurt could play an important role in improving the nutritional health of older adults when combined with a healthy diet (El-Abbadi et al, 2014).*
- Encourage high-protein foods for the older client, unless medically contraindicated by organ failure. EB: *A study found protective effects against weight loss in healthy older adults who had protein intakes greater than 1 g/kg per day (Gray-Donald et al, 2014). Anorexia of aging has been found to have an independent association with sarcopenia (Landi et al, 2013). A study showed that an intervention of a vitamin D- and leucine-enriched whey protein ONS resulted in improvements in muscle mass and lower extremity function among sarcopenic older adults. This study shows proof of principle that specific nutritional supplementation alone might benefit geriatric patients, which is especially relevant for those who are unable to exercise (Bauer et al, 2015).*
- Encourage physical activity throughout the day as tolerated. EB: *A systemic review found that nutritional supplementation is effective in the treatment of sarcopenia in old age, and its positive effects increase when associated with physical exercise (Malafarina et al, 2013).*

- Recognize the implications of malnutrition on client strength and mobility. EB: *Malnutrition is associated with an increased risk of falling and impaired activity in older long-term care residents; malnourished residents were able to decrease their risk for fall after receiving nutritional intervention (Neyens et al, 2013).*
- Monitor for onset of depression. EB: *A systematic review of the literature found that depression, impaired function, and poor oral intake were factors consistently associated with increased likelihood of weight loss, low BMI, and poor nutrition (Tamura et al, 2013).*
- Consider offering nutritional supplement drinks served in a glass rather than with a straw inserted directly into the container. EBN: *A study found that among people with dementia who are able to feed themselves, they drank statistically significantly more when a nutritional supplement was served in a glass than when consumed directly from the container (Allen et al, 2014).*
- Advise families that enteral nutrition may not be indicated for clients with dementia. EB: *A study found that insertions of a percutaneous endoscopic gastrostomy (PEG) tube for enteral nutrition did not improve short-term or long-term mortality (Ayman et al, 2016).* For strategies for feeding clients with dementia, please refer to the ESPEN Guidelines on nutrition in dementia (Volkert et al, 2015). Note: If the client is unable to feed self, refer to Nursing Interventions and *Rationales* for Feeding **Self-Care** deficit. If client has impaired physical function, malnutrition, depression, or cognitive impairment, refer to care plan for **Frail Elderly** syndrome.
- Emphasize the importance of good oral care in the older client. EB: *Poor oral health was found to be strongly associated with malnutrition in older hospitalized clients (Poisson et al, 2016).*
- Consult the dietitian if the client has pressure ulcers. EBN: *A study found that an interdisciplinary approach including nutrition intervention improved pressure ulcer wound healing and decreased both hospital LOS for treatment of pressure ulcer and total hospital LOS in geriatric clients who were admitted with or developed a pressure ulcer from stage 2 to 3 during hospitalization (Allen, 2013).*

Home Care

- The preceding interventions may be adapted for home care use.
- Screen for malnutrition using the MUST, which is easy and simple. Recognize that the client may also use MUST as a self-screening tool in the home setting. EB: *A study demonstrated a high percentage of patients with unrecognized malnutrition risk using the MUST screening tool. The patient-directed nutrition*

● = Independent;   ▲ = Collaborative;   EBN = Evidence-Based Nursing;   EB = Evidence-Based

screening using the MUST screening tool is a reliable approach. Almost all patients reported self-screening as either very easy or easy to use, and all patients were able to self-screen (Sandhu et al, 2016).

- Monitor food intake. Instruct the client in the intake of small frequent meals of foods with increased calories and protein.
- Assess the client's willingness and ability to eat. EB: *Poor intake among older adults has been found to be associated with lack of self-feeding ability, poor dining environment, inadequate time to eat, poor sensory properties of the food, and lack of choice and variety of the food (Keller, 2015).*
- Consider social factors that may interfere with nutrition (e.g., lack of transportation, inadequate income, lack of social support).
- Continue to encourage intake of oral nutritional support to help optimize oral intake. EB: *A meta-analysis of randomized controlled trials suggested that oral nutritional support may be considered for older malnourished medical and surgical clients after discharge from the hospital (Beck et al, 2013).*
- ▲ Recognize that the client on home parenteral nutrition requires regularly scheduled lab work for electrolyte monitoring, increased risk of catheter-related complication, parenteral nutrition-associated liver disease (PNALD), and metabolic bone disease. *Clients should also be educated regarding home parenteral nutrition before discharge from the hospital (Winkler & Smith, 2014).*

 Client/Family Teaching and Discharge Planning

- Help the client/family identify the area to change that will make the greatest contribution to improved nutrition.
- Build on the strengths in the client/family's food habits. Adapt changes to their current practices.
- Select appropriate teaching aids for the client/family's background.
- Implement instructional follow-up to answer the client/family's questions.
- Recommend that clients discuss with their primary health care provider before taking any supplements such as vitamins and minerals.
- Suggest community resources, such as Meals on Wheels and community centers as suitable food sources.
- Teach the client and family how to manage tube feedings or parenteral therapy at home as needed.

REFERENCES

Allard, J. P., et al. (2016). Malnutrition at hospital admission—Contributors and effect on length of stay: a prospective cohort study from the Canadian malnutrition task force. *Journal of Parenteral and Enteral Nutrition, 40*(4), 487–497.

Allen, B. (2013). Effects of a comprehensive nutritional program on pressure ulcer healing, length of hospital stay, and charges to patients. *Clinical Nursing Research, 22*(2), 186–205.

Allen, V. J., et al. (2014). Impact of serving method on the consumption of nutritional supplement drinks: Randomized trial in older adults with cognitive impairment. *Journal of Advanced Nursing, 70*(6), 1323–1333.

Ayman, R. A., et al. (2016). PEG insertion in patients with dementia does not improve nutritional status and has worse outcomes as compared with PEG insertion for other indications. *Journal of Clinical Gastroenterology, 51*(5), 417–420.

Bauer, J. M., et al. (2015). Effects of a vitamin D and leucine-enriched whey protein nutritional supplement on measures of sarcopenia in older adults, the PROVIDE study: A randomized, double-blind, placebo-controlled trial. *Journal of the American Medical Directors Association, 16*(9), 740–747.

Beck, A. M., et al. (2013). Oral nutritional support for older (65 years+) medical and surgical patients after discharge from hospital: Systematic review and meta-analysis of randomized controlled trial. *Clinical Rehabilitation, 27*(1), 19–27.

Carron, S., et al. (2015). Oropharyngeal dysphagia is a prevalent risk factor for malnutrition in a cohort of older patients admitted with an acute disease to a general hospital. *Clinical Nutrition, 34*, 436–442.

El-Abbadi, N. H., Dao, M. C., & Meydani, S. N. (2014). Yogurt: Role in healthy and active aging. *The American Journal of Clinical Nutrition, 99*(5), 1263S–1270S.

Gallinger, Z. R., et al. (2017). Frequency and variables associated with fasting orders in inpatients with ulcerative colitis: The Audit of Diet Orders—Ulcerative Colitis (ADORE-UC) study. *Inflammatory Bowel Disease, 23*, 1790–1795.

Garber, A. K., et al. (2013). Higher calorie diets increase rate of weight gain and shorten hospital stay in hospitalized adolescents with anorexia nervosa. *Journal of Adolescent Health, 53*(5), 579–584.

Gomes, F., et al. (2016). Risk of malnutrition is an independent predictor of mortality, length of hospital stay, and hospitalization costs in stroke patients. *Journal of Stroke and Cerebrovascular Diseases, 25*(4), 799–806.

Gray-Donald, K., et al. (2014). Protein intake protects against weight loss in healthy community-dwelling older adults. *Journal of Nutrition, 144*(3), 321–326.

Keller, H. H., et al. (2015). Improving food and fluid intake for older adults living in long-term care: a research agenda. *JAMDA, 16*, 93–100.

Kinoshita, K., et al. (2013). The measurement of axillary moisture for the assessment of dehydration among older patients: A pilot study. *Experimental Gerontology, 48*(2), 255–258.

Landi, F., et al. (2013). Association of anorexia with sarcopenia in a community-dwelling elderly population: Results from the ilSIRENTE study. *European Journal of Nutrition, 52*(3), 1261–1268.

Malafarina, V., et al. (2013). Effectiveness of nutritional supplementation on muscle mass in treatment of sarcopenia in old age: A systematic review. *Journal of the American Medical Directors Association, 14*(1), 10–17.

McClave, S. A., et al. (2009). Guidelines for the provision and assessment of nutrition support therapy in the adult critically ill patient: Society of Critical Care Medicine (SCCM) and American

● = Independent;   ▲ = Collaborative;   EBN = Evidence-Based Nursing;   EB = Evidence-Based

N

Society for Parenteral and Enteral Nutrition (A.S.P.E.N). *JPEN. Journal of Parenteral and Enteral Nutrition, 33*(3), 277–316.

McClave, S. A., et al. (2016). Guidelines for the provision and assessment of nutrition support therapy in the adult critically ill patient: Society of Critical Care Medicine (SCCM) and American Society for Parenteral and Enteral Nutrition (A.S.P.E.N). *Journal of Parenteral and Enteral Nutrition, 40*(2), 159–211.

Minocho, P., et al. (2018). Subjective Global Nutritional Assessment: A reliable screening tool for nutritional assessment in cerebral palsy children. *Indian Journal of Pediatrics, 85*(1), 15–19.

Mosselman, M. J., et al. (2013). Malnutrition and risk of malnutrition in patients with stroke: Prevalence during hospital stay. *Journal of Neuroscience Nursing, 45*(4), 194–204.

Neyens, J., et al. (2013). Malnutrition is associated with an increased risk of falls and impaired activity in elderly patients in Dutch residential long-term care (LTC): A cross-sectional study. *Archives of Gerontology and Geriatrics, 56*(1), 265–269.

Philipson, T. J., et al. (2013). Impact of oral nutritional supplementation on hospital outcomes. *The American Journal of Managed Care, 19*(2), 121–128.

Poisson, P., Laffond, T., Campos, S., et al. (2016). Relationships between oral health, dysphagia and undernutrition in hospitalised elderly patients. *Gerodontology, 33*(2), 161–168.

Roberts, H. C., et al. (2017). The impact of trained volunteer mealtime assistants on the dietary intake of older female in-patients: The Southampton Mealtime Assistance Study. *Journal of Nutrition Health Aging, 21*(3), 320–328.

Sandhu, A., et al. (2016). Self-screening for malnutrition risk in outpatient inflammatory bowel disease patients using the Malnutrition Universal Screening Tool (MUST). *Journal of Parenteral and Enteral Nutrition, 40*(4), 507–510.

Sharma, Y., et al. (2017). Validity of the Malnutrition Universal Screening Tool (MUST) in Australian hospitalized acutely unwell elderly patients. *Asia Pacific Journal Clinical Nutrition, 26*(6), 994–1000.

Stratton, R. J., Hebuterne, X., & Elia, M. (2013). A systematic review and meta-analysis of the impact of oral nutritional supplements on hospital readmissions. *Ageing Research Reviews, 12*(4), 884–897.

Tamura, B. K., et al. (2013). Factors associated with weight loss, low BMI, and malnutrition among nursing home patients: A systematic review of the literature. *Journal of the American Medical Directors Association, 14*(9), 649–655.

Tappenden, K. A., et al. (2013). Critical role of nutrition in improving quality of care: An interdisciplinary call to action to address adult hospital malnutrition. *Journal of the Academy of Nutrition and Dietetics, 113*(9), 1219–1237.

Uusi-Rasi, K., et al. (2017). A 2-year follow-up after a 2-year RCT with vitamin D and exercise: effects on falls, injurious falls and physical functioning among older women. *Journal of Gerontology. Series A, Biological Sciences and Medical Sciences, 72*(9), 1239–1245.

Volkert, D., et al. (2015). ESPEN guideline on nutrition in dementia. *Clinical Nutrition, 34*, 1052–1073.

Wakefield, B., et al. (2002). Monitoring hydration status in elderly veterans. *Western Journal of Nursing Research, 24*, 132.

Wall, B. T., & van Loon, L. J. (2013). Nutritional strategies to attenuate muscle disuse atrophy. *Nutrition Reviews, 71*(4), 195–208.

White, J., Guenter, P., & Gordon, J. (2012). Consensus statement of the Academy of Nutrition and Dietetics/American Society for Parenteral and Enteral Nutrition: Characteristics recommended for the identification and documentation of adult malnutrition. *Journal of the Academy of Nutrition and Dietetics, 112*, 730–738.

Williams, T. A., et al. (2013). Reducing interruptions to continuous enteral nutrition in the intensive care unit: A comparative study. *Journal of Clinical Nursing, 22*(19–20), 2838–2848.

Winkler, M. F., & Smith, C. E. (2014). Clinical, social, and economic impacts of home parenteral nutrition dependence in short bowel syndrome. *Journal of Parenteral and Enteral Nutrition, 38*(1), 32S–37S.

Young, A. M., Kidston, S., Banks, M. D., et al. (2013). Malnutrition screening tools: Comparison against two validated nutrition assessment methods in older medical inpatients. *Nutrition (Burbank, Los Angeles County, Calif.), 29*(1), 101–106.

Impaired Oral Mucous Membrane integrity   *Morgan Nestingen, MS, AGCNS, ONS*

NANDA-I

Definition

Injury to the lips, soft tissue, buccal cavity, and/or oropharynx.

Defining Characteristics

Bad taste in mouth; bleeding; cheilitis; coated tongue; decrease in taste sensation; desquamation; difficulty eating; difficulty speaking; enlarged tonsils; exposure to pathogen; geographic tongue; gingival hyperplasia; gingival pallor; gingival pocketing deeper than 4 mm; gingival recession; halitosis; hyperemia; impaired ability to swallow; macroplasia; mucosal denudation; oral discomfort; oral edema; oral fissure; oral lesion; oral mucosal pallor; oral nodule; oral pain; oral papule; oral ulcer; oral vesicles; presence of mass; purulent oral-nasal drainage; purulent oral–nasal exudates; smooth atrophic tongue; spongy patches in mouth; stomatitis; white patches in mouth; white plaque in mouth; white, curdlike oral exudate; xerostomia

Related Factors

Alcohol consumption; barrier to dental care; barrier to oral self-care; chemical injury agent; decrease in salivation; dehydration; depression; inadequate nutrition; inadequate oral hygiene; insufficient knowledge of oral hygiene; malnutrition; mouth breathing; smoking; stressors

● = Independent;   ▲ = Collaborative;   **EBN** = Evidence-Based Nursing;   **EB** = Evidence-Based

At-Risk Population

Economically disadvantaged

Associated Condition

Allergy; alteration in cognitive functioning; autoimmune disease; autosomal disorder; behavioral disorder; chemotherapy; cleft lip; cleft palate; decrease in hormone level in women; decrease in platelets; immunodeficiency; immunosuppression; infection; loss of oral support structure; mechanical factor; nil per os (NPO) >24 hours; oral trauma; radiation therapy; Sjogren's syndrome; surgical procedure; trauma; treatment regimen

NOC   (Nursing Outcomes Classification)

Suggested NOC Outcomes

Oral Health; Oral Hygiene; Tissue Integrity: Skin and Mucous Membranes

Example NOC Outcome with Indicators
Oral Health as evidenced by the following indicators: Cleanliness of mouth and teeth/Moisture of oral mucosa and tongue/Color of mucous membranes/Oral mucosa/tongue/gum integrity. (Rate the outcome and indicators of **Oral Health:** 1 = severely compromised, 2 = substantially compromised, 3 = moderately compromised, 4 = mildly compromised, 5 = not compromised [see Section I].)

Client Outcomes

Client Will (Specify Time Frame)

- Maintain intact, moist oral mucous membranes that are free of ulceration, inflammation, infection, and debris
- Demonstrate measures to maintain or regain intact oral mucous membranes
- Demonstrate oral hygiene knowledge and skills

NIC   (Nursing Interventions Classification)

Suggested NIC Intervention

Oral Health Restoration

Example NIC Activities—Oral Health Restoration
Monitor condition of client's mouth including character of abnormalities; Instruct client to avoid commercial mouthwashes

Nursing Interventions and *Rationales*

- ▲ Inspect the oral cavity/teeth/gingiva at least once daily and note any discoloration; presence of debris; amount of plaque buildup; presence of lesions such as white lesions or patches, edema, or bleeding; and intactness of teeth. Refer to a dentist or periodontist as appropriate. *Inspection is a critical diagnostic tool; observations can identify impending problems. Leukoplakia is the presence of uncharacterized white lesions, which can be a precursor to squamous cell carcinoma. If leukoplakia is observed, prompt referral for diagnosis and potential biopsy is indicated (van Der Waal, 2015; American Dental Association [ADA], 2017b).*
- If the client is free of bleeding disorders and able to swallow, encourage toothbrushing with a soft toothbrush using fluoride-containing toothpaste at least two times per day. EB: *The toothbrush is the most effective method for reducing plaque and controlling periodontal disease (Barnes, 2014; ADA, 2017a).*
- Recommend the use of a power, rotation-oscillation toothbrush for removal of dental plaque and prevention of gingivitis. EB: *Two systematic reviews found the powered/oscillating toothbrush to be safe for use on both hard and soft dental tissues and more effective in cleaning teeth (Grender et al, 2013; Slade, 2013; Yaacob et al, 2014).*
- Use foam sticks to moisten the oral mucous membranes, clean out debris, and swab out the mouth of the edentulous client. **Do not use foam sticks to clean the teeth** unless the platelet count is very low and the client is prone to bleeding gums. Foam sticks are useful for cleansing the oral cavity of a client who is edentulous. EB: *Foam sticks are not effective for removing plaque. The toothbrush is much more effective at mechanically removing plaque (Chen, 2014a).*
- If the client does not have a bleeding disorder, encourage the client to floss once per day or use an interdental cleaner. EB: *Floss is useful to remove plaque buildup between the teeth and prevent gingivitis*

● = Independent;   ▲ = Collaborative;   EBN = Evidence-Based Nursing;   EB = Evidence-Based

(ADA, 2017a). Removal of existing plaque buildup is critical to resolving gingivitis (Fiorellini & Stathopoulou, 2015).

- Use an antimicrobial mouthwash as ordered or tap water or saline only for a mouth rinse. Do not use commercial mouthwashes containing alcohol or hydrogen peroxide. Also, do not use lemon-glycerin swabs. *Some antimicrobial mouthwashes have demonstrated effective action in decreasing bacterial counts in plaque and decreasing gingivitis (ADA, 2017a).* CEB/EB: *Hydrogen peroxide can cause mucosal damage and is extremely foul-tasting to clients (Tombes & Gallucci, 1993; Zanelli, Ragazzi, & De Marco, 2017). Use of lemon-glycerin swabs can result in decreased salivary amylase and oral moisture, as well as erosion of tooth enamel; instead ice-cold water sprays/swabs and menthol moisturizers may be effective at decreasing thirst without damaging tissue (Puntillo et al, 2014). Chlorhexidine mouthwash and sodium bicarbonate appropriately diluted may be used during oral care (Chen, 2014b).*
- Provide oral hygiene if the client is unable to care for himself or herself. The nursing diagnosis Bathing **Self-Care** deficit is then applicable.
- If the client is unable to brush own teeth, follow this procedure:
  - ○ Position the client sitting upright or on side.
  - ○ Use a soft bristle toothbrush.
  - ○ Use fluoride toothpaste and tap water or saline as a solution.
  - ○ Brush teeth in an up-and-down manner.
  - ○ Suction as needed.

Each client must receive oral care including toothbrushing two times every day to maintain healthy teeth and mouth and to prevent complications associated with periodontitis (the advanced form of gum disease that can cause tooth loss), which is associated with health problems, such as cardiovascular disease, stroke, and bacterial pneumonia (ADA, 2017d).

- Monitor the client's nutritional and fluid status to determine whether it is adequate. Refer to the care plan for Deficient **Fluid** volume or Imbalanced **Nutrition:** less than body requirements if applicable. *Dehydration and malnutrition predispose clients to impaired oral mucous membranes.*
- Encourage fluid intake of up to 3000 mL/day if not contraindicated by the client's medical condition. *Fluids help increase moisture in the mouth, which protects the mucous membranes from damage.*
- ▲ Determine the client's usual method of oral care and address any concerns regarding oral hygiene. If the client has a dry mouth (xerostomia):
  - ○ Recognize that more than 50 classes of medications may cause xerostomia, which is often exacerbated by polypharmacy. When feasible, medications can be discontinued or replaced to increase the client's comfort (Villa et al, 2015).
  - ○ Provide saliva substitutes as ordered. *Saliva substitutes are helpful to decrease the discomfort of dry mouth and may help prevent stomatitis (ADA, 2017c).*
  - ○ Suggest the client chew sugarless gum or sugarless sour candy to promote salivary flow. *Both sugarless gum and candy stimulate the formation of saliva (ADA, 2017c).*
  - ○ Examine the oral cavity for signs of caries, dental plaque, infection, mucositis ulceration, and oral candidiasis. *Untreated xerostomia may result in these conditions (Gil-Montoya et al, 2016).*
- Recommend that the client decrease or preferably stop intake of soft drinks. Sugar-containing soft drinks can cause cavities, and the low pH of the drink can cause erosion in teeth (*ADA, 2017a*).
- If client has halitosis, review good oral care with the client including brushing teeth, using floss, and brushing the tongue. Halitosis can be a beginning sign of gingivitis and can be eradicated by a good program of dental hygiene (*ADA, 2017b*).
- Instruct the client with halitosis to clean the tongue when performing oral hygiene; brush tongue with tongue scraper or toothbrush and follow with a mouth rinse. EB: A meta-analysis found that tongue cleaning in addition to toothbrushing was effective for short-term control of halitosis (*Kuo et al, 2013; ADA 2017b*).
- ▲ Assess the client for underlying medical condition that may be causing halitosis. *Causes of halitosis can be subdivided into three categories: oral origin in which good mouth care can help prevent halitosis; halitosis from the upper respiratory tract including the sinuses and nose; and halitosis from systemic diseases that are blood-borne, volatilized in the lungs, and expelled from the lower respiratory tract. Potential sources of blood-borne halitosis are some systemic diseases, metabolic disorders, medication, and certain foods such as onions and garlic (ADA, 2017b).*
- Keep the lips well lubricated using a water based or aloe based lip balm. *This is a comfort measure (Radvansky, Pace, & Siddiqui, 2013; Puntillo et al, 2014).*

● = Independent;   ▲ = Collaborative;   EBN = Evidence-Based Nursing;   EB = Evidence-Based

Client Receiving Chemotherapy/Radiation

- Ensure that the client receives a comprehensive oral examination before initiation of chemotherapy or radiation, with aggressive preventive dental care given as needed (Radvansky, Pace, & Siddiqui, 2013; Maria, Eliopoulos, & Muanza, 2017).
- Provide both verbal and written instruction about the need for and method of providing frequent oral care to the client before radiation therapy or chemotherapy. Assess the condition of the oral cavity daily in the client receiving radiation or chemotherapy (Radvansky, Pace, & Siddiqui, 2013).
- For measurement of presence or severity of mucositis, use the Oral Mucositis Assessment Scale (OMAS). EBN: *This is an instrument that has two components: clinician's assessment of presence and severity of mucositis and client report about pain, difficulty swallowing, and ability to eat. Scores indicating the presence of a more severe oral mucositis are associated with decreased quality of life (Franco et al, 2017).*
- Use a protocol to prevent/treat mucositis that includes the following:
  - ○ Use a soft toothbrush that is replaced on a regular basis; brush teeth at least two times a day and for at least 90 seconds.
  - ○ Continue to floss teeth daily.
  - ○ Use a bland, alcohol-free rinse to remove debris and moisten the oral cavity. Rinse the mouth often (every 2 hours while awake) if the client has mouth sores.
  - ○ Avoid tobacco, alcohol, and irritating foods (hot, rough, acidic, or spicy).
  - ○ Use a valid and reliable pain assessment tool and treatment of pain as needed.

EB: *Use of an oral care protocol helps to decrease oral mucositis in clients receiving treatment for cancer (Radvansky, Pace, & Siddiqui, 2013; Eilers et al, 2014; Maria, Eliopoulos, & Muanza, 2017).*

- Help the client use a mouth rinse of normal saline or salt and soda every 1 to 2 hours for prevention and treatment of stomatitis. A typical mixture is 1 teaspoon of salt or sodium bicarbonate per pint of water. Clients are directed to take a tablespoon of the rinse and swish it in the mouth for 30 seconds, then expectorate. EB: *Rinses are helpful to remove debris and hydrate the oral mucous membranes; sodium bicarbonate can discourage yeast colonization (Maria, Eliopoulos, & Muanza, 2017).*
- ▲ If the mouth is severely inflamed and it is painful to swallow, contact the health care provider for a topical anesthetic or analgesic order. Modification of oral intake (e.g., soft or liquid diet) may also be necessary to prevent friction trauma. *The nursing diagnosis Imbalanced **Nutrition:** less than body requirements may apply.*
- If the client's platelet count is lower than 50,000/mm³ or the client has a bleeding disorder, use a specially made toothbrush designed for sensitive or diseased tissue, or a toothette that is not soaked in glycerin or flavorings; if the client cannot tolerate a toothbrush or a toothette, a piece of gauze wrapped around a finger can be used to remove plaque and debris (Radvansky, Pace, & Siddiqui, 2013).

Critical Care—Client on a Ventilator

- Use a soft toothbrush to brush teeth to clean the client's teeth at least every 12 hours; use suction to remove secretions. Provide oral moisturizer to oral mucosa and lips every 4 hours. Recognize that good oral care is paramount in the prevention of ventilator-associated events (VAE) and ventilator-associated pneumonia (VAP). EBN: *Increased plaque on the teeth is associated with increased contamination of the mouth and incidence of VAP (de Lacerda et al, 2017). An integrative review of the literature found that consistently performing frequent oral care along with other interventions (e.g., head of bed >30 degrees, adequate endotracheal tube cuff pressure to reduce aspiration, daily evaluation of client's readiness for extubation) and oral moisturizing reduced VAP and decreased overall health care expenses (Alhazzani et al, 2013; Hillier et al, 2013; Parsons et al, 2013; Chu, 2014).*
- ▲ Apply chlorhexidine gluconate mouthwash or gel in the oral cavity after performing tooth brushing, which may reduce the risk of the client developing VAE and VAP. EB: *The use of chlorhexidine gluconate has been associated with a 40% reduction in the odds of a client developing VAP (Shi et al, 2013). Routine oral care with chlorhexidine gluconate in the care of the mechanically ventilated cardiac surgery clients reduces the risk of VAP (Klompas et al, 2014; Xue, 2015; de Lacerda et al, 2017).*

 Geriatric

- Determine the functional ability of the client to provide his or her own oral care. Refer to Bathing **Self-Care** deficit. *Interventions must be directed toward both treatment of the functional loss and care of oral health.*

● = Independent;   ▲ = Collaborative;   EBN = Evidence-Based Nursing;   EB = Evidence-Based

- Provide appropriate oral care to older adults with a self-care deficit, brushing the teeth after breakfast and in the evening. EBN: *Oral care is often poor for older clients and clients with dementia.* EB: *Several studies have shown that the rate of pneumonia was decreased by providing oral care (van Der Maarel-Wierink et al, 2013; Le, 2015).*
- If the client has dementia or delirium and exhibits care-resistant behavior, such as fighting, biting, or refusing care, then use the following method:
  - ❍ Ensure client is in a quiet environment such as own bathroom, sitting or standing at the sink to prime memory for appropriate actions.
  - ❍ Approach the client at eye level within his or her range of vision.
  - ❍ Approach with a smile and begin conversation with a touch of the hand and gradually move up.
  - ❍ Use mirror–mirror technique, standing behind the client, and brush and floss teeth.
  - ❍ Use respectful adult speech, not "elder speak" (sing-song voice, or diminutive terms such as "dearie" or "honey"). *Elder speak is a documented trigger for care-resistant behavior (Williams et al, 2017).*
  - ❍ Promote self-care in which client brushes own teeth if possible.
  - ❍ Use distractors when needed: talking, reminiscing, singing. EBN: *Use of specific techniques can decrease resistance to nursing care and increase the effectiveness of nurses providing oral care to clients. Additional research is needed to examine oral care in the client with dementia (Mohammadi, Franks, & Hines, 2015; Rozas, Sadowsky, & Jeter, 2017).*
- Carefully observe the oral cavity and lips for abnormal lesions such as white or red patches, masses, ulcerations with an indurated margin, or a raised granular lesion. *Malignant lesions are more common in older adults than in younger persons, especially if there is a history of smoking or alcohol use (Le, 2015; ADA, 2017e).*
- Ensure that dentures are removed and cleaned regularly, preferably after every meal and before bedtime. *Dentures left in the mouth at night may impede circulation to the palate and predispose the client to oral lesions.*

Home Care

- The interventions described previously may be adapted for home care use.
- Instruct the client in ways to soothe the oral cavity (e.g., cool beverages, popsicles, viscous lidocaine).
- ▲ If necessary, refer for home health aide services to support the family in oral care and observation of the oral cavity.

Client/Family Teaching and Discharge Planning

- Teach the client how to inspect the oral cavity and monitor for signs and symptoms of infection or complications, and when to call the health care provider (Radvansky, Pace, & Siddiqui, 2013; Eilers et al, 2014).
- Recommend the client not smoke, use chewing tobacco, or drink excessive amounts of alcohol. *Tobacco use, either smoking or chewing, is a common cause of leukoplakia. Also, alcohol and human papillomavirus have been associated with squamous cell carcinoma in the oral cavity (van Der Waal, 2015; ADA, 2017e).*
- Teach the client and family, if necessary, how to perform appropriate mouth care. Use the motivational interviewing technique. EB: *A systematic review demonstrated improved dental hygiene, including interdental cleaning, when motivational interviewing compared with the usual teaching session on oral hygiene techniques (Kopp et al, 2017). See Appendix C on Evolve for motivational interviewing.*

REFERENCES

Alhazzani, W., Smith, O., Muscedere, J., et al. (2013). Toothbrushing for critically ill mechanically ventilated patients: A systematic review and meta-analysis of randomized trials evaluating ventilator-associated pneumonia. *Critical Care Medicine, 41,* 646–655.

American Dental Association (ADA). (2017a). *Oral health topics: Home oral care.* Retrieved from http://www.ada.org/en/member-center/oral-health-topics/home-care. (Accessed 3 February 2018).

American Dental Association (ADA). (2017b). *Mouth healthy: halitosis.* Retrieved from http://www.mouthhealthy.org/en/az-topics/h/Halitosis. (Accessed February 3, 2018).

American Dental Association (ADA). (2017c). *Oral health topics: Xerostomia (dry mouth).* Retrieved from http://www.ada.org/en/member-center/oral-health-topics/xerostomia. (Accessed 3 February 2018).

American Dental Association (ADA). (2017d). *Oral health topics: Oral-systemic health.* Retrieved from http://www.ada.org/en/member-center/oral-health-topics/oral-systemic-health. (Accessed 3 February 2018).

American Dental Association (ADA). (2017e). *Evaluation of potentially malignant disorders in the oral cavity clinical practice guideline*

● = Independent;   ▲ = Collaborative;   EBN = Evidence-Based Nursing;   EB = Evidence-Based

(2017). Retrieved from http://ebd.ada.org/en/evidence/guidelines/oral-cancer. (Accessed 3 February 2018).

Barnes, C. M. (2014). Dental hygiene intervention to prevent nosocomial pneumonias. *The Journal of Evidence-based Dental Practice, 145,* 103–114.

Chen, Z. (2014a). *Oral care.* Adelaide, Australia: Joanna Briggs Institute.

Chen, Z. (2014b). *Mouth wash.* Adelaide, Australia: Joanna Briggs Institute.

Chu, V. (2014). *Ventilator-associated pneumonia: Clinician information.* Adelaide, Australia: Joanna Briggs Institute.

de Lacerda Vidal, C. F., Vidal, A. K. D. L., Monteiro, J. G. D. M., et al. (2017). Impact of oral hygiene involving toothbrushing versus chlorhexidine in the prevention of ventilator-associated pneumonia: A randomized study. *BMC Infectious Diseases, 17.* doi:10.1186/s12879-017-2188-0.

Eilers, J., Harris, D., Henry, K., et al. (2014). Evidence-based interventions for cancer treatment-related mucositis: Putting evidence into practice. *Clinical Journal of Oncology Nursing, 18*(6), 80–96.

Fiorellini, J. P., & Stathopoulou, P. G. (2015). Clinical features of gingivitis. In *Carranza's clinical periodontology* (pp. 224–231). Philadelphia: Saunders.

Franco, P., Martini, S., Di Muzio, J., et al. (2017). Prospective assessment of oral mucositis and its impact on quality of life and patient-reported outcomes during radiotherapy for head and neck cancer. *Medical Oncology, 34*(5), 81. doi:10.1007/s12032-017-0950-1.

Gil-Montoya, J.-A., Silvestre, F.-J., Barrios, R., et al. (2016). Treatment of xerostomia and hyposalivation in the elderly: A systematic review. *Medicina Oral, Patología Oral y Cirugía Bucal, 21*(3), 355–366.

Grender, J., Williams, K., Walters, P., et al. (2013). Plaque removal efficacy of oscillating-rotating power toothbrushes: Review of six comparative clinical trials. *American Journal of Dentistry, 26*(2), 68–74.

Hillier, B., Wilson, C., Chamberlain, D., et al. (2013). Preventing ventilator-associated pneumonia through oral care, product selection, and application method: A literature review. *AACN Advanced Critical Care, 24*(1), 38–58.

Klompas, M., Speck, K., Howell, M. D., et al. (2014). Reappraisal of routine oral care with chlorhexidine gluconate for patients receiving mechanical ventilation: Systematic review and meta-analysis. *JAMA: The Journal of the American Medical Association, 174,* 751–761.

Kopp, S. L., Ramseier, C. A., Ratka-Krüger, P., et al. (2017). Motivational interviewing as an adjunct to periodontal therapy—A systematic review. *Frontiers in Psychology, 8,* 279. doi:10.3389/fpsyg.2017.00279.

Kuo, Y. W., Yen, M., Fetzer, S., et al. (2013). Toothbrushing versus toothbrushing plus tongue cleaning in reducing halitosis and tongue coating: A systematic review and meta-analysis. *Nursing Research, 62*(6), 422–429.

Le, L. K. D. (2015). *Oral assessment tools: Older adults.* Adelaide, Australia: Joanna Briggs.

Maria, O. M., Eliopoulos, N., & Muanza, T. (2017). Radiation-induced oral mucositis. *Frontiers in Oncology, 7,* 89. doi:10.3389/fonc.2017.00089.

Mohammadi, J. J., Franks, K., & Hines, S. (2015). Effectiveness of professional oral health care intervention on the oral health of residents with dementia in residential aged care facilities: A systematic review protocol. *JBI Database of Systematic Reviews and Implementation Reports, 13*(10), 110–122. doi:10.11124/jbisrir-2015-2330.

Parsons, S., Lee, C. A., Strickert, D., et al. (2013). Oral care and ventilator-associated pneumonia: An integrated review of the literature. *Dimensions of Critical Care Nursing, 3193,* 138–145.

Puntillo, K., Arai, S., Cooper, B., et al. (2014). A randomized clinical trial of an intervention to relieve thirst and dry mouth in intensive care unit patients. *Intensive Care Medicine, 40*(9), 1295–1302. doi:10.1007/s00134-014-3339-z.

Radvansky, L. J., Pace, M. B., & Siddiqui, A. (2013). Prevention and management of radiation-induced dermatitis, mucositis, and xerostomia. *American Journal of Health-System Pharmacy, 70,* 1025–1032.

Rozas, N. S., Sadowsky, J. M., & Jeter, C. B. (2017). Strategies to improve dental health in elderly patients with cognitive impairment: A systematic review: A systematic review. *The Journal of the American Dental Association, 148*(4), 236–245.e233. doi:10.1016/j.adaj.2016.12.022.

Shi, Z., Xie, H., Wang, P., et al. (2013). Oral hygiene care for critically ill patients to prevent ventilator-associated pneumonia. *Cochrane Database of Systematic Reviews,* (8), CD008367.

Slade, S. (2013). *Oral health: manual and powered toothbrushing.* Adelaide, Australia: Joanna Briggs Institute.

Tombes, M. B., & Gallucci, B. (1993). The effects of hydrogen peroxide rinses on the normal oral mucosa. *Nursing Research, 42*(6), 332.

van Der Maarel-Wierink, C. D., Vanobbergen, J. N. O., Bronkhorst, E. M., et al. (2013). Oral health care and aspiration pneumonia in frail older people: A systematic literature review. *Gerodontology, 30*(1), 3. doi:10.1111/j.1741-2358.2012.00637.x.

van Der Waal, I. (2015). Oral leukoplakia, the ongoing discussion on definition and terminology. *Medicina Oral, Patología Oral y Cirugía Bucal, 20*(6), e685. doi:10.4317/medoral.21007.

Villa, A., Wolff, A., Aframian, D., et al. (2015). World Workshop on Oral Medicine VI: A systematic review of medication-induced salivary gland dysfunction: Prevalence, diagnosis, and treatment. *Clinical Oral Investigations, 19*(7), 1563–1580. doi:10.1007/s00784-015-1488-2.

Williams, K., Shaw, C., Lee, A., et al. (2017). Voicing ageism in nursing home dementia care. *Journal of Gerontological Nursing, 43*(9), 16. doi:10.3928/00989134-20170523-02.

Xue, Y. (2015). *Ventilator associated pneumonia: oral hygiene care.* Adelaide, Australia: Joanna Briggs Institute.

Yaacob, M., Worthington, H. V., Deacon, S. A., et al. (2014). Powered versus manual toothbrushing for oral health. *The Cochrane Database of Systematic Reviews,* (6), CD002281.

Zanelli, M., Ragazzi, M., & De Marco, L. (2017). Chemical gastritis and colitis related to hydrogen peroxide mouthwash. *British Journal of Clinical Pharmacology, 83*(2), 427–428. doi:10.1111/bcp.13100.

Risk for impaired Oral Mucous Membrane integrity
Mary Beth Flynn Makic, PhD, RN, CCNS, FAAN, FNAP

NANDA-I

Definition

Susceptible to injury to the lips, soft tissues, buccal cavity, and/or oropharynx, which may compromise health.

Risk Factors

Alcohol consumption; barrier to dental care; barrier to oral self-care; chemical injury agent; decrease in salivation; dehydration; depression; inadequate nutrition; inadequate oral hygiene; insufficient knowledge of oral hygiene; malnutrition; mouth breathing; smoking; stressors

At-Risk Population

Economically disadvantaged

Associated Condition

Allergy; alteration in cognitive functioning; autoimmune disease; autosomal disorder; behavioral disorder; chemotherapy; cleft lip; cleft palate; decrease in hormone level in women; decrease in platelets; immunodeficiency; immunosuppression; infection; loss of oral support structure; mechanical factor; Nil per os (NPO) >24 hours; oral trauma; radiation therapy; surgical procedure; Sjogren's syndrome; trauma; treatment regimen

NIC, Client Outcomes, Nursing Interventions and *Rationales,* Client/Family Teaching, and References

Refer to care plan for Impaired **Oral Mucous Membrane** integrity.

O

Obesity   *Marina Martinez-Kratz, MS, RN, CNE*

NANDA-I

Definition

A condition in which an individual accumulates excessive fat for age and gender that exceeds overweight.

Defining Characteristics

Adult: Body mass index (BMI) >30 kg/m^2; Child <2 years: term not used with children at this age; Child 2 to 18 years: BMI >30 kg/m^2 or >95th percentile or 30 kg/m^2 for age and gender

Related Factors

Average daily physical activity is less than recommended for gender and age; consumption of sugar-sweetened beverages; disordered eating behaviors; disordered eating perceptions; energy expenditure below energy intake based on standard assessment; excessive alcohol consumption; fear regarding lack of food supply; frequent snacking; high frequency of eating restaurant or fried food; low dietary calcium intake in children; portion sizes larger than recommended; sedentary behavior occurring for ≥2 hours/day; shortened sleep time; sleep disorder; solid foods as major food source at >5 months of age

At-Risk Population

Economically disadvantaged; formula- or mixed-fed infants; heritability of interrelated factors; high disinhibition and restraint eating behavior score; maternal diabetes mellitus; maternal smoking; overweight in infancy; paternal obesity; premature pubarche; rapid weight gain during childhood; rapid weight gain during infancy, including the first week, first 4 months, and first year

Associated Condition

Genetic disorder

● = Independent;   ▲ = Collaborative;   EBN = Evidence-Based Nursing;   EB = Evidence-Based

NOC   (Nursing Outcomes Classification)

Suggested NOC Outcomes

Nutritional Status; Nutritional Status: Food and Fluid Intake; Nutrient Intake; Weight Control

> **Example NOC Outcome with Indicators**
>
> **Nutritional Status** as evidenced by the following indicators: Food and fluid intake/Hydration/Body mass index/Weight-height ratio/Hematocrit. (Rate the outcome and indicators of **Nutritional Status:** 1 = severe deviation from normal range, 2 = substantial deviation from normal range, 3 = moderate deviation from normal range, 4 = mild deviation from normal range, 5 = no deviation from normal range [see Section I].)

Client Outcomes

Client Will (Specify Time Frame)

- Explain how to eat according to the US Dietary Guidelines
- Design dietary modifications to meet individual long-term goal of health, using principles of variety, balance, and moderation
- Maintain weight within normal range for height and age

NIC   (Nursing Interventions Classification)

Suggested NIC Interventions

Nutrition Management; Nutritional Counseling; Weight Reduction Assistance

> **Example NIC Activities—Nutrition Management**
>
> Determine the client's motivation for changing eating habits; Develop with the client a method to keep a daily record of intake

Nursing Interventions and *Rationales*

- Assess the meaning and importance of food in the client's life. EB: *Recent research found strong associations between the different domains of food meanings and behavioral outcomes (Arbit et al, 2017).*
- Assess client readiness to determine whether the client is ready to discuss weight loss and/or would like weight loss information. EB: *Client motivation is a key component of success in a weight loss program and a prerequisite for weight loss therapy (Raynor & Champagne, 2016).*
- Use a motivational interviewing technique when working with clients to promote healthy eating and weight loss. EB: *Research shows significant weight loss for clients when motivational interviewing techniques were used (Barnes et al, 2018).*
- Counsel the client to measure regularly consumed foods periodically. Help the client learn usual portion sizes. Measuring food alerts the client to normal portion sizes. Estimating amounts can be extremely inaccurate. EB: *A randomized controlled trial of 278 overweight and obese participants was conducted to increase portion size awareness with results that demonstrated the intervention improved portion control behavior and in turn influenced BMI (Poelman et al, 2015).*
- Assist the client to develop a system of self-management, which may include self-monitoring of weight and BMI; realistic goal setting, planning, and action planning for improved dietary intake and physical activity; problem-solving; and tracking dietary intake and exercise. EB: *A key component of successful weight loss and maintenance is regular self-monitoring (Thomason et al, 2016).*
- Document the client's height and weight and teach the significance of his or her BMI in relationship to current health. Use a chart or a website such as http://www.cdc.gov/healthyweight/assessing/bmi/index.html (Centers for Disease Control and Prevention [CDC], 2015). EB: *Successful treatment of overweight and obesity in adults requires adoption and maintenance of effective self-monitoring (Raynor & Champagne, 2016).*
- Encourage the client to engage in vigorous-intensity physical activity for at least 150 minutes weekly or moderate-intensity physical activity for at least 300 minutes weekly. EB: *Research evidence suggested that regular physical activity is critical for weight loss and weight loss maintenance (Ostendorf et al, 2018).*

● = Independent;   ▲ = Collaborative;   EBN = Evidence-Based Nursing;   EB = Evidence-Based

- Recommend that the client avoid eating in fast-food restaurants. CEB: *A 15-year study demonstrated that people who frequently eat fast foods gain an average of 10 pounds more than those who eat fast food less often and were two times more likely to develop insulin resistance, which can lead to diabetes (Pereira et al, 2005).*
- Assist the client to reframe slips in weight loss or physical activity behavior as lapses that are a single event and not a full return to previous unhealthy behaviors. Relapse prevention strategies include managing lapses in healthy behavior, identifying high-risk situations for relapses, self-monitoring, providing social support, enhancing skills for coping, and increasing self-efficacy for avoiding relapse. EB: *A study of a weight maintenance intervention, delivered primarily by telephone, modestly slowed the rate of weight regain (Voils et al, 2017).*
- Assist clients to engage their social support systems either digitally or face to face in ways that facilitate weight loss, healthy eating, and physical activity behavior change. EB: *Significant others, family, friends, and coworkers can facilitate or hinder weight loss success (Romo, 2018).*
- Assist the client to reframe the goal from a focus on outcome (weight loss) to a focus on process (eating behaviors) for weight loss. EB: *A study showed that there were self-regulatory benefits from mental simulations used in the weight loss process (Marszał-Wiśniewska & Jarczewska-Gerc, 2014).*
- Assist the client to implement informal and formal mindfulness-based interventions (MBIs). Informal MBIs include mindful eating, increasing awareness of hunger and satiety cues, taste satisfaction, and decreasing impulsive tendencies to overeat when experiencing negative emotions. Meditation practice is a formal MBI. EB: *Results of a research review suggested that a combination of formal and informal MBIs are effective in reducing weight and improving obesity-related eating behaviors among individuals with overweight and obesity (Carrière et al, 2018).*
- Assist the client to develop stimulus control techniques designed to reduce environmental cues associated with eating behaviors. Specifically clients should be taught to limit the presence of high-calorie/high-fat foods in the home; to reduce the visibility of unhealthy food choices in the home; to limit where and when they eat; to avoid distractions like reading, using the computer, or watching television when eating; and to eat more slowly. EB: *Stimulus control strategies are a key to successful weight loss and weight maintenance in conjunction with other weight loss strategies (Butryn et al, 2017).*
- Encourage 7.5 to 8.5 hours of sleep nightly. EB: *Recent evidence suggested weight management is hindered when attempted in the context of sleep restriction because there is an upregulation of reward, pleasure, and salience networks in response to food stimuli (St-Onge, 2017).*
- Refer the client to a weight-loss–related therapy group. EBN: *A study found there were significant changes in BMI, waist circumference, body fat percentage, and strength of the lower limbs for weight-loss group therapy participants (Ferrari et al, 2017).*
- *Recommend that clients use dietary supplements such as vitamins and minerals after consulting with their primary health care provider.* EB: *Research shows micronutrient deficits are prevalent in weight-loss plans, especially vitamin B_{12}, calcium, and vitamin D (Engel et al, 2018).*
- Incorporate the following recommendations from the Academy of Nutrition and Dietetics: Interventions for the Treatment of Overweight and Obesity in Adults (Raynor & Champagne, 2016):
  - Assess food- and nutrition-related history; anthropometric measures; biochemical data, medical tests, and procedures; nutrition-focused physical findings; and client history.
  - Assess the energy intake and nutrient content of the diet.
  - Use height and weight to calculate BMI; and waist circumference to determine risk of cardiovascular disease (CVD), type 2 diabetes, and all-cause mortality.
  - Use a measured resting metabolic rate (RMR) to determine energy needs.
  - Set a realistic weight-loss goal such as one of the following: up to 2 pounds/week, up to 10% of baseline body weight, or a total of 3% to 5% of baseline weight if cardiovascular risk factors (hypertension, hyperlipidemia, and hyperglycemia) are present.
  - To achieve weight loss, use an individualized diet, including patient preferences and health status, to achieve and maintain nutrient adequacy and reduce caloric intake, based on one of the following caloric reduction strategies: 1200 to 1500 kcal/day for women and 1500 to 1800 kcal/day for men, with an energy deficit of approximately 500 or 750 kcal/day.

Pediatric

- Offer obese or overweight adolescents healthy methods for weight loss. EB: *A recent study showed statistically significant health behavior improvements after implementing a developmentally informed intervention to increase positive health diet and exercise behaviors (Issner et al, 2017).*

● = Independent;   ▲ = Collaborative;   EBN = Evidence-Based Nursing;   EB = Evidence-Based

- Offer families of obese or overweight children prejudice-free, individually accepting, and supportive interventions to address weight loss. EBN: *Obese children treated with motivational interviewing showed significant improvement in their weight-related behavior and obesity-related anthropometric measures (Wong & Cheng, 2013).*
- Recommend that families eat together for at least one meal per day. EB: *Findings from a review provide clear evidence that family meals (among youth) and shared meals (among adults) are associated with better dietary intake, and that these findings transcend the life span (Fulkerson et al, 2014).*
- Recommend involving the family in planning meals and food preparation. Children can learn about nutrition as they help plan and make meals. EB: *The Healthy Home Offerings via the Mealtime Environment Plus program showed increased cooking skills among the children participating (Fulkerson et al, 2018).*
- Assist parents at being good role models of healthy eating. EB: *The Healthy Home Offerings via the Mealtime Environment Plus program showed significantly improved parental self-efficacy for identifying appropriate portion sizes (Fulkerson et al, 2018).*
- Recommend that the family try new foods, either a new food or recipe every week. EB: *The Healthy Home Offerings via the Mealtime Environment Plus program showed decreasing child neophobia scores over time that were developmentally appropriate (Fulkerson et al, 2018).*

 ### Geriatric

- Determine the risks and benefits of weight loss in the older client. A BMI greater than 30 in the older client suggests a moderate weight loss approach. EB: *Recommendations for treating obesity in the elderly include ensuring a balanced and appropriately distributed intake of high-quality nutrients, particularly of high-quality protein (i.e., 1.2 to 1.5 g/kg of body weight), limiting the intake of simple carbohydrates and saturated fats, providing sufficient intake of calcium and vitamin D_3 (Blaz, 2016).*
- Observe for social, psychological, and economic factors that influence diet quality. EB: *An exploratory study of diet quality influences in community-dwelling older individuals revealed the following influences: food experiences, retirement, bereavement, medical conditions, food environment, food-related habits, social engagement, personal/psychological factors, and transportation (Bloom et al, 2017).*

 ### Multicultural

- Tailor nutritional interventions to be consistent with cultural beliefs, norms, and values. EB: *A systemic review of culturally tailored interventions for Hispanic women included literacy modification, Hispanic foods/recipes, cultural diabetes beliefs, family/friend participation, structured community input, and innovative experiential learning (McCurley et al, 2016).*
- Offer tailored lifestyle counseling via the telephone. EBN: *Investigators have included biweekly and/or monthly health coach calls for African American participants with significant weight gain prevention (Goode et al, 2017).*
- Integrate weight loss and weight maintenance interventions with church faith-based concepts for cultural congruence with African American clients. EB: *Recent research suggested that integrating faith themes into a weight loss maintenance program may increase its long-term effect on participants' health behavior change (Seale et al, 2013).*

 ### Client/Family Teaching and Discharge Planning

- The majority of the preceding interventions involve teaching.
- Work with the family members regarding information on how to support and promote weight loss and healthy intakes.

REFERENCES

Arbit, N., et al. (2017). Development and validation of the meaning of food in life questionnaire (MFLQ): Evidence for a new construct to explain eating behavior. *Food Quality and Preference, 59*, 35–45. Retrieved from http://doi.org.proxy.lib.umich.edu/10.1016/j.foodqual.2017.02.002.

Barnes, R. D., et al. (2018). Examining motivational interviewing plus nutrition psychoeducation for weight loss in primary care. *Journal of Psychosomatic Research, 104*, 101–107. Retrieved from http://doi.org.proxy.lib.umich.edu/10.1016/j.jpsychores.2017.11.013.

Blaz, M. K. (2016). Obesity in the elderly, weight loss yes or no? *Clinical Nutrition ESPEN, 14*, 56. Retrieved from http://doi.org.proxy.lib.umich.edu/10.1016/j.clnesp.2016.04.025.

Bloom, I., et al. (2017). What influences diet quality in older people? A qualitative study among community-dwelling older adults from the Hertfordshire Cohort Study, UK. *Public Health Nutrition, 20*(15), 2685–2693. doi:10.1017/S1368980017001203.

Butryn, M. L., et al. (2017). Efficacy of environmental and acceptance-based enhancements to behavioral weight loss treatment: The ENACT trial. *Obesity, 25*(5), 866–872. doi:10.1002/oby.21813.

Carrière, K., et al. (2018). Mindfulness-based interventions for weight loss: A systematic review and meta-analysis. *Obesity Reviews, 19*(2), 164–177. doi:10.1111/obr.12623.

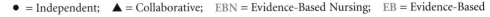 ● = Independent;   ▲ = Collaborative;   EBN = Evidence-Based Nursing;   EB = Evidence-Based

Centers for Disease Control and Prevention (2015). *Healthy weight— It's not a diet, it's a lifestyle!* Retrieved from http://www.cdc.gov/healthyweight/assessing/bmi/index.html. (Accessed 21 June 2015).

Engel, M. G., et al. (2018). Micronutrient gaps in three commercial weight-loss diet plans. *Nutrients, 10*(1), 108. Retrieved from http://doi.org.proxy.lib.umich.edu/10.3390/nu10010108.

Ferrari, G. D., et al. (2017). A multidisciplinary weight-loss program: The importance of psychological group therapy. *Motriz: Revista de Educacao Fisica, 23*(1), 47–52. doi:10.1590/s1980-6574201700010007.

Fulkerson, J. A., et al. (2018). Family home food environment and nutrition-related parent and child personal and behavioral outcomes of the healthy Home Offerings via the Mealtime Environment (HOME) Plus program: A randomized controlled trial. *Journal of the Academy of Nutrition and Dietetics, 118*(2), 240–251. Retrieved from http://doi.org.proxy.lib.umich.edu/10.1016/j.jand.2017.04.006.

Fulkerson, J. A., et al. (2014). A review of associations between family or shared meal frequency and dietary and weight status outcomes across the lifespan. *Journal of Nutrition Education and Behavior, 46*(1), 2–19. Retrieved from http://doi.org.proxy.lib.umich.edu/10.1016/j.jneb.2013.07.012.

Goode, R. W., et al. (2017). African Americans in standard behavioral treatment for obesity, 2001–2015: What have we learned? *Western Journal of Nursing Research, 39*(8), 1045–1069. Retrieved from http://doi.org.proxy.lib.umich.edu/10.1177/0193945917692115.

Issner, J. H., et al. (2017). Increasing positive health behaviors in adolescents with nutritional goals and exercise. *Journal of Child and Family Studies, 26*(2), 548–558. Retrieved from http://doi.org.proxy.lib.umich.edu/10.1007/s10826-016-0585-4.

Marszał-Wiśniewska, M., & Jarczewska-Gerc, E. (2014). Role of mental simulations in the weight loss process. *The Journal of Psychology, 150*(1), 1–14. doi:10.1080/00223980.2014.987102.

McCurley, J. L., et al. (2016). Diabetes prevention in U.S. Hispanic adults: A systematic review of culturally tailored interventions. *American Journal of Preventive Medicine, 52*(4), 519–529. Retrieved from http://doi.org.proxy.lib.umich.edu/10.1016/j.amepre.2016.10.028.

Ostendorf, D. M., et al. (2018). Objectively measured physical activity and sedentary behavior in successful weight loss maintainers. *Obesity, 26*(1), 53–60. doi:10.1002/oby.22052.

Pereira, M., et al. (2005). Fast-food habits, weight gain, and insulin resistance (the CARDIA study): 15-year prospective analysis. *Lancet, 365*(9453), 36–42.

Poelman, M. P., et al. (2015). PortionControl@HOME: Results of a randomized controlled trial evaluating the effect of a multi-component portion size intervention on portion control behavior and body mass index. *Annals of Behavioral Medicine, 49*(1), 18–28. Retrieved from http://doi.org.proxy.lib.umich.edu/10.1007/s12160-014-9637-4.

Raynor, H. A., & Champagne, C. M. (2016). Position of the academy of nutrition and dietetics: Interventions for the treatment of overweight and obesity in adults. *Journal of the Academy of Nutrition and Dietetics, 116*(1), 129–147.

Romo, L. K. (2018). An examination of how people who have lost weight communicatively negotiate interpersonal challenges to weight management, health communication. *Health Communication, 33*(4), 469–477. doi:10.1080/10410236.2016.1278497.

Seale, J. P., Fifield, J., Davis-Smith, Y. M., et al. (2013). Developing culturally congruent weight maintenance programs for African American church members. *Ethnicity & Health, 18*(2), 152–167.

St-Onge, M. P. (2017). Sleep-obesity relation: Underlying mechanisms and consequences for treatment. *Obesity Reviews, 18*(S1), 34–39. doi:10.1111/obr.12499.

Thomason, D. L., et al. (2016). A systematic review of adolescent self-management and weight loss. *Journal of Pediatric Health Care, 30*(6), 569–582. Retrieved from http://doi.org.proxy.lib.umich.edu/10.1016/j.pedhc.2015.11.016.

Voils, C. I., et al. (2017). Maintenance of weight loss after initiation of nutrition training: A randomized trial. *Annals of Internal Medicine, 166*(7), 463–471. doi:10.7326/M16-2160.

Wong, E. M., & Cheng, M. M. (2013). Effects of motivational interviewing to promote weight loss in obese children. *Journal of Clinical Nursing, 22*(17/18), 2519–2530.

Overweight   *Marina Martinez-Kratz, MS, RN, CNE*

NANDA-I

Definition

A condition in which an individual accumulates abnormal or excessive fat for age and gender.

Defining Characteristics

Adult: Body mass index (BMI) >25 kg/m^2; Child <2 years: Weight-for-length >95th percentile; Child 2 to 18 years: BMI >85th percentile or 25 kg/m^2 but <95th percentile or 30 kg/m^2 for age and gender

Related Factors

Average daily physical activity is less than recommended for gender and age; consumption of sugar-sweetened beverages; disordered eating behaviors disordered eating perceptions; energy expenditure below energy intake based on standard assessment; excessive alcohol consumption; fear regarding lack of food supply; frequent snacking; high frequency of restaurant or fried food; insufficient knowledge of modifiable factors; low dietary calcium intake in children; portion sizes larger than recommended; sedentary behavior occurring for >2 hours/day; shortened sleep time; sleep disorder; solid foods as major food source of <5 months of age

● = Independent;   ▲ = Collaborative;   EBN = Evidence-Based Nursing;   EB = Evidence-Based

At-Risk Population

Adult: BMI approaching 25 kg/m²; Child <2 years: Weight-for-length approaching 95th percentile; Child 2 to 18 years: BMI approaching 85th percentile or 25 kg/m²; children who are crossing BMI percentiles upward; children with high BMI percentiles; economically disadvantaged; formula-fed or mixed-fed infants; heritability of interrelated factors; high disinhibition and restraint eating behavior score; maternal diabetes mellitus; maternal smoking; obesity in childhood; paternal obesity; premature pubarche; rapid weight gain during childhood; rapid weight gain during infancy, including the first week, first 4 months, and first year

NOC   (Nursing Outcomes Classification)

Suggested NOC Outcomes

Nutritional Status; Nutritional Status: Food and Fluid Intake; Nutrient Intake; Weight Control

Example NOC Outcome with Indicators
Nutritional Status as evidenced by the following indicators: Food and fluid intake/Hydration/Body mass index/Weight-height ratio/Hematocrit. (Rate the outcome and indicators of **Nutritional Status:** 1 = severe deviation from normal range, 2 = substantial deviation from normal range, 3 = moderate deviation from normal range, 4 = mild deviation from normal range, 5 = no deviation from normal range [see Section I].)

Client Outcomes

Client Will (Specify Time Frame)

- Explain how to eat according to the US Dietary Guidelines
- Design dietary modifications to meet individual long-term goal of health, using principles of variety, balance, and moderation
- Maintain weight within normal range for height and age

NIC   (Nursing Interventions Classification)

Suggested NIC Interventions

Nutrition Management; Nutritional Counseling; Weight Reduction Assistance

Example NIC Activities—Nutrition Management
Determine the client's motivation for changing eating habits; Develop with the client a method to keep a daily record of intake

Nursing Interventions and *Rationales*

- Assess the meaning and importance of food in the client's life. EB: *Recent research found strong associations between the different domains of food meanings and behavioral outcomes (Arbit et al, 2017).*
- Assess client readiness to determine whether the client is ready to discuss weight loss and/or would like weight-loss information. EB: *Client motivation is a key component of success in a weight-loss program and a prerequisite for weight-loss therapy (Raynor & Champagne, 2016).*
- Use a motivational interviewing technique when working with clients to promote healthy eating and weight loss. EB: *Research shows significant weight loss for clients when motivational interviewing techniques were used (Barnes et al, 2018).*
- Counsel the client to measure regularly consumed foods periodically. Help the client learn usual portion sizes. Measuring food alerts the client to normal portion sizes. Estimating amounts can be extremely inaccurate. EB: *A randomized controlled trial of 278 overweight and obese participants was conducted to increase portion size awareness with results that demonstrated the intervention improved portion control behavior and in turn influenced BMI (Poelman et al, 2015).*
- Assist the client to develop a system of self-management, which may include self-monitoring of weight and BMI; realistic goal setting, planning, and action planning for improved dietary intake and physical activity; problem-solving; and tracking dietary intake and exercise. EB: *A key component of successful weight loss and maintenance is regular self-monitoring (Thomason et al, 2016).*

● = Independent;   ▲ = Collaborative;   EBN = Evidence-Based Nursing;   EB = Evidence-Based

- Document the client's height and weight and teach the significance of his or her BMI in relationship to current health. Use a chart or a website such as http://www.cdc.gov/healthyweight/assessing/bmi/index.html (Centers for Disease Control and Prevention [CDC], 2015). **EB:** *Successful treatment of overweight and obesity in adults requires the adoption and maintenance of effective self-monitoring (Raynor & Champagne, 2016).*

- Encourage the client to engage in vigorous-intensity physical activity for at least 150 minutes weekly or moderate-intensity physical activity for at least 300 minutes weekly. **EB:** *Research evidence suggests that regular physical activity is critical for weight loss and weight-loss maintenance (Ostendorf et al, 2018).*

- Recommend the client avoid eating in fast-food restaurants. **CEB:** *A 15-year study demonstrated that people who frequently eat fast foods gain an average of 10 pounds more than those who eat fast food less often and were two times more likely to develop insulin resistance, which can lead to diabetes (Pereira et al, 2005).*

- Assist the client to reframe slips in weight loss or physical activity behavior as lapses that are a single event and not a full return to previous unhealthy behaviors. Relapse prevention strategies include managing lapses in healthy behavior, identifying high-risk situations for relapses, self-monitoring, providing social support, enhancing skills for coping, and increasing self-efficacy for avoiding relapse. **EB:** *A study of a weight maintenance intervention, delivered primarily by telephone, modestly slowed the rate of weight regain (Voils et al, 2017).*

- Assist clients to engage their social support systems either digitally or face to face in ways that facilitate weight loss, healthy eating, and physical activity behavior change. **EB:** *Significant others, family, friends, and coworkers can facilitate or hinder weight-loss success (Romo, 2018).*

- Assist the client to reframe the goal from a focus on outcome (weight loss) to a focus on process (eating behaviors) for weight loss. **EB:** *A study showed that there were self-regulatory benefits from mental simulations used in the weight-loss process (Marszał-Wiśniewska & Jarczewska-Gerc, 2014).*

- Assist the client to implement informal and formal mindfulness-based interventions (MBIs). Informal MBIs include mindful eating, increasing awareness of hunger and satiety cues, taste satisfaction, and decreasing impulsive tendencies to overeat when experiencing negative emotions. Meditation practice is a formal MBI. **EB:** *Results of a research review suggest that a combination of formal and informal MBIs are effective in reducing weight and improving obesity-related eating behaviors among individuals with overweight and obesity (Carrière et al, 2018).*

- Assist the client to develop stimulus control techniques designed to reduce environmental cues associated with eating behaviors. Specifically clients should be taught to limit the presence of high-calorie/high-fat foods in the home; to reduce the visibility of unhealthy food choices in the home; to limit where and when they eat; to avoid distractions like reading, using the computer, or watching television when eating; and to eat more slowly. **EB:** *Stimulus control strategies are the key to successful weight loss and weight maintenance in conjunction with other weight-loss strategies (Butryn et al, 2017.*

- Encourage 7.5 to 8.5 hours of sleep nightly. **EB:** *Recent evidence suggests weight management is hindered when attempted in the context of sleep restriction because there is an upregulation of reward, pleasure, and salience networks in response to food stimuli (St-Onge, 2017).*

- Refer the client to a weight-loss–related therapy group. **EBN:** *A study found there were significant changes in BMI, waist circumference, body fat percentage, and strength of the lower limbs for weight-loss group therapy participants (Ferrari et al, 2017).*

- Recommend that clients use dietary supplements such as vitamins and minerals after consulting with their primary health care provider. **EB:** *Research shows micronutrient deficits are prevalent in weight-loss plans, especially vitamin B_{12}, calcium, and vitamin D (Engel et al, 2018).*

- Incorporate the following recommendations from the Academy of Nutrition and Dietetics: Interventions for the Treatment of Overweight and Obesity in Adults (Raynor & Champagne, 2016):
  - Assess food- and nutrition-related history; anthropometric measures; biochemical data, medical tests, and procedures; nutrition-focused physical findings; and client history.
  - Assess the energy intake and nutrient content of the diet.
  - Use height and weight to calculate BMI and waist circumference to determine risk of cardiovascular disease (CVD), type 2 diabetes, and all-cause mortality.
  - Use a measured resting metabolic rate (RMR) to determine energy needs.
  - Set a realistic weight-loss goal such as one of the following: up to 2 pounds/week, up to 10% of baseline body weight, or a total of 3% to 5% of baseline weight if cardiovascular risk factors (hypertension, hyperlipidemia, and hyperglycemia) are present.

● = Independent;   ▲ = Collaborative;   EBN = Evidence-Based Nursing;   EB = Evidence-Based

○ To achieve weight loss, use an individualized diet, including patient preferences and health status, to achieve and maintain nutrient adequacy and reduce caloric intake, based on one of the following caloric reduction strategies: 1200 to 1500 kcal/day for women and 1500 to 1800 kcal/day for men, and energy deficit of approximately 500 or 750 kcal/day.

Pediatric

- Offer obese or overweight adolescents healthy methods for weight loss. **EB:** A recent study showed statistically significant health behavior improvements after implementing a developmentally informed intervention to increase positive health diet and exercise behaviors (Issner et al, 2017).
- Offer families of obese or overweight children prejudice-free, individually accepting, and supportive interventions to address weight loss. **EBN:** *Obese children treated with motivational interviewing showed significant improvement in their weight-related behavior and obesity-related anthropometric measures (Wong & Cheng, 2013).*
- Recommend that families eat together for at least one meal per day. **EB:** *Findings from a review provide clear evidence that family meals (among youth) and shared meals (among adults) are associated with better dietary intake and that these findings transcend the life span (Fulkerson et al, 2014).*
- Recommend involving the family in planning meals and food preparation. Children can learn about nutrition as they help plan and make meals. **EB:** *The Healthy Home Offerings via the Mealtime Environment Plus program showed increased cooking skills among the children participating (Fulkerson et al, 2018).*
- Assist parents at being good role models of healthy eating. **EB:** The Healthy Home Offerings via the Mealtime Environment Plus program showed significantly improved parental self-efficacy for identifying appropriate portion sizes *(Fulkerson et al, 2018).*
- Recommend that the family try new foods, either a new food or recipe every week. **EB:** *The Healthy Home Offerings via the Mealtime Environment Plus program showed decreasing child neophobia scores over time that were developmentally appropriate (Fulkerson et al, 2018).*

Geriatric

- Determine the risks and benefits of weight loss in the older client. A BMI greater than 30 in the older client suggests a moderate weight-loss approach. **EB:** *Recommendations for treating obesity in the elderly include ensuring a balanced and appropriately distributed intake of high-quality nutrients, particularly of high-quality protein (i.e., 1.2 to 1.5 g/kg of body weight), limiting the intake of simple carbohydrates and saturated fats, and providing sufficient intake of calcium and vitamin D_3 (Blaz, 2016).*
- Observe for social, psychological, and economic factors that influence diet quality. **EB:** *An exploratory study of diet quality influences in community-dwelling older individuals revealed the following influences: food experiences, retirement, bereavement, medical conditions, food environment, food-related habits, social engagement, personal/psychological factors, and transportation (Bloom et al, 2017).*

Multicultural

- Tailor nutritional interventions to be consistent with cultural beliefs, norms, and values. **EB:** *A systemic review of culturally tailored interventions for Hispanic women included literacy modification, Hispanic foods/recipes, cultural diabetes beliefs, family/friend participation, structured community input, and innovative experiential learning (McCurley et al, 2016).*
- Offer tailored lifestyle counseling via the telephone. **EBN:** *Investigators have included biweekly and/or monthly health coach calls for African American participants with significant weight gain prevention (Goode et al, 2017).*
- Integrate weight loss and weight maintenance interventions with church faith-based concepts for cultural congruence with African American clients. **EB:** *Recent research suggested that integrating faith themes into a weight-loss maintenance program may increase its long-term effect on participants' health behavior change (Seale et al, 2013).*

Client/Family Teaching and Discharge Planning

- The majority of the preceding interventions involve teaching.
- Work with the family members regarding information on how to support and promote weight loss and healthy intakes.

● = Independent;   ▲ = Collaborative;   **EBN** = Evidence-Based Nursing;   **EB** = Evidence-Based

REFERENCES

Arbit, N., et al. (2017). Development and validation of the meaning of food in life questionnaire (MFLQ): Evidence for a new construct to explain eating behavior. *Food Quality and Preference*, 59, 35–45. Retrieved from http://doi.org.proxy.lib.umich.edu/10.1016/j.foodqual.2017.02.002.

Barnes, R. D., et al. (2018). Examining motivational interviewing plus nutrition psychoeducation for weight loss in primary care. *Journal of Psychosomatic Research*, 104, 101–107. Retrieved from http://doi.org.proxy.lib.umich.edu/10.1016/j.jpsychores.2017.11.013.

Blaz, M. K. (2016). Obesity in the elderly, weight loss yes or no? *Clinical Nutrition ESPEN*, 14, 56. Retrieved from http://doi.org.proxy.lib.umich.edu/10.1016/j.clnesp.2016.04.025.

Bloom, I., et al. (2017). What influences diet quality in older people? A qualitative study among community-dwelling older adults from the Hertfordshire Cohort Study, UK. *Public Health Nutrition*, 20(15), 2685–2693. doi:10.1017/S1368980017001203.

Butryn, M. L., et al. (2017). Efficacy of environmental and acceptance-based enhancements to behavioral weight loss treatment: the ENACT trial. *Obesity*, 25(5), 866–872. doi:10.1002/oby.21813.

Carrière, K., et al. (2018). Mindfulness-based interventions for weight loss: A systematic review and meta-analysis. *Obesity Reviews*, 19(2), 164–177. doi:10.1111/obr.12623.

Centers for Disease Control and Prevention (2015). *Healthy weight—It's not a diet, it's a lifestyle!* Retrieved from http://www.cdc.gov/healthyweight/assessing/bmi/index.html. (Accessed 21 June 2015).

Engel, M. G., et al. (2018). Micronutrient gaps in three commercial weight-loss diet plans. *Nutrients*, 10(1), 108. Retrieved from http://doi.org.proxy.lib.umich.edu/10.3390/nu10010108.

Ferrari, G. D., et al. (2017). A multidisciplinary weight-loss program: The importance of psychological group therapy. *Motriz: Revista de Educacao Fisica*, 23(1), 47–52. doi:10.1590/s1980-6574201700010007.

Fulkerson, J. A., et al. (2018). Family home food environment and nutrition-related parent and child personal and behavioral outcomes of the healthy Home Offerings via the Mealtime Environment (HOME) Plus program: A randomized controlled trial. *Journal of the Academy of Nutrition and Dietetics*, 118(2), 240–251. Retrieved from http://doi.org.proxy.lib.umich.edu/10.1016/j.jand.2017.04.006.

Fulkerson, J. A., et al. (2014). A review of associations between family or shared meal frequency and dietary and weight status outcomes across the lifespan. *Journal of Nutrition Education and Behavior*, 46(1), 2–19. Retrieved from http://doi.org.proxy.lib.umich.edu/10.1016/j.jneb.2013.07.012.

Goode, R. W., et al. (2017). African Americans in standard behavioral treatment for obesity, 2001–2015: What have we learned? *Western Journal of Nursing Research*, 39(8), 1045–1069. Retrieved from http://doi.org.proxy.lib.umich.edu/10.1177/0193945917692115.

Issner, J. H., et al. (2017). Increasing positive health behaviors in adolescents with nutritional goals and exercise. *Journal of Child and Family Studies*, 26(2), 548–558. Retrieved from http://doi.org.proxy.lib.umich.edu/10.1007/s10826-016-0585-4.

Marszał-Wiśniewska, M., & Jarczewska-Gerc, E. (2014). Role of mental simulations in the weight loss process. *The Journal of Psychology*, 150(1), 1–14. doi:10.1080/00223980.2014.987102.

McCurley, J. L., et al. (2016). Diabetes prevention in U.S. Hispanic adults: A systematic review of culturally tailored interventions. *American Journal of Preventive Medicine*, 52(4), 519–529. Retrieved from http://doi.org.proxy.lib.umich.edu/10.1016/j.amepre.2016.10.028.

Ostendorf, D. M., et al. (2018). Objectively measured physical activity and sedentary behavior in successful weight loss maintainers. *Obesity*, 26(1), 53–60. doi:10.1002/oby.22052.

Pereira, M., et al. (2005). Fast-food habits, weight gain, and insulin resistance (the CARDIA study): 15-year prospective analysis. *Lancet*, 365(9453), 36–42.

Poelman, M. P., et al. (2015). PortionControl@HOME: Results of a randomized controlled trial evaluating the effect of a multi-component portion size intervention on portion control behavior and body mass index. *Annals of Behavioral Medicine*, 49(1), 18–28. Retrieved from http://doi.org.proxy.lib.umich.edu/10.1007/s12160-014-9637-4.

Raynor, H. A., & Champagne, C. M. (2016). Position of the academy of nutrition and dietetics: Interventions for the treatment of overweight and obesity in adults. *Journal of the Academy of Nutrition and Dietetics*, 116(1), 129–147.

Romo, L. K. (2018). An examination of how people who have lost weight communicatively negotiate interpersonal challenges to weight management. *health communication*. *Health Communication*, 33(4), 469–477. doi:10.1080/10410236.2016.1278497.

Seale, J. P., Fifield, J., Davis-Smith, Y. M., et al. (2013). Developing culturally congruent weight maintenance programs for African American church members. *Ethnicity & Health*, 18(2), 152–167.

St-Onge, M.-P. (2017). Sleep-obesity relation: Underlying mechanisms and consequences for treatment. *Obesity Reviews*, 18(S1), 34–39. doi:10.1111/obr.12499.

Thomason, D. L., et al. (2016). A systematic review of adolescent self-management and weight loss. *Journal of Pediatric Health Care*, 30(6), 569–582. Retrieved from http://doi.org.proxy.lib.umich.edu/10.1016/j.pedhc.2015.11.016.

Voils, C. I., et al. (2017). Maintenance of weight loss after initiation of nutrition training: A randomized trial. *Annals of Internal Medicine*, 166(7), 463–471. doi:10.7326/M16-2160.

Wong, E. M., & Cheng, M. M. (2013). Effects of motivational interviewing to promote weight loss in obese children. *Journal of Clinical Nursing*, 22(17/18), 2519–2530.

Risk for Overweight* *Marina Martinez-Kratz, MS, RN, CNE*

*Previously Risk for Imbalanced Nutrition: more than body requirements.

NANDA-I

Definition

Susceptible to excessive fat accumulation for age and gender, which may compromise health.

Risk Factors

Average daily physical activity is less than recommended for gender and age; consumption of sugar-sweetened beverages; disordered eating behaviors; disordered eating perceptions; energy expenditure below energy intake

● = Independent;   ▲ = Collaborative;   EBN = Evidence-Based Nursing;   EB = Evidence-Based

based on standard assessment; excessive alcohol consumption; fear regarding lack of food supply; frequent snacking; high frequency of eating restaurant or fried food; insufficient knowledge of modifiable factors; low dietary calcium intake in children; portion sizes larger than recommended; sedentary behavior occurring for more than 2 hours/day; shortened sleep time; sleep disorder; solid foods as major food sources of less than 5 months of age

At-Risk Population

Adult: Body mass index (BMI) approaching 25 kg/m^2; Child <2 years: Weight for length approaching 95th percentile; Child: 2 to 18 years: BMI approaching 85th percentile, or 25 kg/m^2 (whichever is smaller); children who are crossing BMI percentiles upward; children with high BMI percentiles; economically disadvantaged; formula or mixed-fed infants; heritability of interrelated factors; high disinhibition and restraint eating behavior score; maternal diabetes mellitus; maternal smoking; obesity in childhood; parental obesity; premature pubarche; rapid weight gain during childhood; rapid weight gain during infancy, including the first week, first 4 months, and the first year

Associated Condition

Genetic disorder

NOC   (Nursing Outcomes Classification)

Suggested NOC Outcomes

Nutritional Status; Nutritional Status: Food and Fluid Intake; Nutrient Intake; Weight Control

Example NOC Outcome with Indicators

Nutritional Status as evidenced by the following indicators: Food and fluid intake/Hydration/Body mass index/Weight-height ratio/Hematocrit. (Rate the outcome and indicators of **Nutritional Status:** 1 = severe deviation from normal range, 2 = substantial deviation from normal range, 3 = moderate deviation from normal range, 4 = mild deviation from normal range, 5 = no deviation from normal range [see Section I].)

Client Outcomes

Client Will (Specify Time Frame)

- Explain how to eat according to the US Dietary Guidelines
- Design dietary modifications to meet individual long-term goal of health, using principles of variety, balance, and moderation
- Maintain weight within normal range for height and age

NIC   (Nursing Interventions Classification)

Suggested NIC Interventions

Nutrition Management; Nutritional Counseling; Weight Reduction Assistance

Example NIC Activities—Nutrition Management

Determine the client's motivation for changing eating habits; Develop with the client a method to keep a daily record of intake

Nursing Interventions and *Rationales*

- Assess the meaning and importance of food in the client's life. EB: *Recent research found strong associations between the different domains of food meanings and behavioral outcomes (Arbit et al, 2017).*
- Assess client readiness to determine whether the client is ready to discuss weight loss and/or would like weight-loss information. EB: *Client motivation is a key component of success in a weight-loss program and a prerequisite for weight-loss therapy (Raynor & Champagne, 2016).*
- Use a motivational interviewing technique when working with clients to promote healthy eating and weight loss. EB: *Research shows significant weight loss for clients when motivational interviewing techniques were used (Barnes et al, 2018).*
- Counsel the client to measure regularly consumed foods periodically. Help the client learn usual portion sizes. Measuring food alerts the client to normal portion sizes. Estimating amounts can be extremely

• = Independent;   ▲ = Collaborative;   EBN = Evidence-Based Nursing;   EB = Evidence-Based

inaccurate. EB: *A randomized controlled trial of 278 overweight and obese participants was conducted to increase portion size awareness with results that demonstrated the intervention improved portion control behavior and in turn influenced BMI (Poelman et al, 2015).*

- Assist the client to develop a system of self-management, which may include self-monitoring of weight and BMI; realistic goal setting, planning, and action planning for improved dietary intake and physical activity; problem-solving; and tracking dietary intake and exercise. EB: *A key component of successful weight loss and maintenance is regular self-monitoring (Thomason et al, 2016).*
- Document the client's height and weight and teach significance of his or her BMI in relationship to current health. Use a chart or a website such as http://www.cdc.gov/healthyweight/assessing/bmi/index.html (Centers for Disease Control and Prevention [CDC], 2015). EB: *Successful treatment of overweight and obesity in adults requires adoption and maintenance of effective self-monitoring (Raynor & Champagne, 2016).*
- Encourage the client to engage in vigorous-intensity physical activity for at least 150 minutes weekly or moderate-intensity physical activity for at least 300 minutes weekly. EB: *Research evidence suggested that regular physical activity is critical for weight loss and weight-loss maintenance (Ostendorf et al, 2018).*
- Recommend that the client avoid eating in fast-food restaurants. CEB: *A 15-year study demonstrated that people who frequently eat fast foods gain an average of 10 pounds more than those who eat fast food less often and were two times more likely to develop insulin resistance, which can lead to diabetes (Pereira et al, 2005).*
- Assist the client to reframe slips in weight loss or physical activity behavior as lapses that are a single event and not a full return to previous unhealthy behaviors. Relapse prevention strategies include managing lapses in healthy behavior, identifying high-risk situations for relapses, self-monitoring, providing social support, enhancing skills for coping, and increasing self-efficacy for avoiding relapse. EB: *A study of a weight maintenance intervention, delivered primarily by telephone, modestly slowed the rate of weight regain (Voils et al, 2017).*
- Assist clients to engage their social support systems either digitally or face to face in ways that facilitate weight loss, healthy eating, and physical activity behavior change. EB: *Significant others, family, friends, and coworkers can facilitate or hinder weight-loss success (Romo, 2018).*
- Assist the client to reframe the goal from a focus on outcome (weight loss) to a focus on process (eating behaviors) for weight loss. EB: *A study showed that there were self-regulatory benefits from mental simulations used in the weight-loss process (Marszał-Wiśniewska & Jarczewska-Gerc, 2014).*
- Assist the client to implement informal and formal mindfulness-based interventions (MBIs). Informal MBIs include mindful eating, increasing awareness of hunger and satiety cues, taste satisfaction, and decreasing impulsive tendencies to overeat when experiencing negative emotions. Meditation practice is a formal MBI. EB: *Results of a research review suggested that a combination of formal and informal MBIs are effective in reducing weight and improving obesity-related eating behaviors among individuals with overweight and obesity (Carrière et al, 2018).*
- Assist the client to develop stimulus control techniques designed to reduce environmental cues associated with eating behaviors. Specifically, clients should be taught to limit the presence of high-calorie/high-fat foods in the home; to reduce the visibility of unhealthy food choices in the home; to limit where and when they eat; to avoid distractions like reading, using the computer, or watching television when eating; and to eat more slowly. EB: *Stimulus control strategies are a key to successful weight loss and weight maintenance in conjunction with other weight-loss strategies (Butryn et al, 2017).*
- Encourage 7.5 to 8.5 hours of sleep nightly. EB: *Recent evidence suggested weight management is hindered when attempted in the context of sleep restriction because there is an upregulation of reward, pleasure, and salience networks in response to food stimuli (St-Onge, 2017).*
- Refer the client to a weight-loss–related therapy group. EBN: *A study found there were significant changes in BMI, waist circumference, body fat percentage, and strength of the lower limbs for weight-loss group therapy participants (Ferrari et al, 2017).*
- Recommend that clients use dietary supplements such as vitamins and minerals after consulting with their primary health care provider. EB: *Research shows micronutrient deficits are prevalent in weight-loss plans, especially vitamin B_{12}, calcium, and vitamin D (Engel et al, 2018).*
- Incorporate the following recommendations from the Academy of Nutrition and Dietetics: Interventions for the Treatment of Overweight and Obesity in Adults (Raynor & Champagne, 2016):
  - Assess food- and nutrition-related history; anthropometric measures; biochemical data, medical tests, and procedures; nutrition-focused physical findings; and client history.

• = Independent;   ▲ = Collaborative;   EBN = Evidence-Based Nursing;   EB = Evidence-Based

○ Assess the energy intake and nutrient content of the diet.

○ Use height and weight to calculate BMI and waist circumference to determine risk of cardiovascular disease (CVD), type 2 diabetes, and all-cause mortality.

○ Use a measured resting metabolic rate (RMR) to determine energy needs.

○ Set a realistic weight-loss goal such as one of the following: up to 2 pounds/week, up to 10% of baseline body weight, or a total of 3% to 5% of baseline weight if cardiovascular risk factors (hypertension, hyperlipidemia, and hyperglycemia) are present.

○ To achieve weight loss, use an individualized diet, including patient preferences and health status, to achieve and maintain nutrient adequacy and reduce caloric intake, based on one of the following caloric reduction strategies: 1200 to 1500 kcal/day for women and 1500 to 1800 kcal/day for men and energy deficit of approximately 500 or 750 kcal/day.

 Pediatric

• Offer obese or overweight adolescents healthy methods for weight loss. EB: *A recent study showed statistically significant health behavior improvements after implementing a developmentally informed intervention to increase positive health diet and exercise behaviors (Issner et al, 2017).*

• Offer families of obese or overweight children prejudice-free, individually accepting, and supportive interventions to address weight loss. EBN: *Obese children treated with motivational interviewing showed significant improvement in their weight-related behavior and obesity-related anthropometric measures (Wong & Cheng, 2013).*

• Recommend that families eat together for at least one meal per day. EB: *Findings from a review provided clear evidence that family meals (among youth) and shared meals (among adults) are associated with better dietary intake and that these findings transcend the life span (Fulkerson et al, 2014).*

• Recommend involving the family in planning meals and food preparation. Children can learn about nutrition as they help plan and make meals. EB: *The Healthy Home Offerings via the Mealtime Environment Plus program showed increased cooking skills among the children participating (Fulkerson et al, 2018).*

• Assist parents at being good role models of healthy eating. EB: *The Healthy Home Offerings via the Mealtime Environment Plus program showed significantly improved parental self-efficacy for identifying appropriate portion sizes (Fulkerson et al, 2018).*

• Recommend that the family try new foods, either a new food or recipe every week. EB: *The Healthy Home Offerings via the Mealtime Environment Plus program showed decreasing child neophobia scores over time that were developmentally appropriate (Fulkerson et al, 2018).*

 Geriatric

• Determine the risks and benefits of weight loss in the older client. A BMI greater than 30 in the older client suggests a moderate weight-loss approach. EB: *Recommendations for treating obesity in the elderly include ensuring a balanced and appropriately distributed intake of high-quality nutrients, particularly of high-quality protein (i.e., 1.2 to 1.5 g/kg of body weight), limiting the intake of simple carbohydrates and saturated fats, and providing sufficient intake of calcium and vitamin D_3 (Blaz, 2016).*

• Observe for social, psychological, and economic factors that influence diet quality. EB: *An exploratory study of diet quality influences in community-dwelling older individuals revealed the following influences: food experiences, retirement, bereavement, medical conditions, food environment, food-related habits, social engagement, personal/psychological factors, and transportation (Bloom et al, 2017).*

 Multicultural

• Tailor nutritional interventions to be consistent with cultural beliefs, norms, and values. EB: *A systemic review of culturally tailored interventions for Hispanic women included literacy modification, Hispanic foods/recipes, cultural diabetes beliefs, family/friend participation, structured community input, and innovative experiential learning (McCurley et al, 2016).*

• Offer tailored lifestyle counseling via the telephone. EBN: *Investigators have included biweekly and/or monthly health coach calls for African American participants with significant weight gain prevention (Goode et al, 2017).*

• Integrate weight loss and weight maintenance interventions with church faith-based concepts for cultural congruence with African American clients. EB: *Recent research suggested that integrating faith themes into a weight-loss maintenance program may increase its long-term effect on participants' health behavior change (Seale et al, 2013).*

• = Independent;   ▲ = Collaborative;   EBN = Evidence-Based Nursing;   EB = Evidence-Based

Client/Family Teaching and Discharge Planning

- The majority of the preceding interventions involve teaching.
- Work with the family members regarding information on how to support and promote weight loss and healthy intakes.

REFERENCES

Arbit, N., et al. (2017). Development and validation of the meaning of food in life questionnaire (MFLQ): Evidence for a new construct to explain eating behavior. *Food Quality and Preference*, 59, 35–45. Retrieved from http://doi.org.proxy.lib.umich.edu/10.1016/j.foodqual.2017.02.002.

Barnes, R. D., et al. (2018). Examining motivational interviewing plus nutrition psychoeducation for weight loss in primary care. *Journal of Psychosomatic Research*, 104, 101–107. Retrieved from http://doi.org.proxy.lib.umich.edu/10.1016/j.jpsychores.2017.11.013.

Blaz, M. K. (2016). Obesity in the elderly, weight loss yes or no? *Clinical Nutrition ESPEN*, 14, 56. Retrieved from http://doi.org.proxy.lib.umich.edu/10.1016/j.clnesp.2016.04.025.

Bloom, I., et al. (2017). What influences diet quality in older people? A qualitative study among community-dwelling older adults from the Hertfordshire Cohort Study, UK. *Public Health Nutrition*, 20(15), 2685–2693. doi:10.1017/S1368980017001203.

Butryn, M. L., et al. (2017). Efficacy of environmental and acceptance-based enhancements to behavioral weight loss treatment: The ENACT trial. *Obesity*, 25(5), 866–872. doi:10.1002/oby.21813.

Carrière, K., et al. (2018). Mindfulness-based interventions for weight loss: A systematic review and meta-analysis. *Obesity Reviews*, 19(2), 164–177. doi:10.1111/obr.12623.

Centers for Disease Control and Prevention (2015). *Healthy weight—It's not a diet, it's a lifestyle!* Retrieved from http://www.cdc.gov/healthyweight/assessing/bmi/index.html. (Accessed 25 March 2018).

Engel, M. G., et al. (2018). Micronutrient gaps in three commercial weight-loss diet plans. *Nutrients*, 10(1), 108. Retrieved from http://doi.org.proxy.lib.umich.edu/10.3390/nu10010108.

Ferrari, G. D., et al. (2017). A multidisciplinary weight-loss program: The importance of psychological group therapy. *Motriz: Revista de Educacao Fisica*, 23(1), 47–52. doi:10.1590/s1980-6574201700010007.

Fulkerson, J. A., et al. (2018). Family home food environment and nutrition-related parent and child personal and behavioral outcomes of the Healthy Home Offerings via the Mealtime Environment (HOME) Plus program: A randomized controlled trial. *Journal of the Academy of Nutrition and Dietetics*, 118(2), 240–251. Retrieved from http://doi.org.proxy.lib.umich.edu/10.1016/j.jand.2017.04.006.

Fulkerson, J. A., et al. (2014). A review of associations between family or shared meal frequency and dietary and weight status outcomes across the lifespan. *Journal of Nutrition Education and Behavior*, 46(1), 2–19. Retrieved from http://doi.org.proxy.lib.umich.edu/10.1016/j.jneb.2013.07.012.

Goode, R. W., et al. (2017). African Americans in standard behavioral treatment for obesity, 2001–2015: What have we learned? *Western Journal of Nursing Research*, 39(8), 1045–1069. Retrieved from http://doi.org.proxy.lib.umich.edu/10.1177/0193945917692115.

Issner, J. H., et al. (2017). Increasing positive health behaviors in adolescents with nutritional goals and exercise. *Journal of Child and Family Studies*, 26(2), 548–558. Retrieved from http://doi.org.proxy.lib.umich.edu/10.1007/s10826-016-0585-4.

Marszał-Wiśniewska, M., & Jarczewska-Gerc, E. (2014). Role of mental simulations in the weight loss process. *The Journal of Psychology*, 150(1), 1–14. doi:10.1080/00223980.2014.987102.

McCurley, J. L., et al. (2016). Diabetes prevention in U.S. Hispanic adults: A systematic review of culturally tailored interventions. *American Journal of Preventive Medicine*, 52(4), 519–529. Retrieved from http://doi.org.proxy.lib.umich.edu/10.1016/j.amepre.2016.10.028.

Ostendorf, D. M., et al. (2018). Objectively measured physical activity and sedentary behavior in successful weight loss maintainers. *Obesity*, 26(1), 53–60. doi:10.1002/oby.22052.

Pereira, M., et al. (2005). Fast-food habits, weight gain, and insulin resistance (the CARDIA study): 15-year prospective analysis. *Lancet*, 365(9453), 36–42.

Poelman, M. P., et al. (2015). PortionControl@HOME: Results of a randomized controlled trial evaluating the effect of a multi-component portion size intervention on portion control behavior and body mass index. *Annals of Behavioral Medicine*, 49(1), 18–28. Retrieved from http://doi.org.proxy.lib.umich.edu/10.1007/s12160-014-9637-4.

Raynor, H. A., & Champagne, C. M. (2016). Position of the academy of nutrition and dietetics: Interventions for the treatment of overweight and obesity in adults. *Journal of the Academy of Nutrition and Dietetics*, 116(1), 129–147.

Romo, L. K. (2018). An examination of how people who have lost weight communicatively negotiate interpersonal challenges to weight management, health communication. *Health Communication*, 33(4), 469–477. doi:10.1080/10410236.2016.1278497.

Seale, J. P., Fifield, J., Davis-Smith, Y. M., et al. (2013). Developing culturally congruent weight maintenance programs for African American church members. *Ethnicity & Health*, 18(2), 152–167.

St-Onge, M.-P. (2017). Sleep-obesity relation: Underlying mechanisms and consequences for treatment. *Obesity Reviews*, 18(S1), 34–39. doi:10.1111/obr.12499.

Thomason, D. L., et al. (2016). A systematic review of adolescent self-management and weight loss. *Journal of Pediatric Health Care*, 30(6), 569–582. Retrieved from http://doi.org.proxy.lib.umich.edu/10.1016/j.pedhc.2015.11.016.

Voils, C. I., et al. (2017). Maintenance of weight loss after initiation of nutrition training: A randomized trial. *Annals of Internal Medicine*, 166(7), 463–471. doi:10.7326/M16-2160.

Wong, E. M., & Cheng, M. M. (2013). Effects of motivational interviewing to promote weight loss in obese children. *Journal of Clinical Nursing*, 22(17/18), 2519–2530.

O

Acute Pain *Denise Sullivan, MSN, ANP-BC and Maureen F. Cooney, DNP, FNP-BC*

NANDA-I

Definition

Unpleasant sensory and emotional experience associated with actual or potential tissue damage, or described in terms of such damage (International Association for the Study of Pain); sudden or slow onset of any intensity from mild to severe with an anticipated or predictable end, and with a duration of less than 3 months.

Defining Characteristics

Appetite change; change in physiological parameter; diaphoresis; distraction behavior; evidence of pain using standardized pain behavior checklist for those unable to communicate verbally; expressive behavior; facial expression of pain; guarding behavior; hopelessness; narrowed focus; positioning to ease pain; protective behavior; proxy report of pain behavior/activity changes; pupil dilation; self-focused; self-report of intensity using standardized pain scale; self-report of pain characteristics using standardized pain instrument

Related Factors

Biological injury agent; chemical injury agent; physical injury agent

NOC (Nursing Outcomes Classification)

Suggested NOC Outcomes

Pain Control; Pain Level; Pain: Adverse Psychological Response

Example NOC Outcome

Pain Level as evidenced by severity of observed or reported pain

Note: **Pain Level** is the NOC Outcome label; this text recommends use of the self-report numerical pain rating scale in place of the NOC indicator scales because of the amount of research supporting its use.

Client Outcomes

Client Will (Specify Time Frame)

For the Client Who Is Able to Provide a Self-Report
- Use a self-report pain tool to identify current pain intensity level and establish a comfort-function goal
- Report that the pain management regimen achieves comfort-function goal without side effects
- Describe nonpharmacological methods that can be used to help achieve comfort-function goal
- Perform activities of recovery or activities of daily living (ADLs) easily
- Describe how unrelieved pain will be managed
- State ability to obtain sufficient amounts of rest and sleep
- Notify member of the health care team promptly for pain intensity level that is consistently greater than the comfort-function goal, or occurrence of side effects

For the Client Who Is Unable to Provide a Self-Report
- Decrease in pain-related behaviors
- Perform activities of recovery or ADLs easily as determined by client condition
- Demonstrate the absence of side effects of analgesics
- No pain-related behaviors will be evident in the client who is completely unresponsive; a reasonable outcome is to demonstrate the absence of side effects related to the prescribed pain treatment plan

NIC (Nursing Interventions Classification)

Suggested NIC Interventions

Analgesic Administration; Pain Management; Patient-Controlled Analgesia (PCA) Assistance

● = Independent;   ▲ = Collaborative;   EBN = Evidence-Based Nursing;   EB = Evidence-Based

Example NIC Activities—Pain Management

Ensure client-attentive analgesic care; Perform a comprehensive assessment of pain to include location, characteristics, onset/duration, frequency, quality, intensity or severity of pain, and precipitating factors

Nursing Interventions and *Rationales*

- During the initial assessment and interview if the client is experiencing pain, or when pain first occurs, conduct and document a comprehensive pain assessment, using appropriate pain assessment tools. CEB/EBN: *Determining location, temporal aspects, pain intensity, characteristics, and the effect of pain on function and quality of life are critical to determine the underlying cause of pain and effectiveness of treatment (McCaffery, 1968; Drew & Peltier, 2018). The initial assessment includes all pain information that the client can provide for the development of the individualized pain management plan (Drew & Peltier, 2018).*

- Implement or request orders to implement pain management interventions to achieve a satisfactory level of comfort. Components of this initial assessment include location, quality, onset/duration, temporal profile, intensity, aggravating and alleviating factors, and effects of pain on function and quality of life.

- Assess if the client is able to provide a self-report of pain intensity, and if so, assess pain intensity level using a valid and reliable self-report pain tool, such as the 0 to 10 numerical pain rating scale. EBN: *Self-report is considered the single most reliable indicator of pain presence and intensity, and single-dimension pain ratings are valid and reliable as measures of pain intensity level (Drew & Peltier, 2018). EB: Regularly and routinely assess the client for pain presence during activity and rest and with interventions or procedures likely to cause pain. EB: Acute pain should be reliably assessed both at rest (important for comfort) and during movement (important for function and decreased client risk for cardiopulmonary and thromboembolic events) (Chou et al, 2016; Drew & Peltier, 2018).*

- Ask the client to describe prior experiences with pain, effectiveness of pain management interventions, responses to analgesic medications including occurrence of side effects, and concerns about pain and its treatment (e.g., fear about addiction, worries, anxiety) and informational needs. EBN: *Obtaining an individualized pain history helps identify potential factors that may influence the client's willingness to report pain, as well as factors that may influence pain intensity, the client's response to pain, anxiety, and pharmacokinetics of analgesics (Drew & Peltier, 2018). EB: Anxiety and fear may intensify pain, and pain may trigger emotional responses such as fear and anxiety (Zhuo, 2016).*

- Using a self-report pain tool, ask the client to identify a comfort-function goal that will allow the client to perform necessary or desired activities easily. EBN: *The comfort-function goal provides the basis for individualized pain management plans and assists in determining effectiveness of pain management interventions (Drew & Peltier, 2018).*

- Use the Hierarchy of Pain Measures as a framework for pain assessment (Herr et al, 2011; Drew & Peltier, 2018): (1) attempt to obtain the client's self-report of pain; (2) consider the client's condition and search for possible causes of pain (e.g., presence of tissue injury, pathological conditions, exposure to procedures/interventions that are thought to result in pain); (3) observe for behaviors that may indicate pain presence (e.g., facial expressions, crying, restlessness, changes in activity); (4) evaluate physiological indicators, with the understanding that these are the least sensitive indicators of pain and may be related to conditions other than pain (e.g., shock, hypovolemia, anxiety); and (5) conduct an analgesic trial. EBN: *When a client is unable to use a self-report tool (e.g., cognitively impaired, critically ill, anesthetized or sedated), the presence of pain may be assessed by observing specific client behaviors using a valid and reliable behavioral tool (e.g., Critical Care Observation Tool in the critically ill or Checklist of Nonverbal Pain Indicators in cognitively impaired older adults) (Puntillo et al, 2014; Drew & Peltier, 2018). In a study involving turning of neurocritically ill clients after elective brain surgery, self-report was obtained when possible, behaviors were found to be valid indicators of pain, and fluctuations in vital signs suggested the presence of pain, but their validity for such use was not supported, suggesting they should only be used in combination with other validated pain assessment tools (Kapoustina, Echegaray-Benites, & Gelinas, 2014).*

- Assume that pain is present if the client is unable to provide a self-report and has tissue injury, a pathological condition, or has undergone a procedure that is thought to produce pain, and conduct an analgesic trial. EBN: *Pain is associated with actual or potential tissue damage such as pathological conditions (e.g., cancer) and procedures (e.g., surgery or trauma, fractures). In the absence of self-report (e.g., anesthetized, critically ill, or cognitively impaired client), the health care provider should use clinical judgment and assume pain is present, and then implement pain management interventions accordingly (Drew & Peltier, 2018).*

● = Independent;   ▲ = Collaborative;   EBN = Evidence-Based Nursing;   EB = Evidence-Based

P

▲ Obtain and review an accurate and complete list of medications the client is taking or has taken. **EB:** *Accurate medication reconciliation can guide analgesic plan development and prevent errors associated with incorrect medications, dosages, omission of components of the home medication regimen, drug–drug interactions, and toxicity that can occur when incompatible drugs are combined or when allergies are present (Ignatavicius, 2013).*

▲ Describe the adverse effects of unrelieved pain. **EBN:** *Unrelieved acute pain can have physiological and psychological consequences that facilitate negative client outcomes. Ineffective management of acute pain has the potential for neurohumoral changes; neuronal remodeling; an impact on immune function; and long-lasting physiological, psychological, and emotional distress, and it may lead to persistent pain syndromes (Eksterowicz & DiMaggio, 2018).*

▲ Explain to the client the pain management approach, including pharmacological and nonpharmacological interventions, the assessment and reassessment process, potential side effects, and the importance of prompt reporting of unrelieved pain. **EB:** *One of the most important steps toward improved control of pain is a better client understanding of the nature of pain, its treatment, and the role the client needs to play in pain control (Ignatavicius, 2013).*

▲ Discuss the client's fears of undertreated pain, side effects, and opioid use disorder (OUD), and reassure the client that there will be regular assessment and treatment of pain, and assessment for side effects and signs of OUD. **EBN:** *Cogan et al (2014) reported that among 379 clients scheduled for cardiac surgery, 31% stated that it is easy to become addicted to pain medication, 20% report that "good patients" do not talk about their pain, and 35% believe that pain medication should be "saved in case the pain worsens."*

● Teach the client about pain and pharmacological and nonpharmacological interventions when pain is relatively well controlled. **EB:** *Pain causes cognitive impairment (Baker et al, 2017).*

▲ Regularly reassess the client for the presence of pain and response to pain management interventions, including effectiveness and the presence of adverse effects related to pain management interventions. Review the client's pain flow sheet and medication administration record to evaluate effectiveness of pain relief, previous 24-hour opioid requirements, and occurrence of side effects. **EBN:** *Systematic tracking of pain is an important factor in improving pain management and making adjustments to the pain management regimen (Eksterowicz & DiMaggio, 2018).*

▲ Advocate for and manage acute pain using a multimodal, opioid-sparing approach. **EB:** *A multimodal approach (combining two or more drugs that act by different mechanisms for providing analgesia) enhances pain relief and allows the lowest effective dose of each drug to be administered, resulting in fewer or less severe side effects, such as nausea, sedation, and respiratory depression (The Joint Commission [TJC], 2012; Chou et al, 2016; Jungquist et al, 2016; Behm, Leinum, & Peltier, 2018).*

▲ Select the route for administration of analgesics based on client condition and pain characteristics. **EB:** *Routes have different rates of onset and duration. The oral route is preferred because of its convenience and the resulting relatively steady blood levels, the rectal route may be used when the oral route is not feasible, the intravenous (IV) route is preferred for rapid control of severe pain and would therefore not generally be used for chronic pain, and intramuscular injections are avoided because of variable absorption and the potential for nerve injury and tissue damage (American Pain Society [APS], 2016; Chou et al, 2016).*

▲ Provide perineural infusions and intraspinal analgesia when appropriate and available. **CEBN:** Superior analgesia can be provided through regional analgesic techniques compared with systemic opioids (Nishimori et al, 2012). **EB:** *Use of preoperative continuous femoral nerve blockade reduced morphine side effects in patients with hip fracture (Chaudet et al, 2016).*

▲ Use diverse analgesic delivery methods such as PCA to increase client's satisfaction with pain management, to lower cost, and to decrease occurrence of adverse reactions. **EBN:** *IV PCA provides superior analgesia compared with IV injection in the first 12 hours after total hysterectomy (Hong & Lee, 2014).*

▲ Administer a nonopioid analgesic for mild to moderate pain and add an opioid analgesic if indicated for moderate to severe acute pain. **EB:** *Nonopioids, such as acetaminophen and nonsteroidal antiinflammatory drugs, are first-line analgesics for the treatment of mild and some moderate acute pain, whereas opioids are included for the treatment of moderate to severe acute pain (American Society of Anesthesiologists [ASA], 2012; APS, 2016; Chou et al, 2016).*

● Avoid administering analgesics based solely on a client's pain intensity rating. **EB:** Administering opioid doses based solely on pain intensity disregards the other essential elements of the pain assessment and may contribute to adverse patient outcomes such as excessive sedation and respiratory depression as a result of overmedication, or result in poorly controlled pain from undermedication (Pasero et al, 2016).

● = Independent;   ▲ = Collaborative;   **EBN** = Evidence-Based Nursing;   **EB** = Evidence-Based

- Administer analgesics around the clock for continuous pain (expected to be present approximately 50% of the day, such as postoperative pain) and as needed (PRN) for intermittent or breakthrough pain. **EB:** *If pain is present most of the day, the use of PRN medications alone will lead to periods of undermedication and poor pain control and periods of excessive medication and adverse effects (APS, 2016).*

- Prevent pain by administering analgesia before painful procedures whenever possible (e.g., endotracheal suctioning, wound care, heel puncture, venipunctures, and peripherally inserted IV catheters). **EB:** *Adult clients in the intensive care setting experience numerous sources of procedural pain, and chest tube removal, wound drain removal, and arterial line insertion are identified as the most painful procedures (Puntillo et al, 2014). The use of topical lidocaine 1% before removal of extremity vacuum-assisted closure wound dressings results in reduced pain and opioid use (Christensen, Thorum, & Kubiak, 2013).*

- Perform nursing care during the peak effect of analgesics to optimize client comfort and participation in care. **EB:** *Providing care such as mobilization and bathing should be performed when analgesics have reached peak effect: oral medications peak in 60 minutes, subcutaneous opioids in 30 minutes, and IV analgesics in 15 to 30 minutes (APS, 2016; Eksterowicz & DiMaggio, 2018).*

- Advocate for the use of "as needed" opioid range orders to provide effective and appropriate pain relief. **EB:** *Correctly prescribed range orders for the delivery of IV opioids give nurses the flexibility needed to treat clients' pain in a timely manner while allowing for differences in client response to pain and to analgesia (Drew et al, 2014; APS, 2016).*

- Choose analgesic and dose based on orders that reflect the client's report of pain severity and response to the previous dose in terms of pain relief, occurrence of side effects, and ability to perform the activities of recovery or ADLs. **EB:** *Safe and effective pain management requires opioid dose adjustment based on individualized adequate pain and sedation assessment, opioid administration, and evaluation of the response to treatment (Ignatavicius, 2013).*

- ▲ When converting opioids from parenteral doses to oral doses (the preferred route when the client can tolerate and absorb oral medications), use equianalgesic dosing charts and carefully monitor the client's response to the new medication route and dose. **EB:** *Equianalgesic dosing calculations should be used cautiously to guide dose conversion of an opioid from one route to another to avoid the toxicity associated with overdosing and the inadequate pain control caused by under dosing (APS, 2016).*

- ▲ Clients who are receiving opioids for acute pain require frequent assessment for effectiveness of opioids and assessment for serious opioid-related adverse effects. This includes respiratory assessment (rate, rhythm, noisiness, and depth) and systematic assessment of sedation level using a sedation scale (Eksterowicz & DiMaggio, 2018). **EB:** *Opioid-induced respiratory depression occurs with the greatest frequency in postoperative clients during the first 24 hours after surgery, and factors contributing to postoperative respiratory depression include the intervention of multiple prescribers (33%), concurrent administration of nonopioid sedating medications (34%), and inadequate nursing assessments or response (31%) (Jarzyna et al, 2011; ASA, 2012; Lee et al, 2015; Jungquist et al, 2016).*

- ▲ When opioids are included in the multimodal analgesic plan, clients need regular assessment for common side effects such as constipation, nausea, pruritus, lack of appetite, and changes in rest and sleep, and preventive measures are implemented when possible.

- Monitor frequency of bowel movements and provide the client with adequate hydration, a stool softener, and stimulant to prevent/treat opioid-related constipation. **EB:** *Opioid-induced constipation significantly affects quality of life. First-line treatment includes lifestyle changes such as increasing activity and the administration of stool softeners and laxatives (Dorn, Lembo, & Cremonini, 2014).*

- ▲ Support the client's use of nonpharmacological methods to supplement pharmacological analgesic approaches to help control pain, such as distraction, imagery, music therapy, simple massage, relaxation, and application of heat and cold. **EBN:** *Although more evidence is needed to conclude effectiveness, nonpharmacological methods (which are low cost and low risk) can be used to complement pharmacological treatment of pain (Ignatavicius, 2013). The use of structured touch and guided imagery has shown reduction in pain and anxiety among adults who underwent elective joint replacements (Forward et al, 2015). Evidence suggests efficacy and satisfaction when complementary therapies are integrated into pain treatment plans of older adults (Bruckenthal, Marino, & Snelling, 2016).*

- ▲ Assist client to identify resources for coping with psychological impact of pain. **EB:** *Cognitive behavioral (mind–body) strategies can restore the client's sense of self-control, personal efficacy, and active participation in his or her own care (Broderick et al, 2014).* **EB:** *Nurses should advocate for cognitive behavioral therapy as first-line therapy and especially when medications are contraindicated, not well tolerated, or refused and when patients are exhibiting ineffective coping skills (O'Connor-Von & Heck, 2018).*

● = Independent;   ▲ = Collaborative;   **EBN** = Evidence-Based Nursing;   **EB** = Evidence-Based

Pediatric

- Assess for the presence of pain using a valid and reliable pain scale based on age, cognitive development, and the child's ability to provide a self-report. EBN: *Scales that depict faces at various levels of pain intensity are commonly used in young children and have been shown to be reliable and valid in children as young as 3 years old (Tobias, 2014).* EB: *Behavioral tools such as the Face, Legs, Activity, Cry, Consolability (FLACC) Scale may be used to assess pain in infants and children who cannot provide a self-report (Crellin et al, 2015).*
- ▲ Administer prescribed analgesics using a multimodal approach to treat pain in children, infants, and neonates. EB: *Multimodal analgesia improves pain control and reduces side effects in postoperative pediatric patients (Jitpakdee & Mandee, 2014).*
- Prevent procedural pain in neonates, infants, and children by using opioid analgesics and anesthetics, as indicated, in appropriate dosages. EBN: *Czarnecki et al (2014) found that several barriers exist to the treatment of procedural pain in children including insufficient medication orders before procedures, insufficient time to premedicate children before procedures, the perception of low priority given to pain management by medical staff, and parents' reluctance to have their children medicated.*
- Use a topical local anesthetic treatment or other nonpharmacologic treatment before performing venipuncture in neonates, infants, and children. EBN: *Mechanical vibration with use of Buzzy, a US Food and Drug Administration (FDA)-approved device shaped like a bee that vibrates and has removable "wings" that can be frozen placed proximally to the expected IV insertion site has been shown to be as effective as topical lidocaine (Bahorski et al, 2015).*
- For the neonate, use oral sucrose and nonnutritional sucking (NNS) or human milk for pain of short duration such as heel stick or venipuncture. Neonates, especially preterm neonates, are more sensitive to pain than older children. EBN: *In an integrated literature review, Naughton (2013) found that the combination of oral sucrose and NNS is a safe and effective method of relieving pain in neonates and increases the calming effect in infants undergoing painful procedures.*
- Recognize that breastfeeding has been shown to reduce behavioral indicators of pain. EB: *Breastfeeding has not been shown to have a better analgesic effect than sucrose in late preterm infants (Simonse, Mulder, & Van Beek, 2012).*
- As with adults, use nonpharmacological analgesic interventions to supplement, not replace, pharmacological interventions in pediatric clients. EB: *Infants who underwent upper limb massage prior to venipuncture had significantly less pain with venipuncture than when massage was not used (Chik, Ip, & Choi, 2017). Pain and distress in children receiving immunizations were significantly reduced when live music therapy was used during the immunization procedure (Sundar et al, 2016).*

Geriatric

- Refer to the Nursing Interventions and *Rationales* in the care plan for Chronic **Pain.**

Multicultural

- Refer to the Nursing Interventions and *Rationales* in the care plan for Chronic **Pain.**

Home Care

- ▲ Develop the treatment plan with the client and caregivers. EB: *Client education and motivation play important roles in self-management of clients with pain. Self-management is influenced by client–provider communication (Dorflinger, Kerns, & Auerbach, 2013).*
- ▲ Assess the client's full medication profile, including medications prescribed by all health care providers and all over-the-counter medications for drug interactions, and instruct the client to refrain from mixing medications without health care provider approval. EB: *Pain medications may significantly affect or be affected by other medications and may cause severe side effects; in a study of diabetic pregabalin and duloxetine users, potential duloxetine drug–drug interactions and drug–condition interactions were associated with significant increases in mean health care costs (Johnston et al, 2013).*
- ▲ Assess the client/family's knowledge of side effects and safety precautions associated with pain medications. EB: *Educational activities related to pain medications are necessary to ensure that clients are knowledgeable about opioid side effects and safety. McCarthy et al (2015) found that clients who read and a one-page information sheet they were given about hydrocodone-acetaminophen safety had better knowledge of precautions related to acetaminophen dosing, and they were less likely to drive a car within 6 hours of taking the medication than those who did not receive this educational intervention.*

- If medication is administered using highly technological methods, assess the home for the necessary resources (e.g., electricity) and ensure that there will be responsible caregivers available to assist the client with administration. EB: *With appropriate assessment of home resources, it is possible to provide home management of clients with complex pain management technologies as demonstrated in a study of children with cleft palate repair who received home infusion of local anesthetic via peripheral nerve block catheter (Visoiu, 2014).*
- Assess the knowledge base of the client and family regarding highly technological medication administration and provide necessary education, including the procedure to follow if analgesia is unsatisfactory. EB: *With appropriate education and training, outpatient families can successfully manage infusions of local anesthetics through peripheral nerve catheters for analgesia in clients recovering from cleft palate surgery (Visoiu, 2014).*

 Client/Family Teaching and Discharge Planning

Note: To avoid the negative connotations associated with the words "drugs" and "narcotics," use the term "pain medicine" when teaching clients.

- Discuss the various discomforts encompassed by the word "pain" and ask the client to give examples of previously experienced pain. Explain the pain assessment process and the purpose of the pain rating scale. EB: *It is often difficult for clients to understand the concept of pain and describe their pain experience. Using alternative words and providing a complete description of the assessment process, including the use of scales, ensures that an accurate treatment plan is developed (Drew & Peltier, 2018).*
- Teach the client to use the self-report pain tool to rate the intensity of past or current pain. Ask the client to set a comfort-function goal by selecting a pain level on the self-report tool that will allow performance of desired or necessary activities of recovery with relative ease (e.g., turn, cough, deep breathe, ambulate, participate in physical therapy). If the pain level is consistently above the comfort-function goal, the client should take action that decreases pain or notify a member of the health care team so that effective pain management interventions may be implemented promptly. EB: *The use of comfort-function goals provides the basis for the direction and modification of the treatment plan (Eksterowicz & DiMaggio, 2018).*
- Provide written educational materials on various aspects of pain control to improve client understanding of pain and pain-related interventions. EB: *Written materials and other educational tools assist in improving clients' knowledge related to pain management. In knee replacement clients, the use of an educational pamphlet and a compact disc was associated with decreased postoperative pain and increased participation in physical rehabilitation (Chen et al, 2014).*
- Discuss and evaluate the client's understanding about the total plan for pharmacological and nonpharmacological treatment, including the medications prescribed and their indication, proper dosing schedule, and adverse events and what to do should they occur. EB: *Appropriate instruction increases the accuracy and safety of medication administration (Drew & Peltier, 2018).*
- Teach basic principles of pain management using a variety of educational strategies, and evaluate learning. EB: *Client educational strategies that have been shown to increase knowledge, decrease anxiety, and increase satisfaction include the use of computer technology, audiotapes and videotapes, written materials, and demonstrations, or combinations of these strategies (Curtiss & Wrona, 2018).*
- ▲ Reinforce the importance of taking pain medications to maintain the comfort-function goal. EB: *Teaching clients to stay on top of their pain and prevent it from getting out of control will improve the ability to accomplish the goals of recovery (APS, 2016; Eksterowicz & DiMaggio, 2018).*
- ▲ Reinforce that short-term use of opioids for acute pain relief is an appropriate part of their multimodal pain treatment plan. EB: *Taking opioids only as directed, avoiding alcohol, and talking with the health care provider when pain is poorly controlled are strategies that will lessen the risks for OUD or major opioid-related adverse effects such as respiratory depression and arrest (Costello, 2015).*
- ▲ Reinforce the importance of safe storage of opioid medications out of the reach of others, and to responsibly dispose of any unused opioids. EB: *Community medication "take back" days and drop boxes are becoming increasingly popular. Encourage clients/families to check community resources.*
- ▲ Demonstrate the use of appropriate nonpharmacological approaches in addition to pharmacological approaches to help control pain, such as application of heat and/or cold, distraction techniques, relaxation breathing, visualization, rocking, stroking, listening to music, and watching television. EB: *Nonpharmacological interventions are used to complement, not replace, pharmacological interventions (Bruckenthal, Marino, & Snelling, 2016).*

● = Independent; ▲ = Collaborative; EBN = Evidence-Based Nursing; EB = Evidence-Based

REFERENCES

American Pain Society. (2016). *Principles of analgesic use* (7th ed.). Chicago: Author.

American Society of Anesthesiologists (ASA). (2012). Practice guidelines for acute pain management in the perioperative setting. An updated report by the American Society of Anesthesiologists Task Force on Acute Pain Management. *Anesthesiology, 116,* 248–273.

Bahorski, J. S., Hauber, R. P., Hanks, C., et al. (2015). Mitigating procedural pain during venipuncture in a pediatric population: A randomized factorial study. *International Journal of Nursing Studies, 52*(10), 1553–1563.

Baker, K. S., Georgiou-Karistianis, N., Gibson, S. J., et al. (2017). Optimizing cognitive function in persons with chronic pain. *The Clinical Journal of Pain, 33*(5), 462–472.

Behm, L. B., Leinum, C. J., & Peltier, C. H. (2018). Overview of pain management pharmacology. In M. L. Czarnecki & H. N. Turner (Eds.), *Core curriculum for pain management nursing.* St. Louis: Mosby Elsevier.

Broderick, J. E., Keefe, F. J., Bruckenthal, P., et al. (2014). Nurse practitioners can effectively deliver pain coping skills training to osteoarthritis patients with chronic pain: A randomized, controlled trial. *Pain, 155*(9), 1743–1754.

Bruckenthal, P., Marino, M. A., & Snelling, L. (2016). Complementary and integrative therapies for persistent pain management in older adults: A review. *Journal of Gerontological Nursing, 42*(12), 40–48.

Chaudet, A., Bouhours, G., Rineau, E., et al. (2016). Impact of preoperative continuous femoral blockades on morphine consumption and morphine side effects in hip-fracture patients: A randomized, placebo-controlled study. *Anaesthesia, Critical Care & Pain Medicine, 35*(1), 37–43.

Chen, S. R., Chen, C. S., & Lin, P. C. (2014). The effect of educational intervention on the pain and rehabilitation performance of patients who undergo a total knee replacement. *Journal of Clinical Nursing, 23*(1–2), 279–287.

Chik, Y. M., Ip, W. Y., & Choi, K. C. (2017). The effect of upper limb massage on infants' venipuncture pain. *Pain Management Nursing, 18*(1), 50–57.

Chou, R., Gordon, D. B., de Leon-Casasola, O. A., et al. (2016). Management of postoperative pain: A clinical practice guideline from the American Pain Society, the American Society of Regional Analgesia and Pain Medicine, and the American Society of Anesthesiologists' Committee on Regional Anesthesia, Executive Committee, and Administrative Council. *Journal of Pain, 17*(2), 131–157.

Christensen, T. J., Thorum, T., & Kubiak, E. (2013). Lidocaine analgesia for removal of wound vacuum-assisted closure dressings: A randomized double-blinded placebo-controlled trial. *Journal of Orthopedic Trauma, 27*(2), 107–112.

Cogan, J., Ouimette, M. F., Vargas-Schaffe, G., et al. (2014). Patient attitudes and beliefs regarding pain medication after cardiac surgery: Barriers to adequate pain management. *Pain Management Nursing, 15*(3), 574–579.

Costello, M. (2015). Prescription opioid analgesics: Promoting patient safety with better patient education. *American Journal of Nursing, 115*(11), 50–56.

Crellin, D. J., Harrison, D., Santamaria, N., et al. (2015). Systematic review of the face, legs, activity, cry, and consolability scale for assessing pain in infants and children: Is it reliable, valid and feasible for use? *Pain, 156*(11), 2132–2151.

Curtiss, C. P., & Wrona, S. (2018). Pain management education. In M. L. Czarnecki & H. N. Turner (Eds.), *Core curriculum.* St Louis: Mosby Elsevier.

Czarnecki, M. L., Salamon, K. S., Thompson, J. J., et al. (2014). Do barriers to pediatric pain management as perceived by nurses change over time? *Pain Management Nursing, 15*(1), 292–305.

Dorflinger, L., Kerns, R. D., & Auerbach, S. M. (2013). Providers' roles in enhancing patients' adherence to pain self management. *Translational Behavioral Medicine, 3*(1), 39–46.

Dorn, S., Lembo, A., & Cremonini, F. (2014). Opioid-induced bowel dysfunction: Epidemiology, pathophysiology, diagnosis, and initial therapeutic approach. *The American Journal of Gastroenterology Supplements, 2*(1), 31–37.

Drew, D. J., & Peltier, C. H. (2018). Pain assessment. In M. L. Czarnecki & H. N. Turner (Eds.), *Core curriculum.* St Louis: Mosby Elsevier.

Drew, D., Gordon, D., Renner, L., et al. (2014). The use of "as-needed" range orders for opioid analgesics in the management of pain: A consensus statement of the American Society of Pain Management Nurses and the American Pain Society. *Pain Management Nursing, 15*(2), 551–554.

Eksterowicz, N., & Dimaggio, T. J. (2018). Acute pain management. In M. L. Czarnecki & H. N. Turner (Eds.), *Core curriculum.* St Louis: Mosby Elsevier.

Forward, J. B., Greuter, N. E., Crisall, S. J., et al. (2015). Effect of structured touch and guided imagery for pain and anxiety in elective joint replacement patients—A randomized controlled trial: M-TIJRP. *The Permanente Journal, 19*(4), 18.

Herr, K., Coyne, P. J., McCaffrey, M., et al. (2011). Pain assessment in the patient unable to self-report: Position statement with clinical practice recommendations. *Pain Management Nursing, 12*(4), 230–250.

Hong, S. J., & Lee, E. (2014). Comparing effects of intravenous patient-controlled analgesia and intravenous injection in patients who have undergone total hysterectomy. *Journal of Clinical Nursing, 23,* 967–975.

Ignatavicius, D. (2013). Pain—The 5th vital sign. In D. Ignatavicius & M. L. Workman (Eds.), *Medical-surgical nursing: Patient-centered collaborative care* (7th ed., pp. 39–64). St. Louis: W.B. Saunders Company.

International Association for the Study of Pain (IASP). (2012). *IASP taxonomy.* Retrieved from http://www.iasp-pain.org/Taxonomy.

Jarzyna, D., et al. (2011). American Society for Pain Management Nursing evidence-based consensus guideline on monitoring of opioid-induced sedation and respiratory depression. *Pain Management Nursing, 12*(3), 118–145.

Jitpakdee, T., & Mandee, S. (2014). Strategies for preventing side effects of systemic opioid in postoperative pediatric patients. *Pediatric Anesthesia, 24*(6), 561–568.

Johnston, S. S., Udall, M., Cappelleri, J. C., et al. (2013). Cost comparison of drug–drug and drug–condition interactions in patients with painful diabetic peripheral neuropathy treated with pregabalin versus duloxetine. *American Journal of Health-System Pharmacy, 70*(24), 2207–2217.

Jungquist, C. R., Correll, D. J., Fleisher, L. A., et al. (2016). Avoiding adverse events secondary to opioid-induced respiratory depression: Implications for nurse executives and patient safety. *Journal of Nursing Administration, 46*(2), 87–94.

Kapoustina, O., Echegaray-Benites, C., & Gelinas, C. (2014). Fluctuations in vital signs and behavioral responses of brain surgery patients in the intensive care unit: Are they valid indicators of pain? *Journal of Advanced Nursing, 70*(11), 2562–2576.

Lee, L. A., Caplan, R. A., Stephens, L. S., et al. (2015). Postoperative opioid-induced respiratory depression: A closed claims analysis. *Anesthesiology, 122*(3), 659–665.

McCaffery, M. (1968). *Nursing practice theories related to cognition, bodily pain, and man-environment interactions.* Los Angeles: University of California at Los Angeles Students' Store.

● = Independent;   ▲ = Collaborative;   EBN = Evidence-Based Nursing;   EB = Evidence-Based

McCarthy, D. M., Wolf, M. S., McConnell, R., et al. (2015). Improving patient knowledge and safe use of opioids: A randomized controlled trial. *Academic Emergency Medicine, 22*(3), 331–339.

Naughton, K. A. (2013). The combined use of sucrose and nonnutritive sucking for procedural pain in both term and preterm neonates: An integrative review of the literature. *Advances in Neonatal Care, 13*(1), 9–19.

Nishimori, M., Low, J. H. S., Zheng, H., et al. (2012). Epidural pain relief versus systemic opioid-based pain relief for abdominal aortic surgery. *Cochrane Database of Systematic Reviews,* (7), CD005059.

O'Connor-Von, S. K., & Heck, C. R. (2018). Complementary and integrative therapies for pain management. In M. L. Czarnecki & H. N. Turner (Eds.), *Core curriculum.* St Louis: Mosby Elsevier.

Pasero, C., Quinlan-Colwell, A., Rae, D., et al. (2016). American Society for Pain Management Nursing position statement: Prescribing and administering opioid doses based solely on pain intensity. *Pain Management Nursing, 17*(3), 170–180.

Puntillo, K. A., Max, A., Timsit, J.-F., et al. (2014). Determinants of procedural pain intensity in the intensive care unit. The European study. *American Journal of Respiratory and Critical Care Medicine, 189*(1), 39–47.

Simonse, E., Mulder, P. G., & Van Beek, R. H. (2012). Analgesic effect of breast milk versus sucrose for analgesia during heel lance in late preterm infants. *Pediatrics, 129*(4), 657–663.

Sundar, S., Ramesh, B., Dixit, P. B., et al. (2016). Live music therapy as an active focus of attention for pain and behavioral symptoms of distress during pediatric immunization. *Clinical Pediatrics, 55*(8), 745–748.

The Joint Commission. (2012). *Sentinel event alert issue 49: Safe use of opioids in hospitals.* Retrieved from http://www.jointcomission.org/sea_issue_49/. (Accessed 1 November 2017).

Tobias, J. D. (2014). Acute pain management in infants and children—Part 1: Pain pathways, pain assessment, and outpatient pain management. *Pediatric Annals, 43*(7), e163–e168.

Visoiu, M. (2014). Outpatient analgesia via paravertebral peripheral nerve block catheter and On-Q pump—a case series. *Pediatric Anesthesia, 24*(8), 875–878.

Zhuo, M. (2016). Neural mechanisms underlying anxiety-chronic pain interactions. *Trends in Neurosciences, 39*(3), 136–145.

Chronic Pain   *Denise Sullivan, MSN, ANP-BC and Maureen F. Cooney, DNP, FNP-BC*

NANDA-I

Definition

Unpleasant sensory and emotional experience associated with actual or potential tissue damage, or described in terms of such damage (International Association for the Study of Pain); sudden or slow onset of any intensity from mild to severe, constant or recurring without an anticipated or predictable end, and a duration of greater than 3 months.

Defining Characteristics

Alteration in ability to continue previous activities; alteration in sleep pattern; anorexia; evidence of pain using standardized pain behavior checklist for those unable to communicate verbally; facial expression of pain; proxy report of pain behavior/activity changes; self-focused; self-report of intensity using standardized pain scale; self-report of pain characteristics using standardized pain instrument

Related Factors

Alteration in sleep pattern; emotional distress; fatigue; increase in body mass index; ineffective sexuality pattern; injury agent; malnutrition; nerve compression; prolonged computer use; repeated handling of heavy loads; social isolation; whole-body vibration

At-Risk Population

Age >50 years; female gender; history of abuse; history of genital mutilation; history of over indebtedness; history of static work postures; history of substance misuse; history of vigorous exercise

Associated Condition

Chronic musculoskeletal condition; contusion; crush injury; damage to the nervous system; fracture; genetic disorder; imbalance of neurotransmitters, neuromodulators, and receptors; immune disorder; impaired metabolic functioning; ischemic condition; muscle injury; post-trauma related condition; prolonged increase in cortisol level; spinal cord injury; tumor infiltration

NOC   (Nursing Outcomes Classification)

Suggested NOC Outcomes

Comfort Level; Pain Control; Pain: Disruptive Effects; Pain Level

● = Independent;   ▲ = Collaborative;   EBN = Evidence-Based Nursing;   EB = Evidence-Based

Example NOC Outcome with Indicators

Pain Level as evidenced by use of a numerical pain rating scale (NRS), asking the client to rate the level of pain from 0 to 10. Self-report is considered the single most reliable indicator of pain presence and intensity (American Pain Society [APS], 2016)

Note: **Pain Level** is the NOC Outcome label; this text recommends use of the self-report NRS in place of the NOC indicator scales because of the amount of research supporting its use.

Client Outcomes

Client Will (Specify Time Frame)

For the Client Who Is Able to Provide a Self-Report
- Provide a description of the pain experience including physical, social, emotional, and spiritual aspects
- Use a self-report pain tool to identify current pain level and establish a comfort-function goal
- Report that the pain management regimen achieves comfort-function goal without the occurrence of side effects
- Describe nonpharmacological methods that can be used to supplement, or enhance, pharmacological interventions and help achieve the comfort-function goal
- Perform necessary or desired activities at a pain level less than or equal to the comfort-function goal
- Demonstrate the ability to pace activity, taking rest breaks before they are needed
- Describe how unrelieved pain will be managed
- State the ability to obtain sufficient amounts of rest and sleep
- Notify a member of the health care team for pain level consistently greater than the comfort-function goal or occurrence of side effect

For the Client Who Is Unable to Provide a Self-Report
- Demonstrate decrease or resolved pain-related behaviors
- Perform desired activities as determined by client condition
- Demonstrate the absence of side effects
- No pain-related behaviors will be evident in the client who is completely unresponsive; a reasonable outcome is to demonstrate the absence of side effects related to the prescribed pain treatment plan

NIC   (Nursing Interventions Classification)

Suggested NIC Interventions

Analgesic Administration; Pain Management

Example NIC Activities—Pain Management

Ensure that the client receives attentive analgesic care; Perform comprehensive assessment of pain, including location, characteristics, onset and duration, frequency, quality, intensity or severity, and precipitating factors

Nursing Interventions and *Rationales*

▲ During the initial assessment and interview, if the client is experiencing pain, conduct and document a comprehensive pain assessment, using appropriate pain assessment tools. EBN: *Determining location, temporal aspects, pain intensity, characteristics, and the effect of pain on function and quality of life are critical to determine the underlying cause of pain and effectiveness of treatment (McCaffery, 1968; Drew & Peltier, 2018). The initial assessment includes all pain information that the client can provide for the development of the individualized pain management plan (Drew & Peltier, 2018).*

▲ Determine the quality of the pain and whether the pain has persisted beyond the usual duration for tissue healing. EB: *Chronic pain is persistent, lasting beyond the expected time or usual time of tissue healing (usually 3 months). Descriptors such as "sharp," "shooting," or "burning" assist in discriminating neuropathic pain from nociceptive pain (APS, 2016; Elliot, Simpson, & DiMaggio, 2018).* Please refer to the Acute **Pain** section for the Hierarchy of Pain Measures for assessment approach in clients who are unable to provide self-report of pain.

▲ Perform a pain assessment using a reliable self-report pain tool. EB: *Tools such as the 0 to 10 NRS or faces pain scale (FPS) assess pain intensity. Multidimensional tools such as the Brief Pain Inventory (BPI), McGill*

● = Independent; ▲ = Collaborative; EBN = Evidence-Based Nursing; EB = Evidence-Based

Pain Questionnaire (MPQ), the Pain Relief Scale (PRS), or the Chronic Pain Grade Scale (CPGS) provide a comprehensive evaluation of the client with persistent pain assessing the characteristics and quality of pain; satisfaction with pain control; and how pain affects mood, activity, sleep, and diet (Fillingim et al, 2016; Drew & Peltier, 2018). Lee et al (2014) reported that the NRS together with the PRS increased the objectivity of pain assessment in chronic spinal pain compared with the use of either scale alone.

▲ Ask the client to describe prior experiences with pain, effectiveness of pain management interventions, responses to analgesic medications including occurrence of side effects, and concerns about pain and its treatment (e.g., fear about addiction, worries, anxiety) and informational needs. EBN: *Obtaining an individualized pain history helps identify potential factors that may influence the client's willingness to report pain, as well as factors that may influence pain intensity, the client's response to pain, anxiety, and pharmacokinetics of analgesics (Drew & Peltier, 2018).*

● Using a self-report tool, ask the client to identify a comfort-function goal that will allow the client to perform necessary or desired activities easily. EBN: *The comfort-function goal provides the basis for individualized pain management plans and assists in determining effectiveness of pain management interventions (Drew & Peltier, 2018).* Assess the client for the presence of acute pain (see care plan for Acute **Pain**).

▲ Assess chronic pain regularly including the impact of chronic pain on activity; sleep; eating habits; and social conditions including relationships, finances, and employment. CEB: *Regular assessment of clients with chronic pain is critical because changes in the underlying pain condition, presence of comorbidities, and changes in psychosocial circumstances can affect pain intensity and characteristics and require revision of the pain management plan (Turk et al, 2016).* EB: *Sleep disturbance and decreased physical activity are adverse effects of people with chronic pain. Tang and Sanborn (2014) found clients with chronic pain who had a better night's sleep spontaneously engaged in more physical activity the following day.*

▲ Assess the client for the presence of psychiatric conditions, including anxiety and depression. EB: *Among chronic pain clients, 30% to 50% have been found to have depression as a comorbidity, and there is a fourfold higher risk of suicide attempt than in the general population (Breivik et al, 2014). Anxiety and fear may intensify pain, and pain may trigger emotional responses such as fear and anxiety (Turk et al, 2016; Zhuo, 2016). The coexistence of major depressive disorder and persistent pain has been reported to be 30% to 60% (Maletic & DeMuri, 2016).*

▲ If opioid therapy is considered, assist the provider with aspects of an opioid risk assessment, which includes a comprehensive client interview and examination with a pain focus, mental health screening, use of an opioid risk assessment tool, examination of prescription drug monitoring program results, and urine drug screening. EB: *Although prevalence rates vary, there is evidence of opioid misuse and substance use disorder (SUD) among those who are prescribed opioids, thus to reduce risk and optimize safe opioid use, risk assessment and stratification are recommended (APS, 2016; Dowell, Haegerich, & Chou, 2016; Hudspeth, 2016).*

▲ For the client who is receiving outpatient opioid therapy, at each visit, assess effect of opioids on pain status, function, goal achievement, and presence of side effects including sleep disturbance and sexual dysfunction; assessment for signs of misuse and SUD should be included, which may involve the use of random urine drug toxicology screening, pill counts, and review of prescription monitoring database. EB: *Opioid therapy is associated with risk for misuse and SUD and overdose, whereas the evidence for the long-term use of opioid therapy in chronic pain is inconclusive. To minimize risk, a number of risk mitigation practices, including careful assessment of the client response to opioid therapy, are recommended (APS, 2016; Dowell, Haegerich, & Chou, 2016).*

● Ask the client to maintain a diary (if able) of pain ratings, timing, precipitating events, medications, and effectiveness of pain management interventions. EBN: *Systematic tracking of pain has been demonstrated to be an important factor in improving pain management (Fillingim et al, 2016). In a study of smartphone-based interventions with diaries among women with chronic widespread pain, it was found that the use of the smartphone intervention with diaries and personalized feedback reduced catastrophizing and prevented increases in functional impairment and symptoms (Kristjánsdóttir et al, 2013). Franco et al (2015) suggested the use of a smartphone-based electronic pain diary via telemedicine may be a reliable method for conducting remote assessments of chronic pain clients over time, thus improving clinical monitoring, differential diagnosis, and treatment of pain.*

▲ Obtain and review an accurate and complete list of medications the client is taking or has taken. CEB: *Accurate medication reconciliation can guide analgesic plan development and prevent errors associated with incorrect medications, dosages, omission of components of the home medication regimen, drug–drug interactions, and toxicity that can occur when incompatible drugs are combined or when allergies are present (Ignatavicius,*

● = Independent;   ▲ = Collaborative;   EBN = Evidence-Based Nursing;   EB = Evidence-Based

2013). **EBN:** *Young et al (2015), in an examination of transition-related medication discrepancies in a rural community, found that 55% of the medication discrepancies involved medications for pain control.*

▲ Explain to the client the pain management approach that has been ordered or revised, including therapies, medication administration, side effects, and complications. **EB:** *One of the most important steps toward improved control of pain is a better client understanding of the nature of pain, its treatment, pain management goals, and the role the client needs to play in pain control (Curtiss & Wrona, 2018).*

● Discuss the client's fears of undertreated pain, side effects, opioid use disorder (OUD), and overdose and reassure the client that there will be regular assessment and treatment of pain and assessment for side effects and signs of OUD. **EBN:** *Cogan et al (2014) reported that among 379 clients scheduled for cardiac surgery, 31% stated that it is easy to become addicted to pain medication, 20% report that "good patients" do not talk about their pain, and 35% believe that pain medication should be "saved in case the pain worsens."*

▲ Manage chronic pain using an individualized, multimodal nonopioid or opioid-sparing approach. **EB:** *A multimodal approach (combining two or more drugs that act by different mechanisms for providing analgesia) such as acetaminophen, an anticonvulsant, antidepressant, and opioid in chronic pain enhances pain relief and allows the lowest effective dose of each drug to be administered, resulting in fewer or less severe side effects such as nausea, sedation, and respiratory depression. Nonopioid therapy is the treatment of choice in chronic noncancer pain. Opioids may be considered when all other reasonable attempts at analgesia have failed; however, evidence for long-term effectiveness is not clear (The Joint Commission [TJC], 2012; Dowell, Haegerich, & Chou, 2016; Jungquist et al, 2016; Elliot, Simpson, & DiMaggio, 2018).*

▲ Select the route of administration of analgesics based on client condition and pain characteristics. **CEB:** *The least invasive route of administration capable of providing adequate pain control is recommended. The oral route is preferred because of its convenience and the resulting relatively steady blood levels; the rectal route or transdermal route may be used when the oral route is not feasible; the intravenous route is preferred for rapid control of severe pain, and would therefore not generally be used for chronic pain; and intramuscular injections are avoided because of variable absorption and the potential for nerve injury and tissue damage (APS, 2016; Behm, Leinum, & Peltier, 2018).*

▲ When chronic pain has a neuropathic component, treat with adjuvant analgesics, such as anticonvulsants, antidepressants, and topical local anesthetics. **EB:** *First-line analgesics for neuropathic pain belong to the adjuvant analgesic group and include anticonvulsants, antidepressants, and some topical local anesthetics. Analgesic efficacy with opioids in chronic neuropathic pain is inconclusive (Gilron, Baron, & Jensen, 2015; Dowell, Haegerich, & Chou, 2016; Elliot, Simpson, & DiMaggio, 2018).*

▲ Administer a nonopioid analgesic for mild to moderate chronic pain and as a component of the treatment for all levels of pain for clients with cancer pain. **CEB:** *Nonopioids, such as acetaminophen and nonsteroidal antiinflammatory drugs (NSAIDs), are first-line analgesics for the treatment of mild and moderate pain conditions (e.g., osteoarthritis pain) (Dowell, Haegerich, & Chou, 2016). Consider adding nonopioid analgesics such as acetaminophen and NSAIDs for cancer pain, provided comorbidities and other risks do not prevent the use of these analgesics; NSAIDs are used cautiously, especially when used chronically, because many cancer patients may be at high risk for renal, gastrointestinal (GI), or cardiac toxicities; thrombocytopenia; or bleeding problems (National Comprehensive Cancer Network [NCCN], 2017).*

▲ Recognize that opioid therapy may be indicated for some clients experiencing chronic pain. **EB:** *Opioids are often used in the management of moderate to severe chronic cancer pain. Opioid initiation for chronic, noncancer pain is controversial because of the limited data on long-term efficacy and safety. Opioid therapy may be considered with careful client selection when the benefits for pain control and function outweigh client risk (Chou et al, 2015; APS, 2016; Dowell, Haegerich, & Chou, 2016; Pasero et al, 2016).*

▲ Administer analgesics around the clock for continuous pain and as needed (PRN) for intermittent or breakthrough pain as may be experienced by clients with cancer pain. **EB:** *More than one in two clients with cancer pain also experience breakthrough cancer pain, and if pain is present most of the day, the use of PRN medications alone will lead to periods of undermedication and poor pain control and to periods of excessive medication and adverse effects (Deandrea et al, 2014; APS, 2016).*

▲ Long-acting or extended release opioids may be indicated for patients with cancer or with chronic non-cancer pain if patients require the regular use of short-acting opioids, and receive adequate relief with them. **EB:** *Controlled-release preparations are helpful because the long duration lessens the severity of end-of-dose pain, decreases analgesic gaps, and allows patients to sleep during the night (APS, 2016).*

▲ At regular intervals, assess inpatient clients with chronic pain for opioid-related adverse events and include frequent assessment of pain level, assessment of respiratory status (including rate, rhythm, noisiness, and depth), and systematic assessment of sedation level using a sedation scale. **EB:** *Tolerance to opioid-induced*

● = Independent; ▲ = Collaborative; **EBN** = Evidence-Based Nursing; **EB** = Evidence-Based

respiratory depression usually develops within a week of regular daily opioid dosing, making this side effect less likely to occur in those who are opioid tolerant than those who are not tolerant; however, opioid-tolerant clients are at similar risk for respiratory depression when they misuse opioids, are admitted to the hospital for surgery, or receive more than their usual opioid dose to treat an acute condition, or receive concomitant sedating medications (APS, 2016; Jungquist et al, 2016).

▲ During outpatient follow-up, assess clients receiving opioids for risk factors that may increase opioid-related harm. **EB:** *Clients who are receiving higher opioid doses, prescribed concurrent benzodiazepines, have cognitive impairment that could lead to accidental ingestion of excess opioids, mental health disorders that place a client at greater risk for suicide, or a history of SUD are at greater risk for opioid overdose. Take-home naloxone for the treatment of opioid-induced respiratory depression is recommended by numerous federal, state, and professional organizations (Coe & Walsh, 2015).*

▲ Provide the client with a stool softener and stimulant to prevent/treat opioid-related constipation. Ask about other opioid-related side effects including nausea, pruritus, lack of appetite, and changes in rest and sleep. **EB:** *Although clients may develop tolerance to nausea, pruritus, and other opioid side effects, they do not develop tolerance to opioid-induced constipation. A study of 489 people on long-term opioids revealed varying utilization and responses to laxatives continues to add to the burden of chronic pain (Coyne et al, 2015; Coyne, Bobb, & DiMaggio, 2018).*

▲ In addition to administering analgesics, support the client's use of nonpharmacological methods to help control pain, such as distraction, imagery, relaxation, and application of heat and cold. **EBN:** *Evidence suggested efficacy and satisfaction when complementary therapies are integrated into pain treatment plans of older adults (Bruckenthal, Marino, & Snelling, 2016).*

▲ **EB:** Cognitive behavioral (mind–body) strategies can restore the client's sense of self-control, personal efficacy, and active participation in his or her own care (Broderick et al, 2014). **EB:** *Motivational interviewing, a counseling method that aims to resolve a client's ambivalence about behavior change, may improve chronic pain treatment adherence, but more study is needed to determine whether it will improve pain intensity and function (Alperstein & Sharpe, 2016).* **EB:** *Interdisciplinary outpatient rehabilitation using physical therapy, occupational therapy, and cognitive behavioral therapy can significantly improve function in people with chronic pain (Kurklinsky et al, 2016).*

● Teach and implement nonpharmacological interventions when pain is relatively well controlled with pharmacological interventions. **EB:** *Pain causes cognitive impairment (Baker et al, 2017).*

▲ Encourage the client to plan activities around periods of greatest comfort whenever possible. **EB:** *Some literature supported the use of pacing (a cognitive behavioral therapy strategy), which is an active self-management strategy in which individuals learn to balance activity and rest for the purpose of increasing function (Andrews et al, 2015).*

▲ Explore appropriate resources for management of pain on a long-term basis (e.g., hospice, pain care center). **EB:** *Outpatient pain management resources must be identified to ensure appropriate chronic pain management. A telecare collaborative management study demonstrated that participants with chronic musculoskeletal pain who received telecare management monthly for 1 year experienced at least 30% improvement in pain scores after 12 months and improved secondary pain (Kroenke et al, 2014).*

▲ If the client has progressive cancer pain, assist the client and family with handling issues related to death and dying and provide access to palliative care programs and hospice services. **CEB:** *In a study by Temel et al (2010), clients with non-small cell lung cancer who received early palliative care intervention had significant improvements in quality of life and mood, less aggressive care at the end of life, and longer survival.* **EB:** *Hui et al (2014) reported that in a study of advanced cancer clients, those who were referred to outpatient palliative care had improved end-of-life care compared with those who received inpatient palliative care.*

 Pediatric

● Assess for the presence of pain using a valid and reliable pain scale based on age, cognitive development, and the child's ability to provide a self-report. **EBN:** *Scales that depict faces at various levels of pain intensity are commonly used in young children and have been shown to be reliable and valid in children as young as 3 years old (Tobias, 2014).* **CEB:** *Behavioral tools such as the Face, Legs, Activity, Cry, Consolability (FLACC) Scale may be used to assess pain in infants and children who cannot provide a self-report (Crellin et al, 2015).*

▲ Manage chronic pain children, infants, and neonates with an interdisciplinary and multimodal approach. **EB:** *There is a lack of randomized controlled trials among pediatric patients to identify the best approach to the treatment of pain in this age group. Expert consensus recommends treatment using an interdisciplinary*

● = Independent;   ▲ = Collaborative;   EBN = Evidence-Based Nursing;   EB = Evidence-Based

approach, including physical therapies and cognitive behavioral therapy, and when pharmacological approaches are needed, a multimodal pharmacological approach, using medications from a variety of classes, is recommended (Mathew, Kim, & Zempsky, 2016; Bruce et al, 2017).

- Use a variety of nonpharmacological analgesic interventions to address chronic pain in pediatric clients. **EBN:** *Complementary therapies such as cognitive behavioral strategies, mindfulness-based approaches, and other nonpharmacological approaches may play an important role in chronic pain management in children and adolescents (van der Veek et al, 2013; Song et al, 2014; Bruce et al, 2017).*

 Geriatric

▲ An older client's report of pain should be taken seriously and assessed and treated. **EB:** *Chronic pain decreases quality of life, and elderly people with chronic pain report poorer health and decreased mobility and feel more sadness, loneliness, and fatigue, than those without chronic pain (Rapo-Pylkkö, Haanpää, & Liira, 2016). Chronic pain in the elderly is associated with an increase in physical, social, and psychological frailty (Coelho et al, 2017).* **EBN:** *Among the elderly, the presence of severe daily pain is positively correlated with the presence of depression and the frequency of falls and fatigue (Crowe et al, 2017).*

- When assessing pain, speak clearly, slowly, and loudly enough for the client to hear, ensure hearing aids and glasses are in place as appropriate; enlarge pain scales and written materials, and repeat information as needed. **EB:** *Older clients often have multiple sensory deficits, including vision and hearing difficulties, which can affect cognition, lead to loneliness and isolation, and contribute to declines in social interactions and relationships (Correia et al, 2016; Humes & Young, 2016; Stephan et al, 2017).*

- Handle the client's body gently and allow the client to move at his or her own speed. **EB:** *Older adults are particularly susceptible to injury during care activities. Age-related skeletal muscle changes result in weakness and muscle loss, placing patients at risk for injuries. Slow walking and turns may preserve muscle mass and strength in the trunk and limbs, which may enable continued independence (Araki et al, 2017).*

▲ Use nonpharmacological approaches including physical therapy, exercise, or other movement-based programs as the core components to persistent pain management in the older adult. **EB:** *Physical and occupational rehabilitation, behavioral approaches, and movement-based interventions tailored to the older person's needs and capabilities have been shown to be effective and should be used to treat chronic pain when possible (Makris et al, 2014; Reid, Eccleston, & Pillemer, 2015).*

▲ When pharmacological measures are needed to address chronic pain in the elderly, use a multimodal approach, including nonopioid analgesics for mild to moderate pain. **CEB:** *Acetaminophen (maximum dosage 3000 mg/day) is preferred and recommended, unless contraindicated, as first-line therapy for older persons with persistent pain; NSAIDs (preferably in topical form because there is less system absorption than in the oral form) should be used short term and with extreme caution because of the higher GI, cardiovascular, and renal adverse effects; if a systemic NSAID is needed, naproxen has the safest cardiac profile (Makris et al, 2014; Reid, Eccleston, & Pillemer, 2015).*

▲ Use opioids cautiously in the older client with moderate to severe pain. **CEB:** *When pain is not responsive to other treatment modalities, or when persistent pain is associated with increased functional impairment or decreased quality of life, an opioid trial may be initiated, starting with a short-acting low-dose opioid, carefully and slowly titrating to attain therapeutic goal, with assessment of response and effectiveness (Makris et al, 2014; Reid, Eccleston, & Pillemer, 2015).*

▲ Monitor for signs of depression in older clients and refer to specialists with relevant expertise. **EB:** *Depression is often associated with pain and decreased levels of independence with activities of daily living in the older client. Treatment has been demonstrated to decrease pain and improve functional abilities (Tarakci, Zenginler, & Kaya Mutlu, 2015).*

 Multicultural

▲ Assess for pain disparities among racial and ethnic minorities. **EB:** *Individuals of ethnic and racial minorities often receive fewer treatment options and less effective pain treatment than others because of barriers imposed by health care professionals and health care systems (Tait & Chibnall, 2014).*

▲ Assess for the influence of cultural beliefs, norms, and values on the client's perception and experience of pain. **EB:** *The large variations in chronic back pain prevalence and prognosis across different countries may be influenced by culturally determined health beliefs (Henschke et al, 2016).*

▲ Use a family-centered approach to care. **EB:** *Involving the family in care through early regular communication and decision-making may reduce anxiety, alleviate uncertainty, and improve coping strategies (Michael et al, 2014).*

●	= Independent;	▲	= Collaborative;	**EBN** = Evidence-Based Nursing;	**EB** = Evidence-Based

▲ Use culturally relevant pain scales to assess pain in the client. CEB: *Clients from minority cultures may express pain differently than clients from the majority culture. The FPS-Revised was shown to be preferred over other self-report pain rating tools in older minority adults (Ware et al, 2006) and in Chinese adults (Li, Herr, & Chen, 2009). A later study demonstrated that the Iowa Pain Thermometer was the preferred tool in older Chinese adults (Li, Herr, & Chen, 2009).*

Home Care

- The interventions previously described may be adapted for home care use. Refer to the Nursing Interventions and *Rationales* in the care plan for Acute **Pain.**

Client/Family Teaching and Discharge Planning

Note: To avoid the negative connotations associated with the words "drugs" and "narcotics," use the term "pain medicine" when teaching clients.

- Discuss the various discomforts encompassed by the word "pain" and ask the client to give examples of previously experienced pain. Explain the pain assessment process and the purpose of the pain rating scale. EB: *It is often difficult for clients to understand the concept of pain and describe their pain experience. In a survey, must participants were able to recognize the term narcotic, but very few recognized or understood the term "opioid"(Wallace et al, 2013).*
- Teach the client that if the pain level is consistently above the comfort-function goal, the client should take action that decreases pain or should notify a member of the health care team so that effective pain management interventions may be implemented promptly. (See information on teaching clients to use the pain rating scale.) EB: *The use of comfort-function goals provides direction for the treatment plan. Changes are made according to the client's response and achievement of the goals of recovery or rehabilitation (Boswell & Hall, 2017).*
- Provide educational materials on various aspects of pain control to improve client understanding of pain and pain-related interventions. EB: *Written materials and other educational tools assist in improving clients' knowledge related to pain management. In knee replacement clients, the use of an educational pamphlet and a compact disc was associated with decreased postoperative pain and increased participation in physical rehabilitation (Chen et al, 2014).*
- Discuss and evaluate the client's understanding about the total plan for pharmacological and nonpharmacological treatment, including the medication plan, the maintenance of a pain diary, and the use of supplies and equipment. CEB: *Appropriate instruction increases the accuracy and safety of medication administration (Vaismoradi, Jordan, & Kangasniemi, 2015).*
- Reinforce the importance of taking pain medications to maintain the comfort-function goal. EBN: *Teaching clients to stay on top of their pain and prevent it from getting out of control will improve the ability to accomplish the goals of recovery (APS, 2016; Eksterowicz & DiMaggio, 2018).*
- ▲ Reinforce that when prescribed, opioids for pain relief are an appropriate part of their multimodal pain treatment plan. EB: *Taking opioids only as directed, avoiding alcohol, and talking with the health care provider when pain is poorly controlled are strategies that will lessen the risks for OUD or major opioid-related adverse effects such as respiratory depression and arrest (Costello, 2015).*
- ▲ Reinforce the importance of safe storage of opioid medications out of the reach of others, and to responsibly dispose of any unused opioids. EB: *Community medication "take back" days and drop boxes are becoming increasingly popular. Encourage clients/families to check community resources (Hawk, Vaca, & D'Onofrio, 2015).*
- Demonstrate the use of appropriate nonpharmacological approaches in addition to pharmacological approaches for helping control pain, such as application of heat and/or cold, distraction techniques, relaxation breathing, visualization, rocking, stroking, listening to music, and watching television. Teach these methods when pain is relatively well controlled, because pain interferes with cognition. EB: *Nonpharmacological interventions are used to complement pharmacological interventions (Bruckenthal, Marino, & Snelling, 2016).*
- ▲ Emphasize to the client the importance of participating in a structured, individualized pacing activity and taking rest breaks before they are needed. EB: *In a study of adults with chronic pain and overactive behavior, a two-week inpatient program involving education on pain neurophysiology, pacing, activity scheduling, and gym sessions showed that tailored activity pacing intervention provides more pain relief and less fatigue (Andrews et al, 2015).*
- Teach nonpharmacological methods when pain is relatively well controlled. EB: *Pain interferes with cognition (Baker et al, 2017).*

● = Independent;   ▲ = Collaborative;   EBN = Evidence-Based Nursing;   EB = Evidence-Based

REFERENCES

Alperstein, D., & Sharpe, L. (2016). The efficacy of motivational interviewing in adults with chronic pain: A meta-analysis and systematic review. *The Journal of Pain, 17*(4), 393–403.

Andrews, N. E., Strong, J., Meredith, P. J., et al. (2015). "It's very hard to change yourself": An exploration of overactivity in people with chronic pain using interpretative phenomenological analysis. *Pain, 156*(7), 1215–1231.

American Pain Society (APS). (2016). *Principles of analgesic use* (7th ed.). Chicago, IL: American Pain Society.

Araki, M., Hatamoto, Y., Higaki, Y., et al. (2017). "Slow walking with turns" increases quadriceps and erector spinae muscle activity. *Journal of Physical Therapy Science, 29*(3), 419–424.

Baker, K. S., Georgiou-Karistianis, N., Gibson, S. J., et al. (2017). Optimizing cognitive function in persons with chronic pain. *The Clinical Journal of Pain, 33*(5), 462–472.

Behm, L. B., Leinum, C. J., & Peltier, C. H. (2018). Overview of pain management pharmacology. In M. L. Czarnecki & H. N. Turner (Eds.), *Core curriculum for pain management nursing*. St Louis: Mosby Elsevier.

Breivik, H., Reme, S. E., & Linton, S. J. (2014). High risk of depression and suicide attempt among chronic pain patients: Always explore catastrophizing and suicide thoughts when evaluating chronic pain patients. *Scandinavian Journal of Pain, 5*(1), 1–3.

Boswell, C., & Hall, M. (2017). Engaging the patient through comfort-function levels. *Nursing, 47*(10), 68–69.

Broderick, J. E., Keefe, F. J., Bruckenthal, P., et al. (2014). Nurse practitioners can effectively deliver pain coping skills training to osteoarthritis patients with chronic pain: A randomized, controlled trial. *Pain, 155*(9), 1743–1754.

Bruce, B. K., Ale, C. M., Harrison, T. E., et al. (2017). Getting back to living: Further evidence for the efficacy of an interdisciplinary pediatric pain treatment program. *The Clinical Journal of Pain, 33*(6), 535–542.

Bruckenthal, P., Marino, M. A., & Snelling, L. (2016). Complementary and integrative therapies for persistent pain management in older adults: A review. *Journal of Gerontological Nursing, 42*(12), 40–48.

Chen, S. R., Chen, C. S., & Lin, P. C. (2014). The effect of educational intervention on the pain and rehabilitation performance of patients who undergo a total knee replacement. *Journal of Clinical Nursing, 23*(1–2), 279–287.

Chou, R., Turner, J. A., Devine, E. B., et al. (2015). The effectiveness and risks of long-term opioid therapy for chronic pain: A systematic review for a National Institutes of Health Pathways to Prevention Workshop. *Annals of Internal Medicine, 162*(4), 276–286.

Coe, M. A., & Walsh, S. L. (2015). Distribution of naloxone for overdose prevention to chronic pain patients. *Preventive Medicine, 80*, 41–43.

Coelho, T., Paúl, C., Gobbens, R. J., et al. (2017). Multidimensional frailty and pain in community dwelling elderly. *Pain Medicine, 18*(4), 693–701.

Cogan, J., Ouimette, M. F., Vargas-Schaffe, G., et al. (2014). Patient attitudes and beliefs regarding pain medication after cardiac surgery: Barriers to adequate pain management. *Pain Management Nursing, 15*(3), 574–579.

Correia, C., Lopez, K. J., Wroblewski, K. E., et al. (2016). Global sensory impairment in older adults in the United States. *Journal of the American Geriatrics Society, 64*(2), 306–313.

Costello, M. (2015). Prescription opioid analgesics: Promoting patient safety with better patient education. *American Journal of Nursing, 115*(11), 50–56.

Coyne, P. J., Bobb, B. T., & DiMaggio, T. J. (2018). Pain management and palliative care. In M. L. Czarnecki & H. N. Turner (Eds.), *Core curriculum for pain management nursing*. St Louis: Mosby Elsevier.

Coyne, K. S., Margolis, M. K., Yeomans, K., et al. (2015). Opioid-induced constipation among patients with chronic noncancer pain in the United States, Canada, Germany, and the United Kingdom: Laxative use, response and symptom burden over time. *Pain Medicine (Malden, Mass.), 16*(8), 1551–1565.

Crellin, D. J., Harrison, D., Santamaria, N., et al. (2015). Systematic review of the face, legs, activity, cry, and consolability scale for assessing pain in infants and children: Is it reliable, valid and feasible for use? *Pain, 156*(11), 2132–2151.

Crowe, M., Jordan, J., Gillon, D., et al. (2017). The prevalence of pain and its relationship to falls, fatigue and depression in a cohort of older people living in the community. *Journal of Advanced Nursing, 73*(11), 2642–2651.

Curtiss, C. P., & Wrona, S. (2018). Pain management education. In M. L. Czarnecki & H. N. Turner (Eds.), *Core curriculum for pain management nursing*. St Louis: Mosby Elsevier.

Deandrea, S., Corli, O., Consonni, D., et al. (2014). Prevalence of breakthrough cancer pain: A systematic review and a pooled analysis of published literature. *Journal of Pain and Symptom Management, 47*(1), 57–76.

Dowell, D., Haegerich, T. M., & Chou, R. (2016). CDC guideline for prescribing opioids for chronic pain—United States, 2016. *MMWR. Recommendations and Reports, 65*(1), 1–50.

Drew, D. J., & Peltier, C. H. (2018). Pain assessment. In M. L. Czarnecki & H. N. Turner (Eds.), *Core curriculum for pain management nursing*. St Louis: Mosby Elsevier.

Eksterowicz, N., & Dimaggio, T. J. (2018). Acute pain management. In M. L. Czarnecki & H. N. Turner (Eds.), *Core curriculum*. St Louis: Mosby Elsevier.

Elliott, J., Simpson, M., & DiMaggio, T. J. (2018). Persistent pain management. In M. L. Czarnecki & H. N. Turner (Eds.), *Core curriculum for pain management nursing*. St Louis: Mosby Elsevier.

Fillingim, R. B., Loeser, J. D., Baron, R., et al. (2016). Assessment of chronic pain: Domains, methods, and mechanisms. *Journal of Pain, 17*(9), T10–T20.

Franco, G., Delussi, M., Sciruicchio, V., et al. (2015). The use of electronic pain diaries via telemedicine for managing chronic pain. *The Journal of Headache and Pain, 16*(Suppl. 1), A190.

Gilron, I., Baron, R., & Jensen, T. (2015). Neuropathic pain: Principles of diagnosis and treatment. *Mayo Clinic Proceedings*.

Hawk, K. F., Vaca, F. E., & D'Onofrio, G. (2015). Focus: Addiction: Reducing fatal opioid overdose: Prevention, treatment and harm reduction strategies. *The Yale Journal of Biology and Medicine, 88*(3), 235.

Henschke, N., Lorenz, E., Pokora, R., et al. (2016). Understanding cultural influences on back pain and back pain research. *Best Practice & Research. Clinical Rheumatology, 30*(6), 1037–1049.

Hudspeth, R. S. (2016). Safe opioid prescribing for adults by nurse practitioners: Part 1. Patient history and assessment standards and techniques. *The Journal for Nurse Practitioners, 12*(3), 141–148.

Hui, D., Kim, S. H., Roquemore, J., et al. (2014). Impact of timing and setting of palliative care referral on quality of end-of-life care in cancer patients. *Cancer, 120*(11), 1743–1749.

Humes, L. E., & Young, L. A. (2016). Sensory–cognitive interactions in older adults. *Ear and Hearing, 37*, 52S–61S.

Ignatavicius, D. (2013). Pain—The 5th vital sign. In D. Ignatavicius & M. L. Workman (Eds.), *Medical-surgical nursing: Patient-centered collaborative care* (7th ed., pp. 39–64). St. Louis: W.B. Saunders Company.

International Association for the Study of Pain (IASP). (2012). *IASP taxonomy*. Retrieved from http://www.iasp-pain.org/Taxonomy.

Jungquist, C. R., Correll, D. J., Fleisher, L. A., et al. (2016). Avoiding adverse events secondary to opioid-induced respiratory depression:

● = Independent; ▲ = Collaborative; **EBN** = Evidence-Based Nursing; **EB** = Evidence-Based

Implications for nurse executives and patient safety. *Journal of Nursing Administration*, 46(2), 87–94.

Kristjánsdóttir, Ó. B., Fors, E. A., Eide, E., et al. (2013). A smartphone-based intervention with diaries and therapist-feedback to reduce catastrophizing and increase functioning in women with chronic widespread pain: Randomized controlled trial. *Journal of Medical Internet Research*, 15(1), e5.

Kroenke, K., Krebs, E. E., Wu, J., et al. (2014). Telecare collaborative management of chronic pain in primary care: A randomized clinical trial. *JAMA: The Journal of the American Medical Association*, 312(3), 240–248.

Kurklinsky, S., Perez, R. B., Lacayo, E. R., et al. (2016). The efficacy of interdisciplinary rehabilitation for improving function in people with chronic pain. *Pain Research and Treatment*. Retrieved from http://dx.doi.org.lproxy.nymc.edu/10.1155/2016/7217684.

Lee, J. J., Lee, M. K., Kim, J. E., et al. (2014). Pain relief scale is more highly correlated with numerical rating scale than with visual analogue scale in chronic pain patients. *Pain Physician*, 18(2), E195–E200.

Li, L., Herr, K., & Chen, P. (2009). Postoperative pain assessment with three intensity scales in Chinese elders. *Journal of Nursing Scholarship*, 41(3), 241–249.

Makris, U. E., Abrams, R. C., Gurland, B., et al. (2014). Management of persistent pain in the older patient: A clinical review. *JAMA: The Journal of the American Medical Association*, 312(8), 825–836.

Maletic, V., & DeMuri, B. (2016). Chronic pain and depression: Understanding two culprits in common: First of two parts. *Current Psychiatry*, 15(3), 41–50, 52.

Mathew, E., Kim, E., & Zempsky, W. (2016, August). Pharmacologic treatment of pain. In *Seminars in pediatric neurology* (Vol. 23, No. 3, pp. 209–219). Philadelphia: W.B. Saunders.

McCaffery, M. (1968). *Nursing practice theories related to cognition, bodily pain, and man—Environment interactions*. Los Angeles: University of California at Los Angeles Students' Store.

Michael, N., O'Callaghan, C., Baird, A., et al. (2014). Cancer caregivers advocate a patient- and family-centered approach to advance care planning. *Journal of Pain and Symptom Management*, 47(6), 1064–1077.

National Comprehensive Cancer Network. (2017). NCCN clinical practice guidelines in oncology. *Adult Cancer Pain. Version 2.2017*.

Pasero, C., Quinlan-Colwell, A., Rae, D., et al. (2016). American Society for Pain Management nursing position statement: Prescribing and administering opioid doses based solely on pain intensity. *Pain Management Nursing*, 17(3), 170–180.

Rapo-Pylkkö, S., Haanpää, M., & Liira, H. (2016). Chronic pain among community-dwelling elderly: A population-based clinical study. *Scandinavian Journal of Primary Health Care*, 34(2), 159–164.

Reid, M. C., Eccleston, C., & Pillemer, K. (2015). Management of chronic pain in older adults. *BMJ (Clinical Research Ed.)*, 350, h532.

Song, Y., Lu, H., Chen, H., et al. (2014). Mindfulness intervention in the management of chronic pain and psychological comorbidity: A meta-analysis. *International Journal of Nursing Sciences*, 1(2), 215–223.

Stephan, Y., Sutin, A. R., Bosselut, G., et al. (2017). Sensory functioning and personality development among older adults. *Psychology and Aging*, 32(2), 139.

Tait, R. C., & Chibnall, J. T. (2014). Racial/ethnic disparities in the assessment and treatment of pain: Psychosocial perspectives. *The American Psychologist*, 69(2), 131.

Tarakci, E., Zenginler, Y., & Kaya Mutlu, E. (2015). Chronic pain, depression symptoms and daily living independency level among geriatrics in nursing home. *Journal of the Turkish Society of Algology*, 27(1), 35–41.

Tang, N. K. Y., & Sanborn, A. N. (2014). Better quality sleep promotes daytime physical activity in patients with chronic pain? A multilevel analysis of the within-person relationship. *PLoS ONE*, 9(3), e92158. Retrieved from https://doi.org/10.1371/journal.pone.0092158.

Temel, J. S., Greer, J. A., Muzikansky, M. A., et al. (2010). Early palliative care for patients with metastatic non-small-cell lung cancer. *The New England Journal of Medicine*, 363(8), 733–742.

The Joint Commission. (2012). *Sentinel Event Alert Issue 49: Safe use of opioids in hospitals*. Retrieved from http://www.jointcommission.org/sea_issue_49/. (Accessed 1 November 2017).

Tobias, J. D. (2014). Acute pain management in infants and children—Part 1: Pain pathways, pain assessment, and outpatient pain management. *Pediatric Annals*, 43(7), e163–e168.

Turk, D., Fillingim, R., Ohrbach, R., et al. (2016). Assessment of psychosocial and functional impact of chronic pain. *Journal of Pain*, 17(9 Suppl.), T21–T49.

van der Veek, S. M., Derkx, B. H., Benninga, M. A., et al. (2013). Cognitive behavior therapy for pediatric functional abdominal pain: A randomized controlled trial. *Pediatrics*, 132(5), e1163–e1172.

Vaismoradi, M., Jordan, S., & Kangasniemi, M. (2015). Patient participation in patient safety and nursing input–a systematic review. *Journal of Clinical Nursing*, 24(5–6), 627–639.

Wallace, L. S., Keenum, A. J., AbdurRaqeeb, O., et al. (2013). Terminology matters: Patient understanding of "opioids" and "narcotics." *Pain Practice*, 13(2), 104–108.

Ware, L. J., et al. (2006). Evaluation of the Revised Faces Pain Scale, Verbal Descriptor Scale, Numeric Rating Scale, and Iowa Pain Thermometer in older minority adults. *Pain Management Nursing*, 7(3), 117–125.

Young, L., Barnason, S., Hays, K., et al. (2015). Nurse practitioner-led medication reconciliation in critical access hospitals. *The Journal for Nurse Practitioners*, 11(5), 511–518.

Zhuo, M. (2016). Neural mechanisms underlying anxiety-chronic pain interactions. *Trends in Neurosciences*, 39(3), 136–145.

P

Chronic Pain syndrome   *Mary Beth Flynn Makic, PhD, RN, CCNS, FAAN, FNAP*

NANDA-I

Definition

Recurrent or persistent pain that has lasted at least 3 months and that significantly affects daily functioning or well-being.

Defining Characteristics

Anxiety (00146); constipation (00011); deficient knowledge (00126); disturbed sleep pattern (00198); fatigue (00093); fear (00148); impaired mood regulation (00241); impaired physical mobility (00085); insomnia (00095); obesity (00232); social isolation (00053); stress overload (00177)

● = Independent;   ▲ = Collaborative;   **EBN** = Evidence-Based Nursing;   **EB** = Evidence-Based

Related Factors

To be developed

NIC, NOC, Client Outcomes, Nursing Interventions and *Rationales,* Client/Family Teaching and Discharge Planning, and References

Refer to care plan for Acute **Pain** and Chronic **Pain.**

Labor Pain   *Nichol Chesser, RN, CNM, DNP*

NANDA-I

Definition

Sensory and emotional experience that varies from pleasant to unpleasant, associated with labor and childbirth.

Defining Characteristics

Alteration in blood pressure; alteration in heart rate; alteration in muscle tension; alteration in neuroendocrine functioning; alteration in respiratory rate; alteration in sleep pattern; alteration in urinary functioning; decrease in appetite; diaphoresis; distraction behavior; expressive behavior; facial expression of pain; increase in appetite; narrowed focus; nausea; pain; perineal pressure; positioning to ease pain; protective behavior; pupil dilation; self-focused; uterine contraction; vomiting

Related Factors

To be developed

Associated Condition

Cervical dilation; fetal expulsion

NOC   (Nursing Outcomes Classification)

Suggested NOC Outcomes

Client Satisfaction: Pain Management, Comfort Status; Knowledge: Pain Management, Pain Control, Pain Level

---

Example NOC Outcomes with Indicators

Labor pain management as evidenced by the following indicators: recognizes pain onset, discusses pain treatment options with health care professional, monitors therapeutic effects of analgesic, uses effective coping strategies, reports changes in pain symptoms to health care provider. (Rate the outcome and indicators of **Labor Pain:** 1 = never demonstrated, 2 = rarely demonstrated, 3 = sometimes demonstrated, 4 = often demonstrated, 5 = consistently demonstrated [see Section I].)

Client Outcomes

Client Will (Specify Time Frame)

- Recognize pharmacological and nonpharmacological interventions to address labor pain
- Demonstrate coping strategies to address labor pain
- Verbalize pain relief effectiveness throughout the labor process

NIC   (Nursing Intervention Classification)

Suggested NIC Outcomes

Acute, Analgesic Administration: Intraspinal, Analgesic Administration, Aromatherapy, Dance Therapy, Distraction, Environmental Management: Comfort, Guided Imagery, Massage, Medication Administration: Intraspinal, Meditation Facilitation, Relaxation Therapy, Transcutaneous Electrical Nerve Stimulation

● = Independent;   ▲ = Collaborative;   EBN = Evidence-Based Nursing;   EB = Evidence-Based

Example NIC Activity—Acute Pain Management

Explore the client's knowledge and beliefs about labor pain including cultural influences; monitor pain using a valid and reliable rating tool

Nursing Intervention and *Rationales*

- Initial assessment and interview, if the client is experiencing pain, conduct and document a comprehensive pain assessment, using appropriate pain assessment tools. **EB/CEB:** *A pain assessment tool consists of obtaining all the information that a client can provide to help individualize a pain management plan of care. Information includes location, intensity, characteristics, coping, and desire for pharmacological or nonpharmacological interventions. Pain level, as evidenced by client self-report of coping or not coping with pain from labor contractions, is considered the best indicator of pain presence and intensity (McCaffery, Herr, & Pasero, 2011; Merskey 1979). Use an evidence-based coping algorithm to help the client find the best means available to cope well with labor pain (Roberts et al, 2010).*
- *Observe for nonverbal pain assessment such as grimacing, lackluster eyes, and fixed or scattered movements.*
- Assess pain on pain level tool such as the 0 to 10 numerical pain rating scale (NRS) if appropriate or alternatively use the Coping with Labor Algorithm (Roberts et al, 2010). Discuss with client the desire for pain management for this labor, past experiences with labor and effectiveness of pain management techniques employed at that time, concerns about pain and its treatment, and information needs (e.g., pain coping techniques that are both analgesic and nonpharmaceutical). **EBN:** *Obtaining individualized history and goals for coping with pain during labor and birth helps identify how to better guide a client through childbirth and increase client satisfaction with the process. Women's satisfaction with the childbirth process is not directly correlated with pharmacological pain relief, but it is greatly enhanced by continuity of care and care provider presence (Van der Gucht & Lewis, 2015).*
- Goal is for the client to manage labor pain from admission until delivery of infant with either natural childbirth and associated pain management techniques, or pharmaceutical measures to reduce pain experience. **EB:** *For the client who is able to self-report, when using a self-report pain tool, caution must be used because a high or low score is not always associated with lack of coping or suffering when used for labor pain (Simkin & Klein, 2017).*
- Based on the client's ability to cope with labor pain, discuss with client pain management options, including pharmacological and nonpharmacological interventions. **EB:** *Implement strategies or request orders to help client cope with labor pain. This may include massage, movement (such as rocking or swaying, sitting on birthing ball, and position changes), rhythmic breathing, relaxation techniques, aromatherapy, intradermal water blocks, intravenous (IV) narcotics, transcutaneous electrical nerve stimulus (TENS), nitrous oxide, hydrotherapy, and neuraxial anesthesia (Gilbert, 2017).* **CEBN:** *A study found patients self-identified nonpharmacological coping strategies, such as relaxation techniques, distraction, imagery, and breathing techniques, to assist with labor pain (Niven & Gijsbers, 1996).*
- Based on the client's ability to cope, assess the physiological-natural process of labor, physical environment, and emotional/psychosocial dynamics (Roberts et al, 2010). **CBE:** *Labor pain is a physical sensation of pain but also psychoemotional and spiritual (Simkin & Bolding, 2004). Determining the best way to help a laboring woman cope encompasses physiological, physical, emotional, spiritual, and psychosocial assessments (Roberts et al, 2010).*
- Based on the client's ability to cope, offer intervention (either nonpharmacological or pharmacological). **EBN:** *Nonpharmacological pain interventions are low cost and low risk. They are also directed at increasing comfort during labor, preventing suffering, and allowing women to cope with labor pain (Simkin & Klein, 2017). Nonpharmacological pain measures can be used by themselves or in combination with pharmacological intervention during labor. If the client is unable to cope with labor by using nonpharmacological pain relief measures, offering pharmacological pain relief measures is appropriate. A client may be able to proceed through labor and delivery without pain medication but should never be denied medication if she requests it (Simkin & Klein, 2017).*
- Nonpharmacological pain relief measures are low-risk and low-resource interventions (Simkin & Klein, 2017). These approaches can encompass the physical sensation of pain and the psychoemotional and spiritual components of care. By addressing all aspects of client needs (physical, emotional, and spiritual), suffering can be reduced during labor (Simkin & Klein, 2017).

● = Independent;   ▲ = Collaborative;   **EBN** = Evidence-Based Nursing;   **EB** = Evidence-Based

○ Ambulation/rocking/swaying is a safe and effective coping measure for labor pain. This is usually a client-initiated response to labor pain; however, caregivers can encourage women to ambulate or change position to ease pain or allow clients to cope better with labor pain.

○ Hydrotherapy either as immersion in water or bathing can be used to promote relaxation, decrease anxiety, help client cope with pain, and to possibly correct uterine contraction dystocia (Benfield et al, 2010). **CEBN/EBN:** *Water labor may be indicated for women to help with relaxation during labor. This may enable the client to proceed through labor without pharmacological intervention because it may reduce anxiety around labor and contraction pain (Benfield et al, 2010; Nutter et al, 2014). Water temperature must be regulated to stay between 34°C and 45°C and ideally be at 37°C to have the least effect on the maternal cardiovascular and endocrine system (Benfield et al, 2010).*

○ TENS is a small, handheld device that transmits low-voltage electrical impulses to the skin (Simkin & Klein, 2017). The device suppresses the conduction of pain through pain fibers by using small electrical impulses (Shahoei et al, 2017). **EBN:** *The use of this device is controlled by the client herself and can vary the pattern and intensity of the cutaneous electrical impulse depending on the contraction pattern and pain (Simkin & Klein, 2017). The use of TENS has no adverse side effects and can improve overall satisfaction with the labor and birth experience when used correctly (Shahoei et al, 2017).*

● Pharmacological measures for pain relief are high resource and high risk; they require professional training for administration, incur cost, and have a greater risk to mother and baby (Simkin & Klein, 2017).

● Nitrous oxide is a blend of 50% nitrous oxide with 50% oxygen. The use of nitrous oxide may not alleviate pain, but it may help with satisfaction of the birth experience (American College of Nurse-Midwives [ACNM], 2010). **EBN:** *Nitrous should be avoided in clients with vitamin B_{12} deficiency or MHFR mutation/deficiency (Hays, 2017). Most common side effects of nitrous oxide are nausea and vomiting and respiratory depression (Likis et al, 2014). Correct usage of nitrous is needed for optimum efficacy; it must be initiated prior to contraction pain because the peak onset is 50 seconds from initial inhalation (Collins et al, 2018).*

● IV medications for pain management are an alternative for some women who do not desire an epidural; IV medications are generally opioids. These are advantageous because they are easy to administer, are widely available, and are less invasive than neuraxial techniques of pain relief (i.e., an epidural) *(Collins et al, 2018).* **EBN:** *Side effects are common and include nausea, vomiting, and drowsiness (Collins et al, 2018).*

● Epidural, combined spinal-epidural (CSE), and dural puncture epidural (DPE) are appropriate for laboring women when requested by the client (unless there is a contraindication). **CBE:** *Contraindications to neuraxial anesthesia include coagulopathy, infection of the lower back, and increased intracranial pressure (Leffert, Lee, & Schweamm, 2013).* **EBN:** *During placement of neuraxial anesthesia maternal oxygen saturation and heart rate should be measured continuously. Blood pressure should be measured every 5 minutes, and fetal heart rate should be monitored at least before and after administration according to institution guidelines. Continue to monitor maternal blood pressure, pain control, motor function, and sensory levels at regular intervals to make sure the anesthesia is working properly. Also, continue to document patient's vital signs and pain assessment (Collins et al, 2018).*

● Account for clients' abilities to cope with labor pain regarding their psychosocial, cultural, and spiritual backgrounds. A woman's positive perceptions of how she will be able to cope with labor are associated with reduced anxiety, pain, and intervention during labor (Van der Gucht & Lewis, 2015; Simkin & Klein, 2017). **CBE:** *Coping has many facets, including cognitive, behavioral, and emotional aspects (Abushaikha, 2007). How a woman copes with pain during labor includes factors such as personality traits, type of stress, and personal preference; coping methods encompass physiological, psychological, cognitive, and spiritual methods (Abushaikha, 2007). Each method of coping is an individual decision. Culturally learned values and attitudes may greatly influence how women cope with acute labor pain (Lowe, 2002).*

● *Document pain assessment and interventions and coping assessment and interventions to facilitate labor pain management through the continuum of the women's labor experience (Chajut et al, 2014).*

REFERENCES

Abushaikha, L. (2007). Methods of coping with labor pain used by Jordanian women. *Journal of Transcultural Nursing, 18*(1), 35–40.

American College of Nurse-Midwives. (2010). Position statement: Nitrous oxide for labor analgesia. *Journal of Midwifery and Women's Health, 55*(3).

Benfield, R., et al. (2010). The effects of hydrotherapy on anxiety, pain, neuroendocrine response, and contraction dynamics during labor. *Biological Research for Nursing, 12*(1), 18–36.

Chajut, E., Caspi, A., Chen, R., et al. (2014). In pain thou shalt bring forth children: The peak-and-end rule in recall of labor pain. *Psychological Science, 25*(12), 2266–2271.

● = Independent;   ▲ = Collaborative;   **EBN** = Evidence-Based Nursing;   **EB** = Evidence-Based

Collins, S., Fiore, A. T., Boudreau, J. A., et al. (2018). Nitrous oxide for the management of labor analgesia. *AANA Journal, 86*(1), Retrieved from https://www.aana.com/docs/default-source/aana-journal-web-documents-1/journal-course-6-nitrous-oxide-for-the-management-of-labor-anesthesia-february-2018.pdf?sfvrsn=442d42b1_6.

Gilbert, G. (2017). Pharmacologic management of pain during labor and delivery. *UpToDate*. Retrieved from https://www.uptodate.com/contents/pharmacologic-management-of-pain-during-labor-and-delivery?source=search_result&search=pharmacological%20managemet%20of%20pain%20during%20labor&selectedTitle=1~150. (Accessed 1 January 2018).

Hays, S. (2017). Inhalation anesthetic agents: clinical effects and uses. *UpToDate*. Retrieved from https://www.uptodate.com/contents/inhalation-anesthetic-agents-clinical-effects-and-uses?source=search_result&search=INhalation%20anasthetic%20agents&selectedTitle=1~150. (Accessed 1 January 2018).

Leffert, L. R., Lee, H., & Schweamm, M. D. (2013). Neuraxial anesthesia in parturients with intracranial pathology: A comprehensive review and re assessment of risk. *Anesthesiology, 119*, 703–718.

Likis, F. E., Andrews, J. C., Collins, M. R., et al. (2014). Nitrous oxide for the management of labor pain: A systematic review. *Anesthesia & Analgesia, 118*, 153–167.

Lowe, N. (2002). The nature of labor pain. *America Journal of Obstetrics and Gynecology, 186*, S16–S24.

McCaffery, M., Herr, K., & Pasero, C. (2011). Assessment. In C. Pasero & M. McCaffery (Eds.), *Pain assessment and pharmacologic management* (p. 13176). St. Louis: Mosby Elsevier.

Merskey, H. (1979). Pain terms; a list with definitions and a note on usage. Recommended by the International Association for the Study of Pain (IASP) Subcommittee on Taxonomy. *Pain, 6*, 149–152.

Niven, C. A., & Gijsbers, K. (1996). Coping with labor pain. *Journal of Pain and Symptom Management, 11*(2), 116–125.

Nutter, E., Meyer, S., Shaw-Battista, J., et al. (2014). Waterbirth: An integrative analysis of peer-reviewed literature. *Journal of Midwifery and Women's Health, 59*, 286–319.

Roberts, L., Gulliver, B., Fisher, J., et al. (2010). The coping with labor algorithm: An alternative pain assessment tool for the laboring woman. *Journal of Midwifery and Women's Health, 55*(2), 107–116.

Shahoei, R., Shahghebi, S., Rezaei, M., et al. (2017). The effect of transcutaneous electrical nerve stimulation on the severity of labor pain among nulliparous women: A clinical trial. *Complementary Therapies in Clinical Practice, 28*, 176–180.

Simkin, P., & Bolding, A. (2004). Update on nonpharmacologic approaches to relieve labor pain and prevent suffering. *Journal of Midwifery and Women's Health, 49*(6), 489–504.

Simkin, P., & Klein, M. (2017). Nonpharmacological approaches to management of labor pain. *UpToDate*. Retrieved from https://www.uptodate.com/contents/nonpharmacologic-approaches-to-management-of-labor-pain?source=search_result&search=pharmacological%20managemet%20of%20pain%20during%20labor&selectedTitle=2~150. (Accessed 1 January 2018).

Van der Gucht, N., & Lewis, K. (2015). Women's experience of coping with pain during childbirth: A critical review of qualitative research. *Midwifery, 31*, 349–358.

Impaired Parenting   *Kimberly Silvey, MSN, RN, RAC-CT*

NANDA-I

P

Definition

Inability of the primary caregiver to create, maintain, or regain an environment that promotes the optimum growth and development of the child.

Defining Characteristics

Infant or Child

Behavioral disorders; delay in cognitive development; diminished separation anxiety; failure to thrive; frequent accidents; frequent illness; history of abuse; history of trauma; impaired social functioning; insufficient attachment behavior; low academic performance; run away from home

Parental

Abandonment of child; failure to provide safe home environment; decrease in ability to manage child; decrease in cuddling; deficient parent-child interaction; frustration with child; hostility; inadequate child health maintenance; inappropriate care-taking skills; inappropriate child care arrangements; inappropriate stimulation; inconsistent behavior management; inconsistent care; inflexibility in meeting needs of child; neglects needs of child; perceived inability to meet child's needs; perceived role inadequacy; punitive; rejection of child; speaks negatively about child

Related Factors

Infant or Child

Prolonged separation from parent; temperament conflicts with parental expectations

Parental

Alteration in sleep pattern; conflict between partners; depression; failure to provide safe home environment; father of child uninvolved; inability to put child's needs before own; inadequate child care arrangements;

● = Independent;   ▲ = Collaborative;   EBN = Evidence-Based Nursing;   EB = Evidence-Based

ineffective communication skills; ineffective coping strategies; insufficient access to resources; insufficient family cohesiveness; insufficient knowledge about child development; insufficient knowledge about child health maintenance; insufficient knowledge about parenting skills; insufficient parental role model; insufficient prenatal care; insufficient problem-solving skills; insufficient resources; insufficient response to infant cues; insufficient social support; insufficient transportation; insufficient valuing of parenthood; late-term prenatal care; low self-esteem; mother of child uninvolved; nonrestorative sleep pattern; preference for physical punishment; role strain; sleep deprivation; social isolation; stressors; unrealistic expectations

At-Risk Population

Infant or Child

Developmental delay; difficult temperament; gender other than desired; prematurity

Parental

Change in family unit; closely spaced pregnancies; difficult birthing process; economically disadvantaged; high number of pregnancies; history of abuse; history of being abusive; history of mental illness; history of substance misuse; insufficient cognitive readiness for parenting; legal difficulty; low education level; multiple births; relocation; single parent; unemployment; unplanned pregnancy; work difficulty; young parental age

Associated Condition

Infant or Child

Alteration in perceptual abilities; behavioral disorder; chronic illness; disabling condition

Parental

Alteration in cognitive functioning; disabling condition; physical illness

NOC (Nursing Outcomes Classification)

Suggested NOC Outcomes

Abuse Cessation; Abuse Protection; Abuse Recovery: Abusive Behavior Self-Restraint; Child Development (all); Coping; Family Functioning; Family Social Climate; Knowledge: Child Physical Safety; Neglect Recovery; Parent-Infant Attachment; Parenting Performance; Psychosocial Safety; Role Performance; Social Support

Example **NOC** Outcome with Indicators
Parenting Performance: Psychosocial Safety as evidenced by the following indicators: Fosters open communication/Recognizes risks for abuse/Uses strategies to eliminate risks for abuse/Selects appropriate supplemental caregivers/Uses strategies to prevent high-risk social behaviors/Provides required level of supervision/Sets clear rules for behavior/Maintains structure and daily routine in child's life. (Rate the outcome and indicators of **Parenting Performance: Psychosocial Safety:** 1 = never demonstrated, 2 = rarely demonstrated, 3 = sometimes demonstrated, 4 = often demonstrated, 5 = consistently demonstrated [see Section I].)

Client Outcomes

Client Will (Specify Time Frame)

- Initiate appropriate measures to develop a safe, nurturing environment
- Acquire and display attentive, supportive parenting behaviors and child supervision
- Identify appropriate strategies to manage a child's inappropriate behaviors
- Identify strategies to protect child from harm and/or neglect and initiate action when indicated

NIC (Nursing Interventions Classification)

Suggested NIC Interventions

Abuse Protection Support: Child; Attachment Promotion; Caregiver Support; Developmental Enhancement: Adolescent, Child; Environmental Management: Family Integrity Promotion; Impulse Control Training; Infant Care; Parent Education: Adolescent, Childrearing Family, Infant; Parenting Promotion; Role Enhancement; Substance Use Prevention, Treatment; Teaching: Infant Stimulation; Toddler Nutrition; Toddler Safety

● = Independent; ▲ = Collaborative; EBN = Evidence-Based Nursing; EB = Evidence-Based

Example NIC Activities—Family Integrity Promotion
Identify typical family coping mechanisms; Determine typical family relationships for each family; Counsel family members on additional effective coping skills for their own use; Assist family with conflict resolution; Monitor current family relationships; Facilitate a tone of togetherness within and among the family; Encourage family to maintain positive relationships; Refer for family therapy, as indicated

Nursing Interventions and *Rationales*

- Use the Parenting Sense of Competence (PSOC) scale to measure parental self-efficacy. EB: *The PSOC contains three useful factors that reflect satisfaction with the parental role, parenting efficacy, and interest in parenting. Mothers and fathers will differ in parenting of their children and their sense of competence (Karp et al, 2015).*

- Examine the characteristics of parenting style and behaviors. Consider dysfunctional child-centered and parent-centered cognitions as potentially critical correlates of abusive behavior. EBN: *Identifying possible risk factors for abuse can help nursing and parents reduce the risk of abusive behavior (Ben-Natan et al, 2014).*

- ▲ Institute abuse/neglect protection measures if evidence exists of an inability to cope with family stressors or crisis, signs of parental substance abuse are observed, or a significant level of social isolation is apparent. EBN: *Encouraging parents to be involved with social networking can help reduce stressors and assist with coping in a crisis (Bennett et al, 2017).*

- ▲ For a mother with a toddler, assess maternal depression. Make the appropriate referral. EB: *Helping mothers identify systems of depression through self-assessment or home visits is beneficial for both mother and toddler (Suplee et al, 2014).*

- Appraise the parent's resources and the availability of social support systems. Determine the single mother's particular sources of support, especially the availability of her own mother and partner. Encourage the use of healthy, strong support systems. EB: *Clinicians should help mothers evaluate what resources and support they have and encourage healthy relationships (Letourneau et al, 2013). Provide education to at-risk parents on behavioral management techniques such as looking ahead, giving good instructions, providing positive reinforcement, redirecting, planned ignoring, and instituting time-outs. EB: Parents with mental health issues need education to help them better care for their children (Houlihan et al, 2013).*

- Promotion of better quality relationships between parents and children is an effective strategy that can lead to enhanced learning. Good quality parenting leads to improved cognitive and social skills for children. EB: *Promoting quality relationships promotes optimal health and development (Titze et al, 2014).*

- Support parents' competence in appraising their infant's behavior and responses and aim supportive interventions to minimize parents' experiences of strain or stress. EBN: *Encourage and support the presence of the parents with the care of the infant (Ottosson & Lantz, 2017).*

- Model age-appropriate and cognitively appropriate caregiver skills by doing the following: communicating with the child at an appropriate cognitive level of development, giving the child tasks and responsibilities appropriate for age or functional age/level, instituting safety considerations such as the use of assistive equipment, and encouraging the child to perform activities of daily living as appropriate. EBN: *Children learn from the interactions with family, parents, and even medical staff (Rich et al, 2014).*

- Encourage mothers to understand and capitalize on their infant's capacity to interact, particularly in the early months of life. EBN: *Mother–infant bonding is very important during the first months of life (Lee et al, 2013).*

- ▲ Provide programs for homeless mothers with severe mental illness who have lost physical custody of their children. EB: *Providing education and support to homeless mothers helps empower them (Sleed et al, 2013).*

- ▲ Provide a recovery program that includes instruction in parenting skills and child development for mothers who are addicted to cocaine. EB: *Women need additional assistance for recovery from substance abuse and need to understand the effect that it will have on their child (McKeever et al, 2014).*

- Refer to Readiness for enhanced **Parenting** for additional interventions.

 Multicultural

- Acknowledge that value conflicts from acculturation stresses may contribute to increased anxiety and significant conflict with children. CEBN: *Help parents develop a plan to address conflicts within the family (Kim, 2011).*

● = Independent;   ▲ = Collaborative;   EBN = Evidence-Based Nursing;   EB = Evidence-Based

P

- Clarify parents' feelings, expectations, perceptions, and availability regarding participation in the care of their sick child. **EBN:** *Cultural differences regarding parent participation in the care of ill or hospitalized children should be considered (Mutair et al, 2014).*
- Carefully assess the meaning of terms used to describe health status when working with Native Americans. **EB:** *Health care providers should allow clients to participate in spiritual care according to their beliefs (Hodge & Wolosin, 2014).*
- Provide support for Chinese families caring for children with disabilities. **EBN:** *The care of the sick in China is based on Old World beliefs. It is important to ensure that all aspects of cultural beliefs are included in care (Zhang et al, 2014).*
- Facilitate modeling and role playing to help the family improve parenting skills. **EB:** *Families need to be able to practice parenting in a safe setting (Franks et al, 2013).*

Home Care

- The interventions previously described may be adapted for home care use.
- Assess parenting stress at each home visit to provide appropriate support and anticipatory guidance to families of children with a chronic disease. **EB:** *Assessing parental stress in the home assists the health care provider in identifying interventions that can be implemented at home (Gabler et al, 2014).*
- ▲ Assess the single mother's history regarding childhood and partner abuse and current status regarding depressive symptoms, abusive parenting attitudes (lack of empathy, favorable opinion of corporal punishment, parent–child role reversal, and inappropriate expectations). Refer for mental health services as indicated. **EB:** *A mother's history can contribute to the stress and the care of her children (Boeckel et al, 2014).*

Client/Family Teaching and Discharge Planning

- Consider individual and/or group-based parenting programs for teenaged mothers. **EB:** *Offering parenting programs to teenaged parents helps them to better care for their child (Mills et al, 2013).*
- Consider group-based parenting programs for parents of children younger than 3 years with emotional and behavioral problems. **EBN:** *A study shows that group-based parenting programs assist both the parent and the children (Kendall et al, 2013).*
- Consider group-based parenting programs for parents with anxiety, depression, and/or low self-esteem. **EBN:** *Parenting programs assist parents in identifying issues they may have and learn through others about goals they can set and ways to achieve them (Roose et al, 2014).*
- ▲ Refer adolescent parents for comprehensive psychoeducational parenting classes. **EBN:** *Adolescent parenting class helps teens to learn the best ways to care for their infant (Allen et al, 2014).*
- Parent training is one of the most effective interventions for behavior problems in young children. **EBN:** *Parent training programs assist with improving family functioning and interactions (Arkan et al, 2013). Encourage positive parenting: respect for children, understanding of normal development, and creative and loving approaches to meet parenting challenges rather than using anger, manipulation, punishment, and rewards.* **EBN:** *Parenting programs assist parents in identifying issues they may have and learn through others about goals they can set and ways to achieve them (Roose et al, 2014).*
- ▲ Initiate referrals to community agencies, parent education programs, stress management training, and social support groups. Consider the use of technology and the media. **EB:** *Family use of technology to interact with health care providers can broaden the support that the family can receive (Hanlon-Dearman et al, 2014).*
- Provide information regarding available telephone counseling services and Internet support. **EBN:** *Using the Internet allows parents to communicate with and gain support from others all over the world (Niela-Vilén et al, 2014). Refer to the care plans for Risk for disproportionate* **Growth**, *Risk for delayed* **Development**, *Risk for impaired* **Attachment**, *and Readiness for enhanced* **Parenting** *for additional teaching interventions.*

REFERENCES

Allen, K., El-Beshti, R., et al. (2014). An integrative adlerian approach to creating a teen parenting program. *Journal of Individual Psychology*, 70(1), 6–20.

Arkan, B., ÜstÜn, B., et al. (2013). An analysis of two evidence-based parent training programmes and determination of the

characteristics for a new programme model. *Journal of Psychiatric & Mental Health Nursing*, 20(2), 176–185.

Ben-Natan, M., Sharon, I., et al. (2014). Risk factors for child abuse: Quantitative correlational design. *Journal of Pediatric Nursing*, 29(3), 220–227.

Bennett, C. T., Buchan, J. L., et al. (2017). A realist synthesis of social connectivity interventions during transition to parenthood: The value of relationships. *Applied Nursing Research*, 34(Suppl. C), 12–23.

Boeckel, M. G., Blasco-Ros, C., et al. (2014). Child abuse in the context of intimate partner violence against women: The impact of women's depressive and posttraumatic stress symptoms on maternal behavior. *Journal of Interpersonal Violence*, 29(7), 1201–1227.

Franks, S. B., Mata, F. C., et al. (2013). The effects of behavioral parent training on placement outcomes of biological families in a state child welfare system. *Research on Social Work Practice*, 23(4), 377–382.

Gabler, S., Bovenschen, I., et al. (2014). Foster children's attachment security and behavior problems in the first six months of placement: Associations with foster parents' stress and sensitivity. *Attachment & Human Development*, 16(5), 479–498.

Hanlon-Dearman, A., Edwards, C., et al. (2014). 'Giving voice': Evaluation of an integrated telehealth community care model by parents/guardians of children diagnosed with fetal alcohol spectrum disorder in manitoba. *Telemedicine & e-Health*, 20(5), 478–484.

Hodge, D. R., & Wolosin, R. J. (2014). American Indians and spiritual needs during hospitalization: Developing a model of spiritual care. *The Gerontologist*, 54(4), 683–692.

Houlihan, D., Sharek, D., et al. (2013). Supporting children whose parent has a mental health problem: An assessment of the education, knowledge, confidence and practices of registered psychiatric nurses in Ireland. *Journal of Psychiatric & Mental Health Nursing*, 20(4), 287–295.

Karp, S., Lutenbacher, M., et al. (2015). Evaluation of the parenting sense of competence scale in mothers of infants. *Journal of Child and Family Studies*, 24(11), 3474–3481.

Kendall, S., Bloomfield, L., et al. (2013). Efficacy of a group-based parenting program on stress and self-efficacy among Japanese mothers: A quasi-experimental study. *Nursing & Health Sciences*, 15(4), 454–460.

Kim, E. (2011). Intergenerational acculturation conflict and Korean American parents' depressive symptoms. *Issues in Mental Health Nursing*, 32(11), 687–695.

Lee, G., McCreary, L., et al. (2013). Promoting mother-infant interaction and infant mental health in low-income Korean families: Attachment-based cognitive behavioral approach. *Journal for Specialists in Pediatric Nursing*, 18(4), 265–276.

Letourneau, N., Morris, C. Y., et al. (2013). Social support needs identified by mothers affected by intimate partner violence. *Journal of Interpersonal Violence*, 28(14), 2873–2893.

McKeever, A. E., Spaeth-Brayton, S., et al. (2014). The role of nurses in comprehensive care management of pregnant women with drug addiction. *Nursing for Women's Health*, 18(4), 284–293.

Mills, A., Schmied, V., et al. (2013). Someone to talk to: Young mothers' experiences of participating in a young parents support programme. *Scandinavian Journal of Caring Sciences*, 27(3), 551–559.

Mutair, A. S. A., Plummer, V., et al. (2014). Providing culturally congruent care for Saudi patients and their families. *Contemporary Nurse: A Journal for the Australian Nursing Profession*, 46(2), 254–258.

Niela-Vilén, H., Axelin, A., et al. (2014). Internet-based peer support for parents: A systematic integrative review. *International Journal of Nursing Studies*, 51(11), 1524–1537.

Ottosson, C., & Lantz, B. (2017). Parental participation in neonatal care. *Journal of Neonatal Nursing*, 23(3), 112–118.

Rich, C., Goncalves, A., et al. (2014). Teen advisory committee: Lessons learned by adolescents, facilitators, and hospital staff. *Pediatric Nursing*, 40(6), 289–296.

Roose, R., Mirecki, R. M., et al. (2014). Parents supporting parents: Implementing a peer parent program for perinatal loss. *Journal of Obstetric, Gynecologic & Neonatal Nursing*, 43(Suppl. 1), S46.

Sleed, M., James, J., et al. (2013). A psychotherapeutic baby clinic in a hostel for homeless families: Practice and evaluation. *Psychology and Psychotherapy*, 86(1), 1–18.

Suplee, P. D., Bloch, J. R., et al. (2014). Focusing on maternal health beyond breastfeeding and depression during the first year postpartum. *Journal of Obstetric, Gynecologic & Neonatal Nursing*, 43(6), 782–791.

Titze, K., Schenck, S., et al. (2014). Assessing the quality of the parent-child relationship: Validity and reliability of the child-parent relationship test (ChiP-C). *Journal of Child & Family Studies*, 23(5), 917–933.

Zhang, Y., Wei, M., et al. (2014). Chinese family management of chronic childhood conditions: A cluster analysis. *Journal for Specialists in Pediatric Nursing*, 19(1), 39–53.

P

Readiness for enhanced Parenting   Kimberly Silvey, MSN, RN, RAC-CT

NANDA-I

Definition

A pattern of providing an environment for children to nurture growth and development, which can be strengthened.

Defining Characteristics

Children express desire to enhance home environment; parent expresses desire to enhance parenting; parent expresses desire to enhance emotional support of children; parent expresses desire to enhance emotional support of other dependent person

NOC   (Nursing Outcomes Classification)

Suggested NOC Outcomes

Child Development; Knowledge: Child Physical Safety; Parenting Performance; Parenting: Psychosocial Safety

● = Independent;   ▲ = Collaborative;   EBN = Evidence-Based Nursing;   EB = Evidence-Based

Parenting Performance as evidenced by the following indicators: Provides preventive and episodic health care/Stimulates cognitive and social development/Stimulates emotional and spiritual growth/Empathizes with child/Expresses satisfaction with parental role/Expresses positive self-esteem. (Rate the outcome and indicators of **Parenting Performance:** 1 = never demonstrated, 2 = rarely demonstrated, 3 = sometimes demonstrated, 4 = often demonstrated, 5 = consistently demonstrated [see Section I].)

Client Outcomes

Client/Family Will (Specify Time Frame)

- Affirm desire to improve parenting skills to further support growth and development of children
- Demonstrate loving relationship with children
- Provide a safe, nurturing environment
- Assess risks in home/environment and take steps to prevent possibility of harm to children
- Meet physical, psychosocial, and spiritual needs or seek appropriate assistance

NIC   (Nursing Interventions Classification)

Suggested NIC Interventions

Anticipatory Guidance; Attachment Promotion; Developmental Enhancement: Adolescent; Child; Family Integrity Promotion: Childbearing Family; Infant Care; Newborn Care; Parent Education: Adolescent, Childrearing Family, Infant; Parenting Promotion; Teaching: Infant Stimulation

Example NIC Activities—Parenting Promotion

Assist parents to have realistic expectations appropriate to developmental and ability level of child; Assist parents with role transition and expectations of parenthood

Nursing Interventions and *Rationales*

- Use family-centered care and role modeling for holistic care of families. **EBN:** *Incorporating family-centered care helps enhance the parents' role in caring for their child (Cady et al, 2015).*
- Assess parents' feelings when dealing with a child who has a chronic illness. **EB:** *Nursing should assist parents (Byczkowski et al, 2014) in identifying their feelings about their child to help the parents develop coping mechanisms.*
- Promote low-technology interventions, such as massage and multisensory interventions (maternal voice, eye-to-eye contact, and rocking) and music to reduce maternal and infant stress and improve mother–infant relationship. **EB:** *When mother sing to their infants it can calm the infant and make them feel safe (de l'Etoile et al, 2017).* Support kangaroo care for infants at risk at birth; keep infants in an upright position in skin-to-skin contact. **EB:** *Kangaroo care helps the mother and infant to not only start bonding but also assist in the infant's growth and development (Shourangiz Beiranvand et al, 2014; Gavhane, Eklare, & Mohammad, 2016).*
- When the person who is ill is the parent, use family-centered assessment skills to determine the effect of an adult's illness on the child, and then guide the parent through those topics that are most likely to be of concern. **EB:** *Ill parents can have a negative effect on the life of a child. It is important to help the parent to continue in their role as parent the best way possible (Razaz et al, 2014). Provide practical and psychological assistance for parents of clients with psychiatric diagnoses, such as schizophrenia.* **EBN:** *Help parents understand the diagnosis of mental illness and the things they can do to help their child and also help themselves. Parents need to know that they do not have to deal with this alone (Hsiao & Tsai, 2014).*
- Refer to the care plan for Impaired **Parenting** for additional interventions.

 Multicultural

- Assess the influence of cultural beliefs, norms, and values on the client's perception of parenting. **EB:** *Understanding the cultural beliefs of the family will assist in parental satisfaction with care (Hamilton et al, 2013).*
- Acknowledge racial and ethnic differences at the onset of care and provide appropriate health information and social support. **EB:** *Acknowledgment of racial and ethnicity issues enhances communication, establishes rapport, and promotes treatment outcomes (Tavallali et al, 2014).*

● = Independent;   ▲ = Collaborative;   **EBN** = Evidence-Based Nursing;   **EB** = Evidence-Based

- Support programs for parents of young children in specific cultural communities. EBN: *Parents and children benefit when a support group is incorporated in the care (Thomson-Salo et al, 2017). Clarify parents' feelings, expectations, perceptions, and availability regarding participation in the care of their sick child.* EBN: *Cultural differences regarding parent participation in the care of ill or hospitalized children should be considered and incorporated into the care of the child and their parents (Majdalani et al, 2014).*
- Acknowledge and praise parenting strengths noted. EBN: *Parents see what they are doing right and are encouraged to continue the behavior (Ludmer et al, 2017).*

Home Care

- The nursing interventions previously described should be used in the home environment with adaptations as necessary. EB: *Clinicians should help educate parents on the care the child will need at home and modify to meet the family's needs (Thrasher et al, 2017).*
- ▲ Refer to a parenting program to facilitate learning of parenting skills. EBN: *The study shows that parenting programs can increase parental knowledge and confidence (Kendall et al, 2013).*

Client/Family Teaching and Discharge Planning

- Refer to Client/Family Teaching and Discharge Planning for Impaired **Parenting** for suggestions that may be used with minor adaptations.
- Teach parents home safety: reduction of hot water temperature, proper poison storage, use of smoke alarms, and installation of safety gates for stairs. EB: *Education may reduce injury and promote children's home safety (Lehna et al, 2014).*
- Teach parents and young teens conflict resolution by using a hypothetical conflict solution with and without a structured conflict resolution guide. Support self-direction of the families with minimal therapist intervention. EB: *Encouraging parent participation in positive-parenting programs can decrease the conflict for parents and teens (Salari et al, 2013).*
- Refer mothers of children with type 1 diabetes for community support in babysitting, child care, or respite. EB: *Families raising children with diabetes need to have support and interventions to assist with the care of the child to help reduce the burden of care on the parents (Kobos & Imiela, 2015).*
- Teach families the importance of monitoring television viewing, social media, video gaming, and so forth to limit exposure to violence. EBN: *Media violence can be hazardous to children's health, and studies overwhelmingly point to a causal connection between media violence and aggressive attitudes, values, and behaviors in some children (Aragon Neely et al, 2013).* Promotion of better quality relationships between parents and children is an effective strategy that can lead to enhanced learning. Good quality parenting leads to improved cognitive and social skills for children. EBN: *Parents have a positive effect on their children, which can lead to improved self-confidence and a stronger parent–child relationship (Kim et al, 2015).*
- See Impaired **Parenting** for additional references.

P

REFERENCES

Aragon Neely, J., Hudnut-Beumler, J., et al. (2013). The effect of primary care interventions on children's media viewing habits and exposure to violence. *Academic Pediatrics*, 13(6), 531–539.

Byczkowski, T. L., Munafo, J. K., et al. (2014). Family perceptions of the usability and value of chronic disease web-based patient portals. *Health Informatics Journal*, 20(2), 151–162.

Cady, R. G., Looman, W. S., Lindeke, L. L., et al. (2015). Pediatric care coordination: Lessons learned and future priorities. *Online Journal of Issues in Nursing*, 20(3), 30.

de l'Etoile, S., Behura, S., et al. (2017). Acoustic parameters of infant-directed singing in mothers of infants with down syndrome. *Infant Behavior and Development*, 49(Suppl. C), 151–160.

Gavhane, S., Eklare, D., & Mohammad, H. (2016). Long term outcomes of kangaroo mother care in very low birth weight infants. *Journal of Clinical and Diagnostic Research: JCDR*, 10(12).

Hamilton, L., Lerner, C., et al. (2013). Effects of a medical home program for children with special health care needs on parental perceptions of care in an ethnically diverse patient population. *Maternal & Child Health Journal*, 17(3), 463–469.

Hsiao, C.-Y., & Tsai, Y.-F. (2014). Caregiver burden and satisfaction in families of individuals with schizophrenia. *Nursing Research*, 63(4), 260–269.

Kendall, S., Bloomfield, L., et al. (2013). Efficacy of a group-based parenting program on stress and self-efficacy among Japanese mothers: A quasi-experimental study. *Nursing & Health Sciences*, 15(4), 454–460.

Kim, J., Thompson, E. A., et al. (2015). Trajectories of parent–adolescent relationship quality among at-risk youth: Parental depression and adolescent developmental outcomes. *Archives of Psychiatric Nursing*, 29(6), 434–440.

Kobos, E., & Imiela, J. (2015). Factors affecting the level of burden of caregivers of children with type 1 diabetes. *Applied Nursing Research*, 28(2), 142–149.

Lehna, C., Janes, E. G., et al. (2014). Community partnership to promote home fire safety in children with special needs. *Burns: Journal of the International Society for Burn Injuries*, 40(6), 1179–1184.

Ludmer, J. A., Salsbury, D., et al. (2017). Accounting for the impact of parent internalizing symptoms on parent training benefits: The role

● = Independent;   ▲ = Collaborative;   EBN = Evidence-Based Nursing;   EB = Evidence-Based

of positive parenting. *Behaviour Research and Therapy, 97*(Suppl. C), 252–258.

Majdalani, M. N., Doumit, M. A. A., et al. (2014). The lived experience of parents of children admitted to the pediatric intensive care unit in Lebanon. *International Journal of Nursing Studies, 51*(2), 217–225.

Razaz, N., Hertzman, C., et al. (2014). Children of chronically ill parents: The silence of research. *Child: Care, Health and Development, 40*(5), 753–754.

Salari, R., Fabian, H., et al. (2013). The Children and Parents in Focus project: A population-based cluster-randomised controlled trial to prevent behavioural and emotional problems in children. *BMC Public Health, 13*(1), 225–241.

Tavallali, A. G., Kabir, Z. N., et al. (2014). Ethnic Swedish parents' experiences of minority ethnic nurses' cultural competence in Swedish paediatric care. *Scandinavian Journal of Caring Sciences, 28*(2), 255–263.

Thomson-Salo, F., Kuschel, C. A., et al. (2017). A fathers' group in NICU: Recognising and responding to paternal stress, utilising peer support. *Journal of Neonatal Nursing, 38*, 114–121.

Thrasher, J., Baker, J., et al. (2017). Hospital to home: A quality improvement initiative to implement high-fidelity simulation training for caregivers of children requiring long-term mechanical ventilation. *Journal of Pediatric Nursing.*

Risk for impaired Parenting   *Gail B. Ladwig, MSN, RN*

NANDA-I

Definition

Susceptible to primary caregiver difficulty in creating, maintaining, or regaining an environment that promotes the optimum growth and development of the child, which may compromise the well-being of the child.

Risk Factors

Infant or Child

Prolonged separation from parent; Temperament conflicts with parental expectations

Parental

Alteration in sleep pattern; conflict between partners; depression; failure to provide safe home environment; father of child uninvolved; inability to put child's needs before own; inadequate child care arrangements; ineffective communication skills; ineffective coping strategies; insufficient access to resources; insufficient family cohesiveness; insufficient knowledge about child development; insufficient knowledge about child health maintenance; insufficient knowledge about parenting skills; insufficient parental role model; insufficient parental care; insufficient problem-solving skills; insufficient resources; insufficient response to infant cues; insufficient social support; insufficient transportation; insufficient valuing of parenthood; late-term parental care; low self-esteem; mother of child uninvolved; nonrestorative sleep pattern; preference for physical punishment; role strain; sleep deprivation; social isolation; stressors; unrealistic expectations

At-Risk Population

Infant or Child

Developmental delay; difficult temperament; gender other than desired; prematurity

Parental

Change in family unit; closely spaced pregnancies; difficult birthing process; economically disadvantaged; high number of pregnancies; history of abuse; history of being abusive; history of mental illness; history of substance misuse; insufficient cognitive readiness for parenting; legal difficulty; low educational level; multiple births; relocation; single parent; unemployment; unplanned pregnancy; unwanted pregnancy; work difficulty; young parental age

Associated Condition

Infant or Child

Alteration in perceptual abilities; behavioral disorder; chronic illness; disabling condition

Parental

Alteration in cognitive functioning; disabling condition; physical illness

NOC, NIC, Client Outcomes, Nursing Interventions and *Rationales,* Client/Family Teaching and Discharge Planning, and References

Refer to care plans for Readiness for enhanced **Parenting** and Impaired **Parenting**

● = Independent;   ▲ = Collaborative;   EBN = Evidence-Based Nursing;   EB = Evidence-Based

Risk for Perioperative Positioning injury   *Catherine Kleiner, PhD, MSN, BSN*

NANDA-I

Definition

Susceptible to inadvertent anatomical and physical changes as a result of posture or positioning equipment used during an invasive/surgical procedure, which may compromise health.

Risk Factors

Immobilization

Associated Condition

Disorientation; edema; emaciation; muscle weakness; obesity; sensoriperceptual disturbance from anesthesia

NOC   (Nursing Outcomes Classification)

Suggested NOC Outcomes

Circulation Status; Immobility Consequences: Physiological; Joint Movement; Neurological Status; Respiratory Status; Risk Control; Sensory Function; Skeletal Function; Tissue Integrity: Skin and Mucous Membranes; Tissue Perfusion: Peripheral

---

Example NOC Outcome with Indicators

Tissue Perfusion: Peripheral as evidenced by the following indicators: Peripheral edema/Localized extremity pain/Skin breakdown/Muscle cramps/Peripheral pulses/Numbness/Tingling/Necrosis. (Rate the outcome and indicators of **Tissue Perfusion: Peripheral:** 1 = severe, 2 = substantial, 3 = moderate, 4 = mild, 5 = none [see Section I].)

Client Outcomes

Client Will (Specify Time Frame)

* Demonstrate unchanged skin condition, with exception of the incision, throughout the perioperative experience
* Demonstrate resolution of redness of the skin at points of pressure within 30 minutes after pressure is eliminated
* Remain injury-free related to surgical positioning, including intact skin and absence of pain and/or numbness associated with surgical positioning
* Demonstrate unchanged or improved physical mobility from preoperative status
* Demonstrate unchanged or improved peripheral sensory integrity from preoperative status

NIC   (Nursing Interventions Classification)

Suggested NIC Interventions

Circulatory Precautions; Fall Prevention; Neurological Monitoring; Peripheral Sensation Management; Positioning: Intraoperative; Pressure Ulcer Prevention; Risk Identification; Skin Surveillance; Surgical Precautions

---

Example NIC Activities—Positioning: Intraoperative

Use an adequate number of personnel to transfer client; Maintain client's proper body alignment

---

Nursing Interventions and *Rationales*

General Interventions for Any Surgical Client

* Assess the client's skin integrity throughout the perioperative process to avoid skin breakdown during surgical/invasive procedures. EB: *Developing skin breakdown manifested as a skin tear, pressure ulcer, deep tissue injury, or burn is a significant client complication affected by the duration of surgery and client positioning (National Pressure Ulcer Advisory Panel [NPUAP] and European Pressure Ulcer Advisory Panel [EPUAP], 2014; Van Wicklin, 2017).*

● = Independent;   ▲ = Collaborative;   EBN = Evidence-Based Nursing;   EB = Evidence-Based

- Recognize that surgery increases a patients risk for skin injury because of the time the patient is immobile for the procedure (Spruce, 2017).

Prevention of Pressure Injuries

- Complete a preoperative assessment to identify patient factors that will increase a patients risk for pressure injuries. This includes physical alterations that may require additional precautions for procedure-specific positioning and to identify specific procedural positioning needs, type of anesthesia, and so on. **EBN:** *Factors to consider when assessing the surgical client to plan for proper positioning are preexisting conditions such as vascular disease or diabetes, range of motion, presence of prostheses and/or fractures, skin condition, advanced age, nutritional status, weight, American Society of Anesthesiologists (ASA) physical status classification, and the presence of moisture (Spruce, 2017; Van Wicklin, 2017). Use resources (e.g., positioning aids, padding, transfer devices) to reduce the risk of tissue injury in the care of the older client (Association of periOperative Registered Nurses [AORN], 2015).*

- Identify procedure risk factors such as length and type of surgery, potential for intraoperative hypotensive episodes, low core temperatures, and decreased mobility on postoperative day 1. **EB:** *Assess the client for additional risk factors to include the duration of immobilization before and during the surgical procedure, client severity of illness, preoperative nutritional status, position for the procedure, and type of anesthesia (NPUAP & EPUAP, 2014; Van Wicklin, 2017). Surgeries lasting more than 4 hours provide a significant risk for pressure ulcer development (Sterner et al, 2011).* **CEBN:** *A recent study showed that vasopressor use is a significant risk factor for pressure ulcer development. The study also showed that the number of surgeries a client has during his or her inpatient stay and the length of surgery (over 1 hour), body mass index, Braden score, mortality risk, and history of diabetes are also risk factors for pressure ulcer development. This study did not show that age was related to pressure ulcer development (Tschannen et al, 2012).*

- Recognize that all surgical clients should be considered at high risk for pressure ulcer development, because pressure ulcers can develop in as little as 20 minutes in the operating room. **EBN:** *Operating room mattresses, the patient support surface, should be chosen for its pressure redistribution (Spruce, 2017). Support surfaces that redistribute pressure are recommended; however, which type is most effective is not clear (de Oliveira et al, 2017).*

- Remove all patient jewelry and accessories. **EBN:** *Jewelry and accessories, such as body piercings and hair devices, can get caught and torn out causing skin injury and the patient can lie on them and develop a pressure injury or the patient can experience a burn from cautery equipment (Van Wicklin, 2017).*

- Protect the heels during surgery by elevating the heels completely. **EB:** *Ensure the heels are free of the surface of the operating table (NPUAP & EPUAP, 2014). Heel pressure ulcers are one of the most common sites for pressure injury during surgery. Traditional devices such as egg crates, booties, and heel pads do not decrease the pressure. It is recommended that a device is used to elevate the heels and distribute the weight of the patient's leg along the calf (Van Wicklin, 2017).*

- Use pressure-reducing devices and pressure-relieving mattresses as necessary to prevent pressure injury. **EB:** *Use a high-specification reactive or alternating pressure support surface on the operating table for all individuals identified as being at risk for pressure ulcer development (NPUAP & EPUAP, 2014). Additional support surfaces may be indicated to offload pressure points on the face and body when the client is placed in a prone position (NPUAP & EPUAP, 2014; Van Wicklin, 2017). Support surfaces may be made of foam, gel, air, fluid, or a combination of these surfaces. The goal is to have pressure distributed over the largest area possible. This is accomplished by having the surface envelope the patient (de Oliveira et al, 2017; Van Wicklin, 2017). Assess for shearing forces that may cause tissue injury when placing the client in the Trendelenburg position for selected robotic surgical procedures (Sutton, Link, & Makic, 2013).*

- Avoid using rolled sheets and towels as positioning devices because they tend to produce high and inconsistent pressures. Special positioning devices are available that redistribute pressure. **EBN:** *Towels and rolled sheets contribute to friction injuries and increase pressure on the patient. Pillows are an acceptable alternative when other positioning devices are unavailable (Van Wicklin, 2017).*

- Avoid covering positioning devices or placing extra blankets on top of a pressure-reducing surface. **EB/ CEB:** *Adding material to a pressure reduction surface actually increases the pressure, producing a negative result (Van Wicklin, 2017). Use of rolled sheets and towels beneath overlays decreases the overlay's effectiveness and causes pressure (Van Wicklin, 2017).*

- The nurse should demonstrate knowledge not only of the equipment but also of anatomy and the application of physiological principles to properly position the client. **EBN:** *Preplanning ensures that the correct positioning devices are available and in good working condition, and that appropriate numbers of personnel are available* *to position the client safely and appropriately. High-specification reactive foam mattresses should be used for patients at high risk for pressure injury (Van Wicklin, 2017).*

- Monitor patient position and pressure being applied to the client intraoperatively by staff, equipment, and/or instruments. *Patients may move slightly or shift during surgery, especially during long procedures or when new equipment is introduced, requiring that the patient be repositioned to avoid pressure or nerve injury (Van Wicklin, 2017).*
- Use additional pressure-redistributing padding on all bony prominences. EB: *Additional padding increases patient comfort, helps redistribute pressure, and decreases the chance for development of pressure or nerve injuries (Van Wicklin, 2017). Some positioning devices are solid and can increase pressure over bony prominences (Sutton, Link, & Makic, 2013).*
- Recognize that reddened areas or areas injured by pressure should not be massaged. EB: *Rubbing causes friction that can lead to damage to skin/tissue (NPUAP & EPUAP, 2014; Van Wicklin, 2017).*
- Implement measures to prevent inadvertent hypothermia. *Anesthesia can compromise perfusion by causing hypotension and hypothermia. When coupled with the client being immobile on a noncompliant surface for an extended time period, hypothermia increases vulnerability for pressure ulcer development during surgery.*
- Many surgical clients have medical devices placed as a part of the surgical procedure. Avoid positioning the client on the medical device and perform frequent assessments of the skin under and around the device (Apold & Rydrych, 2012; NPUAP & EPUAP, 2014).

Positioning the Perioperative Client

- Ensure that linens on the operating room table are free of wrinkles. *Wrinkles may cause pressure/injury to the skin if the client is unable to move for prolonged periods of time. Layers of linens or blankets between the patient and the support surface decrease the pressure-redistributing effect of the support surface (Van Wicklin, 2017).*
- Lock the operating room table, cart, or bed and stabilize the mattress before transfer/positioning the client. Monitor the client while on the operating room table at all times. EB: *Studies showed that a lack of clear communication about who should be watching the client has contributed to falls (Van Wicklin, 2017).*
- Lift rather than pull or slide the client when positioning to reduce the incidence of skin injury from shearing and/or friction. EB: *Sliding or pulling the client can cause shearing force and/or friction (NPUAP & EPUAP, 2014; Van Wicklin, 2017).*
- Ensure that appropriate numbers of personnel are present to assist in positioning the client. EBN: *A minimum of two people should assist an awake client to transfer from a cart/bed to the operating room table: one person on the stretcher side to assist the client onto the table and a second person on the far side of the table to prevent the client from falling off (Van Wicklin, 2017). A minimum of four persons are necessary when transferring/positioning an anesthetized, unconscious, obese, or weak client (Van Wicklin, 2017).*
- Recognize that, optimally, clients (especially those with limited range of motion/mobility) should be asked to position themselves under the nurse's guidance before induction of anesthesia so that he or she can verify that a position of comfort has been obtained.
- Ensure that nerves are protected by positioning extremities carefully. EB: *Nerves can be injured by stretching and compression, which is caused by a loss of protective muscle tone and pressure between two fixed points. Careful attention to proper body alignment and padding is necessary to prevent peripheral nerve injury (Bouyer-Ferullo, 2013; Van Wicklin, 2017).*
- Use slow and smooth movements during positioning to allow the circulatory system to readjust.
- Reassess the client after positioning and periodically during the procedure to maintain proper alignment and skin integrity. EBN: *Changes in position can expose or injure body parts (e.g., shearing, friction, compression) that were originally protected, and the safety strap can shift and apply increased pressure. If possible, after 3 or 4 hours of surgery the patient should be checked, under the drapes, to make sure the patient remains in alignment (Van Wicklin, 2017).*
- Frequently assess the eyes and/or monitor intraocular pressure, especially when client is in the prone, Trendelenburg, or knee-chest position. CEB/EB: *The cornea can easily be injured during surgery because of a decrease in lacrimation, failure of the eyes to fully close and/or improperly applied face masks, or prolonged prone positioning (Spruce & Van Wicklin, 2014; Van Wicklin, 2017).*
- Position hips in proper alignment with knees flexed. Unaligned hips can cause pressure to the low back and hip joints. EB: *Proper body alignment needs to be maintained to prevent nerve and pressure injuries (Van Wicklin, 2017).*

● = Independent; ▲ = Collaborative; EBN = Evidence-Based Nursing; EB = Evidence-Based

- Position the arms extended on arm boards so that they do not extend beyond a 90-degree angle. The arms should be at the level of the bed and should not be allowed to hang off the bed. Do not position arms at sides unless surgically necessary. **EB:** *Positioning at less than a 90-degree angle, with elbows slightly flexed and hands supine, decreases the risk of a stretching injury to the brachial plexus and possible compression or occlusion injury to the subclavian and axillary arteries (de Oliveira et al, 2017; Van Wicklin, 2017). When positioning arms at the sides is necessary, place the arms beneath the sheet and bring the sheet over the top of the arm and then tuck the sheet beneath the mattress so that the arm cannot fall off the mattress and hang over the metal edge of the table, where the surgical team could lean against it (Van Wicklin, 2017).*
- Protect the client's skin surfaces from injury by preventing pooling of preparative solutions, blood, irrigation, urine, and feces. **EBN:** *Prep solutions may change the pH of the skin and remove protective oils, making the skin more susceptible to pressure and friction. Pooling also increases the risk of maceration (Van Wicklin, 2017).*
- Keep the client appropriately covered and limit traffic in the room during the procedure. Reducing unnecessary exposure provides privacy and dignity for the client during positioning and helps prevent hypothermia (Van Wicklin, 2017).
- When positioning the client prone, care should be taken to ensure the head and neck are properly positioned. In addition, 5- to 10-degree reverse Trendelenburg should be used, if possible, to reduce intraocular pressure and decrease facial edema. **EB:** *Inappropriate positioning of the head and neck in the prone position can lead to vertebral artery obstruction and possible stroke. Standard foam prone pillows should be used because they stabilize the neck in neutral, and the endotracheal tube can be positioned away from the face to decrease excessive pressure (Spruce & Van Wicklin, 2014; Spruce, 2017; Van Wicklin, 2017).*
- Recognize that clients positioned in the lithotomy position should be kept in this position for as short a time as possible. **EB:** *One research review suggested that the client's legs be removed from lithotomy positioning devices every 2 hours when the procedure is expected to last 4 hours or longer. Reported complications from extended time in this position include muscle contusion, compartment syndrome, and acute renal failure (Van Wicklin, 2017).*
- The lowest heel position should be used in the lithotomy position. **EB:** *When possible the legs should be at or lower than the level of the heart to prevent complications (Van Wicklin, 2017).*
- Maintain normal body alignment. *Misalignment, flexion, extension, and rotation may cause muscle and nerve damage and airway interference; pressure on the carotid sinus can cause arrhythmias; and restricted venous outflow can occur with extreme rotation of the head (Van Wicklin, 2017).*
- When applying body supports and restraint straps (safety belt), apply loosely and secure over waist or midthigh at least 2 inches above the knees, avoiding bony prominences by placing a blanket between the strap and the client. **EB:** *Belts positioned directly over the knees cause compression of the peroneal nerve against the fibula (Van Wicklin, 2017).*
- Assess the client's skin integrity immediately postoperatively. **EB:** *Assess and document postoperative skin/tissue integrity focusing on areas with constant pressure during the procedure and limb function for nerve damage (Sutton, Link, & Makic, 2013; NPUAP & EPUAP, 2014).*
- Ensure that complete, concise, accurate documentation of client assessment and use of positioning devices is in the client's medical record.

REFERENCES

AORN. (2015). *Position statement on the care of the older adult in perioperative settings.* Retrieved from http://www.aorn.org/Clinical_Practice/Position_Statements/Position_Statements.aspx. (Accessed 9 January 2018).

Apold, J., & Rydrych, D. (2012). Preventing device-related pressure ulcers: Using data to guide statewide change. *Journal of Nursing Care Quality, 27*(1), 28–34.

Bouyer-Ferullo, S. (2013). Preventing perioperative peripheral nerve injuries. *AORN Journal, 97*(1), 111–121.

de Oliveira, K. F., Nascimento, K. G., Nicolussi, A. C., et al. (2017). Support surfaces in the prevention of pressure ulcers in surgical patients: An integrative review. *International Journal of Nursing Practice, 23*(4), doi:10.1111/ijn.12553.

National Pressure Ulcer Advisory Panel (NPUAP) and European Pressure Ulcer Advisory Panel (EPUAP). (2014). In E. Haesler (Ed.), *Prevention and Treatment of Pressure Ulcers.* Perth, Australia: Cambridge Media.

Spruce, L. (2017). Back to basics: Preventing perioperative pressure injuries. *AORN Journal, 105*(1), 92–99. doi:10.1016/j.aorn.2016.10.018.

Spruce, L., & Van Wicklin, S. A. (2014). Back to basics: Positioning the patient. *AORN Journal, 100*(3), 299–302.

Sterner, E., et al. (2011). Category I pressure ulcers—How reliable is clinical assessment? *Orthopedic Nursing, 30*(3), 194–205.

Sutton, S., Link, T., & Makic, M. B. F. (2013). A quality improvement project for safe and effective patient positioning during robot-assisted surgery. *AORN Journal, 97*(4), 448–456.

Tschannen, D., et al. (2012). Patient-specific and surgical characteristics in the development of pressure ulcers. *American Journal of Critical Care, 21*(2), 116–124.

Van Wicklin, S. A. (2017). Guideline for positioning the patient. In R. Conner (Ed.), *Guidelines for perioperative practice* (Vol. 1). Denver, CO: AORN, Inc.

● = Independent;   ▲ = Collaborative;   **EBN** = Evidence-Based Nursing;   **EB** = Evidence-Based

Risk for Peripheral Neurovascular dysfunction   *Krystal Chamberlain, BSN, RN, CCRN*

NANDA-I

Definition

Susceptible to disruption in the circulation, sensation, and motion of an extremity, which may compromise health.

Risk Factors

To be developed

Associated Condition

Burns injury; fracture; immobilization; mechanical compression; orthopedic surgery; trauma; vascular obstruction

NOC   (Nursing Outcomes Classification)

Suggested NOC Outcomes

Circulation Status; Neurological Status: Spinal Sensorimotor Function; Tissue Perfusion: Peripheral

---

Example NOC Outcome with Indicators

Tissue Perfusion: Peripheral as evidenced by the following indicators: Radial or pedal pulse strength/Capillary refill in fingers or toes/Extremity skin temperature/Localized extremity pain/Numbness/Tingling/Skin color/Muscle strength/Skin integrity/Peripheral edema. (Rate the outcome and indicators of **Tissue Perfusion: Peripheral:** 1 = severe deviation from normal range, 2 = substantial deviation from normal range, 3 = moderate deviation from normal range, 4 = mild deviation from normal range, 5 = no deviation from normal range [see Section I].)

Client Outcomes

Client Will (Specify Time Frame)

- Maintain circulation, sensation, and movement of an extremity within client's own normal limits
- Explain signs of neurovascular compromise

NIC   (Nursing Interventions Classification)

Suggested NIC Interventions

Exercise Therapy: Joint Mobility; Peripheral Sensation Management

---

Example NIC Activities—Peripheral Sensation Management

Monitor for paresthesia: numbness, tingling, hyperesthesia, and hypoesthesia; Monitor for thrombophlebitis and deep vein thrombosis

---

Nursing Interventions and *Rationales*

- Recognize the risk factors that may result in peripheral neurovascular dysfunction. EB: *Conditions that diminish limb perfusion from excessive pressure (e.g., tight-fitting cast, brace, restrictive dressing, compression stockings, prolonged immobility, intraoperative positioning, edema) can result in peripheral neurovascular dysfunction with wide-ranging effects on overall functional ability (Peters, 2017). Compartment syndrome also can occur and is an elevation of pressure within a compartment, which impairs circulation (Garner et al, 2014).*
- Assess for the early onset of compartment syndrome, and report to provider promptly. Perform neurovascular assessment as ordered or as needed based on client's condition. Use the "five Ps" of assessment as outlined in the following list. *The goal is to prevent ischemia and necrosis (cell death). Delay in recognizing compartment syndrome can lead to chronic pain, paralysis, rhabdomyolysis, contracture, amputation of the limb, and death. Compartment syndrome is primarily diagnosed by physical examination, and because of the devastating*

● = Independent;   ▲ = Collaborative;   EBN = Evidence-Based Nursing;   EB = Evidence-Based

consequences of a missed compartment syndrome, a fasciotomy should be considered. Assess for the presence of any of the five Ps (Donaldson, Haddad, & Khan, 2014; Garner et al, 2014; Peters, 2017).

○ Pain: Assess severity (using an appropriate pain scale), quality, radiation, and relief by medications. *Pain "out of proportion" to the injury, requiring strong opiates, often described as burning, feeling deep in the muscle or structure, and elicited with passive stretching of the compartment are the most reliable signs of compartment syndrome and peripheral neurovascular dysfunction (Donaldson, Haddad & Khan, 2014).*

○ Pulses: Check the pulses distal to the injury and compare with the unaffected limb. *Pulselessness is a late sign of compartment syndrome (Garner et al, 2014).*

○ Pallor: Check color and temperature changes below the injury site and compare with unaffected limb. Check capillary refill. *A cold, pale, or bluish extremity indicates poor arterial perfusion or venous congestion. If pallor, cyanosis, mottling, or changes in temperature are present, report to provider promptly and record your assessment findings (Garner et al, 2014; Le, 2016).*

○ Paresthesia (change in sensation): Check by lightly touching the skin proximal and distal to the injury. Ask if the client has any unusual sensations such as hypersensitivity, tingling, prickling, decreased feeling, or numbness. Check nerve function (e.g., whether the client can feel a touch to the area of concern, such as the first web space of the foot [deep peroneal nerve] with tibial fracture). *Paresthesia may occur as an early sign of compartment syndrome caused by ischemia of peripheral nerves (Garner et al, 2014).*

○ Paralysis: Ask the client to perform appropriate range-of-motion exercises in the unaffected and then the affected extremity. *Loss of movement (paralysis) is a late symptom of compartment syndrome. Decreased range of motion and loss of movement can indicate impending muscle, nerve, and cellular death (Donaldson et al, 2014).*

○ In addition to the five Ps, assess for swelling or increase in compartment pressure by feeling the extremity; note new onset of firmness or swelling of the extremity, and a firm "wooden" feeling on deep palpation. Intercompartmental pressures may also be measured with proprietary monitoring devices. *Internal pressure or external confinement or restriction can proceed to the point at which cellular exchange is diminished. Swelling and tightness of the involved compartment are indications of increased pressure. Not only are surgical or trauma clients at risk for neurovascular compromise, but they also are clients on bed rest because of changes in blood flow through the cardiovascular system (Donaldson et al, 2014).*

▲ All the Ps may not be present, and they are not specific for compartment syndrome. Have a high index of suspicion for any of the Ps. Noting two or more of the Ps increases the probability of compartment syndrome. Monitor the client for compartment syndrome of the nonoperative leg and the operative leg. *Cases of compartment syndrome to the nonoperative side related to patient positioning during surgical procedure, resulting in compression and hypoperfusion, have been reported (Garner et al, 2014).*

● Monitor appropriate application and function of corrective device (e.g., cast, splint, traction) as needed. *Compartment syndrome can result from restrictive pressure from the device or swelling of injured tissue (The Joanna Briggs Institute, 2016). After immobilization (casting or splinting), if pain worsens or there is any tingling or numbness, swelling, delayed capillary refill, or change in color of exposed digits, immediate evaluation is needed.*

● For prevention of deep vein thrombosis (DVT), nursing care of DVT, and pulmonary embolism, refer to the interventions on DVT prevention and treatment in the care plan for Ineffective peripheral **Tissue Perfusion.**

REFERENCES

Donaldson, J., Haddad, B., & Khan, W. S. (2014). The pathophysiology, diagnosis and current management of acute compartment syndrome. *The Open Orthopaedics Journal, Suppl 1*(8), 185–193. PMCID: PMC4110398. Published online Jun 27, 2014.

Garner, M. R., et al. (2014). Compartment syndrome: Diagnosis, management, and unique concerns in the twenty-first century. *HSS Journal, 10*(2).

The Joanna Briggs Institute. (2016). *Recommended Practice. Care of a cast: Older person.* The Joanna Briggs Institute EBP Database, JBI@ Ovid. Retrieved from http://ovidsp.tx.ovid.com.proxy.hsl.ucdenver.edu/sp-3.27.1a/ovidweb.cgi?&S=FJGIFPGMBPDDJAEBNCGKGAIBFLEOAA00&Link+Set=S.sh.58%7c36%7csl_190.

Le, L. K.-D. (2016). *Evidence summary. Neurovascular assessment: Clinician information.* The Joanna Briggs Institute EBP Database. Retrieved from http://ovidsp.tx.ovid.com.proxy.hsl.ucdenver.edu/sp-3.27.1a/ovidweb.cgi?&S=FJGIFPGMBPDDJAEBNCGKGAIBFLEOAA00&Link+Set=S.sh.47%7c1%7csl_190.

Peters, M. D. J. (2017). *Neurovascular assessment: Clinician information.* The Joanna Briggs Institute, JBI Evidence Summary. Retrieved from http://ovidsp.tx.ovid.com.proxy.hsl.ucdenver.edu/sp-3.27.1a/ovidweb.cgi?&S=OEHBFPIIEODDGOFGNCFKGCIBJCHAAA00&Link+Set=S.sh.43%7c3%7csl_190.

Risk for Poisoning   *Melodie Cannon, DNP, MSc/FNP, BHScN, RN (EC), NP-PHC, CEN, GNC(C)*

NANDA-I

Definition

Susceptible to accidental exposure to, or ingestion of, drugs or dangerous products in sufficient doses, which may compromise health.

Risk Factors

External

Access to dangerous product; access to illicit drugs potentially contaminated by poisonous additives; access to pharmaceutical agent; occupational setting without adequate safeguards

Internal

Emotional disturbance; inadequate precautions against poisoning; insufficient knowledge of pharmacological agents; insufficient knowledge of poisoning prevention; insufficient vision

Associated Condition

Alteration in cognitive functioning

NOC   (Nursing Outcomes Classification)

Suggested NOC Outcomes

Knowledge: Child Physical Safety, Medication, Personal Safety; Parenting Performance; Risk Control; Risk Control: Alcohol Use, Drug Use; Risk Detection; Safe Home Environment

> **Example NOC Outcome with Indicators**
>
> **Knowledge: Child Physical Safety** as evidenced by the following indicators: Appropriate activities for child's developmental level/Strategies to prevent medication misuse/Strategies to prevent exposure to toxic chemicals or substances. (Rate the outcome and indicators of **Knowledge: Child Physical Safety:** 1 = no knowledge, 2 = limited knowledge, 3 = moderate knowledge, 4 = substantial knowledge, 5 = extensive knowledge [see Section I].)

Client Outcomes

Client Will (Specify Time Frame)

- Prevent inadvertent ingestion of or exposure to toxins or poisonous substances
- Explain and undertake appropriate safety measures to prevent ingestion of or exposure to toxins or poisonous substances
- Verbalize appropriate response to apparent or suspected toxic ingestion or poisoning

NIC   (Nursing Interventions Classification)

Suggested NIC Interventions

Environmental Management: Safety, First Aid; Health Education; Medication Management; Surveillance; Surveillance: Safety

> **Example NIC Activities—Environmental Management: Safety**
>
> Identify safety hazards in the environment (i.e., physical, biological, chemical); Remove hazards from the environment, when possible

Nursing Interventions and *Rationales*

- When a client comes to the hospital with possible poisoning, begin care following the ABCs (airway, breathing and circulation) and administer oxygen if needed. EB: *Poisoning is a major cause of morbidity/ mortality worldwide. Initial evaluation should include vital signs, mental status, pupil size, oxygenation,*

● = Independent;   ▲ = Collaborative;   EBN = Evidence-Based Nursing;   EB = Evidence-Based

P

finger-stick glucose, and cardiac monitoring. Management is geared to supportive care, prevention of poison absorption, antidote use, and elimination techniques (Rhyee, 2013).

▲ It is important for the triage nurse to call the poison control center. *The poison control hotline is 1-800-222-1222. Poison centers are a valuable tool for medical consultations. They are staffed by nurses, pharmacists, toxicologists, and other specialists in poisons and toxins who can recommend treatment advice (American Association of Poison Control Centers, 2018).*

● Obtain a thorough history of what was ingested, how much, and when, and ask to look at the containers. Note the client's age, weight, medications, medical conditions, and any history of vomiting, choking, coughing, or change in mental status. Also take note of any interventions performed before seeking treatment. **EB:** *The history is important to confirm the diagnosis and is often unreliable when provided by clients with intentional ingestion. Additional information should be obtained from paramedics, police, family, and friends when possible (Rhyee, 2013).*

▲ Note results of toxicology screens, arterial blood gases, blood glucose levels, and any other ordered laboratory tests. *If information about what was ingested is incomplete or inaccurate, laboratory tests may be needed to determine treatment. The poison control center will provide valuable information regarding appropriate laboratory tests and investigations specific to the suspected toxin.*

▲ Initiate any ordered treatment for poisoning quickly. The poison control center will specify any treatment or medications that need to be administered. **EB:** *Some poisoning deaths may be preventable. Substances ingested in preventable deaths have delayed gastrointestinal (GI) absorption or require metabolic activation to produce severe toxicity. This allows a time frame for recognition and successful intervention. Early poison center consultation may improve outcomes and decrease deaths (Srisuma et al, 2016).*

▲ *Ensure that recommendations from the poison control center are clearly documented and readily accessible in the client's chart.*

▲ *If the client's condition deteriorates, contact the poison control center again for further direction and notify the most responsible provider.*

Safety Guidelines for Medication Administration

● Prevent iatrogenic harm to the hospitalized client by following these guidelines for administering medications:
  ○ Use at least two methods to identify the client before administering medications or blood products, such as the client's name and medical record number or birth date. Do not use the client's room number. Use the bar code scanning system for client identification if used by your facility.
  ○ When taking verbal or telephone orders, the orders should be written down and read back for verification to the individual giving the order. The health care provider who gave the orders for the medication then needs to confirm the information that was read back.

● Standardize use of abbreviations, acronyms, symbols, and dose designations and eliminate those that are prone to cause errors. (Refer to The Joint Commission, Critical Access Hospital National Patient Safety Goals for list of abbreviations, acronyms, symbols, and dose designations that should not be used [The Joint Commission, 2014].)
  ○ Be aware of the medications that look/sound alike and ensure that the correct medication is ordered and administered.
  ○ Use the eight rights of medication administration to decrease the potential for error: right client, right medication, right reason, right dose, right frequency, right route, right site, and right time (College of Nurses of Ontario, 2014).
  ○ Take high-alert medications off the nursing unit, such as potassium chloride. Standardize concentrations of medications such as morphine in patient-controlled analgesia pumps.
  ○ Follow agency policy/procedures for medications that require a two-person check and co-signature.
  ○ Label all medications and medication containers or other solutions that are on or off a sterile field for a procedure. Label them when they are first taken out of the original packaging to another container. Label with medication name, strength, amount, and expiration date/time. Review the labels whenever there is a change of personnel.
  ○ Use only intravenous (IV) pumps that prevent free flow of IV solution when the tubing is taken out of the pump.

● Identify all the client's current medications on admission to a health care facility and compare the list with the current ordered medications. Reconcile any differences in medications. Use the expertise of the pharmacy department if there is any uncertainty regarding the accuracy of the client's medications.

● = Independent;   ▲ = Collaborative;   **EBN** = Evidence-Based Nursing;   **EB** = Evidence-Based

Reconcile the list of medications if the client is transferred from one unit to another, when there is a hand off to the next provider of care, and when the client is discharged.

- *Adverse drug events occur with disturbing frequency in health care settings. These events can be reduced by comparing the patient's medication list to any admission, transfer, or discharge orders, and identifying and bringing forward any discrepancies to the prescribers' attention for clarification. Document any discussions and resulting changes (Canadian Patient Safety Institute, 2016).*
- Detect possible interactions and cumulative or other adverse effects among prescribed medications, self-administered over-the-counter products, culturally based home treatments, herbal remedies, and foods. Medication reconciliation is an important safety issue because of the number of people taking multiple medications and involves determining what medications the person should be taking, medications they are actually taking, and resolving discrepancies (Aronson, 2017).

 Pediatric

▲ Evaluate lead exposure risk and consult the health care provider regarding lead screening measures as indicated (public/ambulatory health). EB: *High levels of lead can cause anemia, multiorgan damage, seizures, and death in children. Chronic low lead levels can result in physical, cognitive, and neurobehavioral impairment. Sources of lead exposure include lead industries, leaded petrol, lead-based paint, water pipes, paint, dust, soil, and water. Children at risk for lead exposure include those living in deteriorating or renovated older homes with lead-based paint, living in areas with lead-based industry, and socioeconomic disadvantage (Nussbaumer-Streit et al, 2016).*

- Provide guidance for parents and caregivers regarding age-related safety measures, including the following:
  ○ Store prescription and over-the-counter medications, vitamins, herbs, and alcohol in a locked cabinet far from children's reach.
  ○ Do not take medications in front of children (Rodgers et al, 2012).
  ○ Store cleaning products including things like dishwashing liquids in a high cabinet, out of children's reach.
  ○ Use safety latches on cabinets that contain poisonous substances.
  ○ Store potentially harmful substances in the original containers with safety closures intact.
  ○ Recognize that no container is completely childproof.
  ○ Do not store medications or toxic substances in food containers or near or with food products.
  ○ Do not leave alcoholic drinks, cosmetics, or toiletries where children can reach them.
  ○ Remove poisonous houseplants from the home. Teach children not to put leaves or berries in their mouths (Oerther, 2011).
  ○ Do not suggest that medications are candy.
  ○ If interrupted when using a harmful product, take it with you; children can get into it within seconds.
  ○ Store poisonous automotive or gardening supplies in a locked area.
  ○ Use extreme caution with pesticides and gardening materials close to children's play areas.
  ○ When visitors enter the home, place their handbags or backpacks up high where children are unable to reach them, and ask about any potential poisonous substances.
- *Pediatric poisoning deaths most commonly come from ingestion of opioids, other analgesics, cardiovascular medications, antihistamines, and sedatives (Tadros et al, 2016).*

EB: *A multicenter case-control study found that there were increased odds of poisoning in children aged 0 to 4 years when medicines were not locked away or stored out of reach and household products and medicines were not put away immediately after use (Kendrick et al, 2017).*

- Advise families that syrup of ipecac is no longer recommended to be kept and used in the home. *If potential poisoning occurs, contact emergency services or a poison control center (Theurer & Bhavsar, 2013).* Advise families that over-the-counter cough and cold suppressant medications are not recommended and are no longer considered safe for children 2 or younger (US Food and Drug Administration, 2014). *Colds are self-limiting and improve on their own; over-the-counter medications may help relieve symptoms in older children, but they will not change the natural course of the illness (US Food and Drug Administration, 2014).* EB: *Since the US Food and Drug Administration advised against the use of cough/cold medicines in children younger than 2 in 2008, there has been a decline in childhood poisonings in this category and a decrease in infant emergency department (ED) visits with adverse events caused by cough/cold medications (Spiller et al, 2013).*
- Recognize that some children may have been exposed to methamphetamines or the components used to make methamphetamines. *Home-based methamphetamine manufacturing may represent significant hazards*

● = Independent; ▲ = Collaborative; EBN = Evidence-Based Nursing; EB = Evidence-Based

and exposures to those who manufacture the drug but also to others living in the home. Children are most susceptible to these hazards and these exposures may result in immediate and long-term adverse health effects (Wright, Edwards, & Walker, 2016).

- *Advise families to contact state or local government agencies or pharmacies to ask about safe disposal programs for used, excess, or expired medications (US Food and Drug Administration, 2014).*

Geriatric

- Caution the client and family to avoid storing medications with similar appearances close to one another (e.g., nitroglycerin ointment near toothpaste or denture creams). *Confusion and visual impairment can place the older person at risk of incorrectly identifying the contents. Place medications in a medication organizer that indicates when they are to be taken. Failing eyesight, the use of multiple drugs, and difficulty in remembering whether a medication was taken are among the causes of accidental poisoning in older persons.* EB: *For both sexes, poisoning is a common, self-inflicted injury in patients admitted to hospital. Among seniors, there is concern regarding the recognition of intentional harm by self-induced poisoning (Skinner et al, 2016). Remind older clients to store medications out of reach when young children come to visit. Childhood poisonings are common events that involve exposure to both prescription and nonprescription pharmaceuticals in the home, resulting in an increased number of serious outcomes (Spiller et al, 2013).*
- Perform medication reconciliation in all older clients entering the health care system and on discharge. *Older clients do not compare drugs that they have at home with new prescriptions and often take multiple drugs with the same indications, leading to toxicity. Encourage older clients to speak with their pharmacist to ensure their medications are reviewed whenever a change occurs. Pharmacists can assist clients with strategies to differentiate medications such as visual, tactile, or audible labeling (Smith & Bailey, 2014). Encourage the consistent use of a pharmacy to promote understanding of medications and any changes. Advise clients who use dosettes or prepackaged medications that the appropriate changes will need to be made before continuing to use the current administration method.*

Home Care

- The interventions previously described may be adapted for home care use.
- Provide the client and/or family with a poison control poster to be kept on the refrigerator or a bulletin board. Ensure that the telephone number for local poison control information is readily available and/or preprogrammed into household telephones.
- Prepour medications for a client who is at risk for ingesting too much of a given medication because of mistakes in preparation. Delegate this task to the family or caregivers if possible. *Older clients who live alone are at greatest risk of poisoning.*
- Identify poisonous substances in the immediate surroundings of the home, such as a garage or barn, including paints and thinners, fertilizers, rodent and bug control substances, animal medications, gasoline, and oil. Label with the name, a poison warning sign, and a poison control center number. Lock out of the reach of children. *Dangerous poisonous substances can be found in areas other than the internal home setting. Curious children are at risk for ingestion when exploring.*
- Identify the risk of toxicity from environmental activities such as spraying trees or roadside shrubs. Contact local departments of agriculture or transportation to obtain material safety data sheets or to prevent the activity in desired areas. *Very young children, women who are of childbearing age or who are pregnant, and older adults are at greatest risk of poisoning.*
- To prevent carbon monoxide poisoning, instruct the client and family in the importance of using a carbon monoxide detector in the home and changing it every 6 months, having the home heating system serviced every year by a qualified technician, and ensuring proper installation and venting of all combustion equipment. Carbon monoxide results from fumes produced by portable generators, stoves, lanterns, gas ranges, running vehicles, or burning charcoal and wood, which can build up in enclosed or partially enclosed spaces and result in harm or death for people and animals exposed. EB: *Carbon monoxide poisoning may be not be readily identified because many of the effects are similar to various childhood illnesses (Chang et al, 2017).*

Multicultural

- Prompt caregivers to take action to prevent lead poisoning. EB: *Lead knowledge in urban youth is limited and includes misinformation. Some youth demonstrated awareness of specific sources including paint, dust, and water but had limited awareness of prevention strategies (Bogar et al, 2017).*

• = Independent;   ▲ = Collaborative;   EBN = Evidence-Based Nursing;   EB = Evidence-Based

- If children live in a high-lead environment, teach the need for handwashing before each meal, annual blood testing for lead levels, and avoidance of high-lead areas. EB: *Lead industries, leaded petrol, lead-based paint, water pipes, paint, dust, soil, and water are all sources of lead exposure for children (Nussbaumer-Streit et al, 2016).*

Client/Family Teaching and Discharge Planning

- Teach parents that any substance that is absorbed by the body by a variety of means and can affect health and cause mortality is considered a poison. The increasing use of medications and home cleaning products puts children at risk for poison because of the potential for access in the home environment. EB: *Research has shown that 94% of children who were poisoned accessed the agent in their own home or another home (Nalliah et al, 2014).*

Safety Guidelines

- Counsel the client and family members regarding the following points of medication safety:
  - Avoid sharing prescriptions.
  - Always use good light when preparing medication. Do not dispense medication during the night without a light on.
  - Read the label before you open the bottle, after you remove a dose, and again before you give it.
  - Always use child-resistant caps and lock all medications away from your child or confused older adult.
  - Give the correct dose. *Never* guess.
  - Do not increase or decrease the dose without calling the health care provider.
  - Always follow the weight and age recommendations on the label.
  - Avoid making conversions. If the label calls for 2 teaspoons and you have a dosing cup labeled only with ounces, do not use it.
  - Be sure the health care provider knows if you are taking more than one medication at a time.
  - Never let young children take medication by themselves.
  - Read and follow labeling instructions on all products; adjust dosage for age.
  - Avoid excessive amounts and/or frequency of doses. ("If a little does some good, a lot should do more.")
- EB: *Data from the Nationwide Emergency Department Sample (NEDS) from 2006 to 2012 show there were 21,928 pediatric ED visits for prescription opioid poisonings. An increase in adult prescription opioid abuse contributes to unintentional ingestion of medications in children (Tadros et al, 2016).*
- EB: *Unintentional poisoning is the fastest growing cause of childhood fatal injury. As per the Centers for Disease and Prevention (CDC), most of this increase is linked to the inappropriate use of prescription opioids (Johnston & Ebel, 2013; CDC, 2018).*
- EB: *Poisoning in children is common and places a significant burden on health care. Parents of poisoned children were more likely to not have safely stored or locked medicines (Kendrick et al, 2017).*
- Advise the family to post first-aid charts and poison control center instructions in an accessible location. Poison control center telephone numbers should be posted close to each telephone and the number programmed into cell phones. *A poison control center should always be called immediately before initiating any first-aid measures. The national toll-free number is (800) 222-1222.*
- Advise family when calling the poison control center to do the following:
  - Give as much information as possible, including your name, location, and telephone number, so that the poison control operator can call back in case you are disconnected or summon help if needed.
  - Give the name of the potential poison ingested and, if possible, the amount and time of ingestion. If the bottle or package is available, give the trade name and ingredients if they are listed.
  - Be prepared to divulge the child's height, weight, age, and medical history.
  - Describe the state of the poisoning victim. Is the victim conscious? Does he or she have any symptoms? What is the person's general appearance, skin color, respiration, breathing difficulties, mental status (alert, sleepy, unusual behavior)? Is the person vomiting? Having convulsions?
- Rapid initiation of proper treatment reduces mortality and morbidity rates. Consultation with a poison control center is necessary to assess and treat poisoned clients. EB: *Optimal management of the poisoned client depends on the poison, the severity of the symptoms, and time between exposure and presentation. Poison control centers can provide assistance (Rhyee, 2013).*
- Encourage the client and family to take first-aid and other types of safety-related programs. *These programs raise participants' level of emergency preparation.*

P

- = Independent;   ▲ = Collaborative;   EBN = Evidence-Based Nursing;   EB = Evidence-Based

▲ Initiate referrals to peer group interventions, peer counseling, and other types of substance abuse prevention/rehabilitation programs when substance abuse is identified as a risk factor.

● Teach parents and other caregivers that cough and cold medications bought over the counter are not safe for children younger than 2 unless specifically ordered by a health care provider. **EB:** *Analysis of exposures to cough/cold preparations supports the concept that poisoning exposure occurs in children with substances that they can easily access (Spiller et al, 2013).*

● Teach parents about home prevention strategies to prevent accidental poisonings. **EB:** *Poisoning prevention programs (providing free or low cost cabinet locks and poison control stickers) have improved safe storage practices (Theurer & Bhavsar, 2013).*

● Teach parents that they can be a source of lead exposure for their children via contaminated work clothing from a lead-related occupation such as transportation workers or automobile repair or if they engage in certain hobbies such as stained glass or ceramics (Schnur & John, 2014). Precautions should be taken to eliminate the risk of exposure.

REFERENCES

American Association of Poison Control Centers. (2018). *Health care providers*. Retrieved from http://www.aapcc.org/.

Aronson, J. (2017). Medication reconciliation. *BMJ : British Medical Journal* 356. Retrieved from http://dx.doi.org.proxy.lib.umich.edu/10.1136/bmj.i5336.

Bogar, S., Szabo, A., Woodruff, S., et al. (2017). Urban youth knowledge and attitudes regarding lead poisoning. *Journal of Community Health, 42*(6), 1255–1266. doi:10.1007/s10900-017-0378-8.

Canadian Patient Safety Institute. (2016). *Medication reconciliation (MedRec)*. Retrieved from www.patientsafetyinstitute.ca/en/Topic/…/medication-reconciliation-(med-rec).aspx.

Centers for Disease Control and Prevention. (2018). *Carbon monoxide (CO) poisoning prevention*. Retrieved from http://www.cdc.gov/features/copoisoning/.

Chang, Y., Lee, H., Huang, J., et al. (2017). Risk factors and outcome analysis in children with carbon monoxide poisoning. *Pediatrics and Neonatology, 58*, 171–177.

College of Nurses of Ontario. (2014). *Practice standard: Medication*. Retrieved from http://www.cno.org/Global/docs/prac/41007_Medication.pdf.

Johnston, B. D., & Ebel, B. E. (2013). Child injury control: Trends, themes, and controversies. *Academic Pediatrics, 13*(6), 499–507.

Kendrick, D., Majsak-Newman, G., Benford, P., et al. (2017). Poison prevention practices and medically attended poisoning in young children: multicentre case-control study. *Injury Prevention: Journal of the International Society for Child and Adolescent Injury Prevention, 23*, 93–101. doi:10.1136/injuryprev-2015-041828.

Nalliah, R. P., Anderson, I. M., Lee, M. K., et al. (2014). Children in the United States make close to 200,000 emergency department visits due to poisoning each year. *Pediatric Emergency Care, 30*(7), 453–457.

Nussbaumer-Streit, B., Yeoh, B., Griebler, U., et al. (2016). Household interventions for preventing domestic lead exposure in children. *Cochrane Database of Systematic Reviews*, (10), Art. No. CD00607, doi:10.1002/14651858.CD006047.pub5.

Oerther, S. E. (2011). Plant poisonings: Common plants that contain cardiac glycosides. *Journal of Emergency Nursing, 37*(1), 102–103.

Rhyee, S. H. (2013). General approach to drug poisoning in adults. *UptoDate*. Retrieved from http://www.uptodate.com.

Rodgers, G. B., Franklin, R. L., & Midgett, J. D. (2012). Unintentional paediatric ingestion poisonings and the role of imitative behavior.

Injury Prevention, 18(2), 103–108.

Schnur, J., & John, R. M. (2014). Childhood lead poisoning and the new centers for disease control and prevention guidelines for lead exposure. *Journal of the American Association of Nurse Practitioners, 26*, 238–247.

Skinner, R., McFaull, S., Draca, J., et al. (2016). Suicide and self-inflicted injury hospitalizations in Canada (1979 to 2014/15). *Health Promotion and Chronic Disease Prevention in Canada, 36*(11), 243–251.

Smith, M., & Bailey, T. (2014). Identifying solutions to medication adherence in the visually impaired elderly. *The Consultant Pharmacist, 29*(2), 131–134.

Spiller, H. A., Beuhler, M. C., Ryan, M. L., et al. (2013). Evaluation of changes in poisoning in young children 2000–2010. *Pediatric Emergency Care, 29*(5), 635–640.

Srisuma, S., Cao, D., Kleinschmidt, K., et al. (2016). Missed opportunities?: An evaluation of potentially preventable poisoning deaths. *Clinical Toxicology, 54-5*, 441–446. doi:10.3109/15563650.2016.1157721.

Tadros, A., et al. (2016). Emergency department visits by pediatric patients for poisoning by prescription opioids. *The American Journal of Drug and Alcohol Abuse, 42*(5), 550–555. doi-org.proxy.lib.umich.edu/10.1080/00952990.2016.1194851.

The Joint Commission. (2014). *National patient safety goals effective January 1, 2014. Hospital accreditation program*. Retrieved from http://www.jointcommission.org/assets/1/6HAP_NPSG_Chapter_2014.pdf.

Theurer, W. M., & Bhavsar, A. K. (2013). Prevention of unintentional childhood injury. *American Family Physician, 87*(7), 502–509.

US Food and Drug Administration. (2014). *Consumer updates, how to dispose of unused medications*. Retrieved from http://www.fda.gov/Drugs/ResourcesForYou/Consumers/BuyingUsingMedicineSafely/EEnsuringSafeUseofMedicine/SafeDisposalofMedicine.

US Food and Drug Administration. (2014). *Consumer updates: Have a baby or young child with a cold? Most don't need medicines*. Retrieved from http://www.fda.gov/ForConsumers/ConsumerUpdates/ucm422465.htm.

Wright, J., Edwards, J., & Walker, S. (2016). Exposures associated with clandestine methamphetamine drug laboratories in Australia (2016). *Reviews on Environmental Health, 31*(3), 329–352. doi:10.1515/reveh-2016-0017.

Post-Trauma syndrome   *Gail B. Ladwig, MSN, RN and Julianne E. Doubet, BSN, RN, EMT-B*

NANDA-I

Definition

Sustained maladaptive response to a traumatic, overwhelming event.

Defining Characteristics

Aggression; alienation; alteration in concentration; alteration in mood; anger; anxiety (00146); avoidance behaviors; compulsive behavior; denial; depression; dissociative amnesia; enuresis; exaggerated startle response; fear (00148); flashbacks; gastrointestinal irritation; grieving (00136); guilt; headache; heart palpitations; history of detachment; hopelessness (00124); horror; hypervigilance; intrusive dreams; intrusive thoughts; irritability; neurosensory irritability; nightmares; panic attacks; rage; reports feeling numb; repression; shame; substance misuse

Related Factors

Diminished ego strength; environment not conducive to needs; exaggerated sense of responsibility; insufficient social support; perceives event as traumatic; self-injurious behavior; survivor role

At-Risk Population

Destruction of one's home; displacement from home; duration of traumatic event; event outside the range of usual human experience; exposure to disaster; exposure to epidemic; exposure to event involving multiple deaths; exposure to war; history of abuse; history of being a prisoner of war; history of criminal victimization; history of torture; human service occupations; serious accident; serious injury to loved one; serious threat to loved one; serious threat to self; witnessing mutilation; witnessing violent death

NOC   (Nursing Outcomes Classification)

Suggested NOC Outcomes

Abuse Cessation; Abuse Protection; Abuse Recovery: Emotional, Aggression Self-Control, Anxiety Self-Control, Grief Resolution, Impulse Self-Control; Self-Mutilation Restraint; Sleep

P

Example NOC Outcome with Indicators

Abuse Recovery: Emotional as evidenced by the following indicators: Trauma-induced psychoneurotic behaviors, conduct disorders, and learning difficulties. (Rate outcome and indicators of **Abuse Recovery: Emotional:** 1 = extensive, 2 = substantial, 3 = moderate, 4 = limited, 5 = none [see Section I].)

Client Outcomes

Client Will (Specify Time Frame)

- Return to pretrauma level of functioning as quickly as possible
- Acknowledge traumatic event and begin to work with the trauma by talking about the experience and expressing feelings of fear, anger, anxiety, guilt, and helplessness
- Identify support systems and available resources and be able to connect with them
- Return to and strengthen coping mechanisms used in previous traumatic event
- Acknowledge event and perceive it without distortions
- Assimilate event and move forward to set and pursue life goals

NIC   (Nursing Interventions Classification)

Suggested NIC Interventions

Counseling; Support System Enhancement

Example NIC Activities—Counseling

Encourage expression of feelings; Assist client to identify strengths and reinforce them

● = Independent;   ▲ = Collaborative;   EBN = Evidence-Based Nursing;   EB = Evidence-Based

Nursing Interventions and *Rationales*

- Observe for a reaction to a traumatic event in all clients regardless of age or sex. EBN: *Treatment, after a traumatic incident, is usually concentrated on stabilizing the patient physically; what is not always addressed is the emotional and/or psychological damage that can follow a traumatizing event (Frank, Schroeter, & Shaw, 2017).*
- After a traumatic event, assess for intrusive memories, avoidance and numbing, and hyperarousal. EB: *The inability to complete goal-directed behavior by actively maintaining information while inhibiting irrelevant information is specific to symptoms of post-traumatic stress disorder (PTSD) (Bornyea, Amir, & Lang, 2013).*
- Remain with the client and provide support during periods of overwhelming emotions. EB: *Hansen et al (2014) studied the effects of an intervention for female victims of intimate partner violence (IPV) on perceived social support and found the overall aim of the stabilization part of this treatment was to provide the woman with a sense of control over her physical safety and her psychological and social situation.*
- Help the individual to comprehend the trauma if possible. EBN: *In their study of women exposed to IPV, Svavardottir, Orlygsdottir, and Gudmundsdottir (2015) found that appropriate first responses and immediate advocacy for the victims of IPV by the health care professional can be invaluable; these interventions support access to safer environments and the means to connect to continued assistance.*
- Use touch with the client's permission (e.g., a hand on the shoulder, holding a hand). EBN: *The application of appropriate touch has been used historically by nurses as a means of connecting with their patients and promoting restorative and therapeutic well-being (Coakley, Barron, & Annese, 2016).*
- Explore and enhance available support systems. EBN: *A nursing education piece published by the Australian Nursing and Midwifery Journal (Post-traumatic stress disorder, 2015) stated that PTSD is a mental illness and treatment must fit to the individual's needs; this may include referrals to mental health care providers.*
- Help the client regain previous sleeping and eating habits. EB: *In adult patients, interruptions in usual sleep patterns experienced soon after a traumatic event can be linked to an increased likelihood of developing PTSD (Pruitt, 2015).*
- ▲ Provide the client pain medication if he or she has physical pain. EBN: *Bridgeland et al (2014) affirmed other research describing high rates of chronic pain in returning veterans with polytrauma and PTSD; they concluded that a holistic approach is needed to treat these victims.*
- ▲ Assess the need for pharmacotherapy. EB: *Primary care physicians and/or psychiatrists may use medications for symptom relief in PTSD, including appropriate antidepressants and anxiolytics (Johnson, 2017).*
- ▲ Refer for appropriate psychotherapy: cognitive therapy, exposure therapy, eye movement desensitization and reprocessing (EMDR), and cognitive-behavioral therapy (CBT). EB: *These approaches can help the client gain control of the fear and distress that occur after a traumatic event (Mayo Clinic, 2014).* EB: *Chen et al (2014) confirmed that EMDR significantly reduces the symptoms of PTSD.*
- Help the client use positive cognitive restructuring to reestablish feelings of self-worth. EB: *Anke et al (2013) showed that cognitive therapy was well tolerated and led to a very large improvement in PTSD symptoms, depression, and anxiety; most clients showed reliable improvement that was clinically significant.*
- Provide the means for the client to express feelings through therapeutic drawing. EB: *Because traumatic events are many times too difficult to describe in words, art therapy gives victims another avenue by which they can project their emotions (Ramirez, 2016).*
- Encourage the client to return to his or her normal routine as quickly as possible. EBN: *For families following an intensive care unit admission, written information about possible psychological sequelae and psychological follow-up was found to be preferable, complemented by telephone support and guidance (Gledhill et al, 2014).*
- Talk to and assess the client's social support after a traumatic event. EB: *Given the high number of physical, mental, and social problems in trauma clients, identifying and strengthening support sources can be effective in the adaption of the effects of an amputation on an individual and improvement of the quality of their life (Valizadeh et al, 2014).*

 Pediatric

- Refer to nursing care plan Risk for **Post-Trauma** syndrome.
- ▲ Carefully assess children exposed to disasters and trauma. Note behavior specific to developmental age. Refer for therapy as needed. EBN: *Zhang et al (2014) found continuous screening is recommended to identify adolescent earthquake survivors with PTSD symptoms, especially survivors who are prone to adapt passive coping strategies and who own external causal attribution.*

• = Independent;   ▲ = Collaborative;   EBN = Evidence-Based Nursing;   EB = Evidence-Based

Geriatric

- Carefully screen older adults for signs of PTSD, especially after a disaster. EB: *Older persons who have undergone an earlier in life trauma may react in a different manner than younger persons to a disaster; age alone does not presage psychological outcomes (Cherry et al, 2015).*
- Consider using the Horwitz Impact of Event Scale, which is an appropriate instrument to measure the subjective response to stress in the older population. CEB: *The Impact of Event Scale–Revised is one of the most widely used self-report measures in the trauma literature (Beck et al, 2008).*
- ▲ Monitor the client for clinical signs of depression and anxiety; refer to a health care provider for medication if appropriate. EB: *Assessment and treatment of PTSD symptoms in older clients can be a challenging task because many older adults suffer cognitive and/or sensory deterioration and comorbid mental and physical disorders that, according to Dinnen, Simiola, and Cook (2015), may lead to incorrect diagnosis and ineffective treatments.*
- Instill hope. EBN: *Hope was intentionally used in this study as an intervention in a group setting in a nursing home; it was evident that hope is not static and can change over time (Moore, Hall, & Jackson, 2014).*

Multicultural

- Assess the influence of cultural beliefs, norms, and values on the client's ability to cope with a traumatic experience. EB: *When receiving treatment, African Americans may feel differently toward a European American clinician because of cultural mistrust. Furthermore, racism and discrimination experienced before or during the traumatic event may compound post-trauma reactions, affecting the severity of symptoms (Williams et al, 2014).*
- Acknowledge racial and ethnic differences at the onset of care. EBN: *Sabri et al (2014) showed that blacks and Asians were less likely than whites to be knowledgeable about workplace violence resources or use resources to address workplace violence.*
- ▲ Carefully assess refugees for PTSD and refer for treatment as appropriate; encourage them to learn the language of their new residence. EB: *Two possible explanations were found for the persistently high prevalence of PTSD among refugees: one is the late onset of PTSD and the other is the low utilization of mental health care (Lamkaddem et al, 2014).*
- Use a family-centered approach when working with Latin, Asian, African American, and Native American clients. EB: *In their study of the mental well-being of Latina survivors of sexual abuse, Ulibarri, Ulloa, & Salazar (2015) found that health care professionals can benefit from increased knowledge of cultural norms and customs that play such large roles in Latino society.* EB: *Parent and self-reported mental health service use for social anxiety among high school students showed Asian American students endorsed a greater number of social anxiety symptoms than other ethnic groups. There were no differences in parent-reported impairment or service utilization (Brice et al, 2014).*
- When working with Asian American clients, provide opportunities by which the family can save face. EB: *Understanding Asian American beliefs concerning the basis of mental illnesses can assist health care professionals in recognizing the feelings of shame and stigma that prevent this group from seeking mental health treatment (Bignall, Jacquez, & Vaughn, 2015).*
- Incorporate cultural traditions as appropriate. EB: *Awareness of a patient's traditional beliefs in complementary and alternative medicine (CAM) allows the health care professional to provide insightful, culturally sensitive, and patient-centered care (Read et al, 2014).*

Home Care

- ▲ Assess family support and the response to the client's coping mechanisms. Refer the family for medical social services or other counseling as necessary. EBN: *The hospitalization of a loved one after a traumatic event, plus the emerging responsibilities of caregiving, can be acutely stressful, often triggering a family crisis and serving as the basis of psychological distress (Newcomb & Hymes, 2017).*
- Assess the effect of the trauma on family and significant others and provide empathy and caring to them. EBN: *Donaldson-Andersen (2017) affirmed that nurses must continuously assess and reevaluate the needs of patients, and the patient's loved ones, during a traumatic event and provide essential emotional and social support as needed.*

Client/Family Teaching and Discharge Planning

- Teach positive coping skills and avoidance of negative coping skills. EB: *CBT coupled with an exercise intervention was associated with positive results in an intervention for ovarian cancer clients (Moonsammy et al, 2013).*

● = Independent;   ▲ = Collaborative;   EBN = Evidence-Based Nursing;   EB = Evidence-Based

P

- Teach stress reduction methods such as deep breathing, visualization, meditation, and physical exercise. Encourage their use especially when intrusive thoughts or flashbacks occur. EB: *Bormann et al (2013) explored the efficacy of private meditation-based mantra intervention for veterans to enhance spiritual well-being in outpatient veterans diagnosed with military-related PTSD.*
- Encourage other healthy living habits. EB: *Hall et al (2015) found in their study that PTSD is not only an extensive and expensive psychiatric condition, but is also linked to obesity and many cardiometabolic conditions.*
- Refer the client to peer support groups. EB: *Public stereotypes affect help seeking, at least early in the course of illness; peer-based outreach and therapy groups may help veterans engage in treatment and resist stigma (Mittal et al, 2013).*
- Consider the use of complementary and alternative therapies. EB: *Yoga has been found to help those with PTSD in adopting methods that encourage mindfulness and aid in managing emotions (Jindani & Khalsa, 2015).*

REFERENCES

Anke, E., Gray, N., Wild, J., et al. (2013). Implementation of cognitive therapy for PTSD in routine clinical care: Effectiveness and moderators of outcome in a consecutive sample. *Behaviour Research and Therapy*, 51(11), 742–752.

Beck, J. G., et al. (2008). The impact of event scale—Revised: Psychometric properties in a sample of motor vehicle accident survivors. *Journal of Anxiety Disorders*, 22(2), 187–198.

Bignall, W., Jacquez, F., & Vaughn, L. (2015). Attributions of mental illness: An ethnically diverse community perspective. *Community Mental Health Journal*, 51(5), 540–545.

Bormann, J. E., Thorp, S. R., Wetherell, J. T., et al. (2013). Meditation-based intervention for veterans with posttraumatic stress disorder: A randomized trial. *Psychological Trauma: Theory, Research, Practice and Policy*, 5(3), 259–267.

Bornyea, J., Amir, N., & Lang, A. J. (2013). The relationship between cognitive control and posttraumatic stress symptoms. *Journal of Behavior Therapy and Experimental Psychiatry*, 43(2), 844–848.

Brice, C., Warner, C. M., Okazaki, S., et al. (2014). Social anxiety and mental health service use among Asian American high school students. *Child Psychiatry and Human Development*. [Epub ahead of print]; PMID: 25300.

Bridgeland, H., Hartenberger, K., Poppen, A., et al. (2014). Polytrauma in veterans: What does it mean for the medical-surgical nurse. *Medsurg Nursing*, 28(3), 25–29.

Chen, Y. R., Hung, K. W., Tsai, J. C., et al. (2014). Efficacy of eye-movement desensitization and reprocessing for patients with posttraumatic-stress disorder: A meta-analysis of randomized controlled trials. *PLoS ONE*, 9(8), e103676.

Cherry, K., Sampson, L., Nezat, P., et al. (2015). Long-term psychological outcomes in older adults after disaster: Relationships to religiosity and social support. *Aging & Mental Health*, 19(5), 430–443.

Coakley, A., Barron, A., & Annese, C. (2016). Exploring the experience and impact of therapeutic touch treatments for nurse colleagues. *Visions: The Journal of Rogerian Nursing Science*, 22(1), 4–16.

Dinnen, S., Simiola, V., & Cook, J. (2015). Post-traumatic stress disorder in older adults: A systematic review of the psychotherapy literature. *Aging & Mental Health*, 19(2), 144–150.

Donaldson-Andersen, J. (2017). The nurse's role in supporting patients and family in sharing personal accounts of traumatic events: Personal experiences. *Journal of Trauma Nursing*, 24(2), 134–140.

Frank, C., Schroeter, K., & Shaw, C. (2017). Addressing traumatic stress in the acute traumatically injured patient. *Journal of Trauma Nursing*, 24(2), 78–84.

Gledhill, J., Tareen, A., Cooper, M., et al. (2014). Joint pediatric and psychiatric follow-up for families following paediatric intensive care unit admission: An exploratory study. *Advances in Critical Care*, 2014, Article ID 897627.

Johnson, K. (2017). The DMS-5 definition of PTSD. *Journal of Legal Nurse Consulting*, 28(3), 25–29.

Hall, K., Hoerster, K., Yancy, W., et al. (2015). Post traumatic stress disorder, physical activity and eating behaviors. *Epidemiologic Reviews*, 37(1), 103–115.

Hansen, N. B., Ericksen, S. B., & Elklit, A. (2014). Effects of an intervention for female victims of intimate partner violence psychological symptoms and perceived social support. *European Journal of Psychotraumatology*, 5, 24797.

Jindani, F., & Khalsa, G. (2015). A yoga intervention program for patients suffering from symptoms of posttraumatic stress disorder: A qualitative descriptive study. *Journal of Alternative & Complementary Medicine*, 21(7), 401–408.

Lamkaddem, M., Stronks, K., Deville, W. D., et al. (2014). Course of post-traumatic stress disorder and health care utilization among resettled refugees in the Netherlands. *BMC Psychiatry*, 14, 90.

Mayo Clinic. (2014). *PTSD, treatment and drugs*. Retrieved from http://www.mayoclinic.org/diseases-conditions/post-traumatic-stress-disorder/ basics/treatment/con-20022540. (Accessed 24 October 2014).

Mittal, D., Drummond, K. L., Blevins, D., et al. (2013). Stigma associated with PTSD. *Psychiatric Rehabilitation Journal*, 36(2), 89–92.

Moore, S. L., Hall, S. E., & Jackson, J. (2014). Exploring the experience of nursing home residents participation in a hope-focused group. *Nursing Research and Practice*, 2014, Article ID 623082.

Moonsammy, S. H., Guglietti, C. L., Mina, D. S., et al. (2013). A pilot study of an exercise and cognitive behavioral therapy intervention for epithelial ovarian cancer patients. *Journal of Ovarian Research*. Retrieved from www.ovarianresearch.com/content6/1/21.

Newcomb, A., & Hymes, R. (2017). Life interrupted: The trauma caregiver experience. *Journal of Trauma Nursing*, 24(2), 125–133.

Post-traumatic stress disorder. (2015). *Australian Nursing & Midwifery Journal*, (23(5), 32–33.

Pruitt, B. (2015). PTSD's affect on sleep and sleep disorders. *Journal of Respiratory Care Practioners*, 28(1), 19–22.

Ramirez, J. (2016). A review of art therapy among military service members and veterans with posttraumatic stress disorder. *Journal of Military and Veterans' Health*, 24(2), 40–51. Retrieved from jmvh.org/article/a-review-of-art-therapy-among-military-service-members-and-veterans-with-post-traumatic-stress-disorder/.

Read, S., Carrier, M., Whitley, R., et al. (2014). Complementary and alternative medicine use in infertility: Cultural and religious influences in a multicultural Canadian setting. *Journal of Alternative & Complementary Medicine*, 20(9), 686–692.

- = Independent;   ▲ = Collaborative;   EBN = Evidence-Based Nursing;   EB = Evidence-Based

Sabri, B., St. Vil, N. M., Campbell, J. C., et al. (2014). Racial and ethnic differences in factors related to workplace violence victimization. *Western Journal of Nursing Research.* Retrieved from sage.pub.com/journalsPermissions.nav.

Svavardottir, E., Orlygsdottir, B., & Gudmundsdottir, B. (2015). Reaching out to women who are victims of intimate partner violence. *Perspectives in Psychiatric Care, 51*(3), 190–201.

Ulibarri, M., Ulloa, E., & Salazar, M. (2015). Associations between mental health, substance use, and sexual abuse experiences among Latinas. *Journal of Child Sexual Abuse, 24*(1), 35–54.

Valizadeh, S., Dadkhah, B., Mohammadi, E., et al. (2014). The perception of trauma patients from social support in adjustment to lower-limb amputation: A qualitative study. *Indian Journal of Palliative Care, 20*(3), 229–238.

Williams, M. T., Malcoun, E., Sawyer, B. A., et al. (2014). Cultural adaptations of prolonged exposure therapy for treatment and prevention of posttraumatic stress disorder in African Americans. *Behavioral Science, 2014*(4), 102–124.

Zhang, W., Lui, H., Jiang, X., et al. (2014). A longitudinal study of posttraumatic stress disorder symptoms and its relationship with coping skill and locus of control in adolescents after an earthquake in China. *PLoS ONE.*

Risk for Post-Trauma syndrome
Gail B. Ladwig, MSN, RN and Julianne E. Doubet, BSN, RN, EMT-B

NANDA-I

Definition

Susceptible to sustained maladaptive response to a traumatic, overwhelming event, which may compromise health.

Risk Factors

Related Factors

Diminished ego strength; environment not conducive to needs; exaggerated sense of responsibility; insufficient social support; perceives event as traumatic; self-injurious behavior; survivor role

At-Risk Population

Destruction of one's home; displacement from home; duration of traumatic event; event outside the range of usual human experience; exposure to disaster; exposure to epidemic; exposure to event involving multiple deaths; exposure to war; history of abuse; history of being a prisoner of war; history of criminal victimization; history of torture; human service occupations; serious accident; serious injury to loved one; serious threat to loved one; serious threat to self; witnessing mutilation; witnessing violent death

NOC   (Nursing Outcomes Classification)

Refer to the care plan for **Post-Trauma** syndrome for suggested NOC outcomes

Example NOC Outcome with Indicators

Risk Detection as evidenced by the following indicators: Recognizes signs and symptoms that indicate risk/Uses health care services congruent with need. (Rate the outcome and indicators of **Risk Detection:** 1 = never demonstrated, 2 = rarely demonstrated, 3 = sometimes demonstrated, 4 = often demonstrated, 5 = consistently demonstrated [see Section I].)

Client Outcomes

Client Will (Specify Time Frame)

- Identify symptoms associated with post-traumatic stress disorder (PTSD) and seek help
- Acknowledge event and perceive it without distortions
- Identify support systems and available resources and be able to connect with them
- State that he/she is not to blame for the event

NIC   (Nursing Interventions Classification)

Refer to the care plan for **Post-Trauma** syndrome for suggested NIC interventions

● = Independent;   ▲ = Collaborative;   EBN = Evidence-Based Nursing;   EB = Evidence-Based

Nursing Interventions and *Rationales*

- Assess for PTSD in a client who has chronic/critical illness, anxiety, or personality disorder; was a witness to severe injury or death; or experienced sexual molestation. **EBN:** *Current literature validates that early identification and intervention in the treatment of traumatic stress is essential to optimal recovery for trauma patients (Frank, Schroeter, & Shaw, 2017).*
- Consider the use of a self-reported screening questionnaire. **EB:** *PTSD self-screens are questionnaires that may help to identify those who could have PTSD; positive responses might signal that a referral to a mental health professional is be warranted (National Center for PTSD, 2017).*
- Assess for ongoing symptoms of post-traumatic stress such as dissociation, avoidance behavior, hypervigilance, and reexperiencing. **EB:** *The symptoms for individuals with PTSD can vary considerably, but they generally fall into these categories: reexperience, avoidance, negative changes in beliefs and/or feelings, and increased arousal (National Center for PTSD, 2017).*
- Assess for past experiences with traumatic events. **EBN:** *In their study of rural women with a history of trauma, Handley et al (2015) found that these clients may have other psychological and social repercussions, along with the development of PTSD.*
- Consider screening for PTSD in a client who is a high user of medical care. **EB:** *Dorrington et al (2014) showed that despite high rates of exposure to trauma, a middle-income population had lower rates of PTSD than high-income populations; there are high rates of non-PTSD diagnoses associated with trauma exposure that could be considered in interventions for trauma-exposed populations.*
- ▲ Provide deployed combat veterans with previous history of low mental or physical health status before deployment with appropriate referral after deployment. **EB:** *Yang and Burr (2016), in their study of the well-being of older veterans exposed to combat, cited a previous study done of identical and fraternal twin combat veterans. It was surmised in that study that both environmental and genetic components played a role in combat veterans' negative mental and physical health outcomes.*
- Provide peer support to contact coworkers experiencing trauma to remind them that others in the organization are concerned about their welfare. **EB:** *Motivating factors that urged transit workers to seek help with their emotional problems after a traumatic experience included family and peers (Bance et al, 2014).*
- Provide post-trauma debriefings. Effective post-trauma coping skills are taught, and each participant creates a plan for his or her recovery. **EB:** *Fakour et al (2014) showed the effectiveness of psychological debriefing in treatment of PTSD after an earthquake; the means of PTSD symptom frequency and severity of avoidance symptoms were reduced during the 3-month period of the study.*
- Provide post-trauma counseling. Counseling sessions are extensions of debriefings and include continued discussion of the traumatic event and post-trauma consequences and the further development of coping skills. **EB:** *Evidence suggested that the response to cognitive behavioral therapy may be enhanced in PTSD clients by preparing them with emotion regulation skills; however, a high attrition of participants during the study limits the conclusions (Bryant et al, 2013).*
- Consider exposure therapy for civilian trauma survivors after an assault or motor vehicle crash. **CEB:** *Prolonged exposure therapy is a beneficial first-line intervention for PTSD, no matter the manner of trauma (Rauch, Eftekhari, & Rozek, 2012).*

Things to Try: Critical Incident Stress Debriefing

- Instruct the client to use the following critical incident stress management techniques:
  - ○ Within the first 24 to 48 hours, engage in periods of appropriate physical exercise alternating with relaxation to alleviate some of the physical reactions; structure your time; keep busy; you are normal and are having normal reactions; do not label yourself as "crazy"; talk to people; talk is the most healing medicine; be aware of numbing the pain with overuse of drugs or alcohol; you do not need to complicate the stress with a substance abuse problem; reach out; people do care; maintain as normal a schedule as possible; spend time with others; help your coworkers as much as possible by sharing feelings and checking out how they are doing; give yourself permission to feel rotten and share your feelings with others; keep a journal; write your way through those sleepless hours; do things that feel good to you; realize that those around you are under stress; do not make any big life changes; do make as many daily decisions as possible to give yourself a feeling of control over your life (e.g., if someone asks you what you want to eat, answer the person even if you are not sure); get plenty of rest; recurring thoughts, dreams, or flashbacks are normal; do not try to fight them because they will decrease over time and become less painful; eat well-balanced and regular meals (even if you do not feel like it).

● = Independent;   ▲ = Collaborative;   EBN = Evidence-Based Nursing;   EB = Evidence-Based

EB: *Based on interview results with railroad employees exposed to trauma and in conjunction with management, Bardon and Mishara (2015) developed a thorough prevention, support, and care protocol to reduce the negative effect of critical incidents for employees: the protocol includes preventative actions, quick responses, prompt intervention, and long-term assistance as needed.*

▲ Assess for a history of life-threatening illness such as cancer and provide appropriate counseling. EB: *"The physical and psychological effect of having a life-threatening disease, undergoing cancer treatment, and living with recurring threats to physical integrity and autonomy constitute traumatic experiences for many cancer clients" (National Cancer Institute, 2013).* EB: *Problematic postbiopsy symptoms can lead to increased anxiety, distinct from distress related to a diagnosis of prostate cancer (Wade et al, 2013).*

Pediatric

● Children with cancer should continue to be assessed for PTSD into adulthood. EB: *The presence of health outcomes was ascertained using systematic exposure-based medical assessments among adult survivors of childhood cancer; using clinical criteria, the crude prevalence of adverse health outcomes for neurocognitive impairment was 48% (Hudson et al, 2013).*

● Provide protection for a child who has witnessed violence or who has had traumatic injuries. Help the child acknowledge the event and express grief over the event. EB: *Lafta, Aziz, and Al-Obaidi (2014) showed that more than half of the total sample in Baghdad had reported multiple experiences of trauma such as fear and/or terror and the painful recall of traumatic events, pointing to the need for medical educational opportunities.*

● Assess for a medical history of anxiety disorders. EB: *Findings from this study suggested that parents with social anxiety disorder may exhibit a unique pattern of behaviors when interacting with their children, including elevated levels of criticism and low levels of warmth; this parenting style has been linked to an increased risk for development of anxiety (Budinger, Drazdowski, & Ginsburg, 2013).*

▲ Assess children of deployed parents for PTSD and provide appropriate referrals. EB: *Lucier-Greer et al (2016) found in their research that multiple parental deployments are a powerful indicator of detrimental outcomes for adolescents in military families.*

● Consider implementation of a school-based program for children to decrease PTSD after catastrophic events. EB: *Tol et al (2014) used an evidence base from previous studies to draw conclusions about the benefits and risks of school-based intervention in reducing PTSD, anxiety, and depression.*

P

Geriatric and Multicultural

● Refer to the care plan for **Post-Trauma** syndrome.

Home Care

▲ Evaluate the client's response to a traumatic or critical event. If screening warrants, refer to a therapist for counseling/treatment. EB: *In the Osofsky et al (2017) study they found that addressing life stressors is an important function in integrated patient care.*

● Refer to the care plan for **Post-Trauma** syndrome.

Client/Family Teaching and Discharge Planning

● Instruct family and friends to use the following critical incident stress management techniques:

▲ Listen carefully; spend time with the traumatized person; offer your assistance and a listening ear, even if the person has not asked for help; help the person with everyday tasks such as cleaning, cooking, caring for the family, and minding children; and give the person some private time. Do not take the individual's anger or other feelings personally, and do not tell the person that he or she is "lucky it wasn't worse." Such statements do not console traumatized people. Instead, tell the person that you are sorry such an event has occurred and you want to understand and assist him or her (National Interagency Fire Center, CISM Information Sheets, 2014).

▲ After exposure to trauma, teach the client and family to recognize symptoms of PTSD and seek treatment for "recurrent and intrusive distressing recollections of the traumatic event," insomnia, irritability, difficulty concentrating, and hypervigilance. EBN: *Family and significant others will profit from assistance, education, and explanation concerning the likely effects relating to PTSD counseling (Australian Nursing & Midwifery Journal, 2015).*

● Provide education to explain that acute stress disorder symptoms may be common when preparing combatants for their role in deployment. Provide referrals if the symptoms persist. EB: *Because US military*

● = Independent;   ▲ = Collaborative;   EBN = Evidence-Based Nursing;   EB = Evidence-Based

forces have been engaged in overseas conflicts since 2001, service men and women have faced stressors related to combat and long deployments. Most manage this stress successfully, but others struggle with mental health problems (Farmer et al, 2015).

REFERENCES

Bance, S., Links, P., Strike, C., et al. (2014). Help-seeking in transit workers exposed to acute psychological trauma: A qualitative analysis. *Work (Reading, Mass.)*, 48(1), 3–10.

Bardon, C., & Mishara, B. (2015). Development of a comprehensive programme to prevent and reduce the negative impact of in railway employees. *Journal of Occupational Rehabilitation*, 25(3), 557–568.

Bryant, R. A., Mastrodomenico, J., Hopwood, S., et al. (2013). Augmenting cognitive behaviour therapy for post-traumatic stress disorder with emotional tolerance training: A randomized controlled trial. *Focus (San Francisco, Calif.)*, 11, 379–386.

Budinger, M. C., Drazdowski, T. K., & Ginsburg, G. S. (2013). Anxiety-promoting parenting behaviors: A comparison of anxious parents with and without social anxiety disorder. *Child Psychiatry and Human Development*, 44, 412–418.

Dorrington, S., Zavos, H., Ball, H., et al. (2014). Trauma, post-traumatic stress disorder and psychiatric disorders in a middle-income setting: prevalence and comorbidity. *British Journal of Psychiatry*, 205(5), 383–389.

Fakour, Y., Mahmoudi Gharaie, J., Mohammadi, M., et al. (2014). The effect of psychosocial supportive interventions on PTSD symptoms after barn severe earthquake. *European Psychiatry*, 29(Suppl. 1).

Farmer, C., Vaughan, C., Garnett, J., et al. (2015). Pre-deployment stress, mental health and help-seeking behavior among Marines. *Rand Health Quarterly*, 5(1), 23. Retrieved from https://www.rand.org/pubs/periodicals/health-quarterly/issues/v5/n1/23.html.

Frank, C., Schroeter, K., & Shaw, C. (2017). Addressing traumatic stress in the acute traumatically injured patient. *British Journal of Psychiatry*, 24(2), 78–84.

Handley, T., Kelly, B., Lewin, T., et al. (2015). Long term effects on lifetime trauma exposure in a rural community. *BMC Public Health*, 15(1), 1–8.

Hudson, M. M., Ness, K. K., Gurney, J. G., et al. (2013). Clinical ascertainment of health outcomes among adults treated for childhood cancer. *JAMA: The Journal of the American Medical Association*, 309(22), 2371–2381.

Lafta, R. K., Aziz, Z. S., & Al-Obaidi, A. K. (2014). Post-traumatic stress disorder (PTSD) among male adolescents in Baghdad. *Journal of Psychological Abnormalities in Children*, 3, 121.

Lucier-Greer, M., Arnold, A., Grimsley, R., et al. (2016). Parental military service and adolescent well-being: Mental health, social connections and coping youth in the USA. *Child & Family Social Work*, 21(4), 421–432.

National Cancer Institute. (2013). *Posttraumatic stress disorder.* Retrieved from http://www.cancer.gov/cancertopics/pdq/supportivecare/post-traumatic-stress/Patient/page4. (Accessed 23 October 2014).

National Center for PTSD. (2017). *Screening for PTSD in primary care settings.* Retrieved from https://www.ptsd.va.gov/public/ptsd-overview/basics/symptoms_of_ptsd.asp.

National Interagency Fire Center. (2014). *CISM information sheets.* Retrieved from http://gacc.nifc.gov/wgbc/cism/effectsoftrauma.pdf. (Accessed 23 October 2014).

Osofsky, H., Weems, C., Hansel, T., et al. (2017). Identifying trajectories of change to improve understanding of integrated health care outcomes in PTSD symptoms post disaster. *Families, Systems & Health: The Journal of Collaborative Family HealthCare*, 35(2), 155–166.

Post-traumatic stress disorder. (2015). *Australian Nursing & Midwifery Journal*, 23(5), 32–33. Retrieved from http://web.a.ebscohost.com/ehost/pdfviewer/pdfviewer?vid=34&sid=f1ca972c-3537-4a36-ad14-e88421adc9e1%40sessionmgr40102202-7114.

Rauch, S., Eftekhari, A., & Rozek, J. (2012). Review of exposure therapy, a gold standard for PTSD treatment. *Journal of Rehabilitation, Research & Development*, 49(5), 678–687.

Tol, W., Kamproe, I. H., Jordans, M. J. D., et al. (2014). School based mental health intervention for children in war-affected Burundi: A cluster randomized trial. *BMC Medicine*, 12, 56.

Wade, J., Rosario, D. J., Macefield, R. C., et al. (2013). Psychological impact of prostate biopsy: Physical symptoms, anxiety, and depression. *Journal of Clinical Oncology*, 31(33), 4235–4421.

Yang, M., & Burr, J. (2016). Combat exposure, social relationships, and subjective well-being among middle aged and older veterans. *Aging & Mental Health*, 20(6), 637–646.

Readiness for enhanced Power *Marina Martinez-Kratz, MS, RN, CNE*

NANDA-I

Definition

A pattern of participating knowingly in change for well-being, which can be strengthened.

Defining Characteristics

Expresses desire to enhance awareness of possible changes; expresses desire to enhance identification of choices that can be made for change; expresses desire to enhance independence with actions for change; expresses desire to enhance involvement in change; expresses desire to enhance knowledge for participation in change; expresses desire to enhance participation in choices for daily living; expresses desire to enhance participation in choices for health; expresses desire to enhance power

● = Independent;   ▲ = Collaborative;   EBN = Evidence-Based Nursing;   EB = Evidence-Based

NOC   (Nursing Outcomes Classification)

Suggested NOC Outcomes

Health Beliefs: Perceived Control; Participation in Health Care Decisions; Personal Autonomy

> **Example NOC Outcome with Indicators**
>
> **Health Beliefs: Perceived Control** as evidenced by the following indicators: Belief that own actions and decisions control health outcomes/Perceived responsibility for health decisions/Efforts at gathering information. (Rate the outcome and indicators of **Health Beliefs: Perceived Control** as 1 = very weak, 2 = weak, 3 = moderate, 4 = strong, 5 = very strong [see Section I].)

Client Outcomes

Client Will (Specify Time Frame)

- Describe power resources
- Identify realistic perceptions of control
- Develop a plan of action based on power resources
- Seek assistance as needed

NIC   (Nursing Interventions Classification)

Suggested NIC Interventions

Mutual Goal Setting; Self-Esteem Enhancement; Self-Responsibility Facilitation

> **Example NIC Activities—Mutual Goal Setting**
>
> Encourage the identification of specific life values; Identify with client the goals of care; Assist client in examining available resources to meet goals

Nursing Interventions and *Rationales*

- Assess the meaning of the event to the person. EBN: *Assessing meaning gives a voice to clients and makes it more likely that solutions reached will have meaning and be useful to the individual (Bevan, 2013).*
- Collaborate with and encourage the person to identify resources to put a plan into action. EBN: *Collaborating with clients provides opportunities for learning and growth and is a client-empowering behavior that improves client health outcomes (Jerofke, Weiss, & Yakusheva, 2014).*
- Provide support for client families to identify the balance between client care responsibilities and self-care. EBN: *A recent study found that by supporting client families and considering them as resources, family feelings of powerlessness can be reduced (Lindgren, Söderberg, & Skär, 2016).*
- Initiate and facilitate family health conversations between the client and their family. EBN: *Research findings showed that participation in family health conversations mediated consolation, helped identify family members' problems and suffering, and assisted to identify their family's resources and strengths (Dorell & Sundin, 2016).*
- Identify the client's health literacy and provide access to information. EBN: *Providing clients with access to information is a client-empowering behavior that improves client health outcomes (Jerofke, Weiss, & Yakusheva, 2014).*
- Help client to mobilize social supports, which is a power resource. EBN: *Assisting clients with access to resources is a client-empowering behavior that improves client health outcomes (Jerofke, Weiss, & Yakusheva, 2014).*
- Refer client to an empowerment support group. EBN: *A randomized controlled trial found that clients who participated in an empowerment support group showed significant increases in levels of empowerment and self-care behaviors* (Hsiao et al, 2016*).*

Pediatric

- Provide empowerment-based education for parents that includes a focus on caregiving knowledge, caring behaviors, self-efficacy, and indicators of the child's recovery. EBN: *A study of an empowerment-based*

● = Independent;   ▲ = Collaborative;   EBN = Evidence-Based Nursing;   EB = Evidence-Based

health education program for parents caring for children with a congenital heart defect (CHD) after corrective surgery showed parental improvement in caregiving knowledge, caring behaviors, and self-efficacy (Zhihong, Chao, & Xiaoling, 2016).

- Initiate problem-solving opportunities, empowering discussions, and reflection to help families take action to manage their child's illness. **EBN:** *A randomized clinical trial found that implementation of an asthma family empowerment program decreased parental stress, improved family functioning, and increased children's pulmonary function (Yeh et al, 2016).*

Geriatric

- Provide health education for older individuals that is tailored, interactive, structured, continuous, and incorporates motivational and encouragement techniques. **EB:** *A systematic review of the literature showed that use of specific educational interventions for older nursing home residents were empowering strategies that increased self-efficacy and self-care (Shoberer et al, 2016).*

Multicultural

In addition to the preceding interventions as appropriate:

- Assess for the influence of communication patterns, cultural differences in medical consultations, and client perceptions of inequalities in care quality as contributors to client feelings of powerlessness. **EB:** *Understanding and addressing client perceptions of power disparities may decrease clients' feelings of powerlessness (Akhavan & Karlsen, 2013).*
- Provide support and educational interventions that are culturally tailored. **EB:** *A randomized control trial found that Latino families assigned to a culturally sensitive, cognitive-behavioral (CBT) group intervention reported lower neuropsychiatric symptoms in their relative, less caregiver distress, a greater sense of caregiver self-efficacy, and less depressive symptoms over time (Gonyea, Lopez, & Velasquez, 2016).*

Home Care

- The preceding interventions may be adapted for home care use.

REFERENCES

Akhavan, S., & Karlsen, S. (2013). Practitioner and client explanations for disparities in health care use between migrant and non-migrant groups in Sweden: A qualitative study. *Journal of Immigrant & Minority Health, 15*(1), 188–197.

Bevan, A. L. (2013). Creating communicative spaces in an action research study. *Nurse Researcher, 21*(2), 14–17.

Dorell, A., & Sundin, K. (2016). Becoming visible—Experiences from families participating in Family Health Conversations at residential homes for older people. *Geriatric Nursing, 37*(4), 260–265. doi:10.1016/j.gerinurse.2016.02.015.

Gonyea, J. G., Lopez, L. M., & Velasquez, E. H. (2016). The effectiveness of a culturally sensitive cognitive behavioral group intervention for Latino Alzheimer's caregivers. *The Gerontologist, 56*(2), 292–302. doi-org.proxy.lib.umich.edu/10.1093/geront/gnu045.

Hsiao, C., Lin, L. W., Su, Y. W., et al. (2016). The effects of an empowerment intervention on renal transplant recipients: A randomized controlled trial. *Journal of Nursing Research, 24*(3), 201–210.

Jerofke, T., Weiss, M., & Yakusheva, O. (2014). Patient perceptions of patient-empowering nurse behaviours, patient activation and

functional health status in postsurgical patients with life-threatening long-term illnesses. *Journal of Advanced Nursing, 70*(6), 1310–1322.

Lindgren, E., Söderberg, S., & Skär, L. (2016). Being a parent to a young adult with mental illness in transition to adulthood. *Issues in Mental Health Nursing, 37*(2), 98–105. Retrieved from https://doi-org.proxy.lib.umich.edu/10.3109/01612840.2015.1092621.

Shoberer, D., et al. (2016). Educational interventions to empower nursing home residents: A systematic literature review. *Clinical Interventions in Aging, 11*, 1351–1363. doi:10.2147/CIA.S114068.

Yeh, H., et al. (2016). Evaluating the effectiveness of a family empowerment program on family function and pulmonary function of children with asthma: A randomized control trial. *International Journal of Nursing Studies, 60*, 133–144. doi-org.proxy.lib.umich.edu/10.1016/j.ijnurstu.2016.04.013.

Zhihong, N., Chao, Y., & Xiaoling, X. (2016). An empowerment health education program for children undergoing surgery for congenital heart diseases. *Journal of Child Health Care, 20*(3), 354–364. doi-org.proxy.lib.umich.edu/10.1177/1367493515587057.

P

Powerlessness   *Marina Martinez-Kratz, MS, RN, CNE*

NANDA-I

Definition

The lived experience of lack of control over a situation, including a perception that one's actions do not significantly affect an outcome.

● = Independent;   ▲ = Collaborative;   **EBN** = Evidence-Based Nursing;   **EB** = Evidence-Based

Defining Characteristics

Alienation; dependency; depression; doubt about role performance; frustration about inability to perform previous activities; inadequate participation in care; insufficient sense of control; shame

Related Factors

Anxiety; caregiver role; dysfunctional institutional environment; ineffective coping strategies; insufficient interpersonal interactions; insufficient knowledge to manage a situation; insufficient social support; low self-esteem; pain; social marginalization; stigmatization

At-Risk Population

Economically disadvantaged

Associated Condition

Complex treatment regimen; illness; progressive illness; unpredictability of illness trajectory

NOC (Nursing Outcomes Classification)

Suggested NOC Outcomes

Depression Self-Control; Health Beliefs; Health Beliefs: Perceived Ability to Perform, Perceived Control, Perceived Resources; Participation in Health Care Decisions

Example NOC Outcome with Indicators
Health Beliefs: Perceived Control as evidenced by the following indicators: Perceived responsibility for health decisions/Beliefs that own decisions and actions control health outcomes. (Rate the outcome and indicators of **Health Beliefs: Perceived Control:** 1 = very weak belief, 2 = weak belief, 3 = moderately strong belief, 4 = strong belief, 5 = very strong belief [see Section I].)

Client Outcomes

Client Will (Specify Time Frame)

• State feelings of powerlessness and other feelings related to powerlessness (e.g., anger, sadness, hopelessness)
• Identify factors that are uncontrollable
• Participate in planning and implementing care; make decisions regarding care and treatment when possible
• Ask questions about care and treatment
• Verbalize hope for the future and sense of participation in planning and implementing care

NIC (Nursing Interventions Classification)

Suggested NIC Interventions

Cognitive Restructuring; Complex Relationship Building; Mutual Goal Setting; Self-Esteem Enhancement; Self-Responsibility Facilitation

Example NIC Activities—Self-Responsibility Facilitation
Encourage independence but assist client when unable to perform; Assist client to identify areas in which they could readily assume more responsibility

Nursing Interventions and *Rationales*

Note: Before implementation of interventions in the face of client powerlessness, nurses should examine their own philosophies of care to ensure that control issues or lack of faith in client capabilities will not bias the ability to intervene sincerely and effectively.
• Assess powerlessness with tools that are available for general and specific client groups:
  ❍ Measure of Powerlessness for Adult Patients (De Almeida & Braga, 2006)
  ❍ Personal Progress Scale–Revised, tested with women (Johnson, Worell, & Chandler, 2005)

• = Independent; ▲ = Collaborative; EBN = Evidence-Based Nursing; EB = Evidence-Based

○ Life Situation Questionnaire–Powerlessness subscale, tested with stroke caregivers (Larson et al, 2005)
○ Making Decisions Scale, tested in clients with mental illness (Hansson & Bjorkman, 2005)
○ Family Empowerment Scale, tested on parents of children with emotional disorders (Koren, DeChillo, & Friesen, 1992)

- Observe for factors contributing to powerlessness (e.g., immobility, hospitalization, unfavorable prognosis, lack of support system, misinformation about situation, inflexible routine, chronic illness, addiction, history of trauma, gender). Help clients channel their behaviors in an effective manner. EB: *Many studies identify factors contributing to feelings of powerlessness are related to losses of person, place, health, or social relationships; gender; or the effect of trauma (Salomé et al, 2013; Doyle, 2014).*
- Engage with clients using respectful listening and questioning to develop an awareness of clients' most important concerns. EB: *Engaging clients will integrate clinician expertise with client needs and can diminish feelings of powerlessness (Sheridan et al, 2015).*
- Provide support for client families to identify the balance between client care responsibilities and self-care. EBN: *A recent study found that by supporting client families and considering them as resources, family feelings of powerlessness can be reduced (Lindgren, Söderberg, & Skär, 2016).*
- Use a rehabilitative behavioral learning model that assists clients to understand how the mechanisms of habit and ritual work to reinforce powerlessness in their lives. *For clients with addiction, understanding the learning processes and mechanisms of powerlessness is an important part of recovery (Butler et al, 2015).*
- Refer client to an empowerment support group. EBN: *A randomized controlled trial found that clients who participated in an empowerment support group showed significant increases in levels of empowerment and self-care behaviors (Hsiao et al, 2016).*
- Refer to the care plans for **Hopelessness** and **Spiritual** distress.

Pediatric

- Provided empowerment-based educational preparation for parents that includes a focus on caregiving knowledge, caring behaviors, self-efficacy, and indicators of the child's recovery. EBN: *A study of an empowerment-based health education program for parents caring for children with a congenital heart defect (CHD) after corrective surgery showed parental improvement in caregiving knowledge, caring behaviors, and self-efficacy (Zhihong, Chao, & Xiaoling, 2016).*
- Initiate problem-solving opportunities, empowering discussions, and reflection to help families take action to manage their child's illness. EBN: *A randomized clinical trial found that implementation of an asthma family empowerment program decreased parental stress, improved family functioning, and increased children's pulmonary function (Yeh et al, 2016).*
- Provide nursing care that shifts the focus from the illness to the child. EBN: *Research indicates that children with a new diagnosis of cancer feel powerless and can benefit from being viewed as a competent individual who requires information and is able to participate in their care (Darcy et al, 2014).*

Geriatric

- In addition to the preceding interventions as appropriate:
  ○ Initiate and facilitate family health conversations between the older client and their family. EBN: *Research findings showed that participation in family health conversations mediated consolation, helped identify family members' problems and suffering, and assisted to identify their family's resources and strengths (Dorell & Sundin, 2016).*
  ○ Provide health education for older individuals that is tailored, interactive, structured, continuous, and incorporates motivational and encouragement techniques. EB: *A systematic review of the literature showed that use of specific educational interventions for older nursing home residents was empowering strategies that increased self-efficacy and self-care (Shoberer et al, 2016).*

Multicultural

- In addition to the preceding interventions as appropriate:
  ○ Assess for the influence of communication patterns, cultural differences in medical consultations, and client perceptions of inequalities in care quality as contributors to client feelings of powerlessness. EB: *Understanding and addressing client perceptions of power disparities may decrease clients' feelings of powerlessness (Akhavan & Karlsen, 2013).*
  ○ Provide support and educational interventions that are culturally tailored. EB: *A randomized control trial found that Latino families assigned to a culturally sensitive, cognitive-behavioral (CBT) group*

● = Independent; ▲ = Collaborative; EBN = Evidence-Based Nursing; EB = Evidence-Based

intervention reported lower neuropsychiatric symptoms in their relative, less caregiver distress, a greater sense of caregiver self-efficacy, and less depressive symptoms over time (Gonyea, Lopez, & Velasquez, 2016).

Home Care

- In addition to the preceding interventions as appropriate:
  - ○ Assess for denial in clients with cancer and provide support for caregivers. EB: *Although denial may be a protective mechanism for the client with cancer, it can create additional burdens for caregivers who may experience powerlessness and an inability to meet their own needs (Kogan, Dumas, & Cohen, 2013).*

Client/Family Teaching and Discharge Planning

- The preceding interventions may be adapted for home care use.

REFERENCES

Akhavan, S., & Karlsen, S. (2013). Practitioner and client explanations for disparities in health care use between migrant and non-migrant groups in Sweden: A qualitative study. *Journal of Immigrant & Minority Health, 15*(1), 188–197.

Butler, M. H., Meloy, K. C., & Call, M. L. (2015). Dismantling powerlessness in addiction: Empowering recovery through rehabilitating behavioral learning. *Sexual Addiction & Compulsivity, 22*(1), 26–58.

Darcy, L., Knutsson, S., Huus, K., et al. (2014). The everyday life of the young child shortly after receiving a cancer diagnosis, from both children's and parent's perspectives. *Cancer Nursing, 37*(6), 445–456.

De Almeida, L. M., & Braga, C. G. (2006). Construction and validation of an instrument to assess powerlessness. *International Journal of Nursing Terminologies and Classifications, 17*, 67.

Dorell, A., & Sundin, K. (2016). Becoming visible—Experiences from families participating in Family Health Conversations at residential homes for older people. *Geriatric Nursing, 37*(4), 260–265. doi:10.1016/j.gerinurse.2016.02.015.

Doyle, S. (2014). The impact of power differentials on the care experiences of older people. *Journal of Elder Abuse & Neglect, 26*(3), 319–332.

Gonyea, J. G., Lopez, L. M., & Velasquez, E. H. (2016). The effectiveness of a culturally sensitive cognitive behavioral group intervention for Latino Alzheimer's caregivers. *The Gerontologist, 56*(2), 292–302. doi-org.proxy.lib.umich.edu/10.1093/geront/gnu045.

Hansson, L., & Bjorkman, T. (2005). Empowerment in people with a mental illness: Reliability and validity of the Swedish version of an empowerment scale. *Scandinavian Journal of Caring Sciences, 19*, 32.

Hsiao, C., Lin, L. W., Su, Y. W., et al. (2016). The effects of an empowerment intervention on renal transplant recipients: A randomized controlled trial. *Journal of Nursing Research, 24*(3), 201–210.

Johnson, D. M., Worell, J., & Chandler, R. K. (2005). Assessing psychological health and empowerment in women: The personal progress scale revised. *Women and Health, 41*(1), 109.

Kogan, N. R., Dumas, M., & Cohen, S. R. (2013). The extra burdens patients in denial impose on their family caregivers. *Palliative & Supportive Care, 11*(2), 91–99.

Koren, P. E., DeChillo, N., & Friesen, B. J. (1992). Measuring empowerment in families whose children have emotional disabilities: A brief questionnaire. *Rehabilitation Psychology, 37*, 305–321. doi:10.1037/h0079106.

Larson, J., et al. (2005). Spouse's life situation after partner's stroke: Psychometric testing of a questionnaire. *Journal of Advanced Nursing, 52*, 300.

Lindgren, E., Söderberg, S., & Skär, L. (2016). Being a parent to a young adult with mental illness in transition to adulthood. *Issues in Mental Health Nursing, 37*(2), 98–105. Retrieved from https://doi-org.proxy.lib.umich.edu/10.3109/01612840.2015.1092621.

Salomé, G. M., Openheimer, D. G., de Almeida, S. A., et al. (2013). Feelings of powerlessness in patients with venous leg ulcers. *Journal of Wound Care, 22*(11), 628, 630, 632–634.

Sheridan, N. F., Kenealy, T. W., Kidd, J. D., et al. (2015). Patients' engagement in primary care: Powerlessness and compounding jeopardy. A qualitative study. *Health Expectations, 18*(1), 32–43.

Shoberer, D., Leino-Kilpi, H., Breimaier, H. E., et al. (2016). Educational interventions to empower nursing home residents: A systematic literature review. *Clinical Interventions in Aging, 11*, 1351–1363. doi:10.2147/CIA.S114068.

Yeh, H., et al. (2016). Evaluating the effectiveness of a family empowerment program on family function and pulmonary function of children with asthma: A randomized control trial. *International Journal of Nursing Studies, 60*, 133–144. doi-org.proxy.lib.umich.edu/10.1016/j.ijnurstu.2016.04.013.

Zhihong, N., Chao, Y., & Xiaoling, X. (2016). An empowerment health education program for children undergoing surgery for congenital heart diseases. *Journal of Child Health Care, 20*(3), 354–364. doi-org.proxy.lib.umich.edu/10.1177/1367493515587057.

P

Risk for Powerlessness   *Gail B. Ladwig, MSN, RN*

NANDA-I

Definition

Susceptible to the lived experience of lack of control over a situation, including a perception that one's actions do not significantly affect the outcome, which may compromise health.

● = Independent;   ▲ = Collaborative;   EBN = Evidence-Based Nursing;   EB = Evidence-Based

Risk Factors

Anxiety; caregiver role; dysfunctional institutional environment; ineffective coping strategies; insufficient interpersonal interactions; insufficient knowledge to manage a situation; insufficient social support; low self-esteem; pain; social marginalization; stigmatization

At-Risk Population

Economically disadvantaged

Associated Condition

Complex treatment regimen; illness; progressive illness; unpredictability of illness trajectory

NOC, NIC, Client Outcomes, Nursing Interventions and *Rationales,* Client/Family Teaching and Discharge Planning, and References

See the care plan for **Powerlessness**

Risk for Pressure Ulcer   *Jo Ann Coar, BSN, RN-BC, CWOCN, COS-C*

Definition

Susceptible to localized injury to the skin and/or underlying tissue usually over a bony prominence as a result of pressure, or pressure in combination with shear (National Pressure Ulcer Advisory Panel [NPUAP], 2007).

Risk Factors

Decrease in mobility; dehydration; dry skin; extended period of immobility on hard surface; hyperthermia; inadequate nutrition; incontinence; insufficient caregiver knowledge of pressure ulcer prevention; insufficient knowledge of modifiable factors; pressure over bony prominence; scaly skin; self-care deficit; shearing forces; skin moisture; smoking; surface friction; use of linen with insufficient moisture wicking property

At-Risk Population

ADULT: Braden Scale score <17; American Society of Anesthesiologists (ASA) Physical Status classification score ≥1; CHILD: Braden Q Scale ≤15; extremes of age; extremes of weight; female gender; history of cerebral vascular accident; history of pressure ulcer; history of trauma; low score on Risk Assessment Pressure Sore (RAPS) scale; New York Heart Association (NYHA) Functional Classification ≥1

Associated Condition

Alteration in cognitive functioning; alteration in sensation; anemia; cardiovascular disease; decrease in serum albumin level; decrease in tissue oxygenation; decrease in tissue perfusion; edema; elevated skin temperature by 1°C to 2°C; hip fracture; impaired circulation; lymphopenia; pharmaceutical agent; physical immobilization; reduced triceps skinfold thickness

NOC   Outcomes (Nursing Outcomes Classification)

Suggested NOC Outcomes

Tissue Integrity: Skin and Mucous Membranes

Example NOC Outcome with Indicators

Intact Tissue Integrity: Skin and Mucous Membranes as evidenced by the following indicators: Skin intactness/Skin lesions absent/Tissue perfusion/Skin temperature. (Rate the outcome and indicators of **Tissue Integrity: Skin and Mucous Membranes:** I = severely compromised, 2 = substantially compromised, 3 = moderately compromised, 4 = mildly compromised, 5 = not compromised [see Section I].)

● = Independent;   ▲ = Collaborative;   EBN = Evidence-Based Nursing;   EB = Evidence-Based

Client Outcomes

Client Will (Specify Time Frame)

- Report any altered sensation or pain at site of tissue impairment
- Skin, without redness over bony prominences and capillary refill of less than 6 seconds over areas of redness
- Be repositioned off of bony prominences frequently if risk for pressure injuries is high (e.g., Braden scale score ≤18)
- Demonstrate understanding of plan to reduce pressure injury risk
- Describe measures to protect the skin

NIC Interventions (Nursing Interventions Classification)

Suggested NIC Interventions

Pain Management; Pressure Injury Care; Pressure Injury Prevention; Risk Identification; Skin Care: Topical Treatments; Skin Surveillance

Example NIC Activities—Pressure Injury Care

Monitor color of skin, temperature, edema, erythema, moisture, and appearance of surrounding skin; Note characteristics of skin over bony prominences or under/in contact with medical devices

Nursing Interventions and *Rationales*

▲ NPUAP redefined the definition of a pressure ulcer, which is now referred to as pressure injuries, during the NPUAP 2016 Staging Consensus Conference in 2016. The new definitions more accurately define alterations in tissue integrity from pressure. Classify pressure injuries (NPUAP & European Pressure Ulcer Advisory Panel [EPUAP], 2016) using national guidelines and definitions (see http://www.npuap.org/resources/educational-and-clinical-resources/npuap-pressure-injury-stages/).

○ **Pressure Injury:** A pressure injury is localized damage to the skin and underlying soft tissue usually over a bony prominence or related to a medical or other device. The injury can present as intact skin or an open ulcer and may be painful. The injury occurs as a result of intense and/or prolonged pressure or pressure in combination with shear. The tolerance of soft tissue for pressure and shear may also be affected by microclimate, nutrition, perfusion, comorbidities, and condition of the soft tissue (NPUAP & EPUAP, 2016).

○ **Stage 1 Pressure Injury:** Nonblanchable erythema of intact skin
Area of localized nonbleachable erythema that may appear differently in darkly pigmented skin, and changes in sensation, temperature, or firmness may precede visual changes. Color changes do not include purple or maroon discoloration which is more likely to indicate deep tissue pressure injury (NPUAP & EPUAP, 2016).

○ **Stage 2 Pressure Injury:** Partial-thickness skin loss with exposed dermis
Partial-thickness skin loss with exposed dermis in which the wound bed is pink/red and moist and adipose (fat) and deeper tissues are not visible. Granulation tissue, slough, and eschar are not present. A stage 2 pressure injury may also present as an intact or ruptured blister. These injuries commonly result from adverse microclimate and shear in the skin over the pelvis and shear in the heel. This stage should not be used to describe moisture-associated skin damage (MASD) including incontinence-associated dermatitis (IAD), intertriginous dermatitis (ITD), medical adhesive–related skin injury (MARSI), or traumatic wounds (skin tears, burns, and abrasions) (NPUAP & EPUAP, 2016).

○ **Stage 3 Pressure Injury:** Full-thickness skin loss
Full-thickness loss of skin, in which adipose is visible and granulation tissue and epibole (rolled wound edges) are often present and undermining/tunneling may occur. Slough and/or eschar may also be visible. Fascia, muscle, tendon, ligament, cartilage, and/or bone are not exposed. The depth of tissue damage varies by anatomical location, and areas of significant adiposity can develop deep wounds. If slough or eschar obscures the extent of tissue loss, then this is an unstageable pressure injury (NPUAP & EPUAP, 2016).

○ **Stage 4 Pressure Injury:** Full-thickness skin and tissue loss
Full-thickness skin and tissue loss with exposed or directly palpable fascia, muscle, tendon, ligament, cartilage, or bone, and slough and/or eschar may be visible. Epibole, undermining, and/or tunneling

● = Independent;   ▲ = Collaborative;   EBN = Evidence-Based Nursing;   EB = Evidence-Based

often occur and depth varies by anatomical location. If slough or eschar obscures the extent of tissue loss, then this is an unstageable pressure injury (NPUAP & EPUAP, 2016).

- **Deep Tissue Pressure Injury:** Persistent nonblanchable deep red, maroon, or purple discoloration
  Intact or nonintact skin with localized area of persistent nonblanchable deep red, maroon, or purple discoloration or epidermal separation revealing a dark wound bed or blood-filled blister. Pain and temperature change often precedes skin color changes. Discoloration may appear differently in darkly pigmented skin. This injury results from intense and/or prolonged pressure and shear forces at the bone–muscle interface. The wound may evolve rapidly to reveal the actual extent of tissue injury, or it may resolve without tissue loss. If necrotic tissue, subcutaneous tissue, granulation tissue, fascia, muscle, or other underlying structures are visible, then this indicates a full-thickness pressure injury (unstageable, stage 3, or stage 4). Do not use deep tissue pressure injury to describe vascular, traumatic, neuropathic, or dermatological conditions (NPUAP & EPUAP, 2016).
- **Unstageable Pressure Injury:** Obscured full-thickness skin and tissue loss
  Full-thickness skin and tissue loss in which the extent of tissue damage within the ulcer cannot be confirmed because it is obscured by slough or eschar. If slough or eschar is removed, a stage 3 or stage 4 pressure injury will be revealed. Stable eschar (i.e., dry, adherent, intact without erythema or fluctuance) on the heel or ischemic limb should not be softened or removed (NPUAP & EPUAP, 2016).
- Routinely assess clients for risk of pressure injuries using a valid and reliable risk assessment tool (NPUAP & EPUAP, 2014). A validated risk-assessment tool such as the Norton scale or Braden scale should be used to identify clients at risk for pressure-related skin breakdown (NPUAP & EPUAP, 2014). **EB:** *Targeting variables (e.g., Braden scale risk subscale categories, age, severity of illness) can focus assessment on particular risk factors (e.g., pressure, immobility, perfusion) and help guide the plan of prevention and care (NPUAP/ EPUAP, 2014; Ratliff et al, 2017).*
- Pressure injury risk assessment should be completed on admission, daily, and after procedures or changes in the client's condition (NPUAP & EPUAP, 2014; Baranoski & Ayello, 2016).
- Inspect the skin daily, especially bony prominences and dependent areas for pallor, redness, and breakdown. In addition to assessing pressure injury risk, client-specific interventions should be implemented to prevent tissue injury. Implement the following interventions to prevent tissue breakdown:
  - Turn and reposition all individuals at risk for pressure injury, unless contraindicated because of medical condition or medical treatments.
  - Position client properly; use pressure-reducing or pressure-relieving devices (e.g., pillows, gel or foam cushions, alternating pressure mattress, air-fluidized bed, kinetic bed) if indicated. Continue to turn and reposition the individual regardless of the support surface in use. Establish turning frequency based on the characteristics of the support surface and the individual's response (NPUAP & EPUAP, 2014).
  - Lift and move client carefully using a turn sheet and adequate assistance; keep bed linens dry and wrinkle-free.
  - Perform actions to keep client from sliding down in bed (e.g., bend knees slightly when head of bed is elevated 30 degrees or higher) to reduce the risk of skin surface abrasion and shearing. Use the 30-degree tilted side-lying position (alternately, right side, back, left side) or the prone position if the individual can tolerate this and his or her medical condition allows (NPUAP & EPUAP, 2014).
  - Select a seated posture that is acceptable for the individual and minimizes the pressures and shear exerted on the skin and soft tissues (NPUAP & EPUAP, 2014).
  - Keep client's skin clean. Thoroughly dry skin after bathing and as often as needed, paying special attention to skinfolds and opposing skin surfaces (e.g., axillae, perineum, beneath breasts). Pat skin dry rather than rub, and use a mild soap for bathing. Apply moisturizing lotion at least once a day.
  - Protect the skin from contact with urine and feces (e.g., keep perineal area clean and dry, apply a protective ointment or cream to perineal area).
  - Provide and encourage adequate daily fluid intake for hydration for an individual assessed to be at risk of or with a pressure injury (NPUAP & EPUAP, 2016). This must be consistent with the individual's comorbid conditions and goals (NPUAP & EPUAP, 2014).
  - If the individual cannot be moved or is positioned with the head of the bed elevated over 30 degrees, then place a polyurethane foam dressing on the sacrum (NPUAP & EPUAP, 2016). Use heel offloading device or polyurethane foam dressings on individuals at high risk for heel ulcers (NPUAP & EPUAP, 2016).
  - Consult with nutrition/dietary specialist to evaluate client's nutritional status.
  - Increase activity as allowed.

- = Independent; ▲ = Collaborative; EBN = Evidence-Based Nursing; EB = Evidence-Based

▲ EB: *Pressure injuries result in additional pain and treatment for the client and additional health care services and costs. A comprehensive assessment of the client's risk for pressure injuries and proactive interventions is necessary to reduce the risk for tissue injury (NPUAP & EPUAP, 2014; NPUAP & EPUAP, 2016).*

• Medical device–related pressure injuries (MDRPIs) result from the use of devices designed and applied for diagnostic or therapeutic purposes. The resultant pressure injury generally conforms to the pattern or shape of the device. The injury should be staged using the NPUAP pressure injury staging system and the etiology of the pressure injury noted to be caused by the device (NPUAP & EPUAP, 2016).

  ❍ The head/face/neck, heel/ankle/foot, coccyx/buttocks, abdomen, and extremities are common body regions for MDRPI.

  ❍ Common devices associated with pressure-related tissue injury include oxygen delivery and monitoring devices (e.g., face mask, nasal cannula, pulse oximetry, bilevel positive airway pressure [BiPAP] mask), feeding tubes (e.g., nasogastric, gastric, jejunal tubes), endotracheal devices (oral and/or nasal endotracheal tubes, tracheostomy tubes), urinary and bowel elimination equipment (indwelling urinary catheter, fecal containment catheter), and musculoskeletal appliances (cervical collar, splints, braces).

  ❍ Assess and evaluate the purpose and function of the medical device.

  ❍ Assess proper fit of the medical device and securement to prevent rubbing, torque, or pulling on the device and skin.

  ❍ Protect the skin below and around the device to reduce pressure.

▲ EB: *Incorporate daily and frequent skin inspection around and under the medical device. See the NPUAP Best Practice flyer to help provide education about medical device–related ulcers (see http://www.npuap.org/wp-content/uploads/2013/04/BestPractices-CriticalCare1.pdf).*

• Critically ill clients are at increased risk for pressure ulcers, often requiring frequent skin risk assessment and preventive interventions. EB: *Support surfaces are often needed to reduce pressure risk in the critically ill client (Behrendt et al, 2014). Reposition the client often more frequently than every 2 hours (Makic et al, 2014; NPUAP & EPUAP, 2014). Frequently assess skin for shear injury and pressure areas when the client is in prone positioning or lateral rotation therapy is used (NPUAP & EPUAP, 2014).*

• EB: *Efforts must be taken to disseminate evidence-based guidelines and ensure that health care providers, in all settings, are making every effort to identify individuals who are at risk for pressure injuries and implement preventative and treatment interventions (Ratliff et al, 2017). Consider optimizing work procedures at a professional level through the introduction of tailored staff education, role models or designated wound care "champions," nurse-led quality improvement programs, and cues to perform pressure ulcer prevention (NPUAP & EPUAP, 2014).*

• If tissue breakdown occurs, notify a health care provider or wound care specialist. See care plan for Impaired **Skin** integrity for additional interventions if a pressure ulcer occurs.

P

Pediatric

• Perform an age-appropriate pressure injury (NPUAP & EPUAP, 2016) risk assessment using a valid and reliable tool. CEB/EB: *The Braden Q and Glamorgan scales are valid and reliable scales to assess pediatric client risks for compromised skin integrity related to pressure (Anthony, Willock, & Bahrestani, 2010; Galvin & Curley, 2012; Tume et al, 2013). The Neonatal Skin Risk Assessment Scale was developed to assess unique skin breakdown risk in neonates (Dolack et al, 2013).*

• Implement a comprehensive plan to reduce the client's risk of skin breakdown from pressure. Assessment should include the following:

  ❍ Client independent activity and mobility levels

  ❍ Body mass index and/or birth weight; lower weight may increase client risk of pressure-associated skin breakdown

  ❍ Skin maturity

  ❍ Adequate nutritional and hydration status

  ❍ Perfusion and oxygenation

  ❍ Presence of external devices

  ❍ Duration of hospital stay

▲ EB: *Pediatric clients with medical devices are at higher risk for pressure injuries (NPUAP & EPUAP, 2016). Inspect the skin under and around the device at least twice a day. Conduct more frequent (greater than twice daily) skin assessments at the skin–device interface in individuals vulnerable to fluid shifts and/or exhibiting signs of localized or generalized edema (NPUAP & EPUAP, 2014). Frequent (e.g., daily and after procedures) and ongoing assessment of the client's risk for pressure injury (NPUAP & EPUAP, 2016) is an important*

• = Independent;   ▲ = Collaborative;   EBN = Evidence-Based Nursing;   EB = Evidence-Based

prevention intervention. Carefully assess the skin on the client's occiput as part of the assessment (NPUAP & EPUAP, 2014).

- Select an age-appropriate support surface for premature neonates and pediatric clients at high risk for pressure ulcers. **CEBN:** *A longitudinal study found that the use of continuous and reactive low-pressure mattresses reduced the observed incidence of pressure ulcers (Garcia-Molina et al, 2012). Select a support surface to prevent occipital pressure ulcers for at-risk clients (NPUAP & EPUAP, 2014).*
- *Engage the client/family/legal guardian in the development of a client-specific plan of care to reduce pressure-related risk for skin breakdown (NPUAP & EPUAP, 2014).*
- Document risk assessment and interventions implemented to reduce the client's risk for pressure injury (NPUAP, 2016) development.

 Geriatric

- Consider the older client's cognitive status when assessing the skin and in developing a comprehensive plan of care to prevent pressure injuries (NPUAP & EPUAP, 2014; NPUAP & EPUAP, 2016).
- Aging skin, medications (e.g., steroids), and moisture place the older client at increased risk for pressure-associated skin breakdown. **EB:** *Assess the client for pressure injury (NPUAP & EPUAP, 2016) risk, skin tear, and moisture-associated skin breakdown. It is important to differentiate the cause of the older client's skin breakdown to effectively implement prevention and treatment strategies. Frequently interventions complement each other in the overall goal to prevent a compromise in the client's skin integrity (Holmes et al, 2013; NPUAP & EPUAP, 2014).*
- *Use atraumatic wound dressings to prevent and treat pressure injuries (NPUAP & EPUAP, 2016) to reduce further injury to frail older client's skin (NPUAP & EPUAP, 2014).*
- For older clients with continence concerns, develop and implement an individualized continence management program (NPUAP & EPUAP, 2014). **EB:** *Use skin barrier products and moisture wicking pads to reduce moisture-associated skin irritation that increases the risk for pressure injury (NPUAP & EPUAP, 2016) development; avoid the use of diapers except when the client is ambulating (NPUAP & EPUAP, 2014; Willson et al, 2014).*
- *Regularly reposition the older client who is unable to reposition independently. Consider pressure redistribution support surface for clients assessed to be at high risk for pressure injuries (NPUAP & EPUAP, 2014; Makic et al, 2014; NPUAP & EPUAP, 2016).*

 Home Care

- The interventions described previously may be adapted for home care use.
- Instruct and assist the client and caregivers in how to assess the skin for excessive pressure. Provide written instructions for actions they can implement to reduce the risk of pressure injury (NPUAP, 2016) development.
- Educate client and caregivers on proper nutrition and when to call the agency and/or health care provider with concerns.
- ▲ It may be beneficial to initiate a consultation in a case assignment with a wound, ostomy, continence nurse (or wounds specialist) to establish a comprehensive plan for pressure ulcer risk reduction for clients at high risk for skin breakdown.

REFERENCES

Anthony, D., Willock, J., & Baharestani, M. (2010). A comparison of Braden Q, Garvin, and Glamorgan risk assessment scales in paediatrics. *Journal of Tissue Viability, 19,* 98–105.

Baranoski, S., & Ayello, E. A. (Eds.), (2016). *Wound care essentials: Practice principles* (4th ed.). Ambler, PA: Lippincott Williams & Wilkins.

Behrendt, R., Ghaznavi, A., Mahan, M., et al. (2014). Continuous bedside pressure mapping and rates of hospital-associated pressure ulcers in a medical intensive care unit. *American Journal of Critical Care, 23*(2), 127–133.

Dolack, M., Huffines, B., Stikes, R., et al. (2013). Updated neonatal skin risk assessment scale. *Kentucky Nurse, 61*(4), 6.

Galvin, P. A., & Curley, M. A. Q. (2012). The braden Q+P: A pediatric perioperative pressure ulcer risk assessment and intervention tool. *AORN Journal, 96*(3), 261–270.

Garcia-Molina, P., Balaguer-Lopez, E., Torra, I., et al. (2012). A prospective, longitudinal study to assess use of continuous and reactive low-pressure mattresses to reduce pressure ulcer incidence in a pediatric intensive care unit. *Ostomy/Wound Management, 58*(7), 32–39.

Holmes, R., Davidson, M., Thompson, B., et al. (2013). Skin tears: Care and management of the older adult at home. *Home Healthcare Nurse, 31*(2), 90–101.

Makic, M. B. F., Rauen, C., Watson, R., et al. (2014). Examining the evidence to guide practice: Challenging practice habits. *Critical Care Nurse, 34,* 28–46.

National Pressure Ulcer Advisory Panel (NPUAP) and European Pressure Ulcer Advisory Panel (EPUAP). (2014). *Prevention and treatment of pressure ulcers.* Perth, Australia: Cambridge Media.

● = Independent;   ▲ = Collaborative;   **EBN** = Evidence-Based Nursing;   **EB** = Evidence-Based

National Pressure Ulcer Advisory Panel (NPUAP) and European Pressure Ulcer Advisory Panel (EPUAP). (2016). *Pressure injury stages*. Retrieved from http://www.npuap.org/resources/educational-and-clinical-resources/npuap-pressure-injury-stages/. (Accessed 5 December 2017).

Ratliff, C. R., Droste, L. R., Bonham, P., et al. (2017). WOCN 2016 guidelines for prevention and management of pressure injuries (ulcers). An executive summary. Wound, Ostomy and Continence

Nurses Society-Wound Guidelines Task Force. *Journal of Wound, Ostomy, and Continence Nursing, 44*(3), 241–246.

Tume, L. N., Siner, S., Scott, E., et al. (2013). The prognostic ability of early Braden Q scores in critically ill children. *Nursing in Crit Care, 19*(2), 98–103.

Willson, M. M., Angyus, M., Beals, D., et al. (2014). Executive summary: A quick reference guide for managing fecal incontinence. *Journal of Wound, Ostomy, and Continence Nursing, 41*(1), 61–69.

Ineffective Protection   *Ruth M. Curchoe, RN, BSN, MSN, CIC*

NANDA-I

Definition

Decrease in the ability to guard self from internal or external threats such as illness or injury.

Defining Characteristics

Altered in clotting; alteration in perspiration; anorexia; chilling; coughing; deficient immunity; disorientation; dyspnea; fatigue; immobility; insomnia; itching, maladaptive stress response; neurosensory impairment; pressure ulcer; restlessness; weakness

Related Factors

Inadequate nutrition; substance abuse

At-Risk Population

Extremes of age

Associated Condition

Abnormal blood type; cancer; immune disorder; pharmaceutical agent; treatment regimen

NOC   (Nursing Outcomes Classification)

Suggested NOC Outcomes

Health-Promoting Behavior; Blood Coagulation; Endurance; Immune Status

> **Example NOC Outcome with Indicators**
>
> **Immune Status** as evidenced by the following indicators: Recurrent infections/Tumors/Weight loss. (Rate the outcome and indicators of **Immune Status:** 1 = severe, 2 = substantial, 3 = moderate, 4 = mild, 5 = none [see Section I].)

Client Outcomes

Client Will (Specify Time Frame)

- Remain free of infection while in contact during contact with health care
- Remain free of any evidence of new bleeding as evident by stable vital signs
- Explain precautions to take to prevent infection including hand hygiene
- Explain precautions to take to prevent bleeding including fall prevention

NIC   (Nursing Interventions Classification)

Suggested NIC Interventions

Bleeding Precautions; Infection Prevention; Infection Protection

● = Independent;   ▲ = Collaborative;   **EBN** = Evidence-Based Nursing;   **EB** = Evidence-Based

Example **NIC** Activities—Infection Protection
Monitor for systemic and localized signs and symptoms of infection; Inspect skin and mucous membranes for redness, extreme warmth, or drainage

Nursing Interventions and *Rationales*

- Take temperature, pulse, and blood pressure (e.g., every 1–4 hours). **EBN:** *Changes in vital signs can indicate the onset of bleeding or infection. Rectal and oral temperature measurements are more accurate than other methods of temperature measurement such as temporal or axillary measurement (Perry & Potter, 2014).*
- ▲ Observe nutritional status (e.g., weight, serum protein and albumin levels, muscle mass, and usual food intake). Work with the dietitian to improve nutritional status if needed. **EB:** *Clients diagnosed with asthma or repeated respiratory infections should have a nutritional assessment.* **EB:** *Vitamin D influences the body's immune system by influencing the production of endogenous antimicrobial peptides and regulating the inflammatory cascade (Gunville, Mourani, & Ginde, 2013).*
- Observe the client's sleep pattern; if altered, see Nursing Interventions and *Rationales* for Disturbed **Sleep** pattern.
- Identify stressors in the client's life. If stress is uncontrollable, see Nursing Interventions and *Rationales* for Ineffective **Coping.** **EB:** *Nearly 30% of older clients experience delirium during hospitalization; the incidence is higher in intensive care units. Among older clients who have had surgery, the risk for delirium varies from 10% to more than 50% (Sternicuk, Rusak, & Rockwood, 2014).*

Prevention of Infection

- ▲ Monitor for and report any signs of infection (e.g., fever, chills, flushed skin, drainage, edema, redness, abnormal laboratory values, pain) and notify the health care provider promptly. **EBN:** *Although the white blood cell count may be in the normal range, an increased number of immature bands may be present (Perry & Potter, 2014).* **CEBN:** *A neutropenic client with fever represents an absolute medical emergency (Klastersky et al, 2016). If the client's immune system is depressed, notify the health care provider of elevated temperature, even in the absence of other symptoms of infection.* **EB:** *Clients with depressed immune function are unable to mount the usual immune responses to the onset of infection; fever may be the only sign of infection. A neutropenic client with fever represents an absolute medical emergency.* **CEBN:** *A neutropenic client with fever represents an absolute medical emergency (EB Medicine, 2013).*
- If white blood cell count is severely decreased (i.e., absolute neutrophil count of less than 1000/mm³), initiate the following precautions:
  ○ Take vital signs every 2 to 4 hours
  ○ Complete a head-to-toe assessment twice daily, including inspection of oral mucosa, invasive sites, wounds, urine, and stool; monitor for onset of new reports of pain
- ▲ Avoid any invasive procedures, including catheterization, injections, or rectal or vaginal procedures unless absolutely necessary. **EBN:** *Classic organisms such as influenza cause infections in the immunocompromised host; often their presentation is different and more serious (Flood, 2014).*
  ○ Consider warming the client before elective surgery. Normothermia is associated with low postoperative infection rates (Moucha, 2016)
- ▲ Administer granulocyte growth factor as ordered. **EB:** *Clients most likely to benefit from therapy would be those with profound neutropenia or neutropenia with infections not responding to antimicrobial therapy (Flood, 2014).* **EB:** *Granulocyte macrophage colony-stimulating factor is mostly well tolerated, although some cancer and kidney disease clients have demonstrated significant complications such as leukopenia (McDowell, 2017).*
  ○ Take meticulous care of all invasive sites; use chlorhexidine gluconate for cleansing. **EB:** *Use of chlorhexidine gluconate for vascular catheter site care reduces catheter-related bloodstream infections and catheter colonization (Centers for Disease Control and Prevention [CDC], 2011b).*
  ○ Provide frequent oral care. **EBN:** *The effects of chemotherapy or radiation can cause changes in taste and smell resulting in pain and nutritional deficiencies (Poirier, 2013).*
  ○ Follow Standard Precautions, especially performing hand hygiene to prevent health care–associated infections. **EBN:** *Hands of health care workers are the most common cause of health care–associated infections (CDC, 2011a; Haas, 2014).*
- ▲ Refer for appropriate prophylactic antifungal treatment and avoid pathogen exposure (through air filtration, regular hand hygiene, and avoidance of plants and flowers). *Practical measures can be taken to avoid*

● = Independent; ▲ = Collaborative; **EBN** = Evidence-Based Nursing; **EB** = Evidence-Based

exposing the client to fungi (Flood, 2014). EB: *Highly active imidazoles have had a major effect on human fungal infections (Ferrara, MacDougall, & Gallagher, 2011).*

○ Have the client wear a mask when leaving the room. EB: *To prevent health care–acquired pulmonary aspergillosis during hospital construction, neutropenic clients may be at lesser risk if masked when leaving their room (Thom, Kleinberg, & Roghmann, 2013). Limit and screen visitors to minimize exposure to contagion.*

○ Help the client bathe daily.

○ Practice food safety; a neutropenic diet may not be necessary. EBN: *No clear evidence exists that the neutropenic diet makes a difference in overall rates of infection (Thom, Kleinberg, & Roghmann, 2013).*

○ Ensure that the client is well nourished. Provide food with protein, and consider vitamin supplements. If appetite is suppressed, institute a dietary referral. Keep track of serum albumin levels and transferrin and prealbumin levels. CEB: *Levels of the visceral proteins (albumin, transferrin, and prealbumin) are an indirect measure of nutritional status (Geismar, 2014).*

○ Help the client cough and practice deep breathing regularly. Maintain an appropriate activity level.

○ Obtain a private room for the client. Use high-energy particulate air filters if available and appropriate. Protective isolation is not recommended. Recognize that cotton cover gowns may not be effective in decreasing infection. EBN: *Complete an infection control risk assessment (ICRA) considering such issues as the type of transplant performed, the environment, and prior infection rates. Use the ICRA to decide the types of infections, processes, practices, and risk to be monitored (American Society for Healthcare Engineering [ASHE], 2014; Harris, 2014).*

▲ Watch for signs of sepsis, including change in mental status, fever, shaking, chills, and hypotension. If present, notify the health care provider promptly. *Change in mental status, fever, shaking, chills, and hypotension are indicators of sepsis (Curchoe, 2013).*

• Refer to care plan for Risk for **Infection.**

• Refer to care plan for Readiness for enhanced **Nutrition** for additional interventions.

Pediatric

• Suggest kangaroo care (KC), frequent and exclusive or nearly exclusive breastfeeding, and early discharge from hospital for low-birth-weight infants. EBN: *The practice of KC decreases the incidence of nosocomial infection. Early KC likely increases the chance of the infant being colonized with maternal flora rather than the flora in the nursery, which may include antibiotic-resistant organisms and coagulase-negative staphylococcus. Because KC is only undertaken between individual infant–mother dyads, it should not increase the spread of infection from one infant to another during infectious outbreaks (Jefferies, 2012).*

• Assess postoperative fever in pediatric oncology clients promptly. EB: *Fever is a physiological mechanism that has beneficial effects in fighting infection. There is no evidence that fever itself worsens the course of an illness or that it causes long-term neurological complications (Sullivan & Farrer, 2011).*

• For hand hygiene with low-birth-weight infants, use alcohol hand rub and gloves. EBN: *Audit programs to track compliance with hand hygiene identified a drop in the incidence of health care–associated infections in very low-birth-weight infants in the neonatal intensive care unit (Helder et al, 2014).*

Geriatric

▲ If not contraindicated, promote exercise to promote improved quality of life in older adults. EB: *A study of 95 healthy adults 65 years and older suggested that the effects of resistance-type exercise training can counteract the loss of muscle mass and strength with aging (Buckines, 2017). Give older clients with imbalanced nutrition a vitamin D supplement to reduce risk of fracture.* EB: *Vitamin D deficiency has been correlated with increased risk and greater severity of infection, particularly of the respiratory tract. Vitamin D influences the body's immune system by influencing the production of endogenous antimicrobial peptides and regulating the inflammatory cascade (Dankers et al, 2016).*

• Refer to the care plan for Risk for **Infection** for more interventions related to the prevention of infection.

Prevention of Bleeding

▲ Monitor the client's risk for bleeding; evaluate results of clotting studies and platelet counts. *Laboratory studies give a good indication of the seriousness of the bleeding disorder.*

• Watch for hematuria, melena, hematemesis, hemoptysis, epistaxis, bleeding from mucosa, petechiae, and ecchymoses. EBN: *A study of 200 clients with idiopathic thrombocytopenic purpura revealed that 57% had*

• = Independent;   ▲ = Collaborative;   EBN = Evidence-Based Nursing;   EB = Evidence-Based

ecchymoses, 42% had petechiae, 23% had bleeding from the gums, and 31.5% had epistaxis; 8% had two or more signs and symptoms and 73% were asymptomatic when the diagnosis was established (Garcia-Stivalet et al, 2014).

▲ Give medications orally or intravenously only; avoid giving intramuscularly, subcutaneously, or rectally.

● Apply pressure for a longer time than usual to invasive sites, such as venipuncture or injection sites. *Additional pressure is needed to stop bleeding of invasive sites in clients with bleeding disorders.*

● Take vital signs often; watch for changes associated with fluid volume loss. Excessive bleeding causes decreased blood pressure and increased pulse and respiratory rates (Ackley & Ladwig, 2014).

● Monitor menstrual flow if relevant; have the client use pads instead of tampons. **EB:** *Menstruation can be excessive in clients with bleeding disorders. Adolescents presenting with heavy menstrual bleeding at or near menarche assessment should include bleeding disorders (Rydz & Jamieson, 2013; Singh et al, 2013).*

● Have the client use a moistened toothette or a very soft child's toothbrush instead of an adult toothbrush. Follow the dentist's recommendation for flossing and appropriate rinses to use. Control gum bleeding by applying pressure to gums with gauze pad soaked in ice water. *These actions help prevent trauma to the oral mucosa, which could result in bleeding (National Institute of Dental and Craniofacial Research [NIDCR], 2015).*

● Ask the client either to not shave or to use only an electric razor. *This helps prevent any unnecessary trauma that could result in bleeding (Perry & Potter, 2014).*

▲ To decrease risk of bleeding, avoid administering salicylates or nonsteroidal antiinflammatory drugs (NSAIDs) if possible. **CEB:** *Gastrointestinal bleeding caused by NSAIDs, acetylsalicylic acid, or warfarin was the most common adverse drug reaction (ADR) that resulted in hospital admission and represented 40% of all ADRs (12 of 30), according to the World Health Organization (WHO) causality criteria (Tennant, 2015).*

Home Care

● Some of the interventions previously described may be adapted for home care use.

▲ Consider using a nurse-led patient-centered medical home (PCMH) for monitoring anticoagulant therapy. **EBN:** *Establishment of nurse-led medical homes to monitor anticoagulation therapy management clinics leads to improvements in quality of care in terms of improved control of international normalized ratio and reduced complications. Data support a conclusion that PCMHs do improve quality, access, and cost (Scudder, 2011).*

● For terminally ill clients, teach and institute all of the previously mentioned noninvasive precautions that maintain quality of life. Discuss with the client, family, and health care provider the consequences of contracting infection. Determine which precautions do not maintain quality of life and should not be used (e.g., physical assessment twice daily or multiple vital sign assessments). **CEB:** *Multiple assessments and other invasive procedures are recovery-based and cure-focused activities. The client and provider must agree on an approach to care for the clients during their remaining life (Periyakoil, Stevens, & Kraemer, 2013).*

Client/Family Teaching and Discharge Planning

Depressed Immune Function

● Teach the client and family how to take a temperature. Encourage the family to take the client's temperature between 3 and 7 p.m. at least once daily. **EBN:** *For most people, the difference between high and low values throughout the day is approximately 2°F (1.1°C) (97°F–99°F [36.1°C–37.2°C]), with the lowest value typically occurring in the early morning hours (2 a.m.–5 a.m.) and the highest values commonly occurring in the evening (Medline Plus, 2011; Fetzer, 2013).* Teach precautions to use to decrease the chance of infection (e.g., avoiding uncooked fruits and vegetables, using appropriate self-care including good hand hygiene ensuring a safe environment). Teach the client to avoid crowds and contact with persons who have infections. Teach the need for good nutrition, avoidance of stress, and adequate rest to maintain immune system function. **CEBN:** *Approaches to avoiding infection at home for the client with neutropenia include good hand hygiene and careful management of food, drink, and the client's environment (Yeung, 2014).*

Bleeding Disorder

● Teach the client to wear a medical alert bracelet and notify all health care personnel of his or her bleeding disorder. **CEB:** *Emergency identification schemes such as medical alert bracelets use emblems that alert health*

● = Independent;   ▲ = Collaborative;   **EBN** = Evidence-Based Nursing;   **EB** = Evidence-Based

care professionals to potential problems and can ensure appropriate and prompt treatment (*Medical and Scientific Advisory Council [MASAC], 2017*). Teach the client and family the signs of bleeding, precautions to take to prevent bleeding, and action to take if bleeding begins. Caution the client to avoid taking over-the-counter medications without the permission of the health care provider. *Medications containing salicylates can increase bleeding.*

- Teach the client to wear loose-fitting clothes and avoid physical activity that might cause trauma.

REFERENCES

Ackley, B., & Ladwig, G. (2014). Risk for bleeding. In *Nursing diagnosis handbook* (pp. 156–161). Maryland Height, MO: Mosby Elsevier.

ASHE. (2014) *2014 FGI Guidelines update.* American Society for Healthcare Engineering. Retrieved from www.ashe.org/education.Pdf.

Buckines, S. (2017). *Weightlifting for people over 60.* Retrieved from https://livestrong.com. (Accessed 18 October 2017).

Centers for Disease Control and Prevention (CDC). (2011a). Guideline for hand hygiene in health-care settings. Recommendations of the Healthcare Infection Control Practices Advisory Committee and the HICPAC/SHEA/APIC/IDSA Hand Hygiene Task Force. *MMWR. Recommendations and Reports, 51*(RR–16), 1–45. Retrieved from http://www.cdc.gov/handhygiene/Guidelines.html. (Accessed August 14, 2017; updated 2014).

Centers for Disease Control and Prevention (CDC). (2011b). *Guideline for the prevention of intravascular catheter related infections.* Retrieved from http://www.cdc.gov/hicpac. (Accessed September 5, 2017; updated 2014).

Curchoe, R. M. (2013). Infection prevention and control. In Potter, P. A., Perry, A. G., Stockert, P., et al. (Eds.), *Fundamentals of nursing* (8th ed.). St. Louis: Elsevier.

Dankers, W., Colin, E. M., van Hamburg, J. P., et al. (2016). Vitamin D in autoimmunity: Molecular mechanisms and therapeutic potential. *Frontiers in Immunology, 7,* 697.

EB Medicine. (2013). *Oncologic emergencies.* Retrieved from https://www.ebmedicine.net. (Accessed 17 August 2017).

Ferrara, J., MacDougall, C., & Gallagher, J. (2011). Empiric antifungal therapy in patients with febrile neutropenia. *Pharmacotherapy, 31*(4), 369–385.

Fetzer, S. J. (2013). Vital signs. In Potter, P. A., Perry, A. G., Stockert, P., et al. (Eds.), *Fundamentals of nursing* (8th ed.). St. Louis: Elsevier.

Flood, A. (2014). The immunocompromised host. In *APIC text of infection control and epidemiology* (4th ed.). Washington, DC: Association for Professionals in Infection Control and Epidemiology, Inc (APIC).

Garcia-Stivalet, L. A., Munoz-Flores, A., Montiel-Jarquin, A. J., et al. (2014). Clinical analysis of 200 cases of idiopathic thrombocytopenia purpura. *Revista Medica del Instituto Mexicano del Seguro Social, 52*(3), 322–325.

Geismar, K. (2014). Nutrition and immune function. In *APIC text of infection control and epidemiology* (4th ed.). Washington, DC: Association for Professionals in Infection Control and Epidemiology (APIC). (Accessed 1 September 2017; last revised 6 June 2014).

Gunville, C. F., Mourani, P. M., & Ginde, A. A. (2013). The role of vitamin D in prevention and treatment of infection. *Inflammation and Allergy Drug Targets, 12*(4), 239–245.

Haas, J. (2014). Hand hygiene. In *APIC text of infection control and epidemiology* (4th ed.). Washington, DC: Association for Professionals in Infection Control and Epidemiology (APIC). Last revised 6/6/14. (Accessed 4 September 2017; last revised 6 June 2014).

Harris, P. L. (2014). Solid organ transplantation. In *APIC text of infection control and epidemiology* (4th ed.). Washington, DC: Association for Professionals in Infection Control and Epidemiology (APIC). (Accessed 1 September 2017; last revised 6 June 2014).

Helder, O. K., Brug, J., vanGoudoever, J., et al. (2014). Sequential hand hygiene prevention contributes to a reduced nosocomial bloodstream infection rate among very low birth weight infants: An interrupted time series over a 10 year period. *American Journal of Infection Control, 42*(7), 718–722.

Jefferies, A. (2012). Kangaroo care for preterm infants and family. *Pediatrics Child Health, 17*(3), 141–143.

Klastersky, J., deNaurois, K., et al. (2016). Management of febrile neutropenia: ESMO clinical practice guidelines. *Annals of Oncology, 27*(Suppl. 5), V111–V118.

MASAC. (2017). *Guidelines foe emergency department management of individuals with hemophilia and other bleeding disorders.* National Hemophilia Foundation. Retrieved from https://www.hemophilia.org. (Accessed 17 September 2017).

McDowell, S. (2017). What is leukopenia. *Healthline.*

Medline Plus. (2011). *Bleeding gums.* Retrieved from http://www.nlm.nih.gov/medlineplus/ency/article/003062.htm. (Accessed 31 August 2017).

Moucha, C. (2016). *Patient warming and surgical site infections: a critical analysis of the data.* Retrieved from www.medscape.org. (Accessed 10 June 2016).

NIDCR. (2015). *Oral complications of cancer treatment.* Retrieved from https://NIDCR.nih.gov/oralhealth.

Periyakoil, V. S., Stevens, M., & Kraemer, H. (2013). Multicultural long-term care nurses' perceptions of factors influencing patient dignity at the end-of-life. *Journal of American Geriatrics Society, 61*(3), 440–446.

Perry, P., & Potter, A. (2014). *Essentials for nursing practice—E book* (p. 775). Retrieved from https://books.google.com.

Poirier, P. (2013). Nursing-led management of side effects of radiation: Evidence-based recommendations for practice. *Nursing Research and Reviews, 3,* 47–57.

Rydz, N., & Jamieson, M. A. (2013). Managing heavy menstrual bleeding in adolescents. *Contemporary OBGYN.* Retrieved from http://modernmedicine.com.

Scudder, L. (2011). *Nurse-led medical homes: current status and future plans.* Medscape Nurses.

Singh, S., Best, C., Dunn, S., et al. (2013). Abnormal uterine bleeding in pre-menopausal women. *Journal of Obstetrics and Gynaecology Canada, 35*(5), 473–475.

Sternicuk, R., Rusak, B., & Rockwood, K. (2014). Sleep disturbance in older ICU patients. *Clinical Interventions in Aging, 2014*(9), 969–977.

Sullivan, J., & Farrer, H. (2011). Fever and antipyretic use in children. *Pediatrics, 127*(3), 580–587.

Tennant, F. (2015). GI bleeding and NSAIDs. *Practical pain management.* Retrieved from https://www.practical pain management.com/patient/treatment.

Thom, K. A., Kleinberg, M., & Roghmann, M. C. (2013). Infection prevention in the cancer center. *Clinical Infectious Diseases.* Retrieved from www.cid.oxford.org/content/early/2013/06/06/cid.cit290. (Accessed 31 August 2017).

Yeung, C. (2014). Home care: infection prevention for practice settings. In *APIC text of infection control and epidemiology* (4th ed., Chapter 56). Washington, DC: Association for Professionals in Infection Control and Epidemiology (APIC).

P

● = Independent; ▲ = Collaborative; **EBN** = Evidence-Based Nursing; **EB** = Evidence-Based

Rape-Trauma syndrome   *Julianne E. Doubet, BSN, RN, EMT-B*

NANDA-I

Definition

Sustained maladaptive response to a forced, violent, sexual penetration against the victim's will and consent.

Defining Characteristics

Aggression; agitation; alteration in sleep pattern; anger; anxiety; change in relationship(s); confusion; denial; dependency; depression; disorganization; dissociative identity disorder; embarrassment; fear (00148); guilt; helplessness; history of suicide attempt; humiliation; hyperalertness; impaired decision-making; low self-esteem; mood swings; muscle spasm; muscle tension; nightmares; paranoia; phobias; physical trauma; powerlessness (00125); self-blame; sexual dysfunction; shame; shock; substance misuse; thoughts of revenge

Related Factors

To be developed

At-Risk Population

Rape

NOC   (Nursing Outcomes Classification)

Suggested NOC Outcomes

Abuse Cessation; Abuse Protection; Abuse Recovery: Emotional, Sexual, Coping; Impulse Self-Control; Self-Mutilation Restraint

Example **NOC** Outcome with Indicators
Abuse Recovery: Sexual as evidenced by the following indicators: Acknowledgment of right to disclose abusive situation/ Expression of right to have been protected from abuse. (Rate the outcome and indicators of **Abuse Recovery: Sexual:** 1 = none, 2 = limited, 3 = moderate, 4 = substantial, 5 = extensive [see Section I].)

R

Client Outcomes

Client Will (Specify Time Frame)

- Share feelings, concerns, and fears
- Recognize that the rape or attempt was not client's own fault
- State that, no matter what the situation, no one has the right to assault another
- Describe medical/legal treatment procedures and reasons for treatment
- Report absence of physical complications or pain
- Identify support resources and attend psychotherapy/group assistance in coping with the trauma and effects of the traumatic experience
- Function at same level as before crisis, including sexual functioning
- Recognize that it is normal for full recovery to take a minimum of 1 year

NIC   (Nursing Interventions Classification)

Suggested NIC Interventions

Abuse Protection Support; Counseling; Crisis Intervention; Sexual Counseling; Infection Protection; Rape-Trauma Treatment

Example **NIC** Activities—Rape-Trauma Treatment
Explain rape protocol and obtain consent to proceed through protocol; Implement crisis intervention counseling

● = Independent;   ▲ = Collaborative;   EBN = Evidence-Based Nursing;   EB = Evidence-Based

Nursing Interventions and *Rationales*

- Escort the client to a treatment room immediately on arrival to the emergency department. Stay with (or have a trusted person stay with) the client. EBN: *Victims of sexual assault require special attention from caregivers so they do not feel victimized a second time in the medical facility (Durieux, 2014).*
- Assure the client of confidentiality. EB: *According to Ogunwale and Oshiname (2017), rape is a traumatic experience, which has known physical and psychosocial destructive effects, but survivors rarely seek support to escape being stigmatized.*
- ▲ Provide a sexual assault response team (SART), if available, that includes a sexual assault nurse examiner (SANE), rape counseling advocate, and representative of law enforcement for best possible outcomes. EB: *According to a study by Patterson and Tringali (2015), a team of forensic nurses and victim advocates partner together to provide treatment not only for the necessary physical and medical requirements of sexual assault survivors, but also for dealing with the complex legal and mental health needs that necessitate follow-up.*
- Observe for signs of physical injury. CEB: *Some locations to assess for obvious genital injuries would include tears or abrasions of the posterior labia, abrasion or bruising of the labia minora and fossa navicularis, and ecchymosis or tears of the hymen; document these injuries as evidence for any future legal proceedings (Linden, 2011).*
- Document the client's chief complaint and request an event history of the sexual assault in his or her own words. EBN: *Participants felt cared for and emotionally supported when they were probed about what had happened to them (Selenga & Jooste, 2015).*
- Encourage the client to verbalize his or her feelings. EBN: *Research by Thomas, Scott Tilley, and Esquibel (2015) indicated that survivors want nonjudgmental attitudes from health care providers, acknowledgment of the violence they have suffered, and that their stories are heard and believed.*
- Make sure that the victim understands everything you are doing. EBN: *The preservation of client dignity must be maintained, not only for the victim's protection, but also to show respect and caring; respecting dignity is one of the essential behaviors that nurtures caring (Gustafsson, Wingerblad, & Lindwall, 2013).*
- Explain to the client that all or some of the client's clothing may be kept for evidential purposes and photographs may be taken (with consent) to document the client's injuries. CEB: *Assessment and treatment of victims of sexual assault, as well as the precise collection and documentation of evidence, are critical for a solid case (Fitzpatrick et al, 2012).*
- ▲ If a law enforcement interview is permitted, provide support by staying with the client at his or her request. EB: *A study authorized by the Bureau of Justice (Kruttschnitt, Kalseek, & House, 2014) surmised that we must take into consideration the frequency and environment under which rape and sexual assault are committed because this is vital information in targeting resources for law enforcement and support for victims.*
- Use the sexual assault evidence collection kits that have been reviewed by the SART members and provided by your state to collect adequate and accurate evidence for analysis by a forensic laboratory. EB: *The health care provider who examines victims of sexual assault must be responsible to act in accordance with state and local statutory or policy requirements for the use of evidence-gathering kits (American College of Obstetrics and Gynecology [ACOG], 2014).*
- ▲ Discuss the possibility of pregnancy and sexually transmitted infections (STIs) and the treatments available. EB: *Victims of sexual assault should be advised that they are at risk for pregnancy, STIs, and posttraumatic stress disorder (PTSD); as a victim of sexual assault, he or she should be monitored and offered emergency contraception and STI prophylaxis (American College of Obstetrics and Gynecology, 2014).*
- ▲ Encourage the client to report the sexual assault to a law enforcement agency. EB: *Sexual assault survivors often feel apprehensive about involvement in the criminal justice system; therefore many do not report their sexual assault to law enforcement (Patterson & Tringali, 2015).*
- ▲ For those interested in a spiritual connection, make the appropriate recommendation. EBN: *According to Hellman (2014), research should be introduced to develop theory using religious and spiritual beliefs to aid in the recovery process of sexual assault victims.*
- ▲ Stress the necessity of follow-up care with a mental health professional to recognize and intervene with problems associated with the effects of rape-trauma/sexual assault. EB: *Price et al (2014) stated that although sexual assault increases the risk for psychiatric disorders and although there is treatment available, few victims choose mental health care after their attack.*
- Stress the importance of awareness throughout the community of the scope and severity of the effects of sexual abuse as a means of additional healing empowerment. EB: *Recovery from sexual assault/rape is*

● = Independent; ▲ = Collaborative; EBN = Evidence-Based Nursing; EB = Evidence-Based

frequently hindered by the public's failure to believe the victim and the need to obtain justice (Chapleau & Oswald, 2014).

Geriatric

- Build a trusting relationship with the client. **EBN:** *A patient-centered communication style by the nurse can have positive outcomes in the patient–nurse relationship (Selenga & Jooste, 2015).*
- All examinations should be done on older adults as they would be done on any adult client after sexual assault, with modifications for comfort if necessary. **EB:** *In a study by Nobrega et al (2014) of the forensic assessment of older victims of sexual assault, the forensic evaluation was found to be essential in positive judicial outcomes and invaluable in identifying physical and biological confirmation of sexual assault.*
- Assess for mobility limitations and cognitive impairment. **EB:** *As the aging population swells, a rise in morbidity can be validated, and with it, not only an increase in chronic illnesses, but also the recognition of significant cognitive changes and physical disabilities (Kizie et al, 2014).*
- Explain and encourage the client to report sexual abuse. **EBN:** *It is of the utmost importance that the client's wishes, feelings, and beliefs are taken into consideration prior to any action being taken (Andrews, 2017).*
- Observe for psychosocial distress. **EBN:** *The elderly are often isolated and mistreated, leaving them insecure and vulnerable and without support of family and/or friends (Sena Damasceno, de Sousa, & Moura, 2016).*
- ▲ Consider arrangements for safe housing victim of abuse. **EB:** *In Dakin's (2014) study involving a diverse group of older women who were given scenarios in which the scenario subjects, because of circumstances, had the option of choosing autonomy or protection, the majority picked protection over autonomy.*

Male Rape

- ▲ **EB:** *According to Javaid (2015), there appears to be three barriers to police acknowledgement of male rape: statistics, underreporting of male rape, and "the masculine police subculture."*
- ▲ Assess to determine whether physically abused women are also victims of sexual assault. **EBN:** *According to a study by Santos de Oliveira et al (2016), there is a need for primary care professionals to focus on women who are involved in relationships in which they experience sexual violence.*

Multicultural

- ▲ Assess for the influence of cultural beliefs, norms, and values on the client's ability to cope with the trauma of the rape experience. **EBN:** *Rejection by family and community after a rape remains an enormous concern among survivors of sexual violence (Kohli et al, 2013).*

Home Care

- Some of the interventions described previously may be adapted for home care use.
- Corroborate the client's feelings of self-worth. Posttraumatic disorders were the most common consequences in women victims of violence. **EB:** *Mason and Lodrick (2013) concluded in their study, that sexual violence can have long-lasting and destructive consequences including that of PTSD.*
- Assist the client with realistically assessing the home setting for safety and/or selecting a safe environment in which to live. **CEB:** *The protection or safeguarding of vulnerable adults must be an integral part of everyday nursing practice (Straughair, 2011).*
- ▲ Ensure that the client has systems in place for long-term support. **EBN:** *When treating a victim of sexual assault, the health care provider should not only treat the survivor's physical injuries, but understand and support the emotional needs of the survivor and follow-up with them during the period of recovery (Reis, Lopes, & Osis, 2017).*
- ▲ Design a practical discharge plan to include a safe shelter if needed, follow-up care for physical injury, and follow-up referral for psychological support. **EBN:** *It is vital to abused older adults to be sheltered in a safe, protected, violence-free, and medically suitable environment (Heck & Gillespie, 2013).*
- ▲ Assess for other client vulnerabilities, such as mental health issues or addiction, and refer the client to social agencies for implementation of a therapeutic regimen. **EB:** *Those who have the dual diagnosis of addiction and mental illness are highly prone to sexual victimization, and actions should be taken to reduce their vulnerability (de Waal, Decker, & Gouariaan, 2017).*

Client/Family Teaching and Discharge Planning

- Emphasize the client's needs for safety and to decrease the opportunities for repeat attacks. Recognize the vulnerability of the client. **EBN:** *In a qualitative study by Arend et al (2013) involving survivors of sexual*

● = Independent; ▲ = Collaborative; EBN = Evidence-Based Nursing; EB = Evidence-Based

assault in South Africa, it was found that nurses have numerous opportunities to improve the quality of post–sexual assault care, which in turn advances the clients' emotional and psychosocial outcomes.

- Note: PTSD has a high probability of being a psychological sequela to rape. Research demonstrated two effective treatments for the improvement of PTSD in rape victims: prolonged exposure and stress inoculation training. Prolonged exposure involves reliving the rape experience by imagining it as vividly as possible, describing it aloud in the present tense, taping this description, and listening to the tape at least once daily. Stress inoculation training uses breathing exercises to diminish anxiety and instruction in coping skills, thought stopping, cognitive restructuring, self-dialog, and role playing. Research suggests that a combination of both treatments may provide the optimal effect. Furthermore, for those who reported the assault to police, lower levels of legal system success and satisfaction were linked to higher levels of perceived control over present recovery.

REFERENCES

American College of Obstetrics and Gynecology. (2014). Committee on health care for underserved women. *Obstetrics and Gynecology, 123,* 726–730.

Andrews, J. (2017). Abuse of older people: the responsibilities of community nurses. *British Journal of Community Nursing, 22*(5), 224–225.

Arend, E., Maw, A., deSwardt, C., et al. (2013). South African sexual assault survivors' experiences of post-exposure prophylaxis and individualized nursing care: a qualitative study. *Journal of the Association of Nurses in AIDS Care, 24,* 154–165.

Chapleau, K., & Oswald, D. (2014). A system justification view of sexual violence: legitimizing gender inequality and reduced moral outrage are connected to greater rape myth acceptance. *Journal of Trauma and Dissociation, 15,* 204–218.

Dakin, E. (2014). Protection as care: moral reasoning and moral orientation among ethnically and socioeconomically diverse older women. *The Journal of Aging Studies, 28,* 44–56.

de Waal, M., Dekker, J., & Gouariaan, A. (2017). Prevalence of victimization in patients with dual diagnosis. *Journal of Dual Diagnosis, 13*(2), 119–123.

Durieux, J. (2014). Nursing care of victims of sexual violence. *Revue de L'infirmiere, 201,* 39–41.

Fitzpatrick, M., Ta, A., Lenchus, J., et al. (2012). Sexual assault forensic examiners' training and assessment using simulation technology. *Journal of Emergency Nursing, 38,* 85–90.

Gustafsson, L., Wingerblad, A., & Lindwall, L. (2013). Respecting dignity in forensic cases: the challenge faced by nurses of maintaining patient's dignity in clinical caring situations. *Journal of Psychiatric and Mental Health Nursing, 20,* 1–8.

Heck, L., & Gillespie, G. (2013). Interprofessional program to provide emergency shelter to abused elders. *Advanced Emergency Nursing Journal, 35,* 170–181. Retrieved from http://dx.doi.org.ezproxy.jccmi.edu/10.1097/TME0b013e31828ecc06.

Hellman, A. (2014). Examining sexual assault survival of adult women: responses, mediators and current theories. *Journal of Forensic Nursing, 10,* 175–184.

Javaid, A. (2015). Police responses to, and attitudes toward male rape, issues and concerns. *International Journal of Police Science and Management, 17*(2), 81–90.

Kizie, C., daSilva Talmelli, L., Diniz, M., et al. (2014). Assessment of cognitive status and frailty of older elderly living at home. *Cienc Cuid Saude, 13,* 120–127.

Kohli, A., Tosha, M., Ramazani, P., et al. (2013). Family and community rejection and a Congolese led mediation intervention to reintegrate rejected survivors of sexual violence in Eastern Democratic Republic of Congo. *Health Care for Women International, 34*(9), 736–756.

Kruttschnitt, C., Kalsbeek, W., & House, C. (2014). *Estimating the incidence of rape and sexual assaults.* Committee on National Statistics; Division on Behavioral and Social Sciences and Education; National Research Council. Washington, DC: National Academies Press.

Linden, J. (2011). Care of the adult patient after sexual assault. *New England Journal of Medicine, 365,* 834–841.

Mason, F., & Lodrick, Z. (2013). Psychological consequences of sexual assault. *Best Practice and Research. Clinical Obstetrics and Gynaecology, 21*(1), 27–37.

Nobrega, P., Rodrigues, F., Dinis-Oliveria, R., et al. (2014). Sexual offenses against elderly people: Forensic evaluation and judicial outcome. *Journal of Elder Abuse and Neglect, 26,* 189–204.

Ogunwale, A., & Oshiname, F. (2017). Exploration of date rape survivors' physical and psycho-social experiences in a Nigerian university. *Journal of Interpersonal Violence, 32*(2), 227–248.

Patterson, D., & Tringali, B. (2015). Understanding how advocates can affect sexual assault victim engagement in the criminal justice process. *Journal of Interpersonal Violence, 30*(12), 1987–1997.

Price, M., Davidson, T., Ruggiero, K., et al. (2014). Predictors of using mental health services after sexual assault. *Journal of Trauma Stress, 27,* 331–337.

Reis, M., Lopes, M., & Osis, M. (2017). It's much worse than dying: The experience of female victims of sexual violence. *Journal of Clinical Nursing, 25*(15/16), 2353–2361.

Santos de Oliveira, P., Palmarella Rodriques, V., Laise Gomez Leite Morais, R., et al. (2016). Health professionals assistance to women in situation of sexual violence: An integrated review. *Journal of Nursing UFPE, 10*(5), 1828–1839. Retrieved from doi:10.5205/reuo l.9003-78704-1-SM.1005201632.

Selenga, M., & Jooste, K. (2015). The experience of youth victims of physical violence attending a community health center: A phenomenological study. *African Journal of Nursing and Midwifery,* (Suppl. 2015), S529–S542.

Sena Damasceno, C., deSousa, M., & Moura, M. (2016). Violence against older people registered in specialized police station for security and protection to elderly. *Journal of Nursing UFPE, 10*(3), 949–957. Retrieved from doi:10.5205/reuol.8702-76273-4-SM .1003201602.

Straughair, C. (2011). Safeguarding vulnerable adults: The role of the registered nurse. *Nursing Standard, 25,* 49–56.

Thomas, L., Scott Tilley, D., & Esquibel, K. (2015). Sexual assault: Where are mid-life women in this research. *Perspectives in Psychiatric Care, 51*(2), 86–97.

● = Independent;   ▲ = Collaborative;   EBN = Evidence-Based Nursing;   EB = Evidence-Based

Ineffective Relationship   *Gail B. Ladwig, MSN, RN*

NANDA-I

Definition

A pattern of mutual partnership that is insufficient to provide for each other's needs.

Defining Characteristics

Delay in meeting of developmental goals appropriate for family life cycle stage; dissatisfaction with complementary relationship between partners; dissatisfaction with emotional need fulfillment between partners; dissatisfaction with idea sharing between partners; dissatisfaction with information sharing between partners; dissatisfaction with physical need fulfillment between partners; inadequate understanding of partner's compromised functioning; insufficient balance in autonomy between partners; insufficient balance in collaboration between partners; insufficient mutual respect between partners; insufficient mutual support in daily activities between partners; partner not identified as support person; unsatisfying communication with partner

Related Factors

Ineffective communication skills; stressors; substance misuse; unrealistic expectations

At-Risk Population

Developmental crisis; history of domestic violence; incarceration of one partner

Associated Condition

Alteration in cognitive functioning in one partner

NOC, NIC, Client Outcomes, Nursing Interventions and *Rationales,* Client/Family Teaching and Discharge Planning, and References

Refer to care plan Readiness for enhanced **Relationship**

R

Readiness for enhanced Relationship   *Marina Martinez-Kratz, MS, RN, CNE*

NANDA-I

Definition

A pattern of mutual partnership to provide for each other's needs, which can be strengthened.

Defining Characteristics

Expresses desire to enhance autonomy between partners; expresses desire to enhance collaboration between partners; expresses desire to enhance communication between partners; expresses desire to enhance emotional need fulfillment for each partner; expresses desire to enhance mutual respect between partners; expresses desire to enhance satisfaction with complementary relationship between partners; expresses desire to enhance satisfaction with emotional need fulfillment for each partner; expresses desire to enhance satisfaction with idea sharing between partners; expresses desire to enhance satisfaction with information sharing between partners; expresses desire to enhance satisfaction with physical need fulfillment for each partner; expresses desire to enhance understanding of partner's functional deficit

NOC   (Nursing Outcomes Classification)

Suggested NOC Outcomes

Coping; Family Functioning/Integrity; Role Performance; Social Support

● = Independent;   ▲ = Collaborative;   EBN = Evidence-Based Nursing;   EB = Evidence-Based

Example NOC Outcome with Indicators
Family Integrity as evidenced by the following indicators: Members share thoughts, feelings, interests, concerns/Members communicate openly and honestly with one another/Members encourage individual autonomy and independence/Members assist one another in performing roles and daily tasks. (Rate the outcome and indicators of **Family Integrity**: I = never demonstrated, 2 = rarely demonstrated, 3 = sometimes demonstrated, 4 = often demonstrated, 5 = consistently demonstrated [see Section I].)

Client Outcomes

Family/Client Will (Specify Time Frame)

- Share thoughts and feelings with each other
- Communicate openly with each other
- Assist in performing family roles and tasks
- Provide support for each other
- Obtain appropriate assistance

NIC (Nursing Interventions Classification)

Suggested NIC Interventions

Coping Enhancement; Family Integrity Promotion; Role Enhancement

Example NIC Activities—Family Integrity Promotion
Facilitate a tone of togetherness within/among the family; Encourage family to maintain positive relationships; Facilitate open communication among family members

Nursing Interventions and *Rationales*

- Assess the ways in which the relationship has been altered (communication, sexuality, intimacy, etc.) from both partner's perspective. EB: *A recent review found that when involving both partners in marital interventions, it is necessary to assess both views of the relationship (Albuquerque, Pereira, & Narciso, 2016).*
- Assess relationship quality using the Relationship Flourishing Scale. EB: *The Relationship Flourishing Scale is a 12-item measure of eudaimonic relationship quality that assesses meaning, personal growth, relational giving, and goal sharing (Fowers et al, 2016).*
- Focus on helping couples maintain or develop marital closeness. EB: *A recent review found that marital closeness is a protective factor that may prevent relationship breakdown (Albuquerque, Pereira, & Narciso, 2016).*
- Assist couples to identify sources of their own perceived *dyadic* empathy in the relationship. EB: *Higher perceived empathy toward the relationship partner is associated with relationship satisfaction (Kimmes et al, 2014).*
- Assist families to identify sources of gratitude in their lives. EB: *Research showed that gratitude fostered all facets of posttraumatic growth, such as relationships, personal strengths, and awareness of meaningful possibilities (Ruini & Vescovelli, 2013).*
- Assist clients to identify sources of gratitude in their lives using a future-oriented focus. EB: *Research shows that clients with a regulatory focus of promotion were more likely to express gratitude, which inspired them to strengthen their relationships with helpful and responsive partners (Mathews & Shook, 2013).*
- Encourage couples to engage in reappraisal of conflict in their relationship. EB: *A study demonstrated that a reappraisal of conflict in their marriages protected participants against declines in marital quality over time (Finkel et al, 2017).*
- Encourage the use of positive relational humor and humor evaluation between partners. EB: *Relational humor, which is created and shared between partners, and humor evaluation, which is one partner's judgment of the other partner's sense of humor, were both strongly associated with relationship satisfaction in a meta-analysis (Hall, 2017).*
- Provide support resources to provide military members and their families with assistance in preparation for deployments and education about the importance of maintaining communication during deployment. EBN: *Veterans who have been deployed report that dedicated resources are needed to successfully reestablish their social connections with family and reclaim their place within the family (Messecar, 2017).*

R

● = Independent;   ▲ = Collaborative;   EBN = Evidence-Based Nursing;   EB = Evidence-Based

- Encourage couples to participate together in leisure activities like dance. EB: *This study demonstrated that a light-intensity ballroom dancing intervention improved the life of cancer survivors and the relationship with loved ones (Pisu, Demark-Wahnefried, & Kenzik, 2017).*
- Refer to care plans Readiness for enhanced **Family** processes and Readiness for enhanced family **Coping.**

Pediatric

- Encourage guidance and information on communication for parents of seriously ill children. EBN: *The findings of this study suggested that parents are an important focus of care, and enhancing couples' communication is a way to address changes in marital relationships (Silva-Rodrigues et al, 2016).*

Geriatric

- Assess geriatric spousal caregivers for positive and negative consequences of providing medical care. EB: *A recent study found that more medical/nursing tasks were linked to greater caregiving gains. Spouses who assist with more medical/nursing tasks feel they are directly benefiting their partner, which further enhances perceptions of gains and promotes positive feelings among spousal caregivers (Polenick et al, 2017).*
- Assess sexuality needs and support consensual sexual expression. EB: *Older adult participants in an Australian study made suggestions related to the visibility and normalization of sex in later life, cultural representations of sex and older people, and the need to provide sex-positive aged care and retirement home facilities (Fileborn et al, 2017).*
- Facilitate and increase opportunities for social connectedness for older individuals through the use of technology training. EBN: *A recent study demonstrated that computer training at a senior citizens club helped participants build group cohesion and to form tiered connections with partners, family, and friends with whom they no longer live (Burmeister et al, 2016).*

Multicultural

- Provide a relationship-focused intervention to enhance communication for multicultural couples. EB: *A Korean study found that a relationship-focused communication intervention improved couples' abilities to communicate effectively and to resolve conflicts, and it enhanced intimacy (Kim et al, 2016).*
- Use culturally tailored cognitive behavioral techniques to promote communication, problem-solving, self-disclosure, empathic response skills, and sexual education and counseling. EB: A review of 39 studies found that interventions to promote communication, problem-solving, self-disclosure, empathic responses, and sexual education could enhance marital intimacy and strengthen family bonds and stability. Health care providers need to individualize interventions that are appropriate to the couple characteristics and their relationship (Kardan-Souraki et al, 2016).

R

REFERENCES

Albuquerque, S., Pereira, M., & Narciso, I. (2016). Couple's relationship after the death of a child: A systematic review. *Journal of Child and Family Studies, 25*(1), 30–53. doi:10.1007/s10826-015-0219-2.

Burmeister, O. K., et al. (2016). Enhancing connectedness through peer training for community-dwelling older people: A person centred approach. *Issues in Mental Health Nursing, 37*(6), 406–411. doi:10.3109/01612840.2016.1142623.

Fileborn, B., et al. (2017). Improving the sexual lives of older Australians: Perspectives from a qualitative study. *Australasian Journal of Ageing, 36*, E36–E42. doi:10.1111/ajag.12405.

Finkel, E. J., et al. (2017). A brief intervention to promote conflict reappraisal preserves marital quality over time. *Psychological Science, 24*(8), 1595–1601. doi:10.1177/0956797612474938.

Fowers, B. J., et al. (2016). Enhancing relationship quality measurement: The development of the Relationship Flourishing Scale. *Journal of Family Psychology, 30*(8), 997–1007. doi:10.1037/fam0000263.

Hall, J. A. (2017). Humor in romantic relationships: A meta-analysis. *Personal Relationships, 24*(2), 306–322. doi:10.1111/pere.12183.

Kardan-Souraki, M., et al. (2016). A review of marital intimacy-enhancing interventions among married individuals. *Global Journal of Health Science, 8*(8), 74–93. doi:10.5539/gjhs.v8n8p74.

Kim, G., et al. (2016). Relationship-focused intervention to enhance marriage communication for multicultural couples. *Korean Family Relations Journal, 21*(2), 97–127. doi:10.21321/jfr.21.2.97.

Kimmes, J. G., Edwards, A. B., Wetchler, J. L., et al. (2014). Self and other ratings of dyadic empathy as predictors of relationship satisfaction. *American Journal of Family Therapy, 42*(5), 426–437.

Mathews, M. A., & Shook, N. J. (2013). Promoting or preventing thanks: Regulatory focus and its effect on gratitude and indebtedness. *Journal of Research in Personality, 47*, 191–195.

Messecar, D. C. (2017). Finding their way back in: Family reintegration following guard deployment. *Military Medicine, 182*(S1), 266–273. doi:10.7205/MILMED-D-16-00109.

Pisu, M., Demark-Wahnefried, W., & Kenzik, K. M. (2017). A dance intervention for cancer survivors and their partners (RHYTHM). *Journal of Cancer Survivorship, 11*(3), 350. doi:10.2196/resprot.6489.

Polenick, C. A., et al. (2017). In sickness and in health: Spousal caregivers and the correlates of caregiver outcomes. *The American Journal of Geriatric Psychiatry, 25*(10), 1094–1096. doi:10.1016/j.jagp.2017.05.001.

● = Independent;   ▲ = Collaborative;   EBN = Evidence-Based Nursing;   EB = Evidence-Based

Ruini, C., & Vescovelli, F. (2013). The role of gratitude in breast cancer: Its relationships with post-traumatic growth, psychological well-being and distress. *Journal of Happiness Studies, 14,* 263–274.

Silva-Rodrigues, F. M., et al. (2016). Childhood cancer: Impact on parents' marital dynamics. *European Journal of Oncology Nursing, 23,* 34–42. doi:10.1016/j.ejon.2016.03.002.

Risk for ineffective Relationship   *Gail B. Ladwig, MSN, RN*

NANDA-I

Definition

Susceptible to developing a pattern that is insufficient for providing a mutual partnership to provide for each other's needs.

Risk Factors

Ineffective communications skills; stressors; substance misuse; unrealistic expectations

At-Risk Population

Developmental crisis; history of domestic violence; incarceration of one partner

Associated Condition

Alteration in cognitive functioning in one partner

NOC, NIC, Client Outcomes, Nursing Interventions and *Rationales,* and References

Refer to care plan for Ineffective **Relationship**

Impaired Religiosity   *Barbara Baele Vincensi, PhD, RN, FNP*

NANDA-I

Definition

Impaired ability to exercise reliance on beliefs and/or participate in rituals of a particular faith tradition.

Defining Characteristics

Desire to reconnect with previous belief pattern; desire to reconnect with previous customs; difficulty adhering to prescribed religious beliefs; difficulty adhering to prescribed religious rituals; distress about separation from faith community; questioning of religious belief patterns; questioning of religious customs

Related Factors

Anxiety; cultural barrier to practicing religion; depression; environmental barrier to practicing religion; fear of death; ineffective caregiving; ineffective coping strategies; insecurity; insufficient social support; insufficient sociocultural interaction; insufficient transportation; pain; spiritual distress

At-Risk Population

Aging; end-stage life crisis; history of religious manipulation; hospitalization; life transition; personal crisis; spiritual crisis

Associated Condition

Illness

NOC   (Nursing Outcomes Classification)

Suggested NOC Outcomes

Client Satisfaction: Cultural Needs Fulfillment

● = Independent;   ▲ = Collaborative;   EBN = Evidence-Based Nursing;   EB = Evidence-Based

---

Example NOC Outcome with Indicators

Client Satisfaction: Cultural Needs Fulfillment as evidenced by the following indicators: Respect for religious beliefs/Respect for cultural health behaviors/Incorporation of cultural beliefs in health teaching/Respect for personal values. (Rate each indicator of **Client Satisfaction: Cultural Needs Fulfillment:** 1 = not at all satisfied, 2 = somewhat satisfied, 3 = moderately satisfied, 4 = very satisfied, 5 = completely satisfied [see Section I].)

Client Outcomes

Client Will (Specify Time Frame)

- Express satisfaction with the ability to express religious practices
- Express satisfaction with access to religious materials and rituals
- Demonstrate balance between religious practices and healthy lifestyles
- Avoid high-risk, controlling religious relationships that inflict physical, sexual, or emotional harm and/or exploitation

NIC   (Nursing Interventions Classification)

Suggested NIC Interventions

Religious Ritual Enhancement; Culture Brokerage; Religious Addiction Prevention

Example NIC Activities–Religious Ritual Enhancement

Encourage the use of and participation in usual religious rituals that are not detrimental to health

Nursing Interventions and *Rationales*

- Recognize when clients integrate religious practices in their life. **EB:** *In a prospective study, of 110 patients pre-, during, and post chemotherapy, Kaliampos and Roussi (2017) found that use of religious coping significantly predicted a positive affect 7 months later.* **EB:** *In a mixed-methods study, those who were homeless (N = 500) and had difficulty with alcohol and substance abuse but participated in religious ceremonies or rituals were found to have better outcomes related to the quantity of abuse (Torchalla et al, 2014).*
- Encourage and/or coordinate the use of and participation in usual religious rituals or practices that support coping. **EBN:** *In a cross-sectional descriptive study (Akgül & Karadag, 2016) fecal ostomies were found to be a barrier to incorporating specific religious practices of salat, fasting, and pilgrimage in the lives of 150 Muslims postoperatively, providing an opportunity for nurses to assist patients in meeting their religious needs through adaptation or facilitation around this barrier.* **EB:** *In a secondary analysis, Ellison et al (2014) discovered that the introduction of prayer was helpful in shaping positive mental health in those who had a nonanxious and comfortable relationship with God; however, this did always have the same outcome for those who did not have a similar relationship with God or the Transcendent when using prayer in a similar manner.*
- Encourage the use of prayer or meditation as appropriate. **EB:** *In a cross-sectional cohort study of 132 participants, Watkins et al (2013) identified that encouraging religious practices, such as prayer and meditation, improved specific self-care activities in hard to control type II diabetics.* **EBN:** *In a qualitative study by Woods-Giscombé and Gaylord (2015) with 15 African American participants who had mindfulness meditation experience, the results indicated that mindfulness meditation was helpful in managing stress but it also had several concepts in common with African American religious concepts, suggesting this type of meditation could be used within a religious framework with this population.*
- Promote family coping using religious practices to help cope with loss, as appropriate. **EBN:** *In a longitudinal qualitative study by Nilmanat et al (2015) of 15 Thai patients dying of cancer, three themes emerged to help cope with the dying process: surrounded by love from family, moving beyond suffering, and reconnecting to religious faith to counter suffering.*
- ▲ Refer to a religious leader, professional counseling, or support group as needed. **EB:** *A cross-sectional survey by Ghesquiere et al (2015) of 591 hospices in the United States, found complicated grief or depression related to death can be assessed and managed by most hospices in varying degrees with the use of transdisciplinary teams, support groups, individual counseling, or group therapy.* **EBN:** *In a descriptive study by Brelsford et al (2016) of 52 neonatal intensive care unit (NICU) parents, family cohesiveness decreased with the use of negative religious and spiritual coping, providing an indicator to nurses of a need for potential referral or support.*

● = Independent;   ▲ = Collaborative;   EBN = Evidence-Based Nursing;   EB = Evidence-Based

Geriatric

- Promote established religious practices in older adults. EB: *In a systematic review by Agli, Bailly, and Ferrand (2015), the effects of encouraging spiritual and religious practices on older adults with dementia were increased positive coping strategies, increased cognitive function, and increased quality of life.* EBN: *Using a pre-post control group with 66 older patients admitted to an ICU, Elham et al (2015) found a significant inverse relationship between groups regarding spiritual well-being (SWB) and anxiety when patient concerns were met after an adequate assessment of spiritual/religious needs was completed and interventions implemented.*

 Multicultural

- Promote religious practices that are culturally appropriate:
  - **African American.** EB: *Salas-Wright et al (2015) found an inverse relationship between religious involvement and violent and nonviolent antisocial behaviors in adolescent African American females residing in high-risk communities.* EB: *In a cross-sectional survey of 1013 African American women, Ludema et al (2015) found that those who highly identified with organized religion, nonorganized religion, and spirituality had less risky sexual behaviors for potential HIV exposure than those who had no affiliation.* EBN: *In a qualitative study by Woods-Giscombé and Gaylord (2015) with 15 African American participants who had mindfulness meditation experience, the results indicated that mindfulness meditation was helpful in managing stress. They also found several concepts that mindfulness meditation had in common with African American religious concepts, suggesting meditation could be used within a religious framework with this population for health concerns.*
  - **Korean.** EB: *A focused ethnographic research approach by Choi et al (2014) of middle and older aged Korean women identified that immigration experiences tended to be difficult; engaging in religion, prayer, and church community were found to be important supports for these women.*
  - **African.** EBN: *In a qualitative study of 10 participants addressing the challenges and resources of living with multiple sclerosis (MS) in the Western Cape area of Africa, Pretorius and Joubert (2014) found religion as one of the major themes for resources along with social support, mobility aids, and knowledge/education.*
  - **Jordanian.** EBN: *Using a cross-sectional and correlational design, Musa, Pevalin, and Shahin (2016) found that spiritual well-being and religiosity had a positive correlation with self-rated health in a convenience sample of 340 Jordanian Arab Christians who make up only 3% of the population of this country.*
  - **Hispanic.** EB: *With diabetes having a high prevalence in the Hispanic population, Riveria-Hernandez (2016) found a positive relationship between religiosity with diabetes care and blood sugar control in a sample of 2216 Hispanics 50 years and older living in Mexico.*
  - **Sexual Minority Individuals (Lesbian, Gay, Bisexual, Transgender, Queer).** EB: *Brewster et al (2016) found religious coping strategies may or may not promote psychological well-being or relieve psychological symptoms of distress caused by internalization of specific thoughts and experiences in a sample of self-identified sexual minority participants (N = 143), in which sexual discrimination and harassment had occurred within and outside of the religious/church establishment. Therefore promotion of religious coping or practices for this minority should be approached carefully.*

REFERENCES

Agli, O., Bailly, N., & Ferrand, C. (2015). Spirituality and religion in older adults with dementia: A systematic review. *International Psychogeriatrics, 27*(5), 715–725. doi:10.1017/S1041610214001665.

Akgül, B., & Karadag, A. (2016). The effect of colostomy and ileostomy on acts of worship in the islamic faith. *Journal of Wound, Ostomy, and Continence Nursing, 43*(4), 392–397. doi:10.1097/WON.0000000000000237.

Brelsford, B., Ramirez, J., Veneman, K., et al. (2016). Religious and secular coping and family relationships in the neonatal intensive care unit. *Advances in Neonatal Care, 16*(4), 315–322. doi:10.1097/ANC.0000000000000263.

Brewster, M., Velez, B., Foster, A., et al. (2016). Minority stress and the moderating role of religious coping among religious and spiritual sexual minority individuals. *Journal of Counseling Psychology, 63*(1), 119–126. doi:10.1037/cou0000121.

Choi, J., Kushner, K. E., Mill, J., et al. (2014). The experience of Korean immigrant women adjusting to Canadian society. *Journal of Cross-cultural Gerontology, 29*(3), 277–297. doi:10.1007/s10823-014-9235-8.

Elham, H., Hazrati, M., Momennasab, M., et al. (2015). The effect of need-based spiritual/religious intervention on spiritual well-being and anxiety of elderly people. *Holistic Nursing Practice, 29*(3), 136–143. doi:10.1097/HNP.0000000000000083.

Ellison, C., Bradshaw, M., Flannelly, K., et al. (2014). Prayer, attachment to God, and symptoms of anxiety-related disorders among U.S. adults. *Sociology of Religion, 75*(2), 208–233. doi:10.1093/socrel/srt079.

● = Independent;   ▲ = Collaborative;   EBN = Evidence-Based Nursing;   EB = Evidence-Based

Ghesquiere, A., Aldridge, M., Johnson-Hurzeler, R., et al. (2015). Hospice services for complicated grief and depression: Results from a national survey. *Journal of the American Geriatric Society*, 63(10), 2173–2180.

Kaliampos, A., & Roussi, P. (2017). Religious beliefs, coping, and psychological well-being among Greek cancer patients. *Journal of Health Psychology*, 22(6), 754–764. doi:10.1177/13591053156114995.

Ludema, C., Doherty, I., White, B., et al. (2015). Religiosity, spirituality, and HIV risk behaviors among African American women from four rural counties in the Southeastern U.S. *Journal of Health Care for the Poor and Underserved*, 26(1), 168–181. doi:10.1353/hpu .2015.0005.

Musa, A., Pevalin, D., & Shahin, F. (2016). Impact of spiritual well-being, spiritual perspective, and religiosity on the self-rated health of Jordanian Arab Christians. *Journal of Transcultural Nursing*, 27(6), 550–557. doi:10.1177/1043659615587590.

Nilmanat, K., Promnoi, C., Phungrassami, T., et al. (2015). The experiences of Thai persons with advanced cancer. *Cancer Nursing*, 38(3), 224–231. doi:10.1097/NCC.0000000000000169.

Pretorius, C., & Joubert, N. (2014). The experiences of individuals with Multiple Sclerosis in the Western Cape, South Africa. *Health South Africa Gesondheid*, 19(1), 1–12. doi:10.4102/hsag.v19i1.756.

Riveria-Hernandez, M. (2016). Religiosity, social support and care associated with health in older Mexicans with diabetes. *Journal of Religion and Health*, 55, 1394–1410. doi:10.1007/s10943-015 -0150-7.

Salas-Wright, C., Tirmazi, T., Lombe, M., et al. (2015). Religiosity and antisocial behavior: Evidence from young African American women in public housing communities. *Social Work Research*, 39(2), 82–93. doi:10.1093/swr/svv010.

Torchalla, I., Li, K., Strehlau, V., et al. (2014). Religious participation and substance use behaviors in a Canadian sample of homeless people. *Community Mental Health Journal*, 50, 862–869. doi:10.1007/s10597-014-9705-z.

Watkins, Y., Quinn, L., Ruggeiero, L., et al. (2013). Spiritualt and religious beliefs and practices and social support's relationship to ciabetes self-care activities in African Americans. *The Diabetes Educator*, 39(2), 231–239. doi:10.1177/0145721713475843.

Woods-Giscombé, C., & Gaylord, S. (2015). The cultural relevance of mindfulness meditation as a health intervention for African Americans: Implications for reducing stress-related health disparities. *Journal of Holistic Nursing*, 32(3), 147–160. doi:10.1177/ 0898010113519010.

Readiness for enhanced Religiosity

Lisa Burkhart, PhD, RN, ANEF and Barbara Baele Vincensi, PhD, RN, FNP

NANDA-I

Definition

A pattern of reliance on religious beliefs and/or participation in rituals of a particular faith tradition, which can be strengthened.

Defining Characteristics

Expresses desire to enhance belief patterns used in the past; expresses desire to enhance connection with a religious leader; expresses desire to enhance forgiveness; expresses desire to enhance participation in religious experiences; expresses desire to enhance participation in religious practices (e.g., ceremonies, regulations, clothing, prayer, services, holiday observances); expresses desire to enhance religious customs used in the past; expresses desire to enhance religious options; expresses desire to enhance use of religious material

NIC, NOC, Client Outcomes, Nursing Interventions and *Rationales,* Client/Family and Discharge Planning, and References

See care plan for Impaired **Religiosity.**

Pediatric

- Provide spiritual care for children based on developmental level. Theory: When nurses are comfortable providing spiritual care, they can implement numerous spiritual care activities and interventions to meet the spiritual needs of the child and family. After determining the child's spiritual beliefs and spiritual needs, a plan of care is developed based on the child's developmental age (Fowler, 1981, 1987; Elkins & Cavendish, 2004).
  - ○ **Parents:** Incorporate religious traditions and faith practices for parents with hospitalized and chronically ill children. **EB:** *A qualitative study indicated that religion was a positive coping mechanism for parents with infants in the neonatal intensive care unit (NICU) (Huenink & Porterfield, 2017).* **EBN:** *In a quantitative descriptive study, parents of children with cancer demonstrated an increase in spiritual faith (Wiener et al, 2016).*
  - ○ **School-age:** Encourage faith community involvement and religious attendance with parent(s). **EB:** *In a review of literature, studies consistently indicated that school-aged children who attend church with*

● = Independent;   ▲ = Collaborative;   EBN = Evidence-Based Nursing;   EB = Evidence-Based

their parents demonstrated higher psychological well-being and greater spiritual closeness with parents in adolescence (Mahoney & Cano, 2014).

○ **School Age:** Encourage children to participate in faith community health programs. EBN: *An ethnographic study indicated that faith communities provide a forum for healthy nutrition as part of the faith culture (Opalinski, Dyess, & Gropper, 2017).* EB: *A participatory action research study of African American churches in developing Focus on Youth programs indicated the importance of integrating faith and health to prevent disease and promote health (Lightfoot et al, 2014).*

○ **Adolescents:** Encourage religious coping in the adolescent population EBN: *Qualitative research indicates urban African American youth have multifaceted dimensions of their spirituality, including the role of prayer in their lives, an unwavering faith in a higher power, and the importance of giving back to their communities (Dill, 2017).* EB: *Access to religious resources may be a powerful factor that helps protect teens from turning to alcohol, marijuana, and cigarettes to cope with harsh parenting and poor self-control (Kim-Spoon et al, 2014).*

○ **Adolescents:** Encourage prayer, particularly within the African American community. EB: *In a qualitative study, prayer was a positive coping mechanism and supported an intrinsic motivation for positive change (Breland-Noble et al, 2015).*

○ **Adults:** Encourage centering prayer or other forms of mediation to promote mental and spiritual health. EB: *In a small sample, centering prayer demonstrated positive effects on emotional and spiritual health (Fox et al, 2016).*

○ **Interprofessional:** Chaplain referral when individuals engage in religious coping mechanisms. EB: When individuals engage in religious coping, additional religious struggles follow, which may benefit from chaplain expertise to promote spiritual well-being (Fox et al, 2016). EB: *In a grounded theory study of hospitalized patients, patients look for a relationship with the chaplain, and the role of the chaplain in helping patients to discover and express meaning in their experiences to promote spiritual wellness (McCormick & Hildebrand, 2015).*

○ **African American:** Collaborate with faith communities to promote wellness. EB: *In a qualitative participatory action study with church leaders, findings indicated medical distrust and self-management and suggested incorporating a religious orientation to rebuild trust within the African American community (Lew et al, 2015).* EB: *A program to decrease HIV stigma was developed with African American faith communities incorporating sermons and HIV testing (Derose et al, 2014).* EB: *A participatory action research study of African American churches in developing Focus on Youth programs indicated the importance of integrating faith and health to prevent disease and promote health (Lightfoot et al, 2014).*

○ **African American:** Incorporate faith traditions in coping with chronic disease. EBN: *In an ethnographic study of African American parents of children with autism, faith in God was a positive theme and can support culturally congruent health care (Burkett et al, 2017).*

○ **Latino:** Collaborate with faith communities to promote wellness. EB: *A program to decrease HIV stigma was developed with Latino faith communities incorporating sermons and HIV testing (Derose et al, 2014).*

○ **Latino:** Incorporate faith traditions among patients and families in pediatric settings. EBN: *In an ethonursing study with Latino families and health care providers to develop a culturally competent model of care on a medical-surgical unit, findings indicated that five care factors as most valuable: family, faith, communication, care integration, and meeting basic needs (Mixer et al, 2015).*

○ **Uninsured/low income:** Explore faith community nurses to provide wellness services and care monitoring. EB: *Faith Community Nursing is a nursing specialty focusing on integration of faith and health while providing wellness care within faith communities (Morris, 2015; Young et al, 2015).*

○ **Geriatrics:** *Encourage listening to religious music.* EB: *In a national quantitative study, frequency of listening to religious music was associated with decreases in death anxiety and increases in life satisfaction, self-esteem, and sense of control (Bradshaw et al, 2015).*

R

REFERENCES

Bradshaw, M., Ellison, C. G., Fang, Q., et al. (2015). Listening to religious music and mental health in later life. *The Gerontologist*, 55(6), 961–971. doi:10.1093/geront/gnu020.

Breland-Noble, A. M., Wong, M. J., Childers, T., et al. (2015). Spirituality and religious coping in African-American youth with depressive illness. *Mental Health, Religion & Culture, 18*(5), 330–341. doi:10.1080/13674676.2015.1056120.

Burkett, K., Morris, E., Anthony, J., et al. (2017). Parenting African American children with autism: The influence of respect and faith in mother, father, single-, and two-parent care. *Journal of Transcultural Nursing, 28*(5), 496–504.

Derose, K. P., Bogart, L. M., Kanouse, D. E., et al. (2014). An intervention to reduce HIV-related stigma in partnership with African-American and Latino churches. *AIDS Education & Prevention, 26*(1), 28–42.

● = Independent;   ▲ = Collaborative;   EBN = Evidence-Based Nursing;   EB = Evidence-Based

Dill, L. J. (2017). "Wearing my spiritual Jacket": The role of spirituality as a coping mechanism among African American youth. *Health Education & Behavior, 44*(5), 696–704. doi:10.1177/1090198117729398.

Elkins, M., & Cavendish, R. (2004). Developing a plan for pediatric spiritual care. *Holistic Nursing Practice, 18*(4), 179–184.

Fowler, J. (1981). *Stages of faith: The psychology of human development and quest for meaning.* San Francisco: Harper & Row.

Fowler, J. (1987). *Faith development and pastoral care.* Philadelphia: Fortress Press.

Fox, J., Gutierrez, D., Haas, J., et al. (2016). Centering prayer's effects on psycho-spiritual outcomes: A pilot outcome study. *Mental Health, Religion & Culture, 19*(4), 379–392. doi:10.1080/13674676.2016.1203299.

Huenink, E., & Porterfield, S. (2017). Parent Support Programs and coping mechanisms in NICU parents. *Advances in Neonatal Care, 17*(2), E10–E18. doi:10.1097/ANC.0000000000000359.

Kim-Spoon, J., Farley, J. P., Holmes, C. J., et al. (2014). Does adolescents' religiousness moderate links between harsh parenting and adolescent substance use? *Journal of Family Psychology, 28,* 739–748. doi:10.1037/a0037178.

Lew, K. N., Arbauh, N., Banach, P., et al. (2015). Diabetes: Christian worldview, medical distrust and self-management. *Journal of Religion and Health, 54,* 1157–1172.

Lightfoot, A. F., Taggart, T., Woods-Jaeger, B. A., et al. (2014). Where is the faith? Using a CBPR approach to propose adaptations to an evidence-based HIV prevention intervention for adolescents in African American faith settings. *Journal of Religion and Health, 53,* 1223–1235. doi:10.1007/s10943-014-9846-y.

Mahoney, A., & Cano, A. (2014). Introduction to the special section on religion and spirituality in family life: Pathways between relational spirituality, family relationships and personal well-being. *Journal of Family Psychology, 28*(6), 735–738. doi:10.1037/fam0000041.

McCormick, S., & Hildebrand, A. A. (2015). A qualitative study of patient and family perceptions of chaplain presence during post-trauma care. *Journal of Health Care Chaplaincy, 21*(2), 60–75. doi:10.1080/08854726.2015.1016317.

Mixer, S. J., Carson, E., McArthur, P. M., et al. (2015). Nurses in action: A response to cultural care challenges in a pediatric acute care setting. *Journal of Pediatric Nursing, 30*(6), 896–907. doi:10.1016/j.pedn.2015.05.001.

Morris, S. (2015). Holistic health care for the medically uninsured: The church health center of memphis. *Ethnicity & Disease, 25*(4), 507–510.

Opalinski, A. S., Dyess, S. M., & Gropper, S. S. (2017). Food culture of faith communities and potential impact on childhood obesity. *Public Health Nursing, 34*(5), 437–443.

Wiener, L., Viola, A., Kearney, J., et al. Lone Parent Study Group. (2016). Impact of caregiving for a child with cancer on parental health behaviors, relationship quality, and spiritual faith: Do lone parents fare worse? *Journal of Pediatric Oncology Nursing, 33*(5), 378–386. doi:10.1177/1043454215616610.

Young, S., Patterson, L., Wolff, M., et al. (2015). Empowerment, leadership, and sustainability in a faith-based partnership to improve health. *Journal of Religion and Health, 54,* 2086–2098. doi:10.1007/s10943-014-9911-6.

Risk for impaired Religiosity   *Gail B. Ladwig, MSN, RN*

NANDA-I

R

Definition

Susceptible to an impaired ability to exercise reliance on religious beliefs and/or participate in rituals of a particular faith tradition, which may compromise health.

Risk Factors

Insufficient transportation; pain; anxiety; depression; fear of death; ineffective caregiving; ineffective coping strategies; insecurity; insufficient social support; cultural barrier to practicing religion; environmental barrier to practicing religion; insufficient sociocultural interaction; spiritual distress

At-Risk Population

Aging; end-stage life crisis; life transition; history of religious manipulation; hospitalization; personal crisis; spiritual crisis

Associated Condition

Illness

NOC, NIC, Client Outcomes, Nursing Interventions and *Rationales,* and References

Refer to care plan for Impaired **Religiosity**

● = Independent;   ▲ = Collaborative;   EBN = Evidence-Based Nursing;   EB = Evidence-Based

Relocation stress syndrome
Mary Beth Flynn Makic, PhD, RN, CCNS, FAAN, FNAP, Rebecca Johnson, PhD, RN, FAAN, FNAP, and Jessica Bibbo, MA

NANDA-I

Definition

Physiological and/or psychosocial disturbance following transfer from one environment to another.

Defining Characteristics

Alienation; aloneness; alteration in sleep pattern; anger; anxiety (00146); concern about relocation; dependency; depression; fear (00148); frustration; increase in illness; increase in physical symptoms; increase in verbalization of needs; insecurity; loneliness; loss of identity; loss of self-worth; low self-esteem; pessimism; preoccupation; unwillingness to move; withdrawal

Related Factors

Ineffective coping strategies; insufficient predeparture counseling; insufficient support system; language barrier; move from one environment to another; powerlessness; significant environmental change; social isolation; unpredictability of experience

At-Risk Population

History of loss

Associated Condition

Compromised health status; deficient mental competence; impaired psychosocial functioning

NOC (Nursing Outcomes Classification)

Suggested NOC Outcomes

Relocation Adaptation; Anxiety Self-Control; Child Adaptation to Hospitalization; Coping; Depression Level; Depression Self-Control; Loneliness Severity; Psychosocial Adjustment: Life Change, Quality of Life; Stress Level

R

Example NOC Outcome with Indicators

Relocation Adaptation as evidenced by the following indicators: Recognizes reason for change in living environment/ Participates in decision-making in new environment/Expresses satisfaction with daily routine/Expresses satisfaction with level of independence/Compares care needs with available resources/Expresses satisfaction with social relationships/Expresses satisfaction with variety of food/Expresses satisfaction with food preparation/Expresses satisfaction with retained personal belongings/Expresses satisfaction with living arrangements/Exhibits positive mood/Appears content/Respects others' rights/Maintains positive relationships with family/Maintains positive relationships with friends/Maintains positive relationships with others in new environment/ Participates in social activities/Seeks information to reduce anxiety/Plans coping strategies for stressful situations/Uses effective coping strategies/Uses relaxation techniques to reduce anxiety/Maintains social relationships/Maintains adequate sleep/Controls anxiety response. (Rate the outcome and indicators of **Relocation Adaptation:** 1 = never demonstrated, 2 = rarely demonstrated, 3 = sometimes demonstrated, 4 = often demonstrated, 5 = consistently demonstrated [see Section I].)

Client Outcomes

Client Will (Specify Time Frame)

- Recognize and know the name of at least one staff member or new neighbor within 1 week of relocating
- Express concern about move when encouraged to do so during individual contacts within 24 hours of awareness of impending relocation
- Perform activities of daily living (ADLs) in usual manner
- Maintain previous mental and physical health status (e.g., nutrition, elimination, sleep, social interaction, physical activity) within 2 months of relocating

• = Independent;   ▲ = Collaborative;   EBN = Evidence-Based Nursing;   EB = Evidence-Based

| NIC | (Nursing Interventions Classification) |

Suggested NIC Interventions

Anxiety Reduction; Coping Enhancement; Discharge Planning; Hope Instillation; Self-Responsibility Facilitation; Animal-Assisted Therapy; Art Therapy; Music Therapy; Massage; Mood Management; Active Listening

Example NIC Activities—Anxiety Reduction

Stay with client to promote safety and reduce fear; Provide objects that symbolize safeness to the client

Nursing Interventions and *Rationales*

- Be aware that relocation to retirement communities may be a positive change. EBN: *A cross-sectional study of older individuals relocating to retirement communities found the older individual experienced less stress when they had more relocation controllability, positive cognitions, and adjustment resources (Bekhet & Zauszniewski, 2013).*
- Begin relocation planning as early in the decision process as possible. EBN: *Having a well-organized plan for the move with support and advocacy through the process may reduce anxiety (Sörensen, Mak, & Pinquart, 2011).*
- Obtain a history, including the reason for the move, the client's usual coping mechanisms, history of losses, and family support for the client. EBN: *A history helps the nurse determine the amount of support needed and appropriate interventions to decrease relocation stress (Brownie, Horstmanshof, & Garbutt, 2014).*
- Identify to what extent the client can participate in the relocation decisions and advocate for this participation. EBN: *Engaging older adults in the decision-making process is likely to increase the level of adjustment after the relocation (Bekhet & Zauszniewski, 2013) and promote psychological well-being (Street & Burge, 2012; Ewen & Chahal, 2013; Hertz et al, 2016).* EB: *A study of highly dependent older adults who were relocated were found to have a higher use of new antidepressant agents and new antibiotics orders, suggesting the need for vigilant planning to reduce the stress of the move (Mello & O'Connor, 2016).*
- Assess client's readiness to relocate and relocation self-efficacy. EB: *Relocation is a complex process that requires careful consideration and planning before the move (prelocation) and adjustment to the new home after the move (postrelocation) to promote the older client's adjustment (Hertz et al, 2016).*
- Consult an evidence-based practice guide for relocation. EBN: *Researchers compiled the latest findings to develop a protocol to assist in relocating older adults (Hertz et al, 2016).*
- Assess family members' perceptions of client's ability to participate in relocation decisions. Particularly in cases of dementia, be alert to care workers' involvement in making the decision to relocate. They may need support and encouragement through the process. CEB: *Care workers were found to be highly stressed during the relocation decision-making process and "walking a tightrope" between the older adult's needs and those of the person's family members (Hortana, Fahlstrom, & Ahlstrom, 2010).*
- Consider the cultural and ethnic values of the client and family as much as possible when choosing roommates, foods, and other aspects of care. EBN: *Nurses need to be aware of the differences in values and practices of different cultures and ensure that they give culturally appropriate care that is respectful of older adults and family caregivers' beliefs about elder care (Bekhet & Zauszniewski, 2013).*
- Promote clear communication between all participants in the relocation process. EB: *A narrative study exploring older client's transitions found communication and exploring unspoken fears helped reduce concerns of loss of control and uncertainty (Lee, Simpson, & Froggatt, 2013).*
- Observe the following procedures if the client is being transferred to an extended care facility or assisted living facility:
  - Facilitate the client's participation in decisions and choice of placement, and arrange a preadmission visit if possible.
  - If the client cannot visit the new facility, arrange for a visit or telephone call by a member of the staff to welcome the client and show a videotape or at least provide pictures of the new care facility.
  - Have a familiar person accompany the client to the new facility. This lessens client and family anxiety, confusion, and dissatisfaction.
  - Recommend that the caregiver write a journal of thoughts and feelings regarding the relocation of his or her loved one.

● = Independent;   ▲ = Collaborative;   EBN = Evidence-Based Nursing;   EB = Evidence-Based

○ Continue to assess caregiver psychological distress during a 6-month period after relocation. Caregivers experience distress because of the responsibility of moving their loved one. **EB:** *Caregivers may begin to resolve conflicted feelings during this time and need support (Smit et al, 2011).*

- Identify previous routines for ADLs. Try to maintain as much continuity with the previous schedule as possible. **EB:** *Continuity of client's everyday personal care by care aides that is both empathetic and nurturing is perceived as supportive and compassionate and eases relocation stress (Andersen & Spiers, 2016).*
- Bring in familiar items from home (e.g., pictures, clocks, afghans). Familiarity eases transition and symbolizes safeness.
- Establish the way the client would like to be addressed (Mr., Mrs., Miss, first name, or nickname). *Calling clients by their desired name shows respect.*
- Thoroughly orient the client and the family to the new environment and routines; repeat directions as needed. **EB:** *Providing honest answers to client questions and supporting the individual adjustment to the new location will be necessary for at least 6 months until the client feels at home (Hertz et al, 2016).*
- Spend one-to-one time with the client. Allow the client to express feelings and convey acceptance of them; emphasize that the client's feelings are real and individual and that it is acceptable to be sad or angry about moving. **EB:** *Interventions should recognize personal values; allow adequate time to listen to and respect the views and needs of the older adult (Hertz et al, 2016).*
- Allocate a caring staff member to help the client adjust to the move. Assign the same staff members to the client for care if compatible with client; maintain consistency in the personnel with whom the client interacts.
- Ask the client to state one positive aspect of the new living situation each day. Helping the client focus on the positive aspects of the move can help change attitude and reframe the situation in a positive fashion. **EBN:** *Assisting the client to focus on positive thinking has been found to promote their ability to manage daily activities and adapt to change. Clients with greater resourcefulness have been found to be able to adapt to challenging situations in a more constructive and successful manner (Bekhet & Zauszniewski, 2013).*
- Ask the client to state one positive aspect of the new living situation each day. *Helping the client focus on the positive aspects of the move can help change attitude and reframe the situation in a positive fashion (Bekhet & Zauszniewski, 2013; Hertz et al, 2016).*
- Monitor the client's health status and provide appropriate interventions for problems with social interaction, nutrition, sleep, new onset of infection, or elimination problems. **EB:** *Older clients and lower socioeconomic status are associated with greater risk of maladjustment after relocation (Hertz et al, 2016). A study found a significant increase in morbidity before and after transfer. Residents who transferred had increased rates of illness and greater antibiotic and antidepressant medication prescription rates in the months before and after relocation (Mello & O'Connor, 2016).*
- If the client is being transferred within a facility, have staff members from the new unit visit the client before transfer.
- Work with the caregivers and family members helping them deal with stages of "making the best of it," "making the move," and "making it better." **EBN:** *Provide opportunities for family to visit, encourage engagement in facility social events, and provide electronic access for the client to maintain ties with loved ones and friends (Hertz et al, 2016).*
- If a client is being transferred from the intensive care unit (ICU), have previous staff make occasional visits until the client is comfortable in the new surroundings. Ensure that the family is told relevant information. **EB:** *Providing an individualized transfer plan from the ICU to the medical-surgical unit that addresses patient and family questions prior to transfer reduces relocation stress (Lee et al, 2017).*
- Watch for coping problems (e.g., withdrawal, regression, angry behavior, impaired sleeping, refusal to eat, flat affect, anxiety) and intervene immediately. **EB:** *Loss of independence with transfer to a nursing home may manifest in anxiety, anger, and depression (Bekhet & Zauszniewski, 2013).*
- Encourage the client to express grief for the loss of the old situation; explain that it is normal to feel sadness over change and loss.
- Assess the client's psychological needs along with physiological needs. **EB:** *Although physical care may predicate the relocation, meeting psychosocial care needs must be individualized via careful assessment (Hertz et al, 2016).*
- Encourage the client to participate in care as much as possible and make his or her own decisions when possible (e.g., placement of the bed, choice of roommate, bathing routines). *Having choices helps prevent feelings of powerlessness that may lead to depression (Hertz et al, 2016).*

R

● = Independent;   ▲ = Collaborative;   EBN = Evidence-Based Nursing;   EB = Evidence-Based

Pediatric

- Assess family history and contact information from children relocated to rescue shelters. EB: *Efforts have been made to develop systematic processes to reunite children that are separated from families during disasters. Current guidelines established by the Federal Emergency Management Agency (FEMA), the Red Cross, the Centers for Disease Control and Prevention (CDC), and the National Center for Missing and Exploited Children focus on providing effective, efficient action through:*
  ○ *A shared understanding of local and national resources and capabilities,*
  ○ *Collaboration, coordination, effective communication for children with disabilities and other access and functional needs, and needs assessments during disasters, and*
  ○ *Shared operational procedures and technologies (FEMA, 2013).*
- Be aware that community relocation may be beneficial for children and assess community resources of new location.
- Provide support for a child and family who must relocate to be near a transplant center.
- In divorce situations, recommend alternative dispute resolution versus traditional litigated settlement. EBN: *This non-adversarial approach may mitigate some of the trauma of divorce experienced by children (Stein & Oler, 2010).*
- Assess presence of allergies before and after relocation.
- If the client is an adolescent, try to avoid a move in the middle of the school year, find a newcomers' club for the adolescent to join, and refer for counseling if needed. EB: *Most adolescents who relocate suffer a brief period of loss of companionship and intimacy with close friends (McBride, 2015).*
- Assess adolescents' perceptions of their acceptance by peers. EB: *Poor perceptions of peer acceptance have been related to less initiation of social interactions in new settings (McBride, 2015).*
- Help parents recognize that relocation stress syndrome may persist for prolonged periods (e.g., 2 years) in adolescents. EB: *Adolescents were found to commonly express their ideology of the relocation (Nuttman-Shwartz, Huss, & Altman, 2010).*
- Be aware that young people may cope with the transition by exerting control in particular domains. EBN: *Adolescents may be at risk of developing eating disorders after a major transition (Berge et al, 2012).*
- The effects of frequent relocation may not manifest immediately and may have long-term effects on physical and mental health. EBN: *Longitudinal analysis found that frequent relocation in adolescence was associated with higher rates of stress and physical exhaustion in adulthood (Lin, Twisk, & Huang, 2012).*

 Geriatric

- Monitor the need for transfer and transfer only when necessary. EB: *Older adults often experience loss of function after relocation (Bekhet & Zauszniewski, 2013; Lee, Simpson, & Froggatt, 2013).*
- Implement discharge planning early and engage the older adult in decisions about relocation decisions. EB: *Engaging the older adult in decision-making is key to successful relocation (Hertz et al, 2016).*
- Use technologies, such as sensing devices, to measure average in-home gait speed (AIGS) as a predictor of fall risk. EBN: *AIGS was found to be a more reliable and valid predictor of fall risk than traditional physical performance assessments (Stone et al, 2015).*
- Implement a registered nurse (RN) care coordination model to restore older adults' health, maintain their independence, and reduce care costs. EBN: *RN care coordination was found to significantly and positively affect older adult outcome variables and to result in lesser costs of care (Rantz et al, 2014).*
- After the transfer, determine the client's mental status. Document and observe for any new onset of confusion. Confusion can follow relocation because of the overwhelming stress and sensory overload.
- Facilitate visits from companion animals. EB: *Pet therapy has been found to improve depressive symptoms and cognitive function in residents of long-term care facilities with mental illness (Moretti et al, 2011).*

 Client/Family Teaching and Discharge Planning

- Teach family members and remind direct care staff about relocation stress syndrome. Encourage them to monitor for signs of the syndrome.
- Help significant others learn how to support the client in the move by setting up a schedule of visits, arranging for holidays, bringing familiar items from home, and establishing a system for contact when the client needs support. EBN: *Social support of family and friends was significantly related to relocation adjustment (Hertz et al, 2016).*

● = Independent;   ▲ = Collaborative;   EBN = Evidence-Based Nursing;   EB = Evidence-Based

- Assist family members and the relocating older adult to use Internet/webcam technology for interaction to supplement in-person visits. EB: *When older adults in a care facility have less than one visitor per week, interaction can be supplemented with technological "visits" (Meyer, Marx, & Ball-Seiter, 2011; Hertz, 2016).*

REFERENCES

Andersen, E. A., & Spiers, J. (2016). Care Aides' relational practices and caring contributions. *Journal of Gerontological Nursing, 42*(11), 24–30.

Bekhet, A. K., & Zauszniewski, J. A. (2013). Resourcefulness, positive cognitions, relocation controllability and relocation adjustment among older people: A cross-sectional study of cultural differences. *International Journal of Older People Nursing, 8*(3), 244–252.

Berge, J. M., Loth, K., Hanson, C., et al. (2012). Family life cycle transitions and the onset of eating disorders: A retrospective grounded theory approach. *Journal of Clinical Nursing, 21*, 1355–1363.

Brownie, S., Horstmanshof, L., & Garbutt, R. (2014). Factors that impact residents' transition and psychological adjustment to long-term aged care: A systematic literature review. *International Journal of Nursing Studies, 51*(12), 1654–1666.

Ewen, H. H., & Chahal, J. (2013). Influence of late life stressors on the decisions of older women to relocate into congregate senior housing. *Journal of Housing for the Elderly, 27*(4), 392–408.

FEMA (2013) *Post-Disaster Reunification of Children: A Nationwide Approach.* Retrieved from https://rems.ed.gov/docs/24post-disaster-reunification-of-children-a-nationwide-approach.pdf. (Accessed 10 March 2018).

Hertz, J. E., Koren, M. E., Rossetti, J., et al. (2016). Evidence-Based Practice Guideline: Management of relocation in cognitively intact older adults. *Journal of Gerontological Nursing, 42*(11), 14–23.

Hortana, B., Fahlstrom, G., & Ahlstrom, G. (2010). Experiences of relocation in dementia care workers. *International Journal of Older People Nursing, 6*(2), 93–101.

Lee, S., Oh, H., Suh, Y., et al. (2017). A tailored relocation stress intervention programme for family caregivers of patients transferred from a surgical intensive care unit to a general ward. *Journal of Clinical Nursing, 26*(5–6), 784–794. doi:10.1111/jocn.13568.

Lee, V. S. P., Simpson, J., & Froggatt, K. (2013). A narrative exploration of older people's transitions into residential care. *Aging & Mental Health, 17*(1), 48–56.

Lin, K. C., Twisk, J. W. R., & Huang, H. C. (2012). Longitudinal impact of frequent geographic relocation from adolescence to adulthood

on psychological stress and vital exhaustion at ages 32 and 42 years: The Amsterdam growth and health longitudinal study. *Journal of Epidemiology, 22*(5), 469–476.

McBride, M. E. (2015). Beyond butterflies: Generalized anxiety disorder in adolescents. *The Nurse Practitioner, 40*(3), 29–36.

Mello, S., & O'Connor, K. A. (2016). Morbidity and mortality following relocation of highly dependent long-term care residents: A retrospective analytical study. *Journal of Gerontological Nursing, 42*(11), 34–38.

Meyer, D., Marx, T., & Ball-Seiter, V. (2011). Social isolation and telecommunication in the nursing home: A pilot study. *Gerontechnology, 10*(1), 51–58.

Moretti, F., De Ronchi, D., Bernabei, V., et al. (2011). Pet therapy in elderly patients with mental illness. *Psychogeriatrics., 11*(2), 125–129. doi:10.1111/j.1479-8301.2010.00329.x.

Nuttman-Shwartz, O., Huss, E., & Altman, A. (2010). The experience of forced relocation as expressed in children's drawings. *Clinical Social Work Journal, 38*, 397–407.

Rantz, M., et al. (2014). The continued success of registered nurse care coordination in a state evaluation of aging in place in senior housing. *Nursing Outlook, 62*(4), 237–246.

Smit, D., et al. (2011). The long-term effect of group living homes versus regular nursing homes for people with dementia on psychological distress of informal caregivers. *Ageing and Mental Health, 15*(5), 557–561.

Sörensen, S., Mak, W., & Pinquart, M. (2011). Planning and decision making for care transitions. *Annual Review of Gerontology and Geriatrics, 31*(1), 142–173.

Stein, S., & Oler, C. (2010). Emotional and legal considerations in divorce and relocation: A call for alternative dispute resolution. *Journal of Individual Psychology, 66*(3), 290–301.

Stone, E., Skubic, M., Rantz, M., et al. (2015). Average in-home gait speed: Investigation of a new metric for mobility and fall risk assessment of elders. *Gait and Posture, 41*(1), 57–62.

Street, D., & Burge, S. W. (2012). Residential context, social relationships, and subjective well-being in assisted living. *Research on Aging, 34*(3), 1–30.

R

Risk for Relocation stress syndrome *Marina Martinez-Kratz, MS, RN, CNE*

NANDA-I

Definition

Susceptible to physiological and/or psychosocial disturbance following transfer from one environment to another, which may compromise health.

Risk Factors

Ineffective coping strategies; insufficient predeparture counseling; insufficient support system; language barrier; move from one environment to another; powerlessness; significant environmental change; social isolation; unpredictability of experience

At-Risk Population

History of loss

● = Independent;   ▲ = Collaborative;   EBN = Evidence-Based Nursing;   EB = Evidence-Based

Associated Condition

Compromised health status; deficient mental competence; impaired psychosocial functioning

NIC, NOC, Client Outcomes, Nursing Interventions and *Rationales,* Client/Family Teaching and Discharge Planning, and References

Refer to care plan for **Relocation** stress syndrome.

Impaired Resilience   *Gail B. Ladwig, MSN, RN and Julianne E. Doubet, BSN, RN, EMT-B*

NANDA-I

Definition

Decreased ability to recover from perceived adverse or changing situations, through a dynamic process of adaptation.

Defining Characteristics

Decreased interest in academic activities; decreased interest in vocational activities; depression; guilt; impaired health status; ineffective coping strategies; ineffective integration; ineffective sense control; low self-esteem; renewed elevation of distress; shame; social isolation

Related Factors

Community violence; disruption in family rituals; disruption in family roles; disturbance in family dynamics; dysfunctional family processes; inadequate resources; inconsistent parenting; ineffective family adaptation; insufficient impulse control; insufficient resources; insufficient social support; multiple coexisting adverse situations; perceived vulnerability; substance misuse

At-Risk Population

Chronicity of existing crisis; demographics that increase chance of maladjustment; economically disadvantaged; ethnic minority status; exposure to violence; female gender; large family size; low intellectual ability; low maternal educational level; new crisis; parental mental illness

R

Associated Condition

Psychological disorder

NOC   (Nursing Outcomes Classification)

Suggested NOC Outcomes

Personal Resiliency; Coping; Decision-Making; Self-Esteem

Example NOC Outcome with Indicators

Personal Resiliency as evidenced by the following indicators: Adapts to adversities as challenges. (Rate the outcome and indicators of **Personal Resiliency:** 1 = never demonstrated, 2 = rarely demonstrated, 3 = sometimes demonstrated, 4 = often demonstrated, 5 = consistently demonstrated [see Section I].)

Client Outcomes

Client Will (Specify Time Frame)

- Demonstrate reduced or cessation of drug and alcohol usage
- State effective life events on feelings about self
- Seek help when necessary
- Verbalize or demonstrate cessation of abuse
- Adapt to unexpected crises or challenges
- Verbalize positive outlook on illness, family, situation, and life

• = Independent;   ▲ = Collaborative;   EBN = Evidence-Based Nursing;   EB = Evidence-Based

- Use available resources to meet coping needs
- Identify role models
- Identify available assets and resources
- Be able to verbalize meaning of one's life

NIC (Nursing Interventions Classification)

Suggested NIC Interventions

Resiliency Promotion; Coping Enhancement; Counseling; Emotional Support; Self-Esteem Enhancement; Support Group; Support System Enhancement

Example NIC Activities—Resiliency Promotion

Encourage positive health-seeking behaviors; Facilitate family communication

Nursing Interventions and *Rationales*

- Encourage positive, health-seeking behaviors. **EB:** *Johansson et al (2016) concluded in their study of diabetic health, that caregivers should establish an atmosphere of open learning that generates interactions, in a climate that establishes and encourages contemplation to promote health and well-being.*
- Ensure access to biological, psychological, and spiritual resources. **EBN:** *Identifying and linking persons to available resources will foster engagement in resources that enhance protective factors and resilience (Tuck & Anderson, 2014).*
- Foster communication skills through basic communication skill training. **CEB:** *Individuals who are skilled communicators have fewer problems with family relationships and can articulate their own viewpoint (Szanton & Gill, 2010).*
- Foster cognitive skills in decision-making. **EB:** *Patient's comprehension of pertinent information is an essential part of the standard that allows for informed decisions (Gerstenecker et al, 2015).*
- Assist client in cognitive restructuring of negative thought processes. **EBN:** *Positive thinking has been associated with increased feelings of coherence and resourcefulness when dealing with adversity (Everly et al, 2014).*
- Facilitate supportive family environments and communication. **EBN:** *Individuals found to be resilient if raised in families with greater levels of parental supervision and consistent expectations, rules, and consequences for problem behaviors, and effective systems for monitoring children and adolescents (Schofield, Conger, & Neppl, 2014).*
- Promote engagement in positive social activities. **EB:** *In their study of persons with learning disabilities, Howarth et al (2016) ascertained that taking part in various social activities provided a key opportunity for individuals to expand their social connections.*
- Assist client to identify strengths, and reinforce these. **EB:** *According to McMahon, Kenyon, and Carter (2013), in their study of American Indian youth, interventions that promoted their strengths, as opposed to their problems, showed increased promise in combating stress.*
- Help the client identify positive emotions during adverse situations**. EB:** *Even though positive emotions may be the transitory, their benefits stockpile and intensify to forecast resilience and anticipate thriving mental well-being (Ruthig, Trisko, & Chipperfield, 2013).*
- Build on supportive counseling and therapy. **EBN:** *Education and counseling are important interventions in patient care, but patients can also gain a feeling of well-being and control using their own inner strengths and methods of coping (Sandruddin et al, 2017).*
- Identify protective factors such as assets and resources to enhance coping. **CEB:** *According to the protective factor model of resilience, a protective factor that interacts with a stressor reduces the likelihood of negative outcomes (Vahia et al, 2011).*
- Provide positive reinforcement and emotional support during the learning process. **EB:** *Clients with positive, supportive educational environments show self-efficacy in attaining goals during adverse situations (Masten, 2014).*
- Encourage mindfulness, a conscious attention, and awareness of self. **EBN:** *Key elements that promote the alleviation of stress and encourage resilience are mindfulness and meditation (Savel & Munro, 2017).*
- Educate and encourage the use of stress-reduction techniques, such as guided imagery, in which the client focuses on positive images and emotions. **EB:** *Negative thoughts influence both emotions and behaviors. Positive imagery has been shown to reduce subjective feelings of stress (Park et al, 2013).*

● = Independent; ▲ = Collaborative; **EBN** = Evidence-Based Nursing; **EB** = Evidence-Based

- Enhance knowledge and use of self-care strategies. **EB:** *Promoting stress reduction and enhancing self-care has been shown to positively affect quality of life (Bryant & Nickerson, 2014).*
- Assist the client to have an optimistic world view. **EBN:** *Stagman-Tyrer (2014), in her study of the importance of optimism in nurse leaders, found that optimism can be initiated, cultivated, and achieved with enterprise and determination.*

 Pediatric

- The preceding interventions may be adapted for the pediatric client.
- Promote nurturing, supportive relationships with family. **EB:** *According to the National Scientific Council on the Developing Child (2015), "Supportive relationships with adults help children develop resilience, or the set of skills needed to respond to adversity and thrive."*
- Support the seeking of opportunities to improve cognitive abilities, such as tutoring and other resources; the development of positive and supportive relations, such as family, community members, or mentors; and the improvement of general health. **CEB:** *These activities help encourage the promotion of protective factors of adolescent resilience such as positive coping and positive self-esteem (Lau & van Niekerk, 2011).*
- Promote the development of positive mentor relationships. **EB:** *DeWit et al (2016) found in their study of supported mentoring that girls and boys involved in long-term, supported mentoring connections, experienced beneficial outcomes.*
- ▲ Consider referral to appropriate community resources, such as faith-based communities for children who have had adverse childhood experiences. *There is a critical need to identify cost-effective community resources that optimize stress resilience. Faith-based communities may promote forgiveness rather than retaliation, opportunities for cathartic emotional release, and social support, all of which have been related to neurobiology, behavior, and health outcomes. Although spirituality and religion can be related to guilt, neurotic, and psychotic disorders, they also can be powerful sources of hope, meaning, peace, comfort, and forgiveness for the self and others (Brewer-Smyth & Koenig, 2014).*

REFERENCES

Brewer-Smyth, K., & Koenig, H. G. (2014). Could spirituality and religion promote stress resilience in survivors of childhood trauma? *Issues in Mental Health Nursing, 35*(4), 251–256.

Bryant, R. A., & Nickerson, A. (2014). Acute intervention. In L. A. Zollner & N. C. Feeny (Eds.), *Facilitating resilience and recovery following trauma.* New York: Guilford Press.

Everly, G. S., McCabe, L., Sermon, N., et al. (2014). The development of a model of psychological first aid for non-mental health trained public health personnel: The Johns Hopkins RAPID-PFA. *Journal of Public Health Management and Practice, 20*(5), S24–S29.

DeWit, D., DuBois, D., Erdem, G., et al. (2016). The role of program-supported mentoring relationships in promoting youth mental health, behavioral and developmental outcomes. *Prevention Science, 17*(5), 646–657.

Gerstenecker, A., Meneses, K., Duff, K., et al. (2015). Cognitive predictors of understanding treatment decisions in patients with newly diagnosed brain metastasis. *Cancer, 121*(12), 2013–2019.

Howarth, S., Morris, D., Newlin, M., et al. (2016). Health and social care interventions which promote social participation for adults with learning disabilities: A review. *British Journal of Learning Disabilities, 44*(1), 3–15.

Johansson, K., Osterberg, S., Leskell, J., et al. (2016). Patients' experience of support for learning to live with diabetes to promote health and well-being: A lifeworld phenomenological study. *International Journal of Qualitative Studies on Health and Well-Being, 11*, 1–10. Retrieved from http://dx.doi.org/10.3402/ghw.v11.31330.

Lau, U., & van Niekerk, A. (2011). Restoring the self: An exploration of young burn survivors' narratives of resilience. *Qualitative Health Research, 21*(9), 1165–1181.

Masten, A. (2014). *Ordinary magic: Resilience in development.* New York: Guilford Press.

McMahon, T., Kenyon, D., & Carter, J. (2013). My culture, my family, my school, me: Identifying strengths and challenges in the lives and communities of American Indian youths. *Journal of Child & Family Studies, 22*(5), 694–706.

National Scientific Council on the Developing Child (2015). *Supportive relationships and active skill-building strengthen the foundations of resilience. Working Paper No. 13.* Retrieved from www.developingchild.harvard.edu.

Park, E. R., Traeger, L., Vranceanu, A., et al. (2013). The development of a patient-centered program based on the relaxation response: The Relaxation Response Resiliency Program (3RP). *Psychosomatics, 54*(2), 165–174.

Ruthig, J., Trisko, J., & Chipperfeld, J. (2013). Shifting positivity ratios: Emotions and psychological health in later life. *Aging & Mental Health, 18*(5), 547–553.

Sandruddin, S., Rafat, J., Jabber, A., et al. (2017). Patient education and mind diversion in supportive care. *British Journal of Nursing, 26*(10), 514–519.

Savel, R., & Munro, C. (2017). Quiet the mind: Mindfulness, meditation, and search for inner peace. *American Journal of Critical Care, 26*(6), 433–436. Retrieved from http://dx.doi.org/10.4037/ajcc2017914.

Stagman-Tyrer, D. (2014). Resiliency and the nurse leader: The importance of equanimity, optimism, and perseverance. *Nursing Management, 46*(6), 46–50. Retrieved from http://dx.doi.org/10.1097/01.NUMA.0000449763.99370.7f.

Schofield, T. J., Conger, R. D., & Neppl, T. K. (2014). Positive parenting, beliefs about parental efficacy, and active coping: Three sources of intergenerational resilience. *Journal of Family Psychology.* Retrieved from http://dx.doi.org/10.1037/fam000002.

● = Independent;   ▲ = Collaborative;   **EBN** = Evidence-Based Nursing;   **EB** = Evidence-Based

Szanton, S. L., & Gill, J. M. (2010). Facilitating resilience using a society-to-cells framework: A theory of nursing essentials applied to research and practice. *Advances in Nursing Science, 33*(4), 329–343.

Tuck, I., & Anderson, L. (2014). Forgiveness, flourishing, and resilience: The influences of expressions of spirituality on mental health recovery. *Issues in Mental Health Nursing, 35*(4), 277–282.

Vahia, I. V., Chattillion, E., Kavirajan, H., et al. (2011). Psychological protective factors across the lifespan: Implications for psychiatry. *Psychiatric Clinics of North America, 34*(1), 231–248.

Readiness for enhanced Resilience
Gail B. Ladwig, MSN, RN and Julianne E. Doubet, BSN, RN, EMT-B

NANDA-I

Definition

A pattern of ability to recover from perceived adverse or changing situations, through a dynamic process of adaption, which can be strengthened.

Defining Characteristics

Expresses desire to enhance available resources; expresses desire to enhance communication skills; expresses desire to enhance environmental safety; expresses desire to enhance goal-setting; expresses desire to enhance involvement in activities; expresses desire to enhance own responsibility for action; expresses desire to enhance positive outlook; expresses desire to enhance progress toward goal; expresses desire to enhance relationships with others; expresses desire to enhance resilience; expresses desire to enhance self-esteem; expresses desire to enhance sense of control; expresses desire to enhance support system; expresses desire to enhance use of conflict management strategies; expresses desire to enhance use of coping skills; expresses desire to enhance use of resource

NOC   (Nursing Outcomes Classification)

Suggested NOC Outcomes

Personal Resiliency; Family Resiliency; Quality of Life

Example NOC Outcome with Indicators
Personal Resiliency as evidenced by the following indicator: Adapts to adversities and challenges. (Rate the outcome and indicators of **Personal Resiliency:** 1 = never demonstrated, 2 = rarely demonstrated, 3 = sometimes demonstrated, 4 = often demonstrated, 5 = consistently demonstrated [see Section I].)

Client Outcomes

Client Will (Specify Time Frame)

- Adapt to adversities and challenges
- Communicate clearly and appropriately for age
- Take responsibility for own actions
- Make progress towards goals
- Use effective coping strategies
- Express emotions

NIC   (Nursing Interventions Classification)

Suggested NIC Interventions

Resiliency Promotion; Self-Efficacy Enhancement; Counseling; Emotional Support

Example NIC Activities—Self-Efficacy Enhancement
Explore individual's perception of his or her capability to perform the desired behavior

● = Independent;   ▲ = Collaborative;   EBN = Evidence-Based Nursing;   EB = Evidence-Based

Nursing Interventions and *Rationales*

- Listen to and encourage expressions of feelings and beliefs. **EBN:** *Communication assists individuals and families resolve conflicts and facilitate potential for growth, identify inherent strengths, and problem-solve effectively (Doherty & Thompson, 2014).*
- Establish a therapeutic relationship based on trust and respect. **EBN:** *Schwind et al (2014), in their study of how best to advance nursing students toward person-centered care (PCC), found that PCC is based on the principles of respect, autonomy, and empowerment and necessitates the establishment of interpersonal relationships.*
- Assist client in rating current level of resilience. **EBN:** *Although there are many excellent theories that can be used to measure resilience, it remains a complex task that involves "person-level perspectives, individual resources, processes of adaptation, and emotional well-being" (Rosenberg, Starks, & Jones, 2014).*
- Facilitate supportive family environments and communication. **EBN:** *Individuals were found to be resilient if raised in families with greater levels of parental supervision and consistent expectations, rules, and consequences for problem behaviors, and effective systems for monitoring children and adolescents (Schofield, Conger, & Neppl, 2014).*
- Assist client to identify and reinforce strengths. **EB:** *Fostering the use of protective factors promotes the ability of an individual to overcome adverse situations (Poteat, Scheer, & Mereish, 2014).*
- Enhance skills associated with social and executive functioning. **EB:** *Research has shown that social and self-regulation skills enhance one's ability to respond sensitively and are associated with better school adjustment, increased competence, and life success (Masten, 2014).*
- Provide positive reinforcement and emotional support during implementation of care. **EB:** *Providing positive reinforcement and emotional support will enhance a client's self-esteem, which is a key component of physical and mental health; individuals with higher self-esteem are more likely to be resilient than peers with less self-esteem (Masten, 2014).*
- ▲ Facilitate the development of mentorship and volunteer opportunities. **EB:** *Mentoring programs have been shown to prevent negative outcomes and foster a sense of social and community engagement for clients across the life span (Klinedinst & Resnick, 2014).*
- Determine how family behavior affects the client. **EB:** *Resilience models are based on the presupposition that individuals and families are connected to each other and their community and have collective strengths, which help them compensate for their adversity (Masten, 2014).*
- Promote use of mindfulness and other stress-reduction techniques. **EB:** *In their study of the use of mindfulness-based stress reduction (MBSR) in Parkinson's disease, McClean et al (2017) noted that the use of MBSR as an intervention has increased and improved outcomes in a mix of long-term conditions, including stress and depression.*
- Establish individual/family/community goals. **EBN:** *Individuals, families, and communities that set goals will focus on attaining or achieving positive outcomes despite adversity (Masten, 2014).*

 ### Pediatric

- The preceding interventions may be adapted for the pediatric client.
- Encourage the promotion of protective factors by fostering the seeking of opportunities to improve cognitive abilities, such as tutoring and other resources; the development of positive and supportive relations such as family, community members, or mentors; and the improvement of general health. **EB:** *According to Lehrer et al (2017), adolescents who experience positive emotions and receive social support will develop an increased sense of well-being.*

 ### Multicultural

- Use teaching strategies that are culturally and age appropriate. **EBN:** *In their study of nurses' cultural competency, Norton and Marks-Maran (2014) found that the nurses must frame education and skills training into a culturally appropriate design, if they are to be of any value to the recipients.*

REFERENCES

Doherty, M., & Thompson, H. (2014). Enhancing person-centered care through the development of the therapeutic relationship. *British Journal of Community Nursing, 19*(10), 502–507.

Klinedinst, N. J., & Resnick, B. (2014). Resilience and volunteering: A critical step to maintaining function among older adults with depressive symptoms and mild cognitive impairment. *Topics in Geriatric Rehabilitation, 30*(3), 181–187.

Lehrer, M., Janus, K., Gloria, C., et al. (2017). Personal and environmental resources mediate the positivity-emotional dysfunction relationship. *American Journal of Health Behavior, 41*(2), 186–193.

● = Independent;   ▲ = Collaborative;   EBN = Evidence-Based Nursing;   EB = Evidence-Based

R

Masten, A. (2014). *Ordinary magic: Resilience in development.* New York: Guilford Press.

McClean, G., Lawrence, M., Simpson, R., et al. (2017). Mindfulness-based stress reduction in Parkinson's disease: A systematic review. *BMC Neurology, 17,* 1–7.

Norton, D., & Marks-Maran, D. (2014). Developing cultural sensitivity and awareness in nursing overseas. *Nursing Standard, 28*(44), 39–43. Retrieved from http://dx.doi.org/10.7748/ns.28.44.39.e8417.

Poteat, V. P., Scheer, J. R., & Mereish, E. H. (2014). Factors affecting academic achievement among sexual minority and gender-variant youth. *Advances in Child Development and Behavior, 47,* 261–300.

Rosenberg, A., Starks, S., & Jones, B. (2014). The complexities of measuring resilience among parents of children with cancer. *Supportive Care in Cancer, 22*(10), 2661–2668.

Schofield, T. J., Conger, R. D., & Neppl, T. K. (2014). Positive parenting, beliefs about parental efficacy, and active coping: Three sources of intergenerational resilience. *Journal of Family Psychology.* Retrieved from http://dx.doi.org/10.1037/fam000002.

Schwind, J., Beanlands, H., Lapum, J., et al. (2014). Fostering person-centered care among nursing students: Creative pedagogical approaches to developing personal knowing. *Journal of Nursing Education, 53*(6), 343–347.

Risk for impaired Resilience   *Gail B. Ladwig, MSN, RN and Julianne E. Doubet, BSN, RN, EMT-B*

NANDA-I

Definition

Susceptible to decreased ability to recover from perceived adverse or changing situations, through a dynamic process of adaptation, which may compromise health.

Risk Factors

Community violence; disruption in family rituals; disruption in family roles; disturbance in family dynamics; dysfunctional family processes; inadequate resources; inconsistent parenting; ineffective family adaptation; insufficient impulse control; insufficient resources; insufficient social support; multiple coexisting adverse situations; perceived vulnerability; substance misuse

At-Risk Population

Chronicity of existing crisis; demographics that increase chance of maladjustment; economically disadvantaged; ethnic minority status; exposure to violence; female gender; large family size; low intellectual ability; low maternal educational level; new crisis; parental mental illness

Associated Condition

Psychological disorder

R

NOC   (Nursing Outcomes Classification)

Suggested NOC Outcomes

Personal Resiliency; Family Resiliency; Knowledge: Health Resources

> **Example NOC Outcome with Indicators**
>
> **Personal Resiliency** as evidenced by the following indicator: Takes responsibility for own actions. (Rate the outcome and indicators of **Personal Resiliency:** 1 = never demonstrated, 2 = rarely demonstrated, 3 = sometimes demonstrated, 4 = often demonstrated, 5 = consistently demonstrated [see Section I].)

Client Outcomes

Client Will (Specify Time Frame)

- Identify available community resources
- Propose practical, constructive solutions for disputes
- Identify and access community resources for assistance
- Accept assistance with activities of daily living from family and friends
- Verbalize an enhanced sense of control
- Verbalize meaningfulness of one's life

● = Independent;   ▲ = Collaborative;   EBN = Evidence-Based Nursing;   EB = Evidence-Based

| NIC | (Nursing Interventions Classification) |

Suggested NIC Interventions

Resiliency Promotion; Assertiveness Training; Values Clarification; Parenting Promotion

Example NIC Activities—Resiliency Promotion

Encourage family involvement with child's schoolwork and activities; Assist family in providing atmosphere conducive to learning

Nursing Interventions and *Rationales*

- Determine how family behavior affects client. **EBN:** *The model of resilience is based on the presupposition that individuals and families are connected to each other and their community and have collective strengths, which will help them compensate for their adversity (Deist & Greeff, 2015).*
- Help identify personal rights, responsibilities, and conflicting norms. **EBN:** *All nurses have a responsibility to actively promote both mental and physical health and well-being for their clients, so stated Patrick and Robertson (2016) in their study of men's health.*
- Encourage consideration of values underlying choices and consequences of the choice. **EBN:** *It was found in a study by Finderup et al (2016) that acceptance of responsibility must take place before one can make lifestyle choices and/or feel satisfaction for these choices.*
- Help client practice conversational and social skills. **EBN:** *Children who are found to have poor speech, language, and communications skills require prompt intervention and support because these skills are crucial to other areas of childhood development (Crichton, 2013).*
- Assist client to prioritize values. **EBN:** *Evidence-based practice merges cutting-edge research with clinical proficiency and patient values to implement objective interventions for favorable patient outcomes and improvement in quality of life (Butcher, 2016).*
- Help to create an accepting, nonjudgmental atmosphere. **EB:** *The results of a study by Usaite and Cameron (2015) found that active participation in pleasurable, but structured pastimes, can enrich the lives of children and their families by promoting "a positive sense of self, constructive relationships, roles, routines and responsibilities."*
- Help identify self-defeating thoughts. **EBN:** *Cognitive reframing is a tool that assists individuals in reflecting and shifting negative thinking toward positive perspectives (Resnick, 2014).*
- ▲ Refer to community resources/social services as appropriate. **EB:** *Social support is assistance provided by others in the community that promotes and maintains a client's well-being and resilience (Fuentes-Pelaez et al, 2016).*
- ▲ Help clarify problem areas in interpersonal relationships. **EBN:** *Individuals who were socially connected to their environment, family, and sense of self can maintain a supportive mindset and experience a decent quality of life despite compromising health conditions, serious diagnosis, and poor prognosis (Stuckey et al, 2014).*
- ▲ Promote a sense of an individual's autonomy and control over choices to be made in one's environment. **EBN:** *Autonomy promotes a sense of self-efficacy and has been linked to increased quality of life and positive health outcomes for clients (Resnick, 2014).*
- ▲ Identify and enroll high-risk families in follow-up programs. **EBN:** *Families with adequate resources and positive relationships have a better chance of managing stress and restoring balance in the presence of adversity and limited resources (Lester et al, 2013).*

REFERENCES

Butcher, H. (2016). Development and use of gerontological evidence-based practice guidelines. *Journal of Gerontological Nursing, 42*(7), 25–32.

Crichton, S. (2013). Understanding, identifying, and supporting speech, language, and communication needs of children. *Community Practitioner, 86*(12), 44–47. Retrieved from ebscohost.com/login.aspx?direct=true&profile=ehost.

Deist, M., & Greeff, A. P. (2015). Resilience in family members caring for a family member diagnosed with dementia. *Educational Gerontology, 41*(2), 93–105.

Finderup, J., Bjerre, T., Soendergaad, A., et al. (2016). Developing skills in haemodialysis using the guided self-determination method: A qualitative study. *Journal of Renal Care, 42*(2), 83–92.

Fuentes-Pelaez, N., Balsells, M., & Fernandez, J. (2016). The social support in kinship foster care: A way to enhance resilience. *Child & Family Social Work, 21*(4), 581–590.

Lester, P., Stein, J. A., Saltzman, W., et al. (2013). Psychological health of military children: Longitudinal evaluation of a family-centered prevention program to enhance family resilience. *Military Medicine, 178*(8), 838–845.

● = Independent;   ▲ = Collaborative;   **EBN** = Evidence-Based Nursing;   **EB** = Evidence-Based

Patrick, S., & Robertson, S. (2016). Mental health and well-being: Focus on men's health. *British Journal of Nursing, 25*(21), 1163–1169.

Resnick, B. (2014). Resilience in older adults. *Topics in Geriatric Rehabilitation, 30*(3), 155–163.

Stuckey, H. L., Mullan-Jensen, C. B., Reach, G., et al. (2014). Personal accounts of the negative and adaptive psychosocial experiences of

people with diabetes in the second diabetes attitudes, wishes and needs (DAWN2) study. *Diabetes Care, 37*(9), 2466–2474.

Usaite, K., & Cameron, J. (2015). Participation in enjoyable activities can promote resilience in young people. *British Journal of Occupational Therapy, 78*(Suppl.), 2–3.

Parental Role conflict   *Kimberly Silvey, MSN, RN*

NANDA-I

Definition

Parental experience of role confusion and conflict in response to crisis.

Defining Characteristics

Anxiety; concern about change in parental role; concern about family; disruption in caregiver routines; fear; frustration; guilt; perceived inadequacy to provide for child's needs; perceived loss of control over decisions relating to child; reluctance to participate in usual caregiver activities

Related Factors

Interruptions in family life due to home care regimen; intimidated by invasive modalities; intimidation by restrictive modalities; parent–child separation

At-Risk Population

Change in marital status; home care of a child with special needs; living in nontraditional setting

NOC   (Nursing Outcomes Classification)

Suggested NOC Outcomes

Caregiver Emotional Health; Caregiver Well-Being; Caregiver Lifestyle Disruption; Coping; Parenting Performance; Role Performance; Family Coping

> #### Example NOC Outcome with Indicators
>
> **Family Coping** as evidenced by the following indicators: Establishes role flexibility/Manages family problems/Uses family-centered stress reduction activities. (Rate the outcome and indicators of **Family Coping:** 1 = never demonstrated, 2 = rarely demonstrated, 3 = sometimes demonstrated, 4 = often demonstrated, 5 = consistently demonstrated [see Section I].)

Client Outcomes

Client Will (Specify Time Frame)

- Express feelings and perceptions regarding effects of illness, disability, and/or hospitalization on parental role
- Participate in hospital and home care as much as able given the availability of resources and support systems
- Exhibit assertiveness and responsibility in active family decision-making regarding care of the child
- Describe and select available resources to support parental management of the needs of the child and family

NIC   (Nursing Interventions Classification)

Suggested NIC Interventions

Caregiver Support; Counseling; Decision-Making Support; Family Process Maintenance; Family Therapy; Parenting Promotion; Role Enhancement

● = Independent;   ▲ = Collaborative;   EBN = Evidence-Based Nursing;   EB = Evidence-Based

R

Example NIC Activities—Role Enhancement
Teach new behaviors needed by client/parent to fulfill a role; Serve as role model for learning new behaviors as appropriate

Nursing Interventions and *Rationales*

- Assess and support parent's previous coping behaviors. EBN: *Understanding what experience a parent has with coping will enable the nurse to support the parents in the current situation (Senger, 2016).*
- Determine parent/family sources of stress, usual methods of coping, and perceptions of illness/condition. Maximize the identified strengths. EB: *Helping to identify stressors in a family's life can help parents better cope with theirs child's illness (Pritchard & Montgomery-Hönger, 2014).*
- Evaluate the family's perceived strength of its social support system, including religious beliefs. Encourage the family to use social support. EB: *Parents use their support from their family to help reduce anxiety (Nabors et al, 2013).*
- Determine the older childbearing woman's support systems and expectations for motherhood. EBN: *Supporting mothers during their transition into parenthood can assist with the bonding of the mother and the infant (Gilmer, 2016).*
- Consider the use of family-centered theory as the conceptual foundation to help guide interventions. EB: *When planning care for a child, family is always the constant in their lives and should be included in all decision-making (King & Chiarello, 2014).*
- Be available to accept and support parents by listening and discussing concerns. EBN: *The nurse's ability to observe and listen to parents helps parents gain confidence in caring for their child (Panicker, 2013).*
- ▲ Maintain parental involvement in shared decision-making regarding care by using the following steps: incorporate parents' information concerning the child's typical routines, behaviors, fears, likes, and dislikes; provide clear and direct firsthand information concerning the child's condition and progress; normalize the home/hospital environment as much as possible; collaborate in care by providing choices when possible. EB: *Understanding the ways decisions are made by the parents will help the nurse better care for the child (Schmidt, 2014).*
- Seek and support parental participation in care. EBN: *Nurses should support the parents in whatever way they choose to participate in care and involve them in as much as the parents feel comfortable (Romaniuk et al, 2014).*
- Provide support for each parent's primary coping strategies and needs. EBN: *Parent support at home can enhance parents' confidence in caring for their child (Callery et al, 2013).*
- ▲ Inform parents of financial resources, respite care, and home support to assist them in maintaining sufficient energy and personal resources to continue caregiving responsibilities. EB: *There can be a financial burden on parents of children with chronic illness and a need to help the family identify their resources (Stewart et al, 2016).*
- Encourage the parent to meet his or her own needs for rest, nutrition, and hygiene. Provide bed space so that the parent may stay with the sick child. EB: *Children with an illness can have an effect on parent sleep, which in turn can cause parental fatigue and lead to other health problems (Mörelius & Hemmingsson, 2014).*
- Provide family-centered care: allow parents to touch and talk to the child, and assist in the handling of medical equipment; offer a comfortable chair, preferably a rocking chair. Provide opportunities and offer praise for successful caregiving. EBN: *Allowing the parents to participate in care as they feel comfortable enhances family-centered care (Romaniuk et al, 2014).*
- Refer parents to available telephone and/or Internet support groups. EB: *Many parents find that Internet support groups help in coping with their child's illness (Clifford & Minnes, 2013).*
- Involve new mother's partner or parents in clinical encounters and invite family members to discuss their expectations and parenting experiences. EBN: *Health care providers realize the importance of family-centered care of the infant to help the mother and her partner care for the infant (Dzubaty, 2016).*

Multicultural

- Acknowledge racial/ethnic differences at the onset of care. EBN: *Providing culturally competent care is important to health care equality and is important for nurses to understand the importance of identifying the cultural differences that their patients will require (Dzubaty, 2016).*

● = Independent;   ▲ = Collaborative;   EBN = Evidence-Based Nursing;   EB = Evidence-Based

- Assess for the influence of cultural beliefs, norms, and values on the client's perceptions of the parental role. EBN: *Understanding the cultures and beliefs of parents can enhance the interactions between nurse and family and assist the nurse to better care for the child and their family (Xiong et al, 2016).*
- Acknowledge that value conflicts arising from acculturation stresses may contribute to increased anxiety and significant conflict with the parental role. EBN: *Nurses should assess for any care that may interfere with a family's cultural beliefs and practices (Majdalani et al, 2014).*
- Promote the female parenting role by providing a treatment environment that is culturally based and woman centered. EBN: *Mothers should be the main focus for shorter hospital stays and better infant bonding (Miah, 2013).*
- Support the client's parenting role in her usual setting via social exchange, including online support. EBN: *Online messaging boards can be very helpful and support the client's parenting role (Porter & Ispa, 2013).*

Home Care

- The interventions described previously may be adapted for home care use.
- Assess family adjustment prenatally and postpartum; assist new parents to renegotiate parenting roles and responsibilities with coparenting. Encourage the father to take an active role in infant care with the mother's support. EBN: *Home visits can have a positive effect on both the mother and father (Ferguson & Vanderpool, 2013).*

Client/Family Teaching and Discharge Planning

- Offer family-led education interventions to improve participants' knowledge about their condition and its treatment and decreasing their information needs. EBN: *Education of client and family on the condition can improve self-care at home (Swerczek et al, 2013).*
- For children and their parents involved in bereavement support groups, identify the family's positive way of coping. EB: *Support groups and bereaving programs can help parents better cope with the death of a child (Ayers et al, 2013).*
- ▲ Refer parents of children with behavioral problems to parenting programs. EB: *Parenting programs can help parents identify and reduce problem behaviors in children (Salari et al, 2013).*
- Involve parents in formal and/or informal social support situations, such as Internet support groups. EBN: *Online support groups can allow families to receive support from their peers from around the world and share the knowledge and problems of their child (Mo & Coulson, 2014).*
- Teach the client about available community resources (e.g., therapists, ministers, counselors, self-help groups). EBN: *Community-based resources can support caregivers and ensure that they can identify needed services (Tallon et al, 2017).*
- Encourage parents with chronic illnesses to identify areas of family conflicts and assist to integrate interventions into the family. EBN: *Supporting chronically ill parents to identify conflicts will help the parents to better care for the child (Popp et al, 2014).*

REFERENCES

Ayers, T. S., Wolchik, S. A., et al. (2013). The family bereavement program: Description of a theory-based prevention program for parentally-bereaved children and adolescents. *Omega: Journal of Death & Dying, 68*(4), 293–314.

Callery, P., Kyle, R. G., et al. (2013). Enhancing parents' confidence to care in acute childhood illness: Triangulation of findings from a mixed methods study of community children's nursing. *Journal of Advanced Nursing, 69*(11), 2538–2548.

Clifford, T., & Minnes, P. (2013). Logging on: Evaluating an online support group for parents of children with autism spectrum disorders. *Journal of Autism & Developmental Disorders, 43*(7), 1662–1675.

Dzubaty, D. R. (2016). Providing family-centered care in maternal-newborn settings: A case study. *Newborn and Infant Nursing Reviews, 16*(2), 55–57.

Ferguson, J., & Vanderpool, R. (2013). Impact of a Kentucky maternal, infant, and early childhood home-visitation program on parental risk factors. *Journal of Child & Family Studies, 22*(4), 551–558.

Gilmer, C., Buchan, J. L., et al. (2016). Parent education interventions designed to support the transition to parenthood: A realist review. *International Journal of Nursing Studies, 59*(Suppl. C), 118–133.

King, G., & Chiarello, L. (2014). Family-centered care for children with cerebral palsy: Conceptual and practical considerations to advance care and practice. *Journal of Child Neurology, 29*(8), 1046–1054.

Majdalani, M. N., Doumit, M. A. A., et al. (2014). The lived experience of parents of children admitted to the pediatric intensive care unit in Lebanon. *International Journal of Nursing Studies, 51*(2), 217–225.

Miah, R. (2013). Does transitional care improve neonatal and maternal health outcomes? A systematic review. *British Journal of Midwifery, 21*(9), 634–646.

Mo, P. K. H., & Coulson, N. S. (2014). Are online support groups always beneficial? A qualitative exploration of the empowering and disempowering processes of participation within HIV/AIDS-related online support groups. *International Journal of Nursing Studies, 51*(7), 983–993.

● = Independent; ▲ = Collaborative; EBN = Evidence-Based Nursing; EB = Evidence-Based

Mörelius, E., & Hemmingsson, H. (2014). Parents of children with physical disabilities-perceived health in parents related to the child's sleep problems and need for attention at night. *Child: Care, Health & Development, 40*(3), 412–418.

Nabors, L. A., Kichler, J. C., et al. (2013). Factors related to caregiver state anxiety and coping with a child's chronic illness. *Families, Systems & Health: The Journal of Collaborative Family HealthCare, 31*(2), 171–180.

Panicker, L. (2013). Nurses' perceptions of parent empowerment in chronic illness. *Contemporary Nurse: A Journal for the Australian Nursing Profession, 45*(2), 210–219.

Popp, J. M., Robinson, J. L., et al. (2014). Parent adaptation and family functioning in relation to narratives of children with chronic illness. *Journal of Pediatric Nursing, 29*(1), 58–64.

Porter, N., & Ispa, J. M. (2013). Mothers' online message board questions about parenting infants and toddlers. *Journal of Advanced Nursing, 69*(3), 559–568.

Pritchard, V. E., & Montgomery-Hönger, A. (2014). A comparison of parent and staff perceptions of setting-specific and everyday stressors encountered by parents with very preterm infants experiencing neonatal intensive care. *Early Human Development, 90*(10), 549–555.

Romaniuk, D., O'Mara, L., et al. (2014). Are parents doing what they want to do? Congruency between parents' actual and desired participation in the care of their hospitalized child. *Issues in Comprehensive Pediatric Nursing, 37*(2), 103–121.

Salari, R., Fabian, H., et al. (2013). The children and parents in focus project: A population-based cluster-randomised controlled trial to prevent behavioural and emotional problems in children. *BMC Public Health, 13*(1), 225–241.

Schmidt, J. (2014). Primary care decision making among first-time parents in Aotearoa/New Zealand. *Women's Studies Journal, 28*(1), 18–35.

Senger, B. A., Ward, L. D., et al. (2016). Stress and coping of parents caring for a child with mitochondrial disease. *Applied Nursing Research, 29*(Suppl. C), 195–201.

Stewart, M., Evans, J., et al. (2016). Low-income children, adolescents, and caregivers facing respiratory problems: Support needs and preferences. *Journal of Pediatric Nursing, 31*(3), 319–329.

Swerczek, L. M., Banister, C., et al. (2013). A telephone coaching intervention to improve asthma self-management behaviors. *Pediatric Nursing, 39*(3), 125–145.

Tallon, M. M., Kendall, G. E., et al. (2017). Barriers to addressing social determinants of health in pediatric nursing practice: An integrative review. *Journal of Pediatric Nursing, 37*(Suppl. C), 51–56.

Xiong, S., Degroote, N., et al. (2016). Engaging in culturally informed nursing care with Hmong children and their families. *Journal of Pediatric Nursing, 31*(1), 102–106.

Ineffective Role performance   *Marina Martinez-Kratz, MS, RN, CNE*

NANDA-I

Definition

A pattern of behavior and self-expression that does not match the environmental context, norms, and expectations.

Defining Characteristics

Alteration in role perceptions; anxiety; change in capacity to resume role; change in other's perception of role; change in self-perception of role; change in usual patterns of responsibility; depression; discrimination; domestic violence; harassment; inappropriate developmental expectations; ineffective adaptation to change; ineffective coping strategies; ineffective role performance; insufficient confidence; insufficient external support for role enactment; insufficient knowledge of role requirements; insufficient motivation; insufficient opportunity for role enactment; insufficient self-management; insufficient skills; pessimism; powerlessness; role ambivalence; role conflict; role confusion; role denial; role dissatisfaction; role strain; system conflict; uncertainty

Related Factors

Alteration in body image; conflict; depression; domestic violence; fatigue; inadequate role model; inappropriate linkage with the health care system; insufficient resources; insufficient rewards; insufficient role preparation; insufficient role socialization; insufficient support system; low self-esteem; pain; stressors; substance misuse; unrealistic role expectations

At-Risk Population

Developmental level inappropriate for role expectation; economically disadvantaged; high demands of job schedule; low educational level; young age

Associated Condition

Neurological defect; personality disorder; physical illness; psychosis

● = Independent;   ▲ = Collaborative;   EBN = Evidence-Based Nursing;   EB = Evidence-Based

NOC (Nursing Outcomes Classification)

Suggested NOC Outcomes

Coping; Psychosocial Adjustment: Life Change; Role Performance

Example NOC Outcome with Indicators

Role Performance as evidenced by the following indicators: Knowledge of role transition periods/Reported comfort with role changes. (Rate the outcome and indicators of **Role Performance:** 1 = not adequate, 2 = slightly adequate, 3 = moderately adequate, 4 = substantially adequate, 5 = totally adequate [see Section I].)

Client Outcomes

Client Will (Specify Time Frame)

- Identify realistic perception of role
- State personal strengths
- Acknowledge problems contributing to inability to perform usual role
- Accept physical limitations regarding role responsibility and consider ways to change lifestyle to accomplish goals associated with role performance
- Demonstrate knowledge of appropriate behaviors associated with new or changed role
- State knowledge of change in responsibility and new behaviors associated with new responsibility
- Verbalize acceptance of new responsibility

NIC (Nursing Interventions Classification)

Suggested NIC Intervention

Role Enhancement

Example NIC Activities—Role Enhancement

Assist client to identify behaviors needed for role development; Assist client to identify positive strategies for managing role changes

Nursing Interventions and *Rationales*

- Assess the client's level of resilience and implement nursing actions that increase client resilience and sense of coherence. EBN: *A study of individuals with chronic obstructive pulmonary disease indicated that high levels of a sense of coherence and resilience were negatively associated with symptoms of anxiety and depression and perceived illness-specific disability (Keil et al, 2016).*
- Assess the effect of uncertainty on the client's role and provide support and education. EBN: *A study of caregivers with hospitalized children showed that levels of uncertainty and stress decreased, and role performance improved after an educational intervention (Jeon & Kwon, 2016).*
- Assess the client's social support system. EB: *A recent study showed that clients with good social support are more likely to change their lifestyle and make more changes (Clementi et al, 2016).*
- Assess for the presence of shame related to current health situation. EBN: *A Greek study of intensive care unit (ICU) families found family members who live with the client and have low educational levels are prone to feel shame, which could interfere with coping and caregiving (Koulouras, 2017).*
- Assess for the characteristics of role stress. EB: *A recent study showed that a lack of role clarity was significantly linked to emotional exhaustion (Portoghese, 2017).*
- Assess male military members for gender role stressors with the Male Gender Role Stressor Inventory (MGRSI). EB: *Research piloting the MGRSI found that honor, strength, and achievement were the most commonly reported sources of male gender role stress and may be associated with suicidal behaviors (Sterling et al, 2016).*
- Ask the client what they need to feel prepared for the tasks and demands of their role. EB: *A study of caregivers found that preparedness was significantly associated with higher levels of hope and reward and with a lower level of anxiety (Henriksson & Arestad, 2013).*

● = Independent;   ▲ = Collaborative;   EBN = Evidence-Based Nursing;   EB = Evidence-Based

R

▲ Refer the client to Acceptance and Commitment Therapy (ACT). **CEB:** *ACT is a therapy that focuses on the development of psychological flexibility through acceptance of what is out of personal control and a commitment to action that improves and enriches one's life (Hayes, Strosahl, & Wilson, 2011).*

● Support the client's spirituality practices. **EB:** *Spiritual care was found to reduce care strain in caregivers of elderly patients with Alzheimer's disease (Mahdavi et al, 2017).*

● Refer to the care plans for Readiness for enhanced family **Coping,** Readiness for enhanced **Decision-Making,** Impaired **Home** maintenance, Impaired **Parenting,** Risk for **Loneliness,** Readiness for enhanced community **Coping,** Readiness for enhanced **Self-Care,** and Ineffective **Sexuality** pattern.

 Pediatric

▲ Provide parents of disabled children with information about and referrals to educational and social resources available to assist their child. **EB:** *A longitudinal study found that parents' educational expectations shape academic development and changes in self-concept among young people with different types of disabilities (McCoy et al, 2016).*

● Assist new parents to adjust to changes in workload associated with childbirth. Mothers may need additional support. **EBN:** *A Brazilian study found that women in the postpartum period experience multiple stressors that affect their role performance (Cavalcanti et al, 2014).*

● Assess mothers who present with depressive symptoms in the postpartum period for evidence of role performance distress. **EBN:** *Nursing research indicates that role performance disturbances are correlated with depressive symptoms in the postpartum period (Cavalcanti et al, 2014).*

● Provide parents with information about mindfulness-based interventions (MBIs) to enhance coping when the role change is associated with a critically and chronically ill child. **EB:** *Research found that MBI is a culturally adaptable, acceptable, and effective method to improve quality of life and positive stress reappraisal coping in parents of children with autism spectral disorder (Rayun & Ahmad, 2016).*

● Provide parents with information to increase their awareness of their child's psychological and social needs after a critical illness. **EBN:** *Childhood survivors of critical illness face a complex trajectory of recovery with enduring psychosocial adversity. Parents and families are fundamental in shaping psychological and social well-being of survivors (Manning et al, 2014).*

 Geriatric

● Assess older adults' choices regarding their care and enable them to live as they wish and receive the help they want by carefully listening to their stories. **EB:** *A recent study found that complementing standardized assessment data with informal interviews provided information that older adults and their families believed was important to their care (Lafortune et al, 2017).*

● Assess older adults for a sense of competence in their daily life. **EB:** *A French study showed that increased competence was associated with a decrease of depressive symptoms and apathy (Souesme et al, 2016).*

● Provide support and practice for older adults to use technology. **EB:** *A recent study found that participants used information and communication technology (ICT) to connect with friends and family. ICT use predicted higher well-being across outcomes (Sims et al, 2017).*

● Support the client's spiritual beliefs and activities and provide appropriate spiritual support persons. **EB:** *Spiritual care was found to reduce care strain in caregivers of elderly patients with Alzheimer's disease (Mahdavi et al, 2017).*

● Explore community needs after assessing the client's strengths. Encourage older adults to participate in volunteer programs. **EB:** *Research indicated an association between volunteering and reductions in symptoms of depression, better overall health, fewer functional limitations, feeling appreciated and needed, and greater longevity with vulnerable seniors benefiting the most (Anderson et al, 2014).*

 Multicultural

● Assess for the influence of cultural beliefs, norms, values, and expectations on the individual's role. **CEB:** *The individual's role may be based on cultural perceptions (Leininger & McFarland, 2002).*

● Assess for conflicts between the caregiver's cultural role, obligations, and competing factors, such as employment or school. **EB:** *A study found that it is important to identify and understand culturally and geographically influenced barriers to cancer treatment and symptom management (Itty, Hodge, & Martinez, 2014).*

● Negotiate with the client regarding the aspects of their role that can be modified and still honor cultural beliefs. **CEB:** *Give-and-take with the client will lead to culturally congruent care (Leininger & McFarland, 2002).*

● = Independent;   ▲ = Collaborative;   **EBN** = Evidence-Based Nursing;   **EB** = Evidence-Based

- Identify perceived barriers to family to use support groups or other service programs to assist with role changes. **EB:** *A systematic review identified that assessment for support resources, home care, or community assistance was needed prior to discharge and at routine intervals throughout the care situation (Greenwood et al, 2015).*
- The preceding interventions may be adapted for home care use.

 Client/Family Teaching and Discharge Planning

- ▲ Refer client to comprehensive services to assist with transition needs at discharge. **EB:** *A study found no 30-day rehospitalizations for participants in the Kentucky Care Coordination for Community Transitions ([KCT]-T-3) program, which provided access to medical, social, and environmental services to support community transitions (Kitzman et al, 2017).*
- Provide educational materials to family members on client behavior management plus caregiver stress-coping management. **EB:** *Research has identified multiple components to provide education, support, counseling, care continuity, and linkage to community resources to ease transitions can improve caregiver health and coping (Naylor et al, 2017).*
- Help the client identify resources for assistance in caring for a disabled or aging parent (e.g., adult day care, nursing home placement). **EB:** *A systematic review identified assessment for support resources, home care, or community assistance was needed prior to discharge and at routine intervals throughout the care situation (Greenwood et al, 2015).*

REFERENCES

Anderson, N. D., et al. (2014). The benefits associated with volunteering among seniors: A critical review and recommendations for future research. *Psychological Bulletin, 140*(6), 1505–1533. doi:10.1037/a0037610.

Cavalcanti, B., Marques, D., Guimarães, F., et al. (2014). "Ineffective role performance" nursing diagnosis in postpartum women: A descriptive study. *Online Brazilian Journal of Nursing, 13*(2), 246–254.

Clementi, S., et al. (2016). The role of psychosocial status in the change of lifestyles in patients with colorectal cancer in follow up. *Annals of Oncology, 27*(S4), iv81. doi:10.1093/annonc/mdw339.06.

Greenwood, N., Habibi, R., Smith, R., et al. (2015). Barriers to access and minority ethnic carers' satisfaction with social care services in the community: A systematic review of qualitative and quantitative literature. *Health & Social Care in the Community, 23*(1), 64–78. doi:10.1111/hsc.12116.

Hayes, S., Strosahl, K., & Wilson, K. (2011). *Acceptance and commitment therapy, second edition: The process and practice of mindful change* (2nd ed.). New York: Guilford.

Henriksson, A., & Arestad, K. (2013). Exploring factors and caregiver outcomes associated with feelings of preparedness for caregiving in family caregivers in palliative care: A correlational, cross-sectional study. *Palliative Medicine, 27*(7), 639–646. doi:10.1177/0269216313486954.

Itty, T. L., Hodge, F. S., & Martinez, F. (2014). Shared and unshared barriers to cancer symptom management among urban and rural American Indians. *Journal of Rural Health, 30*(2), 206–213. doi:10.1111/jrh.12045.

Jeon, E., & Kwon, I. S. (2016). Effect of caregiver's role improvement program on the uncertainty, stress, and role performance of caregivers with hospitalized children. *Child Health Nursing Research, 23*(1), 70–80. doi:10.4094/chnr.2017.23.1.70.

Kitzman, P., et al. (2017). Care coordination for community transitions for individuals post-stroke returning to low-resource rural communities. *Journal of Community Health, 42*(3), 565–572. doi:10.1007/s10900-016-0289-0.

Keil, D. C., et al. (2016). With the strength to carry on: The role of sense of coherence and resilience for anxiety, depression and disability in chronic obstructive pulmonary disease. *Chronic Respiratory Disease, 14*(1), 11–21. doi:10.1177/1479972316654286.

Koulouras, V., et al. (2017). Shame feeling in the Intensive Care Unit patient's family members. *Intensive and Critical Care Nursing, 41*, 84–89. doi:10.1016/j.iccn.2017.03.011.

Lafortune, C., et al. (2017). The rest of the story: A qualitative study of complementing standardized assessment data with informal interviews with older patients and families. *The Patient - Patient-Centered Outcomes Research, 10*(2), 215–224. doi:10.1007/s40271-016-0193-9.

Leininger, M. M., & McFarland, M. R. (2002). *Transcultural nursing: Concepts, theories, research and practices* (3rd ed.). New York: McGraw-Hill.

Mahdavi, B., Fallahi-Khoshknab, M., Mohammadi, F., et al. (2017). Effects of spiritual group therapy on caregiver strain in home caregivers of the elderly with Alzheimer's disease. *Archives of Psychiatric Nursing, 31*(3), 269–273. doi:10.1016/j.apnu.2016.12.003.

Manning, J. C., et al. (2014). Long-term psychosocial impact reported by childhood critical illness survivors: A systematic review. *Nursing in Critical Care, 19*, 145–156. doi:10.1111/nicc.12049.

McCoy, S., et al. (2016). The role of parental expectations in understanding social and academic well-being among children with disabilities in Ireland. *European Journal of Special Needs Education, 31*(4), 535–552. doi:10.1080/08856257.2016.1199607.

Naylor, M. D., et al. (2017). Components of comprehensive and effective transitional care. *Journal of the American Geriatrics Society, 65*(6), 1119–1125. doi:10.1111/jgs.14782.

Portoghese, I., et al. (2017). Role stress and emotional exhaustion among health care workers: The buffering effect of supportive coworker climate in a multilevel perspective. *Journal of Occupational and Environmental Medicine, 59*(10), e187–e193. doi:10.1097/JOM.0000000000001122.

Rayun, A., & Ahmad, M. (2016). Effectiveness of mindfulness-based interventions on quality of life and positive reappraisal coping among parents of children with autism spectrum disorder. *Research in Developmental Disabilities, 55*, 185–196. doi:10.1016/j.ridd.2016.04.002.

R

● = Independent;   ▲ = Collaborative;   **EBN** = Evidence-Based Nursing;   **EB** = Evidence-Based

Sims, T., et al. (2017). Information and communication technology use is related to higher well-being among the oldest-old. *Journals of Gerontology Series B—Psychological Sciences and Social Sciences*, 72(5), 761–770. doi:10.1093/geronb/gbw130.

Souesme, G., et al. (2016). Perceived autonomy support, psychological needs satisfaction, depressive symptoms and apathy in French hospitalized older people. *Archives of Gerontology and Geriatrics*, 65, 70–78. doi:10.1016/j.archger.2016.03.001.

Sterling, A. G., et al. (2016). Perspectives of suicide bereaved individuals on military suicide decedents' life stressors and male gender role stress. *Archives of Suicide Research*, 21(1), 155–168. doi:10.1080/13811118.2016.1166087.

Sedentary lifestyle   *Marina Martinez-Kratz, MS, RN, CNE*

NANDA-I

Definition

A habit of life that is characterized by a low physical activity level.

Defining Characteristics

Average daily physical activity is less than recommended for gender and age; physical deconditioning; preference for activity low in physical activity

Related Factors

Insufficient interest in physical activity; insufficient knowledge of health benefits associated with physical exercise; insufficient motivation for physical activity; insufficient resources for physical activity; insufficient training for physical exercise

NOC   (Nursing Outcomes Classification)

Suggested NOC Outcomes

Ambulation; Activity Tolerance; Endurance; Exercise Participation; Health Promoting Behavior; Lifestyle Balance; Personal Health Status; Physical Fitness; Exercise Promotion

Example NOC Outcome with Indicators

Ambulation as evidenced by the following indicators: Walks with effective gait/Walks at moderate pace/Walks up and down steps/Walks moderate distance. (Rate the outcome and indicators of **Ambulation:** 1 = severely compromised, 2 = substantially compromised, 3 = moderately compromised, 4 = mildly compromised, 5 = not compromised [see Section I].)

Client Outcomes

Client Will (Specify Time Frame)

- Engage in purposeful moderate-intensity cardiorespiratory (aerobic) exercise for 30 to 60 minutes/day on 5 or more days per week for a total of 2 hours and 30 minutes (150 minutes) per week
- Increase exercise to 20 minutes/day (<150 minutes/week); light to moderate intensity exercise may be beneficial in deconditioned persons
- Increase pedometer step counts by 1000 steps per day every 2 weeks to reach a daily step count of at least 7000 steps per day, with a daily goal for most healthy adults of 10,000 steps per day
- Perform resistance exercises that involve all major muscle groups (legs, hips, back, chest, abdomen, shoulders, and arms) performed 2 to 3 days/week
- Perform flexibility exercise (stretching) for each of the major muscle-tendon groups 2 days/week for 10 to 60 seconds to improve joint range of motion; greatest gains occur with daily exercise
- Engage in neuromotor exercise 20 to 30 minutes/day including motor skills (e.g., balance, agility, coordination, and gait), proprioceptive exercise training, and multifaceted activities (e.g., Tai chi and yoga) to improve and maintain physical function and reduce falls in those at risk for falling (older persons)

NIC   (Nursing Interventions Classification)

Suggested NIC Interventions

Exercise Therapy: Ambulation; Joint Mobility; Positioning; Exercise Promotion; Activity Therapy; Energy Management

● = Independent;   ▲ = Collaborative;   EBN = Evidence-Based Nursing;   EB = Evidence-Based

Example NIC Activities—Exercise Therapy: Ambulation
Assist the client to use footwear that facilitates walking and prevents injury; Instruct in availability of assistive devices, if appropriate

Nursing Interventions and *Rationales*

- Observe the client for sedentary behaviors such as prolonged sitting, physical inactivity, and prolonged sleep. **EB:** *Prolonged sitting, physical inactivity, and prolonged sleep were identified as lifestyle health risk behaviors in an Australian study (Ding et al, 2015).* See care plans for Ineffective **Coping** or **Hopelessness.**

- Use the Self-Efficacy for Exercise Scale (Resnick & Jenkins, 2000) and the Outcome Expectation for Exercise Scale (Resnick et al, 2001) to determine client's self-efficacy and outcome expectations toward exercise (Resnick & D'Adamo, 2011). **CEB:** *Interventions most effective in promoting physical activity were those that focused only on the targeted behavior of physical activity and those that used behavioral strategies (e.g., rewards, contracts, goal setting, feedback and cueing) and self-monitoring (e.g., tracking physical activity using logs or websites). Supervised exercise, tailoring, contracting, exercise prescription, intensity recommendations, behavioral cueing, and fitness testing were also effective, although only modestly supported (Ruppar & Conn, 2010).*

- Assess client with exercise preparticipation health screening prior to implementing physical activity interventions. **EB:** *The American College of Sports Medicine (ACSM) has made recommendations to identify individuals (1) who should receive medical clearance before initiating an exercise program or increasing the frequency, intensity, and/or volume of their current program; (2) with clinically significant disease(s) who may benefit from participating in a medically supervised exercise program; and (3) with medical conditions that may require exclusion from exercise programs. The specific ACSM guidelines can be accessed at: http:// certification.acsm.org/docs/default-source/files-for-resource-library/acsm-101-prescreeninginfographiccolorlegal-2015-12-15-v02.pdf?sfvrsn=cd75273d_4 (Riebe et al, 2015).*

- Recommend the client enter an exercise program with an active person who supports exercise behavior (e.g., friend or exercise buddy). **EB:** *A 12-week pilot controlled trial of a physical activity buddy program found that the active buddy group (P = 0.005) showed significantly higher step changes than the inactive buddy group (Choi, 2017).*

- Recommend the client use a mobile fitness application for customizing, cueing, tracking, and analyzing an exercise program. **EB:** *A study showed exercise app users were more likely to exercise during their leisure time, and the data suggest exercise apps may increase exercise levels and health outcomes, such as body mass index (BMI), by making it easier for users to overcome barriers to exercise, leading to increased self-efficacy (Litman et al, 2015).*

- Recommend participation in group physical activity programs. **EBN:** *A nurse-monitored 7-week group exercise training program (ETP) with obese women improved adherence to some type of physical activity program 1 year after the intervention period, and the likelihood of adherence increased with the number of ETP sessions attended (del Rey-Moya et al, 2013).*

- Recommend client begin performing resistance exercises for additional health benefits. **EB:** *A research review found that resistance training is effective in controlling and improving cholesterol levels (Mann, 2014).*

- Encourage prescriptive resistance exercise of each major muscle group (hips, thighs, legs, back, chest, shoulders, and abdomen) using a variety of exercise equipment. **EB:** *Equipment such as free weights, bands, stair climbing, or machines should be used 2 to 3 days/week. Involve the major muscle groups for 8 to 12 repetitions to improve strength and power in most adults, 10 to 15 repetitions to improve strength in middle-aged and older persons starting exercise, and 15 to 20 repetitions to improve muscular endurance. Intensity should be between moderate (5 to 6) and hard (7 to 8) on a scale of 0 to 10 (ACSM, 2014).*

- Encourage gradual progression of greater resistance, more repetitions per set, and/or increasing frequency. **EB:** *A study found that a global progressive resistance strength training program was effective for improving the functional capacity of patients with rheumatoid arthritis (Lourenzi et al, 2015).*

 Multicultural

- Assess for reasons why the client would be unable to participate in regular physical activity; address reasons and refer to resources as needed. **EB:** *A systematic integrative literature review to identify barriers to physical activity among African American women found intrapersonal barriers (lack of time, knowledge, and motivation; physical appearance concerns; health concerns; monetary cost of exercise facilities; and tiredness/ fatigue), interpersonal barriers (family/caregiving responsibilities; lack of social support; and lack of a physical activity partner), and environmental barriers (safety concerns; lack of facilities; weather concerns; lack of sidewalks, and lack of physically active African American role models) (Jackson et al, 2015).*

● = Independent;   ▲ = Collaborative;   **EBN** = Evidence-Based Nursing;   **EB** = Evidence-Based

- Assess for their perceptions of the neighborhood they reside in. **EB:** *A study found that negative neighborhood environment perceptions were associated with greater sedentary time for individuals living in lower socioeconomic areas (Ahuja et al, 2017).*

Pediatric

- Assess the child's current activity status using the Pediatric Inactivity Triad (Faigenbaum et al, 2018). **EB:** *Components of the Pediatric Inactivity Triad include (1) exercise deficit disorder (less than 60 minutes of recommended physical activity daily), (2) pediatric dynapenia (decreased muscle strength and power), and (3) physical illiteracy (low competence and confidence). Addressing these components collectively will enhance effective change (Faigenbaum et al, 2018).*
- Children and adolescents should participate in 60 minutes (1 hour) or more of physical activity daily.
  - Aerobic: Sixty or more minutes a day should be either moderate-intensity or vigorous-intensity aerobic physical activity, and should include vigorous-intensity physical activity at least 3 days a week.
  - Muscle-strengthening: As part of daily physical activity, children and adolescents should include muscle-strengthening physical activity on at least 3 days of the week.
  - Bone-strengthening: As part of daily physical activity, children and adolescents should include bone-strengthening physical activity on at least 3 days of the week.
  - Providing activities that are age appropriate, enjoyable, and offer a variety will encourage young people to participate in physical activities (US Department of Health and Human Services, 2018).
- Assist families to develop family-based interventions to increase child physical activity. **EB:** *A meta-analysis of family-based interventions found a small effect on physical activity when interventions were tailored to the ethnicity, motivation, and time constraints of the family; combined goal-setting and reinforcement techniques were used; educational strategies were used to increase knowledge as needed; and consideration of the family psychosocial environment (Brown et al, 2016).*
- Encourage parents and caregivers to adhere to the following American Academy of Pediatrics guidelines for children's media use (Chassiakos et al, 2016):
  - For children younger than 18 months, avoid use of screen media other than video-chatting.
  - Parents of children 18 to 24 months of age who want to introduce digital media should choose high-quality programming and watch it with their children to help them understand what they are seeing.
  - For children ages 2 to 5 years, limit screen use to 1 hour/day of high-quality programs. Parents should co-view media with children to help them understand what they are seeing and apply it to the world around them.
  - For children ages 6 and older, place consistent limits on the time spent using media, and the types of media, and make sure media does not take the place of adequate sleep, physical activity, and other behaviors essential to health.
  - Designate media-free times together, such as dinner or driving, and media-free locations at home, such as bedrooms.
  - Have ongoing communication about online citizenship and safety, including treating others with respect online and off-line.
  - Encourage parents and caregivers to create their personalized family media plan (see https://www.healthychildren.org/English/media/Pages/default.aspx).

Geriatric

- Use valid and reliable criterion-referenced standards for fitness testing (e.g., Senior Fitness Test) designed for older adults that can predict the level of capacity associated with maintaining physical independence into later years of life (e.g., get up and go test). *Interventions can subsequently be designed to target weak areas and therefore help reduce the risk of immobility and dependence (Bhattacharya, Deka, & Roy, 2016).*
- Recommend the client begin a regular exercise program, even if generally active. **EB:** *A meta-analysis of the association between time in sedentary behavior and hospitalizations, mortality, cardiovascular disease, cancer, and diabetes found prolonged sedentary time associated as an independent risk factor for poor health outcomes despite engagement in physical activity (Biswas et al, 2015).*
- ▲ Refer the client to physical therapy for resistance exercise training, as able, involving all major muscle groups. **CEB:** *A Cochrane review found that progressive resistance-strength training for physical disability in older clients resulted in increased strength and positive improvements in some limitations (Liu & Latham, 2009).*

- Implement progressive resistance training plus balance exercise for older adults as indicated. **EB:** *A cluster randomized controlled trial showed that the Sunbeam Program of progressive resistance training in conjunction with balance exercise significantly reduced the rate of falls and improved physical performance in clients of residential care (Hewitt et al, 2018).*
- Use the Function-Focused Care (FFC) rehabilitative philosophy of care with older adults in residential nursing facilities to prevent avoidable functional decline. **EBN:** *The primary goals of FFC are to alter how direct care workers provide care to residents to maintain and improve time spent in physical activity and improve or maintain function. Residents receiving FFC had less functional decline, and a greater percentage who were not ambulating returned to ambulatory status for short functional distances. Residents with dementia also had a significant decrease in falls (28% versus 50% in the control group) (Galik et al, 2013).*
- Recommend the older client practice Tai chi. **EBN:** *A study of older community dwelling stroke survivors found that Tai chi led to improved aerobic endurance and was more effective in reducing fall rates than other interventions (Taylor-Pilae et al, 2014).*
- Prior to surgery, refer clients to a personalized prehabilitation program that includes a warm-up followed by aerobic, strength, flexibility, neuromotor, and functional task work. **EB:** *A study of major surgery clients assigned to personalized prehabilitation programs showed enhanced aerobic capacity and reduction in postoperative complications by 51% (Barbaren-Garcia et al, 2018).*

Home Care

- The preceding interventions may be adapted for home care use.
- ▲ Assess home environment for factors that create barriers to mobility. Refer to physical and occupational therapy services if needed to assist the client in restructuring home environment and daily living patterns.

Client/Family Teaching and Discharge Planning

- Work with the client using theory-based interventions (e.g., social, cognitive, theoretical components such as self-efficacy; transtheoretical model). **EBN:** *Residents living in senior housing who attended a 12-week intervention including education, motivational modalities, and exercise classes reported stronger outcome expectations for exercise, less pain, and decreased intake of fat and salt (Resnick et al, 2014).*
- Consider using motivational interviewing techniques when working with both children and adult clients to increase their activity. **EB:** *A study to increase physical activity among patients with rheumatoid arthritis found that at posttreatment and 6-months follow-up, significantly more clients met current physical activity recommendations (Knittle et al, 2015).*

REFERENCES

Ahuja, C., et al. (2017). Unfavorable perceptions of neighborhood environment are associated with greater sedentary time—Data from the Washington, D.C. Cardiovascular Health and Needs Assessment. *Circulation*, *135*(Suppl. 1, AMP002). Retrieved from http://circ.ahajournals.org/content/135/Suppl_1/AMP025.

American College of Sports Medicine (ACSM). (2014). *American College of Sports Medicine's guidelines for exercise testing and prescription* (9th ed.). Philadelphia: Lippincott Williams & Wilkins.

Barbaren-Garcia, A., et al. (2018). Personalised prehabilitation in high-risk patients undergoing elective major abdominal surgery: A randomized blinded controlled trial. *Annals of Surgery*, *267*(1), 50–56. doi:10.1097/SLA.0000000000002293.

Bhattacharya, P. K., Deka, K., & Roy, A. (2016). Assessment of inter-rater variability of the Senior Fitness Test in the geriatric population: A community based study. *International Journal of Biomedical and Advance Research*, *7*(5), 208–212. doi:10.7439/ijbar.

Biswas, A., Oh, P., Faulkner, G., et al. (2015). Sedentary time and its association with risk for disease incidence, mortality, and hospitalization in adults. *Annals of Internal Medicine*, *162*, 123–132.

Brown, H. E., et al. (2016). Family-based interventions to increase physical activity in children: A systematic review, meta-analysis and realist synthesis. *Obesity Reviews: An Official Journal of the International Association for the Study of Obesity*, *17*(4), 345–360. doi:10.1111/obr.12362.

Chassiakos, L. R., et al. (2016). Children and adolescents and digital media. *Pediatrics*, *138*(5), e1–e18. doi:10.1542/peds.2016-2593.

Choi, J. (2017). Active exercise buddies help women with young children improve physical activity. *Circulation*, *135*(Suppl. 1, AMP002). Retrieved from http://circ.ahajournals.org/content/135/Suppl_1/AMP002.short.

del Rey-Moya, L., Alvarez, C., Pichiule-Castaneda, M., et al. (2013). Effect of a group intervention in the primary healthcare setting on continuing adherence to physical exercise routines in obese women. *Journal of Clinical Nursing*, *22*, 2114–2121.

Ding, D., et al. (2015). Traditional and emerging lifestyle risk behaviors and all-cause mortality in middle-aged and older adults: Evidence from a large population-based Australian cohort. *PLoS Medicine*, *12*(12), e1001917. Retrieved from https://doi.org/10.1371/journal.pmed.1001917.

Faigenbaum, A. D., et al. (2018). Pediatric inactivity triad: A risky PIT. *Current Sports Medicine Reports*, *17*(2), 45–47. doi:10.1249/JSR.0000000000000450.

Galik, E., Resnick, B., Hammersla, M., et al. (2013). Optimizing function and physical activity among nursing home residents with dementia: Testing the impact of function-focused care. *The Gerontologist*, *54*(6), 930–943.

Hewitt, J., et al. (2018). Progressive resistance and balance training for falls prevention in long-term residential aged care: A cluster

S

randomized trial of the Sunbeam Program. *Journal of the American Medical Directors Association*, *19*(4), 361–369. doi:10.1016/j.jamda.2017.12.014.

Jackson, R. P., et al. (2015). Barriers to physical activity among African American women: An integrative review of the literature. *Women and Health*, *55*(6), 679–699. doi:10.1080/03630242.2015.1039184.

Knittle, K., et al. (2015). Targeting motivation and self-regulation to increase physical activity among patients with rheumatoid arthritis: A randomised controlled trial. *Clinical Rheumatology*, *34*(2), 231–238. doi:10.1007/s10067-013-2425-x.

Litman, L., et al. (2015). Mobile exercise apps and increased leisure time exercise activity: A moderated mediation analysis of the role of self-efficacy and barriers. *Journal of Medical Internet Research*, *17*(8), e195. doi:10.2196/jmir.4142.

Liu, C. J., & Latham, N. K. (2009). Progressive resistance strength training for improving physical function in older adults. *The Cochrane Database of Systematic Reviews*, (3), CD002759.

Lourenzi, F., Jones, A., Pereira, D., et al. (2015). *FRI0611-HPR global progressive resistance training improved functional capacity in patients with rheumatoid arthritis. Annals of the Rheumatic Diseases*, 74, 1323. Retrieved from http://dx.doi.org/10.1136/annrheumdis-2015-eular.2451.

Mann, S. (2014). Differential effects of aerobic exercise, resistance training and combined exercise modalities on cholesterol and the lipid profile: Review, synthesis and recommendations. *Sports Medicine*, *44*(2), 211–221. doi:10.1007/s40279-013-0110-5.

Resnick, B., & D'Adamo, C. (2011). Factors associated with exercise among older adults in a continuing care retirement community. *Rehabilitation Nursing*, *36*(2), 47–53, 82.

Resnick, B., & Jenkins, L. S. (2000). Testing the reliability and validity of the self-efficacy for exercise scale. *Nursing Reviews*, *49*(3), 154–159.

Resnick, B., Hammersla, M., Michael, K., et al. (2014). Changing behavior in senior housing residents: Testing of phase I of the PRAISEDD-2 Intervention. *Applied Nursing Research*, *27*(3), 162–169.

Resnick, B., Zimmerman, S., & Orwig, D. (2001). Model testing for reliability and validity of the outcome expectations for exercise scale. *Nursing Research*, *50*(5), 293.

Riebe, D., et al. (2015). Updating ACSM's recommendations for exercise preparticipation health screening. *Medicine & Science in Sports & Exercise*, *47*(11), 2473–2479. doi:10.1249/MSS.0000000000000664.

Ruppar, T. M., & Conn, V. S. (2010). Interventions to promote physical activity in chronically ill adults. *The American Journal of Nursing*, *110*(7), 30–37.

Taylor-Pilae, R. E., et al. (2014). Effect of Tai Chi on physical function, fall rates and quality of life among older stroke survivors. *Archives of Physical Medicine and Rehabilitation*, *95*(5), 816–824. doi:10.1016/j.apmr.2014.01.001.

US Department of Health and Human Services. (2018). *Physical activity guidelines for Americans: Youth physical activity recommendations*. Washington, DC: US Department of Health and Human Services.

Readiness for enhanced Self-Care

Ruth A. Wittmann-Price, PhD, RN, CNS, CNE, CHSE, ANEF, FAAN

NANDA-I

Definition

A pattern of performing activities for oneself to meet health-related goals, which can be strengthened.

Defining Characteristics

Expresses desire to enhance independence with health; expresses desire to enhance independence with life; expresses desire to enhance independence with personal development; expresses desire to enhance independence with well-being; expresses desire to enhance knowledge of self-care strategies; expresses desire to enhance self-care

NOC   (Nursing Outcomes Classification)

Suggested NOC Outcomes

Adherence Behavior; Health-Seeking Behavior; Self-Care Status

Example NOC Outcome with Indicators
Health-Seeking Behavior as evidenced by the following indicators: Completes health-related tasks/Performs self-screening/Obtains assistance from health professionals. (Rate the outcome and indicators of **Health-Seeking Behavior:** 1 = never demonstrated, 2 = rarely demonstrated, 3 = sometimes demonstrated, 4 = often demonstrated, 5 = consistently demonstrated [see Section I].)

Client Outcomes

Client Will (Specify Time Frame)

- Evaluate current levels of self-care as optimum for abilities
- Express the need or desire to continue to enhance levels of self-care

● = Independent;   ▲ = Collaborative;   EBN = Evidence-Based Nursing;   EB = Evidence-Based

- Seek health-related information as needed
- Identify strategies to enhance self-care
- Perform appropriate interventions as needed
- Monitor level of self-care
- Evaluate the effectiveness of self-care interventions at regular intervals

NIC   (Nursing Interventions Classification)

Suggested NIC Interventions

Coping Enhancement; Energy Management; Learning Facilitation; Multidisciplinary Care Conference; Mutual Goal Setting; Self-Care Assistance

Example NIC Activity—Self-Care Assistance

Encourage person to perform normal activities of daily living to level of ability

Nursing Interventions and *Rationales*

- For assessment of self-care, use a valid and reliable screening tool if available for specific characteristics of the person, such as arthritis, diabetes, stroke, heart failure (HF), or dementia. **EBN:** *Bryant (2017) developed a Self-Care to Success toolkit that supports nurse practitioners to empower patients with HF and promote self-care behaviors (SCBs) successfully.* **EBN:** *Researchers completed a systematic review of self-care instruments (N = 26) and found seven instruments based on Orem's Self-Care Theory, but none of the instruments reviewed were fully recommended because of deficits in methodological quality and measurement properties (Matarese, Lommi, & DeMarinis, 2017). Conduct mutual goal setting with the person.* **EBN:** *Todhunter (2017) explored self-administered compression therapy for patients with chronic edema from venous and lymphatic impairment and found that by including patients in their treatment decisions they were empowered and more likely to be accountable.* **EBN:** *Researchers explored outcomes for patients with diabetic foot ulcers and found that the majority of focus was on patient compliance (adherence) rather than on self-care management. Researchers suggested that shifting focus to self-care will improve outcomes (Costa, del Pilar Camargo Plazas, & Tregunno, 2017).*
- Support the person's awareness that enhanced self-care is an achievable, desirable, and positive life goal. **EBN:** *Crown and Vogel (2017) completed a mixed-method pilot study of patients receiving hemodialysis in relation to self-care about dietary fluid restrictions. Researchers used motivational interviewing to promote self-care fluid management, and participants deemed it as helpful.* **EBN:** *Kauric-Klein, Peters, and Yarandi (2017) examined how educational sessions and individual counseling effected blood pressure self-efficacy and self-care outcomes in adults (N = 118) receiving hemodialysis, and results demonstrated that self-efficacy was related to SCBs such as decreased salt intake, lower weight gain, increased adherence to medications, and fewer missed appointments.*
- Show respect for the person, regardless of characteristics and/or background. **EBN:** *Marzband and Zakayi (2017) explored the concept of self-care from Islamic texts and found that self-care is participating in responsible activities to God for health promotion, preventive disease, and treatment. Self-care included physical, mental, spiritual, and social dimensions.* **EBN:** *Gowani, Gul, and Dhakam (2017) explored, using a cross-sectional survey, SCB among patients with HF in Karachi, Pakistan. The survey was the European Heart Failure Self-Care Behavior Scale, and of six variables, only three factored into self-care for this population, including education, income, and chronicity of the HF, suggesting that different populations define self-care differently.*
- Promote trust and enhanced communication between the person and health care providers. **EBN:** *Reb et al (2017) studied a Self-Management Survivorship Care Planning intervention in colorectal and lung cancer survivors (N = 30) with pretest and posttest and results revealing significant differences in depression, anxiety, self-efficacy, physical functioning, role limitations (physical, pain, general health, health transition, physical health summary), and total quality of life. Participants also expressed that they felt empowered from the nurse-driven intervention.* **EBN:** *Researchers studied the patient–provider relationships (communication, integration, collaboration, and empowerment) in pregnant patients (N = 139) in relation to better patient self-care and women's perceptions of better communication, collaboration, and empowerment from their midwives, which were associated with more frequent SCBs (Nicoloro-SantaBarbara et al, 2017).*

● = Independent;   ▲ = Collaborative;   **EBN** = Evidence-Based Nursing;   **EB** = Evidence-Based

- Promote opportunities for spiritual care and growth. **EBN:** *Salamizadeh, Mirzaei, and Ravari (2017) studied the effects of a spiritual care educational intervention with caretakers (N = 60) of Alzheimer's patients using a random group pretest–posttest method and concluded that spiritual care enhanced the self-efficacy of the caregivers.*
- Promote social support through facilitation of family involvement. **EB:** *Morgan et al (2017) performed a literature review regarding social support for self-management for patients to manage their chronic condition(s) in terms of disease control and found the two elements that were most important for self-care were commitment and empowerment.* **EB:** *Campbell et al (2017) examined the social adaptability index (SAI) with patients (N = 615) and its applicability to self-care and diabetes outcomes and revealed that the SAI was correlated with quality of life but not SCBs, suggesting that five items alone are not enough to explain self-care in relation to social adaptability for patients with type 2 diabetes.*
- Provide opportunities for ongoing group support through establishment of self-help groups on the Internet. **EB:** *Nickel, Trojan, and Kofahl (2017) studied the outcomes of a health care initiative "Self-Help Friendliness (SHF) and Patient-Centeredness in Health Care" to describe (1) how patients were involved in the development of SHF and (2) to test the survey. The study results identified the following important aspects of SHF: cooperation and involvement in establishing the quality criteria and it appears to be a good fit to study self-care groups.* **EB:** *Researchers completed a meta-analysis (N = 47) review to determine the effectiveness of group-based interventions compared with individual interventions for improving clinical, lifestyle, and psychosocial outcomes in people with type 2 diabetes. They found that group-based interventions are more effective than individual education at improving clinical, lifestyle, and psychosocial outcomes in people with type 2 diabetes (Odgers-Jewell et al, 2017).*
- Help the person identify and reduce the barriers to self-care. **EBN:** *Woith et al (2017) qualitatively explored homeless people's (N = 15) perceptions of their interactions with nurses and identified three major themes: (1) nurses should be civil, (2) SCBs, and (3) barriers to care indicating that homeless people find nurses uncivil toward them and this becomes a self-care barrier.* **EBN:** *Restorick Roberts, Betts Adams, and Beckette Warner (2017) used a mixed-methods study to look at the experience of living with chronic illness and identified barriers to self-care in older women (N = 130) and found that barriers to self-care included pain, lack of financial resources, and worry.*
- Provide literacy-appropriate education for self-care activities. **EBN:** *Lelorain et al (2017) studied health care professionals' perception of therapeutic patient education for promoting self-care and found that nurses often lack skills and knowledge, and are disillusioned about the effectiveness of therapeutic patient education and that* patient-centered care is needed *in many places to promote education that can increase self-care.* **EB:** *Hayward et al (2017) completed a pilot study in people with liver cirrhosis (N = 50) and found that only 54% of patients could recall being given written information and 64% had self-sought Internet information. In addition patients reported difficulties understanding the written material.*
- Facilitate self-efficacy by ensuring the adequacy of self-care education. **EBN:** *Grafton and Bassett (2017) studied HF patients' (N = 40) confidence in relation to self-care and found that confidence is an important element in successful self-care activities.* **EBN:** *Researchers used a correlation (a descriptive design to examine the relationship between glycemic control and SCBs in patients with type 2 diabetes) and found that patients with poor glycemic control had poorer self-efficacy and SCBs (D'Souza et al, 2017).*
- Provide alternative mind–body therapies such as reiki, guided imagery, yoga, and self-hypnosis. **EBN:** *Orellana-Rios et al (2017) piloted an "on the job" mindfulness and compassion-oriented meditation training for interdisciplinary team members (N = 27) designed to reduce distress, foster resilience, and strengthen a prosocial motivation in the clinical encounter. Improvements were realized in two burnout components (emotional exhaustion and personal accomplishment), and overall improvement of self-care.* **EB:** *Rothberg and Friedman (2017) completed a literature review about low back pain (LBP) and complementary therapies (spinal manipulation, massage, exercise, or yoga), and found that for patients with LBP evidence does not support the use of spinal manipulation or exercise therapy.*
- Promote the person's hope to maintain self-care. **EB:** *Anderson, Turner, and Clyne (2017) developed a self-management intervention called the Help to Overcome Problems Effectively (HOPE: MS) to improve the physical and psychological well-being of people living with multiple sclerosis (MS) and found that the HOPE: MS was helpful and useful to patients living with MS and covered the parameters needed to identify self-care needs.* **EB:** *Ritholz, MacNeil, and Weinger (2017) investigated how adults (N = 148) with diabetes were educated about microvascular complications and found the first discussions focused on prevention, but when complications occurred, 78% of participants perceived the provider-provided comprehensive interactive education; specific self-care guidance; reassuring messages; and referrals, follow-ups, and results indicated that training*

● = Independent;   ▲ = Collaborative;   **EBN** = Evidence-Based Nursing;   **EB** = Evidence-Based

is needed to help providers discuss complications with honest but positive messages so diabetic patients can remained informed and maintain hope.

Pediatric

- Assess and evaluate a child's level of self-care and adjust strategies as needed. **EBN:** *Sawin et al (2017) developed a theory-based conversation guide to assist parents of hospitalized chronically ill children better prepare for self-management of home care for the child and found the theory-based intervention operationalized self-management was well-received.* **EB:** *Burns-Nader, Joe, and Pinion (2017) studied using computer tablets with children who were burned during treatments, and nurses reported significantly less pain and anxiety for the tablet distraction group compared with the control group.*
- Assist families to engage in and maintain social support networks. **EB:** *Pumar-Mendez et al (2017) interviewed stakeholders (N = 90) in six countries about the support for self-care for patients with chronic illness (SSSC) and investigated the stakeholders' roles. The stakeholders described the ideal SSSC as inclusive, interdependent, and patient-centered and needed support was from patients, governments, health care professionals, associations, private companies, and the media. The recommendations were to continue to promote SSSC with stakeholders and health professionals to improve care.* **EB:** *Researchers qualitatively studied a parenting intervention, Circle of Security, for mothers with mood and anxiety disorders at a pediatric clinic and through surveys and medical records found that the intervention is feasible and will assist with pediatric care (Kimmel et al, 2017).*
- Encourage activities that support or enhance spiritual care. **EBN:** *O'Shea et al (2017) completed a qualitative descriptive study about meeting the physical, emotional, and spiritual needs of parents with seriously ill children and found there was a need among providers to enhance both basic education and advanced skills in pediatric palliative and end-of-life care education statewide.* **EB:** *Campos, Soria, and Liz (2016) studied pediatric complex chronic conditions (CCC) by developing a multidisciplinary team (called the PRINCEP program) that included a pediatrician, nurse, social worker, and psychospiritual specialist to offer patient-centered care. The program assisted with family's needs being met and better satisfaction.*

Multicultural

- Identify cultural beliefs, values, lifestyle practices, and problem-solving strategies when assessing the client's level of self-care. **EB:** *Oh, Ell, and Palinkas (2017) studied SCBs (healthy diet, exercise, self-blood glucose monitoring, and foot care) to see if changes in them predicted depression in low-income Hispanic patients with diabetes. Results supported that poor diet and lack of exercise are indicators of depression.* **EB:** *Researchers evaluated the validity and reliability of the Danish version of the European Heart Failure Self-Care Behavior Scale (EHFScBS-9) on a Danish population of patients (N = 147) and found it a valid and reliable instrument to assess HF self-care behaviors in a Danish population (Ostergaard et al, 2017). Enhance cultural knowledge by seeking out information regarding different cultural or ethnic groups.* **EBN:** *Researchers studied the COM-B model (consisting of capability, opportunity, and motivation) to explore SCBs and examine the self-care confidence on Chinese patients (N = 321) with chronic HF and found that Chinese patients have poor SCBs caused by lack of confidence, functional capacity, knowledge, and health literacy (Zou et al, 2017).*
- Recognize the effect of culture on SCBs. **EB:** *Researchers studied the elements that effect self-care in HF patients (N = 226) in Jordan by looking at knowledge, sociodemographics, and SCBs. Results revealed that knowledge, income, and educational levels; shorter duration of disease; fewer people living at home; older age; and being unemployed were significant predictors of low self-care scores (Tawalbeh et al, 2017).*
- Provide culturally competent care. **EBN:** *Labore et al (2017) culturally explored the meaning of transition to self-care in sickle cell disease patients using an existential framework, and meaning was found in lived time, space, body, and human relationship.* **EB:** *DiZazzo-Miller et al (2017) completed a qualitative study to examine providers' perspectives on cultural barriers and facilitators to diabetes self-management in Arab Americans, and results identified that the main barriers are the disease itself and patients' denial or refusal to recognize the diabetes. These findings reflect the cultural stigma associated with diabetes by many Arab Americans.*
- Support independent self-care activities. **EBN:** *Teppala et al (2017) studied post-acute rehabilitation for patients with hip fracture by examining the variation in mobility and self-care using a retrospective cohort study and found variation in discharge mobility and self-care related to health care organization differences.* **EB:** *Researchers investigated self-care deficits, health behaviors, and management of patients (N = 12) with chronic systemic sclerosis because it affects a person's physical, emotional, psychosocial, and spiritual dimensions. They found Thai patients developed specific self-care agencies to improve their health and well-being.*

● = Independent;   ▲ = Collaborative;   **EBN** = Evidence-Based Nursing;   **EB** = Evidence-Based

The study assists in the understanding of how patients live and cope with systemic sclerosis (Hornboonherm et al, 2017).

 Home Care

- The nursing interventions described previously may also be used in home care settings. **EBN:** *Revell (2017) studied nausea and vomiting in pregnancy and patients' coping mechanisms and found that many women self-manage and the condition affects both psychological and physiological well-being. Nausea and vomiting interrupt activities of daily living and self-care should be augmented by provider-implemented management.* **EBN:** *Lee et al (2017) studied rural residents (N = 580) with HF to explore the variables (health literacy, psychosocial status, current symptom status, and aging status) related to self-care and found that depressive symptoms, lower perceived control, better symptom status, and annual income of <$20,000 were negatively associated with self-care. Support the new sense of self that may occur with complex health problems.* **EBN:** *Kao, Chuang, and Chen (2017) studied chronic disease self-management using smartphone applications that support patient self-management of chronic disease, facilitating health management, and health promotion, which have been shown to assist health care professionals and patients manage their diseases.* **EB:** *Chang et al (2017) explored depression's effect on self-care, self-care confidence, and resilience in stable outpatients (N = 201) with HF and found depression reduced self-care by decreasing self-care confidence for patients with moderate and high levels of resilience.*

- Assist individuals and families to prevent exacerbations of chronic illness symptoms so rehospitalization is not necessary. **EB:** *Blashill et al (2017) studied the relationship of body image, self-care, and depression in HIV-positive minority men (N = 44) comparing cognitive behavioral therapy as a mediator and found that it assisted in improving body image and HIV SCBs.* **EB:** *Patel et al (2017) studied African American women (N = 422), asthmatics, and a telephone-based self-regulation intervention and compared the results with a control group. Findings demonstrated that patients who completed a culturally responsive self-care program had improvements in asthma outcomes when compared with the control group, even when comorbidities were present. In complex chronic illnesses such as HF, individuals and families should be helped to accept continued functional disabilities and work toward maintenance of optimum functional status, considering the reality of illness status.* **EB:** *Reid et al (2017) studied cognitive-behavioral pain self-management by older adults (N = 588) with activity-limiting pain living at home in a randomized control trial and found no significant result differences in the treatment and control groups, indicating other variables should be explored.* **EBN:** *Lai, Ching, and Wong (2017) studied experiences of patients (N = 10) with breast cancer using a mixed-methods approach and found that chemotherapy affected the patients in different ways. Most women adopted behavioral, social, cognitive, and emotional strategies to cope, and researchers found that chemotherapy can be equated to going on a hike.*

- Use educational guidelines for stroke survivors. **EB:** *Murdolo et al (2017) studied the Graded Repetitive Arm Supplementary Program (GRASP) with patients who experienced a stroke. Patients perceived the program as helpful in activities of daily living during the acute stroke phase.* **EB:** *Atler et al (2017) completed a study about yoga as an intervention in poststroke patients (N = 13), and five themes were identified from qualitative analysis: (1) improved abilities, (2) gained new knowledge, (3) enhanced engagement in activities, (4) improved relaxation, and (5) increased confidence.*

- Ensure appropriate *interdisciplinary communication to support client safety.* **EB:** *Johnson et al (2017) explored the consensus of an expert panel related to over-the-counter (OTC) proton pump inhibitors (PPIs) for gastroesophageal reflux disease and found that although OTC PPI would probably not mask gastric cancer, effect bone density, Clostridium difficile infection, or cardiovascular adverse events, they may be associated with slightly increased risks for infectious diarrhea, certain idiosyncratic reactions, and cirrhosis-related spontaneous bacterial peritonitis.*

- For public safety health *care professionals and consumers should participate in decision-making when managing reflux-related symptoms in the self-care setting.* **EBN:** *Mackintosh et al (2017) explored the experiences of women (N = 22) with pregnancy complications and found that women and relatives used self-diagnosis, self-care, and seeking triage, but they also found that health care providers did not pay attention to their needs as they saw appropriate and therefore did not encompass "safety partnerships."*

- Enhance individual and family coping with chronic illnesses. **EBN:** *Kim and Kim (2017) studied elements that effected health-related quality of life (HRQOL) in elderly patients (N = 365) with diabetes and found that gender (male) and depression were negatively correlated with diabetic self-care.* **EB:** *Kessing et al (2017) investigated quality of life in patients (N = 459) with HF in relation to self-care and found that quality of life and degree of self-care was affected by depression and could be affected poorly by increased anxiety.*

● = Independent;   ▲ = Collaborative;   **EBN** = Evidence-Based Nursing;   **EB** = Evidence-Based

- Implement a community care management program. EBN: *Merius and Rohan (2017) completed a literature review (N = 14) related to adult attrition from community programs on diabetes self-care and found barriers for retention included transportation, family obligations, and scheduling conflicts.*

 Client/Family Teaching and Discharge Planning

- Teach clients how to regularly assess their level of self-care.
- Instruct clients that a variety of interventions may be needed to enhance self-care.
- Help clients to understand that enhanced self-care is an achievable goal.
- Empower clients.
- Teach clients about the decision-making process and self-care activities needed to manage their illness state and promote well-being.
- Continuously stress that all self-care activities must be regularly evaluated to ensure that enhanced levels of self-care can be maintained.

REFERENCES

Anderson, J. K., Turner, A., & Clyne, W. (2017). Development and feasibility of the Help to Overcome Problems Effectively (HOPE) self-management intervention for people living with multiple sclerosis. *Disability & Rehabilitation, 39*(11), 1114–1121. Retrieved from http://dx.doi.org.fmarion.idm.oclc.org/10.1080/09638288.2016.1181211.

Atler, K. E., Van Puymbroeck, M., Portz, J. D., et al. (2017). Participant-perceived outcomes of merging yoga and occupational therapy: Self-management intervention for people post stroke. *British Journal of Occupational Therapy, 80*(5), 294–301. Retrieved from http://dx.doi.org.fmarion.idm.oclc.org/10.1177/0308022617690536.

Blashill, A. J., Safren, S. A., Wilhelm, S., et al. (2017). Cognitive behavioral therapy for body image and self-care (CBT-BISC) in sexual minority men living with HIV: A randomized controlled trial. *Health Psychology, 36*(10), 937–946. Retrieved from http://dx.doi.org.fmarion.idm.oclc.org/10.1037/hea0000505.

Bryant, R. (2017). Heart failure: Self-care to success: Development and evaluation of a program toolkit. *Nurse Practitioner, 42*(8), 1–8. Retrieved from http://dx.doi.org.fmarion.idm.oclc.org/10.1097/01.NPR.0000520833.22030.d0.

Burns-Nader, S., Joe, L., & Pinion, K. (2017). Computer tablet distraction reduces pain and anxiety in pediatric burn patients undergoing hydrotherapy: A randomized trial. *Burns: Journal of the International Society for Burn Injuries, 43*(6), 1203–1211. Retrieved from http://dx.doi.org.fmarion.idm.oclc.org/10.1016/j.burns.2017.02.015.

Campbell, J. A., Walker, R. J., Smalls, B. L., et al. (2017). Use of social adaptability index to explain self-care and diabetes outcomes. *BMC Endocrine Disorders, 17*, 1–9. Retrieved from http://dx.doi.org.fmarion.idm.oclc.org/10.1186/s12902-017-0185-3.

Campos, S. R., Soria, E. L., & Liz, A. A. (2016). PRINCEP program: Clinical program for specialized and integrated care of paediatric patients with complex chronic conditions. *International Journal of Integrated Care, 16*(6), 1–2. Retrieved from http://dx.doi.org.fmarion.idm.oclc.org/10.5334/ijic.2669.

Chang, L., Wu, S., Chiang, C., et al. (2017). Depression and self-care maintenance in patients with heart failure: A moderated mediation model of self-care confidence and resilience. *European Journal of Cardiovascular Nursing, 16*(5), 435–443. Retrieved from http://dx.doi.org.fmarion.idm.oclc.org/10.1177/1474515116687179.

Costa, I. G., del Pilar Camargo Plazas, P. M. P., & Tregunno, D. (2017). Rethinking self-care management for individuals with diabetic foot ulcers. *Wounds International, 8*(2), 22–26.

Crown, S., & Vogel, J. A. (2017). Enhancing self-care management of interdialytic fluid weight gain in patients on hemodialysis: A pilot study using motivational interviewing. *Nephrology Nursing Journal, 44*(1), 49–56. MEDLINE Info: *NLM UID:* 100909377.

DiZazzo-Miller, R., Pociask, F. D., Bertran, E. A., et al. (2017). Diabetes is devastating, and insulin is a death sentence: Provider perspectives of diabetes self-management in Arab-American patients. *Clinical Diabetes, 35*(1), 43–50. Retrieved from http://dx.doi.org.fmarion.idm.oclc.org/10.2337/cd15-0030.

D'Souza, M. S., Karkada, S. N., Parahoo, K., et al. (2017). Self-efficacy and self-care behaviours among adults with type 2 diabetes. *Applied Nursing Research, 36*, 25–32. Retrieved from http://dx.doi.org.fmarion.idm.oclc.org/10.1016/j.apnr.2017.05.004.

Gowani, A., Gul, R., & Dhakam, S. (2017). Self-care and its predictors among patients with heart failure in Karachi, Pakistan. *British Journal of Cardiac Nursing, 12*(7), 333–338. Retrieved from http://dx.doi.org.fmarion.idm.oclc.org/10.12968/bjca.2017.12.7.333.

Grafton, T., & Bassett, A. (2017). The role of confidence in self-care of patients with a diagnosis of heart failure. *Medsurg Nursing, 26*(4), 263–268. MEDLINE Info: *NLM UID:* 9300545.

Hayward, K. L., Horsfall, L. U., Ruffin, B. J., et al. (2017). Optimising care of patients with chronic disease: Patient-oriented education may improve disease knowledge and self-management. *Internal Medicine Journal, 47*(8), 952–955. Retrieved from http://dx.doi.org.fmarion.idm.oclc.org/10.1111/imj.13505.

Hornboonherm, P., Nanagara, R., Kochamat, A., et al. (2017). Self-care behaviours and trajectory management by people with scleroderma in northeastern Thailand. *International Journal of Nursing Practice, 23*(3). Retrieved from http://dx.doi.org.fmarion.idm.oclc.org/10.1111/ijn.12523.

Johnson, D., Katz, P., Armstrong, D., et al. (2017). The safety of appropriate use of over-the-counter proton pump inhibitors: An evidence-based review and Delphi consensus. *Drugs, 77*(5), 547–561. Retrieved from http://dx.doi.org.fmarion.idm.oclc.org/10.1007/s40265-017-0712-6.

Kao, C., Chuang, H., & Chen, T. (2017). The utilization of health-related applications in chronic disease self-management. *Journal of Nursing, 64*(4), 19–25. Retrieved from http://dx.doi.org.fmarion.idm.oclc.org/10.6224/JN.000050.

Kauric-Klein, Z., Peters, R. M., & Yarandi, H. N. (2017). Self-efficacy and blood pressure self-care behaviors in patients on chronic hemodialysis. *Western Journal of Nursing Research, 39*(7), 886–905. Retrieved from http://dx.doi.org.fmarion.idm.oclc.org/10.1177/0193945916661322.

Kessing, D., Denollet, J., Widdershoven, J., et al. (2017). Self-care and health-related quality of life in chronic heart failure: A longitudinal analysis. *European Journal of Cardiovascular Nursing, 16*(7), 605–613. Retrieved from http://dx.doi.org.fmarion.idm.oclc.org/10.1177/1474515117702021.

Kim, H., & Kim, K. (2017). Health-related quality-of-life and diabetes self-care activity in elderly patients with diabetes in Korea. *Journal*

S

- = Independent; ▲ = Collaborative; EBN = Evidence-Based Nursing; EB = Evidence-Based

of Community Health, 42(5), 998–1007. Retrieved from http://dx.doi.org.fmarion.idm.oclc.org/10.1007/s10900-017-0347-2.

Kimmel, M. C., Cluxton-Keller, F., Frosch, E., et al. (2017). Maternal experiences in a parenting group delivered in an urban general pediatric clinic. *Clinical Pediatrics, 56*(1), 13–19. Retrieved from http://dx.doi.org.fmarion.idm.oclc.org/10.1177/0009922816675012.

Labore, N., Mawn, B., Dixon, J., et al. (2017). Exploring transition to self-management within the culture of sickle cell disease. *Journal of Transcultural Nursing, 28*(1), 70–78. Retrieved from http://dx.doi.org.fmarion.idm.oclc.org/10.1177/1043659615609404.

Lai, X. B., Ching, S. S. Y., & Wong, F. K. Y. (2017). A qualitative exploration of the experiences of patients with breast cancer receiving outpatient-based chemotherapy. *Journal of Advanced Nursing, 73*(10), 2339–2350. Retrieved from http://dx.doi.org.fmarion.idm.oclc.org/10.1111/jan.13309.

Matarese, M., Lommi, M., & DeMarinis, M. G. (2017). Systematic review of measurement properties of self-reported instruments for evaluating self-care in adults. *Journal of Advanced Nursing, 73*(6), 1272–1287. Retrieved from http://dx.doi.org.fmarion.idm.oclc.org/10.1111/jan.13204.

Lee, K. S., Moser, D. K., Pelter, M. M., et al. (2017). Self-care in rural residents with heart failure: What we are missing. *European Journal of Cardiovascular Nursing, 16*(4), 326–333. Retrieved from http://dx.doi.org.fmarion.idm.oclc.org/10.1177/1474515116666439.

Lelorain, S., Bachelet, A., Bertin, N., et al. (2017). French healthcare professionals' perceived barriers to and motivation for therapeutic patient education: A qualitative study. *Nursing & Health Sciences, 19*(3), 331–339. Retrieved from http://dx.doi.org.fmarion.idm.oclc.org/10.1111/nhs.12350.

Mackintosh, N., Rance, S., Carter, W., et al. (2017). Working for patient safety: A qualitative study of women's help-seeking during acute perinatal events. *BMC Pregnancy and Childbirth, 17*, 1–13. Retrieved from http://dx.doi.org.fmarion.idm.oclc.org/10.1186/s12884-017-1401-x.

Marzband, R., & Zakayi, A. A. (2017). A concept analysis of self-care based on Islamic sources. *International Journal of Nursing Knowledge, 28*(3), 153–158. Retrieved from http://dx.doi.org.fmarion.idm.oclc.org/10.1111/2047-3095.12126.

Merius, H. N., & Rohan, A. J. (2017). An integrative review of factors associated with patient attrition from community health worker programs that support diabetes self-care. *Journal of Community Health Nursing, 34*(4), 214–228. Retrieved from http://dx.doi.org.fmarion.idm.oclc.org/10.1080/07370016.2017.1369811.

Morgan, H. M., Entwistle, V. A., Cribb, A., et al. (2017). We need to talk about purpose: A critical interpretive synthesis of health and social care professionals' approaches to self-management support for people with long-term conditions. *Health Expectations, 20*(2), 243–259. Retrieved from http://dx.doi.org.fmarion.idm.oclc.org/10.1111/hex.12453.

Murdolo, Y., Brown, T., Fielding, L., et al. (2017). Stroke survivors' experiences of using the Graded Repetitive Arm Supplementary Program (GRASP) in an Australian acute hospital setting: A mixed-methods pilot study. *Australian Occupational Therapy Journal, 64*(4), 305–313. Retrieved from http://dx.doi.org.fmarion.idm.oclc.org/10.1111/1440-1630.12363.

Nickel, S., Trojan, A., & Kofahl, C. (2017). Involving self-help groups in health-care institutions: The patients' contribution to and their view of 'self-help friendliness' as an approach to implement quality criteria of sustainable co-operation. *Health Expectations, 20*(2), 274–287. Retrieved from http://dx.doi.org.fmarion.idm.oclc.org/10.1111/hex.12455.

Nicoloro-SantaBarbara, J., Rosenthal, L., Auerbach, M., et al. (2017). Patient-provider communication, maternal anxiety, and self-care in pregnancy. *Social Science & Medicine, 190*, 133–140. Retrieved from http://dx.doi.org.fmarion.idm.oclc.org/10.1016/j.socscimed.2017.08.011.

Odgers-Jewell, K., Ball, L. E., Kelly, J. T., et al. (2017). Effectiveness of group-based self-management education for individuals with Type 2 diabetes: A systematic review with meta-analyses and meta-regression. *Diabetic Medicine, 34*(8), 1027–1039. Retrieved from http://dx.doi.org.fmarion.idm.oclc.org/10.1111/dme.13340.

Oh, H., Ell, K., & Palinkas, L. A. (2017). Self-care behavior change and depression among low-income predominantly Hispanic patients in safety-net clinics. *Social Work in Health Care, 56*(8), 714–732. Retrieved from http://dx.doi.org.fmarion.idm.oclc.org/10.1080/00981389.2017.1333972.

Orellana-Rios, C. L., Radbruch, L., Kern, M., et al. (2017). Mindfulness and compassion-oriented practices at work reduce distress and enhance self-care of palliative care teams: A mixed-method evaluation of an "on the job" program. *BMC Palliative Care, 17*, 1–15. Retrieved from http://dx.doi.org.fmarion.idm.oclc.org/10.1186/s12904-017-0219-7.

O'Shea, E. R., Lavallee, M., Doyle, E. A., et al. (2017). Assessing palliative and end-of-life educational needs of pediatric health care professionals: Results of a statewide survey. *Journal of Hospice & Palliative Nursing, 19*(5), 468–473. Retrieved from http://dx.doi.org.fmarion.idm.oclc.org/10.1097/NJH.0000000000000374.

Ostergaard, B., Mahrer-Imhof, R., Lauridsen, J., et al. (2017). Validity and reliability of the Danish version of the 9-item European Heart Failure Self-Care Behavior Scale. *Scandinavian Journal of Caring Sciences, 31*(2), 405–412. Retrieved from http://dx.doi.org.fmarion.idm.oclc.org/10.1111/scs.12342.

Patel, M. R., Song, P. X. K., Sanders, G., et al. (2017). A randomized clinical trial of a culturally responsive intervention for African American women with asthma. *Annals of Allergy, Asthma & Immunology, 118*(2), 212–219. Retrieved from http://dx.doi.org.fmarion.idm.oclc.org/10.1016/j.anai.2016.11.016.

Pumar-Mendez, M. J., Muika, A., Regaira, E., et al. (2017). Stakeholders in support systems for self-care for chronic illness: The gap between expectations and reality regarding their identity, roles and relationships. *Health Expectations, 20*(3), 434–447. Retrieved from http://dx.doi.org.fmarion.idm.oclc.org/10.1111/hex.12471.

Reb, A., Ruel, N., Marwan, L. L., et al. (2017). Empowering survivors after colorectal and lung cancer treatment: Pilot study of a Self-Management Survivorship Care Planning intervention. *European Journal of Oncology Nursing, 29*, 125–134. Retrieved from http://dx.doi.org.fmarion.idm.oclc.org/10.1016/j.ejon.2017.06.003.

Reid, M. C., Henderson, C. R., Trachtenberg, M. A., et al. (2017). Implementing a pain self-management protocol in home care: A cluster-randomized pragmatic trial. *Journal of the American Geriatrics Society, 65*(8), 1667–1675. Retrieved from http://dx.doi.org.fmarion.idm.oclc.org/10.1111/jgs.14836.

Restorick Roberts, A., Betts Adams, K., & Beckette Warner, C. (2017). Effects of chronic illness on daily life and barriers to self-care for older women: A mixed-methods exploration. *Journal of Women & Aging, 29*(2), 126–136. Retrieved from http://dx.doi.org.fmarion.idm.oclc.org/10.1080/08952841.2015.1080539.

Revell, M. A. (2017). Self-care of nausea and vomiting in the first trimester of pregnancy. *International Journal of Childbirth Education, 32*(1), 35–38. MEDLINE Info: *NLM UID:* 8712412.

Ritholz, M. D., MacNeil, T., & Weinger, K. (2017). Difficult conversations: Adults with diabetes and the discussion of microvascular complications. *Diabetic Medicine, 34*(10), 1447–1455. Retrieved from http://dx.doi.org.fmarion.idm.oclc.org/10.1111/dme.13419.

Rothberg, S., & Friedman, B. W. (2017). Complementary therapies in addition to medication for patients with nonchronic, nonradicular low back pain: A systematic review. *The American Journal of Emergency Medicine, 35*(1), 55–61. Retrieved from http://dx.doi.org.fmarion.idm.oclc.org/10.1016/j.ajem.2016.10.001.

Tawalbeh, L. I., Al Qadire, M., Ahmad, M. M., et al. (2017). Knowledge and self-care behaviors among patients with heart failure in Jordan.

● = Independent; ▲ = Collaborative; **EBN** = Evidence-Based Nursing; **EB** = Evidence-Based

Research in Nursing & Health, 40(4), 350–359. Retrieved from http://dx.doi.org.fmarion.idm.oclc.org/10.1002/nur.21805.

Salamizadeh, A., Mirzaei, T., & Ravari, A. (2017). The impact of spiritual care education on the self-efficacy of the family caregivers of elderly people with Alzheimer's disease. *International Journal of Community Based Nursing & Midwifery*, 5(3), 231–238. MEDLINE Info: NLM UID: 101615484.

Sawin, K. J., Weiss, M. E., Johnson, N., et al. (2017). Development of a self-management theory-guided discharge intervention for parents of hospitalized children. *Journal of Nursing Scholarship*, 49(2), 202–213. Retrieved from http://dx.doi.org.fmarion.idm. oclc.org/10.1111/jnu.12284.

Teppala, S., Ottenbacher, K. J., Eschbach, K., et al. (2017). Variation in functional status after hip fracture: Facility and regional influence on mobility and self-care. *Journals of Gerontology Series A: Biological*

Sciences & Medical Sciences, 72(10), 1376–1382. Retrieved from http://dx.doi.org.fmarion.idm.oclc.org/10.1093/gerona/glw249.

Todhunter, J. (2017). Empowering patients to self-care with a Velcro wrap compression device. *Journal of Community Nursing*, 31(4), 28–33. MEDLINE Info: NLM UID: 101090738.

Woith, W. M., Kerber, C., Astroth, K. S., et al. (2017). Lessons from the homeless: Civil and uncivil interactions with nurses, self-care behaviors, and barriers to care. *Nursing Forum*, 52(3), 211–220. Retrieved from http://dx.doi.org.fmarion.idm.oclc.org/10.1111/nuf.12191.

Zou, H., Chen, Y., Fang, W., et al. (2017). Identification of factors associated with self-care behaviors using the COM-B model in patients with chronic heart failure. *European Journal of Cardiovascular Nursing*, 16(6), 530–538. Retrieved from http://dx.doi.org.fmarion.idm.oclc.org/10.1177/1474515117695722.

Bathing Self-Care deficit   Linda S. Williams, RN, MSN

NANDA-I

Definition

Inability to independently complete cleansing activities.

Defining Characteristics

Impaired ability to access bathroom; impaired ability to access water; impaired ability to dry body; impaired ability to gather bathing supplies; impaired ability to regulate bath water; impaired ability to wash body

Related Factors

Anxiety; decrease in motivation; environmental barrier; pain; weakness

Associated Condition

Alteration in cognitive functioning; impaired ability to perceive body part; impaired ability to perceive spatial relationships; musculoskeletal impairment; neuromuscular impairment; perceptual disorders

NOC   (Nursing Outcomes Classification)

Suggested NOC Outcomes

Self-Care: Activities of Daily Living (ADLs); Self-Care: Bathing; Self-Care: Hygiene

> **Example NOC Outcome with Indicators**
>
> **Self-Care: ADLs** as evidenced by the following indicators: Bathing/Hygiene. (Rate outcome and indicators of **Self-Care: ADLs**: 1 = severely compromised, 2 = substantially compromised, 3 = moderately compromised, 4 = mildly compromised, 5 = not compromised [see Section I].)

Client Outcomes

Client Will (Specify Time Frame)

- Remain free of body odor and maintain intact skin
- State satisfaction with ability to use adaptive devices to bathe
- Use methods to bathe safely and effectively with minimal difficulty
- Bathe with assistance of caregiver as needed and report satisfaction and dignity maintained during bathing experience
- Bathe with assistance of caregiver as needed without exhibiting defensive (aggressive) behaviors

● = Independent;   ▲ = Collaborative;   EBN = Evidence-Based Nursing;   EB = Evidence-Based

NIC (Nursing Interventions Classification)

Suggested NIC Intervention

Self-Care Assistance: Bathing/Hygiene

Example NIC Activities—Self-Care Assistance: Bathing/Hygiene
Determine amount and type of assistance needed; Consider the culture of the client when promoting self-care activities; Provide assistance until client is fully able to assume self-care

Nursing Interventions and *Rationales*

- QSEN (Patient-Centered): Ask patients about their bathing preferences, which can increase patient privacy and satisfaction. **EBN:** *Perceptions of patients (N = 71) after an acute myocardial infarction who received bed baths were not as positive as those of patients who took showers (Lopes, Nogueira-Martins, & Barros, 2013).*
- QSEN (Safety): Warm bathing area above 25.1°C (77.18°F) while bathing, especially on cold days. **EB:** *Bathing and ambient temperature decreasing from 25.1°C can be a trigger for increasing occurrence of out-of-hospital cardiac arrest (Nishiyama et al, 2011).*
- QSEN (Safety): Use chlorhexidine-impregnated cloths rather than soap and water for daily patient bathing. **EB:** *Chlorhexidine reduces hospital-acquired infection risk from the potentially harmful pathogens methicillin-resistant* Staphylococcus aureus *(MRSA) and vancomycin-resistant enterococcus (VRE) (Kassakian et al, 2011).*
- QSEN (Safety): Consider using a prepackaged bath, especially for patients at high risk for infection (older adult, immunocompromised, invasive procedures, wounds, catheters, drains), to avoid patient exposure to multidrug-resistant pathogens from contaminated bath basins. **EB:** *In a 44-month study by Marchaim et al (2012), hospital bath basins (N = 1103) were found 62.2% of the time to be contaminated with hospital-acquired pathogens.*
- QSEN (Safety): Use chlorhexidine gluconate for bath basin bathing. **EBN:** *Powers et al (2012) found in a study (N = 90) that when patients are bathed with chlorhexidine gluconate the bacterial growth in the bath basin is significantly reduced.*
- QSEN (Patient-Centered): Use patient-centered bathing interventions: plan for patient's comfort and bathing preferences, show respect in communications, critically think to solve issues that arise, and use a gentle approach. **CEB:** *Focusing on the patient rather than the task of bathing results in greater comfort and fewer aggressive behaviors, which are likely defensive behaviors that result from feeling threatened or anxious, and increase with shower (especially) and tub bathing (Hoeffer et al, 2006).*
- ▲ Provide pain relief measures, such as ice packs, heat, and analgesics for sore joints 45 minutes before bathing; move extremities slowly and carefully; and inform the client before movements associated with pain occur (walking; transferring to a new location; moving joints; and washing genitals, face, and between toes and under arms). Have the client wash painful areas; recognize indicators of pain and apologize for any pain caused. **CEB:** *Pain relief and client participation reduce discomfort, preserve dignity, and give a sense of control (Rader et al, 2006).*
- Use a comfortable padded shower chair with foot support, or adapt a chair: pad it with towels/washcloths, cover the cold back with dry towels, and cover the arms with foam pipe insulation. **CEB:** *Unpadded shower chairs with large openings and no foot support contribute to pain by allowing clients to sink into the opening with their feet unsupported (Rader et al, 2006).*
- Ensure that bathing assistance preserves client dignity through use of privacy with a traffic-free bathing area and posted privacy signs, timeliness of personal care, and conveyance of honor and recognition of the deservedness of respect and esteem of all persons. **CEBN:** *Older adults report that dignity is promoted via respect, independence, exerting control, timeliness, privacy for the body, cleanliness, independence and sufficient time from staff, attitudes toward older people, and communication (Webster & Bryan, 2009).*
- For cognitively impaired clients, avoid upsetting factors associated with bathing: instead of using the terms *bath, shower,* or *wash,* use comforting words, such as *warm, relaxing,* or *massage.* Start at the client's feet and bathe upward; bathe the face last after washing hands and using a clean cloth. Use a beautician/barber or wash hair at another time to avoid water dripping in the face. **CEB:** *Some words are associated*

● = Independent;   ▲ = Collaborative;   **EBN** = Evidence-Based Nursing;   **EB** = Evidence-Based

with unpleasant bathing experiences, whereas others convey a pleasant bathing experience. Starting with the face or hair is distressing, because water drips on the face and the head becomes cold and wet (Rader et al, 2006).

- Use towel bathing to bathe client in bed, a bath blanket, and warm towels to keep the client covered the entire time. Warm and moisten towels/washcloths and place in plastic bags to keep them warm. Use the towels to massage large areas (front, back) and one washcloth for facial areas and another one for genital areas. No rinsing or drying is needed as is commonly thought for bathing. **CEB:** *Towel bathing is a gentle experience with less discomfort that significantly reduces aggression as well as bathing time and soap residue after showering without accumulation of pathogenic bacteria (Hoeffer et al, 2006).*

- QSEN (Patient-Centered): For shower bathing use patient-centered techniques, keep patient covered with towels and cleanse under the towels, use no-rinse products, use favorite bathing items, and use a handheld shower with adjustable spray. **CEB:** *Covering the patient is an easy means to maintain dignity, reduce embarrassment, and keep the patient warm and unexposed without increasing bathing time (Rader et al, 2006).*

▲ QSEN (Teamwork and Collaboration): Request referral of patient who has had a stroke to rehabilitation services. **EB:** *In a systematic review of 19 studies, Mehrholz et al (2012) found that electromechanical and robot-assisted arm training devices used in rehabilitation may assist in improving arm function after stroke, which is important for ADLs such as bathing.*

▲ QSEN (Patient-Centered): Use a wrapped warm footbath for relaxation in patients with cancer. **EBN:** *Yamamoto and Nagata (2011) found in a randomized controlled trial that the wrapped warm footbath in patients with cancer can increase relaxation and provide pain relief.*

 ## Geriatric

- QSEN (Patient-Centered, Safety): Advocate for the use of the Bathing Without a Battle educational program for patients with dementia. **EB:** *In a randomized crossover diffusion study, the Bathing Without a Battle educational program that trains caregivers in methods for improving the bathing experience of patients with dementia in nursing homes was found to be effective in reducing the rate of aggressive and agitated behaviors (Gozalo et al, 2014).*

- QSEN (Patient-Centered): Provide nighttime bathing options for nursing home residents. **EBN:** *Hashimoto (2014), in an interview survey of administrators of nursing homes (N = 3), found that nighttime bathing options provided more flexibility for bathing needs, improved sleep, and quality of life for the residents, and for caregivers it provided improved care quality and ability to provide patient-centered care.*

- Design the bathing environment for comfort: **Visual.** Reduce clutter and use partitions to hide equipment storage. Laminate and put artwork or decorative objects in bather's view, or place cue cards to bathing process (wall, ceiling, shower). Stand or sit in bather's position to experience what he or she sees. Decrease glare from tiles, white walls, and artificial lights. Use contrasting colors and soft but adequate lighting on a dimming switch for adjustment. *Bathing rooms are sterile, institutional, and frightening spaces filled with unfamiliar equipment—tubs with sides that open up and look like they might swallow you, or gurneys with arms that look like construction cranes. Overhead lights can be bright and shine into the bather's eyes. Glare can cause visual discomfort, especially in clients with visual changes or cataracts (Calkins, 2005).*

- Arrange the bathing environment to promote sensory comfort: **Auditory.** Reduce noise of voices and water. Do not allow traffic into bathing room. Add fabric to absorb sound (three to four times the width of the opening for sound-absorbing folds). Play soft music. **CEB:** *Noise discomfort can result from high-echo tiled walls, loud voices, and running water. Traffic can compromise privacy. Absorb negative sounds, and add positive sounds through music (Calkins, 2005).* **EBN:** *In an observational study (N = 53) by Joosse (2012), sound was a predictor of agitation for those with dementia.*

- Design the bathing environment for comfort: **Tactile.** Use heat lamps or radiant heat panels to keep the room warm. Use powder-coated grab bars in decorative colors with nonslip grip. Provide a soft rug to stand on. Ensure that flooring is not slippery (a high coefficient of friction, ideally above 80, is desired and obtained through flooring coatings). **CEB:** *If the caregiver is warm to the point of sweating, room temperature is about right for an older person being bathed. Appealing, stable grab bars are needed for balance. Preventing the floor from becoming slippery from water is essential (Calkins, 2005).*

- Use music during shower for clients with dementia. *Music may reduce agitation and improve moods to increase job satisfaction (Ray & Fitzsimmons, 2014).*

- Train caregivers bathing clients with dementia to avoid behaviors that can trigger assault: confrontational communication, invalidation of the resident's feelings, failure to prepare a resident for a task, initiating

• = Independent;   ▲ = Collaborative;   **EBN** = Evidence-Based Nursing;   **EB** = Evidence-Based

shower spray or touch during bathing without verbal prompts beforehand, washing the hair and face, speaking disrespectfully to the client, and hurrying the pace of the bath. CEB: *During bathing, assaults (defensive behavior) by nursing home residents with dementia are frequently triggered by caregiver actions that startle, frighten, hurt, or upset the resident. This might happen when caregivers spray water on a resident without warning or when they touch a resident's feet, axilla, or perineum, which is possibly caused by the startle reflex (Somboontanont et al, 2004).*

- Develop awareness of the ethics of presence during bathing to better meet clients' needs. Raholm (2012) found in a phenomenological study of nurses in elder care (*N* = 7) who discussed bathing that one must go beyond being physically present and enter into a caring relationship in which there is no indifference to the client's unique needs.
- Focus on the abilities of the client with dementia to obtain client's participation in bathing. EBN: *The use of an abilities-focused approach increases the ability of people with dementia to participate in their care (Sidani, Streiner, & LeClerc, 2012).*
- QSEN (Patient-Centered): Use a Chinese herb formula in bath water to reduce paraplegia spasm. EB: *In a randomized controlled trial by Liu et al (2014), Chinese herbs placed in bath water (N = 160) reduced paraplegia spasticity.*

Multicultural

- QSEN (Patient-Centered): Ask the patient for input on bathing habits and cultural bathing preferences. CEB: *Bathing is a personal experience with variability in attitudes, preferences, and adaptations to disability to be considered when developing interventions for bathing (Ahluwalia et al, 2010).*

Home Care

- If in a typical bathing setting for the client, assess the client's ability to bathe self via direct observation using physical performance tests for ADLs. *Observation of bathing performed in an atypical bathing setting may result in false data.*
- QSEN (Safety): Turn down temperature of water heater and recommend use of a water temperature-sensing shower valve to prevent scalding. *Older or disabled people have slower reflexes to respond to hot water and may be unable to regulate water temperature, yet they may be left unattended. Water at 130°F produces a first-degree burn in 20 seconds; at 135°F to 140°F, exposure for 5 to 6 seconds causes third-degree burns (Fathers, 2004).*

Client/Family Teaching and Discharge Planning

- Inform clients with extremity casts or bandages of inexpensive options to protect these devices during showering such as with plastic newspaper bags or bread bags. In a case study, Naram, Makhijani, and Chao (2011) reported on the use of inexpensive or free cast and bandage protector bags.

REFERENCES

Ahluwalia, S. C., et al. (2010). Perspectives of older persons on bathing and bathing disability: A qualitative study. *Journal of American Geriatric Society, 58*, 450–456.

Calkins, M. (2005). Designing bathing rooms that comfort. *Nursing Homes, 54*(1), 54–55.

Fathers, B. (2004). Bathing safety for the elderly and disabled. *Nursing Homes, 53*(9), 50–52.

Gozalo, P., Prakash, S., Qato, D. M., et al. (2014). Effect of the bathing without a battle training intervention on bathing-associated physical and verbal outcomes in nursing home residents with dementia: A randomized crossover diffusion study. *Journal of the American Geriatrics Society, 62*(5), 797–804.

Hashimoto, T. (2014). Investigation into the actual conditions of night bathing for the elderly in nursing homes [Japanese]. *Journal of the Japanese Society of Balneology, Climatology & Physical Medicine, 77*(4), 314–323.

Hoeffer, B., et al. (2006). Assisting cognitively impaired nursing home residents with bathing: Effects of two bathing interventions on caregiving. *The Gerontologist, 46*(4), 524–532.

Joosse, L. L. (2012). Do sound levels and space contribute to agitation in nursing home residents with dementia? *Research in Gerontological Nursing, 5*(3), 174–184.

Kassakian, S. Z., et al. (2011). Impact of chlorhexidine bathing on hospital-acquired infections among general medical patients. *Infection Control and Hospital Epidemiology, 32*(3), 238–243.

Liu, X., Meng, Q., Yu, D., et al. (2014). Novel medical bathing with traditional Chinese herb formula alleviates paraplegia spasticity. *International Journal of Nursing Practice, 20*(3), 227–232.

Lopes, J., Nogueira-Martins, L. A., & Barros, A. L. (2013). Bed and shower baths: Comparing the perceptions of patients with acute myocardial infarction. *Journal of Clinical Nursing, 22*(5/6), 733–740.

Marchaim, D., Taylor, A. R., Hayakawa, K., et al. (2012). Hospital bath basins are frequently contaminated with multidrug-resistant human pathogens. *American Journal of Infection Control, 40*(6), 562–564.

Mehrholz, J., Hädrich, A., Platz, T., et al. (2012). Electromechanical and robot-assisted arm training for improving generic activities of daily living, arm function, and arm muscle strength after stroke. *The Cochrane Database of Systematic Reviews*, (6), CD006876.

● = Independent;　▲ = Collaborative;　EBN = Evidence-Based Nursing;　EB = Evidence-Based

Naram, A., Makhijani, S. N., & Chao, J. D. (2011). Inexpensive alternatives for extremity cast and bandage protection. *Orthopaedic Nursing, 30*(2), 117–118.

Nishiyama, C., Iwami, T., Nichol, G., et al. (2011). Association of out-of-hospital cardiac arrest with prior activity and ambient temperature. *Resuscitation, 82*(8), 1008–1012.

Powers, J., Peed, J., Burns, L., et al. (2012). Chlorhexidine bathing and microbial contamination in patients' bath basins. *American Journal of Critical Care, 21*(5), 338–343.

Rader, J., et al. (2006). The bathing of older adults with dementia: Easing the unnecessarily unpleasant aspects of assisted bathing. *American Journal of Nursing, 106*(4), 4–49.

Raholm, M.-B. (2012). The ethics of presence when bathing patients in a nursing home. *International Journal for Human Caring, 16*(4), 30–35.

Ray, K. D., & Fitzsimmons, S. (2014). Music-assisted bathing: Making shower time easier for people with dementia. *Journal of Gerontological Nursing, 40*(2), 9–13.

Sidani, S., Streiner, D., & LeClerc, C. (2012). Evaluating the effectiveness of the abilities-focused approach to morning care of people with dementia. *International Journal of Older People Nursing.*

Somboontanont, W., et al. (2004). Assaultive behavior in Alzheimer's disease: Identifying immediate antecedents during bathing. *Journal of Gerontological Nursing, 30*(9), 22–29.

Webster, C., & Bryan, K. (2009). Older people's views of dignity and how it can be promoted in a hospital environment. *Journal of Clinical Nursing, 18*(12), 1784–1792.

Yamamoto, K., & Nagata, S. (2011). Physiological and psychological evaluation of the wrapped warm footbath as a complementary nursing therapy to induce relaxation in hospitalized patients with incurable cancer: A pilot study. *Cancer Nursing, 34*(3), 185–192.

Dressing Self-Care deficit   Linda S. Williams, RN, MSN

NANDA-I

Definition

Impaired ability to perform or complete dressing activities for self.

Defining Characteristics

Impaired ability to choose clothing; impaired ability to fasten clothing; impaired ability to gather clothing; impaired ability to maintain appearance; impaired ability to pick up clothing; impaired ability to put clothing on lower body; impaired ability to put clothing on upper body; impaired ability to put on various items of clothing; impaired ability to remove clothing item; impaired ability to use assistive device; impaired ability to use zipper

Related Factors

Anxiety; decrease in motivation; discomfort; environmental barrier; fatigue; pain; weakness

NOC (Nursing Outcomes Classification)

Suggested NOC Outcomes

Self-Care: Activities of Daily Living (ADLs), Dressing, Hygiene

Example NOC Outcome with Indicators

Self-Care: Dressing as evidenced by the following indicators: Gets clothing from drawer and closet/Puts clothing on upper body and lower body. (Rate outcome and indicators of **Self-Care: Dressing**: 1 = severely compromised, 2 = substantially compromised, 3 = moderately compromised, 4 = mildly compromised, 5 = not compromised [see Section I].)

Client Outcomes

Client Will (Specify Time Frame)

- Dress and groom self to optimal potential
- Use assistive technology to dress and groom
- Explain and use methods to enhance strengths during dressing and grooming
- Dress and groom with assistance of caregiver as needed

NIC (Nursing Interventions Classification)

Suggested NIC Intervention

Self-Care Assistance: Dressing/Grooming

● = Independent;   ▲ = Collaborative;   EBN = Evidence-Based Nursing;   EB = Evidence-Based

Example NIC Activities—Self-Care Assistance: Dressing/Grooming
Be available for assistance in dressing, as necessary; Reinforce efforts to dress self; Maintain privacy while the client is dressing

Nursing Interventions and *Rationales*

▲ QSEN (Patient-Centered): Assess independence in dressing and bathing skills after rehabilitation to determine the need for follow-up care. EB: *It was found that dressing and bathing independence at rehabilitation discharge were predictors of independence at 5 years after stroke (De Wit et al, 2014).*

▲ QSEN (Teamwork and Collaboration): Assess functional impairment and report functional changes to health care provider to aid in earlier cancer diagnosis. EB: *Functional impairments were found to be symptoms during the diagnostic phase that occurred in clusters based on cancer site: head/neck—impairments in dressing, eating/feeding, bathing, toileting, and walking (Fodeh et al, 2013).*

▲ QSEN (Teamwork and Collaboration): Refer patients after stroke to occupational therapy for ADL rehabilitation. EB: *A systematic review of nine studies (N = 994) found low-quality evidence that occupational therapy improves ADL performance after stroke and reduces risk of ADL deterioration (Legg et al, 2017).*

● QSEN (Patient-Centered): For clients with spinal cord injury, encourage their self-efficacy and involve them in decision-making. EBN: *A systematic review of 6 studies (N = 84) showed that rehabilitation is influenced by resilience, which can be enhanced with encouragement by nurses (Kornhaber et al, 2018).*

● QSEN (Patient-Centered): Use adaptive dressing and grooming equipment as needed (e.g., button hooks, dressing stick, elastic shoelaces, long-handled shoehorn, reacher, sock application devices, Velcro clothing and shoes, zipper pull, long-handled brushes, soap-on-a-rope, suction holders). *Use of adaptive clothing and devices for dressing and grooming can improve self-care ability and promote independence.*

● QSEN (Patient-Centered): Provide client analgesics prior to dressing as needed, sufficient time for dressing, and assist as needed. *Analgesics, adequate time, and assistance if tiring can promote independence in dressing.*

 ### Geriatric

▲ QSEN (Teamwork and Collaboration): Refer older cognitively impaired patients to physical and/or occupational therapy for functional rehabilitation with ADLs. EB: *An observational study using the Barthel ADL tool found that even those with moderate cognitive ability improved ADL function with rehabilitation (Poynter, Kwan, & Vassallo, 2013).*

● QSEN (Patient-Centered): Offer residents choices in what to wear and ensure staff is trained to do so. EBN: *A controlled study by Schnelle et al (2013) provided training of nursing aides on how to offer long-term care residents (N = 169) morning care choices that resulted in increased frequency of choice being offered in timing for getting out of bed, clothing selection, and incontinence care.*

● QSEN (Patient-Centered): Allow post stroke patients who are cognitively impaired, especially if unimanual, to practice dressing. CEB: *Fletcher-Smith, Walker, and Drummon (2012) found that bimanual cognitively impaired stroke survivors did better with dressing skills than those who are unimanual, although with practice those with arm paresis improved significantly.*

● QSEN (Patient-Centered): Inform patient that a winter coat with a funnel sleeve design can be easier to put on. CEB: *Green et al (2011) found that older adults (N = 8) required less shoulder range of motion in putting on a winter coat with a funnel sleeve design, which could reduce social isolation in winter.*

 ### Multicultural

● Consider use of assistive technology versus personal care assistance for Native Americans. CEB: *Older American Indians use more assistive technology for assistance with ADLs than the general same-age population (Goins et al, 2010).*

 ### Home Care

● QSEN (Patient-Centered): Teach assisted living staff the philosophy and methods to increase resident participation in dressing. EBN: *Staff awareness and knowledge increased significantly after a training program to encourage residents to participate more in dressing themselves (Walker, Harrington, & Cole, 2013).*

● = Independent;   ▲ = Collaborative;   EBN = Evidence-Based Nursing;   EB = Evidence-Based

Client/Family Teaching and Discharge Planning

- QSEN (Teamwork and Collaboration): Include caregiver's perceptions of client rehabilitation needs after stroke. EB: *A meta-analysis of 66 studies of stroke survivors needs as perceived by their caregivers found three areas of need themes whose outcomes may be improved by including caregivers in rehabilitation planning (Krishnan et al, 2017).*

REFERENCES

De Wit, L., Putman, K., Devos, H., et al. (2014). Long-term prediction of functional outcome after stroke using single items of the Barthel Index at discharge from rehabilitation centre. *Disability & Rehabilitation, 36*(5), 353–358.

Fletcher-Smith, J., Walker, M. F., & Drummond, A. (2012). The influence of hand use on dressing outcome in cognitively impaired stroke survivors. *British Journal of Occupational Therapy, 75*(1), 2–9.

Fodeh, S. J., Lazenby, M., Bai, M., et al. (2013). Functional impairments as symptoms in the symptom cluster analysis of patients newly diagnosed with advanced cancer. *Journal of Pain & Symptom Management, 46*(4), 500–510.

Goins, R. T., et al. (2010). Assistive technology use of older American Indians in a southeastern tribe: The native elder care study. *Journal of the American Geriatrics Society, 58*(11), 2185–2190.

Green, S., Boger, J., & Mihailidis, A. (2011). Toward enabling winter occupations: Testing a winter coat designed for older adults. *Canadian Journal of Occupational Therapy, 78*(1), 57–64.

Kornhaber, R., Mclean, L., Betihavas, V., et al. (2018). Resilience and the rehabilitation of adult spinal cord injury survivors: A qualitative systematic review. *Journal of Advanced Nursing, 74*, 23–33. doi:10.1111/jan.13396.

Krishnan, S., Pappadis, M. R., Weller, S., et al. (2017). Needs of stroke survivors as perceived by their caregivers: A scoping review. *American Journal of Physical Medicine & Rehabilitation, 96*(7), 487–505. doi:10.1097/PHM.0000000000000717.

Legg, L. A., Lewis, S. R., Schofield-Robinson, O. J., et al. (2017). Occupational therapy for adults with problems in activities of daily living after stroke. *The Cochrane Database of Systematic Reviews*, (7), CD003585. doi:10.1002/14651858.CD003585.pub3.

Poynter, L., Kwan, J., & Vassallo, M. (2013). How does cognitive impairment impact on functional improvement following the rehabilitation of elderly patients? *International Journal of Clinical Practice, 67*(8), 811–815. doi:10.1111/ijcp.12161.

Schnelle, J. F., Rahman, A., Durkin, D. W., et al. (2013). A controlled trial of an intervention to increase resident choice in long term care. *Journal of the American Medical Directors Association, 14*(5), 345–351.

Walker, B. L., Harrington, S. S., & Cole, C. S. (2013). Teaching philosophy and methods of restorative care to assisted living owners and staff. *Educational Gerontology, 39*(1), 28–36.

Feeding Self-Care deficit Linda S. Williams, RN, MSN

NANDA-I

Definition

Inability to eat independently.

Defining Characteristics

Impaired ability to bring food to the mouth; impaired ability to chew food; impaired ability to get food onto utensils; impaired ability to handle utensils; impaired ability to manipulate food in mouth; impaired ability to open containers; impaired ability to pick up cup; impaired ability to prepare food; impaired ability to self-feed a complete meal; impaired ability to self-feed in an acceptable manner; impaired ability to swallow food; impaired ability to swallow sufficient amount of food; impaired ability to use assistive device

Related Factors

Anxiety; decrease in motivation; discomfort; environmental barrier; fatigue; pain; weakness

Associated Condition

Alteration in cognitive functioning; musculoskeletal impairment; neuromuscular impairment; perceptual disorders

NOC (Nursing Outcomes Classification)

Suggested NOC Outcomes

Self-Care: Activities of Daily Living (ADLs), Eating

● = Independent;   ▲ = Collaborative;   EBN = Evidence-Based Nursing;   EB = Evidence-Based

S

Example NOC Outcome with Indicators
Self-Care: Eating as evidenced by the following indicators: Opens containers/Uses utensils/Completes a meal. (Rate the outcome and indicators of **Self-Care: Eating:** 1 = severely compromised, 2 = substantially compromised, 3 = moderately compromised, 4 = mildly compromised, 5 = not compromised [see Section I].)

Client Outcomes

Client Will (Specify Time Frame)

- Feed self safely and effectively
- State satisfaction with ability to use adaptive devices for feeding
- Use assistance with feeding when necessary (caregiver)

NIC   (Nursing Interventions Classification)

Suggested NIC Intervention

Self-Care Assistance: Feeding

Example NIC Activities—Self-Care Assistance: Feeding
Provide adaptive devices to facilitate client's feeding self (e.g., long handles, handle with large circumference, or small strap-on utensils), as needed; Provide frequent cueing and close supervision as appropriate

Nursing Interventions and *Rationales*

- QSEN (Safety): Consider assessment of patients in the intensive care unit (ICU) and stepdown patients or of patients with acute stroke for readiness of an oral diet with a 3-ounce water swallow challenge by a trained provider. EB: *If a 3-ounce water swallow challenge, administered by a trained provider to a patient in ICU or to a stepdown patient, is passed, then an individualized diet plan can be made safely (Leder et al, 2011). EB: Leder et al (2012) studied (N = 75) patients with acute stroke who were given a 90-mL water swallow challenge and found that specific oral diets could be successfully recommended after passing the 90-mL water swallow challenge.*
- QSEN (Patient-Centered): Conduct repeat structured observations of patients at mealtime after a stroke to detect patients with eating difficulties to prevent possible social and functional consequences. EBN: *In a longitudinal and comparative study (N = 36), Medin et al (2012) found eating difficulties continued among clients 3 months after stroke despite improvement in other physical functions, indicating that factors such as psychological well-being should be assessed.*
- ▲ QSEN (Patient-Centered): Develop an overriding guideline for assisted feeding so it is less dependent on a caregiver's own beliefs, time pressures, and organizational characteristics. EBN: *Martinsen and Norlyk (2012a) conducted a qualitative study interviewing caregivers (N = 12) on their experience with assisted feeding and found a focus on nutrition blended with their own beliefs and societal norms about eating.*
- ▲ QSEN (Patient-Centered): Prioritize assisted feeding as important in a caregiver's assignment to allow adequate dedicated time to the activity. EBN: *The experience of assisted feeding for clients with language impairment (N = 42) depends on the caregiver's availability and goal for efficiency rather than the relational and affective aspects of meals, which institutions could address with flexible feeding assistance times that are free from other responsibilities (Martinsen & Norlyk, 2012b).*
- ▲ QSEN (Teamwork and Collaboration): Give priority to continuity in the cooperation between the parties involved in assisted feeding for those who are completely dependent. CEBN: *The continuity in the cooperation between the parties involved in assisted feeding is significant in creating a new eating pattern (Martinsen, Harder, & Biering-Sorensen, 2008).*
- QSEN (Patient-Centered): Consult patient on the benefit or desire to use assistive devices for feeding. CEBN: *The value of a particular assistive device can only be determined by the patient who may feel that it is insulting (Martinsen, Harder, & Biering-Sorensen, 2008).*
- QSEN (Safety): Presentation of feeding: provide 1 teaspoon of solid food or 10 to 15 mL of liquid at a time; wait until patient has swallowed the prior food/liquid. CEB: *Feeding large volumes and feeding quickly occurred commonly because caregivers lacked knowledge that this could exacerbate dysphagia and increase*

● = Independent;   ▲ = Collaborative;   EBN = Evidence-Based Nursing;   EB = Evidence-Based

the risk of health problems (Pelletier, 2004). **EBN:** *For a water swallow to accurately identify dysphagia, it is critical to administer 10 teaspoons (Martino, Maki, & Diamant, 2014).*

- QSEN (Safety): Ensure oral care is provided to all patients regardless of type of feeding. **EBN:** *Patients receiving tube feedings had inferior oral hygiene compared with those receiving oral feeding, creating a higher risk for aspiration pneumonia for patients receiving tube feedings (Maeda et al, 2011).*

Geriatric

- QSEN (Safety): Assess for tooth loss in older patients prior to feeding. **EB:** *Tooth loss contributes to swallowing difficulties that can increase risk of aspiration in the older patient (Okamoto et al, 2012).*
- QSEN (Patient-Centered): Assess the ability of patients with dementia to self-feed, and supervise the feeding of those with moderate dependency by providing verbal or physical assistance. **CEBN:** *Although low-dependency patients can self-feed, and those with severe dependency are fed, food intake among residents with moderate dependence is often ignored (Lin, Watson, & Wu, 2010).*
- QSEN (Patient-Centered): Implement Montessori interventions for patients with dementia who have eating problems, such as playing music to signal learning session start for hand-eye coordination, scooping, pouring, and squeezing activities. **EBN:** *In an experimental crossover design, Lin et al (2011) confirmed that use of a Montessori intervention method for those with dementia helps maintain self-feeding ability and can reduce caregiver feeding frequency.*
- ▲ QSEN (Patient-Centered): Reduce interruptions during mealtimes and provide additional feeding assistance for older patients, especially those with cognitive impairment. **EB:** *Additional assistance with feeding and protected mealtimes while hospitalized can improve nutritional intake in older clients (Young et al, 2013).*
- QSEN (Patient-Centered): Use high-calorie oral supplements for patients with advanced dementia. **EB:** *Desirable weight gain has been shown with the use of high-calorie oral supplements in patients with dementia who have feeding problems (Hanson et al, 2011).*
- QSEN (Patient-Centered): Provide nutritional supplement drinks in a glass to older adults with cognitive impairment. **EBN:** *Allen, Methven, and Gosney (2014) conducted a nonblind randomized control trial that identified that the best method to provide nutritional supplement drinks to older adults with cognitive impairment is in a glass/beaker rather than using a straw in the container.*
- QSEN (Patient-Centered): Allow a resident an average of 42 minutes of staff time per meal and 13 minutes per between-meal snack to improve oral intake. **CEB:** *When these time frames are provided for staff to assist with meals and snacks, improved oral intake and weight gain in residents at risk for weight loss results (Simmons et al, 2008).*
- QSEN (Patient-Centered): Discuss meaningful life topics, as identified by family members, with residents with dementia during mealtimes. **EB:** *Cleary et al (2012) found that conversations during meals that generated reminiscence may improve food intake during the reminiscence state for residents with dementia.*
- QSEN (Patient-Centered): Encourage family visits at mealtimes for patients with dementia. **EB:** *Family participation at mealtimes increased feeding assistance and helped promote satisfactory adaptation to the nursing home environment, which was found by Durkin, Shotwell, and Simmons (2014) in a study of 74 residents and their visitors during mealtimes.*
- QSEN (Patient-Centered): Play familiar music during meals for clients with dementia. **EB:** *Agitation often increases at mealtimes in patients with dementia, which seems to be reduced by music (Whear et al, 2014).*
- Use aromatherapy with the smell of baking bread for those with dementia. **CEB:** *The smell of baking bread increased intake of food and self-feeding in those with dementia (Cleary et al, 2008).*
- ▲ QSEN (Teamwork and Collaboration): Provide feeding training and education programs for nursing home staff. **EBN:** *Liu, Cheon, and Thomas (2014) did a systematic review of the literature about interventions for mealtime difficulties in older adults with dementia and found that training and education programs for professionals demonstrated moderate evidence to increase eating time and decrease feeding difficulty.*

Multicultural

- QSEN (Patient-Centered): For those with impaired hand function who use chopsticks, suggest adapted chopsticks. **CEB:** *In a pilot equipment study, adapted chopsticks, which can be inexpensive and easily constructed, for those with lower cervical spinal cord injury and residual gross grasp were found to convert gross grasp into 2-point pinch (Chang et al, 2006).*
- QSEN (Patient-Centered): Use the simplified Chinese Edinburgh Feeding Evaluation in Dementia scale to measure feeding problems in people with dementia from Mainland China and other Chinese cultural

S

• = Independent;   ▲ = Collaborative;   **EBN** = Evidence-Based Nursing;   **EB** = Evidence-Based

groups. EBN: *Identifying patient behaviors during feeding allows development of effective interventions for feeding (Liu, Watson, & Lou, 2014).*

Home Care

- QSEN (Teamwork and Collaboration): Request referral for physical therapy and occupational therapy to assess client's ability to position and self-feed and provide client and caregiver support with feeding. EB: *Ingestive skill difficulties are frequent among acutely hospitalized frail elderly patients (Hansen, Lambert, & Farber, 2012).*

Client/Family Teaching and Discharge Planning

- QSEN (Teamwork and Collaboration): Discuss with family caregivers, who are involved in the feeding of a family member with advanced dementia, the feeding experience to provide support to ensure that the mealtime purpose is preserved. EBN: *Lopez and Amella (2011) in a phenomenological study interviewed family caregivers (N = 16) of those with advanced dementia who indicated that the feeding assistance experience was like living in a time warp with an uncertain future.*
- ▲ QSEN (Patient-Centered): Educate family members that neither insertion of a feeding tube nor timing of its insertion affects client survival for those with advanced dementia who have eating problems. EB: *Teno et al (2012) studied all nursing home residents with advanced dementia who had eating problems from 1999 to 2007 (N = 36,492) and found that survival was not affected by insertion of or timing of insertion of a percutaneous endoscopic gastrostomy feeding tube.*

REFERENCES

Allen, V. J., Methven, L., & Gosney, M. (2014). Impact of serving method on the consumption of nutritional supplement drinks: Randomized trial in older adults with cognitive impairment. *Journal of Advanced Nursing, 70*(6), 1323–1333.

Chang, B., Huang, B., Chou, C., et al. (2006). A new type of chopsticks for patients with impaired hand function. *Archives of Physical Medicine & Rehabilitation, 87*(7), 1013–1015.

Cleary, S., Hopper, T., & Van Soest, D. (2012). Reminiscence therapy, mealtimes and improving intake in residents with dementia. *Canadian Nursing Home, 23*(2), 8–13.

Cleary, S., Van Soest, D., Milke, D., et al. (2008). Using the smell of baking bread to facilitate eating in residents with dementia. *Canadian Nursing Home, 19*(1), 6.

Durkin, D. W., Shotwell, M. S., & Simmons, S. F. (2014). The impact of family visitation on feeding assistance quality in nursing homes. *Journal of Applied Gerontology, 33*(5), 586–602.

Hansen, T., Lambert, H. C., & Faber, J. (2012). Ingestive skill difficulties are frequent among acutely-hospitalized frail elderly patients, and predict hospital outcomes. *Physical & Occupational Therapy in Geriatrics, 30*(4), 271–287.

Hanson, L. C., Ersek, M., Gilliam, R., et al. (2011). Oral feeding options for people with dementia: A systematic review. *Journal of the American Geriatrics Society, 59*(3), 463–472.

Leder, S. B., Suiter, D. M., Warner, H. L., et al. (2012). Success of recommending oral diets in acute stroke patients based on passing a 90-cc water swallow challenge protocol. *Topics in Stroke Rehabilitation, 19*(1), 40–44.

Leder, S., Suiter, D., Warner, H., et al. (2011). Initiating safe oral feeding in critically ill intensive care and step-down unit patients based on passing a 3-ounce (90 milliliters) water swallow challenge. *Journal of Trauma, 70*(5), 1203–1207.

Lin, L., Huang, Y., Watson, R., et al. (2011). Using a Montessori method to increase eating ability for institutionalised residents with dementia: A crossover design. *Journal of Clinical Nursing, 20*(21/22), 3092–3101.

Lin, L., Watson, R., & Wu, S. (2010). What is associated with low food intake in older people with dementia? *Journal of Clinical Nursing, 19*(1–2), 53–59.

Liu, W., Cheon, J., & Thomas, S. A. (2014). Interventions on mealtime difficulties in older adults with dementia: A systematic review. *International Journal of Nursing Studies, 51*(1), 14–27.

Liu, W., Watson, R., & Lou, F. (2014). The Edinburgh feeding evaluation in dementia scale (EdFED): Cross-cultural validation of the simplified Chinese version in mainland China. *Journal of Clinical Nursing, 23*(1/2), 45–53.

Lopez, R. P., & Amella, E. J. (2011). Time travel: The lived experience of providing feeding assistance to a family member with dementia. *Research in Gerontological Nursing, 4*(2), 127–134.

Maeda, E., Nakamoto, S., Ikeda, T., et al. (2011). Oral microorganisms in the homebound elderly: A comparison between oral feeding and tube feeding. *Journal of Japan Academy of Nursing Science, 31*(2), 34–41.

Martino, R., Maki, E., & Diamant, N. (2014). Identification of dysphagia using the Toronto Bedside Swallowing Screening Test: Are 10 teaspoons of water necessary? *International Journal of Speech-Language Pathology, 16*(3), 193–198.

Martinsen, B., & Norlyk, A. (2012a). Caregivers' lived experience of assisted feeding. *Journal of Clinical Nursing, 21*(19/20), 2966–2974.

Martinsen, B., & Norlyk, A. (2012b). Observations of assisted feeding among people with language impairment. *Journal of Clinical Nursing, 21*(19/20), 2949–2957.

Martinsen, B., Harder, I., & Biering-Sorensen, F. (2008). The meaning of assisted feeding for people living with spinal cord injury: A phenomenological study. *Journal of Advanced Nursing, 62*(5), 533–540.

Medin, J., Windahl, J., von Arbin, M., et al. (2012). Eating difficulties among patients 3 months after stroke in relation to the acute phase. *Journal of Advanced Nursing, 68*(3), 580–589.

Okamoto, N., Tomioka, K., Saeki, K., et al. (2012). Relationship between swallowing problems and tooth loss in community-dwelling independent elderly adults: The Fujiwara-Kyo study. *Journal of the American Geriatrics Society, 60*(5), 849–853.

Pelletier, C. (2004). What do certified nurse assistants actually know about dysphagia and feeding nursing home residents? *American Journal of Speech-Language Pathology, 13*(2), 99–113.

● = Independent;   ▲ = Collaborative;   EBN = Evidence-Based Nursing;   EB = Evidence-Based

Simmons, S. F., Keeler, E., Zhuo, X., et al. (2008). Prevention of unintentional weight loss in nursing home residents: A controlled trial of feeding assistance. *Journal of American Geriatric Society*, *56*(8), 1466–1473.

Teno, J. M., Gozalo, P. L., Mitchell, S. L., et al. (2012). Does feeding tube insertion and its timing improve survival? *Journal of the American Geriatrics Society*, *60*(10), 1918–1921.

Whear, R., Abbott, R., Thompson-Coon, J., et al. (2014). Effectiveness of mealtime interventions on behavior symptoms of people with

dementia living in care homes: A systematic review. *Journal of the American Medical Directors Association*, *15*(3), 185–193.

Young, A. M., Mudge, A. M., Banks, M. D., et al. (2013). Encouraging, assisting and time to EAT: Improved nutritional intake for older medical patients receiving protected mealtimes and/or additional nursing feeding assistances. *Clinical Nutrition: Official Journal of the European Society of Parenteral and Enteral Nutrition*, *32*(4), 543–549.

Toileting Self-Care deficit   Linda S. Williams, RN, MSN

NANDA-I

Definition

Impaired ability to perform or complete self-toileting activities.

Defining Characteristics

Impaired ability to complete toilet hygiene; impaired ability to flush toilet; impaired ability to manipulate clothing for toileting; impaired ability to reach toilet; impaired ability to rise from toilet; impaired ability to sit on toilet

Related Factors

Alteration in cognitive functioning; anxiety; decrease in motivation; environmental barrier; fatigue; impaired ability to transfer; impaired mobility; musculoskeletal impairment; neuromuscular impairment; pain; perceptual impairment; weakness

NOC   (Nursing Outcomes Classification)

Suggested NOC Outcomes

Self-Care: Activities of Daily Living (ADLs), Toileting

Example NOC Outcome with Indicators

Self-Care: Toileting as evidenced by the following indicators: Responds to full bladder and urge to have a bowel movement in a timely manner/Gets to toilet between urge and passage of urine/Between urge and evacuation of stool. (Rate the outcome and indicators of **Self-Care: Toileting:** 1 = severely compromised, 2 = substantially compromised, 3 = moderately compromised, 4 = mildly compromised, 5 = not compromised [see Section I].)

Client Outcomes

Client Will (Specify Time Frame)

- Remain free of incontinence and impaction with no urine or stool on skin
- State satisfaction with ability to use adaptive devices for toileting
- Explain and demonstrate use of methods to be safe and independent in toileting

NIC   (Nursing Interventions Classification)

Suggested NIC Interventions

Environmental Management; Self-Care Assistance: Toileting

Example NIC Activities—Self-Care Assistance: Toileting

Assist client to toilet/commode/bedpan/fracture pan/urinal at specified intervals; Institute a toileting schedule, as appropriate

● = Independent;   ▲ = Collaborative;   EBN = Evidence-Based Nursing;   EB = Evidence-Based

Nursing Interventions and *Rationales*

- QSEN (Safety): Assess patients for fall risk using established and valid fall risk assessment tools (Morse and Heindrich) and implement fall prevention interventions for those at risk for falling or in physical restraints. **EBN:** *In a retrospective study of 3 years of acute care fall incident reports (N = 547), Huey-Ming and Chang-Yi (2012) found 45.2% of falls were related to toileting, and that predictors of toileting-related falls were having a previous fall, being physically restrained, and being a fall risk.*
- QSEN (Patient-Centered): Assess patient's prior use of incontinence briefs and avoid use for hospitalized continent but limited mobility patient. **EBN:** *Use of adult incontinence briefs for low-mobility continent clients versus self-toileting occurs more frequently for females and can be associated with adverse outcomes (Zisberg, 2011).*
- QSEN (Patient-Centered): Assess patients who have had sphincter-saving surgery for self-care strategies to manage bowel symptoms to help support these strategies. **EBN:** *In a quantitative descriptive study of self-care strategies used by patients who had sphincter-saving surgery and bowel symptoms (N = 143), the strategy of proximity and knowing the location of a toilet at all times was used most by those with more bowel symptoms (Landers et al, 2014).*
- QSEN (Safety): Make assistance call button readily available to the client and answer call light promptly. **CEBN:** *Falls often occur related to toileting, and individualized planning for safe transfer to toilet is essential to safety (Tzeng, 2010).*
- QSEN (Safety): Provide folding commode chairs in client bathrooms/at bedside. **EBN:** *Availability of a folding commode chair as part of a fall prevention program can increase accessibility and efficiency in patient care (Tzeng, 2011).*
- QSEN (Patient-Centered): Before use of a bedpan, discuss its use with clients. **CEBN:** *When nurses facilitate discussion about bedpan use with orthopedic patients, they may be less anxious about its use (Cohen, 2009).*
- QSEN (Patient-Centered): Use necessary assistive toileting equipment. **EB:** *Amyotrophic lateral sclerosis clients reported satisfaction and usefulness of all bathroom assistive technology such as elevated toilet seat and arm rails by the toilet (Gruis, Wren, & Huggins, 2011).*
- QSEN (Safety): Close toilet lid before flushing toilet and teach patient to do so. **EB:** *A literature review of studies of toilet plume aerosols found that potential infectious aerosols during toilet flushing are produced, which can continue to expose toilet users later when some of the aerosols become droplet nuclei in air currents (Johnson et al, 2013).* **EB:** *A study revealed viral contamination of aerosol and surfaces through toilet use (Verani, Bigazzi, & Carducci, 2014).*

Geriatric

- Assess residents without dementia for risk factors associated with toileting disability (such as rating health as fair or poor; living in a residence with four or less residents or that is for-profit, incontinence; physical, visual, or hearing impairment; and need for ADL or transferring assistance) to guide prevention interventions. **EBN:** *In a cross-sectional analysis of adults 65 years or older without dementia in residential care facilities (N = 2395), 15% were found to have toileting disability that was associated with rating health as fair or poor; living in a residence with four or fewer residents or that is for-profit; incontinence; physical, visual, or hearing impairment; and need for ADL or transferring assistance (Talley et al, 2014).*
- QSEN (Patient-Centered): Consider use of urine alarm systems for patients with dementia. **EB:** *Caregivers preferred use of urine alarms over time toileting to reduce urinary accidents (Lancioni et al, 2011).*
- QSEN (Patient-Centered): Assess the patient's functional ability to manipulate clothing for toileting, and if necessary modify clothing with Velcro fasteners, elastic waists, drop-front underwear, or slacks. *For clients with impaired dexterity or weakness, wearing dresses, athletic bottoms, or skirts with a stretch waistband makes it easier to use the toilet than wearing clothing with buttons and zippers (Cohen, 2008).*
- QSEN (Patient-Centered): Provide patients with dementia access to regular exercise. **EBN:** *ADL performance improved with a regular exercise program of stretching, walking, and leg weight bearing (Chang et al, 2011).*

Multicultural

- QSEN (Patient-Centered): Remove barriers to toileting, support patient's cultural beliefs, and preserve dignity. **CEB:** *The physical and sociocultural environments in long-term care require older patients to overcome greater physical and cognitive challenges to maintain their participation, autonomy, and dignity in toileting than if they were at home (Sacco-Peterson & Borell, 2004).*

Home Care

- **QSEN** (Patient-Centered): To design a bathroom for an older adult, consider adaptable bath fixtures/furniture and safety needs. **EB:** *Poor bathroom design requires use of assistive adaptive devices, reduces quality of life, and contributes to safety concerns such as falls (Burton, Reed, & Chamberlain, 2011).*

Client/Family Teaching and Discharge Planning

- Teach men who perform routine clean intermittent catheterization that a 40-cm intermittent catheter was found to provide ease of use, instill confidence in bladder emptying, and draining of urine into a receptacle. **EB:** *Costa et al (2013) found in a randomized controlled study of self-catheterizing wheelchair-using men (N = 81) that a 40-cm intermittent catheter was preferred over one that was 30 cm.*
- Have the family install a toilet seat of a contrasting color. **CEB:** *Visualization of the toilet is aided by installing a toilet seat of a contrasting color (Gerdner, Buckwalter, & Reed, 2002).*
- Explain to family and caregivers of clients with dementia that toilet self-care activities decrease when self-awareness is lost. *An observational study of toileting self-care in older adults with dementia revealed that toilet activities are affected and decline when self-awareness is lost (composed of theory of mind, self-evaluation, and self-consciousness) (Uchimoto et al, 2013).*

REFERENCES

Burton, M., Reed, H., & Chamberlain, P. (2011). Age-related disability and bathroom use. *International Journal of Integrated Care, 19*(1), 37–43.

Chang, S. H., Chen, C. Y., Shen, S. H., et al. (2011). The effectiveness of an exercise programme for elders with dementia in a Taiwanese day-care centre. *International Journal of Nursing Practice, 17*(3), 213–220.

Cohen, D. (2008). Providing an assist. *Rehabilitation Management, 21*(8), 16–19.

Cohen, S. (2009). Orthopaedic patient's perceptions of using a bed pan. *Journal of Orthopedic Nursing, 13*(2), 78–84.

Costa, J. A., Menier, M., Doran, T. J., et al. (2013). Catheter length preference in wheelchair-using men who perform routine clean intermittent catheterization. *Spinal Cord, 51*(10), 772–775.

Gerdner, L. A., Buckwalter, K. C., & Reed, D. (2002). Impact of a psychoeducational intervention on caregiver response to behavioral problems. *Nursing Research, 51*(6), 363.

Gruis, K., Wren, P., & Huggins, J. (2011). Amyotrophic lateral sclerosis patients' self-reported satisfaction with assistive technology. *Muscle and Nerve, 43*(5), 643–647.

Huey-Ming, T., & Chang-Yi, Y. (2012). Toileting-related inpatient falls in adult acute care settings. *Medsurg Nursing, 21*(6), 372–377.

Johnson, D. L., Mead, K. R., Lynch, R. A., et al. (2013). Lifting the lid on toilet plume aerosol: A literature review with suggestions for future research. *American Journal of Infection Control, 41*(3), 254–258.

Lancioni, G., Singh, N., O'Reilly, M., et al. (2011). Persons with mild or moderate Alzheimer's disease learn to use urine alarms and prompts to avoid large urinary accidents. *Research in Developmental Disabilities, 32*(5), 1998–2004.

Landers, M., McCarthy, G., Livingstone, V., et al. (2014). Patients' bowel symptom experiences and self-care strategies following sphincter-saving surgery for rectal cancer. *Journal of Clinical Nursing, 23*(15/16), 2343–2354.

Sacco-Peterson, M., & Borell, L. (2004). Struggles for autonomy in self-care: The impact of the physical and socio-cultural environment in a long-term care setting. *Scandinavian Journal of Caring Science, 18*(4), 376–386.

Talley, K. C., Wyman, J. F., Bronas, U. G., et al. (2014). Factors associated with toileting disability in older adults without dementia living in residential care facilities. *Nursing Research, 63*(2), 94–104.

Tzeng, H. (2010). Understanding the prevalence of inpatient falls associated with toileting in adult acute care settings. *Journal of Nursing Care Quality, 25*(1), 22–30.

Tzeng, H. (2011). A feasibility study of providing folding commode chairs in patient bathrooms to reduce toilet-related falls in an adult acute medical-surgical unit. *Journal of Nursing Care Quality, 26*(1), 61–68.

Uchimoto, K., Yokoi, T., Yamashita, T., et al. (2013). Investigation of toilet activities in elderly patients with dementia from the viewpoint of motivation and self-awareness. *American Journal of Alzheimer's Disease & Other Dementias, 28*(5), 459–468.

Verani, M., Bigazzi, R., & Carducci, A. (2014). Viral contamination of aerosol and surfaces through toilet use in health care and other settings. *American Journal of Infection Control, 42*(7), 758–762.

Zisberg, A. (2011). Incontinence brief use in acute hospitalized patients with no prior incontinence. *Journal of Wound Ostomy Continence Nursing, 38*(5), 559–564.

S

Readiness for enhanced Self-Concept   *Marina Martinez-Kratz, RN, MS, CNE*

NANDA-I

Definition

A pattern of perceptions or ideas about the self, which can be strengthened.

● = Independent;   ▲ = Collaborative;   **EBN** = Evidence-Based Nursing;   **EB** = Evidence-Based

Defining Characteristics

Acceptance of limitations; acceptance of strengths; actions are congruent with verbal expression; confidence in abilities; expresses desire to enhance role performance; expresses desire to enhance self-concept; expresses satisfaction with body image; expresses satisfaction with personal identity; expresses satisfaction with sense of worth; expresses satisfaction with thoughts about self

NOC (Nursing Outcomes Classification)

Suggested NOC Outcomes

Self-Esteem; Personal Well-Being; Psychosocial Adjustment Life Change

> **Example NOC Outcome with Indicators**
>
> **Self-Esteem** as evidenced by the following indicators: Verbalizations of self-acceptance/Open communication/Confidence level/ Description of pride in self. (Rate the outcome and indicators of **Self-Esteem:** 1 = never positive, 2 = rarely positive, 3 = sometimes positive, 4 = often positive, 5 = consistently positive [see Section I].)

Client Outcomes

Client Will (Specify Time Frame)

- State willingness to enhance self-concept
- State satisfaction with thoughts about self, sense of worthiness, role performance, body image, and personal identity
- Demonstrate actions that are congruent with expressed feelings and thoughts
- State confidence in abilities
- Accept strengths and limitations

NIC (Nursing Interventions Classification)

Suggested NIC Intervention

Self-Esteem Enhancement

> **Example NIC Activities—Self-Esteem Enhancement**
>
> Encourage client to identify strengths; Assist client in setting realistic goals to achieve higher self-esteem

Nursing Interventions and *Rationales*

- Encourage client to express feelings through songwriting. EB: *Study findings suggested that people who find songwriting has strong meaning for them might be more likely to start accepting their emotions and as a result experience decreases in anxiety and depression (Baker, 2016).*
- Refer to nutritional and exercise programs to support weight loss. EB: *Study findings suggested that weight-loss treatments emphasize changes in self-perception (Annesi & Porter, 2015).*
- Offer client complementary and alternative medicine (CAM) interventions like acupressure, aromatherapy, compress, and massage. EBN: *A recent study reviewed the development of a complex nursing intervention including CAM for breast and gynecological cancer patients during chemotherapy to improve quality of life (Klafke et al, 2016).*
- Support homeless individuals to identify and endorse a positive self-concept. EB: *A study found that assumption of positive identity meanings, even a stigmatized identity such as being a homeless person, may provide support for a more general sense of self-esteem (Parker et al, 2016).*
- Support unemployed individuals to cope with identity threats and support individual identity growth. EB: *Research shows that to cope with self-definition threats, mature-aged workers protect and restructure their self-definitions with alternative goals of either remaining in paid employment or opting out from it (Kira & Klehe, 2016).*
- Support establishing community-based partnerships to address health needs. EBN: *To prevent suicide and substance abuse, a community-based participatory research approach was used to obtain community input,*

• = Independent; ▲ = Collaborative; EBN = Evidence-Based Nursing; EB = Evidence-Based

which led to the development of a strengths-based intervention incorporating the Gathering of Native Americans' curriculum (Holliday et al, 2016).

- For clients with a history of trauma, offer a mindfulness-based intervention of hatha yoga. **EB:** *A qualitative study explored the experiences of women with posttraumatic stress disorder (PTSD) who participated in a 10-week Trauma Sensitive Yoga (TSY) class. It was found that they specifically perceived changes in symptoms and feelings of gratitude and compassion, relatedness, acceptance, centeredness, and empowerment (West et al, 2017).*

 Pediatric

- Consider the development of a Healthy Kids Mentoring Program that has four components: (1) relationship building, (2) self-esteem enhancement, (3) goal setting, and (4) academic assistance (tutoring). Mentors met with students twice each week for 1 hour each session on school grounds. During each meeting, mentors devoted time to each program component. **CEB:** *The Healthy Kids Mentoring Program results indicated that students' overall self-esteem, school connectedness, peer connectedness, and family connectedness were significantly higher at posttest than at pretest (Kelly et al, 2011).*
- Facilitate healthy relationships with teachers, coaches, and other supportive adults in the adolescents' lives. **EB:** *Research found that the presence of supportive teachers and coaches in an adolescents' social network is associated with healthier self-concept and decreased substance use (Dudovitz et al, 2017).*
- Provide parents with information designed to promote body satisfaction, healthy eating, and weight management in early childhood. **EB:** *Research evaluated Confident Body, Confident Child (CBCC), which is an intervention for parents of 2- to 6-year-old children and found significant increases in parents' intentions to use positive behaviors and knowledge of child body image and healthy eating patterns (Hart et al, 2016).*
- Promote the adoption of a recovery identity through online interactions and support groups for individuals with eating disorders. **EB:** *A study found that an eating disorder identity is seen as problematic and most interventions are targeted at changing an individual's self-concept. The study suggested that interventions could instead focus on identity resources to support a transition to a recovery identity (McNamara & Parsons, 2016).*
- Provide activities to bolster physical self-concept. **EB:** *A meta-analytic review found that physical activity interventions increased positive self-concept in adolescents (Spruit et al, 2016).*
- ▲ Consider wheelchair dancing for disabled adolescents. **EB:** *A wheelchair dancing intervention was associated with an improvement in self-esteem among disabled adolescents (de Villiers et al, 2013).*
- ▲ Provide overweight adolescents access to group-based weight control interventions. **EB:** *A 12-week group-based exergaming intervention was associated with positive effects on overweight and obese adolescent girls' television viewing, self-efficacy, and intrinsic motivation (Staiano et al, 2016).*
- Provide an alternative school-based program for pregnant and parenting adolescents. **EB:** *Despite Title IX legislation mandating equal educational opportunities for pregnant and parenting teens, only 50% of adolescent parents graduate high school. A study found themes of struggle, support, hope, perseverance, and transformation in a cohort of young mothers' descriptions of finishing high school (Watson et al, 2016).*

 Geriatric

- Assess for depression as needed. **EB:** *A study found that self-concept, particularly physical self-concept, was an important predictor of psychosocial well-being in elderly residents (Grace & Toukhsati, 2014).*
- Encourage clients to consider a web-based support program when they are in a caregiving situation. **EBN:** *Research found participation in a web-based family support network provided a venue to share experiences, to be informed, and to gain insights into care issues. Participation reinforced the caregiver's sense of competence, helped them meet caregiving demands, and allowed them to identify the positive aspects of their situation (Andersson et al, 2016).*
- Encourage activity and a strength, mobility, balance, and endurance training program. **EB:** *Older participants in a fitness training trial demonstrated beneficial effects on muscular strength, functionality, and confidence (Schreier et al, 2016).*
- Support meaning and purpose in the lives of older adults through a focus on everyday well-being and facilitation of personally treasured activities. **EBN:** *An exploratory study found four key experiences that promote meaning and purpose in life: (1) physical and mental well-being, (2) belonging and recognition, (3) personally treasured activities, and (4) spiritual closeness and connectedness (Drageset et al, 2017).*
- Use an approach that reduces the emphasis put on ageist self-concept attributions when working with older clients. **EB:** *Ageism includes cognitive, behavioral, and emotional manifestations. Ageism tends to*

S

● = Independent;   ▲ = Collaborative;   **EBN** = Evidence-Based Nursing;   **EB** = Evidence-Based

reinforce social inequalities because it is more pronounced toward older women, poor people, or those with dementia (Ayalon et al, 2017).

Multicultural

- Carefully assess each client and allow families to participate in providing care that is acceptable based on the client's cultural beliefs. **EBN:** *What the client considers normal and abnormal health behavior may be based on cultural perceptions (Itty, Hodge, & Martinez, 2014).*
- Refer to the care plans Disturbed **Body Image,** Readiness for enhanced **Coping,** Chronic low **Self-Esteem,** and Readiness for enhanced **Spiritual** well-being.

Home Care

- Previously discussed interventions may be used in the home care setting.

REFERENCES

Andersson, S., et al. (2016). The experiences of working carers of older people regarding access to a web-based family care support network offered by a municipality. *Scandinavian Journal of Caring Sciences, 31,* 487–496. doi:10.1111/scs.12361.

Annesi, J. J., & Porter, K. J. (2015). Reciprocal effects of exercise and nutrition treatment-Induced weight loss with improved body image and physical self-concept. *Behavioral Medicine, 41*(1), 18–24. Retrieved from http://doi.org.proxy.lib.umich.edu/10.1080/08964289.2013.856284.

Ayalon, L., et al. (2017). Taking a closer look at ageism: Self- and other-directed ageist attitudes and discrimination. *European Journal of Ageing, 14*(1), 1–4. Retrieved from http://doi.org.proxy.lib.umich.edu/10.1007/s10433-016-0409-9.

Baker, F. (2016). Mechanisms of change in self-concept and well-being following songwriting interventions for people in the early phase of neurorehabilitation. *Nordic Journal of Music Therapy, 25,* 10–11.

de Villiers, D., van Rooyen, F. C., Beck, V. V., et al. (2013). Wheelchair dancing and self-esteem in adolescents with physical disabilities. *South African Journal of Occupational Therapy, 43*(2), 23–27.

Drageset, J., et al. (2017). Crucial aspects promoting meaning and purpose in life: Perceptions of nursing home residents. *BMC Geriatrics, 17*(1), 1–9. doi:10.1186/s12877-017-0650-x.

Dudovitz, R. N., et al. (2017). Teachers and coaches in adolescent social networks are associated with healthier self-concept and decreased substance use. *Journal of School Health, 87*(1), 12–20. doi:10.1111/josh.12462.

Grace, N., & Toukhsati, S. R. (2014). Psychosocial functioning in the elderly: An assessment of self-concept and depression. *International Journal of Psychological Research, 7*(1), 12–18.

Holliday, C. E., et al. (2016). A CBPR approach to finding community strengths and challenges to prevent youth suicide and substance abuse. *Journal of Transcultural Nursing, 29*(1), 64–73. Retrieved from http://doi.org.proxy.lib.umich.edu/10.1177/1043659616679234.

Hart, L. M., et al. (2016). Confident body, confident child: A randomized controlled trial evaluation of a parenting resource for promoting healthy body image and eating patterns in 2- to 6-year old children. *International Journal of Eating Disorders, 49*(5), 458–472. doi:10.1002/eat.22494.

Itty, T. L., Hodge, F. S., & Martinez, F. (2014). Shared and unshared barriers to cancer symptom management among urban and rural American Indians. *Journal of Rural Health, 30*(2), 206–213. doi:10.1111/jrh.12045.

Kelly, S., et al. (2011). Correlates among healthy lifestyle cognitive beliefs, healthy lifestyle choices, social support, and healthy behaviors in adolescents: Implications for behavioral change strategies and future research. *Journal of Pediatric Health Care, 25*(4), 216–223.

Kira, M., & Klehe, U. (2016). Self-definition threats and potential for growth among mature-aged job-loss victims. *Human Resource Management Review, 26*(3), 242–259. Retrieved from http://doi.org.proxy.lib.umich.edu/10.1016/j.hrmr.2016.03.001.

Klafke, N., et al. (2016). Developing and implementing a complex Complementary and Alternative (CAM) nursing intervention for breast and gynecologic cancer patients undergoing chemotherapy—Report from the CONGO (Complementary Nursing in Gynecologic Oncology) study. *Supportive Care in Cancer, 24*(5), 2341–2350. Retrieved from http://doi.org.proxy.lib.umich.edu/10.1007/s00520-015-3038-5.

McNamara, N., & Parsons, H. (2016). 'Everyone here wants everyone else to get better': The role of social identity in eating disorder recovery. *British Journal of Social Psychology, 55*(4), 662–680. doi:10.1111/bjso.12161.

Parker, J., et al. (2016). Preserving and protecting well-being among homeless men. *Sociological Perspectives, 59*(1), 201–218. Retrieved from http://doi.org.proxy.lib.umich.edu/10.1177/0731121415591096.

Schreier, M. M., et al. (2016). Fitness training for the old and frail. *Zeitschrift für Gerontologie und Geriatrie, 49*(2), 107–114. Retrieved from http://doi.org.proxy.lib.umich.edu/10.1007/s00391-015-0966-0.

Spruit, A., et al. (2016). The effects of physical activity interventions on psychosocial outcomes in adolescents: A meta-analytic review. *Clinical Psychology Review, 45,* 56–71. Retrieved from http://doi.org.proxy.lib.umich.edu/10.1016/j.cpr.2016.03.006.

Staiano, A. E., et al. (2016). Twelve weeks of dance exergaming in overweight and obese adolescent girls: Transfer effects on physical activity, screen time, and self-efficacy. *Journal of Sport and Health Science, 6*(1), 4–10. doi:10.1016/j.jshs.2016.11.005.

Watson, L. L., et al. (2016). Educational resiliency in teen mothers. *Cogent Education, 4*(1), 1–22. Retrieved from http://doi.org.proxy.lib.umich.edu/10.1080/2331186X.2016.1276009.

West, J., et al. (2017). Trauma sensitive yoga as a complementary treatment for posttraumatic stress disorder: A qualitative descriptive analysis. *International Journal of Stress Management, 24*(2), 173–195. doi:10.1037/str0000040.

Chronic low Self-Esteem   *Marina Martinez-Kratz, MS, RN, CNE*

NANDA-I

Definition

Negative evaluation and/or feelings about one's own capabilities, lasting at least three months.

Defining Characteristics

Dependent on others' opinions; exaggerates negative feedback about self; excessive seeking of reassurance; guilt; hesitant to try new experiences; indecisive behavior; nonassertive behavior; overly conforming; passivity; poor eye contact; rejection of positive feedback; repeatedly unsuccessful in life events; shame; underestimates ability to deal with situation

Related Factors

Cultural incongruence; inadequate affection received; inadequate belonging; inadequate group membership; inadequate respect from others; ineffective coping with loss; receiving insufficient approval from others; spiritual incongruence

At-Risk Population

Exposure to traumatic situation; pattern of failure; repeated negative reinforcement

Associated Condition

Psychiatric disorder

NOC   (Nursing Outcomes Classification)

Suggested NOC Outcome

Self-Esteem

Example NOC Outcome with Indicators

Demonstrates improved **Self-Esteem** as evidenced by the following indicators: Verbalizations of acceptance of self and limitations/Open communication. (Rate the outcome and indicators of **Self-Esteem**: 1 = never positive, 2 = rarely positive, 3 = sometimes positive, 4 = often positive, 5 = consistently positive [see Section I].)

Client Outcomes

Client Will (Specify Time Frame)

- Demonstrate improved ability to interact with others (e.g., maintains eye contact, engages in conversation, expresses thoughts/feelings)
- Verbalize increased self-acceptance through positive self-statements about self
- Identify personal strengths, accomplishments, and values
- Identify and work on small, achievable goals
- Improve independent decision-making and problem-solving skills

NIC   (Nursing Interventions Classification)

Suggested NIC Intervention

Self-Esteem Enhancement

Example NIC Activities—Self-Esteem Enhancement

Encourage patient to identify strengths; Assist in setting realistic goals to achieve higher self-esteem

---

Nursing Interventions and *Rationales*

- Actively listen to and respect the client. EB: *This study described active listening as essential in uncovering patients' emotions (Del Piccolo et al, 2014).*

● = Independent;   ▲ = Collaborative;   EBN = Evidence-Based Nursing;   EB = Evidence-Based

S

- Assess the client's environmental and everyday stressors, including physical health concerns and the potential for abusive relationships. **EB:** *Findings in this study suggested that early adverse conditions have lasting implications for physical health and that continued exposure to increased levels of both social and nonsocial stress in adolescence, as well as the presence of depression, might be important mechanisms by which early adversity affects later physical health (Raposa et al, 2014).*
- Assess existing strengths and coping abilities, and provide opportunities for their expression and recognition. **CEB:** *Persons with psychiatric illness need help to stop their "negative self-image" and become more conscious of affirmative self-evaluation (Kunikata, 2010).*
- Assess the client's self-esteem using valid and established tools like the Rosenberg Self-Esteem Scale. **EBN:** *The use of valid and established measures of self-esteem will facilitate the identification of appropriate nursing interventions that strengthen self-esteem (McMullen & Resnick, 2013).*
- Assess the client for addictive use of social media. **EB:** *Results from a recent study demonstrated that lower age, being a woman, not being in a relationship, being a student, lower education, lower income, lower self-esteem, and narcissism were associated with higher scores on the Bergen Social Media Addiction Scale (BSMAS) (Andreasson et al, 2017).*
- Reinforce the personal strengths and positive self-perceptions that a client identifies. **EB:** *A recent study found that self-esteem mediates the relationship between hope and life satisfaction (Du et al, 2015).*
- Encourage self-affirmations by reflecting on values and strengths, in response to daily threats. **EB:** *A study found that engaging in spontaneous self-affirmation was related to greater happiness, hopefulness, optimism, subjective health, personal health efficacy, and less anger and sadness (Emanuel et al, 2016).*
- Identify client's negative self-assessments. **EB:** *Body image was found to have significant effects on both self-esteem and depression (You et al, 2017).*
- Assess individuals with low self-esteem for nonsuicidal self-injury (NSSI). **EB:** *A systemic review indicated a significant negative relationship between self-esteem and NSSI (Forrester et al, 2017).*
- Assess individuals with low self-esteem for symptoms of depression. **EB:** *Self-esteem is related to depressive symptoms and interpersonal problems. Improvement of self-esteem during psychotherapy correlates with improvements of symptoms and interpersonal problems (Dinger et al, 2017).*
- Encourage realistic and achievable goal setting and resources and identify impediments to achievement. **EB:** *A combined decision support and goal-setting intervention improved diet quality, diabetes-related self-efficacy, and empowerment, and reduced diabetes-related distress and depressive symptoms (Swoboda et al, 2017).*
- Assist client to challenge negative perceptions of self and performance. **EB:** *A study found that more often than not, self-critical thoughts were viewed as facts and would rarely be seen as distorted or biased (Kolubinski et al, 2016).*
- Encourage the client's usual religious or spiritual practices. **EB:** *Research supports a positive association between religious involvement and self-esteem (Schieman et al, 2017).*
- Promote maintaining a level of functioning in the community and a sense of community feeling. **EB:** *Research found that the community feeling is positively connected with self-esteem and psychological well-being (Kałużna-Wielobób, 2017).*

 Pediatric

- Assess children/adolescents with chronic illness for evidence of reduced self-esteem and make needed referrals. **EB:** *Children and adolescents with chronic illness have lower levels of self-esteem compared with their healthy peers; experiences of success and positive peer relations are important sources of self-esteem (Pinquart, 2013).*
- Encourage mothers of premature infants to use kangaroo care for at least 30 minutes/day. **EBN:** *A recent study found kangaroo care showed significantly positive effects on stabilizing infant physiological functions such as respiration rate, increasing maternal–infant attachment, and reducing maternal stress (Cho et al, 2016).*
- Implement interventions that promote and maintain positive peer relations for adolescent patients. **EB:** *Peer relationships had the greatest effect on self-esteem for adolescent patients (Farineau et al, 2013).*
- Encourage attendance at social support groups. **EB:** *A study found that lesbian, gay, bisexual, transgender, and queer (LGBTQ) youth who attended a Hatch group-level intervention that consisted of unstructured social time, consciousness-raising (education), and a youth-led peer support group had higher levels of self-esteem (Wilkerson et al, 2016).*
- Encourage parents to praise children in ways that are not overly positive or inflated. **EB:** *A study found that parents' inflated praise predicted lower self-esteem in children (Brummelman et al, 2017).*

● = Independent; ▲ = Collaborative; EBN = Evidence-Based Nursing; EB = Evidence-Based

- Provide parents with information designed to promote body satisfaction, healthy eating, and weight management in early childhood. **EB:** *Research evaluated Confident Body, Confident Child (CBCC), which is an intervention for parents of 2- to 6-year-old children, and found significant increases in parents' intentions to use positive behaviors and knowledge of child body image and healthy eating patterns (Hart et al, 2016).*
- Assess children/adolescents that express a body image of self-perceived underweight, self-perceived overweight (OW), and/or frustration with appearance for evidence of bullying. **EB:** *Research indicated that self-perceived underweight, self-perceived OW, and frustration with appearance were positively associated with being bullied (Lin et al, 2017).*
- ▲ Provide bully prevention programs and include information on cyberbullying. **EB:** *A moderate and statistically significant relationship exists between low self-esteem and experiences with cyberbullying (Lin et al, 2017).*

Geriatric

- Support client in identifying and adapting to functional changes. **EBN:** *A study outlined the importance of enquiring about feelings of uselessness, which is linked to both psychological and physical health status, especially in older people who need help in daily activities (Curzio et al, 2017).*
- Use reminiscence therapy and productive activities. **EB:** *This study suggested that productive activities with reminiscence therapy may alleviate depressive symptoms and improve task performance of older people with dementia (Nakamae et al, 2014).*
- Encourage older adult clients to participate in flexibility, toning, and balance exercise. **EB:** *Older participants in a fitness training trial demonstrated beneficial effects on muscular strength, functionality, and confidence (Schreier et al, 2016).*
- Encourage regular physical activity with prerecorded workouts. **EB:** *Research found that a DVD-delivered exercise intervention for older adults was associated with improved and maintained levels of self-esteem (Awick et al, 2017).*
- Encourage participation in intergenerational social activities. **EB:** *Older adults reported that their participation in the "Time after Time" intergenerational program enhanced their confidence, self-esteem, and social skills; contributed to their emotional and overall health and well-being; and enabled them to learn about others and feel connected to their community (Teater, 2016).*
- Encourage activities in which a client can support/help others. **EB:** *Research indicated an association between volunteering and reductions in symptoms of depression, better overall health, fewer functional limitations, feeling appreciated and needed, and greater longevity with vulnerable seniors benefitting the most (Anderson et al, 2014).*

Multicultural

- Assess for the influence of cultural beliefs, norms, and values on the client's sense of self-esteem. **EB:** *A study of Latino youth suggested that specific cultural orientations were associated with increased global self-worth, and increased levels of acculturation risk factors were associated with decreased global self-worth (Kapke, 2017).*
- Assess individuals with low self-esteem for symptoms of depression. **EB:** *Research found that low self-esteem and high depressive symptoms are more closely associated among blacks than whites (Assari, 2017).*
- Validate the client's feelings regarding ethnic or racial identity. **EB:** *A study found high ethnic identity was found to be protective against perceived stress (Espinosa et al, 2017).*

Home Care

- Assess a client's immediate support system/family for relationship patterns and content of communication. **EB:** *A recent study supported the beneficial effects of perceived family support on mental and physical health after surgery (Cardoso-Moreno & Tomás-Aragones, 2017).*
- ▲ Refer to continuous support and help from medical social services to assist the family in care of the client and support the caregiver's well-being. **EB:** *A recent study found that caregiving stress showed a significant positive correlation with depression and with economic and psychological stress, and it showed a significant negative correlation with self-esteem (Kim, 2017).*
- ▲ If a client is involved in counseling or self-help groups, monitor and encourage attendance. Help the client identify the value of group participation after each group encounter. *Discussion about group participation clarifies and reinforces group feedback and support.*

● = Independent;   ▲ = Collaborative;   **EBN** = Evidence-Based Nursing;   **EB** = Evidence-Based

S

Client/Family Teaching and Discharge Planning

▲ Refer to community agencies for psychotherapeutic counseling. **EB:** *Self-esteem is related to depressive symptoms and interpersonal problems. Improvement of self-esteem during psychotherapy correlates with improvements of symptoms and interpersonal problems (Dinger et al, 2017).*

▲ Refer to psychoeducational groups on stress reduction and coping skills. **EB:** *Research findings indicated that participants reported improved self-esteem and knowledge of healthy relationship dynamics after enrollment in psychoeducation groups (Marrs Fuchsel, 2014).*

▲ Refer to self-help support groups specific to needs. **EB:** *Research shows that client participation in support groups increases self-esteem (Seebohm et al, 2013).*

REFERENCES

Anderson, N. D., et al. (2014). The benefits associated with volunteering among seniors: A critical review and recommendations for future research. *Psychological Bulletin*, 140(6), 1505–1533. doi:10.1037/a0037610.

Andreasson, C. S., et al. (2017). The relationship between addictive use of social media, narcissism, and self-esteem: Findings from a large national survey. *Addictive Behaviors*, 64, 287–293. Retrieved from http://doi.org.proxy.lib.umich.edu/10.1016/j.addbeh.2016.03.006.

Assari, S. (2017). Association between self-esteem and depressive symptoms is stronger among black than white older adults. *Journal of Racial and Ethnic Health Disparities*, 4(4), 687–695. Retrieved from http://doi.org.proxy.lib.umich.edu/10.1007/s40615-016-0272-6.

Awick, E. A., et al. (2017). Effects of a home-based DVD-delivered physical activity program on self-esteem in older adults: Results from a randomized controlled trial. *Psychosomatic Medicine*, 79(1), 71–80. doi:10.1097/PSY.0000000000000358.

Brummelman, E., et al. (2017). When parents' praise inflates, children's self-esteem deflates. *Child Development*, 88(6), 1799–1809. doi:10.1111/cdev.12936.

Cardoso-Moreno, M. J., & Tomás-Aragones, L. (2017). The influence of perceived family support on post surgery recovery. *Psychology, Health & Medicine*, 22(1), 121–128.

Cho, E., et al. (2016). The effects of kangaroo care in the neonatal intensive care unit on the physiological functions of preterm infants, maternal–infant attachment, and maternal stress. *Journal of Pediatric Nursing: Nursing Care of Children and Families*, 31(4), 430–438. doi:10.1016/j.pedn.2016.02.007.

Curzio, O., et al. (2017). Feelings of uselessness and 3-year mortality in an Italian community older people: The role of the functional status. *Psychogeriatrics*, 17(5), 300–309. doi:10.1111/psyg.12238.

Del Piccolo, L., Danzi, O., Fattori, N., et al. (2014). How psychiatrist's communication skills and patient's diagnosis affect emotions disclosure during first diagnostic consultations. *Patient Education & Counseling*, 96(2), 151–158.

Dinger, U., et al. (2017). Change in self-esteem predicts depressive symptoms at follow-up after intensive multimodal psychotherapy for major depression. *Clinical Psychology & Psychotherapy*, 24, 1040–1046. Retrieved from http://doi.org.proxy.lib.umich.edu/10.1002/cpp.2067.

Du, H., et al. (2015). Locus-of-hope and life satisfaction: The mediating roles of personal self-esteem and relational self-esteem. *Personality and Individual Differences*, 83, 228–233. Retrieved from http://doi.org.proxy.lib.umich.edu/10.1016/j.paid.2015.04.026.

Emanuel, A. S., et al. (2016). Spontaneous self-affirmation is associated with psychological well-being: Evidence from a US national adult survey sample. *Journal of Health Psychology*, 23(1), 95–102. Retrieved from http://doi.org.proxy.lib.umich.edu/10.1177/1359105316643595.

Espinosa, A., et al. (2017). Ethnic identity and perceived stress among ethnically diverse immigrants. *Journal of Immigrant Minority Health*, 20(1), 155–163. Retrieved from http://doi.org.proxy.lib.umich.edu/10.1007/s10903-016-0494-z.

Farineau, H. M., Stevenson Wojciak, A., & McWey, L. M. (2013). You matter to me: Important relationships and self-esteem of adolescents in foster care. *Child & Family Social Work*, 18(2), 129–138.

Forrester, R. L., et al. (2017). Self-esteem and non-suicidal self-injury in adulthood: A systematic review. *Journal of Affective Disorders*, 221, 172–183. doi:10.1016/j.jad.2017.06.027.

Hart, L. M., et al. (2016). Confident body, confident child: A randomized controlled trial evaluation of a parenting resource for promoting healthy body image and eating patterns in 2- to 6-year old children. *International Journal of Eating Disorders*, 49(5), 458–472. doi:10.1002/eat.22494.

Kałużna-Wielobób, A. (2017). The community feeling versus anxiety, self-esteem and well-being—introductory research. *Polish Psychological Bulletin*, 48(2), 167–174. doi:10.1515/ppb-2017-0020.

Kapke, T. L. (2017). Global self-worth in Latino youth: The role of acculturation and acculturation risk factors. *Child Youth Care Forum*, 46(3), 307–333. Retrieved from http://doi.org.proxy.lib.umich.edu/10.1007/s10566-016-9374-x.

Kim, D. (2017). Relationships between caregiving stress, depression, and self-esteem in family caregivers of adults with a disability. *Occupational Therapy International*, 1–9. Retrieved from http://doi.org.proxy.lib.umich.edu/10.1155/2017/1686143.

Kolubinski, D. C., et al. (2016). The role of metacognition in self-critical rumination: An investigation in individuals presenting with low self-esteem. *Journal of Rational-Emotive & Cognitive-Behavior Therapy*, 34(1), 73–85. Retrieved from http://doi.org.proxy.lib.umich.edu/10.1007/s10942-015-0230-y.

Kunikata, H. (2010). Psychiatric illness persons' structure of mind, body and behavior when they felt low self-esteem [Japanese]. *Journal of Japan Academy of Nursing Science*, 30(4), 36–45.

Lin, Y., et al. (2017). Poor health and experiences of being bullied in adolescents: Self-perceived overweight and frustration with appearance matter. *Obesity*, 26, 397–404. doi:10.1002/oby.22041.

Marrs Fuchsel, C. L. (2014). Exploratory evaluation of Sí, Yo Puedo: A culturally competent empowerment program for immigrant Latina women in group settings. *Social Work With Groups*, 37(4), 279–296.

McMullen, T., & Resnick, B. (2013). Self-esteem among nursing assistants: Reliability and validity of the Rosenberg Self-Esteem Scale. *Journal of Nursing Measurement*, 21(2), 335–344.

Nakamae, T., Yotsumoto, K., Tatsumi, E., et al. (2014). Effects of productive activities with reminiscence in occupational therapy for people with dementia: A pilot randomized controlled study. *Hong Kong Journal of Occupational Therapy*, 24(1), 13–19.

Pinquart, M. M. (2013). Self-esteem of children and adolescents with chronic illness: A meta-analysis. *Child: Care, Health & Development*, 39(2), 153–161.

Raposa, E., Hammen, C., O'Callaghan, F., et al. (2014). Early adversity and health outcomes in young adulthood: The role of ongoing stress. *Health Psychology*, 33(5), 410–418.

S

● = Independent;   ▲ = Collaborative;   **EBN** = Evidence-Based Nursing;   **EB** = Evidence-Based

Seebohm, P., Chaudhary, S., Boyce, M., et al. (2013). The contribution of self-help/mutual aid groups to mental well-being. *Health & Social Care in the Community, 21*(4), 391–401.

Schreier, M. M., et al. (2016). Fitness training for the old and frail. *Zeitschrift für Gerontologie und Geriatrie, 49*(2), 107–114. Retrieved from http://doi.org.proxy.lib.umich.edu/10.1007/s00391-015-0966-0.

Schieman, S., et al. (2017). Love thy self? How belief in a supportive God shapes self-esteem. *Review of Religious Research, 59*(3), 293–318. Retrieved from http://doi.org.proxy.lib.umich.edu/10.1007/s13644-017-0292-7.

Swoboda, C. M., et al. (2017). Impact of a goal setting and decision support telephone coaching intervention on diet, psychosocial, and decision outcomes among people with type 2 diabetes. *Patient*

Education and Counseling, 100(7), 1367–1373. Retrieved from http://doi.org.proxy.lib.umich.edu/10.1016/j.pec.2017.02.007.

Teater, B. (2016). Intergenerational programs to promote active aging: The experiences and perspectives of older adults. *Activities, Adaptation & Aging, 40*(1), 1–19. Retrieved from http://doi.org.proxy.lib.umich.edu/10.1080/01924788.2016.1127041.

Wilkerson, J. M., et al. (2016). Social support, depression, self-esteem, and coping among LGBTQ adolescents participating in Hatch Youth. *Health Promotion Practice, 18*(3), 58–365. Retrieved from http://doi.org.proxy.lib.umich.edu/10.1177/152483991665446.

You, S., et al. (2017). Body image, self-esteem, and depression in Korean adolescents. *Child Indicators Research, 10*(1), 231–245. Retrieved from http://doi.org.proxy.lib.umich.edu/10.1007/s12187-016-9385-z.

Situational low Self-Esteem   Marina Martinez-Kratz, MS, RN, CNE

NANDA-I

Definition

Development of a negative perception of self-worth in response to a current situation.

Defining Characteristics

Helplessness; indecisive behavior; nonassertive behavior; purposelessness; self-negating verbalizations; situational challenge to self-worth; underestimates ability to deal with situation

Related Factors

Alteration in body image; alteration in social role; behavior inconsistent with values; decrease in control over environment; inadequate recognition; pattern of helplessness; unrealistic expectations

At-Risk Population

Developmental transition; history of abandonment; history of abuse; history of loss; history of neglect; history of rejection; pattern of failure

Associated Condition

Functional impairment; physical illness

NOC   (Nursing Outcomes Classification)

Refer to Chronic low **Self-Esteem** for suggested NOC outcomes

Client Outcomes

Client Will (Specify Time Frame)

- State effect of life events on feelings about self
- State personal strengths
- Acknowledge presence of guilt and not blame self if an action was related to another person's appraisal
- Seek help when necessary
- Demonstrate self-perceptions are accurate given physical capabilities
- Demonstrate separation of self-perceptions from societal stigmas

NIC   (Nursing Interventions Classification)

Refer to Chronic low **Self-Esteem** for suggested NIC interventions

Nursing Interventions and *Rationales*

▲ Assess the client for signs and symptoms of depression and potential for suicide and/or violence. If present, immediately notify the appropriate personnel of symptoms. EB: *Recent research supported the vulnerability model of low self-esteem and depression with findings that indicated that individuals with high self-esteem*

● = Independent;   ▲ = Collaborative;   EBN = Evidence-Based Nursing;   EB = Evidence-Based

have a lower risk for developing depression (Orth et al, 2016). See care plans for Risk for other-directed **Violence** and Risk for **Suicide**.

- Assess the client's environmental and everyday stressors, including evidence of abusive relationships. **EB:** *Research showed dysfunctional forms of self-esteem were significantly associated with the number of negative events reported and an increased risk of developing stress-related symptoms (Alessandri et al, 2016).*

- ▲ Assess the client's self-esteem using valid and established tools like the Rosenberg Self-Esteem Scale. **EBN:** *The use of valid and established measures of self-esteem will facilitate the identification of appropriate nursing interventions that strengthen self-esteem (McMullen & Resnick, 2013).*

- Assess for unhealthy coping mechanisms, such as substance abuse, and make appropriate referrals. **EB:** *Numerous factors influence the onset and continuation of alcohol use, including the complex ways that genes interact with one another and with the environment (Faye et al, 2015).*

- Encourage expressions of gratitude through a gratitude journal or kind acts. **EB:** *Research shows that gratitude is significantly and positively associated with several domains of life satisfaction and overall life satisfaction in both the United States and Japan (Robustelli & Whisman, 2018).*

- Use a cognitive approach like problem-solving education (PSE) to assist in the identification of problems and situational factors that contribute to problems and offer options for resolution. **EB:** *A recent study found that supplementing drug abuse treatment with PSE reduced relapse rates and enhanced self-efficacy and self-esteem among patients (Habibi et al, 2016).*

- Mutually identify strengths, resources, and previously effective coping strategies. **EB:** *A recent study showed that a behavioral intervention focusing on the individual's strengths showed a reduction of psychological distress and improvement of self-esteem, optimism, and quality of life compared with the control group (Victor, Teismann, & Willutzki, 2017).*

- Encourage self-affirmations by reflecting on values and strengths, in response to daily threats. **EB:** *A study found that engaging in spontaneous self-affirmation was related to greater happiness, hopefulness, optimism, subjective health, personal health efficacy, and less anger and sadness (Emanuel et al, 2016).*

- Accept client's own pace in working through grief or crisis situations. **EB:** *Rigid adherence to stage or time line models of grief models is too simplistic and limited; they fail to represent the complex emotions and processes of grief and grieving (Stroebe et al, 2017).*

- Encourage the client to accept their own defenses, feelings, and urges in dealing with the crisis. **EB:** *Acceptance and commitment therapy (ACT) is an intervention that enhances well-being and reduces distress (Wersebe et al, 2018).*

- Provide information about support groups of people who have common experiences or interests. **EBN:** *Research shows that client participation in support groups increases self-esteem (Seebohm et al, 2013).*

- Teach the client mindfulness techniques to cope more effectively with strong emotional responses. **EB:** *Mindfulness training has direct positive effects on self-esteem (Pepping et al, 2013).*

- Encourage objective appraisal of self and life events and challenge negative or perfectionist expectations of self. **EB:** *Self-critical perfectionism has been reliably associated with poor goal progress (Moore et al, 2018).*

- Provide psychoeducation to client and family. **EB:** *Research findings indicated that participants reported improved self-esteem and knowledge of healthy relationship dynamics after enrollment in psychoeducation groups (Marrs Fuchsel, 2014).*

- Acknowledge the presence of societal stigma. Teach management tools. **EBN:** *Stigma toward mental illness affects both self-esteem and recovery and treatment adherence (Vass et al, 2017).*

- Validate the effect of negative past experiences on self-esteem and work on corrective measures. **EB:** *Negative life events influence current self-esteem (Tetzner et al, 2016).*

Geriatric and Multicultural

- See care plan for Chronic low **Self-Esteem.**

Home Care

- Establish an emergency plan and contract with the client for its use. Having an emergency plan is reassuring to the client. Establishing a contract validates the worth of the client and provides a caring link between the client and society.

- Access supplies that support a client's success at independent living.

- See care plan for Chronic low **Self-Esteem.**

● = Independent;   ▲ = Collaborative;   EBN = Evidence-Based Nursing;   EB = Evidence-Based

Client/Family Teaching and Discharge Planning

- Assess the person's support system (family, friends, and community) and involve them if desired. **CEB:** Teach client and family that the crisis is temporary. Knowing that the crisis is temporary provides a sense of hope for the future.
- ▲ Refer to self-help support groups specific to needs. **EB:** *Research showed that client participation in support groups increases self-esteem (Seebohm et al, 2013).*
- ▲ Refer to appropriate community resources or crisis intervention centers.
- ▲ Refer to resources for handicap and/or disability services.
- See care plan for Chronic low **Self-Esteem.**

REFERENCES

Alessandri, G., et al. (2016). The costly burden of an inauthentic self: Insecure self-esteem predisposes to emotional exhaustion by increasing reactivity to negative events. *Anxiety, Stress & Coping, 30*(6), 630–646. doi:10.1080/10615806.2016.1262357.

Emanuel, A. S., et al. (2016). Spontaneous self-affirmation is associated with psychological well-being: Evidence from a US national adult survey sample. *Journal of Health Psychology, 23*(1), 95–102. Retrieved from http://doi.org.proxy.lib.umich.edu/10.1177/1359105316643595.

Faye, C., et al. *NIAAA's strategic plan to address health disparities.* Retrieved from http://www.niaaa.nih.gov/-publications/HealthDisparities/Strategic.html. (Accessed 2 January 2015).

Habibi, R., et al. (2016). The effects of family-centered problem-solving education on relapse rate, self efficacy and self esteem among substance abusers. *International Journal of High Risk Behaviors & Addiction, 5*(1), e24421. Retrieved from http://doi.org.proxy.lib.umich.edu/10.5812/ijhrba.24421.

Marrs Fuchsel, C. L. (2014). Exploratory evaluation of Sí, Yo Puedo: A culturally competent empowerment program for immigrant Latina women in group settings. *Social Work With Groups, 37*(4), 279–296.

McMullen, T., & Resnick, B. (2013). Self-esteem among nursing assistants: Reliability and validity of the Rosenberg Self-Esteem Scale. *Journal of Nursing Measurement, 21*(2), 335–344.

Moore, E., et al. (2018). Perfectionism and the pursuit of personal goals: A self-determination theory analysis. *Motivation and Emotion, 42*(1), 37–49. Retrieved from http://doi.org.proxy.lib.umich.edu/10.1007/s11031-017-9654-2.

Orth, U., et al. (2016). Refining the vulnerability model of low self-esteem and depression: Disentangling the effects of genuine self-esteem and narcissism. *Journal of Personality and Social Psychology, 110*(1), 133–149. doi:10.1037/pspp0000038.

Pepping, C. A., O'Donovan, A., & Davis, P. J. (2013). The positive effects of mindfulness on self-esteem. *Journal Of Positive Psychology, 8*(5), 376–386.

Robustelli, B. L., & Whisman, M. A. (2018). Gratitude and life satisfaction in the United States and Japan. *Journal of Happiness Studies, 19*(1), 41–55. Retrieved from https://doi.org.proxy.lib.umich.edu/10.1007/s10902-016-9802-5.

Seebohm, P., Chaudhary, S., Boyce, M., et al. (2013). The contribution of self-help/mutual aid groups to mental well-being. *Health & Social Care in the Community, 21*(4), 391–401.

Stroebe, M., et al. (2017). Cautioning health-care professionals: Bereaved persons are misguided through the stages of grief. *Omega, 74*(4), 455–473. Retrieved from http://doi.org.proxy.lib.umich.edu/10.1177/0030222817691870.

Tetzner, J., et al. (2016). Still Doing Fine? The interplay of negative life events and self-esteem during young adulthood. *European Journal of Personality, 30*(4), 358–373. doi:10.1002/per.2066.

Vass, V., et al. (2017). How stigma gets under the skin: The role of stigma, self-stigma and self-esteem in subjective recovery from psychosis. *Psychosis, 9*(3), 235–244. doi:10.1080/17522439.2017.1300184.

Victor, P., Teismann, T., & Willutzki, U. (2017). A pilot evaluation of a strengths-based CBT intervention module with college students. *Behavioural and Cognitive Psychotherapy, 45*(4), 427–431. doi:10.1017/S1352465816000552.

Wersebe, H., et al. (2018). The link between stress, well-being, and psychological flexibility during an Acceptance and Commitment Therapy self-help intervention. *International Journal of Clinical and Health Psychology, 18*(1), 60–68. Retrieved from http://doi.org.proxy.lib.umich.edu/10.1016/j.ijchp.2017.09.002.

S

Risk for chronic low Self-Esteem   *Gail B. Ladwig, MSN, RN*

NANDA-I

Definition

Susceptible to longstanding negative self-evaluating/feelings about self or self-capabilities, which may compromise health.

Risk Factors

Cultural incongruence; inadequate affection received; inadequate belonging; inadequate group membership; inadequate respect from others; ineffective coping with loss; receiving insufficient approval from others; spiritual incongruence

● = Independent;   ▲ = Collaborative;   **EBN** = Evidence-Based Nursing;   **EB** = Evidence-Based

At-Risk Population

Exposure to traumatic situation; pattern of failure; repeated negative reinforcement

Associated Condition

Psychiatric disorder

NOC, NIC, Client Outcomes, Nursing Interventions and *Rationales,* and References

Refer to care plan for Chronic low **Self-Esteem**

Risk for situational low Self-Esteem   *Marina Martinez-Kratz, MS, RN, CNE*

NANDA-I

Definition

Susceptible to developing a negative perception of self-worth in response to a current situation, which may compromise health.

Risk Factors

Alteration in body image; alteration in social role; behavior inconsistent with values; decrease in control over environment; inadequate recognition; pattern of helplessness; unrealistic self-expectations

At-Risk Population

Developmental transition; history of abandonment; history of abuse; history of loss; history of neglect; history of rejection; pattern of failure

Associated Condition

Functional impairment; physical illness

NOC   (Nursing Outcomes Classification)

See Chronic low **Self-Esteem** for suggested NOC outcomes

Client Outcomes

Client Will (Specify Time Frame)

- State accurate self-appraisal
- Demonstrate the ability to self-validate
- Demonstrate the ability to make decisions independent of primary peer group
- Express effects of media on self-appraisal
- Express influence of substances on self-esteem
- Identify strengths and healthy coping skills
- State life events and change as influencing self-esteem

NIC   (Nursing Interventions Classification)

See Chronic low **Self-Esteem** for suggested NIC interventions

Nursing Interventions and *Rationales*

- Assist client to challenge negative perceptions of self and performance. EB: *A study found that more often than not, self-critical thoughts were viewed as facts and would rarely be seen as distorted or biased (*Kolubinski et al, 2016*).*
- Assess the client's self-esteem using valid and established tools like the Rosenberg Self-Esteem Scale. EBN: *The use of valid and established measures of self-esteem will facilitate the identification of appropriate nursing interventions that strengthen self-esteem (McMullen & Resnick, 2013).*
- Encourage client to maintain highest level of community functioning. EB: *Research found that the community feeling is positively connected with self-esteem and psychological well-being (Kałużna-Wielobób, 2017).*

● = Independent;   ▲ = Collaborative;   EBN = Evidence-Based Nursing;   EB = Evidence-Based

- Encourage self-affirmations by reflecting on values and strengths, in response to daily threats. **EB:** *A study found that engaging in spontaneous self-affirmation was related to greater happiness, hopefulness, optimism, subjective health, personal health efficacy, and less anger and sadness (Emanuel et al, 2016).*
- Encourage realistic and achievable goal setting and resources and identify impediments to achievement. **EB:** *A combined decision support and goal-setting intervention improved diet quality, diabetes-related self-efficacy, and empowerment, and reduced diabetes-related distress and depressive symptoms (Swoboda et al, 2017).*
- ▲ Assess the client for symptoms of depression and anxiety. Refer to specialist as needed. Prompt and effective treatment can prevent exacerbation of symptoms or safety risks. **EB:** *Recent research supported the vulnerability model of low self-esteem and depression with findings that indicated that individuals with high self-esteem have a lower risk for developing depression (Orth et al, 2016).*
- See care plans for Disturbed personal **Identity,** Situational low **Self-Esteem,** and Chronic low **Self-Esteem.**

Pediatric

- Assess children/adolescents with chronic illness for evidence of reduced self-esteem and make needed referrals. **EB:** *Children and adolescents with chronic illness have lower levels of self-esteem compared with their healthy peers; experiences of success and positive peer relations are important sources of self-esteem (Pinquart, 2013).*
- Identify environmental and/or developmental factors that increase risk for low self-esteem, especially in children/adolescents, to make needed referrals. **EB:** *A study found that relative to other students, risk for internalizing problems and low self-esteem was elevated for aggressive adolescents, students who were hassled or bullied at school, and those who were rejected by peers or in conflict with their parents (Cicchetti et al, 2014).*
- Encourage attendance at social support groups. **EB:** *A study found that lesbian, gay, bisexual, transgender, and queer (LGBTQ) youth who attended a Hatch group-level intervention that consisted of unstructured social time, consciousness-raising (education), and a youth-led peer support group had higher levels of self-esteem (Wilkerson et al, 2016).*
- Assess children/adolescents who are either a victim or an offender of cyberbullying for low self-esteem. **EB:** *A moderate and statistically significant relationship exists between low self-esteem and experiences with cyberbullying (Lin et al, 2017).*
- ▲ Encourage a combination of extracurricular activity for adolescents in a safe, supportive, and empowering environment. **EB:** *Research suggested that enabling relations within the family, school, peer, and community are factors related to youth self-satisfaction (Simon, 2018).*

Geriatric

- Support humor as a coping mechanism. **EB:** *This paper identified that humor has a positive effect on all of these issues with an increasing sense of well-being and life satisfaction for the elder (Lurie & Monahan, 2015).*
- Support client in identifying and adapting to functional changes. **EBN:** *A study outlined the importance of enquiring about feelings of uselessness, which is linked to both psychological and physical health status, especially in older people who need help in daily activities (Curzio et al, 2017).*
- Encourage participation in intergenerational social activities. **EB:** *Older adults reported that their participation in the "Time after Time" intergenerational program enhanced their confidence, self-esteem, and social skills; contributed to their emotional and overall health and well-being; and enabled them to learn about others and feel connected to their community (Teater, 2016).*
- Assist the client in life review and identifying positive accomplishments. *Life review is a developmental task that increases a person's sense of peace and serenity.*
- Help client establish a peer group and structured daily activities. *Social isolation and lack of structure increase a client's sense of feeling lost and worthless.*
- See care plans for Situational low **Self-Esteem** and Chronic low **Self-Esteem.**

Home Care

- Assess current environmental stresses and identify community resources. *Accessing resources to help decrease environmental stress will increase the client's ability to cope.*
- Encourage family members to acknowledge and validate the client's strengths. *Validation allows the client to increase self-reliance and to trust personal decisions.*

● = Independent; ▲ = Collaborative; **EBN** = Evidence-Based Nursing; **EB** = Evidence-Based

S

- Assess the need for establishing an emergency plan. *Openly assessing safety risks increases the client's sense of limits, boundaries, and safety.*
- See care plans for Situational low **Self-Esteem** and Chronic low **Self-Esteem**.

 Client/Family Teaching and Discharge Planning

▲ Refer the client/family to community-based self-help and support groups. **EB:** *Research showed that clients who participate in support groups show increased self-esteem (Seebohm et al, 2013).*

▲ Refer to psychoeducational groups on stress reduction and coping skills. **EB:** *Research findings indicated that participants reported improved self-esteem and knowledge of healthy relationship dynamics after enrollment in psychoeducation groups (Marrs Fuchsel, 2014).*

▲ Refer the client to community agencies that offer support and environmental resources. Make referrals as needed.

- See care plans for Situational low **Self-Esteem** and Chronic low **Self-Esteem**.

REFERENCES

Cicchetti, D., et al. (2014). Multilevel risk factors and developmental assets for internalizing symptoms and self-esteem in disadvantaged adolescents: Modeling longitudinal trajectories from the rural adaptation project. *Development and Psychopathology, 26*(4), 1495–1513. Retrieved from http://doi.org.proxy.lib.umich.edu/10.1017/S0954579414001163.

Curzio, O., et al. (2017). Feelings of uselessness and 3 year mortality in an Italian community older people: The role of the functional status. *Psychogeriatrics, 17*(5), 300–309. doi:10.1111/psyg.12238.

Emanuel, A. S., et al. (2016). Spontaneous self-affirmation is associated with psychological well-being: Evidence from a US national adult survey sample. *Journal of Health Psychology, 23*(1), 95–102. Retrieved from http://doi.org.proxy.lib.umich.edu/10.1177/1359105316643595.

Kałużna-Wielobób, A. (2017). The community feeling versus anxiety, self-esteem and well-being—Introductory research. *Polish Psychological Bulletin, 48*(2), 167–174. doi:10.1515/ppb-2017-0020.

Kolubinski, D. C., et al. (2016). The role of metacognition in self-critical rumination: An investigation in individuals presenting with low self-esteem. *Journal of Rational-Emotive & Cognitive-Behavior Therapy, 34*(1), 73–85. Retrieved from http://doi.org.proxy.lib.umich.edu/10.1007/s10942-015-0230-y.

Lin, Y., et al. (2017). Poor health and experiences of being bullied in adolescents: Self-perceived overweight and frustration with appearance matter. *Obesity, 26*, 397–404. doi:10.1002/oby.22041.

Lurie, A., & Monahan, K. (2015). Humor, aging, and life review: Survival through the use of humor. *Social Work in Mental Health, 13*(1), 82–91. doi:10.1080/15332985.2014.884519.

Marrs Fuchsel, C. L. (2014). Exploratory evaluation of Sí, Yo Puedo: A culturally competent empowerment program for immigrant Latina women in group settings. *Social Work With Groups, 37*(4), 279–296.

McMullen, T., & Resnick, B. (2013). Self-esteem among nursing assistants: Reliability and validity of the Rosenberg Self-Esteem Scale. *Journal of Nursing Measurement, 21*(2), 335–344.

Orth, U., et al. (2016). Refining the vulnerability model of low self-esteem and depression: Disentangling the effects of genuine self-esteem and narcissism. *Journal of Personality and Social Psychology, 110*(1), 133–149. doi:10.1037/pspp0000038.

Pinquart, M. M. (2013). Self-esteem of children and adolescents with chronic illness: A meta-analysis. *Child: Care, Health & Development, 39*(2), 153–161.

Seebohm, P., Chaudhary, S., Boyce, M., et al. (2013). The contribution of self-help/mutual aid groups to mental well-being. *Health & Social Care in the Community, 21*(4), 391–401.

Simon, P. (2018). Enabling relations as determinants of self-satisfaction in the youth: The path from self-satisfaction to prosocial behaviors as explained by strength of inner self. *Current Psychology, 37*, 1–9. Retrieved from http://doi.org.proxy.lib.umich.edu/10.1007/s12144-018-9791-0.

Swoboda, C. M., et al. (2017). Impact of a goal setting and decision support telephone coaching intervention on diet, psychosocial, and decision outcomes among people with type 2 diabetes. *Patient Education and Counseling, 100*(7), 1367–1373. Retrieved from http://doi.org.proxy.lib.umich.edu/10.1016/j.pec.2017.02.007.

Teater, B. (2016). Intergenerational programs to promote active aging: The experiences and perspectives of older adults. *Activities, Adaptation & Aging, 40*(1), 1–19. Retrieved from http://doi.org.proxy.lib.umich.edu/10.1080/01924788.2016.1127041.

Wilkerson, J. M., et al. (2016). Social support, depression, self-esteem, and coping among LGBTQ adolescents participating in Hatch Youth. *Health Promotion Practice, 18*(3), 58–365. Retrieved from http://doi.org.proxy.lib.umich.edu/10.1177/152483991665446.

S

Risk for Self-Mutilation   Kathleen L. Patusky, MA, PhD, RN, CNS

NANDA-I

Definition

Susceptible to deliberate self-injurious behavior causing tissue damage with the intent of causing nonfatal injury to attain relief of tension.

Risk Factors

Absence of family confidant; alteration in body image; dissociation; disturbance in interpersonal relationships; eating disorder; emotional disturbance; feeling threatened with loss of significant relationship; impaired

● = Independent;   ▲ = Collaborative;   **EBN** = Evidence-Based Nursing;   **EB** = Evidence-Based

self-esteem; impulsiveness; inability to express tension verbally; ineffective communication between parent and adolescent; ineffective coping strategies; irresistible urge for self-directed violence; irresistible urge to cut self; isolation from peers; labile behavior; loss of control over problem-solving situation; low self-esteem; mounting tension that is intolerable; negative feeling; pattern of inability to plan solutions; pattern of inability to see long-term consequences; perfectionism; requires rapid stress reduction; substance misuse; use of manipulation to obtain nurturing relationship with others

At-Risk Population

Adolescence; battered child; childhood illness; childhood surgery; developmental delay; family divorce; family history of self-destructive behavior; family substance misuse; history of childhood abuse; incarceration; living in nontraditional setting; loss of significant relationship; peers who self-mutilate; sexual identity crisis; violence between parental figures

Associated Condition

Autism; borderline personality disorder; character disorder; depersonalization; psychotic disorder

NOC   (Nursing Outcomes Classification)

See care plan for **Self-Mutilation** for suggested NOC outcomes

Client Outcomes

Client Will (Specify Time Frame)

- Refrain from self-injury
- Identify triggers to self-mutilation
- State appropriate ways to cope with increased psychological or physiological tension
- Express feelings
- Seek help when having urges to self-mutilate
- Maintain self-control without supervision
- Use appropriate community agencies when caregivers are unable to attend to emotional needs

NIC   (Nursing Interventions Classification)

See care plan for **Self-Mutilation** for suggested NIC interventions

Nursing Interventions and *Rationales*

Note: Before implementing interventions in the face of self-injury, nurses should examine their own knowledge base and emotional responses to incidents of self-injury to ensure that interventions will not be based on countertransference reactions. EBN: *Lack of educational background on self-harm can influence response to self-harm clients. Nurses' tendency to focus on physical care, especially when working under stressful conditions, can hinder awareness of and response to psychosocial issues (Cleaver, 2014).*

- A nonjudgmental approach to clients is critical. EBN: *A qualitative study of nurses' experiences caring for patients who self-harmed indicated the need for acceptance of the client (Moola, 2017).*
- Assess for history of self-harm behavior. EB: *A meta-analysis of self-harm risk factors revealed prior history as a strong predictor of current self-harm behavior (Fox et al, 2015).*
- Assess client's ability to regulate his or her own emotional states. These states may be influenced by the client's perception of his or her body or by the presence of a psychiatric disorder. EB: *Clients who self-injure are more likely to be lower in emotional self-regulation and regulation of affect than persons who do not self-injure, especially in adolescents and young adults. They may use self-harm to increase or decrease feelings. Self-injury has been associated with low body regard (Muehlenkamp et al, 2013; Sadeh et al, 2014).*
- Assess client's perception of powerlessness. Refer to the care plan for **Powerlessness.** EBN: *Involve clients in clinical decision-making (Moola, 2017).*
- Assessment data from the client and family members may have to be gathered at different times; allowing a family member or trusted friend with whom the client is comfortable to be present during the assessment may be helpful. CEBN: *Self-mutilation sometimes occurs if clients have been victims of abuse or other types of adverse family experiences (Catledge, Scharer, & Fuller, 2012). Clients or family members may be more willing to disclose the presence of abuse if greater privacy is afforded them, or if presence of a trusted family member or friend helps clients to respond more comfortably to the interview situation.*

● = Independent;   ▲ = Collaborative;   EBN = Evidence-Based Nursing;   EB = Evidence-Based

S

- Perform a thorough skin assessment at least annually and check for behavioral cues of self-harm. CEBN: *Skin assessment must cover body areas normally clothed. Signs of self-harm include scratches, burns, lacerations, objects embedded under the skin (e.g., razor blades), multiple scars, or carved words. Scars may vary in age and depth. Behavioral cues include wearing long sleeves and pants, wristbands or bulky bracelets, and avoiding situations that would result in exposed skin (e.g., physical education class) (Catledge, Scharer, & Fuller, 2012).*
- Assess for co-occurring disorders that require response, especially childhood abuse, substance abuse, and suicide attempts. Implement reporting or referral as indicated. EB: *Self-mutilation has been associated with multiple psychiatric disorders (Moller, Tait, & Byrne, 2013; Sadeh et al, 2014).*
- Assess family dynamics and the need for family therapy and community support. EBN: *A comprehensive assessment of needs should address social, psychological, and motivational elements of the client and family members (Moola, 2017).*
- Assess for the presence of medical disorders, mental retardation, medication effects, or disorders such as autism that may include self-mutilation. Initiate referral for evaluation and treatment as appropriate. *Self-mutilation has been reported as a presenting or ongoing symptom with medical disorders.*
- Be alert to other risk factors of self-mutilation in clients with psychosis, including acute intoxication, dramatic changes in body appearance, preoccupation with religion and sexuality, and anticipated or perceived object loss. *Many psychiatric disorders have shown a connection with self-mutilation. Command hallucinations occurring in schizophrenia or brief psychotic episodes may direct the client to hurt himself or herself or others.*
- Monitor the client's behavior closely by using engagement and support as elements of safety checks while avoiding intrusive overstimulation. Offer activities that will serve as a distraction. *When lack of control exists, client safety is an important issue and close observation is essential.* EBN: *Clients may feel overstimulated by intrusive close observation, resulting in agitation (Moola, 2017).*
- Focus on understanding the function that self-harm serves for the client and on managing the client's distress. EB: *Self-harm is a form of distress management. A qualitative study of mental health staff interventions and efficacy suggested individualized care highlighting management of distress and identification of obstacles to interventions are more effective. If clients are unable to self-harm, prevention can lead to power struggles and the use of more harmful methods (Thomas & Haslam, 2017).*
- Establish trust, show a caring attitude and hope for recovery, listen to client, convey safety, promote client's verbal expression, and assist in developing positive goals for the future. Assist client to identify triggers and identify prevention activities. EBN: *A qualitative study of nursing interventions focused on identifying and dealing with triggers, and promoting person-centered nursing (Tofthagen, Talseth, & Fagerstrom, 2014).*
- Refer to mental health counseling. Multiple therapeutic modalities are available for treatment.
▲ Case finding and referral by school nurses for psychological or psychiatric treatment is critical. Treatment includes starting therapy and medications, increasing coping skills, facilitating decision-making, encouraging positive relationships, and fostering self-esteem. EB: *Although the repeat rate of self-harm is around 21%, clients may have a very low treatment follow-up rate. Access to care must be a consideration (Hunter et al, 2018).*
- Inform the client of expectations for appropriate behavior and consequences within the unit. Emphasize that the client must comply with the rules. Give positive reinforcement for compliance and minimize attention paid to disruptive behavior while setting limits. *Clients benefit from clear guidance regarding behavioral expectations and consequences, providing much needed structure. It is important to reinforce appropriate behavior to encourage repetition.* EB: *Treatment should involve assisting the client to learn healthier affective regulation skills (Sadeh et al, 2014).*
- Clients need to learn to recognize distress as it occurs and express it verbally rather than as a physical action against the self. CEB: *Treatment should involve assisting the client to learn healthier affective regulation skills (Sadeh et al, 2014).*
- Assist the client to identify the motives/reasons for self-mutilation that have been perceived as positive. Self-harm serves as a defense mechanism. CEB: *Persecutory self-criticism and limited coping skills are linked with self-harm.*
- Assist clients to identify ways to soothe themselves and generate hopefulness when faced with painful emotions. *Generating hopefulness is an important self-comforting intervention.*
- Reinforce alternative ways of dealing with depression and anxiety, such as exercise, engaging in unit activities, or talking about feelings. *Goal direction enhances self-efficacy, which is an important antecedent of empowerment.*

● = Independent; ▲ = Collaborative; EBN = Evidence-Based Nursing; EB = Evidence-Based

- Keep the environment safe; remove all harmful objects from the area. Use of unbreakable glass is recommended for the client at risk for self-injury. *Client safety is a nursing priority. Unbreakable glass would eliminate this type of injury.*
- Anticipate trigger situations and intervene to assist the client in applying alternatives to self-mutilation. *When triggers occur, client stress level may obstruct the ability to apply recent learning. Cognitive strategies can be useful to correct irrational beliefs that are part of the trigger.*
- If self-mutilation does occur, use a calm, nonpunitive approach. Whenever possible, assist the client to assume responsibility for consequences (e.g., dress self-inflicted wound). Refer to the care plan for **Self-Mutilation.** *This approach does not promote inappropriate attention-getting behavior, may decrease repetition of behavior, and reinforces self-responsibility and self-care management.*
- If the client is unable to control self-mutilation behavior, provide interactive supervision, not isolation. *Isolation and deprivation take away the individual's coping abilities and place him or her at risk for self-harm. Implementing seclusion for clients who have injured themselves in the past may actually facilitate self-injury. Clients are extraordinarily resourceful at identifying environmental objects with which to self-mutilate.*
- ▲ Refer to protective services if evidence of abuse exists. *It is the nurse's legal responsibility to report abuse.*
- Refer to the care plan for **Self-Mutilation.**

Pediatric

- The same dynamics described previously applies to adolescents. **CEBN:** *Self-harm is a major public health issue arising in persons aged 12 to 24 years, and most often in females (Catledge, Scharer, & Fuller, 2012).*
- Maintaining a therapeutic relationship with teens requires explicit assurances of confidentiality, consistency of clinical routines, and a nonjudgmental communication style. **CEB:** *Even adolescents younger than age 18 years need assurances that confidentiality will be maintained unless there is a serious risk of harm to themselves or others. However, teens of all ages should be advised that parental notification will be made to ensure the teen's safety and to implement a treatment plan (Derouin & Bravender, 2004).*
- Encourage expression of painful experiences and provide supportive counseling. **CEBN:** *Among female adolescents, themes from a qualitative study included living with childhood trauma, feeling abandoned, being an outsider, loathing self, silently screaming, releasing the pressure, feeling alive, being ashamed, and being hopeful (Lesniak 2010; Rissanen, Kylma, & Laukkanen, 2011).*
- Assess for the presence of an eating disorder, history of sexual abuse and/or substance abuse, or nascent psychiatric disorders. Attend to the themes that preoccupy teens with eating disorders who self-mutilate. **EB:** *Self-harmers with a history of childhood sexual abuse reported more eating disorders (Sadeh et al, 2014).*
- Be mindful of possible social influences on self-harm behaviors. **EB:** *A systematic review of 86 studies considering positive associations between self-harm and suicidal behaviors among peer group members supported the finding that young people were more likely to engage in such behaviors when peers had also done so (Quigley, Rasmussen, & McAlaney, 2017).*
- Evaluate for suicidal ideation/suicide risk. Refer to the care plan for **Suicide** for additional information. **CEB:** *Adolescents who attempted suicide by overdose admitted to some method of self-mutilation. The self-mutilators were significantly more likely than non–self-mutilators to be diagnosed with oppositional defiant disorder, major depression, and dysthymia and had higher scores on measures of hopelessness, loneliness, anger, risk-taking, and alcohol use (Guertin et al, 2001).*
- Be aware that there is no complete overlap between self-mutilation and suicidal behavior. The motivation may be different (coping with difficult feelings rather than ending life), and the method is usually different.
- Use treatment approaches detailed in nursing interventions, with modifications as appropriate for this age group.

Geriatric

- Provide hand or back rubs and calming music when older clients experience anxiety. *Calming music or hand massage can soothe agitation for up to 1 hour. No additional benefit was found from combining the two interventions.*
- Provide soft objects for older clients to hold and manipulate when self-mutilation occurs as a function of delirium or dementia. Apply mitts, splints, helmets, or restraints as appropriate. *Delirious or demented clients may scratch or pick at themselves. Soft objects may provide a substitute object to pick at; mitts or restraints may be necessary if the client is unable to exercise self-restraint. They should only be used for a limited amount of time because they may contribute to delirium.*

● = Independent;　▲ = Collaborative;　EBN = Evidence-Based Nursing;　EB = Evidence-Based

- Be aware that older adults may demonstrate self-neglect. Older adults who show self-destructive behaviors should be evaluated for dementia. **EB:** *In a qualitative study of unsupervised assisted living residents, more than half of the participants showed self-neglect behaviors (Caspi, 2014).*

Home Care

- Communicate degree of risk to family/caregivers; assess the family and caregiving situation for ability to protect the client and to understand the client's self-mutilative behavior. Provide family and caregivers with guidelines on how to manage self-harm behaviors in the home environment. *Client safety between home visits is a nursing priority. Appropriate family/caregiver support is important to the client. Appropriate support will only be forthcoming if all parties understand the basis of the behavior and how to respond to it.*
- Establish an emergency plan, including when to use hotlines and 911. Develop a contract with the client and family for use of the emergency plan. Role-play access to the emergency resources with the client and caregivers. *Having an emergency plan reassures the client and caregivers and promotes client safety. Contracting gives guided control to the client and enhances self-esteem.*
- Assess the home environment for harmful objects. Have family remove or lock objects as able. *Client safety is a nursing priority.*
- ▲ If client behaviors intensify, institute an emergency plan for mental health intervention. The degree of disturbance and the ability to manage care safely at home determine the level of services needed to protect the client.
- ▲ Refer for homemaker or psychiatric home health care services for respite, client reassurance, and implementation of therapeutic regimen. *Responsibility for a person at high risk for self-mutilation provides high caregiver stress. Respite decreases caregiver stress. The presence of caring individuals is reassuring to both the client and caregivers, especially during periods of client anxiety. A client with self-mutilative behavior, especially if accompanied by depression, can benefit from the interventions described previously that are modified for the home setting.*
- ▲ If the client is on psychotropic medications, assess client and family knowledge of medication administration and side effects. *Teach as necessary. Knowledge of the medical regimen promotes compliance and promotes safe use of medications.*
- ▲ Evaluate the effectiveness and side effects of medications. Accurate clinical feedback improves health care provider's ability to prescribe an effective medical regimen specific to client needs.

Client/Family Teaching and Discharge Planning

- Explain all relevant symptoms, procedures, treatments, and expected outcomes for self-mutilation that are illness based (e.g., borderline personality disorder, autism). *Participation in treatment enhances a sense of control.*
- Assist family members to understand the complex issues of self-mutilation. Provide instruction on relevant developmental issues and on actions that parents can take to avoid media that glorify self-harm behaviors. *Family members need to understand the behaviors they are dealing with, receive positive reinforcement that will promote their patience and perseverance, and know that they can take positive action to remove media triggers for self-mutilation.*
- Provide written instructions for treatments and procedures for which the client will be responsible. *A written record provides a concrete reference so that the client and family can clarify any verbal information that was given.*
- Instruct the client in coping strategies (assertiveness training, impulse control training, deep breathing, and progressive muscle relaxation). *Clients who self-mutilate have difficulty dealing with stress and painful emotions, which serve as triggers to self-harm. Once clients are able to identify these triggers, they need to learn how to respond to them more effectively through assertiveness, impulse control, or relaxation, as appropriate.*
- Role-play responses to stressful situations (e.g., say, "Tell me how you will respond if someone ignores you"). *Role-playing is the most commonly used technique in assertiveness training. It deconditions the anxiety that arises from interpersonal encounters by allowing the client to practice how he or she might respond in a given situation. Anxiety levels tend to be higher in situations that are unfamiliar.*
- Teach cognitive-behavioral activities, such as active problem-solving, reframing (reappraising the situation from a different perspective), or thought-stopping (in response to a negative thought, picture a large stop sign and replace the image with a prearranged positive alternative). Teach the client to confront his or her own negative thought patterns (or cognitive distortions), such as catastrophizing (expecting the very

S

worst), dichotomous thinking (perceiving events in only one of two opposite categories), or magnification (placing distorted emphasis on a single event). *Cognitive-behavioral activities address clients' assumptions, beliefs, and attitudes about their situations, fostering modification of these elements to be as realistic and optimistic as possible. Through cognitive-behavioral interventions, clients become more aware of their cognitive choices in adopting and maintaining their belief systems, exercising greater control over their own reactions.*

▲ Provide the client and family with phone numbers of appropriate community agencies for therapy and counseling. Continuous follow-up care should be implemented; therefore the method to access this care must be given to the client.

▲ Give the client positive things on which to focus by referring to appropriate agencies for job-training skills or education. *Clients benefit from the desire for goals they could aim for as a means of regaining a positive view of the future.*

REFERENCES

Caspi, E. (2014). Does self-neglect occur among older adults with dementia when unsupervised in assisted living? An exploratory, observational study. *Journal of Elder Abuse & Neglect, 26*(2), 123–149.

Catledge, C. B., Scharer, K., & Fuller, S. (2012). Assessment and identification of deliberate self-harm in adolescents and young adults. *Journal for Nurse Practitioners, 8*(4), 299–305.

Cleaver, K. (2014). Attitudes of emergency care staff towards young people who self-harm: A scoping review. *International Emergency Nursing, 22*, 52–61.

Derouin, A., & Bravender, T. (2004). Living on the edge: The current phenomenon of self-mutilation in adolescents. *MCN. The American Journal of Maternal Child Nursing, 29*(1), 12.

Fox, K. R., et al. (2015). Meta-analysis of risk factors for nonsuicidal self-injury. *Clinical Psychology Review, 42*, 156.

Guertin, T., et al. (2001). Self-mutilative behavior in adolescents who attempt suicide by overdose. *Journal of the American Academy of Child and Adolescent Psychiatry, 40*(9), 1062.

Hunter, J., Maunder, R., Kurdyak, P., et al. (2018). Mental health follow-up after deliberate self-harm and risk for repeat self-harm and death. *Psychiatry Research, 259*, 333–339.

Lesniak, R. G. (2010). The lived experience of adolescent females who self-injure by cutting. *Advanced Emergency Nursing Journal, 32*(2), 137.

Moller, C. I., Tait, R. J., & Byrne, D. G. (2013). Deliberate self-harm, substance use, and negative affect in nonclinical samples: A systematic review. *Substance Abuse, 34*(2), 188–207.

Moola, S. (2017). *Evidence summary. Self-harm (inpatient mental health ward): Assessment, prevention, and treatment.* The Joanna Briggs Institute EBP Database, JBI@Ovid, JBI18050.

Muehlenkamp, J. J., Bagge, C. L., Tull, M. T., et al. (2013). Body regard as a moderator of the relation between emotion dysregulation and nonsuicidal self-injury. *Suicide & Life-Threatening Behavior, 43*(5), 479–493.

Quigley, J., Rasmussen, S., & McAlaney, J. (2017). The associations between children's and adolescent's suicidal and self-harming behaviors, and related behaviors within their social networks: A systematic review. *Archives of Suicide Research, 21*, 185.

Rissanen, M., Kylma, J., & Laukkanen, E. (2011). A systematic literature review: Self-mutilation among adolescents as a phenomenon and help for it—What kind of knowledge is lacking? *Issues in Mental Health Nursing, 32*, 575.

Sadeh, M., et al. (2014). Functions of non-suicidal self-injury in adolescents and young adults with borderline personality disorder symptoms. *Psychiatry Research, 216*(2), 217.

Thomas, J. B., & Haslam, C. O. (2017). How people who self-harm negotiate the inpatient environment: The mental healthcare workers perspective. *Journal of Psychiatric and Mental Health Nursing, 24*(7), 480–490.

Tofthagen, R., Talseth, A. G., & Fagerstrom, L. (2014). Mental health nurses' experiences of caring for patients suffering from self-harm. *Nursing Research Practice, 2014*, 905741. doi:10.1155/2014/905741.

S

Self-Mutilation   *Kathleen L. Patusky, MA, PhD, RN, CNS*

NANDA-I

Definition

Deliberate self-injurious behavior causing tissue damage with the intent of causing nonfatal injury to attain relief of tension.

Defining Characteristics

Abrading; biting; constricting a body part; cuts on body; hitting; ingestion of harmful substances; inhalation of harmful substances; insertion of object into body orifice; picking at wounds; scratches on body; self-inflicted burn; severing of a body part

Related Factors

Absence of family confidant; alteration in body image; dissociation; disturbance in interpersonal relationships; eating disorder; emotional disorder; feeling threatened with loss of significant relationship; impaired

● = Independent;   ▲ = Collaborative;   EBN = Evidence-Based Nursing;   EB = Evidence-Based

self-esteem; impulsiveness; inability to express tension verbally; ineffective communication between parent and adolescent; ineffective coping strategies; irresistible urge for self-directed violence; irresistible urge to cut self; isolation from peers; labile behavior; loss of control over problem solving; low self-esteem; mounting tension that is intolerable; negative feeling; pattern of inability to plan solutions; pattern of inability to see long-term consequences; perfectionism; requires rapid stress reduction; substance misuse; use of manipulation to obtain nurturing relationship with others

At-Risk Population

Adolescence; battered child; childhood illness; childhood surgery; developmental delay; family divorce; family history of self-destructive behavior; family substance misuse; history of childhood abuse; history of self-directed violence; incarceration; living in nontraditional setting; peers who self-mutilate; sexual identity crisis; violence between parental figures

Associated Condition

Autism; borderline personality disorder; character disorder; depersonalization; psychotic disorder

NOC   (Nursing Outcomes Classification)

Suggested NOC Outcomes

Self-Control; Distorted Thought Self-Control; Impulse Self-Control; Mood Equilibrium; Risk Detection; Self-Mutilation Restraint

> **Example NOC Outcome with Indicators**
>
> **Self-Mutilation Restraint** as evidenced by the following indicators: Refrains from gathering means for self-injury/Obtains assistance as needed/Upholds contract not to harm self/Maintains self-control without supervision/Refrains from injuring self. (Rate the outcome and indicators of **Self-Mutilation Restraint:** 1 = never demonstrated, 2 = rarely demonstrated, 3 = sometimes demonstrated, 4 = often demonstrated, 5 = consistently demonstrated [see Section I].)

Client Outcomes

Client Will (Specify Time Frame)

- Have injuries treated
- Refrain from further self-injury
- State appropriate ways to cope with increased psychological or physiological tension
- Express feelings
- Seek help when having urges to self-mutilate
- Maintain self-control without supervision
- Use appropriate community agencies when caregivers are unable to attend to emotional needs

NIC   (Nursing Interventions Classification)

Suggested NIC Interventions

Active Listening; Anger Control Assistance; Behavior Management: Self-Harm; Calming Technique; Environmental Management: Safety; Limit Setting; Mood Management; Mutual Goal Setting; Risk Identification; Self-Responsibility Facilitation

> **Example NIC Activities—Behavior Management: Self-Harm**
>
> Anticipate trigger situations that may prompt self-harm and intervene to prevent it; Teach client and reinforce effective coping behaviors and appropriate expression of feelings

Nursing Interventions and *Rationales*

Note: Before implementing interventions in the face of self-mutilation, nurses should examine their own knowledge base and emotional responses to incidents of self-harm to ensure that interventions will not be based on countertransference reactions. EBN/EB: *Lack of educational background on self-harm can influence*

● = Independent;   ▲ = Collaborative;   EBN = Evidence-Based Nursing;   EB = Evidence-Based

response to self-harm clients. Nurses' tendency to focus on physical care, especially when working under stressful conditions, can hinder awareness of and response to psychosocial issues (Cleaver, 2014).

- A nonjudgmental approach to clients is critical. EBN: *A qualitative study of nurses' experiences caring for patients who self-harmed indicated the need for acceptance of the client (Moola, 2017).*
- Consider using a measure of self-harm risk that is available for clients: EB: *The Ottawa Self-Injury Inventory addresses both functions and potential addictive elements of self-harm (Martin et al, 2013). EBN: A systematic review of multiple instruments rated most of their support as Grade B. The Suicide Attempt Self-Injury Interview (SASII) was reviewed as Level 3, although its length was noted as an issue (Borschmann et al, 2012; Li, 2017).*
- ▲ Provide medical treatment for injuries. Use aseptic technique when caring for wounds. Care for the wounds in a matter-of-fact manner. CEBN: *A significant impediment to wound healing is infection. A matter-of-fact approach avoids positive reinforcement and may decrease repetition of behavior. Recognize that the distress behind self-harm can motivate a response to psychological intervention (Catledge, Scharer, & Fuller, 2012).*
- Assess for risk of suicide or other self-damaging behaviors. EBN: *Although self-mutilation should not be viewed simply as failed suicide, it is a significant indicator of suicide risk. Clients may also engage in other self-damaging behaviors, including substance abuse or eating disorders (Moller, Tait, & Byrne, 2013; Cleaver, 2014). Refer to the care plan for Risk for* **Suicide.**
- Assess for signs of psychiatric disorders, including depression, anxiety, borderline personality disorder, dissociative disorders, eating disorders, and impulsivity. EB: *Self-mutilation has been associated with multiple psychiatric disorders (Moller, Tait, & Byrne, 2013).*
- Assess for the presence of hallucinations. Ask specific questions: "Do you hear voices that other people do not hear?" "Are they telling you to hurt yourself?" *Command hallucinations occurring with schizophrenia or brief psychotic episodes may direct the client to hurt himself or herself or others.*
- ▲ Assure the client that he or she will be safe during hallucinations, and engage supportively. Provide referrals for medication. *Hallucinations can be very frightening; therefore clients need reassurance that they will be kept safe while avoiding a sense of intrusion that overstimulates clients.*
- ▲ Assess for the presence of medical disorders, mental retardation, medication effects, or disorders such as autism that may include self-mutilation. Initiate referral for evaluation and treatment as appropriate. *Self-mutilation has been reported as a presenting or ongoing symptom with medical disorders.*
- ▲ Case finding and referral by school nurses for psychological or psychiatric treatment is critical. *Treatment includes starting therapy and medications, increasing coping skills, facilitating decision-making, encouraging positive relationships, and fostering self-esteem.* EB: *Although the repeat rate of self-harm is around 21%, clients may have a very low treatment follow-up rate. Access to care must be a consideration (Hunter et al, 2018).*
- Monitor the client's behavior closely, using engagement and support as elements of safety checks while avoiding intrusive overstimulation. *When lack of control exists, client safety is an important issue, and close observation is essential.* EBN: *Clients may feel overstimulated by intrusive close observation, resulting in agitation (Moola, 2017).*
- Focus on understanding the function that self-harm serves for the client and on managing the client's distress. EB: *Self-harm is a form of distress management. A qualitative study of mental health staff interventions and efficacy suggested individualized care highlighting management of distress and identification of obstacles to interventions are more effective. If clients are unable to self-harm, prevention can lead to power struggles and the use of more harmful methods by the client (Thomas & Haslam, 2017).*
- Establish trust, listen to client, convey safety, and assist in developing positive goals for the future. EBN: *A qualitative study of nursing interventions focused on identifying and dealing with triggers, and promoting person-centered nursing (Tofthagen, Talseth, & Fagerstrom, 2014).*
- Problem-solving therapy, access to emergency contacts, and long-term psychological therapy may be helpful. Although some studies suggest interventions that may be helpful, findings should be used with caution. EB: *A Cochrane Review found some usefulness of problem-solving therapy, access to emergency contacts, and long-term psychological therapy with female patients with borderline personality disorder (Hawton et al, 2015a).*
- ▲ Use a collaborative approach for care. A collaborative approach to care is more helpful to the client.
- Refer to the care plan for Risk for **Self-Mutilation** for additional information.

🐻 Pediatric

- Self harm is a major concern in children and adolescents, although few interventions have been adequately tested. EB: *An updated Cochrane Review concluded that studies have not supported group therapy as an*

- = Independent;   ▲ = Collaborative;   EBN = Evidence-Based Nursing;   EB = Evidence-Based

effective treatment for children and adolescents; mentalization and dialectical behavior therapy (DBT) show some promise (Hawton et al, 2015b).

Home Care and Client/Family Teaching and Discharge Planning

- See the care plan for Risk for **Self-Mutilation.**

REFERENCES

Borschmann, R., Hogg, J., Phillips, R., et al. (2012). Measuring self-harm in adults: A systematic review. *European Psychiatry, 27,* 176.

Catledge, C. B., Scharer, K., & Fuller, S. (2012). Assessment and identification of deliberate self-harm in adolescents and young adults. *The Journal for Nurse Practitioners: JNP, 8*(4), 299–305.

Cleaver, K. (2014). Attitudes of emergency care staff towards young people who self-harm: A scoping review. *International Emergency Nursing, 22,* 52–61.

Hawton, K., Townsend, E., Arensman, E., et al. (2015a). Psychosocial and pharmacological treatments for deliberate self harm. *The Cochrane Database of Systematic Reviews,* (10), CD001764. doi:10.1002/14651858.CD001764.pub2.

Hawton, K., Witt, K. G., Taylor Salisbury, T. L., et al. (2015b). Interventions for self-harm in children and adolescents. *The Cochrane Database of Systematic Reviews,* (12), CD012013. doi:10.1002/14651858.CD012013.

Hunter, J., Maunder, R., Kurdyak, P., et al. (2018). Mental health follow-up after deliberate self-harm and risk for repeat self-harm and death. *Psychiatry Research, 259,* 333–339.

Li, Y. (2017). *Evidence summary. Self-harm (adults): Validated measurement instruments.* The Joanna Briggs Institute EBP Database, JBI@Ovid. JBI7927.

Martin, J., Cloutier, P. F., Levesque, C., et al. (2013). Psychometric properties of the functions and addictive features scales of the Ottawa Self-Injury Inventory: A preliminary investigation using a university sample. *Psychological Assessment, 25*(3), 1013.

Moller, C. I., Tait, R. J., & Byrne, D. G. (2013). Deliberate self-harm, substance use, and negative affect in nonclinical samples: A systematic review. *Substance Abuse, 34*(2), 188–207.

Moola, S. (2017). *Evidence summary. Self-harm (inpatient mental health ward): Assessment, prevention, and treatment.* The Joanna Briggs Institute EBP Database, JBI@Ovid, JBI18050.

Thomas, J. B., & Haslam, C. O. (2017). How people who self-harm negotiate the inpatient environment: The mental healthcare workers perspective. *Journal of Psychiatric and Mental Health Nursing, 24*(7), 480–490.

Tofthagen, R., Talseth, A. G., & Fagerstrom, L. (2014). Mental health nurses' experiences of caring for patients suffering from self-harm. *Nursing Research Practice, 2014,* 905741. doi:10.1155/2014/905741.

Self-Neglect

Susanne W. Gibbons, PhD, C-ANP/GNP and Mary Rose Day, DN, MA, PGDip PHN, BSc, Dip Management (RCSI), RPHN, RM, RGN

NANDA-I

S

Definition

A constellation of culturally framed behaviors involving one or more self-care activities in which there is a failure to maintain a socially accepted standard of health and well-being (Gibbons, Lauder, & Ludwick, 2006).

Defining Characteristics

Insufficient environmental hygiene; insufficient personal hygiene; nonadherence to health activity

Related Factors

Deficient executive function; fear of institutionalization; inability to maintain control; lifestyle choice; stressors; substance misuse

Associated Condition

Alteration in cognitive functioning; Capgras syndrome; frontal lobe dysfunction; functional impairment; learning disability; malingering; psychiatric disorder; psychotic disorder

NOC (Nursing Outcomes Classification)

Suggested NOC Outcomes

Cognitive Function; Executive Function; Depression; Alcohol and Other Substance Use; Activities of Daily Living (ADLs), Instrumental Activities of Daily Living (IADLs); Safety; Nutritional Status; Social Support, Medication Safety Assessment

● = Independent;   ▲ = Collaborative;   **EBN** = Evidence-Based Nursing;   **EB** = Evidence-Based

Examples of NOC Outcome with Indicators

Self-Neglect Status as evidenced by the following indicators: Maintains personal cleanliness and health/Recognizes safety needs in the home. (Rate outcome and indicators of **Self-Neglect Status:** 1 = severely compromised, 2 = substantially compromised, 3 = moderately compromised, 4 = mildly compromised, 5 = not compromised [see Section I].)

Client Outcomes

Client Will (Specify Time Frame)

- Reveal improvement in cognition (e.g., if reversible and treatable)
- Show improvement in mental health problems
- Show improvement in chronic medical problems
- Demonstrate improvement in functional status (e.g., basic and IADLs)
- Demonstrate adherence to health activities (e.g., medications and medical appointments)
- Exhibit improved personal hygiene
- Exhibit improved environmental hygiene
- Have fewer hospitalizations and emergency room visits
- Increase safety of client
- Increase safety of community in which client lives
- Agree to necessary personal and environmental changes that eliminate risk/endangerment to self or others (e.g., neighbors)
- Improve social networks
- Identify eligibility for public services and other benefits

Note: Because self-neglect is present along a continuum of severity and includes an array of behavioral and environmental issues, a change in a client's status must occur in such a way that it balances obligation for protection and respects individual rights (e.g., autonomy and self-determination) while ensuring individual health and well-being. This is accomplished through a client–provider partnership that keeps the door open even though the client may initially decline help. Building a relationship with the client will improve trust and assist in developing an individually tailored care plan to address problems contributing to self-neglect. Interdisciplinary collaboration and teamwork, and in some instances assistance of next of kin and/or adult protective services (APS), may be needed (e.g., a state agency or local social services program).

NIC (Nursing Interventions Classification)

Suggested NIC Interventions

Self-Neglect; Self-Care Assistance: Activities of Daily Living; Support System Enhancement

Example NIC Activities—Self-Care Assistance: Instrumental Activities of Daily Living

Determine individual's need for assistance with IADLs (e.g., shopping, cooking, housekeeping, laundry, use of transportation, managing money, managing medications, use of communication, and use of time)

Nursing Interventions and *Rationales*

- Monitor individuals with acute or chronic mental and physical illness for defining characteristics for self-neglect. **EBN/CEB:** *Holistic assessment includes medical and social history, cognitive status, state of mental health, well-being, physical function, social networks, medication, alcohol use, and data on factors that limit individual coping and self-care ability (Pavlou & Lachs, 2008; Mulcahy, Leahy-Warren, & Day, 2018).*
- Assist individuals with complex mental and physical health issues to adopt positive health behaviors so that they may maintain their health status in the community. **EB:** *Greater severity self-neglect was associated with an increased 30-day hospital readmission rate (Dong & Simon, 2014).*
- Assist individuals with reconnecting with family, friends, and other social networks available to them. **EBN:** *Social isolation is a risk for self-neglect (Mulcahy, Leahy-Warren, & Day, 2018).*
- Assist individuals whose self-care is failing with managing their medications regimen. **EB:** *Individuals who exhibit self-neglect may have difficulty managing medications because of complex medication regimens, and low adherence is significant among older adults who self-neglect (Alpert, 2014).*

● = Independent;   ▲ = Collaborative;   EBN = Evidence-Based Nursing;   EB = Evidence-Based

- Assist persons with self-care deficits caused by ADL or IADL impairments. **CEB:** *Individuals with self-care deficits may have difficulty with ADLs and IADLs because greater self-neglect severity has been associated with lower levels of physical function among older adults (Lachs et al, 2002; Hildebrand, Taylor, & Bradway, 2014).*
- Assess persons with failing self-care for changes in cognitive function (e.g., dementia or delirium). **EB:** *Individuals with failing self-care may have changes in cognition. Decline in executive function has been associated with risk of reported and confirmed elder self-neglect, and decline in global cognitive function has been associated with risk of greater self-neglect severity (Mackay, 2017; Mills & Naik, 2018).*
- Refer persons with failing self-care to appropriate specialists (e.g., psychologist, psychiatrist, social worker) and therapists (e.g., physical therapy, occupational therapy). **EBN/EB:** *Individuals with self-care deficits may need assistance from other health professionals using an interprofessional team approach, open communication, and collaboration (Burnett et al, 2014; Braye, Orr, & Preston-Shoot, 2014).*
- Use behavioral modification as appropriate to bring about client changes that lead to improvement in personal hygiene, environmental hygiene, and adherence to medical regimen. **CEB:** *Behavioral modification approaches have been effective in reversing self-neglect in older adults who had triggers or events that brought about the behavior (Thibault, 2008).*
- Monitor persons with substance abuse problems (i.e., drugs, alcohol, smoking) for adequate safety. **EBN/EB:** *Because mental health and substance use disorders can go unrecognized and untreated in this population, identified self-neglecting clients should be screened as appropriate (Hansen et al, 2016; Alpert et al, 2014).*
- ▲ Refer persons with failing self-care who are significantly impaired cognitively (e.g., executive function, dementia) or functionally and/or who are suspected victims of abuse to APS. **EB/CEB:** *Self-neglect has been associated with mistreatment in older adults, especially those who live alone (Dyer et al, 2007; Pavlou & Lachs, 2008).*

Geriatric

- ▲ Assess client's socioeconomic status and refer for appropriate support. **EBN/EB:** *Providers are advised to assess available financial and other resources to help older adults and their families obtain essential goods and services (Zhao et al, 2017; Mulcahy, Leahy-Warren, & Day, 2018).*
- ▲ Refer persons demonstrating a significant decline in self-care abilities (e.g., posing a threat to themselves or to their community) for formal evaluation of capacity and executive function. **CEB:** *Current evidence indicates that executive dyscontrol contributes to self-neglect in the older adult population, in which it is considered a geriatric syndrome (Dyer et al, 2007; Pavlou & Lachs, 2006).*

Multicultural

- Deliver health care that is sensitive to the culture and philosophy of individuals whose self-care appears inadequate. **EBN:** *Providers must be careful not to prematurely judge clients' health choices or living arrangements because personal values and beliefs that might appear as self-neglect do not necessarily indicate self-neglect. However, when client behavior poses a risk to self and/or others, providers have an ethical obligation to intervene (Gibbons, Lauder, & Ludwick, 2006; Braye, Orr, & Preston-Shoot, 2018).*

REFERENCES

Alpert, P. T. (2014). Alcohol abuse in older adults: An invisible population. *Home Health Care Management & Practice, 26*(4), 269–272.

Braye, S., Orr, D., & Preston-Shoot, M. (2014). *Self-neglect policy and practice: Building an evidence base for adult social care.* London: Social Care Institute for Excellence.

Burnett, J., Dyer, C. B., Halphen, J. M., et al. (2014). Four subtypes of self-neglect in older adults: Results of a latent class analysis. *Journal of the American Geriatrics Society, 62*(6), 1127–1132. doi:10.1111/jgs.12832.

Dong, X., & Simon, M. A. (2014). Elder self-neglect is associated with an increased rate of 30-day hospital readmission: Findings from the Chicago Health and Aging Project. *Gerontology, 61*(1), 41–50.

Dyer, C. B., Goodwin, J. S., Pickens, S., et al. (2007). Self-neglect among the elderly: A model based on more than 500 patients seen by a geriatric medicine team. *American Journal of Public Health, 97*(9), 1671–1676.

Gibbons, S., Lauder, W., & Ludwick, R. (2006). Self-neglect: A proposed new NANDA diagnosis. *International Journal of Nursing Terminologies and Classifications, 17*(1), 10–18.

Hansen, M. C., Flores, D. V., Coverdale, J., et al. (2016). Correlates of depression in self-neglecting older adults: A cross-sectional study examining the role of alcohol abuse and pain in increasing vulnerability. *Journal of Elder Abuse & Neglect, 28*(1), 41–56.

Hildebrand, C., Taylor, M., & Bradway, C. (2014). Elder self-neglect: The failure of coping because of cognitive and functional impairments. *Journal of the American Association of Nurse Practitioners, 26,* 452–462.

Lachs, M. S., Williams, C. S., O'Brien, S., et al. (2002). Adult protective service use and nursing home placement. *The Gerontologist, 42,* 734–739.

Mackay, K. (2017). Choosing to live with harm? A presentation of two case studies to explore the perspective of those who experienced

S

adult safeguarding interventions. *Ethics and Social Welfare*, *11*(1), 33–46.

Mills, W. L., & Naik, A. D. (2018). Making and executing decisions for safe and independent living (MED-SAIL): A screening tool for community-dwelling older adults. In M. R. Day, G. McCarthy, & J. J. Fitzpatrick (Eds.), *Self-neglect in older adults: A global, evidence-based resource for nurses and other healthcare providers* (Chapter 21, pp. 303–314). New York: Springer.

Mulcahy, H., Leahy-Warren, P., & Day, M. R. (2018). Health and social care professionals' perspectives of self-neglect. In M. R. Day, G. McCarthy, & J. J. Fitzpatrick (Eds.), *Self-neglect in older adults: A global, evidence-based resource for nurses and other healthcare providers* (Chapter 13, pp. 163–174). New York: Springer.

Pavlou, M. P., & Lachs, M. S. (2006). Could self-neglect in older persons be a geriatric syndrome? *Journal of the American Geriatrics Society*, *54*, 831–842.

Pavlou, M. P., & Lachs, M. S. (2008). Self-neglect in older adults: A primer for physicians. *Journal of General Internal Medicine*, *23*(11), 1841–1846.

Thibault, J. M. (2008). Analysis and treatment of self-neglectful behaviors in three elderly female patients. *Journal of Elder Abuse & Neglect*, *19*(3/4), 151–166.

Zhao, Y., Hu, C., Feng, F., et al. (2017). Associations of self-neglect with quality of life in older people in rural China: A cross-sectional study. *International Psychogeriatric*, *29*(6), 1015–1026.

Sexual dysfunction   *Elaine E. Steinke, PhD, APRN, CNS-BC, FAHA, FAAN*

NANDA-I

Definition

A state in which an individual experiences a change in sexual function during the sexual response phases of desire, arousal, and/or orgasm, which is viewed as unsatisfying, unrewarding, or inadequate.

Defining Characteristics

Alteration in sexual activity; alteration in sexual excitation; alteration in sexual satisfaction; change in interest toward others; change in self-interest; change in sexual role; decrease in sexual desire; perceived sexual limitation; seeking confirmation of desirability; undesired change in sexual function

Related Factors

Absence of privacy; inadequate role model; insufficient knowledge about sexual function; misinformation about sexual function; presence of abuse; psychosocial abuse; value conflict; vulnerability

At-Risk Population

Absence of significant other

Associated Condition

Alteration in body function; alteration in body structure

NOC   (Nursing Outcomes Classification)

Suggested NOC Outcomes

Abuse Recovery: Sexual; Knowledge: Sexual Functioning, Physical Aging; Psychosocial Adjustment: Life Change; Risk Control: Sexually Transmitted Diseases (STDs); Sexual Functioning; Sexual Identity

---

Example NOC Outcome with Indicators

Sexual Functioning as evidenced by the following indicators: Expresses comfort with sexual expression/Expresses comfort with body/Expresses sexual interest. (Rate the outcome and indicators of **Sexual Functioning:** 1 = never demonstrated, 2 = rarely demonstrated, 3 = sometimes demonstrated, 4 = often demonstrated, 5 = consistently demonstrated [see Section I].)

Client Outcomes

Client Will (Specify Time Frame)

- Identify individual cause of sexual dysfunction
- Identify stressors that contribute to dysfunction
- Discuss alternative, satisfying, and acceptable sexual practices for self and partner
- Identify the degree of sexual interest by the client and partner

● = Independent;   ▲ = Collaborative;   EBN = Evidence-Based Nursing;   EB = Evidence-Based

- Adapt sexual technique as needed to cope with sexual problems
- Discuss with partner concerns about body image and sex role

NIC   (Nursing Interventions Classification)

Suggested **NIC** Interventions

Sexual Counseling; Teaching: Sexuality

Example **NIC** Activities—Sexual Counseling
Provide privacy and ensure confidentiality; Discuss necessary modifications in sexual activity, as appropriate; Provide referral/consultation with other members of the health care team, as appropriate

Nursing Interventions and *Rationales*

- Gather the client's sexual history, noting normal patterns of functioning and the client's vocabulary, and encouraging clients to ask questions or discuss sexual problems experienced. **EB:** *In a nationally representative sample of women in the United States, those who were sexually active had greater relationship satisfaction, better communication, and higher ratings of the importance of sexual activity, illustrating the importance of assessing sexual activity and encouraging discussion of any sexual concerns or problems (Thomas, Hess, & Thurston, 2015).* **EB:** *In a large cross-sectional study of men, the prevalence of erectile dysfunction (ED) increased for those with comorbidities such as hypertension, diabetes mellitus, depression, or benign prostatic hypertrophy (BPH) (Mulhall et al, 2016).*
- ▲ Assess duration and risk factors for sexual dysfunction and explore potential causes such as medications, medical problems, aging process, or psychosocial issues. **EBN:** *In a population-based sample comparing those with a cardiac condition to those without a cardiac condition, those with coronary artery disease, angina, and myocardial infarction reported significantly less sexual activity, as did those who smoked, had a weight problem, had lung problems, had depression, had shortness of breath or chest pain with exertion, or took certain medications. This illustrated that multiple factors affect sexual activity and may contribute to sexual dysfunction (Steinke, Mosack, & Hill, 2017).*
- ▲ Assess for history of sexual abuse. **EB:** *Men who were forced to have sex by a woman had greater risks such as higher number of lifetime partners and greater alcohol and drug use, compared with nonvictimized men, putting them at increased risk of sexually transmitted infections (Cook et al, 2016).*
- ▲ Assess and provide treatment for sexual dysfunction, involving the person's partner in the process, and evaluating pharmacological and nonpharmacological interventions. **EB:** *Results of a systematic review of men and women found that dehydroepiandrosterone (DHEA) improved sexual interest, pain, arousal, lubrication, orgasm, and frequency of sexual activity, particularly for women and those with sexual dysfunction, whereas some men had improved erectile function, but others did not (Peixoto et al, 2017).* **EB:** *Phosphodiesterase type 5 (PDE5) inhibitors are first-line therapies for ED in men with several drugs available. Tadalafil as a once daily treatment was found to be well tolerated and provides an alternative to as needed dosing of PDE5 inhibitors (Kim et al, 2015).*
- Assess risk factors for sexual dysfunction, especially with varying sexual partners. **EB:** *In substance-dependent men who were polydrug users, having occasional sexual partners resulted in 14 times the risk of ED compared with married men, illustrating the importance of a complete sexual history and evaluation of risks for sexual dysfunction (Clemente et al, 2017).*
- Observe for stress and anxiety as possible causes of dysfunction. **EBN:** *In men with diabetes mellitus type 2, 82% experienced ED and overall mild anxiety; thus both physical and psychological causes of sexual dysfunction should be routinely evaluated (Erden & Kaya, 2015).* **EB:** *In women, fibromyalgia significantly affected sexual function, and the severity and duration of fibromyalgia, the duration of the sexual partnership, and severity of anxiety significantly increased the degree of sexual dysfunction (Hayta & Mert, 2017).*
- ▲ Assess for depression as a possible cause of sexual dysfunction, and institute appropriate treatment. **EBN:** *In women who had given birth in the prior 12 months, 24% reported postnatal depression, which was significantly associated with sexual dysfunction, not initiating partnered sexual activity, and relationship dissatisfaction, illustrating the importance of assessment and early intervention for both depression and sexual dysfunction (Khajehei & Doherty, 2017).*
- Observe for grief-related loss (e.g., amputation, mastectomy, ostomy) because a change in body image often precedes sexual dysfunction. See care plan for Disturbed **Body Image.** **EBN:** *In men after lower*

S

• = Independent;   ▲ = Collaborative;   EBN = Evidence-Based Nursing;   EB = Evidence-Based

anterior resection for rectal cancer, ED occurred in 97% compared with 76% in those undergoing colectomy, and worse overall sexual function for those with lower anterior resection, particularly for those with a stoma. This illustrates the importance of discussing sexual function and loss in those diagnosed with rectal cancer (Shieh et al, 2016).

▲ Explore physical causes of sexual dysfunction such as diabetes, cardiovascular disease, arthritis, or BPH. **EB:** *In men and women with heart failure, approximately 60% experienced sexual problems related to performance, overall sexual function, and decreased sexual pleasure and satisfaction; contributing factors included lack of energy, decreased exercise capacity, and depressed mood (Jaarsma, Fridlund, & Mårtensson, 2014).*

▲ Consider that ED may indicate the presence of cardiovascular disease, and screening and referral of men is recommended. **EB:** *Vasculogenic ED may be a sign of silent or future cardiovascular disease; thus cardiovascular risk stratification using the Framingham Risk Score is indicated. Management of those men with ED of low cardiovascular risk focuses on risk factor control, whereas men at high risk should be referred to a cardiologist (Miner et al, 2014).*

• Certain chronic diseases such as cancer often have significant effects on sexual function, and both the disease process and treatment can contribute to sexual dysfunction. **EBN:** *Although women after gynecological cancer were sexually active, 54% had impaired sexual satisfaction and experienced problems such as vaginal dryness and discomfort with vaginal penetration during sexual activity (Sekse, Hufthammer, & Vika, 2016).*

• Consider that neurological diseases can affect sexual function directly, with secondary effects caused by disability related to the illness and social and emotional effects. **EB:** *In men and women with a diagnosis of muscular dystrophy, spinal cord injury, or postpolio syndrome, only 37.8% reported engaging in sexual activity in the past 30 days, and sexual dysfunction was a significant predictor of sexual satisfaction regardless of type of disability, and depression was also a significant predictor in women (Smith et al, 2015).*

• Explore behavioral or other causes of sexual dysfunction, such as smoking, dietary factors, or obesity. **EB:** *Although smoking and ED have been linked in men, a study of women supported prior findings that women smokers were not at increased risk for sexual dysfunction, although nicotine dependence might negatively affect libido (Costa & Peres, 2015).*

▲ Consider medications as a cause of sexual dysfunction. **EB:** *Cardiovascular drug effects on sexual function include overall negative effects of beta blockers (with the exception of nebivolol), cardiac glycosides, antiarrhythmics, and diuretics; neutral effects with alpha blockers, angiotensin-converting enzyme inhibitors, vasodilators, and calcium channel blockers; and positive effects from angiotensin receptor blockers, although there are mixed results for some of these drug classes (La Torre et al, 2015).* **EB:** *A meta-analysis from 63 studies of second-generation antidepressants in clients with major depressive disorder showed that bupropion conferred a significantly lower risk of sexual dysfunction, and citalopram and paroxetine were significantly associated with higher risk of sexual dysfunction compared with other second-generation drugs (Reichenpfader et al, 2014).*

▲ Refer to appropriate medical providers for consideration of medication for premature ejaculation, ED, or orgasmic problems. **EB:** *A combination treatment with a selective serotonin reuptake inhibitor and a PDE5 inhibitor was superior in treating men with premature ejaculation (Bai et al, 2015).* **EB:** *Treatment response for the ED drug sildenafil was better than placebo in men with no comorbidity and for those with cardiovascular disease/hypertension only, diabetes only, or depression only, regardless of age (Goldstein, Stecher, & Carlsson, 2017).*

• Refer to the care plan Ineffective **Sexuality** pattern for additional interventions.

 Geriatric

▲ Carefully assess the sexuality needs and sexual dysfunction of older adults and refer for counseling if needed. **EBN:** *Treatment approaches for ED in older adults include behavioral and lifestyle changes (e.g., smoking cessation, healthy diet, physical activity, limiting alcohol intake), pelvic floor muscle exercises, PDE5 inhibitors, psychotherapy, and assistive devices (Marchese, 2017).*

• Teach about normal changes that occur with aging that may be perceived as sexual dysfunction, such as reduction in vaginal lubrication and reduction in duration and resolution of orgasm for women; for men these changes include increased time required for erection and for subsequent erections, erection without ejaculation, less firm erection, and decreased volume of seminal fluid. **EBN:** *Results of a phenomenological study revealed that older men showed sexual interest regardless of age, health, or sexual function, although anxiety was increased when biomedical interventions for ED were unsuccessful; nurses and health care professionals must proactively assess and discuss sexual function with older adults (Gledhill & Schweitzer, 2014).*

• = Independent;   ▲ = Collaborative;   EBN = Evidence-Based Nursing;   EB = Evidence-Based

- If prescribed, instruct clients with chronic pain to take pain medication before sexual activity. EB: *In a randomized controlled trial of estrogen-deficient breast cancer survivors who had severe dyspareunia with vaginal penetration, compared with saline, the use of 4% aqueous lidocaine to the vulvar vestibule for three minutes prior to vaginal penetration resulted in less pain during intercourse, decreased sexual distress, and improved sexual function (Goetsch, Lim, & Caughey, 2015).*
- See care plan for Ineffective **Sexuality** pattern.

Multicultural

- Evaluate culturally influenced risk factors for sexual function and dysfunction. EBN: *Bisexual women had greater sexual coercion, more lifetime partners, physical and sexual violence, traded sex for resources, and had posttraumatic stress disorder symptoms, illustrating the importance of history-taking, screening protocols, and counseling, taking into account race, ethnicity, gender, class, and sexual identity (Alexander et al, 2016).*
- Validate client feelings and emotions regarding the changes in sexual behavior by letting the client know that the nurse heard and understands what was said, promoting the nurse–client relationship. EB: *Culturally sensitive approaches with older adults includes discussing sexual function and dysfunction regardless of culture, sexual orientation, age, gender, or marital status, and inquiring about culture in a nonjudgmental way (Atallah, 2016).*

Home Care

- Previously discussed interventions may be adapted for home care use.
- ▲ Identify specific sources of concern about sexual dysfunction and provide reassurance and instruction on appropriate expectations as indicated. EB: *Clients with schizophrenia and sexual dysfunction had significantly worse subjective quality of life, and aspects of physical arousal such as vaginal lubrication and penile erection were commonly affected; it is important to address causes of sexual dysfunction and implement management strategies tailored to the client (Bushong, Nakonezny, & Byerly, 2013).*
- ▲ Confirm that physical reasons for dysfunction have been addressed, and refer for therapy and/or support groups if appropriate. EB: *Most individuals with sexual problems would benefit from both pharmacologic and psychological treatment, including sexual counseling and therapy (Almås, 2016).*
- See care plan for Ineffective **Sexuality** pattern.

Client/Family Teaching and Discharge Planning

- Provide accurate information for clients regarding interventions for sexual dysfunction. EB: *To address sexual problems in those with cancer, psychosexual counseling should be offered to both men and women. Women may benefit from pelvic floor physiotherapy, hormonal therapy for vasomotor symptoms (if safe), and vaginal lubricants, whereas men might be offered PDE5 inhibitors, vacuum erectile devices, and intracavernosal injection (Barbera et al, 2017).*
- *Include the partner/family in discharge instructions because partner concerns are often overlooked regarding sexual issues.* EB: *Women as cervical cancer survivors wanted both information and practical advice in dealing with sexual dysfunction; physical functioning, sexual distress, relationship satisfaction, and partner perspectives should be assessed, with interventions tailored to the particular needs of the couple (Vermeer et al, 2016).*
- Teach the client and partner about condom use, for those at risk. EB: *In couples, feelings of commitment to the sexual partner resulted in reduced perceived sexual risk, illustrating that interventions for couples should include discussion of sexual risk, prevention of HIV risk, including condom use, and monogamy agreements before condoms are discontinued (Agnew et al, 2017).*
- ▲ Refer to appropriate community resources, such as a clinical specialist, family counselor, or cardiac rehabilitation, including the partner if appropriate; for complex issues, a referral to a sex counselor, urologist, gynecologist, or other specialist may be needed. EB: *College students stated a preference for help-seeking related to sexual problems from gynecologists, urologists, and family physicians, with the next preference being sex therapists, psychologists, and counselors (Bergvall & Himelein, 2014).* EB: *Men and their partners need comprehensive information before and after treatment for prostate cancer, including support groups to help patients and partners gain education and support (Albaugh et al, 2017).*
- ▲ Refer for medical advice when ED lasts longer than 2 months or is recurring. EB: *ED can be treated, and underlying causes need to be investigated through a thorough medical and sexual history (Glina, Cohen, & Vieira, 2014).*
- Teach the following interventions to decrease the likelihood of ED: limit or avoid the use of alcohol, stop smoking, exercise regularly, reduce stress, get enough sleep, deal with anxiety or depression, and see a

S

● = Independent;   ▲ = Collaborative;   EBN = Evidence-Based Nursing;   EB = Evidence-Based

health care provider for regular checkups and medical screening tests. **EB:** *In a study of nondiabetic men with cardiovascular risk factors, those with ED were more likely to be smokers, sedentary, and consumed more alcohol, whereas those consuming more nuts and vegetables had less ED, illustrating the importance of counseling regarding lifestyle and its effect on ED (Ramírez et al, 2016).*
- See care plan for Ineffective **Sexuality** pattern.

REFERENCES

Agnew, C. R., Harvey, S. M., VanderDrift, L. E., et al. (2017). Relational underpinnings of condom use: Findings from the project on partner dynamics. *Health Psychology*, 36(7), 713–720. doi:10.1037/hea0000488.

Albaugh, J. A., Sufrin, N., Lapin, B. R., et al. (2017). Life after prostate cancer treatment: A mixed methods study of the experiences of men with sexual dysfunction and their partners. *BMC Urology*, 17(1), 1–9. doi:10.1186/s12894-017-0231-5.

Alexander, K. A., Volpe, E. M., Abboud, S., et al. (2016). Reproductive coercion, sexual risk behaviours and mental health symptoms among young low-income behaviourally bisexual women: Implications for nursing practice. *Journal of Clinical Nursing*, 25(23–24), 3533–3544. doi:10.1111/jocn.13238.

Almås, E. (2016). Psychological treatment of sexual problems. Thematic analysis of guidelines and recommendations, based on a systematic literature review 2001–2010. *Sexual and Relationship Therapy*, 31(1), 54–69. doi:10.1080/14681994.2015.1086739.

Atallah, S. (2016). Cultural aspects of sexual function and dysfunction in the geriatric population: A review of the current literature and clinical overview of clinical interventions with efficacy. *Topics in Geriatric Rehabilitation*, 32(3), 156–166. doi:10.1097/TGR.0000000000000105.

Bai, U., Pu, C., Han, P., et al. (2015). Selective serotonin reuptake inhibitors plus phosphodiesterase-5 inhibitors for premature ejaculation: A systematic review and meta-analysis. *Urology*, 86(4), 758–764. doi:10.1016/j.urology.2015.06.045.

Barbera, L., Zwaal, C., Elterman, D., et al. (2017). Interventions to address sexual problems in people with cancer. *Current Oncology*, 24(3), 192–200. doi:10.3747/co.24.3583.

Bergvall, L., & Himelein, M. J. (2014). Attitudes toward seeking help for sexual dysfunctions among US and Swedish college students. *Sexual and Relationship Therapy*, 29(2), 215–228.

Bushong, M. E., Nakonezny, P. A., & Byerly, M. J. (2013). Subjective quality of life and sexual dysfunction in outpatients with schizophrenia or schizoaffective disorder. *Journal of Sex & Marital Therapy*, 39(4), 336–346. doi:10.1080/0092623X.2011.606884.

Clemente, J., Diehl, A., Santana, P. R., et al. (2017). Erectile dysfunction symptoms in polydrug dependents seeking treatment. *Substance Abuse & Misuse*, 52(12), 1565–1574. doi:10.1080/10826084.2017.1290114.

Cook, M. C., Morisky, D. E., Williams, J. K., et al. (2016). Sexual risk behaviors and substance use among men sexually victimized by women. *American Journal of Public Health*, 106(7), 1263–1269. doi:10.2105/AJPH.2016.303136.

Costa, R. M., & Peres, L. (2015). Smoking is unrelated to female sexual function. *Substance Abuse & Misuse*, 50(2), 189–194. doi:10.3109/10826084.2014.962054.

Erden, S., & Kaya, H. (2015). Sexual dysfunction and anxiety levels of type 2 male diabetics. *Applied Nursing Research*, 28(3), 239–243. doi:10.1016/j.apnr.2015.04.014.

Gledhill, S., & Schweitzer, R. D. (2014). Sexual desire, erectile dysfunction and the biomedicalization of sex in older heterosexual men. *Journal of Advanced Nursing*, 70(4), 894–903. doi:10.1111/jan.12256.

Glina, S., Cohen, D. J., & Vieira, M. (2014). Diagnosis of erectile dysfunction. *Current Opinion in Psychiatry*, 27(6), 394–399. doi:10.1097/YCO.0000000000000097.

Goetsch, M. F., Lim, J. Y., & Caughey, A. B. (2015). A practical solution for dyspareunia in breast cancer survivors: A randomized controlled trial. *Journal of Clinical Oncology*, 33(30), 3394–3400. doi:10.1200/JCO.2014.60.7366.

Goldstein, I., Stecher, V., & Carlsson, M. (2017). Treatment response to sildenafil in men with erectile dysfunction relative to concomitant comorbidities and age. *The International Journal of Clinical Practice*, 71(3/4), e12939. doi:10.1111/ijcp.12939.

Hayta, E., & Mert, D. G. (2017). Potential risk factors increasing the severity of sexual dysfunction in women with fibromyalgia. *Sexuality and Disability*, 35(2), 147–155. doi:10.1007/s11195-016-9472-6.

Jaarsma, T., Fridlund, B., & Mårtensson, J. (2014). Sexual dysfunction in heart failure patients. *Current Heart Failure Reports*, 11(3), 330–336. doi:10.1007/s11897-014-0202-z.

Khajehei, M., & Doherty, M. (2017). Exploring postnatal depression, sexual dysfunction and relationship dissatisfaction in Australian women. *British Journal of Midwifery*, 25(3), 162–172. doi:10.12968/bjom.2017.25.3.162.

Kim, E., Seftel, A., Goldfischer, E., et al. (2015). Comparative efficacy of tadalafil once daily in men with erectile dysfunction who demonstrated previous partial responses to as-needed sildenafil, tadalafil, or vardenafil. *Current Medical Research & Opinion*, 31(2), 379–389. doi:10.1185/03007995.2014.989317.

La Torre, A., Giupponi, G., Duffy, D., et al. (2015). Sexual dysfunction related to drugs: A critical review. Part IV: Cardiovascular drugs. *Pharmacopsychiatry*, 48(1), 1–6. doi:10.1055/s-0034-1395515.

Marchese, K. (2017). An overview of erectile dysfunction in the elderly population. *Urologic Nursing*, 37(3), 157–170. doi:10.7257/1053-816X.2017.37.3.157.

Miner, M., Nehra, A., Jackson, G., et al. (2014). All men with vasculogenic erectile dysfunction require a cardiovascular workup. *The American Journal of Medicine*, 127(3), 174–182. doi:10.1016/j.amjmed.2013.10.013.

Mulhall, J. P., Luo, X., Zou, K. H., et al. (2016). Relationship between age and erectile dysfunction diagnosis or treatment using real-world observational data in the USA. *International Journal of Clinical Practice*, 70(12), 1012–1018. doi:10.1111/ijcp.12908.

Peixoto, C., Carrilho, C. G., Barros, J. A., et al. (2017). The effects of dehydroepiandrosterone one sexual function: A systematic review. *Climacteric: The Journal of the International Menopause Society*, 20(2), 129–137. doi:10.1080/13697137.2017.1279141.

Ramírez, R., Pedro-Botet, J., Garcia, M., et al. (2016). Erectile dysfunction and cardiovascular risk factors in a Mediterranean diet cohort. *Internal Medicine Journal*, 46(1), 52–56. doi:10.1111/imj.12937.

Reichenpfader, U., Gartlehner, G., Morgan, L. C., et al. (2014). Sexual dysfunction associated with second-generation antidepressants in patients with major depressive disorder: Results from a systematic review with network meta-analysis. *Drug Safety*, 37(1), 19–31. doi:10.1007/s40264-013-0129-4.

Sekse, R. J., Hufthammer, K. O., & Vika, M. E. (2016). Sexual activity and functioning in women treated for gynaecological cancers. *Journal of Clinical Nursing*, 26(3–4), 400–410. doi:10.1111/jocn.13407.

S

● = Independent;   ▲ = Collaborative;   **EBN** = Evidence-Based Nursing;   **EB** = Evidence-Based

Shieh, S. I., Lin, Y. H., Huang, C. Y., et al. (2016). Sexual dysfunction in males following low anterior resection. *Journal of Clinical Nursing*, 25(15–16), 2348–2356. doi:10.1111/jocn.13172.

Smith, A. E., Molton, I. R., McMullen, K., et al. (2015). Sexual function, satisfaction, and use of aids for sexual activity in middle-aged adults with long-term physical disability. *Topics in Spinal Cord Injury Rehabilitation*, 21(3), 227–232. doi:10.1310/sci2103-227.

Steinke, E. E., Mosack, V., & Hill, T. J. (2017). The influence of comorbidities, risk factors, and medications on sexual activity in individuals aged 40 to 59 years with and without cardiac conditions: US National Health and Nutrition Examination Survey, 2011–2012. *Journal of Cardiovascular Nursing*. doi:10.1097/JCN.0000000000000433. June 28.

Thomas, H. N., Hess, R., & Thurston, R. C. (2015). Correlates of sexual activity and satisfaction in midlife and older women. *Annals of Family Medicine*, 13(4), 336–342. doi:10.1370/afm.1820.

Vermeer, W. M., Bakker, R. M., Kenter, G. G., et al. (2016). Cervical cancer survivors' and partners' experiences with sexual dysfunction and psychosexual support. *Supportive Care in Cancer*, 24(4), 1679–1687. doi:10.1007/s00520-015-2925-0.

Ineffective Sexuality pattern   *Elaine E. Steinke, PhD, APRN, CNS-BC, FAHA, FAAN*

NANDA-I

Definition

Expressions of concern regarding own sexuality.

Defining Characteristics

Alterations in relationship with significant other; alteration in sexual activity; alteration in sexual behavior; change in sexual role; difficulty with sexual activity; difficulty with sexual behavior; value conflict

Related Factors

Conflict about sexual orientation; conflict about variant preference; fear of pregnancy; fear of sexually transmitted infection; impaired relationship with a significant other; inadequate role model; insufficient knowledge about alternatives related to sexuality; skill deficit about alternatives related to sexuality; absence of privacy

At-Risk Population

Absence of significant other

NOC   (Nursing Outcomes Classification)

Suggested NOC Outcomes

Abuse Recovery: Sexual; Body Image; Child Development: Middle Childhood/Adolescence; Client Satisfaction: Teaching; Knowledge: Pregnancy and Postpartum Sexual Functioning; Knowledge: Sexual Functioning; Psychosocial Adjustment: Life Change; Risk Control: Sexually Transmitted Diseases (STDs); Risk Control: Unintended Pregnancy; Role Performance; Self-Esteem; Sexual Functioning; Sexual Identity

> ### Example NOC Outcome with Indicators
>
> **Risk Control: Sexually Transmitted Diseases (STDs)** as evidenced by the following indicators: Acknowledges personal risk factors for STD/Uses strategies to prevent STD transmission. (Rate the outcome and indicators of **Risk Control: Sexually Transmitted Diseases (STDs):** 1 = never demonstrated, 2 = rarely demonstrated, 3 = sometimes demonstrated, 4 = often demonstrated, 5 = consistently demonstrated [see Section I].)

Client Outcomes

Client Will (Specify Time Frame)

- State knowledge of difficulties, limitations, or changes in sexual behaviors or activities
- State knowledge of sexual anatomy and functioning
- State acceptance of altered body structure or functioning
- Describe acceptable alternative sexual practices
- Identify importance of discussing sexual issues with significant other
- Describe practice of safe sex with regard to pregnancy and avoidance of sexually transmitted infections (STIs)

● = Independent;   ▲ = Collaborative;   EBN = Evidence-Based Nursing;   EB = Evidence-Based

NIC   (Nursing Interventions Classification)

Suggested NIC Interventions

Abuse Protection Support: Child; Abuse Protection Support: Domestic Partner; Abuse Protection Support: Elder; Abuse Protection Support: Religious; Behavior Management: Sexual; Sexual Counseling; Teaching: Safe Sex; Teaching: Sexuality

Example NIC Activities—Sexual Counseling

Provide privacy and ensure confidentiality; Provide information about sexual functioning, as appropriate

Nursing Interventions and *Rationales*

- After establishing rapport or therapeutic relationship, give the client permission to discuss issues dealing with sexuality, for example, "Have you been or are you concerned about functioning sexually because of your health status?" EB: *Use the PLISSIT model (permission, limited information, specific suggestions, referral to intensive therapy) to uncover additional concerns and begin with more general questions and then those more personal, such as discussing exercise recommendations and then sexual activity as another form of exercise (Steinke et al, 2013); use of the model has been shown to improve sexual function in women with multiple sclerosis (MS) (Khakbazan et al, 2016).*
- Use assessment questions and standardized instruments to assess sexual problems, where possible. EBN: *Use specific assessment questions to obtain information on current level of sexual activity, changes in sexual satisfaction, the nature of any problems experienced, underlying causes, medication review, and beliefs and misconceptions (Steinke, Mosack, & Hill, 2015).*
- ▲ Assess any risks associated with sexual activity, particularly coronary risks. EB: *Cardiac patients without angina or with mild angina who can exercise at a rate of at least 3 to 5 METs (amount of energy expenditure), and without experiencing angina, ischemic ST segment changes, or excess dyspnea are generally at low risk for cardiac events with sexual activity. For those at high risk or if a risk classification has not been determined, exercise stress testing is recommended (Lange & Levine, 2014). EB: If a cardiac patient is able to engage in physical activity at the rate of 3 to 5 METs or 3 to 4 miles per hour on a treadmill, or climb two flights of stairs briskly, sexual activity can generally be resumed (Steinke & Jaarsma, 2015).*
- Assess knowledge about sexual functioning and return to sexual activity after experiencing a health problem with both patients and partners. EBN: *Information provided to partners is often inadequate, and discussing sexual issues increases partner understanding and may minimize overprotectiveness by the partner; in post myocardial infarction (MI) patients and partners, patient knowledge about sex after MI improved at 1 year, whereas partners' knowledge did not change (Brännström et al, 2014).*
- Encourage the client to discuss concerns with his or her partner. EB: *Not communicating sexual concerns as a couple can lead to stress and deterioration in the relationship, whereas open and honest discussions with one's partner can promote sexual intimacy; an ideal time for such discussions might be during a daily walk together (Steinke et al, 2013).*
- Explore attitudes about sexual intimacy and changes in sexuality patterns. EBN: *Women with hematopoietic cell transplantation reported absent to low sexual desire, inadequate lubrication, problems with orgasm, pain with vaginal penetration, and overall sexual dissatisfaction, although quality of life scores improved in the first year, particularly for those with decreased psychosocial and physical symptoms, and there was improved sexual satisfaction (Tierney, Palesh, & Johnston, 2015). EBN: After breast cancer, women had reduced sexual desire, frequency, and satisfaction, with no association between sexual performance and body image (de Morais et al, 2016).*
- Assess psychosocial function such as anxiety, fear, depression, and low self-esteem. EBN: *Coronary heart disease patients who screened positive for moderate to high risk of depression while in acute care later had greater depression and anxiety, and less well-being and social support, emphasizing the importance of screening for psychological sequelae (Ski et al, 2015). EBN: In a population-based study, men who had sex with men had greater depressive symptoms compared with those with partners of the opposite sex (Scott, Lasiuk, & Norris, 2016).*
- Discuss alternative sexual expressions for altered body functioning or structure, including closeness and sexual and nonsexual touching as other forms of expression. EBN: *Women with fibromyalgia experienced pain with sexual activity, postcoital stiffness, anxiety about sex, and altered body image, although maintaining*

● = Independent;   ▲ = Collaborative;   EBN = Evidence-Based Nursing;   EB = Evidence-Based

an active sex life was important; therefore discussion of sexual concerns, individual symptoms, and psychoemotional needs can assist in developing approaches for sexual activity, such as changes in position or alternatives to sexual intercourse when symptom burden is high (Jiménez et al, 2017). EB: For some clients with severe heart failure, activities such as mutual masturbation, oral sex, or sexual intercourse may not be possible if exercise capacity is compromised, making other expressions of intimacy of greater importance (Steinke, 2013a).

- Assess the client's sexual orientation and usual pattern of sexual activities, and discuss prevention of illnesses for which the client may be at increased risk (e.g., anorectal cancer), asking specific questions about sexual orientation, for example, "Do you have sexual relationships with men, women, or both?" Assess use of safer sex practices (e.g., condom use); the frequency of anal intercourse; number of sexual partners in the last year; last HIV screening/results; and use of medications, alcohol, and illicit drugs. **EBN:** *Transgender women had low levels of HIV risk perception and knowledge about HIV risk and transmission, illustrating the importance of assessing transgender women's sexual health care needs and educating regarding risks (De Santis et al, 2017).*
- Specific guidelines for sexual activity for clients who have had total hip arthroplasty (THA) include the following: sexual activity can be generally resumed 1 to 2 months after surgery, and positioning to avoid hip dislocation, e.g., a supine position ("missionary") at maximum abduction in extension, or the man and woman standing, with the woman's legs slightly bent and the man approaching the woman from behind (McFadden, 2013). **EB:** *In a systematic review of THA and sexual activity, 76% of individuals identified hip arthritis as contributing to sexual problems, whereas post-THA, 44% reported improvement in sexual satisfaction, 27% reported increased intercourse frequency, and most returned to sexual activity at 4 months post-THA. Health care professionals and surgeons should discuss return to sexual activity after THA, including the best positions postsurgery (Harmsen et al, 2017; Issa et al, 2017).*
- Specific guidelines for those who have had an MI include the following: sexual activity can generally be resumed 1 week after MI unless complications are experienced, such as arrhythmias or cardiac arrest, if the client does not have cardiac symptoms during mild to moderate physical activity; begin with activities that require less exertion, such as fondling or kissing, building confidence in tolerance for sexual activity prior to sexual intercourse; engage in sexual activity in familiar surroundings with the usual partner; have a comfortable room temperature, and be well rested to minimize cardiac stress; avoid heavy meals or alcohol for 2 to 3 hours before sexual activity; and choose a position of comfort to minimize stress of the cardiac client (Steinke et al, 2013). **EB:** *Among younger individuals experiencing MI in the United States and Spain, 72% of women and 86% of men reported return to sexual activity at 1 month post MI, and the majority rated sexual activity as important, illustrating the importance of providing sexual education while hospitalized and during the early recovery period (Lindau et al, 2014).*
- Specific guidelines include that those who have had complete coronary revascularization, in addition to those mentioned with MI, including those with successful percutaneous cardiovascular revascularization without complication, can resume sex within a few days, and those who have had standard coronary artery bypass grafting (CABG) or noncoronary open heart surgery may resume sex in 6 to 8 weeks. Incisional pain with sexual activity can be managed by premedicating with a mild pain reliever, and reassurance should be provided to the partner that sexual activity will not harm the sternum as long as direct pressure is avoided (Steinke et al, 2013). **EB:** *Women, particularly those with large breasts, may report more issues related to pain in the breast, chest numbness, and difficulty healing; therefore encourage these women to choose a position of comfort, support with pillows, and take a pain reliever such as acetaminophen before sexual activity (Steinke & Jaarsma, 2015).*
- Specific guidelines for those with an implantable cardioverter defibrillator (ICD) include returning to sexual activity is generally safe after ICD implantation if moderate physical activity does not precipitate arrhythmias; avoid strain on the incision at the implant site; assure the client and partner that fears about being shocked during sexual activity are normal; if the ICD discharges with sexual activity, the client should stop, rest, and later notify the health care provider that the device fired so that a determination can be made if this was an appropriate shock or not; and report any dyspnea, chest pain, or dizziness with sexual activity (Steinke et al, 2013). **EB:** *Although most clients with ICD reported the ability to engage in sexual activity (64.6%), 51% chose to avoid sexual activity, citing reasons such as fear of shock, fear of increased heart rate, and no desire, illustrating the importance of evaluating and discussing both psychological and physical aspects of return to sexual activity (Cutitta et al, 2014).*
- Specific guidelines for those with chronic lung disease include planning for sexual activity when energy level is highest; use of controlled breathing techniques; avoiding physical exertion prior to sexual activity; using positions that minimize shortness of breath, such as a semireclining position; engaging in sexual

● = Independent; ▲ = Collaborative; **EBN** = Evidence-Based Nursing; **EB** = Evidence-Based

activity when medications are at peak effectiveness; use of an oxygen cannula, if prescribed, to provide oxygen before, during, or after sex; and use of continuous positive airway pressure (CPAP) therapy, if prescribed (Steinke, 2013b). **EB:** *For patients and families participating in exercise training and psychoeducational support, family members reported significantly greater improvement in sexual relationships and psychological distress compared with the control group, demonstrating the importance of psychoeducational sexual interventions (Marques et al, 2015).* **EB:** *In a systematic review of sexual dysfunction and obstructive sleep apnea in men, CPAP improved daytime sleepiness and erectile and orgasmic dysfunction, although sildenafil was superior to CPAP in improving erectile dysfunction; intervention studies for women were not available (Steinke et al, 2016).*

- Specific guidelines for those with MS include treatment of symptoms with prescribed medications, assessing changes in body image, and supportive therapies to assist with a more satisfying sexual experience, including treatment of neuropathic pain, sexual positions that are most supportive, discussing changes in sensation and stimulation with the partner, use of stretching exercise for tight muscles prior to sexual activity, and avoiding a distended bowel or bladder that may cause discomfort. **EB:** *Women with MS attending a 12-week sexual therapy program significantly improved sexual desire, arousal, lubrication, orgasm, satisfaction, overall quality of life, energy, cognitive function, and social function; designing targeted educational and sexual interventions are important to improve sexual and overall quality of life (Zamani et al, 2017).*

- Refer to the care plan **Sexual** dysfunction for additional interventions.

 Pediatric

- Initiate discussions regarding sexual health, attitudes, and knowledge about sexual behavior, and sexual abstinence, providing information that is age-appropriate and accurate regarding sexual activity and risky sexual behaviors. **EBN:** *In a small intervention study of African American girls between the ages of 12 and 14 years, mother and daughter dyads that completed the sexual communication intervention had improved sexual knowledge, confidence to discuss sexual issues, and openness to communication, illustrating the importance of initiating these conversations with adolescents and their families (Aronowitz et al, 2015).* **EB:** *Focus groups conducted in black churches with senior pastors, youth ministers, parents of youth, and youth ages 13 to 19 years, on the topic of youth sexual and reproductive health, resulted in the themes of engaging stakeholders, the authenticity of the curriculum, making the curriculum relevant to youth, discussion of relationships, and adaptation, providing an example that implementing sexual health programs in new settings can be successful in reaching youth and the community (Weeks et al, 2016).*

- Provide age-appropriate information for adolescents regarding HIV/AIDS and sexual behavior, and discuss STIs, particularly human papillomavirus, including the risks of perinatal transmission and methods to reduce risks among HIV-infected adolescents. **EB:** *African American female adolescents who participated in an HIV prevention intervention with specific sexual health telephone counseling contacts had greater improvement in depressive symptoms than the comparison group. More than 40% had moderate to severe depression at baseline, illustrating the importance of addressing depression in intervention programs (Brown et al, 2014).*

- Provide age-appropriate information regarding potential for sexual abuse. **EBN:** *A structured teaching program on prevention of sexual abuse with high school students resulted in improved knowledge of prevention strategies, illustrating the importance of education and directly addressing this sensitive issue (Fulgen, 2017).*

 Geriatric

- Carefully assess the sexuality needs of the older client and refer for counseling if needed; the ability to form satisfying social relationships and to be intimate with others, including building strong emotional intimate connections, contributes to adaptation and successful aging (Steinke, 2013b). **EB:** *Positive affect and life satisfaction was associated with increased sexual behavior in community-dwelling older men and women, regardless of depressive symptoms, physical health, and chronic diseases, whereas unpartnered adults' life satisfaction was linked with more physical tenderness and less sexual behavior, demonstrating the importance of sexual assessment of all older adults and in promoting psychological and sexual well-being (Freak-Poli et al, 2017a).*

▲ Explore possible changes in sexuality related to health status, menopause, medications, and sexual risk, and make appropriate referrals. **EB:** *Although two-thirds of older adults had experienced some sexual problems, most were not distressed by it, reporting positive sexual well-being, with positive sexual self-esteem and attitudes toward sex, high sexual satisfaction and interest, and frequently engaging in sexual activity,* *illustrating that although some older adults may experience challenges regarding sexual activity, many report positive sexual health (Santos-Iglesias, Byers, & Moglia, 2016).* **EB:** *Sexual risk-taking was prevalent among older adults, with 49% reporting engaging in vaginal sex and 43% engaging in oral sex without a condom in the prior 6 months, although 65.5% of the sample believed they were not susceptible to STIs, revealing the need for assessment, education, and intervention related to sexual risk (Syme, Cohn, & Barnack-Tavlaris, 2017).*

- Allow the client to verbalize feelings regarding loss of sexual partner, and acknowledge problems such as disapproving children, lack of available partner for women, and environmental variables that make forming new relationships difficult. **EB:** *Health status, frequency of sexual activity, and importance of sexual behavior were important predictors of quality of life, and these findings were independent of the presence of a spouse/ partner, illustrating the importance of health care providers evaluating sexual activity as a component of quality of life with all clients (Flynn & Gow, 2015).*

- ▲ Provide a milieu that allows for discussion of sexual issues and a higher level of sexual satisfaction, including allowing couples to room together and the provision of privacy. **EBN:** *Sexual expression and consent should be openly addressed in long-term care settings, and results from a qualitative study of directors of long-term care facilities revealed the common themes of addressing the issue, making environmental changes, identifying staff expertise, providing education and training, assessing sexuality initially and recurrently, establishing policies and procedures for sexual expression management, developing assessment tools, and clarifying legal issues. These are all important areas that staff in long-term care facilities can use to improve the sexual health of their residents (Syme, Lichtenberg, & Moye, 2016).*

- See care plan for **Sexual** dysfunction.

Multicultural

- Assess for the influence of cultural beliefs, norms, and values on client's perceptions of sexual behavior. **EBN:** *Among Hispanic men who had sex with men, parental knowledge and rejection of their sexual orientation contributed to greater depressive symptoms and no effect on safer sex behaviors, although acculturation (Americanism) may have had a protective role. These findings emphasized the importance of educating and supporting both the individual and family, including assessing mental health (Mitrani et al, 2017).*

Home Care

- Previously discussed interventions may be adapted for home care use. Also see care plan for **Sexual** dysfunction.

- Help the client and significant other identify a place and time in the home and daily living for privacy in sharing sexual or relationship activity, and, if necessary, help the client communicate the need for privacy to family members. **EB:** *In community-dwelling older adults, most reported experiencing physical tenderness and about half engaged in sexual activity, with sexual activity more likely in those of younger age, those with greater social support, those with healthier behaviors, and those with better psychological and physical health, illustrating the importance of maintaining sexual quality of life regardless of setting, not assuming that the older person is not interested in sexual pleasure, and having health care professionals proactively address sexuality and sexual health (Freak-Poli et al, 2017b).*

- Confirm that physical reasons for dysfunction have been addressed, and provide support for coping behaviors, including participation in support groups or therapy if appropriate. **EB:** *A pilot study using a psychoeducational group intervention in women with MS and spinal cord injury resulted in improved sexual functioning, particularly for sexual desire and arousal, demonstrating the importance of supportive interventions to improve sexual functioning (Hocaloski et al, 2016).*

Client/Family Teaching and Discharge Planning

- ▲ Refer to appropriate community agencies (e.g., certified sex counselor, Reach to Recovery, Ostomy Association, American Association of Sex Educators, Counselors, and Therapists). **EBN:** *Sexuality concerns should be addressed with all clients for whom sexual function might be affected because of an acute or chronic condition (Steinke, 2013a).*

- ▲ Sexuality education is important to all populations, whether hearing or deaf, sighted or blind, disabled or not disabled; discuss contraceptive choices as appropriate, safer sexual practices, and refer to a health professional (e.g., gynecologist, urologist, nurse practitioner). **EB:** *Sexuality education of older adults is often overlooked, and they may have inaccurate perceptions regarding sexual risk behaviors and STIs (Syme, Cohn, & Barnack-Tavlaris, 2017).*

• = Independent;   ▲ = Collaborative;   EBN = Evidence-Based Nursing;   EB = Evidence-Based

REFERENCES

Aronowitz, T., Ogunlade, I. J., Nwosu, C., et al. (2015). Sexual communication intervention for African American mothers and daughters. *Applied Nursing Research*, 28(3), 229–234. doi:10.1016/j.apnr.2015.04.017.

Brännström, M., Kristofferzon, M. L., Ivarsson, B., et al. (2014). Sexual knowledge in patients with myocardial infarction and their partners. *Journal of Cardiovascular Nursing*, 29(4), 332–339. doi:10.1097/JCN.0b013e318291ede6.

Brown, J. L., Sales, J. M., Swartzendruber, A. L., et al. (2014). Added benefits: Reduced depressive symptom levels among African-American female adolescents participating in an HIV prevention intervention. *Journal of Behavioral Medicine*, 37(5), 912–920. doi:10.1007/s10865-013-9551-4.

Cutitta, K. E., Woodrow, L. K., Ford, J., et al. (2014). Shocktivity: Ability and avoidance of daily activity behaviors in ICD patients. *Journal of Cardiopulmonary Rehabilitation and Prevention*, 34(4), 241–247. doi:10.1097/HCR0000000000000055.

de Morais, F. D., Freitas-Junior, R., Rahal, R. M., et al. (2016). Sociodemographic and clinical factors affecting body image, sexual function and sexual satisfaction in women with breast cancer. *Journal of Clinical Nursing*, 25(11–12), 1557–1565. doi:10.1111/jocn.13125.

De Santis, J. P., Hauglum, S. D., Deleon, D. A., et al. (2017). HIV risk perception, HIV knowledge, and sexual risk behaviors among transgender women in South Florida. *Public Health Nursing*, 34(3), 210–218. doi:10.1111/phn.12309.

Flynn, T. J., & Gow, A. J. (2015). Examining associations between sexual behaviours and quality of life in older adults. *Age and Ageing*, 44(5), 823–828. doi:10.1093/ageing/afv083.

Freak-Poli, R., De Castro Lima, G., Direk, N., et al. (2017a). Happiness, rather than depression, is associated with sexual behaviour in partnered older adults. *Age and Ageing*, 46(1), 101–107. doi:10.1093/ageing/afw168.

Freak-Poli, R., Kirkman, M., De Castro Lima, G., et al. (2017b). Sexual activity and physical tenderness in older adults: Cross-sectional prevalence and associated characteristics. *Journal of Sexual Medicine*, 14(7), 918–927. doi:10.1016/j.jsxm.2017.05.010.

Fulgen, F. (2017). Effectiveness of structured teaching programme on knowledge of high school children regarding prevention of sexual abuse. *International Journal of Nursing Education*, 9(2), 61–65. doi:10.5958/0974-9357.2017.00037.X.

Harmsen, R. T. E., Nicolai, M. P. J., Den Oudsten, B. L., et al. (2017). Patient sexual function and hip replacement surgery: A survey of surgeon attitudes. *International Orthopaedics*. doi:10.1007/s00264-017-3473-7.

Hocaloski, S., Elliott, S., Brotto, L. A., et al. (2016). A mindfulness psychoeducational group intervention targeting sexual adjustment for women with multiple sclerosis and spinal cord injury: A pilot study. *Sexuality and Disability*, 34(2), 183–198. doi:10.1007/s11195-016-9426z.

Issa, K., Pierce, T. P., Brothers, A., et al. (2017). Sexual activity after total hip arthroplasty: A systematic review of outcomes. *Journal of Arthroplasty*, 32(1), 336–340. doi:10.1016/j.arth.2016.07.052.

Jiménez, T. M., Fernández-Sola, C., Hernández-Padilla, J. M., et al. (2017). Perceptions about the sexuality of women with fibromyalgia syndrome: A phenomenological study. *Journal of Advanced Nursing*, 73(7), 1646–1656. doi:10.1111/jan.13262.

Khakbazan, Z., Daneshfar, F., Behboodi-Moghadam, Z., et al. (2016). The effectiveness of the Permission, Limited Information, Specific Suggestions, Intensive Therapy (PLISSIT) model based sexual counseling on the sexual function of women with multiple sclerosis who are sexually active. *Multiple Sclerosis and Related Disorders*, 8, 113–119. doi:10.1016/j.msard.2016.05.007.

Lange, R. A., & Levine, G. N. (2014). Sexual activity and ischemic heart disease. *Current Cardiology Reports*, 16(2), 445. doi:10.1007/s11886-013-0445-4.

Lindau, S. T., Abramsohn, E. M., Bueno, H., et al. (2014). Sexual activity and counseling in the first month after acute myocardial infarction among younger adults in the United States and Spain. *Circulation*, 130, 2302–2309. doi:10.1161/CIRCULATIONAHA.114.012709.

Marques, A., Jácome, C., Cruz, J., et al. (2015). Family-based psychosocial support and education as part of pulmonary rehabilitation in COPD: A randomized controlled trial. *Chest*, 147(3), 662–672. doi:10.1378/chest.14-1488.

McFadden, B. (2013). Is there a safe coital position after a total hip arthroplasty? *Orthopaedic Nursing*, 32(4), 223–226. doi:10.1097/NOR.0b013e31829b0349.

Mitrani, V. B., De Santis, J. P., McCabe, B. E., et al. (2017). The impact of parenteral reaction to sexual orientation on depressive symptoms and sexual risk behavior among Hispanic men who have sex with men. *Archives of Psychiatric Nursing*, 31(4), 352–358. doi:10.1016/j.apnu.2017.04.004.

Santos-Iglesias, P., Byers, E. S., & Moglia, R. (2016). Sexual well-being of older men and women. *The Canadian Journal of Human Sexuality*, 25(2), 86–98. doi:10.3138/cjhs.252-A4.

Scott, R. L., Lasiuk, G., & Norris, C. (2016). The relationship between sexual orientation and depression in a national population sample. *Journal of Clinical Nursing*, 25(23–24), 3522–3532. doi:10.1111/jocn.13286.

Ski, C. F., Worrall-Carter, L., Cameron, J., et al. (2015). Depression screening and referral in cardiac wards: A 12-month patient trajectory. *European Journal of Cardiovascular Nursing*, 16(2), 157–166. doi:10.1177/1474515115583617.

Steinke, E. E. (2013a). How can heart failure patients and their partners be counseled on sexual activity? *Current Heart Failure Reports*, 10(3), 262–269. doi:10.1007/s11897-013-0138-8.

Steinke, E. E. (2013b). Sexuality and chronic illness. *Journal of Gerontological Nursing*, 39(11), 18–27. doi:10.3928/00989134-20130916-01.

Steinke, E. E., Jaarsma, T., Barnason, S. A., et al. (2013). Sexual counseling for individuals with cardiovascular disease and their partners: A consensus document from the American Heart Association and the ESC Council on Cardiovascular Nursing and Allied Health Professionals (CCNAP). *Circulation*, 128(18), 2075–2096. doi:10.1161/CIR.0b013e31829c2e53.

Steinke, E. E., & Jaarsma, T. (2015). Sexual counseling and cardiovascular disease: Practical approaches. *Asian Journal of Andrology*, 17(1), 32–39. doi:10.4103/1008-682X.135982.

Steinke, E. E., Johansen, P. P., Fridlund, B., et al. (2016). Determinants of sexual dysfunction and interventions for patients with obstructive sleep apnoea: A systematic review. *The International Journal of Clinical Practice*, 70(1), 5–19. doi:10.1111/ijcp.12751.

Steinke, E. E., Mosack, V., & Hill, T. J. (2015). Change in sexual activity after a cardiac event: The role of medications, comorbidity, and psychosocial factors. *Applied Nursing Research*, 28(3), 244–250. doi:10.1016/j.apnr.2015.04.011.

Syme, M. L., Lichtenberg, P., & Moye, J. (2016). Recommendations for sexual expression management in long-term care: A qualitative needs assessment. *Journal of Advanced Nursing*, 72(10), 2457–2467. doi:10.1111/jan.13005

Syme, M. L., Cohn, T. J., & Barnack-Tavlaris, J. (2017). A comparison of actual and perceived sexual risk among older adults. *The Journal of Sex Research*, 54(2), 149–160. doi:10.1080/00224499.2015.1124379.

Tierney, D. K., Palesh, O., & Johnston, L. (2015). Sexuality, menopausal symptoms, and quality of life in premenopausal women in the first

S

year following hematopoietic cell transplantation. *Oncology Nursing Forum*, 42(5), 488–497. doi:10.1188/15.ONF.488-497.

Weeks, F. H., Powell, T. W., Illangasekare, S., et al. (2016). Bringing evidence-based sexual health programs to adolescents in black churches: Applying knowledge from systematic adaptation frameworks. *Health Education & Behavior*, 43(6), 699–704. doi:10.1177/1090198116633459.

Zamani, M., Tavoli, A., Khasti, B. Y., et al. (2017). Sexual therapy for women with multiple sclerosis and its impact on quality of life. *Iranian Journal of Psychiatry*, 12(1), 56–65.

Risk for Shock   *Tara Cuccinelli, RN, MS, AGCNS-BC*

NANDA-I

Definition

Susceptible to an inadequate blood flow to the body's tissues that may lead to life-threatening cellular dysfunction, which may compromise health.

Risk Factors

To be developed

Associated Condition

Hypotension; hypovolemia; hypoxemia; hypoxia; infection; sepsis; systemic inflammatory response syndrome (SIRS)

NOC   (Nursing Outcomes Classification)

Suggested NOC Outcomes

Cardiac Pump Effectiveness; Fluid Balance; Infection Severity; Respiratory Status: Gas Exchange; Neurological Status: Autonomic; Tissue Perfusion: Cellular

Example **NOC** Outcome with Indicators
Neurological Status: Autonomic as evidenced by the following indicators: Apical heart rate/Systolic blood pressure/Urinary elimination pattern/Thermoregulation. (Rate the outcome and indicators of **Neurological Status: Autonomic:** 1 = severely compromised, 2 = substantially compromised, 3 = moderately compromised, 4 = mildly compromised, 5 = not compromised [see Section I].)

Client Outcomes

Client Will (Specify Time Frame)

- Discuss precautions to prevent complications of disease
- Maintain adherence to agreed-on medication regimens
- Maintain adequate hydration
- Monitor for infection signs and symptoms
- Maintain a mean arterial pressure (MAP) above 65 mm Hg
- Maintain a heart rate between 60 and 100 with a normal rhythm
- Maintain urine output greater than 0.5 mL/kg/hr
- Maintain warm, dry skin

NIC   (Nursing Intervention Classification)

Suggested NIC Interventions

Admission Care; Allergy Management; Cardiac Care; Cerebral Perfusion Promotion; Electrolyte Monitoring; Fever Treatment; Fluid Management; Hemodynamic Regulation; Infection Precaution; Medication Management; Oxygen Therapy; Postanesthesia Care; Risk Identification; Shock Prevention; Teaching: Disease Process; Temperature Regulation; Vital Signs Monitoring

● = Independent;   ▲ = Collaborative;   EBN = Evidence-Based Nursing;   EB = Evidence-Based

Example **NIC Activities—Shock Prevention**
Monitor circulatory status; Monitor for signs of inadequate tissue oxygenation; Administer oxygen and/or mechanical ventilation, as appropriate; Instruct client and/or family on precipitating factors of shock

Nursing Interventions and *Rationales*

- Review data pertaining to client risk status including age, primary diseases, immunosuppression, antibiotic use, and presence of hemodynamic alterations such as tachycardia, tachypnea, and decrease in blood pressure (BP). **EB:** *Many clients who develop shock have underlying circumstances that predispose them to shock states as evidenced by hypotension and inadequate organ perfusion (Kalil, 2014; Kleinpell, Schorr, & Balk, 2016).*

- Review client's medical and surgical history, noting conditions that place the client at higher risk for shock, including trauma, myocardial infarction, pulmonary embolism, head injury, dehydration, infection, endocrine problems, certain medications, and pregnancy. **EB:** *Certain clinical conditions place clients at higher risk for shock, which requires prompt identification and treatment to improve morbidity and mortality outcomes (Delgado et al, 2013; American Heart Association [AHA], 2016).*

- Complete a full nursing physical examination. *A full nursing physical examination is crucial in identifying all factors that might place that client at risk for the development of shock, such as hypoperfusion of internal organs (manifesting as decreased urinary output and shortness of breath) and tissue hypoperfusion (manifesting as cool, clammy, mottled skin and diminished pulses).* **EB:** *The use of extremity skin temperatures alone, as a predictor of decreased cardiac output (CO), cannot be validated or supported because of a lack of consensus in the literature (Hiemstra et al, 2017).* However, the presence of skin mottling, especially over the knees, ears, and fingers, suggests tissue hypoperfusion states often seen in shock (Contou & de Prost, 2016).

- Monitor circulatory status (e.g., BP, MAP, skin color, skin temperature, heart sounds, heart rate and rhythm, presence and quality of peripheral pulses, pulse oximetry, and end-tidal carbon dioxide monitoring [$EtCO_2$]). **EB:** *The initial phase of shock is characterized by decreased CO and tissue perfusion, which results in immediate compensatory changes evidenced by a drop in BP, increased heart rate, and shunting of blood away from the periphery, resulting in pale, cooler, damp skin, and mottling with reduced peripheral pulses (Kalil, 2014; Contou & de Prost, 2016; Kleinpell, Schorr, & Balk, 2016).*

- Maintain intravenous (IV) access and provide isotonic IV fluids such as 0.9% normal saline or Ringer's lactate as ordered; these fluids are commonly used in the prevention and treatment of shock. **EB:** *Restrictive fluid resuscitation and permissive hypotension (achievement of systolic pressure around 90 mm Hg) may have an advantage over standard higher volume fluid resuscitation regarding overall and early intraoperative survival benefit in trauma patients experiencing shock (Sweeney, 2013; Carrick et al, 2016).* **EB:** *Septic shock hypoperfusion should be initially managed with a 30 mL/kg bolus of crystalloid fluid for patients who have no underlying comorbidities (e.g., congestive heart failure or chronic renal conditions) (Rhodes et al, 2017).*

- Monitor for inadequate tissue oxygenation (e.g., apprehension, increased anxiety, altered mental status, agitation, oliguria, cool/mottled periphery) and determinants of tissue oxygen delivery (e.g., PaO_2, SpO_2, $ScvO_2/SvO_2$, MAP, hemoglobin levels, lactate levels, CO). *Assessment of tissue oxygen delivery and oxygenation patterns provides data to assess trends in client's status and evaluates treatment responses (Kalil, 2014). Changes in client mental status are highly sensitive to changes in perfusion and oxygenation (Singer, 2016).* **EB:** *Invasive monitoring has not been shown to improve overall mortality. Many clinicians are using noninvasive monitoring even for hemodynamically unstable patients including the use of bedside ultrasonography and infrared spectroscopy (Seymour & Rosengart, 2015; Rhodes et al, 2017).* **EB:** *Reduction in mortality was observed with interventions aimed at lactate-guided resuscitation (Rhodes et al, 2017).*

▲ Maintain vital signs (BP, pulse, respirations, and temperature) and pulse oximetry within normal parameters. **EB:** *Trending of vital signs using an early warning score (EWS) is a quick cost-effective way to identify early patients at risk of deterioration and intervene in a timely manner (Albur, Hamilton, & MacGowan, 2016).* **EB:** *Increased heart rate (above 90 beats per minutes), hypotension (BP below 90 mm Hg systolic), tachypnea (greater than 20 breaths per minute), hypoxia (SpO_2 below 90%), lactate levels (above 2 mmol/L), and change in mentation are indicators of shock (Dellinger et al, 2013, Kalil, 2014; Singer, 2016; Rhodes et al, 2017). Temperature greater than 38°C or less than 36°C with white blood cell count greater than 12,000/mm^3 or less than 4000/mm^3 plus symptoms listed earlier are indicators of SIRS (Dellinger et al, 2013; Rhodes et al, 2017).* **EB:** *Quick Sequential Organ Failure Assessment (qSOFA), which looks at altered mentation, systolic BP of 100 mm Hg or less, and respiratory rate greater than 22 breaths per minute has shown to identify patients who are likely to have poor outcomes (Singer, 2016).*

● = Independent;   ▲ = Collaborative;   EBN = Evidence-Based Nursing;   EB = Evidence-Based

S

▲ Administer oxygen immediately to maintain SpO$_2$ greater than 90%, and antibiotics and other medications as prescribed to any client presenting with symptoms of early shock. **EBN:** *The experienced nurse has an important role in the implementation of the Surviving Sepsis Campaign (SSC), which includes specific early goal-directed therapies that enhance client survival (Kleinpell, Aitken, & Schorr, 2013; Turi & Von Ah, 2013; Kleinpell, Schorr, & Balk, 2016).* **EB:** *Early goal-directed therapy protocols focusing on administration of oxygen, fluid resuscitation, antibiotics administered within an hour, and vasoactive medications provide early correction of risks for shock and improve survival of shock. Antibiotics as prescribed administered within 1 hour of diagnosis of a sepsis state facilitates a better rate of survival. For each hour in delayed antibiotic administration, survival decreases by 7.6% (Seymour & Rosengart, 2015; Rhodes et al, 2017).*

▲ Monitor trends in noninvasive hemodynamic parameters (e.g., MAP) as appropriate. **EB:** *A MAP less than 60 to 65 mm Hg for any extended time period is associated with poor outcomes (Leone et al, 2015)* **EB:** *Restoring MAP to desired levels (above 65 mm Hg) facilitates adequate perfusion to organs; (Dellinger et al, 2013; Rhodes et al, 2017; Singer, 2016).* **EB:** *An overarching goal of cardiovascular support is optimization of blood flow to tissues; however, there is no single optimum MAP that can be applied to all. In patients with chronic arterial hypertension, a higher MAP (75–85 mm Hg) may be preferable (Leone et al, 2015; Rhodes et al, 2017). Monitor hydration status including daily weights, postural BP changes, serum electrolytes (sodium, potassium, chloride, bilirubin, creatinine, and blood urea nitrogen), intake and output, and skin turgor. Consider insertion of an indwelling urinary catheter as ordered to measure hourly output for a goal of 0.5 mL/kg/hr (Kleinpell, Schorr, & Balk, 2016).*

▲ Monitor serum lactate levels and interpret them within the context of each client. **EB:** *Elevations in serum lactate (above 2 mmol/L) may indicate circulatory failure and resultant tissue hypoxia from anaerobic metabolism that results in toxin accumulation, cellular inflammation, and cellular death with higher lactate levels predictive of higher mortality (Casserly et al, 2015).* **EB:** *Progression to septic shock may result as characterized by the onset of SIRS (Rhodes et al, 2017). Two or more of the following indicators suggest SIRS: altered temperatures; heart rates above 90 beats per minute; tachypnea or hypocarbia; and/or leukocytosis/leukopenia, which may or may not be related to infection as other causative factors exist (Kaplan & Pinsky, 2014; Rhodes et al, 2017). The degree of serum lactate elevation correlates with morbidity and mortality in sepsis; early detection facilitates early treatment and is a more accurate triage tool than vital signs (Casserly et al, 2015). Monitor blood glucose levels frequently and administer insulin as prescribed to targeted blood glucose levels of <180 mg/dL (Rhodes et al, 2017).*

Critical Care

▲ Prepare the client for the placement of an additional IV line, central line, and/or a pulmonary artery catheter as prescribed. *Adequate IV and central line access may be required for fluid resuscitation and medication delivery. Maintaining more than one IV access ensures rapid IV medication and fluid delivery in a crisis situation. Large amounts of fluid can be delivered more efficiently through centrally placed vascular access sites. Most vasoactive agents, especially vasopressors, should be delivered only through central lines because of risk of tissue sloughing.* **EB:** *A Cochrane systematic review of 13 studies on 5686 clients found no difference in mortality rates or days spent in an intensive care unit (ICU) between those clients with a pulmonary artery catheter and those without (Rajaram et al, 2013).*

▲ Monitor trends in hemodynamic parameters (e.g., central venous pressure [CVP], CO, cardiac index [CI], systemic vascular resistance [SVR], pulmonary artery pressure [PAP], MAP) as appropriate. *Hemodynamic indices will be altered depending on the underlying form of shock (hypovolemic, distributive, or cardiogenic). Dehydration will result in reduced CVP, CO, PAP, and ultimately MAP because of hypovolemia. Vasodilation as seen in distributive shock patterns (forms of third spacing as in neurogenic, anaphylactic, and septic shock states) will decrease BP and CVP (a surrogate for intravascular volume) and other hemodynamic indices. Cardiogenic shock will result in low CO and MAP with higher PAP and CVP indices caused by heart failure and subsequent congestion of the cardiopulmonary systems. Compensatory mechanisms to address reductions in CO and MAP include tachycardia and reduced urinary output (less than 0.5 mL/kg/hr). Both CO and SVR may temporarily increase with the onset of shock because of compensatory mechanisms; however, as shock progresses, both CO and SVR decline (Dellinger et al, 2013; Kalil, 2014).*

▲ Monitor electrocardiography. Tachycardia may be present as a result of decreased fluid volume, which will be seen before a decrease in BP as a compensatory mechanism. **EB:** *As oxygen demands increase, tachycardia and cardiac dysrhythmias may be evident, such as premature ventricular contractions (Dellinger et al, 2013).*

● = Independent;   ▲ = Collaborative;   **EBN** = Evidence-Based Nursing;   **EB** = Evidence-Based

▲ Monitor arterial blood gases, coagulation, blood chemistries, blood glucose, cardiac enzymes, blood cultures, and hematology labs. EB: *Abnormalities can identify the cause of the perfusion deficits and identify complications related to the decreased perfusion or shock state. Cardiogenic shock may be identified by elevations in cardiac enzymes as a result of myocardial infarction in association with low MAP. Elevation/reductions in white blood cell counts may be indicative of septic shock when associated with alterations in MAP (Kalil, 2014; Rhodes et al, 2017).*

▲ Administer vasopressor agents as prescribed. EB: *Norepinephrine is the vasopressor of choice for septic shock (Avni et al, 2015; Rhodes et al, 2017). Norepinephrine should be administered through a central line.* EB: *Low-dose dopamine should not be started for renal protection (Rhodes et al, 2017).*

• If the client is in shock, refer to the following care plans: Risk for ineffective **Renal** perfusion, Risk for ineffective **Gastrointestinal** perfusion, Impaired **Gas** exchange, and Decreased **Cardiac** output.

 ## Client/Family Teaching and Discharge Planning

▲ *Teach client and family or significant others about any medications prescribed. Instruct the client to report any adverse side effects to his or her health care provider. Medication teaching includes the drug name, purpose, administration instructions (e.g., with or without food), and any side effects. Provision of such information using clear communication principles and with an understanding of what the health literacy level of the client/family/significant others may be can facilitate appropriate adherence to the therapeutic regimen (Balentine, 2014; National Institutes of Health [NIH], 2016).*

• Instruct the client and family on disease process and rationale for care. EB: *Tailored interventions targeted to the level of the learner enhance client activation (Hibbard & Greene, 2013). Knowledge empowers clients and family members, allowing them to be active participants in their care (Finchman, 2013).* EB: *When clients and their family members have sufficient understanding of their disease process, they can participate more fully in care and healthy behaviors (Finchman, 2013).*

• Instruct clients and their family members on the signs and symptoms of low BP to report to their health care provider (dizziness, lightheadedness, fainting, dehydration and unusual thirst, lack of concentration, blurred vision, nausea, cold, clammy, pale skin, rapid and shallow breathing, fatigue, and depression). EBN: *Teach-back methods were found to be significantly associated with self-care activities and fewer hospitalizations in a sample of 276 clients with heart failure (White et al, 2013).* EB: *Use of the teach-back method enhances an individual's knowledge and adherence behaviors (Negarandeh et al, 2013). Early recognition and treatment of these symptoms may avoid more serious sequelae (AHA, 2016).*

• Promote a culture of client safety and individual accountability. EB: *Organizations that promote a just culture of safety help to reduce or prevent errors and improve overall health care quality (Agency for Healthcare Research and Quality [AHRQ], 2017). Include health literacy strategies into all aspects of client-centered care and weave into organizational values (Koh et al, 2013).*

S

REFERENCES

Agency for Healthcare Research and Quality. (2017). *Culture of safety.* Retrieved from https://psnet.ahrq.gov/primers/primer/5/safety-culture. (Accessed 31 October 2017).

Albur, M., Hamilton, F., & MacGowan, A. P. (2016). Early warning score: A dynamic marker of severity and prognosis in patients with Gram-negative bacteraemia and sepsis. *Annals of Clinical Microbiology and Antimicrobials, 15,* 23.

American Heart Association (AHA). (2016). *When is blood pressure too low?* Retrieved from https://www.heart.org/HEARTORG/Conditions/HighBloodPressure/GettheFactsAboutHighBloodPressure/Low-Blood-Pressure. (Accessed 17 October 2017).

Avni, T., Lador, A., Lev, S., et al. (2015). Vasopressors for the treatment of septic shock: Systematic review and meta-analysis. *PLoS ONE, 10*(8), e0129305.

Balentine, J. (2014). *Sepsis (blood infection).* Retrieved from http://www.emedicinehealth.com/sepsis_blood_infection/article_em.htm. (Accessed 17 October 2017).

Carrick, M., Leonard, J., Slone, D., et al. (2016). Hypotensive resuscitation among trauma patients. *BioMed Research International.*

Casserly, B., Phillips, G., Schorr, C., et al. (2015). Lactate measurements in sepsis induced tissur hypoperfusion: Results from the Surviving Sepsis Campaign database. *Critical Care Medicine, 43*(3), 567–573.

Contou, D., & de Prost, N. (2016). Skin mottling. *The New England Journal of Medicine, 375,* 2187. doi:10.1056/NEJMicm1602055.

Delgado, M. K., Liu, V., Pines, J. M., et al. (2013). Risk factors for unplanned transfer to intensive care within 24 hours of admission from the emergency department in an integrated healthcare system. *Journal of Hospital Medicine, 8,* 13–19.

Dellinger, R. P., Levy, M. M., Rhodes, A., et al. (2013). Surviving Sepsis Campaign: International guidelines for management of severe sepsis and septic shock, 2012. *Intensive Care Medicine, 39,* 165–228.

Finchman, J. (2013). The public health importance of improving health literacy. *American Journal of Pharmaceutical Education, 77,* 41.

Hibbard, J. H., & Greene, J. (2013). What the evidence shows about patient activation: Better health outcomes and care experiences; fewer data on costs. *Health Affairs, 32,* 207–214.

• = Independent;   ▲ = Collaborative;   EBN = Evidence-Based Nursing;   EB = Evidence-Based

Hiemstra, B., Eck, R., Keus, F., et al. (2017). Clinical examination for diagnosing circulatory shock. *Current Opinion in Critical Care, 23*, 293–301.

Kalil, A. (2014). *Septic shock, 2014. Medscape reference: Drugs, disease, and procedures.* Retrieved from http://emedicine.medscape.com/article/168402-overview. (Accessed October 31, 2014).

Kaplan, L., & Pinsky, M. (2014). *Systemic inflammatory response syndrome.* Retrieved from http://emedicine.medscape.com/article/1168943-overview. (Accessed 30 October 2014).

Kleinpell, R., Aitken, L., & Schorr, C. A. (2013). Implications of the new international sepsis guidelines for nursing care. *American Journal of Critical Care, 22*, 212–222.

Kleinpell, R. M., Schorr, C. A., & Balk, R. A. (2016). The new sepsis definitions: Implications for critical care practitioners. *American Journal of Critical Care: An Official Publication, American Association of Critical-Care Nurses, 25*(5), 457–464. doi:10.4037/ajcc2016574.

Koh, H. K., Brach, C., Harris, L. M., et al. (2013). A proposed 'health literate care model' would constitute a systems approach to improving patients' engagement in care. *Health Affairs, 32*, 357–367.

Leone, M., Asfar, P., Radermacher, P., et al. (2015). Optimizing mean arterial pressure in septic shock: A critical reappraisal of the literature. *Critical Care: The Official Journal of the Critical Care Forum, 19*(1), 101.

National Institutes of Health (NIH). (2016). *Clear communication: an NIH health literacy initiative.* Retrieved from http://www.nih.goc/clearcommunication. (Accessed from 17 October 2017).

Negarandeh, R., Mahmoodi, H., Noktehdan, H., et al. (2013). Teach back and pictorial image educational strategies on knowledge about diabetes and medication/dietary adherence among low health literate patients with type 2 diabetes. *Primary Care Diabetes, 7*, 111–118.

Rajaram, S., Desai, N., Kalra, A., et al. (2013). Pulmonary artery catheter for adults in intensive care. *The Cochrane Database of Systematic Reviews*, (2), CD003408.

Rhodes, A., Evans, L., Alhazzani, W., et al. (2017). Surviving Sepsis Campaign: International guidelines for management of sepsis and septic shock: 2016. *Intensive Care Medicine, 43*, 307–377.

Seymour, C., & Rosengart, M. (2015). Septic shock advances in diagnosis and treatment. *JAMA: The Journal of the American Medical Association, 314*(7), 708–717.

Singer, M. (2016). The new sepsis consensus definitions (Sepsis-3): The good, the not-so-bad, and the actually-quite-pretty. *Intensive Care Medicine, 42*(12), 2027–2029. doi:10.1007/s00134-016-4600-4.

Sweeney, J. (2013). Mass transfusion to combat trauma's lethal triad. *Journal of Emergency Nursing, 39*, 37–39.

Turi, S. K., & Von Ah, D. (2013). Implementation of early goal-directed therapy for septic patients in the emergency department: A review of the literature. *Journal of Emergency Nursing, 39*, 13–19.

White, M., Garbez, R., Carroll, M., et al. (2013). Is "teach-back" associated with knowledge retention and hospital readmission in hospitalized heart failure patients? *Journal of Cardiovascular Nursing, 28*, 137–146.

Impaired Sitting   *Ruth A. Wittmann-Price, PhD, RN, CNS, CNE, CHSE, ANEF, FAAN*

NANDA-I

S

Definition

Limitation of ability to independently and purposefully attain and/or maintain a rest position that is supported by the buttocks and thighs, in which the torso is upright.

Defining Characteristics

Impaired ability to adjust position of one or both lower limbs on uneven surface; impaired ability to attain a balanced position of the torso; impaired ability to flex or move both hips; impaired ability to flex or move both knees; impaired ability to maintain the torso in balanced position; impaired ability to stress torso with body weight

Related Factors

Insufficient endurance; insufficient energy; insufficient muscle strength; malnutrition; pain; self-imposed relief posture

Associated Condition

Alteration in cognitive functioning; impaired metabolic functioning; neurological disorder; orthopedic surgery; prescribed posture; psychological disorder; sarcopenia

NOC   Outcomes (Nursing Outcomes Classification)

Suggested NOC Outcomes

Activity Tolerance; Balance; Body Mechanics Performance; Body Positioning: Self-Initiated; Endurance; Tissue Perfusion: Peripheral; Self Care Status; Skeletal Function

● = Independent;   ▲ = Collaborative;   EBN = Evidence-Based Nursing;   EB = Evidence-Based

Example NOC Outcome with Indicators
Body Mechanics Performance: as evidenced by the following indicators: Uses correct sitting posture; Uses supportive devices correctly. (Rate outcome and indicators of **Body Mechanics Performance:** 1 = never demonstrated, 2 = rarely demonstrated, 3 = sometimes demonstrated, 4 = often demonstrated, 5 = consistently demonstrated].)

Client Outcomes

Client Will (Specify Time Frame)

- Verbalize importance of being able to sit as a method to engage in activities of daily living
- Understand somatic physiology of posture control
- Choose health care options that enhance ability to sit
- Engage in physical conditioning exercises to enhance sitting ability
- Understand relationship of posture and emotions
- Control pain to increase ability to sit

NIC   Interventions (Nursing Interventions Classification)

Suggested NIC Interventions

Activity Therapy; Body Mechanics Promotion; Fall Prevention; Energy Management; Exercise Promotion: Strength Training; Exercise Therapy: Balance, Joint Mobility, Muscle Control; Functional Ability Enhancement; Positioning; Pressure Ulcer Prevention

Example NIC Activities—Exercise Therapy: Sitting
Assist client to use chair that facilitates sitting and prevents injury; Transfer safely from bed to chair; Encourage to sit in chair, as tolerated; Provide activities that can be completed while sitting

Nursing Interventions and *Rationales*

- Acknowledge the importance of being able to sit as a method to engage in activities of daily living. EB: *Junhyuck, Jihwan, and Jongeun (2017) investigated upper limb function, balance, gait, and quality of life in two groups of stroke patients (N = 26) before and after a sitting boxing program and found that the Stroke-Specific Quality of Life questionnaire (SS-QOL) scores were significantly improved in the boxing group concluding that the sitting boxing program group had positive effects on upper extremity function, balance, gait, and quality of life.* EB: *Swinton, Cooper, and Hancock (2017) performed a literature review (N = 12) about how workplace interventions improved workers' sitting posture and found limited evidence to indicate that ergonomic workplace interventions improved gross sitting posture. Additional research is needed about proper sitting conditions in workplaces so patients can better participate in activities of daily living.*
- Understand the somatic physiology of posture control. EB: *DongGeon et al (2017) studied trunk muscle activities in four types of seated postures, including cross-legged, long, side, and W-shaped in adults (N = 8), and found that trunk muscle activity did not significantly differ between the four types of sitting postures.* EB: *Researchers studied the effect of different sitting positions on hip joint loading by examining three different sitting positions, such as a simple chair, a car seat, and a kneeling chair, and found that the kneeling chair was the best ergonomic sitting position for hip joints (Van Houcke et al, 2017).*
- Choose the musculoskeletal options that enhance ability to sit properly. EB: *Milosevic et al (2017) studied patients (N = 25) with thoracic spinal cord injury (SCI) in relation to unsupported sitting and found that patients with high- and low-thoracic SCI swayed more with unsupported sitting. Recommendations include providing patients with different postural regulation strategies to enhance proper sitting.* EB: *Lee, Lee, and Shin (2017) studied forward head posture in seven different posture conditions in patients (N = 20) including sitting comfortably and sitting with the back straight and found that head posture evaluation is a reliable assessment for evaluating proper sitting conditions.*
- Engage in physical conditioning exercises to enhance proper sitting ability. EB: *Molik et al (2017) investigated disabled patients playing volleyball in a sitting position and found that the vertical sitting position and degree of disability directly related to performance, but the exercise was beneficial.* EB: *Sanchez et al (2017) studied full trunk control (head-trunk alignment) in sitting with patients (N = 10) with neuromotor disability using*

S

• = Independent;   ▲ = Collaborative;   EBN = Evidence-Based Nursing;   EB = Evidence-Based

the Segmental Assessment of Trunk Control (SATCo) and used video for clinical evaluation to determine whether the upper limbs were free. This study shows promise in developing the first stages of a clinically friendly, fully automated method to assess proper sitting and understand the relationship of posture and somatic functioning. EB: *Alghdir, Zafar, and Iqbal (2017) studied the effects of upright and slouch sitting postures and voluntary teeth clenching on hand grip strength (HGS) in patients (N = 100) and found that HGS was actually stronger during slouching than sitting upright and HGS had no effect on teeth clenching, indicating that sitting posture may matter when testing HGS in a physical assessment evaluation.* EB: *Nutritional researchers studied protein digestion in patients sitting in an upright position compared with a recumbent position and found increased gastric emptying and increased postprandial elevation in plasma amino acid availability when patients are sitting (Holwerda et al, 2017).*

- Understand the relationship of posture and emotions. EB: *Shinpei et al (2017) investigated physical and psychological effects of the Shiatsu Stimulation (SS) (finger pressure) in a sitting position on patients (N = 20). The SS demonstrated significant change in all six mood states (tension-anxiety, depression-dejection, fatigue, and confusion decreased while vigor elevated).* EB: *Researchers examined sitting and the use of social media in patients (N = 1120) with physiological and psychological conditions (cardiovascular disease, type 2 diabetes, obesity, and poorer mental health status) and found that patients with high social media use had significantly greater sitting times especially on nonworkdays for leisure, but the negative affect on health was not correlated and the study indicated that a longitudinal study is needed (Alley et al, 2017).*

- Maintain pain levels below 3 to 4 on a 0 to 10 scale to increase ability to sit. EB: *Joshi et al (2017) studied neuropathy of the posterior femoral cutaneous nerve, which can cause pain while sitting, and performed magnetic resonance (MR)-guided cryoablation to successfully treat sitting pain caused by neuropathy.* EB: *Researchers studied the relationship between office workers (N = 35) and musculoskeletal pain by comparing the ergonomic, physical, and psychosocial factors and found that computer office workers who reported pain had worse ergonomics for their chair workstation, but psychosocial factors did not demonstrate a difference (Santana et al, 2017).*

Pediatric

- Increase cognitive and physical functioning by promoting proper sitting ability. EB: *Researchers studied the change of sagittal spinal curvatures in children (N = 56) with generalized joint hypermobility (GJH) who were instructed with the "straighten your back" (SYB) command and found that it did not improve standing and sitting positioning; this command is recommended but not to be used (Czaprowski et al, 2017).* EBN: *Hitchcock (2017) reviewed the research regarding safe infant sleeping and addressed the fact that sitting devices are not recommended. Nurses should model recommended behaviors for safe infant sleep and teach parents about safe infant sleep throughout the hospital stay.*

Geriatric

- Increase cognitive and physical functioning by promoting prober sitting ability. EB: *Researchers studied the effects of aging on patients' (N = 39) muscle control during transition from lying to sitting positions using myotonometry measurements of tone, stiffness, and elasticity; results suggested that increased age increases stiffness and tone and decreases the elasticity of muscles (Kocur et al, 2017).* EB: *Bell et al (2017) studied elderly patients (age 65 and older) in the hospital and community in relation to their ability to open food packages in a sitting and laying down position and found that while laying down greater strength was required to open packages and that sitting improved eating overall.*

Multicultural

- Understand the importance of unimpaired sitting to different populations. EB: *A case study analyzed in Japan discussed the researchers' novel "hip prosthesis in the sitting posture" on a patient who was an amputee and found that implanting a hip prosthesis in a sitting position enabled the patient to better stand, walk, and begin balance training (Yukiyo et al, 2017).* EB: *Lazennec et al (2017) completed a study in France that investigated the effect of spinal fusion effects on sitting in patients (N = 93) and found that the fusion assisted in patients' ability to position themselves from standing to sitting.*

Home Care

- Encourage proper sitting posture in the home environment to promote health. EB: *Chun-Ting et al (2017) studied patients (N = 16) in four modes of reclining wheelchairs with and without different sitting devices*

- = Independent;   ▲ = Collaborative;   EBN = Evidence-Based Nursing;   EB = Evidence-Based

and found the lumbar support with femur upward with back reclined mode provided the most significant reduction in stress load on the ischial area. **EB:** *Eriksson et al (2017) explored activation of a range of trunk muscles using intramuscular electromyography in patients (N = 13) and results revealed muscles demonstrated a directional preference and the least muscular energy was spent in an upright sitting position.*

REFERENCES

Alghdir, A., Zafar, H., & Iqbal, Z. A. (2017). Effect of upright and slouch sitting postures and voluntary teeth clenching on hand grip strength in young male adults. *Journal of Back & Musculoskeletal Rehabilitation, 30*(5), 961–965. Retrieved from http://dx.doi.org.fmarion.idm.oclc.org/10.3233/BMR-150278.

Alley, S., Wellens, P., Schoeppe, S., et al. (2017). Impact of increasing social media use on sitting time and body mass index. *Health Promotion Journal of Australia, 28*(2), 91–95. Retrieved from http://dx.doi.org.fmarion.idm.oclc.org/10.1071/HE16026.

Bell, A., Tapsell, L., Walton, K., et al. (2017). Accessing hospital packaged foods and beverages: The importance of a seated posture when eating. *Journal of Human Nutrition & Dietetics, 30*(3), 394–402. Retrieved from http://dx.doi.org.fmarion.idm.oclc.org/10.1111/jhn.12430.

Chun-Ting, L., Kuo-Yuan, H., Chien-Feng, K., et al. (2017). Evaluation of the effect of different sitting assistive devices in reclining wheelchair on interface pressure. *Biomedical Engineering Online, 16*, 1–10. Retrieved from http://dx.doi.org.fmarion.idm.oclc.org/10.1186/s12938-017-0398-8.

Czaprowski, D., Pawlowska, P., Kolwicz-Ganko, A., et al. (2017). The influence of the "Straighten Your Back" command on the sagittal spinal curvatures in children with generalized joint hypermobility. *BioMed Research International*, 1–7. Retrieved from http://dx.doi.org.fmarion.idm.oclc.org/10.1155/2017/9724021.

DongGeon, L., SeoJeong, Y., SunHae, S., et al. (2017). Comparison of trunk electromyographic muscle activity depends on sitting postures. *Work (Reading, Mass.), 56*(3), 491–495. Retrieved from http://dx.doi.org.fmarion.idm.oclc.org/10.3233/WOR-172515.

Eriksson, C. M., Tucker, K., Holford, C., et al. (2017). Directional preference of activation of abdominal and paraspinal muscles during position-control tasks in sitting. *Journal of Electromyography & Kinesiology, 35*, 9–16. Retrieved from http://dx.doi.org.fmarion.idm.oclc.org/10.1016/j.jelekin.2017.05.002.

Hitchcock, S. C. (2017). An update on safe infant sleep. *Nursing for Women's Health, 21*(4), 307–311. Retrieved from http://dx.doi.org.fmarion.idm.oclc.org/10.1016/j.nwh.2017.06.007.

Holwerda, A. M., Lenaerts, K., Bierau, J., et al. (2017). Food ingestion in an upright sitting position increases postprandial amino acid availability when compared with food ingestion in a lying down position. *Applied Physiology, Nutrition & Metabolism, 42*(7), 738–743. Retrieved from http://dx.doi.org.fmarion.idm.oclc.org/10.1139/apnm-2016-0522.

Joshi, D., Thawait, G., Del Grande, F., et al. (2017). MRI-guided cryoablation of the posterior femoral cutaneous nerve for the treatment of neuropathy-mediated sitting pain. *Skeletal Radiology, 46*(7), 983–987. Retrieved from http://dx.doi.org.fmarion.idm.oclc.org/10.1007/s00256-017-2617-6.

Junhyuck, P., Jihwan, G., & Jongeun, Y. (2017). Effects of a sitting boxing program on upper limb function, balance, gait, and quality of life in stroke patients. *Neurorehabilitation, 40*(1), 77–86. Retrieved from http://dx.doi.org.fmarion.idm.oclc.org/10.3233/NRE-161392.

Kocur, P., Grzeskowiak, M., Wiernicka, M., et al. (2017). *Archives of Gerontology & Geriatrics, 70*, 14–18. Retrieved from http://dx.doi.org.fmarion.idm.oclc.org/10.1016/j.archger.2016.12.005.

Lazennec, J. Y., Clark, I. C., Folinais, D., et al. (2017). What is the impact of a spinal fusion on acetabular implant orientation in functional standing and sitting positions? *Journal of Arthroplasty, 32*(10), 3184–3190. Retrieved from http://dx.doi.org.fmarion.idm.oclc.org/10.1016/j.arth.2017.04.051.

Lee, C., Lee, S., & Shin, G. (2017). Reliability of forward head posture evaluation while sitting, standing, walking and running. *Human Movement Science, 55*, 81–86. Retrieved from http://dx.doi.org.fmarion.idm.oclc.org/10.1016/j.humov.2017.07.008.

Milosevic, A., Gagnon, D. H., Gourdow, P., et al. (2017). Postural regulatory strategies during quiet sitting are affected in individuals with thoracic spinal cord injury. *Gait and Posture, 58*, 446–452. Retrieved from http://dx.doi.org.fmarion.idm.oclc.org/10.1016/j.gaitpost.2017.08.032.

Molik, B., Morgulec-Adamowicz, N., Marzalek, J., et al. (2017). Evaluation of game performance in elite male sitting volleyball players. *Adapted Physical Activity Quarterly, 34*(2), 104–124. Retrieved from http://dx.doi.org.fmarion.idm.oclc.org/10.1123/apaq.2015-0028.

Sanchez, M. B., Loram, I., Darby, J., et al. (2017). The potential of an automated system to identify the upper limb component of a controlled sitting posture. *Gait and Posture, 58*, 223–228. Retrieved from http://dx.doi.org.fmarion.idm.oclc.org/10.1016/j.gaitpost.2017.08.002.

Santana, R. M., Veraldi, L. R. D., Maira, L. C., et al. (2017). Differences in ergonomic and workstation factors between computer office workers with and without reported musculoskeletal pain. *Work (Reading, Mass.), 57*(4), 563–572. Retrieved from http://dx.doi.org.fmarion.idm.oclc.org/10.3233/WOR-172582.

Shinpei, O., Koichi, O., Mayumi, W., et al. (2017). Physical and psychological effects of the Shiatsu Stimulation in the sitting position. *Health, 9*(8), 1264–1272. Retrieved from http://dx.doi.org.fmarion.idm.oclc.org/10.4236/health.2017.98091.

Swinton, P. A., Cooper, K., & Hancock, E. (2017). Workplace interventions to improve sitting posture: A systematic review. *Preventive Medicine, 101*, 204–212. Retrieved from http://dx.doi.org.fmarion.idm.oclc.org/10.1016/j.ypmed.2017.06.023.

Van Houcke, J., Schouten, A., Steenackers, G., et al. (2017). Computer-based estimation of the hip joint reaction force and hip flexion angle in three different sitting configurations. *Applied Ergonomics, 63*, 99–105. Retrieved from http://dx.doi.org.fmarion.idm.oclc.org/10.1016/j.apergo.2017.04.008.

Yukiyo, S., Hirotaka, M., Takayuki, M., et al. (2017). Hip prosthesis in sitting posture for bilateral transfemoral amputee after burn injury: A case report. *Prosthetics & Orthotics International, 41*(5), 522–526. Retrieved from http://dx.doi.org.fmarion.idm.oclc.org/10.1177/0309364616682384.

S

● = Independent;   ▲ = Collaborative;   **EBN** = Evidence-Based Nursing;   **EB** = Evidence-Based

Impaired Skin integrity   *Jo Ann Coar, BSN, RN-BC, CWOCN, COS-C*

NANDA-I

Definition

Altered epidermis and/or dermis.

Defining Characteristics

Acute pain; alteration in skin integrity; bleeding; foreign matter piercing skin; hematoma; localized area hot to touch; redness

Related Factors

External

Chemical injury agent; excretions; humidity; hyperthermia; hypothermia; moisture; pressure over bony prominence; secretions

Internal

Alteration in fluid volume; inadequate nutrition; psychogenic factor

At-Risk Population

Extremes of age

Associated Condition

Alteration in metabolism; alteration in pigmentation; alteration in sensation; alteration in skin turgor; arterial puncture; hormonal change; immunodeficiency; impaired circulation; pharmaceutical agent; radiation therapy; vascular trauma

NOC   (Nursing Outcomes Classification)

Suggested NOC Outcomes

Tissue Integrity: Skin and Mucous Membranes; Wound Healing: Primary Intention, Secondary Intention

---

Example NOC Outcome with Indicators

Tissue Integrity: Skin and Mucous Membranes will be intact as evidenced by the following indicators: Skin integrity/Skin lesions not present/Tissue perfusion/Skin temperature/Skin thickness. (Rate the outcome and indicators of **Tissue Integrity: Skin and Mucous Membranes:** 1 = severely compromised, 2 = substantially compromised, 3 = moderately compromised, 4 = mildly compromised, 5 = not compromised [see Section I].)

Client Outcomes

Client Will (Specify Time Frame)

- Regain integrity of skin surface
- Report any altered sensation or pain at site of skin impairment
- Demonstrate understanding of plan to heal skin and prevent reinjury or complications
- Describe measures to protect and heal the skin and to care for any skin lesion

NIC   (Nursing Interventions Classification)

Suggested NIC Interventions

Incision Site Care; Pain Management; Pressure Ulcer Care (currently referred to as Pressure Injury Care [National Pressure Ulcer Advisory Panel (NPUAP), 2016]); Pressure Ulcer Prevention (Pressure Injury Prevention [NPUAP, 2016]); Risk Identification; Skin Care: Topical Treatments; Skin Surveillance; Wound Care; Wound Irrigation

● = Independent;   ▲ = Collaborative;   EBN = Evidence-Based Nursing;   EB = Evidence-Based

Example NIC Activities—Pressure Ulcer Care (Pressure Injury Care [NPUAP, 2016])
Monitor color of wound bed, temperature, edema, erythema, moisture, and appearance of surrounding skin; Note characteristics of any drainage

Nursing Interventions and *Rationales*

- NPUAP redefined the definition of a pressure ulcer, now referred to as pressure injuries, during the NPUAP 2016 Staging Consensus Conference. The new definitions more accurately define alterations in tissue integrity from pressure as the following: *A pressure injury is localized damage to the skin and underlying soft tissue usually over a bony prominence or related to a medical or other device. The injury can present as intact skin or an open ulcer and may be painful. The injury occurs as a result of intense and/or prolonged pressure or pressure in combination with shear. The tolerance of soft tissue for pressure and shear may also be affected by microclimate, nutrition, perfusion, comorbidities, and condition of the soft tissue (NPUAP, 2016).*

- Pressure ulcer is no longer a current clinical term; rather, pressure injury is used to describe an alteration in tissue integrity from pressure (NPUAP, 2016). Similarly, hospital-acquired pressure ulcers (HAPUs) are currently referred to as hospital-acquired pressure injury (HAPIs).

- Assess site of skin impairment and determine cause or type of wound (e.g., acute or chronic wound, burn, dermatological lesion, pressure injury, skin tear). EB: *Identification of etiological factors, or what is causing the impairment, is the first step, and requires a thorough assessment of the individual, not only the impairment. The assessment should include the medical history, current medical status, medications, and family history (Baranoski & Ayello, 2016; Murphree, 2017). Skin and tissue assessment is important in pressure injury prevention, classification, diagnosis, and treatment (NPUAP, European Pressure Ulcer Advisory Panel [EPUAP], 2014; NPUAP, 2016).*

- Use a risk assessment tool to systematically assess client risk factors for skin breakdown caused by pressure. EB: *A validated risk assessment tool such as the Norton scale or Braden scale should be used to identify clients at risk for immobility-related skin breakdown (NPUAP/EPUAP, 2014). An individual identified at risk for pressure injury development or who has healed pressure injuries will need to be evaluated for pressure redistributing surfaces (Murphree, 2017). Targeting variables (e.g., age and Braden Scale Risk Category) can focus assessment on particular risk factors (e.g., pressure) and help guide the plan of prevention and care (NPUAP/EPUAP, 2014).*

- Determine the extent of the skin impairment caused by pressure using the revised classification system and definition for pressure injuries (NPUAP, 2016).
  - **Stage 1 Pressure Injury:** Nonblanchable erythema of intact skin
    Area of localized nonblanchable erythema that may appear differently in darkly pigmented skin, and changes in sensation, temperature, or firmness may precede visual changes. Color changes do not include purple or maroon discoloration, which is more likely to indicate deep tissue pressure injury (NPUAP, 2016).
  - **Stage 2 Pressure Injury:** Partial-thickness skin loss with exposed dermis
    Partial-thickness skin loss with exposed dermis in which the wound bed is pink/red and moist and adipose (fat) and deeper tissues are not visible. Granulation tissue, slough, and eschar are not present. A stage 2 pressure injury may also present as an intact or ruptured blister. These injuries commonly result from adverse microclimate and shear in the skin over the pelvis and shear in the heel. This stage should not be used to describe moisture-associated skin damage (MASD) including incontinence-associated dermatitis (IAD), intertriginous dermatitis (ITD), medical adhesive–related skin injury (MARSI), or traumatic wounds (skin tears, burns, and abrasions) (NPUAP, 2016).
  - **Stage 3 Pressure Injury**: Full-thickness skin loss
    Full-thickness loss of skin, in which adipose is visible and granulation tissue and epibole (rolled wound edges) are often present and undermining/tunneling may occur. Slough and/or eschar may also be visible. Fascia, muscle, tendon, ligament, cartilage, and/or bone are not exposed. The depth of tissue damage varies by anatomical location, and areas of significant adiposity can develop deep wounds. If slough or eschar obscures the extent of tissue loss this is an unstageable pressure injury (NPUAP, 2016).
  - **Stage 4 Pressure Injury**: Full-thickness skin and tissue loss
    Full-thickness skin and tissue loss with exposed or directly palpable fascia, muscle, tendon, ligament, cartilage or bone, and slough and/or eschar may be visible. Epibole, undermining, and/or tunneling

S

● = Independent;   ▲ = Collaborative;   EBN = Evidence-Based Nursing;   EB = Evidence-Based

often occur, and depth varies by anatomical location. If slough or eschar obscures the extent of tissue loss, this is an unstageable pressure injury (NPUAP, 2016).

○ **Deep Tissue Pressure Injury:** Persistent nonblanchable deep red, maroon, or purple discoloration Intact or nonintact skin with localized area of persistent nonblanchable deep red, maroon, or purple discoloration or epidermal separation revealing a dark wound bed or blood-filled blister. Pain and temperature change often precede skin color changes. Discoloration may appear differently in darkly pigmented skin. This injury results from intense and/or prolonged pressure and shear forces at the bone–muscle interface. The wound may evolve rapidly to reveal the actual extent of tissue injury, or it may resolve without tissue loss. If necrotic tissue, subcutaneous tissue, granulation tissue, fascia, muscle, or other underlying structures are visible, this indicates a full-thickness pressure injury (unstageable, stage 3, or stage 4). Do not use the term deep tissue pressure injury to describe vascular, traumatic, neuropathic, or dermatological conditions (NPUAP, 2016).

○ **Unstageable Pressure Injury:** Obscured full-thickness skin and tissue loss Full-thickness skin and tissue loss in which the extent of tissue damage within the ulcer cannot be confirmed because it is obscured by slough or eschar. If slough or eschar is removed, a stage 3 or stage 4 pressure injury will be revealed. Stable eschar (i.e., dry, adherent, intact without erythema or fluctuance) on the heel or ischemic limb should not be softened or removed (NPUAP, 2016).

○ **Mechanical device–related pressure injury** is used to describe alterations in tissue integrity caused by pressure from mechanical devices used in the care of clients (e.g., indwelling urinary catheters, endotracheal tubes, nasogastric tubes, drains). The pressure injury typically conforms to the shape of the device (NPUAP, 2016).

○ **Mucosal Membrane Pressure Injury:** Mucosal membrane pressure injury is found on mucous membranes with a history of a medical device in use at the location of the injury. Because of the anatomy of the tissue, these ulcers cannot be staged (NPUAP, 2016).

- Inspect and monitor site of skin impairment at least once a day for color changes, redness, swelling, warmth, pain, or other signs of infection. Determine whether the client is experiencing changes in sensation or pain. Closely assess high-risk areas such as bony prominences, skinfolds, the sacrum, and heels. *Systematic inspection can identify impending problems early (NPUAP/EPUAP, 2014; Baranoski & Ayello, 2016). When conducting a skin assessment in an individual with darkly pigmented skin prioritize assessment of skin temperature, presence of edema, and change in tissue consistency in relation to surrounding tissue (NPUAP/ EPUAP, 2014).*

- Monitor the client's skin care practices, noting type of soap or other cleansing agents used, temperature of water, and frequency of skin cleansing. *Cleansing should not compromise the skin (Baranoski & Ayello, 2016).* **EB:** *Keep the skin clean and dry. Use a pH balanced skin cleanser. Consider using a skin moisturizer to hydrate dry skin to reduce risk of skin damage. Protect the skin from exposure to excessive moisture with a barrier product to reduce the risk of pressure damage (NPUAP/EPUAP, 2014). Products to promote healthy skin in the elderly include cleansers that are pH balanced, preferably no-rinse in soft disposable cloths and superfatted nonalkaline soaps (Murphree, 2017).*

- Consider using normal saline to clean the pressure injury or as ordered by the health care provider, but if necessary tap water suitable for drinking may be used to clean the wound. **EB:** *A Cochrane review found no evidence that using tap water to cleanse acute wounds in adults or children increases or reduces infection (Fernandez & Griffiths, 2012). Cleanse most pressure injuries with potable water (i.e., water suitable for drinking) or normal saline (NPUAP/EPUAP, 2014; NPUAP, 2016).*

- Maintain good skin hygiene, using mild nondetergent soap, drying gently, and lubricating with lotion or emollient to reduce the risk of dermal trauma; improve circulation; and promote comfort. Provide client education on good skin hygiene practices (Doenges, Moorhouse, & Murr, 2016).

- Urinary and fecal incontinence can cause skin breakdown. **EB:** *Develop and implement an individualized continence management plan. Cleanse the skin promptly after episodes of incontinence. Protect the skin from exposure to excessive moisture with a barrier product to reduce the risk of pressure damage (NPUAP/EPUAP, 2014).* **EB:** *Implementing an incontinence prevention plan with the use of a skin protectant or a cleanser protectant can significantly decrease skin breakdown and pressure injury formation (Scemons, 2013).*

- For clients with limited mobility and activity, use a risk assessment tool to systematically assess immobility and activity-related risk factors. **EB:** *A validated risk assessment tool such as the Norton scale or Braden scale should be used to identify clients at risk for immobility-related skin breakdown (NPUAP/EPUAP, 2014).* **EBN:** *A study found that the most commonly reported interventions to reduce skin breakdown in acutely ill patients were protocol development, staff education, new use of a risk assessment tool, performance monitoring,*

● = Independent;   ▲ = Collaborative;   **EBN** = Evidence-Based Nursing;   **EB** = Evidence-Based

development of a team approach, use of new beds/support surfaces, implementation of guidelines, providing feedback to staff, and linking staff with resources (Stotts et al, 2013).

- Do not position the client on site of skin impairment. If consistent with overall client management goals, reposition the client as determined by individualized tissue tolerance and overall condition. Reposition and transfer the client with care to protect against the adverse effects of external mechanical forces such as pressure, friction, and shear. EB: *Do not position an individual directly on a pressure injury. Continue to turn/reposition the individual regardless of the support surface in use. Establish turning frequency based on the characteristics of the support surface and the individual's response (NPUAP & EPUAP, 2014). If the goal of care is to keep the client (e.g., a terminally ill client) comfortable, turning and repositioning may not be appropriate (NPUAP & EPUAP, 2014).*
- Evaluate for use of support surfaces (specialty mattresses, beds), chair cushions, or devices as appropriate. Maintain the head of the bed at the lowest possible degree of elevation to reduce shear and friction, and use lift devices, pillows, foam wedges, and pressure-reducing devices in the bed (Brienza et al, 2016; NPUAP & EPUAP, 2014).
- Implement a written treatment plan for topical treatment of the site of skin impairment. *A written plan ensures consistency in care and documentation (Baranoski & Ayello, 2016).*
- Select a topical treatment that will maintain a moist wound-healing environment (stage 2) that is balanced with the need to absorb exudate. Stage 1 pressure injuries may be managed by keeping the client off of the area and using a protective dressing (Baranoski & Ayello, 2016). EBN: *Choose dressings that provide a moist environment, keep periwound skin dry, and control exudate and eliminate dead space (NPUAP & EPUAP, 2014). Select a wound dressing based on the ability to keep the wound bed moist; need to address bacterial bioburden; nature and volume of wound exudate; condition of the tissue in the ulcer bed; condition of periulcer skin; ulcer size, depth, and location; presence of tunneling and/or undermining; and goals of the individual with the ulcer (NPUAP & EPUAP, 2014).*
- Avoid massaging around the site of skin impairment and over bony prominences. EB: *Research suggested that massage may lead to deep tissue trauma (NPUAP & EPUAP, 2014).*
- Assess the client's nutritional status. Refer for a nutritional consult and/or institute dietary supplements as necessary. EB: *Optimizing nutritional intake, including calories, fatty acids, protein, and vitamins, is needed to promote wound healing. Both the EPUAP and NPUAP (NPUAP & EPUAP, 2014) endorse the application of reasonable nutritional assessment and treatment for clients at risk for and with pressure ulcers.*
- Identify the client's phase of wound healing (inflammation, proliferation, or maturation) and stage of injury. EBN: *The selection of the dressing is based on the tissue in the ulcer bed (wound bed), the condition of the skin around the ulcer bed, and the goals of the person with the ulcer. Generally, maintaining a moist ulcer bed is the ideal when the ulcer bed is clean and granulating to promote healing and closure (NPUAP & EPUAP, 2014). No single wound dressing is appropriate for all phases of wound healing.*

 Home Care

- The interventions described previously may be adapted for home care use.
- Instruct and assist the client and caregivers in how to change dressings and maintain a clean environment. Provide written instructions and observe the client completing the dressing change before hospital discharge and in the home setting.
- Educate client and caregivers on proper nutrition, signs and symptoms of infection, and when to call the agency and/or health care provider with concerns.
- It may be beneficial to initiate a consultation in a case assignment with a wound, ostomy, continence nurse (or wounds specialist) to establish a comprehensive plan for complex wounds (Vrtis, 2013).

 Client/Family Teaching and Discharge Planning

- Teach skin and wound assessment and ways to monitor for signs and symptoms of infection, complications, and healing. Early assessment and intervention help prevent serious problems from developing. EB: *A home visit by a wound care specialist can provide essential in-home education, client specific plan of care, and reduce health care costs (Vrtis, 2013).*
- Teach the client why a topical treatment has been selected. EBN: *The type of dressing needed may change over time as the wound heals and/or deteriorates (NPUAP & EPUAP, 2014).*
- If consistent with overall client management goals, teach how to reposition as client condition warrants. EB: *If the goal of care is to keep a client (e.g., terminally ill client) comfortable, turning and repositioning may not be appropriate (NPUAP & EPUAP, 2014).*

● = Independent;   ▲ = Collaborative;   EBN = Evidence-Based Nursing;   EB = Evidence-Based

- Teach the client to use pillows, foam wedges, chair cushions, and pressure-redistribution devices to prevent pressure injury (Brienza et al, 2016). *Individualize the selection and periodic reevaluation of a seating support surface and associated equipment for posture and pressure redistribution with consideration of body size and configuration, the effects of posture and deformity on pressure distribution, and mobility and lifestyle needs (NPUAP & EPUAP, 2014).*

REFERENCES

Baranoski, S., & Ayello, E. A. (Eds.), (2016). *Wound care essentials: Practice principles* (4th ed.). Ambler, PA: Lippincott Williams & Wilkins.

Brienza, D. M., et al. (2016). Pressure redistribution: Seating, positioning, and support surfaces. In S. Baranoski & E. A. Ayello (Eds.), *Wound care essentials: Practice principles* (4th ed.). Ambler, PA: Lippincott Williams & Wilkins.

Doenges, M. E., Moorhouse, M. F., & Murr, A. C. (2016). *A nurse's pocket guide: Diagnoses, prioritized interventions and rationales* (14th ed.). Philadelphia, PA: Davis Company.

Fernandez, R., & Griffiths, R. (2012). Water for wound cleansing. *The Cochrane Database of Systematic Reviews*, (2), CD003861.

Murphree, R. W. (2017). Impairments in skin integrity. *The Nursing Clinics of North America, 52*(3), 405–417.

National Pressure Ulcer Advisory Panel, European Pressure Ulcer Advisory Panel, and Pan Pacific Pressure Injury Alliance. (2014). In

Haesler, E. (Ed.), *Prevention and treatment of pressure ulcers: Quick reference guide*. Osborne Park, Australia: Cambridge Media.

National Pressure Ulcer Advisory Panel (NPUAP). (2016). *Pressure injury stages*. Retrieved from http://www.npuap.org/resources/educational-and-clinical-resources/npuap-pressure-injury-stages/. (Accessed 28 November 2017).

Scemons, D. (2013). Urinary incontinence in adults. *Nursing, 43*(11), 52–60.

Stotts, N. A., Brown, D. S., Donaldson, N. E., et al. (2013). Eliminating hospital-acquired pressure ulcers: Within our reach. *Advances in Skin & Wound Care, 26*(1), 13–18.

Vrtis, M. C. (2013). The economic impact of complex wound care on home health agencies. *Journal of Wound, Ostomy, and Continence Nursing, 40*(4), 360–363.

Risk for impaired Skin integrity   *Jo Ann Coar, BSN, RN-BC, CWOCN, COS-C*

NANDA-I

Definition

Susceptible to alteration in epidermis and/or dermis, which may compromise health.

Risk Factors

External

Chemical injury agent; excretions; humidity; hyperthermia; hypothermia; moisture; secretions

Internal

Alteration in fluid volume; inadequate nutrition; pressure over bony prominence; psychogenetic factor

At-Risk Population

Extremes of age

Associated Condition

Alteration in metabolism; alteration in pigmentation; alteration in sensation; alteration in skin turgor; arterial puncture; hormonal change; immunodeficiency; impaired circulation; pharmaceutical agent; radiation therapy; vascular trauma

NOC   (Nursing Outcomes Classification)

Suggested NOC Outcomes

Immobility Consequences: Physiological; Tissue Integrity: Skin and Mucous Membranes

Example NOC Outcome with Indicators
Tissue Integrity: Skin and Mucous Membranes will be intact as evidenced by the following indicators: Skin intactness/Skin lesions not present/Tissue perfusion/Skin temperature. (Rate the outcome and indicators of **Tissue Integrity: Skin and Mucous Membranes:** 1 = severely compromised, 2 = substantially compromised, 3 = moderately compromised, 4 = mildly compromised, 5 = not compromised [see Section I].)

• = Independent;   ▲ = Collaborative;   EBN = Evidence-Based Nursing;   EB = Evidence-Based

Client Outcomes

Client Will (Specify Time Frame)

- Report altered sensation or pain at risk areas as soon as noted
- Demonstrate understanding of personal risk factors for impaired skin integrity
- Verbalize a personal plan for preventing impaired skin integrity

NIC (Nursing Interventions Classification)

Suggested NIC Interventions

Positioning: Pressure Management; Pressure Ulcer Care (currently referred to as Pressure Injury Care [National Pressure Ulcer Advisory Panel (NPUAP), 2016]); Pressure Ulcer Prevention (Pressure Injury Prevention [NPUAP, 2016]; Skin Surveillance

Example NIC Activities—Pressure Ulcer Care

Monitor color of wound bed, temperature, edema, erythema, moisture, and appearance of surrounding skin; Note characteristics of any drainage

Nursing Interventions and *Rationales*

- The NPUAP redefined the definition of a pressure ulcer, which is now referred to as a pressure injury, during the NPUAP 2016 Staging Consensus Conference in 2016. The new definition more accurately defines alterations in tissue integrity from pressure as the following: A pressure injury is localized damage to the skin and underlying soft tissue usually over a bony prominence or related to a medical or other device. The injury can present as intact skin or an open ulcer and may be painful. The injury occurs as a result of intense and/or prolonged pressure or pressure in combinations with shear. The tolerance of soft tissue for pressure and shear may also be affected by microclimate, nutrition, perfusion, comorbidities, and conditions of the soft tissue (NPUAP, 2016).
- Identify clients at risk for impaired skin integrity as a result of immobility, chronological age, malnutrition, incontinence, compromised perfusion, immunocompromised status, or chronic medical condition, such as diabetes mellitus, spinal cord injury, or renal failure. EB: *These client populations are known to be at high risk for impaired skin integrity (Baranoski & Ayello, 2016). Targeting variables (e.g., age and Braden Scale Risk Category) can focus assessment on particular risk factors (e.g., pressure) and help guide the plan of prevention and care (NPUAP & European Pressure Ulcer Advisory Panel [EPUAP], 2014).*
- Inspect and monitor skin condition at least once a day for color or texture changes, redness, localized heat, edema or induration, pressure damage, dermatological conditions, or lesions and any incontinence-associated dermatitis. Determine whether the client is experiencing loss of sensation or pain. *Systematic inspection can identify impending problems early (NPUAP & EPUAP, 2014; Baranoski & Ayello, 2016). When conducting a skin assessment in an individual with darkly pigmented skin prioritize assessment of skin temperature, presence of edema, and change in tissue consistency in relation to surrounding tissue (NPUAP & EPUAP, 2014).*
- Monitor the client's skin care practices, noting type of soap or other cleansing agents used, temperature of water, and frequency of skin cleansing. *Individualize plan according to the client's skin condition, needs, and preferences (Baranoski & Ayello, 2016).*
- Keep skin clean and dry. Cleanse the skin gently with pH-balanced cleansers. Consider use of skin moisturizers to hydrate skin to reduce risk of skin damage. Protect skin from exposure to excessive moisture with a barrier product to reduce the risk of pressure-related damage (NPUAP & EPUAP, 2014).
- ▲ Develop and implement an individualized continence management plan. Cleanse the skin promptly after episodes of incontinence. Use incontinence skin barriers including creams, ointments, pastes, or film-forming skin protectants as needed to protect skin and maintain intact skin (Ratliff et al, 2017). EB: *Implementing an incontinence prevention plan with the use of a skin protectant or a cleanser protectant can significantly decrease skin breakdown and pressure ulcer formation (NPAUP & EPUAP 2014; Baranoski & Ayello, 2016).*
- For clients with limited mobility, inspect and monitor condition of skin covering bony prominences. *Pressure injuries usually occur over bony prominences, such as the sacrum, coccyx, trochanter, and heels, as*

● = Independent;   ▲ = Collaborative;   EBN = Evidence-Based Nursing;   EB = Evidence-Based

a result of unrelieved pressure between the prominence and support surface, or with shearing and friction (Wound, Ostomy, and Continence Nurses Society [WOCN], 2010; NPUAP & EPUAP, 2014; Baranoski & Ayello, 2016). Position individuals in the sitting position with special attention to anatomy, weight distribution, postural alignment, and support of feet (Ratliff et al, 2017).

- Implement and communicate a client-specific prevention plan. **EB:** *A plan of care clearly documented in the client's electronic health record will assist in ensuring consistency in care and documentation (Baranoski & Ayello, 2016).*

- At-risk clients should be frequently repositioned. Frequency of repositioning will be influenced by variables concerning the individual's independent mobility and the support surface in use. Frequency of repositioning should be determined by the individual's tissue tolerance and medical condition (NPUAP & EPUAP, 2014). Use of heel suspension devices can remove pressure from the heels and support the lower extremity of individuals who are unable to keep pressure off the heels, without placing pressure on the Achilles tendon (Ratliff et al, 2017).

- Evaluate for use of specialty mattresses, beds, or devices as appropriate (Lippoldt et al, 2014; Brienza et al, 2016). *Maintain the head of the bed at the lowest possible degree of elevation to reduce shear and use lift devices, pillows, foam wedges, and pressure-reducing devices in the bed (Lippoldt et al, 2014). If the goal of care is to keep the client (e.g., a terminally ill client) comfortable, turning and repositioning may not be appropriate; reposition the client for position of comfort and provide pain relief measures (Horn & Irion, 2014). Pressure redistributing devices are adjuncts and not replacements for regular repositioning (Ratliff et al, 2017).*

- Avoid massaging or vigorously rubbing over bony prominences. *Massage may lead to deep tissue trauma (NPUAP & EPUAP, 2014).*

- ▲ Assess the client's nutritional status; refer for a nutritional consult, and/or institute dietary supplements. **EB:** *Meeting nutritional needs of the client is important to prevention of skin breakdown and preventing complications of illness. Adequate nutrition is important for maintaining overall homeostasis and health (O'Hanlon, Dowsett, & Smyth, 2015).*

 Geriatric

- Limit the number of complete baths to two or three per week, and alternate them with partial baths. Use a tepid water temperature (between 90°F and 105°F) for bathing or use a no-rinse alternative product. **EB:** *Excessive bathing, especially in hot water, depletes aging skin of moisture and increases dryness. The ability to retain moisture is decreased in aging skin because of diminished amounts of dermal proteins. One of the most common age-related changes to the skin is damage to the stratum corneum (Baranoski & Ayello, 2016).*

- Use lotions and moisturizers to prevent skin from drying out, especially in the winter. **EB:** *Avoid skin care products that contain allergens such as lanolin, latex, and dyes (Baranoski & Ayello, 2016). Use barrier products to protect aged skin from exposure to excessive moisture to reduce the risk of pressure damage (NPUAP & EPUAP, 2014).*

- Increase fluid intake within cardiac and renal limits to a minimum of 1500 mL/day. *Dry skin is caused by loss of fluid; increasing fluid intake hydrates the skin (Baranoski & Ayello, 2016). Recommend individuals with nutritional and pressure injury risks a minimum of 30 to 35 kcal/kg body weight per day, 1.25 to 1.5 g of protein/kg body weight per day, and 1 mL of fluid intake per kilocalorie per day, if there are no contraindications (Ratliff et al, 2017).*

- Increase humidity in the environment, especially during the winter, by using a humidifier or placing a container of water on a warm object. *Increasing the moisture in the air helps keep moisture in the skin.*

 Home Care

- Assess client and caregiver ability to recognize potential risk for skin breakdown. Provide resources for client/caregiver to contact health care provider with questions/concerns related to skin and incontinence care as needed (Vrtis, 2013). Engage family, caregivers, or legal guardian when establishing goals of care and validate their understanding of these goals. Educate the individual and his or her caregiver regarding skin changes in aging and at end of life (NPUAP & EPUAP, 2014).

- ▲ Initiate a consultation in a case assignment with a wound care specialist or wound, ostomy, and continence nurse to establish a comprehensive plan as soon as possible (Vrtis, 2013).

- See the care plan for Impaired **Skin** integrity.

● = Independent;   ▲ = Collaborative;   **EBN** = Evidence-Based Nursing;   **EB** = Evidence-Based

Client/Family Teaching and Discharge Planning

- Teach the client skin assessment and ways to monitor for impending skin breakdown. Early assessment and intervention help prevent the development of serious problems. EB: *Basic elements of a skin assessment are assessment of temperature, color, moisture, turgor, and intact skin (Baranoski & Ayello, 2016). Seek information from the health care team to address individual pressure injury prevention and treatment needs (NPUAP & EPUAP, 2014).*
- If consistent with overall client management goals, teach how to turn and reposition the client. EB: *Do not position an individual directly on a pressure ulcer. Continue to turn/reposition the individual even if a low-airloss support surface is in use. Establish turning frequency based on the characteristics of the support surface and the individual's response (NPUAP & EPUAP, 2014). If the goal of care is to keep the client (e.g., a terminally ill client) comfortable, turning and repositioning may not be appropriate (Horn & Irion, 2014; NPUAP & EPUAP, 2014).*
- Teach the client and/or caregivers to use pillows, foam wedges, and pressure-reducing devices to prevent pressure injury (NPUAP & EPUAP, 2014). CEB: *The use of effective pressure-reducing seat cushions for older wheelchair users may significantly prevent sitting-acquired pressure injuries (Brienza et al, 2016). Pressure redistribution devices serve as adjuncts to prevention and do not replace repositioning (Ratliff et al, 2017).*

REFERENCES

Baranoski, S., & Ayello, E. A. (2016). Skin an essential organ. In S. Baranoski & E. A. Ayello (Eds.), *Wound care essentials: Practice principles* (4th ed.). Ambler, PA: Lippincott, Williams & Wilkins.

Brienza, D. M., et al. (2016). Pressure redistribution: Seating, positioning, and support surfaces. In S. Baranoski & E. A. Ayello (Eds.), *Wound care essentials: Practice principles* (4th ed.). Ambler, PA: Lippincott Williams & Wilkins.

Horn, J., & Irion, G. L. (2014). The integument: Current concepts in care at end of life. *Journal of Acute Care Physical Therapy*, 5(1), 11–16.

Lippoldt, J., & Staudinger, T. (2014). Interface pressure at different degrees of backrest elevation with various types of pressure redistribution surfaces. *American Journal of Critical Care*, 23(2), 119–126.

National Pressure Ulcer Advisory Panel (NPUAP). (2016). *Pressure injury stages*. Retrieved from http://www.npuap.org/resources/educational-and-clinical-resources/npuap-pressure-injury-stages/. (Accessed 28 November 2017).

National Pressure Ulcer Advisory Panel (NPUAP) and European Pressure Ulcer Advisory Panel (EPUAP). (2014). In Haesler, E. (Ed.), *Prevention and treatment of pressure ulcers*. Perth, Australia: Cambridge Media.

O'Hanlon, C., Dowsett, J., & Smyth, N. (2015). Nutrition assessment of the intensive care unit patient. *Topics in Clinical Nutrition*, 30(1), 47–70.

Ratliff, C. R., Droste, L. R., Bonham, P., et al. (2017). WOCN 2016 guideline for prevention and management of pressure injuries (ulcers). An executive summary, Wound, Ostomy and Continence Nurses Society—Wound Guidelines Task Force. *Journal of Wound, Ostomy, and Continence Nursing*, 44(3), 241–246.

Vrtis, M. C. (2013). The economic impact of complex wound care on home health agencies. *Journal of Wound, Ostomy, and Continence Nursing*, 40(4), 360–363.

Wound, Ostomy, and Continence Nurses Society (WOCN). (2010). *Guideline for prevention and management of pressure ulcers*. WOCN clinical practice guideline series no. 2. Mount Laurel, NJ.

S

Sleep deprivation   *Judith Ann Floyd, PhD, RN, FNAP, FAAN*

NANDA-I

Definition

Prolonged periods of time without sustained natural, periodic suspension of relative consciousness that provides rest.

Defining Characteristics

Agitation, alteration in concentration, anxiety, apathy, combativeness, confusion, decrease in functional ability, decrease in reaction time, drowsiness, fatigue, fleeting nystagmus, hallucinations, hand tremors, heightened sensitivity to pain, irritability, lethargy, malaise, perceptual disorders, restlessness, transient paranoia

Related Factors

Age-related sleep stage shifts; average daily physical activity less than recommended for gender and age; environmental barrier; late day confusion; nonrestorative sleep pattern; overstimulating environment; prolonged discomfort; sleep terror; sleep walking; sustained circadian asynchrony; sustained inadequate sleep hygiene

● = Independent;   ▲ = Collaborative;   EBN = Evidence-Based Nursing;   EB = Evidence-Based

At-Risk Population

Familial sleep paralysis

Associated Condition

Conditions with periodic limb movement; dementia; idiopathic central nervous system hypersomnolence; narcolepsy; nightmares; sleep apnea; sleep-related enuresis; sleep-related painful erections; treatment regimen

NOC (Nursing Outcomes Classification)

Suggested NOC Outcomes

Rest; Sleep; Symptom Severity

Example NOC Outcome with Indicators

Sleep as evidenced by the following indicators: Hours of sleep/Sleep pattern/Sleep quality/Sleep efficiency/Feels rejuvenated after sleep/Sleeps through the night consistently. (Rate the outcome and indicators of **Sleep:** 1 = severely compromised, 2 = substantially compromised, 3 = moderately compromised, 4 = mildly compromised, 5 = not compromised [see Section I].)

Client Outcomes

Client Will (Specify Time Frame)

- Verbalize plan that provides adequate time for sleep
- Identify actions that can be taken to ensure adequate sleep time
- Awaken refreshed once adequate time is spent sleeping
- Be less sleepy during the day once adequate time is spent sleeping

NIC (Nursing Interventions Classification)

Suggested NIC Intervention

Sleep Enhancement

Example NIC Activities—Sleep Enhancement

Monitor/record client's sleep pattern and number of sleep hours; Encourage client to establish a schedule that allows age-appropriate hours of sleep with minimal environmental and personal disruptions

---

Nursing Interventions and *Rationales*

- Assess the amount of sleep obtained each night compared with the amount of sleep needed. EB: *A national survey of 444,306 American adults found that more than one-third (34.8%) slept less than 7 hours per night, an amount at which physiological and neurobehavioral deficits manifest and become progressively worse under chronic conditions (Liu et al, 2016).*
- Assess the extent to which patients can be provided three to four consecutive hours of sleep time that is free from disturbance. CEB: *A meta-analysis using data from 159 studies found the deepest stages of sleep occurred during the first 3 to 4 hours of the sleep period followed by several 90- to 110-minute sleep cycles that consisted of increasingly lower percentages of deep sleep (Floyd, 2002).* EB: *Sleep hygiene education focuses on teaching healthy sleep habits such as avoiding caffeine, exercising regularly, eliminating noise from the sleeping environment, and maintaining a regular sleep schedule. However, research exploring direct links to these actions and subsequent sleep as a treatment for insomnia has been limited and inconclusive (Irish et al, 2015).*
  - ○ Minimize environmental factors that deprive clients of sleep. See Nursing Interventions and *Rationales* for Disturbed **Sleep** pattern.
  - ○ Minimize personal factors that deprive clients of sleep. See Nursing Interventions and *Rationales* for **Insomnia.**
- When required nighttime care leaves patients sleep deprived, schedule a specific time for rest and sleep during the day. EBN: *An action research study based on an evidence review, plus experiences of 22 intensive*

● = Independent;   ▲ = Collaborative;   EBN = Evidence-Based Nursing;   EB = Evidence-Based

care unit (ICU) patients, and suggestions from approximately 250 health-setting personnel led to the development of an ICU clinical practice guideline that included planned daytime rest/sleep periods (Elliot & McKinley, 2014).

- Assess for hypersensitivity to pain. EB: *In a laboratory experiment using 14 healthy adults, sleep restriction protocols altered processes of pain habituation and sensitization, which may help explain why chronic pain conditions often accompany insufficient sleep (Simpson et al, 2017).* EB: *In an observational study of postoperative orthopedic surgery patients (N = 50), a significant correlation was found between increased self-reported pain scores and decreased total sleep time (Miller et al, 2015).*
- When daytime drowsiness occurs despite adequate periods of undisturbed nighttime sleep, consider sleep apnea as a possible cause. EB: *In a household survey of more than 7000 adults, unexplained excessive daytime sleepiness was identified as a predictor of undiagnosed sleep apnea (Dosman et al, 2014).*
- Monitor caffeine intake (amounts and time of day) in sleep-deprived clients who may overuse caffeinated drinks to ward off daytime drowsiness. EB: *An experimental study of 12 participants found that caffeine (400 mg), even when consumed 6 hours before bedtime, had a disruptive effect on both objective and subjective sleep measures (Drake et al, 2013).*
- If evidence-based interventions are inadequate, consider and carefully evaluate unstudied but commonly used countermeasures for fighting drowsiness. CEB: *A descriptive study of 77 middle-aged adults identified the following unstudied strategies as possibly effective interrupters of drowsiness: (1) change physical position, (2) improve ventilation (e.g., get fresh air, turn on fan, open window), (3) reduce air temperature (e.g., turn on air conditioning, turn on fan), (4) increase auditory stimulation (e.g., play music, sing, engage in conversation, listen to debate), and (5) engage in interesting visual activity (e.g., board games, watching TV sports events, watching serial TV dramas) (Davidsson, 2012).*

Pediatric

- Assess the amount of sleep obtained each night compared with the amount of sleep needed to avoid daytime drowsiness. EB: *Using data from a nationally representative survey (N = 2832), normal sleep times were found to vary by several hours at each age from birth to 18 years (Williams, Zimmerman, & Bell, 2013).*
- Encourage daily schedules that allow for late awakening times for adolescents. EB: *A review of evidence from 38 reports showed that delaying school start time increased sleep duration among adolescents, primarily by delaying rise times (Wheaton, Chapman, & Croft, 2016).*
- See the Pediatric section of Nursing Interventions and *Rationales* for Disturbed **Sleep** pattern.

Geriatric

- ▲ If an older client has daytime symptoms of sleep deprivation despite long nighttime sleep, refer to a sleep laboratory to evaluate the client for sleep apnea. *Older adults with heart failure, pulmonary disease, and dementia have a higher risk of sleep apnea, which may be undiagnosed (Gooneratne & Vitiello, 2014).*
- Assess the amount of sleep obtained each night compared with the amount of sleep needed to function well during the day. EB: *An integrative review of research published since 2000 suggested that sleep need in adults does not change across the life span, but obtaining adequate sleep becomes more difficult for older adults because of gradual changes in circadian functioning and sleep structure (Rybarczyk et al, 2013).*
- Assess how much time the client spends in bed unable to sleep and client's comfort with low sleep efficiency. EBN: *A meta-analysis of results from samples representing 5061 general-population adults showed a steady increase after age 50 in the amount of time set aside for nighttime sleep, which contributed to a steady decline in sleep efficiency over the life span (Floyd, 2017).*
- If a client is obtaining less sleep than required for optimal daytime function, explore if daytime napping will supplement, rather than replace, nighttime sleep. CEB: *In a pretest/posttest study of 22 older adults, a consistent regimen of daily napping for 45 minutes enhanced waking function without negatively affecting nighttime sleep (Campbell et al, 2011).*
- See the Geriatric section of Nursing Interventions and *Rationales* for disturbed **Sleep** pattern and **Insomnia.**

Multicultural

- Be aware of racial and ethnic disparities in sleep deprivation. EB: *A national survey of 444,306 American adults found that non-Hispanic black, American Indian/Alaska Native, Native Hawaiian/Pacific Islander, and multiracial populations reported a higher prevalence of sleeping less than 7 hours sleep compared with the rest of the US adult population (Liu et al, 2016).*

● = Independent;   ▲ = Collaborative;   EBN = Evidence-Based Nursing;   EB = Evidence-Based

Home Care

- Teach family members about the short-term and long-term consequences of inadequate amounts of sleep for both clients and family caregivers. CEB: *In an integrative review of 10 studies, insufficient sleep was associated with poor attention, decreased performance, increased mortality and morbidity, and cardiovascular risk factors, including hypertension, insulin resistance, hormonal deregulation, and inflammation (Mullington et al, 2009).*
- Teach client/family caregivers about the need for those with medical conditions to avoid schedules and commitments that interfere with obtaining adequate amounts of sleep. EB: *Critical appraisal of 22 studies provided evidence that sleep disturbance was common in critically ill patients up to 12 months after hospital discharge (Altman, Knauert, & Pisani, 2017).* CEB: *In a study of 21 subjects with left ventricular assist devices, nurse researchers found they obtained inadequate sleep persisting up to 6 months after surgery (Casida et al, 2011).*
- Promote adoption of behaviors that ensure adequate amounts of sleep for all family members. See Nursing Interventions and *Rationales* for Readiness for enhanced **Sleep.**
- Teach family members ways to avoid chronic sleep loss. See Nursing Interventions and *Rationales* for Disturbed **Sleep** pattern.
- Advise against chronic use of caffeinated drinks to overcome daytime fatigue and drowsiness while focusing on elimination of factors that lead to chronic sleep loss. CEB: *In an integrative review of 26 controlled laboratory studies of adult subjects, caffeine was found helpful in the temporary management of sleepiness, but overuse and late-day use contributed to subsequent sleep disruption and caffeine habituation (Roehrs & Roth, 2008).*

REFERENCES

Altman, M. T., Knauert, M. P., & Pisani, M. A. (2017). Sleep disturbance after hospitalization and critical illness: A systematic review. *Annals of the American Thoracic Society, 14*(9), 1457–1468. doi:10.1513/AnnalsATS.201702-148SR.

Campbell, S. S., Stanchina, M. D., Schlang, J. R., et al. (2011). Effects of a month-long napping regimen in older individuals. *Journal of the American Geriatric Society, 59*(2), 224–232. doi:10.1111/j.1532-5415.2010.03264.x.

Casida, J. M., Davis, J. E., Brewer, R. J., et al. (2011). Sleep and daytime sleepiness of patients with left ventricular assist devices: A longitudinal pilot study. *Progress in Transplantation, 21*(2), 131–136.

Davidsson, S. (2012). Countermeasure drowsiness by design: Using common behaviour. *Work (Reading, Mass.), 41*, 5062–5067. doi:10.3233/WOR-2012-0798-5062.

Dosman, J., Gjevre, J., Karunanayake, C., et al. (2014). Predicting sleep apnea in the clinic. *Chest, 145*(3), Suppl–595A.

Drake, C., Roehrs, T., Shambroom, B. S., et al. (2013). Caffeine effects on sleep taken 0, 3, or 6 hours before going to bed. *Journal of Clinical Sleep Medicine: JCSM: Official Publication of the American Academy of Sleep Medicine, 9*(11), 1195–1200. doi:10.5664/jcsm.3170.

Elliot, R., & McKinley, S. (2014). The development of a clinical practice guideline to improve sleep in intensive care patients: A solution focused approach. *Intensive and Critical Care Nursing, 30*, 246–256. doi:10.1016/j.iccn.2014.04.003.

Floyd, J. A. (2002). Sleep and aging. *Nursing Clinics of North America, 37*(4), 719–731.

Floyd, J. A. (2017). Patterns of decline in sleep efficiency over the adult lifespan: Clarification via use of smoothing splines. *International Journal of Sleep Disorders, 1*(1), 1–6.

Gooneratne, N. S., & Vitiello, M. V. (2014). Sleep in Vitiello older adults: Normative changes, sleep disorders, and treatment options. *Clinics in Geriatric Medicine, 30*(3), 591–627. doi:10.1016/j.cger.2014.04.007.

Irish, L. A., Klein, C. E., Gunn, H. E., et al. (2015). The role of sleep hygiene in promoting public health: A review of empirical evidence. *Sleep Medicine Reviews, 22*, 23–36.

Liu, Y., Wheaton, A. G., Chapman, D. P., et al. (2016). Prevalence of healthy sleep duration among adults United States, 2014. *MMWR. Morbidity and Mortality Weekly Report, 65*(6), 137–141. doi:10.15585/mmwr.mm6506a1.

Miller, A., Roth, T., Roehrs, T., et al. (2015). Correlation between sleep disruption on postoperative pain. *Otolaryngology–Head and Neck Surgery: Official Journal of American Academy of Otolaryngology—Head and Neck Surgery, 152*(5), 964–968. doi:10.1177/0194599815572127.

Mullington, J. M., Haack, M., Toth, M., et al. (2009). Cardiovascular, inflammatory, and metabolic consequences of sleep deprivation. *Progress in Cardiovascular Diseases, 51*(4), 294–302. doi:10.1016/j.pcad.2008.10.003.

Roehrs, T. A., & Roth, T. (2008). Caffeine: Sleep and daytime sleepiness. *Sleep Medicine Review, 12*(2), 153–162. doi:10.1016/j.smrv.2007.07.004.

Rybarczyk, B., Lund, H. G., Garroway, A. M., et al. (2013). Cognitive behavioral therapy for insomnia in older adults: Background, evidence, and overview of treatment protocol. *Clinical Gerontologist, 36*, 70–93. doi:10.1080/07317115.2012.731478.

Simpson, N. S., Scott-Sutherland, J., Gautam, S., et al. (2017). Chronic exposure to insufficient sleep alters processes of pain habituation and sensitization. *Pain, 158*(9), N.PAG-N.PAG. doi:10.1097/j.pain.0000000000001053.

Wheaton, A. G., Chapman, D. P., & Croft, J. B. (2016). School start times, sleep, behavioral, health, and academic outcomes: A review of the literature. *Journal of School Health, 86*(5), 363–381. doi:10.1111/josh.12388.

Williams, J. A., Zimmerman, F. J., & Bell, J. F. (2013). Norms and trends of sleep time among US children and adolescents. *JAMA Pediatrics, 167*(1), 55–60. doi:10.1001/jamapediatrics.2013.423.

● = Independent;   ▲ = Collaborative;   EBN = Evidence-Based Nursing;   EB = Evidence-Based

Readiness for enhanced sleep   *Judith Ann Floyd, PhD, RN, FNAP, FAAN*

NANDA-I

Definition

A pattern of natural, periodic suspension of relative consciousness to provide rest and sustain a desired lifestyle, which can be strengthened.

Defining Characteristics

Expresses desire to enhance sleep

NOC   (Nursing Outcomes Classification)

Suggested NOC Outcomes

Personal Well-Being; Rest; Sleep

> **Example NOC Outcome with Indicators**
>
> **Sleep** as evidenced by the following indicators: Hours of sleep/Sleep pattern/Sleep quality/Sleep efficiency/Feels rejuvenated after sleep/Napping appropriate for age. (Rate each indicator of **Sleep:** 1 = severely compromised, 2 = substantially compromised, 3 = moderately compromised, 4 = mildly compromised, 5 = not compromised [see Section I].)

Client Outcomes

Client Will (Specify Time Frame)

- Verbalize a current interest in what constitutes normal sleep
- Reflect on own experiences and beliefs about sleep
- Verbalize an interest in nonpharmacological approaches to sleep promotion
- Take concrete steps to establish an environment conducive to sleep initiation and maintenance

NIC   (Nursing Interventions Classification)

Suggested NIC Intervention

Sleep Enhancement

> **Example NIC Activities—Sleep Enhancement**
>
> Assess client's sleep/activity pattern; Assist/encourage client to create an environment that facilitates sleep; Assist/encourage client to adopt personal practices that enhance sleep

Nursing Interventions and *Rationales*

- Assess client's current knowledge and beliefs about sleep need and factors affecting sleep quantity and quality. **EB:** *In a descriptive study of 1707 subjects from nine primary care practices, assessment of knowledge and beliefs about sleep were identified as an essential first step in patient education programs (Phillips et al, 2014). **EB:** In an observational study of 229 subjects, false beliefs about sleep requirements were associated with sleep disorders (Cronlein et al, 2014).*
- Whenever there is a lack of knowledge or false beliefs about sleep requirements, provide information regarding sleep need and encourage clients to identify their personal sleep requirements. **CEB:** *In a meta-analysis (N = 180 studies), a nurse researcher found that normal-population adults averaged 7.5 to 9.0 hours of sleep per night (range of 6.5–10.0 hours) and fell asleep within 20 minutes initially and more quickly if awakened during the night; daytime was characterized by no naps or regularly scheduled brief naps, and little fatigue or sleepiness (Floyd, 2002). **EB:** In a review of research by a panel of 15 sleep experts, sleep need was found to be highly variable among adults, but 7 or more hours of sleep on a regular basis was found to promote optimal health and reduce risk of adverse health outcomes; it was unclear if averaging more than 9 hours was associated with health risk (Watson et al, 2015).*

● = Independent;   ▲ = Collaborative;   EBN = Evidence-Based Nursing;   EB = Evidence-Based

- Based on assessment, focus on one or more of the following sleep hygiene strategies, choosing the most relevant. **EBN:** *An experimental study involving 40 community-based adults living with HIV/AIDS found that a sleep hygiene educational program focused on changing the interpersonal system was effective for changing beliefs and behavior and for improving sleep patterns (Webel et al, 2013).* **EBN:** *An experimental study of 79 college students with complaints of insomnia found that sleep hygiene strategies improved sleep (Lillehei et al, 2015). Sleep hygiene strategies include:*
  ○ Regular scheduling of the nighttime sleep period, daytime exposure to light, exercise, napping, and mealtimes characterized by (1) vigorous exercise during the day, (2) avoidance of long periods of daytime sleep (unless a night-shift worker), (3) avoidance of large meals before bed, and (4) arising at the same time each day even if sleep was poor during the previous night. *Experts have concluded that regular schedules of rest/activity and light/dark promote sleep initiation and sleep maintenance by maintaining a circadian rhythm of alertness/drowsiness (Gooneratne & Vitiello, 2014; Meltzer, Moreno, & Johnson, 2014).* **EB:** *An experimental study of 173 young adults suggested interactions among rest/activity, light/dark, sleep, and other physiological parameters (body temperature, blood pressure, and heart rate) are complex and require more study, but factors that suppress or stimulate melatonin secretion likely play a key role in circadian rhythm interactions (Gubin et al, 2017).*
  ○ Relaxing bedtime routine that includes (1) activities that calm the mind (e.g., mindfulness or other types of meditation, listening to music, prayer) and (2) activities that relax the body (e.g., warm baths, massage, progressive muscle relaxation). *Both mental and physical relaxation practices are believed to facilitate sleep initiation (Gooneratne & Vitiello, 2014; Meltzer, Moreno, & Johnson, 2014).* **EBN:** *A review of evidence from nine intervention studies suggested relaxation, meditation, guided imagery, or a combinations of these strategies resulted in better sleep and less fatigue in heart-failure patients (Kwekkeboom & Bratzke, 2016).*
  ○ Oil of lavender. **EBN:** *An experimental study of 79 college students with complaints of insomnia found that adding the scent of lavender to the sleep environment as part of a sleep hygiene program improved sleep duration beyond the improvements achieved by other hygiene practices (Lillehei et al, 2015).*
  ○ Creation of an environment conducive to sleep including (1) comfortable sleepwear, sleep surface, and room temperature; (2) low or masked levels of light and noise; and (3) a sleep space as free as possible from interruptions from others including pets. *A quiet, dark, physically comfortable sleep setting free from interruptions is believed best for promoting sleep (Gooneratne & Vitiello, 2014; Meltzer, Moreno, & Johnson, 2014).* **CEB:** *In an experimental study of 122 sociodisadvantaged new mothers, nurse researchers found that sleep hygiene measures, including infant proximity, noise masking, and dim lighting, improved sleep quality during the postpartum period (Lee and Gay, 2011).*
  ○ Management of any sources of pain as needed prior to sleep. **EB:** *In a national survey of 1029 noninstitutionalized adults aged 18 years or older, pain was associated with lower sleep quality, more sleep disruption, and greater sleep deprivation (National Sleep Foundation, 2015). (See further Nursing Interventions and Rationales for Acute **Pain** and Chronic **Pain**.)*
  ○ Avoidance of late-day electronic device-use. **EB:** *A descriptive study of 1674 adults found participants with more screen time from TV watching and use of computers and other electronic devises reported more difficulty falling asleep and staying asleep (Vallance et al, 2015).* **EB:** *A representative survey of 1508 adults found that 90% of Americans used some type of electronics at least a few nights per week before bedtime and also found that adults who reported use of e-readers had reduced evening sleepiness, took longer to fall asleep, and reported reduced next-morning alertness compared with adults who read printed books at bedtime (Chang et al, 2015).*
  ○ Monitoring of late-day intake of caffeine from all sources including energy drinks, coffee, colas, teas, and chocolate. *Many common beverages and foodstuffs contain large enough doses of caffeine to affect nighttime sleep (Gooneratne & Vitiello, 2014; Meltzer, Moreno, & Johnson, 2014).* **EB:** *In an experimental study (N = 12) researchers found that caffeine consumption (400 mg) up to 6 hours before bedtime had a disruptive effect on objectively measured and self-reported symptoms of insomnia (Drake et al, 2013).*
  ○ Avoidance of alcoholic beverages to induce sleep. *Experts have concluded that alcoholic drinks before bed interfere with overall sleep quality (Gooneratne & Vitiello, 2014; Lenz, 2014).* **CEB:** *In a descriptive study of 50 oncology outpatients, nurse researchers found that limited alcohol use (one to two drinks) was related to shortened time to falling asleep and increased depth of sleep the first 2 hours, as well as suppressed rapid eye movement (REM) sleep, which sometimes led to REM rebound (i.e., lighter, more fragmented sleep later in the night) (Dean et al, 2010).*

• = Independent;   ▲ = Collaborative;   **EBN** = Evidence-Based Nursing;   **EB** = Evidence-Based

○ Avoidance of nicotine. *Experts have concluded that nicotine use interferes with overall sleep quality (Gooneratne & Vitiello, 2014; Lenz, 2014).* **CEB:** *In a national survey of 6400 participants, cigarette smokers took longer to fall asleep and had shorter and lighter nighttime sleep than nonsmokers; however, acute nicotine withdrawal caused even more sleep disruption (Zhang et al, 2006).*

○ Avoidance of a sedentary lifestyle. **EB:** *In a national survey of 1000 representative adults aged 23 to 60, excessive sitting during waking hours was associated with poor sleep quality (Buman et al, 2015).*

 Geriatric

• Interventions discussed previously can all be adapted for use with geriatric clients.

• Counsel the older client regarding normal age-related sleep changes. *Older adults may be unaware of which age-related sleep changes are typical versus symptoms of a sleep disorder (Gooneratne & Vitiello, 2014).* **CEB:** *In a meta-analysis (N = 180 studies), a nurse researcher discovered that as adults aged, they increased time needed to fall asleep, increased the frequency and duration of waking after sleep onset, and decreased nighttime sleep amount (Floyd, 2002).*

• Elicit the older client's beliefs about sleep and correct any misconceptions, which may manifest as undue concern for some, but too little concern for others. *Experts have concluded that the older adult may be unduly concerned about normal age-related changes in sleep patterns (Gooneratne & Vitiello, 2014).* **EB:** *In a descriptive study comparing sleep beliefs and behaviors of 41 black and 24 white older women, the majority of women, regardless of race/ethnicity, incorrectly stated that poor sleep did not have negative effects on other health conditions (Grandner et al, 2013).*

• Review older client's prescription medications; use of over-the-counter (OTC) medications; and use of caffeine, tobacco, and alcohol. *Older adults may be unaware of how their medications and commonly used psychoactive substances affect sleep (Allen et al, 2013).* **EB:** *A double-blind cross-over study (N = 46) of adults in their fifties compared with young adults found caffeine interfered with initiation of deep sleep in all and that the older adults experienced even more sensitivity to caffeine intake than the younger adults (Robillard et al, 2015).*

• Assess and refer as appropriate if coexisting conditions may be affecting older client's sleep. *Depression, sleep apnea, and restless leg syndrome are commonly missed coexisting conditions in older adults (Allen et al, 2013; Gooneratne & Vitiello, 2014).*

• Expand older client's awareness of sleep hygiene behaviors for improving sleep. **EB:** *In a descriptive study of 195 older adults, only three strategies were heavily used by elders to address sleep concerns: ignoring the symptoms, staying in bed or resting, and praying (Sandberg et al, 2014).* **EBN:** *A meta-analysis of results from samples representing 5061 general-population adults showed a steady increase after age fifty in the amount of time spent in bed with the intent to sleep, which contributed to a steady decline in sleep efficiency with aging (Floyd, 2017).*

• Encourage the older client to walk and engage in other exercise outside unless contraindicated. *Experts have concluded that exercise and exposure to natural light reinforce circadian rhythms that control sleep (Gooneratne & Vitiello, 2014; Meltzer, Moreno, & Johnson, 2014).* **EB:** *In an evidence review of 34 research reports, exercise increased sleep efficiency and duration in healthy older adults regardless of the mode and intensity of activity, and even more so in the elderly with chronic conditions such as hypertension, obesity, diabetes, rheumatoid arthritis, or sleep disorders (Dolezal et al, 2017).*

 Home Care

• All interventions discussed previously can be adapted for home care use.

• Assess family caregivers' readiness for enhancing sleep. **EB:** *A qualitative study of 12 people with dementia and their family caregivers found that family members need guidance with balancing their own sleep requirements with those of homecare recipients (Gibson, Gander, & Jones, 2014).* **EB:** *A secondary analysis of quantitative data from 395 family caregivers of hospice patients found nearly one-third experienced clinically noteworthy levels of sleep problems and/or anxiety that can interfere with sleep initiation (Washington et al, 2018).*

• Assess the conduciveness of the home environment for promoting both caregiver and client sleep and the resources needed to improve the sleep environment. **EB:** *A qualitative study of 12 people with dementia and their family caregivers found many factors in the home can promote or interfere with creating an environment conducive to sleep (Gibson et al, 2014).* **CEB:** *In an experimental study of 122 sociodisadvantaged new mothers, nurse researchers found approximately two-thirds of homes incorporated sleep hygiene recommendations consistently over three months (Lee & Gay, 2011).*

• = Independent;   ▲ = Collaborative;   **EBN** = Evidence-Based Nursing;   **EB** = Evidence-Based

REFERENCES

Allen, A. M., Coon, D. W., Uriri-Glover, J., et al. (2013). Factors associated with sleep disturbance among older adults in inpatient rehabilitation facilities. *Rehabilitation Nursing, 38*, 221–230. doi:10.1002/rnj.88.

Buman, M. P., Kline, C. E., Youngstedt, S. D., et al. (2015). Sitting and television viewing: Novel risk factors for sleep disturbance and apnea risk? Results from the 2013 National Sleep Foundation Sleep in America Poll. *Chest, 147*(3), 728–734.

Chang, A. M., Aeschbacha, D., Duffya, J. F., et al. (2015). Evening use of light-emitting eReaders negatively affects sleep, circadian timing, and next-morning alertness. *Proceedings of the National Academy of Sciences of the United States of America, 112*(4), 1232–1237. doi:10.1073/pnas.1418490112.

Cronlein, T., Wagner, S., Langguth, B., et al. (2014). Are dysfunctional attitudes and beliefs about sleep unique to primary insomnia? *Sleep Medicine, 15*(12), 1463–1467.

Dean, G. E., Finnell, D. S., Scribner, M., et al. (2010). Sleep in lung cancer: The role of anxiety, alcohol and tobacco. *Journal of Addictions Nursing, 21*, 130–137. doi:10.3109/10884601003777620.

Dolezal, B. A., Neufeld, E. V., Boland, D. M., et al. (2017). Interrelationship between sleep and exercise: A systematic review. *Advances in Preventive Medicine, 2017*, Article ID 1364387, 14 pages. Retrieved from https://doi.org/10.1155/2017/1364387. (Accessed 29 January 2018).

Drake, C., Roehrs, T., Shambroom, B. S., et al. (2013). Caffeine effects on sleep taken 0, 3, or 6 hours before going to bed. *Journal of Clinical Sleep Medicine: JCSM: Official Publication of the American Academy of Sleep Medicine, 9*(11), 1195–1200. doi:10.5664/jcsm.3170.

Floyd, J. A. (2002). Sleep and aging. *Nursing Clinics of North America, 37*(4), 719–731.

Floyd, J. A. (2017). Patterns of decline in sleep efficiency over the adult lifespan: Clarification via use of smoothing splines. *International Journal of Sleep Disorders, 1*(1), 1–6.

Gibson, R. H., Gander, P. H., & Jones, L. M. (2014). Understanding the sleep problems of people with dementia and their family caregivers. *Dementia (Basel, Switzerland), 13*(3), 350–365. doi:10.1177/1471301212473884.

Gooneratne, N. S., & Vitiello, M. V. (2014). Sleep in older adults: Normative changes, sleep disorders, and treatment options. *Clinics in Geriatric Medicine, 30*, 591–627. doi:10.1016/j.cger.2014.04.007.

Grandner, M. A., Patel, N. P., Girardin, J. L., et al. (2013). Sleep-related behaviors and beliefs associated with race/ethnicity in women. *Journal of the National Medical Association, 105*, 4–15.

Gubin, D. G., Weinert, D., Rybina, S. V., et al. (2017). Activity, sleep and ambient light have a different impact on circadian blood pressure, heart rate and body temperature rhythms. *Chronobiology International, 34*(5), 632–649. doi:10.1080/07420528.2017.1288632.

Kwekkeboom, K., & Bratzke, L. C. (2016). A systematic review of relaxation, meditation, and guided imagery strategies for symptom management in heart failure. *Journal of Cardiovascular Nursing, 31*(5), 457–468. doi:10.1097/JCN.0000000000000274.

Lee, K. A., & Gay, C. L. (2011). Can modifications to the bedroom environment improve the sleep of new parents? Two randomized controlled trials. *Research in Nursing & Health, 34*, 7–19. doi:10.1002/nur.20413.

Lenz, T. L. (2014). Drugs that negatively affect sleep. *American Journal of Lifestyle Medicine, 8*(6), 383–385. doi:10.1177/1559827614544436.

Lillehei, A. S., Halcon, L. L., Savik, K., et al. (2015). Effect of inhaled lavender and sleep hygiene on self-reported sleep issues: A randomized controlled trial. *The Journal of Alternative and Complementary Medicine, 21*(7), 430–438. doi:10.1089/acm.2014.0327.

Meltzer, L. J., Moreno, J. P., & Johnson, C. A. (2014). Behavioral medicine review: Sleep is not for slackers. *American Journal of Lifestyle Medicine, 8*(6), 380–382. doi:10.1177/1559827614545314.

National Sleep Foundation. (2015). *2015 Sleep in America poll: Sleep and pain—Summary of findings*. Arlington, VA: Author. Retrieved from https://sleepfoundation.org/sleep-polls-data/sleep-in-america-poll/2015-sleep-and-pain. (Accessed 29 January 2018).

Phillips, S. M., Glasgow, R. E., Bello, G., et al. (2014). Frequency and prioritization of patient health risks from a structured health risk assessment. *Annuals of Family Medicine, 12*, 505–513. doi:10.1370/afm.1717.

Robillard, R., Bouchard, M., Cartier, A., et al. (2015). Sleep is more sensitive to high doses of caffeine in the middle years of life. *Journal of Psychopharmacology, 29*(6), 688–697. doi:10.1177/0269881115575535.

Sandberg, K. T., Parker Oliver, D., Smith, J. B., et al. (2014). Self-reported sleep difficulties and self-care. *Journal of Evidence-Based Complementary & Alternative Medicine, 19*(1), 36–42. doi:10.1177/2156587213510005.

Vallance, J. K., Buman, M. P., Stevinson, C., et al. (2015). Associations of overall sedentary time and screen time with sleep outcomes. *American Journal of Health Behavior, 39*(1), 62–67. doi:10.5993/AJHB.39.1.7.

Washington, K. T., Parker Oliver, D., Smith, J. B., et al. (2018). Sleep problems, anxiety, and global self-rated health among hospice family caregivers. *The American Journal of Hospice & Palliative Medicine, 35*(2), 244–249. doi:10.1177/1049909117703643.

Watson, N. F., Badr, M. S., Belenky, G., et al. (2015). Recommended amount of sleep for a healthy adult: A joint consensus statement of the American Academy of Sleep Medicine and Sleep Research Society. *Sleep, 38*(6), 843–844. doi:10.5665/sleep.4716.

Webel, A. R., Moore, S. M., Hanson, J. E., et al. (2013). Improving sleep hygiene behavior in adults living with HIV/AIDS: A randomized control pilot study of the SystemCHANGETM–HIV intervention. *Applied Nursing Research, 26*, 85–91. doi:10.1016/j.apnr.2012.10.002.

Zhang, L., Samet, J., Caffo, B., et al. (2006). Cigarette smoking and nocturnal sleep architecture. *American Journal of Epidemiology, 164*(6), 529–537. doi:10.1093/aje/kwj231.

Disturbed Sleep pattern   *Judith Ann Floyd, PhD, RN, FNAP, FAAN*

NANDA-I

Definition

Time-limited awakenings due to external factors.

● = Independent;   ▲ = Collaborative;   **EBN** = Evidence-Based Nursing;   **EB** = Evidence-Based

Defining Characteristics

Difficulty in daily functioning; difficulty initiating sleep; difficulty maintaining sleep state; dissatisfaction with sleep; feeling unrested; unintentional awakening

Related Factors

Disruption caused by sleep partner; environmental barrier; immobilization; insufficient privacy; nonrestorative sleep pattern

NOC   (Nursing Outcomes Classification)

Suggested NOC Outcomes

Personal Well-Being; Rest; Sleep

Example NOC Outcome with Indicators
Sleep as evidenced by the following indicators: Hours of sleep/Sleep pattern/Sleep quality/Sleep efficiency/Feels rejuvenated after sleep. (Rate the outcome and indicators of **Sleep:** 1 = severely compromised, 2 = substantially compromised, 3 = moderately compromised, 4 = mildly compromised, 5 = not compromised [see Section I].)

Client Outcomes

Client Will (Specify Time Frame)

- Verbalize plan to implement sleep promotion routines
- Maintain a regular schedule of sleep and waking
- Fall asleep without difficulty
- Remain asleep throughout the night
- Awaken naturally, feeling refreshed and is not fatigued during day

NIC   (Nursing Interventions Classification)

Suggested NIC Intervention

Sleep Enhancement

Example NIC Activities—Sleep Enhancement
Determine external factors leading to sleep fragmentation; Reduce environmental disrupters of sleep

Nursing Interventions and *Rationales*

- Obtain a sleep history to identify (1) noise, temperature, and light levels in the sleep environment; (2) activities occurring in the sleep environment during hours of sleep including use of handheld technology; (3) number of times awakened during the sleep period; and (4) when during the sleep period, time is available for undisturbed sleep. **EBN:** *A qualitative study of hospital staff and patients (N = 24) showed environmental disturbances during hospitalization were caused by noise, light, and provision of care (Ding et al, 2017).* **EB:** *A descriptive study of environmental characteristics in a 12-bed rehabilitation unit found that average temperatures and noise levels were above the recommended levels, and abrupt increases of light and noise levels were high enough to cause sleep fragmentation (Yelden et al, 2015).*
- Negotiate use of handheld technology whenever clients have access to electronic devises in the care setting. **EB:** *A representative survey of 1508 adults found that that 90% of Americans used some type of electronics at least a few nights per week before bedtime and also found that adults who reported use of e-readers had reduced evening sleepiness, took longer to fall asleep, and reported reduced next-morning alertness compared with adults who read printed books at bedtime (Chang et al, 2015).*
- Keep environment quiet during sleep periods. **EB:** *Recorded intensive care unit (ICU) noise led to more fragmented sleep, less slow-wave (deep) sleep, more arousals, and more time awake when played during sleep (N = 17) (Perrson-Waye et al, 2013).* **EBN:** *An evidence review of 51 papers showed that noise remains a persistent disruption to sleep at night in hospitals and continues to register as a concern on patient satisfaction surveys (Fillary et al, 2015).*

● = Independent;   ▲ = Collaborative;   **EBN** = Evidence-Based Nursing;   **EB** = Evidence-Based

S

- Consider masking hospital noise that cannot be eliminated. **CEB:** *In a systematic review of nine experimental studies, nurse researchers found that recorded natural sounds, music, and music videos were effective for masking noise in health care settings (Hellstrom, Fagerstrom, & Willman, 2011).*
- Offer earplugs when feasible. **EB:** *The English-language abstract of a foreign-language research paper reported better sleep when earplugs were used alone or with other sleep promoting interventions (N = 80) (Eliyasianfar et al, 2016).* **EBN:** *Results from an experimental study of patients in intensive care (N = 50) showed that perceptions of nighttime noise decreased significantly in patients who used earplugs (Hu et al, 2015).*
- Dim the lights during sleep periods. **EB:** *A sequential prestudy/poststudy (N = 171) found the number of awakenings decreased when monitored lighting levels were part of a multicomponent program to decrease sleep disruption in intensive care (Patel et al, 2014).*
- Offer eye covers when lighting cannot be dimmed. **EB:** *The English-language abstract of a foreign-language research paper reported that hospitalized cardiac care patients (N = 80) had better sleep when eye covers were used alone or with other sleep-promoting interventions (Eliyasianfar et al, 2016).* **EBN:** *A combination of nonpharmacological interventions that included eye covers was useful for promoting sleep in ICU adult patients (Hu et al, 2015).*
- Be aware that use of eye covers in intubated clients may lead to sensory deprivation and anxiety. **CEB:** *An experimental study of eye cover use in ICU patients (N = 18) reported less sleep fragmentation, but 72% of intubated patients refused eye covers or removed them prematurely because of restlessness (30%), discomfort (20%), or anxiety (11%) (Simons, van den Boogaard, & de Jager, 2012).*
- Consolidate essential care to provide the opportunity for uninterrupted sleep the first 3 to 4 hours of the sleep period. Follow with periods of 90 to 110 minutes between interruptions. **CEB:** *In a meta-analysis using data from 159 studies a nurse researcher found that the deepest stages of sleep occurred during the first 3 to 4 hours of the sleep period followed by several 90- to 110-minute sleep cycles that consisted of increasingly lower percentages of deep sleep (Floyd, 2002).*
- If the client must be disturbed the first 3 to 4 hours of the sleep period, attempt to protect 90- to 110-minute blocks of time between awakenings. **CEB:** *In three studies of hospitalized patients, nurse researchers found that the high frequency of nocturnal care interactions left patients with no 90-minute blocks of uninterrupted time for sleep (Missildine, 2008; Missildine et al, 2010a,b).* **EB:** *In an experimental study that included protocols for consolidating care, the number of patient nights that contained a 3-hour window of uninterrupted sleep was increased (Patel et al, 2014).*
- Assess for medications and other stimulants that fragment sleep. Use caution when administering sleep medications. See Nursing Interventions and *Rationales* for **Insomnia.**
- Schedule newly ordered medications to avoid the need to wake the client the first few hours of the night. **CEB:** *A survey of sleep promotion protocols (N = 68) conducted by nurse researchers identified the need for nurses to plan ahead when initiating new medication regimens to help ensure uninterrupted sleep periods (Hofhuis et al, 2012).*
- Combine the previously mentioned interventions as feasible to create a sleep-promotion care bundle. **EBN:** *A combination of nonpharmacological interventions that included earplugs, eye covers, and relaxing music was useful for promoting sleep in ICU adult patients (Hu et al, 2015).* **EBN:** *A qualitative study of how experienced nurses promote sleep in hospitals (N = 8) identified use of a comprehensive set of cost-effective sleep-promoting measures that adapted the hospital environment for sleep and also reduced the use of sedative drugs (Salzmann-Erikson, Lagerqvist, & Pousette, 2016).*

 Pediatric

- Assess use of nighttime texting and consider limiting as needed to protect sleep. **EBN:** *A study of 278 community-based teens found that sending and/or receiving text messages at night was significantly associated with later bedtimes, shorter time in bed, daytime tiredness, and irregular sleep habits (Garmy & Ward, 2017).*
- Adapt interventions for pediatric clients with caution because of limited empirical evidence regarding the effects of their use. **EB:** *A survey of 341 pediatric critical care providers worldwide found that use of earplugs, eye masks, noise reduction, and lighting optimization for sleep promotion was uncommon (Kudchadkar, Yaster, & Punjabi, 2014).* **EBN:** *During a focus-group study, nurses (N = 30) working on general and critical-care pediatric units identified several interrelated factors that create challenges to promoting children's sleep in hospitals and highlighted the need for formal policy and mentoring related to provision of nursing care at night in pediatric settings (Stremler, Adams, & Dryder-Palmer, 2015).*

● = Independent; ▲ = Collaborative; **EBN** = Evidence-Based Nursing; **EB** = Evidence-Based

Geriatric

- Most interventions discussed previously can all be adapted for use with geriatric clients.
- Use of earplugs and eye covers with ataxic clients and clients with dementia may contribute to disorientation. CEB: *A case report and integrative review of the literature suggested sensory deficits in patients with dementia, which can be augmented by use of earplugs and eye covers, decrease their quality of life, increase their risk for delirium and falls, and pose a higher risk for poor outcomes (Haque, Abdelrehman, & Alavi, 2012).*

Multicultural

- Be aware that cultural sleep practices may alter the kinds of environmental sleep disruptors that require management. CEB: *As the result of an integrative review of the literature on family sleep practices, nurses found that bed sharing and other aspects of the sleep environment were influenced most by ethnic factors (Jain, Romack, & Jain, 2011).*

Home Care

- Consider the unique characteristics of each home sleep environment when addressing sleep disruption. EBN: *A longitudinal study of postpartum women (N = 142) showed that new mothers' sleep was disturbed 56% of the time by their infant's cries, but other environmental disrupters included (1) family, friends, and pets in the home; (2) sleeping with the television on; (3) traffic sounds; and (4) other outside noise from neighbors (Doering, 2013).*
- In addition, see the Home Care section of Nursing Interventions and *Rationales* for Readiness for enhanced **Sleep**.

REFERENCES

Chang, A. M., Aeschbacha, D., Duffya, J. F., et al. (2015). Evening use of light-emitting eReaders negatively affects sleep, circadian timing, and next-morning alertness. *Proceedings of the National Academy of Sciences of the United States of America, 112*(4), 1232–1237. doi:10.1073/pnas.1418490112.

Ding, Q., Redeker, N. S., Pisani, M. A., et al. (2017). Factors influencing patients' sleep in the intensive care unit: Perceptions of patients and clinical staff. *American Journal of Critical Care, 26,* 278–286. doi:10.4037/ajcc2017333.

Doering, J. J. (2013). The physical and social environment of sleep in socioeconomically disadvantaged postpartum women. *Journal of Obstetric, Gynecologic, & Neonatal Nursing, 42,* E33–E43. doi: 10.1111/j.1552-6909.2012.01421.x.

Eliyasianfar, S., Khazaei, H., Khatoni, A., et al. (2016). The effect of blindfolds and earplugs on sleep quality of patients admitted to the cardiac intensive care unit. *Journal of Clinical Research in Paramedical Sciences, 5*(1), 15–22.

Floyd, J. A. (2002). Sleep and aging. *Nursing Clinics of North America, 37*(4), 719–731.

Fillary, J., Chaplin, H., Jones, G., et al. (2015). Noise at night in hospital general wards: A mapping of the literature. *British Journal of Nursing, 24*(10), 536–540. doi:10.12968/bjon.2015.24.10.536.

Garmy, P., & Ward, T. M. (2017). Sleep habits and nighttime texting among adolescents. *The Journal of School Nursing, 34*(2), 121–127. doi:10.1177/1059840517704964.

Hellstrom, A., Fagerstrom, C., & Willman, A. (2011). Promoting sleep by nursing interventions in health care settings: A systematic review. *Worldviews on Evidence-Based Nursing, 8*(3), 128–142. doi: 10.1111/j.1741-6787.2010.00203.x.

Hofhuis, J. G. M., Langevoort, G., Rommes, J. H., et al. (2012). Sleep disturbances and sedation practices in the intensive care unit: A postal survey in the Netherlands. *Intensive Care Critical Care Nursing, 28,* 141–149. doi:10.1016/j.iccn.2011.10.006.

Hu, R. F., Jiang, X. Y., Hegadoren, K. M., et al. (2015). Effects of earplugs and eye masks combined with relaxing music on sleep, melatonin and cortisol levels in ICU patients: A randomized controlled trial. *Critical Care: The Official Journal of the Critical Care Forum, 19,* 115–123. doi:10.1186/s13054-015-0855-3.

Haque, R., Abdelrehman, N., & Alavi, Z. (2012). "There's a monster under my bed": Hearing aids and dementia in long-term care settings. *The Annals of Long-Term Care, 20*(8), 28–33.

Jain, S., Romack, B. S., & Jain, R. (2011). Bed sharing in school-age children—clinical and social implications. *Journal of Child and Adolescent Psychiatric Nursing, 24,* 185–189. doi:10.1111/j.1744-6171.2011.00293.x.

Kudchadkar, S. R., Yaster, M., & Punjabi, N. M. (2014). Sedation, sleep promotion, and delirium screening practices in the care of mechanically ventilated children: A wake-up call for the pediatric critical care community. *Critical Care Medicine, 42*(7), 1592–1600. doi:10.1097/CCM.0000000000000326.

Missildine, K. (2008). Sleep and the sleep environment of older adults in acute care settings. *Journal of Gerontological Nursing, 34*(6), 15–21. doi:10.3928/00989134-20080601-06.

Missildine, K., Bergstrom, N., Meininger, J., et al. (2010a). Case studies: Is the sleep of hospitalized elders related to delirium? *Medsurg Nursing, 19*(1), 39–46.

Missildine, K., Bergstrom, N., Meininger, J., et al. (2010b). Sleep in hospitalized elders: A pilot study. *Geriatric Nursing, 31*(4), 263–272. doi:10.1016/j.gerinurse.2010.02.013.

Patel, J., Baldwin, J., Bunting, P., et al. (2014). The effect of a multicomponent multidisciplinary bundle of interventions on sleep and delirium in medical and surgical intensive care patients. *Anaesthesia, 69,* 540–549. doi:10.1111/anae.12638.

Perrson-Waye, K., Elmenhorst, E. M., Croy, I., et al. (2013). Improvement of intensive care using sound environment and analysis of consequences on sleep: An experimental study. *Sleep Medicine, 14*(12), 1334–1340. doi:10.1016/j.sleep.2013.07.011.

Salzmann-Erikson, M., Lagerqvist, L., & Pousette, S. (2016). Keep calm and have a good night: Nurses' strategies to promote inpatients' sleep in the hospital environment. *Scandinavian Journal of Caring Science, 30,* 356–364. doi:10.1111/scs.12255.

● = Independent;   ▲ = Collaborative;   EBN = Evidence-Based Nursing;   EB = Evidence-Based

S

Simons, K. S., van den Boogaard, M., & de Jager, C. P. C. (2012). Reducing sensory input in critically ill patients: Are eye-masks a blind spot? *Critical Care: The Official Journal of the Critical Care Forum*, 16, 439. doi:10.1186/cc11402.

Stremler, R., Adams, S., & Dryder-Palmer, K. (2015). Nurses' views of factors affecting sleep for hospitalized children and their families: A focus group study. *Research in Nursing and Health*, 38(4), 311–322. doi:10.1002/nur.21664.

Yelden, K., Duport, S., Kempny, A., et al. (2015). A rehabilitation unit at night: Environmental characteristics of patient rooms. *Disability & Rehabilitation*, 37(1), 91–96. doi:10.3109/09638288.2014.906662.

Impaired Social interaction   *Marina Martinez-Kratz, MS, RN, CNE*

NANDA-I

Definition

Insufficient or excessive quantity or ineffective quality of social exchange.

Defining Characteristics

Discomfort in social situations; dissatisfaction with social engagement; dysfunctional interaction with others; family reports change in interaction; impaired social functioning

Related Factors

Communication barrier; disturbance in self-concept; disturbance in thought process; environmental barrier; impaired mobility; insufficient knowledge about how to enhance mutuality; insufficient skills to enhance mutuality; sociocultural dissonance

At-Risk Population

Absence of significant other

Associated Condition

Therapeutic isolation

NOC   (Nursing Outcomes Classification)

Suggested NOC Outcomes

Child Development: Middle Childhood, Adolescence; Play Participation; Role Performance; Social Interaction Skills; Social Involvement

Example NOC Outcome with Indicators

Social Involvement as evidenced by the following indicator: Interacts with close friends, neighbors, family members, and members of work groups. (Rate the outcome and indicators of **Social Involvement:** 1 = never demonstrated, 2 = rarely demonstrated, 3 = sometimes demonstrated, 4 = often demonstrated, 5 = consistently demonstrated [see Section I].)

Client Outcomes

Client Will (Specify Time Frame)

- Identify barriers that cause impaired social interactions
- Discuss feelings that accompany impaired and successful social interactions
- Use available opportunities to practice interactions
- Use successful social interaction behaviors
- Report increased comfort in social situations
- Communicate, state feelings of belonging, demonstrate caring and interest in others
- Report effective interactions with others

NIC   (Nursing Interventions Classification)

Suggested NIC Intervention

Socialization Enhancement

● = Independent;   ▲ = Collaborative;   EBN = Evidence-Based Nursing;   EB = Evidence-Based

Example NIC Activities—Socialization Enhancement
Encourage patience in developing relationships; Help client increase awareness of strengths and limitations in communicating with others

Nursing Interventions and *Rationales*

- Monitor the client's use of defense mechanisms and support healthy defenses (e.g., the client focuses on the present and avoids placing blame on others for personal behavior). CEBN: *Solution-focused techniques have been demonstrated to be beneficial. Therapy focuses on the client's present and future, capitalizing on the strengths and resources of the client and significant others around them (Wand, 2010).*
- Encourage the client to keep a gratitude journal. EB: *A recent study demonstrated that study participants who participated in a gratitude journal intervention experienced more positive emotions during the social interactions (Drążkowski, Kaczmarek, & Kashdan, 2017).*
- Encourage dancing with Parkinson's programs for individuals with Parkinson's disease. EB: *Research demonstrated that dance programs provide opportunities for social interaction and nonverbal communication (Bognar et al., 2017).*
- Model appropriate social interactions and use focused imitation interventions. Give positive verbal and nonverbal feedback for appropriate behavior (e.g., make statements such as, "I'm proud that you made it to work on time and did all the tasks assigned to you"; make eye contact). If not contraindicated, touch the client's arm or hand when speaking. CEBN: *Use of focused imitation interventions improved social functioning in children with autism spectrum disorders (ASDs) (Ingersoll, 2012).*
- Consider use of social cognition and interaction training (SCIT) combined with social mentoring to improve social functioning. EB: *A randomized controlled trial using SCIT and social mentoring demonstrated improved social cognition and social functioning in individuals with severe mental illness living in the community (Hasson-Ohayon et al, 2014).*
- Consider use of animal-assisted therapy (AAT). EB: *An AAT-treatment group showed improvement in negative symptoms of schizophrenia such as apathy, asociality, anhedonia, and alogia (Calvo et al., 2016).*
- ▲ Refer client for social cognition training to increase social skills. EB: *Social cognition training using targeted programs are most effective at improving social functioning in clients with a diagnosis of psychosis or schizophrenia (Henderson, 2013).*
- ▲ Refer rehabilitation clients for assistive technologies to increase therapeutic engagement and promote social engagement. EB: *Rehabilitation clients' desire to use mainstream technologies (cell phones, tablets, and computers) underscores the need for accessible options that will provide opportunities to engage in therapeutically meaningful activities and promote social interaction (Fager & Burnfield, 2014).*
- Refer to care plans for Risk for **Loneliness** and **Social** isolation for additional interventions.

 ### Pediatric

- Provide supervised interaction opportunities for children of chronically ill parents. EBN: *Research has identified that social isolation is a challenge for children with parents who experience chronic disabling pain (Umberger, Risko, & Covington, 2015).*
- Encourage family style dining (FSD) for preschool children to promote social interactions during mealtimes. EB: *The current study showed that rates of interactions were increased during FSD (Lochetta, Barton, & Kaiser, 2017).*
- Use peer-mediated interaction (PMI) to increase social interactions of children on the autistic spectrum. EB: *A review of studies showed that PMI was an effective intervention to increase social interaction intervention for promoting social interaction between students with ASD and their peers (Watkins et al., 2015).*
- Provide computers and Internet access to children with chronic disabilities that limit socialization. EB: *Children with autism showed more active other-awareness using technology with a supportive interface and when collaborating with a peer (Holt & Yuill, 2014).*
- ▲ Refer children with autism for family-centered music therapy (FCMT). EB: *Research demonstrated that family participation in FCMT improved social interactions in the home and community and the parent–child relationship (Thompson, McFerran, & Gold, 2014).*
- Consider the use of animal-assisted activities for children on the autistic spectrum. EB: *Research demonstrated significant improvements in social functioning and decreases in social withdrawal behaviors after 8 weeks of animal exposure in a school classroom in addition to 16 20-minute animal-interaction sessions (O'Haire et al, 2014).*

● = Independent; ▲ = Collaborative; EBN = Evidence-Based Nursing; EB = Evidence-Based

S

Geriatric

- Assess for depression in clients with impaired social functioning. **EB:** *Research shows higher depressive symptoms were associated with smaller numbers of close, inner circle relationships (Shouse, Rowe, & Mast, 2013).*
- Assess older clients for hearing loss and refer for hearing aids as needed. **EB:** *A recent study demonstrated that hearing aid fitting was associated with a subsequent improvement in older person-specific quality of life (Yamada, Švejdíková, & Kisvetrová, 2017).*
- Assess the communication patterns of clients with verbal domain problems for enactment strategies, paralinguistic features, and nonvocal communication. **EBN:** *Research has demonstrated that clients with semantic dementia spontaneously use enactment (acting out scenes), paralinguistic features (pitch and volume of tone), and nonvocal communication (e.g., body posture, pointing, facial expression) to compensate for loss of verbal abilities (Kindell et al, 2013).*
- Encourage socialization through physical activity and meaningful activities incorporated into normal daily care practices. **EB:** *The current study shows that when activities are performed, residents of a green care farm were more engaged and had more social interaction (de Boer et al., 2017).*
- Provide live concert music for clients with dementia. **EB:** *A recent study showed that clients with mild to midstage dementia had increased levels of cooperation, interaction, and conversation after a live music concert (Shibazaki & Marshall, 2015).*
- ▲ Refer depressed clients to services for cognitive-behavioral therapy (CBT). **EB:** *A systematic review indicated that CBT was likely to be efficacious for depression and accompanying symptoms such as impaired social functioning in older people (Jayasekara et al, 2015).*
- Refer to care plans for **Frail Elderly** syndrome, Risk for **Loneliness,** and **Social** isolation for additional interventions.

Multicultural

- Approach individuals of color with respect, warmth, and professional courtesy. **EBN:** *To provide client- and family-centered care, nurses must acknowledge their cultural differences, be willing to incorporate their beliefs within the health care treatment plan, and respect their values and lifeways of differing cultures (Hart & Mareno, 2015).*
- Use interpreters as needed. **EB:** *Primary care nurses act as gatekeepers to interpreting services (McCarthy et al, 2013).*
- Refer to care plan for **Social** isolation for additional interventions.

Home Care

- Previously discussed interventions may be adapted for home care use.

Client/Family Teaching and Discharge Planning

- Previously discussed interventions may be adapted for client/family teaching and discharge planning.

REFERENCES

Bognar, S., et al. (2017). More than just dancing: Experiences of people with Parkinson's disease in a therapeutic dance program. *Disability and Rehabilitation, 39*(11), 1073–1078. Retrieved from http://doi.org.proxy.lib.umich.edu/10.1080/09638288.2016.1175037.

Calvo, P., et al. (2016). Animal assisted therapy (AAT) program as a useful adjunct to conventional psychosocial rehabilitation for patients with schizophrenia: Results of a small-scale randomized controlled trial. *Frontiers in Psychology, 7*, 1–13. Retrieved from http://doi.org.proxy.lib.umich.edu/10.3389/fpsyg.2016.00631.

de Boer, B., et al. (2017). Green care farms as innovative nursing homes, promoting activities and social interaction for people with dementia. *Journal of the American Medical Directors Association, 18*(1), 40–46. doi:10.1016/j.jamda.2016.10.013.

Drążkowski, D., Kaczmarek, L. D., & Kashdan, T. B. (2017). Gratitude pays: A weekly gratitude intervention influences monetary decisions, physiological responses, and emotional experiences during a trust-related social interaction. *Personality and Individual Differences, 110,* 148–153. Retrieved from https://doi.org/10.1016/j.paid.2017.01.043.

Fager, S. K., & Burnfield, J. M. (2014). Patients' experiences with technology during inpatient rehabilitation: Opportunities to support independence and therapeutic engagement. *Disability & Rehabilitation. Assistive Technology, 9*(2), 121–127.

Hart, P. L., & Mareno, N. (2015). Cultural challenges and barriers through the voices of nurses. *Journal of Clinical Nursing, 23*(15/16), 2223–2233. *CINAHL Plus with Full Text,* EBSCO*host* (Accessed 27 June 2015).

Hasson-Ohayon, I., Mashiach-Eizenberg, M., Avidan, M., et al. (2014). Social cognition and interaction training: Preliminary results of an RCT in a community setting in Israel. *Psychiatric Services, 65*(4), 555–558.

● = Independent;   ▲ = Collaborative;   EBN = Evidence-Based Nursing;   EB = Evidence-Based

Henderson, A. R. (2013). The impact of social cognition training on recovery from psychosis. *Current Opinion in Psychiatry*, 26(5), 429–432.

Holt, S. 1., & Yuill, N. (2014). Facilitating other-awareness in low-functioning children with autism and typically-developing preschoolers using dual-control technology. *Journal of Autism and Developmental Disorders*, 44(1), 236–248.

Ingersoll, B. (2012). Brief report: Effect of a focused imitation intervention on social functioning in children with autism. *Journal of Autism & Developmental Disorders*, 42(8), 1768–1773.

Jayasekara, R., Procter, N., Harrison, J., et al. (2015). Cognitive behavioural therapy for older adults with depression: A review. *Journal of Mental Health*, 24(3), 168–171.

Kindell, J., Sage, K., Keady, J., et al. (2013). Adapting to conversation with semantic dementia: Using enactment as a compensatory strategy in everyday social interaction. *International Journal of Language & Communication Disorders*, 48(5), 497–507.

Lochetta, B. M., Barton, E. E., & Kaiser, A. (2017). Using family style dining to increase social interactions in young children. *Topics in Early Cildhood Special Education*, 37(1), 54–64. Retrieved from http://doi.org.proxy.lib.umich.edu/10.1177/0271121416678078.

McCarthy, J., Cassidy, I., Graham, M. M., et al. (2013). Conversations through barriers of language and interpretation. *British Journal of Nursing*, 22(6), 335–339.

O'Haire, M. E., McKenzie, S. J., McCune, S., et al. (2014). Effects of classroom animal-assisted activities on social functioning in children with autism spectrum disorder. *Journal of Alternative & Complementary Medicine*, 20(3), 162–168.

Shibazaki, K., & Marshall, N. A. (2015). Exploring the impact of music concerts in promoting well-being in dementia care. *Aging & Mental Health*, 21(5), 468–476. Retrieved from http://doi.org.proxy.lib.umich.edu/10.1080/13607863.2015.1114589.

Shouse, J. N., Rowe, S. V., & Mast, B. T. (2013). Depression and cognitive functioning as predictors of social network size. *Clinical Gerontologist*, 36(2), 147–161.

Thompson, G. A., McFerran, K. S., & Gold, C. (2014). Family-centred music therapy to promote social engagement in young children with severe autism spectrum disorder: A randomized controlled study. *Child: Care, Health and Development*, 40(6), 840–852.

Umberger, W. A., Risko, J., & Covington, E. (2015). The forgotten ones: Challenges and needs of children living with disabling parental chronic pain. *Journal of Pediatric Nursing*, 30(3), 498–507.

Wand, T. (2010). Mental health nursing from a solution focused perspective. *International Journal of Mental Health Nursing*, 19(3), 210–219.

Watkins, L., O'reilly, M., Kuhn, M., et al. (2015). A review of peer-mediated social interaction interventions for students with autism in inclusive settings. *Journal of Autism and Developmental Disorders*, 45(4), 1070–1083. Retrieved from http://dx.doi.org.proxy.lib.umich.edu/10.1007/s10803-014-2264-x.

Yamada, Y., Švejdíková, B., & Kisvetrová, H. (2017). Improvement of older-person-specific QOL after hearing aid fitting and its relation to social interaction. *Journal of Communication Disorders*, 67, 14–21. doi:10.1016/j.jcomdis.2017.05.001.

Social isolation *Julianne E. Doubet, BSN, RN, EMT-B*

NANDA-I

Definition

Aloneness experienced by the individual and perceived as imposed by others and as a negative or threatening state.

Defining Characteristics

Absence of support system; aloneness imposed by others; cultural incongruence; desire to be alone; development delay; disabling condition; feeling different from others; flat affect; history of rejection; hostility; illness; inability to meet expectations of others; insecurity in public; meaningless actions; member of a subculture; poor eye contact; preoccupation with own thoughts; purposelessness; repetitive actions; sad affect; values incongruent with cultural norms; withdrawn

Related Factors

Developmentally inappropriate interests; difficulty establishing relationships; inability to engage in satisfying personal relationships; insufficient personal resources; social behavior incongruent with norms; values incongruent with cultural norms

Associated Condition

Alteration in mental status; alteration in physical appearance; alteration in wellness

NOC (Nursing Outcomes Classification)

Suggested NOC Outcomes

Loneliness Severity; Mood Equilibrium; Personal Well-Being; Play Participation; Social Anxiety Level; Social Interaction Skills; Social Involvement; Social Support

● = Independent;   ▲ = Collaborative;   EBN = Evidence-Based Nursing;   EB = Evidence-Based

Example NOC Outcome with Indicators

Social Involvement as evidenced by the following indicator: Interacts with close friends, neighbors, family members, and members of work groups. (Rate the outcome and indicators of **Social Involvement:** I = never demonstrated, 2 = rarely demonstrated, 3 = sometimes demonstrated, 4 = often demonstrated, 5 = consistently demonstrated [see Section I].)

Client Outcomes

Client Will (Specify Time Frame)

- Identify feelings of isolation
- Practice social and communication skills needed to interact with others
- Initiate interactions with others; set and meet goals
- Participate in activities and programs at level of ability and desire
- Describe feelings of self-worth

NIC   (Nursing Interventions Classification)

Suggested NIC Intervention

Socialization Enhancement

Example NIC Activities—Socialization Enhancement

Encourage patience in developing relationships; Help patient increase awareness of strengths and limitations in communicating with others

Nursing Interventions and *Rationales*

- Establish a therapeutic relationship with the client. **EBN:** *In her study, Skingley (2013) suggested that many of the circumstances that contribute to social isolation are amendable and that the community nurse is in the position to affect changes.*
- Observe for barriers to social interaction. **EBN:** *A study by Drury (2014) stated that social isolation can be measured by objective indicators, such as the client's social network, his or her participation in community activities, and by subjective indicators, including a client's self-rating of loneliness and perception of support.*
- Discuss/assess causes of perceived or actual isolation. **EBN:** *Some variables that were recognized by Nicholson, Dixon, and McCorkle (2014) as precursors to diminished social interaction included severe health problems, symptoms of depression, smoking, and decreased religious participation.*
- Allow the client opportunities to describe his or her daily life and to introduce any issues that may be of concern. **EBN:** *McDonald (2014) surmised that the biggest problem in health care today is lack of communication skills, which can then be related to poor client outcome, and maintained that the nurse of today must be proficient in effective communication.*
- Promote social interactions. **EB:** *Positive social interactions may act as a basis for the client to establish new social group relationships (Cruwys et al, 2014).*
- Assist the client in identifying specific health and social problems and involve him or her in their resolution. **EBN:** *Pearce (2013) maintained that interventions customized to fit a client's disorganized lifestyle reduced his or her social isolation.*
- Assist the client in identifying activities that encourage socialization. **EB:** *According to this study, the sooner the older client is supported in mobility and social participation, the sooner he or she will be able to experience a sense of well-being and lessening of the feelings of social isolation (Elbasan et al, 2013).*
- Identify available support systems and involve those individuals in the client's care. **EBN:** *According to Mattila et al (2014), nurse support of clients and their families is effective in establishing a positive outlook, mental well-being, and thoughts of getting well.* **EB:** *"Clinicians should be aware of social isolation and loneliness in late life and discuss nonpharmacological treatment options with their aging patients" (Canham, 2014).*
- ▲ Refer clients and caregivers to support groups as necessary. **EB:** *Caring for a family member who is physically and/or mentally challenged can be a drain on caregivers, causing a negative effect both on the client and the caregiver: effective outside assistance might be a factor in modifying the challenges confronted by these families (Thompson et al, 2014).*

● = Independent;   ▲ = Collaborative;   EBN = Evidence-Based Nursing;   EB = Evidence-Based

- Encourage interactions with others with similar interests. **EBN:** *According to this research study, a community integrative therapy program will allow those involved to form new relationships, gather emotional support, reinforce ties, and reduce social isolation (da Roche et al, 2013).*
- See the care plan for Risk for **Loneliness.**

Pediatric

▲ Refer obese adolescents for diet, exercise, and psychosocial support. **EB:** *Nesbit et al (2014) suggested that to combat adolescent obesity interventions should target sedentary behavior and promote the increase of physical activity. Interventions should also address parental concerns about neighborhood safety and access to safe areas for physical activity development.* **EBN:** *This study found that family meals two to three times per week during adolescence are an important factor in preventing obesity in young adulthood (Berge et al, 2015).*

▲ Assess socially isolated adolescents. Refer to appropriate rehabilitation programs as needed. **EB:** *A study by Plaiser and Konijn (2013) implied that both peers and media have a firm influence on adolescents and that peer rejection may be why adolescents turn to antisocial media content.*

Geriatric

▲ Assess physical and mental status to establish an early baseline for referring at-risk individuals to community resources. **CBE:** *In this study, Nicholson (2012) stated that health professionals can take measures that will allow early detection of social isolation in at-risk, older clients and match them to suitable community resources; this may serve to prevent negative health outcomes.* **EB:** *Older individuals should be routinely screened for depression because it may be a crucial factor in giving rise to later social isolation (Pritchard et al, 2014).*

- Assess for hearing. **EB:** *It is well documented that hearing loss is common in older adults; it is also considered a known factor in the cause of social isolation, depression, and dementia (Genther et al, 2014).*

- Involve client in planning activities. **EBN:** *According to Drury (2014), programs for the socially isolated should be planned and coordinated with contributions from various community groups and those of the recipients.*

- Involve nonprofessionals in activities and projects with the client. **EB:** *Pettigrew et al (2014) wrote that both group activities and a focused approach to those clients who are at risk for social isolation may be the way to manage the problem.*

- Suggest varied social activities that would decrease isolation and encourage participation. **EB:** *Leisure activities can play a significant part in an older person's social life and improve their quality of life; these could include volunteer work, cultural activities, sports, reading books, hobbies, and shopping (Toepoel, 2013).*

▲ Consider the use of simulated presence therapy (see the care plan for **Hopelessness**). **EB:** *Obdrzalek et al (2013) promoted an automated exercise coaching system for older adults living in assisted homes: this technique is designed to allow remote interaction with a coach and to strengthen the social aspects of exercise.*

- Consider using computers and the Internet to alleviate or reduce loneliness and social isolation. **EB:** *The use of technology that is tailored to older people may aid in better self-management of health conditions; thus it may produce an increased improvement in social connectedness (Morris et al, 2014).*

Multicultural

- Acknowledge racial/ethnic differences at the onset of care. **EB:** *Every client has a unique culture that has many aspects, is vibrant, and cannot be labeled by race or language group (Hawes & Viera, 2014).*

- Assess for the influence of cultural beliefs, norms, values, and the client's personal cultural needs. **EBN:** *Culturally responsive caregiver involvement is necessary to make certain that people of culturally and linguistically dissimilar backgrounds have the proper skills to self-manage their multifaceted medical conditions (Williams et al, 2014).*

- Use a culturally competent, professional approach when working with clients of various ethnic groups. **EBN:** *Today's professional nurse must be aware of the role of cultural competency and cultural safety in his or her practice (Rowan et al, 2013).*

- Promote a sense of ethnic attachment. **EB:** *According to Enguidanos et al (2014), there is a need for client-centered intervention and prevention standards that incorporate the client's cultural background, health care requirements, and individual preferences.*

- Assess the client's feelings regarding social isolation. **EBN:** *Feelings that contribute to the client's perception of social isolation may include loneliness, anger, fear, despair, and sadness (Hadi & Hadi, 2017).*

● = Independent;   ▲ = Collaborative;   **EBN** = Evidence-Based Nursing;   **EB** = Evidence-Based

- Assist those ethnic minorities who are underserved to access essential health care. EBN: *Jeffreys and Dogan (2013) maintained that a comprehensive nursing assessment is the first step necessary in providing culturally specialized care, recognition of high-risk groups, and reduction of health care inequality.* EBN: *According to Waite, Nardi, and Killian (2014), it is vital that clinicians recognize the necessity of cultural competence in their practice to both improve and maintain health care for their clients.*

 ### Home Care

- The interventions described previously may be adapted for home care use.
- Confirm that the home setting has health-safety systems in place. EB: *The medical and safety goals for older adults should be taken into account when redesigning an approach for home care delivery (Depuccio & Hoff, 2014).*
- Consider the use of the computer and Internet to decrease isolation social interaction. EBN: *A study by Culley et al (2013) illustrated the ability of technology to develop connectedness and diminish the feeling of isolation in community-dwelling older adults.*
- Assess options for living that allow the client privacy but not isolation. EBN: *Rulliere (2014) explained that a person's dignity and privacy must be preserved, regardless of his or her cognitive ability, not only when receiving nursing care but also in all phases of life.*
- Assist clients to interact with neighbors in the community when they move to supported housing. EB: *Those clients transferring to supported housing will be placed in an unfamiliar environment that necessitates the need to develop skills to successfully adapt to their new surroundings (Kirchen & Hersch, 2015).*

 ### Client/Family Teaching and Discharge Planning

- Assist the client in initiating contacts with self-help groups, counselors, and therapists. EBN: *Seebohm et al (2013) advised, as a result of their study, that policy-makers might partner with the local population to provide support for diverse types of residents to facilitate their own self-help/mutual aid groups.*
- Provide information to the client about senior citizen services and community resources. EB: *Senior centers are excellent locations to deliver evidence-based health support programs that will bolster this rapidly growing age group in remaining healthy and independent (Felix et al, 2014).*
- Refer socially isolated caregivers to appropriate support groups. EBN: *Eriksson, Sandberg, and Hellstrom (2013) maintained that woman who are 24/7 caregivers need choices that can be recommended by health care professionals who will not disregard their ethical concerns.*
- See the care plan for **Caregiver Role Strain**.

REFERENCES

Berge, J. M., Wall, M., Hsueh, T. F., et al. (2015). The protective role of family meals for youth obesity: 10 years longitudinal associations. *Journal of Pediatrics, 166*(2), 296–301.

Canham, S. L. (2014). What's loneliness got to do with it? Older woman who use benzodiazepines. *Australian Journal on Ageing, 26.* [Epub ahead of print].

Cruwys, T., Dingle, G. A., Hornsby, M. J., et al. (2014). Social isolation schema responds to positive social experiences: Longitudinal evidence from vulnerable populations. *British Journal of Clinical Psychology, 53*, 265–280. [Epub 2014 Jan 13].

Culley, J. M., Herman, J., Smith, D., et al. (2013). Effects of technology and connectedness in community dwelling older adults. *On-Line Journal of Nursing Informatics, 17*, 1–6.

da Roche, I. A., al Sa, A. N., Braga, L. A., et al. (2013). Community integrative therapy: Situations of emotional suffering and patients' coping strategies. *Revista Gaúcha de Enfermagem, 34*, 135–162.

Depuccio, M. J., & Hoff, T. J. (2014). Medical home interventions and quality outcomes for older adults: A systematic review. *Quality Management in Health Care, 23*, 226–239.

Drury, R. (2014). Social Isolation and loneliness in the elderly: an exploration of some of the issues. *British Journal of Community Nursing, 19*, 125–128.

Elbasan, B., Yilmaz, G. D., Cirak, Y., et al. (2013). Cultural adaption of the friendship scale and health-related quality of life and functional mobility parameters in the elderly living at home and

in the nursing home. *Topics in Geriatric Rehabilitation, 29*, 265–280.

Enguidanos, S. M., Deliema, M., Aguilar, I., et al. (2014). Multicultural voices: Attitudes of older adults in the United States about elder mistreatment. *Ageing and Society, 34*, 877–903.

Eriksson, H., Sandberg, J., & Hellstrom, I. (2013). Experience of long-term home care as an informa; care giver to a spouse: Gendered meanings in everyday life for female caregivers. *International Journal of Older People Nursing, 8*, 159–165.

Felix, H. C., Adams, B., Cornell, C., et al. (2014). Barriers and facilitators to senior center participating in translational research. *Research on Aging, 36*, 22–39.

Genther, D. J., Betz, J., Pratt, S., et al. (2014). Association of hearing impairment and morbidity in older adults. *The Journals of Gerontology, 14.*

Hadi, H., & Hadi, S. (2017). Social isolation—A current reality in the corridors of our society. *Journal of Nursing, 7*(1), 29–33.

Hawes, E. M., & Viera, A. J. (2014). Immigrant and refugee health: Cross cultural communication. *FP Essentials, 423*, 30–39.

Jeffreys, M., & Dogan, E. (2013). Evaluating cultural competence in the clinical practicum. *Nursing Education Perspectives, 34*, 88–94.

Kirchen, T., & Hersch, G. (2015). Understanding person and environment factors that facilitate veteran adaption to long-term care. *Physical and Occupational Therapy in Geriatrics, 33*(3), 204–219.

• = Independent;   ▲ = Collaborative;   EBN = Evidence-Based Nursing;   EB = Evidence-Based

Mattila, E., Kaunonen, M., Aalto, P., et al. (2014). The method of nursing support in hospital and patients' and family members' experiences of the effectiveness of the support. *Scandinavian Journal of Caring Sciences, 28,* 305–314.

McDonald, A. M. (2014). *Simulation education of communication skills and the effects on nurse empowerment* (p. 201). Teachers College, Columbia University, EdD.

Morris, M. E., Adair, B., Ozanne, E., et al. (2014). Smart technologies to enhance social connectiveness in older people who live at home. *Australasian Journal on Ageing, 33,* 142–152 [Epub 2014 Apr 15].

Nesbit, K. C., Kolobe, T. H., Sisson, S. B., et al. (2014). A model of environment correlates of adolescent obesity in the United States. *Journal of Adolescent Health, 55,* 394–401. Retrieved from http://dx.doi.org.ezproxy.jccmi.edu/10.1016/j.jadohealth.2014.02.022.

Nicholson, N. R. (2012). A review of social isolation: An important but underassessed condition in older adults *Journal of Primary Prevention, 33,* 137–152.

Nicholson, R., Dixon, J. K., & McCorkle, A. U. (2014). Predictions of dementia levels of social integration in older adults. *Research in Gerontological Nursing, 7,* 33–43. [Epub 2013 Sep 25].

Obdrzalek, S., Kurillo, G., Seto, E., et al. (2013). Architecture of an automated coaching system for elderly populations. *Studies in Health Technologies and informatics, 184,* 309–311.

Pearce, L. (2013). Self care success. *Nursing Standard, 27,* 19.

Pettigrew, S., Donavon, R., Boldy, D., et al. (2014). Older people's perceived causes of and strategies for dealing with social isolation. *Aging and Mental Health, 18,* 914–920. [Epub 2014 Mar 31].

Plaiser, X. S., & Konijn, A. (2013). Rejected by peers-attracted to antisocial media content: Rejection-based anger impairs moral judgment among adolescents. *Developmental Psychology, 49,* 1105–1173. [Epub 2012 Jul 16].

Pritchard, E., Barker, A., Day, L., et al. (2014). Factors impacting the recreation participation of older adults living in the community. *Disability and Rehabilitation, 24.*

Rowan, M. S., Ruckholm, E., Bourque-Bearskin, L., et al. (2013). Cultural competence and cultural safety in Canadian schools of nursing: A mixed methods study. *International Journal of Nursing Education Scholarship, 10,* 1–10.

Rulliere, N. (2014). Privacy and dignity in nursing homes. *Revue de L'infirmiere, 200,* 37–38.

Seebohm, P., Chaudnary, S., Boyce, M., et al. (2013). The contribution of self help/mutual aid groups to mental well-being. *Health and Social Care in the Community, 21,* 391–401.

Skingley, A. (2013). Older people, isolation and loneliness: Implications for community nursing. *British Journal of Community Nursing, 18,* 84–90.

Thompson, R., Kerr, M., Glynn, M., et al. (2014). Caring for a family with intellectual disability and epilepsy: Practical, social and emotional perspectives. *Seizure: The Journal of the British Epilepsy Association, 19.* [Epub ahead of print].

Toepoel, V. (2013). Ageing, leisure, and social connectedness: How could leisure help reduce social isolation of older people? *Social Indicators Research, 113,* 355–372.

Waite, R., Nardi, D., & Killian, P. (2014). Examination of cultural knowledge and provider sensitivity in nurse managed health centers. *Journal of Cultural Diversity, 21,* 74–79.

Williams, A., Manias, E., Cross, W., et al. (2014). Motivational interviewing to explore culturally and linguistically diverse people's medication self-efficacy. *The Journal of Clinical Nursing, 30* [Epub ahead of print].

Chronic Sorrow   Tracy P. George, DNP, APRN-BC, CNE

NANDA-I

S

Definition

Cyclical, recurring, and potentially progressive pattern of pervasive sadness experienced (by parent, caregiver, individual with chronic illness or disability) in response to continual loss throughout the trajectory of an illness or disability.

Defining Characteristics

Feeling that interferes with well-being; overwhelming negative feelings; sadness

Related Factors

Crisis in disability management; crisis in illness management; missed milestones; missed opportunities

At-Risk Population

Death of significant other; developmental crisis; length of time as a caregiver

Associated Condition

Chronic disability; chronic illness

NOC   (Nursing Outcomes Classification)

Suggested NOC Outcomes

Acceptance: Health Status; Depression Level; Depression Self-Control; Grief Resolution; Hope; Mood Equilibrium

● = Independent; ▲ = Collaborative; **EBN** = Evidence-Based Nursing; **EB** = Evidence-Based

Example NOC Outcome with Indicators
Grief Resolution with plans for a positive future as evidenced by the following indicators: Describes meaning of loss or death/Reports decreased preoccupation with loss/Reports adequate nutritional intake/Reports adequate sleep/Expresses positive expectations about the future. (Rate the outcome and indicators of **Grief Resolution:** 1 = never demonstrated, 2 = rarely demonstrated, 3 = sometimes demonstrated, 4 = often demonstrated, 5 = consistently demonstrated [see Section I].)

Client Outcomes

Client Will (Specify Time Frame)

- Express appropriate feelings of guilt, fear, anger, or sadness
- Identify problems associated with sorrow (e.g., changes in appetite, insomnia, nightmares, loss of libido, decreased energy, alteration in activity levels)
- Seek help in dealing with grief-associated problems
- Plan for the future one day at a time
- Function at normal developmental level

NIC   (Nursing Interventions Classification)

Suggested NIC Interventions

Grief Work Facilitation; Grief Work Facilitation: Perinatal Death

Example NIC Activities—Grief Work Facilitation
Encourage client to verbalize memories of loss, both past and current; Assist client in identifying personal coping strategies

Nursing Interventions and *Rationales*

- Determine the client's degree of sorrow. EBN: *Use the Adapted Burke Questionnaire for the individual or caregiver, which assesses eight mood states including grief, shock, anger, disbelief, sadness, hopelessness, fear, and guilt on a four-point scale (Whittingham et al, 2013).*
- Assess for the four discrete stages of grieving in chronic obstructive pulmonary disease (COPD) clients. EB: *The four stages of grief for clients with COPD can be assessed by the Acceptance of Disease and Impairments Questionnaire (Boer et al, 2014).*
- Provide coping strategies for caregivers who may experience chronic sorrow. EBN: *Coping strategies for the caregivers of clients with schizophrenia may include discussing their feelings about the situation with others, reading, praying, being physically active; emotional strategies such as crying; and cognitive strategies such as thinking positively about the situation (Olwit et al, 2015). See care plan for* **Caregiver Role Strain.**
- Assess clients for chronic sorrow and provide them with coping strategies. CEB: *Clients who come to the emergency department frequently may be at an increased risk for chronic sorrow (Joseph, 2012).*
- Develop a trusting relationship to care for clients with chronic sorrow. EBN: *Creating rapport and a close connection is helpful when caring for clients experiencing chronic sorrow (Johnson, 2015).* EBN: *Nurses should offer compassion, empathy, consideration, and knowledge to those experiencing chronic sorrow (Glenn, 2015).*
- Help the client understand that sorrow may be ongoing. CEB: *Studies have demonstrated that feelings of sadness, guilt, anger, frustration, and fear occur periodically throughout the lives of people experiencing chronic loss, resulting in chronic sorrow (Isaksson & Ahlström, 2008).*
- Urge the client to use positive coping techniques:
  - EBN: *Encourage the client to participate in a support group, talk with others, or communicate via an online support group (Vitale & Falco, 2014).* EBN: *Support groups, counseling, and participating in activities are strategies that can be used with clients who are experiencing chronic sorrow (Marcella-Brienza, 2015).*
  - EBN: *Encourage the client to engage in a hobby or physical activity (Vitale & Falco, 2014).*
  - EBN: *Encourage the client to think positively about the situation (Vitale & Falco, 2014).*
  - EBN: *Encourage the client to discuss his or her situation with a provider, such as a nurse, physician, or social worker (Vitale & Falco, 2014).*
  - EBN: *Discuss the need for the client to anticipate triggers that may increase chronic sorrow (Vitale & Falco, 2014).* EB: *Triggers for parents of children with cerebral palsy may include times in which there is*

- = Independent;   ▲ = Collaborative;   EBN = Evidence-Based Nursing;   EB = Evidence-Based

awareness of the actual versus expected achievements of the child or during times of medical intervention (Whittingham et al, 2013).

○ **EB:** *Refer for professional counseling if needed (Hottensen, 2013).*

▲ Refer the client for mental health services if needed. **EB:** *There may be an increase in depression among patients with chronic sorrow, so the nurse may need to refer the patient for mental health care (Ghesquiere et al, 2016).*

○ Refer clients for financial assistance if needed. **EB:** *Bereavement may be associated with financial burdens caused by the loss of income (Ghesquiere et al, 2016).*

Pediatric

- Encourage the parents of children with uncommon diseases to use online resources to manage their chronic sorrow. **EBN:** *In a study of 16 mothers of children with a rare disease, online communication was used effectively to manage chronic sorrow (Glenn, 2015).*
- Educate parents that an increase in chronic sorrow can occur after stressful events. **EB:** *An increase in chronic sorrow was noted in parents with children who have cerebral palsy after triggering events, indicating that recurring grieving can occur after the diagnosis is made. Triggers can include when the child would have met a developmental milestone or started school (Whittingham et al, 2013).*
- Nurses should assess for chronic sorrow and discuss coping strategies for parents of children who have been in the neonatal intensive care unit (NICU). **EBN:** *Chronic sorrow is a useful framework for families affected by a NICU stay (Vitale & Falco, 2014).*
- Allow children the opportunity to talk about the impending death of a parent or loved one. **CEB:** *In a qualitative study of seven children whose parent was dying, children often were not encouraged to discuss their feelings, and they developed anxiety and ways to deal with the stress (Buchwald, Delmar, & Schantz-Laursen, 2012).*
- Encourage parents to listen to their child's expression of grief. **EB:** *It is important for parents whose child is grieving to listen to their child's concerns and create a balance between making new memories while holding onto the old memories (Bugge et al, 2014).*
- Educate parents that children may grieve differently than adults. **EB:** *Children may grieve intermittently for short periods of time in "grief puddles," certain children may grieve at each developmental stage, and some children may try to console their parents instead of going through the grieving process themselves (Gao & Slaven, 2017).*
- ▲ Refer grieving children to peer support groups. **EB:** *Peer support groups with other children who are grieving are important for children with chronic sorrow (Gao & Slaven, 2017).*
- Encourage children experiencing grief to participate in bereavement activities and camps. **EB:** *In children who participated in a ropes course as activities-based counseling during bereavement camp, five themes were noted: grief as a process, expression of feelings, support, coping, and empowerment and hope (Swank, 2013).*
- Encourage children who are grieving to participate in other forms of therapy, in addition to individual counseling and psychotherapy. **EB:** *Art therapy, play therapy, music therapy, and bibliotherapy are useful for children with chronic sorrow (Gao & Slaven, 2017).*
- Help the adolescent with chronic sorrow determine sources of support and refer for counseling if needed. **EB:** *Cognitive-behavioral therapy along with parental counseling has been useful in adolescents who experience prolonged grief (Spuij, Dekovic, & Boelen, 2015).*
- Provide family-centered care to parents of children with disabilities, and encourage parents to attend support groups. **EB:** *Caring for a child with cerebral palsy affects the quality of life for families and is related to anticipatory grieving among parents (Al-Gamal, 2013).*
- Encourage parents with chronic sorrow to participate in an online support group and learn coping strategies. **EB:** *Online bereavement support groups for parents who have lost children can be a convenient and anonymous way to obtain coping support (Elder & Burke, 2015).*
- Recognize that mothers who have a miscarriage or lose an infant often grieve and experience sorrow. **EB:** *Telephone hotlines staffed 24-hours a day by peer volunteers can be an effective way to provide support for women who have experienced the loss of a pregnancy (Boyle et al, 2015).* **EBN:** *It is important for providers to offer compassionate care to women after the loss of an infant (McGuinness, Coughlan, & Power, 2014).*

Geriatric

- Identify previous losses and assess the client for depression. **EB:** *Bereavement may result in major depression in some older adults, and participation support groups can be helpful in depression management (Ghesquiere, Shear, & Duan, 2013).*

- Evaluate the social support system of the older client and refer for bereavement counseling if needed. **EB:** *In a study of 28 geriatric clients who had recently experienced a death, older adults often used family and friends as a support network after death, but community-based organizations also play an important role in bereavement support (Bellamy et al, 2014).*

 Home Care

- In-home bereavement follow-up by nurses should be considered if available. **EBN:** *In Australia, home health nurses provide bereavement visits in which they provide comfort, counseling, client education, and encouragement and also evaluate the client who has recently experienced a loss (Brownhill et al, 2013).*
- Assess the client for depression and refer for mental health services if appropriate. **EB:** *Clients experiencing bereavement are at risk for depression, so assessing for depression is necessary (Ghesquiere, Shear, & Duan, 2013).*
- Encourage the client to participate in activities that are diversionary and uplifting as tolerated (e.g., outdoor activities, hobby groups, church-related activities, pet care). **EBN:** *Diversionary activities decrease the time spent in sorrow, can give meaning to life, and provide a sense of well-being (Vitale & Falso, 2014).*
- Encourage the client to participate in support groups appropriate to the area of loss or illness. **EBN:** *Support groups can increase an individual's sense of belonging (Vitale & Falco, 2014).*
- Provide empathetic communication for family/caregivers. **EB:** *Nurses should offer compassion and empathy to those experiencing chronic sorrow (Glenn, 2015).*
- The interventions described previously may be adapted for home care use.
- See the care plans for Chronic low **Self-Esteem,** Risk for **Loneliness,** and **Hopelessness.**

REFERENCES

Al-Gamal, E. (2013). Quality of life and anticipatory grieving among parents living with a child with cerebral palsy. *International Journal of Nursing Practice,* 19(3), 288–294.

Bellamy, G., Gott, M., Waterworth, S., et al. (2014). But I do believe you've got to accept that that's what life's about': Older adults living in New Zealand talk about their experiences of loss and bereavement support. *Health & Social Care in the Community,* 22(1), 96–103.

Boer, L., Daudey, L., Peters, J., et al. (2014). Assessing the stages of the grieving process in chronic obstructive pulmonary disease (COPD): Validation of the acceptance of disease and impairments questionnaire (ADIQ). *International Journal of Behavioral Medicine,* 21(3), 561–570.

Boyle, F. M., Mutch, A. J., Barber, E. A., et al. (2015). Supporting parents following pregnancy loss: A cross-sectional study of telephone peer supporters. *BMC Pregnancy and Childbirth,* 15, 291. doi:10.1186/s12884-015-0713-y.

Brownhill, S., Chang, E., Bidewell, J., et al. (2013). A decision model for community nurses providing bereavement care. *British Journal of Community Nursing,* 18(3), 133–139.

Buchwald, D., Delmar, C., & Schantz-Laursen, B. (2012). How children handle life when their mother or father is seriously ill and dying. *Scandinavian Journal of Caring Sciences,* 26(2), 228–235.

Bugge, K. E., Darbyshire, P., Røkholt, E. G., et al. (2014). Young children's grief: Parents' understanding and coping. *Death Studies,* 38(1), 36–43.

Elder, J., & Burke, L. A. (2015). Parental grief expression in online cancer support groups. *Illness, Crises, and Loss,* 23(2), 175–190. doi:10.1177/1054137315576617.

Gao, M., & Slaven, M. (2017). Best practices in children's bereavement: A qualitative analysis of needs and services. *Journal of Pain Management,* 10(1), 119–126.

Ghesquiere, A. R., Bazelais, K. N., Berman, J., et al. (2016). Associations between recent bereavement and psychological and financial burden in homebound older adults. *Omega,* 73(4), 326–339. doi:10.1177/0030222815590709.

Ghesquiere, A., Shear, M. K., & Duan, N. (2013). Outcomes of bereavement care among widowed older adults with complicated grief and depression. *Journal of Primary Care & Community Health,* 4(4), 256–264.

Glenn, A. D. (2015). Using online health communication to manage chronic sorrow: Mothers of children with rare diseases speak. *Journal of Pediatric Nursing,* 30(1), 17–24.

Hottensen, D. (2013). Bereavement: Caring for families and friends after a patient dies. *Omega,* 67(1–2), 121–126.

Isaksson, A., & Ahlström, G. (2008). Managing chronic sorrow: Experiences of patients with multiple sclerosis. *Journal of Neuroscience Nursing,* 40(3), 180–191.

Johnson, A. (2015). Role of district and community nurses in bereavement care: A qualitative study. *British Journal of Community Nursing,* 20(10), 494–501.

Joseph, H. A. (2012). Recognizing chronic sorrow in the habitual ED patient. *Journal of Emergency Nursing: JEN,* 38(6), 539–540.

Marcella-Brienza, S. (2015). Back to work: Manager support of nurses with chronic sorrow. *Creative Nursing,* 21(4), 206–210. doi:10.1891/1078-4535.21.4.206.

McGuinness, D., Coughlan, B., & Power, S. (2014). Empty arms: Supporting bereaved mothers during the immediate postnatal period. *British Journal Of Midwifery,* 22(4), 246–252.

Olwit, C., Musisi, S., Leshabari, S., et al. (2015). Chronic sorrow: Lived experiences of caregivers of patients diagnosed with schizophrenia in Butabika Mental Hospital, Kampala, Uganda. *Archives of Psychiatric Nursing,* 29(1), 43–48.

Spuij, M., Dekovic, M., & Boelen, P. A. (2015). An open trial of 'grief-help': A cognitive-behavioural treatment for prolonged grief in children and adolescents. *Clinical Psychology & Psychotherapy,* 22(2), 185–192.

Swank, J. M. (2013). Obstacles of grief: The experiences of children processing grief on the ropes course. *Journal of Creativity in Mental Health,* 8(3), 235–248.

Vitale, S. A., & Falco, C. (2014). Children born prematurely: Risk of parental chronic sorrow. *Journal of Pediatric Nursing,* 29(3), 248–251.

Whittingham, K., Wee, D., Sanders, M. R., et al. (2013). Sorrow, coping and resiliency: Parents of children with cerebral palsy share their experiences. *Disability & Rehabilitation,* 35(17), 1447–1452.

S

Spiritual distress   *Barbara Baele Vincensi, PhD, RN, FNP and Elizabeth Burkhart, PhD, RN, ANEF*

NANDA-I

Definition

A state of suffering related to the impaired ability to experience meaning in life through connections with self, others, the world, or a superior being.

Defining Characteristics

Connections to Self

Anger; decrease in serenity; feeling unloved; guilt; inadequate acceptance; ineffective coping strategies; insufficient courage; perceived insufficient meaning in life

Connections with Others

Alienation; refuses to interact with spiritual leader; refuses to interact with significant other; separation from support system

Connections with Art, Music, Literature, Nature

Decrease in expression of previous pattern of creativity; disinterest in nature; disinterest in reading spiritual literature

Connections with Power Greater Than Oneself

Anger toward power greater than self; feeling abandoned; hopelessness; inability for introspection; inability to experience the transcendent; inability to participate in religious activities; inability to pray; perceived suffering; request for a spiritual leader; sudden change in spiritual practice

Related Factors

Anxiety; barrier to experiencing love; change in religious ritual; change in spiritual practice; cultural conflict; depression; environmental change; inability to forgive; increasing dependence on another; ineffective relationships; loneliness; low self-esteem; pain; perception of having unfinished business; self-alienation; separation from support system; social alienation; sociocultural deprivation; stressors; substance misuse

At-Risk Population

Aging; birth of a child; death of significant other; exposure to death; exposure to natural disaster; life transition; loss; racial conflict; receiving bad news; unexpected life event

Associated Condition

Actively dying; chronic illness; illness; imminent death; loss of body part; loss of function of a body part; physical illness; treatment regimen

NOC   (Nursing Outcomes Classification)

Suggested NOC Outcomes

Coping; Dignified Life Closure; Grief Resolution; Hope; Spiritual Health; Stress Level

> **Example NOC Outcome with Indicators**
>
> **Spiritual Health** as evidenced by the following indicators: Quality of faith, hope, meaning, and purpose in life/ Connectedness with inner-self and with others to share thoughts, feelings, and beliefs. (Rate each indicator of **Spiritual Health:** 1 = severely compromised, 2 = substantially compromised, 3 = moderately compromised, 4 = mildly compromised, 5 = not compromised [see Section I].)

Client Outcomes

Client Will (Specify Time Frame)

- Express meaning and purpose in life
- Express sense of hope in the future

● = Independent;   ▲ = Collaborative;   EBN = Evidence-Based Nursing;   EB = Evidence-Based

- Express sense of connectedness with self
- Express sense of connectedness with family/friends
- Express ability to forgive
- Express acceptance of health status
- Find meaning in relationships with others
- Find meaning in relationship with Higher Power
- Find meaning in personal and health care treatment choices

NIC   (Nursing Interventions Classification)

Suggested NIC Interventions

Active Listening, Forgiveness Facilitation, Grief Work Facilitation, Hope Inspiration, Humor, Music Therapy, Presence, Referral, Reminiscence Therapy, Self-Awareness Enhancement, Simple Guided Imagery, Simple Massage, Simple Relaxation Therapy, Spiritual Support, Therapeutic Touch, Touch

Example NIC Activities—Spiritual Support

Encourage use of spiritual resources if desired; Be available to listen to client's feelings

Nursing Interventions and *Rationales*

- Observe clients for cues indicating difficulties in finding meaning, purpose, or hope in life. EB: *In a correlational study of 132 participants with American Heart Association (AHA)/American College of Cardiology (ACC) classification of stage B heart failure, Mills et al (2015) found that spiritual well-being was associated with fewer depressive episodes, especially when focusing on increasing meaning and peace in patient's lives.* EB: *In a state of the science consensus report, spirituality included meaning and peace, hope, forgiveness, and gratitude (Steinhauser et al, 2017).*
- Observe clients with chronic illness, poor prognosis, or life-changing conditions for loss of meaning, purpose, and hope in life. EBN: *In a clinical validation study using logistic regression, Caldeira, Carvalho, and Vieira (2014) were able to identify significant correlations between patient variables of lower education levels and previous treatment with antidepressants, to the presence of spiritual distress in the 45 study participants of elderly cancer patients.*
- Promote a sense of love, caring, and compassion in nursing encounters. EBN: *In a cross-sectional, descriptive study of 202 cognitively intact nursing home residents, the nurse–patient interaction had a significant effect on the development of meaning in life, hope, and self-transcendence, potentially promoting health and well-being in this population (Haugan et al, 2014).*
- Be physically present and actively listen to the client. EBN: *In a cross-sectional correlational study by Haugan et al (2014), nurses were found to facilitate both interpersonal and intrapersonal transcendence for long-term nursing home residents by their presence and by encouraging connections with oneself and others in meaningful ways.*
- Help the client find a reason for living, be available for support, and promote hope. EBN: *A cross-sectional descriptive study in 44 different nursing homes found nurse–resident interaction was a resource for hope, meaning in life, and self-transcendence for residents (Haugan et al, 2014). Listen to the client's feelings about suffering and/or death. Be nonjudgmental and allow time for grieving.* EB: *Swinton et al (2017) conducted 208 semistructured interviews with 70 dying patients, 76 family members, and 150 health care providers in an intensive care unit (ICU) to describe how spirituality was expressed during the dying process. The outcome was the development of a program to support the expressions of spirituality during the dying process (i.e., peace, connections, spiritually enhanced environments, and specific expressions of spirituality).*
- Respect the client's beliefs; avoid imposing your own spiritual beliefs on the client. Be aware of your own belief systems and accept the client's spirituality. EB: *In a state of the science consensus report, spirituality is not a monoism phenomenon but is holistic and infuses all aspects of being human and requires honoring individuality, promoting conversations, and capturing the breadth of experience (Steinhauser et al, 2017).*
- Monitor and promote supportive social contacts. EB: *In a meta-analytic review, Sherman et al (2015) found that those with greater spiritual and religious involvement have a greater ability to maintain satisfying social roles and relationships in individuals with cancer.*
- Integrate and assist family in searching for meaning in the client's health care situation. EB: *A scoping review indicated spirituality and spiritual practices can support resilience and coping with life-altering conditions, including spinal cord injury (Jones et al, 2015) and palliative care (Balboni et al, 2017).*

● = Independent;   ▲ = Collaborative;   EBN = Evidence-Based Nursing;   EB = Evidence-Based

- Offer spiritual support to family and caregivers. EB: *In a state of the science report, patients and families who experience serious illness have spiritual needs (Balboni et al, 2017).*
- *Screen for spiritual needs and if a need arises, offer chaplain referral.* EB: *In a state of the science report, spiritual screening is an initial assessment for spiritual need, whereas chaplains provide a more in-depth assessment (Balboni et al, 2017).*
- Support mind–body interventions (e.g., meditation, guided imagery, relaxation, massage). Support outdoor activities. EB: *In a state of the science report, mind–body interventions are encouraged to promote spiritual healing (Balboni et al, 2017).*
- Encourage journaling. EB: *In a scoping review, Jones et al (2015) found use of narratives helpful in coping with spinal cord injury.* EB: *In a state of the science report, journaling was a spiritual care intervention (Balboni et al, 2017).*
- Provide privacy or a "sacred space." EB: *In a state of the science report, meditation and life review were spiritual care interventions that may require privacy (Balboni et al, 2017).*
- Integrate spiritual care in interprofessional palliative care teams. EB: *A state of the science report indicated that multidisciplinary palliative care teams incorporate a spiritual care component (Balboni et al, 2017).*
- Encourage life review at end of life, including recalling, evaluating, and integrating life experiences. EB: *A state of the science report indicated that life review enhanced a personal sense of legacy and promoted dignity when facing terminal illness (Balboni et al, 2017).*

Geriatric

- Identify client's past spiritual practices that have been helpful. Help the client explore his or her life and identify those experiences that are noteworthy. EBN: *A cross-sectional study of 202 cognitively intact nursing home residents revealed a significant relationship between promotion of intrapersonal and interpersonal self-transcendence and meaning in life for the resident and the type of nurse–resident interaction (Haugan et al, 2014).*
- Offer opportunities to practice one's religion. EBN: *In a descriptive cross-sectional study of older adult patients admitted to a coronary care unit, Elham et al (2015) found a significant difference in the means between those who received spiritual care interventions by nurses regarding state-trait anxiety levels, but not in the control group.*

Pediatric

- ○ Offer adolescents opportunities for reflection and storytelling to express their spirituality. EB: *In a longitudinal study of 46 adolescents with cystic fibrosis, Reynolds et al (2014) found those who used positive spiritual coping strategies, such as reframing/rethinking difficult situations from a spiritual perspective, had slowing of disease progression over a 5-year period.*
- ○ Foster spiritual activities among adolescents. EB: *Mirghafourvand et al (2016) found that in a sample of 520 Iranian adolescent girls, spiritual well-being was highly correlated with health-related quality of life (r = .60, p < .001).*

Multicultural

- Recognize the importance of spirituality and provide culturally competent spiritual care to specific populations:
  - ○ Muslims. EBN: *In a cross-sectional descriptive study (Akgül & Karadag, 2016) fecal ostomies were found to be a barrier to incorporating specific religious practices of salat, fasting, and pilgrimage in the lives of 150 Muslims postoperatively, providing an opportunity for nurses to assist patients in meeting their religious needs through adaptation or facilitation around this barrier.*
  - ○ Hispanic. EB: *With diabetes having a high prevalence in the Hispanic population, Rivera-Hernandez (2016) found a positive relationship between religiosity/spirituality with diabetes care and blood sugar control in a sample of 2216 Hispanics 50 years and older living in Mexico.*
  - ○ African Americans (AAs). EBN: *One of four themes identified in analyzing secondary data with content analysis indicated spirituality for AA women was a source of inner peace, joy, strength, hope, comfort, calm, coping, and other positive aspects contributing to well-being and potentially supportive of health-promoting behaviors (Conway-Phillips & Janusek, 2016).*
  - ○ Veterans of Armed Services. Recognize the unique spiritual needs of veterans and provide spiritual support or appropriate referrals. EB: *An exploratory study by Ganocy et al (2016), found an inverse relationship to suicidal ideation, posttraumatic stress disorder (PTSD), and alcohol use with existential and spiritual well-being for National Guard who had ever been deployed overseas at least once.*

• = Independent;   ▲ = Collaborative;   EBN = Evidence-Based Nursing;   EB = Evidence-Based

S

Home Care

- All of the nursing interventions described previously apply in the home setting.

REFERENCES

Akgül, B., & Karadag, A. (2016). The effect of colostomy and ileostomy on acts of worship in the islamic faith. *Journal of Wound, Ostomy, and Continence Nursing, 43*(4), 392–397. doi:10.1097/WON.0000000000000237.

Balboni, T. A., Fitchett, G., Handzo, G. F., et al. (2017). State of the Science of spirituality and palliative care research. Part II: Screening, assessment, and interventions. *Journal of Pain and Symptom Management, 54*(3), 441–453.

Caldeira, S., de Carvalho, E., & Vieira, M. (2014). Between spiritual wellbing and spiritual distress: Possible related factors in elderly patients with cancer. *Revista Latino-Americana de Enfermagem, 22*(1), 28–34. doi:10.1590/0104-1169.2382.

Conway-Phillips, R., & Janusek, L. (2016). Exploring spirituality among African American women: Implications for promoting breast health behaviors. *Holistic Nursing Practice, 20*(6), 322–329. doi:10.1097/HNP.000000000173.

Elham, H., Hazrati, M., Momennasab, M., et al. (2015). The effect of need-based spiritualt/religious intervention on spiritual well-being and anxiety of elderly people. *Holistic Nursing Practice, 29*(3), 136–143. doi:10.1097/HNP.0000000000000083.

Ganocy, S., Goto, T., Chan, P., et al. (2016). Association of spirituality with mental health conditions in Ohio National Guard soldiers. *The Journal of Nervous and Mental Disease, 204*(7). doi:10.1097/NMD.000000000000519.

Haugan, G., Rannestad, T., Hammervold, R., et al. (2014). The relationships between self-transcendence and spiritual well-being in cognitively intact nursing home patients. *International Journal of Older People Nursing, 9*, 65–78.

Jones, K., Simpson, G. K., Briggs, L., et al. (2015). Does spirituality facilitate adjustment and resilience among individuals and families after SCI? *Disability and Rehabilitation, 38*(10), 921–935.

Mills, P., Wilson, K., Iqbal, N., et al. (2015). Depressive symptoms and spiritual wellbeing in asymptomatic heart failure patients. *Journal of Behavioral Medicine, 38*, 407–416. doi:10.1007/s10865-014-9615-0.

Mirghafourvand, M., Charandabi, S. M., Sharajabad, F. A., et al. (2016). Spiritual well-being and health-related quality of life in Iranian adolescent girls. *Community Mental Health Journal, 52*, 484–492. doi:10.1007/s10597-016-9988-3.

Reynolds, N., Mrug, S., Britton, L., et al. (2014). Spiritual coping predicts 5-year health outcomes in adolescents with cystic fibrosis. *Journal of Cystic Fibrosis, 13*, 593–600. doi:10.1016/j.jcf.2014.01.013.

Rivera-Hernandez, M. (2016). Religiosity, social support and care associated with health in older Mexicans with diabetes. *Journal of Religion and Health, 55*, 1394–1410. doi:10.1007/s10943-015-0150-7.

Sherman, A. C., Merluzzi, T. V., Pustejovsky, J. E., et al. (2015). A meta-analytic review of religious or spiritual involvement and social health among cancer patients. *Cancer, 121*, 3779–3788.

Steinhauser, K. E., Fitchett, G., Handzo, G. F., et al. (2017). State of the science of spirituality and palliative care research. Part I: Definitions, measurement, and outcomes. *Journal of Pain and Symptom Management, 54*(3), 428–440.

Swinton, M., Giacomini, M., Toledo, F., et al. (2017). Experiences and expressions of spirituality at the end of life in the intensive care unit. *Journal of Respiratory and Critical Care in Medicine, 195*(2), 198–204. Retrieved from https://doi.org/10.1164/rccm.201606-1102OC.

Risk for Spiritual distress *Gail B. Ladwig, MSN, RN*

S

NANDA-I

Definition

Susceptible to an impaired ability to experience and integrate meaning and purpose in life through connectedness within self, literature, nature, and/or a power greater than oneself, which may compromise health.

Risk Factors

Anxiety; barrier to experiencing love; change in religious ritual; change in spiritual practice; cultural conflict; depression; environmental change; inability to forgive; increasing dependence on another; ineffective relationships; loneliness; low self-esteem; pain; perception of having unfinished business; self-alienation; separation from support system; social alienation; sociocultural deprivation; stressors; substance misuse

At-Risk Population

Aging; birth of a child; death of significant other; exposure to death; life transition; loss; exposure to natural disaster; racial conflict; receiving bad news; unexpected life event

Associated Condition

Actively dying; chronic illness; illness; imminent death; loss of a body part; loss of function of a body part; physical illness; treatment regimen

● = Independent;   ▲ = Collaborative;   EBN = Evidence-Based Nursing;   EB = Evidence-Based

NIC, NOC, Client Outcomes, Nursing Interventions and *Rationales,* and References

Refer to care plan for **Spiritual Distress**

Readiness for enhanced Spiritual well-being
Elizabeth Burkhart, PhD, RN, ANEF and Barbara Baele Vincensi, PhD, RN, FNP

NANDA-I

Definition

A pattern of experiencing and integrating meaning and purpose in life through connectedness with self, others, art, music, literature, nature, and/or a power greater than oneself that is sufficient for well-being and can be strengthened.

Defining Characteristics

Connections to Self

Expresses desire for enhanced acceptance; expresses desire for enhanced coping; expresses desire for enhanced courage; expresses desire for enhanced hope; expresses desire for enhanced joy; expresses desire for enhanced love; expresses desire for enhanced meaning in life; expresses desire for enhanced purpose in life; expresses desire for enhanced satisfying philosophy of life; expresses desire for enhanced self-forgiveness; expresses desire for enhanced serenity (e.g., peace); expresses desire for enhanced surrender; meditation

Connections with Others

Provides service to others; requests forgiveness of others; requests interactions with significant others; requests interaction with spiritual leaders

Connections with Art, Music, Literature, Nature

Displays creative energy (e.g., writing, poetry, singing); listens to music; reads spiritual literature; spends time outdoors

Connection with Power Greater Than Self

Expresses awe; expresses reverence; participates in religious activities; prays; reports mystical experiences

NOC   (Nursing Outcomes Classification)

Suggested NOC Outcomes

Personal Health Status; Coping; Dignified Life Closure; Grief Resolution; Hope; Personal Health Status; Psychosocial Adjustment: Life Change; Quality of Life; Social Involvement; Spiritual Health

Example NOC Outcome with Indicators
Hope as evidenced by the following indicators: Expresses expectation of a positive future/Faith/Optimism/Belief in self/Sense of meaning in life/Belief in others/Inner peace. (Rate each indicator of **Hope:** 1 = never demonstrated, 2 = rarely demonstrated, 3 = sometimes demonstrated, 4 = often demonstrated, 5 = constantly demonstrated [see Section I].)

Client Outcomes

Client Will (Specify Time Frame)

- Express hope
- Express sense of meaning and purpose in life
- Express peace and serenity
- Express love
- Express acceptance
- Express surrender
- Express forgiveness of self and others

● = Independent;   ▲ = Collaborative;   EBN = Evidence-Based Nursing;   EB = Evidence-Based

- Express satisfaction with philosophy of life
- Express joy
- Express courage
- Describe being able to cope
- Describe use of spiritual practices
- Describe providing service to others
- Describe interaction with spiritual leaders, friends, and family
- Describe appreciation for art, music, literature, and nature

| NIC | (Nursing Interventions Classification) |

Suggested NIC Interventions

Active Listening, Coping Enhancement, Counseling, Crisis Intervention, Decision-Making Support, Grief Work Facilitation, Hope Instillation, Meditation Facilitation, Mutual Goal Setting, Presence, Religious Ritual Enhancement, Imagery, Simple Relaxation Therapy, Socialization Enhancement, Spiritual Growth Facilitation, Spiritual Support, Support System Enhancement, Touch, Values Clarification

| Example NIC Activities—Spiritual Support |

Encourage use of spiritual resources if desired; Be available to listen to client's expression of feelings

Nursing Interventions and *Rationales*

- Perform a spiritual assessment that includes the client's relationship with God, meaning and purpose in life, religious affiliation, and any other significant beliefs. EBN: *In a pre/post non-randomized interventional study, researchers Vlasblom et al (2015) found referrals to spiritual caregivers (chaplains) increased after implementing a spiritual assessment instrument by nurses at patient admission, in spite of nurse hesitancy in using the tool.*
- Be present and actively listen to the client. EB: *In a state of the science report, spirituality requires observations and understanding of human experience (Steinhauser et al, 2017).*
- Encourage the client to engage in other spiritual meditative or mind–body practices. EBN: *In a quasi-experimental interprofessional study with nursing, Sun et al (2015) discovered that religious affiliation and practices improved coping, comfort, and faith in palliative care patients. EB: In a state of the science report, mind–body interventions are encouraged to promote spiritual healing (Balboni et al, 2017).*
- Coordinate or encourage nurses to attend spiritual retreats or courses. EBN: *Attard, Baldacchino, and Camilleri (2014), using a pre/post methodology, found that nurses who received specific education on spiritual care in Malta had higher overall competency scores on spiritual caregiving. This supported the intentionality of spiritual care, which the authors stated was something that needs to be "taught" and not "caught" in practice.*
- Promote hope. EBN: *Using a cross-sectional descriptive design, Haugan (2014) found important factors for health in cognitively intact nursing home patients were nurse–patient interactions, which promoted hope and self-transcendence.*
- Encourage clients to reflect on what is meaningful to them in life. EBN: *In a descriptive, cross-sectional design of 202 cognitively intact nursing home patients, the ability to use reflection to discover meaning in life was enhanced by the patient's interactions with the nurse (Haugan, 2014).*
- Offer spiritual support to family and caregivers. EB: *In a state of the science report, patients and families who experience serious illness have spiritual needs (Balboni et al, 2017).*
- Assist the client in identifying religious or spiritual beliefs that encourage integration of meaning and purpose in the client's life. EBN: *Haugan (2014) discovered in a cross-sectional descriptive study that nurse's interactions with the patient positively affected hope, meaning in life, and intrapersonal self-transcendence of the patient.*
- Support spiritual practices, including meditation, guided imagery, journaling, relaxation, and involvement in art, music, or poetry. EB: *In a meta-analysis, Oh and Kim (2014) found spiritual interventions that focused on meaning-centered meditation, psychotherapy, or counseling had a significant but moderate effect on spiritual well-being, meaning of life, and depression. EB: In a state of the science report, mind–body interventions are encouraged to promote spiritual healing (Balboni et al, 2017).*
- Encourage expressions of spirituality. EB: *Swinton et al (2017) conducted 208 semistructured interviews with 70 dying patients, 76 family members, and 150 health care providers in an intensive care unit (ICU) to describe how spirituality was expressed during the dying process. The outcome of these interviews was the*

S

● = Independent;   ▲ = Collaborative;   EBN = Evidence-Based Nursing;   EB = Evidence-Based

development of the 3 Wishes Program to support the expressions of spirituality during the dying process (i.e., peace, connections, spiritually enhanced environments, and specific expressions of spirituality).

- Encourage integration of spirituality in healthy lifestyle choices. EBN: *In a phenomenological study of African-Caribbean women poststroke, Moorley, Cahill, and Corcoran (2016) identified one of three themes, which included the use of faith, spirituality, and church, to promote choices for healthy behaviors.*
- Encourage forgiveness. EB: *Park et al (2014) found that, in a sample of 111 patients with chronic heart failure, forgiveness was related to less subsequent depression.*

Geriatric

- Offer opportunities to practice one's religion. EB: *Freeze & DiTommaso (2014) identified in their descriptive study and development of a structural equation model (SEM) that a secure connection to God through religious behaviors and prayers lessened emotional distress and increased a sense of purpose in life.* EB: *Soriano et al (2016) found in a sample of 200 Filipino older adults living in a community and institutional setting that regular visits with chaplains and religious practices enhanced older adult's spiritual contentment and religion and culture quality of life. Encourage social relationships and connections with family for institutionalized older adults.* EB: *Soriano et al (2016) found that the loss of familial and peer relationships on admission to a nursing home was associated with lower religion and culture quality of life and quality of life overall.*
- For those with chronic disease, encourage individual spiritual practices that promote meaning and peace. EB: *Mills et al (2015), in a sample of 132 men and women with asymptomatic stage B heart failure, found that spiritual well-being, particularly meaning and peace, was associated with less depression.* EB: *Park et al (2014) found that, in a sample of 111 patients with advanced chronic heart failure, daily spiritual experiences were linked with higher existential well-being and predicted less subsequent spiritual strain.*
- For those with chronic illness, encourage patients to attend meaning-centered meditation programs, therapy, or counseling. EB: *In a meta-analysis, Oh and Kim (2014) found spiritual interventions that focused on meaning-centered meditation, psychotherapy, or counseling had a significant but moderate effect on spiritual well-being, meaning of life, and depression.*
- Promote spiritual activities for those receiving palliative care. EB: *Chaiviboontham (2014) found that, in a sample of 240 patient with advanced cancer, patients with higher spiritual well-being significantly responded better to palliative care strategies.*
- During bereavement, encourage bereavement life review to promote spiritual well-being and alleviate depression. EB: *In a sample of 20 bereaved Hawaiian Americans, Ando et al (2015) found that participating in bereavement life review statistically significantly increased spiritual well-being and decreased depression.*

Pediatric

- Offer adolescents opportunities for reflection and storytelling to express their spirituality. EB: *In a longitudinal study of 46 adolescents with cystic fibrosis Reynolds et al (2014) found those who used positive spiritual coping strategies, such as reframing/rethinking difficult situations from a spiritual perspective, had slowing of disease progression over a 5-year period.*
- Foster spiritual activities among adolescents. EB: *Mirghafourvand et al (2016) found that, in a sample of 520 Iranian adolescent girls, spiritual well-being was highly correlated with health-related quality of life (r = .60, p < .001).*

Multicultural

- Recognize the importance of spirituality and provide culturally competent spiritual care to specific populations:
  - Muslims. EB: *In a cross-sectional study with 223 Iranian patients with type 2 diabetes, Jafari et al (2014) found those with a higher spiritual well-being had significantly better diabetes control, improved quality of life, and less depression related to their disease.*
  - Thai. EB: *In a 4-year longitudinal study of Thai elders (N = 3537), Hsu (2014) used hierarchical linear modeling for analysis and found that certain religious activities helped to reduce depressive symptoms and increase coping over time.*
  - Latinos. EBN: *In a cross-sectional secondary analysis of a longitudinal study, Prince et al (2015) found that Hispanic stem cell transplant survivors (N = 171) had greater spiritual well-being and quality of life than non-Hispanic survivors, even at ≥3 years posttransplant.*
  - African Americans (AAs). EBN: *One of four themes identified in analyzing secondary data with content analysis indicated spirituality for AA women was a source of inner peace, joy, strength, hope, comfort, calm,*

S

coping, and other positive aspects contributing to well-being and potentially supportive of health-promoting behaviors (Conway-Phillips & Janusek, 2016). **EB:** In a cross-sectional survey of 1013 AA women, Ludema et al (2015) found that those who identified with high organizational religion, high nonorganizational religion, and high spirituality had less risky sexual behaviors for potential HIV exposure.

○ Sheltered Homeless. **EBN:** In a cross-sectional correlational study examining the relationship between spiritual resources and life attitudes in 160 sheltered homeless AA women, a significant relationship was found between a potential for moving out of homelessness and higher levels of faith, instrumental religion and spiritual resources, and increased coping skills (Gash et al, 2014).

○ Chinese. **EB:** Leung et al (2015) used a pretest/posttest methodology with 160 Chinese patients diagnosed with chronic disease to study the effects of a psychoeducational death preparation intervention. The findings indicated that there was significant improvement in psychological, behavioral, and spiritual dimensions over time related to fear of death and preparation for death.

○ Armed Forces. **EB:** An exploratory study by Ganocy et al (2016) found an inverse relationship to suicidal ideation, posttraumatic stress disorder (PTSD), and alcohol use with existential and spiritual well-being for National Guard who had ever been deployed overseas at least once.

• Integrate spiritual practices in health-promoting programs, particularly within the AA community. **EB:** In a cross-sectional study (N = 144) using regression analysis, spirituality was found to be a protective factor within a culturally informed risk-protective framework for AA women of lower socioeconomic status living in disordered neighborhoods with parenting stress (Lamis et al, 2014).

 Home Care

• All of the nursing interventions described previously apply in the home setting.

REFERENCES

Ando, M., Marquez-Wong, F., Simon, G. B., et al. (2015). Bereavement life review improves spiritual well-being and ameliorates depression among American caregivers. *Palliative and Supportive Care, 13,* 319–325. doi:10.1017/S1478951514000030.

Attard, J., Baldacchino, D., & Camilleri, L. (2014). Nurses' and midwives' acquisition of competency in spiritual care: A focus on education. *Nurse Education Today, 34,* 1460–1466. Retrieved from http://doi.org.10.1016.j.nedt.2014.015.

Balboni, T. A., Fitchett, G., Handzo, G. F., et al. (2017). State of the science of spirituality and palliative care research. Part II: Screening, assessment, and interventions. *Journal of Pain and Symptom Management, 54*(3), 441–453.

Chaiviboontham, S. (2014). Factors predicting the effectiveness of palliative care in patients with advanced cancer. *Palliative and Supportive Care.* doi:10.1017/S1478951514000856.

Conway-Phillips, R., & Janusek, L. (2016). Exploring spirituality among African American women: Implications for promoting breast health behaviors. *Holistic Nursing Practice, 20*(6), 322–329. doi:10.1097/HNP.000000000173.

Freeze, T., & DiTommaso, E. (2014). An examination of attachment, religiousness, spirituality and well-being in a Baptist faith sample. *Mental Health, Religion and Culture, 17*(7), 690–702.

Ganocy, S., Goto, T., Chan, P., et al. (2016). Association of spirituality with mental health conditions in Ohio National Guard soldiers. *The Journal of Nervous and Mental Disease, 204*(7), 524–529. doi:10.1097/NMD.000000000000519.

Gash, J., Washington, O., Moxley, D., et al. (2014). The relationships between spiritual respources and life attitudes of African American homeless women. *Issues in Mental Health Nursing, 35*(4), 238–250. doi:10.3109/01612840.2013.797062.

Haugan, G. (2014). Nurse-patient interaction is a resource for hope, meaning in life and self-transcendence in nursing home patients. *Scandinavian Journal of Caring Sciences, 28,* 74–88.

Hsu, H.-C. (2014). Effects of religiousness on depressive symptoms among elderly persons in Taiwan. *Clinical Gerontologist, 37,* 446–457. doi:10.1080/07317115.2014.937549.

Jafari, N., Farajzadegan, Z., Loghmani, A., et al. (2014). Spiritual well-being and quality of life of Iranian adults with type 2 diabetes. *Evidence-Based Complementary and Alternative Medicine, 2014.* doi:10.1155/2014/619028. Retrieved from https://www.ncbi.nlm.nih.gov/pmc/articles/PMC3926225/pdf/ECAM2014-619028.pdf.

Lamis, D., Wilson, C., Tarantino, N., et al. (2014). Neighborhood disorder, spiritual well-being and parenting stress in African American women. *Journal of Family Psychology, 28*(6), 769–778. doi:10.1037/a0036373.

Leung, P., Wan, A., Lui, J., et al. (2015). The effects of a positive death education group on psycho-spiritual outcomes for Chinese with chronic illness: A quasi-experimental study. *Illness, Crises, and Loss, 23*(1), 5–19. Retrieved from http://dx.doi.org/10.2190/IL.23.1.b.

Ludema, C., Doherty, I., White, B., et al. (2015). Religiosity, spirituality, and HIV risk behaviors among African American women from four rural counties in the Southeastern U.S. *Journal of Health Care for the Poor and Underserved, 26*(1), 168–181. Retrieved from https://doi.org/10.1353/hpu.2015.0005.

Mills, P. J., Wilson, K., Iqbal, N., et al. (2015). Depressive symptoms and spiritual wellbeing in asymptomatic heart failure patients. *Journal of Behavioral Medicine, 38,* 407–415. doi:10.1007/s10865-014-9615-0.

Mirghafourvand, M., Charandabi, S. M., Sharajabad, F. A., et al. (2016). Spiritual well-being and health-related quality of life in Iranian adolescent girls. *Community Mental Health Journal, 52,* 484–492. doi:10.1007/s10597-016-9988-3.

Moorley, C., Cahill, S., & Corcoran, N. (2016). Life after stroke: Coping mechanisms among African Caribbean women. *Health and Social Care in the Community, 24*(6), 769–778. doi:10.1111/hsc.12256.

Oh, P. J., & Kim, S. H. (2014). The effects of spiritual interventions in patients with cancer: A meta-analysis. *Oncology Nursing Forum, 41*(5), E298–E301. doi:10.1188/14.ONF.E290-E301.

Park, C. L., Lim, H., Newlon, M., et al. (2014). Dimensions of religiousness and spirituality as predictors of well-being in advanced chronic heart failure patients. *Journal of Religion and Health, 53,* 579–590. doi:10.1007/s10943-013-9714-1.

● = Independent; ▲ = Collaborative; **EBN** = Evidence-Based Nursing; **EB** = Evidence-Based

Prince, P., Mitchell, S., Wehlen, L., et al. (2015). Spiritual well-being in hispanic and non-hispanic survivors of alogeneic hematopoeitic stem cell transplantation. *Journal of Psychosocial Oncology, 33*(6), 635–654. doi:10.1080/07347332.2015.1082167.

Reynolds, N., Mrug, S., Britton, L., et al. (2014). Spiritual coping predicts 5-year health outcomes in adolescents with cystic fibrosis. *Journal of Cystic Fibrosis, 13,* 593–600. doi:10.1016/j.jcf.2014.01.013.

Soriano, C. A. F., Sarmiento, W. D., Songco, F. J. G., et al. (2016). Socio-demographics, spirituality, and quality of life among community-dwelling and institutionalized older adults: A structural equation model. *Archives of Gerontology and Geriatrics, 66,* 176–182.

Steinhauser, K. E., Fitchett, G., Handzo, G. F., et al. (2017). State of the science of spirituality and palliative care research. Part I: Definitions, measurement, and outcomes. *Journal of Pain and Symptom Management, 54*(3), 428–440.

Sun, V., Kim, J., Irish, T., et al. (2015). Palliative care and spiritual well-being in lung cancer patients and family caregivers. *Psycho-Oncology.* doi:10.1002/pon.3987. Retrieved from https://www.researchgate.net/profile/Tami_Borneman/publication/282038483_Palliative_care_and_spiritual_well-being_in_lung_cancer_patients_and_family_caregivers/links/5707f1a508aea66081331e67.pdf.

Swinton, M., Giacomini, M., Toledo, F., et al. (2017). Experiences and expressions of spirituality at the end of life in the intensive care unit. *Journal of Respiratory and Critical Care in Medicine, 195*(2), 198–204. Retrieved from https://doi.org/10.1164/rccm.201606-1102OC.

Vlasblom, J., Van der Steen, J., Walton, M., et al. (2015). Effects of nurses' screening of spiritual needs of hospitalized patients on consultation and perceived nurses' support and patients' spiritual well-being. *Holistic Nursing Practice, 29*(6), 346–356. doi:10.1097/HNP.0000000000000111.

Impaired Standing   *Tracy P. George, DNP, APRN-BC, CNE*

NANDA-I

Definition

Limitation of ability to independently and purposefully attain and/or maintain the body in an upright position from feet to head.

Defining Characteristics

Impaired ability to adjust position of one or both lower limbs on uneven surface; impaired ability to attain a balanced position of the torso; impaired ability to extend one or both hips; impaired ability to extend one or both knees; impaired ability to flex one or both hips; impaired ability to flex one or both knees; impaired ability to maintain the torso in balanced position; impaired ability to stress torso with body weight

Related Factors

Emotional disturbance; insufficient endurance; insufficient energy; insufficient muscle strength; malnutrition; obesity; pain; self-imposed relief posture

Associated Condition

Circulatory perfusion disorder; impaired metabolic functioning; injury to lower extremity; neurological disorder; prescribed posture; sarcopenia; surgical procedure

NOC   Outcomes (Nursing Outcomes Classification)

Suggested NOC Outcomes

Activity Tolerance; Balance; Body Mechanics Performance; Body Positioning: Self-Initiated; Comfort Status: Physical; Endurance; Mobility; Risk Control: Hypotension; Skeletal Function

Example NOC Outcome with Indicators
Mobility as evidenced by the following indicators: Balance/Coordination/Body positioning performance. (Rate outcome and indicators of **Mobility:** 1 = severely compromised, 2 = substantially compromised, 3 = moderately compromised, 4 = mildly compromised, 5 = not compromised [see Section I].)

Client Outcomes

Client Will (Specify Time Frame)

- Demonstrate optimal independence and safety when standing
- Demonstrate the proper use of assistive devices
- State benefits of standing

● = Independent;   ▲ = Collaborative;   **EBN** = Evidence-Based Nursing;   **EB** = Evidence-Based

| NIC | Interventions (Nursing Interventions Classification) |

Suggested NIC Interventions

Body Mechanics Promotion

| Example NIC Activities |

Instruct client on structure and functional spine and optimal posture for moving and using the body

Nursing Interventions and *Rationales*

- Encourage clients to stand at intervals throughout the day. EB: *In a randomized control trial of overweight or obese Australian office workers, participants who completed work while alternating between sitting and standing at 30-minute intervals throughout the day demonstrated a 11.1% decrease in glucose levels after meals (Thorp et al, 2014). EB: Patients who engaged in standing, walking, or cycling during an 8-hour work period had lower 24-hour and postprandial blood sugars than those who sat (Crespo et al, 2016). Advise patients of the physical and psychological benefits of being upright and active. EB: In patients 1 to 3 years after suffering a stroke, depression, left hemisphere infarction, visual neglect, and difficulty with mobility and balance were associated with being less active (Kunkel et al, 2015).*
- Educate patients about the health risks of sitting. EB: *In a study of 221,240 adults ages 45 and older in Australia, standing less than 2 hours/day was associated with a greater mortality rate from all causes compared with standing from 2 to 5 hours, 5 to 8 hours, or greater than 8 hours/day (van der Ploeg et al, 2014).*

 Geriatric

- Advise older clients who have difficulty standing to use assistive devices. EB: *In a Swedish study using the Psychosocial Impact of Assistive Devices Scale, Nordström et al (2014) found that the frequent use of standing assistive devices was associated with higher psychosocial scores in older adults.*
- Encourage trunk exercises after clients have had strokes. EB: *In a meta-analysis of six randomized controlled studies, trunk exercises were associated with improvements in standing and walking for clients after strokes (Sorinola, Powis, & White, 2014).*
- Encourage clients who are unable to stand to consider chair exercises. EB: *In a study of 100 older adults with lower extremity osteoarthritis, the 40 adults who participated in chair yoga twice a week for 8 weeks reported less pain than the 60 participants who participated in a health education program two times per week for 8 weeks (Park et al, 2016).*
- Encourage clients poststroke to participate in rehabilitation interventions that promote standing. EB: *In a meta-analysis using 11 studies, interventions used after strokes to improve standing were associated with faster sitting-to-standing position times and improved lateral symmetry during sitting-to-standing position changes (Pollock et al, 2014). EB: A study of seven participants found that a home-based intervention, Rehab@ home, can be used effectively to improve the rehabilitation of balance and the movement from the sitting to standing position in patients with neurological deficits, without the presence of a physical therapist (Faria, Silva, & Campilho, 2015).*
- Raise the height of the bed and encourage the use of the client's hands when an older adult is rising from a sitting to standing position. EB: *In a study of 24 older clients, Lindemann et al (2014) found that raising the bed height and using the hands while transferring from a sitting to standing position resulted in less effort.*
- Educate older adults who have fallen about the need for balance and muscle training of the ankle joint. EB: *In a randomized controlled trial of 26 older clients who were at risk of falling and had fallen previously, Jung-Hyun and Nyeon-Jun (2015) found that balance and ankle muscle training resulted in improvements in the gait of older adults.*
- Educate adults older than age 80 years on the need for vitamin D. EB: *Low serum 25-hydroxyvitamin D (25OHD) levels were associated with orthostatic hypotension in a study involving community-dwelling clients 80 years of age and older (N = 329) (Annweiler et al, 2014).*
- Advise older clients who are at risk for falls to avoid doing multiple tasks at one time while standing. EB: *In a study of 243 adults ages 65 years and older, older participants' standing balance was worse than that seen in younger participants; the standing balance was worse when clients were performing a second task, which is important when considering the risk of falls (Coelho et al, 2016).*

• = Independent;   ▲ = Collaborative;   EBN = Evidence-Based Nursing;   EB = Evidence-Based

Client/Family Teaching and Discharge Planning

- Educate clients that standing can be beneficial for their health. **EB:** *In a Canadian prospective cohort study in which participants were followed for a mean duration of 12 years, Katzmarzyk (2014) found that increased daily standing times were associated with decreased cardiovascular and all-cause mortality rates.* **EB:** *In a study of participants with chronic pain (N = 18) and participants without chronic pain (N = 19), Raijmakers et al (2015) found that patients with chronic pain spent more time lying and less time sitting and standing over a 1-week period.*
- Teach clients about the need to take frequent breaks when standing for long periods. **EB:** *With 45 minutes of standing to 15 minutes of sitting (3:1 ratio), 55% of participants experienced low back pain while standing, so this ratio may be not be adequate, and alternate rest activities may be needed (Gallagher, Campbell, & Callaghan, 2014).*
- Instruct clients about the use of yoga for individuals who have difficulty with standing balance. **EB:** *In a randomized control of obese adults with poor standing balance, participation in yoga classes three times per week was associated with improved static and dynamic standing balance (Chaiyong et al, 2015).*

REFERENCES

Annweiler, C., Schott, A., Rolland, Y., et al. (2014). Vitamin D deficiency is associated with orthostatic hypotension in oldest-old women. *Journal of Internal Medicine, 276*(3), 285–295.

Chaiyong, J., Jutaluk, K., Chiraprapa, P., et al. (2015). Effect of yoga training on one leg standing and functional reach tests in obese individuals with poor postural control. *Journal of Physical Therapy Science, 27*(1), 59–62.

Coelho, T., Fernandes, Â., Santos, R., et al. (2016). Quality of standing balance in community-dwelling elderly: Age-related differences in single and dual task conditions. *Archives of Gerontology and Geriatrics, 67,* 34–39.

Crespo, N. C., Mullane, S. L., Zeigler, Z. S., et al. (2016). Effects of standing and light-intensity walking and cycling on 24-h glucose. *Medicine & Science in Sports & Exercise, 48*(12), 2503–2511. doi:10.1249/MSS.0000000000001062.

Faria, C., Silva, J., & Campilho, A. (2015). Rehab@home: A tool for home-based motor function rehabilitation. *Disability & Rehabilitation. Assistive Technology, 10*(1), 67–74.

Gallagher, K. M., Campbell, T., & Callaghan, J. P. (2014). The influence of a seated break on prolonged standing induced low back pain development. *Ergonomics, 57*(4), 555–562 [Epub 2014 Mar 19].

Jung-Hyun, C., & Nyeon-Jun, K. (2015). The effects of balance training and ankle training on the gait of elderly people who have fallen. *Journal of Physical Therapy Science, 27*(1), 139–142.

Katzmarzyk, P. T. (2014). Standing and mortality in a prospective cohort of Canadian adults. *Medicine & Science in Sports & Exercise, 46*(5), 940–946.

Kunkel, D., Fitton, C., Burnett, M., et al. (2015). Physical inactivity post-stroke: A 3-year longitudinal study. *Disability & Rehabilitation, 37*(4), 304–310.

Lindemann, U., van Oosten, L., Evers, J., et al. (2014). Effect of bed height and use of hands on trunk angular velocity during the sit-to-stand transfer. *Ergonomics, 57*(10), 1536–1540.

Nordström, B., Nyberg, L., Ekenberg, L., et al. (2014). The psychosocial impact on standing devices. *Disability & Rehabilitation. Assistive Technology, 9*(4), 299–306.

Park, J., Newman, D., McCaffrey, R., et al. (2016). The effect of chair yoga on biopsychosocial changes in English- and Spanish-speaking community-dwelling older adults with lower-extremity osteoarthritis. *Journal of Gerontological Social Work, 59*(7/8), 604–626. doi:10.1080/01634372.2016.1239234.

Pollock, A., Gray, C., Culham, E., et al. (2014). Interventions for improving sit-to-stand ability following stroke. *The Cochrane Database of Systematic Reviews,* (5), CD007232.

Raijmakers, B. G., Nieuwenhuizen, M. G., Beckerman, H., et al. (2015). Differences in the course of daily activity level between persons with and without chronic pain. *American Journal of Physical Medicine & Rehabilitation, 94*(2), 101–167.

Sorinola, I., Powis, I., & White, C. (2014). Does additional exercise improve trunk function recovery in stroke patients? A meta-analysis. *Neurorehabilitation, 35*(2), 205–213.

Thorp, A. A., Kingwell, B. A., Sethi, P., et al. (2014). Alternating bouts of sitting and standing attenuate postprandial glucose responses. *Medicine & Science in Sports & Exercise, 46*(11), 2053–2061.

van der Ploeg, H. P., Chey, T., Ding, D., et al. (2014). Standing time and all-cause mortality in a large cohort of Australian adults. *Preventive Medicine, 69,* 187–191. doi:10.1016/j.ypmed.2014.10.004.

S

Stress overload   *Gail B. Ladwig, MSN, RN*

NANDA-I

Definition

Excessive amounts and types of demands that require action.

Defining Characteristics

Excessive stress; feeling of pressure; impaired decision-making; impaired functioning; increase in anger; increase in anger behavior; increase in impatience; negative impact from stress; tension

● = Independent;   ▲ = Collaborative;   **EBN** = Evidence-Based Nursing;   **EB** = Evidence-Based

Related Factors

Insufficient resources; repeated stressors; stressors

NOC   (Nursing Outcomes Classification)

Suggested NOC Outcomes

Anxiety Level; Caregiver Stressors; Stress Level; Health-Promoting Behavior; Knowledge: Stress Management

Example NOC Outcome with Indicators
Stress Level as evidenced by the following indicators: Increased blood pressure, restlessness, emotional outbursts, anxiety, diminished attention to detail. (Rate the outcome and indicators of **Stress Level:** 1 = severe, 2 = substantial, 3 = moderate, 4 = mild, 5 = none [see Section I].)

Client Outcomes

Client Will (Specify Time Frame)

- Review the amounts and types of stressors in daily living
- Identify stressors that can be modified or eliminated
- Mobilize social supports to facilitate lower stress levels
- Reduce stress levels through use of health promoting behaviors and other strategies

NIC   (Nursing Interventions Classification)

Suggested NIC Interventions

Active Listening; Anger Control Assistance; Anxiety Reduction; Aroma Therapy; Counseling; Crisis Intervention; Emotional Support; Family Integrity Promotion; Presence; Support System Enhancement

Example NIC Activities—Support System Enhancement
Identify psychological response to situation and availability of support system; Determine adequacy of social networks; Explain to concerned others how they can help; Refer to a self-help group or Internet-based resource as appropriate; Provide services in a caring and supportive manner

Nursing Interventions and *Rationales*

- Assist client in identification of stress overload during vulnerable life events. EBN: *Research suggested that role overload, associated with high stress levels, among nurses and volunteer caregivers may negatively affect health, well-being, and job performance (Akintola, Hlengwa, & Dageid, 2013; Kath et al, 2013). EB: In a systematic review of 40 studies it was found that at least 33% of surrogates experience stressful emotional burden on making treatment decisions for others (Wendler & Rid, 2011). CEB: Women with breast cancer who were involved in group therapy focusing on stress reduction and muscle relaxation were 56% less likely to succumb to the disease and 45% less likely to experience a recurrence (Andersen et al, 2008). Men with high stress have higher all-cause mortality, and the effects are more pronounced among middle-aged men (Nielsen et al, 2008).*
- Listen actively to descriptions of stressors and the stress response. EBN: *In a recent longitudinal study of clients with heart failure, researchers found that clients with high anxiety experienced shorter periods of event-free (hospitalization, mortality) survival than those with lower anxiety (P = .03) (Dejong et al, 2011). EB: Adolescents exposed to daily stress demonstrate increased risky decision-making compared with those with low stress (Galván & McGlennen, 2012).*
- In younger adult women, assess interpersonal stressors. EB: *In a sample of 127 spouse caregivers of clients with Alzheimer's disease who were predominantly female (71%), greater stress was associated with more depressive symptoms, and these symptoms were significantly associated with decreased personal mastery (P = .006), self-efficacy (P < .001), increased avoidance coping (P < .001), and activity restriction (P = .040) (Mausbach et al, 2012). CEB: A systematic review and meta-analysis of 30 studies found that maternal exposure to the stress of domestic violence results in significantly increased risk of low birth weight and preterm birth (Shah & Shah, 2010).*

● = Independent;   ▲ = Collaborative;   EBN = Evidence-Based Nursing;   EB = Evidence-Based

- Categorize stressors as modifiable or nonmodifiable. EB: *Strategizing on nonavoidance coping and increased socialization along with enhanced personal mastery and self-efficacy in use of problem-solving coping may minimize depression symptoms in Alzheimer's disease caregivers (Mausbach et al, 2012). CEBN: Removing or minimizing some stressors, changing responses to stressors, and modifying the long-term effects of stress are all actions that can assist those with chronic illnesses and stress (Upton & Solowiej, 2010).*

- Help clients modify or mitigate stressors identified as modifiable. EBN: *In a sample of 480 nurse managers from 36 hospitals in the southwestern United States, role overload was found to be the most significant predictor of work-related stress followed by organizational constraints and role conflict (all P < .01 [two-tailed]); all three are areas that organizational leaders need to be aware of to mitigate stress overload in managerial staff (Kath et al, 2013). CEB: There are numerous possible strategies to modify stressors, including time management, improved organizational skills, problem-solving, changing perceptions of stress, breathing, relaxation techniques, visual imagery, and soothing rituals (Lloyd, Smith, & Weinger, 2005).*

- Help clients distinguish among short-term, chronic, and secondary stressors. EB: *Cellular aging, identified by leukocyte telomere length (TL), was found to be different in a sample of 36 ethnically diverse, older adults between four pain/stress groups (P = .01) in which those with chronic pain/higher stress had the shortest TL indicative of cellular aging (Sibille et al, 2012). CEBN: Social support is a critical dimension of health and health promotion and serves as a buffer in the stress response (Pender, Murtaugh, & Parsons, 2010).*

- Provide information as needed to reduce stress responses to acute and chronic illnesses. EBN: *Nursing interventions including strategies to deal with child behavior, a focus on physical health, and planning to meet resource needs may enhance the well-being of African American grandmothers raising grandchildren (Kelley, Whitley, & Campos, 2013). Proactive nursing interventions including assessment of caregiver needs for support and preparedness including early psychoeducational interventions can enhance caregiver ability to navigate the challenges associated with caring for a relative with Alzheimer's disease (Ducharme et al, 2011).*

- ▲ Explore possible therapeutic approaches such as cognitive-behavioral therapy, biofeedback, neurofeedback, acupuncture, pharmacological agents, and complementary and alternative therapies. EBN: *Nonpharmacological nursing interventions through the use of nature-based sounds played through headsets was found to effectively decrease the stress response in mechanically ventilated clients in a sample of 60 Iranian clients aged 18 to 65 (Saadatmand et al, 2013). EB: In a sample of 111 healthy adults, those who exercised regularly were more resistant to acute stress (Childs & de Wit, 2014). Mindfulness techniques have been suggested as an effective means of reducing stress in adolescents (Broderick & Jennings, 2012), nursing personnel (Zeller & Levin, 2013), and older adults (Gallegos et al, 2013).*

- Help the client to reframe his or her perceptions of some of the stressors. EBN: *A study on 335 Thai nursing students found that coping mediated the effects of stress on physical and psychological health (Klainin-Yobas et al, 2014). Researchers found that nursing students with higher anxiety states were 62% less optimistic, with findings supporting that individuals with pessimistic outlooks perceive situations as more threatening (Warning, 2011).*

- Assist the client to mobilize social supports for dealing with recent stressors. CEBN: *Emotional support in Taiwanese caregivers is suggested as a moderator of stressors experienced by caregivers of clients with Alzheimer's disease or stroke, particularly in caregivers with lower household incomes (Huang et al, 2009). EB: In a sample of 79 German adults a predicted association between needed and received emotional support and well-being was found in younger adults (aged 23–34) (Wolff et al, 2013).*

 Pediatric

- With children, nurses should work with parents to help them to reduce children's stressors. EB: *A longitudinal study on 115 children aged 7 to 12 suggested that early life stress and trauma may result in increased limbic activity, which is a biomarker that may have implications as a risk for later psychiatric diagnoses (Suzuki et al, 2014). A study on 181 18 to 20 year olds suggested that more positive parenting behaviors are statistically significantly (P < .01) associated with more adaptive cognitions in the emerging adult, which may affect stress/health outcomes (Donnelly, Renk, & McKinney, 2013).*

- Help children to manage their feelings related to self-concept. CEB: *Perceived isolation as experienced in high school associated with victimization results in higher stress and longer lasting negative psychological outcomes (Newman, Holden, & Delville, 2005).*

- Help children to deal with bullies and other sources of violence in schools and neighborhoods. EB: *In a sample of 1420 children and adolescents the number of times that the individual was bullied predicted higher levels of C-reactive protein (CRP) (a risk factor for negative health consequences later in life) in which those who bullied had lower levels of CRP (Copeland et al, 2014). Violence in schools and neighborhoods has*

● = Independent;   ▲ = Collaborative;   EBN = Evidence-Based Nursing;   EB = Evidence-Based

significant effects on children's stress. In a recent study of college-aged respondents (N = 1339), researchers found that a history of being bullied (victimized) was associated with both increased stress and use of avoidant behaviors (Newman, Holden, & Delville, 2011).

• Help children to manage the complexities of chronic illnesses. **EB:** *Individuals who grow up with a chronic illness have lower odds of graduating college, being employed, having a good income, and have a higher need for public assistance, although they do succeed socially, which is evident by similar odds of marriage, having children, and living with their parents compared with those without chronic illness (Maslow et al, 2011). **CEB:** Teenagers who had recently been diagnosed with diabetes described high levels of stress that often related to the complexities of managing the illness (Davidson et al, 2004).*

Geriatric

• Assess for chronic stress with older adults and provide a variety of stress relief techniques. **EB:** *In a sample of over 9000 American adults over the age of 60, lifetime posttraumatic stress disorder (PTSD) was found to be associated with greater odds of being diagnosed with hypertension, angina pectoris, tachycardia, other heart disease, stomach ulcer, gastritis, and arthritis (Pietrzak et al, 2012).*

▲ Encourage older adults to seek appropriate counseling. **EB:** *Treatment modalities for PTSD in older adults may vary depending on whether the PTSD was experienced early or late in life; however, trauma confrontation and cognitive restructuring combined with age-specific life review in cognitive-behavioral therapy may hold the most promise (Böttche, Kuwert, & Knaevelsrud, 2012). **CEB:** Bereavement-related major depression differs from major depression seen in other stressful life events only in relation to older age at onset. Individuals are more likely to be female; have lower levels of treatment-seeking; and have higher levels of guilt, fatigue, and loss of interest; therefore they should not be excluded from a diagnosis of major depression (Kendler, Myers, & Zisook, 2008).*

Multicultural

• Review cultural beliefs and acculturation level in relation to perceived stressors. **EBN:** *A study done to assess how the type of premigration trauma, postmigration stressors, and resources predicted PTSD and major depressive disorder (MDD) symptoms found that postmigration-related stressors greatly increased the odds (nearly 16-fold) of being in a comorbid group (PTSD or MDD) (Norris, Aroian, & Nickerson, 2011). **EB:** A review of qualitative studies found that organizational constraints, work overload, and interpersonal conflict were universally experienced stressors in studies that assessed occupational stress on an international perspective (Mazzola, Schonfeld, & Spector, 2011). Assess families for whether they experience high stress or low stress. **EB:** In a sample of 97 native Norwegian adolescents and 59 immigrant adolescents from an urban Norwegian secondary school, global victimization was found to be higher in the immigrant group compared with the native group, although there was no difference in the report of depressive symptoms (Fandrem, Strohmeier, & Jonsdottir, 2012). **CEB:** Stress related to racial microaggressions experienced by African Americans may have a negative cumulative effect on health outcomes (Sue et al, 2007).*

S

Home Care

• The preceding interventions may be adapted for home care use.
• Develop community-based programs for stress management as needed for groups with increased risk of stress overload (e.g., firefighters, policemen, military personnel, nurses). **CEB:** *Some situations have higher risks of stress overload. Stress management interventions may prevent or modify the experience of stress overload (McNulty, 2005).*
• Support and encourage neighborhood stability. **CEB:** *A "significant proportion of health differentials across neighborhoods is due to disparate stress levels across [Detroit] neighborhoods," and neighborhood stability was a buffer to reduce the negative effects of high stress (Boardman, 2004).*

Client/Family Teaching and Discharge Planning

• Diagnose the possibility of stress overload before teaching.
• Establish readiness for learning.
• Provide manageable amounts of information at the appropriate educational level.
• Evaluate the need for additional teaching and learning experiences.

• = Independent;   ▲ = Collaborative;   **EBN** = Evidence-Based Nursing;   **EB** = Evidence-Based

REFERENCES

Akintola, O., Hlengwa, W., & Dageid, W. (2013). Perceived stress and burnout among volunteer caregivers working in AIDS care in South Africa. *Journal of Advanced Nursing, 69,* 2738–2749.

Andersen, B., et al. (2008). Psychologic intervention improves survival for breast cancer. *Cancer, 113*(12), 3450–3458.

Boardman, J. (2004). Stress and physical health: The role of neighborhoods as mediating and moderating mechanisms. *Social Science & Medicine, 58*(12), 2473–2483.

Böttche, M., Kuwert, P., & Knaevelsrud, C. (2012). Posttraumatic stress disorder in older adults: An overview of characteristics and treatment approaches. *International Journal of Geriatric Psychiatry, 27,* 230–239.

Broderick, P. C., & Jennings, P. A. (2012). Mindfulness for adolescents: A promising approach to supporting emotion regulation and preventing risky behavior. *New Directions for Youth Development, 2012,* 111.

Childs, E., & de Wit, H. (2014). Regular exercise is associated with emotional resilience to acute stress in healthy adults. *Frontiers in Physiology, 5,* 161.

Copeland, W. E., Wolke, D., Lereya, S. T., et al. (2014). Childhood bullying involvement predicts low-grade systemic inflammation into adulthood. *Proceedings of the National Academy of Sciences of the United States of America, 111,* 7570–7575.

Davidson, M., et al. (2004). Stressors and self-care challenges faced by adolescents living with type 1 diabetes. *Applied Nursing Research, 2,* 72–80.

Dejong, M., et al. (2011). Linkages between anxiety and outcomes in heart failure. *Heart and Lung: The Journal of Critical Care, 40,* 393–404.

Donnelly, R., Renk, K., & McKinney, C. (2013). Emerging adults' stress and health: The role of parent behaviors and cognitions. *Child Psychiatry and Human Development, 44,* 19–38.

Ducharme, F., Lévesque, L., Lachance, L., et al. (2011). Challenges associated with transition to caregiver role following diagnostic disclosure of Alzheimer disease: A descriptive study. *International Journal of Nursing Studies, 48,* 1109–1119.

Fandrem, H., Strohmeier, D., & Jonsdottir, K. A. (2012). Peer groups and victimisation among native and immigrant adolescents in Norway. *Emotional & Behavioural Difficulties, 17,* 273–285.

Gallegos, A. M., Hoerger, M., Talbot, N. L., et al. (2013). Emotional benefits of mindfulness-based stress reduction in older adults: The moderating roles of age and depressive symptom severity. *Aging & Mental Health, 17,* 823–829.

Galván, A., & McGlennen, K. M. (2012). Daily stress increases risky decision-making in adolescents: A preliminary study. *Developmental Psychobiology, 54,* 433–440.

Huang, C., et al. (2009). Stressors, social support, depressive symptoms and general health status of Taiwanese caregivers of persons with stroke or Alzheimer's disease. *Journal of the Clinics in Nursing, 18*(4), 502–511.

Kath, L. M., Stichler, J. F., Ehrhart, M. G., et al. (2013). Predictors of nurse manager stress: A dominance analysis of potential work environment stressors. *International Journal of Nursing Studies, 50,* 1474–1480.

Kelley, S. J., Whitley, D. M., & Campos, P. E. (2013). Psychological distress in African American grandmothers raising grandchildren: The contribution of child behavior problems, physical health, and family resources. *Research in Nursing & Health, 36,* 373–385.

Kendler, K., Myers, J., & Zisook, M. (2008). Does bereavement-related major depression differ from major depression associated with other stressful life events? *American Journal of Psychiatry, 165*(11), 1449–1455.

Klainin-Yobas, P., Keawkerd, O., Pumpuang, W., et al. (2014). The mediating effects of coping on the stress and health relationships among nursing students: A structural equation modelling approach. *Journal of Advanced Nursing, 70,* 1287–1298.

Lloyd, C., Smith, J., & Weinger, K. (2005). Stress and diabetes: A review of the links. *Diabetes Spectrum, 18*(2), 121–127.

Maslow, G. R., Haydon, A., McRee, A.-L., et al. (2011). Growing up with a chronic illness: Social success, educational/vocational distress. *Journal of Adolescent Health, 49,* 206–212.

Mausbach, B. T., Roepke, S. K., Chattillion, E. A., et al. (2012). Multiple mediators of the relations between caregiving stress and depressive symptoms. *Aging & Mental Health, 16,* 27–38.

Mazzola, J., Schonfeld, I., & Spector, P. (2011). What qualitative research has taught us about occupational stress. *Stress Health, 27,* 93–110.

McNulty, P. (2005). Reported stressors and health care needs of active duty Navy personnel during three phases of deployment in support of the war in Iraq. *Military Medicine, 170,* 530–535.

Newman, M., Holden, G., & Delville, Y. (2005). Isolation and the stress of being bullied. *Journal of Adolescence, 28,* 343–357.

Newman, M., Holden, G., & Delville, Y. (2011). Coping with the stress of being bullied: Consequences of coping strategies among college students. *Social Psychological Perspectives in Science, 2,* 205–211.

Nielsen, N., et al. (2008). Perceived stress and cause-specific mortality among men and women: Results from a prospective cohort study. *American Journal of Epidemiology, 168*(5), 481–491.

Norris, A. E., Aroian, K. J., & Nickerson, D. M. (2011). Premigration persecution, postmigration stressors and resources, and postmigration mental health: A study of severely traumatized U.S. Arab immigrant women. *Journal of the American Psychiatric Nurses Association, 17,* 283–293.

Pender, N., Murtaugh, C., & Parsons, M. (2010). *Health promotion in nursing practice* (6th ed.). Upper Saddle River NJ: Prentice Hall.

Pietrzak, R. H., Goldstein, R. B., Southwick, S. M., et al. (2012). Physical health conditions associated with posttraumatic stress disorder in U.S. older adults: Results from wave 2 of the National Epidemiologic Survey on Alcohol and Related Conditions. *Journal of the American Geriatrics Society, 60,* 296–303.

Saadatmand, V., Rejeh, N., Heravi-Karimooi, M., et al. (2013). Effect of nature-based sounds' intervention on agitation, anxiety, and stress in patients under mechanical ventilator support: A randomised controlled trial. *International Journal of Nursing Studies, 50,* 895–904.

Shah, P., & Shah, J. (2010). Maternal exposure to domestic violence and pregnancy and birth outcomes: A systematic review and meta-analysis. *Journal of Womens Health, 19,* 2017–2031.

Sibille, K. T., Langaee, T., Burkley, B., et al. (2012). Chronic pain, perceived stress, and cellular aging: An exploratory study. *Molecular Pain, 8,* 12.

Sue, D., et al. (2007). Racial microaggressions in everyday life. *American Psychologist, 62*(4), 271–286.

Suzuki, H., Luby, J. L., Botteron, K. N., et al. (2014). Early life stress and trauma and enhanced limbic activation to emotionally valenced faces in depressed and healthy children. *Journal of the American Academy of Child and Adolescent Psychiatry, 53,* 800–813, e810.

Upton, D., & Solowiej, K. (2010). Pain and stress as contributors to delayed wound healing. *Wound Practice & Research, 18,* 114–122.

Warning, L. (2011). Are you positive? The influence of life orientation on the anxiety levels of nursing students. *Holistic Nursing Practice, 25,* 254–257.

● = Independent;   ▲ = Collaborative;   **EBN** = Evidence-Based Nursing;   **EB** = Evidence-Based

Wendler, D., & Rid, A. (2011). Systematic review: The effect on surrogates of making treatment decisions for others. *Annals of Internal Medicine, 154,* 336–346.

Wolff, J. K., Schmiedek, F., Brose, A., et al. (2013). Physical and emotional well-being and the balance of needed and received

emotional support: Age differences in a daily diary study. *Social Science & Medicine, 91,* 67–75.

Zeller, J. M., & Levin, P. F. (2013). Mindfulness interventions to reduce stress among nursing personnel: An occupational health perspective. *Workplace Health & Safety, 61,* 85–89.

Acute Substance Withdrawal syndrome   *Marina Martinez-Kratz, MS, RN, CNE*

NANDA-I

Definition

Serious, multifactorial sequelae following abrupt cessation of an addictive compound.

Defining Characteristics

Acute confusion (00128); anxiety (00146); disturbed sleep pattern (00198); nausea (00134); risk for electrolyte imbalance (00195); risk for injury (00035)

Related Factors

Developed dependence to alcohol or other addictive substance; heavy use of an addictive substance over time; malnutrition; sudden cessation of an addictive substance

At-Risk Population

History of previous withdrawal symptoms; older adults

Associated Condition

Comorbid mental disorder; comorbid serious physical illness

NOC   (Nursing Outcomes Classification)

Suggested NOC Outcomes

Anxiety Level; Comfort Status; Drug Abuse Cessation Behavior; Electrolyte Balance; Seizure Severity; Substance Addiction Consequences; Substance Withdrawal Severity; Symptom Severity; Vital Signs

Example NOC Outcome with Indicators
Substance Withdrawal Severity as evidenced by the following indicators: Substance cravings/Change in vital signs/ Irritability/Nausea. (Rate the outcome and indicators of **Substance Withdrawal Severity:** 1 = severe deviation from normal range, 2 = substantial deviation from normal range, 3 = moderate deviation from normal range, 4 = mild deviation from normal range, 5 = no deviation from normal range [see Section I].)

Client Outcomes

Client Will (Specify Time Frame)

- Will stabilize and remain free from physical injury
- Verbalizes effects of substances on body
- Maintain vital signs and lab values within normal range
- Verbalizes importance of adequate nutrition

NIC   (Nursing Interventions Classification)

Suggested NIC Interventions

Behavior Management; Drug Withdrawal; Electrolyte Monitoring; Emotional Support; Nausea Management; Seizure Precautions; Smoking Cessation Assistance; Substance Use Treatment: Alcohol Withdrawal; Substance Use Treatment: Anxiety Reduction

• = Independent;   ▲ = Collaborative;   EBN = Evidence-Based Nursing;   EB = Evidence-Based

Example NIC Activities—Substance Use Treatment: Alcohol Withdrawal

Monitor vital signs during withdrawal, Monitor for delirium tremens, Administer medications, Provide symptom management, Implement seizure precautions

Nursing Interventions and *Rationales*

Alcohol-Induced Withdrawal Syndrome

- Assess for client's pattern of alcohol use, last drink, and current blood alcohol levels. EB: *Because of ethanol's short action, withdrawal symptoms begin within 6 to 8 hours after blood alcohol levels decrease, peak at 72 hours, and are markedly reduced by days 5 through 7 (Schuckit, 2014; Long, Long, & Koyfman, 2017).*
- Implement seizure precautions. EB: *Clients in alcohol withdrawal are at risk for developing withdrawal seizures related to central nervous system (CNS) hyperstimulation caused by loss of gamma-aminobutyric acid (GABA) inhibitory effect (Long, Long, & Koyfman, 2017). The development of acute symptomatic seizures during an alcohol withdrawal episode is associated with a fourfold increase in the mortality rate that is caused by complications of severe alcohol use disorder (Jesse et al, 2017).*
- Rule out other causes of symptoms. EB: *The presence of other disease processes requires immediate treatment and stabilization (Long, Long, & Koyfman, 2017). Other assessments should include a check of blood gases, a review of glucose and electrolyte laboratory panels, a review of potential medication reactions, presence for infection, and other conditions.*
- Monitor vital signs. EB: *Tachycardia and hypertension are among the broad symptoms of alcohol withdrawal (Long, Long, & Koyfman, 2017).*
- Assess for progression of withdrawal symptoms such as insomnia, anxiety, nausea/vomiting, tremulousness, headache, diaphoresis, palpitations, increased body temperature, tachycardia, and hypertension. EBN: *These are the broad symptoms of alcohol withdrawal that can progress in intensity without treatment (Makic, 2017).*
- Monitor severity of withdrawal symptoms with the Clinical Institute Withdrawal Assessment (CIWA-Ar). CEB: *The CIWA-Ar is a 10-item scale for clinical quantification of the severity of the alcohol withdrawal syndrome (Sullivan et al, 1989; Kattimani & Bharadwaj, 2013). The CIWA-Ar scale is available at http://www.cbhallc.com/documents/4a-detox%20guidelines.pdf.*
- Evaluate the client for progression to the delirium tremens (DTs). EB: *The DTs are severe and life-threatening withdrawal symptoms that occur in 3% to 5% of patients on about the third day of withdrawal. DT symptoms have a rapid onset and include the broad alcohol withdrawal symptoms, fluctuating levels of cognition and attention, and autonomic instability. Associated risk factors are previous DTs, untreated seizures, CIWA-Ar score > 15, heart rate > 100, history of sustained drinking, systolic blood pressure > 150 mm Hg, alcohol intake > 2 days, age > 30 years, recent misuse of benzodiazepines, and concurrent medical illness (Long, Long, & Koyfman, 2017).*
- Assess nutritional status for risk of malnutrition. Assess for thiamine (B_1) deficiency, which is associated with chronic alcohol abuse, folate deficiency, and vitamin D deficiency associated with a history of inadequate exposure to sunlight. Consult with health care provider as needed for supplement order. EB: *Alcoholism is a major cause of malnutrition in the United States. Thiamine deficiencies contribute to the development of Korsakoff's syndrome and Wernicke's encephalopathy, which are neurological complications of alcohol abuse (Manzo et al, 2014; Dugum & McCullough, 2015). Vitamin D insufficiency is associated with cognitive impairment (Goodwill & Szoeke, 2017).*
- Address hydration needs. EB: *Clients in alcohol withdrawal require administration of fluids to correct dehydration (Mirijello et al, 2015; Long, Long, & Koyfman, 2017).*
- Determine hepatic and renal functioning prior to administration of medications. EB: *Hepatic or renal disease can slow the clearance of medications and lead to complications or toxicities (Long, Long, & Koyfman, 2017).*

Opioid-Induced Withdrawal Syndrome

- Assess for client's opioid of choice, last use, and current withdrawal symptoms. EB: *The onset of withdrawal symptoms depends on the half-life of the opioid used. Heroin withdrawal occurs 6 to 8 hours after the last use, and methadone and fentanyl withdrawal occurs 1 to 3 days after the last dose (Donroe et al, 2017).*
- Monitor severity of withdrawal symptoms with the Clinical Opiate Withdrawal Scale (COWS). EB: *A standardized assessment tool is necessary for evaluating and treating opioid withdrawal. The COWS is scored*

● = Independent;   ▲ = Collaborative;   EBN = Evidence-Based Nursing;   EB = Evidence-Based

numerically based on severity, with values summed to give a cumulative score. A threshold score indicates when treatment should be initiated (Wesson & Ling, 2003).

- Nurses should wait to administer the first dose of buprenorphine to opioid-dependent patients until clients are experiencing mild to moderate opioid withdrawal symptoms. **EB:** *The American Society of Addiction Medicine (ASAM) National Practice Guidelines recommended waiting to administer the first dose of buprenorphine until clients are experiencing mild to moderate opioid withdrawal symptoms to reduce the risk of precipitated withdrawal (Kampman & Jarvis, 2015).*
- Assess and manage early opioid withdrawal symptoms (agitation, anxiety, insomnia, muscle aches, increased lacrimation, rhinorrhea, sweating, and yawning) and late opioid withdrawal symptoms (abdominal cramping, diarrhea, pupillary dilation, nausea, vomiting, and piloerection) of opioid withdrawal. **EBN:** *Severe withdrawal can lead to fluid and electrolyte imbalances, cardiac dysrhythmias, acute kidney injury, or rhabdomyolysis. A failure to treat could result in client injury or in clients leaving the clinical setting against medical advice (Turner et al, 2018).*
- Monitor vital signs. **EBN:** *Parameters for blood pressure should be followed especially for patients treated with clonidine or other alpha-2 agonists, which can cause hypotension (Turner et al, 2018).*
- Teach the client about the anticipated withdrawal symptoms and opioid cravings while offering support and encouragement. **EBN:** *A lack of knowledge in conjunction with decreased nurse empathy and engagement are barriers to treatment (Worley, 2017).*
- ▲ Monitor laboratory reports and report to health care provider. **EBN:** *Serum electrolytes are closely evaluated for abnormalities and replaced as indicated (Turner et al, 2018).*
- ▲ Refer patient for buprenorphine, methadone, or naltrexone treatment. **EB:** *Using medications for opioid withdrawal management is recommended over abrupt cessation of opioids. Abrupt cessation of opioids may lead to strong cravings, which can lead to continued use (Kampman & Jarvis, 2015). A recent study showed that emergency department–initiated buprenorphine was associated with increased engagement in addiction treatment and reduced illicit opioid use during the 2-month interval when buprenorphine was continued in primary care (D'Onofrio et al, 2017).*

Benzodiazepine-Induced Withdrawal Syndrome

- Assess for client's last benzodiazepine use, and current withdrawal symptoms. **EB:** *The onset of withdrawal symptoms occurs within 1 to 3 days of drug cessation. Common withdrawal symptoms include any of the following: autonomic instability (tachycardia, elevated blood pressure), tremulousness, diaphoresis, insomnia, anxiety, depression, psychosis (hallucinations, delusions), sensory hypersensitivity (photophobia, hyperacusis), perceptual distortions, depersonalization, agoraphobia, flulike symptoms, paresthesias, muscle stiffness, ataxia, visual disturbances, DTs, and seizures (Puening et al, 2016).*
- Implement seizure precautions. **EB:** *Clients withdrawing from benzodiazepines may also experience seizures on withdrawal (Puening et al, 2016).*
- Rule out delirium from other causes or other withdrawal syndromes. **EB:** *The symptoms of benzodiazepine withdrawal appear similar to delirium, as well as barbiturate or alcohol withdrawal (Puening et al, 2016).*
- ▲ Anticipate use of the same treatment protocols as for alcohol withdrawal and use of a long-acting benzodiazepine in tapering doses over time. **EB:** *A tapering schedule will assist with prevention of relapse (Donroe et al, 2017).*

Cocaine/Methamphetamine-Induced Withdrawal Syndrome

- Assess for client's last stimulant use, and current withdrawal symptoms. **EB:** *The onset of withdrawal symptoms occurs within 24 hours after abrupt discontinuation of using high amounts of amphetamine-type substances over a prolonged period of time. Common stimulant withdrawal symptoms include depressed mood with any of the following: fatigue, vivid dreams, insomnia, increased appetite, psychomotor retardation, and agitation. Cocaine withdrawal is mild and treated supportively. Methamphetamine use can result in significant psychiatric withdrawal symptoms and intense craving after abrupt cessation (Donroe et al, 2017).*

Cannabis-Induced Withdrawal Syndrome

- Assess for client's last cannabis use, and current withdrawal symptoms. **EB:** *The onset of withdrawal symptoms occurs within a week of cannabis cessation. Common cannabis withdrawal symptoms include any of the following: anxiety, irritability, malaise, dysphoria, decreased appetite, restlessness, and sleep disturbances (Zehra et al, 2018).*

- Direct nursing actions to address anxiety, irritability, sleep disturbances, and decreased appetite. **EB:** *Nursing care should target the specific symptoms of cannabis withdrawal as part of a treatment that targets cannabis use reduction and prevention of relapse (Zehra et al, 2018).*

Nicotine-Induced Withdrawal Syndrome

- Assess for client's last nicotine use, and current withdrawal symptoms. **EB:** *The onset of withdrawal symptoms occurs within hours of last use. Common nicotine withdrawal symptoms include craving for nicotine, irritability, anger, frustration, anxiety, difficulty concentrating, restlessness, decreased heart rate, increased appetite, weight gain, tremor, headaches, craving, delirium, and sleep disturbance (Ginige, 2016).*
- Rule out nicotine withdrawal as the cause of delirium in critically ill clients. **EB:** *Chronic consumption of nicotine can cause desensitization and upregulation of acetylcholine receptors. In an acute nicotine withdrawal state, the lack of sufficient nicotinic stimulation leads to acetylcholine deficiency, which is associated with delirium (Ginige, 2016).*

All Withdrawal Syndromes

- Obtain a drug and/or alcohol history using a tool such as the AUDIT-C or the DAST-10. **EB:** *The Audit-C is a simple 3-question screen for hazardous or harmful drinking that can stand alone or be incorporated into general health history questionnaires. The DAST-10 is a 10-item, yes/no self-report instrument that takes less than 8 minutes to complete (Mulvaney-Day et al, 2018).*
- Implement and follow institutional withdrawal protocols. **EB:** *A recent study suggested that using a protocol for treatment of critical care patients with alcohol withdrawal leads to decreased intensive care unit (ICU) length of stay and reduced ICU cost (Tavani et al, 2017).*
- Assess for signs of recent trauma or head injury. **EB:** *A study found that trauma patients that present to the hospital in a delayed fashion have unique characteristics and are more likely to suffer negative outcomes including substance withdrawal (Kao et al, 2017).*
- Assess client's level of consciousness, monitor for changes in behavior, and orient to reality as needed. **EB:** *Reality orientation will support the client with changes in level of consciousness or behavior and may indicate progression of withdrawal (Mirijello et al, 2015).*
- Assess vital signs and monitor for existing medical conditions and current medications. **EB:** *Withdrawal symptoms can be exacerbated or masked by existing medical conditions, medications, or treatments (Long, Long, & Koyfman, 2017).*
- Assess and monitor for expression of psychological distress. **EB:** *Withdrawal can cause or exacerbate current emotional, psychological, or mental problems (Harford et al, 2018).*
- Collect urine/serum samples for laboratory tests. **EB:** *Routine treatment for substance withdrawal should include serum (or breath) alcohol concentrations, complete blood count, renal function tests, electrolytes, glucose, liver enzymes, urinalysis, and urine toxicology screening (Mirijello et al, 2015).*
- Address craving for substances with mindfulness-based techniques. **EB:** *Compared with those receiving usual care, a study found mindfulness-based addiction treatment participants reported lower anxiety, concentration difficulties, craving, and dependence, as well as higher self-efficacy for managing negative affect without smoking (Spears et al, 2017).*
- Respond to agitated behavior with deescalation techniques. **EBN:** *Research shows staff intervention can modify processes and reduce further conflict (Berring, Pedersen, & Buus, 2016).*
- Administer as needed (PRN) medications for agitation and symptom control as ordered. **EB:** *A study found symptom-triggered treatment for alcohol withdrawal syndrome individualizes treatment, is safe, decreases treatment duration and the use of benzodiazepines, and consequently reduces health care costs (Soravia et al, 2018).*
- Provide a quiet room without dark shadows, noises, or other excessive stimuli. **EB:** *Supportive care includes controlling environmental stimuli that may increase client agitation or irritability (Mirijello et al, 2015).*
- Provide suicide precautions and 1:1 staffing for clients that are delirious or who may present a danger to themselves or others. **EB:** *A recent study showed that substance use disorders are associated with self- and other-directed violence (Harford et al, 2018).*

 ### Client/Family Teaching and Discharge Planning

- ▲ After withdrawal symptoms have subsided, refer client to substance use treatment. **EB:** *Collaborative discharge planning can increase the likelihood of the patient's success with substance abstinence. Referral to appropriate services can reduce discharges against medical advice and increase follow-up in postdischarge addiction treatment centers (Donroe et al, 2017).*

● = Independent;   ▲ = Collaborative;   **EBN** = Evidence-Based Nursing;   **EB** = Evidence-Based

▲ Refer for smoking cessation services that target nicotine craving. **EB:** *A recent study found that nicotine craving may be a useful therapeutic target for increasing the effectiveness of smoking-cessation treatment (Magee, Lewis, & Winhusen, 2016).*

REFERENCES

Berring, L. L., Pedersen, L., & Buus, N. (2016). Coping with violence in mental health care settings: Patient and staff member perspectives on de-escalation practices. *Archives of Psychiatric Nursing, 30*(5), 499–507. doi-org.proxy.lib.umich.edu/10.1016/j.apnu.2016.05.005.

D'Onofrio, G., et al. (2017). Emergency department-initiated buprenorphine for opioid dependence with continuation in primary care: Outcomes during and after intervention. *Journal of General Internal Medicine, 32*(6), 660–666. doi-org.proxy.lib.umich.edu/10.1007/s11606-017-3993-2.

Donroe, J. H., et al. (2017). Substance use, intoxication, and withdrawal in the critical care setting. *Critical Care Clinics, 33*(3), 543–558.

Dugum, M., & McCullough, A. (2015). Diagnosis and management of alcoholic liver disease. *Journal of Clinical Translational Hepatolgy, 3*(2), 109–116.

Ginige, S. (2016). Nicotine withdrawal: An often overlooked and easily reversible cause of terminal restlessness. *European Journal of Palliative Care, 23*(3), 128–129.

Goodwill, A. M., & Szoeke, C. (2017). A systematic review and meta-analysis of the effect of low vitamin D on cognition. *Journal of the American Geriatric Society, 65*(10), 2161–2168. doi:10.1111/jgs.15012.

Harford, T. C., et al. (2018). Substance use disorders and self- and other-directed violence among adults: Results from the National Survey on Drug Use and Health. *Journal of Affective Disorders, 225*, 365–373. Retrieved from http://dx.doi.org/10.1016/j.jad.2017.08.021.

Jesse, S., et al. (2017). Alcohol withdrawal syndrome: Mechanisms, manifestations, and management. *Acta Neurologica Scandinavica, 135*(1), 4–16. doi:10.1111/ane.12671.

Kampman, K., & Jarvis, M. (2015). American Society of Addiction Medicine (ASAM) national practice guideline for the use of medications in the treatment of addiction involving opioid use. *Journal of Addiction Medicine, 9*, 358–367.

Kattimani, S., & Bharadwaj, B. (2013). Clinical management of alcohol withdrawal: A systematic review. *Industrial Psychiatry Journal, 22*(2), 100–108. doi:10.4103/0972-6748.132914.

Kao, M. J., et al. (2017). Trauma patients who present in a delayed fashion: A unique and challenging population. *Journal of Surgical Research, 208*, 204–210. doi-org.proxy.lib.umich.edu/10.1016/j.jss.2016.09.037.

Long, D., Long, B., & Koyfman, A. (2017). The emergency medicine management of severe alcohol withdrawal. *The American Journal of Emergency Medicine, 35*(7), 1005–1011. http://doi.org.proxy.lib.umich.edu/10.1016/j.ajem.2017.02.002.

Magee, J. C., Lewis, D. F., & Winhusen, T. (2016). Evaluating nicotine craving, withdrawal, and substance use as mediators of smoking cessation in cocaine- and methamphetamine-dependent patients. *Nicotine & Tobacco Research: Official Journal of the Society for Research on Nicotine and Tobacco, 18*(5), 1196–1201. doi-org.proxy.lib.umich.edu/10.1093/ntr/ntv121.

Manzo, G., De Gennaro, A., Cozzolino, A., et al. (2014). MR imaging findings in alcoholic and nonalcoholic acute Wernicke's encephalopathy: A review. *BioMed Research International, 2014*, 503596. doi:10.1155/2014/503596.

Makic, M. B. F. (2017). Alcohol withdrawal syndrome. *Journal of Perianesthesia Nursing, 32*(2), 140–141. Retrieved from https://doi-org.proxy.lib.umich.edu/10.1016/j.jopan.2017.01.007.

Mirijello, A., D'Angelo, C., Ferrulli, A., et al. (2015). Identification and management of alcohol withdrawal syndrome. *Drugs, 75*(4), 353–365. doi-org.proxy.lib.umich.edu/10.1007/s40265-015-0358-1.

Mulvaney-Day, N., et al. (2018). Screening for behavioral health conditions in primary care settings: A systematic review of the literature. *Journal of General Internal Medicine, 33*(3), 335–346. Retrieved from https://doi.org/10.1007/s11606-017-4181-0.

Puening, S. E., et al. (2016). Psychiatric emergencies for clinicians: Emergency department management of benzodiazepine withdrawal. *The Journal of Emergency Medicine, 52*(1), 66–69. doi-org.proxy.lib.umich.edu/10.1016/j.jemermed.2016.05.035.

Schuckit, M. A. (2014). Recognition and management of withdrawal delirium (delirium tremens). *New England Journal of Medicine, 371*(22), 2109–2113. doi:10.1056/NEJMra1407298.

Soravia, L. M., et al. (2018). Symptom-triggered detoxification using the alcohol-withdrawal-scale reduces risks and healthcare costs. *Alcohol and Alcoholism, 53*(1), 71–77. doi-org.proxy.lib.umich.edu/10.1093/alcalc/agx080.

Spears, C. A., et al. (2017). Mechanisms underlying mindfulness-based addiction treatment versus cognitive behavioral therapy and usual care for smoking cessation. *Journal of Consulting and Clinical Psychology, 85*(11), 1029–1040. doi:10.1037/ccp0000229.

Sullivan, J. T., Sykora, K., Schneiderman, J., et al. (1989). Assessment of alcohol withdrawal: The revised clinical institute withdrawal assessment for alcohol scale. *British Journal of Addiction, 84*(11), 1353–1357.

Tavani, L., et al. (2017). A protocol for the management of alcohol withdrawal in the intensive care unit: A pilot study. *Critical Care Medicine, 46*(1 Suppl. 1), 357. doi:10.1097/01.ccm.0000528755.55400.b6.

Turner, C. C., et al. (2018). Opioid use disorder: Challenges during acute hospitalization. *The Journal for Nurse Practitioners, 14*(2), 61–67. Retrieved from https://doi.org/10.1016/j.nurpra.2017.12.009.

Wesson, D. R., & Ling, W. (2003). The clinical opiate withdrawal scale (COWS). *Journal of Psychoactive Drugs, 35*(2), 253–259.

Worley, J. (2017). A primer on heroin and fentanyl. *Journal of Psychosocial Nursing & Mental Health Services, 55*(6), 16–20. doi.org.proxy.lib.umich.edu/10.3928/02793695-20170519-02.

Zehra, A., et al. (2018). Cannabis addiction and the brain: A review. *Journal of Neuroimmune Pharmacology: The Official Journal of the Society on NeuroImmune Pharmacology, 13*(4), 438–452. Retrieved from https://doi.org/10.1007/s11481-018-9782-9.

S

● = Independent;   ▲ = Collaborative;   **EBN** = Evidence-Based Nursing;   **EB** = Evidence-Based

Risk for acute Substance Withdrawal syndrome   *Marina Martinez-Kratz, MS, RN, CNE*

NANDA-I

Definition

Susceptible to serious, multifactorial sequelae following abrupt cessation of an addictive compound, which may compromise health.

Risk Factors

Developed dependence to alcohol or other addictive substance, heavy use of an addictive substance over time, malnutrition, sudden cessation of an addictive substance

At-Risk Population

History of previous withdrawal symptoms; older adults

Associated Condition

Comorbid mental disorder; comorbid serious physical illness

NOC   (Nursing Outcomes Classification)

Suggested NOC Outcomes

Anxiety Level; Comfort Status; Drug Abuse Cessation Behavior; Electrolyte Balance; Seizure Severity; Substance Addiction Consequences; Substance Withdrawal Severity; Symptom Severity; Vital Signs

Example NOC Outcome with Indicators

Substance Withdrawal Severity as evidenced by the following indicators: Substance cravings/Change in vital signs/Irritability/Nausea. (Rate the outcome and indicators of **Substance Withdrawal Severity:** 1 = severe deviation from normal range, 2 = substantial deviation from normal range, 3 = moderate deviation from normal range, 4 = mild deviation from normal range, 5 = no deviation from normal range [see Section I].)

Client Outcomes

Client Will (Specify Time Frame)

- Will stabilize and remain free from physical injury
- Verbalizes effects of substances on body
- Maintain vital signs and lab values within normal range
- Verbalizes importance of adequate nutrition

NIC   (Nursing Interventions Classification)

Suggested NIC Interventions

Anxiety Reduction; Behavior Management; Electrolyte Monitoring; Emotional Support; Nausea Management; Seizure Precautions; Smoking Cessation Assistance; Substance Use Treatment: Alcohol Withdrawal; Substance Use Treatment: Drug Withdrawal

Example NIC Activities—Substance Use Treatment: Alcohol Withdrawal

Monitor vital signs during withdrawal, Monitor for delirium tremens, Administer medications, Provide symptom management, Implement seizure precautions

Nursing Interventions and *Rationales*

Risk for Alcohol-Induced Withdrawal Syndrome

- Assess for client's pattern of alcohol use, last drink, and current blood alcohol levels. EB: *Because of ethanol's short action, withdrawal symptoms begin within 6 to 8 hours after blood alcohol levels decrease, peak at 72 hours, and are markedly reduced by days 5 through 7 (Schuckit, 2014; Long, Long, & Koyfman, 2017).*

● = Independent;   ▲ = Collaborative;   EBN = Evidence-Based Nursing;   EB = Evidence-Based

S

- Implement seizure precautions. **EB:** *Clients in alcohol withdrawal are at risk for developing withdrawal seizures related to central nervous system (CNS) hyperstimulation caused by loss of gamma-aminobutyric acid (GABA) inhibitory effect (Long, Long, & Koyfman, 2017). The development of acute symptomatic seizures during an alcohol withdrawal episode is associated with a fourfold increase in the mortality rate caused by complications of severe alcohol use disorder (Jesse et al, 2017).*
- Rule out other causes of symptoms. **EB:** *The presence of other disease processes requires immediate treatment and stabilization (Long, Long, & Koyfman, 2017). Other assessments should include a check of blood gases, a review of glucose and electrolyte laboratory panels, a review of potential medication reactions, presence for infection, and other conditions.*
- Monitor vital signs. **EB:** *Tachycardia and hypertension are among the broad symptoms of alcohol withdrawal (Long, Long, & Koyfman, 2017).*
- Assess for progression of withdrawal symptoms such as insomnia, anxiety, nausea/vomiting, tremulousness, headache, diaphoresis, palpitations, increased body temperature, tachycardia, and hypertension. **EBN:** *These are the broad symptoms of alcohol withdrawal that can progress in intensity without treatment (Makic, 2017).*
- Monitor severity of withdrawal symptoms with the Clinical Institute Withdrawal Assessment (CIWA-Ar). **CEB:** *The CIWA-Ar is a 10-item scale for clinical quantification of the severity of the alcohol withdrawal syndrome (Sullivan et al, 1989; Kattimani & Bharadwaj, 2013). The CIWA-Ar scale is available at http://www.cbhallc.com/documents/4a-detox%20guidelines.pdf.*
- Evaluate the client for progression to the delirium tremens (DTs). **EB:** *The DTs are severe and life-threatening withdrawal symptoms that occur in 3% to 5% of patients on about the third day of withdrawal. DT symptoms have a rapid onset and include the broad alcohol withdrawal symptoms, fluctuating levels of cognition and attention, and autonomic instability. Associated risk factors are previous DTs, untreated seizures, CIWA-Ar score > 15, heart rate > 100, history of sustained drinking, systolic blood pressure > 150 mm Hg, alcohol intake > 2 days, age > 30 years, recent misuse of benzodiazepines, and concurrent medical illness (Long, Long, & Koyfman, 2017).*
- Assess nutritional status for risk of malnutrition, thiamine (B_1) deficiency associated with chronic alcohol abuse, folate deficiency, and vitamin D deficiency–associated history of inadequate exposure to sunlight. Consult with health care provider as needed for supplement order. **EB:** *Alcoholism is a major cause of malnutrition in the United States. Thiamine deficiencies contribute to the development of Korsakoff's syndrome and Wernicke's encephalopathy, which are neurological complications of alcohol abuse (Manzo et al, 2014; Dugum & McCullough, 2015). Vitamin D insufficiency is associated with cognitive impairment (Goodwill & Szoeke, 2017).*
- Address hydration needs. **EB:** *Clients in alcohol withdrawal require administration of fluids to correct dehydration (Mirijello et al, 2015; Long, Long, & Koyfman, 2017).*
- Determine hepatic and renal functioning prior to administration of medications. **EB:** *Hepatic or renal disease can slow the clearance of medications and lead to complications or toxicities (Long, Long, & Koyfman, 2017).*

Risk for Opioid-Induced Withdrawal Syndrome

- Assess for client's opioid of choice, last use, and current withdrawal symptoms. **EB:** *The onset of withdrawal symptoms depends on the half-life of the opioid used. Heroin withdrawal occurs 6 to 8 hours after the last use, and methadone and fentanyl withdrawal occurs 1 to 3 days after the last dose (Donroe et al, 2017).*
- Monitor severity of withdrawal symptoms with the Clinical Opiate Withdrawal Scale (COWS). **EB:** *A standardized assessment tool is necessary for evaluating and treating opioid withdrawal. The COWS is scored numerically based on severity, with values summed to give a cumulative score. A threshold score indicates when treatment should be initiated (Wesson & Ling, 2003).*
- Assess and manage early opioid withdrawal symptoms (agitation, anxiety, insomnia, muscle aches, increased lacrimation, rhinorrhea, sweating, and yawning) and late opioid withdrawal symptoms (abdominal cramping, diarrhea, pupillary dilation, nausea, vomiting, and piloerection) of opioid withdrawal. **EBN:** *Severe withdrawal can lead to fluid and electrolyte imbalances, cardiac dysrhythmias, acute kidney injury, or rhabdomyolysis. A failure to treat could result in client injury or in clients leaving the clinical setting against medical advice (Turner et al, 2018).*
- Monitor vital signs. **EBN:** *Parameters for blood pressure should be followed especially for patients treated with clonidine or other alpha-2 agonists, which can cause hypotension (Turner et al, 2018).*
- Clients should be taught about risk of relapse and other safety concerns from using opioid withdrawal management as stand-alone treatment for opioid use disorder. **EB:** *Opioid withdrawal management on its own is not a treatment method (Kampman & Jarvis, 2015).*

● = Independent;　▲ = Collaborative;　**EBN** = Evidence-Based Nursing;　**EB** = Evidence-Based

- Teach the client about the anticipated withdrawal symptoms and opioid cravings, while offering support and encouragement. EBN: *A lack of knowledge in conjunction with decreased nurse empathy and engagement are barriers to treatment (Worley, 2017).*
▲ Monitor laboratory reports and report to health care provider. EBN: *Serum electrolytes are closely evaluated for abnormalities and replaced as indicated (Turner et al, 2018).*
▲ Refer patient for buprenorphine or methadone treatment. EB: *Using medications for opioid withdrawal management is recommended over abrupt cessation of opioids. Abrupt cessation of opioids may lead to strong cravings, which can lead to continued use (Kampman & Jarvis, 2015). A recent study showed that emergency department–initiated buprenorphine was associated with increased engagement in addiction treatment and reduced illicit opioid use during the 2-month interval when buprenorphine was continued in primary care (D'Onofrio et al, 2017).*

Risk for Benzodiazepine-Induced Withdrawal Syndrome

- Assess for client's last benzodiazepine use, and current withdrawal symptoms. EB: *The onset of withdrawal symptoms occurs within 1 to 3 days of drug cessation. Common withdrawal symptoms include any of the following: autonomic instability (tachycardia, elevated blood pressure), tremulousness, diaphoresis, insomnia, anxiety, depression, psychosis (hallucinations, delusions), sensory hypersensitivity (photophobia, hyperacusis), perceptual distortions, depersonalization, agoraphobia, flulike symptoms, paresthesia, muscle stiffness, ataxia, visual disturbances, DTs, and seizures (Puening et al, 2016).*
- Implement seizure precautions. EB: *Clients withdrawing from benzodiazepines may also experience seizures on withdrawal (Puening et al, 2016).*
- Rule out delirium from other causes or other withdrawal syndromes. EB: *The symptoms of benzodiazepine withdrawal appear similar to delirium, as well as barbiturate or alcohol withdrawal (Puening et al, 2016).*
▲ Anticipate use of the same treatment protocols as for alcohol withdrawal and use of a long-acting benzodiazepine in tapering doses over time. EB: *A tapering schedule will assist with prevention of relapse (Donroe et al, 2017).*

Risk for Cocaine/Methamphetamine-Induced Withdrawal Syndrome

- Assess for client's last stimulant use, and current withdrawal symptoms. EB: *The onset of withdrawal symptoms occurs within 24 hours after abrupt discontinuation of using high amounts of amphetamine-type substances over a prolonged period of time. Common stimulant withdrawal symptoms include depressed mood with any of the following: fatigue, vivid dreams, insomnia, increased appetite, psychomotor retardation, and agitation. Cocaine withdrawal is mild and treated supportively. Methamphetamine use can result in significant psychiatric withdrawal symptoms and intense craving after abrupt cessation (Donroe et al, 2017).*

Risk for Cannabis-Induced Withdrawal Syndrome

- Assess for client's last cannabis use, and current withdrawal symptoms. EB: *The onset of withdrawal symptoms occurs within a week of cannabis cessation. Common cannabis withdrawal symptoms include any of the following: anxiety, irritability, malaise, dysphoria, decreased appetite, restlessness, and sleep disturbances (Zehra et al, 2018).*
- Direct nursing actions to address anxiety, irritability, sleep disturbances, and decreased appetite. EB: *Nursing care should target the specific symptoms of cannabis withdrawal as part of a treatment that targets cannabis use reduction and prevention of relapse (Zehra et al, 2018).*

Risk for Nicotine-Induced Withdrawal Syndrome

- Assess for client's last nicotine use, and current withdrawal symptoms. EB: *The onset of withdrawal symptoms occurs within hours of last use. Common nicotine withdrawal symptoms include craving for nicotine, irritability, anger, frustration, anxiety, difficulty concentrating, restlessness, decreased heart rate, increased appetite, weight gain, tremor, headaches, craving, delirium, and sleep disturbance (Ginige, 2016).*
- Rule out nicotine withdrawal as the cause of delirium in critically ill clients. EB: *Chronic consumption of nicotine can cause desensitization and upregulation of acetylcholine receptors. In an acute nicotine withdrawal state, the lack of sufficient nicotinic stimulation leads to acetylcholine deficiency, which is associated with delirium (Ginige, 2016).*

All Withdrawal Syndromes

- Obtain a drug and/or alcohol history using a tool such as the AUDIT-C or the DAST-10. EB: *The Audit-C is a simple 3-question screen for hazardous or harmful drinking that can stand alone or be incorporated into*

● = Independent;   ▲ = Collaborative;   EBN = Evidence-Based Nursing;   EB = Evidence-Based

general health history questionnaires. The DAST-10 is a 10-item, yes/no self-report instrument that takes less than 8 minutes to complete (Mulvaney-Day et al, 2018).

- Implement and follow institutional withdrawal protocols. **EB:** *A recent study suggested that using a protocol for treatment of critical care patients with alcohol withdrawal leads to decreased intensive care unit (ICU) length of stay and reduced ICU cost (Tavani et al, 2017).*
- Assess for signs of recent trauma or head injury. **EB:** *A study found that trauma patients that present to the hospital in a delayed fashion have unique characteristics and are more likely to suffer negative outcomes including substance withdrawal (Kao et al, 2017).*
- Assess client's level of consciousness, monitor for changes in behavior, and orient to reality as needed. **EB:** *Reality orientation will support the client with changes in level of consciousness or behavior and may indicate progression of withdrawal (Mirijello et al, 2015).*
- Assess vital signs and monitor for existing medical conditions and current medications. **EB:** *Withdrawal symptoms can be exacerbated or masked by existing medical conditions, medications, or treatments (Long, Long, & Koyfman, 2017).*
- Assess and monitor for expression of psychological distress. **EB:** *Withdrawal can cause or exacerbate current emotional, psychological, or mental problems (Harford et al, 2018).*
- Collect urine/serum samples for laboratory tests. **EB:** *Routine treatment for substance withdrawal should include serum (or breath) alcohol concentrations, complete blood count, renal function tests, electrolytes, glucose, liver enzymes, urinalysis, and urine toxicology screening (Mirijello et al, 2015).*
- Address craving for substances with mindfulness-based techniques. **EB:** *Compared with those receiving usual care, a study found mindfulness-based addiction treatment participants reported lower anxiety, concentration difficulties, craving, and dependence, as well as higher self-efficacy for managing negative affect without smoking (Spears et al, 2017).*
- Respond to agitated behavior with deescalation techniques. **EBN:** *Research shows staff intervention can modify processes and reduce further conflict (Berring, Pedersen, & Buus, 2016).*
- Administer as needed (PRN) medications for agitation and symptom control as ordered. **EB:** *A study found symptom-triggered treatment for alcohol withdrawal syndrome individualizes treatment, is safe, decreases treatment duration and the use of benzodiazepines, and consequently reduces health care costs (Soravia et al, 2018).*
- Provide a quiet room without dark shadows, noises, or other excessive stimuli. **EB:** *Supportive care includes controlling environmental stimuli that may increase client agitation or irritability (Mirijello et al, 2015).*
- Provide suicide precautions and 1:1 staffing for clients that are delirious or who may present a danger to themselves or others. **EB:** *A recent study showed that substance use disorders are associated with self- and other-directed violence (Harford et al, 2018).*

 Client/Family Teaching and Discharge Planning

- ▲ After withdrawal symptoms have subsided, refer client to substance use treatment. **EB:** *Collaborative discharge planning can increase the likelihood of the patient's success of substance abstinence. Referral to appropriate services can reduce discharges against medical advice and increase follow-up in postdischarge addiction treatment centers (Donroe et al, 2017).*
- ▲ Refer for smoking cessation services that target nicotine craving. **EB:** *A recent study found that nicotine craving may be a useful therapeutic target for increasing the effectiveness of smoking-cessation treatment (Magee, Lewis, & Winhusen, 2016).*

REFERENCES

Berring, L. L., Pedersen, L., & Buus, N. (2016). Coping with violence in mental health care settings: Patient and staff member perspectives on de-escalation practices. *Archives of Psychiatric Nursing, 30*(5), 499–507. doi-org.proxy.lib.umich.edu/10.1016/j.apnu.2016.05.005.

D'Onofrio, G., et al. (2017). *Journal of General Internal Medicine, 32*(6), 660–666. doi-org.proxy.lib.umich.edu/10.1007/s11606-017-3993-2.

Donroe, J. H., et al. (2017). Substance use, intoxication, and withdrawal in the critical care setting. *Critical Care Clinics, 33*(3), 543–558.

Dugum, M., & McCullough, A. (2015). Diagnosis and management of alcoholic liver disease. *Journal of Clinical Translational Hepatology, 3*(2), 109–116.

Ginige, S. (2016). Nicotine withdrawal: An often overlooked and easily reversible cause of terminal restlessness. *European Journal of Palliative Care, 23*(3), 128–129.

Goodwill, A. M., & Szoeke, C. (2017). A systematic review and meta-analysis of the effect of low vitamin D on cognition. *Journal of the American Geriatric Society, 65*(10), 2161–2168. doi:10.1111/jgs.15012.

Harford, T. C., et al. (2018). Substance use disorders and self- and other-directed violence among adults: Results from the National Survey on Drug Use And Health. *Journal of Affective Disorders, 225*, 365–373. Retrieved from http://dx.doi.org/10.1016/j.jad.2017.08.021.

● = Independent; ▲ = Collaborative; **EBN** = Evidence-Based Nursing; **EB** = Evidence-Based

Jesse, S., et al. (2017). Alcohol withdrawal syndrome: Mechanisms, manifestations, and management. *Acta Neurologica Scandinavica, 135*(1), 4–16. doi:10.1111/ane.12671.

Kampman, K., & Jarvis, M. (2015). American Society of Addiction Medicine (ASAM) national practice guideline for the use of medications in the treatment of addiction involving opioid use. *Journal of Addiction Medicine, 9*, 358–367.

Kattimani, S., & Bharadwaj, B. (2013). Clinical management of alcohol withdrawal: A systematic review. *Industrial Psychiatry Journal, 22*(2), 100–108. doi:10.4103/0972-6748.132914.

Kao, M. J., et al. (2017). Trauma patients who present in a delayed fashion: A unique and challenging population. *Journal of Surgical Research, 208*, 204–210. doi-org.proxy.lib.umich.edu/10.1016/j.jss.2016.09.037.

Long, D., Long, B., & Koyfman, A. (2017). The emergency medicine management of severe alcohol withdrawal. *The American Journal of Emergency Medicine, 35*(7), 1005–1011. Retrieved from http://doi.org.proxy.lib.umich.edu/10.1016/j.ajem.2017.02.002.

Magee, J. C., Lewis, D. F., & Winhusen, T. (2016). Evaluating nicotine craving, withdrawal, and substance use as mediators of smoking cessation in cocaine- and methamphetamine-dependent patients. *Nicotine & Tobacco Research: Official Journal of the Society for Research on Nicotine and Tobacco, 18*(5), 1196–1201. doi-org.proxy.lib.umich.edu/10.1093/ntr/ntv121.

Manzo, G., De Gennaro, A., Cozzolino, A., et al. (2014). MR imaging findings in alcoholic and nonalcoholic acute Wernicke's encephalopathy: A review. *BioMed Research International, 2014*, 503596. doi:10.1155/2014/503596.

Makic, M. B. F. (2017). Alcohol withdrawal syndrome. *Journal of Perianesthesia Nursing, 32*(2), 140–141. Retrieved from https://doi-org.proxy.lib.umich.edu/10.1016/j.jopan.2017.01.007.

Mirijello, A., D'Angelo, C., Ferrulli, A., et al. (2015). Identification and management of alcohol withdrawal syndrome. *Drugs, 75*(4), 353–365. doi-org.proxy.lib.umich.edu/10.1007/s40265-015-0358-1.

Mulvaney-Day, N., et al. (2018). Screening for behavioral health conditions in primary care settings: a systematic review of the literature. *Journal of General Internal Medicine, 33*(3), 335–346. Retrieved from https://doi.org/10.1007/s11606-017-4181-0.

Puening, S. E., et al. (2016). Psychiatric emergencies for clinicians: Emergency department management of benzodiazepine withdrawal. *The Journal of Emergency Medicine, 52*(1), 66–69. doi-org.proxy.lib.umich.edu/10.1016/j.jemermed.2016.05.035.

Schuckit, M. A. (2014). Recognition and management of withdrawal delirium (delirium tremens). *New England Journal of Medicine, 371*(22), 2109–2113. doi:10.1056/NEJMra1407298.

Soravia, L. M., et al. (2018). Symptom-triggered detoxification using the alcohol-withdrawal-scale reduces risks and healthcare costs. *Alcohol and Alcoholism, 53*(1), 71–77. doi-org.proxy.lib.umich.edu/10.1093/alcalc/agx080.

Spears, C. A., et al. (2017). Mechanisms underlying mindfulness-based addiction treatment versus cognitive behavioral therapy and usual care for smoking cessation. *Journal of Consulting and Clinical Psychology, 85*(11), 1029–1040. doi:10.1037/ccp0000229.

Sullivan, J. T., Sykora, K., Schneiderman, J., et al. (1989). Assessment of alcohol withdrawal: The revised clinical institute withdrawal assessment for alcohol scale. *British Journal of Addiction, 84*(11), 1353–1357.

Tavani, L., et al. (2017). A protocol for the management of alcohol withdrawal in the intensive care unit: A pilot study. *Critical Care Medicine, 46*(1 Suppl. 1), 357. doi:10.1097/01.ccm.0000528755.55400.b6.

Turner, C. C., et al. (2018). Opioid use disorder: challenges during acute hospitalization. *The Journal for Nurse Practitioners, 14*(2), 61–67. Retrieved from https://doi.org/10.1016/j.nurpra.2017.12.009.

Wesson, D. R., & Ling, W. (2003). The clinical opiate withdrawal scale (COWS). *Journal of Psychoactive Drugs, 35*(2), 253–259.

Worley, J. (2017). A primer on heroin and fentanyl. *Journal of Psychosocial Nursing & Mental Health Services, 55*(6), 16–20. doi.org.proxy.lib.umich.edu/10.3928/02793695-20170519-02.

Zehra, A., et al. (2018). Cannabis addiction and the brain: A review. *Journal of Neuroimmune Pharmacology: The Official Journal of the Society on NeuroImmune Pharmacology*, 1–15. Retrieved from https://doi.org/10.1007/s11481-018-9782-9.

Risk for Sudden Infant Death *Marina Martinez-Kratz, MS, RN, CNE*

NANDA-I

Definition

Susceptible to unpredicted death of an infant.

Risk Factors

Delay in prenatal care; exposure to secondhand smoke; infant overheating; infant overwrapping; infant placed in prone position to sleep; infant placed in side-lying position to sleep; insufficient prenatal care; soft sleep surface; soft, loose objects placed near infant; infant less than 4 months, placed in sitting devices for routine sleep

At-Risk Population

African American ethnicity; age 2 to 4 months; infant not breastfed exclusively or fed with expressed breast milk; low birth weight; male gender; maternal smoking during pregnancy; Native American ethnicity; postnatal exposure to alcohol; postnatal exposure to elicit drug; prematurity; prenatal exposure to alcohol; prenatal exposure to elicit drug; young parental age

Associated Condition

Cold weather

● = Independent;   ▲ = Collaborative;   EBN = Evidence-Based Nursing;   EB = Evidence-Based

NOC (Nursing Outcomes Classification)

Suggested NOC Outcomes

Knowledge: Infant Care; Parenting Performance; Safe Home Environment; Safe Sleep Environment

---
Example NOC Outcome with Indicators

Knowledge: Infant Care as evidenced by the following indicators: Proper infant positioning/Age-appropriate cardiopulmonary resuscitation techniques. (Rate the outcome and indicators of **Knowledge: Infant Care:** 1 = no knowledge, 2 = limited knowledge 3 = moderate knowledge, 4 = substantial knowledge, 5 = extensive knowledge [see Section I].)

Client Outcomes

Client Will (Specify Time Frame)

- Explain appropriate measures to prevent sudden infant death syndrome (SIDS)
- Demonstrate correct techniques for positioning and blanketing the infant, protecting the infant from harm

NIC (Nursing Interventions Classification)

Suggested NIC Interventions

Infant Care; Teaching: Infant Safety 0 to 3 Months

Example NIC Activities—Teaching: Infant Safety

Instruct parent/caregiver to place infant on back to sleep and keep loose bedding, pillows, and toys out of crib; Instruct parent/caregiver to avoid holding infant while smoking or holding hot liquids

---

Nursing Interventions and *Rationales*

- Position the infant supine to sleep during naps and night; do not position in the prone position or side-lying position (American Academy of Pediatrics [AAP], 2014a). **EB:** *In a research review, evidence shows sleeping prone or in a side-lying position is associated with an increased risk of SIDS (Carlin & Moon, 2017).*
- Avoid use of bedding, such as blankets and loose sheets, for sleeping. Also keep quilts, pillows, bumpers, sheepskins, and soft toys out of the infant's bed. Dress the child in one-piece sleepers or wearable blankets (AAP, 2014b). *Infants can suffocate from close proximity to these soft items.*
- Avoid over bundling, overheating, and swaddling the infant. The infant should not feel hot to touch. **EB:** *Swaddling increases the risk of SIDS twofold in infants 6 months or younger (Pease et al, 2016). Swaddling has been associated with infant death, especially when the infant has shown the ability to roll over (Carlin & Moon, 2017).*
- Provide the infant a certain amount of time in the prone position while the infant is awake and observed. Change the direction that the baby lies in the crib from one week to the next; avoid too much time in car seats and carriers. *Prolonged time in the supine position can result in a flat head shape and decreased strength of the neck and shoulder muscles (AAP, 2014a).*

Home Care

- Most of the interventions and client teaching information are relevant to home care.
- Evaluate home for potential safety hazards, such as inappropriate cribs, cradles, or strollers.
- Determine where and how the child sleeps, and provide instructions on safe sleeping positions and environments as needed.

Multicultural

- Encourage pregnant American Indian mothers and native Alaskan Indian mothers to avoid drinking alcohol and to avoid wrapping infants in excessive blankets or clothing. **EB:** *A study of the death rate of infants of Indian mothers found an increased rate of SIDS compared with the white population, which was*

● = Independent; ▲ = Collaborative; **EBN** = Evidence-Based Nursing; **EB** = Evidence-Based

thought to be associated with alcohol ingestion and excessive clothing and blankets used by the mothers (Wong et al, 2014).

- Encourage Hispanic and black mothers to find alternatives to bed sharing or placing infants for sleep on adult beds, sofas, or cots, and to avoid placing pillows, soft toys, and soft bedding in the sleep environment. **EB:** *A study found that both Hispanic and black mothers were more likely to share a bed with an infant, and as a result there is an increasing rate of SIDS in their infants (Colson et al, 2013).*

 ### Client/Family Teaching and Discharge Planning

- Teach the safety guidelines for infant care in the previous interventions.
- Provide parents of both term and preterm infants with verbal and written education about SIDS and ways to reduce the risk of SIDS before discharge to home. **EBN:** *Study results demonstrated that providing current written material along with modeling safe sleep practices in the hospital prior to discharge to home can help further reduce the incidence of SIDS (Dufer & Godfrey, 2017).*
- Recommend breastfeeding. **EB:** *A review identified breast feeding as a protective factor (Carlin & Moon, 2017).*
- Teach parents the need to obtain a crib that conforms to the safety standards of the Consumer Product Safety Commission (CPSC). *Drop-side rail cribs are now prohibited; cribs need stronger slats and mattress supports and better quality hardware (CPSC, 2013).*
- Teach the need to stop smoking during pregnancy and to not smoke around the infant. Do not allow the infant to be exposed to any secondhand smoke. **EB:** *Maternal smoking remains the strongest prenatal modifiable risk factor for SIDS (Friedmann et al, 2017).*
- Teach parents, especially mothers, not to use alcohol, medications, or illicit drugs while caring for or bed sharing with an infant. **EB:** *Research has shown that mothers who were previously diagnosed with alcoholism had infants with a significant risk for SIDS (O'Leary et al, 2013).*
- Teach parents not to sleep in the same bed with the infant, regardless of alcohol, medications, smoking, or illicit drug use. **EB:** *A study of more than 1000 SIDS cases found that bed sharing with an infant resulted in an increased incidence of SIDS even without illicit drugs, alcohol, or smoking (Carpenter et al, 2013).*
- Teach parents not to place the infant on a cushion to sleep, or a sofa chair or other soft surface. Infants should sleep in a crib *(AAP, 2014a).*
- Recommend an alternative to sleeping with an infant of placing the infant's crib near their bed to allow for more convenient breastfeeding and parent contact. *Parents should be advised to place the baby in his or her own crib next to the parent's bed (AAP, 2014a).*
- Recommend that parents with infants in child care make it very clear to the employees that the infant must always be placed in the supine position to sleep, not prone or in a side-lying position (AAP, 2014a).

REFERENCES

American Academy of Pediatrics (AAP). (2014a). *Preventing SIDS.* Retrieved from http://www.healthychildren.org/English/ages-stages/baby/sleep/Pages/Preventing-SIDS.aspx.

American Academy of Pediatrics (AAP). (2014b). *Winter safety tips.* Retrieved from http://www.aap.org/en-us/about-the-aap/aap-press-room/news-features-and-safety-tips/Pages/Winter-Safety-Tips.aspx.

Carlin, R. F., & Moon, R. Y. (2017). Risk factors, protective factors, and current recommendations to reduce sudden infant death syndrome: A review. *Journal of the American Medical Association Pediatrics, 171*(2), 175–180. doi:10.1001/jamapediatrics.2016.3345.

Carpenter, R., et al. (2013). Bed sharing when parents do not smoke: Is there a risk of SIDS? An individual level analysis of five major case-control studies. *BMJ Open, 3*(5), pii, e002299.

Colson, R. R., et al. (2013). Trends and factors associated with infant bed sharing, 1993–2010: The National Infant Sleep Position Study. *JAMA Pediatrics, 167*(11), 1032–1037

Consumer Product Safety Commission (CPSC). (2013). *The new crib standard: Questions and answers.* Retrieved from http://www.cpsc.gov/onsafety/2011/06/the-new-crib-standard-questions-and-answers/.

Dufer, H., & Godfrey, K. (2017). Integration of safe sleep and sudden infant death syndrome (SIDS) education among parents of preterm infants in the Neonatal Intensive Care Unit (NICU). *Journal of Neonatal Nursing, 23*(2), 103–108. doi:10.1016/j.jnn.2016.09.001.

Friedmann, I., Dahdouh, E. M., Kugler, P., et al. (2017). Maternal and obstetrical predictors of sudden infant death syndrome (SIDS). *Journal of Maternal-Fetal & Neonatal Medicine, 30*(19), 2315–2323.

O'Leary, C. M., et al. (2013). Maternal alcohol use and sudden infant death syndrome and infant mortality excluding SIDS. *Pediatrics, 131*(3), e770–e778.

Pease, A. S., et al. (2016). Swaddling and the risk of sudden infant death syndrome: A meta-analysis. *Pediatrics,* e20153275. doi:10.1542/peds.2015-3275.

Wong, C. A., et al. (2014). American Indian and Alaska native infant and pediatric mortality, United States, 1999–2009. *American Journal of Public Health, S3*(Suppl. 3), S320–S328.

S

• = Independent;   ▲ = Collaborative;   **EBN** = Evidence-Based Nursing;   **EB** = Evidence-Based

Risk for Suffocation
Melodie Cannon, DNP, MSc/FNP, BHScN, RN(EC), NP-PHC, CEN, GNC(C)

NANDA-I

Definition

Vulnerable to inadequate air availability for inhalation, which may compromise health.

Risk Factor

Access to empty refrigerator/freezer; eating large mouthfuls of food; emotional disturbance; gas leak; insufficient knowledge of safety precautions; low-strung clothesline; pacifier around infant's neck; playing with plastic bag; propped bottle placed in infant's crib; small object in airway; smoking in bed; soft underlayment; unattended in water; unvented fuel-burning heater; vehicle running in closed garage

Associated Condition

Alteration in cognitive functioning; alteration in olfactory function: face/neck disease; face/neck injury; impaired motor functioning

NOC   (Nursing Outcomes Classification)

Suggested NOC Outcomes

Knowledge: Infant Care; Parenting: Adolescent Physical Safety, Early/Middle Childhood Physical Safety, Infant/Toddler Physical Safety; Personal Safety; Risk Control; Risk Detection; Safe Home Environment; Substance Addiction Consequences

> #### Example NOC Outcome with Indicators
>
> **Knowledge: Infant Care** as evidenced by the following indicators: Strategies to prevent choking/Appropriate activities for child's developmental level/First aid techniques. (Rate the outcome and indicators of **Knowledge: Infant Care:** 1 = no knowledge, 2 = limited knowledge, 3 = moderate knowledge, 4 = substantial knowledge, 5 = extensive knowledge [see Section I].)

Client Outcomes

Client Will (Specify Time Frame)

- Undertake appropriate measures to prevent suffocation
- Demonstrate correct techniques for emergency rescue maneuvers (e.g., Heimlich maneuver, rescue breathing, cardiopulmonary resuscitation [CPR]) and describe situations that require them

NIC   (Nursing Interventions Classification)

Suggested NIC Interventions

Aspiration Precautions; Environmental Management: Safety; Infant Care; Positioning; Security Enhancement; Surveillance; Surveillance: Safety; Teaching: Infant Safety

> #### Example NIC Activities—Environmental Management: Safety
>
> Identify safety hazards in the environment (i.e., physical, biological, and chemical); Remove hazards from the environment, when possible

Nursing Interventions and *Rationales*

- Identify hospitalized clients at particular risk for suffocation, including the following:
  - ○ Clients with altered levels of consciousness
  - ○ Infants or young children
  - ○ Clients with developmental delays
  - ○ Clients with mental illness, especially schizophrenia
  - ○ Clients who have been physically or chemically restrained

● = Independent;   ▲ = Collaborative;   EBN = Evidence-Based Nursing;   EB = Evidence-Based

Restraint use has been associated with mortality.

EB: *A review of restraint use in nursing home patients found evidence of physical restraint associated deaths. Neck compression was found to be the most common mechanism that resulted in asphyxia (Bellenger et al, 2017).*

Institute safety measures such as proper positioning and feeding precautions. See the care plans for Risk for **Aspiration** and Impaired **Swallowing** for additional interventions. Vigilance and special protective measures are necessary for clients at greater risk for suffocation. **EB:** *Swallowing disorders are common in schizophrenia with associated morbidity and mortality from either acute asphyxia from airway obstruction or from aspiration and pneumonia. The death rate from acute asphyxia is significantly higher in these patients (up to 100 times greater than the general population) (Kulkarni, Kamath, & Stewart, 2017).*

Pediatric

- Counsel families on the following for care of an infant:
  - ○ Position infants on their back to sleep; do not position them on their side or prone (Registered Nurses' Association of Ontario, 2014).
  - ○ Position infants on their back to sleep; do not position them on their side or prone. Obtain a new crib that conforms to the safety standards of the Federal Safety Commission. *Ensure cribs/playpens are properly assembled to prevent collapse. Only the original size mattress should be used to prevent gaps in which the child could potentially become wedged. Cribs/playpens that do not conform to current safety standards should not be used (Theurer & Bhavsar, 2013).* Place the infant in the crib with a properly fitted mattress, only to sleep, not on an adult bed, sofa, chair, baby seats, swings, slings, or playpen. *The safest infant sleep surface is a firm, tight-fitting mattress. Cribs, bassinets, and playpens that meet these criteria may be acceptable. Soft bedding, bumper pads, pillows, blankets, positioning devices, and sheepskins are associated with an increase in sudden infant death syndrome. Soft bedding also increases the risk of unintentional suffocation and asphyxia (Carlin & Moon, 2017).* **EB:** *A study demonstrated that the sofa as a sleep surface is extremely hazardous and increases the risk of sudden and unexplained infant deaths. Sofa deaths were associated with surface sharing, being found in the side position, a change in sleep location, and prenatal tobacco exposure (Rechtman et al, 2014).*
  - ○ Avoid use of loose bedding, such as blankets and sheets, for sleeping. If blankets are used, they should be tucked in around the crib mattress so the infant's face is less likely to become covered by bedding. The blanket should end at the level of the infant's chest. **EB:** *A study of sleep-related infant deaths found that infants from 0 to 3 months were more likely to die while sharing a bed surface, whereas infants 4 months up to 364 days were more likely to die having been found in the prone position with blankets and stuffed animals in the area (Colvin et al, 2014).* See care plan Risk for **Sudden Infant Death** for further interventions.
- Assess for signs and symptoms of abuse such as Munchausen syndrome by proxy (MSBP). **CEB:** *Suffocation in MSBP is one important differential diagnosis in suspected cases of SIDS (Vennemann et al, 2005).*
- Conduct risk factor identification, noting special circumstances in which preventive or protective measures are indicated. Note the presence of environmental hazards, including plastic bags; cribs with slats wider than 2 inches; ill-fitting crib mattresses that can allow the infant to become wedged between the mattress and crib; pillows/loose bedding in cribs; placement of crib near windows with blinds or cords; co-sleeping; abandoned large appliances such as refrigerators, dishwashers, or freezers; clothing with cords or hoods that can become entangled; bibs; pacifiers on a string; necklaces in infants and children; drapery cords; and pull-toy strings. *Suffocation by airway obstruction is a leading cause of death in children younger than 6 years of age. Families need to be taught child protection. Cribs should not be near walls, furniture, or any object that could result in entrapment should the child get out of the crib. Items with cords and strings should also be removed (Theurer & Bhavsar, 2013).* **EB:** *Bed sharing is associated with accidental suffocation and strangulation and sudden infant death. The risk of infant bed sharing is increased in infants who have no identified place to sleep, have health or care issues, and are breast fed. Education should support breastfeeding without bed sharing, highlight the need for safe sleep places, and address the risk factors for sleep-related deaths (Heere et al, 2017).*
- Counsel families to evaluate household furniture for safety, including large dressers, televisions, book shelves, and appliances, which may need to be anchored to the wall to prevent the child from climbing on the furniture and it falling forward and suffocating the child.
- *Strategies to prevent suffocation should essentially include removing any item from the child's sleep or play area that could potentially cause harm or even death caused by entrapment or entanglement (Theurer & Bhavsar, 2013).* **EB:** *Injuries to children by falling televisions have become more frequent. Dressers and other furniture not designed for holding televisions were commonly involved. Toddlers ages 1 to 3 most frequently*

S

● = Independent;   ▲ = Collaborative;   **EBN** = Evidence-Based Nursing;   **EB** = Evidence-Based

suffer head and neck injuries. Small children may suffer secondary brain injuries or death by mechanical asphyxia because of their small size compared with the size of the television (Cusimano & Parker, 2016).

- Counsel families not to serve these foods to the child younger than 5 years of age: nuts, seeds, hot dogs, popcorn, pretzels, chips, chunks of meat, hard pieces of fruit or vegetables, raisins, whole grapes, hard candies, gum, chewable vitamins, fish with bones, snacks on toothpicks, and marshmallows. **EB:** *A review of the literature demonstrated that seeds, nuts, and legumes were the most commonly aspirated food items. There is legislation by the Consumer Product Safety Commission regarding labeling of toy parts, but there are no similar guidelines for food products (Sidell et al, 2013).*

- Counsel families to keep the following items away from the sight and reach of infants and toddlers: buttons, beads, jewelry, pins, nails, marbles, coins, stones, magnets, and balloons. Choose age appropriate toys and games for children and check for any small parts that may be a choking hazard because children have the need to put everyday objects in their mouths (Safekids.org, 2015). *Reviews of foreign body injuries found that pearls, balls, coins, nuts, seeds, and toy parts were common objects ingested by children and resulted in increased morbidity and mortality (choking) (Passali et al, 2015).*

- Stress water and pool safety precautions, including vigilant, uninterrupted parental supervision. *Children can drown quickly in various water sources including tubs, buckets, pools, ponds, and lakes. Open water drowning is prevalent in older teens and young adults and prevention strategies should include the need for personal flotation devices and education regarding impaired judgment with alcohol use (Johnston & Ebel, 2013).* **EB:** *The majority of pediatric immersion-related deaths could be prevented with supervision (Bamber et al, 2014). Pools should be surrounded completely by fencing that is difficult to climb, is regularly assessed for structural defects, and has self-closing latches. Four-sided isolation fencing has been found to significantly reduce the risk of drowning (Johnston & Ebel, 2013).*

- Underscore the necessity of not allowing children to play with or near electric garage doors and of keeping garage door openers out of the reach of young children. *Children close to the ground may not be large enough to trigger reversal mechanisms on the door and may become trapped.*

- For adolescents, watch for signs of depression that could result in suicide by suffocation. **EB:** *Suicide in adolescents and young adults is increasing. According to 2014 data, for males and females in all age groups (including adults), the rate of suicide by suffocation has increased over the years (Curtin, Warner, & Hedegaard, 2016).* **EB:** *A surveillance data review of suicide in children and early adolescents found that compared with adolescents who commit suicide, in death by suicide in children, the victims were commonly male, black, and died by hanging, strangulation, or suffocation. Children who died by suicide often experienced relationship problems with family, girlfriends, or boyfriends (Sheftall et al, 2016).*

 Geriatric

- Assess the status of the swallow reflex. Offer appropriate foods and beverages accordingly. Older adults, especially those receiving antipsychotic medications, have an increased incidence of choking. Refer to Impaired **Swallowing**. **EB:** *Dysphagia is a common problem in adults with mental health illness and has a significant mortality risk because of choking asphyxiation (Aldridge & Taylor, 2012).*

- A swallowing assessment by a speech-language pathologist is recommended in patients with suspected or confirmed dysphagia to ensure the appropriate type and consistency of diet to mitigate choking and aspiration risk. **EBN:** *Safe nursing care includes a consultation with a speech-language pathologist whenever doubts arise regarding a client's ability to tolerate oral-supported nutrition in any form (Teasell et al, 2015).*

- Ensure proper positioning during and after feeding to decrease the risk of aspiration. *Dysphagia in the elderly results in increased morbidity and mortality. It is important to recognize the relationship between dysphagia and aspiration pneumonia in the elderly because of the high mortality rate associated with this (Smukalla et al, 2017).*

- Use care in pillow placement when positioning frail older clients who are on bed rest. *Frail older clients are at risk for suffocation if the head becomes lodged against pillows and the client cannot reposition himself or herself because of weakness. Older adults who are cognitively impaired require assessment of the safety of their sleep environment for potential hazards similar to sleeping risks for the very young (Byard & Gilbert, 2011).*

- Recognize that older adults in depression may use hanging, strangulation, and suffocation as a means of suicide. **EB:** *Suicide attempts in seniors often result in death. Social isolation, poor health, frailty, loneliness, and depression are thought to be possible contributing factors. Regardless of age, suffocation, which includes hanging and strangulation, accounted for almost half of the suicides in Canada in 2012 (Skinner et al, 2016).*

● = Independent;   ▲ = Collaborative;   **EBN** = Evidence-Based Nursing;   **EB** = Evidence-Based

Home Care

- Assess the home for potential safety hazards in systems that are not likely to be fixed (e.g., faulty pilot lights or gas leaks in gas stoves, carbon monoxide release from heating systems, kerosene fumes from portable heaters).
- Assist the family in having these areas assessed and making appropriate safety arrangements (e.g., installing detectors, making repairs, home safety inspections). *Assessment and correction of system problems prevent accidental suffocation.*
- Advise the family to have a safety plan for potential escape routes from the home in the event of detectors going off, fire, or other emergencies.

Client/Family Teaching and Discharge Planning

- Recommend that families who are seeking day care or in-home care for children, geriatric family members, or at-risk family members with developmental or functional disabilities inspect the environment for hazards and examine the first aid preparation and vigilance of providers. *Many working families must trust others to care for family members.*
- Recommend to families that they advise any caregivers of specific food consistency, types, and any feeding precautions and strategies required to decrease risk of choking and aspiration in high-risk children or adults.
- Ensure family members learn and practice rescue techniques, including treatment of choking and lack of breathing, as well as CPR. *Family members need preparation to deal with emergency situations and should take part in the American Heart Association Basic Lifesaving Course or the American Red Cross Infant/Child CPR Course.*
- *Use client/family encounters to provide age appropriate anticipatory guidance for safety precautions for infants and children and education regarding risk reduction for suffocation for vulnerable older adults or clients with physical or mental disabilities.*

REFERENCES

Aldridge, K. J., & Taylor, N. F. (2012). Dysphagia is a common and serious problem for adults with mental illness: A systematic review. *Dysphagia, 27,* 124–137.

Bamber, A. R., Pryce, J. W., Ashworth, M. T., et al. (2014). Immersion-related deaths in infants and children: Autopsy experience from a specialist center. *Forensic Science Medicine Pathology, 10,* 363–370.

Bellenger, E. N., Ibrahim, J. E., Lovell, J. J., et al. (2018). The nature and extent of physical restraint-related deaths in nursing homes: A systematic review. *Journal of Aging Health, 30*(7), 1042–1061. doi:10.1177/0898264317704541.

Byard, R. W., & Gilbert, J. D. (2011). Sleeping accidents in the elderly. *Journal of Forensic Sciences, 56*(6), 1645–1647.

Carlin, R. F., & Moon, R. Y. (2017). Risk factors, protective factors, and current recommendations to reduce sudden infant death syndrome: A review. *Journal of the American Medical Association Pediatrics, 171*(2), 175–180. doi:10.1001/jamapediatrics.2016.3345.

Colvin, J. D., Collie-Akers, V., Schunn, C., et al. (2014). Sleep environment risks for younger and older infants. *Pediatrics, 134*(2).

Curtin, S. C., Warner, M., & Hedegaard, H. (2016). *Increase in suicide in the United States, 1999–2014. NCHS data brief, no 241,* Hyattsville, MD: National Center for Health Statistics.

Cusimano, M. D., & Parker, N. (2016). Toppled television sets and head injuries in the pediatric population: A framework for prevention. *Journal of Neurosurgery. Pediatrics, 17*(1), 3–12. doi:10.3171/2015.2. PEDS14472.

Heere, M., Moughan, B., Alfonsi, J., et al. (2017). Factors associated with infant bed-sharing. *Global Pediatric Health, 4,* 2333794X17690313. doi:10.1177/2333794X17690313.

Johnston, B. D., & Ebel, B. E. (2013). Child injury control: Trends, themes, and controversies. *Academic Pediatrics, 13*(6), 499–507.

Kulkarni, D. P., Kamath, V. D., & Stewart, J. T. (2017). Swallowing disorders in schizophrenia. *Dysphagia, 32*(4), 467–471. doi:10.1007/s00455-017-9802-6.

Passali, D., Gregor, D., Lorenzoni, G., et al. (2015). Foreign body injuries in children: A review. *Acta Otorhinolaryngologica Italica, 35*(4), 265–271. Retrieved from https://www.ncbi.nlm.nih.gov/pmc/articles/PMC47381891/.

Rechtman, L. R., Colvin, J. D., Blair, P. S., et al. (2014). Sofas and infant mortality. *Pediatrics, 134*(5), e1293–e1300. doi:10.1542/peds.2014-154.

Registered Nurses' Association of Ontario. (2014). *Working with families to promote safe sleep for infants 0–12 months of age.* Toronto, ON: Registered Nurses' Association of Ontario. Retrieved from http://www.rnao.ca/bpg/guidelines.

Safekids.org. (2015). *Choking and strangulation prevention tips.* Retrieved from https://www.safekids.org/safetytips/field_risks/choking_and_strangulation.

Sheftall, A. H., Asti, L., Horowitz, L. M., et al. (2016). Suicide in elementary school-aged children and early adolescents. *Pediatrics, 138*(4).

Sidell, D. R., Kim, I. A., Coker, T. R., et al. (2013). Food choking hazards in children. *International Journal of Pediatric Otorhinolaryngology, 77,* 140–1946.

Skinner, R., McFaull, S., Draca, J., et al. (2016). Suicide and self-inflicted injury hospitalizations in Canada (1979 to 2014/15). *Health Promotion and Chronic Disease Management in Canada, 36*(11), 243–251.

Smukalla, S. M., Dimitrova, I., Feintuch, J. M., et al. (2017). Dysphagia in the elderly. *Current Treatment Options in Gastroenterology, 15,* 382–396. doi:10.10007/s11938-017-0144-0.

• = Independent; ▲ = Collaborative; EBN = Evidence-Based Nursing; EB = Evidence-Based

Teasell, R. W., et al. (2015). Dysphagia and aspiration following stroke. In *2015 Evidence-based review of stroke rehabilitation*. Retrieved from http://www.ebrsr.com/.

Theurer, W. M., & Bhavsar, A. K. (2013). Prevention of unintentional childhood injury. *American Family Physician, 87*(7), 502–509.

Vennemann, B., Bajanowski, T., Karger, B., et al. (2005). Suffocation and poisoning-the hard hitting side of Munchausen syndrome by proxy. *International Journal of Legal Medicine, 119*, 98–102.

Risk for Suicide   *Kathleen L. Patusky, MA, PhD, RN, CNS*

NANDA-I

Definition

Susceptible to self-inflicted, life threatening injury.

Related Factors

Behavioral

Changing a will; giving away possessions; impulsiveness; making a will; marked change in attitude; marked change in behavior; marked change in school performance; purchase of a gun; stockpiling medication; sudden euphoric recovery from major depression

Psychological

Guilt (substance misuse)

Situational

Access to weapon; loss of autonomy; loss of independence

Social

Cluster suicides; disciplinary problems; disrupted family life; grieving; helplessness; hopelessness; insufficient social support; legal difficulty; loneliness; loss of significant relationship; social isolation

Verbal

Reports desire to die; threats of killing self

Other

Chronic pain

At-Risk Population

Adolescence; adolescents living in nontraditional settings; Caucasian ethnicity; divorced status; economically disadvantaged; older adults; family history of suicide; history of childhood abuse history of suicide attempt; homosexual youth; institutionalization; living alone; male gender; Native American ethnicity; relocation; retired; widowed; young adult males

Associated Condition

Physical illness; psychiatric disorder; terminal illness

NOC   (Nursing Outcomes Classification)

Suggested NOC Outcomes

Depression Level; Impulse Self-Control; Loneliness Severity; Mood Equilibrium; Risk Detection; Suicide Self-Restraint

• = Independent;   ▲ = Collaborative;   EBN = Evidence-Based Nursing;   EB = Evidence-Based

Example NOC Outcome with Indicators

Suicide Self-Restraint as evidenced by the following indicators: Expresses feelings/Refrains from attempting suicide/ Verbalizes suicidal ideas/Controls impulses. (Rate the outcome and indicators of **Suicide Self-Restraint:** 1 = never demonstrated, 2 = rarely demonstrated, 3 = sometimes demonstrated, 4 = often demonstrated, 5 = consistently demonstrated [see Section I].)

Consider using one of the measures of suicide risk that are available for clients: Nurses' Global Assessment of Suicide Risk (Cutcliffe & Barker, 2004); Center for Epidemiological Studies Depression Scale measures depressed mood level (Chiu et al, 2010); Beck Suicide Intent Scale identifies a strong intent to die (Astruc et al, 2004); Suicide Assessment Checklist (Rogers, Lewis, & Subich, 2002)

Client Outcomes

Client Will (Specify Time Frame)

- Not harm self
- Maintain connectedness in relationships
- Disclose and discuss suicidal ideas if present; seek help
- Express decreased anxiety and control of impulses
- Talk about feelings; express anger appropriately
- Refrain from using mood-altering substances
- Obtain no access to harmful objects
- Yield access to harmful objects
- Maintain self-control without supervision

NIC (Nursing Interventions Classification)

Suggested NIC Interventions

Anxiety Reduction; Coping Enhancement; Crisis Intervention; Delusion Management; Mood Management; Substance Use Prevention; Suicide Prevention; Support System Enhancement; Surveillance

Example NIC Activities—Suicide Prevention

Determine presence and degree of suicidal risk; Encourage patient to seek out care providers to talk as urge to harm self occurs

Nursing Interventions and *Rationales*

The American Psychiatric Nurses Association (APNA, 2015) has adapted a set of essential competencies for psychiatric nurses, all of which can be useful for generalist nurses. These competencies have been incorporated in the following sections.

- Before implementing interventions in the face of suicidal behavior, nurses should examine their own emotional responses to incidents of suicide to ensure that interventions will not be based on counter-transference reactions. EBN: *Understanding of nurses' responses to suicidal clients can facilitate suicide prevention and recovery (Talseth & Gilje, 2011; APNA, 2015).*
- Pursue an understanding of suicide as a phenomenon at all levels of nursing practice. Elements to be considered include the terminology used with suicidality and self-harm phenomena, the epidemiology of suicide, the risk and protective influences on suicide, and the evidence-based best practices in preventing and responding to suicidality (APNA, 2015).
- Assess for suicidal ideation when the history reveals the following: depression, substance abuse; bipolar disorder, schizophrenia, anxiety disorders, posttraumatic stress disorder, dissociative disorder, eating disorders, substance use disorders, antisocial or other personality disorders; attempted suicide, current or past; recent stressful life events (divorce and/or separation, relocation, problems with children); recent unemployment; recent bereavement; adult or childhood physical or sexual abuse; gay, lesbian, or bisexual gender orientation; family history of suicide; and history of chronic trauma. *Clinicians should be alert for suicide when the previously mentioned factors are present in asymptomatic persons (Li et al, 2011; American Psychiatric Association [APA], 2015). EB: In a 10-year longitudinal study, 83% of persons who committed suicide received health care within the previous year; only 24% had been diagnosed with a mental disorder*

S

• = Independent; ▲ = Collaborative;   EBN = Evidence-Based Nursing;   EB = Evidence-Based

in the 4 weeks prior to death. Medical specialty and primary care accounted for the most common visits (Ahmedani et al, 2014). Assess all medical clients and clients with chronic illnesses, traumatic injuries, or pain for their perception of health status and suicidal ideation. *Medical clients who perceived their health to be poor or who were in chronic pain were significantly more likely to report current suicidal ideation.* EB: *Research, including systematic review, supported the association of both type 1 and type 2 diabetes with an increase in suicidal ideation (Ceretta et al, 2012; Pompili et al, 2014). Myocardial infarction has been connected with higher suicide rates, especially during the first month after discharge, and with impaired prognosis (Larsen, 2013). Persons living with HIV/AIDS who had depressive symptoms and low life satisfaction were at significantly higher risk of suicide (Davis et al, 2011).*

- Assess the client's ability to enter into a no-suicide contract. Contract (verbally or in writing) with the client for no self-harm if the client is appropriate for a contract; recontract at appropriate intervals. *Discussing feelings of self-harm with a trusted person provides relief for the client. A contract gets the subject out in the open and places some of the responsibility for safety with the client.* CEB: *Some clients are not appropriate for a contract, such as those under the influence of drugs or alcohol or unwilling to abstain from substance use, and those who are isolated or alone without assistance to keep the environment safe (Hauenstein, 2002). If the client will not contract, the risk of suicide should be considered higher.* CEBN: *Note: Although contracting is a common practice in psychiatric care settings, research has suggested that self-harm is not prevented by contracts. Thorough, ongoing assessment of suicide risk is necessary, whether or not the client has entered into a no-self-harm contract. Contracts may not be appropriate in a community setting (McMyler & Pryjmachuk, 2008).*

- Be alert for the following warning signs of suicide: making statements such as, "I can't go on," "Nothing matters anymore," "I wish I were dead"; becoming depressed or withdrawn; behaving recklessly; getting affairs in order and giving away valued possessions; showing a marked change in behavior, attitudes, or appearance; abusing drugs or alcohol; and suffering a major loss or life change. *Suicide is rarely a spontaneous decision. In the days and hours before people kill themselves, clues and warning signs usually appear.*

- Take suicide notes seriously and ask if a note was left in any previous suicide attempts. Consider themes of notes in determining appropriate interventions. *Clients who leave a suicide note may be at higher risk of completed suicide in the future. A note should be viewed as an indication of a failed but serious attempt.*

- Question family members regarding the preparatory actions mentioned. *Clinicians should be alert for suicide when these factors are present in asymptomatic persons (APA, 2015).*

- Determine the presence and degree of suicidal risk. A number of questions will elicit the necessary information: Have you been thinking about hurting or killing yourself? How often do you have these thoughts and how long do they last? Do you have a plan? What is it? Do you have access to the means to carry out that plan? How likely is it that you could carry out the plan? Are there people or things that could prevent you from hurting yourself? What do you see in your future a year from now? Five years from now? What do you expect would happen if you died? What has kept you alive up to now? CEB: *Using the acronym SAL, the nurse can evaluate the client's suicide plan for its specificity (how detailed and clear is the plan), availability (does the client have immediate access to the planned means), and lethality (could the plan be fatal, or does the client believe it would be fatal). Assessment of reasons for living is another important part of evaluating suicidal clients (Malone et al, 2000).*

- Observe, record, and report any changes in mood or behavior that may signify increasing suicide risk and document results of regular surveillance checks. EB: *Suicidal ideation often is not continuous; it may decrease and then increase in response to negative thinking or exposure to stressors (e.g., family visits). Documentation of surveillance will alert all members of the health care team to changes in the clients' potential risk for suicide so they may be prepared to respond in the event of suicidal behavior (APNA, 2015).*

- Develop a positive therapeutic relationship with the client; do not make promises that may not be kept. *Be aware that some clients may offer to self-disclose if the nurse will promise not to tell anyone what they have said. Clarify with the clients that anything they share will be communicated only to other staff but that secrets cannot be kept.* EBN: *Nurses reconnect suicidal clients with humanity by guiding the client, helping them learn how to live, and helping them connect appropriately with others. Positive support can buffer against suicide, whereas conflictual interactions can increase suicide risk (Hirsch & Barton, 2011; APNA, 2015).*

- Express desire to help client. Provide education about suicide and the effectiveness of intervention. Validate the client's experience of psychological pain while maintaining a safe environment for the client. *The nurse must reconcile their goal of preventing suicide with recognition of the client's goal to alleviate their psychological pain (APNA, 2015).*

● = Independent;   ▲ = Collaborative;   EBN = Evidence-Based Nursing;   EB = Evidence-Based

▲ Refer for mental health counseling and possible hospitalization if evidence of suicidal intent exists, which may include evidence of preparatory actions (e.g., obtaining a weapon, making a plan, putting affairs in order, giving away prized possessions, preparing a suicide note). **EB:** *Clients vary in the preparation for suicide attempts, and professional assessment is required to determine the need for hospitalization (APA, 2015). The following interventions may be instituted.*

● Perform risk assessment for possible suicidality on admission to the hospital and thereafter during hospitalization. Alert treatment team to level of risk. *Risk assessment includes evaluating each client's risk factors, ameliorating factors, stated suicidal intent, mental status, history of physical or psychological trauma, triggers that prompt distress, tendency to minimize or exaggerate symptoms, sources of assistance, warning signs of acute risk, and history of previous suicidal or self-harm behavior (APNA, 2015).*

● Determine client's need for supervision and assign a hospitalized client to a room located near the nursing station. *Close assignment increases ease of observation and availability for a rapid response in the event of a suicide attempt (APNA, 2015).*

● Search the newly hospitalized client and the client's personal belongings for weapons or potential weapons and hoarded medications during the inpatient admission procedure, as appropriate. Remove dangerous items. *Clients who are intent on suicide may bring the means with them. Action is necessary to maintain a hazard-free environment and client safety (APNA, 2015).*

● Limit access to windows and exits unless locked and shatterproof, as appropriate. *Suicidal behavior may include attempts to jump out of windows or to escape the unit to find other means of suicide (e.g., gaining roof access for a jump). Hospitals should ensure that exits are secure.*

● Monitor the client during the use of potential weapons (e.g., razor, scissors). *Clients with suicidal intent may take advantage of any opportunity to harm themselves (APNA, 2015).*

● Increase surveillance of a hospitalized client at times when staffing is predictably low (e.g., staff meetings, change of shift report, periods of unit disruption). *Clients who remain intent on suicide will be watchful of periods when staff surveillance lessens to permit completion of a suicide plan.*

● Ensure that all oncoming staff members have adequate information to assist the client, using the acronym SBARR: situation (current status, observations), background (relevant client history), assessment (including nurse's current risk assessment and relevant lab findings), recommendations (what the nurse believes is necessary going forward), and response feedback (verification of oncoming staff members' understanding) (APNA, 2015).

▲ If imminent suicide is suspected or an attempt has occurred, call for assistance and do not leave the client alone. Client and staff safety will be served by assistance in the response. The client may attempt additional self-harm if left alone.

● Place the client in the least restrictive, safe, and monitored environment that allows for the necessary level of observation. Assess suicidal risk at least daily and more frequently as warranted. *Close observation of the client is necessary for safety as long as intent remains high. Suicide risk should be assessed at frequent intervals to adjust suicide precautions and limitations on the client's freedom of movement and to ensure that restrictions continue to be appropriate.* **EB:** *Inpatient root cause analyses of suicide attempts and environmental safety checklists for units can be helpful in maintaining safety (Mills et al, 2008; APNA, 2015).*

● Consider strategies to decrease isolation and opportunity to act on harmful thoughts (e.g., use of a sitter). **CEB:** *Clients have reported feeling safe and having their hope restored in response to close observation (Bowers & Park, 2001).*

● Explain suicide precautions and relevant safety issues to the client and family (e.g., purpose, duration, behavioral expectations, and behavioral consequences). **CEB:** *Suicide precautions may be viewed as restrictive. Clients have reported the loss of privacy as distressing (Bowers & Park, 2001).*

▲ Refer for treatment and participate in the management of any psychiatric illness or symptoms that may be contributing to the client's suicidal ideation or behavior. *Psychiatric disorders have been associated with suicidal behavior. Symptoms of the disorder may require treatment with antidepressant, antipsychotic, or antianxiety medications.* **EB:** *A systematic review has shown a highly significant effect for cognitive behavior therapy in reducing suicidal behavior (Tarrier, Taylor, & Gooding, 2008).*

▲ Verify that the client has taken medications as ordered (e.g., conduct mouth checks after medication administration). *The client may attempt to hoard medications for a later suicide attempt.*

▲ Maintain increased surveillance of the client whenever use of an antidepressant has been initiated or the dose increased. Antidepressant medications take anywhere from 2 to 6 weeks to achieve full efficacy. *During that period the client's energy level may increase, although the depression has not yet lifted, which increases the potential for suicide.*

● = Independent;   ▲ = Collaborative;   **EBN** = Evidence-Based Nursing;   **EB** = Evidence-Based

- Involve the client in treatment planning and self-care management of psychiatric disorders. *Self-care management promotes feelings of self-efficacy, particularly for clients with depression. Suicidal ideation may occur in response to a sense of hopelessness, or a sense that the client has no control over life circumstances. The more clients participate in their own care, the less powerless and hopeless they feel. Refer to the care plan for* **Powerlessness.**
- Explore with the client all circumstances and motivations related to the suicidality. Listen to the client's own views on his or her problems. **EB:** *Primary reasons for suicide attempts were found to be feelings of loneliness or hopelessness and mental illness/psychological problems (APA, 2015).*
- Explore with the client all perceived consequences that could act as a barrier to suicide (e.g., effect on family, religious beliefs). **CEB:** *The most common barrier to suicide is consequences to family members (Bell, 2000).*
- Keep discussion oriented to the present and future. *Clients under stress have difficulty focusing their thoughts, which leads to a sense of being overwhelmed by problems. Focusing on the present and future helps the client to address problem-solving regarding current stressors.*
- Discuss plans for dealing with suicidal ideation in the future (e.g., how to identify precipitating factors, who to contact, where to go for help, and how to respond to desire for self-harm). *Clients are supported in self-care management when they are helped to identify actions they can take if suicidal ideation recurs.*
- Assist the client in identifying a network of supportive persons and resources (e.g., clergy, family, care providers). **EB:** *Social support and positive events were found to have a protective support against suicidal ideation (Kleiman, Riskind, & Schaefer, 2014).*
- ▲ Refer family members and friends to local mental health agencies and crisis intervention centers if the client has suicidal ideation or a suspicion of suicidal thoughts exists. *Clients at risk should receive evaluation and help (APA, 2015).*
- ▲ Document client behavior in detail to support outpatient commitment or an overnight psychiatric observation program for an actively suicidal client. *Involuntary outpatient commitment can improve treatment, reduce the likelihood of hospital readmission, and reduce episodes of violent behavior in persons with severe psychiatric illnesses. Overnight psychiatric observation followed by outpatient referral also can be an effective alternative to traditional hospitalization without leading to an increase in suicide gestures or attempts.*
- Use cognitive-behavioral techniques that help the client to modify thinking styles that promote depression, hopelessness, and a belief that suicide is a valid means of escaping the current situation. *Suicide has been shown to be associated with constriction in cognitive style, leading to decreased problem-solving and information processing.* **EB:** *Cognitive-behavioral therapy has been shown to be effective in decreasing suicide attempts with improvement in problem-solving skills (Ghahramanlou-Holloway et al, 2012).*
- Engage the client in group interventions that can be useful to address recurrent suicide attempts. *Group therapy was shown to decrease suicidality.*
- With the client's consent, facilitate family-oriented crisis intervention. Family-oriented crisis intervention can clarify stresses and allow assessment of family dynamics. **EBN:** *An educational intervention addressing ability to care, stress levels, and attitudes toward the suicidal family member was effective in promoting attitudes toward and ability to care for a suicidal family member (Sun et al, 2014).*
- Involve the family in discharge planning (e.g., illness/medication teaching, recognition of increasing suicidal risk, client's plan for dealing with recurring suicidal thoughts, community resources). *Suicidal clients often are ambivalent about hurting themselves; they may not want to die so much as to escape an intolerable situation. Consequently, they often leave clues about their state of mind.* **EBN:** *Family members must learn before clients leave the hospital how to respond to clues early, support the treatment regimen, and encourage the client to initiate the emergency plan. Nurses help in guiding families through the process (Sun et al, 2014).*
- ▲ Before discharge from the hospital, ensure that the client has a supply of ordered medications, has a plan for outpatient follow-up, understands the plan or has a caregiver able and willing to follow the plan, and has the ability to access outpatient treatment. *Clients may be discharged before they have recovered substantial functional ability and may have difficulty concentrating on the plan for follow-up. They may need the assistance of others to ensure that prescriptions are filled, that they attend appointments, or that they have transportation to the outpatient care setting.*
- ▲ In the event of successful suicide, refer the family to a therapy group for survivors of suicide. Recommended clinical interventions include addressing psychological distress, normalizing denial as an effective coping strategy, working with concerns about family disintegration, and helping families deal with stigmatization. **EB:** *Psychoeducational support group participants found relief in sharing a personal narrative of their suicide bereavement with others (Feigelman & Feigelman, 2011a,b).*

● = Independent;   ▲ = Collaborative;   EBN = Evidence-Based Nursing;   EB = Evidence-Based

- See the care plans for Risk for self-directed **Violence, Hopelessness,** and Risk for **Self-Mutilation.** *Clients with suicidal ideation often are reacting to a feeling of hopelessness.*

Pediatric

- The previously mentioned interventions may be appropriate for pediatric clients.
- Use brief self-report measures to improve clinical management of at-risk cases. **CEBN:** *The Home, Education, Activities, Drug use and abuse, Sexual behavior, and Suicidality and depression (HEADSS) instrument has been found useful in suicide risk assessment of adolescents (Biddle et al, 2010).*
- Recognize that the developmental issues of childhood and adolescence may heighten suicide risks and involve different issues from those with adults. Assess specific stressors for the pediatric client, including bullying. **EBN:** *The experience of being bullied can contribute to suicidality (Cooper, Clements, & Holt, 2012).* **CEBN:** *A model accounting for 41.9% of adolescents' suicide risk showed that negative life events and rumination contributed to suicidal risk behaviors, whereas resilience and social support could decrease the risk (Thanoi et al, 2010).*
- Assess for exposure to suicide of a significant other. **CEB:** *Among risk factors of previous psychiatric history, poor psychosocial function, dysphoric mood, and psychomotor restlessness, suicide of a significant other was shown to create risk for adolescents diagnosed with adjustment disorder (Pelkonen et al, 2005).*
- Be alert to the presence of school victimization around lesbian, gay, bisexual, and transgender (LGBT) issues and be prepared to advocate for the client. **EBN/EB:** *Male adolescents experience greater levels of depression and suicidal ideation in response to high rates of LGBT school victimization (Hatzenbuehler, 2011; Russell et al, 2011; Lea, deWit, & Reynolds, 2014).*
- Evaluate for the presence of self-mutilation and related risk factors. Refer to care plan for Risk for **Self-Mutilation** for additional information. *Self-mutilation and suicidality may co-occur.*
- Be aware that complete overlap does not exist between suicidal behavior and self-mutilation. The motivation may be different (ending life rather than coping with difficult feelings), and the method is usually different. **CEB:** *In one study, about half of the participants reported both attempted suicide and self-mutilation; in the other half there was no overlap in types of acts (Bolognini et al, 2003).*
- Involve the adolescent in multimodal treatment programs. **CEBN:** *A systematic review identified that individual, family, group, and psychopharmacological therapies are used for treatment; however, limited research exists to determine which therapy is most effective (Pryjmachuk & Trainor, 2010). Cognitive behavior therapy was cited as showing promise in one study included in a systematic review, but further study was recommended (Robinson, Hetrick, & Martin, 2011).*
- Before discharge from the hospital, ensure that the client's parent has a supply of ordered medications, has a plan for outpatient follow-up, has a caregiver who understands the plan or is able and willing to follow the plan, and has the ability to access outpatient treatment. **CEB:** *A compliance enhancement intervention (including contracting interviews with parent and adolescent and telephone contacts) improved attendance at follow-up appointments only when barriers to service were controlled (e.g., delays in getting appointments, placement on a waiting list, inability to switch therapists, problems with insurance coverage) (Spirito et al, 2002).*
- Parental education groups can influence suicide risk factors. **CEB:** *A program of parent education groups focused on improved communication skills and relationships with adolescents. Students in the intervention group reported increased maternal care, decreased conflict with parents, decreased substance abuse, and decreased delinquency (Toumbourou & Gregg, 2002).*
- Support the implementation of school-based suicide prevention programs. *School nurses can be key to early intervention.* **EB:** *School-based suicide prevention programs have been shown in systematic review to improve knowledge, attitude, and help-seeking behavior, with some reports of decreased suicidal ideation (Cusimano & Sameem, 2011). A randomized controlled trial including more than 11,000 students in the European Union were divided into the following three groups: a question and refer group, a mental health awareness group, and a professional screening group. No differences between the groups showed up at 3 months. At 12 months the mental health awareness group showed significant reduction in suicide attempts and severe suicidal ideation (Wasserman et al, 2015).*

Geriatric

- Evaluate the older client's mental and physical health status and financial stressors. **EB:** *Depression in particular is more prevalent in persons with chronic medical conditions, including cardiac disease, diabetes mellitus, cancer, and so forth. Psychological distress, daily hassles, and marital status, along with chronic*

● = Independent;   ▲ = Collaborative;   **EBN** = Evidence-Based Nursing;   **EB** = Evidence-Based

illnesses and substance abuse, have been associated with suicidal ideation (Bosse et al, 2011; Shelef et al, 2014).

- Explore with the client any concerns or pressures (physical and financial) regarding the ability to secure support of medical care, especially perceived pressures about being a burden on family. **EB:** *"Perceived burdensomeness" has been found to be a risk factor of older adults' suicidality, whether clinical depression is present or not, accounting for 68.3% variance of suicidal ideation (Jahn et al, 2011). The presence of stressful life events in the previous year and the presence of untreated major depression were also found to increase suicidal behavior (Pompili et al, 2014).*

- Conduct a thorough assessment of clients' medications. **EB:** *The use of psychotropic medications, especially long-term use and high doses of benzodiazepines, has been significantly associated with suicidal ideation or death thoughts (Bosse et al, 2011).*

- When assessing suicide risk factors, incorporate a higher degree of risk for older men and for some older adults who have lost a loved one in the previous year. **CEB:** *Although mortality for oldest old adults (80+) has increased, the suicide mortality has not decreased. In one study, oldest old men had the highest increase in suicide risk after death of a partner (more so than oldest old women) and took a longer time to recover from the death of a spouse (Erlangsen et al, 2004). Suicide rate may be rising among men older than age 65, and marriage may no longer be the protective factor it was once considered to be (Lamprecht et al, 2005).*

- Explore triggers of and barriers to suicidal behavior, with particular attention to real and perceived losses (e.g., professional role, health). **EB:** *A qualitative study found that older adults' reflections preceding their suicide attempt included loss of a significant other, loneliness, loss of control, and unwillingness to live under these conditions (Bonnewyn et al, 2014). "Perceived burdensomeness" has been found to be a risk factor of older adults' suicidality, whether clinical depression is present or not, accounting for 68.3% variance of suicidal ideation (Jahn et al, 2011).*

- An older adult who shows self-destructive behaviors should be evaluated for dementia. **EB:** *Reviews of older adult psychiatric care for both the medical and psychiatric communities emphasize the possible overlap of depression, dementia, and suicidality (DeMers, Dinsio, & Carlson, 2014).*

- ▲ Advocate for the older client with other professionals in securing treatment for suicidal states. Primary care providers have been noted to under recognize and undertreat older adult clients with depression. **EB:** *In a 10-year longitudinal study, 83% of persons who committed suicide received health care within the previous year; only 24% had been diagnosed with a mental disorder in the 4 weeks prior to death. Medical specialty and primary care accounted for the most common visits (Ahmedani et al, 2014).*

- Encourage physical activity in older adults. **EB:** *Suicide and sleep disturbances have been linked. Exercise has been associated with improved sleep and lower suicide risk (Davidson et al, 2013).*

- ▲ Refer older adults in primary care settings for care management. **EBN:** *The Depression Care for Patients at Home (Depression CAREPATH) program provided assistance for medical and surgical homebound clients as a routine part of clinical practice (Bruce et al, 2011).*

- Consider telephone contacts as an effective intervention for suicidal older adults. **EB:** *One study predicted that, over a 10-year period, telephone and chat services could help to avoid about 36% of suicides and attempts in a high-risk population with a modest effect on quality-adjusted-life-years (Pil et al, 2013).*

 Multicultural

- Assess for the influence of cultural beliefs, norms, and values on the client's perceptions of suicide and on the nurse's perception and approach to suicide. **EBN:** *A qualitative study of suicidal ideation in Korean college students found that the facilitators of suicidal ideation included physical, psychological, and societal factors. Inhibitors were religious and cultural factors. Buddhism and Confucianism influenced reasons not to attempt suicide (Jo, An, & Sohn, 2011).* **EB:** *A systematic review of psychological autopsies across multiple countries concluded that cultural influences in the diagnosis of a mental disorder might account for the variance in cases without a psychiatric diagnosis (Milner, Sveticic, & DeLeo et al, 2013).*

- Identify and acknowledge the stresses unique to culturally diverse individuals. *Financial difficulties and maintaining cultural values are two of the most common family stressors in women of color.* **EB:** *Acculturative stress and perceived discrimination, moderated by hopelessness, can increase vulnerability to suicide. A strong ethnic identity can serve as a buffer (Polanco-Roman & Miranda, 2013).*

- Identify and acknowledge unique cultural responses to stressors in determining sensitive interventions to prevent suicide. **CEB:** *In a randomized controlled trial, the Mexican American Problem Solving (MAPS) program addressed depression symptoms of immigrant Mexican women and their fourth- and fifth-grade children using home visits and afterschool programs. Family problem-solving communication improved, and*

● = Independent;   ▲ = Collaborative;   EBN = Evidence-Based Nursing;   EB = Evidence-Based

children's depression symptoms decreased (Cowell et al, 2009). Encourage family members to demonstrate and offer caring and support to each other. EB: *Connectedness had been identified as a culture-based protective factor against suicide among young Alaska natives (Mohatt et al, 2011).*

- Validate the individual's feelings regarding concerns about the current crisis and family functioning. *Validation lets the client know that the nurse has heard and understood what was said, and it promotes the nurse–client relationship (APNA, 2015).*

Home Care

- Communicate the degree of risk to family and caregivers; assess the family and caregiving situation for the ability to protect the client and to understand the client's suicidal behavior. Provide the family and caregivers with guidelines on how to manage self-harm behaviors in the home environment. *Client safety between home visits is a nursing priority. Family and caregivers may become frightened by the client's suicidal ideation, may be angry at the client's perceived lack of self-control, or may feel as if they are walking on eggshells awaiting another suicide attempt.*
- Assess risk factors in the home. *The presence of a gun must be determined. Safe gun ownership should address the five Ls: locked, loaded, little children, feeling low, and learned owner (Pinholt et al, 2014).*
- If the client's suicidal ideation intensifies, or if a suicide plan with access to means becomes evident, institute an emergency plan for mental health intervention. CEB: *More than a quarter (29%) of clients who had previously self-harmed died within 3 months of discharge from psychiatric care and 36% had missed their last service appointment. Measures that may prevent suicide pacts in the mentally ill include the effective treatment of depression and closer supervision in both inpatient and community settings (Hunt et al, 2009).*
- Identify the client's concerns and implement interventions to address the consequences of disability in a client with medical illness. EB: *Depression, perceived social support, and disability have been found to be predictors of suicidal ideation. Lower levels of family support have been implicated in higher levels of suicidal ideation (Park et al, 2014).* Refer to the care plans for **Hopelessness** and **Powerlessness.**
- ▲ Refer for homemaker or psychiatric home health care services for respite, client reassurance, and implementation of a therapeutic regimen. *Respite decreases the high degree of caregiver stress that goes with the responsibility of caring for a person at risk for suicide.* EBN: *The Depression CAREPATH program provided assistance for medical and surgical homebound clients as a routine part of clinical practice (Bruce et al, 2011).*
- ▲ If the client is on psychotropic medications, assess the client's and family's knowledge of medication administration and side effects. Teach as necessary. *Knowledge of the medical regimen promotes compliance and promotes safe use of medications.*
- ▲ Evaluate the effectiveness and side effects of medications and adherence to the medication regimen. Review with the client and family all medications kept in the home; encourage discarding of old prescriptions. Monitor the amount of medications ordered/provided by the health care provider; limiting the amount of medications to which the client has access may be necessary. *Accurate clinical feedback improves the health care provider's ability to prescribe an effective medical regimen specific to the client's needs. At home, clients may have greater access to medications, including old prescriptions that may be used to overdose.*

Client/Family Teaching and Discharge Planning

- Establish a supportive relationship with family members. EBN: *Family members experience a great deal of stress around suicidal ideation and benefit from nurses' support (Sun et al, 2014).*
- Explain all relevant symptoms, procedures, treatments, and expected outcomes for suicidal ideation that is illness based (e.g., depression, bipolar disorder). CEBN: *The Health Belief Model identifies perceived barriers and perceived susceptibility to disease as powerful predictors of clients' motivation in taking action to prevent disease and participate in self-care management (Pender, Murdaugh, & Parsons, 2010).*
- Teach the family how to recognize that the client is at increased risk for suicide (changes in behavior and verbal and nonverbal communication, withdrawal, depression, or sudden lifting of depression). EBN: *A client may be at peace because a suicide plan has been made and the client has the energy to carry it out. Therefore when depression lifts, increased vigilance is necessary (Sun et al, 2014).*
- Provide written instructions for treatments and procedures for which the client will be responsible. EBN: *A written record provides a concrete reference so that the client and family can clarify any verbal information that was given (Sun et al, 2014).*
- Instruct the client in coping strategies (assertiveness training, impulse control training, deep breathing, progressive muscle relaxation). CEBN: *Suicidal ideation may be triggered by stress and painful emotions.*

● = Independent; ▲ = Collaborative; EBN = Evidence-Based Nursing; EB = Evidence-Based

S

Once clients are able to identify these triggers, they need to learn how to respond to them more effectively through assertiveness, impulse control, or relaxation techniques, as appropriate (Lakeman & FitzGerald, 2008).

- Teach cognitive-behavioral activities, such as active problem-solving, reframing (reappraising the situation from a different perspective), or thought stopping (in response to a negative thought, picturing a large stop sign and replacing the image with a prearranged positive alternative). Teach the client to confront his or her own negative thought patterns (or cognitive distortions), such as catastrophizing (expecting the very worst), dichotomous thinking (perceiving events in only one of two opposite categories), or magnification (placing distorted emphasis on a single event). *Cognitive-behavioral activities address clients' assumptions, beliefs, and attitudes about their situations and foster modification of these elements to be as realistic and optimistic as possible. Through cognitive-behavioral interventions, clients become more aware of their cognitive choices in adopting and maintaining their belief systems, exercising greater control over their own reactions (Hagerty & Patusky, 2011).*

- Provide the client and family with phone numbers of appropriate community agencies for therapy and counseling. The National Alliance on Mental Illness (NAMI) is an excellent resource for client and family support. *Continuous follow-up care should be implemented; therefore the method to access this care must be given to the client (NAMI, 2012).*

REFERENCES

Ahmedani, B. K., Simon, G. E., Stewart, C., et al. (2014). Health care contacts in the year before suicide death. *Journal of General Internal Medicine, 29*(6), 870–877 [Epub 2014 Feb 25].

American Psychiatric Association (APA). (2015). *Practice guidelines for the treatment of psychiatric disorders: Compendium.* Retrieved from http://psychiatryonline.org/guidelines.

American Psychiatric Nurses Association. (2015). *Psychiatric-mental health nurse essential competencies for assessment and management of individuals at risk for suicide.* Retrieved from http://www.apna.org/i4a/pages/index.cfm?pageid=5684.

Astruc, B., et al. (2004). A history of major depressive disorder influences intent to die in violent suicide attempters. *The Journal of Clinical Psychiatry, 65*, 690.

Bell, M. A. (2000). *Losing connections: a process of decision-making in late-life suicidality.* [Doctoral dissertation]. Tucson: University of Arizona.

Biddle, V. S., et al. (2010). Identification of suicide risk among rural youth: Implications for the use of HEADSS. *Journal of Pediatric Health Care, 24*(3), 152.

Bolognini, M., et al. (2003). Adolescents' self-mutilation: Relationship with dependent behaviour. *Swiss Journal of Psychology, 62*(4), 241.

Bonnewyn, C. A., Shah, C. A., Bruffaerts, R., et al. (2014). Reflections of older adults on the process preceding their suicide attempt: A qualitative approach. *Death Studies, 38*(6–10), 612–618.

Bosse, C., et al. (2011). Suicidal ideation, death thoughts, and use of benzodiazepines in the elderly population. *Canadian Journal of Community Mental Health, 30*, 1.

Bowers, L., & Park, A. (2001). Special observation in the care of psychiatric inpatients: A literature review. *Issues in Mental Health Nursing, 22*, 769.

Bruce, M. L., et al. (2011). Depression care for patients at home (Depression CAREPATH): Intervention development and implementation, part 1. *Home Healthcare Nurse, 29*, 416.

Ceretta, L. B., Reus, G. Z., Abelaira, H. M., et al. (2012). Increased prevalence of mood disorders and suicidal ideation in type 2 diabetic patients. *Acta Diabetologica, 49*(Suppl. 1), S227–S234.

Chiu, S., et al. (2010). Validation of the center for epidemiologic studies depression scale in screening for major depressive disorder among retired firefighters exposed to the world trade center disaster. *Journal of Affective Disorders, 121*(3), 212–219.

Cooper, G. D., Clements, P. T., & Holt, K. E. (2012). Examining childhood bullying and adolescent suicide: Implications for school nurses. *Journal of School Nursing, 28*(4), 275–283.

Cowell, J. M., et al. (2009). Clinical trial outcomes of the Mexican American Problem Solving Program (MAPS). *Hispanic Health Care International, 7*, 178.

Cusimano, M. D., & Sameem, M. (2011). The effectiveness of middle and high school-based suicide prevention programmes for adolescents: A systematic review. *Injury Prevention, 17*, 43–49.

Cutcliffe, J. R., & Barker, P. (2004). The nurses' global assessment of suicide risk (NGASR): Developing a tool for clinical practice. *Journal of Psychiatric and Mental Health Nursing, 11*(4), 393.

Davidson, C. L., Babson, K. A., Bonn-Miller, M. O., et al. (2013). The impact of exercise on suicide risk: Examining pathways through depression, PTSD, and sleep in an inpatient sample of veterans. *Suicide & Life-Threatening Behavior, 43*(3), 279–289.

Davis, S. J. (2011). Recognizing suicide risk in consumers with HIV/AIDS. *Journal of Rehabilitation, 77*, 14.

DeMers, S., Dinsio, K., & Carlson, W. (2014). Psychiatric care of the older adults: An overview for primary care. *Medical Clinics of North America, 98*(5), 1145–1168.

Erlangsen, A., et al. (2004). Loss of partner and suicide risks among oldest old: A population-based register study. *Age and Ageing, 33*(4), 378–383.

Feigelman, B., & Feigelman, W. (2011a). Suicide survivor groups: Comings and goings, part I. *Illness, Crises, and Loss, 19*, 57.

Feigelman, B., & Feigelman, W. (2011b). Suicide survivor groups: Comings and goings, part II. *Illness, Crises, and Loss, 19*, 165.

Ghahramanlou-Holloway, M., Bhar, S. S., Brown, G. K., et al. (2012). Changes in problem-solving appraisal after cognitive therapy for the prevention of suicide. *Psychological Medicine, 42*(6), 1185–1193.

Hagerty, B., & Patusky, K. (2011). Mood disorders: Depression and mania. In K. M. Fortinash & P. A. Holoday-Worret (Eds.), *Psychiatric mental health nursing* (5th ed.). St Louis: Mosby.

Hatzenbuehler, M. L. (2011). The social environment and suicide attempts in lesbian, gay, and bisexual youth. *Pediatrics, 127*, 896.

Hauenstein, E. J. (2002). Case finding and care in suicide: Children, adolescents, and adults. In M. A. Boyd (Ed.), *Psychiatric nursing: Contemporary practice* (2nd ed.). Philadelphia: Lippincott Williams & Wilkins.

● = Independent;   ▲ = Collaborative;   EBN = Evidence-Based Nursing;   EB = Evidence-Based

Hirsch, J., & Barton, A. (2011). Positive social support, negative social exchanges, and suicidal behavior in college students. *Journal of American College Health: J of ACH, 59*(5), 393–398.

Hunt, I. M., While, D., Windfuhr, K., et al. (2009). Suicide pacts in the mentally ill: A national clinical survey. *Psychiatry Research, 167*(1–2), 131–138.

Jahn, D. R., et al. (2011). The mediating effect of perceived burdensomeness on the relation between depressive symptoms and suicide ideation in a community sample of older adults. *Aging and Mental Health, 15*, 214.

Jo, K., An, G. J., & Sohn, K. (2011). Qualitative content analysis of suicidal ideation in Korean college students. *Collegian (Royal College of Nursing, Australia), 18*, 87.

Kleiman, E. M., Riskind, J. H., & Schaefer, K. E. (2014). Social support and positive events as suicide resiliency factors: Examination of synergistic buffering effects. *Archives of Suicide Research, 18*(2), 144–155.

Lakeman, R., & FitzGerald, M. (2008). How people live with or get over being suicidal: A review of qualitative studies. *Journal of Advanced Nursing, 64*, 114.

Lamprecht, H. C., et al. (2005). Deliberate self-harm in older people revisited. *International Journal of Geriatric Psychiatry, 20*, 1090.

Larsen, K. K. (2013). Depression following myocardial infarction—An overseen complication with prognostic importance. *Danish Medical Journal, 60*(8), B4689.

Lea, T., deWit, J., & Reynolds, R. (2014). Minority stress in lesbian, gay, and bisexual young adults in Australia: Associations with psychological distress, suicidality, and substance use. *Archives of Sexual Behavior, 43*(8), 1571–1578.

Li, Z., et al. (2011). Attributable risk of psychiatric and socio-economic factors for suicide from individual-level, population-based studies: A systematic review. *Social Science and Medicine, 72*, 608.

Malone, K. M., et al. (2000). Protective factors against suicidal acts in major depression: Reasons for living. *The American Journal of Psychiatry, 157*, 1084.

McMyler, C., & Pryjmachuk, S. (2008). Do "no-suicide" contracts work? *Journal of Psychiatric and Mental Health Nursing, 15*, 512.

Mills, P. D., et al. (2008). National patient safety goals. Inpatient suicide and suicide attempts in Veterans Affairs hospitals. *Joint Commission Journal on Quality and Patient Safety, 34*, 482.

Milner, A., Sveticic, J., & DeLeo, D. (2013). Suicide in the absence of mental disorder? A review of psychological autopsy studies across countries. *International Journal of Social Psychiatry, 59*(6), 545–554.

Mohatt, N. V., Fok, C. C., Burket, R., et al. (2011). Assessment of awareness of connectedness as a culturally-based protective factor for Alaska native youth. *Cultural Diversity and Ethnic Minority Psychology, 17*(4), 444–455.

National Alliance on Mental Illness (NAMI). Retrieved from http://www.nami.org/. (Accessed 11 October 2012).

Park, J., Han, M., Kim, M., et al. (2014). Predictors of suicidal ideation in older individuals receiving home-care services. *International Journal of Geriatric Psychiatry, 29*(4), 367–376.

Pelkonen, M., et al. (2005). Suicidality in adjustment disorder: Clinical characteristics of adolescent outpatients. *European Child and Adolescent Psychiatry, 14*, 174.

Pender, N. J., Murdaugh, C. L., & Parsons, M. A. (2010). *Health promotion in nursing practice* (6th ed.). Upper Saddle River, NJ: Prentice-Hall.

Pil, L., Pauwels, K., Muijzers, E., et al. (2013). Cost effectiveness of a helpline for suicide prevention. *Journal of Telemedicine & Telecare, 19*(5), 273–281.

Pinholt, E. M., Mitchell, J. D., Butler, J. H., et al. (2014). "Is there a gun in the home?" Assessing the risks of gun ownership in older adults. *Journal of the American Geriatrics Society, 62*(6), 1142–1146.

Polanco-Roman, L., & Miranda, R. (2013). Culturally related stress, hopelessness, and vulnerability to depressive symptoms and suicidal ideation in emerging adulthood. *Behavior Therapy, 44*, 74–87.

Pompili, M., Forte, A., Lester, D., et al. (2014). Suicide risk in type 1 diabetes mellitus: A systematic review. *Journal of Psychosomatic Research, 76*(5), 352–360.

Pompili, M., Innamorati, M., DiVottorio, C., et al. (2014). Sociodemographic and clinical differences between suicide ideators and attempters: A study of mood disordered patients 50 years and older. *Suicide & Life-Threatening Behavior, 44*, 34–45.

Pryjmachuk, S., & Trainor, G. (2010). Helping young people who self-harm: Perspectives from England. *Journal of Child and Adolescent Psychiatric Nursing, 23*(2), 52.

Robinson, J., Hetrick, S. E., & Martin, C. (2011). Preventing suicide in young people: Systematic review. *The Australian and New Zealand Journal of Psychiatry, 45*, 3–26.

Rogers, J. R., Lewis, M. M., & Subich, L. M. (2002). Validity of the suicide assessment checklist in an emergency crisis center. *Journal of Counseling and Development, 80*, 493.

Russell, S. T., et al. (2011). Lesbian, gay, bisexual, and transgender adolescent school victimization: Implications for young adult health and adjustment. *The Journal of School Health, 81*(5), 223.

Shelef, A., Hiss, J., Cherkashin, G., et al. (2014). Psychosocial and medical aspects of older adult suicide completers in Israel: A 10-year survey. *International Journal of Geriatric Psychiatry, 29*(8), 846–851.

Spirito, A., et al. (2002). An intervention trial to improve adherence to community treatment by adolescents after a suicide attempt. *Journal of the American Academy of Child and Adolescent Psychiatry, 41*(4), 435.

Sun, F., Chiang, C., Lin, Y., et al. (2014). Short-term effects of a suicide education intervention for family caregivers of people who are suicidal. *Journal of Clinical Nursing, 23*(102), 91–102.

Talseth, A., & Gilje, F. L. (2011). Nurses' responses to suicide and suicidal patients: A critical interpretive synthesis. *Journal of Clinical Nursing, 20*, 1651.

Tarrier, N., Taylor, K., & Gooding, P. (2008). Cognitive-behavioral interventions to reduce suicidal behavior. *Behavior Modification, 32*, 77.

Thanoi, W., et al. (2010). The adolescent suicide risk behaviors: A model of negative life events, rumination, emotional distress, resilience, and social support. *Pacific Rim International Journal of Nursing Research, 14*, 187.

Toumbourou, J. W., & Gregg, M. E. (2002). Impact of an empowerment-based parent education program on the reduction of youth suicide risk factors. *Journal of Adolescent Health, 31*, 277.

Wasserman, D., Hoven, C. W., Wasserman, C., et al. (2015). School-based suicide prevention programmes: The SEYLE cluster-randomized, controlled trial. *The Lancet*. Retrieved from http://www.mdlinx.com/internal-medicine/print-preview.cfm/5874195.

S

● = Independent;   ▲ = Collaborative;   **EBN** = Evidence-Based Nursing;   **EB** = Evidence-Based

Delayed Surgical Recovery
Mary Beth Flynn Makic, PhD, CNS, CCNS, FAAN, FNAP

NANDA-I

Definition

Extension of the number of postoperative days required to initiate and perform activities that maintain life, health, and well-being.

Defining Characteristics

Discomfort; evidence of interrupted healing of surgical area; excessive time required for recuperation; impaired mobility; inability to resume employment; loss of appetite; postpones resumption of work; requires assistance for self-care

Related Factors

Malnutrition; obesity; pain; postoperative emotional response

At-Risk Population

Extremes of age; history of delayed wound healing

Associated Condition

American Society of Anesthesiologists (ASA) Physical Status classification score ≥ 2; diabetes mellitus; edema at surgical site; extensive surgical procedure; impaired mobility; perioperative surgical site infection; persistent nausea; persistent vomiting; pharmaceutical agent; prolonged surgical procedure; psychological disorder in postoperative period; surgical site contamination; trauma at surgical site

NOC   (Nursing Outcomes Classification)

Suggested NOC Outcomes

Endurance; Infection Severity; Mobility; Pain Control; Self-Care: Activities of Daily Living (ADLs); Surgical Recovery: Convalescence/Immediate Postoperative; Wound Healing: Primary Intention

Example NOC Outcome with Indicators

Surgical Recovery: Convalescence as evidenced by the following indicators: Extent of physiological, psychological, and role function after discharge from postanesthesia care to the final postoperative clinic visit/Vital signs/Performance of normal activities, self-care activities. (Rate the outcome and indicators of **Surgical Recovery: Convalescence** 1 = severe deviation from normal range, 2 = substantial deviation from normal range, 3 = moderate deviation from normal range, 4 = mild deviation from normal range, 5 = no deviation from normal range [see Section I].)

Client Outcomes

Client Will (Specify Time Frame)

- Have surgical area that shows evidence of healing: no redness, induration, draining, or immobility
- State that appetite is regained
- State that no nausea is present
- Demonstrate ability to move about
- Demonstrate ability to complete self-care activities
- State that no fatigue is present
- State that pain is controlled or relieved after nursing interventions
- Resume employment activities/ADLs
- State no depression or anxiety related to surgical procedure

NIC   (Nursing Interventions Classification)

Suggested NIC Interventions

Incision Site Care; Nutrition Management; Pain Management; Self-Care Assistance; Surgical Assistance

● = Independent;   ▲ = Collaborative;   EBN = Evidence-Based Nursing;   EB = Evidence-Based

S

Example NIC Activities—Incision Site Care
Teach the client and/or the family how to care for the incision, including signs and symptoms of infection; Inspect the incision site for redness, swelling, or signs of dehiscence or evisceration

Nursing Interventions and *Rationales*

- Encourage smoking cessation prior to surgery. EB: *Smoking cessation improves tissue oxygenation and improves pulmonary function. Clients who smoke are at higher risk of developing blood clots (venous thromboembolism) postoperatively and may experience delayed surgical wound healing (Wechter, 2016).*

- Preoperatively, perform a thorough assessment of the client, including risk factors. Allow time to be with the client, and actively listen to client's concerns and questions about care, functional status, and recovery. EB: *Assessment of clients preoperatively is an important part of the surgical intervention, and ensuring health care literacy is addressed during this assessment is important for postoperative education and surgical recovery (Ross, 2013).* EB: *Clients with higher presurgery levels of emotional distress appear to be at greater risk for experiencing higher levels of postsurgery side effects (Sadati et al, 2013).*

- Assess for the presence of medical conditions and treat appropriately before surgery. If the client is diabetic, maintain normal blood glucose levels before surgery. EB: *High blood glucose levels slow healing and increase risk of infection. The American Diabetes Association (ADA) recommended that blood glucose should be less than 180 mg/dL for people in the hospital or having surgery. For some, the goal is less than 140 mg/dL (ADA, 2014; Sudhakaran & Surani, 2015).*

- Carefully assess client's use of dietary supplements such as feverfew, fish oil, ginkgo biloba, garlic, ginseng, ginger, valerian, kava, St. John's wort, ephedra (Ma huang or metabolite), and *Echinacea.* It is recommended that all clients be advised to stop all dietary supplements at least 1 week before major surgical or diagnostic procedures. EB: *Because of the increasingly complicated medication regimens and polypharmacy, it is important to assess client's use of herbal and dietary supplements because they can cause medication reactions or have unintended medical side effects (Nieva et al, 2012).* EB: *Herbal remedies are common in clients presenting for anesthesia. Because of the potential interactions between anesthetic drugs or techniques and such medication, it is important for anesthetists to be aware of their use (Bajwa & Panda, 2012; Kaye, 2014).*

- Assess and treat for depression and anxiety in a client before surgery and postoperatively. CEB/EB: *Clients with higher levels of preoperative anxiety and depression report increased postoperative pain, nausea, fatigue, and morbidity (Ghoneim & O'Hara, 2016; Manworren, Gordon, & Montgomery, 2018).* EB: *Early identification of clients with preoperative depression and anxiety allows the nurse to prepare postoperative interventions and support systems that may facilitate postoperative recovery (Ghoneim & O'Hara, 2016).*

- Play music of the client's choice preoperatively, intraoperatively, and postoperatively. EBN: *Listening to self-selected music during the preoperative period can effectively reduce anxiety levels and should be a useful tool for preoperative nursing (Ni et al, 2012; McClurkin & Smith, 2016).* CEBN: *Results of this research provided evidence to support the use of music and/or a quiet rest period to decrease pain and anxiety. The interventions pose no risks and have the benefits of improved pain reports and decreased anxiety (Pittman & Kridli, 2011).*

- Consider using healing touch and other mind-body-spirit interventions such as stress control, therapeutic massage, and imagery in the perianesthesia setting. EBN: *Research shows that use of holistic therapies in the perioperative setting can decrease pain, surgical trauma, and anesthesia complications, leading to increased client satisfaction with health care (Selimen & Andsoy, 2011).* EB: *Therapeutic touch may help restore client's integrity by providing consolation and a sense of safety (Airosa et al, 2013).*

- Use reflective blankets to reduce heat loss during surgery. EBN: *A randomized control trial found that reflective blankets were a more effective method of passive warming than warm blankets (Koenen, Passey, & Rolf, 2017).*

- Postoperatively, discuss with the surgeon vital sign parameters, signs, and symptoms that could indicate early postoperative infection. EB: *Surgical site infections are a leading cause of prolonged hospitalization, which increase cost of care and are associated with poorer outcomes (Tanner et al, 2013).*

- Use careful aseptic technique when caring for wounds. EBN: *Handwashing continues to be the most important factor in reducing health care–associated infection, but the use of an aseptic technique will further cut the risk of infection (Harrington, 2014).* EBN: *Dressings should be changed by nurses who are trained in antiseptic, nontouch technique.*

● = Independent;   ▲ = Collaborative;   EBN = Evidence-Based Nursing;   EB = Evidence-Based

S

- Clients should be allowed to shower after surgery to maintain cleanliness if not contraindicated because of the presence of pacemaker wires. EB: *In an analysis of existing studies, it was determined that there was no statistically significant increase in wound infection related to early bathing. Avoiding washing may have an adverse effect on the wound because of accumulation of sweat or dirt at the site. The decision to bathe the client immediately postoperatively should be specific to surgical type and site (Toon et al, 2013).*
- Promote early ambulation and deep breathing. EBN: *A quality improvement study found that early ambulation improved client and nurse satisfaction, decreased postoperative ileus events, and there was noted improvement in postoperative client progress and discharge readiness (Kilber et al, 2012)*
- The client should be provided with a complete, balanced therapeutic diet after the immediately postoperative period (24–48 hours). EBN: *Optimal wound healing requires adequate nutrition. Nutrition deficiencies impede the normal processes that allow progression through stages of wound healing. Malnutrition has also been related to decreased wound tensile strength and increased infection rates (Collins & Sloan, 2013).*
- Encourage the client to use prayer as a form of spiritual coping if this is comfortable for the client. EB: *Prayer has been shown to reduce pain intensity and provide a stabilizing effect on cardiovascular measurements (Jegindø et al, 2013).*
- Carefully assess functional status of client postoperatively using a fall-risk stratification tool, such as the Morse Fall Scale, to identify clients at high risk for fall. EBN: *The Morse Fall Scale has been validated in numerous studies, and it helps identify clients at high risk for falls. All clients identified as high risk should have increased monitoring and nursing and be placed under increased safety precautions until discharge, regardless of functional improvement (Baek et al, 2014).*
- See the care plans for **Anxiety,** Acute **Pain, Fatigue,** Risk for deficient **Fluid** volume, Risk for **Perioperative Positioning** injury, Impaired physical **Mobility,** and **Nausea.**

 ### Pediatric

- Encourage children to ask questions about their procedures and postoperative expectations regarding pain, function, and long-term social and emotional care needs. EBN: *Children often report having little input or understanding of their medical conditions and requirements for surgical and functional interventions. Parents and children report higher levels of satisfaction, decreased preoperative anxiety, and better experiences if they are given the opportunity preoperatively to discuss all aspects of the surgery, including realistic postoperative expectations (Bray, Callery, & Kirk, 2012; Alanazi, 2014).*
- Teach imagery and encourage distraction for children for postsurgical pain relief. EBN: *Distraction decreases pain in children undergoing painful procedures (Helgadottir & Wilson, 2014; Ha & Kim, 2013).*

 ### Geriatric

- Perform a thorough preoperative assessment, including a cardiac, social support, and skin assessment. EB: *The condition of the client' skin should be noted before and after the procedure and should be fully documented using an objective evaluation tool, such as the Braden scale, to allow early identification of older clients at higher risk for developing surgical site infections or other types of skin breakdown (Cohen et al, 2012).*
- Older clients are at increased risk of delayed surgical recovery associated with physical and psychological postsurgical stress, nutritional deficits, aging immune system, and comorbid disease states. EB: *Older clients requiring surgical procedures need individualized assessments that explore nutrition, frailty and functional status, and cognitive assessment in addition to preexisting comorbid diseases (Kim, Brooks, & Groban, 2014).*
- Routinely assess pain in postoperative clients using a pain scale that is appropriate for clients with impaired cognition or inability to verbalize. CEB: *The Pain Assessment in Advanced Dementia (PAINAD) and Pain Assessment Checklist for Seniors with Limited Ability to Communicate (PACSLAC) have been validated for reliability (Herr, 2011).*
- Serially evaluate the client's vital signs, including temperature. Know what is normal and abnormal for each client. Check baseline vital signs and monitor trends. EB: *Physiological changes of aging often result in lower baseline body temperatures and decreased heart rates, and prevent the older client from developing fever. Medications, such as blood pressure agents, may prevent client from having an increased heart rate (Chester & Rudolph, 2011).*
- Ongoing evaluation of the older client for signs and symptoms of delirium should be incorporated into each assessment. Provide tools such as clocks, calendars, and other orientation tools to help reduce the risk of delirium in the postoperative area. Ensure that hearing aids and glasses are also available as needed. EBN: *A quality improvement project that continuously reviewed the older clients' physiological recovery and*

● = Independent;   ▲ = Collaborative;   EBN = Evidence-Based Nursing;   EB = Evidence-Based

implemented frequent assessment for delirium and reorientation strategies reduced delirium events (Brooks et al, 2014).

- Offer spiritual support. EB: *Religiousness is related to significantly fewer depressive symptoms, better quality of life, less cognitive impairment, and less perceived pain. Clinicians should consider taking a spiritual history and ensuring that spiritual needs are addressed among older clients in rehabilitation settings (Lucchetti et al, 2011).*

Home Care

- The preceding interventions may be adapted for the home setting.
- Provide supportive telephone calls from nurse to client as a means of decreasing anxiety and providing the psychosocial support necessary for recovery from surgery. EBN: *A systematic review of qualitative studies found that clients report being motivated to participate in recovery but face challenges with symptoms (e.g., pain, nausea, weakness). Postoperative follow-up and phone calls provide much needed encouragement and additional assistance to facilitate recovery (Sibbern et al, 2017).*

Client/Family Teaching and Discharge Planning

- Provide discharge planning and teaching in a language that is appropriate to the client and caregiver's education and literacy level. EBN: *Do not use technical or medical jargon, and be aware that clients and caregivers may to be reluctant to ask for explanation or clarification because of embarrassment and may verbalize dishonestly understanding. Allow the client to repeat their understanding of the discharge plan (Ross, 2013).*
- Meet with client and caregivers to create a discharge plan that includes measurable goals for functional ADLs and pain levels, discuss expectations for recovery, and address signs and symptoms of postoperative complications. EBN: *In a study on successful discharge planning, it was found that plans that were detailed and precise, and addressed client and caregiver feedback, situations, preferences, and agreement with the care plan had greater satisfaction and plan adherence (Tomura et al, 2011).*
- Provide individualized teaching plans for the client with an ostomy. Assess client's ability to manage basic needs such as (1) maintenance of a pouching seal for a consistent, predictable wear time; (2) maintenance of peristomal skin integrity; and (3) social and professional support. Referrals for home wound care or nursing visits may be necessary to help client maintain hygiene and prevent readmission for complications. EBN: *Careful assessment of client's ability to manage colostomy will help the nurse anticipate possible problems with routine care requiring close follow-up and referrals for skilled care after discharge (Walker & Lachman, 2013).*

REFERENCES

Airosa, F., Falkenberg, T., Ohlen, G., et al. (2013). Tactile massage or healing touch: Caring touch for patients in emergency care—A qualitative study. *European Journal of Integrative Medicine, 5*(4), 374–381.

Alanazi, A. (2014). Reducing anxiety in preoperative patients: A systematic review. *British Journal of Nursing, 23*(7), 387–393.

ADA: American Diabetes Association. (2014). Standards of medical care in diabetes—2014. *Diabetes Care, 37*(s.1).

Baek, S., Piao, J., Jinshi, J., et al. (2014). Validity of the morse fall scale implemented in an electronic medical record system. *Journal of Clinical Nursing, 23*(17/18), 2434–2441.

Bajwa, S. J., & Panda, A. (2012). Alternative medicine and anesthesia: Implications and considerations in daily practice. *Ayu, 33*(4), 475–480.

Bray, L., Callery, P., & Kirk, S. (2012). A qualitative study of the pre-operative preparation of children, young people and their parents' for planned continence surgery: Experiences and expectations. *Journal of Clinical Nursing, 21*(13/14), 1964–1973.

Brooks, P., Spillane, J. P., Dick, K., et al. (2014). Developing a strategy to identify and treat older patients with postoperative delirium. *AORN Journal, 99*(2), 257–275.

Chester, J. G., & Rudolph, J. L. (2011). Vital signs in older patients: Age-related changes. *Journal of the American Medical Directors Association, 12*(5), 337–343.

Cohen, R., Lagoo-Deenadayalan, S. A., Heflin, M. T., et al. (2012). Exploring predictors of complication in older surgical patients: A deficit accumulation index and the Braden Scale. *Journal of the American Geriatrics Society, 60*(9), 1609–1615.

Collins, N., & Sloan, C. (2013). Back to basics: Nutrition as part of the overall wound treatment plan. *Ostomy/Wound Management, 59*(4), 16–19.

Ghoneim, M. M., & O'Hara, M. W. (2016). Depression and postoperative complications: An overview. *BMC Surgery, 16*, 5. doi:10.1186/s12893-016-0120-y. Retrieved from https://bmcsurg.biomedcentral.com/track/pdf/10.1186/s12893-016-0120-y?site=bmcsurg.biomedcentral.com. (Accessed 9 March 2018).

Ha, Y., & Kim, H. (2013). The effects of audiovisual distraction on children's pain during laceration repair. *International Journal of Nursing Practice, 19*(Suppl. 3), 20–27.

Harrington, P. (2014). Prevention of surgical site infection. *Nursing Standard, 28*(48), 50–58.

Helgadottir, H., & Wilson, M. (2014). A randomized controlled trial of the effectiveness of educating parents about distraction to decrease

S

postoperative pain in children at home after tonsillectomy. *Pain Management Nursing, 15*(3), 632–640.

Herr, K. (2011). Pain assessment strategies in older patients. *The Journal of Pain, 15*(11), 1069–1202.

Jegindø, E., Vase, L., Skewes, J., et al. (2013). Expectations contribute to reduced pain levels during prayer in highly religious participants. *Journal of Behavioral Medicine, 36*(4), 413–426.

Kaye, A. (2014). Critical care medicine and the emerging challenges of dietary supplements, including herbal products. *Critical Care Medicine, 42*(4), 1014–1016.

Kilber, V., Hayes, R. M., Johnson, D. E., et al. (2012). Early postoperative ambulation: Back to basics. *American Journal of Nursing, 112*(4), 63–69.

Kim, S., Brooks, A. K., & Groban, L. (2014). Preoperative assessment of the older surgical patient: Honing in on geriatric syndromes. *Clinical Interventions in Aging, 10*, 13–27. Retrieved from https://www.dovepress.com/preoperative-assessment-of-the-older-surgical-patient-honing-in-on-ger-peer-reviewed-article-CIA. (Accessed 9 March 2018).

Koenen, M., Passey, M., & Rolf, M. (2017). "Keeping them warm"—A randomized controlled trial of two passive perioperative warming methods. *Journal of Perianesthesia Nursing, 32*(3), 188–198.

Lucchetti, G., Lucchetti, A., Granero, L., et al. (2011). Religiousness affects mental health, pain and quality of life in older people in an outpatient rehabilitation setting. *Journal of Rehabilitation Medicine, 43*(4), 316–322.

Manworren, R., Gordon, D., & Montgomery, R. (2018). Managing postoperative pain. *American Journal of Nursing, 118*(1), 36–43. doi:10.1097/01.NAJ.0000529695.38192.67.

McClurkin, S. L., & Smith, C. D. (2016). The duration of self-selected music needed to reduce preoperative anxiety. *Journal of Perianesthesia Nursing, 31*(3), 196–208.

Ni, C., Tsai, W., Lee, L., et al. (2012). Minimising preoperative anxiety with music for day surgery patients—a randomised clinical trial. *Journal of Clinical Nursing, 21*(5), 620–625.

Nieva, R., Safavynia, S., Lee Bishop, K., et al. (2012). Herbal, vitamin, and mineral supplement use in patients enrolled in a cardiac rehabilitation program. *Journal of Cardiopulmonary Rehabilitation and Prevention, 32*(5), 270–277.

Pittman, S., & Kridli, S. (2011). Music intervention and preoperative anxiety: An integrative review. *International Nursing Review, 58*(2), 157–163.

Ross, J. (2013). Preoperative assessment and teaching of postoperative discharge instructions: The importance of understanding health literacy. *Journal of PeriAnestheisa Nursing, 38*(5), 318–320.

Sadati, L., Pazouki, A., Mehdizadeh, A., et al. (2013). Effect of preoperative nursing visit on preoperative anxiety and postoperative complications in candidates for laparoscopic cholecystectomy: A randomized clinical trial. *Scandinavian Journal of Caring Sciences, 27*(4), 994–998.

Selimen, D., & Andsoy, I. (2011). The importance of a holistic approach during the perioperative period. *AORN Journal, 93*(4), 482–490.

Sibbern, T., Bull Sellevold, V., & Steindal, S. A. (2017). Patients' experiences of enhanced recovery after surgery: A systematic review of qualitative studies. *Journal of Clinical Nursing, 26*(9–10), 1172–1188. doi:10.1111/jocn.13456.

Sudhakaran, S., & Surani, S. R. (2015). Guidelines for perioperative management of the diabetic patient surgery. *Research and Practice, 2015*, Article ID 284063, 8 pages. Retrieved from http://dx.doi.org/10.1155/2015/284063, Retrieved from https://www.ncbi.nlm.nih.gov/pmc/articles/PMC4452499/pdf/SRP2015-284063.pdf. (Accessed 9 March 2018).

Tanner, J., Padley, W., Kiernan, M., et al. (2013). A benchmark too far: findings from a national survey of surgical site infection surveillance. *Journal of Hospital Infection, 83*(2), 87–91.

Tomura, H., Yamamoto-Mitani, N., Nagata, S., et al. (2011). Creating an agreed discharge: Discharge planning for clients with high care needs. *Journal of Clinical Nursing, 20*(3/4), 444–453.

Toon, C. D., Sinha, S., Davidson, B. R., et al. (2013). Early versus delayed post-operative bathing or showering to prevent wound complications. *The Cochrane Library.* Retrieved from http://onlinelibrary.wiley.com/doi/10.1002/14651858.CD010075.pub2/pdf/standard.

Walker, C., & Lachman, V. (2013). Gaps in the discharge process for patients with an ostomy: An ethical perspective. *Medsurg Nursing, 22*(1), 61–64.

Wechter, D. G. (2016). *Smoking and surgery.* MedlinePlus. Retrieved from https://medlineplus.gov/ency/patientinstructions/000437.htm. (Accessed 8 March 2018).

S

Risk for delayed Surgical recovery
Gail B. Ladwig, MSN, RN and Mary Beth Flynn Makic, PhD, CNS, CCNS, FAAN, FNAP

NANDA-I

Definition

Susceptible to an extension of the number of postoperative days required to initiate and perform activities that maintain life, health, and well-being, which may compromise health.

Risk Factors

Malnutrition, obesity, pain, postoperative emotional response

At-Risk Population

Extremes of age, history of delayed wound healing

Associated Conditions

American Society of Anesthesiologists (ASA) >2, diabetes mellitus, edema at surgical site, extensive surgical procedure, impaired mobility, perioperative surgical site infection, persistent nausea, persistent vomiting,

● = Independent;   ▲ = Collaborative;   EBN = Evidence-Based Nursing;   EB = Evidence-Based

pharmaceutical agent, prolonged surgical procedures, psychological disorder in postoperative period, surgical site contamination, trauma at surgical site

NIC, NOC, Client Outcomes, Nursing Interventions and *Rationales,* Client/Family Teaching and Discharge Planning and References

See the care plan for Delayed **Surgical** recovery.

Impaired Swallowing   *Mary E. Oesterle, MA, CCC-SLP and Marina Martinez-Kratz, MS, RN, CNE*

NANDA-I

Definition

Abnormal functioning of the swallowing mechanism associated with deficits in oral, pharyngeal, or esophageal structure or function.

Defining Characteristics

First Stage: Oral

Abnormal oral phase of swallow study; choking prior to swallowing; coughing prior to swallowing; drooling; food falls from mouth; food pushed out of mouth; gagging prior to swallowing; inability to clear oral cavity; incomplete lip closure; inefficient nippling; inefficient suck; insufficient chewing; nasal reflux; piecemeal deglutition; pooling of bolus in lateral sulci; premature entry of bolus; prolonged bolus formation; prolonged mealtime with inefficient consumption; tongue action ineffective in forming bolus

Second Stage: Pharyngeal

Abnormal pharyngeal phase of swallow study; alteration in head position; choking; coughing; delayed swallowing; fevers of unknown etiology; food refusal; gagging sensation; gurgling voice quality; inadequate laryngeal elevation; nasal reflux; recurrent pulmonary infection; repetitive swallowing

Third Stage: Esophageal

Abnormal esophageal phase of swallow study; acidic-smelling breath; bruxism; difficulty swallowing; epigastric pain; food refusal; heartburn; hematemesis; hyperextension of head; nighttime awakening; nighttime coughing; odynophagia; regurgitation; repetitive swallowing; reports "something stuck"; unexplained irritability surrounding mealtimes; volume limiting; vomiting; vomitus on pillow

Related Factors

Behavioral feeding problem; self-injurious behavior

At-Risk Population

Behavioral feeding problem; failure to thrive; history of enteral feeding; self-injurious behavior; developmental delay and prematurity

Associated Condition

Abnormality; achalasia; acquired autonomic defects; brain injury; cerebral palsy; conditions with significant hypotonia; congenital heart disease; cranial nerve involvement; esophageal reflux disease; laryngeal abnormality; laryngeal defect; mechanical obstruction; nasal defect; nasopharyngeal cavity defect; neurological problems; neuromuscular impairment; protein-energy malnutrition; respiratory condition; tracheal defect; trauma; upper airway anomaly

NOC   (Nursing Outcomes Classification)

Suggested NOC Outcomes

Swallowing Status: Esophageal Phase, Oral Phase, Pharyngeal Phase

● = Independent;   ▲ = Collaborative;   EBN = Evidence-Based Nursing;   EB = Evidence-Based

---

Example NOC Outcome with Indicators
Swallowing Status as evidenced by the following indicators: Delivery of bolus to hypopharynx is timed with swallow reflex/Ability to clear oral cavity/Number of swallows appropriate for bolus size and texture/Voice quality/Choking, coughing, gagging/Normal swallow effort. (Rate the outcome and indicators of **Swallowing Status:** 1 = severely compromised, 2 = substantially compromised, 3 = moderately compromised, 4 = mildly compromised, 5 = not compromised [see Section I].)

Client Outcomes

Client Will (Specify Time Frame)

- Demonstrate effective swallowing without signs of aspiration (see the section Defining Characteristics)
- Remain free from aspiration (e.g., lungs clear, temperature within normal range)

NIC (Nursing Interventions Classification)

Suggested NIC Interventions

Aspiration Precautions; Swallowing Therapy

Example NIC Activities—Swallowing Therapy
Assist client to sit in erect position (as close to 90 degrees as possible) for feeding/exercise; Instruct client not to talk during eating, if appropriate

Nursing Interventions and *Rationales*

- Complete swallow screen per facility protocol. **EBN:** *Nurse-initiated dysphagia screening with formal guidelines for the identification and management of dysphagia may have a significant effect on serious adverse outcomes such as chest infections and death (Hines, Kynoch, & Munday, 2016).*
- ▲ Do not feed clients with impaired swallowing orally until an appropriate diagnostic workup is completed. **EBN:** *Impaired swallow function or dysphagia places a patient at greater risk for dehydration and malnutrition Dehydration thickens secretions, increasing the risk for certain respiratory problems, and aspiration may lead to pneumonia and death (Mauk, 2017, p 578).*
- ▲ Ensure proper nutrition by consulting with a health care provider regarding alternative nutrition and hydration when oral nutrition is not safe/adequate. **EBN:** *The decision to proceed with tube feeding should be made as early as possible after admission, usually within the first 3 days of admission in collaboration with the patient, family (or substitute decision maker), and interprofessional team. Enteral nutrition via intravenous, nasogastric, or percutaneous endoscopic gastrostomy (PEG) tube could substantially reduce risks of aspiration and choking while providing patients with needed hydration and nutrients.*
- ▲ Refer to a speech-language pathologist for evaluation and diagnostic evaluation of swallowing to determine swallowing problems and solutions as soon as oral and/or pharyngeal dysphagia is suspected. **EBN:** *Safe nursing care includes a consultation with a speech-language pathologist whenever doubts arise regarding a client's ability to tolerate oral-supported nutrition in any form (Teasell et al, 2016). Video fluoroscopic swallow study (VSS, VFSS, or MBS), or fiberoptic endoscopic examination of swallowing (FEES), should be performed on all patients considered at risk for pharyngeal dysphagia or poor airway protection based on results from the bedside swallowing assessment (Gomes et al, 2013).*
- ▲ To manage impaired swallowing, use a multidisciplinary dysphagia team composed of a speech pathologist, dietitian, nursing, health care provider, and medical staff. A comprehensive assessment from a multidisciplinary dysphagia team can lead to personalized therapeutic interventions that can help the client learn to swallow safely and maintain a good nutritional status. **EBN:** *Elderly patients with dysphagia require a multidisciplinary team working closely together to perform feeding management. Nurses have more opportunities to contact patients in clinical work, so they must learn the correct guidance of safe eating and feeding for elderly patients with dysphagia (Li et al, 2015).*
- ▲ Observe the following feeding guidelines:
  - ○ Before giving oral feedings, determine the client's readiness to eat (e.g., alert, able to hold head erect, follow instructions, move tongue in mouth, and manage oral secretions). *If one of these elements is missing, it may be advisable to withhold oral feeding and use enteral feeding for nourishment.*

● = Independent;　▲ = Collaborative;　**EBN** = Evidence-Based Nursing;　**EB** = Evidence-Based

○ Monitor client during oral feedings and provide cueing as needed to ensure client follows swallowing guidelines/aspiration precautions recommended by speech-language pathologist or dysphagia specialist. Note: General aspiration precautions include the following: sit at 90 degrees for all oral feedings, take small bites/sips, eat at a slow rate, and no straws. However, client-specific strategies will be determined via bedside and/or instrumental swallowing evaluation performed by dysphagia specialist. *Postural changes, sensory enhancements, swallow maneuvers, or voluntary controls exerted over the swallow can improve swallow, but the use and effectiveness of these treatments will vary systematically with the client's medical diagnosis (Logemann & Larsen, 2012).*

○ Keep bolus size to 5 mL or smaller. **EB:** *Evidence gathered from the appraised studies generally supports the clinical hypothesis that a small bolus size (5 mL or smaller) decreases the risk of penetration or aspiration of liquids during swallowing events (Rizzo et al, 2016).*

○ *If the client is older or has gastroesophageal reflux disease, ensure the client is kept in an upright posture for an hour after eating.* **CEB:** *An upright posture after eating has been associated with a decreased incidence of pneumonia in older adults (Coleman, 2004). Because the trachea is in front of the esophagus while sitting up straight and the trachea is above the esophagus while leaning back or lying down, aspiration into the trachea can be reduced because of gravity (Logemann & Larsen, 2012).*

• During meals and all oral intake, observe for signs associated with swallowing problems such as coughing, choking, spitting of food, drooling, difficulty handling oral secretions, double swallowing or delay in swallowing, watering eyes, nasal discharge, wet or gurgling voice, decreased ability to move the tongue and lips, decreased mastication of food, decreased ability to move food to the back of the pharynx, and slow or scanning speech. **CEB:** *Perceptual judgments of a clear postswallow voice quality provided reasonable evidence that aspiration and dysphagia were absent as measured by video fluoroscopy (Waito et al, 2011).*

▲ Watch for uncoordinated chewing or swallowing; coughing immediately after eating or delayed coughing; pocketing of food; wet-sounding voice; sneezing when eating; delay of more than 1 second in swallowing; or a change in respiratory patterns. If any of these signs of dysphagia and/or aspiration is present, remove all food from the oral cavity, stop feedings, and consult with speech-language pathologist and dysphagia team. *Placing a client with suspected dysphagia on nothing by mouth (NPO) status is the strongest measure that can be taken to prevent choking and aspiration (Tanner & Culbertson, 2014).*

▲ If signs of aspiration or pneumonia are present, auscultate lung sounds after feeding. Note new onset of crackles or wheezing, or elevated temperature. **CEB:** *Bronchial auscultation of lung sounds was shown to be specific in identifying clients at risk for aspiration (Shaw et al, 2004).*

▲ Assess for signs of malnutrition and dehydration and keep a record of food intake. **EB:** *A recent study showed that patients with diagnosed high-risk dysphagia had significantly lower scores on the geriatric nutritional risk index (Saito et al, 2017).*

▲ Evaluate nutritional status daily. Weigh the client weekly to help evaluate nutritional status. If the client is not adequately nourished, work with the dysphagia team to determine whether the client needs therapeutic feeding only or needs enteral feedings until the client can swallow adequately. **CEB:** *PEG feedings are preferable to nasogastric tube (NGT) feedings when longer term feeding is required (Geeganage et al, 2012).*

▲ *Assist client in following dysphagia specialist's recommendations and provide open, accurate, and effective communication with dysphagia team regarding client's diet tolerance. Understanding and following dysphagia specialist's recommendations is a pivotal role that nurses play in helping ensure positive dysphagia management outcomes (Tanner & Culbertson, 2014).*

▲ Document and notify the health care provider and dysphagia team of changes in medical, nutritional, or swallowing status. *Many negative dysphagia management outcomes can be avoided by ensuring dysphagia communication is accurate, complete, and disseminated among and between health care professionals; nurses are pivotal in this process (Tanner & Culbertson, 2014).*

▲ Work with the client on swallowing exercises prescribed by the dysphagia team. **EB:** *Exercise programs can improve airway closure, the range of oral or pharyngeal structure movement during swallow, cricopharyngeal opening, and tongue strength (Logemann & Larsen, 2012).*

▲ If needed, provide meals in a quiet environment away from excessive stimuli, such as a community dining room, for some clients who are easily distracted. *A noisy environment can be an aversive stimulus and can decrease effective chewing and swallowing.*

▲ For many adult clients, avoid the use of straws if recommended by the speech pathologist. *Use of straws can increase the risk of aspiration, because straws can result in spilling of a bolus of fluid rapidly in the posterior pharynx.*

• = Independent; ▲ = Collaborative; **EBN** = Evidence-Based Nursing; **EB** = Evidence-Based

▲ Recognize that the client can aspirate oral feedings, even if there are no symptoms of coughing or distress. This phenomenon is called silent aspiration and is common. **EB:** *In a study of elderly long-term residents, dementia was the best predictor of silent aspiration (Sakai et al, 2016).*

▲ Ensure oral hygiene is maintained. **EB:** *Oral health care including toothbrushing after each meal, cleaning dentures once a day, and consistent professional oral health care reduces the incidence of aspiration pneumonia (van der Maarel-Wierink et al, 2013).*

▲ Check the oral cavity for proper emptying after the client swallows and after the client finishes the meal. Provide oral care at the end of the meal. It may be necessary to manually remove food from the client's mouth. If this is the case, use gloves and keep the client's teeth apart with a padded tongue blade. *Food may become pocketed on the affected side and cause stomatitis, tooth decay, and possible later aspiration.*

▲ Praise the client for successfully following directions and swallowing appropriately. *Praise reinforces behavior and sets up a positive atmosphere in which learning takes place.*

▲ Keep the client in an upright position for 45 minutes to an hour after a meal. **CEB:** *Matsui et al (2002) found the number of older clients who developed a fever was significantly reduced when clients were kept sitting upright after eating.*

▲ Recognize that impaired swallowing may be caused by the medications the client is taking. Side effects of medications include xerostomia (antidepressants, anticholinergics, antihistamines, bronchodilators, antineoplastic, and anti-Parkinson), central nervous system depression (anticonvulsants, benzodiazepines, antispasmodics, antidepressants, and antipsychotics), myopathy (corticosteroids, lipid-lowering agents, and colchicines), and decreased esophageal sphincter tone (antihistamines, diuretics, opiates, antipsychotics, antihypertensives, and anticholinergics). *Medications can cause impaired swallowing in multiple ways.*

▲ For clients receiving mechanical ventilation with a tracheostomy tube or after postextubation, request a referral to a speech-language pathologist or dysphagia specialist for an instrumental swallowing evaluation before beginning oral diet. **EB:** *Objective swallowing studies and early intervention are the best ways to determine the safest oral intake and rule out silent aspiration in these clients (Rodrigues et al, 2015).*

Pediatric

▲ Refer a child who has difficulty swallowing and symptoms such as difficulty manipulating food, delayed swallow response, and pocketing of a bolus of food to a speech-language pathologist (or dysphagia specialist) and a dietitian. *Adequate nutrition is extremely important for children to ensure sufficient growth and development of all body systems.*

▲ Consult with a speech-language pathologist or dysphagia specialist regarding modifications to nipple, appropriate positioning and feeding strategies, and other therapeutic activities deemed most appropriate based on bedside and instrumental swallowing evaluation. *Speech-language pathologists are trained to evaluate and treat pediatric dysphagia. Consultation with a speech-language pathologist or feeding therapist with pediatric expertise improves the diagnostic utility of a feeding assessment and can result in better outcomes.*

▲ The following are general feeding guidelines. Specific strategies to eliminate aspiration and maximize intake should be individualized and determined by a swallowing specialist through bedside and instrumental swallowing evaluation.

• Attempt feedings when infant is in an optimal behavioral feeding state (e.g., awake, alert, not agitated) and halt feedings if infant is not able to maintain or regain a proper feeding state. *Infants' feeding state can fluctuate rapidly and caregiver's attention to this state can influence feedings (Lau, 2014).*

• In a preterm infant, provide opportunities for patterned nonnutritive sucking (NNS). **EB:** *Although adequate NNS is not sufficient to predict adequacy of oral feeding (Lau, 2014), providing skilled training in patterned NNS has been demonstrated to accelerate the transition from NNS to oral feeding (Lau et al, 2012).*

• In a preterm infant, alter nipple flow rate to one that is easily managed by infant to facilitate intake while achieving physiological stability. **CEB:** *Increased flow rate should only be considered when doing so assists the infant in obtaining adequate intake while maintaining physiological stability. Aspiration risk is increased with faster flow rates.*

• Watch for indicators of aspiration and physiological instability during feeding: coughing, a change in vocal quality or wet vocal quality, perspiration and color changes, sneezing, apnea, and/or increased heart rate and breathing. Infants and children with silent aspiration may only have indicators of increased respiratory mucous, congestion and chronic wheeze or rhonchi, recurrent bronchitis, or recurrent pneumonia (Tutor & Gosa, 2012).

• Watch for warning signs of reflux such as sour-smelling breath after eating, sneezing, lack of interest in feeding, crying and fussing extraordinarily when feeding, pained expressions when feeding, and

S

• = Independent;   ▲ = Collaborative;   **EBN** = Evidence-Based Nursing;   **EB** = Evidence-Based

excessive chewing and swallowing after eating. *Many premature and medically fragile children experience growth deficits and respiratory problems from an underlying dysphagia. Some infants may need to work harder to breathe than others and as a result develop a decreased tolerance for food intake. They also demonstrate inconsistent arousal and poor/uncoordinated suck-swallow-breath synchrony. Many of these infants require supplemental tube feedings and the use of special nipples or bottles to boost oral intake.*

- Observe infant's behavior and cues and adjust feeding to promote a safe pleasurable feeding experience while eliminating aspiration and maximizing intake. *Individualize interventions based on infant's cues related to swallowing, breathing, physiological stability, postural control, and state regulation to help infant maintain or regain stability. Some approaches include reducing noise/light levels, adjusting feeding position, letting infant regulate milk flow, and varying number and/or duration of feedings to reduce adverse events (Lau, 2014).*

Geriatric

▲ Recognize that age-related changes can affect swallowing and these changes have a more pronounced effect when superimposed on disease such as neurological and other chronic medical problems. *Subtle motor changes and age-related decrements in oral moisture, taste, and smell can contribute to less efficient and effective swallowing in older adults (Sura et al, 2012).*

▲ Evaluate medications the client is presently taking and consult with the pharmacist for assistance in monitoring for incorrect doses and drug interactions that could result in dysphagia. *Most older clients take numerous medications, which when taken individually can slow motor function, cause anxiety and depression, and reduce salivary flow. When taken together, these medications can interact, resulting in impaired swallowing function.*

▲ Ensure all nursing home residents are screened for swallowing problems. *It is estimated that up to 40% to 60% of nursing home residents have swallowing problems (Tanner, 2013).*

▲ Encourage and provide good oral hygiene when indicated. **EB:** *Good oral health care reduces the incidence of aspiration pneumonia (van der Maarel-Wierink et al, 2013).*

▲ Consult with occupational therapist for adaptive equipment when appropriate. *The use of adaptive equipment such as cups without rims and angled utensils can improve outcomes for older clients with dysphagia (Sura et al, 2012).*

▲ Recognize that the older client with dementia may need a longer time to eat and is often easily distracted. Help optimize hydration and nutrition using the following techniques:
  ○ Encourage six small meals and hydration breaks per day.
  ○ Offer foods that are sweet, spicy, or sour to increase sensory input.
  ○ Allow clients to touch food and self-feed, if necessary (Tanner, 2013).
  ○ Eliminate from the tray or table nonfoods such as salt and pepper, or anything that can be distracting. *Dementia clients are often impulsive and easily distracted.*
  ○ Keep desserts out of sight until the end of the meal.
  ○ Offer finger foods to the client who has trouble holding still to eat.
  ○ Allow clients to eat immediately when they come for the meal.
  ○ Recognize that the client with advanced dementia, who is unable to swallow, may or may not benefit from enteral tube feedings. *Some dementia clients enter into a catabolic state with negative protein balance, and it may be irreversible. In addition, there is often an increased risk for aspiration pneumonia in the tube-fed client.*

Home Care

▲ Refer to speech therapy. Speech-language pathologists can work with clients to enhance swallowing ability and teach compensatory strategies.

Client/Family Teaching and Discharge Planning

▲ Teach the client and family exercises prescribed by the dysphagia team.

▲ Teach the client a systematic method of swallowing effectively as prescribed by the dysphagia team.

- Educate the client, family, and all caregivers about rationales for food consistency and choices. *It is common for family members to disregard necessary dietary restrictions and give the client inappropriate foods that predispose to aspiration.*

- Teach the family how to monitor the client to prevent and detect aspiration during eating.

• = Independent; ▲ = Collaborative; **EBN** = Evidence-Based Nursing; **EB** = Evidence-Based

REFERENCES

Coleman, P. R. (2004). Pneumonia in the long-term care setting: Etiology, management, and prevention. *Journal of Gerontological Nursing, 30*(4), 14.

Geeganage, C., Beavan, J., Elender, S., et al. (2012). Interventions for dysphagia and nutritional support in acute and subacute stroke. *The Cochrane Database of Systematic Reviews,* (10), CD000323.

Gomes, F., et al. (2013). Royal College of Physicians Intercollegiate Stroke Working Party evidence-based guidelines for the nutritional support of patients who have had a stroke. *Journal of Human Nutrition and Dietetics, 27*(2), 107–121.

Hines, S., Kynoch, K., & Munday, J. (2016). Nursing interventions for identifying and managing acute dysphagia are effective for improving patient outcomes: A systematic review update. *Journal of Neuroscience Nursing, 48*(4), 215–223.

Lau, C., Fucille, S., & Gisel, E. G. (2012). Impact of nonnutritive oral motor stimulation and infant massage therapy on oral feeding skills of preterm infants. *Journal of Neonatal-Perinatal Medicine, 5,* 311–317.

Lau, C. (2014). Interventions to improve oral feeding performance of preterm infants. *SIG 13 Perspectives on Feeding and Swallowing (Dysphagia), 23,* 23–25.

Li, M., Wang, Z., Han, W.-J., et al. (2015). Effect of feeding management on aspiration pneumonia in elderly patients with dysphagia. *Chinese Nursing Research, 2,* 40–44. doi:10.1016/j.cnre.2015.09.004.

Logemann, J. A., & Larsen, K. (2012). Oropharyngeal dysphagia: Pathophysiology and diagnosis for the anniversary issue of diseases of the esophagus. *Diseases of the Esophagus, 25*(4), 299–304.

Matsui, T., Yamaya, M., Ohrui, T., et al. (2002). Sitting position to prevent aspiration in bed-bound patients. *Gerontology, 48*(3), 194.

Mauk, K. L. (2017). *Gerontological nursing: Competencies for care* (4th ed.). Burlington, MA: Jones and Bartlett Learning.

Rizzo, K., et al. (2016). Effects of bolus size on swallow safety: A systematic review of external evidence. *EBP Briefs, 11*(3), 1–12.

Rodrigues, K. A., et al. (2015). Swallowing rehabilitation of dysphagic tracheostomized patients under mechanical ventilation in intensive care units: A feasibility study. *Revista Brasiliera de Terapia Intensiva, 27*(1), 64–71. doi:10.5935/0103-507X.20150011.

Saito, T., et al. (2017). A significant association of malnutrition with dysphagia in acute patients. *Dysphagia.* doi:10.1007/s00455-017-9855-6.

Sakai, K., et al. (2016). An examination of factors related to aspiration and silent aspiration in older adults requiring long-term care in rural Japan. *Journal of Oral Rehabilitation, 43*(2), 103–110. doi:10.1111/joor.12349.

Shaw, J. L., et al. (2004). Bronchial auscultation: An effective adjunct to speech and language therapy bedside assessment when detecting dysphagia and aspiration? *Dysphagia, 19*(4), 211.

Sura, L., Madhavan, A., Carnaby, G., et al. (2012). Dysphagia in the elderly: Management and nutritional considerations. *Clinical Interventions in Aging, 7,* 287–298.

Teasell, R. W., et al. (2016). Dysphagia and aspiration following stroke. In *2015 Evidence-Based Review of Stroke Rehabilitation.* Retrieved from http://www.ebrsr.com. (Accessed 13 October 2016).

Tutor, J. D., & Gosa, M. M. (2012). Dysphagia and aspiration in children. *Pediatric Pulmonology, 47*(4), 321–337.

Tanner, D. (2013). CNA observations could save a resident: An interview. Nursing assistant. *Cengage Learning, 18*(8).

Tanner, D. C., & Culbertson, W. R. (2014). Avoiding negative dysphagia outcomes. *Online Journal of Issues in Nursing, 19*(2), 6.

van der Maarel-Wierink, C. D., Vanobbergen, J. N. O., Bronkhorst, E. M., et al. (2013). Oral healthcare and aspiration pneumonia in frail older people: A systematic literature review. *Gerodontology, 30*(1), 3–9.

Waito, A., Bailey, G. L., Molfenter, S. M., et al. (2011). Voice-quality abnormalities as a sign of dysphagia: Validation against acoustic and videofluoroscopic data. *Dysphagia, 26*(2), 125.

Risk for Thermal injury   *Wendie A. Howland, MN, RN-BC, CRRN, CCM, CNLCP, LNCC*

NANDA-I

T

Definition

Susceptible to extreme temperature damage to skin and mucous membranes, which may compromise health.

Risk Factors

Fatigue; inadequate protective clothing; inadequate supervision; inattentiveness; insufficient caregiver knowledge of safety precautions; insufficient knowledge of safety precautions; smoking; unsafe environment

At-Risk Population

Extremes of age; extremes of environmental temperature

Associated Condition

Alcohol intoxication; drug intoxication; alteration in cognitive functioning; neuromuscular impairment; neuropathy; treatment regimen

NOC   (Nursing Outcomes Classification)

Suggested NOC Outcomes

Safe Home Environment; Parenting: Early/Middle/Adolescent; Physical Safety

● = Independent;   ▲ = Collaborative;   EBN = Evidence-Based Nursing;   EB = Evidence-Based

Client Outcomes

Client Will (Specify Time Frame)

- Be free of thermal injury to skin or tissue
- Explain actions can take to protect self and others from thermal injury
- Explain actions can take to protect self and others in the work environment

NIC   (Nursing Interventions Classification)

Suggested NIC Intervention

Environmental Management: Safety

Example NIC Activities—Environmental Management: Safety
Identify safety hazards in the environment; Modify the environment to minimize hazards and risk

Nursing Interventions and *Rationales*

- Teach the following interventions to prevent fires in the home, to handle any possible fire, and to have a readily available exit from the home:
  - Avoid plugging several appliance cords into the same electrical socket.
  - Do not use open candles or allow smoking in the home.
  - Keep a fire extinguisher within reach in case a fire should occur.
  - Install smoke alarms on every level of the home and in every sleeping area.
  - Keep furniture and other heavy objects out of the way of doors and windows.
  - Develop a fire escape plan that includes two ways out of every room and an outside meeting place. Practice the escape plan at least twice a year.
- Teach clients about home grill safety to prevent thermal injury (propane and charcoal grills). EB: *The National Fire Protection Association (NFPA) suggested that grills should be inspected annually, especially when not used frequently; complete the "soapy bubble" test with propane grills to look for leaks that may result in fires; keep children and pets at a safe distance from the grill; and only grill outdoors (NFPA, 2016).*
- Apply sunscreen as directed on the container when out in the sun. Also use sun-blocking clothing, and stay in the shade if possible. EB: *Sunburn is a clear indicator of overexposure to ultraviolet (UV) radiation and increases the risk of skin cancer. The estimated prevalence of sunburn in the United States is high; 37.1% of adults and 55.8% of youth reported one or more sunburns in the past 12 months. Emergency room costs for sunburn nationally are considerable (Guy, Berkowitz, & Watson, 2017).*
- Teach clients safety measures to prevent fires in the home in which medical oxygen is in use:
  - **Never smoke** in a home in which medical oxygen is in use. "No smoking" signs should be posted inside and outside the home. EB: *There is considerable morbidity and mortality from burns secondary to smoking while using home oxygen. Ongoing education and careful consideration of prescribing home oxygen therapy for known smokers is highly encouraged (Carlos et al, 2016).*
  - Do not wear oxygen near an ignition source (e.g., open flame, gas stove, fireplace, candles, cigarettes, matches, lighters). Note that petroleum jelly, lip balm, skin lotion, or the like will not spontaneously combust in the presence of supplemental oxygen without an ignition source (e.g., flame or spark) and are safe to use on the face and in bed in the presence of oxygen (Winslow & Jacobsen, 1998; Hadjiliadis, 2016).
  - Homes with medical oxygen must have working smoke alarms that are tested monthly.
  - Test fire extinguishers every 3 to 6 months. Keep a fire extinguisher within reach. If a fire occurs, turn off the oxygen, leave the home, and summon the fire department.
  - Develop a fire escape plan that includes two ways out of every room and an outside meeting place. Practice the escape plan at least twice a year.
- Be aware that thermal injury also includes injury from cold materials and environmental conditions, including freezing injury, nonfreezing injury, and hypothermia. *Frostbite is classified in the same way as burns and can inflict similar damage on tissue (Handford, Thomas, & Imray, 2016; Fabian, Taljaard, & Perry, 2017).*
- Provide adequate environmental temperatures. Older clients and others at risk for temperature dysregulation can easily become hypothermic in air-conditioned environments (e.g., a surgical suite), with inadequate

● = Independent;   ▲ = Collaborative;   EBN = Evidence-Based Nursing;   EB = Evidence-Based

clothing, inhaling cold gases, or when exposed to room temperature or chilled fluids (e.g., intravenous, gastric lavage, bowel prep, continuous renal replacement therapy (CRRT), dialysis). *Inadvertent hypothermia is common in surgical procedures, affecting 70% of surgical patients, and can predispose to infection, blood loss, pressure injury, cardiac events, and shivering that increases metabolic demands (Giuliano & Hendricks, 2017).*

- Monitor temperature in vulnerable clients. Core temperature is the best measure to assess for hypothermia. If a pulmonary artery catheter is not available, use a thermometer calibrated for lower body temperature such as a distal esophageal probe or rectal or bladder temperature probe (Leon & Bouchama, 2015).
- Use active warming measures to help clients maintain body temperature (e.g., warming blankets, warmed fluids, forced warm air warming devices, foil wraps, radiant warmers) as indicated. Be aware that passive devices (e.g., socks or blankets) do not add heat to body tissues.
- Ensure that exposed skin is protected from cold with adequate clothing.
- Monitor for developing cold thermal injury by checking peripheral circulation, temperature, and sensation. Be aware that fine motor coordination decreases as a very early sign of hypothermia. *Preventing progression of thermal injury is critical to client outcomes. Shivering is the body's attempt to generate heat through muscle activity; it consumes considerable metabolic energy, and is a late sign of hypothermia.*
- Check the temperature of all equipment and other materials before allowing them to contact client skin, especially if client has increased risk factors for thermal injury.

 Pediatric

- Teach the following activities to homes with small children:
  - Lock up matches and lighters out of sight and reach.
  - Never leave a hot stove unattended.
  - Do not allow small children to use the microwave until they are at least 7 or 8 years of age.
  - Keep all portable heaters out of children's reach and at least 3 feet away from anything that can burn.
  - Teach fire prevention and safety to older children.
- Install thermostatic mixer valves in a hot water system to prevent extreme hot water causing scalding burns. **EB:** *Scald injuries in children can be decreased by parental education on risk factors (Stewart et al, 2016). Risk factors for residential fire death are common in urban pediatric emergency department patients (Wood et al, 2016). The majority of pediatric burn injuries are scald burns that occur at home and primarily affect the lower extremities in Caucasian and African American males. Among Caucasian teenagers flame burns predominate. The results of this study highlight the need for primary prevention programs focusing on avoiding home scald injuries in the very young and fire safety training for teenagers (Lee et al, 2016).*

REFERENCES

Carlos, W. G., Baker, M. S., McPherson, K. A., et al. (2016). Smoking-related home oxygen burn injuries: Continued cause for alarm. *Respiration; International Review of Thoracic Diseases, 91,* 151–155.

Fabian, J. C., Taljaard, M., & Perry, J. (2017). A retrospective cohort study examining treatments and operative interventions for frostbite in a tertiary care hospital. *Canadian Journal of Emergency Medicine, 19*(2), 88–95.

Giuliano, K., & Hendricks, J. (2017). Inadvertent perioperative hypothermia: Current nursing knowledge. *AORN, 105*(5), 453–463.

Guy, G. P., Berkowitz, Z., & Watson, M. (2017). Estimated cost of sunburn-associated visits to us hospital emergency departments. *JAMA Dermatol, 153*(1), 90–92.

Handford, C., Thomas, O., & Imray, C. (2016). Frostbite. *Emergency Medicine Clinics, 35*(2), 281–299.

Hadjiliadis, D. (2016). *Oxygen safety. MedlinePlus.* Retrieved from https://medlineplus.gov/ency/patientinstructions/000049.htm. (Accessed 30 January 2018).

Lee, C. J., Mahendraraj, K., et al. (2016). Pediatric burns: A single institution retrospective review of incidence, etiology, and outcomes in 2273 burn patients (1995–2013). *Journal of Burn Care & Research, 37*(6), e579–e585.

Leon, L. R., & Bouchama, A. (2015). Heat stroke. *Comprehensive Physiology, 5,* 611–647. doi:10.1002/cphy.c140017.

National Fire Protection Association. (2016). *Grilling safety.* Retrieved from https://www.nfpa.org/-/media/Files/Public-Education/Resources/Safety-tip-sheets/Grilling_safety_Tips.pdf. (Accessed 30 January 2018).

Stewart, J., Benford, P., et al. (2016). Modifiable risk factors for scald injury in children under 5 years of age: A multi-centre case-control study. *Burns: Journal of the International Society for Burn Injuries, 42*(8), 1831–1843.

Winslow, E. H., & Jacobson, A. F. (1998). Dispelling the petroleum jelly myth. *American Journal of Nursing, 98*(11), 16.

Wood, R., Teach, S., et al. (2016). Home fire safety practices and smoke detector program awareness in an urban pediatric emergency department population. *Pediatric Emergency Care, 32*(11), 763–767.

T

● = Independent;   ▲ = Collaborative;   **EBN** = Evidence-Based Nursing;   **EB** = Evidence-Based

Ineffective Thermoregulation   *Rosemary Timmerman, DNP, APRN, CCNS, CCRN-CSC-CMC*

NANDA-I

Definition

Temperature fluctuation between hypothermia and hyperthermia.

Defining Characteristics

Cyanotic nail beds; flushed skin; hypertension; increase in body temperature above normal range; increase in respiratory rate; mild shivering; moderate pallor; piloerection; reduction in body temperature below normal range; seizure; skin cool to touch; skin warm to touch; slow capillary refill; tachycardia

Related Factors

Dehydration; fluctuating environmental temperature; inactivity; inappropriate clothing for environmental temperature; increase in oxygen demand; vigorous activity

At-Risk Population

Extremes of age; extremes of weight; extremes of environmental temperature; increased body surface area to weight ration; insufficient supply of subcutaneous fat

Associated Condition

Alteration in metabolic rate; brain injury; condition affecting temperature regulation; decrease in sweat response; illness; inefficient nonshivering thermogenesis; pharmaceutical agent; sedation; sepsis; trauma

NOC   (Nursing Outcomes Classification)

Suggested NOC Outcomes

Thermoregulation; Thermoregulation: Newborn

Example NOC Outcome with Indicators
Thermoregulation as evidenced by the following indicators: Body temperature/Skin temperature/Skin color changes/ Hydration/Reported thermal comfort. (Rate the outcome and indicators of **Thermoregulation:** 1 = severely compromised, 2 = substantially compromised, 3 = moderately compromised, 4 = mildly compromised, 5 = not compromised [see Section I].)

Client Outcomes

Client Will (Specify Time Frame)

- Maintain temperature within normal range
- Explain measures needed to maintain normal temperature
- Describe two to four symptoms of hypothermia or hyperthermia
- List two or three self-care measures to treat hypothermia or hyperthermia

NIC   (Nursing Interventions Classification)

Suggested NIC Interventions

Temperature Regulation; Temperature Regulation: Inoperative

Example NIC Activities—Temperature Regulation
Institute use of a continuous core temperature-monitoring device, as appropriate; Promote adequate fluid and nutritional intake

Nursing Interventions and *Rationales*

Temperature Measurement

- Measure and record the client's temperature using a consistent method of temperature measurement every 1 to 4 hours depending on the severity of the situation or whenever a change in condition occurs (e.g.,

● = Independent;   ▲ = Collaborative;   EBN = Evidence-Based Nursing;   EB = Evidence-Based

T

chills, change in mental status). **CEB:** *Errors in accurate temperature measurement are most often associated with instrument-related errors, choice of temperature site chosen for monitoring, and operator error (Makic et al, 2011).* **CEB/EBN:** *A consistent mode of temperature measurement for accurate trending of body temperature is important for accurate treatment decisions; if different devices are used to obtain temperature measurements, the results should not vary more than 0.3°C to 0.5°C (Makic et al, 2011; Munro, 2014).*

- Select core, near core, or peripheral temperature monitoring mode based on ability to obtain an accurate temperature from that site and clinical situation dictating the need for mode of temperature monitoring required for clinical treatment decisions. **CEB/EB:** *Core temperature is obtained by pulmonary artery catheter and distal esophagus; near core temperature measurements include oral, bladder, rectal, tympanic membrane, and temporal artery; and peripheral measurements are obtained by skin surface measurements such as measurement in the axilla (Munro, 2014; Niven et al, 2015).*
- Caution should be taken in interpreting extreme values of temperature (less than 35°C or greater than 39°C) from a near core temperature site device. **CEB/EBN:** *Accurate oral temperature measurement requires the probe to be placed in the posterior sublingual pocket to provide a reliable near core temperature measurement (Makic et al, 2011; El-Radhi, 2013).* **EBP:** *Research has demonstrated that the accuracy of temperature measurement from most accurate to least accurate are intravascular (pulmonary artery), distal esophageal, bladder thermistor, rectal, and oral (Niven & Laupland, 2016); axillary temperature is accurate in neonates but is not well supported in adults (Smith, Alcock, & Usher, 2013).* **EB/EBN:** *Tympanic membrane and temporal artery measurements and chemical dot thermometers are least accurate and should be avoided in caring for the acutely ill adult client. Evidence is limited in testing the accuracy of temperature measurement devices outside of normal temperature ranges (Bijur, Shah, & Esses, 2016; Kiekkas et al, 2016).*
- Evaluate the significance of a decreased or increased temperature. *Normal adult temperature is usually identified as 98.6°F (37°C), but in actuality the normal temperature fluctuates throughout the day; in the early morning it may be as low as 96.4°F (35.8°C) and in the late afternoon or evening as high as 99.1°F (37.3°C); disease, injury, or pharmacological agents may cause an adaptive increase in the hypothalamic set point resulting in fever (Hooper et al, 2010; Niven & Laupland, 2016).*
- ▲ Notify the health care provider of temperature according to institutional standards or written orders, or when temperature reaches 100.5°F (38.3°C) and above; use a lower threshold for immunocompromised clients who will be less likely to exhibit a fever when seriously ill (Niven & Laupland, 2016). Also notify the health care provider of the presence of a change in mental status and temperature greater than 100.5°F (38.3°C) or less than 96.8°F (36°C). *A change in mental status may indicate the onset of septic shock (Rhodes et al, 2017).*

Fever (Pyrexia)

- Recognize that fever is characterized as a temporary elevation in internal body temperature 1°C to 2°C higher than the client's normal body temperature. *A rise in body temperature is an innate immune response to a perceived threat and is regulated by the hypothalamus. Hyperthermia may occur when a client gains heat through either an increase in the body's heat production or is unable to effectively dissipate heat, and hypothermia occurs when a client loses heat or cannot generate heat (Rehman & deBoisblanc, 2014; Leon & Bouchama, 2015).*
- Recognize that fever is a normal physiological response to a perceived threat by the body, frequently in response to an infection. **EB:** *Fever is a deliberate, active thermoregulatory defense action by the body; metabolic heat accelerates the body's antibody production to defend the body and assists the body's cellular repair processes (nursing care should focus on supporting the body's normal physiological response [fever], locating the cause for the fever, and providing comfort) (Munro, 2014; Rehman & deBoisblanc, 2014).*
- ▲ Review client history to include current medical diagnosis, medications, recent procedures/interventions, recent travel, environmental exposure to infectious agents, recent blood product administration, and review of laboratory analysis for cause of ineffective thermoregulation. **EB:** *Changes in body temperature (fever) should be explored for possible problems associated with a client's health status (Munro, 2014; Rehman & deBoisblanc, 2014).*
- Recognize that fever may be low grade (96.8°F–100.4°F [36°C–38°C]) in response to an inflammatory process such as infection, allergy, trauma, illness, or surgery; moderate to high-grade fever (100.4°F–104°F [38°C–40°C]) indicates a more concerted inflammatory response from a systemic infection; hyperpyrexia (40°C and higher) occurs as a result of damage of the hypothalamus, bacteremia, or an extremely overheated room (Munro, 2014; Niven & Laupland, 2016). **EB:** *Interventions to treat fever focus on client comfort, allowing*

● = Independent;   ▲ = Collaborative;   **EBN** = Evidence-Based Nursing;   **EB** = Evidence-Based

the body to progress through the natural course of fever; exceptions may exist for the client with hyperpyrexia or when oxygen consumption threatens to exhaust metabolic reserves (Munro, 2014; Rehman & deBoisblanc, 2014).

- Recognize that fever has a predictable physiological pattern; *the initial phase (cold or chill stage) presents with an increased heart rate, respiratory rate, shivering, pale, cold skin, absence of sweat, and piloerection. As the hypothalamus adjusts, the body temperature shivering ceases, skin becomes warm, and heart rate and respiratory rate remain elevated. The client may complain of thirst, poor appetite, painful muscles, exhaustion, and lethargy. The resolution phase presents with warm, flushed, sweaty skin, reduced shivering, and possible signs of dehydration (Adam, 2013; Rehman & deBoisblanc, 2014).*
- Monitor and intervene to provide comfort during a fever by:
  - Obtaining vital signs and accurate intake and output
  - Checking laboratory analysis trends of white blood cell counts and other markers of infection
  - Providing blankets when the client complains of being cold, but removing surplus of blankets when the client is too warm
  - Encouraging fluid and nutrition
  - Limiting activity to conserve energy
  - Providing frequent oral care
  - Adjust room temperature for client comfort
- ▲ **EBN/EB:** *Current evidence that examined the evidence of antipyretic therapies used to treat fever, such as administration of antipyretic medications, cooling blankets, and sponge baths, found these therapies did not reduce the duration of illness and may even prolong it (Munro, 2014; Niven et al, 2013).*

Hypothermia

- Take vital signs frequently, noting changes associated with hypothermia, such as increased blood pressure, pulse, and respirations, that then advance to decreased values as hypothermia progresses. *Mild hypothermia activates the sympathetic nervous system, which can increase the levels of vital signs; as hypothermia progresses, the heart becomes suppressed, with decreased cardiac output, heart rate, blood pressure, and respiratory rate (Paal et al, 2016; Zafren, 2017).*
- Monitor the client for signs of hypothermia (e.g., shivering, cool skin, piloerection, pallor, slow capillary refill, cyanotic nailbeds, decreased mentation, dysrhythmias) (Paal et al, 2016; Zafren, 2017).
- See the care plan for **Hypothermia** as appropriate.

Hyperthermia

- Recognize that hyperthermia is a different etiology than fever so the cause of the elevated body temperature should be explored for definitive treatment. *Hyperthermia is a condition in which an environmental (e.g., heat stroke), pharmacological (malignant hyperthermia), or endocrine (e.g., thyrotoxicosis) stimulus results in an increase in body temperature without a corresponding increase in the hypothalamic set point (Leon & Bouchama, 2015; Niven & Laupland, 2016).*
- Note changes in vital signs associated with hyperthermia, such as rapid, bounding pulse; increased respiratory rate; and decreased blood pressure, accompanied by orthostatic hypotension; and signs and symptoms of dehydration (Gaudio & Grissom, 2016; Niven & Laupland, 2016). *Consistent monitoring promotes prevention and early intervention in clients with altered cardiopulmonary status associated with hyperthermia (Gaudio & Grissom, 2016; Rehman & deBoisblanc, 2014).*
- Monitor the client for signs of hyperthermia (e.g., headache, nausea and vomiting, weakness, extreme fatigue, delirium, coma). *Monitoring for the defining characteristics of hyperthermia allows for early intervention.*
- Adjust clothing to facilitate passive warming or cooling as appropriate.
- See the care plan for **Hyperthermia** as appropriate.

 Pediatric

- For routine measurement of temperature, use an electronic thermometer in the axilla in infants younger than 4 weeks; for a child up to 5 years of age, use an electronic thermometer in the axilla or an infrared temporal artery thermometer. **EB:** *Oral and rectal routes should not be used routinely to measure the temperature of infants to children of 5 years of age (National Institute for Health and Clinical Excellence [NICE], 2017). Tympanic thermometers often provide inaccurate temperature from incorrect placement in the ear canal and presence of cerumen adversely affecting temperature reading; fever strips and pacifier thermometers often provide inaccurate readings (Adam, 2013; Zhen et al, 2014).*

● = Independent;   ▲ = Collaborative;   EBN = Evidence-Based Nursing;   EB = Evidence-Based

- Recognize that pediatric clients have a decreased ability to adapt to temperature extremes. Take the following actions to maintain body temperature in the infant/child:
  - ❍ Keep the head covered.
  - ❍ Use blankets to keep the client warm.
  - ❍ Keep the client covered during procedures, transport, and diagnostic testing.
  - ❍ Keep the room temperature at 72°F (22.2°C).

The combination of a relatively smaller body surface area, smaller body fluid volume, less well-developed temperature control mechanisms, and smaller amount of protective body fat limits the ability of the infant and child to maintain normal temperatures (NICE, 2017).

- Recognize that the infant and small child are both vulnerable to develop heat stroke in hot weather; ensure that they receive sufficient fluids and are protected from hot environments. *Infants and young children are at risk for heat stroke for many reasons, including a decreased thermoregulatory ability in the young body and the inability to obtain their own fluids (Leon & Bouchama, 2015).*
- Antipyretic treatments typically are not indicated unless the child's temperature is higher than 38.3°C and may be given to provide comfort. EB: *The use of antipyretics in febrile children should be examined in light of the therapeutic goal for treatment, which may be primarily to improve the child's discomfort; acetaminophen and ibuprofen are the only antipyretic medications recommended for pediatric clients; both agents should not be administered simultaneously because of concern for inaccurate dosing; alternating doses may be considered only if client distress is not relieved before the next dose is due (Chiappini et al, 2017; NICE, 2017).*

 Geriatric

- Do not allow an older client to become chilled; keep the client covered when giving a bath and offer socks to wear in bed; be aware of factors such as room temperature (heating/air conditioning), clothing (layered/loose), and fluid intake. *Older adults have a decreased ability to adapt to temperature extremes and need protection from extreme environmental temperatures; the response to cold environment is also compromised with the cutaneous vasoconstrictor response, the shivering process being less effective, decreased ability to feel cold, and medications commonly used to treat chronic age-associated diseases (Leon & Bouchama, 2015).*
- Recognize that the older client may have an infection without a significant rise in body temperature. EB: *Febrile response to infection was found to be reduced with increasing age, and baseline temperatures were generally lower in older clients; therefore this blunted febrile response may lead to delayed diagnosis and treatment necessitating review of all data to include a change in temperature, rather than fever (Munro, 2014; Rehman & deBoisblanc, 2014).*
- Fever does not put the older adult at risk for long-term complications; thus fever should not be treated with antipyretic agents or other external methods of cooling, unless there is serious heart disease present. CEB: *Exceptions in treating fever should be considered in some older clients with significant cardiovascular disease, because fever may increase metabolic rate by 10% and shivering may double the metabolic rate, greatly increasing the oxygen consumption requirements of the body and creating significant stress on the cardiovascular system (Outzen, 2009).*
- Ensure that older clients receive sufficient fluids during hot days and stay out of the sun. *Older adults may have trouble walking independently to obtain fluids, have decreased thirst sensation, and have chronic illnesses that predispose them to heat stroke, which is a hyperthermic condition (Leon & Bouchama, 2015).*
- Assess the medication profile for the potential risk of drug-related altered body temperature. *Anesthetics, barbiturates, salicylates, nonsteroidal antiinflammatory drugs, diuretics, antihistamines, anticholinergics, beta-blockers, and thyroid hormones have been linked to decreased body temperature (American Geriatrics Society, 2015; Beers Criteria Update Expert Panel, 2015).*

 Home Care

Treating Fever

- Instruct client/parents on the physiological benefits of fever and provide interventions to treat fever symptoms, avoiding antipyretic agents and external cooling interventions.
- Ensure that client/parents know when to contact a health care provider for fever-related concerns.

Prevention of Hypothermia in Cold Weather

See the care plan **Hypothermia.**

• = Independent; ▲ = Collaborative; EBN = Evidence-Based Nursing; EB = Evidence-Based

Prevention of Hyperthermia in Hot Weather

See the care plan **Hyperthermia.**

 Client/Family Teaching and Discharge Planning

- Teach the client and family the signs of fever, hypothermia, and hyperthermia and appropriate actions to take if either condition develops.
- Teach the client and family an age-appropriate method for taking the temperature.
- Teach the client to avoid alcohol and medications that depress cerebral function. *When the client is sedated or under the influence of alcohol, mentation is depressed, which results in decreased activities to maintain an adequate body temperature.*

REFERENCES

Adam, H. M. (2013). Fever: Measuring and managing. *Pediatrics in Review, 34*, 368–370. doi:10.1542/pir.34-8-368.

American Geriatrics Society 2015 Beers Criteria Update Expert Panel. (2015). American Geriatrics Society 2015 updated Beers criteria for potentially inappropriate medication use in older adults. *Journal of the American Geriatrics Society, 63*, 2227–2246. doi:10.1111/jgs.13702.

Bijur, P. E., Shah, P. D., & Esses, D. (2016). Temperature measurement in the adult emergency department: Oral tympanic membrane and temporal artery temperatures versus rectal temperature. *Emergency Medicine Journal, 33*, 843–847. doi:10.1136/emermed-2015-205122.

Chiappini, E., Venturini, E., Remaschi, G., et al. (2017). 2016 Update of the Italian Pediatric Society guidelines for management of fever in children. *The Journal of Pediatrics, 180*, 177–183. doi:10.1016/j.jpeds.2016.09.043.

El-Radhi, A. S. (2013). Temperature measurement: The right thermometer and site. *British Journal of Nursing, 22*(4), 208–210.

Gaudio, F. G., & Grissom, C. K. (2016). Cooling methods in heat stroke. *The Journal of Emergency Medicine, 50*, 607–616. doi:10.1016/j.jemermed.2015.09.014.

Hooper, V. D., Chard, R., Clifford, T., et al. (2010). ASPAN's evidence-based linical practice guideline for the promotion of perioperative normothermia: Second edition. *Journal of Perianesthesia Nursing, 25*, 346–365. doi:10.1016/j.jopan.2010.10.006.

Kiekkas, P., Stefanopoulos, N., Bakalis, N., et al. (2016). Agreement of infrared temporal artery thermometry with other thermometry methods in adults: A systematic review. *Journal of Clinical Nursing, 25*, 894–905. doi:10.1111/jocn.13117.

Leon, L. R., & Bouchama, A. (2015). Heat stroke. *Comprehensive Physiology, 5*, 611–647. doi:10.1002/cphy.c140017.

Makic, M. B. F., et al. (2011). Evidence-based practice habits: Putting more sacred cows out to pasture. *Critical Care Nurse, 31*, 38–62. doi:10.4037/ccn2011908.

Munro, N. (2014). Fever in acute and critical care: A diagnostic approach. *AACN Advanced Critical Care, 25*, 237–248. doi:10.1097/NCI.0000000000000041.

National Institute for Health and Clinical Excellence (NICE). (2017). *Fever in under 5s: Assessment and initial management*. Retrieved from https://www.nice.org.uk/guidance/cg160.

Niven, D. J., Gaudet, J. E., Laupland, K. B., et al. (2015). Accuracy of peripheral thermometers for estimating temperature: A systematic review and meta-analysis. *Annals of Internal Medicine, 163*, 768–777. doi:10.7326/M15-1150.

Niven, D. J., & Laupland, K. B. (2016). Pyrexia: Aetiology in the ICU. *Critical Care, 20*, 247. doi:10.1186/s13054-016-1406-2.

Niven, D. J., Stelfox, H. T., & Laupland, K. B. (2013). Antipyretic therapy in febrile critically ill adults: A systematic review and meta-analysis. *Journal of Critical Care, 28*, 303–310. doi:10.1016/j.jcrc.2012.09.009.

Outzen, M. (2009). Management of fever in older adults. *Journal of Gerontological Nursing, 35*(5), 17–23.

Paal, P., Gordon, L., Strapazzon, G., et al. (2016). Accidental hypothermia—An update. *Scandinavian Journal of Trauma, Resuscitation and Emergency Medicine, 24*, 111. doi:10.1186/s13049-016-0303-7.

Rehman, T., & deBoisblanc, B. P. (2014). Persistent fever in the ICU. *Chest, 145*(1), 158–165. doi:10.1378/chest.12-2843.

Rhodes, A., Evans, L., Alhazzani, W., et al. (2017). Surviving sepsis campaign: International guidelines for management of sepsis and septic shock: 2016. *Critical Care Medicine, 45*, 486–552. doi:10.1097/CCM.0000000000002255.

Smith, J., Alcock, G., & Usher, K. (2013). Temperature measurement in the preterm and term neonate: A review of the literature. *Neonatal Network, 32*(1), 16–25. doi:10.1891/0730-0832.32.1.16.

Zafren, K. (2017). Out-of-hospital evaluation and treatment of accidental hypothermia. *Emergency Medicine Clinics of North America, 35*, 261–279. doi:10.1016/j.emc.2017.01.003.

Zhen, C., Xia, Z., Long, L., et al. (2014). Accuracy of infrared ear thermometry in children: A meta-analysis and systematic review. *Clinical Pediatrics, 53*, 1158–1165. doi:10.1177/0009922814536774.

T

Risk for ineffective Thermoregulation   *Mary Beth Flynn Makic, PhD, RN, CCNS, FAAN, FNAP*

NANDA-I

Definition

Susceptible to temperature fluctuation between hypothermia and hyperthermia, which may compromise health.

● = Independent;   ▲ = Collaborative;   **EBN** = Evidence-Based Nursing;   **EB** = Evidence-Based

Risk Factors

Dehydration; fluctuating environmental temperature; inactivity; inappropriate clothing for environmental temperature; increase in oxygen demand; vigorous activity

At-Risk Population

Extremes of age; extremes of weight; extremes of environmental temperature; increase body surface area to weight ration; insufficient supply of subcutaneous fat

Associated Condition

Alteration in metabolic rate; brain injury; condition affecting temperature regulation; decrease in sweat response; illness; inefficient nonshivering thermogenesis; pharmaceutical agent; sedation; sepsis; trauma

NOC, NIC, Client Outcomes, Nursing Interventions and *Rationales,* Client/Family Teaching and Discharge Planning, and References

Refer to care plans for Ineffective **Thermoregulation** (fever), **Hyperthermia,** or **Hypothermia.**

Impaired Tissue integrity   *Jo Ann Coar, BSN, RN-BC, CWOCN, COS-C*

NANDA-I

Definition

Damage to the mucous membrane, cornea, integumentary system, muscular fascia, muscle, tendon, bone, cartilage, joint capsule, and/or ligament.

Defining Characteristics

Acute pain, bleeding, destroyed tissue, hematoma, localized area hot to touch, redness, tissue damage

Related Factors

Chemical injury agent, excessive fluid volume, humidity, imbalanced nutritional state, insufficient fluid volume, insufficient knowledge about maintaining tissue integrity, insufficient knowledge about protecting tissue integrity

At-Risk Population

Extremes of age, extremes of environmental temperature, exposure to high-voltage power supply

Associated Condition

Alteration in metabolism; alteration in sensation; arterial puncture; impaired circulation; impaired mobility; peripheral neuropathy; pharmaceutical agent; radiation therapy; surgical procedure; vascular trauma

NOC   (Nursing Outcomes Classification)

Suggested NOC Outcomes

Tissue Integrity: Skin and Mucous Membranes; Wound Healing: Primary Intention, Secondary Intention

Example NOC Outcome with Indicators
Intact **Tissue Integrity: Skin and Mucous Membranes** as evidenced by the following indicators: Skin intactness/ Skin lesions absent/Tissue perfusion/Skin temperature. (Rate the outcome and indicators of **Tissue Integrity: Skin and Mucous Membranes:** 1 = severely compromised, 2 = substantially compromised, 3 = moderately compromised, 4 = mildly compromised, 5 = not compromised [see Section I].)

● = Independent;   ▲ = Collaborative;   EBN = Evidence-Based Nursing;   EB = Evidence-Based

Client Outcomes

Client Will (Specify Time Frame)

- Report any altered sensation or pain at site of tissue impairment
- Demonstrate understanding of plan to heal tissue and prevent reinjury
- Describe measures to protect and heal the tissue, including wound care
- Experience a wound that decreases in size and has increased granulation tissue

NIC   (Nursing Interventions Classification)

Suggested NIC Interventions

Incision Site Care; Pain Management; Pressure Ulcer Care; Risk Identification; Skin Care: Topical Treatments; Skin Surveillance; Wound Care; Wound Irrigation

Example NIC Activities—Pressure Ulcer Care
Monitor color of wound bed, temperature, edema, erythema, moisture, and appearance of surrounding skin; Note characteristics of any drainage

Nursing Interventions and *Rationales*

- The National Pressure Ulcer Advisory Panel (NPUAP) redefined the definition of a pressure ulcer, which is now referred to as a pressure injury, during the NPUAP 2016 Staging Consensus Conference. The new definitions more accurately define alterations in tissue integrity from pressure as follows: A pressure injury is localized damage to the skin and underlying soft tissue usually over a bony prominence or related to a medical device or other device. The injury can present as intact skin or an open ulcer and may be painful. The injury occurs as a result of intense and/or prolonged pressure or pressure in combination with shear. The tolerance of soft tissue for pressure and shear may also be affected by microclimate, nutrition, perfusion, comorbidities, and condition of the soft tissue (NPUAP/European Pressure Ulcer Advisory Panel [EPUAP], 2016).
- The first step is to identify etiological factors or what is causing the impairment. A thorough assessment of the individual, not only the impairment, is crucial. This includes a comprehensive medical history, current medical status, medications, and family history (Murphree, 2017). Differentiate pressure injuries form other types of wounds such as moisture-associated skin damage (MASD) (Ratliff et al, 2017). A comprehensive assessment helps identify specific risk factors and systemic factors, which aids the clinician in a more successful wound management approach (Murphree, 2017).
- Determine the size (length, width) and depth of the wound. Select a uniform, consistent method for measuring wound length, width or wound area, and depth to facilitate meaningful comparisons of wound measurements over time. A careful assessment should be performed to avoid causing injury when probing the depth of a wound bed or determining the extent of undermining or tunneling (NPUAP/EPUAP, 2014).
- ▲ Classify pressure injuries (NPUAP, 2016) using national guidelines and definitions (see http://www.npuap.org/resources/educational-and-clinical-resources/npuap-pressure-injury-stages/).
  - ○ **Pressure Injury:**
    A pressure injury is localized damage to the skin and underlying soft tissue usually over a bony prominence or related to a medical or other device. The injury can present as intact skin or an open ulcer and may be painful. The injury occurs as a result of intense and/or prolonged pressure or pressure in combination with shear. The tolerance of soft tissue for pressure and shear may also be affected by microclimate, nutrition, perfusion, comorbidities, and condition of the soft tissue (NPUAP, 2016).
  - ○ **Stage 1 Pressure Injury:** Nonblanchable erythema of intact skin
    Area of localized nonblanchable erythema that may appear differently in darkly pigmented skin, and changes in sensation, temperature, or firmness may precede visual changes. Color changes do not include purple or maroon discoloration, which is more likely to indicate deep tissue pressure injury (NPUAP, 2016).
  - ○ **Stage 2 Pressure Injury:** Partial-thickness skin loss with exposed dermis
    Partial-thickness skin loss with exposed dermis in which the wound bed is pink/red and moist and adipose (fat) and deeper tissues are not visible. Granulation tissue, slough, and eschar are not present.

● = Independent;   ▲ = Collaborative;   EBN = Evidence-Based Nursing;   EB = Evidence-Based

A stage 2 pressure injury may also present as an intact or ruptured blister. These injuries commonly result from adverse microclimate and shear in the skin over the pelvis and shear in the heel. This stage should not be used to describe MASD including incontinence-associated dermatitis (IAD), intertriginous dermatitis (ITD), medical adhesive–related skin injury (MARSI), or traumatic wounds (skin tears, burns, and abrasions) (NPUAP, 2016).

○ **Stage 3 Pressure Injury:** Full-thickness skin loss
Full-thickness loss of skin, in which adipose is visible and granulation tissue and epibole (rolled wound edges) are often present, and undermining/tunneling may occur. Slough and/or eschar may also be visible. Fascia, muscle, tendon, ligament, cartilage, and/or bone are not exposed. The depth of tissue damage varies by anatomical location, and areas of significant adiposity can develop deep wounds. If slough or eschar obscures the extent of tissue loss this is an unstageable pressure injury (NPUAP. 2016).

○ **Stage 4 Pressure Injury:** Full-thickness skin and tissue loss
Full-thickness skin and tissue loss with exposed or directly palpable fascia, muscle, tendon, ligament, cartilage, or bone and slough and/or eschar may be visible. Epibole, undermining, and/or tunneling often occur and depth varies by anatomical location. If slough or eschar obscures the extent of tissue loss, this is an unstageable pressure injury (NPUAP, 2016).

○ **Deep Tissue Pressure Injury:** Persistent nonblanchable deep red, maroon, or purple discoloration
Intact or nonintact skin with localized area of persistent nonblanchable deep red, maroon, or purple discoloration or epidermal separation revealing a dark wound bed or blood-filled blister. Pain and temperature change often precede skin color changes. Discoloration may appear differently in darkly pigmented skin. This injury results from intense and/or prolonged pressure and shear forces at the bone–muscle interface. The wound may evolve rapidly to reveal the actual extent of tissue injury, or it may resolve without tissue loss. If necrotic tissue, subcutaneous tissue, granulation tissue, fascia, muscle, or other underlying structures are visible, this indicates a full-thickness pressure injury (unstageable, stage 3, or stage 4). Do not use deep tissue pressure injury to describe vascular, traumatic, neuropathic, or dermatological conditions (NPUAP, 2016).

○ **Unstageable Pressure Injury:** Obscured full-thickness skin and tissue loss
Full-thickness skin and tissue loss in which the extent of tissue damage within the ulcer cannot be confirmed because it is obscured by slough or eschar. If slough or eschar is removed, a stage 3 or stage 4 pressure injury will be revealed. Stable eschar (i.e., dry, adherent, intact without erythema or fluctuance) on the heel or ischemic limb should not be softened or removed (NPUAP, 2016).

- Inspect and monitor the site of impaired tissue integrity at least once daily for color changes, redness, swelling, warmth, pain, or other signs of infection or per facility/agency policy. Monitor the status of the skin around the wound. Pay special attention to all high-risk areas such as bony prominences, skinfolds, sacrum, and heels. There is evidence that stage 1 pressure injuries are under detected in individuals with darkly pigmented skin because areas of redness are not easily identified. *Systematic inspection can identify impending problems early (NPUAP/EPUAP, 2014).* EB: Determine whether the client is experiencing changes in sensation or pain. *An initial pain assessment, using a validated tool, should include the following four elements: a detailed pain history including the character, intensity, and duration of pressure ulcer pain; a physical examination that includes a neurological component; a psychosocial assessment; and an appropriate diagnostic workup to determine the type and cause of the pain. Select a wound dressing that requires less frequent changing, is nonadherent, and maintains a moist wound environment (NPUAP/EPUAP, 2014).*

- *Individualizing plans for bathing frequency, pH-balanced soaps, and applying moisturizing products while skin is still damp can help improve skin integrity (Murphree, 2017).*

- Assess for incontinence and implement an individualized plan for management. Differentiate wounds caused by incontinence from other types of wounds. Cleanse the skin promptly after episodes of incontinence and use pH-balanced cleansers (NPUAP/EPUAP, 2014). Use incontinence skin barriers including creams, ointments, pastes, or film-forming skin protectants as needed to protect and maintain skin integrity with incontinent individuals (Ratliff et al, 2017).

- Monitor for correct placement of tubes, catheters, and other devices. Assess the skin and tissue affected by the pressure of the devices and tape used to secure these devices. EB: *Reposition the individual and/or the medical device to redistribute pressure and decrease shear forces. Keep skin clean and dry under medical devices. Moisture underneath a medical device can create an environment in which the skin is more vulnerable to alterations in skin integrity, including irritant dermatitis and ulceration (NPUAP/EPUAP, 2014).*

● = Independent;   ▲ = Collaborative;   EBN = Evidence-Based Nursing;   EB = Evidence-Based

- Medical device–related pressure injury describes an etiology. Medical device–related pressure injuries result from the use of devices designed and applied for diagnostic or therapeutic purposes. The resultant pressure injury generally conforms to the pattern or shape of the device. The injury should be staged using the previously discussed staging system (NPUAP, 2016).
- Assess frequently for correct placement of foot boards, restraints, traction, casts, or other devices, and assess skin and tissue integrity. Frequently assess for signs and symptoms of compartment syndrome (refer to the care plan for Risk for **Peripheral Neurovascular** dysfunction). Reposition the individual and/or the medical device to redistribute pressure and decrease shear force (NPUAP/EPUAP, 2014).
- Implement and communicate a comprehensive treatment plan for the topical treatment of the skin impairment site. *To improve care and outcomes for individuals with or at risk for skin impairments, evidence-based guidelines must be disseminated to ensure that health care providers are making every effort to identify individuals with or at risk for skin alterations and implement appropriate preventative and treatment interventions (Ratliff et al, 2017).*
- ▲ Identify a plan for debridement if necrotic tissue (eschar or slough) is present and if consistent with overall client management goals (i.e., curative versus palliative care). **EB:** *Debride devitalized tissue within the wound bed or edge of pressure injuries (NPUAP, 2016) when appropriate to individual's condition and consistent with overall goals of care. Do not debride stable, hard, dry eschar in ischemic limbs or heels (NPUAP/EPUAP, 2014).*
- Select a topical treatment that maintains a moist, wound-healing environment and also allows absorption of exudate and filling of dead space. *No single wound care product provides the optimal environment for healing all wounds.* **EB:** *Choose dressings that provide a moist healing environment, keep periwound skin dry, and control exudate and eliminate dead space NPUAP/EPUAP, 2014).*
- Avoid positioning the client on the site of impaired tissue integrity. **EB:** *If it is consistent with overall client management goals, reposition the client based on level of tissue tolerance and overall condition, and transfer or reposition the client carefully to avoid adverse effects of external mechanical forces (pressure, friction, and shear) (NPUAP/EPUAP, 2014).*
- Evaluate for the use of support surfaces (specialty mattresses, beds) chair cushion, or devices as appropriate (Lippoldt, Pernicka, & Staudinger, 2014). Before replacing the existing mattress evaluate the effectiveness of previous and current prevention and treatment plans and set treatment goals consistent with the individual's goals and lifestyle (NPUAP/EPUAP, 2014). Continued repositioning of individuals placed on a pressure redistribution support surface is paramount (NPUAP/EPUAP, 2014).
- If the goal of care is to keep the client comfortable (e.g., for a terminally ill client), repositioning may not be appropriate. *Position the client in position of optimal comfort (Horn & Irion, 2014). Reposition and turn the individual, periodically, in accordance with the individual's wishes, comfort, and tolerance (NPUAP/EPUAP, 2014). Maintain the head of the bed at the lowest degree of elevation possible to reduce shear and friction and use lift devices, pillows, foam wedges, and pressure-reducing devices in the bed (NPUAP/EPUAP, 2014; Baranoski & Ayello, 2016).*
- ▲ Assess the client's nutritional status. Refer for a nutritional consult and/or institute dietary supplements as necessary. *Optimizing nutritional intake, including calories, fatty acids, protein, and vitamins, is needed to promote wound healing (NPUAP/EPUAP, 2014; O'Hanlon, Dowsett, & Smyth, 2015).* Review client nutrition plan evaluating for the intake of 1.25 to 1.5 g of protein per kilogram body weight daily, unless medically contraindicated, for adults at risk of a pressure injury or with existing pressure injuries. Offer 1 mL of fluid intake per kilocalorie per day, unless medically contraindicated (Ratliff et al, 2017). Reassess as condition changes (NPUAP/EPUAP, 2014).
- ▲ Develop a comprehensive plan of care that includes a thorough wound assessment, treatment interventions, support surfaces, nutritional products, adjunctive therapies, and evaluation of the outcome of care. *Documentation of these essential elements is paramount to establishing a framework for quality care.*

Home Care

- Some of the interventions previously described may be adapted for home care use.
- ▲ Assess the client's current phase of wound healing (inflammation, proliferation, or maturation) and stage of injury; initiate appropriate wound management. **EB:** *A holistic assessment is required to guide correct dressing selection. Underlying pathophysiological factors need to be addressed to improve outcomes.*
- Instruct and assist the client and caregivers in understanding how to change dressings and in the importance of maintaining a clean environment. Provide written instructions and observe them completing the dressing change.

● = Independent;   ▲ = Collaborative;   **EBN** = Evidence-Based Nursing;   **EB** = Evidence-Based

▲ Initiate a consultation in a case assignment with a wound specialist or wound, ostomy, and continence nurse to establish a comprehensive plan as soon as possible. Plan case conferencing to promote optimal wound care. *Case conferencing ensures that cases are regularly reviewed to discuss and implement the most effective wound care management to meet client needs.*

▲ Consult with other health care disciplines to provide a thorough, comprehensive assessment. *Consider referring to a dietitian, physical therapist, occupational therapist, and social worker/case manager as needed. Early engagement of wound care specialists can enhance overall care and reduce health care costs (Vrtis, 2013).*

 Client/Family Teaching and Discharge Planning

• Teach skin and wound assessment and ways to monitor for signs and symptoms of infection, complications, and healing. *Early assessment and intervention help prevent serious problems from developing.*

• Teach the client why a topical treatment has been selected. Explain wound bed changes that the caregiver can expect to see. Instruct on when the dressing needs to be changed. Assess pressure injuries with each wound dressing change and confirm the appropriateness of the current dressing regimen (NPUAP/EPUAP, 2014). **EB:** *The type of wound dressing needed may change over time as the wound heals and/or deteriorates (NPUAP/EPUAP, 2014; Baranoski & Ayello, 2016).*

▲ Teach the use of pillows, foam wedges, and pressure-reducing devices, on beds and chairs to prevent pressure injury. Pressure redistributing surfaces serve as adjuncts and not replacements to regular repositioning (Ratliff et al, 2017).

REFERENCES

Baranoski, S., & Ayello, E. A. (Eds.), (2016). *Wound care essentials: Practice principles* (4th ed.). Ambler, PA: Lippincott Williams & Wilkins.

Horn, J., & Irion, G. L. (2014). The integument: Current concepts in care at end of life. *Journal of Acute Care Physical Therapy, 5*(1), 11–16.

Lippoldt, J., Pernicka, E., & Staudinger, T. (2014). Interface pressure at different degrees of backrest elevation with various types of pressure redistribution surfaces. *American Journal of Critical Care, 23*(2), 119–126.

Murphree, R. W. (2017). Impairments in skin integrity. *Nursing Clinics of North America, 52*(3), 405–417.

National Pressure Ulcer Advisory Panel (NPUAP) and European Pressure Ulcer Advisory Panel (EPUAP). (2014). In E. Haesler (Ed.), *Prevention and treatment of pressure ulcers*. Perth, Australia: Cambridge Media.

National Pressure Ulcer Advisory Panel (NPUAP) and European Pressure Ulcer Advisory Panel (EPUAP). (2016). *Pressure Injury Stages*. Retrieved from http://www.npuap.org/resources/educational-and-clinical-resources/npuap-pressure-injury-stages/. (Accessed 5 December 2017).

O'Hanlon, C., Dowsett, J., & Smyth, N. (2015). Nutrition assessment of the intensive care unit patient. *Topics in Clinical Nutrition, 30*(1), 47–70.

Ratliff, C. R., Droste, L. R., Bonham, P., et al. (2017). WOCN 2016 Guidelines for Prevention and Management of Pressure Injuries (Ulcers), An executive summary, Wound, Ostomy and Continence Nurses Society-Wound Guidelines Task Force. *Journal of Wound, Ostomy, and Continence Nursing, 44*(3), 241–246.

Vrtis, M. C. (2013). The economic impact of complex wound care on home health agencies. *Journal of Wound, Ostomy, and Continence Nursing, 40*(4), 360–363.

T

Risk for impaired Tissue integrity   *Mary Beth Flynn Makic, PhD, RN, CCNS, FAAN, FNAP*

NANDA-I

Definition

Susceptible to damage to the mucous membrane, cornea, integumentary system, muscular fascia, muscle, tendon, bone, cartilage, joint capsule, and/or ligament, which may compromise health.

Risk Factors

Chemical injury agent; excessive fluid volume; humidity; imbalanced nutritional state; insufficient fluid volume; insufficient knowledge about maintaining tissue integrity; insufficient knowledge about protecting tissue integrity

At-Risk Population

Extremes of age; extremes of environmental temperature; exposure to high-voltage power supply

● = Independent;   ▲ = Collaborative;   EBN = Evidence-Based Nursing;   EB = Evidence-Based

Associated Condition

Alteration in metabolism; alteration in sensation; arterial puncture; impaired circulation; impaired mobility; peripheral neuropathy; pharmaceutical agent; radiation therapy; surgical procedure; vascular trauma

NOC, NIC, Client Outcomes, Nursing Interventions and *Rationales,* Client/Family Teaching and Discharge Planning, and References

Refer to care plan for Impaired **Tissue** integrity

Ineffective peripheral Tissue Perfusion   *Lorraine Duggan, MSN, ACNP-BC*

NANDA-I

Definition

Decrease in blood circulation to the periphery, which may compromise health.

Defining Characteristics

Absence of peripheral pulses; alteration in motor function; altered skin characteristics; ankle-brachial index <0.90; capillary refill time >3 seconds; color does not return to lowered limb after 1 minute of leg elevation; decrease in blood pressure in extremities; decrease in pain-free distances during a 6-minute walk test; decrease in peripheral pulses; delay in peripheral wound healing; distance in the 6-minute walk test below normal range; edema; extremity pain; femoral bruit; intermittent claudication; paresthesia; skin color pales with limb elevation

Related Factors

Excessive sodium intake; insufficient knowledge of disease process; insufficient knowledge of modifiable factors; sedentary lifestyle; smoking

Associated Condition

Diabetes mellitus; endovascular procedure; hypertension; trauma

NOC   (Nursing Outcomes Classification)

Suggested NOC Outcomes

Circulation Status; Fluid Balance; Hydration; Tissue Perfusion: Peripheral

---

Example NOC Outcome with Indicators

Demonstrates adequate **Circulation Status** as evidenced by the following indicators: Peripheral pulses strong/Peripheral pulses symmetrical/Skin color and temperature/Peripheral edema not present. (Rate the outcome and indicators of **Circulation Status:** 1 = severely compromised, 2 = substantially compromised, 3 = moderately compromised, 4 = mildly compromised, 5 = not compromised [see Section I].)

Client Outcomes

Client Will (Specify Time Frame)

- Demonstrate adequate tissue perfusion as evidenced by palpable peripheral pulses, warm and dry skin, adequate urine output, and absence of respiratory distress
- Verbalize knowledge of treatment regimen, including appropriate exercise and medications and their actions and possible side effects
- Identify changes in lifestyle needed to increase tissue perfusion

NIC   (Nursing Interventions Classification)

Suggested NIC Intervention

Circulatory Care: Arterial Insufficiency

● = Independent;   ▲ = Collaborative;   EBN = Evidence-Based Nursing;   EB = Evidence-Based

T

Example NIC Activities—Circulatory Care: Areterial Insufficiency
Evaluate peripheral edema and pulses; Inspect skin for arterial ulcers and tissue breakdown

Nursing Interventions and *Rationales*

▲ Check the brachial, radial, dorsalis pedis, posterior tibial, and popliteal pulses bilaterally. If unable to find them, use a Doppler stethoscope and notify the health care provider immediately if new onset of absence of pulses along with a cold extremity. EB/QSEN: *Audible handheld Doppler ultrasound proved to be a reliable, simple, rapid, and inexpensive bedside test of peripheral arterial disease in diabetic and nondiabetic patients (Alavi et al, 2015).*

● Note skin color and feel the temperature of the skin. Check capillary refill.

● Assess for pain in the extremities, noting severity, quality, timing, and exacerbating and alleviating factors. Differentiate venous from arterial disease. EB: *When peripheral artery disease (PAD) involves the lower extremities it produces signs and symptoms like claudication, ischemic rest pain, or skin ulceration (Wei et al, 2017).*

● Note skin texture and the presence of hair, ulcers, or gangrenous areas on the legs or feet. EB: *A chronic wound is defined as an area in which the skin is not intact that fails to heal within 8 weeks. Chronic wounds often develop on the lower limbs as a complication of diabetes, venous insufficiency, or inadequate arterial perfusion (Ruttermann et al, 2013; Bosanquet & Harding, 2014).*

● Note the presence of edema in the extremities and rate severity on a four-point scale. Measure the circumference of the ankle and calf at the same time each day in the early morning (Busti, 2016).

▲ Prepare for vascular lab. EB: *Evaluation for PAD if signs and symptoms are present frequently involves a non-invasive vascular lab assessment as a next step in diagnosis (Wei et al, 2017).*

Arterial Insufficiency

▲ Monitor peripheral pulses. If there is new onset of loss of pulses with bluish, purple, or black areas and extreme pain, notify the health care provider immediately. *These are symptoms of arterial obstruction that can result in loss of a limb if not immediately reversed.* EB: *Risks of peripheral disease increased proportionally with the number of absent peripheral pulses, with the highest risks observed in patients with three or four absent pulses. Every additional absent pulse increases the risk of all outcome (Mohammedi et al, 2016).*

▲ Measure ankle-brachial index (ABI) via Doppler imaging. EB: *Measurement of the ABI via a palpatory method offers an inexpensive, readily available alternative approach for early disease detection of PAD. Normal ABI is >0.9 (Orellana-Barrios et al, 2014).*

● Avoid elevating the legs above the level of the heart. With arterial insufficiency, leg elevation decreases arterial blood supply to the legs.

▲ For early arterial insufficiency, encourage exercise such as walking or riding an exercise bicycle from 30 to 60 minutes per day as ordered by the health care provider. EB: *Regardless of exercise length and modality, regularly intensive walking exercise improves walking ability in PAD patients more than usual care (Lyu et al, 2016).*

● Keep the client warm and have the client wear socks and shoes or sheepskin-lined slippers when mobile. Do not apply heat. Clients with arterial insufficiency report being constantly cold; keep extremities warm to maintain vasodilation and blood supply. Heat application can easily damage ischemic tissues.

▲ Pay meticulous attention to foot care. Refer to a podiatrist if the client has a foot or nail abnormality. Ischemic feet are vulnerable to injury; meticulous foot care can prevent further injury. EB: *Symptoms or signs of PAD can be observed in up to 50% of the patients with a diabetic foot ulcer and is a risk factor for poor healing and amputation (Hinchliffe et al, 2016).*

● If the client has ischemic arterial ulcers, refer to the care plan for Impaired **Tissue** integrity.

▲ If the client smokes, aggressively counsel the client to stop smoking and refer to the health care provider for medications to support nicotine withdrawal and a smoking withdrawal program. EB: *Smoking is a particularly strong risk factor for PAD, and several newer risk markers have shown independent associations with PAD (Criqui & Aboyans, 2015).*

▲ Educate on use and safety of antiplatelet medications. EB: *Dual antiplatelet therapy is associated with reduced rates of major adverse cardiovascular events and mortality among patients with severe symptomatic PAD (Armstrong et al, 2015).*

● = Independent;   ▲ = Collaborative;   EBN = Evidence-Based Nursing;   EB = Evidence-Based

Venous Insufficiency

▲ Elevate edematous legs as ordered and ensure no pressure under the knee and heels to prevent pressure ulcers. **EB:** *Patients who are inactive (sedentary) for long periods may have leg edema because the calf muscle pump is underused or ineffective. Elevating the ankles above the level of the heart can help relieve this type of swelling (Evans & Ratchford, 2016).*

▲ Apply graduated compression stockings as ordered. Ensure proper fit by measuring accurately. Remove the stockings at least twice a day, in the morning with the bath and in the evening, to assess the condition of the extremity, then reapply. Knee length is preferred rather than thigh length. **EB:** *Hosiery is a dominant treatment; that is, on average it results in higher quality-adjusted life years and lower costs than bandages (Rebecca, 2014).*

● Encourage the client to walk with compression stockings on and perform toe-up and point-flex exercises. *Exercise helps increase venous return, builds up collateral circulation, and strengthens the calf muscles.* **EBN:** *Physical therapy modalities improve ABI, Doppler flow velocity, and blood parameters in clients with type 2 diabetes (Castro-Sanchez, 2013).*

● If the client is overweight, encourage weight loss to decrease venous disease.

● If the client has venous leg ulcers, encourage the client to avoid prolonged sitting, standing, and elevation of the involved leg. Encourage proper use of compression stockings. Pain may prevent compliance. **EBN:** *A study shows a high incidence of ulcer pain, confirming that pain has a great effect on clients with venous leg ulcers (Akessonrut et al, 2014).*

▲ If the client is mostly immobile, consult with the health care provider regarding use of a calf-high pneumatic compression device for prevention of deep venous thrombosis (DVT). **EB:** *Below-the-knee devices have demonstrated the most efficacy with multiple guidelines recommending usage (Pierce et al, 2015; Kearon et al, 2016).*

● Observe for signs of DVT, including pain, tenderness, swelling in the calf and thigh, and redness in the involved extremity. Take serial leg measurements of the thigh and calf circumferences. In some clients a tender venous cord can be felt in the popliteal fossa. Do not rely on Homan's sign. **EBN:** *Screening and detection of DVT must be as accurate as possible. Failing to diagnose a DVT can contribute to a fatal pulmonary embolism (PE), whereas false-positive screening can result in costly diagnostics or the patient's unnecessary anticoagulation (Anthony, 2013).*

▲ Note the results of a D-dimer test and ultrasounds. **EB:** *A study suggested that the D-dimer test be used during the initial workup for all patients who present to the emergency department (ED) for suspected DVT (Mousa et al, 2017).*

● If DVT is present, observe for symptoms of a PE. **EB:** *PE is a significant risk of a DVT. Signs and symptoms range from sudden onset, acute chest pain of a sharp stabbing nature, anxiety, and cough (Kearon et al, 2016).*

▲ Educate on use and safety of anticoagulant medications. **EB:** *DVT and PE are two manifestations of venous thromboembolism (VTE). The mainstay of therapy for DVT is anticoagulation, provided there is no contraindication (Lip & Hull, 2017). Clients need to be aware of adverse effects of anticoagulant medications, wear a medical alert bracelet, and be aware of food–drug interactions (Kearon et al, 2016).*

 Geriatric

● Complete a thorough lower extremity assessment, documenting the smallest change from previous assessment, and implement a plan immediately. **EB:** *Complete and accurate assessment is essential to guide health care providers in formulating efficacious plans of care. The prevalence of peripheral arterial disease increases with age. The elevated risk of ulcerations leading to amputation among older adults reflects not only increased rates of PAD and diabetic pathologies but also age-related changes of the integument (Hakim & Heitzman, 2013).*

● Recognize that older adults have an increased risk for development of PE. **EB:** *PE is associated with high short-term mortality in elderly patients, even when hemodynamically stable (Castelli et al, 2014).*

 Home Care

● The interventions previously described may be adapted for home care use.

● If arterial disease is present and the client smokes, aggressively encourage smoking cessation.

● Examine the feet carefully at frequent intervals for changes and new ulcerations. Encourage the client to perform regular assessment of the feet.

▲ Assess the client's nutritional status, paying special attention to obesity, hyperlipidemia, and malnutrition. Refer to a dietitian if appropriate.

● Monitor for development of gangrene, venous ulceration, and symptoms of cellulitis (redness, pain, and increased swelling in an extremity).

● = Independent;   ▲ = Collaborative;   EBN = Evidence-Based Nursing;   EB = Evidence-Based

Client/Family Teaching and Discharge Planning

- Explain the importance of good foot care. Teach the client and family to wash and inspect the feet daily. Recommend that the diabetic client wear comfortable shoes and break them in slowly, watching for blisters (Oliveira et al, 2014).
- ▲ Teach the diabetic client that he or she should have a comprehensive foot examination at least annually (which includes an analysis for predicting foot ulceration risk), which includes assessment of sensation using the Semmes–Weinstein monofilaments. If good sensation is not present, refer to a footwear professional for fitting of therapeutic shoes and inserts, the cost of which is covered by Medicare.
- For arterial disease, stress the importance of not smoking, following a weight loss program (if the client is obese), carefully controlling a diabetic condition, controlling hyperlipidemia and hypertension, maintaining intake of antiplatelet therapy, and reducing stress.
- Teach the client to avoid exposure to cold; limit exposure to brief periods if going out in cold weather and wear warm clothing.
- For venous disease, teach the importance of wearing compression stockings as ordered, elevating the legs at intervals, and watching for skin breakdown on the legs.
- Teach the client to recognize the signs and symptoms that should be reported to a health care provider (e.g., change in skin temperature, color or sensation, or the presence of a new lesion on the foot).
- Provide clear, simple instructions about plan of care.
- Instruct and provide emotional support for client undergoing hyperoxygenation treatment. **EB:** *Hyperbaric oxygen may be associated with ulcer healing in selected diabetic foot ulcers (Oliveira et al, 2014).*

REFERENCES

Akessonrut, N., ÖienHenrik, F., & Forssell, C. (2014). Ulcer pain in patients with venous leg ulcers related to antibiotic treatment and compression therapy. *British Journal of Community Nursing.* Retrieved from http://dx.doi.org/10.12968/bjcn.2014.19.Sup9.S6.

Alavi, A., Sibbald, R., & Nabavizadeh, R. (2015). Peripheral arterial disease. *Vascular, 23*(6), 622–629.

Anthony, M. (2013). Nursing assessment of DVT. *Medsurg Nursing, 22*(2), 95–98.

Armstrong, E., et al. (2015). Association of dual-antiplatelet therapy with reduced major adverse cardiovascular events in patients with symptomatic peripheral arterial disease. *Journal of Vascular Surgery, 62*(1), 157–165.

Bosanquet, D. C., & Harding, K. G. (2014). Wound duration and healing rates: Cause or effect? *Wound Repair and Regeneration, 22*(2), 143–150.

Busti, A. (2016). *Pitting edema assessment.* Retrieved from www.ebmconsult.com.

Castelli, R., Bucciarelli, P., Porroc, F., et al. (2014). Pulmonary embolism in elderly patients: Prognostic impact of the Cumulative Illness Rating Scale (CIRS) on short term mortality. *Thrombosis Research, 134*(2), 326–330.

Castro-Sanchez, A. (2013). A program of 3 physical therapy modalities improves peripheral arterial disease in diabetes type 2 patients: A randomized controlled trial. *Journal of Cardiovascular Nursing, 28*(1), 74–82.

Criqui, M., & Aboyans, V. (2015). Epidemiology of peripheral artery disease. *Circulation Research, 116*(9), 1509–1526.

Evans, N., & Ratchford, E. (2016). The swollen leg. *Vascular Medicine, 21*(6).

Hakim, E., & Heitzman, J. (2013). Wound management in the presence of peripheral arterial disease. *Topics in Geriatric Rehabilitation, 29*(3), 187–194.

Hinchliffe, R., et al. (2016). Effectiveness of revascularization of the ulcerated foot in patients with diabetes and peripheral artery disease: A systematic review. *Diabetes Metabolisim Research and Reviews, 32*(S1), 136–144.

Kearon, C., Akl, E. A., Omelas, J., et al. (2016). Antithrombotic therapy for VTE disease. Chest Guideline and expert panel report. *Chest, 149*, 315–352.

Lip, G., & Hull, R. (2017). *Overview of the treatment of lower extremity deep vein thrombosis (DVT). UpToDate.* Retrieved from www.uptodate.com.

Lyu, X., et al. (2016). Intensive walking exercise for lower extremity peripheral arterial disease: A systematic review and meta-analysis. *Journal of Diabetes, 8*(3), 363–377.

Mohammedi, K., et al. (2016). Absence of peripheral pulses and risk of major vascular outcomes in patients with type 2 diabetes. *Diabetes Care, 39*(12), 2270–2277.

Mousa, A., Morkos, R., De Wit, D., et al. (2017). Utilization of D-Dimer along with clinical probability testing in determining the magnitude and location of deep vein thrombosis in a high-volume tertiary practice. *Journal of Vascular Surgery: Venous and Lymphatic disorders, 5*(1), 170–171.

Oliveira, N., Rosa, P., Borges, L., et al. (2014). Treatment of diabetic foot complications with hyperbaric oxygen therapy: A retrospective experience. *Foot and Ankle Surgery, 20*(2), 104–143.

Orellana-Barrios, M., et al. (2014). Abstract 286: Concordance between ankle-brachial index measurement methods (palpatory versus doppler). *Arteriosclerosis, Thrombosis, and Vascular Biology, 34*, A286.

Pierce, T. D., Cherian, J. J., Jauregui, J. J. (2015). A current review of mechanical compression and its role in venous thromboembolic prophylaxis in total knee and total hip arthroplasty. *The Journal of Arthroplasty, 30*(12), 2279–2284.

Rebecca, L. (2014). Clinical and cost-effectiveness of compression hosiery verus compression bandages in treatment of venous leg ulcers (Venous Leg Ulcer Study IV, VenUS IV): A randomised controlled trial. *The Lancet, 383*(9920), 871–879.

Ruttermann, M., et al. (2013). Local treatment of chronic wounds in patients with peripheral vascular disease, chronic venous insufficiency and diabetes. *Dtsch Arztebl International, 110*(3), 25–31.

Wei, B., Qian, C., Fang, Q., et al. (2016). The prognostic value of peripheral artery disease in heart failure: Insights from a meta-analysis. *Heart, Lung Circulation, 25*(12), 1195–1202. doi:10.1016/j.hlc.2016.04.002.

• = Independent;   ▲ = Collaborative;   EBN = Evidence-Based Nursing;   EB = Evidence-Based

Risk for ineffective peripheral Tissue Perfusion
Mary Beth Flynn Makic, PhD, RN, CCNS, FAAN, FNAP

NANDA-I

Definition

Susceptible to a decrease in blood circulation to the periphery, which may compromise health.

Risk Factors

Excessive sodium intake; insufficient knowledge of disease process; insufficient knowledge of modifiable Factors; sedentary lifestyle; smoking

Associated Condition

Diabetes mellitus; endovascular procedure; hypertension; trauma

NOC, NIC, Client Outcomes, Nursing Interventions and *Rationales,* Client/Family Teaching and Discharge Planning, and References

Refer to care plan for Ineffective peripheral **Tissue Perfusion**

Impaired Transfer ability   *Kerri J. Reid, RN, MS, CNS, CCRN-K*

NANDA-I

Definition

Limitation of independent movement between two nearby surfaces.

Defining Characteristics

Impaired ability to transfer between bed and chair; impaired ability to transfer between bed and standing position; impaired ability to transfer between car and chair; impaired ability to transfer between chair and floor; impaired ability to transfer between chair and standing position; impaired ability to transfer between floor and standing position; impaired ability to transfer between uneven levels; impaired ability to transfer in or out of bath tub; impaired ability to transfer in or out of shower; impaired ability to transfer on or off a commode; impaired ability to transfer on or off a toilet

Related Factors

Environmental barrier; impaired balance; insufficient knowledge of transfer techniques; insufficient muscle strength; obesity; physical deconditioning; pain

Associated Condition

Alteration in cognitive functioning; impaired vision; musculoskeletal impairment; neuromuscular impairment

NOC   (Nursing Outcomes Classification)

Suggested NOC Outcomes

Balance; Body Positioning: Self-Initiated; Transfer Performance

Example NOC Outcome with Indicators
Transfer Performance as evidenced by the following indicators: Transfers from bed to chair and back/Transfers from wheelchair to toilet and back/Transfers from wheelchair to vehicle and back. (Rate the outcome and indicators of **Transfer Performance:** 1 = severely compromised, 2 = substantially compromised, 3 = moderately compromised, 4 = mildly compromised, 5 = not compromised [see Section I].)

• = Independent;   ▲ = Collaborative;   EBN = Evidence-Based Nursing;   EB = Evidence-Based

Client Outcomes

Client Will (Specify Time Frame)

- Transfer from bed to chair and back successfully
- Transfer from chair to chair successfully
- Transfer from wheelchair to toilet and back successfully
- Transfer from wheelchair to car and back successfully

NIC (Nursing Interventions Classification)

Suggested NIC Interventions

Exercise Promotion: Strength Training; Exercise Therapy: Muscle Control

Example NIC Activities—Exercise Promotion: Strength Training
Obtain medical clearance for initiating a strength-training program, as appropriate; Assist to set realistic short- and long-term goals and to take ownership of the exercise plan

Nursing Interventions and *Rationales*

- Specify level of independence using a standardized functional scale. **EB:** *Use a nurse-driven bedside assessment tool to evaluate the patient's mobility status. Continuous surveillance of patients by nurses and using a mobility evaluation tool allows more awareness of the knowledge and skill needed for safe patient handling and mobility, reducing the risk for fall and potential injury to the nursing staff (Boynton et al, 2014).*
- Assess level of patient ability to perform specific tasks prior to transfer of patient. **EB:** *Valid and reliable assessment tools such as The Bedside Mobility Assessment Tool provides assessment of a patient using "levels of activity" to indicate safe patient handling and mobility (Boynton et al, 2014; Boynton, Kelly, & Perez, 2014; Hillrom, 2018).*
- ▲ Complications associated with immobility and resultant muscle loss begins within 48 hours of onset or injury and is greatest during the first 2 to 3 weeks (Cameron et al, 2015). Request consult for a physical and/or occupational therapist (PT and OT) to develop plan of care for safe patient handling and mobility. **EB:** *Progressive mobility, or mobility that starts earlier and more aggressively during a patient's hospital stay, even as early as in the intensive care unit (ICU), decreases mechanical ventilation days and decreases complications such as weakness from disuse and contractures (Kalisch, Dabney, & Lee, 2013). Early exercise in the ICU improved patients' abilities to complete activities of daily living (bathing, dressing, eating, grooming, transferring from bed to chair, and using the toilet) and increased the distances they were able to walk (Schubert 2011; Stiller 2013).*
- Assess client's dependence, weight, strength, balance, tolerance to position change, cooperation, fatigue level, and cognition plus available equipment and staff ratio/experience to decide whether to do a manual or device-assisted transfer (Cohen et al, 2010; American Nurses Association [ANA] 2013).
- ▲ Obtain a consult for a PT, OT, or orthotist to evaluate and fit clients with proper orthoses, braces, collars, and walking aids before helping them stand. **CEB:** *Equipment helps clients move and function safely, comfortably, and independently (Hoeman, Liszner, & Alverzo, 2008).*
- ▲ Help client put on/take off collars, braces, prostheses in bed, and put on/take off antiembolism stockings and abdominal binders. If applying antiembolism stockings is prescribed to reduce the risk of DVT, apply while the client is in bed for ease of application. **EB:** *In patients with diagnosed acute DVT of the leg, compression stockings may not be routinely used to prevent postthrombotic syndrome (PST). PST is a complication that may occur after a DVT develops from venous insufficiency producing symptoms of pain, edema, and venous ulcers. Current guidelines recommend not routinely using compression stockings with patients who have a DVT (Kearon et al, 2017).*
- ▲ Collaborate with PT and OT to use algorithms to identify technological aids to handle and transfer dependent and obese clients. Use assistive mobility devices such as gait belts, lifts, and transport devices to move obese clients to avoid harm to both client and health care professional (Choi & Brings, 2015). *Assess the client for appropriate use of assistive devices to include powered stand-assist devices, mechanical lifts, stretchers to chairs, and friction-reducing devices to prevent musculoskeletal injuries of staff and allow safe client handling (ANA, 2013; Centers for Disease Control and Prevention, 2015; Choi & Brings, 2015).*

• = Independent;   ▲ = Collaborative;   **EBN** = Evidence-Based Nursing;   **EB** = Evidence-Based

- Implement and document type of transfer (e.g., slide board, pivot), weight-bearing status (non–weight-bearing, partial), equipment (walker, sling lift), and level of assistance (standby, moderate) on care plan, white board in room, and/or electronic medical record.
- Apply a gait belt with handles before transferring clients with partial weight-bearing abilities; keep the belt and client close to provider during the transfer. *If used incorrectly, such as at arm's length, it prevents support of client and places staff at risk for back and arm injuries (Kalisch, Dabney, & Lee, 2013; Choi & Brings, 2015; Hallmark, Meachan, & Shores, 2015).*
- Help clients when wearing shoes with nonskid soles and socks/hose. *Proper shoes help prevent slips/pain/pressure and improve balance.* CEB: *Suggest trying a running shoe that is comfortable and lightweight. A recent study found that participants, who were unable to see the type of shoe (control shoe, running shoe, or orthopedic shoe), chose the running shoe based on comfort and weight (Riskowski, Dufour, & Hannan, 2011).*
- Remove or swivel wheelchair armrests, leg rests, and footplates to the side, especially with squat or slide board transfers. *This gives clients and nurses feet space in which to maneuver and provides fewer obstacles to trip over.*
- Adjust transfer surfaces so they are similar in height. For example, lower a hospital bed to about an inch higher than commode height. EB: *Similar heights between seat surfaces require less upper extremity muscular effort during transfers (Darragh et al, 2015).*
- Place wheelchair and commode at a slight angle toward the surface onto which the client will transfer. *The two surfaces are close together yet allow room for the caregiver to adjust the client's movements during the transfer (Darragh et al, 2015).*
- Teach client to consistently lock brakes on wheelchair/commode/shower chair before transferring. *Wheels will roll if not locked, creating risk for falls. Pneumatic wheelchair tires must be adequately inflated for brakes to lock effectively (Choi & Brings, 2015; Darragh et al, 2015).*
- Give clear, simple instructions, allow client time to process information, and let him or her do as much of the transfer as possible. *Over-assistance by staff and family may decrease client learning, independence, self-care, and self-esteem.*
- ▲ Remind clients to comply with weight-bearing restrictions ordered by their health care provider. *Weight-bearing may retard healing in fractured bones.*
- Place client in set position before standing him or her, for example, sitting on edge of surface with bilateral weight-bearing on buttocks and hips, with knees flexed, balls of feet aligned under knees, and head in midline. *This position prepares individuals for bearing weight and permits shifting of weight from pelvis to feet as the center of gravity changes while rising.*
- Support and stabilize client's weak knees by placing one or both of your knees next to or encircling client's knees, rather than blocking them. *This allows client to flex his or her knees and lean forward to stand and transfer.*
  - Squat transfer: client leans well forward, slightly raises flexed hips off the surface, pivots, and sits down on new surface. *This is beneficial for clients with slight weight-bearing ability.*
  - Standing pivot transfer: client leans forward with hips flexed and pushes up with hands from seat surface (or arms of chair), then stands erect, pivots, and sits down on new surface. *This is beneficial for clients who have fair weight-bearing ability.*
  - Slide board transfer: client should have on pants or have a pillowcase over the board. Remove arm and leg rest from wheelchair on one side, then slightly angle chair toward new surface. Help client lean sideways, shifting his or her weight so the transfer board can be placed well under the upper thigh of the leg next to new surface. Make sure the board is safely angled across both surfaces. Help client to sit upright and place one hand on the board and the other hand on the surface. Remind and help client perform a series of pushups with arms while leaning slightly forward and lifting (not sliding) hips in small increments across the board with each pushup. *This benefits clients with little to no weight-bearing ability (Hoeman, Lizner, & Alverzo, 2008; Cameron et al, 2012; Hallmark, Mechan, & Shores, 2015; Darragh et al, 2015).*
- Position walking aids appropriately so a standing client can grasp and use them once he or she is upright. *These aids help provide support, balance, and stability to help client stand and step safely (Kalisch, Dabney, & Lee, 2013; Mayeda-Letourneau, 2014).*
- Reinforce to clients who use walkers to place one hand on walker and push with opposite hand against chair arm or surface from which they are arising to stand up. *Placing both hands on the walker may cause it to tip and the client to lose balance and fall.*

● = Independent;   ▲ = Collaborative;   EBN = Evidence-Based Nursing;   EB = Evidence-Based

- Use ceiling-mounted or bedside mechanical bariatric lifts to transfer dependent bariatric (extremely obese) clients. *Equipment prevents client/staff injury and is essential for clients who require a moderate/maximum assist transfer (Cohen et al, 2010; ANA 2013; Choi & Brings, 2015).*
- Use bariatric devices and use available safe client handling equipment for lifting, transferring, positioning, and sliding client (Cohen et al, 2010; ANA 2013; Choi & Brings, 2015).
- Place a mechanical lift sling in the wheelchair preventively. Place two transfer sheets or a slide board under the bariatric client. *Reinforce that head should be leaning forward and that knees should be level with hips; help hold wheelchair in place as therapist directs/helps client with a scoot transfer. Client may be too fatigued to do a manual transfer back to bed after sitting, so sling/lift can be used.*
- Perform initial and subsequent fall risk assessment. *Use standardized tools for fall risk assessment and interdisciplinary multifactorial interventions to reduce falls and risk of falling in hospitals.* **EB:** *Best practice in falls reduction occurs when fall risk assessment; visual identification of individuals at high risk for falls; falls risk factor directed interventions; and standardized multifactorial education, including visual tools for staff, families, and, patients are implemented (Degelau et al, 2012; Low et al, 2015).*
- ▲ Collaborate with PT, OT, and pharmacist for individualized preventive/postfall plans; for example, scheduled toileting, balance and strength training, removal of hazards, chair alarms, call system/phone in reach, and review of medications. **EB:** *A systematic review of the evidence found low-intensity exercise and incontinence care in residents in nursing homes reduced falls (Low et al, 2015; Hopkins, Mitchell, Thomsen, et al. (2016).*
- Coordinate a follow-up encounter within 30 days of discharge from any inpatient facility with a licensed provider to perform a medication reconciliation to include all medications the client has been taking or receiving prior to the outpatient visit to provide quality care and improve quality of communication related to medications (Agency for Healthcare Research and Quality [AHRQ], 2015). **EB:** *Review of medications, especially new medications added to a client plan of care, can place the individual at risk for falls, changes in mentation, or mobility limitations (AHRQ, 2015).*
- Encourage an exercise component such as Tai chi, physical therapy, or other exercise for balance, gait, and strength training in group programs or at home.
- Integrate structured and progressive exercise protocols into a client's plan of care and innovative partnerships with other providers to create longer duration interventions for clients at risk of falling. *This promotes strength and aids in increasing confidence and will then reduce the risk for falling (Schubert, 2011; Low et al, 2015).*
- Modify the environment for safety; recommend vision assessment and consideration for cataract removal.
- To reduce the risk of falling, assess the physical environment (e.g., poor lighting, high bed position, improper equipment). *Continuous and intentional observational assessment of the environment promotes safety by reducing potential fall hazards (Low et al, 2015).*
- Recommend polypharmacy assessment with special consideration to sedatives, antidepressants, and drugs affecting the central nervous system; recommend evaluation for orthostatic hypotension and irregular heartbeats; and recommend vitamin D supplementation 800 IU/day (AHRQ, 2015).

 Home Care

- ▲ Obtain referral for OT and PT to teach home exercises and balance and fall prevention and recovery. They also evaluate for potential modifications such as an entry ramp, elevated toilet seat/toilevator (raised base under toilet), tub seat or shower chair, need for shower stall with built-in seat or wheel-in shower stall without a curb/threshold, handheld flexible shower head, lever-type facets, pull-out drawers with loop handles versus cupboards, standing lift, and so on. **EB:** *A study found that evaluating the home environment that facilitated assistive devices was necessary for safe and successful mobility of clients within the dwelling and outdoors (Clark, 2014).*
- Develop a multifactorial/multicomponent interventions risk strategy to reduce the risk for falls that include adaptation or modification of the home environment; withdrawal or minimization of psychoactive medications; withdrawal of minimization of other medications; management of postural hypotension; management of foot problems and footwear; and exercise, particularly balance, strength, and gait training (AHRQ, 2013; Skelton et al, 2013).
- Assess for adequate lighting and hazards such as throw/area rugs, clutter, cords, and unfitted bedspreads. Suggest safe floor surfaces, such as use of adhesive nonslip strips in tubs/thresholds/areas in which floor height changes; removal of wax from slippery floors; and installing low-pile carpet/nonglazed or nonglossy tiles/wood/linoleum coverings. Stress relocating commonly used items to shelves/drawers in reach; applying remote controls to appliances; and optimizing furniture placement for function, maneuverability, and

T

● = Independent;   ▲ = Collaborative;   **EBN** = Evidence-Based Nursing;   **EB** = Evidence-Based

stability. *Barrier removal promotes safety and accessibility; steady furniture can be used to steady or pull oneself up if a fall occurs (Chase et al, 2012; Skelton et al, 2013).*

- Assess clients for impairment of vision because this can result in a loss of function in activities of daily living and, consequently, result in impaired functional capacity and is an important risk factor for falls. **EB:** *Possible mechanisms to reduce activity restriction and improve mobility include environmental and behavioral interventions delivered by multiple types of health professionals, including OTs (Skelton et al, 2013).*

- Nurses can provide further safety assessments by suggesting installing hand rails in bathrooms and by stairs, ensuring client's slippers and clothes fit properly, and recommending repairing or discarding broken equipment in the home (Taylor et al, 2011).

- ▲ Involve social worker or case manager to educate clients about potential assistive technology, financial cost and benefits, regulations of payers, and local resources. *Information helps clients understand options and cost of services and aids to make informed decisions.*

- ▲ Implement approaches for home care staff and family to safely handle and transfer clients. *Risk of injury is high because people often work alone, without mechanical aids or adjustable beds and in crowded spaces, while giving care (Mayeda-Letourneau, 2014).*

- For further information, refer to care plans for Impaired physical **Mobility** and Impaired **Walking.**

 Client/Family Teaching and Discharge Planning

- Assess for readiness to learn and use teaching modalities conducive to personal learning styles, including written instructions for home use.

- Supervise practice sessions in which client and family apply items such as gait belts, braces, and orthoses. Check skin once aids are removed. *Repetition reinforces motor learning for safety and sound skin integrity.*

- Teach and monitor client/family for consistent use of safety precautions for transfers (e.g., nonskid shoes, correctly placed equipment/chairs, locked brakes, leg rests swiveled away) and for correct performance of transfer or use of lifts/slings. *Promotes safety.*

- Teach client/family how to check brakes on chairs to ensure they engage and how to check tires for adequate air pressure; advise routine inspection and annual tune-up of devices. *Long-term use may loosen brakes or cause them to slip; brakes work only if they make sound contact with tire or wheel. Pneumatic tires must be adequately inflated.*

- Offer information on safe use of shower and commode chairs to prevent discomfort, pressure, and falls during transfer, transport, care, and hygiene.

- For further information, refer to the care plans for Impaired physical **Mobility,** Impaired **Walking,** and Impaired wheelchair **Mobility.**

REFERENCES

Agency for Healthcare Research and Quality, U.S. Department of Health and Human Services. (2013). *Geriatrics: Percentage of patients aged 65 and older with a history of falls who had a plan of care for falls documented within 12 months.* Retrieved from https://www.guidelinecentral.com/share/quality-measures/49449. (Accessed 20 January 2019).

Agency for Healthcare Research and Quality, U.S. Department of Health and Human Services. (2015). *Geriatrics: Percentage of patients aged 65 and older discharged from any inpatient facility (e.g., hospital, skilled nursing facility, or rehabilitation facility) and seen within 30 days of discharge in the office by the physician, prescribing practitioner, registered nurse, or clinical pharmacist who had reconciliation of the discharge medications with the current medication list in the outpatient medical record documented.* Retrieved from https://www.guidelinecentral.com/share/quality-measures/49444#h2_measure-domain. (Accessed 20 January 2019).

American Nurses Association. (2013). *Safe patient handling and mobility: Interprofessional national standards.* Spring Field, MD. Nursebooks. Retrieved from http://www.nursesbooks.org/ebooks/download/SPHM-Standards.pdf. (Accessed 1 January 2018).

Boynton, T., Kelly, L., & Perez, A. (2014). Implementing a mobility assessment tool for nurses. *Am Nurse Today, 9*(9), 13–16.

Cameron, I. D., Murray, G. R., Gillespie, L. D., et al. (2012). Interventions for preventing falls in older people in nursing care facilities and hospitals. *Cochrane Database of Systematic Reviews,* (1), CD005465.

Cameron, S., Ball, I., Cepinskas, G., et al. (2015). Early mobilization in the critical care unit: A review of adult and pediatric literature. *Journal of Critical Care, 30,* 664–672.

Centers for Disease Control and Prevention. (2015). *Safe patient handling.* Retrieved from http://www.cdc.gov/niosh/topics/safepatient/. (Accessed January 2, 2018).

Chase, C., Mann, K., Wasek, S., et al. (2012). Systematic review of the effect of home modification and fall prevention programs on falls and the performance of community-dwelling older adults. *American Journal of Occupational Therapy, 66*(3), 284–291.

Choi, S. D., & Brings, K. (2015). Work-related musculoskeletal risks associated with nurses and nursing assistants handling overweight and obese patients: A literature review. *Work (Reading, Mass.), 53*(2), 439–448.

• = Independent;   ▲ = Collaborative;   **EBN** = Evidence-Based Nursing;   **EB** = Evidence-Based

Clark, P. J. (2014). The Role of the Built Environment and Assistive Devices for Outdoor Mobility in Later Life. *Journals of Gerontology, Series B: Psychological Sciences and Social Sciences, 69*(7), S8–S15.

Cohen, M. H., et al. (2010). *Patient handling and movement assessments: a white paper,* The Facility Guideline Institute. Retrieved from http://www.wsha.org/wp-content/uploads/Worker-Safety_4-Equipment-needs-FGI_PHAMA_whitepaper_042810.pdf. (Accessed 2 January 2018).

Darragh, A., Shiyko, M., Margulis, H., et al. (2015). Effects of a safe patient handling and mobility program on patient self-care outcomes. *The American Journal of Occupational Therapy, 68*(5), 589–596.

Degelau, J., Belz, M., Bungum, L., et al. (2012). *Prevention of falls (acute care): Health care protocol.* Bloomington, MN: Institute for Clinical Systems Improvement (ICSI). Retrieved from file:///C:/Users/mbfma/Downloads/Falls-Interactive0412.pdf. (Accessed 2 January 2018).

Hallmark, B., Mechan, P., & Shores, L. (2015). Ergonomics: Safe patient handling and mobility. *The Nursing Clinics of North America, 50,* 153–166.

Hillrom. (2018). *Bedside mobility assessment tool.* Retrieved from https://library.hill-rom.com/Clinical-Programs/Safe-Transfers-and-Movement-Program/Design-Your-Program/BMAT--Bedside-Mobility-Assessment-Tool-For-Nurses/. (Accessed January 2, 2018).

Hoeman, S. P., Liszner, L., & Alverzo, J. (2008). Functional mobility with activities of daily living. In S. P. Hoeman (Ed.), *Rehabilitation nursing: Process, application, and outcomes* (4th ed.). St Louis: Mosby.

Hopkins, R. O., Mitchell, L., Thomsen, G. E., et al. (2016). Implementing a mobility program to minimize post-intensive care syndrome. *AACN Advanced Critical Care, 27*(2), 187–203.

Kalisch, B. J., Dabney, B. W., & Lee, S. (2013). Safety of mobilizing hospitalized adults: Review of the literature. *Journal of Nursing Care Quality, 28*(2), 162–168.

Kearon, C., et al. (2017). Antithrombotic Therapy for VTE Disease: CHEST Guideline and Expert Panel Report. *CHEST 2016, 149*(2), 315–352.

Low, F., Fletcher, J., Goodenough, B., et al. (2015). A systematic review of interventions to change staff care practices in order to improve resident outcomes in nursing homes. *PLoS ONE, 10*(11), e0140711. doi:10.1371/journal.pone.0140711. Retrieved from https://www.ncbi.nlm.nih.gov/pmc/articles/PMC4641718/pdf/pone.0140711.pdf. (Accessed January 2, 2018).

Mayeda-Letourneau, J. (2014). Safe patient handling and movement: A literature review. *Rehabilitation Nursing, 39,* 123–129.

Riskowski, J., Dufour, A. B., & Hannan, M. T. (2011). Arthritis, foot pain and shoe wear. *Current Opinion in Rheumatology, 23*(2), 148–155.

Schubert, T. E. (2011). Evidence-based exercise prescription for balance and falls prevention: A current review of the literature. *Journal of Geriatric Physical Therapy (2001), 34*(3), 100–108.

Skelton, D. A., et al. (2013). Environmental and behavioural interventions for reducing physical activity limitation in community-dwelling visually impaired older people. *Cochrane Database of Systematic Review,* (6), CD009233. doi:10.1002/14651858.CD009233.pub2.

Stiller, K. (2013). Physiotherapy in intensive care: An updated systematic review. *Chest, 144,* 825–847.

Taylor, C. R., et al. (2011). Safety, security and emergency preparedness. In C. R. Taylor, et al. (Eds.), *Fundamentals of nursing: The art and science of nursing care* (7th ed.). Philadelphia: Lippincott Williams & Wilkins.

Risk for physical Trauma   *Julianne E. Doubet, BSN, RN, EMT-B*

NANDA-I

Definition

Vulnerable to accidental tissue injury (e.g., wound, burn, fracture), which may compromise health.

Risk Factors

External

Absence of call for aid device; absence of stairway gate; absence of window guard; access to weapon; bathing in very hot water; bed in high position; children riding in front seat of car; defective appliance; delay in ignition of gas appliance; dysfunctional call for aid device; electrical hazard (e.g., faulty plug, frayed wire, overloaded outlet/fuse box); exposure to corrosive product; exposure to dangerous machinery; exposure to radiation; exposure to toxic chemical; extremes of environmental temperature; flammable object (e.g., clothing, toys); gas leak; grease on stove; high-crime neighborhood; icicles hanging from roof; inadequate stair rails; inadequately stored combustible (e.g., matches, oily rags); inadequately stored corrosive (e.g., lye); insufficient lighting; insufficient protection from heat source; misuse of headgear (e.g., hard hat, motorcycle helmet); misuse of seat restraint; insufficient antislip material in bathroom; nonuse of seat restraints; obstructed passageway; playing with dangerous object; playing with explosive; pot handle facing front of stove; proximity to vehicle pathway (e.g., driveway, railroad track); slippery floor; smoking in bed; smoking near oxygen; struggling with restraints; unanchored electric wires; unsafe operation of heavy equipment (e.g., excessive speed while intoxicated with required eyewear); unsafe road; unsafe walkway; use of cracked dishware; use of throw rugs; use of unstable chair; use of unstable ladder; wearing loose clothing around open flame

● = Independent;   ▲ = Collaborative;   EBN = Evidence-Based Nursing;   EB = Evidence-Based

Internal

Alteration in cognitive functioning; alteration in sensation (e.g., resulting from spinal cord injury, diabetes mellitus); decrease in eye–hand coordination; decrease in muscle coordination; economically disadvantaged; emotional disturbance; history of trauma (e.g., physical, psychological, sexual); impaired balance; insufficient knowledge of safety precautions; insufficient vision; weakness

NOC (Nursing Outcomes Classification)

Suggested NOC Outcomes

Risk Control; Fall Prevention Behavior

Example NOC Outcome with Indicators

Accomplishes **Risk Control** as evidenced by the following indicators: Acknowledges risk/Develops effective risk-control strategies/Follows selected risk control strategies. (Rate the outcome and indicators of **Risk Control:** 1 = never demonstrated; 2 = rarely demonstrated; 3 = sometimes demonstrated; 4 = often demonstrated; 5 = consistently demonstrated [see Section I].)

Client Outcomes

Client Will (Specify Time Frame)

- Remain free from trauma
- Explain actions that can be taken to prevent trauma

NIC (Nursing Interventions Classification)

Suggested NIC Interventions

Environmental Management: Safety; Skin Surveillance

Example NIC Activities—Environmental Management

Provide family/significant other with information about making home environment safe for client; Remove harmful objects from the environment

---

Nursing Interventions and *Rationales*

- Provide vision aids for visually impaired clients. EB: *Low-vision rehabilitation enables people to restart and/or maintain the capability of performing the tasks of daily living (Virgili et al, 2013).*
- Assist the client with ambulation. Encourage the client to use assistive devices in activities of daily living (ADLs) as needed. EB: *Studies reviewed by Edelstein (2013) have shown the advantages, if used correctly, of using time-honored assistive devices (e.g., crutches, walker).*
- Evaluate client's risk for burn injury. EBN: *Grant (2013) stated that the very young and the elderly are at an increased risk for burn injuries compared with any other age group.* EBN: *It is apparent to Goodarzi et al (2014) in their research that there is a continuing need for further safety education and the utilization of environmental safety measures to reduce burn trauma.*
- Assess the client for causes of impaired cognition. EB: *Adults with intellectual disabilities are likely to have an elevated risk for traumatic injury compared with the general populace (Finlayson et al, 2014).*
- Provide assistive devices in the home. EBN: *According to Johnston et al (2014), shared conclusions between the health care giver and the client with disabilities allows the client to choose the best assistive devices and services that are vital to achieving their goals of education, community living, and employment.*
- ▲ Question the client concerning his or her sense of safety. EBN: *In their study, Edwards et al (2014) stated that clients who wish to remain at home at the end of life are at increased risk for trauma caused by declining cognitive and/or physical capabilities, environmental dangers, and concerns with caregivers.*
- ▲ Assess for a substance abuse problem and refer to appropriate resources for drug and alcohol education. EB: *According to Choi, DiNitto, and Marti (2014), older adults who abuse alcohol and/or illicit drugs should be sent to the most appropriate service that meets his or her needs, both for rehabilitation and any mental health challenges that may be involved.* EB: *Although drinking and driving among student drivers has declined in*

● = Independent;   ▲ = Collaborative;   EBN = Evidence-Based Nursing;   EB = Evidence-Based

recent years, driving after the use of marijuana has increased; therefore O'Malley and Johnston (2013) believed that more attention should be focused on preventing those under the influence of illicit drugs from driving.

- Review drug profile for potential side effects that may inhibit performance of ADLs. *In their study of pain management in the elderly, Veal and Peterson (2015) found that older adults are at increased risk for detrimental medication side effects caused by changes in drug metabolism and to polypharmacy that may put them at risk for drug interactions.*
- See care plans for Risk for **Aspiration,** Risk for **Falls,** Impaired **Home** maintenance, Risk for **Injury,** Risk for **Poisoning,** and Risk for **Suffocation.**

 ### Pediatric

- Assess the client's socioeconomic status. EB: *The presently used evaluations that measure evidence of adverse childhood experiences (ACEs) may be insufficient to recognize the extent of adversity to which low-income urban children are exposed (Wade et al, 2014).*
- Never leave young children unsupervised. EB: *According to van Beelen et al (2014), the death, disability, and loss of quality of life among young children is directly related to injuries that occur in the home.*
- Keep flammable and potentially flammable articles out of reach of young children. EB: *Infants and toddlers who scald themselves by spilling hot liquids on themselves or touching irons and hair straighteners are a main cause for concern for targeted prevention (Kemp et al, 2014).* EBN: *Hollywood and O'Neill (2014) maintained that nurses working with children in hospitals, schools, and the community can connect with parents, families, school staff, and children to offer professional advice and health and safety guidance for burn prevention.*
- Lock up harmful objects such as guns. EB: *Easy access to firearms in the home is responsible for injury to thousands of children in the United States (Barton & Kologi, 2014).* EB: *There is an increased risk for childhood injury when firearms are left loaded and unlocked (Schwebel et al, 2014).*

 ### Geriatric

- Assess the geriatric client's cognitive level of functioning. EB: *Patel et al (2014) agreed that the occurrence of neurocognitive disorders can be an obstacle to the capability of older adults to perform ADLs and this deficit will continue to escalate with age.*
- Assess for routine eye examinations. EBN: *The older client may find it difficult to adjust to vision loss and aging because of the psychological, functional, social, and health implications that play a significant role in the process (Mac Cobb, 2013).*
- Perform a home safety assessment and recommend the following preventive measures: keep electrical cords out of the flow of traffic; remove small rugs or make sure they are slip resistant; increase lighting in hallways and other dark areas; place a light in the bathroom; keep towels, curtains, and other items that might catch fire away from the stove; store harmful products away from food products; provide at least one grab bar in tubs and showers; check prescribed medications for appropriate labels; store medications in original containers or in a dispenser of some type (e.g., egg carton, 7-day plastic dispenser). If the client cannot administer medications according to directions, secure someone to administer medications. Mark stove knobs with bright colors (yellow or red) and outline the borders of steps. EBN: *As part of a person-centered, evidenced-based approach, a professional case manager/care coordinator can perform a thorough assessment of the client's needs and will design and put into operation an all-inclusive care plan to meet the clinical, psychosocial, and environmental requirements of the client (Johansson & Harkey, 2014).*
- Discourage driving at night. EB: *Gruber et al (2013) suggested that there is an increasing number of older adults who continue to drive, and the population of drivers who are affected by deteriorating night vision is increasing.*
- Encourage the client to participate in resistance and impact exercise programs as tolerated. EB: *In their review of current evidence, Carvalho et al (2014) suggested that physical activity may not only aid in improving cognitive function in older adults, but it could also play a part in delaying the development of cognitive impairment in the older adult.*

 ### Client/Family Teaching and Discharge Planning

- Educate the family regarding age-appropriate child safety precautions, environmental safety precautions, and intervention in an emergency. EB: *Safety education for parents of young children is essential in the prevention of accidental injuries in and/or around the home (van Beelen et al, 2013).* EB: *In their study, Morrongiello, McArthur, and Bell (2014) found that to decrease a child's risk of harm, the child must first understand the safety issue.*

● = Independent;   ▲ = Collaborative;   EBN = Evidence-Based Nursing;   EB = Evidence-Based

- Teach the family to assess the child care provider's knowledge regarding child safety. **EB:** *Home safety interventions not only aid in reducing children's injuries, but they also enhance the general safety of the home (Kendrick et al, 2013).*
- Educate the client and family regarding helmet use during recreation and sports activities. **EB:** *It has been proven time and time again that wearing a bicycle helmet has averted or reduced the risk of serious head injuries (Basch et al, 2014).*
- Encourage the proper use of car seats and safety belts. **EB:** *Himle and Wright (2014) stated that child passenger safety restraint, when used correctly, can diminish the risk of severe injury and/or death in motor vehicle crashes.*
- Teach parents to restrict driving for teens. **EB:** *According to Taubman et al (2014), research studies have shown that parents are the most important influence on young people's driving conduct.*
- Teach parents the importance of monitoring children after school. **EB:** *In a study by Freisthler et al (2014), children who are not supervised appropriately, either by inattentive parents and/or caregivers, could be considered neglected.*
- Teach firearm safety. **EB:** *According to Schwebel et al (2014), firearms in the home that are loaded and unlocked are sources of increased risks for trauma.* **EB:** *Health care professionals must have knowledge and skills to address safe gun ownership in older adults (Pinholt et al, 2014).*
- For further information, refer to care plans for Risk for **Aspiration,** Risk for **Falls,** Impaired **Home** maintenance, Risk for **Injury,** Risk for **Poisoning,** and Risk for **Suffocation.**

REFERENCES

Barton, B. K., & Kologi, S. M. (2014). Why do we keep them there? A qualitative assessment of firearms storage practices. *Journal of Pediatric Nursing*, pii, 14, 208–205.

Basch, C. H., Ethan, D., Rajan, S., et al. (2014). Helmet use among users of the Citi Bike bicycle-sharing program: A pilot study in New York City. *Journal of Community Health*, 39, 503–507.

Carvalho, A., Rea, I. M., Pariman, T., et al. (2014). Physical activity and cognitive function in individuals over 60 years of age: A systematic review. *Journal of Clinical Interventions in Aging*, 12, 661–682. eCollection 2014.

Choi, N. G., DiNitto, D. M., & Marti, C. N. (2014). Risk factors for self-reported driving under the influence of alcohol and illicit drugs among older adults. *The Gerontologist*, 56(2), 282–291.

Edelstein, J. E. (2013). Assistive devices for ambulation. *Physical Medicine and Rehabilitation Clinics of North America*, 29, 291–303.

Edwards, S. B., Galanis, E., McGarvey, K., et al. (2014). Safety issues at the end of life in the home setting. *Home Health Nurse*, 22, 398–401.

Finlayson, J., Jackson, A., Mantry, D., et al. (2014). The provision of aids and adaptations, risk assessments and incident reporting and recording procedures in relation to injury prevention in adults with intellectual disabilities: Cohort study. *Journal of Intellectual Disability Research*, 59(6), 519–529.

Freisthler, B., Johnson-Motoyama, M., & Kepple, N. J. (2014). Inadequate child supervision: The role of alcohol outlet density, parent drinking behaviors, and social support. *Children and Youth Service Review*, 1, 75–84.

Goodarzi, M., Reisi-Dehkordi, N., Darabeigi, R., et al. (2014). An epidemiologic study of burns: Standards of care and patient education. *Iranian Journal of Nursing and Midwifery Research*, 19, 385–389.

Grant, E. J. (2013). Preventing burns in the elderly. *Home Healthcare Nurse*, 31, 561–575.

Gruber, R. M., Mosimann, U. P., Muri, R. M., et al. (2013). Vision and night driving abilities of elderly drivers. *Traffic Injury Prevention*, 14, 477–485.

Himle, M. B., & Wright, K. A. (2014). Behavior skills training to improve installation and use of child passenger safety restraints. *Journal of Implied Behavior Analysis*, 47, 549–559.

Hollywood, E., & O'Neill, T. (2014). Assessment and management of scalds and burns in children. *Nursing Children and Young People*, 26, 28–33.

Johansson, B., & Harkey, J. (2014). Care coordination in long term home- and community-based care. *Home Healthcare Nurse*, 32, 470–475.

Johnston, P., Currie, L. M., Drynan, D., et al. (2014). Getting it "right": How collaborative relationships between people with disabilities and professionals can lead to acquisition of needed assistive technology. *Disability and Rehabilitation: Assistive Technology*, 9, 421–431.

Kemp, A. M., Jones, S., Lawson, Z., et al. (2014). Patterns of burns and scalds in children. *Archives of Diseases in Childhood*, 99, 316–321 [Epub 2014 Feb 3].

Kendrick, D., Mulvaney, C. A., Yee, L., et al. (2013). Parenting interventions for the prevention of unintentional injuries in childhood. *Cochrane Database of Systematic Reviews*, (3), CD006020.

Mac Cobb, S. (2013). Mobility restriction and co-morbidity in vision impaired individuals living in the community. *British Journal of Nursing*, 18, 608–613.

Morrongiello, B. A., McArthur, B. A., & Bell, M. (2014). Managing children's risk of injury in the home: Does parental teaching about home safety reduce young children's hazard interactions? *Accident Analysis and Prevention*, 71, 194–200.

O'Malley, P. M., & Johnson, L. D. (2013). Driving after drug or alcohol use by US high school seniors, 2001-2011. *American Journal of Public Health*, 103, 2027–2034.

Patel, D., Syed, Q., Messenger-Rapport, B. J., et al. (2014). Firearms in frail hands: An ADL or public health crisis. *American Journal of Alzheimer's Disease and Other Dementias*, pii: 1533317514545867.

Pinholt, G. M., Mitchell, J. D., Butler, J. H., et al. (2014). "Is there a gun in the home?" Assessing the risks of gun ownership in older adults. *Journal of the American Geriatric Society*, 62, 1142–1146.

Schwebel, D. C., Lewis, T., Simon, S. R., et al. (2014). Prevalence and correlation of firearm ownership in the homes of fifth graders: Birmingham, Ala., Houston, Tex., and Los Angeles, Ca. *Health Education and Behavior*, 41, 299–306.

Taubman, B. A. O., Musicant, O., Lotan, T., et al. (2014). The contribution of parents' driving behavior, family climate for road

● = Independent;   ▲ = Collaborative;   **EBN** = Evidence-Based Nursing;   **EB** = Evidence-Based

safety, and parent-targeted intervention to young male driving behavior. *Accident Analysis and Prevention, 2*, 296–301.

van Beelen, M. E., Beirens, T. M., den Hartog, P., et al. (2014). Effectiveness of web-based tailored advice on parents' child safety behaviors randomized controlled trial. *Journal of Medical Internet Research, 16*, e17.

van Beelen, M. E., Vogel, I., Bieriens, T. M., et al. (2013). Web-based e health to support counseling in routine well-child care: Pilot study of E-Health4Uth home safety. *Journal of Medical Internet Research, 2*, e9.

Veal, F., & Peterson, G. (2015). Pain in the frail elderly patient: Does tapentadol have a role. *Drugs and Aging, 32*(6), 419–426.

Virgili, G., Acosta, R., Grover, L. L., et al. (2013). Reading aids for adults with low vision. *Cochrane Database of Systematic Reviews*, (10), CD003303.

Wade, R., Shea, J. A., Ruben, D., et al. (2014). Adverse childhood experiences of low-income, urban youth. *Pediatrics, 134*, 13–20.

Unilateral Neglect   *Lori M. Rhudy, PhD, RN, CNRN, ACNS-BC*

NANDA-I

Definition

Impairment in sensory and motor response, mental representation, and spatial attention of the body, and the corresponding environment, characterized by inattention to one side and overattention to the opposite side. Left-side neglect is more severe and persistent than right-side neglect.

Defining Characteristics

Alteration in safety behavior on neglected side; disturbance of sound lateralization; failure to dress neglected side; failure to eat food from portion of plate on neglected side; failure to groom neglected side; failure to move eyes in the neglected hemisphere; failure to move head in the neglected hemisphere; failure to move limbs in the neglected hemisphere; failure to move trunk in the neglected hemisphere; failure to notice people approaching from the neglected side; hemianopsia; impaired performance on line cancellation, line bisection, and target cancellation tests; left hemiplegia from cerebrovascular accident; marked deviation of the eyes to stimuli on the non-neglected side; marked deviation of the trunk to stimuli on the non-neglected side; omission of drawing on the neglected side; perseveration; representational neglect; substitution of letters to form alternative words when reading; transfer of pain sensation to the non-neglected side; unaware of positioning of neglected limb; unilateral visuospatial neglect; use of vertical half of page only when writing

Related Factors

To be developed

Associated Condition

Brain injury

NOC   (Nursing Outcomes Classification)

Suggested NOC Outcomes

Body Image; Body Positioning: Self-Initiated; Mobility; Self-Care: Activities of Daily Living (ADLs)

Example **NOC** Outcome with Indicators
Mobility as evidenced by the following indicators: Balance/Coordination/Gait/Muscle movement. (Rate the outcome and indicators of **Mobility:** 1 = severely compromised, 2 = substantially compromised, 3 = moderately compromised, 4 = mildly compromised, 5= not compromised [see Section I].)

Client Outcomes

Client Will (Specify Time Frame)

- Use techniques that can be used to minimize unilateral neglect (UN)
- Care for both sides of the body appropriately and keep affected side free from harm
- Return to the highest functioning level possible based on personal goals and abilities
- Remain free from injury

● = Independent;   ▲ = Collaborative;   EBN = Evidence-Based Nursing;   EB = Evidence-Based

| NIC | (Nursing Interventions Classification) |

Suggested NIC Intervention

Unilateral Neglect Management

| **Example NIC Activities—Unilateral Neglect Management** |
| Ensure that affected extremities are properly and safely and positioned; Rearrange the environment to use the right or left visual field |

Nursing Interventions and *Rationales*

▲ Assess the client for signs of UN (e.g., not washing, shaving, or dressing one side of the body; sitting or lying inappropriately on affected arm or leg; failing to respond to environmental stimuli contralateral to the side of lesion; eating food on only one side of plate; or failing to look to one side of the body). EB: *Many tests for UN exist, but there is no consensus about which is the most valid. Joint assessments of that include both clinical observation and precise testing perform better than either used alone (Grattan & Woodbury, 2017).* EB: *In one study, 67.8% of patients had UN on admission to inpatient rehabilitation (Chen et al, 2015).*

▲ Collaborate with health care provider for referral to a rehabilitation team (including, but not limited to, rehabilitation clinical nurse specialist, physical medicine and rehabilitation health care provider, neuropsychologist, occupational therapist, physical therapist, and speech and language pathologist) for continued help in dealing with UN. EB: *There is some evidence that rehabilitation for unilateral spatial neglect using tools such as visual scanning and prism adaptation improves function, but their effect on disability is not clear. Further studies are needed (Gillen et al, 2015).*

• Use the principles of rehabilitation to progressively increase the client's ability to compensate for UN by using assistive devices, feedback, and support. EB: *Studies demonstrated that recovery from UN generally resolves within 1 month of stroke, but it can still be detectable after 3 months and/or at discharge from inpatient rehabilitation (Chan & Man, 2013; Chen et al, 2015).*

• Teach the client to be aware of the problem and modify behavior and environment. EB: *Awareness of the environment decreases risk of injury. There is some evidence that use of scanning techniques may decrease visual neglect (Chan & Man, 2013).*

• Set up the environment so that essential activity is on the unaffected side:
  ○ Place the client's personal items within view and on the unaffected side.
  ○ Position the bed so that client is approached from the unaffected side.
  ○ Monitor and assist the client to achieve adequate food and fluid intake.
  Helps in focusing attention and aids in maintenance of safety.

• Implement fall prevention interventions. *Clients with right hemisphere brain damage are twice as likely to fall as those with left hemisphere damage.* EB: *Patients with poor timed up and go (TUG) performance, longer times since stroke onset, and right-hemisphere injury have particularly high fall rates (Pinto et al, 2014).* EB: *UN is significantly related to falls in patients with a neurological diagnosis (Bergman & Papendick, 2014).*

• Position affected extremity in a safe and functional manner. EB: *A study found that musculoskeletal pain, shoulder subluxation, spasticity, and joint contracture were among the most common complications during the first year after stroke (Kuptniratsaikul et al, 2013).* EB: *Clients with neglect had significantly lower functional independence measure (FIM) scores (Chen et al, 2015).*

▲ Collaborate closely with rehabilitation professionals to identify and reinforce therapies aimed at reducing neglect symptoms. *Techniques such as scanning, visual cuing approaches, limb activation strategies, prisms, mirror therapy, and music listening are being used to treat UN (Pernet, Jughters, & Kerckhofs, 2013; Tsai et al, 2013; Pandian et al, 2014), but the evidence is limited and inconclusive on the most effective approach (Azouvi, Jacquin-Courtois, & Luaute, 2017), and the type of neglect may affect outcomes associated with each technique.*

Home Care

• Many of the previously listed interventions may be adapted for use in the home care setting.
• Position bed at home so that client gets out of bed on unaffected side. *Positioning the bed so that the client gets out on the unaffected side can increase safety.*

• = Independent; ▲ = Collaborative; EBN = Evidence-Based Nursing; EB = Evidence-Based

Client/Family Teaching and Discharge Planning

- Engage discharge planning specialists for comprehensive assessment and planning early in the client's stay. EB: *Clients with UN have longer lengths of stay and more difficulty resuming ADLs (Chan & Man, 2013).* EB: *In one study 67.8% of patients on admission and 47.2% on discharge had symptoms of spatial neglect (Chen et al, 2015).* EB: *Neglect scores at admission negatively predicted FIM scores at discharge (Chen et al, 2015).*
- Encourage family participation in care. EB: *Severity of stroke and presence of UN were significant prognostic indicators for inability to gain independence in ADLs (Morone, Paolucci, & Iosa, 2015; Semrau et al, 2015).*
- Explain pathology and symptoms of UN to both the client and family. *Family members may not understand that inattention is a complication of the neurological injury.*
- Teach the client how to scan regularly to check the position of body parts and to regularly turn head from side to side for safety when ambulating, using a wheelchair, or doing self-care tasks. EB: *In one study, incorporating task-specific treatments, such as eating food from a plate and grooming, improved functional outcome and reduced neglect symptoms (Patole et al, 2015).* EB: *One study found that effectiveness of cues depended on severity of neglect (Wansard et al, 2014).*
- Teach caregivers to cue the client to the environment.

REFERENCES

Azouvi, P., Jacquin-Courtois, S., & Luaute, J. (2017). Rehabilitation of neglect: Evidence-based medicine. *Annals of Physical and Rehabilitation Medicine, 60*(3), 191–197. doi:10.1016/j.rehab.2016.10.006.

Bergman, K., & Papendick, L. (2014). Falls in the neurologic illness population. *Journal of Trauma Nursing, 21*(4), 182–185. doi:10.1097/JTN.0000000000000060.

Chan, D. Y. W., & Man, D. W. K. (2013). Unilateral neglect in stroke: A comparative study. *Topics in Geriatric Rehabilitation, 29*(2), 126–134. doi:10.1097/TGR.0b013e31827ea7c9.

Chen, P., Chen, C. C., Hreha, K., et al. (2015). Kessler Foundation Neglect Assessment Process uniquely measures spatial neglect during activities of daily living. *Archives of Physical Medicine and Rehabilitation, 96*(5), 869–876. doi:10.1016/j.apmr.2014.10.023.

Gillen, G., Nilsen, D., Attridge, J., et al. (2015). Effectiveness of interventions to improve occupational performance of people with cognitive impairments after stroke: An evidence-based review. *The American Journal of Occupational Therapy, 69*(1), 1–9. doi:10.5014/ajot.2015.012138.

Grattan, E., & Woodbury, M. L. (2017). Do neglect assessments detect neglect differently? *The American Journal of Occupational Therapy, 71*(3), 1–7. doi:10.5014/ajot.2017.025015.

Kuptniratsaikul, V., Kovindha, A., Suethanapornkul, S., et al. (2013). Long-term morbidities in stroke survivors: A prospective multicenter study of Thai stroke rehabilitation registry. *BMC Geriatrics, 33*(3). doi:10.1186/1471-2318-13-33.

Morone, G., Paolucci, S., & Iosa, M. (2015). In what daily activities do patients achieve independence after stroke? *Journal of Stroke and Cerebrovascular Diseases, 24*(8), 1931–1937. doi:10.1016/j.jstrokecerebrovasdis.2015.05.006.

Pandian, J. D., Arora, R., Kaur, P., et al. (2014). Mirror therapy in unilateral neglect after stroke (MUST trial): A randomized controlled trial. *Neurology, 83*(11), 1012–1017. doi:10.1212/WNL.0000000000000773.

Patole, R. R., Kulkani, V. N., Rairikar, S. A., et al. (2015). Effect of task specific treatment in patients with unilateral neglect. *Indian Journal of Physiotherapy and Occupational Therapy, 9*(1), 74–77. doi:10.5958/0973-5674.2015.00016.7.

Pernet, L., Jughters, A., & Kerckhofs, E. (2013). The effectiveness of different treatment modalities for the rehabilitation of unilateral neglect in stroke patients: A systematic review. *Neurorehabilitation, 33*, 611–620. doi:10.3233/NRE-130986.

Pinto, E. B., Nascimento, C., Marinho, C., et al. (2014). Risk factors associated with falls in adult patients after stroke living in the community: Baseline data from a stroke cohort in Brazil. *Topics in Stroke Rehabilitation, 21*(3), 220–227. Retrieved from http://dx.doi.org/10.1310/tsr2103-220.

Semrau, J. A., Wang, J. C., Herter, T. M., et al. (2015). Relationship between visuospatial neglect and kinesthetic deficits after stroke. *Neurorehabilitation and Neural Repair, 29*(4), 318–328. doi:10.1177/1545968314545173.

Tsai, P.-L., Chen, M.-C., Huang, Y., et al. (2013). Listening to classical music ameliorates unilateral neglect after stroke. *The American Journal of Occupational Therapy, 67*(3), 328–335. doi:10.5014/ajot.2013.006312.

Wansard, M., Barolomeo, P., Vanderaspoilden, V., et al. (2014). Can the exploration of left space be induced implicitly in unilateral neglect? *Consciousness and Cognition, 31*, 115–123. doi:10.1016/j.concog.2014.11.004.

Impaired Urinary elimination

Michelle Acorn, DNP, NP PHC/Adult, BA, BScN/PHCNP, MN/ACNP, GNC(C), CGP

NANDA-I

Definition

Dysfunction in urine elimination.

● = Independent;   ▲ = Collaborative;   EBN = Evidence-Based Nursing;   EB = Evidence-Based

Defining Characteristics

Dysuria; frequent voiding; hesitancy; nocturia; urinary incontinence; urinary retention; urinary urgency

Related Factors

Multiple causality

Associated Condition

Anatomic obstruction; sensory motor impairment; urinary tract infection

NOC   (Nursing Outcomes Classification)

Suggested NOC Outcome

Urinary Elimination

> ### Example NOC Outcome with Indicators
>
> **Urinary Elimination** as evidenced by the following indicators: Urine clarity/urine odor, fluid intake, pain with urination. (Rate the outcome and indicators of **Urinary Elimination:** 1 = severely compromised 2 = substantially compromised, 3 = moderately compromised, 4 = mildly compromised, 5 = not compromised [see Section I].)

Client Outcomes

Client Will (Specify Time Frame)

- State absence of pain or excessive urgency during urination
- Demonstrate voiding frequency no more than every 2 hours

NIC   (Nursing Interventions Classification)

Suggested NIC Intervention

Urinary Elimination Management

> ### Example NIC Activities—Urinary Elimination Management
>
> Monitor urinary elimination, including frequency, consistency, odor, volume, and color, as appropriate; Teach client signs and symptoms of urinary tract infection (UTI)

Nursing Interventions and *Rationales*

- Ask the client about urinary elimination patterns and concerns. Urinary elimination problems have many presenting signs and symptoms. Asking the client questions may help understand the subtle signs and symptoms associated with urinary elimination (Mayo Clinic, 2017).
- Question the client regarding the following:
  - ○ Presence of symptoms such as incontinence, dribbling, frequency, urgency, dysuria, and nocturia
  - ○ Presence of pain in the area of the bladder
  - ○ Pattern of urination and approximate amount
  - ○ Possible aggravating and alleviating factors for urinary problems
- Ask the client to keep a bladder diary/bladder log. EB: *Use of a bladder diary may reduce client discrepancies in recall and is a valuable tool for assessment; short (24-hour) duration of the bladder diary may yield inadequate data, and excessive diary duration reduces compliance (Bright, Drake, & Abrams, 2011).*
- For interventions on urinary incontinence, refer to the following nursing diagnosis care plans as appropriate: Stress urinary **Incontinence,** Urge urinary **Incontinence,** Reflex urinary **Incontinence,** Overflow urinary **Incontinence,** or Functional urinary **Incontinence.**
- ▲ Perform a focused physical assessment including inspecting the perineal skin integrity, percussion, and palpation of the lower abdomen looking for obvious bladder distention or an enlarged kidney. *A palpable kidney or bladder provides direct evidence of a dilated urinary collection system (Policastro, Sinert, & Guerrero, 2014).* If signs of urinary obstruction are present, refer client to a urologist. *Unrelieved obstruction of*

● = Independent;   ▲ = Collaborative;   EBN = Evidence-Based Nursing;   EB = Evidence-Based

urine can result in renal damage, and if severe, renal failure (Policastro, Sinert, & Guerrero, 2014). Refer to the nursing care plan for **Urinary Retention** *if retention is present.*

▲ Check for costovertebral tenderness. *Costovertebral tenderness is seen with pyelonephritis and kidney stones (Gupta & Trautner, 2015; Pietrucha-Dilanchian & Hooton, 2016).*

▲ Review results of urinalysis for the presence of urinary infection such as white blood cells, red blood cells, bacteria, and positive nitrites. If urinalysis results are not available, request a midstream specimen of urine (urine obtained during voiding, discarding the first and last portions) for a urinalysis (Pietrucha-Dilanchian & Hooton, 2016).

▲ If blood or protein is present in the urine, recognize that both hematuria and proteinuria are serious symptoms, and the client should be referred to a urologist to receive a workup to rule out pathology.

● Inquire about the client's history of smoking. **EB:** *Smoking and bladder symptoms in women found that urgency and frequency are three times more common among current than never smokers. Parallel associations suggest dose-related response associations. Nocturia and stress urinary incontinence (SUI) are not associated with smoking. Smoking cessation is recommended (Tahtinen et al, 2011).*

Urinary Tract Infection

▲ Consult the provider for culture and sensitivity testing and antibiotic treatment in the individual with evidence of a symptomatic UTI. *UTI is a transient, reversible condition that is usually associated with urgency or urge urinary incontinence (Nicolle & Norrby, 2016). Eradication of UTI will alleviate or reverse symptoms of suprapubic pressure and discomfort, urgency, daytime voiding frequency, and dysuria (Nicolle & Norrby, 2016).*

▲ Teach the client to recognize symptoms of UTI, such as dysuria that crescendos as the bladder nears complete evacuation; urgency to urinate followed by micturition of only a few drops; suprapubic aching discomfort; malaise; and voiding frequency; sudden exacerbation of urinary incontinence with or without fever, chills, and flank pain. Recognize that a cloudy or malodorous urine, in the absence of other lower urinary tract symptoms, may not indicate the presence of a UTI and that asymptomatic bacteriuria in the older adult does not justify a course of antibiotics. *Asymptomatic bacteriuria may be associated with cloudy or malodorous urine, but these signs alone do not justify antimicrobial therapy when balanced against the potential adverse effects of treatment, including adverse side effects of the various antibiotics and encouragement of colonization of the urine with antibiotic-resistant bacterial strains (Ariathianto, 2011; Nicolle & Norrby, 2016).*

▲ Refer the individual with chronic lower urinary tract pain to a urologist or specialist in the management of pelvic pain. *Bladder pain and storage symptoms, in the absence of an acute urinary infection, may indicate the presence of interstitial cystitis, which is a chronic condition requiring ongoing treatment (Interstitial Cystitis Association, 2017).*

 ### Geriatric

● Evidence for behavioral interventions include the following: (1) prompted voiding is effective in the treatment of daytime symptoms when patients and caregivers comply; (2) prompted voiding is ineffective and should not be used for people who need the assistance of more than one person to transfer, instead manage with "check and change"; (3) promoted voiding should not be continued in people who have less than 20% reduction in wet checks or toilet successfully less than two-thirds of the time after a 3-day trial; and (4) interventions combining toileting, exercise, food, and fluids are effective (Wagg et al, 2014).

● Encourage older women to consume one to two servings of fresh blueberries and consider drinking at least 10 ounces of cranberry juice daily or supplement the diet with cranberry concentrate capsules as ordered. **EB:** *Although the evidence supporting the consumption of cranberry juice or tablets to reduce UTIs is inconclusive (Jepson, Williams, & Craig, 2012; Foxman et al, 2015), some evidence does suggest that the consumption of 8 to 10 ounces of cranberry juice, ascorbic acid (vitamin C) supplement, or an equivalent portion of foods containing whole cranberries or blueberries exerts a bacteriostatic effect on* Escherichia coli, *which is the most common pathogen associated with urinary infection among community-dwelling adult women (Aydin et al, 2014).*

▲ Refer the older woman with recurrent UTIs to her health care provider for possible use of topical estrogen creams for treatment of atrophic vaginal mucosa from decreased hormonal stimulation, which can predispose to UTIs (Aydin et al, 2014; Nicolle & Norrby, 2016).

● Postresidual volumes (PRVs) should be assessed in older women with overactive bladder (OAB). A volume of greater than 200 mL is significant. A history of back or pelvic injury or surgery increases the risk of greater PRV (Park and Palmer, 2015).

▲ Recognize that UTIs in older men are typically associated with prostatic hyperplasia or strictures of the urethra. Refer the client to a urologist (Nicolle & Norrby, 2016).

● Analysis of urinary elimination patterns of clients could help in clinical follow-up of elderly postoperative patients and in the selection of best nursing interventions. **EB:** *A study exploring NOC indictor interrater reliability showed classifications can be useful for monitoring clinical changes related to urinary elimination. High agreements for the indicators of urine odor, leukocytes, nitrates, blood, painful urination, and urinary continence were found (Bitencourt et al, 2016).*

● Practice recommendations when caring for older clients include (1) frailty, not age should guide urinary elimination treatment decisions; (2) caring for individuals with urinary incontinence and cognitive impairment needs to be tailored to the individuals abilities; and (3) be cautious of anticholinergic medications and weigh the risk and benefits for antimuscarinics (Wagg et al, 2014).

 ### Client/Family Teaching and Discharge Planning

● Teach the client/family methods to keep the urinary tract healthy. Refer to Client/Family Teaching in the care plan for Readiness for enhanced **Urinary** elimination.

● Teach the following measures to women to decrease the incidence of UTIs:
  ○ Urinate at appropriate intervals. Do not ignore need to void, which can result in stasis of urine.
  ○ Drink plenty of liquids, especially water. *Drinking water helps dilute the urine, allowing bacteria to be flushed from the urinary tract before an infection can begin (Nicolle & Norrby, 2016).*
  ○ Wipe from front to back. *This helps prevent bacteria in the anal region from spreading to the vagina and urethra.*
  ○ Wear underpants that have a cotton crotch. *This allows air to circulate in the area and decreases moisture in the area, which predisposes to infection.*
  ○ Avoid potentially irritating feminine products. *Using deodorant sprays, bubble baths, or other feminine products, such as douches and powders, in the genital area can irritate the urethra. There are multiple common sense measures that can be used to decrease the incidence of UTIs (Gupta & Trautner, 2015; Mayo Clinic, 2017).*

● Teach the sexually active woman with recurrent UTIs prevention measures including:
  ○ Void after intercourse to flush bacteria out of the urethra and bladder.
  ○ Use a lubricating agent as needed during intercourse to protect the vagina from trauma and decrease the incidence of vaginitis.
  ○ Watch for signs of vaginitis and seek treatment as needed.
  ○ Avoid use of diaphragms with spermicide.

Sexually active women have the highest incidence of UTIs (Nicolle & Norrby, 2016). The vagina and periurethral area can become colonized with organisms from the intestinal flora, such as E. coli, *and increase the risk for UTIs (Gupta & Trautner, 2015; Pietrucha-Dilanchian and Hontoon, 2016).*

● Teach clients with spinal cord injury and neurogenic bladder dysfunction to consider adding cranberry extract tablets or cranberry juice, or fruits containing D-mannose (e.g., apples, oranges, peaches, blueberries) on a daily basis, monitor fluid intake. The client is encouraged to discuss the use of probiotics and antibiotic therapy with the provider for frequent recurrent symptomatic UTIs. **EB:** *Limited evidence suggested that clients who regularly consume cranberry extract tablets experience fewer UTIs than clients who do not routinely consume cranberry extract tablets (Jepson et al, 2012; Keifer, 2013; Foxman et al, 2015). Additionally, clients with spinal cord injury and neurogenic bladder dysfunction are at higher risk for UTI, and more frequent monitoring of symptomatic infection is necessary (Goetz & Klausner, 2014).*

● Teach all persons to recognize hematuria and to promptly seek care if this symptom occurs.

REFERENCES

Ariathianto, Y. (2011). Asymptomatic bacteriuria—Prevalence in the elderly population. *Australian Family Physician, 40*(10), 805–809.

Aydin, A., Ahmed, K., Zaman, I., et al. (2014). Recurrent urinary tract infections in women. *International Urogynecology Journal, 26*(6), 795–804.

Bright, E., Drake, M. J., & Abrams, P. (2011). Urinary diaries: Evidence for the development and validation of diary content, format, and duration. *Neurourology and Urodynamics, 30*(3), 348–352.

Bitencourt, G. R., Alves, L., Santana, F., et al. (2016). Agreement between experts regarding assessment of postoperative urinary elimination nursing outcomes in elderly patients. *International Journal of Nursing Knowledge, 27*(3), 143–147.

Foxman, B., Cronewett, A. E., Spino, C., et al. (2015). Cranberry juice capsules and urinary tract infection after surgery: Results of a randomized trial. *American Journal of Obstetrics and Gynecology, 213*(2), 194.e1–194.e8. doi:10.1016/j.ajog.2015.04.003.

Goetz, L. L., & Klausner, A. P. (2014). Strategies for prevention of urinary tract infections in neurogenic bladder dysfunction. *Physical*

● = Independent;   ▲ = Collaborative;   EBN = Evidence-Based Nursing;   EB = Evidence-Based

Medicine and Rehabilitation Clinics of North America, *25*(3), 605–618, viii.

Gupta, K., & Trautner, B. (2015). Urinary tract infections, pyelonephritis, and prostatitis. In D. L. Longo, et al. (Eds.), *Harrison's principles of internal medicine* (19th ed.). New York: McGraw-Hill.

Interstitial Cystitis Association. (2017). *Pain and IC*. Retrieved from http://www.ichelp.org/Page.aspx?pid=821. (Accessed 31 October 2017).

Jepson, R. G., Williams, G., & Craig, J. C. (2012). Cranberries for preventing urinary tract infections. *Cochrane Database of Systematic Reviews*, (10), CD001321.

Keifer, D. (2013). *Vitamins and supplements: D-mannose*. WebMD. Retrieved from http://www.webmd.com/vitamins-and-supplements/d-mannose-uses-and-risks. (Accessed 31 October 2017).

Mayo Clinic. (2017). *Prevention of urinary tract infections*. Retrieved from http://www.mayoclinic.com/health/urinary-tract-infection/DS00286/DSECTION=prevention. (Accessed 31 October 2017).

Nicolle, L. E., & Norrby, S. R. (2016). Approach to the patient with urinary tract infection. In L. Goldman & A. Schafer (Eds.), *Goldman's Cecil medicine* (25th ed., pp. 1872–1876). St Louis: Saunders/Elsevier.

Park, J., & Palmer, M. (2015). Factors associated with incomplete bladder emptying in older women with overactive bladder symptoms. *Journal of the American Geriatrics Society*, *63*, 1426–1431.

Pietrucha-Dilanchian, P., & Hooton, T. M. (2016). Diagnosis, treatment and prevention of urinary track infection. *Microbiology Spectrum*, *4*(6). doi:10.1128/microbiolspec.UTI-0021-2015.

Policastro, M., Sinert, R. H., & Guerrero, P. (2014). *Urinary obstruction. Medscape Reference*. Retrieved from http://emedicine.medscape.com/article/778456-overview. (Accessed 31 October 2017).

Tahtinen, R. M., Auvinen, A., Cartwithgt, R., et al. (2011). Smoking and bladder symptoms in women. *Obstetrics and Gynecology*, *118*(3), 643–648.

Wagg, A., Gibson, W., Ostaszkiewicz, J., et al. (2014). Urinary incontinence in frail elderly persons: Report from the 5th International Consultation on Incontinence. *Neurourology and Urodynamics*, *34*, 398–406.

Urinary Retention   *Michelle Acorn, DNP, NP PHC-Adult, BA, BScN/PHCNP, MN/ACNP, GNC(C), CAP, CGP*

NANDA-I

Definition

Inability to empty bladder completely.

Defining Characteristics

Absent of urinary output; bladder distention; dribbling of urine; dysuria; frequent voiding; overflow incontinence; residual urine; sensation of bladder fullness; small voiding

Related Factors

To be developed

Associated Condition

Blockage in urinary tract; high urethral pressure; reflex arc inhibition; strong sphincter

NOC   (Nursing Outcomes Classification)

Suggested NOC Outcome

Urinary Elimination

Example NOC Outcome with Indicators
Urinary Elimination as evidenced by the following indicators: Empties bladder completely/Absence of urinary leakage/Urine clarity. (Rate the outcome and indicators of **Urinary Elimination:** 1 = severely compromised, 2 = substantially compromised, 3 = moderately compromised, 4 = mildly compromised, 5 = not compromised [see Section I].)

Client Outcomes

Client Will (Specify Time Frame)

- Demonstrate consistent ability to urinate when desire to void is perceived
- Have measured urinary residual volume of less than 300 mL
- Experience correction or relief from dysuria, nocturia, postvoid dribbling, and voiding frequently
- Be free of a urinary tract infection

● = Independent;   ▲ = Collaborative;   EBN = Evidence-Based Nursing;   EB = Evidence-Based

NIC   (Nursing Interventions Classification)

Suggested NIC Interventions

Urinary Catheterization; Urinary Retention Care

> **Example NIC Activities—Urinary Retention Care**
>
> Perform a comprehensive urinary assessment focusing on incontinence (e.g., urinary output, urinary voiding pattern, cognitive function, and preexistent urinary problems); Use the power of suggestion by running water or flushing toilet

Nursing Interventions and *Rationales*

- Obtain a focused urinary history including questioning the client about episodes of acute urinary retention (UR; complete inability to void) or chronic retention (documented elevated postvoid residual volumes), as well as symptoms such as dysuria, nocturia, postvoid dribbling, and voiding frequently. *A history of difficulty voiding, pain, infection, or decreased urine volume is common in clients with urinary obstruction (Seifter, 2012).*
- Question the client concerning specific risk factors for UR including:
  - Spinal cord injuries
  - Ischemic stroke
  - Metabolic disorders such as diabetes mellitus, chronic alcoholism, and related conditions associated with polyuria and peripheral polyneuropathies
  - Herpetic infection
  - Heavy-metal poisoning (lead, mercury) causing peripheral polyneuropathies
  - Advanced stage HIV infection
  - Medications including antispasmodics/parasympatholytics, alpha-adrenergic agonists, antidepressants, sedatives, narcotics, psychotropic medications, illicit drugs
  - Recent surgery requiring general or spinal anesthesia
  - Vaginal delivery within the past 48 hours
  - Bowel elimination patterns, history of fecal impaction, encopresis
  - Recent surgical procedures
  - Recent prostatic biopsy

UR is related to multiple factors affecting either detrusor contraction strength or urethral resistance to urinary outflow (Policastro et al, 2016).

- Complete a pain assessment including pain intensity using a self-report pain tool, such as the 0 to 10 numerical pain rating scale. Also determine location, quality, onset/duration, intensity, aggravating/alleviating factors, and effects of pain on function and quality of life. **EB:** *Acute onset of obstruction with inability to void is associated with significant pain; partial obstruction causes minimal pain, which may delay diagnosis (Policastro et al, 2016). Bladder distention is associated with pain overlying the bladder (Seifter, 2012).*
- Perform a focused physical assessment including perineal skin integrity and inspection, percussion, and palpation of the lower abdomen, looking for obvious bladder distention or an enlarged kidney. *A palpable kidney or bladder provides direct evidence of a dilated urinary collection system (Policastro et al, 2016).*
- Recognize that unrelieved obstruction of urine can result in kidney damage and, if severe, kidney failure. UR can be a medical emergency and should be reported to the primary provider as soon as possible. **EB:** *As urine backs up in the urinary tract, the pressure increases inside the ureters, which results in pressure on the nephrons, damaging the nephrons and decreasing glomerular blood flow (Policastro et al, 2016).*
- Review laboratory test results including serum electrolytes, blood urea nitrogen (BUN) and creatinine, along with calcium, phosphate, magnesium, uric acid, and albumin. *Serum electrolytes (sodium, potassium, chloride, bicarbonate, BUN, and creatinine) and calcium, phosphate, magnesium, uric acid, and albumin should be measured. Elevations of BUN and creatinine and changes in electrolytes may be caused by kidney failure secondary to obstruction (Policastro et al, 2016).*
- Monitor for signs of dehydration, peripheral edema, elevating blood pressure, and heart failure. *The kidney can develop concentrating defects associated with partial obstruction of urine flow, resulting in symptoms that indicate kidney insufficiency (Policastro et al, 2016).*

- = Independent;   ▲ = Collaborative;   **EBN** = Evidence-Based Nursing;   **EB** = Evidence-Based

Ask the client to complete a bladder diary including patterns of urine elimination, urine loss (if present), nocturia, and volume and type of fluids consumed for a period of 3 to 7 days.

- Consult with the provider concerning eliminating or altering medications suspected of producing or exacerbating UR.
- EB: *Assess for postresidual voids (PVR) greater than 300 mL because it is the minimal volume at which a bladder becomes palpable (American Urological Association, 2016).*
- Both men and women may develop UR from obstruction of the bladder outlet and abnormalities in detrusor contractility. EB: *A common cause of bladder outlet obstruction (BOO) is caused by prostate/bladder neck enlargement, urethral stricture, vaginal vault prolapse, obstructing urethral sling, or impacted stool. Long-term use of medications such as alpha-agonists and tricyclic antidepressants contribute to the problem (American Urological Association, 2016).*
- In clients treated with an indwelling urethral catheter (IUC), complications such as catheter-associated urinary tract infections are common, whereas underuse of IUC may cause harmful UR. EB: *A quality improvement (QI) program aimed at staff ability to identify and manage patient risk, prevention, and treatment of UR optimizes appropriate IUC use (Anderson et al, 2017).*
- Advise the male client with UR related to benign prostatic hyperplasia (BPH) to avoid risk factors associated with acute UR:
  - ○ Avoid over-the-counter (OTC) cold remedies containing a decongestant (alpha-adrenergic agonist) or antihistamine, such as diphenhydramine, which has anticholinergic effects.
  - ○ Avoid taking OTC dietary medications (frequently contain alpha-adrenergic agonists).
  - ○ Discuss voiding problems with a health care provider before beginning new prescription medications.
  - ○ After prolonged exposure to cool weather, and warm the body before attempting to urinate.
  - ○ Avoid overfilling the bladder by regular urination patterns and refrain from excessive intake of alcohol.

EB: *Botulinum toxin injection into the bladder neck is a promising minimally invasive, tolerated, and cost-effective approach for the treatment of UR in patients with benign prostatic obstruction who are not candidates for surgery and for whom medical treatments have failed (Alam et al, 2016).*

These modifiable factors predispose the client to acute UR by over distending the bladder and decreasing muscle contraction (Mayo Clinic, 2017).

- Advise the client who is unable to void of specific strategies to manage this potential medical emergency as follows:
  - ○ Attempt urination in complete privacy.
  - ○ Place the feet solidly on the floor.
  - ○ If unable to void using these strategies, take a warm sitz bath or shower and void (if possible) while still in the tub or shower.
  - ○ Drink a warm cup of caffeinated coffee or tea to stimulate the bladder, which may promote voiding.
- If unable to void within 6 hours or if bladder distention is producing significant pain, seek urgent or emergency care. *Attempting urination in complete privacy and placing the feet solidly on the floor help relax the pelvic muscles and may encourage voiding. Warm water also stimulates the bladder and may produce voiding; the cooling experienced by leaving the tub or shower may again inhibit the bladder (Joanna Briggs Institute, 2013).*
- Perform sterile (in acute care) or clean intermittent catheterization at home as ordered for clients with UR. Refer to care plan for Reflex urinary **Incontinence** for more information about intermittent catheterization.
- ▲ Insert an indwelling catheter only as ordered by a health care provider. Understand the indication for the urinary catheter to be placed as part of client management. Catheter-associated urinary tract infections (CAUTIs) are among the most common health care–associated infections. Each CAUTI episode is estimated to cost $600, rising to $2800 per episode when a CAUTI leads to a bloodstream infection. Although certain conditions among hospitalized clients may require the use of a urinary catheter, limiting their use and decreasing the length of use are the most effective methods of reducing clients' exposure to CAUTIs (Choosing Wisely and the American Academy of Nursing, 2014).
- Nurse-led and computer-based reminders are both successful in reducing how long urinary catheters remain in place (Bernard, Hunter, & Moore, 2012).
- Nurse-driven practice recommendations to reduce CAUTI risk include securing catheters; maintaining drainage bags lower than level of bladder; emptying drainage bags every 8 hours, when two-thirds full,

● = Independent; ▲ = Collaborative; EBN = Evidence-Based Nursing; EB = Evidence-Based

and before any transfer; daily evaluation of catheter indication/need to promote removal; and use of bladder scanner to prevent reinsertion. EB: *Incorporating practice policies that use nurse-driven catheter practices was found to reduce catheter days, decrease length of hospital stay, and decrease reinsertions (Alexaitis & Broome, 2014).*

- Current practice recommendations support aseptic catheter insertions, whereas the use of hydrophilic-coated catheters for clean intermittent catheters can reduce the rate of CAUTIs. Suprapubic catheterization is not more effective than urethral catheterization in reducing the incidence of catheter-related bacteremia. EB: *Evidence does not support routine use of antimicrobial-impregnated catheters to prevent CAUTIs (Tenke, Koves, & Johansen, 2014).*

- For the individual with UR who is not a suitable candidate for intermittent catheterization, recognize that the catheter can be a significant cause of harm to the client through development of a CAUTI or through genitourinary trauma when the catheter is pulled. *An indwelling catheter provides continuous drainage of urine; however, the risks for serious urinary complications, such as chronic CAUTIs, with prolonged use are significant.* EB: *One study found that the risk for genitourinary trauma was as common as symptomatic urinary tract infection when clients were repeatedly catheterized (Leuck et al, 2012).* EBN: *Indwelling urinary catheters are associated with up to 80% of hospital-acquired CAUTIs. Appropriate use of bladder ultrasonography can reduce the rate of bladder damage and the need to use catheters. Incorporating bladder ultrasonography into the client's assessment can lead to decreased use of urinary catheter and rate of CAUTIs, lower risk for spread of multiresistant gram-negative bacteria, and lower hospital costs (Johansson et al, 2013).*

- Advise clients with indwelling catheters that bacteria in the urine is an almost universal finding after the catheter has remained in place for more than 1 week and that only symptomatic infections warrant treatment. *The long-term indwelling catheter is inevitably associated with bacterial colonization, with formation of biofilm on the catheter surfaces (Nicolle & Norrby, 2016).*

- Use the following strategies to reduce the risk for CAUTI whenever feasible:
  - Insert the indwelling catheter with sterile technique, only when insertion is indicated.
  - Remove the indwelling catheter as soon as possible; acute care facilities should institute a policy for regular review of the necessity of an indwelling catheter.
  - Maintain a closed drainage system whenever feasible.
  - Maintain unobstructed urine flow, avoiding kinks in the tubing and keeping the collecting bag below the level of the bladder at all times.
  - Regularly cleanse the urethral meatus with a gentle cleanser to remove apparent soiling.
  - Change the long-term catheter every 4 weeks; more frequent catheter changes should be reserved for clients who experience catheter encrustation and blockage.

- Educate staff about the risks for CAUTI development and specific strategies to reduce these risks. EB: *These strategies are supported by sufficient evidence to recommend routine use (Felix et al, 2014). Numerous nursing studies have demonstrated that nurse-controlled methods to decrease the length of catheterization such as chart reminders and computerized interventions lead to decreased incidences of CAUTI (Andreessen, Wilde, & Herendeen, 2012).*

Postoperative Urinary Retention

- UR is a common complication of surgery, anesthesia, and advancing age. If conservative measures do not help the client pass urine, then the bladder needs to be drained using either an intermittent catheter or IUC, which places the client at risk for development of CAUTI (Steggall, Treacy, & Jones, 2013). EBN: *A study demonstrated increased UR after transurethral resection of the prostate in clients with preoperative increased prostate size, urinary tract infection, and clot retention (McKinnon et al, 2011).*

- Remove the IUC at midnight in the hospitalized postoperative client to reduce the risk for acute UR.

- Perform a bladder scan before considering inserting a catheter to determine PVR volume after surgery. EBN: *A study in postoperative patients demonstrated a significant decrease in the number of catheterizations when ultrasonic bladder scanning was done to monitor postoperative UR (Daurat et al, 2015).* CEB: *Another study found that in hip fracture clients, use of bladder scanning and intermittent catheterization resulted in less retention after surgery than in clients in whom a retention catheter was inserted (Johansson & Christensson, 2010).* CEB: *A meta-analysis found that performing bladder scanning was effective in decreasing urinary catheterization and development of urinary tract infection (Palese et al, 2010).*

- The overall incidence of postoperative urinary catheterization is 40% for total hip and knee arthroplasties. EB: *Spinal anesthesia is a risk factor (Bjerregaard et al, 2015).*

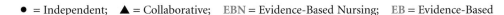

● = Independent;   ▲ = Collaborative;   EBN = Evidence-Based Nursing;   EB = Evidence-Based

Geriatric

- Aggressively assess older clients, particularly those with dribbling urinary incontinence, urinary tract infection, and related conditions for UR. CEB: *Older women and men may experience UR with few or no apparent symptoms; a urinary residual volume and related assessments are necessary to determine the presence of retention in this population (Johansson & Christensson, 2010).*
- Assess older clients for impaction when UR is documented or suspected: Monitor older male clients for retention related to BPH or prostate cancer. *Prostate enlargement in older men increases the risk for acute and chronic UR.*

 Home Care

- Encourage the client to report any inability to void.
- Maintain an up-to-date medication list; evaluate side effect profiles for risk of UR. *New medications or changes in dose may cause UR.*
- Refer the client for health care provider evaluation if UR occurs. *Identification of cause is important. Left untreated, UR may lead to urinary tract infection or kidney failure.*

 Client/Family Teaching and Discharge Planning

- Teach the client with mild to moderate obstructive symptoms to double void by urinating, resting in the bathroom for 3 to 5 minutes, and then trying again to urinate. *Double voiding promotes more efficient bladder evacuation by allowing the detrusor to contract initially and then rest and contract again (Mayo Clinic, 2017).*
- Teach the client with UR and infrequent voiding to urinate by the clock. *Timed or scheduled voiding may reduce UR by preventing bladder over distention (Mayo Clinic, 2017).*
- Teach the client with an indwelling catheter to assess the tube for patency, maintain the drainage system below the level of the symphysis pubis, and routinely cleanse the bedside bag as directed.
- Teach the client with an indwelling catheter or undergoing intermittent catheterization the symptoms of a significant urinary infection, including hematuria, acute-onset incontinence, dysuria, flank pain, fever, or acute confusion.

REFERENCES

Alam, M., Dalati, M., & Khoury, F. (2016). Botulinum toxin A injection in the bladder neck: A promising treatment for urinary retention. *Case Reports in Urology*.

Alexaitis, I., & Broome, B. (2014). Implementation of a nurse-driven protocol to prevent catheter-associated urinary tract infections. *Journal of Nursing Care Quality, 29*(3), 245–252.

American Urological Association. (2016). *White paper: Non-neurogenic chronic urinary retention: Consensus definition, management strategies and future opportunities.*

Anderson, A. C., Johansson, R. M., Elg, M., et al. (2017). Using quality improvement methods to implement guidelines to decrease the proportion of urinary retention in orthopaedic care. *International Archives of Nursing and Health Care, 3*, 1.

Andreessen, L., Wilde, M. H., & Herendeen, P. (2012). Preventing catheter-associated urinary tract infections in acute care: The bundle approach. *Journal of Nursing Care Quality, 27*(3), 209–217.

Bernard, M. S., Hunger, K. F., & Moore, K. N. (2012). A review of strategies to decrease the duration of indwelling urethral catheters and potentially reduce the incidence of catheter-associated urinary tract infections. *Urologic Nursing, 32*(1), 29–37.

Bjerregaard, L., Bogo, S., Raaschou, S., et al. (2015). Incidence of and risk factors for postoperative urinary retention in fast-track hip and knee arthroplasty. *Acta Orthopaedica, 86*(2), 183–188.

Choosing Wisely and the American Academy of Nursing. (2014). *Don't place or maintain a urinary catheter in a patient unless there is a specific indication to do so.* Retrieved from http://www.choosingwisely.org/clinician-lists/american-academy-nursing-urinary-catheters-without-specific-indication/. (Accessed 31 October 2017).

Daurat, A., Choquet, O., Bringuier, S., et al. (2015). Diagnosis of postoperative urinary retention using a simplified ultrasound bladder measurement. *Anesthesia & Analgesia, 120*(5), 1033–1038.

Felix, K., et al. (2014). *Guide to preventing urinary tract infections.* Washington, DC: APIC. Retrieved from http://apic.org/Resource_/Elimination GuideForm/0ff6ae59-0a3a-4640-97b5-eee38b8bed5b/File/CAUTI_06.pdf. (Retrieved 25 November 2017).

Joanna Briggs Institute. (2013). *Trial of void: Post operative.*

Johansson, R. M., & Christensson, L. (2010). Urinary retention in older patients in connection with hip fracture surgery. *Journal of Clinical Nursing, 12*, 2110–2116.

Johansson, R. M., Malmmanvall, B. E., Andersson-Gare, B., et al. (2013). *Journal of Clinical Nursing, 22*(3), 346–355.

Leuck, A. M., et al. (2012). Complications of Foley catheters—Is infection the greatest risk? *The Journal of Urology, 187*(5), 1662–1666.

Mayo Clinic. (2017). *Prostatic gland enlargement: lifestyle and home remedies.* Retrieved from http://www.mayo.edu/research/departments-divisions/department-urology/benign-prostatic-hyperplasia. (Accessed 31 October 2017).

McKinnon, K., et al. (2011). Predictors of acute urinary retention after transurethral resection of the prostate: A retrospective chart audit. *Urologic Nursing, 31*(4), 207–213.

Nicolle, E. L., & Norrby, S. R. (2016). Approach to the patient with urinary tract infection. In L. Goldman & A. Schafer (Eds.), *Goldman's Cecil medicine* (26th ed., pp. 1872–1876). St Louis: Saunders/Elsevier.

 U

● = Independent;   ▲ = Collaborative;   EBN = Evidence-Based Nursing;   EB = Evidence-Based

Palese, A., et al. (2010). The effectiveness of the ultrasound bladder scanner in reducing urinary tract infections: A meta-analysis. *Journal of Clinical Nursing, 19*(21/22), 2970–2979.

Policastro, M., et al. (2016). *Urinary obstruction, Medscape Reference.* Retrieved from https://emedicine.medscape.com/article/778456-overview. (Accessed 25 November 2017).

Seifter, J. (2012). Urinary tract obstruction. In D. L. Longo, et al. (Eds.), *Harrison's principles of internal medicine* (18th ed.). New York: McGraw-Hill.

Steggall, M., Treacy, C., & Jones, M. (2013). Post-operative urinary retention. *Nursing Standard, 28*(5), 43–48.

Tenke, P., Koves, B., & Johansen, T. E. B. (2014). An update on prevention and treatment of CAUTI. *Current Opinion in Infectious Diseases, 27*(1), 102–107.

Risk for Vascular Trauma   *Elyse Bueno, MS, ACCNS-AG, CCRN*

NANDA-I

Definition

Susceptible to damage to vein and its surrounding tissues related to the presence of a catheter and/or infusion solutions, which may compromise health.

Risk Factors

Inadequate available insertion site; prolonged period of time catheter is in place

Associated Condition

Irritating solution; rapid infusion rate

NOC   (Nursing Outcomes Classification)

Suggested NOC Outcomes

Risk Control; Tissue Integrity: Skin and Mucous Membranes

Example NOC Outcome with Indicators
Accomplishes **Risk Control** as evidenced by the following indicators: Monitors environmental risk factors/Develops effective risk control strategies/Modifies lifestyle to reduce risk. (Rate the outcome and indicators of **Risk Control:** 1 = never demonstrated, 2 = rarely demonstrated, 3 = sometimes demonstrated, 4 = often demonstrated, 5 = consistently demonstrated [see Section I].)

Client Outcomes

Client Will (Specify Time Frame)

- Remain free from vascular trauma
- Remain free from signs and symptoms that indicate vascular trauma
- Remain free of signs and symptoms of vascular inflammation or infection
- Remain free from impaired tissue and/or skin
- Maintain skin integrity, tissue perfusion, usual tissue temperature, color, and pigment
- Report any altered sensation or pain
- State site is comfortable

NIC   (Nursing Interventions Classification)

Suggested NIC Interventions

Intravenous Therapy; Medication Administration: Intravenous

Example NIC Activities—Intravenous Therapy
Monitor intravenous (IV) flow rate and IV site during infusion; Perform IV site care according to agency protocol

● = Independent;   ▲ = Collaborative;   EBN = Evidence-Based Nursing;   EB = Evidence-Based

Nursing Interventions and *Rationales*

Client Preparation

▲ Verify objective and estimate duration of treatment. Check health care provider's order. *Verify if client will remain hospitalized during the entire treatment or will go home with the device (Phillips, 2014).*

● Assess client's clinical situation when venous infusion is indicated. *Consider possible clinical conditions that cause changes in temperature, color, and sensitivity of the possible venous access site. Verify situations that alter venous return (e.g., mastectomy, stroke) (Phillips, 2014). The site of catheter insertion influences the risk of infection and phlebitis, such as preexisting catheters, anatomic deformity, and bleeding diathesis (Xue, 2014).*

● Assess if client is prepared for an intravenous (IV) procedure. Explain the procedure if necessary to decrease stress. *Stress may cause vasoconstriction that can interfere in the visualization of the vein and flow of the infused solution (Xue, 2014).*

● Provide privacy and make the client comfortable during the IV insertion. *Privacy and comfort help decrease stress (Phillips, 2014).*

● Teach the client what symptoms of possible vascular trauma he or she should be alert to and to immediately inform staff if any of these symptoms are noticed. *Prompt attention to adverse changes decreases the chance of adverse effects from complications.*

Insertion

● Wash hands before and after touching the client, as well as when inserting, replacing, accessing, repairing, or dressing an intravascular catheter (Infusion Nurses Society [INS], 2016).

● Maintain aseptic technique for the insertion and care of intravascular catheters. *Using an approved antiseptic solution, wearing gloves during insertion of an IV catheter, and immediately covering the insertion site with a transparent sterile semipermeable dressing are important interventions to reduce the risk of infection (McGowan, 2014; Xue, 2014).*

● In preparation, assess the patient's medical history for disease processes such as diabetes and hypertension, frequent venipuncture, variations in skin color, skin alteration, age, obesity, fluid volume deficit, and IV drug use; these factors may lead to difficult vascular visualization (INS, 2016).

● When vascular visualization is difficult, consider the use of visible light devices that provide transillumination of the peripheral veins or ultrasonography (INS, 2016). *Ultrasonography reduces the number of venipuncture attempts and procedure time.*

● Avoid areas of joint flexion or bony prominences. *Movement in these sites can cause mechanical trauma in veins (McGowan, 2014).*

● Avoid the use of the antecubital area, which has high failure rates, and do not use lower extremities unless necessary because of the risk of tissue damage, thrombophlebitis, and ulceration (INS, 2016).

▲ Avoid the dorsal hand, radial wrist, and the volar (inner) wrist, if possible. *These are high-risk areas for venipuncture-related nerve injury (INS, 2016).*

▲ Consider topical anesthetic prior to IV cannula insertion to reduce pain (Porritt, 2015a).

● Choose an appropriate vascular access device (VAD) based on the types and characteristics of the devices and insertion site. Consider the following:
  ○ Peripheral cannulae: these are short devices that are placed into a peripheral vein. They can be straight, winged, or ported and winged.
  ○ Midline catheters or peripherally inserted central catheters (PICCs) that range from 7.5 to 20 cm.
  ○ Central venous access devices (CVADs) are terminated in the central venous circulation and are available in a range of gauge sizes; they can be nontunneled catheters, skin-tunneled catheters, implantable injection ports, or PICCs.
  ○ Polyurethane venous devices and silicone rubber may cause less friction and, consequently, may reduce the risk of mechanical phlebitis (Phillips, 2014).

▲ Choose a device with consideration of the nature, volume, and flow of prescribed solution. **EBN:** *Choosing the right gauge size reduces the risk of vascular trauma (McGowan, 2014). Verify that the osmolarity of the solution to be infused is compatible with the available access site and device (Phillips, 2014; Loubani & Green, 2015).*

● If possible, choose the venous access site considering the client's preference. *Engaging the client in choosing the venous access site, when possible, may facilitate line patency.*

● Select the gauge of the venous device according to the duration of treatment, purpose of the procedure, and size of the vein. **EB:** *Emergency situations require short, large-bore cannulae. Hydration fluids and*

● = Independent;   ▲ = Collaborative;   EBN = Evidence-Based Nursing;   EB = Evidence-Based

antibiotics can be delivered through much smaller cannulae (Loubani & Green, 2015). Select the smallest gauge necessary to achieve the prescribed flow rate (INS, 2013; Vizcarra et al, 2014). The time of infusion of the drug, especially chemotherapy and vasoactive agents, can contribute to the occurrence of phlebitis (Loubani & Green, 2015).

- Verify whether the client is allergic to fixation or device material.
- Disinfect the venipuncture site. Assess that skin is dry before puncturing to *achieve maximal benefit of the disinfection agent.*
- Provide a comfortable, safe, hypoallergenic, easily removable stabilization dressing, allowing for visualization of the access site. *Catheter stabilization should be used to preserve the integrity of the access device, to minimize catheter movement at the hub, and to prevent catheter migration and loss of access (INS, 2013; Vizcarra et al, 2014). Some peripheral cannulae have stabilization wings (which increase the external surface area) and/or ports (which are used to administer bolus medication) incorporated into their design.*
- Use sterile, transparent, semipermeable dressing to cover catheter site. *Replace dressing with catheter change, or at a minimum every 7 days for transparent dressings (INS, 2013; Vizcarra et al, 2014). The use of a transparent occlusive dressing can facilitate regular monitoring by visually inspecting the VAD (McGowan, 2014; Xue, 2014). Use of gauze may be necessary if the client is diaphoretic, if the site is oozing or bleeding, or if it becomes damp; if gauze is used, it should be changed every 2 days (INS, 2013; Vizcarra et al, 2014).*
- Document insertion date, site, type of VAD, number of punctures performed, other occurrences, and measures/arrangements.
- Always decontaminate the device before infusing medication or manipulating IV equipment (Xue, 2014; Helm et al, 2015).
- ▲ Verify the sequence of drugs to be administered. Vesicants should always be administered first in a sequence of drugs (Loubani & Green, 2015).

Monitoring Infusion

- Monitor permeability and flow rate at regular intervals.
- Monitor catheter–skin junction and surrounding tissues at regular intervals, observing possible appearance of burning, pain, erythema, altered local temperature, infiltration, extravasation, edema, secretion, tenderness, or induration. Remove promptly. *The infusion should be discontinued at the first sign of infiltration or extravasation, the administration set disconnected, and all fluid aspirated from the catheter with a small syringe (INS, 2013; Vizcarra et al, 2014).*
- ▲ Replace device according to institution protocol. EBN: *Remove peripheral IV cannula if there are signs of phlebitis, infection, or if the cannula is no longer functioning. There is no need to routinely change the catheter every 72 to 96 hours (Porritt, 2015b).*
- ▲ Flush vascular access according to organizational policies and procedures, and as recommended by the manufacturer. *A pulsating flushing technique should be used (Porritt, 2016). VADs should be flushed after each infusion to clear the infused medication from the catheter lumen, preventing contact between incompatible medications (INS, 2013; Vizcarra et al, 2014). Sodium chloride 0.9% or heparinized sodium chloride has been studied to determine optimal solution for catheter patency. A recent Cochrane review found little difference in catheter patency between either solution; thus given the cost and possible client risks to heparin exposure, sodium chloride flush solution is recommended (López-Briz et al, 2014).* When locking a catheter, use enough fluid to fill the entire catheter and use a positive pressure technique when disconnecting the syringe (Porritt, 2016).
- Remove catheter on suspected contamination, if the client develops signs of phlebitis or infection, the catheter is malfunctioning, or when the catheter no longer required. *VADs should be removed on unresolved complication, therapy discontinuation, or if deemed unnecessary (INS, 2013; Vizcarra et al, 2014). Replace any catheter inserted under emergency conditions within 24 hours because the sterility of the procedure may have been compromised.*
- Encourage clients to report any discomfort such as pain, burning, swelling, or bleeding (Xue, 2014).

Pediatric

- The preceding interventions may be adapted for the pediatric client. *Consider age, culture, development level, health literacy, and language preferences (INS, 2013; Vizcarra et al, 2014; American Nurses Association [ANA], 2015).*
- Inform the client and family about the IV procedure; obtain permissions, maintain client's comfort, and perform appropriate assessment prior to venipuncture. Assess the client for any allergies or sensitivities

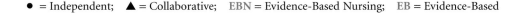

● = Independent;   ▲ = Collaborative;   EBN = Evidence-Based Nursing;   EB = Evidence-Based

V

to tape, antiseptics, or latex. *Choose a healthy vein and appropriate site for insertion of selected device (Abolfotouh et al, 2014).*

- Consider using a two-dimensional ultrasound for venous cannulation. EBN: *Ultrasound has been shown more effective than traditional techniques and should be considered for pediatric patients (Jayasekara, 2017).* EBN: *The cephalic vein in the proximal forearm is the best initial site for ultrasound-guided catheterization when veins are not visible or palpable (Jayasekara, 2017).*
- The use of an appropriate device to obtain blood samples reduces discomfort in the pediatric client. *Accessing a pediatric client's vein successfully can be difficult, and measures to optimize the health care provider's skill are important to ensure successful venous cannulation (Goff et al, 2013).*
- Avoid areas of joint flexion or bony prominences. *Cannulae inserted away from joints remain patent for longer periods of time (McGowan, 2014).*
- ▲ Consider whether sedation or the use of local anesthetic is suitable for insertion of a catheter, taking into consideration the age of the pediatric client. *The use of effective local anesthetic methods and agents before each painful dermal procedure should be discussed with the health care provider (INS, 2013; Vizcarra et al, 2014).*
- ▲ Use diversion while performing the procedure. *Diversion reduces anxiety (Goff et al, 2013).*

Geriatric

- The preceding interventions may be adapted for the geriatric client.
- Consider the physical, emotional, and cognitive changes related to older adults.
- Use strict aseptic technique for venipuncture of older clients. EB: *Older adults are at an increased risk of infection because of decreased immunological function (Azar & Ballas, 2017).*

Home Care

- Some devices may remain after discharge. Provide device-specific education to the client and family members about care of the selected device.
- Help in the choice of actions that support self-care. The nurse can provide valuable information that can be used to guide decision-making to maximize the self-care abilities of clients receiving home infusion therapy.
- Select, with the client, the insertion site most compatible with the development of activities of daily living (ADLs) (McGowan, 2014; Xue, 2014).
- Minimize the use of continuous IV therapy whenever possible. CEBN: *Clients who received intermittent IV therapy via a saline lock were more independent regarding ability to perform self-care ADLs than those who received continuous IV therapy. The need for assistive mobility devices was also an independent predictor of ability to perform self-care ADLs (O'Halloran, El-Masri, & Fox-Wasylyshyn et al, 2008).*

REFERENCES

Abolfotouh, M. A., Salam, M., Bani-Mustafa, A., et al. (2014). Prospective study of incidence and predictors of peripheral intravenous catheter-induced complications. *Therapeutic and Clinical Risk Management, 10,* 993–1001.

American Nurses Association (ANA). (2015). *Pediatric nursing: Scope and standards of practice,* Silver Spring, MD. Retrieved from http://www.nursingworld.org/scopeandstandardsofpractice.

Azar, A., & Ballas, Z. (2017). Immune function in older adults. *UpToDate.* Retrieved from https://www.uptodate.com/contents/immune-function-in-older-adults?source=see_link.

Goff, D. A., Larsen, P., Brinkley, J., et al. (2013). Resource utilization and cost of inserting peripheral intravenous catheters in hospitalized children. *Hospital Pediatrics, 3*(3), 185–191.

Helm, R. E., Klausner, J. D., Klemperer, J. D., et al. (2015). Accepted but unacceptable: Peripheral IV catheter failure. *Journal of Infusion Nursing, 38*(3), 189–201.

Infusion Nurses Society (INS). (2013). *Recommendations for improving safety practices with short peripheral catheters.* Retrieved from http://www.ins1.org/i4a/pages/index.cfm?pageid=3412.

Infusion Nurses Society (INS). (2016). *Infusion therapy standards of practice.* Retrieved from http://ins.tizrapublisher.com/hai13r/.

Jayasekara, R. (2017). *Intravenous cannulation (pediatric): Clinical information.* Joanna Briggs Institute EBP Database. JBI166.

López-Briz, E., Ruiz, G. V., Cabello, J. B., et al. (2014). Heparin versus 0.9% sodium chloride intermittent flushing for prevention of occlusion in central venous catheters in adults. *Cochrane Database of Systematic Reviews,* (10), CD008462.

Loubani, O. M., & Green, R. S. (2015). A systematic review of extravasation and local tissue injury from administration of vasopressors through peripheral intravenous catheters and central venous catheters. *Journal of Critical Care, 30*(3), 653–659.

McGowan, D. (2014). Peripheral intravenous cannulation: What is considered best practice? *British Journal of Nursing, 23*(14), S26–S28.

O'Halloran, L., El-Masri, M. M., & Fox-Wasylyshyn, S. M. (2008). Home intravenous therapy and the ability to perform self-care activities of daily living. *Journal of Infusion Nursing, 31*(6), 367–373.

Phillips, L. D. (2014). *Manual of IV therapeutics: evidence-based practice for infusion therapy* (6th ed.). Philadelphia: F. A. Davis.

Porritt, K. (2015a). *Peripheral intravenous cannula: Insertion.* Joanna Briggs Institute EBP Database. JBI14045.

● = Independent;   ▲ = Collaborative;   EBN = Evidence-Based Nursing;   EB = Evidence-Based

Porritt, K. (2015b). *Peripheral intravenous cannula: Removal.* Joanna Briggs Institute EBP Database. JBI14047.

Porritt, K. (2016). *Intravascular therapy: Maintaining catheter lumen patency.* Joanna Briggs Institute EBP Database. JBI14448.

Vizcarra, C., Cassutt, C., Corbitt, N., et al. (2014). Recommendations for improving safety practices with short peripheral catheters. *Journal of Infusion Nursing, 37*(2), 121–124.

Xue, Y. (2014). *Peripheral intravenous line: Insertion.* Joanna Briggs Institute EBP Database. JB11841.

Risk for Venous Thromboembolism   *Dina M. Hewett, PhD, RN, NEA-BC, CCRN-A*

NANDA-I

Definition

Susceptible to the development of a blood clot in a deep vein, commonly in the thigh, calf or upper extremity, which can break off and lodge in another vessel, which may compromise health.

Risk Factors

Dehydration; impaired mobility; obesity

At-Risk Population

Age > 60; critical care admission; current smoker; first degree relative with history of venous thromboembolism; history of cerebral vascular accident; history of previous venous thromboembolism; less than 6 weeks postpartum

Associated Condition

Cerebral vascular accident; current cancer diagnosis; trauma below the waist; significant medical comorbidity; postoperative for major surgery; postoperative for orthopedic surgery; surgery and total anesthesia time > 90 minutes; thrombophilia; trauma of upper extremity; use of estrogen-containing contraceptives; use of hormone replacement therapy; varicose veins

NOC   (Nursing Outcomes Classification)

Suggested NOC Outcomes

Tissue Perfusion: Peripheral; Tissue Perfusion: Pulmonary Risk Control: Dehydration; Hydration; Knowledge Thrombus Threat Reduction; Risk Control: Thrombus

> **Example NOC Outcome with Indicators**
>
> **Risk Control: Thrombus** as evidenced by the following indicators: Seeks current information about embolus prevention/ Identifies risk factors for thrombus formation/Monitors for warning signs and symptoms of thrombus formation or embolus. (Rate outcome and indicators of **Risk Control: Thrombus:** 1 = never demonstrated, 2 = rarely demonstrated, 3 = sometimes demonstrated, 4 = often demonstrated, 5 = consistently demonstrated [see Section I].)

Client Outcomes

Client Will (Specify Time Frame)

- Not develop a venous thromboembolism (VTE) during hospitalization
- State the relevant risk factors associated with the development of a VTE
- Engage in behaviors or lifestyle changes to reduce risk of developing a VTE

NIC   (Nursing Interventions Classification)

Suggested NIC Interventions

Embolus Precautions; Embolus Care: Peripheral; Embolus Care: Pulmonary; Lower Extremity Monitoring

> **Example NIC Activities**
>
> Obtain a history of the client's present illness and medical history to evaluate the risk of VTE and implement preventative interventions

● = Independent;   ▲ = Collaborative;   EBN = Evidence-Based Nursing;   EB = Evidence-Based

Nursing Interventions and *Rationales*

- It is estimated that 40% of patients with a deep vein thrombosis (DVT) will progress to postthrombotic syndrome (PTS); therefore prevention of DVT is a key component. *PTS is a chronic disorder characterized by pain, swelling, redness (erythema), and ulcerations. The degree will vary from client to client. Individuals with recurrent ipsilateral DVT are considered the highest risk for PTS (Kvamme & Costanzo, 2015; Lenchus et al, 2017).*
- Assess client's risk factors to develop VTE. **EB:** *There are several factors that may predispose a client to DVT. According to Bruni-Fitzgerald (2015), the strongest risk factors include:*
  - ○ Venous stasis as a result of dehydration, immobility, heart failure, or venous compressions from a tumor
  - ○ Hypercoagulable states from disease, obesity, and trauma
  - ○ Immobilization from prolonged bed rest or limb casting
  - ○ Surgery and trauma, especially hip, pelvic, and spinal surgery, and leg amputation; several burns also predispose clients to DVT
  - ○ Pregnancy results in a hypercoagulable state placing these clients at risk; although fatal events are rare
  - ○ Oral contraceptives and estrogen replacement may place clients at risk, which is proportional to the estrogen content; postmenopausal women on hormone replacement therapy are considered at risk
  - ○ In malignancy cases 17% of patients with VTE have a neoplasm with the most frequent occurrence in patients with pancreatic cancer
- *Use a VTE risk assessment tool to determine individual susceptibility to VTE.* **EB:** *Determining a patient's risk may be guided through the use of an assessment tool such as the Wells Criteria or the Caprini Risk Assessment Model. Assessment tools in the acute care setting are developed based on evidence-based research (Modi et al, 2016).*
- ▲ Implement evidence-based prevention methods, both chemical (pharmacological) and/or mechanical. **EB:** *The nurse must be proactive in the assessment of the client for risks for VTE and implementing prophylactic measures as prescribed (Adams, 2015).*
- ▲ Chemical thromboprophylaxis should be anticipated in the postoperative care of critically ill clients. **CEB/EB:** *Research has shown that chemical thromboprophylaxis, when initiated in critically ill and postoperative clients, such as anticoagulants, are not associated with clinically significant bleeding (Makic, 2014). Evidence-based practice guidelines support the use of chemical and mechanical prophylaxis interventions for clients undergoing orthopedic surgery for a minimum of 14 to 35 days to reduce VTE risk (Falck-Ytter et al, 2012).*
- Implement mechanical prophylaxis through use of intermittent pneumatic compression (IPC) devices (Ho & Harahsheh, 2016). **EB:** *IPC is demonstrated to be more effective than no IPC at reducing DVT and is essential when pharmacological therapy is contraindicated because of an increased risk of bleeding (Dunn & Ramos, 2017). IPC devices reduce the risk of venous stasis by increasing the velocity of venous outflow and promoting the emptying of valvular cusps (Muñoz-Figueroa & Ojo, 2015).*
- Ensure proper fit and application of the device. **EB:** *Moore (2012) recommended using a measuring tape to obtain accurate measurements and follow the manufacturer's recommendations for correct sizing. Two fingers should be easily placed between the patient's leg and the sleeve. Monitor for edema and resize as needed.*
- Implement progressive mobility and early ambulation as the client tolerates to reduce risk of VTE. **EB:** *Studies indicate early mobility may reduce patient deconditioning and VTE complications (Booth et al, 2016). One study conducted in a trauma critical care unit revealed a statistically significant (P = .0004) reduced rate of DVT in patients in which early mobility and ambulation were implemented (Booth et al, 2016).*
- Provide education to the client and family about the importance of continued use of IPC after the client is ambulatory. Ensure that IPC is reapplied after ambulation (Corbett & Hannison, 2016; Dunn & Ramos, 2017). **EB:** *IPC should be reapplied after the client ambulates and returns to bed to maintain prevention interventions for VTE (Makic, 2014; Dunn & Ramos, 2017).*
- Perform a skin inspection during the bathing. *It is important to assess the skin with each application of the IPC and during the bath for signs of skin irritation or breakdown from the device.*
- IPC should be applied even when the client is sitting in a chair (Dunn & Ramos, 2017).
- Provide appropriate education or referral to a smoking cessation program. Smoking is a well-established risk factor for atherosclerotic disease that increases the client's risk for VTE. **EB:** *A systematic review and meta-analysis found that smoking increased the risk of VTE and the risk increased by 10.2% for every additional 10 cigarettes smoked per day or by 6.1% for every additional 10 pack-years of smoking. The study also found smokers who were overweight had a higher risk of VTE (Cheng et al, 2013).*

V

● = Independent;   ▲ = Collaborative;   **EBN** = Evidence-Based Nursing;   **EB** = Evidence-Based

- Obesity is an independent risk for VTE. EB: *A study of 27,818 clients who underwent bariatric surgery found significant risk factors to include male gender, operative time greater than 3 hours, type of procedure risk increased as body mass index (BMI) increased, and age (Finks et al, 2012). A systematic review of bariatric surgery clients found that male gender, increased BMI, smoking history, and operative procedure and time were risk factors for VTE (Bartlett, Mauck, & Daniels, 2015). Chemical and mechanical preventative interventions should be implemented to reduce the risk of VTE in the bariatric client population (Bartlett, Mauck, & Daniels, 2015).*
- Patients with cancer are at an increased risk of developing a DVT mainly because of the release of certain chemicals from the tumor and spread of the tumor into blood vessels. Generally, bloodstream cancers such as leukemia carry the highest risk for development of DVT followed by solid tumors of the pancreas, stomach, lungs, ovaries, uterus, bladder, and brain (Udoh, 2016).

Pediatric

- The nurse should be alert to certain diagnoses that increase the pediatric client's risk for VTE. *Diagnoses associated with increased risk of VTE include sepsis, acute infection, oncological malignant growth, surgery/ trauma, congenital heart disease, systemic lupus, obesity, and immobility (Prentiss, 2012).*
- Incidence of VTE in children is low; however, the rate of VTE in hospitalized children is much higher (Austin, Jenkins, & Hines, 2017).
- Risk factors for pediatric development of VTE include use of central venous access devices (Prentiss, 2012). EB: *A study by Austin, Jenkins, and Hines (2017) found that pediatric patients are at risk of a catheter-associated DVT because of the size of the device and resulting damage to the fragile intima, leading to clot formation and dislodgement of the clot.*
- Neonatal and adolescent age groups are at higher risk for VTE compared with other pediatric age groups (Prentiss, 2012). Additional studies are needed to further understand the risks and interventions for this population.

Geriatric

- The risk of VTE increases with age, increasing 90% between the ages of 15 and 80. *Many of the risk factors for VTE are commonly seen in the older patient with heart failure, chronic obstructive pulmonary disease, and malignancy. VTE is also seen in patients on bed rest and those with implantable devices such as pacemakers and hip/knee replacements (Bruni-Fitzgerald, 2015).*
- It is well established that older patients are at a greater risk to develop atrial fibrillation (Heeringa et al, 2006). The Framingham study indicated increasing risk of developing atrial fibrillation with increasing age (Wolf, Abbott, & Kannel, 1991). *Treatment for chronic atrial fibrillation requires the use of anticoagulants to reduce the risk of an embolic event.*

Home Care

- Provide client education on the importance of continued use of compression stockings as directed. *Ensuring the client is aware of the benefit of compression stockings reduces the risk of VTE and may facilitate compliance in wearing the compression stocking. The client may only be required to wear stockings during the day and be allowed to remove them at night (Bonner & Johnson, 2014; Kaur et al, 2016; Pai & Douketis, 2017).*
- Provide education to the client and/or family caregiver about the continued use of anticoagulant pharmacological therapy as directed. *The client and/or family caregiver may need instruction on proper injection technique if the client is not discharged on an oral anticoagulant.* EB: *If the client is discharged home on subcutaneous low-molecular-weight heparin or fondaparinux, the nurse needs to teach the client and or family caregiver how to properly administer the medication by injection (Bonner & Johnson, 2014; Pai & Douketis, 2017).*
- Patients who take the anticoagulant warfarin should have dietary education. Warfarin's effects may be decreased with a diet rich in vitamin K. *Food containing vitamin K includes dark green leafy vegetables such as kale, Brussels sprouts, collard greens, and spinach. Avoid eating large quantities of these vegetables. Cranberry juice and alcohol should be avoided because it enhances the effects of warfarin and may lead to bleeding.*
- The newer anticoagulants, such as rivaroxaban, apixaban, and edoxaban, do not have the same medication–food interactions as warfarin.

V

REFERENCES

Austin, P., Jenkins, S., & Hines, A. (2017). Thromboembolic events in PICU: A descriptive study. *Pediatric Nursing, 43*(3), 132–137.

Adams, A. (2015). Proactivity in VTE prevention: A concept analysis. *British Journal of Nursing, 24*(1), 20–25. Retrieved from https://doi.org/10.12968/bjon.2015.24.1.20.

Bartlett, M. A., Mauck, K. F., & Daniels, D. R. (2015). Prevention of venous thromboembolism in patients undergoing bariatric surgery. *Vascular Health and Risk Management, 11*, 461–477.

Bonner, L., & Johnson, J. (2014). Deep vein thrombosis: Diagnosis and treatment. *Nursing Standard, 28*(21), 51–58. Retrieved from https://doi.org/10.7748/ns2014.01.28.21.51.e8222.

Booth, K., Rivet, J., Flici, R., et al. (2016). Progressive mobility protocol reduces venous thromboembolism rate in trauma intensive care patients: A quality improvement project. *Journal of Trauma Nursing, 23*(5), 284–289. Retrieved from https://doi.org/10.1097/JTN.0000000000000234.

Bruni-Fitzgerald, K. R. (2015). Venous thromboembolism: An overview. *Journal of Vascular Nursing, 33*(3), 95–99.

Cheng, Y. J., Liu, H. O., Yao, F. J., et al. (2013). Current and former smoking and risk for venous thromboembolism: A systematic review and meta-analysis. *PLoS Medicine, 10*(9), e1001515. doi:10.1371/journal.pmed.1001515.

Corbett, K., & Hannison, E. (2016). Non-pharmacological interventions for the prevention of venous thromboembolism: A literature review. *Nursing Standard, 31*(8), 48–57.

Dunn, N., & Ramos, R. (2017). Preventing venous thromboembolism: The role of nursing with intermittent pneumatic compression. *American Journal of Critical Care, 26*(2), 164–167. Retrieved from https://doi.org/10.4037/ajcc2017504.

Falck-Ytter, Y., Francis, C. W., Johanson, N. A., et al. (2012). Prevention of VTE in orthopedic surgery patients antithrombotic therapy and prevention of thrombosis, 9th ed: American College of Chest Physicians Evidence-Based Clinical Practice Guidelines. *Chest, 141*(2), e278S–2325S.

Finks, J. F., English, W. J., Carlin, A. M., et al. (2012). Predicting risk for venous thromboembolism with bariatric surgery: Results from the Michigan bariatric surgery collaborative. *Annals of Surgery, 255*(6), 1100–1104.

Heeringa, J., Deirdre, A. M., van der Kuip, A., et al. (2006). Prevalence, incidence and lifetime risk of atrial fibrillation: The Rotterdam study. *European Heart Journal, 27*(8), 949–953. Retrieved from https://doi.org/10.1093/eurheartj/ehi825.

Ho, K. M., & Harahsheh, Y. (2016). Intermittent pneumatic compression is effective in reducing proximal DVT. *Evidence-Based Nursing, 19*(2), 47.

Kaur, R., Saagi, M. K., & Choudhary, R. (2016). Evaluate the effectiveness of structured teaching program on knowledge regarding prevention and management of deep vein thrombosis (DVT) in patients among nursing staffs. *International Journal of Nursing Education, 8*(1), 123–127. Retrieved from https://doi.org/10.5958/0974-9357.2016.00022.2.

Kvamme, A. M., & Costanzo, C. (2015). Preventing progression of post-thrombotic syndrome for patients post-deep vein thrombosis. *Medsurg Nursing, 24*(1), 27–34.

Lenchus, J. D., Biehl, M., Cabrera, J., et al. (2017). In-hospital management and follow-up treatment of venous thromboembolism: Focus on new and emerging treatments. *Journal of Intensive Care Medicine (Sage Publications Inc.), 32*(5), 299–311. Retrieved from https://doi.org/10.1177/0885066616648265.

Makic, M. B. (2014). Preventing postsurgical venous thromboembolism. *Journal of Perianesthesia Nursing, 29*(4), 317–319.

Modi, S., Deisler, R., Gozel, K., et al. (2016). Wells Criteria for DVT is a reliable clinical tool to assess the risk of deep vein thrombosis in trauma patients. *World Journal of Emergency Surgery, 11*(24), Retrieved from https://doi.org/10.1186/s13017-016-007801.

Moore, C. (2012). Enhancing patient outcomes with sequential compression device therapy. *American Nurse Today, 7*(11). Retrieved from https://www.americannursetoday.com/enhancing-patient-outcomes-with-sequential-compression-device-therapy/. (Accessed 2 March 2018).

Muñoz-Figueroa, G. P., & Ojo, O. (2015). Venous thromboembolism: Use of graduated compression stockings. *British Journal of Nursing, 24*(13), 680–685.

Pai, M., & Douketis, J. D. (2017). Patient education: Deep vein thrombosis (DVT) (beyond the basics). Retrieved from https://www.uptodate.com. (Accessed 6 January 2019).

Prentiss, A. S. (2012). Early recognition of pediatric venous thromboembolism: A risk-assessment tool. *American Journal of Critical Care, 21*(3), 178–183.

Udoh, I. (2016). Understanding venous thromboembolism in patients with cancer. *The Journal for Nurse Practitioners., 12*(1), 53–59.

Wolf, P. A., Abbott, R. D., & Kannel, W. B. (1991). Atrial fibrillation as an independent risk factor for stroke: The Framingham study. *Stroke; a Journal of Cerebral Circulation, 22*, 983–988.

V

Impaired spontaneous Ventilation   *Debra Siela, PhD, RN, CCNS, ACNS-BC, CCRN-K, CNE, RRT*

NANDA-I

Definition

Inability to initiate and/or maintain independent breathing that is adequate to support life.

Defining Characteristics

Apprehensiveness; decrease in arterial oxygen saturation (SaO_2); decrease in cooperation; decrease in partial pressure of oxygen (Po_2); decrease in tidal volume; dyspnea; increase in accessory muscle use; increase in heart rate; increase in metabolic rate; increase in partial pressure of carbon dioxide (Pco_2); restlessness

Related Factors

Respiratory muscle fatigue

● = Independent;   ▲ = Collaborative;   EBN = Evidence-Based Nursing;   EB = Evidence-Based

Associated Condition

Alteration in metabolism

Suggested NOC Outcomes

Neurological Status: Central Motor Control; Respiratory Status: Gas Exchange, Ventilation

Example NOC Outcome with Indicators
Achieves appropriate **Respiratory Status: Ventilation** as evidenced by the following indicators: Respiratory rate/ Respiratory rhythm/Depth of inspiration/Symmetrical chest expansion/Ease of breathing/Moves sputum out of airway/Accessory muscle use not present/Adventitious breath sounds not present/Chest retraction not present/Tidal volume/Vital capacity. (Rate the outcome and indicators of **Respiratory Status: Ventilation:** 1 = severe deviation from normal range, 2 = substantial deviation from normal range, 3 = moderate deviation from normal range, 4 = mild deviation from normal range, 5 = no deviation from normal range [see Section I].)

Client Outcomes

Client Will (Specify Time Frame)

- Maintain arterial blood gases within safe parameters
- Remain free of dyspnea or restlessness
- Effectively maintain airway
- Effectively mobilize secretions

NIC (Nursing Interventions Classification)

Suggested NIC Interventions

Artificial Airway Management; Mechanical Ventilation: Invasive; Respiratory Monitoring; Resuscitation: Neonate; Ventilation Assistance; Mechanical Ventilation Management: Noninvasive

Example NIC Activities—Mechanical Ventilation Management
Monitor for conditions indicating a need for ventilation support (e.g., respiratory muscle fatigue, neurological dysfunction second to trauma, anesthesia, drug overdose, refractory respiratory acidosis); Consult with other health care personnel in selection of a ventilator mode

Nursing Interventions and *Rationales*

▲ Collaborate with the client, family, and health care provider regarding possible intubation and ventilation. Ask whether the client has advanced directives and, if so, integrate them into the plan of care with clinical data regarding overall health and reversibility of the medical condition. EB: *Client preferences and goals of care need to be acknowledged and discussed when planning care. Advanced directives protect client autonomy and help ensure that the client's wishes are respected (You et al, 2014).*

- Assess and respond to changes in the client's respiratory status. Monitor the client for dyspnea, increase in respiratory rate, use of accessory muscles, retraction of intercostal muscles, flaring of nostrils, decrease in O_2 saturation, cyanosis, and subjective complaints (Kjellström & van der Wal, 2013; Gallagher, 2017).

- Have the client use a numerical scale (0–10) or visual analog scale to self-report dyspnea before and after interventions. *The numerical rating scale is a valid measure of dyspnea and has been found to be easiest for clients to use. Incorporating client self-report of dyspnea assists with assessment of symptom intensity, distress, progression, affect, and resolution of dyspnea (Mahler & O'Donnell, 2015). Determine intensity, unpleasantness, or distress of dyspnea using a rating scale such as an intensity-focused modified Borg scale or visual analog scale (Kjellström & van der Wal, 2013).*

- Assess for history of chronic respiratory disorders when administering oxygen. *When managing acute respiratory failure (ARF) in clients with chronic obstructive pulmonary disease (COPD), continually assess the client's oxygenation needs. Long-term administration of oxygen (>15 hours per day) has been shown to increase survival in clients with severe, resting hypoxemia (GOLD, 2017).*

● = Independent;   ▲ = Collaborative;   EBN = Evidence-Based Nursing;   EB = Evidence-Based

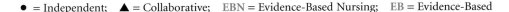

▲ Collaborate with the health care provider and respiratory therapists in determining the appropriateness of noninvasive positive pressure ventilation (NPPV) and noninvasive ventilation (NIV) for the decompensated client with COPD. Ventilatory support in a COPD exacerbation can be provided by either noninvasive or invasive ventilation (GOLD, 2017). NIV improves respiratory acidosis and decreases respiratory rate, severity of breathlessness, incidence of ventilator-associated pneumonia (VAP), and hospital length of stay (Mas & Masip, 2014; American Association of Critical Care Nurses [AACN], 2017a; GOLD, 2017).

▲ Assist with implementation, client support, and monitoring if NPPV/NIV is used. **EB/CEB:** *In a client with exacerbation of COPD, NPPV/NIV can be as effective as intubation with use of a ventilator (Ramsey & Hart, 2013; Lindenauer et al, 2014). NPPV/NIV also has been found to improve outcomes in clients with acute cardiogenic pulmonary edema (Bakke et al, 2014; Mas & Masip, 2014). It also can be used in ARF causes such as asthma, pneumonia, postextubation failure, thoracic trauma, and palliative care (Masclans et al, 2013; Nava et al, 2013; Gifford, 2014; Johnson et al, 2014; Lin et al, 2014; Pallin & Naughton, 2014; Murad et al, 2015). The use of continuous positive airway pressure and bilevel positive airway pressure has been shown to improve oxygenation and decrease the rate of endotracheal intubation in clients with acute pulmonary edema (Frazier, 2017; GOLD, 2017).*

• If the client has apnea, respiratory muscle fatigue, somnolence, hypoxemia, and/or acute respiratory acidosis, then prepare the client for possible intubation and mechanical ventilation. **EB:** *These indicators may predict the need for invasive mechanical ventilation to support the client's respiratory efforts (Gallagher, 2017; Stacy, 2018). The indications for initiating invasive mechanical ventilation during a COPD exacerbation include a failure of an initial trial of NIV (Gallagher, 2017; GOLD, 2017).*

• If a client with ARF has a rapid shallow breathing index (RSBI) >105, endotracheal intubation is likely needed with invasive mechanical ventilation. A client with ARF with an RSBI of <105 may require only noninvasive ventilation (Karthika et al, 2016).

Ventilator Support

▲ Explain the endotracheal intubation and mechanical ventilation process to the client and family as appropriate, and during intubation administer sedation for client comfort according to the health care provider's orders. **EBN:** *Explanation of the procedure decreases anxiety and reinforces information; premedication allows for a more controlled intubation with decreased incidence of insertion problems (Joanna Briggs Institute, 2013; Gallagher, 2017).*

• Secure the endotracheal tube in place using either tape or a commercial available device, auscultate bilateral breath sounds, use a CO_2 detector, and obtain a chest radiograph to confirm endotracheal tube placement. **EBN:** *Security of the tube is needed to prevent inadvertent extubation. Nursing studies have shown conflicting results regarding the preferable way to secure the endotracheal tube (Goodrich, 2017a).* **EB:** *Auscultation alone is an unreliable method for checking endotracheal tube placement. A CO_2 detector can be used to confirm tube placement in the trachea (Goodrich, 2017b; Stacy, 2018); however, correct position of the endotracheal tube in the trachea (3–5 cm above the carina) must be confirmed by chest radiograph (Goodrich, 2017a,b; Stacy, 2018). Calorimetric CO_2 detectors have also been used successfully to detect inadvertent airway intubation during gastric tube placement (Goodrich, 2017a,b).*

• Review ventilator settings with the health care provider and respiratory therapy to ensure support is appropriate to meet the client's minute ventilation requirements (Chacko et al, 2015; Stacy, 2018). *Ventilator settings should be adjusted to prevent hyperventilation or hypoventilation. A variety of new modes of ventilation are currently available that are responsive to client effort (pressure support)(Gallagher, 2017).*

▲ Suction as needed and hyperoxygenate according to facility policy. Refer to the care plan for Ineffective **Airway** clearance for further information on suctioning.

• Check that monitor alarms are set appropriately at the start of each shift. *This action helps ensure client safety (Gallagher, 2017).*

• Respond to ventilator alarms promptly. If unable to immediately locate the source/cause of an alarm, use a manual self-inflating resuscitation bag to ventilate the client while waiting for assistance. *Common causes of a high-pressure alarm include secretions, condensation in the tubing, biting of the endotracheal tube, decreased compliance of the lungs, and compression of the tubing. Common causes of a low-pressure alarm are ventilator disconnection, leaks in the circuit, and changing compliance. Using a manual self-inflating resuscitation bag with supplemental oxygen, the nurse can provide immediate ventilation and oxygenation as needed (Gallagher, 2017).*

• Prevent unplanned extubation by maintaining stability of the endotracheal tube (Goodrich, 2017b). **EB:** *Prevent unplanned extubation with use of weaning protocol (Karthika et al, 2016).*

• = Independent;   ▲ = Collaborative;   EBN = Evidence-Based Nursing;   EB = Evidence-Based

- Drain collected fluid from condensation out of ventilator tubing as needed. *This action reduces the risk for infection by decreasing inhalation of contaminated water droplets (Gallagher, 2017).*
- Note ventilator settings of flow of inspired oxygen, peak inspiratory pressure, tidal volume, and alarm activation at intervals and when removing the client from the ventilator for any reason (Gallagher, 2017). *Checking the settings ensures that safety measures are taken and that the client is not left on 100% oxygen after suctioning (Gallagher, 2017).*
- ▲ Administer analgesics and sedatives as needed to facilitate client comfort and rest. Use behavioral and sedation scales for nonverbal clients to provide a consistent way of monitoring pain and sedation levels and ensuring that therapeutic outcomes are being met (Barr et al, 2013; Dale et al, 2014; Reade & Finfer, 2014). Clients receiving mechanical ventilation frequently require sedation to help attenuate the anxiety, pain, and agitation associated with this intervention (Barr et al, 2013). The overall goal of sedation during mechanical ventilation is to provide physiological stability, ventilator synchrony, and comfort for clients (Makic et al, 2015).
- Tools such as the Riker Sedation-Agitation Scale, the Motor Activity Assessment Scale, the Ramsey Scale, or the Richmond Agitation-Sedation Scale may be useful in monitoring levels of sedation. *Each of these instruments has established reliability and validity and can be used to monitor the effect of sedative therapy (Barr et al, 2013; Dale, 2014).*
- Alternatives to medications for decreasing anxiety should be attempted, such as music therapy with selections of the client's choice played on headphones at intervals. CEB/EBN: *Music therapy has been reported to decrease anxiety and reduce heart and respiratory rate in critically ill and intubated clients (Hunter et al, 2010; Tracy & Chlan, 2011; Gelinas et al, 2013; Hetland, Lindquist, & Chlan, 2015).*
- Analyze and respond to arterial blood gas results, end-tidal CO_2 levels, and pulse oximetry values. *Ventilatory support must be closely monitored to ensure adequate oxygenation and acid-base balance.* EBN: *End-tidal CO_2 monitoring is best used as an adjunct to direct client observation and is used to monitor a client's ventilatory status and pulmonary blood flow (Gallagher, 2017).*
- Use an effective means of verbal and nonverbal communication with the client. Barriers to communication include endotracheal tubes, sedation, and general weakness associated with a critical illness. Basic technologies should be readily available to the client, including eyeglasses and hearing aids. A variety of communication devices are available, including electronic voice output communication aids, alphabet boards, picture boards, computers, and writing slate. Ask the client for input into their care as appropriate (ten Hoorn et al, 2016).
- Move the endotracheal tube from side to side at least every 24 hours, and tape it or secure it with a commercially available device. Assess and document client's skin condition, and ensure correct tube placement at the lip line (National Pressure Ulcer Advisory Panel, 2013; Vollman, Sole, & Quinn, 2017).
- Implement steps to prevent ventilator-associated events (VAE), such as VAP, including continuous removal of subglottic secretions, elevation of the head of bed to 30 to 45 degrees (Patient Safety Movement Foundation, 2017; AACN, 2017a) unless medically contraindicated, change of the ventilator circuit no more than every 48 hours, and handwashing before and after contact with each client.
- *The accumulation of contaminated oropharyngeal secretions above the endotracheal tube may contribute to the risk of aspiration.* Use endotracheal tubes that allow for the continuous aspiration of subglottic secretions (Frost et al, 2013; Vollman, Sole, & Quinn, 2017). EB: *Subglottic secretion drainage during mechanical ventilation results in a significant reduction in VAE, including late-onset VAP (Frost et al, 2013; Vollman, Sole, & Quinn, 2017). Use of continuous subglottic suctioning endotracheal tubes for intubation in clients who are predicted to require more than 48 hours of intubation likely results in decreased incidence of VAP (AACN, 2017b).*
- Position the client in a semirecumbent position with the head of the bed at a 30 to 45 degree angle to decrease the aspiration of gastric, oral, and nasal secretions (Patient Safety Movement Foundation, 2017; AACN, 2017b; Vollman, Sole, & Quinn, 2017). Consider use of kinetic therapy, using a kinetic bed that slowly moves the client with 40 degree turns. *Rotational therapy may decrease the incidence of pulmonary complications in high-risk clients with increasing ventilator support requirements, at risk for VAP, and with clinical indications for acute lung injury or acute respiratory distress syndrome with worsening Pao_2:FiO_2 ratio, presence of fluffy infiltrates via chest radiograph concomitant with pulmonary edema, and refractory hypoxemia (Joanna Briggs Institute, 2014; Klompas, 2014; Makic et al, 2015; Hanneman, 2015; St. Clair et al, 2017).*
- Perform handwashing using both soap and water and alcohol-based solution before and after all mechanically ventilated client contact to prevent spread of infections (Makic et al, 2013; Centers for Disease Control and Prevention, 2014).

V

● = Independent;   ▲ = Collaborative;   EBN = Evidence-Based Nursing;   EB = Evidence-Based

- Provide routine oral care using toothbrushing and oral rinsing with an antimicrobial agent if needed (Joanna Briggs Institute, 2014; AACN, 2017a,b; Vollman, Sole, & Quinn et al, 2017). **EB:** *Reducing bacterial colonization of the oral cavity includes interventions of daily oral assessment, deep suctioning every 4 hours, toothbrushing twice per day with a plaque reducer, and oral tissue cleaning with peroxide every 4 hours. A Cochrane review found that routine oral care that included chlorhexidine mouthwash or gel resulted in a 40% reduction in development of VAP (Shi et al, 2013).*
- Maintain proper cuff inflation for both endotracheal tubes and cuffed tracheostomy tubes with minimal leak volume or minimal occlusion volume to decrease risk of aspiration and reduce incidence of VAP (AACN, 2016; Johnson, 2017; Stacy, 2018).
- Reposition the client as needed. Use rotational bed or kinetic bed therapy in clients for whom side-to-side turning is contraindicated or difficult. **EBN:** *Changing position frequently decreases the incidence of atelectasis, pooling of secretions, and resultant VAP (Johnson, 2017; St. Clair et al, 2017). **EB/EBN:** Continuous, lateral rotational therapy has been shown to improve oxygenation and decrease the incidence of VAP (Joanna Briggs Institute, 2014; St. Clair et al, 2017).*
- ▲ Patients mechanically ventilated for more than 24 hours can benefit from protocolized rehabilitation directed toward early mobilization (Schmidt et al, 2017).
- Assess bilateral anterior and posterior breath sounds every 2 to 4 hours and as needed; respond to any relevant changes (Gallagher, 2017).
- Assess responsiveness to ventilator support; monitor for subjective complaints and sensation of dyspnea (Gallagher, 2017).
- ▲ Collaborate with the interdisciplinary team in treating clients with ARF to meet the client's ventilator care needs and avoid complications (Karthika et al, 2016). **EB:** *A collaborative approach to caring for mechanically ventilated clients has been demonstrated to reduce length of time on the ventilator and length of stay in the intensive care unit (Rose et al, 2014).*
- *Document assessments and interventions according to policy.*

Geriatric

- Recognize that critically ill older adults have a high rate of morbidity when mechanically ventilated.
- ▲ NPPV may be used during acute treatment of older clients with impaired ventilation. **EB:** *A recent study found that older immunocompromised clients admitted with pneumonia had decreased morbidity and mortality when NPPV compared with mechanical ventilation was used to support impaired ventilation (Johnson et al, 2014).*

Home Care

- ▲ Some of the interventions listed previously may be adapted for home care use. Begin discharge planning as soon as possible with the case manager or social worker to assess the need for home support systems, assistive devices, and community or home health services.
- ▲ With help from a medical social worker, assist the client and family to determine the fiscal effect of care in the home versus an extended care facility.
- Assess the home setting during the discharge process to ensure the home can safely accommodate ventilator support (e.g., adequate space and electricity).
- Have the family contact the electric company and place the client residence on a high-risk list in case of a power outage. *Some home-based care requires special conditions for safe home administration.*
- Assess the caregivers for commitment to supporting a ventilator-dependent client in the home.
- Be sure that the client and family or caregivers are familiar with operation of all ventilation devices, know how to suction secretions if needed, are competent in doing tracheostomy care, and know schedules for cleaning equipment. Have the designated caregiver or caregivers demonstrate care before discharge. *Some home-based care involves specialized technology and requires specific skills for safe and appropriate care.*
- Assess client and caregiver knowledge of the disease, client needs, and medications to be administered via ventilation-assistive devices. Avoid analgesics. Assess knowledge of how to use equipment. Teach as necessary. *A client receiving ventilation support may not be able to articulate needs. Respiratory medications can have side effects that change the client's respiration or level of consciousness.*
- Establish an emergency plan and criteria for use. Identify emergency procedures to be used until medical assistance arrives. Teach and role-play emergency care. *A prepared emergency plan reassures the client and family and ensures client safety.*

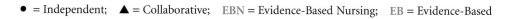

● = Independent; ▲ = Collaborative; EBN = Evidence-Based Nursing; EB = Evidence-Based

Client/Family Teaching and Discharge Planning

- Explain to the client the potential sensations that will be experienced, including relief of dyspnea, the feeling of lung inflations, the noise of the ventilator, and the reality of alarms. **EBN:** *Knowledge of potential sensations and experiences before they are encountered can decrease anxiety. Administration of sedatives and/ or narcotics may be needed to provide adequate oxygenation and ventilation in some clients (Barr et al, 2013; Gallagher, 2017).*
- Explain to the client and family about being unable to speak, and work out an alternative system of communication. See previously mentioned interventions (Gallagher, 2017).
- Demonstrate to the family how to perform simple procedures, such as suctioning secretions in the mouth with a tonsil-tip catheter, providing range-of-motion exercises, and reconnecting the ventilator immediately if it becomes disconnected. *Families are a critical part of the client's care, may be present at the bedside for prolonged periods of time, and need information about the plan of care (Gallagher, 2017).*
- Offer both the client and family explanations about how the ventilator works and answer any questions. *Having questions answered is often cited as an important need of clients and families when a client is on a ventilator (Gallagher, 2017).*

REFERENCES

American Association of Critical Care Nurses. (2016). *AACN Practice Alert—Prevention of aspiration in adults.* Retrieved from https://www.aacn.org/~/media/aacn-website/clincial-resources/practice-alerts/preventionaspirationpracticealert.pdf. (Accessed 10 February 2018).

American Association of Critical Care Nurses. (2017a). *AACN Practice Alert—Prevention of ventilator-associated pneumonia in adults.* Retrieved from https://www.aacn.org/~/media/aacn-website/clincial-resources/practice-alerts/preventingvapinadults2017.pdf. (Accessed 10 February 2018).

American Association of Critical Care Nurses. (2017b). *AACN Practice Alert—Oral care for acutely and critically ill patients.* Retrieved from https://www.aacn.org/~/media/aacn-website/clincial-resources/practice-alerts/oralcarepractalert2017.pdf. (Accessed 10 February 2018).

Bakke, S., et al. (2014). Continuous positive airway pressure and noninvasive ventilation in prehospital treatment of patients with acute respiratory failure: A systematic review of controlled studies. *Scandinavia Journal of Trauma Resuscitation Emergency Medicine,* 22(1).

Barr, J., Fraser, G. L., Puntillo, K., et al. (2013). Clinical practice guidelines for the management of pain, agitation, and delirium in adult patients in the intensive care unit. *Critical Care Medicine,* 41(1), 263–306.

Centers for Disease Control and Prevention. (2014). *Hand hygiene basics.* Retrieved from http://www.cdc.gov/handhygiene/Basics.html. (Accessed 10 February 2018).

Chacko, B., Peter, J. V., Tharyan, P. I., et al. (2015). Pressure-controlled versus volume-controlled ventilation for acute respiratory failure due to acute lung injury (ALI) or acute respiratory distress syndrome (ARDS). *Cochrane Database of Systematic Reviews,* (1), CD008807.

Dale, C., Kannas, D., Fran, V., et al. (2014). Improved analgesia, sedation, and delirium protocol associated with decreased duration of delirium and mechanical ventilation. *Annals of American Thoracic Society,* 11(3), 367–374.

Frazier, K. (2017). Weaning mechanical ventilation. In D. L. Wiegand (Ed.), *AACN procedure manual for high acuity, progressive, and critical care* (7th ed.). Philadelphia: Saunders Elsevier.

Frost, S. A., Azeem, A., Alexandrou, E., et al. (2013). Subglottic secretion drainage for preventing ventilator associated pneumonia: A meta-analysis. *Australian Critical Care,* 26(4), 180–188.

Gallagher, J. (2017). Invasive mechanical ventilation (through an artificial airway): Volume and pressure modes. In D. L. Wiegand (Ed.), *AACN procedure manual for high acuity, progressive, and critical care* (7th ed.). Philadelphia: Saunders Elsevier.

Gelinas, C., Arbour, C., Michaud, C., et al. (2013). Patients and ICU nurses' perspectives of non-pharmacological interventions for pain management. *Nursing in Care Nurse,* 18(6), 307–318.

Gifford, A. (2014). Noninvasive ventilation as a palliative measure. *Current Opinion Support Palliative Care,* 8(3), 218–224.

GOLD. *Global strategy for the diagnosis, management, and prevention of COPD (revised 2017), Global Initiative for Chronic Obstructive Lung Disease.* Retrieved from http://goldcopd.org/wp-content/uploads/2016/12/wms-GOLD-2017-Pocket-Guide.pdf. (Accessed 10 February 2018).

Goodrich, C. (2017a). Endotracheal intubation (assist). In D. L. Wiegand (Ed.), *AACN procedure manual for high acuity, progressive, and critical care* (7th ed.). Philadelphia: Saunders Elsevier.

Goodrich, C. (2017b). Endotracheal intubation (perform). In D. L. Wiegand (Ed.), *AACN procedure manual for high acuity, progressive, and critical care* (7th ed.). Philadelphia: Saunders Elsevier.

Hanneman, S. (2015). Manual vs. automated lateral rotation to reduce preventable pulmonary complications in ventilator patients. *American Journal of Critical Care,* 24, 24–32.

Hetland, B., Lindquist, R., & Chlan, L. (2015). The influence of music during mechanical ventilation and weaning from mechanical ventilation: A review. *Heart and Lung: The Journal of Critical Care,* 44, 416–425.

Hunter, B. C., Oliva, R., Sahler, O. J. Z., et al. (2010). Music therapy as an adjunctive treatment in the management of stress for patients being weaned from mechanical ventilation. *Journal of Music Therapy,* 17(3), 198–219.

Joanna Briggs Institute. (2013). *Endotracheal tube (ventilated patient) care.*

Joanna Briggs Institute. (2014). *Ventilator-associated pneumonia prevention.*

Johnson, C. S., Frei, C. R., Metersky, M. L., et al. (2014). Non-invasive mechanical ventilation and mortality in elderly immunocompromised patients hospitalized with pneumonia: A retrospective cohort study. *BMC Pulmonary Medicine,* 14(7), 1–10. Retrieved from http://www.biomedcentral.com/1471-2466/14/7. (Accessed 23 April 2015).

Johnson, R. (2017). Tracheostomy cuff and tube care. In D. L. Wiegand (Ed.), *AACN procedure manual for high acuity, progressive, and critical care* (7th ed.). Philadelphia: Saunders Elsevier.

● = Independent;   ▲ = Collaborative;   **EBN** = Evidence-Based Nursing;   **EB** = Evidence-Based

Karthika, M., Al Enezi, F. A., Pillai, L. V., et al. (2016). Rapid shallow breathing index. *Annals of Thoracic Medicine, 11*(3), 167–176. Retrieved from http://doi.org/10.4103/1817-1737.176876.

Kjellström, B., & van der Wal, M. H. L. (2013). Old and new tools to assess dyspnea in the hospitalized patient. *Current Heart Failure Reports, 2013*(10), 204–211.

Klompas, B. (2014). Strategies to prevent ventilator-associated pneumonia in acute care hospitals: 2014 update. *Infection Control & Hospital Epidemiology, 35*, 915–936.

Lin, C., et al. (2014). The efficacy of noninvasive ventilation in managing postextubation respiratory failure: A meta-analysis. *Heart and Lung, 43*, 99–104.

Lindenauer, P., et al. (2014). Outcomes associated with invasive and noninvasive ventilation among patients hospitalized with exacerbations of chronic obstructive pulmonary disease. *Journal of American Medical Association Internal Medicine, 174*(2), 1982–1993.

Mahler, D. A., & O'Donnell, D. E. (2015). Recent advances in dyspnea. *Chest, 147*(1), 232–241.

Makic, M., Rauen, C., Jones, K., et al. (2015). Continuing to challenge practice to be evidence based. *Critical Care Nurse, 35*(2), 39–50.

Makic, M. B. F., Martin, S. A., Burns, S., et al. (2013). Putting evidence into nursing practice: Four traditional practices not supported by the evidence. *Critical Care Nurse, 33*(2), 28–42.

Mas, A., & Masip, J. (2014). Noninvasive ventilation in acute respiratory failure. *International Journal of COPD, 9*, 837–852.

Masclans, J., et al. (2013). Early non-invasive ventilation treatment for severe influenza pneumonia. *Clinical Microbiology Infection, 19*(3), 249–256.

Murad, A., et al. (2015). The role of noninvasive positive pressure ventilation in community-acquired pneumonia. *Journal of Critical Care, 30*(1), 49–54.

National Pressure Ulcer Advisory Panel. (2013). *Best practices for prevention of medical device-related pressure ulcers in critical care.* Retrieved from http://www.npuap.org/wp-content/uploads/2013/04/BestPractices-CriticalCare1.pdf. (Accessed 10 February 2018).

Nava, S., et al. (2013). Palliative use of non-invasive ventilation in end-of-life patients with solid tumours: A randomized feasibility trial. *Lancet Oncology, 14*(3), 219–227.

Pallin, M., & Naughton, M. (2014). Noninvasive ventilation in acute asthma. *Journal of Critical Care, 29*, 586–593.

Patient Safety Movement Foundation. (2017). Continuing to challenge practice to be evidence based. *Critical Care Nurse, 35*(2), 39–50.

Retrieved from https://patientsafetymovement.org/wp-content/uploads/2016/02/APSS-2D_-Ventilator-associated-Pneumonia-VAP-copy.pdf. (Accessed 23 November 2018).

Ramsey, M., & Hart, N. (2013). Current opinions on non-invasive ventilation as a treatment for chronic obstructive pulmonary disease. *Current Opinion Pulmonary Medicine, 19*(6), 626–630.

Reade, M., & Finfer, S. (2014). Sedation and delirium in the intensive care unit. *New England Journal of Medicine, 370*, 444–454.

Rose, L., Dainty, K., Jordan, J., et al. (2014). Weaning from mechanical ventilation: A scoping review of qualitative studies. *American Journal of Critical Care, 23*(5), e54–e71.

Schmidt, C., Girard, T., Kress, J., et al. (2017). Official executive summary of an American thoracic Society/American College of chest physicians clinical practice guideline: Liberation from mechanical ventilation in critically ill adults. *American Journal of Respiratory and Critical Care Medicine, 195*(1), 115–119.

Shi, Z., Xie, H., Wang, P., et al. (2013). Oral hygiene care for critically ill patients to prevent ventilator-associated pneumonia. *Cochrane Database of Systematic Reviews*, (8), CD008367.

Stacy, K. M. (2018). Pulmonary therapeutic management. In L. D. Urden, K. M. Stacy, & M. E. Lough (Eds.), *Critical care nursing: diagnosis and management* (8th ed.). Maryland Heights, MO: Elsevier.

St. Clair, J. (2017). Continuous lateral rotation therapy. In D. L. Wiegand (Ed.), *AACN procedure manual for critical care* (7th ed.). Philadelphia: Saunders Elsevier.

ten Hoorn, S., Elbers, P. W., Girbes, A. R., et al. (2016). Communicating with conscious and mechanically ventilated critically ill patients: A systematic review. *Critical Care, 20*, 333. doi:10.1186/s13054-016-1483-2. Retrieved from https://www.ncbi.nlm.nih.gov/pmc/articles/PMC5070186/pdf/13054_2016_Article_1483.pdf. (Accessed 10 February 2018).

Tracy, M. F., & Chlan, L. (2011). Nonpharmacological interventions to manage common symptoms in patients receiving mechanical ventilation. *Critical Care Nurse, 31*(3), 19–28.

You, J. J., Fowler, R. A., & Heyland, D. K. (2014). Just ask: Discussing goals of care with patients in hospital with serious illness. *Canadian Medical Association Journal, 186*(6), 425–432.

Vollman, K., Sole, M., & Quinn, B. (2017). Endotracheal tube care and oral care practices for ventilated and non-ventilated patients. In D. L. Wiegand (Ed.), *AACN procedure manual for high acuity, progressive, and critical care* (7th ed.). Philadelphia: Saunders Elsevier.

Dysfunctional Ventilatory weaning response

Debra Siela, PhD, RN, CCNS, ACNS-BC, CCRN-K, CNE, RRT

NANDA-I

Definition

Inability to adjust to lowered levels of mechanical ventilator support that interrupts and prolongs the weaning process.

Defining Characteristics

Mild

Breathing discomfort; fatigue; fear of machine malfunction; feeling warm; increase in focus on breathing; mild increase in respiratory rate over baseline; perceived need for increased in oxygen; restlessness

● = Independent;   ▲ = Collaborative;   **EBN** = Evidence-Based Nursing;   **EB** = Evidence-Based

Moderate

Abnormal skin color; apprehensiveness; decrease in air entry on auscultation; diaphoresis; facial expression of fear; hyperfocused on activities; impaired ability to cooperate; impaired ability to respond to coaching; increase in blood pressure from baseline (<20 mm Hg); increase in heart rate from baseline (<20 beats/minute); minimal use of respiratory accessory muscles; moderate increase in respiratory rate over baseline

Severe

Abnormal skin color; adventitious breath sounds; agitation; asynchronized breathing with the ventilator; decrease in level of consciousness; deterioration in arterial blood gases from baseline; gasping breaths; increase in blood pressure from baseline (≥20 mm Hg); increase in heart rate from baseline (≥20 beats/minute); paradoxical abdominal breathing; profuse diaphoresis; shallow breathing; significant increase in respiratory rate above baseline; use of significant respiratory accessory muscles

Related Factors

Physiological

Alteration in sleep pattern; inadequate nutrition; ineffective airway clearance; pain

Psychological

Anxiety; decrease in motivation; fear; hopelessness; insufficient knowledge of weaning process; insufficient trust in health care professional; low self-esteem; powerlessness; uncertainty about ability to wean

Situational

Environmental barrier; inappropriate pace of weaning process; insufficient social support; uncontrolled episodic energy demands

Associated Condition

History of unsuccessful weaning attempt; history of ventilator dependence >4 days

 NOC (Nursing Outcomes Classification)

Suggested NOC Outcomes

Respiratory Status: Gas Exchange; Ventilation

Example NOC Outcome with Indicators
Achieves appropriate **Respiratory Status: Ventilation** as evidenced by the following indicators: Respiratory rate/Respiratory rhythm/Depth of inspiration/Symmetrical chest expansion/Ease of breathing/Moves sputum out of airway/Accessory muscle use not present/Adventitious breath sounds not present/Chest retraction not present/Tidal volume/Vital capacity. (Rate the outcome and indicators of **Respiratory Status: Ventilation:** 1 = severe deviation from normal range, 2 = substantial deviation from normal range, 3 = moderate deviation from normal range, 4 = mild deviation from normal range, 5 = no deviation from normal range [see Section I].)

Client Outcomes

Client Will (Specify Time Frame)

- Wean from ventilator with adequate arterial blood gases
- Remain free of unresolved dyspnea or restlessness
- Effectively clear secretions

NIC (Nursing Interventions Classification)

Suggested NIC Interventions

Mechanical Ventilation Management: Invasive; Mechanical Ventilatory Weaning

Example NIC Activities—Mechanical Ventilatory Weaning
Monitor for optimal fluid and electrolyte status; Monitor to ensure client is free of significant infection before weaning

● = Independent;   ▲ = Collaborative;   EBN = Evidence-Based Nursing;   EB = Evidence-Based

Nursing Interventions and *Rationales*

- Assess client's readiness for weaning as evidenced by the following:
  - ○ Physiological and psychological readiness; there has been little research devoted to the study of psychological readiness to wean. EBN: *Assess fears and anxieties that can contribute to prolonged and repeated failure of ventilator weaning (Ward & Fulbrook, 2016).*
  - ○ Resolution of initial medical problem that led to ventilator dependence.
  - ○ Hemodynamic stability.
  - ○ Normal hemoglobin levels.
  - ○ Absence of fever.
  - ○ Normal state of consciousness.
  - ○ Metabolic, fluid, and electrolyte balance.
  - ○ Adequate nutritional status with serum albumin levels >2.5 g/dL.
  - ○ Adequate sleep.
  - ○ Adequate pain management and minimal sedation.

EB: *A rapid shallow breathing index (RSBI) may predict weaning success (Penuelas, Thille, & Esteban, 2015; Karthika et al, 2016). A spontaneous breathing trial (SBT) is often preceded by evaluation of the patient's level of consciousness, physiological and hemodynamic stability, adequacy of oxygenation and ventilation, spontaneous breathing capability, and respiratory rate (RR) and pattern. Routine weaning predictor parameters include negative inspiratory force (NIF), vital capacity (VC), tidal volume (VT), RR, minute volume (VE), and RSBI (Kacmarek, 2013), although, applying these weaning predictors should not delay extubation decisions (Penuelas, Thille, & Esteban, 2015). Decreased heart rate variability and RR variability are associated with weaning/ extubation failure and should be assessed to help predict weaning outcomes (Huang et al, 2014; Seely et al, 2014). Assessment of the percentage of change in diaphragm thickness (Δtdi%) between end-expiration and end-inspiration can reflect diaphragm strength. This measurement is analogous to the ejection fraction of the heart (Matamis et al, 2013; DiNino et al, 2014; Penuelas, Thille, & Esteban, 2015). Predictors of extubation failure include disease severity, secretion burden, higher minute ventilation, and lower oxygenation (Miu et al, 2014).*

- ▲ Noninvasive weaning may be used in place of invasive mechanical support in adults with respiratory failure. EB: *Noninvasive weaning reduces rates of death and pneumonia without increasing the risk of weaning failure or reintubation. In subgroup analyses, mortality benefits were significantly greater in patients with chronic obstructive pulmonary disease (COPD) (Burns et al, 2013; Penuelas, Thille, & Esteban, 2015). After an SBT to extubation high-risk patients receiving mechanical ventilation for more than 24 hours should be placed on noninvasive ventilation (NIV; Schmidt et al, 2017). Early use of NIV as a prophylactic intervention can be used to prevent reintubation for patients considered at high risk (Bajaj et al, 2015).*

- *Patients managed with ventilator liberation protocols spend fewer hours on mechanical ventilation and earlier intensive care unit (ICU) discharge than did patients managed without a protocol. However, ventilator liberation protocols have no significant effect on mortality or reintubation rates (Schmidt et al, 2017).*

- ▲ A spontaneous awakening trial (SAT) in conjunction with a daily weaning assessment has a great effect on ventilator liberation outcomes (Haas & Loik, 2012; Jones et al, 2014, Klompas et al, 2015; Penuelas, Thille, & Esteban, 2015). EB: *Using computerized automated weaning systems based on weaning protocols decreases weaning time, time to successful extubation, ICU length of stay (LOS), and number of patients requiring prolonged mechanical ventilation (Blackwood et al, 2014; Burns et al, 2014; Dale et al, 2014; Rose et al, 2014). EB: Goal-directed weaning decreased ventilator days and ICU and hospital LOS (Zhu et al, 2015). Pairing of an SBT and SAT or sedation interruption reduced ICU and hospital LOS, duration of mechanical ventilation, and ventilator-associated events (Klompas et al, 2015; Rose, 2015).*

- ▲ *The use of lighter sedation resulted in less duration of mechanical ventilation, more ventilator-free days and ICU-free days, and reduced mortality (Dale et al, 2014; Reade & Finfer, 2014; Schmidt et al, 2017).*

- *An early mobility and walking program can promote weaning from ventilator support as a client's overall strength and endurance improve (Balas et al, 2014; Penuelas, Thille, & Esteban, 2015). Acutely hospitalized patients who are mechanically ventilated for greater than 24 hours require early mobilization (Schmidt et al, 2017). When assessing clinical outcomes of survivors of critical illness requiring prolonged mechanical ventilation, the combination of high protein and a mobility-based rehabilitation program leads to increased rates of discharge home and ventilator weaning success (Wappel et al, 2017).*

- *Early mobility and physical rehabilitation can reduce muscle weakness, mechanical ventilation duration, and ICU and hospital stays (Penuelas, Thille, & Esteban, 2015; Spruit et al, 2013). Patients mechanically ventilated for more than 24 hours can benefit from protocolized rehabilitation directed toward early mobilization (Schmidt*

● = Independent;   ▲ = Collaborative;   EBN = Evidence-Based Nursing;   EB = Evidence-Based

et al, 2017). **CEB/EB:** *The Awakening and Breathing Coordination, Delirium Monitoring and Management, and Early Mobility (ABCDE) bundle has criteria to determine when clients are candidates for early mobility (Balas et al, 2012; Costa et al., 2017).*

- Provide adequate nutrition to ventilated clients, using enteral feeding when possible. *When assessing clinical outcomes of survivors of critical illness requiring PMV, the combination of high protein and a mobility-based rehabilitation program leads to increased rates of discharge home and ventilator weaning success (Wappel et al, 2017).*

- Use evidence-based weaning and extubation protocols as appropriate. **EBN/EB:** *The American Thoracic Society recommended use of ventilator liberation protocols to manage patients who have been mechanically ventilated for over 24 hours (Schmidt et al, 2017). The duration of treatment with mechanical ventilation and ventilation utilization ratio (VUR) were reduced in clients who received a SBT protocol (Jones et al, 2014). Protocol-directed weaning has been demonstrated to be safe and effective but not superior to other weaning methods that used structured rounds and other processes that allow for timely and ongoing clinical decision-making by expert nurses and health care providers (Balas et al, 2012; Costa et al, 2017).*

- Identify reasons for previous unsuccessful weaning attempts, and include that information in the development of the weaning plan. **EBN:** *Compared with the Venturi mask, high-flow nasal cannula oxygen use results in better oxygenation for the same set FiO_2 after extubation. Use of high-flow nasal cannula is associated with better comfort, fewer desaturations and interface displacements, and a lower reintubation rate (Maggiore et al, 2014; Penuelas, Thille, & Esteban, 2015). Pressure support reduces respiratory effort compared with T-piece. Continuous positive airway pressure of 0 cm H2O and T-piece more accurately reflect the physiological conditions after extubation (Penuelas, Thille, & Esteban, 2015; Sklar et al, 2017).*

- Reducing the size of artificial airways can increase airway resistance and overly increase energy expenditures of the diaphragm (Penuelas, Thille, & Esteban, 2015). **EB:** *Deflating the tracheal cuff in tracheostomized patients shortens weaning, reduces respiratory infections, and probably improves swallowing (Hernandez et al, 2013; Penuelas, Thille, & Esteban, 2015). A cuff leak test (CLT) should be performed in patients who meet extubation criteria and are at high risk for postextubation stridor (PES). PES may result in reintubation. Systemic steroids may be necessary 4 hours before extubation for patients who failed their CLT (Schmidt et al, 2017).*

- ▲ *Extubation failure may be avoided in patients with neurological disease by using protective ventilation, early enteral nutrition, antibiotic therapy standardization, and systematic testing extubation compared with a conventional strategy (Penuelas, Thille, & Esteban, 2015).*

- ▲ Collaborate with an interdisciplinary team (health care provider, nurse, respiratory therapist, physical therapist, and dietitian) to develop a weaning plan with a time line and goals; revise this plan throughout the weaning period. **CEB/EB:** *Decisions related to weaning trials should be made in conjunction with members of the interdisciplinary team (Balas et al, 2012; Haas & Loik, 2012; Rose et al, 2014; Costa et al, 2017).*

- In clients with COPD who fail extubation, NIV facilitates weaning, prevents reintubation, and reduces mortality. Early NIV after extubation reduces the risk for respiratory failure and lowers 90-day mortality in clients with hypercapnia during an SBT (Burns et al, 2013; Mas & Masip, 2014; Ward & Fulbrook, 2016).

- Assist client to identify personal strategies that result in relaxation and comfort (e.g., music, visualization, relaxation techniques, reading, television, family visits). Support implementation of these strategies. Music intervention can be used to allay anxiety and can be a powerful distractor from distressful sounds and thoughts in the ICU (Tracy & Chlan, 2011; Bradt & Dileo, 2014). **EBN:** *Evidence supports music as an effective intervention that can lessen symptoms related to mechanical ventilation and promote effective weaning (Hetland, Lindquist, & Chlan, 2015). Music therapy increases weaning duration on daily weaning and also decreases RR and dyspnea (Liang et al, 2016). Patients who received a guided imagery intervention had reduced length of hospital stay (1.4 less days) and 4.88 less mechanical ventilation days compared with the comparison group (Spiva et al, 2015).*

- Provide a safe and comfortable environment.

- If unable to stay, make the call light button readily available and assure the client that needs will be met responsively. **EBN:** *Presence entails a focus by the nurse to engage attentively with the client (Tracy & Chlan, 2011).* **EBN:** *Knowing the client in association with objective clinical data helps individualize the weaning process (Rose et al, 2014).*

- ▲ Coordinate pain and sedation medications to minimize sedative effects. Appropriate levels of sedation may be key to successful weaning (Reade & Finfer, 2014). **EBN:** *Nursing-implemented sedation protocols have been used effectively to improve the probability of successful extubation (Balas et al, 2012; Costa et al, 2017). Wake up and breathe protocols that pair daily SATs with daily SBTs result in better outcomes for*

● = Independent;   ▲ = Collaborative;   **EBN** = Evidence-Based Nursing;   **EB** = Evidence-Based

mechanically ventilated clients in intensive care (Balas et al, 2012, 2014; Haas & Loik, 2012; Khan et al, 2014; Klompas et al, 2015; Costa et al, 2017). Daily interruption of sedation (DIS) is safe in mechanically ventilated medical ICU clients. Further information is needed to determine benefits in other client populations. Current practice evidence suggested that sedation should be client specific to avoid overuse of sedating agents. DIS may not reduce the duration of mechanical ventilation (Makic et al, 2015).

- Administer analgesics and sedatives as needed to facilitate client comfort and rest. Use behavioral and sedation scales for nonverbal clients to provide a consistent way of monitoring pain and sedation levels and ensuring that therapeutic outcomes are being met (Barr et al, 2013; Dale et al, 2014; Reade & Finfer, 2014). **EB:** *Clients receiving mechanical ventilation frequently require sedation to help attenuate the anxiety, pain, and agitation associated with this intervention (Balas et al, 2012; Barr et al, 2013; Reade & Finfer, 2014). The overall goal of sedation during mechanical ventilation is to provide physiological stability, ventilator synchrony, and comfort for clients (Balas et al, 2012; Makic et al, 2015).*

- Tools such as the Riker Sedation-Agitation Scale, the Motor Activity Assessment Scale, the Ramsey Scale, or the Richmond Agitation-Sedation Scale may be useful in monitoring levels of sedation (Balas et al, 2012; Barr et al, 2013; Dale et al, 2014).

- Schedule weaning periods for the time of day when the client is most rested. Cluster care activities to promote successful weaning. Avoid other procedures during weaning: keep the environment quiet and promote restful activities between weaning periods.

- Promote a normal sleep-wake cycle, allowing uninterrupted periods of nighttime sleep. *Limit visitors during weaning to close and supportive persons; ask visitors to leave if they are negatively affecting the weaning process.* **EB:** *Communication with a client and/or the client's family is important to assess the client's typical pattern of sleep (Tracy & Chlan, 2011; Ward & Fulbrook, 2016).*

- During weaning, monitor the client's physiological and psychological responses; acknowledge and respond to fears and subjective complaints. Validate the client's efforts during the weaning process.

- Involve the client and family in the weaning plan. Inform them of the weaning plan and possible client responses to the weaning process (e.g., potential feelings of dyspnea). Foster a partnership between clients and nurses in care planning for weaning. **EBN:** *Consider the experience of the client and the client's family members to develop interventions for weaning success (Rose et al, 2014).*

- Coach the client through episodes of increased anxiety. Remain with the client or place a supportive and calm significant other in this role. Give positive reinforcement and, with permission, use touch to communicate support and concern. *It is not unusual for a client with lung disease to experience self-limiting episodes of increased shortness of breath. Supporting and coaching a client through such episodes allows weaning to continue (Tracy & Chlan, 2011; Ward & Fulbrook, 2016).*

- Terminate weaning when the client demonstrates predetermined criteria or when the following signs of weaning intolerance occur:
  - Tachypnea, dyspnea, or chest and abdominal asynchrony
  - Agitation or mental status changes
  - Decreased oxygen saturation: $SaO_2 < 90\%$
  - Increased $Paco_2$ or $EtCO_2$
  - Change in pulse rate or blood pressure or onset of new dysrhythmias

▲ If the dysfunctional weaning response is severe, consider slowing weaning to brief periods (e.g., 5 minutes). Continue to collaborate with the team to determine whether an untreated physiological cause for the dysfunctional weaning pattern remains. Consult with health care provider regarding use of NIV immediately after discontinuing ventilation. Consider an alternative care setting (subacute, rehabilitation facility, or home) for clients with prolonged ventilator dependence as a strategy that can positively affect outcomes.

 Geriatric

- Recognize that older clients may require longer periods to wean. **EBN:** *An integrative review found that nursing interventions that incorporated early mobility, close monitoring of fluid and electrolyte balance, effective pain management minimizing sedation, and early and frequent assessment of readiness to wean can reduce ventilator days. The study also found the assessment of frailty is important in discussing weaning options (Stieff, Lim, & Chen, 2017).*

- Frequently assess the older client for hypodelirium and hyperdelirium states. **EB:** *Delirium in the older client may prolong mechanical ventilation and worsen overall morbidity and mortality risk (Stieff, Lim, & Chen, 2017).*

● = Independent;   ▲ = Collaborative;   **EBN** = Evidence-Based Nursing;   **EB** = Evidence-Based

Home Care

- Weaning from a ventilator at home should be based on client stability and comfort of the client and caregivers under an intermittent care plan. *Generally the client will be safer weaning in a hospital environment.*

REFERENCES

Balas, M. C., Vasilevskis, E. E., Burke, W. J., et al. (2012). Critical care nurses' role in implementing the "ABCDE Bundle" into practice. *Critical Care Nurse, 32*(2), 35–38, 40–48.

Balas, M., Vasilevskis, E., Olsen, K., et al. (2014). Effectiveness and safety of the awakening and breathing coordination, delirium monitoring/management, and early exercise/mobility bundle. *Critical Care Medicine, 42*, 1024–1036.

Bajaj, A., Rathor, P., Sehgal, V., et al. (2015). Efficacy of noninvasive ventilation after planned extubation: A systematic review and meta-analysis of randomized controlled trials. *Heart and Lung: The Journal of Critical Care, 44*, 150–157.

Barr, J., Fraser, G. L., Puntillo, K., et al. (2013). Clinical practice guidelines for the management of pain, agitation, and delirium in adult patients in the intensive care unit. *Critical Care Medicine, 41*(1), 263–306.

Blackwood, B., Burns, K., Cardwell, C., et al. (2014). Protocolized versus non-protocolized weaning for reducing the duration of mechanical ventilation in critically ill adult patients. *Cochrane Database Systematic Review,* (11), CD006904.

Bradt, J., & Dileo, C. (2014). Music interventions for mechanically ventilated patients. *Cochrane Database of Systematic Reviews,* (12), CD006902. doi:10.1002/14651858.CD006902.pub3.

Burns, K., Lellouche, F., Nisenbaum, R., et al. (2014). Automated weaning and SBT systems versus non-automated weaning strategies for weaning time in invasively ventilated critically ill adults. *Cochrane Database Systematic Review,* (9), CD008638.

Burns, K., Meade, M., & Premji, A. (2013). Noninvasive positive-pressure ventilation as a weaning strategy for intubated adults with respiratory failure. *Cochrane Database Systematic Review,* (12), CD004127.

Costa, D. K., White, M. R., Milisa, G., et al. (2017). Identifying barriers to delivering the awakening and breathing coordination, delirium, and early exercise/mobility bundle to minimize adverse outcomes for mechanically ventilated patients a systematic review. *Chest, 152*(2), 304–311.

Dale, C., Kannas, D., Fan, V., et al. (2014). Improved analgesia, sedation, and delirium protocol associated with decreased duration of delirium and mechanical ventilation. *Annals of American Thoracic Society, 11*(3), 367–374.

DiNino, E., Gartman, E., Sethi, J., et al. (2014). Diaphragm ultrasound as a predictor of successful extubation from mechanical ventilation. *Thorax, 2014*(69), 423–427.

Haas, C. F., & Loik, P. S. (2012). Ventilator discontinuation protocols. *Respiratory Care, 57*(10), 1649–1662.

Hernandez, G., Pedrosa, A., Ortiz, R., et al. (2013). The effects of increasing effective airway diameter on weaning from mechanical ventilation in tracheostomized patients: A randomized control trial. *Intensive Care Medicine, 39*, 1063–1070.

Hetland, B., Lindquist, R., & Chlan, L. L. (2015). The influence of music during mechanical ventilation and weaning from mechanical ventilation: A review. *Heart and Lung: The Journal of Critical Care, 44*, 416–425.

Huang, C., Tsai, Y., Lin, J., et al. (2014). Application of heart-rate variability in patients undergoing weaning from mechanical ventilation. *Critical Care, 18*, R21. Retrieved from http://ccforum.com/content/18/1/R21.

Jones, K., Newhouse, R., Johnson, K., et al. (2014). Achieving quality health outcomes through the implementation of a spontaneous awakening and spontaneous breathing trial protocol. *AACN Advanced Critical Care, 25*(1), 33–42.

Kacmarek, R. (2013). Discontinuing ventilatory support. In R. Kacmarek, J. Stoller, & A. Heuer (Eds.), *Egan's fundamentals of respiratory care* (10th ed., pp. 1199–1227). St. Louis: Elsevier.

Karthika, M., Al Enezi, F. A., Pillai, L. V., et al. (2016). Rapid shallow breathing index. *Annals of Thoracic Medicine, 11*(3), 167–176. Retrieved from http://doi.org/10.4103/1817-1737.176876.

Khan, B., Fadel, W., Tricker, J., et al. (2014). Effectiveness of implementing a wake up and breathe program on sedation and delirium in the ICU. *Critical Care Medicine, 42*, e791–e795.

Liang, Z., Ren, D., Choi, J., et al. (2016). Music interventions during daily weaning trials-A 6 day prospective randomized crossover trial. *Complementary Therapies in Medicine, 29*, 72–77.

Klompas, M., Anderson, D., & Trick, W. (2015). The preventability of ventilator-associated events. The CDC prevention epicenters wake up and breathe collaborative. *American Journal of Respiratory and Critical Care Medicine, 191*, 292–301.

Maggiore, S., Idone, F., Vaschetto, R., et al. (2014). Nasal high-flow versus venture mask oxygen therapy after extubation. Effects on oxygenation, comfort, and clinical outcome. *American Journal of Respiratory and Critical Care Medicine, 190*(3), 282–288.

Makic, M. B. F., Rauen, C., Jones, K., et al. (2015). Continuing to challenge practice to be evidence based. *Critical Care Nurse, 35*(2), 39–50.

Mas, A., & Masip, J. (2014). Noninvasive ventilation in acute respiratory failure. *International Journal of COPD, 9*, 837–852.

Matamis, D., Soilmezi, E., Tsagourias, M., et al. (2013). Sonographic evaluation of the diaphragm in critically ill patients. Techniques and clinical applications. *Intensive Care Medicine, 39*, 801–810.

Miu, T., Jofffe, A. M., Yanez, N. D., et al. (2014). Predictors of reintubation in critically ill patients. *Respiratory Care, 59*(2), 178–185.

Penuelas, O., Thille, A., & Esteban, A. (2015). Discontinuation of ventilatory support: New solutions to old dilemmas. *Current Opinion in Critical Care, 21*(1), 74–81.

Reade, M., & Finfer, S. (2014). Sedation and delirium in the intensive care unit. *New England Journal of Medicine, 370*, 444–454.

Rose, L. (2015). Strategies for weaning from mechanical ventilation: A state of the art review. *Intensive and Critical Care Nursing, 31*, 189–195.

Rose, L., Dainty, K. N., Jordan, J., et al. (2014). Weaning from mechanical ventilation: A scoping review of qualitative studies. *American Journal of Critical Care, 23*(5), e54–e71.

Schmidt, G., Girard, T., Kress, J., et al. (2017). Official executive summary of an American thoracic society/American college of chest physicians clinical practice guideline: Liberation from mechanical ventilation in critically ill adults. *American Journal of Respiratory and Critical Care Medicine, 195*(1), 115–119.

Seely, A., Bravi, A., Herry, C., et al. (2014). Do heart and respiratory rate variability improve prediction of extubation outcomes in critically ill patients? *Critical Care, 2014*(18), R65. Retrieved from http://ccforum.com/content/18/2/R65.

● = Independent;   ▲ = Collaborative;   **EBN** = Evidence-Based Nursing;   **EB** = Evidence-Based

Sklar, M., Burns, K., Rittayamai, N., et al. (2017). Effort to breathe with various spontaneous breathing trial techniques. *American Journal of Respiratory and Critical Care Medicine, 195*(11), 1477–1485.

Spiva, L., Hart, P., Gallagher, E., et al. (2015). The effects of guided imagery on patients being weaned from mechanical ventilation. *Evidence-based Complementary and Alternative Medicine, 2015,* 9. Retrieved from http://dx.doi.org/10.1155/2015/802865.

Spruit, M. A., Singh, S. J., Garvey, C., et al. (2013). An official American Thoracic Society/European Respiratory Society statement: Key concepts and advances in pulmonary rehabilitation. *American Journal of Respiratory and Critical Care Medicine, 188*(8), e13–e64.

Stieff, K. V., Lim, F., & Chen, L. (2017). Factors influencing weaning older adults from mechanical ventilation: An integrative review. *Critical Care Nursing Quarterly, 40*(2), 165–177.

Tracy, M. F., & Chlan, L. (2011). Nonpharmacological interventions to manage common symptoms in patients receiving mechanical ventilation. *Critical Care Nurse, 31*(3), 19–29.

Wappel, S., Ali, O., & Verceles, A. (2017). The effects of high protein intake and mobility-based rehabilitation on ventilator weaning and discharge status in survivors of critical illness. *American Journal of Respiratory and Critical Care Medicine, Poster Abstract, 195,* A7575.

Ward, D., & Fulbrook, P. (2016). Nursing strategies for effective weaning of the critically ill mechanically ventilated patient. *Critical Care Nursing Clinics of North America, 28*(4), 499–512.

Zhu, B., Li, Z., Jiang, L., et al. (2015). Effect of a quality improvement program on weaning from mechanical ventilation: A cluster randomized trial. *Intensive Care Medicine, 41,* 1781–1790.

Risk for other-directed Violence   *Kathleen L. Patusky, MA, PhD, RN, CNS*

NANDA-I

Definition

Susceptible to behaviors in which an individual demonstrates that he or she can be physically, emotionally, and/or sexually harmful to others.

Risk Factors

Access to weapon; impulsiveness; negative body; pattern of indirect violence; pattern of other directed violence pattern of threatening violence); pattern of violent antisocial behavior; suicidal behavior

At-Risk Population

History of childhood abuse; history of cruelty to animals; history of fire-setting; history of motor vehicle offense; history of substance misuse; history of witnessing family violence

Associated Condition

Alteration in cognitive functioning; neurological impairment; pathological intoxication; perinatal complications; prenatal complications; psychotic disorder

NOC   (Nursing Outcomes Classification)

Suggested NOC Outcomes

Abuse Cessation; Abusive Behavior Self-Restraint; Aggression Self-Restraint; Distorted Thought Self-Control; Impulse Self-Control; Risk Detection

Example **NOC** Outcome with Indicators

Aggression Self-Restraint as evidenced by the following indicators: Refrains from harming others/Expresses/Vents needs and negative feelings in a nondestructive manner/Identifies when angry. (Rate the outcome and indicators of **Aggression Self-Restraint:** 1 = never demonstrated, 2 = rarely demonstrated, 3 = sometimes demonstrated, 4 = often demonstrated, 5 = consistently demonstrated [see Section I].)

Client Outcomes

Client Will (Specify Time Frame)

- Stop all forms of abuse (physical, emotional, sexual; neglect; financial exploitation)
- Have cessation of abuse reported by victim
- Display no aggressive activity
- Refrain from verbal outbursts
- Refrain from violating others' personal space

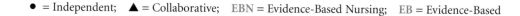

● = Independent;   ▲ = Collaborative;   EBN = Evidence-Based Nursing;   EB = Evidence-Based

- Refrain from antisocial behaviors
- Maintain relaxed body language and decreased motor activity
- Identify factors contributing to abusive/aggressive behavior
- Demonstrate impulse control or state feelings of control
- Identify impulsive behaviors
- Identify feelings/behaviors that lead to impulsive actions
- Identify consequences of impulsive actions to self or others
- Avoid high-risk environments and situations
- Identify and talk about feelings; express anger appropriately
- Express decreased anxiety and control of hallucinations as applicable
- Displace anger to meaningful activities
- Communicate needs appropriately
- Identify responsibility to maintain control
- Express empathy for victim
- Obtain no access or yield access to harmful objects
- Use alternative coping mechanisms for stress
- Obtain and follow through with counseling
- Demonstrate knowledge of correct role behaviors

Victim (and Children if Applicable) Will (Specify Time Frame)

- Have safe plan for leaving situation or avoiding abuse
- Resolve depression or traumatic response

Parent Will (Specify Time Frame)

- Monitor social/play contacts
- Provide supervision and nurturing environment
- Intervene to prevent high-risk social behaviors

NIC   (Nursing Interventions Classification)

Suggested NIC Interventions

Abuse Protection Support; Anger Control Assistance; Behavior Management; Calming Technique; Coping Enhancement; Crisis Intervention; Delusion Management; Dementia Management; Distraction; Environmental Management: Violence Prevention; Mood Management; Physical Restraint; Seclusion; Substance Use Prevention

Example NIC Intervention—Environmental Management: Violence Prevention

Remove other individuals from the vicinity of a violent or potentially violent client; Provide ongoing surveillance of all client access areas to maintain client safety and therapeutically intervene as needed

Nursing Interventions and *Rationales*

Client Violence

- Aggressive/violent behavior may be impulsive, but more commonly it evolves in reaction to the environment (internal or external). In either case, nursing staff must go through specialized training to be prepared for a quick response. EBN: *Aggression management may include the use of physical or chemical restraints (medications), but the former should be used for brief periods only, and the latter should include monitoring for side effects. Music therapy may positively influence the environment (Fong, 2016).*
- Monitor the environment, evaluate situations that could become violent, and intervene early to deescalate the situation. Know and follow institutional policies and procedures concerning violence. Consider that family members or other staff may initiate violence in all settings. Enlist support from other staff rather than attempting to handle situations alone. EBN: *American Psychiatric Nurses Association (APNA) guidelines (2016) warn that workplace violence can occur in all settings and from a variety of sources. Nurses need to be aware and informed of department policies and procedures. Policies should be developed and training programs should be provided in proper use and application of restraints. All nursing units should develop a proactive plan for dealing with violent situations.*

V

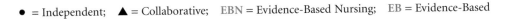 ● = Independent;   ▲ = Collaborative;   EBN = Evidence-Based Nursing;   EB = Evidence-Based

- Assess causes of aggression, such as social versus biological. *Knowing the client, having experience with similar clients, paying attention, and planning interventions are expert practices used by clinicians to predict and respond to aggressive behavior effectively. A nonconfrontational approach is the most effective.*
- Assess the client for risk factors of violence, including those in the following categories: personal history (e.g., past violent behavior, especially violent behavior in the community within 2 weeks of admission); psychiatric disorders (particularly psychoses, paranoid or bipolar disorders, substance abuse, post-traumatic stress disorder [PTSD], antisocial personality, borderline personality disorder); neurological disorders (e.g., head injury, temporal lobe epilepsy, cardiovascular accident, dementia or senility), medical disorders (e.g., hypoxia, hypoglycemia, hyperglycemia), psychological precursors (e.g., low tolerance for stress, impulsivity, hostility), coping difficulties (e.g., inability to plan solutions or see long-term consequences of behavior), younger age, risk of suicide, and childhood or adolescent disorders (e.g., conduct disorders, hyperactivity, autism, learning disability). EBN/EB: *All of these risk factors have been implicated in aggressive, agitated, or violent behavior, with prior history as a key indicator (APNA, 2014a,b; Battaglini, 2014a).*
- Measures of violence may be useful in predicting or tracking behavior, and serving as outcome measures. EBN: *The Broset Violence Checklist (BVC) and the Kennedy Axis V have been shown to help identify clients at risk for seclusion (Sande et al, 2013). CEB: The Alert System identifies potential violent incidents (odds ratio = 7.74, 95% confidence interval [CI] = 4.81–12.47), but they should be combined with resources and procedures to prevent escalation of behavior (Kling et al, 2011).*
- Assess the client with a history of previous assaults, especially violent behavior in the community, within 2 weeks of admission. Listen to and acknowledge feelings of anger, observe for increased motor activity, and prepare to intervene if the client becomes aggressive. EBN/EB: *The most significant risk factor for physical violence is a past history of physically aggressive behavior (Battaglini, 2014a).*
- Assess the client for physiological signs and external signs of anger. Internal signs of anger include increased pulse rate, respiration rate, and blood pressure; chills; prickly sensations; numbness; choking sensation; nausea; and vertigo. External signs include increased muscle tone, changes in body posture (clenched fists, set jaw), eye changes (eyebrows lower and drawn together, eyelids tense, eyes assuming a "hard" appearance), lips pressed together, flushing or pallor, goose bumps, twitching, and sweating. *Anger is an early warning sign of possible violence.*
- Assess for the presence of hallucinations. *Command hallucinations may direct the client to behave violently.*
- Apply STAMPEDAR as an acronym for assessing the immediate potential for violence. CEBN: *A study of nurses experienced in workplace violence identified the following as factors and behaviors indicating the likelihood of a violent episode: staring, tone of voice, anxiety, mumbling, pacing, emotions, disease process, assertive/nonassertive behavior, and access to resources that might be used for violent behavior (STAMPEDAR) (Chapman et al, 2009).*
- Determine the presence and degree of homicidal or suicidal risk. A number of questions will elicit the necessary information: Have you been thinking about harming someone? If yes, who? How often do you have these thoughts, and how long do they last? Do you have a plan? What is it? Do you have access to the means to carry out that plan? What has kept you from hurting the person until now? Refer to the care plan for Risk for **Suicide**. Mental health providers are required to report harm or threats of harm to another person, referred to as the "duty to warn." State laws and mental health codes should be checked to determine local mandates for threat reporting by specific health care professionals.
- Take action to minimize personal risk; use nonthreatening body language. Respect personal space and boundaries. Maintain at least an arm's length distance from the client; do not touch the client without permission (unless physical restraint is the goal). Do not allow the client to block access to an exit. If speaking with the client alone, keep the door to the room open. Be aware of where other staff is at all times. Notify other staff of where you are at all times. Take verbal threats seriously and notify other staff. Wear clothing and accessories that are not restricting and that will not be dangerous (e.g., sandals or shoes with heels can lead to twisted ankles; necklaces or dangling earrings could be grabbed). Ensure staff training to deal with violence. EBN/EB: *Aggression management training has been identified as a critical need (Battaglini, 2014a; Chu, 2014a). Programs for violence prevention have been implemented that reduce workplace violence. For Occupational Safety and Health Association (OSHA) guidelines, see https://www.osha.gov/SLTC/workplaceviolence/index.html.*
- Remove potential weapons from the environment. Be prepared to remove obstructions to staff response from the environment. Search the client and his or her belongings for weapons or potential weapons on admission to the hospital as appropriate. EBN: *Preventive strategies are important (Chu, 2014a; Zhili,*

V

• = Independent;   ▲ = Collaborative;   EBN = Evidence-Based Nursing;   EB = Evidence-Based

2013). Clients prone to violence may use available weapons opportunistically. If client restraint becomes necessary, environmental hazards (e.g., chairs, wastebaskets) should be moved out of the way to prevent injuries.

- Inform the client of unit expectations for appropriate behavior and the consequences of not meeting these expectations. Emphasize that the client must comply with the rules of the unit. Give positive reinforcement for compliance. Increase surveillance of the hospitalized client at smoking, meal, and medication times. CEB/EBN: *Clients benefit from clear guidance and positive reinforcement regarding behavioral expectations and consequences, providing much needed structure and emphasizing client responsibility for his or her own behavior (APNA, 2014a,b). The unit serves as a microcosm of the client's outside world, so adherence to social norms while on the unit models adherence on discharge and provides the client with staff support to learn appropriate coping skills and alternative behaviors.*

- Assign a single room to the client with a potential for violence toward others. The client will be able to take time away from unit stimulation to calm self as needed. Another client will not be placed at risk as a roommate.

- Maintain a calm attitude in response to the client. Provide a low level of stimulation in the client's environment; place the client in a safe, quiet place, and speak slowly and quietly. Anxiety is contagious. EBN/EB: *Maintenance of a calm environment contributes to the prevention of aggression (APNA, 2014a,b). Harmony among staff can help prevent violence, in that disharmony transmits itself to clients' emotional state (Battaglini, 2014a). Music therapy may help (Chu, 2014b).*

- Redirect possible violent behaviors into physical activities (e.g., walking, jogging) if the client is physically able. Using a punching bag or hitting a pillow is not indicated because these are not calming activities and they continue patterning violent behavior. However, activities that distract while draining excess energy help build a repertoire of alternative behaviors for stress reduction.

- Provide sufficient staff if a show of force is necessary to demonstrate control to the client. *When staff respond to an escalating or violent situation, it can reassure clients that they will not be allowed to lose control. On the other hand, leave immediately if the client becomes violent and you are not trained to handle it.*

- Deescalation is the first and most important action in response to anger and hostility. Constant special observation may be implemented. EBN: *Response to hostility should be appropriate, measured, and reasonable. Constant special observation should be used to prevent acutely disturbed clients from harming self or others (Battaglini, 2014a).*

- Protect other clients in the environment from harm. Remove other individuals from the vicinity of a violent or potentially violent client. Follow safety protocols of the department. The risk of a violent client to others in the area (other clients, visitors) should be anticipated, even as efforts proceed to deescalate the situation with the client. EBN: *Clients exposed to violence need timely support and assistance (Chu, 2014a).*

- Maintain a secluded area for the client to be placed when violent. Ensure that staff is continuously present and available to client during seclusion. EBN: *Staff presence is necessary to prevent the harmful effects of social isolation and to honor clients' motivation to connect with staff (APNA, 2014b). Seclusion should be short and should be reviewed at least every 2 hours (Zhili, 2013).*

▲ Recognize legal requirements that the least restrictive alternative of treatment should be used with aggressive clients. The hierarchy of intervention is as follows: promote a milieu that provides structure and calmness, with negotiation and collaboration taking precedence over control; maintain vigilance of the unit and respond to behavioral changes early; talk with client to calm and promote understanding of emotional state; use chemical restraints as ordered; increase to manual restraint if needed; increase to mechanical restraint and seclusion as a last resort. EBN: *APNA guidelines (2014a,b) support early assessment and intervention to prevent aggression, with nursing actions to reduce stimulation, divert client from aggressive thought patterns, set appropriate limits on behavior, and provide medications as needed. Chemical restraints are useful, but clients* must *be monitored for response and side effects (Chu, 2014b). Physical restraints should be avoided and used for short periods when necessary (Battaglini, 2014a; Chu, 2014b).*

▲ Use mechanical restraints if ordered and as necessary. Physical restraint can be therapeutic to keep the client and others safe. EBN: *Physical restraints should be avoided and used for short periods when necessary (Battaglini, 2014a; Chu, 2014b). Restraint skill training, audits of adverse events, and examination of the safe use of restraints and medications are important to safe restraint practices (APNA, 2014a,b).*

▲ Follow the institutional protocol for releasing restraints. Observe the client closely, remain calm, and provide positive feedback as the client's behavior becomes controlled. EBN: *The period during which restraints are removed can be dangerous for staff if they do not recognize that the client may choose to reinitiate violence. Protocols will specify safe procedures for removing restraints (APNA, 2014a,b).*

● = Independent; ▲ = Collaborative; EBN = Evidence-Based Nursing; EB = Evidence-Based

▲ After a violent event on a unit, debriefing and support of both staff and clients should be made available. *Allowing discussion of a violent episode, either individually or in a group, among other clients present reveals clients' responses to the event and provides the opportunity for staff to offer reassurance and support. Clients may have concerns that staff will attempt to restrain them without reason or may feel uncertain whether staff can keep them safe.* EBN: *A study of the effect of serious events on psychiatric units found that staff reported a variety of negative emotional responses, levels of containment increased, the provision of care could be affected, and client reactions were largely ignored (APNA, 2014a,b). Injury after violence has a strong negative influence on staff and calls for treatment (Chu, 2014a).*

● Form a therapeutic alliance with the client, remaining calm, identifying the source of anger as external to both nurse and client, and using the therapeutic relationship to prevent the need for seclusion or restraint. *The development of a therapeutic relationship before aggressive behavior occurs provides an alternative for working through anger and frustration. Assisting the client to identify a source of anger or frustration that is external to both the nurse and client prevents the need for defensiveness by both and directs energy at solving an external problem.* EBN: *A therapeutic environment has a mitigating effect against violence (Zhili, 2013).*

● Allow, encourage, and assist the client to verbalize feelings appropriately either one-on-one or in a group setting. Actively listen to the client; explore the source of the client's anger, and negotiate resolution when possible. Teach healthy ways to express feelings/anger, appropriate gender roles, and how to communicate needs appropriately.

● Identify with client the stimuli that initiate violence and the means of dealing with the stimuli. Have the client keep an anger diary and discuss alternative responses together. Teach cognitive-behavioral techniques. *Assisting the client to identify situations and people that upset him or her provides information needed for problem solving. The client may then identify alternative responses (e.g., leaving the stimulus; using relaxation techniques, such as deep breathing; initiating thought stopping; initiating a distracting activity; responding assertively rather than aggressively).*

▲ Initiate and promote staff attendance at aggression management training programs. EBN: *Aggression management training programs have a positive influence on the ability and confidence of nurses in responding to aggressive or violent behavior (APNA, 2011).*

Intimate Partner Violence/Domestic Violence

Note: Before implementation of interventions in the face of domestic violence, nurses should examine their own emotional responses to abuse, their knowledge base about abuse, and systemic elements within the emergency department (ED) to ensure that interventions will be compassionate and appropriate. EBN: *A meta-synthesis of health care provider studies identified a strong therapeutic relationship and the ability to hear what the client is not saying as facilitators of intimate partner violence (IPV) screening (LoGiudice, 2015).*

● Screen for possible abuse in women or children with a pattern of multiple injuries, particularly if any suspicion exists that the physical findings are inconsistent with the explanation of how the injuries were incurred. *IPV/domestic violence is recognized as a nationwide public health issue.*

▲ Report suspected child abuse to Child Protective Services. Refer women suspected of being in a spousal abuse situation to an area crisis center and provide phone number of area crisis hotline. *Rapid screening tools are helpful to identify IPV. All nurses are required by law to report suspected child abuse.* EBN: *Systematic reviews resulted in best practice recommendations: Positive Parenting Program as a hospital-based educational program, parent–child interaction therapy, cognitive-behavioral therapy, school-based instruction for children and adolescents about protective behaviors in the face of sexual abuse, and community-based group therapy for women in IPV relationships (Le, 2016).*

● Assess for physical and mental concerns of women, including risk of HIV. *Major health needs of women with a history of IPV include chronic pain, chronic diseases, and mental illness, as well as concerns regarding risk of HIV. Barriers to health care created by the IPV may prevent these concerns from being addressed.*

● Assist the client in negotiating the health care system and overcoming barriers. *Victims of IPV experience barriers, including inappropriate responses from providers, when attempting to access health care services.*

● With women who repeatedly experience injuries from domestic violence, maintain a nonjudgmental approach and continue to offer resources/referrals. If the woman voices a willingness to leave her situation, assist with developing an emergency plan that will consider all contingencies possible (e.g., safe location, financial resources, care of children, when to leave safely). A woman in a domestic violence situation may change her mind several times before actually leaving. Proactive organization of an emergency plan helps

● = Independent;   ▲ = Collaborative;   EBN = Evidence-Based Nursing;   EB = Evidence-Based

increase the possibility that women will be able to leave safely. The most dangerous time of a domestic violence situation is when the spouse tries to leave.

- Maintain a nonjudgmental response when clients return to husbands or refuse to leave them. Women have many reasons for remaining in an abusive relationship, including economic concerns (especially with children), socialization about the woman's role, political or legal obstacles, powerlessness, and a realistic fear of retaliation or death. Refer to the care plan for **Powerlessness.** Experienced nurses working with abused women define success as client personal growth over time, rather than the woman leaving the relationship.
- Focus on providing support, ensuring safety, and promoting self-efficacy while encouraging disclosure about IPV events. *Nursing care should focus on providing physical, psychological, and emotional support; ensuring safety of the client and family; and promoting the self-efficacy of the woman.*
- Pregnancy is a particular risk period for interpersonal violence. Screen pregnant women for the potential for domestic violence during pregnancy, especially in teenage pregnancies. EBN: *In a comprehensive review of effective interventions, group interventions with pregnant women have included establishing a social support network, emphasizing a positive perspective and self-care knowledge, teaching goal setting and communication skills, and developing skills in assessing risks in the relationship. Individual interventions have included weekly telephone support sessions, self-help workbooks, empowerment training, and music therapy. In some of the individual approaches, depression improved but the rate of IPV did not. Women preferred to focus on the pregnancy or basic needs, feeling judged when the IPV was a focus (Morales & Records, 2013). CEB: Less educated women, women who reported substance abuse by spouse, and women who reported unwanted pregnancies were at risk for IPV both during and after pregnancy. Violence during pregnancy predicted postpartum violence. American women employed during pregnancy were most likely to leave an abusive partner at 1 year postpartum (Charles & Perreira, 2007).*
- Women with physical or mental disabilities require extended assessment, including a comprehensive functional assessment, with attention to cultural issues, the nature of the disability, and needed resources. Women with disabilities may experience abuse from multiple sources, and particular attention should be paid to the additional emotional stressors present. Difficulties leaving home, physical needs that a shelter may not be able to accommodate, and the undesirability of nursing home placement are just a few stressors. Personal assistance providers may be abusive or take advantage financially.
- ▲ Referral for spiritual counseling may be considered, but be aware that clergy vary in their helpfulness. *Survivors of sexual violence may be able to cope with their situation through spiritual connection, spiritual journey, and spiritual transformation.*
- Evaluate medical and mental illness as precursors to elder abuse. EBN: *Systematic reviews identify the need to address medical and mental illnesses in providing care (Lizarondo, 2016b).*
- Consider risk versus benefit when deciding if, when, and in how great a depth to explore client responses to abuse or violence. EB: *A systematic review of research on violence and abuse concluded that risks and benefits may derive from clients talking about such experiences (McClinton Appollis et al, 2015). Clinical judgment must be exercised in the decision to introduce the topic of abuse. Is the client ready? Will raising the issue now prevent further disclosure? Do the current circumstances allow for sufficient resolution of affect?*
- ▲ When spouse or child abuse accompanies substance abuse, refer the abusive client to a substance abuse treatment program. Refer the spouse receiving abuse to Al-Anon and the children to Alateen. *Use of drugs or alcohol may decrease impulse control and aggravate abusive behavior, depending on the specific drug used and culture.*
- ▲ When an adult reveals a history of unresolved/untreated sexual abuse as a child, referral to a local Adults Molested as Children (AMAC) group may be helpful. *Childhood sexual abuse has been associated with adult depression, attempted suicide, self-harm, and higher risk for later interpersonal violence. Interventions tailored to the AMAC experience may be helpful (AMAC, 2017).* Refer to the care plans for Risk for **Suicide, Self-Mutilation,** and Risk for **Self-Mutilation.**
- ▲ Referral of women for psychiatric/psychological treatment or parenting classes should be considered as an appropriate intervention. *Overcoming shame, building a stable sense of identity, and becoming less dependent on others' approval should be addressed, along with physical health and PTSD symptoms.*
- ▲ Referral of children for psychiatric/psychological treatment should be considered as an appropriate intervention. CEB: *Children living with domestic violence were found to express fear and anxiety, self-esteem issues, ambivalent relationships with the abuser, and a sense of a lost childhood (Buckley et al, 2007).*

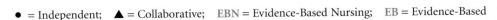

● = Independent;   ▲ = Collaborative;   EBN = Evidence-Based Nursing;   EB = Evidence-Based

▲ Refer to batterer intervention programs that are often available and may be court mandated. *Batterers may believe behaviors toward them are not justified, and their behaviors toward others are justified and minimized. Treatment should include emotional skills training that addresses these areas.*

Social Violence

- Assess for acute stress disorder (ASD) and PTSD among victims of violence. **CEB:** *In the acute phase after an assault, women reported high rates of ASD symptoms. Four months after an attack, dissatisfaction with previous life, prior mental health problems, recent life events, and earlier abuse were risk factors for PTSD (Renck, 2006).*
- ▲ Assess the support network of women who become victims of violent crime and refer for appropriate levels of assistance. Of particular concern would be women who do not have family or friends to provide support or who have difficulty accessing other types of assistance.
- Be aware that hate crime is increasing, particularly toward gay and transgendered individuals, and it requires support and advocacy for victims. **CEB:** *Gay men who experienced antigay abuse reported that the events affected their self-image. In addition to verbal and physical abuse, spiritual abuse emerged as the men internalized schemas of outcast and sinner (Lucies & Yick, 2007).*
- ▲ Victims of violence seen in the ED should receive an assessment for needed services and assignment to case management. *Establishment of linkages with social service agencies can provide important services for referral.*

Rape-Trauma Syndrome

- Brief relationship abuse instruction with counseling in a student health center can be effective in preventing and responding to episodes of sexual coercion. **EB:** *In a randomized control trial (RCT), a student health service provided effective interventions in addressing abusive relationship with adolescents (Miller et al, 2015).*
- Assist client to cope with potential stalking activity. **EBN:** *The usual coping of college students in response to stalking was found to include ignoring or minimizing the problem; distancing or depersonalizing, using verbal escape strategies; attempting to end the relationship; and restricting availability (Amar & Alexy, 2010). Emphasizing the need to take stalking behavior seriously and problem-solving interventions may prevent a rape situation.*
- Approach client with sensitivity. **CEBN:** *Using Peplau's theory of nursing roles, researchers found that the roles of counselor and technical expert were most helpful, with interpersonal sensitivity important to clients (Courey et al, 2008).*
- ▲ Monitor for paradoxical drug reactions, and report any to the health care provider. Violent behavior can be stimulated by a medication intended to calm the client.
- Assess for brain insults, such as recent falls or injuries, strokes, or transient ischemic attacks. Clients with brain injuries may respond to stimulus control, problem-solving, social skills training, relaxation training, and anger management to reduce aggressive behaviors. Brain injuries, lowered impulse control, and reduced coping can cause violent reactions to self or others. Brain injury symptoms may be mistaken for mental illness.
- Decrease environmental stimuli if violence is directed at others. Removal of the client to a quiet area can reduce violent impulses. Use a calm voice to "talk down" the client.
- Assess holistic needs of the client. *Negative mental health outcomes after sexual violence may be low income, low education level, lack of social support, and poor health promotion.*
- Discuss with client her wishes regarding use of an emergency contraceptive.
- ▲ If abuse or neglect of an older client is suspected, report the suspicion to an adult protective services agency with jurisdiction over the geographical area in which the client lives.

 ### Pediatric

- Assess for predictors of anger that can lead to violent behavior. **EBN:** *A correlational study of adolescent anger predictors identified trait anger, anxiety, depression, stress, exposure to violence, and parental drinking behaviors as predictors of anger. Frequency of religious participation was associated with decreased anger (Pullen et al, 2015).*
- Be alert for both shaken baby syndrome and exposure of children to violence. *In homes in which domestic violence exists, children are involved as either witnesses or victims. Such children tend not to seek help and need care providers to elicit actively the need for assistance.*
- Pregnant teens should be assessed for abuse, particularly if they are with an older partner.

● = Independent;   ▲ = Collaborative;   **EBN** = Evidence-Based Nursing;   **EB** = Evidence-Based

▲ In the case of child abuse or neglect, refer for early childhood home visitation. CEB: *Home visits during a child's first 2 years of life may be effective in preventing child abuse and neglect.*

Geriatric

● Be alert to the potential for elder abuse in clients, including the possibility of psychological abuse. EBN: *Abuse may be physical, sexual, psychological, financial, or may appear as neglect. Look for signs of bruising, malnutrition, and fearful responses to or around caregivers (Battaglini, 2014b). Cognitive impairment, behavioral problems, and psychiatric illness in the client are risk factors for becoming recipients of abuse (Battaglini, 2014c). Assess for changes in physiological functions (e.g., constipation, dehydration) or impairment of the ability to meet basic needs (e.g., inadequate toileting, decreased mobility). Observe for signs of fear, anxiety, anger, and agitation, and intervene immediately. In older adults, subtle physiological changes, interruptions of or changes in routine, or fears about medical disorders or potential loss of independence can be transformed into anger, irritability, or agitation. A comprehensive physical exam should include a neurological exam and x-rays as needed (Battaglini, 2014b).*

● Assess for presence or client history of mental illness or treatment. EBN: *There is a high likelihood of elder abuse in the presence of mental illness, even if receiving psychiatric treatment (Battaglini, 2014c).*

● Assess and observe for aggressive behavior in older clients at long-term care facilities. EBN: *Between 25% and 50% of clients with dementia have demonstrated aggressive behavior. Knowledge of the client's history and risk factors is important. Treatment with antipsychotics should be individualized and carefully monitored. Use of restraints should be avoided, used for a short time, and removed at the earliest possible time. Staff should receive training in aggression management (Battaglini, 2014d). Insufficient evidence supports the efficacy of agitation reduction protocols or emotion-oriented care (Lizarondo, 2016a).*

● Observe clients for dementia and delirium. EBN: *Between 25% and 50% of clients with dementia have demonstrated aggressive behavior. Clients with dementia or delirium may strike out if they are frustrated or if they have the sense that their personal space is being violated. The competency of the client should be assessed to determine whether he or she possesses a cognitive capacity that permits discussion of the behavior (Battaglini, 2014c,d).*

● For clients with dementia, provide music therapy. EB: *A systematic review of interventions with aggression in adults with dementia demonstrated significant improvement with music therapy. Patient-centered care, communication skills training, and dementia care matching showed reductions in aggression for up to 6 months (Lizarondo, 2016a).*

● Be aware of laws and regulations in the appropriate jurisdiction in which the client is located. EBN: *Confidentiality, consent, and information sharing are sensitive issues that are determined by federal and local regulation (Battaglini, 2014b; Goh, 2014a).*

● Document and record suspected elder abuse according to mandatory regulations. EBN: *Incidents of abuse should be recorded with date, time, chronology of abuse, family history, potential indicators of abuse, details regarding care planning and decision-making process, and actual care provided. Photographic evidence of abuse should be obtained. The police may be requested to take forensic pictures (Goh, 2014b).*

● Apart from mandated requirements, abide by the older client's wishes regarding action to be taken in response to abuse. Avoid interventions that increase the risk of abuse. EBN: *Discuss with client his or her reasons for refusing to disclose abuse. There may be a fear that the only available caregiver will withdraw, leaving the client helpless. Allow adequate time for the discussion; respect the client's pace and need for a sense of control. Corroborate events as possible (Battaglini, 2014b). Avoid the use of antidepressants or sedatives without a thorough abuse assessment, the recommendation of family counseling without intervention for the abuser, blaming the victim, colluding with the abuser, or minimizing the possible danger (Goh, 2014c).*

● Develop a safety plan and provide referrals to all relevant agencies or services. EBN: *Discuss safety options for both client and provider. Contact police if there is a concern regarding the availability of a gun. The registered nurse should debrief with manager as necessary (Battaglini, 2014c). Multidisciplinary and interagency collaboration is important to meet client needs (Goh, 2014c).*

V

Multicultural

● Exercise cultural competence when dealing with domestic violence. CEBN: *Battered Latina women reported protecting their partner, preventing their mother from worrying, and fear of losing their children as barriers to disclosing IPV (Montalvo-Liendo et al, 2009).*

● Identify and respond to unique needs of immigrant women who experience IPV. CEBN: *A study of Sri Lankan immigrants to Canada revealed that violence prior to the immigration, gender inequity in the marriage,*

● = Independent; ▲ = Collaborative; EBN = Evidence-Based Nursing; EB = Evidence-Based

changes in social networks and supports, and changes in socioeconomic status were identified by the women as factors involved in IPV (Guruge et al, 2010). Filipina women focused on keeping their family together and did not realize that IPV had a negative influence on the mental health of the women and their children (Shoultz et al, 2010).

- Assist with acculturation and activating social support. CEB: *Type of support and acculturation helped promote resiliency and improved mood among Hispanic women in IPV situations (Shoultz & Magnussen, 2009).*

 Home Care

- Be alert to the potential for violent behavior in the home setting. Respond to verbal aggression with interventions to deescalate negative emotional states. Violence is a process that can be recognized early. Deescalation involves reducing client stressors, responding to the client with respect, acknowledging the client's feeling state, and assisting the client to regain control. If deescalation does not work, the nurse should leave the home.
- Assess family members or caregivers for their ability to protect the client and themselves. The safety of the client between home visits is a nursing priority. Caregivers often need assistance with recognizing or admitting fear of or danger from a loved one. EBN: *A qualitative study with home care staff and caregivers of clients with dementia advised that staff use a calm, compassionate approach and minimize controlling strategies such as medications or restraints in dealing with aggressive behavior. A patient-centered approach was recommended (Lizarondo, 2016a).*
- Include an initial and ongoing assessment and evaluation of potential abuse and neglect. Photograph evidence of abuse or neglect when possible. *Victims of abuse perceive themselves to be powerless to change the situation. Indeed, the abuser fosters this perception and may threaten violence or death if the victim attempts to leave. Chronic abuse and neglect by a spouse or other family among older adults is often hidden until home care is actively involved.* Refer to the care plan for **Powerlessness.**
- ▲ If neglect or abuse is suspected, identify an emergency plan that addresses the problem immediately, ensures client safety, and includes a report to the appropriate authorities. Discuss when to use hotlines and 911. Role-play access to emergency resources with the client and caregivers. *Client safety is a nursing priority. An emergency plan should address either immediate removal to a safe environment or identification of appropriate steps to take in the event of abuse and the securing of resources for the anticipated action (e.g., available phone, packed bag, alternative living arrangements). Reporting is a legal requirement for health care workers.*
- Encourage appropriate safety behaviors in abused women; call the client at intervals during a 6-month period to determine whether safety behaviors are being performed. CEB: *A study of telephone contacts to women who sought help through the district attorney's office demonstrated that safety behaviors increased dramatically. Safety behaviors included hiding money; hiding an extra set of house and car keys; establishing a code for abuse occurrence with family or friends; asking neighbors to call police if violence occurs; removing weapons; keeping available family social security numbers, rent and utility receipts, family birth certificates, identification or driver licenses, bank account numbers, insurance policies and numbers, marriage license, valuable jewelry, important phone numbers, and a hidden bag with extra clothing (McFarlane et al, 2002).*
- Assess the home environment for harmful objects. Have the family remove or lock objects as able. *The safety of the client and caregivers is a nursing priority.*
- ▲ Refer for homemaker or psychiatric home health care services for respite, client reassurance, and implementation of a therapeutic regimen. Responsibility for a person who may become violent provides high caregiver stress. Respite decreases caregiver stress. The presence of caring individuals is reassuring to both the client and caregivers, especially during periods of client anxiety. Individuals exhibiting violent behaviors can respond to the interventions described previously, modified for the home setting.
- ▲ If the client is taking psychotropic medications, assess client and family knowledge of medication and its administration and side effects. Teach as necessary. Knowledge of the medical regimen supports compliance.
- ▲ Evaluate effectiveness and side effects of medications. Accurate clinical feedback improves the health care provider's ability to prescribe an effective medical regimen specific to a client's needs.
- If client displays mildly intensifying aggressive behavior, attempt to diffuse anger or violence (e.g., ask for a glass of water to distract client). Later in the visit, explain that aggressive behavior is not acceptable and present consequences of continued aggressive behavior (i.e., right of agency to discontinue services). *Mild aggression can be defused safely. Confronting the client before severe aggression is evident places responsibility on the client and family for respectful partnership in care.*

● = Independent;   ▲ = Collaborative;   EBN = Evidence-Based Nursing;   EB = Evidence-Based

- Document all acts or verbalizations of aggression. Safety of the staff is a primary responsibility of home health agencies. Law enforcement intervention may be necessary.
- ▲ If client verbalizes or displays threatening behavior, notify your supervisor and plan to make joint visits with another staff person or a security escort. *Having a second person at the visit is a show of power and control used to subdue aggressive behavior.*
- If the client's behavior is not overtly threatening but makes the nurse uncomfortable, a meeting may be held outside the home in sight of others (e.g., front porch). *The nurse should trust a "gut" reaction that prompts concern regarding the client's potential for aggressive or violent behavior. Such intuitive reactions are often the result of subliminal cues that are not readily voiced.*
- Never enter a home or remain in a home if aggression threatens your well-being.
- ▲ Never challenge a show of force, such as a gun threat. Leave and notify your supervisor and the appropriate authorities. Document the incident. *Safety of the staff is a primary responsibility of home health agencies. Law enforcement intervention may be necessary.*
- ▲ If client behaviors intensify, refer for immediate mental health intervention. The degree of disturbance and ability to manage care safely at home determines the level of services needed to protect the client.

 ## Client/Family Teaching and Discharge Planning

- Instruct victims of IPV in the dynamics and prognosis of domestic violence behavior, as well as the effect on children who witness or are victims of domestic violence. *Victims of IPV feel alone and isolated. They can begin to take back control of their circumstances once they better understand what is happening within the interpersonal relationship, what their options are, and what the consequences of inaction may be. Do not expect an immediate change in the victim's behavior.*
- Teach relaxation and exercise as ways to release anger and deal with stress.
- Teach cognitive-behavioral activities, such as active problem-solving, reframing (reappraising the situation from a different perspective), or thought stopping (in response to a negative thought, picture a large stop sign and replace the image with a prearranged positive alternative). Teach the client to confront his or her own negative thought patterns (or cognitive distortions), such as catastrophizing (expecting the very worst), dichotomous thinking (perceiving events in only one of two opposite categories), magnification (placing distorted emphasis on a single event), or unrealistic expectations (e.g., "should get what I want when I want it"). *Cognitive-behavioral activities address clients' assumptions, beliefs, and attitudes about their situations, fostering modification of these elements to be as realistic as possible. Through cognitive-behavioral interventions, clients become more aware of their cognitive choices in adopting and maintaining their belief systems, exercising greater control over their own reactions.*
- ▲ Refer to individual or group therapy.
- Teach the adolescent client violence prevention, and encourage him or her to become involved in community service activities. School programs that couple community service with classroom health instruction can have a measurable effect on violent behaviors of young adolescents at high risk for being both the perpetrators and victims of peer violence. Community service programs may be a valuable part of multi-component violence prevention programs.
- Teach the use of appropriate community resources in emergency situations (e.g., hotline, community mental health agency, ED, 911 in most places in the US, the toll-free National Domestic Violence Hotline [1-800-799-SAFE]). Internet resources are increasing and should be made available to clients. It is necessary to get immediate help when violence occurs.
- Encourage the use of self-help groups in nonemergency situations.
- Inform the client and family about any applicable medication actions, side effects, target symptoms, and toxic reactions.

REFERENCES

AMAC. (2017). *Adults molested as children*. Retrieved from https://www.facebook.com/AMACSUPPORTgroup/. (Accessed 12 December 2017).

Amar, A. F., & Alexy, E. M. (2010). Coping with stalking. *Issues in Mental Health Nursing*, *31*, 8.

American Psychiatric Nurses Association (APNA). (2011). *Position statement on staffing inpatient psychiatric units*. Retrieved from https://www.apna.org/i4a/pages/index.cfm?pageID=4662. (Accessed 30 December 2017).

American Psychiatric Nurses Association (APNA). (2014a). *Position statement on seclusion and restraint*. Retrieved from http://www.apna.org/i4a/pages/index.cfm?pageid=3728. (Accessed 30 December 2017).

American Psychiatric Nurses Association (APNA). (2014b). *Seclusion and restraints standards of practice*. Retrieved from http://www.apna.org/i4a/pages/index.cfm?pageid=3730. (Accessed 30 December 2017).

American Psychiatric Nurses Association (APNA). (2016). *Position statement on workplace violence*. Retrieved from https://

● = Independent;   ▲ = Collaborative;   EBN = Evidence-Based Nursing;   EB = Evidence-Based

www.apna.org/i4a/pages/index.cfm?pageID=6081. (Accessed 6 July 2017).

Battaglini, E. (2014a). *Violence management: Acute psychiatric facilities [evidence based recommended practice]*. Retrieved from http://0-connect.jbiconnectplus.org.library.newcastle.edu.au.

Battaglini, E. (2014b). *Domestic elder abuse (persons with mental health problems): Clinical management: Screening, detection/assessment (nurses; rural and remote areas) [evidence based recommended practice]*. Retrieved from http://0-connect.jbiconnectplus.org.library.newcastle.edu.au.

Battaglini, E. (2014c). *Domestic elder abuse (persons with mental health problems): Clinical management: Competency of the elderly and safety issues (nurses; rural and remote areas) [evidence based recommended practice]*. Retrieved from http://0-connect.jbiconnectplus.org.library.newcastle.edu.au.

Battaglini, E. (2014d). *Aggression in the elderly: Risk factors and management [evidence based recommended practice]*. Retrieved from http://0-connect.jbiconnectplus.org.library.newcastle.edu.au.

Buckley, H., et al. (2007). Listen to me! Children's experiences of domestic violence. *Child Abuse Review, 16*, 296.

Chapman, R., et al. (2009). Predicting patient aggression against nurses in all hospital areas. *British Journal of Nursing, 18*, 476.

Charles, P., & Perreira, K. M. (2007). Intimate partner violence during pregnancy and 1-year postpartum. *Journal of Family Violence, 22*, 609.

Chu, V. (2014a). *Healthcare facilities: Patient aggression/violence [evidence based recommended practice]*. Retrieved from http://0-connect.jbiconnectplus.org.library.newcastle.edu.au.

Chu, V. (2014b). *Aggressive behavior management: Acute care [evidence based recommended practice]*. Retrieved from http://0-connect.jbiconnectplus.org.library.newcastle.edu.au.

Courey, T. J., et al. (2008). Hildegard Peplau's theory and the health care encounters of survivors of sexual violence. *Journal of the American Psychiatric Nurses Association, 14*, 136.

Fong, E. (2016). *Aggressive behavior management: Acute care*. Joanna Briggs Institute EBP Database, JBI@Ovid.; JBI1725.

Goh, C. (2014a). *Domestic elder abuse (persons with mental health problems): Clinical management: Confidentiality, consent, information sharing, consultation and supervision (nurses; rural and remote areas) [evidence based recommended practice]*. Retrieved from http://0-connect.jbiconnectplus.org.library.newcastle.edu.au.

Goh, C. (2014b). *Domestic elder abuse (persons with mental health problems): Clinical management: Documentation, reporting, and referral (nurses; rural and remote areas) [evidence based recommended practice]*. Retrieved from http://0-connect.jbiconnectplus.org.library.newcastle.edu.au.

Goh, C. (2014c). *Domestic elder abuse (persons with mental health problems): Clinical management: Planning, interventions and follow-up (nurses; rural and remote areas) [evidence based recommended practice]*. Retrieved from http://0-connect.jbiconnectplus.org.library.newcastle.edu.au.

Guruge, S., et al. (2010). Intimate male partner violence in the immigration process: Intersections of gender, race, and class. *Journal of Advanced Nursing, 66*, 103.

Kling, R. N., Yassi, A., Smailes, E., et al. (2011). Evaluation of a violence risk assessment system (the Alert System) for reducing violence in an acute hospital: A before and after study. *International Journal of Nursing Studies, 48*(5), 534–539.

Le, L. K. D. (2016). *Child and partner abuse: interventions*. Joanna Briggs Institute EBP Database, JBI@Ovid. JBI625.

Lizarondo, L. (2016a). *Evidence summary. Aggression in the elderly with dementia: Non-pharmacological interventions*. Joanna Briggs Institute EBP Database, JBI@Ovid.; JBI1527.

Lizarondo, L. (2016b). *Evidence Summary. Domestic elder abuse: Nursing assessment*. Joanna Briggs Institute EBP Database, JBI@Ovid.JBI8057.

LoGiudice, J. (2015). Prenatal screening for intimate partner violence: A qualitative metasynthesis. *Applied Nursing Research, 28*, 2–9.

Lucies, C., & Yick, A. G. (2007). Images of gay men's experiences with antigay abuse: Object relations theory reconceptualized. *Journal of Theory Construction & Testing, 11*, 55.

McClinton Appollis, T. M., Lund, C., de Vries, P., et al. (2015). Adolescents' and adults' experiences of being surveyed about violence and abuse: A systematic review of harms, benefits, and regrets. *American Journal of Public Health, 105*(2), e31–e45.

McFarlane, J., et al. (2002). An intervention to increase safety behaviors of abused women: Results of a randomized clinical trial. *Nursing Research, 51*, 347.

Miller, E., Goldstein, S., McCauley, H. L., et al. (2015). A school health center intervention for abusive adolescent relationships: A cluster RCT. *Pediatrics, 135*, 81.

Montalvo-Liendo, N., et al. (2009). Factors influencing disclosure of abuse by women of Mexican descent. *Journal of Nursing Scholarship, 41*, 359.

Morales, S., & Records, K. (2013). Interventions to reduce abusive-stress during pregnancy. *International Journal of Childbirth Education, 28*, 34.

Pullen, L., Modrcin, M., McGuire, S. L., et al. (2015). Anger in adolescent communities: How angry are they? *Pediatric Nursing, 41*, 135.

Renck, B. (2006). Psychological stress reactions of women in Sweden who have been assaulted: Acute response and four-month follow-up. *Nursing Outlook, 54*, 312.

Sande, R., Noothroon, E., Wierdsma, A., et al. (2013). Association between short-term structured risk assessment outcomes and seclusion. *International Journal of Mental Health Nursing, 22*(6), 475–484.

Shoultz, J., & Magnussen, L. (2009). Understanding cultural perceptions: Foundation for IPV interventions. *Communicating Nursing Research, 42*, 288.

Shoultz, J., et al. (2010). Listening to Filipina women: Perceptions, responses and needs regarding intimate partner violence. *Issues in Mental Health Nursing, 31*, 54.

Zhili, C. (2013). *Violence: Short-term management [evidence based recommended practice]*. Retrieved from http://0-connect.jbiconnectplus.org.library.newcastle.edu.au.

Risk for self-directed Violence   Kathleen L. Patusky, MA, PhD, RN, CNS

NANDA-I

Definition

Susceptible to behaviors in which an individual demonstrates that he or she can be physically, emotionally, and/or sexually harmful to self.

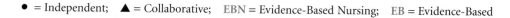

● = Independent;   ▲ = Collaborative;   **EBN** = Evidence-Based Nursing;   **EB** = Evidence-Based

Risk Factors

Behavioral cures of suicidal intent; conflict about sexual orientation; conflict in interpersonal relationship(s); employment concern; engagement in autoerotic sexual acts; history of multiple suicide attempts; insufficient personal resources; social isolation; suicidal ideation; suicidal plan; verbal cues of suicidal intent

At-Risk Population

Age ≥45 years; age 15 to 19 years, history of multiple suicide attempts; marital status; occupation; pattern of difficulties in family background

Associated Condition

Mental health issue; physical health issue; psychological disorder

NOC, NIC, Client Outcomes, Nursing Interventions and *Rationales,* Client/Family Teaching and Discharge Planning, and References

Refer to care plans for Risk for **Suicide, Self-Mutilation,** and Risk for **Self-Mutilation**

Impaired Walking   *Wendie A. Howland, MN, RN-BC, CRRN, CCM, CNLCP, LNCC*

NANDA-I

Definition

Limitation of independent movement within the environment on foot.

Defining Characteristics

Impaired ability to climb stairs; impaired ability to navigate curbs; impaired ability to walk on decline; impaired ability to walk on incline; impaired ability to walk on uneven surface; impaired ability to walk required distance

Related Factors

Alteration in mood; decrease in endurance; environmental barrier; fear of falling; insufficient knowledge of mobility strategies; insufficient muscle strength; obesity; pain; physical deconditioning

Associated Condition

Alteration in cognitive functioning; impaired balance; impaired vision; musculoskeletal impairment; neuromuscular impairment

NOC   (Nursing Outcomes Classification)

Suggested NOC Outcomes

Ambulation, Mobility

Example NOC Outcome with Indicators

Ambulation as evidenced by the following indicators: Walks with effective gait/Walks at moderate pace/Walks up and down steps/Walks moderate distance. (Rate the outcome and indicators of **Ambulation:** 1 = severely compromised, 2 = substantially compromised, 3 = moderately compromised, 4 = mildly compromised, 5 = not compromised [see Section I].)

Client Outcomes/Goals

Client Will (Specify Time Frame)

- Demonstrate optimal independence and safety in walking
- Demonstrate the ability to direct others on how to assist with walking
- Demonstrate the ability to use and care for assistive walking devices properly and safely

● = Independent;   ▲ = Collaborative;   EBN = Evidence-Based Nursing;   EB = Evidence-Based

NIC	(Nursing Interventions Classification)

Suggested NIC Intervention

Exercise Therapy: Ambulation

Example NIC Activities—Exercise Therapy: Ambulation
Assist client to use footwear that facilitates walking and prevents injury; Encourage to sit in bed, on side of bed ("dangle"), or in chair, as tolerated

Nursing Interventions and *Rationales*

- Progressive mobilization as tolerated (gradually raising head of bed [HOB], sitting in reclined chair, standing, with assistance). Progressing mobility gradually from bed rest to increased sit to stand times to short distance walking and timed testing can provide goals for the client and staged mobility successes (Ellison et al, 2016). See also the care plan for Impaired physical **Mobility.**
- Consider and monitor for side effects of prescribed hydration and medications; physical condition; length of immobility contributing to orthostatic hypotension; and/or if lightheadedness, dizziness, syncope, or unexplained falls occur. EB: *Understanding the mechanisms of blood pressure regulation is critical for assessment (Lowry, Windsor, & Ashelford, 2016). Orthostatic hypotension is highly prevalent in patients with unexplained syncope and is associated with the use of antihypertensive drugs (Van Twist et al, 2017).*
- ▲ Assess for orthostatic hypotension if systolic pressure falls 15 mm Hg or diastolic pressure falls 7 mm Hg from sitting to standing within 3 minutes. If this occurs, then replace client in bed and notify prescriber (Arnold & Raj, 2017). *Orthostatic hypotension increases fall risk (Windsor, 2016).*
- Apply thromboembolic deterrent (TED) stockings and/or elastic leg wraps and abdominal binders as prescribed; raise HOB slowly in small increments to sitting, have client move feet/legs up and down, and then stand slowly; avoid prolonged standing. *Movement enhances venous return, improving cardiac output and decreasing syncope.*
- Assess for cognitive, neuromuscular, and sensory deficits that will affect safety when walking (e.g., stroke, diabetic neuropathy, history of falls).
- ▲ Take pulse rate/rhythm, respiratory rate, and pulse oximetry before walking clients, and reassess within 5 minutes of walking, then ongoing as needed. If abnormal, have the client sit 5 minutes, then remeasure. If still abnormal, walk clients more slowly and with more help or for a shorter time, or notify physician. If uncontrolled diabetes/angina/arrhythmias/tachycardia (100 beats per minute or more) or resting systolic blood pressure (SBP) at or above 200 mm Hg or diastolic blood pressure (DBP) at or above 110 mm Hg occurs, do not initiate walking exercise. Refer to the care plan **Activity** intolerance.
- Assist clients to apply orthosis, immobilizers, splints, braces, and compression stockings as prescribed before walking.
- Eat frequent small, low-carbohydrate meals. *Low-carbohydrate meals help prevent postprandial hypotension.*
- Reinforce correct use of prescribed mobility devices, and remind clients of weight-bearing restrictions.
- Emphasize the importance of wearing properly fitting, low-heeled shoes with nonskid soles and socks/hose, and of seeking medical care for foot pain or problems with abnormal toenails, corns, calluses, or diabetes. Refer to podiatric consult if indicated.
- ▲ Use a snug gait belt with handles and assistive devices while walking clients, as recommended by the physical therapist (PT). EB: *A gait belt should be applied before and during all ambulation and functional gait activities; it should be applied securely around the waist and held firmly. Do not rely on clothing for a safe grip (Collins, 2016).*
- Walk clients frequently with an appropriate number of people; have one team member state short, simple motor instructions. *Standing/weight-bearing benefits gut motility, spasticity, and respiratory/bowel/bladder function, and promotes muscle stretching (Collins, 2016).*
- Cue and manually guide clients with neglect as they walk. *Prevents clients bumping into objects/people.*
- Document the number of helpers, level of assistance (maximum, standby, etc.), type of assistance, and devices needed in communication tools (e.g., plan of care, client room signage, verbal report).

Special Considerations: Lower Extremity Amputation

- Teach clients to don stump socks, liner, immediate postoperative prostheses (IPOP), or traditional prosthesis correctly before standing/walking. EB: *IPOPs often reduce pain, healing time, and knee flexion contractures*

• = Independent;   ▲ = Collaborative;   EBN = Evidence-Based Nursing;   EB = Evidence-Based

and promote early ambulation (Samuelsen et al, 2017). A thin nylon sheath prevents the limb from turning in the socket of the prosthesis. A stump sock establishes proper fit between limb and socket. The liner helps prevent pressure ulcers.

- Teach clients the importance of avoiding prolonged hip and knee flexion. If contractures occur, they will affect prosthesis fit and function. EB: *Limit amount of time the client is permitted to sit to no more than 40 minutes of each hour. Ensure that when client sits, stands, or is recumbent, the hip and knee are in extension and periodic prone lying is recommended (Fairchild, 2013).*

Geriatric

- ▲ Assess for swaying, poor balance, weakness, and fear of falling while elders stand/walk. If present, implement fall protection precautions and refer for PT evaluation and recommendations.
- ▲ Review medications for polypharmacy (more than five drugs) and medications that increase the risk of falls, including sedatives, antidepressants, and drugs affecting the central nervous system (CNS). *Consult with pharmacist as part of polypharmacy assessment (Fritsch & Shelton, 2017).*
- Encourage Tai chi, PT, or other exercise for balance, gait, and strength training in group programs or at home.
- Recommend vision assessment and consideration for cataract removal if needed.

Home Care

- Establish a support system for emergency and contingency care (e.g., wearable medical alert alarm; notify local emergency medicine services [EMS] of potential need). *Impaired walking may be life-threatening during a crisis (e.g., fall, fire, orthostatic episode).*
- Assess for and modify any barriers to walking in the home environment.
- ▲ Refer to occupational therapist (OT)/PT for home assessment and evaluation for home assessment for barriers, individualized strength, balance retraining, an exercise plan, and environmental modifications for safety (Peterson et al, 2016).
- ▲ Make referrals for home health services for support and assistance with activities of daily living (ADLs). An activity program pairing trained health care assistants with frail elders resulted in significant improvements in health outcomes and functional activity (Muramatsu et al, 2017).

Client/Family Teaching and Discharge Planning

- Teach clients to check ambulation devices weekly for cracks, loose nuts, or worn tips and to clean dust and dirt on tips.
- Teach diabetics that they are at risk for foot ulcers and teach them preventive interventions. See care plan Risk for ineffective peripheral **Tissue Perfusion.**
- ▲ Instruct clients at risk for osteoporosis or hip fracture to bear weight, walk, engage in resistance exercise (with appropriate adjustments for conditions), ensure good nutrition (especially adequate intake of calcium and vitamin D), drink milk, stop smoking, monitor alcohol intake, and consult a physician for appropriate medications. EB: *Supplementation with vitamin D_3 and calcium reduced the risk of hip fracture by 43%. The National Osteoporosis Foundation recommends daily calcium intake of at least 1200 mg with diet plus supplements, if needed, for postmenopausal women and men age 50 years and older and vitamin D_3 800 to 1000 IU per day (Cosman et al, 2014).*

REFERENCES

Arnold, A., & Raj, S. (2017). Orthostatic hypotension: A practical approach to investigation and management. *Canadian Journal of Cardiology.*, 33(12), 1725–1728.
Collins, D. (2016) *Restorative nursing care plans,* MDS v1.15.1. LTCS Books.
Cosman, F., de Beur, S. J., LeBoff, M. S., et al. (2014). Clinician's guide to prevention and treatment of osteoporosis. *Osteoporosis International,* 25, 2359–2381. Retrieved from https://doi.org/10.1007/s00198-014-2794-2.
Ellison, J., Drummond, M., Dickinson, J., et al. (2016). Short-term intensive rehabilitation induces recovery of physical function after 7 days of bed rest in older adults. *Journal of Acute Care Physical Therapy,* 7(4), 156–163.

Fairchild, S. L. (2013). *Pierson and Fairchild's principles and techniques of patient care.* St. Louis: Elsevier.
Fritsch, M., & Shelton, D. (2017). Geriatric polypharmacy: Pharmacist as key facilitator in assessing falls risk. *Clinics in Geriatric Medicine,* 33(2), 205–223.
Lowry, M., Windsor, J., & Ashelford, S. (2016). Orthostatic hypotension 2: The physiology of blood pressure regulation. *Nursing Times,* 112(43), 17–19.
Muramatsu, N., Yin, L., Berbaum, M., et al. (2017). Promoting seniors' health with home care aides: A pilot. *The Gerontologist,* gnx101. Retrieved from https://doi.org/10.1093/geront/gnx101.
Peterson, M., Goodman, S., et al. (2016). Attitudes and plans for low-income elderly homeowners to age in place. *American Journal*

● = Independent; ▲ = Collaborative; EBN = Evidence-Based Nursing; EB = Evidence-Based

of Occupational Therapy, 70, 7011500074p1. doi:10.5014/
ajot.2016.70S1-PO7023.

Samuelsen, B. T., Andrews, K. L., Houdek, M. T., et al. (2017). The
impact of the immediate postoperative prosthesis on patient
mobility and quality of life after transtibial amputation. *American
Journal of Physical Medicine and Rehabilitation, 96*(2), 116–119.

Van Twist, D., Dinh, T., et al. (2017). Initial orthostatic hypotension
associated with the use of antihypertensive drugs is highly
prevalent in patients with unexplained syncope. *Journal of
Hypertension, 35,* e11.

Windsor, J. (2016). Effect of orthostatic hypotension on falls risk.
Nursing Times, 112(43), 11–13.

Wandering   *Olga F. Jarrín, PhD, RN*

NANDA-I

Definition

Meandering; aimless or repetitive locomotion that exposes the individual to harm; frequently incongruent with boundaries, limits, or obstacles.

Defining Characteristics

Continuous movement from place to place; eloping behavior; frequent movement from place to place; fretful locomotion; haphazard locomotion; hyperactivity; impaired ability to locate landmarks in a familiar setting; locomotion into unauthorized spaces; locomotion resulting in getting lost; locomotion that cannot be easily dissuaded; long periods of locomotion without an apparent destination; pacing; periods of locomotion interspersed with periods of nonlocomotion; persistent locomotion in search of something; scanning behavior; searching behavior; shadowing a caregiver's locomotion; trespassing

Related Factors

Alteration in sleep-wake cycle; desire to go home; overstimulating environment; physiological stage; separation from familiar environment

At-Risk Population

Premorbid behavior

Associated Condition

Alteration in cognitive functioning; cortical atrophy; psychological disorder; sedation

NOC   (Nursing Outcomes Classification)

Suggested NOC Outcomes

Safe Wandering; Safe Home Environment; Safe Health Care Environment; Caregiver Emotional Health; Caregiver-Patient Relationship; Family Normalization: Autism Spectrum Disorder; Family Normalization: Dementia; Community Competence

Example NOC Outcome with Indicators

Safe Wandering as evidenced by the following indicators: Moves about without harming self or others/Sits for more than 5 minutes at a time/Paces a given route/Appears content in environment/Distracts easily/Can be redirected from unsafe activities. (Rate the outcome and indicators of **Safe Wandering:** 1 = never demonstrated, 2 = rarely demonstrated, 3 = sometimes demonstrated, 4 = often demonstrated, 5 = consistently demonstrated [see Section I].)

Client Outcomes

Client Will (Specify Time Frame)

- Maintain psychological well-being and reduce need to wander
- Reduce episodes of wandering in restricted areas/getting lost/elopement
- Maintain appropriate body weight
- Remain safe and free from falls
- Maintain physical activity and remain comfortable and free of pain

● = Independent;   ▲ = Collaborative;   EBN = Evidence-Based Nursing;   EB = Evidence-Based

Caregiver Will (Specify Time Frame)

- Be able to explain interventions he or she can use to provide a safe environment for a care receiver who displays wandering behavior
- Develop strategies to reduce caregiver stress levels

NIC (Nursing Interventions Classification)

Suggested NIC Interventions

Dementia Management: Wandering; Anxiety Reduction; Area Restriction; Exercise Promotion; Environmental Management; Family Mobilization; Family Support; Normalization Promotion

Example NIC Activities—Dementia Management: Wandering
Include family members in planning, providing, and evaluating care to the extent desired; Identify usual patterns of wandering behavior; Alert neighbors and police about the patient's wandering behavior; Provide a secure and safe place for wandering; Encourage physical activity during the daytime; Consider use of electronic devices to locate patient and monitor wandering.

Nursing Interventions and *Rationales*

- Assess for physical distress or unmet needs (e.g., hunger, thirst, pain/discomfort, elimination needs). EBN: *Behavioral signs of unmet need for bowel movement or urination include anxiety, taking off/putting on clothes, restlessness, attempting to go elsewhere, scratching skin, repeated behavior, and making strange sounds (Shih et al, 2015).*
- Assess for emotional or psychological distress, such as anxiety, fear, or feeling lost; considering the situated experience of the client. EB: *Restlessness and wandering may be understood as expressions of existential needs and feelings of anxiety, loneliness, and separation (Solomon & Lawlor, 2018).* CEB: *Triggers for wanderers include being placed in an unfamiliar environment, seeing a coat and hat, experiencing an argumentative or confrontational situation, a change in schedule or routine, and recent relocation to a care facility (Algase et al, 2009).*
- Assess and document the pattern, rhythm, and frequency of wandering over time. EBN: *Wandering should be assessed with one or more of the following scales: Cohen-Mansfield Agitation Inventory (CMAI), the Rating Scale for Aggressive Behavior in the Elderly (RAGE), the Neuropsychiatric Inventory (NPI), the Revised Algase Wandering Scale (RAWS), or its version for community (RAWS-CV) and long-term care settings (RAWS-LTC) (White & Montgomery, 2013; Graham, 2017).*
- Obtain a psychosocial history, including stress-coping behaviors. CEB: *Premorbid personality traits (e.g., history of a physically active job or leisure activities) and behavioral responses to stress (e.g., history of responding to stress with psychomotor activity) may reveal circumstances under which wandering will occur and can aid in interpreting both positive and negative meanings of wandering behavior (Nelson & Algase, 2007).*
- Observe the location and environmental conditions in which wandering is occurring and modify those that appear to induce wandering. EBN: *In a recent observational study, wanderers were less likely to wander from where the likelihood of social interaction was greater (i.e., activities room, dayroom, staff area); where the environment was more soothing (i.e., their own room); or where rooms had a designated purpose (e.g., dayrooms, the wanderer's own room, activities and staff areas), and wandering was less likely when lighting was low and variation in sound levels was small (Algase et al, 2010).*
- Assess the client's environment and advocate for appropriate modifications using a survey such as the Wayfinding Evidence-Based Checklist and Rating (WEBCAR) instrument (Benbow, 2013). EBN: *Residents with dementia depend on meaningful cues at decision points, such as distinctive and colorful architectural features, landmarks, and signs (Davis & Weisbeck, 2016).*
- Use a full-length mirror in front of exit doors to deter elopement. EBN: *Looking in the mirror raises patients' awareness regarding self-care and is effective in decreasing exiting by residents with severe cognitive impairment (Gu, 2015).*
- Use camouflage (a cloth panel or wall hanging) to cover door knobs or locks to prevent elopement (check fire safety code/policy first). EBN: *Covering door knobs and locks is an effective strategy to prevent elopement of residents with advanced dementia (Gu, 2015).*
- Change the floor pattern to create a subjective barrier (illusion of a step, hole, or pit) at exit door. EBN: *Impaired depth perception can cause a sharp contrast in the pattern of the floor (such as black stripes of tape*

• = Independent; ▲ = Collaborative; EBN = Evidence-Based Nursing; EB = Evidence-Based

or black floor tiles in front of door area) to create the illusion of steps, a hole, or pit, reducing elopement for some clients (Gu, 2015; Nelson & Algase, 2007).

- Increase social interaction and offer structured activity and stress-reducing approaches, such as walking and exercise, music, massage, or a rocking chair. EB: *Wandering in restricted areas was reduced 50% to 80% by the use of nonpharmacological multimodal behavioral approaches and cognitive techniques such as problem-solving, behavioral rehearsal, and relaxation training (Nascimento Dourado & Laks, 2016). CEB: Montessori methods and activities using household materials and games can provide a rich social and caring environment to encourage socialization, meaningful activity, and diversion (Padilla, 2011).*

- Create a familiar, low-stress or home-like environment with familiar belongings and regular daily activities. EB: *Environments with low stress or stimuli, home-like, or multi-sensory/transformed environments decrease wandering (Gu, 2015; Lee et al, 2017).*

- Provide safe and secure surroundings that deter and detect accidental elopements, using perimeter control devices or electronic tracking systems (including radiofrequency identification [RFID] tags, *global positioning system* [GPS] locator, smart watch, or cell phone application). CEB: *A review of technology identified boundary alarms activated by wrist bands, alarms alerting caregivers of wandering behavior, and electronic monitoring and tracking systems, such as GPS, as effective in improving client safety (Gu, 2015).*

- When using electronic tracking technologies, an approach emphasizing relationships, respect, and the individual needs of patients and caretakers is best suited to finding solutions that both protect and empower. EB: *Balancing the ethical principles of beneficence and respect in treating cognitively impaired persons goes beyond the necessary step of evaluating decision-making capacity to include partnering with families, caretakers, and cognitively impaired individuals who wander in a collaborative coalition of care (Yang & Kels, 2017). Resistance to surveillance technology is associated with clients feeling stigmatized, missing the company of human supervision, and disliking being "watched" (Niemeijer et al, 2015).*

- Develop and update unit and facility procedures and staff education related to wandering. EBN: *A facility-based risk management approach should include identification of the wanderer, a wandering prevention program, an elopement response plan when patients are missing, and staff mobilization around the problem (Futrell, Devereaux Melillo, & Remington, 2016).*

- Role model person-centered care and provide appropriate supervision, support, and education of direct-care staff. EBN: *Positive work environments for staff are associated with lower prevalence of client escape, restlessness, and wandering behaviors compared with less positive work environments (Gu, 2015).*
  - Establish a caring, calm, friendly, and inviting climate in which relationships are valued.
  - Develop a culture of team spirit in which staff feel valued.
  - Support the development and maintenance of staff competencies in dementia care.
  - Encourage discussion of ethical issues and conflicts that arise during care.

- Help residents find their rooms by placing signs with their names and portraits of themselves at a younger age next to the doorways. EB: *External memory aids in the form of signs with the person's name and portrait photograph can help people with dementia navigate their environment (Jensen & Padilla, 2017).*

- Provide a regularly scheduled and supervised exercise or walking program, particularly if wandering occurs excessively during the night or at times that are inconvenient in the setting *(Jensen & Padilla, 2017).*

- Keep a current client photograph on file to help with identification (see Client/Family Teaching and Discharge Planning section regarding community safe return programs, including AMBER and Silver alerts).

- Refer to the care plan for **Caregiver Role Strain**.

- For clients with dementia, also see care plan for Chronic **Confusion**.

Multicultural

- Assess for the effect of cultural assets, beliefs, life experiences, and values on the family's understanding of wandering behavior and caregiving. CEB: *Wandering behavior is prevalent among people with dementia, regardless of culture, but may be viewed as part of the normal process in some cultures and as abnormal behavior in others; cultural differences may buffer stress and caregiver burden (Nelson & Algase, 2007).*

- Assess client preferences for use of social services and family caregivers' availability and willingness to provide care. EB: *A qualitative study in North Carolina found that service providers assumed that Latino families did not want to use government services and that they preferred to care for their elders; however,*

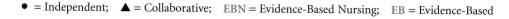

● = Independent;   ▲ = Collaborative;   EBN = Evidence-Based Nursing;   EB = Evidence-Based

Latino participants expressed the need to work and not depend on family members for caregiving and financial support (Larson et al, 2017).

Client/Family Teaching and Discharge Planning

- Use a broad range of descriptions for the term "wandering" to enhance caregivers' understanding. **EB:** *In structured interviews, it was found that informal caregivers rarely used the term "wandering," which could lead to miscommunication with health care providers (Nelson & Algase, 2007).*
- Teach caregivers about AMBER and Silver Alert, Safe Return/Safely Home, and/or Project Lifesaver programs. **CEB:** *The Alzheimer's Association's Medic Alert + Safe Return program (called "Safely Home" in Canada), and Project Lifesaver International (PLI) have assisted in locating numerous persons who have eloped from their homes or other residential care settings (Petonito et al, 2013).* **EB:** *Similar to the AMBER alert emergency response system for missing children, the Silver alert system has been enacted in some but not all states (Gergerich & Davis, 2017).*
- Refer to supportive community and social services, such as a psychiatric home health nurse and companion or respite care, to assist with the impact of caregiving for the wandering client. **CEB:** *Caring for a person at high risk for wandering is associated with high caregiver stress (Nelson & Algase, 2007).*

Home Care

- The previously mentioned interventions may be adapted for home care use.
- Help the caregiver set up a plan to reduce and manage wandering behavior, including a plan of action to use if the client elopes:
  ○ Assess the home environment for modifications that will protect the client and prevent elopement. **EB:** *Security devices are available to notify the caregiver of the client's movements, such as alarms at doors, bed alarms, and ongoing surveillance (Gu, 2015).*
  ○ Assist the family to set up a plan of exercise for the client, including safe walking. **EB:** *Welfare concerns arise when freedom to walk outdoors is restricted; however, the risk of getting lost or injured must be minimized (Bantry White & Montgomery, 2016).*
- Provide information about therapy dog/assistance dog resources. **EB:** *Therapy dogs provide a calming presence and are trained to keep children with autism from straying by circling them and barking to alert family members (Burgoyne et al, 2014).*

REFERENCES

Algase, D. L., Antonakos, C., Beattie, E. R., et al. (2009). Empirical derivation and validation of a wandering typology. *Journal of the American Geriatrics Society*, 57(11), 2037–2045. doi:10.1111/j.1532-5415.2009.02491.x.

Algase, D. L., Beattie, E. R., Antonakos, C., et al. (2010). Wandering and the physical environment. *American Journal of Alzheimer's Disease and Other Dementias*, 25(4), 340–346. doi:10.1177/1533317510365342.

Bantry White, E., & Montgomery, P. (2016). Supporting people with dementia to walkabout safely outdoors: Development of a structured model of assessment. *Health and Social Care in the Community*, 24(4), 473–484. doi:10.1111/hsc.12226.

Benbow, W. (2013). Evidence-based checklist for wayfinding design in dementia care facilities. *Canadian Nursing Home*, 24(1), 4–10.

Burgoyne, L., Dowling, L., Fitzgerald, A., et al. (2014). Parents' perspectives on the value of assistance dogs for children with autism spectrum disorder: A cross-sectional study. *BMJ Open*, 4(6), e004786. doi:10.1136/bmjopen-2014-004786.

Davis, R., & Weisbeck, C. (2016). Creating a supportive environment using cues for wayfinding in dementia. *Journal of Gerontological Nursing*, 42(3), 36–44. doi:10.3928/00989134-20160212-07.

Futrell, M., Devereaux Melillo, K., & Remington, R. (2016). Evidence-based practice guideline: wandering. *Journal of Gerontological Nursing*, 40(11), 16–23.

Gergerich, E., & Davis, L. (2017). Silver alerts: A notification system for communities with missing adults. *Journal of Gerontological Social Work*, 60(3), 232–244. doi:10.1080/01634372.2017.1293757.

Graham, M. E. (2017). From wandering to wayfaring: Reconsidering movement in people with dementia in long-term care. *Dementia (London)*, 16(6), 732–749. doi:10.1177/1471301215614572.

Gu, L. (2015). Nursing interventions in managing wandering behavior in patients with dementia: A literature review. *Archives of Psychiatric Nursing*, 29(6), 454–457. doi:10.1016/j.apnu.2015.06.003.

Jensen, L., & Padilla, R. (2017). Effectiveness of environment-based interventions that address behavior, perception, and falls in people with Alzheimer's disease and related major neurocognitive disorders: A systematic review. *The American Journal of Occupational Therapy*, 71(5), 7105180030p2147483647–7105180030p2147483647. doi:10.5014/ajot.2017.027409.

Larson, K., Mathews, H. F., Torres, E., et al. (2017). Responding to health and social needs of aging Latinos in new-growth communities: A qualitative study. *BMC Health Service Research*, 17(1), 601. doi:10.1186/s12913-017-2551-2.

Lee, K. H., Boltz, M., Lee, H., et al. (2017). Is an engaging or soothing environment associated with the psychological well-being of people with dementia in long-term care? *Journal of Nursing Scholarship*, 49(2), 135–142. doi:10.1111/jnu.12263.

Nascimento Dourado, C. M., & Laks, J. (2016). Psychological interventions for neuropsychiatric disturbances in mild and moderate Alzheimer's disease: Current evidences and future directions. *Current Alzheimer Research*, 13(10), 1100–1111. doi:10.2174/1567205013666160728143123.

Nelson, A. L., & Algase, A. (Eds.), (2007). *Evidence-based protocols for managing wandering behaviors.* New York: Springer.

● = Independent; ▲ = Collaborative; EBN = Evidence-Based Nursing; EB = Evidence-Based

Niemeijer, A. R., Depla, M. F., Frederiks, B. J., et al. (2015). The experiences of people with dementia and intellectual disabilities with surveillance technologies in residential care. *Nursing Ethics*, 22(3), 307–320. doi:10.1177/0969733014533237.

Padilla, R. (2011). Effectiveness of environment-based interventions for people with Alzheimer's disease and related dementias. *The American Journal of Occupational Therapy*, 65(5), 514–522.

Petonito, G., Muschert, G. W., Carr, D. C., et al. (2013). Programs to locate missing and critically wandering elders: A critical review and a call for multiphasic evaluation. *The Gerontologist*, 53(1), 17–25. doi:10.1093/geront/gns060.

Shih, Y. H., Wang, C. J., Sue, E. P., et al. (2015). Behavioral characteristics of bowel movement and urination needs in patients with dementia in Taiwan. *Journal of Gerontological Nursing*, 41(6), 22–29, quiz 30–21. doi:10.3928/00989134-20150414-01.

Solomon, O., & Lawlor, M. C. (2018). Beyond V40.31: Narrative phenomenology of wandering in autism and dementia. *Culture, Medicine and Psychiatry*. doi:10.1007/s11013-017-9562-7.

White, E. B., & Montgomery, P. (2013). A review of "wandering" instruments for people with dementia who get lost. *Research on Social Work Practice*, 24(4), 400–413. doi:10.1177/1049731513514116.

Yang, Y. T., & Kels, C. G. (2017). Ethical considerations in electronic monitoring of the cognitively impaired. *Journal of the American Board of Family Medicine*, 30(2), 258–263. doi:10.3122/jabfm.2017.02.160219.

• = Independent;   ▲ = Collaborative;   EBN = Evidence-Based Nursing;   EB = Evidence-Based

Index

Entries followed by *b*, *t*, or *f* indicate boxes, tables, or figures, respectively. **Boldface** entries indicate care plan titles. Page numbers in *italics* indicate care plan locations.